Vascular Surgery

Principles and Practice

SAMUEL E. WILSON, M.D.
Chairman, Department of Surgery, Harbor-UCLA Medical Center, Torrance, California; Professor of Surgery, UCLA School of Medicine, Los Angeles, California; Surgeon, Wadsworth Veterans Administration Medical Center, Los Angeles, California

FRANK J. VEITH, M.D.
Professor of Surgery, Chief of Vascular Surgical Services, Department of Surgery, Division of Vascular Surgery, Montefiore Medical Center—Albert Einstein College of Medicine, New York, New York

ROBERT W. HOBSON II, M.D.
James Utley Professor of Surgery, Boston University School of Medicine; Chairman, Department of Surgery, Boston University Medical Center, Boston, Massachusetts

RUSSELL A. WILLIAMS, M.D.
Associate Chairman, Department of Surgery, Harbor-UCLA Medical Center, Torrance, California; Staff Surgeon, Vascular Surgery Section, Wadsworth Veterans Administration Medical Center, Los Angeles, California; Associate Professor, Department of Surgery, UCLA School of Medicine, Los Angeles, California

McGRAW-HILL BOOK COMPANY
New York St. Louis San Francisco Auckland Bogotá Hamburg Johannesburg Lisbon London Madrid Mexico Milan Montreal New Delhi Panama Paris San Juan São Paulo Singapore Sydney Tokyo Toronto

Notice

Medicine is an ever-changing science. As new research and clinical experience broaden our knowledge, changes in treatment and drug therapy are required. The editors and the publisher of this work have checked with sources believed to be reliable in their efforts to provide drug dosage schedules that are complete and in accord with the standards accepted at the time of publication. However, readers are advised to check the product information sheet included in the package of each drug they plan to administer to be certain that the information contained in these schedules is accurate and that changes have not been made in the recommended dose or in the contraindications for administration. This recommendation is of particular importance in connection with new or infrequently used drugs.

VASCULAR SURGERY
Principles and Practice

1 2 3 4 5 6 7 8 9 0 HALHAL 8 9 8 7 6

ISBN 0-07-070812-6

This book was set in Times Roman by Waldman Graphics Incorporated; the editors were Robert E. McGrath, Thomas H. Kothman, and Muza Navrozov; the production supervisor was Avé McCracken; the designer was Bob Arnold; the cover was designed by Edward R. Schultheis. Arcata Graphics/Halliday was printer and binder.

Library of Congress Cataloging-in-Publication Data

Vascular surgery.

Includes bibliographies and index.
1. Blood-vessels—Surgery. 2. Blood-vessels—Diseases. I. Wilson, Samuel E., date.
[DNLM: 1. Vascular Surgery. WG 170 V3315]
RD598.5.V388 1987 617'.413 86-10412
ISBN 0-07-070812-6

CONTENTS

Part Four Aneurysms

Part Seven Vascular Disorders of the Upper Extremity

Part Eight Venous and Lymphatic Disease

Part Nine Vascular Trauma

Part Ten Arteriovenous Fistula

Part Eleven Infection, Amputation, Transplantation, and Sexual Function

LIST OF CONTRIBUTORS

Enrico Ascer, M.D.
Head, Vascular Surgery Research Laboratory, Department of Surgery, Division of Vascular Surgery, Montefiore Medical Center; Assistant Professor of Surgery, Albert Einstein College of Medicine, New York, New York

James I. Ausman, M.D., Ph.D.
Chairman, Department of Neurological Surgery, Henry Ford Hospital, Detroit, Michigan

Ronald J. Baird, M.D., F.R.C.S.C., F.A.C.S.
Professor of Surgery, University of Toronto; Head of Cardiovascular Surgery, Toronto General Hospital, Toronto, Ontario, Canada

Robert S. Bennion, M.D.
Assistant Professor of Surgery, Department of Surgery, UCLA School of Medicine, Los Angeles, California

John J. Bergan, M.D.
Magerstadt Professor of Surgery and Chief, Division of Vascular Surgery, Northwestern University Medical School, Chicago, Illinois

Henry D. Berkowitz, M.D.
Associate Professor of Surgery, Director, Peripheral Vascular Laboratory, Hospital University of Pennsylvania, University of Pennsylvania, Philadelphia, Pennsylvania

Victor M. Bernhard, M.D.
Professor of Surgery, Chief, Section of Vascular Surgery, University of Arizona Health Sciences Center, Tucson, Arizona

Eugene F. Bernstein, M.D., Ph.D.
Adjunct Professor of Surgery, Department of Surgery, University of California, San Diego, San Diego, California; Division of Vascular and Thoracic Surgery, Scripps Clinic and Research Foundation, La Jolla, California

F. William Blaisdell, M.D.
Professor and Chairman, Department of Surgery, University of California, Davis, Sacramento, California

David H. Blankenhorn, M.D.
Professor of Medicine, Atherosclerosis Research, Department of Medicine, University of Southern California School of Medicine, Los Angeles, California

Scott J. Boley, A.B., M.D.
Professor of Surgery, Department of Surgery, Montefiore Medical Center—Albert Einstein College of Medicine, New York, New York

Edward B. Borden, M.D.
Assistant Professor of Surgery, Department of Surgery, Montefiore Medical Center—Albert Einstein College of Medicine, New York, New York

Marcello A. Borzatta, M.D.
Chief Resident, Department of Surgery, Harbor-UCLA Medical Center, Torrance, California; Fellow, Surgery, Surgical Service, Royal Prince Alfred Hospital, Camperdown, Sydney, NSW, Australia

Bruce J. Brener, M.D.
Clinical Associate Professor of Surgery, University of Medicine and Dentistry of New Jersey; Director of Vascular Laboratory, Department of Surgery, Newark Beth Israel Medical Center, University of Medicine and Dentistry of New Jersey, Newark, New Jersey

Donald K. Brief, M.D.
Clinical Professor of Surgery and Chief of General Surgery, Department of General Surgery, Newark Beth Israel Medical Center, University of Medicine and Dentistry of New Jersey, Newark, New Jersey

John A. C. Buckels, M.B., Ch.B., F.R.C.S.
Research Fellow, Department of Surgery, Harbor-UCLA Medical Center, Torrance, California; Lecturer, Department of Surgery, Queen Elizabeth Hospital, Birmingham, England

Allan D. Callow, M.D., Ph.D.
Professor of Surgery; Senior Vascular Surgeon, Department of Surgery, New England Medical Center, Boston, Massachusetts

Vern M. Campbell, M.D.
Staff Surgeon, Cardiovascular Surgery, Toronto General Hospital, Toronto, Ontario, Canada

George J. Collins, Jr., M.D.
Chief, Department of Surgery and Peripheral Vascular Surgery Service, Walter Reed Army Medical Center, Washington, D.C.

John Connor, M.D.
Surgery Resident, Department of Surgery, Harbor-UCLA Medical Center, Torrance, California

John D. Corson, M.D.
Associate Professor of Surgery, Department of Surgery, Albany Medical College, Albany, New York

E. Stanley Crawford, M.D.
Professor of Surgery, Department of Surgery, Baylor College of Medicine, Houston, Texas

John L. Crawford, M.D.
Vascular Surgeon, private practice, Ft. Worth, Texas

Pamela J. Curry, M.P.H.
University of Southern California, Los Angeles, California

Richard H. Dean, M.D.
Professor of Surgery, Head, Department of Surgery, Division of Vascular Surgery, Vanderbilt University School of Medicine, Nashville, Tennessee

Ralph G. DePalma, M.D.
Professor and Chairman, Department of Surgery, The George Washington University Medical Center, Washington, D.C.

James A. DeWeese, M.D.
Professor and Chairman, Division of Cardiothoracic Surgery, The University of Rochester School of Medicine and Dentistry, Rochester, New York

Fernando G. Diaz, M.D., Ph.D.
Director of Clinical Research, Department of Neurosurgery, Henry Ford Hospital, Detroit, Michigan

Carlos E. Donayre, M.D.
Vascular Fellow, Department of Surgery, Harbor-UCLA Medical Center, Torrance, California

Hugh J. Donohue, M.D.
Assistant Professor of Surgery, Affiliated (USUHS), Department of Surgery, Uniformed Services University of the Health Sciences, Bethesda, Maryland

William H. Edwards, M.D.
Clinical Professor of Surgery, Department of Surgery, Vanderbilt University Medical Center, Nashville, Tennessee

W. Sterling Edwards, M.D.
Professor and Chairman, Department of Surgery, University of New Mexico School of Medicine, Albuquerque, New Mexico

David J. Effeney, M.D.
Associate Professor of Surgery, Department of Surgery, Division of Vascular Surgery, University of California, San Francisco, San Francisco, California; Professor of Surgery, University of Queensland, Brisbane, Australia

William K. Ehrenfeld, M.D.
Professor of Surgery; Co-Chief, Vascular Surgery, Department of Surgery, University of California, San Francisco, San Francisco, California

Bruce M. Elliott, M.D.
Assistant Professor of Surgery (USUHS), Department of Surgery, Uniformed Services University of the Health Sciences, Bethesda, Maryland

Calvin B. Ernst, M.D.
Clinical Professor of Surgery, University of Michigan, and Head, Division of Vascular Surgery, Henry Ford Hospital, Detroit, Michigan

William E. Evans, M.D.
Chief, Vascular Surgery, Saint Anthony Medical Center, Columbus, Ohio; Clinical Professor of Surgery, The Ohio State University, Columbus, Ohio; Professor of Surgery, Meharry Medical College, Nashville, Tennessee

David V. Feliciano, M.D.
Associate Professor, Cora and Webb Mading Department of Surgery, Baylor College of Medicine, Houston, Texas

William S. Fields, M.D.
Professor of Neurology, University of Texas Medical School, Houston, Texas; Chairman, Department of Neurooncology, University of Texas System Cancer Center, Houston, Texas

William R. Flinn, M.D.
Assistant Professor of Surgery, Division of Vascular Surgery, Northwestern University Medical School, Chicago, Illinois

Thomas J. Fogarty, M.D.
Director, Cardiac Surgery, Department of Surgery, Sequoia Hospital, Redwood City, California

J. Timothy Fulenwider, M.D.
Chief, Vascular Surgery, Department of Surgery, Emory University Medical Center, Atlanta, Georgia; Assistant Chief, Surgery Service, Veterans Administration Medical Center, Decatur, Georgia

Wilson V. Garrett, M.D.
Associate Attending Surgeon; Clinical Instructor, University of Texas Southwestern Medical School at Dallas, Dallas, Texas

Bruce L. Gewertz, M.D.
Associate Professor of Surgery, Department of Surgery, University of Chicago, Chicago, Illinois

James A. Gillespie, M.D., Ch.M., F.R.C.S.
Consultant Surgeon, St. George's Hospital, London, England

Seymour Glagov, M.D.
Professor of Pathology, Department of Pathology, University of Chicago, Chicago, Illinois

Lazar J. Greenfield, M.D.
Stuart McGuire Professor and Chairman, Department of Surgery, School of Medicine, Virginia Commonwealth University Medical College of Virginia, Richmond, Virginia

Verity S. Grinnell, M.D.
Staff Specialist, Department of Radiology, Royal North Shore Hospital, St. Leonard's, NSW, Australia

Sushil K. Gupta, M.D.
Associate Professor of Surgery; Associate Chief of Vascular Surgery, Department of Surgery, Division of Vascular Surgery, Montefiore Medical Center—Albert Einstein College of Medicine, New York, New York

W. Clark Hargrove III, M.D.
Instructor in Surgery, Department of Surgery, Hospital of the University of Pennsylvania, Philadelphia, Pennsylvania

Ronald D. Harris, M.D.
Staff Radiologist, Assistant Clinical Professor, Department of Radiology, University of California, San Diego, San Diego, California; Scripp's Clinic & Research Foundation, La Jolla, California

Carl J. Hauser, M.D.
Regional Trauma Center, Hollywood Presbyterian Medical Center, Los Angeles, California

Herbert B. Hechtman, M.D.
Senior Associate in Surgery, Department of Surgery, Brigham & Women's Hospital, Boston, Massachusetts

Grant B. Hieshima, M.D.
Associate Professor, Department of Radiology, UCLA Center for Health Sciences, Los Angeles, California

Robert W. Hobson II, M.D.
James Utley Professor of Surgery, Boston University School of Medicine; Chairman, Department of Surgery, Boston University Medical Center, Boston, Massachusetts

James W. Holcroft, M.D.
Professor of Surgery, Chief of Vascular Surgery Service, Department of Surgery, University of California, Davis, School of Medicine, Sacramento, California

Lawrence Hollander, M.D.
Assistant Professor of Surgery, Department of Surgery, Chicago Medical School, Chicago, Illinois

K. Wayne Johnston, M.D.
Head of Vascular Surgery, Department of Cardiovascular Surgery, Toronto General Hospital, Toronto, Ontario, Canada

Donald N. Kapsch, M.D.
Surgeon, private practice, Austell, Georgia

Allastair M. Karmody, M.D., Ch.M., F.R.C.S. (Eng. & Ed), F.A.C.S.
Professor of Surgery, Department of Surgery, Albany Medical College, Albany, New York

Stanley R. Klein, M.D.
Assistant Professor of Surgery, Department of Surgery, Division of Vascular Surgery, Harbor-UCLA Medical Center, Torrance, California

William C. Krupski, M.D.
Assistant Professor of Surgery, Division of Vascular Surgery, University of California, San Francisco, San Francisco, California

Deborah A. Lange, M.D.
Clinical Assistant Professor of Surgery, Department of General Surgery, University of Illinois, Chicago, Illinois

Robert P. Leather, M.D.
Professor of Surgery, Department of Surgery, Albany Medical College, Albany, New York

John B. Long, M.D.
Vascular Surgeon, private practice, San Francisco, California

Thomas G. Lynch, M.D.
Associate Professor of Surgery, Section of Vascular Surgery, Department of Surgery, University of Medicine and Dentistry of New Jersey, New Jersey Medical School, Newark, New Jersey; Chief, Section of Vascular Surgery, Veterans Administration Medical Center, East Orange, New Jersey

Herbert I. Machleder, M.D.
Professor of Surgery, Department of Surgery, UCLA School of Medicine, Los Angeles, California

Kenneth E. McIntyre, Jr., M.D.
Assistant Professor of Surgery, Section of Vascular Surgery, Department of Surgery, University of Arizona, Health Sciences Center, Tucson, Arizona

John A. Mannick, M.D.
Moseley Professor of Surgery, Harvard Medical School; Department of Surgery, Brigham & Women's Hospital, Boston, Massachusetts

Kenneth L. Mattox, M.D.
Professor of Surgery, Cora and Webb Mading Department of Surgery, Baylor College of Medicine, Houston, Texas

C. Mark Mehringer, M.D.
Associate Professor, Chief of Diagnostic Radiology, Department of Radiology, Harbor-UCLA Medical Center, Torrance, California

Timothy A. Miller, M.D.
Professor of Surgery, Surgical Service, UCLA School of Medicine, Wadsworth Veterans Administration Medical Center, Los Angeles, California

Jeffrey C. Milliken, M.D.
Chief Resident, Department of Surgery, UCLA School of Medicine, Los Angeles, California

V. K. Mittal, M.D.
Staff Surgeon, Department of Surgery, Section of Transplantation, Mt. Carmel Mercy Hospital, Detroit, Michigan

Wesley S. Moore, M.D.
Professor of Surgery, Chief, Section of Vascular Surgery, Department of Surgery, University of California, Los Angeles, Los Angeles, California

Joseph L. Mulherin, Jr., M.D.
Associate Clinical Professor of Surgery, Department of Surgery, Vanderbilt University Hospitals, Nashville, Tennessee

Aksel G. Nordestgaard, M.D.
Research Fellow in Surgery, Department of Surgery, Harbor-UCLA Medical Center, Los Angeles, California

Marshall J. Orloff, M.D.
Professor of Surgery, Department of Surgery, University of California, San Diego, School of Medicine, San Diego, California

Robert Sanford Ozeran, M.D.
Associate Clinical Professor of Surgery, UCLA School of Medicine, Los Angeles, California

Frank T. Padberg, Jr., M.D.
Assistant Professor of Surgery, Department of Vascular Surgery, University of Medicine and Dentistry of New Jersey, Newark, New Jersey

Bruce A. Perler, M.D.
Department of Surgery, Johns Hopkins University School of Medicine, Baltimore, Maryland

Malcolm O. Perry, M.D.
Professor of Surgery, Chief, Division of Vascular Surgery, Deparment of Surgery, Cornell University Medical College, New York, New York

Alfred V. Persson, M.D.
Head, Section of Peripheral Vascular Surgery, Department of Surgery, Lahey Clinic Medical Center, Burlington, Massachusetts

John M. Porter, M.D.
Professor of Surgery and Head, Division of Vascular Surgery, Oregon Health Sciences University School of Medicine, Portland, Oregon

Luis A. Queral, M.D.
Associate Professor of Surgery, Chief, Division of Vascular Surgery, Department of Surgery, University of Maryland, Baltimore, Maryland

Linda M. Reilly, M.D.
Assistant Professor of Surgery, Department of Surgery, University of California, San Francisco, School of Medicine, San Francisco, California

Norman M. Rich, M.D., F.A.C.S
Professor and Chairman, Department of Surgery; Chief, Division of Vascular Surgery, Uniformed Services University of the Health Sciences, Bethesda, Maryland

Steven P. Rivers, M.D.
Vascular Surgery, Oregon Health Sciences University School of Medicine, Portland, Oregon

Charles G. Rob, M.D.
Professor, Department of Surgery, Uniformed Services University of the Health Sciences, Bethesda, Maryland

Brooke Roberts, M.D.
Emeritus Professor of Surgery, Department of Surgery, University of Pennsylvania, Philadelphia, Pennsylvania

Michael F. Roizen, M.D.
Professor and Chairperson, Department of Anesthesia and Critical Care, University of Chicago, Chicago, Illinois

Russell Ross, Ph.D.
Professor and Chairman of Pathology, Adjunct Professor of Biochemistry, Department of Pathology, University of Washington, Seattle, Washington

James M. Salander, M.D.
Associate Professor of Surgery (USUHS), Department of Surgery, Uniformed Services University of the Health Sciences, Bethesda, Maryland

Russell H. Samson, M.D.
Assistant Professor of Surgery, Director, Vascular Laboratory, Albert Einstein College of Medicine; Vascular Surgeon in Charge, Department of Surgery, Division of Vascular Surgery, Bronx Municipal Hospital Center, New York, New York

Larry A. Scher, M.D.
Associate Professor of Surgery, Albert Einstein College of Medicine; Vascular Surgeon in Charge, Department of Surgery, Hospital of the Albert Einstein College of Medicine, New York, New York

Dhiraj M. Shah, M.D.
Professor of Surgery, Department of Surgery, Division of Vascular Surgery, Albany Medical College, Albany, New York

William C. Shoemaker, M.D.
Professor of Surgery, Department of Surgery, Harbor-UCLA Medical Center, Torrance, California

Donald Silver, M.D.
Professor and Chairman, Department of Surgery, University of Missouri—Columbia School of Medicine, Columbia, Missouri

Bertram L. Smith, M.D.
Associate Attending Surgeon, Department of Surgery, Baylor University Medical Center; Clinical Instructor, University of Texas Southwestern Medical School, Dallas, Texas

G. Jeffrey Smith, M.D.
Surgical Resident, Department of Surgery, University of California, Davis, School of Medicine, Sacramento, California

Robert B. Smith III, M.D.
Professor of Surgery and Head of General Vascular Surgery, Department of Surgery, Emory University School of Medicine, Atlanta, Georgia

Yung J. Sohn, M.D.
Associate Professor of Anesthesia and Pharmacology, Department of Anesthesia, University of California, San Francisco, San Francisco, California

Bruce E. Stabile, M.D.
Associate Professor of Surgery, University of California, San Diego; Chief, Surgical Service, Veterans Administration Medical Center, San Diego, California

Lygia Stewart, M.D.
Surgical Research Fellow, Surgical Service, Wadsworth Veterans Administration Medical Center, Los Angeles, California

Ronald J. Stoney, M.D.
Professor of Surgery and Chief, Vascular Surgery, Department of Surgery, University of California, San Francisco, San Francisco, California

Richard A. Sullivan, M.D.
Associate Professor and Acting Chairman, Department of Rehabilitation Medicine, University of Medicine and Dentistry–New Jersey Medical School, Newark, New Jersey; Medical Director, Kessler Institute for Rehabilitation, West Orange, New Jersey

David S. Sumner, M.D.
Professor of Surgery, Chief, Vascular Surgery, Department of Surgery, St. John's Hospital, Springfield, Illinois

D. Emerick Szilagyi, M.D.
Consultant in Vascular Surgery, Department of Surgery, Henry Ford Hospital, Detroit, Michigan

C. M. Talkington, M.D.
Attending Surgeon, Department of Surgery, Baylor University Medical Center; Clinical Assistant Professor of Surgery, University of Texas Southwestern Medical School, Dallas, Texas

Jesse E. Thompson, M.D.
Chief, Surgery Department, Baylor University Medical Center; Clinical Professor of Surgery, University of Texas Southwestern Medical School, Dallas, Texas

L. H. Toledo-Pereyra, M.D., Ph.D.
Staff Surgeon, Department of Surgery, Section of Transplantation, Mt. Carmel Mercy Hospital, Detroit, Michigan

William D. Turnipseed, M.D.
Associate Professor, Department of Surgery, Section of Vascular Surgery, University of Wisconsin Hospital and Clinics, Madison, Wisconsin

Frank J. Veith, M.D.
Professor of Surgery, Chief of Vascular Surgical Services, Department of Surgery, Division of Vascular Surgery, Montefiore Medical Center—Albert Einstein College of Medicine, New York, New York

Blair D. Vermilion, M.D.
Clinical Assistant Professor, Department of Surgery, Ohio State University Medical Centers, Columbus, Ohio

J. Leonel Villavicencio, M.D.
Professor of Surgery (USUHS), Department of Surgery, Uniformed Services University of the Health Sciences, Bethesda, Maryland

Paul M. Walker, M.D.
Staff Surgeon, Vascular Surgery, Department of Cardiovascular Surgery, Toronto General Hospital, Toronto, Ontario, Canada

Richard D. Weisel, M.D.
Staff Surgeon, Department of Cardiovascular Surgery, Toronto General Hospital, Toronto, Ontario, Canada

Geoffrey H. White, M.B., B.S., F.R.A.C.S.
Vascular Surgeon, Department of Surgery, Harbor-UCLA Medical Center; Assistant Professor of Surgery, UCLA School of Medicine, Chief, Vascular Section, Wadsworth Veterans Administration Medical Center, Los Angeles, California

Rodney A. White, M.D.
Associate Professor of Surgery, Chief, Vascular Surgery, Department of Surgery, Harbor-UCLA Medical Center, Torrance, California

Anthony D. Whittemore, M.D.
Assistant Professor of Surgery, Harvard Medical School; Department of Surgery, Brigham & Women's Hospital, Boston, Massachusetts

Russell A. Williams, M.D.
Associate Chairman, Department of Surgery, Harbor-UCLA Medical Center, Torrance, California; Staff Surgeon, Vascular Surgery Section, Wadsworth Veterans Administration Medical Center, Los Angeles, California; Associate Professor, Department of Surgery, UCLA School of Medicine, Los Angeles, California

Samuel E. Wilson, M.D.
Chairman, Department of Surgery, Harbor-UCLA Medical Center, Torrance, California; Professor of Surgery, UCLA School of Medicine, Los Angeles, California; Surgeon, Wadsworth Veterans Administration Medical Center, Los Angeles, California

Martin A. Winston, M.D.
Assistant Chief, Associate Professor of Medicine, Department of Nuclear Medicine, Wadsworth Veterans Administration Medical Center; Associate Professor of Radiology, Adjunct, University of California, Los Angeles, California

Gerald L. Wolf, M.D.
Professor of Radiology, University of Pittsburgh, Radiology Service, Medical Center, Pittsburgh, Pennsylvania

Creighton B. Wright, M.D.
Professor of Clinical Surgery, Division of Thoracic and Cardiovascular Surgery, University of Cincinnati Medical Center, Cincinnati, Ohio; Clinical Professor of Surgery, Department of Surgery, Uniformed Services University of the Health Sciences, Bethesda, Maryland

Joan Wright, M.D.
Plastic Surgery Resident, Department of Surgery, Harbor-UCLA Medical Center, Torrance, California

James S. T. Yao, M.D., Ph.D.
Professor of Surgery and Director, Blood Flow Laboratory, Division of Vascular Surgery, Northwestern University Medical School, Chicago, Illinois

Richard A. Yeager, M.D.
Assistant Professor and Staff Surgeon, Department of Surgery and Surgical Service, Oregon Health Sciences University and Veterans Administration Medical Center, Portland, Oregon

Jerry R. Youkey, M.D.
Clinical Assistant Professor of Surgery (USUHS), Department of Surgery, University of Uniformed Services of the Health Sciences, Bethesda, Maryland

Christoper K. Zarins, M.D.
Professor of Surgery, Chief of Vascular Surgery, Department of Surgery, University of Chicago, Chicago, Illinois

R. Eugene Zierler, M.D.
Chief, Vascular Surgery Section, Seattle Veterans Administration Medical Center, Seattle, Washington; Assistant Professor of Surgery, Department of Surgery, University of Washington School of Medicine, Seattle, Washington

James J. Zimmerman, M.D.
Vascular Surgeon, Sequoia Hospital, Redwood City, California, and Stanford Medical Center, Stanford, California

PREFACE

Peripheral arterial occlusive disease, with pathology similar to that seen today, has been identified in the Egyptian mummies of a dynasty 3,400 years old. Hippocrates understood that interruption of the arterial blood flow produced local tissue death and ultimately gangrene of the extremity, but it is the greatly extended life expectancy of contemporary humans that gives atherosclerotic arterial occlusive disease the proportions of an epidemic, unknown in earlier societies. Peripheral vascular disease of the extremities is now one of the most common and serious causes of morbidity and disability in the aged.

Vascular surgery's earliest roots grew tentatively; arterial trauma and aneurysm were treated with simple procedures. Particularly notable were Pare's ligation of arterial injuries on the battlefield and Hunter's and Cooper's occlusions of aneurysms. Even the prescient organ transplantation experiments of Alexis Carrel may have had their beginning when he observed his teacher unsuccessfully struggle to repair the transsected portal vein of the French President Carnot.

Reconstruction characterizes modern vascular surgery, which has evolved over only three decades. No other surgical field has had a more accelerated growth. There is now a need to gather in this large body of knowledge, and *Vascular Surgery: Principles and Practice* does exactly this, comprehensively and concisely. The discussion of each topic progresses logically from pathophysiology through critical elements in diagnosis and treatment. Vascular diseases are analyzed with a practical orientation to medical and surgical alternatives for therapy, always substantiated with current data on outcome.

Our goal for *Vascular Surgery* is that it be useful for the surgeon caring for patients with vascular diseases. Contributions are mostly from the "second generation" of vascular surgeons, but we have capitalized on the experience of established leaders. Authors for each chapter have been selected on the basis of their special interests and experience. These experts provide up-to-date and balanced information. Contributions by medical and radiological specialists—conventional and interventional—emphasize today's need for cooperation among physicians treating vascular disease. Although *Vascular Surgery* primarily addresses vascular surgeons, the internist, resident, and allied specialist will also find its approach similarly useful.

A book of this size and depth combines the efforts of many. We sincerely appreciate the generous time and effort of all one hundred and thirty-two authors. Our objectives would not have been accomplished without the unflagging assistance of the Health Professions Division at McGraw-Hill, particularly Robert McGraw, who first broached the idea, and Muza Navrozov, who edited every line of the text; Norma Zimmerman and Astara Mayeda in Los Angeles, Julie Panek-Colon and June Gitstein in New York, and Barbara Edwards in New Jersey provided expert assistance in manuscript preparation.

Samuel E. Wilson, M.D.
Frank J. Veith, M.D.
Robert W. Hobson II, M.D.
Russell A. Williams, M.D.

PART ONE

Assessment of the Disease

Chapter 1

VASCULAR SURGERY: A PROPAEDEUTIC OF ITS PAST, PRESENT, AND FUTURE

D. EMERICK SZILAGYI

Vascular surgery as a self-contained and distinct specialty has a very brief history. Virtually all its development has taken place in the last 35 years.

The Beginnings

Operations on the vascular system have been performed since antiquity. Until the middle of the twentieth century, however, these interventions were not only of limited scope, indeed, usually of extreme simplicity, but the results they achieved were, even on the modest scale of achievement of contemporary surgery in other fields, disappointing. Instead of a discipline of cohesive continuity, they comprised dissociated individual efforts. Their scope was limited since only surface lesions could have been diagnosed, and successful results were rare. This was so since even simple vascular procedures are far more fastidious in their demands for an appropriate operative environment and for technical skills than operations on other anatomic systems. The simple act of suturing and ligating an artery seems to have created enough difficulties to engage the ingenuity of many of the leading surgeons for centuries. The problem of the successful management of aneurysms (almost without exception of the peripheral arteries and most of them traumatic) remained an unanswered challenge until the time of Rudolph Matas, whose active surgical life was quite close to our own.

Even the celebrated contributions to vascular surgery of Rudolph Matas (1,2) failed to broaden the scope of the surgical treatment of vascular disease to a degree that would signal the beginning of a new discipline. Deficiencies in the material environment of contemporary surgery (to be touched upon presently) forced him into a narrow circle of achievement. He performed, according to his own careful account, 620 vascular operations between 1888 and 1940 (principally during the years 1900 to 1930), but over 80 percent of these procedures (519 cases) were arterial ligations, and only about 15 percent (101 cases) included attempts at some form of restoration of the arteries. During his long surgical career, he operated on the diseased abdominal aorta only five times (each time for aneurysm); none of these interventions aimed at reconstruction, and only one patient survived. A measure of the difficulties facing the surgeon who attempted to repair arteries and of the futility of his efforts is the fact that Matas's achievement of lasting importance was the technical development of operations that ensured effective occlusion of peripheral arterial aneurysms, that is, a method of occlusion that would not be followed by hemorrhage or recurrence. This accomplishment—which now appears so simple—in the late nineteenth century required both technical brilliance and intelligent courage.

Matas may well deserve to be called the "father of vascular surgery" in this country, but he was a father without offspring or at least without direct descendants. By his own account (2), between 1902 and 1927 (when he stopped following the world literature), the number of cases using his technique of obliterative, and occasionally, reparative aneurysmorrhaphy was 505 (that is about 20 cases per year) throughout the world. In the following years the reports of cases gradually fell off, and by the late 1940s the various types of aneurysmorrhaphy according to Matas's were infrequently used.

The circumstances that limited the scope of Matas's contributions were the same constraints that were in general responsible for the tardiness of the emergence of vascular surgery as a broad and self-contained endeavor.

These constraints were multiple and interdependent. The most conspicuous deficiencies were the absence of an effective method to prevent clotting and the inability to replace arteries with a serviceable substitute. Another very important, if somewhat indirect, contributing factor to restrict the broadening of the field of vascular surgery was the surgeon's inability to control infection, for the intercurrence of infection after vascular operations had a far more disastrous consequence than it had in operations on other anatomical structures.

But even if all the facilities to control clotting and infection to use arterial substitutes had been on hand, the evolution of vascular surgery would have been critically hampered by the extremely sparse clinical material to which vascular surgical procedures could have been applied. The surgeon was completely unaware of the existence of occlusive arterial lesions suitable for surgical correction, a group of lesions that later became the most receptive ground for the extension of vascular reconstruction.

This ignorance was not as ingenuous as it may appear. The dominant and generally accepted concept of the gross morphology of the arterial disease that we now call atherosclerosis (a designation proposed by Marchand in 1904) was woefully wrong. Known by a variety of names, its etiology completely unknown, and even its microscopic identity often misinterpreted, atherosclerosis was until well into the twentieth century described as a diffuse involvement of the arterial wall of quite uniform and universal distribution. It would have sounded absurd to suggest that surgical correction was applicable to such a systemic disease.

The misconception was the natural consequence of the character of the pathological material and the method of examination then available for the study of the disease. The pathology described was derived from the inspection of arteries in the autopsy room and amputation specimens. At autopsy the pathologist was confined to the study of limited sections of the arterial tree, seldom gaining access to an overall view of the pathological changes of the entire vascular system. As an example, the atherosclerotic pathological involvement of the extracranial carotid arterial system remained poorly understood until the 1940s, since in the routine autopsy technique the carotid arteries were usually not dissected out; they were needed intact for the embalmer.

The essentially segmental nature of the atherosclerotic process did not become obvious until methods were devised to explore the arterial system in its entirety, first by injection methods in the dissecting room and ultimately in the living subject by angiography.

The nearly contemporaneous arrival (all within about a decade!) on the clinical scene of answers to the problems of coagulation, arterial substitution, and the nature of segmental atherosclerosis is one of the most impressive instances of the fundamental law of growth of medical knowledge that great advances do not spring forth from the flash of a genius but germinate slowly in many minds. The example of the coming to life of vascular surgery is particularly telling, since three disparate discoveries had to converge to bring it about.

Before sketching the emergence of the triad of essentials, it will be instructive to note how their absence brought about an oft-quoted historical interlude that has in the past puzzled many historians.

During the first decade of this century, Carrel and Guthrie (3–5) resolved virtually all the problems of vascular reconstruction that were of purely technical character. They refined suturing methods that allowed resection, transplantation, and replacement of autogenic and allogenic arterial segments, and even of organs. They had no anticoagulants, antibiotics, or synthetic arterial substitutes, but they succeeded since their experiments were acute, their technical skill superb, and they understood asepsis. Their work received sufficient recognition to assure for Carrel the distinction of a Nobel Prize (1912), but their work never became a part of clinical practice. Scattered writings in the 1920s and 1930s make reference to attempts at duplicating these technical procedures on the clinical level, but by 1950 the procedures had been forgotten (as had been Carrel's name). The modern pioneers of vascular surgery started their work in the belief that the techniques they used were new and of their own invention.

The brilliantly conceived experimental ideas of Carrel and Guthrie could not survive in the setting of clinical practice owing to the same practical constraints that for so long retarded the advent of vascular surgery as an independent discipline. Their acute experiments performed with superb skill and meticulous asepsis proved too often failures in the less friendly atmosphere of the operating theater.

Among the triad of essentials, the means of exploring the living human arterial tree came first.

As do so many technical advances, contrast angiography followed a tentative, wavering, but eventually successful path of growth. The turning point in this evolution was the introduction in 1929 (6) of water-soluble organic iodides to replace such contrast media as strontium bromide, sodium iodide, and iodized poppyseed oil that had proved to be hazardous. Many methods of introducing the contrast substances into the body were devised (some quite fanciful, such as transesophageal puncture of the thoracic aorta) but eventually three approaches gained general usage: direct transcutaneous needle puncture (when an artery was easily accessible), translumbar abdominal aortic puncture, and transcatheter injection (1953). It was the demonstration by Moniz (7) (in 1927) of the feasibility of obtaining roentgen images of the intracerebral circulation by the carotid injection of sodium iodide that signaled the inception of the acceptance of contrast visualization of the arterial tree as a practical clinical diagnostic tool. The development by Raimundo dos Santos (8) of the method of translumbar aortography (1929) provided a wide scope for the study of the peripheral arterial circulation. Since then remarkable advances have been achieved both in the methods of introduction [notably by the Seldinger technique in 1953 (9)] and in the pharmacologic quality of contrast media.

The second indispensable aid for direct surgical attack on the arteries, a safe agent to control blood coagulation, entered clinical practice in 1937 (10), although it had been available as early as 1933. By the early 1940s, heparin was in wide clinical use in the treatment of venous thrombosis and was ready to be applied to intervention on the arterial tree. With the ability to localize by means of angiography potentially correctable arterial obstructing lesions and the details of the practical administration of a potent anticoagulant well-understood, the stage was set for a direct attack on arterial obliterative disease.

The Years of Maturation

In 1947 Cid dos Santos (11) (the son of Raimundo) was the first to take advantage of this clinical potential and performed what can be regarded as the first reconstructive procedure on a human artery in the modern mode by removing the obstructive atherosclerotic complex from a femoral artery. Wylie (12) extended the use of this technique to the aortoiliac area. In quick succession, arterial homografts for the replacement of diseased arteries came into use, resurrecting the homograft replacement techniques described by Guthrie in laboratory experiments. The first outstanding achievement with the use of human allograft was the successful treatment of coarctation of the thoracic aorta by resection and insertion of arterial homografts in 1949 by Gross (13).

In 1951 Dubost (14) performed the first resection and allograft replacement of an abdominal aortic aneurysm, and the following year Oudot (15) resected an occluded aortic bifurcation and replaced it with an allograft.

The rapid forward march of vascular surgery—now possessed of the three conditions of successful existence: patient material in abundance, an effective anticoagulant method, and the availability of arterial allografts for replacement—was seriously threatened when postoperative follow-up observations proved arterial allografts to be unstable and thus unreliable (16). Providentially, the long-continued search for an artificial replacement for arteries met with success at this critical moment. In 1949 Voorhees (17) reported the successful demonstration of the use of a porous conduit woven of synthetic material for arterial replacement. Then a vigorous search began for the best-suited synthetic arterial substitute, a search that is still continuing.

The early experience with the most popular synthetic textile tube, the one made of Dacron, regardless of minor differences in the details of fabrication among various brands, yielded very satisfactory short-term results in all the anatomical regions in which it was used. Extended postoperative follow-up, however, soon showed that the good results were maintained after the second and third postoperative years only in areas of high flow and high pressure, and under special geometric conditions of the implantation. Grafts less than 8 mm in diameter, extending over distances greater than 30 to 40 cm, and crossing joints showed a consistent tendency for early clotting.

In the mid-1950s reconstructive surgery with synthetic grafts of arteries of the dimensions of the femoral artery or less reached a critical point. Fortunately, the ingenious concept of the utilization of bypass technique with the greater saphenous vein in femoropopliteal reconstruction first proposed in 1949 by Kunlin (18) had proved to be highly successful. When the use of small-bore synthetic arterial substitutes was found to be unsatisfactory, the surgeon now had an excellent alternative in the form of the greater saphenous vein, wider popularity of which earlier was retarded by the considerable technical demands of its insertion.

The decades 1950 to 1970 saw an unprecedented expansion of the clinical use of the newfound surgical techniques. The domain of application, first limited to the abdominal aorta and large peripheral arterial trunks, was extended to all the visceral branches of the abdominal aorta, to the thoracic aorta and its branches, to the carotid arteries, and to the infrapopliteal arterial branches. The specific indications for the suitability of technical modalities, such as endarterectomy or bypass grafting or resection and grafting, for different types of lesions and anatomical environments, were clarified. Aided not only by increased experience but also by improved suture materials and such secondary aids as magnifying loupes, there was great improvement in the technical details. The early and late postoperative success rates rose and were reported with increasingly more stringent statistical methods. In a purely technical sense, by the conclusion of the 1970s there seemed to be relatively small room for advance in the operative technical field of vascular surgery. A good deal of improvement remained to be achieved, however, in the areas of diagnostic methods and vascular substitutes.

Perspectives of Progress

Between 1949 and 1970 traditional contrast angiography for diagnosing vascular disease had been refined and its risk reduced to an acceptable level. Still its disadvantages were not negligible: As a screening examination it was expensive and somewhat risky; its static representation of the vascular disease was at times a drawback; and its availability with the desired high quality of excellence was limited. Thus the advent of the so-called noninvasive diagnostic methods (19) utilizing ultrasound both for hemodynamic analysis and for imaging filled a genuine need. First accepted as an adjunct that simplified sorting out the significant from the unimportant vascular lesions, or as a handy tool for follow-up, the applicability of these methods using harmless forms of radiation from ultrasound to positron emission has widened and deepened the area of diagnostic exploration to a degree where they promised to augment the information about vascular disease never foreseen. Although at this moment the quality of imaging of the arterial lesions by these methods does not equal that of contrast radiology, the pace at which their technology is being refined promises that these deficiencies will soon be corrected and the resolution of these methods will approach or match the resolution of angiography.

Contrast angiography itself has made forward strides in the realms of safety and patient convenience. Digital subtraction angiography, by reducing the concentration of dye in vital organs, has increased the safety factor and significantly reduced the inconvenience of direct aortic injection. The imaging quality of this technique when the intraarterial route of introduction is used is improving with astounding rapidity. Even at the present time it frequently comes close to the quality of traditional contrast angiography.

Progress has been much slower in the second area of need: in the area of improving the small-bore arterial substitutes.

The textile prostheses now available from commercial sources for arterial substitution have shown no substantive change in the last 20 years. As already mentioned, they perform satisfactorily in high-flow, large-bore applications but have had highly limited usefulness in replacing small-bore arteries (those less than 8 mm in diameter). All textile prostheses are, of course, vulnerable to thrombosis even under the most favorable conditions of implantation and would perform better if their thrombogenic propensity could be modified.

The attempts to improve fabric prostheses and to create a satisfactory (''ideal'') arterial substitute have been vigorous and numerous (20). Three directions of search can be distinguished. (1) One line of effort has been aimed at modifying the method of fabrication of the standard knitted or woven Dacron prosthesis. The most widely accepted modification of construction has been the introduction of filamentous velour surface, either external or both internal and external, in knitted Dacron grafts. (2) The second type of alteration has been the introduction of nontextile materials—tanned processed human umbilical vein and expanded Teflon (polytetrafluoroethylene, or PTFE)—both for use in femoropopliteal grafting. (3) The third category of attempts at improvement has concerned the blood-graft interface, that is the modification of the process of thrombogenesis of the inner surface of the graft.

The velour surface has not brought about statistically firmly proven changes in operative results. In small-diameter replacement the late patency rates with the use of nontextile conduits (human umbilical vein and PTFE) have been better than those of textile prostheses, but do not equal the success of autogenous vein grafts. They have, however, proved that the old concept of the essentiality of porous construction is no longer tenable and that the factors that have the greater importance in the maintenance of patency in arterial substitutes are related to the very complex factors of thrombogenicity of the luminal surface.

This observation has been in keeping with the lessons learned from the constantly expanding knowledge of the physiology of the endothelial cells and smooth-muscle elements of the arterial wall. These have placed the problem of maintaining patency in an artificial artery in a new light. Advances in the performance of arterial substitutes will come from this field. Observations of the behavior of endothelial cells seeded on textile prostheses have already altered our concept of many of the details of the role of the inner lining of artificial arteries.

Crisis of Identity; Problems of Practice

While the answers to the problems I have just considered (the refinement of diagnostic techniques and the development of biologically satisfactory arterial substitutes) are slowly emerging from the work of research investigators, two problems, far removed from the laboratory, have recently intruded into the daily life of the vascular surgeon.

These problems concern the conceptual and actual identity of vascular surgery as a specialty, and, closely allied, some mundane details of its practice.

The first problem, the identity of vascular surgery as a specialty, has been a matter of controversy in the United States for over a decade. As the range of the accomplishments of vascular surgery grew from 1961 to 1970, it inevitably assumed the hallmarks of a field of surgical endeavor requiring special skills and therefore special cognitive and technical preparation, that is, the hallmarks of a self-contained specialty. The growth of the diagnostic and therapeutic techniques in the new field placed increasingly greater demands in skill and knowledge on the surgeon undertaking its practice. By the early 1970s it became obvious to the leaders of the two national vascular societies (the Society for Vascular Surgery and the International Society for Cardiovascular Surgery) that a large proportion of the surgeons venturing into the practice of treating vascular disease did not have adequate preparation and that the results of their interventions were unacceptably poor. It was the desire to improve the teaching of vascular surgery within the broad framework of general surgery that prompted the leaders of the vascular societies to approach the American Board of Surgery with the concept of a subsidiary organization for setting standards for and supervising the graduate education in the treatment of vascular diseases (21). It seemed clear that this goal could be accomplished only by lengthening the time of the training program in general surgery, preferably by adding to it a terminal year. It was also clear that owing to lack of adequate clinical material such a readjustment would be difficult to accomplish in some of the accredited general surgical training programs.

When this proposal was first submitted to the American Board of Surgery in 1972, it was summarily rejected. Although in the following years the attitude of the American Board of Surgery became more receptive, no agreement could be reached, and the two vascular societies organized their own method of inspecting graduate training programs purely for the purpose of evaluating the adequacy of teaching. No examination or granting of a diploma was contemplated.

After a series of events, the recounting of which would be lengthy and unprofitable, the attitude of the American Board of Surgery changed, and in 1982 the American Board of General Vascular Surgery was established under the aegis of the American Board of Surgery.

The impartial observer would conclude that this decision of the American Board of Surgery meant the recognition of vascular surgery as a field of surgical endeavor requiring special, strictly defined educational preparation beyond that of general surgery, and that the completion of a general surgical training program would continue to provide familiarity only with the essentials of the surgical treatment of vascular diseases.

In a strangely self-contradictory way, however, at the same time as it began to organize the first examination for special vascular competence, the American Board of Surgery reasserted that "general surgeons are expected to have detailed knowledge . . . of the pre-operative, operative, and post-operative care of the patients with diseases of the . . . vascular system" (22).

This requirement, somewhat less sharply worded, had been on the books for many years, but had in actual practice been loosely interpreted. When the Surgical Residency Review Board began to inspect the vascular training programs, however, it became obvious that the American Board of Surgery now wished the requirement to be enforced in its literal sense. The vascular training programs that were reviewed in 1983 and 1984 were scrutinized principally by the criterion of their "interference" with the opportunity of the general surgical trainees to acquire "adequate exposure" to the whole range of vascular problems and their treatment. By the end of 1984, only 20 of the inspected programs had been approved. In virtually every instance, the reason for rejection was the insufficient vascular experience provided for the general surgical resident. Unfortunately and somewhat inexplicably, the Surgical Residency Review Board never seemed willing to define precisely what "adequate experience" in vascular surgery for the general surgical resident was. Rumors have spoken of the minimum requirement of 30 to 40 independent vascular reconstructive operations, but no firm guideline has been announced.

These events have, of course, created an atmosphere of apprehension and confusion in the ranks of surgeons treating vascular diseases. They find it extremely difficult to assign a rational explanation to the position of the American Board of Surgery as reflected in the process of evaluation pursued by the Surgical Residency Review Committee.*

The circumstance that makes it particularly difficult for the practicing surgeon to see the logic of the Board's position is that there is universal agreement among those acquainted with the demands of vascular surgery that the minimum requirement for gaining competence is a 12-month segment of time, which a standard (five-year) general surgical residency cannot provide without serious curtailment of the time essential for exposure to other subdivisions of general surgical experience. Moreover, the number of independently performed surgical cases required for gaining genuine competence in vascular surgery must be in the range of 80 to 120 (rather than 30 to 40), which is most unlikely to be obtainable in the course of general surgical training.

Since the establishment of the General Vascular Surgical Board by the American Board of Surgery seems to be an overt endorsement of these views, one is at a loss to see clearly the motives behind the contradictory policy now pursued. Unfortunately the American Board of Surgery has not clearly stated the motivating factors behind the decision of insisting on a substantive though incomplete training experience in the treatment of vascular disease for the general surgical resident. One is forced to search for explanation by weighing some assumptions.

The suspicion voiced by some that the American Board of Surgery is motivated by the ideological goal of attempting to maintain the "integrity of the field of general surgery," that is, that it has resolved to stop the so-called fragmentation, cannot be evaluated objectively. This attitude, if it existed, would be rooted in subjective conceptions unsuited to objective analysis, and the validity of its existence could only be ascertained by elimination of other possible motives.

At times members of the policymakers of the American Board of Surgery have informally expressed the view that the purpose of the rotation of the general surgical resident through a number of cognate specialties and general surgical subspecialties is to equip the general surgical resident with skills and knowledge that may be required yet unavailable from specialists in small communities. Today it is difficult to find an acceptable rationale for this view. As far as vascular surgery is concerned, one may hear the argument that vascular emergencies must be handled locally by a general surgeon if a fully trained vascular surgeon is not available. Unfortunately, the life-threatening emergencies of arterial lesions (ruptured aneurysms and acute occlusion or injury of major arteries) require the ultimate in skill and judgment. The general surgeon incompletely trained in vascular surgery cannot properly (and usually is not willing to) handle these problems. Indeed, these cases are best managed by transporting, in the appropriate direction, either the patient or a competent vascular surgeon, as the case may be.

*It is, of course, common knowledge that the Surgical Residency Review Committee is administratively quite separate and independent of the American Board of Surgery. In practice its actions, however, seem to reflect faithfully the requirements that flow from the policy positions of the American Board of Surgery.

The assumption that the American Board of Surgery perceives a shortage of personnel to respond to the needs of the patients requiring treatment for vascular disease seems an unlikely factor in the pursuit of the current policy of the Board. Even if one accepts, for the sake of argument, that such motivation exists and that a shortage indeed is present, the proper remedy would obviously not be the admission to practice of inadequately trained vascular surgeons. (The question of the size of the available personnel for the treatment of vascular disease is to be touched upon presently.)

If, for the sake of argument again, one presumes that the need of the public requires surgical personnel beyond the available number of fully trained vascular surgeons, the question must be answered whether there are at hand sufficient educational resources to provide the training. To answer this question one needs numerical data regarding the available clinical material, its distribution among the surgeons practicing vascular surgery, and the number of residents to be trained. The available data regarding all these parameters are not firm or up-to-date, but they show strong enough trends to allow projections on which acceptable conclusions can be based.

As quoted by Rutkow and Ernst (23), the National Center for Health Statistics (NCHS) has collected reasonably reliable data that show that in 1978 the number of vascular reconstructive operations in the United States was about 340,000. It is also important to note that according to the data of NCHS this figure represented an increase of 117 percent over the total number of operations in 1970. The increase between 1970 and 1978 was at an almost predictable rate of 15 percent per year.

The cohort of surgeons performing these operations must be divided into two subsets: vascular surgeons and general surgeons. According to the estimates of Rutkow and Ernst (23), 1900 surgeons claimed to be regarded as vascular specialists in 1978. An undefinable proportion of these surgeons, however, also practiced general surgery. It is probably correct to assume that as a group they devoted an average of 70 percent of their working time to the management of vascular problems. In such practice environment the caseload of vascular operations for each surgeon of this group would be from 100 to 150 reconstructive procedures per year. Altogether this cadre of vascular surgeons can reasonably be assumed to take care of from 190,000 to 270,000 vascular patients yearly. This would then leave, of the total of 340,000 cases, from 70,000 to 140,000 cases for treatment by general surgeons. The American Medical Association publication *Physician Distribution and Medical Licensure* stated in 1978 that 25,000 physicians classified themselves as general surgeons. There is no firm estimate available of what proportion of the general surgeons also performed vascular operations, but an acceptable and conservative guess would be 25 percent, or about 6000. Relating this estimate to the number of vascular problems not attended to by so-called vascular surgeons (70,000 to 140,000) would leave at the disposal of general surgeons interested in vascular surgery about 12 to 24 cases a year. The disturbing implication of this estimate is that this amount of involvement in vascular reconstruction will not allow the surgeon, regardless of the quality of training, to maintain technical proficiency in a field in which demands on operative skill are of the highest order. There is abundant factual proof that the quality of technical performance seen in this category of surgical practice is well below standard.

To look at the other side of the coin, all the reconstructive vascular procedures now carried out could be without difficulty performed by the cadre of so-called well-trained vascular surgeons at the rate of about 200 to 220 cases per year, the average load of the truly full-time vascular surgeon.

The conclusion is inevitable: The personnel trained to perform vascular surgery is fully adequate for the task of providing the necessary service to the public.

The amount of available personnel and the amount of vascular disease requiring surgical treatment have a serious bearing on graduate education in vascular surgery.

There are currently about 1200 general surgical residents in senior status in about 300 accredited general surgical programs in the United States. To provide them with the kind of vascular experience that seems to be demanded by the American Board of Surgery would require an aggregate of about 48,000 cases a year. These cases would have to come out of the clinical volume of full-time, fully trained vascular surgeons, since the general surgeon with "occasional" vascular practice does not have the interest, time, or opportunity to instruct.* How big is this pool? The answer is a mere guess since even the speculative figures of caseload quoted earlier would be inapplicable to this problem. One would have to know the clinical volume of a very specific type of practice: the volume of vascular surgical cases in major teaching centers. As a crude approximation (with adjustment for increases for the past 5 years), this figure would not exceed 150,000. The required "teaching material" would thus constitute at least about 30 percent of the total caseload of the teaching staff. It is not likely that in the private practice setting that is now universal such a large segment of the clinical volume would be readily released for teaching.

A summation of all these considerations together strongly supports the view shared by the vast majority of the experienced surgeons interested in vascular disease that the American Board of Surgery's current educational goal in the vascular training of the general surgical resident faces extremely serious practical difficulties. It seems very likely that it will not succeed in improving the general quality of the surgical treatment of vascular diseases. On the contrary, it may create two classes of surgeons at different levels of competence dealing with vascular diseases, and such a system of double standard may in fact lower the overall level of quality of the service to patients, particularly since the effect of triage of difficult cases generally observed at the present time would be impeded. The increased number of surgeons with the desire to put to use their assumed newly gained knowledge of vascular surgery will sharpen whatever competition already exists in acquiring cases for surgical treatment, a trend that will inevitably lead to lowering of operative indications and possibly result in unnecessary surgical interventions. Thus the net result will likely be a loss of quality in the service offered to the sick.

*In this regard it is relevant to note that 20 percent of the accredited general surgical residencies are in hospitals with fewer than 400 beds, in which the volume of vascular surgical cases is undoubtedly inadequate for teaching.

Is the Bold New World Too Bold?

A look at the nearly exponential rise in the number of vascular surgical procedures performed during the years 1970 to 1978 (a trend that may since have slowed but has not stopped) raises some disturbing questions.

Has vascular surgery discovered new domains of disease requiring surgical treatment? Have the techniques of vascular surgery been so improved that they can now be applied with success to degrees of vascular disease heretofore unsuited for surgical management? Or are the existing surgical procedures being used under extended, less rigid, perhaps even less critical indications?

On reflection one finds that all these factors contributed to the spectacular growth of numbers, but while the extension of the applicability of the correction of vascular disease into new areas (such as the vertebrobasilar and infrapopliteal anatomical regions) and the technical advances (such as microsurgical techniques) have augmented the value of the service to the sick, the last-named phenomenon (the uncritical relaxation of the restrictions to operate) may serve an unworthy goal and may be damaging to the ethics of medicine.

The danger of broadening operative indications beyond justifiable boundaries is particularly alive in vascular surgery. The philosophy that underlies vascular operative decisions (that is, to save life and limb by all reasonable means) has the widest range in which it can exert its influence and still remain within the bounds of conventional ethics.

The very nature of arterial reconstruction is embedded in variability. The fundamental goal of vascular reconstruction is to make blood flow where it did not flow before. The unbidden forces of nature favor this effort. The blood is impelled to move if the minimal demands of the laws of flow are met. For this reason vascular conduits of complex and even bizarre geometry can be devised and used with at least temporary success. On the other hand, when compelling hydrodynamic forces are not present, even the ideal conduit fails. These contradictory forces lend an element of gambling to arterial operations and encourage audacity. In general, imagination has a wide field in which to play, and if blood flow is even fleetingly maintained, the most unorthodox approach to a problem may be accepted and can even become popular.

An added incentive to adventurousness is that in many instances even the least promising operation can be justified since the alternative is loss of a limb. For the peace of mind of a surgeon, the triumph of immediate salvage, however ephemeral, justifies the effort. It is easy to overlook what happens later.

Finally, not infrequently there are no reliable objective guidelines for the choice of the best way to proceed in face of a complex arterial lesion. Any action seems as justified as any other.

All these, of course, may be and usually are excusable and even honorable sources of motivation. The disenchanting question is the degree to which they are used to serve less honorable goals, such as mere effort of compiling numbers or to ensure commercial gain, or even to fight for turf.

Excluding venal motives, the philosophy of making surgical decisions inevitably is in part a matter of personal temperament, but it must not be wholly or mostly so. Tradition has built a list of precepts in service of the guidance of the vascular surgeon in this regard, which may by some be perceived as a litany of truisms, but which are still worth remembering.

1. It is a grievous error to operate on the basis of the angiogram. Properly made and interpreted angiograms do not lie, but the same pathological lesions as shown in an angiogram may have fundamentally different meaning in another patient. The starting point of the decision-making process is always the patient's history and the physical findings.

2. Failure to acknowledge the limits of one's potential is usually the first step to disaster. One must recognize the share that one has of the ability rationed to human beings to accomplish a difficult goal. To adopt such realism is a matter of tough self-discipline.

3. One must make a thoughtful choice of the statistical figures one believes. The decision to perform a complex operation under unpromising conditions often hinges on the acceptance or disregard of the results that others have reported under similar circumstances. One wants to be guided by the most reliable figures. Very few surgeons who write about their experience lie, but some accept poorly controlled or uncontrolled observations, and a few fudge their results. In general, the closer the reported results are to the observations of a conscientious, well-trained surgeon, the more likely it is that they are correct.

4. One must remember "What price a leg?" in a given case, for the price varies. A below-knee amputation properly rehabilitated and fitted is, at almost any age, one of the lesser disasters of life. Contrariwise, an above-knee amputation in a person over 60 may mean lameness. A double amputation under any conditions means an unhappy and often miserable existence. The patient who has already lost one limb is entitled to rather heroic attempts to salvage the other.

5. These days the problems that the choice of diagnostic methods raises in vascular disease are almost as vexatious as the dilemmas of surgical decision. There was a time when the surgeon took a history, felt the pulses, observed the skin, checked the motor and sensory function, and decided whether an angiogram was necessary and, if so, what kind. Now the methods of examination that have come to be called *noninvasive* (principally ultrasound imaging and flow-velocity measurements) are available in great abundance. If there is a single characteristic that distinguishes the current practice of vascular surgery from the practice of 10 or 15 years ago, it is the great, at times uncritical, reliance on these noninvasive diagnostic methods. It is undeniable that the potential benefits of these methods for the patient are great, but they are subject to easy misuse and even abuse. The most damaging misuse is the substitution of the new methods for a careful history and a thorough physical examination. Used in this preemptive fashion, not only are they uninformative and often unnecessary, but they can be misleading. Their most immediate and most useful function is as an extension of the senses of the examiner. On a more sophisticated level, they represent a less risky and less costly alternative to angiography for a preliminary exploration. And ultimately they add a physiological dimension to the results of the angiographic study of the arterial tree. Keeping these precepts in mind, the so-called flow laboratory can be a fruitful and economical source of solid information.

At the present state of evolution, studies based on ultrasound imagery and ultrasound measurement of flow velocity can very seldom be regarded as the ultimate tools for making surgical decisions. There is little doubt, however, that their capabilities are rapidly enlarging, and ultimately they may become the decisive instrument for operative planning. But by prudent standards that time is not yet.

Epilogue

The young surgeons who have cast their lot with the demanding craft of vascular surgery have the rare chance of solving problems that only a few years ago were unsolvable: they can ease the burden of life of the sick with means out of the reach of an earlier generation. And when their resources seem short of their need, they can take courage in the knowledge that their artful science is still growing and very likely will find answers to the questions now unanswerable. In these, the subtle, almost transcendental, qualities of their work alone, they may find a fair recompense for the sweat and anguish that a conscientious practice of vascular surgery exacts.

References

1. Cohn I: *Rudolph Matas, Biography of the Great Pioneer in Surgery*. New York, Doubleday, 1960.
2. Matas, R.: Personal experiences in vascular surgery. Ann Surg 1940, 112:802.
3. Carrel A: Results of the transplantation of blood vessels, organs and limbs. JAMA 1908, 51:1662.
4. Carrel A: Latent life of arteries. J Exp Med 1910, 12:460.
5. Guthrie CC: *Blood Vessel Surgery and Its Applications* (Reprint). Harbinson SP, Fisher B (eds). Pittsburgh, University of Pittsburgh Press, 1959, p 360.
6. Binz A, et al: Der Wiedergabe von Nieren und Harnwegen im Röntgenbilde durch Jodpyridonderviate. Angew Chem 1930, 43:452.
7. Moniz E: L'encephalographie arterielle; son importance dans la localisation des tumeurs cerebrales. Rev Neurol 1927, 2:72.

8. Dos Santos R, Lamas A, Pereira CJ: L'arteriographie des membres de l'aorte et ses branches abdominales. Bull Soc Nat Chir 1929, 55:587.
9. Seldinger S: Catheter replacement of the needle in percutaneous arteriography. Acta Radiol 1953, 39:368.
10. Murray DWG, Best CH: The use of heparin in thrombosis. Ann Surg 1938, 108:163.
11. Dos Santos JC: Sur la désobstruction des thromboses arterielles anciennes. Mem Acad Chir 1947, 73:409.
12. Wylie EJ, et al: Experimental and clinical experiences with the use of fascia lata applied as a graft about major arteries after thrombo-endarteriectomy and aneurysmorrhaphy. Surg Gynecol Obstet 1951, 93:257.
13. Gross RE, Bill AH Jr, Pierce EC II: Methods for preservation and transplantation of arterial grafts: Observations on arterial grafts in dogs. Report of transplantation of preserved arterial grafts in nine human cases. Surg Gynecol Obstet 1949, 88:689.
14. Dubost C, et al: A propos du traitement des aneurysms de l'aorte; ablation de l'aneurysm: Rétablissement de la continuité par greffe d'aorte conserve. Mem Acad Chir 1951, 77:381.
15. Oudot J: La greffe vasculaire dans les thromboses du carrefour aortique. Presse Med 1951, 59:234.
16. Szilagyi DE, et al: Biologic fate of human arterial homografts. AMA Arch Surg 1957, 75:506 (Oct).
17. Voorhees AB Jr, Jaretzki A III, Blakemore AW: The use of tubes constructed from Vinyon "N" cloth in bridging arterial defects. Ann Surg 1952, 135:332.
18. Kunlin J: Le traitement de l'artérite oblitérante par la greffe veineuse. Arch Mal Coeur 1949, 42:371.
19. Satomura S, Kanecko Z: Ultrasonic blood rheograph. In *Proceedings of the Third International Conference on Medical Electronics*, 1960.
20. Stanley JC, et al (eds): *Biologic and Synthetic Vascular Prostheses*. New York: Grune & Stratton, 1982.
21. Garrett HE: Evaluation and endorsement of vascular training programs and certificate of qualifications in general vascular surgery. Surgery 1982, 92:915.
22. The American Board of Surgery, Inc: Specialty of surgery defined. In *Directory of Medical Specialists*. Chicago, Marquis Who's Who, 1983, p 3835.
23. Rutkow JM, Ernst CB: Vascular surgical manpower. Arch Surg 1982, 117:1537.

Chapter 2

PATHOPHYSIOLOGY OF ATHEROSCLEROSIS

RUSSELL ROSS

The Disease Process

The lesions of atherosclerosis take different forms, depending upon their anatomic site; the age, genetic, and physiological status of the affected individual; and upon the so-called risk factors to which each individual may have been exposed. The examination of atherosclerotic lesions with modern techniques of cell and molecular biology has revealed that each lesion contains significant elements of each of three cellular phenomena. These are smooth-muscle proliferation; the formation by the proliferated cells of large amounts of connective tissue matrix including collagen, elastic fibers, and proteoglycans; and the accumulation of intracellular and extracellular lipid (1). In each instance, the relative degree to which each of the cells responds to different atherogenic stimuli determines the unique combination of these three elements that defines the type and extent of the resulting lesion.

The lesions of atherosclerosis occur principally within the innermost layer of the artery wall, the intima. They include the fatty streak, the fibrous plaque, and the so-called complicated lesions (2). Secondary changes have been noted in the media of the artery underlying the lesion, principally in association with the more advanced lesions of atherosclerosis.

THE LESIONS

The Fatty Streak

The process of atherosclerosis begins in childhood with the development of flat, lipid-rich lesions called fatty streaks. These lesions consist of lipid-laden macrophages together with varying numbers of smooth-muscle cells. Both these cell types contain deposits of cholesterol and cholesterol oleate. Fatty streaks can be found in increasing numbers between the ages of 8 and 18 years. Fatty streaks appear in the coronary arteries at about the age of 15 years and continue to increase in amount in these vessels through the third decade of life (3).

The lesions are yellowish and sessile and cause little or no obstruction of the affected artery and no clinical sequelae. The fatty streak is ubiquitous in young people and even in those populations that do not appear to develop severe atherosclerosis. This observation suggests that lipid deposition does not inevitably lead to the advanced lesions of atherosclerosis, but that a number of other factors are associated with the progression of the lesions and with the development of the more complex form of atherosclerosis, the fibrous plaque.

The Fibrous Plaque

More advanced lesions begin to develop around the age of 25 in those populations in which there is a high incidence of atherosclerosis and its clinical sequelae. The fibrous plaque is grossly white; it becomes elevated and therefore may protrude into the lumen of the artery. If this lesion progresses sufficiently, it can occlude the lumen and compromise the vascular supply of the involved tissue. The principal change that occurs within the arterial intima during the development of the fibrous plaque consists of the proliferation of smooth-muscle cells. These cells usually form a fibrous cap due to the deposition by the cells of new connective tissue matrix and to the accumulation of intracellular and extracellular lipids. The fibrous cap covers a deeper deposit of varying amounts of extracellular lipid and cell debris (4).

It has been suggested that fibrous plaques are derived from fatty streaks that continue the process of cell proliferation, lipid accumulation, and connective tissue formation, and that the deep core of lipid and cell debris results from inadequate blood supply, and cell necrosis. Such a relationship has not been proved, since although fatty streaks in young persons are often found at the same anatomic location in the coronary and extracranial cerebral arteries as fibrous plaques in older persons, fatty streaks can also occur at anatomic sites that are different from those at which fibrous plaques appear. The reasons for these differences are not understood. It has been suggested that in those instances in which their location is different, the fatty streaks have simply regressed and disappeared, whereas in the instances in which the anatomic location is the same, lesion progression has occurred. This remains a matter of controversy (5).

The Complicated Lesion

The complicated lesions of atherosclerosis occur with increasing frequency with increasing age. The fibrous plaque can become vascularized both from the luminal and from its medial aspects.

In the complicated lesion, the necrotic "lipid-rich core" increases in size and often becomes calcified. The lesions may become increasingly complex as a result of hemorrhage and calcification, and the intimal surface may disintegrate and ulcerate and become involved with thrombotic episodes that may lead to occlusive disease. Such thrombi may then organize and further increase the thickness of the plaque while progressively reducing the size of the arterial lumen. Sometimes as the intimal lesions progress, the number of smooth-muscle cells in the underlying media decreases and the media atrophies; this can result in aneurysmal changes rather than lead to thrombotic occlusion of the artery.

There is quite a range in the degree of severity of the atherosclerotic lesions in different arteries. The recognition that smooth-muscle proliferation, connective tissue formation, and lipid accumulation represent the key elements of the developing lesions of atherosclerosis has led to the use of a number of models of experimentally induced atherosclerosis to study this process in different animal species.

STUDIES IN EXPERIMENTAL ANIMALS

Four species have been widely used in studying atherogenesis: rabbits, chickens, swine, and nonhuman primates. Most early work was performed in rabbits; however, swine and nonhuman primates are generally considered to develop lesions that correspond more closely with those that occur in human beings. Atherosclerosis has been induced in most of the animal models by a high-fat, high-cholesterol diet. A principal shortcoming of this approach, however, is that to produce more advanced lesions, it is necessary to maintain animals on such diets for years. Even though it is possible to induce the lesions in a relatively short period (1 to 3 years in the monkey), it is not clear that the lesions produced in this manner actually simulate those that may require 20 to 30 years to form in human beings. On the other hand, the rate at which the lesions form in humans is not entirely clear; some may progress more rapidly than had heretofore been considered to be possible (6).

Other approaches to studying the smooth-muscle proliferative changes associated with atherosclerosis have included endothelial injury resulting from mechanical trauma from various types of intraarterial catheters (7,8), chemically induced injury (from sources such as chronic hypercholesterolemia) (9) or chronic homocystinemia (10), immune-type injury (11) (from exposure to antigen-antibody complexes), and, more recently, virally induced injury in diseases such as Marek's disease (12).

In a recent study of diet-induced hypercholesterolemia in nonhuman primates, Faggiotto et al. (13,14) described the changes that lead to fatty streak development, and the manner in which some fatty streaks progress to become more complicated fibrous plaques. Within 12 days after the induction of high levels of plasma cholesterol (>700 mg/dL), numerous monocytes were observed attached to the surface of the endothelium throughout the arterial tree. These monocytes probe between junctional complexes of the endothelium, migrate, and localize subendothelially, where they accumulate lipid and become foam cells that establish the initial fatty streak. These fatty streaks form at branches and bifurcations and accumulate increasing numbers of macrophages and smooth-muscle cells, and in the process create a markedly uneven surface contour and stretch the overlying endothelium exceedingly thin. After about 5 months, breaks occur between endothelial cells, exposing the lipid-filled macrophages, some of which appear to enter the circulation. Many of the exposed macrophages serve as sites where platelets adhere and form mural thrombi. These sites of platelet-macrophage interactions were first observed in the iliac arteries, and after longer periods of hypercholesterolemia, similar changes occur at higher levels in the abdominal and then the thoracic aorta. Interestingly, the sites that are first involved with platelet-macrophage interactions are the same sites that 1 to 2 months later contain the proliferative smooth-muscle lesions of atherosclerosis. These findings further support observations that endothelial injury and platelet-macrophage interactions may be important in atherogenesis.

Hypotheses of Atherogenesis

Atherosclerosis has been recognized in humans for thousands of years. Lesions of atherosclerosis were identified in Egyptian mummies as early as the fifteenth century B.C. Long (15) has discussed the development of clinical-pathological correlations during the era when autopsy permitted an understanding of the relationship between the degree of atherosclerosis and the incidence of myocardial infarction and stroke. In the mid-nineteenth century, Virchow (16) proposed that some form of injury to the artery wall associated with an inflammatory response results in what was then considered to be the degenerative lesion of atherosclerosis. This idea was subsequently modified by Anitschkow (17) and further included the role of platelets and thrombogenesis in atherosclerosis, as expounded by Duguid (18) in 1948. Many of the modern views of atherogenesis stem from the work of John French (19), who suggested that the structural integrity of the endothelial lining of the artery represents a key element in the maintenance of normal arterial function and that alterations in endothelial integrity may precede a sequence of events that lead to the various lesions in atherosclerosis. Thus over the years a number of theories concerning the etiology and pathogenesis of atherosclerosis have been developed. At least two of these deserve elaboration and comment. There are the response-to-injury hypothesis and the lipogenic hypothesis.

THE RESPONSE-TO-INJURY HYPOTHESIS

One basis for the *response-to-injury hypothesis* of atherosclerosis (1,9,20) lies in the marked similarity, observed by many investigators, between the ubiquitous fibromusculoelastic lesions noted at autopsy and a similar lesion that can be induced in a number of animal species, including nonhuman primates, rabbits, and swine, after different forms of arterial endothelial injury.

This hypothesis states that some form of "injury" to the endothelium results in structural and/or functional alterations in the endothelial cells. Factors such as chronic hypercholesterolemia (9); increased shear stress from the flow of blood over the endothelial cells, as may occur at branch points or bifurcations in arteries in hypertension (21); and dysfunction induced by toxins or other injurious agents may lead to changes in the nature of the permeability barrier established by the endothelial cells. In the normal artery, the endothelial cells form a continuous monolayer that regulates the passage of substances from the plasma to the underlying artery wall. Injury to the endothelial cells may alter their permeability characteristics and change endothelial cell–cell or endothelial cell–connective tissue relationships, permitting hemodynamic forces to induce focal endothelial cell detachment and thus permit interactions to occur between elements from the blood and the wall of the artery.

Not only do the endothelial cells play an important role as a permeability barrier, but they also form a thromboresistant surface that promotes the continuous flow of blood throughout the vascular tree. The thromboresistant character of the endothelium appears to be due principally to two factors produced by the cells. Both of these have been identified, but their physiological roles are relatively poorly understood. They are the glycoproteins and proteoglycans that form the surface coat of the endothelial cells, and a prostaglandin derivative, prostacyclin (PGI_2) (22). PGI_2 is one of the most potent vasodilatory agents thus far isolated and is a potent inhibitor of platelet aggregation. Both endothelial cells and smooth-muscle cells are capable of synthesizing PGI_2; however, endothelial cells appear to make this prostaglandin derivative in greater quantities. This is discussed in greater detail below.

Endothelial injury that results in alterations in permeability would permit plasma constituents such as lipoproteins to have more ready access to the artery wall. Endothelial dysfunction could also alter the thromboresistant character of the lumen of the artery so that platelets could interact directly at the sites of endothelial injury. If the injury were sufficiently severe, the endothelial cells might detach and be lost into the bloodstream, exposing the underlying connective tissue to platelets and to other elements in the circulation. The response-to-injury hypothesis suggests that the interaction between platelets and the subendothelial connective tissue, principally collagen, results in platelet adherence, platelet aggregation, and the release of contents normally stored within the granules of the platelets, in particular, a mitogen, the platelet-derived growth factor. At the sites of injury the exposure of the artery wall to factors derived from the platelets, together with components from the plasma, such as lipoproteins and hormones, would then lead to the focal proliferation of arterial smooth-muscle cells. According to the hypothesis, this smooth-muscle proliferation would be derived from two sources: preexisting intimal smooth-muscle cells and medial smooth-muscle cells that are attracted to, and migrate and proliferate within, the intima at the sites of injury. Such a local stimulus could also lead to the formation of new connective tissue matrix constituents by the proliferating smooth-muscle cells and to the deposition of lipids both within and around the proliferated cells (Figure 2-1).

According to this hypothesis, if the injury to the endothelium were a self-limited event and endothelial integrity were restored, the proliferative lesions might be capable of regressing. If this were the case, the lesions would be reversible, and if they had not reached a critical size, they would be clinically silent. There is evidence both in experimental animals and in human beings that the lesions of atherosclerosis can, under certain conditions, regress (23).

On the other hand, if the injury at focal sites in the artery wall is either long-standing or chronically repeated over periods of many years, the lesions could continue to progress, become increasingly complex in composition, and eventually lead to the principal clinical sequelae of atherosclerosis, myocardial infarction, and cerebral infarction. The capacity of the endothelium to regenerate and to restore endothelial integrity at sites of injury may be critical in determining whether the lesions of atherosclerosis enlarge, remain relatively constant in size, or regress. The superimposition of risk factors possibly affects this balance by providing a chronic source of injury, or by somehow altering the normal balance so that lesions become slowly progressive. As an example, the increased levels of plasma low-density lipoproteins associated with hypercholesterolemia may provide a source of injury to the endothelial cells and may also convert what might otherwise be a limited tissue response to injury to the frank progressive lesions of atherosclerosis.

This hypothesis has stimulated a great deal of experimental work that has led to an increase in our understanding of factors that determine the capacity of the endothelial cells to maintain themselves as an integral continuous cell layer; the hypothesis has also led to studies of those factors that control the growth of endothelium. Of equal importance, many studies have elucidated factors that modify the capacity of arterial smooth-muscle cells to form connective tissue proteins, to synthesize and metabolize lipids and lipoproteins, and to proliferate in response to different mitogenic factors.

One of the most important observations that has resulted from the examination of this hypothesis is the discovery that platelets contain a potent mitogen, the platelet-derived growth factor (24). It has been suggested that this factor may play an important role in inducing the intimal smooth-muscle proliferation seen in experimentally induced atherosclerosis and in atherosclerosis in human beings. This is discussed in greater detail below.

A number of important questions have arisen about the factors that promote the proliferation of smooth-muscle and endothelial cells and about the mechanisms whereby the lesions of atherosclerosis may regress. Relatively little is known about the factors responsible for the turnover of connective tissue matrix within the artery wall or about the mechanisms responsible for removing either this matrix or cholesterol from the lesions. The response-to-injury hypothesis has provided potential explanations for some of these phenomena. However, much remains to be learned, for example, with respect to the capacity of endothelium and smooth muscle to bind and to metabolize the different types of lipoproteins. These topics are discussed below.

THE ROLE OF LIPIDS

In many persons, both the initiation and the progression of atherosclerotic lesions appear somehow to be associated with markedly increased levels of plasma low-density lipoproteins (LDL). The accumulation of lipid within proliferated smooth-muscle cells, within macrophages in the lesions, and within the extracellular

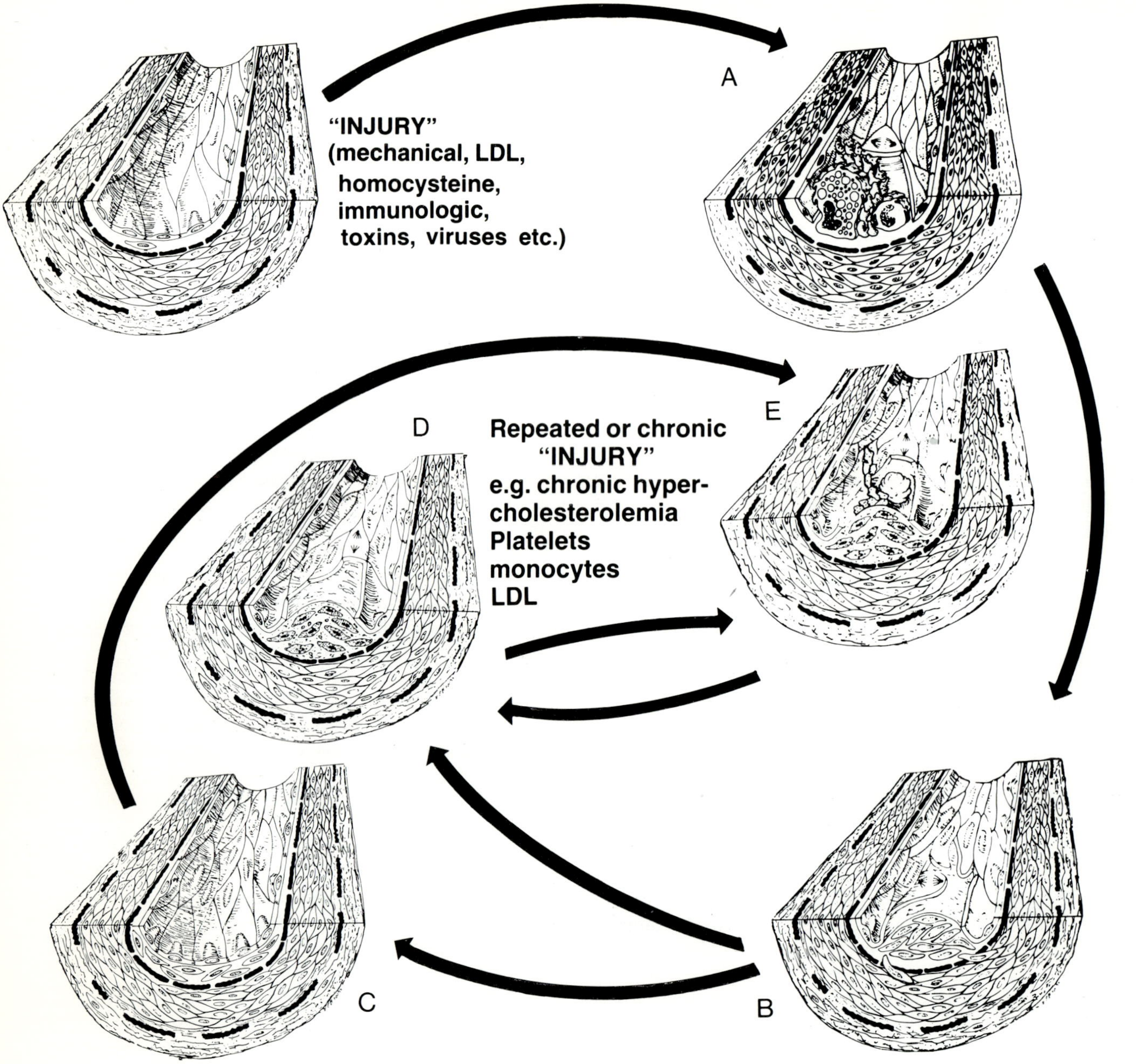

FIGURE 2-1. A diagram of a version of the response-to-injury hypothesis of atherosclerosis, modified from that described by Ross and Glomset (1). According to this hypothesis, endothelial injury results in the exposure of the subendothelium (*A*) and this allows interactions between monocytes, macrophages, and platelets. The endothelial injury in this diagram represents the maximal response in which cell-cell detachment and cell–connective tissue detachment lead to subendothelial denudation. Platelet interactions with the connective tissue or with macrophages may lead to the deposition of a growth factor such as platelet-derived growth factor, which can then induce the migration and proliferation of medial smooth-muscle cells into the intima (*B*). If the injury ceases and the endothelium regenerates, the lesion may be reversible and the result would be a slightly thickened intima (*C*). On the other hand, if the injury continues for a prolonged period of time, there may be a sequence of injury and repair followed by reinjury and repair, leading to proliferative lesions that may compromise the vascular supply (*D*) and (*E*). (Reproduced by permission of Arteriosclerosis, a journal of the American Heart Association.)

connective tissue matrix is a common finding, particularly in the lesions of atherosclerosis (25). The presence of elevated levels of LDL suggests that cholesterol internalization and esterification by cells may be accelerated to such a degree that proliferated smooth-muscle cells within the lesions become filled with cholesterol oleate. Many of the cells may go on to become necrotic and may release their lipid into the extracellular spaces. In the presence of excess plasma LDL, which is relatively rich in cholesterol linoleate, the debris may be a mixture of both types of cholesteryl esters.

Some studies have suggested that in hyperlipemic animals there are factors in LDL that in themselves may promote the proliferation of smooth-muscle cells and the production of new connective tissue components by these cells (26). Thus a sequence of events involving endothelial injury by chronic elevated levels of LDL and the continuing progression of atherosclerotic lesions by exposure to elevated levels of LDL [and presumably to decreased levels of high-density lipoproteins (HDL)] could lead to the development of advanced atherosclerotic lesions. This hypothesis might explain how some fatty streaks could progress to become fibrous plaques but fails to take into account many of the other components of the lesions of atherosclerosis; in particular, it fails to explain, in addition to the proliferative response of smooth-muscle cells, other phenomena such as the stimulation of new connective tissue formation.

It is possible that the different lesions of atherosclerosis may occur by any of the mechanisms suggested in these hypotheses; however, it is also clear that as many aspects of our understanding of the biology of smooth muscle and endothelium continue to be expanded, new unanticipated factors that may play a role in the pathogenesis of atherosclerosis may be revealed.

RISK FACTORS

A number of risk factors of atherosclerosis have become reasonably well established on the basis of their relationship in epidemiologic studies to the incidence of clinically manifest disease. Unfortunately, there is no basis for comparison between risk factors and the severity or extent of the lesions of atherosclerosis. Among many factors that are considered to be important are hyperlipidemia, hypertension, cigarette smoking, male sex, and diabetes mellitus. These have in general been associated with an increased incidence of fibrous plaques and their sequelae. The associations are relatively strong when they are made on a group basis, although all the studies have demonstrated a high degree of variability among individuals within even the most homogeneous groups (27).

Hypercholesterolemia

Dietary lipids are considered to be one of the most important environmental agents responsible for severe atherosclerosis and for the high frequency of atherosclerotic disease in industrially developed parts of the world. Saturated fats became known to be associated with an increased incidence of atherosclerosis when it was found that they elevate the concentration of plasma cholesterol; however, the specific contributions of cholesterol, saturated fats, polyunsaturated fats, and total fats in atherosclerosis are still unclear. It has not been possible to demonstrate an unequivocal association between dietary cholesterol or plasma cholesterol levels and the incidence and prevalence of coronary disease within population groups when they are analyzed on an individual basis. Unfortunately, there is a great deal of daily variation from individual to individual in terms of the dietary intake of fats and plasma cholesterol levels. There is also intrinsic variation in plasma cholesterol levels among individuals who consume the same diet and respond differently to it. This has increased the difficulty of relating this factor to the incidence of atherosclerosis but does not negate the clear association between hyperlipidemia and atherosclerosis that has been demonstrated by numerous epidemiologic studies.

There is little question that dietary cholesterol directly affects the levels of plasma cholesterol (28). However, only recently has it been suggested that dietary cholesterol may affect the incidence of atherosclerosis by altering the profile of plasma lipoproteins and possibly by changing the structural or functional properties of these lipoproteins (29). Increased dietary cholesterol generally results in an increase in LDL cholesterol levels with a lesser increase in HDL cholesterol levels. The role of these two lipoproteins in atherogenesis is not clear, although it has been suggested that elevated HDL levels may be protective, whereas the reverse is true for elevated LDL levels.

Unfortunately, there are many differences in the ways in which animals and humans respond to dietary cholesterol, and there are limits to the extent to which information concerning responses to dietary intake in experimental animals can be applied to human beings. Nevertheless, the epidemiologic association between the increased incidence of atherosclerosis and the increased intake of fat is very strong. The means by which these fats affect the incidence of atherosclerosis at the cellular and molecular levels remain to be elucidated.

Hypertension

Hypertension has been established unequivocally as an associated risk factor in that persons with elevated blood pressure show accelerated atherogenesis, an increased incidence of coronary heart disease, and in particular, an increased incidence of cerebrovascular disease. The effects of hypertension appear to be independent of other risk factors in an epidemiologic sense; however, it does not appear to be a primary cause of advanced atherosclerosis in those populations in which the incidence of clinically manifest atherosclerosis is less than average.

The means by which hypertension induces atherogenesis are not clear, although there are many humoral mediators of blood pressure which may participate in this process. For example, renin and other hypertensive agents may induce cellular changes that lead to atherogenesis. Fry (21) and his colleagues, as well as others, have suggested that the increased shear stress of the flow of blood, particularly in hypertensive persons, at selected anatomic sites within the arterial tree may result in focally altered endothelium and in the development of atherosclerotic lesions very much as suggested in the response-to-injury hypothesis discussed earlier.

Cigarette Smoking

Cigarette smoking provides perhaps the strongest and most consistent correlation with the increased incidence of atherosclerotic disease and appears to be a major contributor to the increased risk of disease, generally in combination with other risk factors. Unfortunately, there is relatively little information about how cigarette smoking exerts an impact at the cellular level. Early studies suggested that carbon monoxide might be a causative agent; however, these studies have not been confirmed. Becker (30) has identified agents derived from cigarette smoke that may be injurious to the artery wall. He has also suggested that the inhalation of cigarette smoke may result in the exposure of arterial cells to mutagens that transform the smooth-muscle cells, which are stimulated to proliferate. Apparently, the cessation of cigarette smoking decreases the risk for the development of the clinical sequelae of atherosclerosis and may augment the regression of lesions. Further research is clearly required to identify the factors in cigarette smoke that are responsible for its cardiovascular effects and to determine the mechanisms by which it alters cellular metabolism.

Male Sex

Perhaps one of the best-documented and most consistent risk factors for coronary atherosclerosis is male sex. This differential is accentuated in nonwhite populations, and it has been suggested that women have a decreased incidence because estrogens exert a protective function. Paradoxically, large doses of estrogenic hormones appear to increase cardiovascular mortality in men who have had one myocardial infarct and in men under treatment for prostatic cancer. Consequently, the reasons for the sex differential are not yet understood.

Diabetes

Another risk factor known to be associated with an increased incidence of atherosclerosis and myocardial infarction is diabetes mellitus. The mechanisms involved are poorly understood. There is, unfortunately, no consistency in the evidence related to whether elevated concentrations of plasma cholesterol and lipoproteins occur in diabetics whose concentrations of blood and urine glucose are carefully regulated. There is some evidence suggesting a decreased concentration of HDL cholesterol in diabetics and a high prevalence of hypertension associated with hyperglycemia. The basic mechanisms associated with the proliferation of smooth-muscle-type cells in the mesangium of the kidney in the renal complication of diabetes and in the increased thickness of capillary basement membranes in diabetics with microvascular disease may bear some similarity to the mechanisms of smooth-muscle proliferation in atherogenesis. However, the alterations in the arterial tree that precede the lesions of atherosclerosis in diabetics are not well-documented and are poorly understood.

Although a great deal is known (see below) about endothelial cells, smooth-muscle cells, platelets, and their interactions, the specific role of each of the risk factors associated with atherosclerosis remains, for the most part, to be investigated. This information is critical if we are to improve the means of diagnosis, prevention, and intervention in this disease process.

Cellular Modifications in Atherosclerosis

ENDOTHELIUM

Endothelial cells provide a selective permeability barrier, a blood-compatible interphase, and a thromboresistant lining to the artery wall; and they are also metabolically active. A number of studies of endothelial permeability using various tracer molecules have demonstrated the presence of pinocytotic vesicles, transendothelial channels, and intracellular clefts in different kinds of endothelium. The junctional complexes between endothelial cells and the artery wall appear to be functionally dynamic structures that can respond to stimuli such as pharmacologic agents and changes in blood pressure. At the molecular level, the surface components of the endothelial cells appear to influence the selective permeability of the endothelium (31,32). Endothelial cells have been shown by the Steins (33) to be capable of transporting plasma lipoproteins of certain sizes into the artery wall via vesicles. Thus molecules like HDL are transported, but larger lipoproteins the size of very-low-density lipoprotein (VLDL) or chylomicrons have difficulty crossing the endothelial barrier without some kind of alteration in these lipid-rich particles.

In a number of experimental animals, the disruption of this barrier has been shown to permit interactions between platelets and the artery wall at the sites of endothelial injury; this interaction results in an intimal smooth-muscle proliferative response. Stemerman and Ross (7) observed that if endothelial cells are removed by abrasion with an intraarterial catheter, the sites of exposure of the subendothelial connective tissue are quickly coated with a "carpet" of degranulated platelets. At such sites of endothelial injury, the interaction of plasma constituents with products released from the platelets is followed by focal smooth-muscle migration and proliferation that eventually lead to the development of a fibromusculoelastic lesion. If this mechanical injury is accompanied by a high-fat, high-cholesterol diet, the hyperlipemic animals develop intimal proliferative lesions essentially identical to fibrous plaques. In the normocholesterolemic animals, such endothelial injury leads to fibromusculoelastic proliferative lesions that, over a period of 6 months, may undergo regression, whereas in hypercholesterolemic animals, the lesions become slowly progressive and show no signs of regression.

Ross and Harker (9) and Faggioto et al. (13,14) observed that monkeys that received no mechanical injury but were only fed a high-fat, high-cholesterol diet for a year or longer showed signs of endothelial injury as determined morphologically and by measurements of endothelial cell turnover at selected sites in the arterial tree (Figure 2-2).

The intimal smooth-muscle proliferation that accompanies the disruption of the endothelial cell barrier has been shown to be associated with the interaction between platelets and the exposed subendothelium at such sites of injury. This is further discussed below.

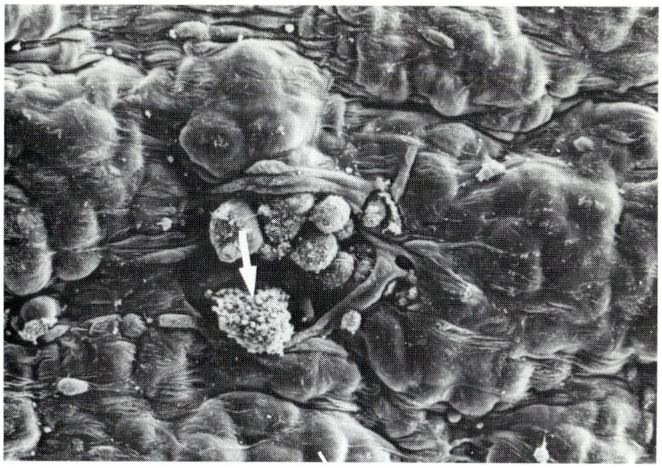

FIGURE 2-2. A scanning electron micrograph demonstrating an area over a fatty streak in the iliac artery of a monkey that had been hypercholesterolemic (600 mg/dL) for 5 months. Several exposed macrophages are visible. One of them is covered by a mural collection of platelets (*arrow*). A lesion such as this is found in the same anatomic site that 1 or 2 months later is occupied by a smooth-muscle proliferative lesion of atherosclerosis.

Endothelial Cell Culture

Arterial endothelial cells have been successfully cultured from a number of species, including the cow, rabbit, swine, nonhuman primate, and human being (34,35). Endothelial cells from each of these species demonstrate a number of common characteristics. They grow, as they do in vivo, in a unique, continuous monolayer, and unlike other cells such as smooth muscle cells or fibroblasts, appear to be truly *contact-inhibited*. That is, the cells become quiescent when they become confluent and remain quiescent as long as they remain in contact. If the monolayer is disrupted, for example, by wounding, the cells are stimulated to synthesize new DNA and to proliferate and restore the continuity of the monolayer. Only those cells next to the margins of the wound appear to undergo DNA synthesis and proliferation, whereas those in the monolayer at a distance from the wound appear to remain relatively quiescent. This peculiar characteristic of the growth of endothelium is so strikingly different from that of smooth-muscle cells that it has been suggested that these two different cell types are under different sets of growth controls and that somehow cell-cell contact is important in determining the state of quiescence of endothelial cells. Endothelial cells grown in a culture have been shown to be capable of forming a number of connective tissue matrix macromolecules including particular types of collagen (36); capable of transporting lipids; capable of synthesizing PGI_2 (37), factor VIII (38), and angiotensin-converting enzyme (39); and capable of maintaining many aspects of their differentiated phenotype through several passages.

Endothelial-Derived Growth Factor

Recently, endothelial cells have been shown to be capable of forming a mitogen, or growth factor, in culture. This substance, termed the endothelial-derived growth factor, appears to be a potent molecule in terms of its capacity to stimulate cells such as fibroblasts and smooth muscle cells to proliferate (40). Endothelial cells in culture release this factor into the medium after they have been exposed to plasma or to serum-free medium. Studies of this factor suggest that it has a number of characteristics different from those of the platelet-derived growth factor (discussed below). It is not yet known whether the endothelial-derived growth factor is formed by endothelial cells in vivo. If it were, this could have potential importance in atherogenesis; however, this is not yet clear.

SMOOTH MUSCLE

Smooth-Muscle Proliferation

Smooth-muscle cells have long been recognized to possess a number of features important to normal arterial function, including their capacity to contract, to maintain arterial tone, and to synthesize connective tissue proteins. Perhaps the most important phenomenon associated with the smooth-muscle cell is cell proliferation in atherogenesis. Since intimal smooth-muscle proliferation is an important early feature in atherogenesis, the factors responsible for this proliferative response are under intensive investigation in vivo and in vitro. In cell culture, it is well known that whole blood serum provides all the factors necessary for smooth-muscle proliferation. Arterial smooth-muscle cells from a large number of species can be grown in culture and are able to maintain their differentiated phenotype under these conditions (41,42).

Ross and coworkers (24) together with several other research groups (43,44) demonstrated that the principal component that is present in whole-blood serum and missing in cell-free, plasma-derived serum and that is responsible for the proliferation of arterial smooth-muscle cells in culture is a mitogen derived from the platelet, the platelet-derived growth factor. The observation that smooth-muscle proliferation in culture is stimulated principally by this mitogen led to a series of studies to examine the role of platelets in smooth-muscle proliferation induced in vivo.

As described above, several forms of endothelial injury result in the adherence of platelets at the sites of injury. Platelet adherence is followed by degranulation and then material stored in the platelet granules is released into the artery wall. Together with plasma constituents, these platelet products have far-reaching effects upon the smooth-muscle cells of the artery wall.

Harker et al. (10) demonstrated that in homocystinuria, a genetic disease of childhood commonly associated with a markedly increased incidence of arteriosclerosis, platelets appear to interact at sites where the endothelium has somehow been injured by increased levels of plasma homocysteine. Harker et al. demonstrated this association by measuring the survival of autologous ^{51}Cr-labeled platelets in homocystinuric children and observed that the greater the levels of plasma homocysteine, the greater the decrease in platelet survival. As a result of these observations, they developed an animal model of homocystinuria by chronically infusing homocysteine in baboons. In this model they showed a similar correlation between elevated levels of plasma homocysteine and decreased rates of platelet survival (or increased rate of platelet utilization). When they maintained the baboons on a homocystinemic regimen for 3 months, they observed an increased incidence of missing endothelial cells by morphometric examination of whole-mount preparations of the aorta. Their studies established a correlation between the amount of injured endothelium, the rate of platelet survival, and the formation of proliferative smooth-muscle atherosclerotic lesions at the sites of endothelial injury. Harker and his colleagues (10) went on to demonstrate that if they administer to the homocystinemic baboons a pharmacologic agent that can inhibit platelet interactions with the injured artery wall, they can prevent the intimal smooth-muscle proliferative lesions that otherwise develop. One agent, dipyridamole, returns platelet survival rates to normal. This drug is known to have the capacity to inhibit platelet phosphodiesterase activity and to inhibit platelet adherence. Another agent, sulfinpyrazone, appears to somehow protect the endothelial cells, since the sulfinpyrazone-treated homocystinemic baboons demonstrate fewer areas of endothelial injury. In both approaches, platelet survival rates are normalized and the proliferative lesions of atherosclerosis are prevented. These were the first data to correlate a requirement for platelet function with experimentally induced atherosclerosis.

Other approaches to examining these same phenomena were taken by Moore and his colleagues (45) and by Friedman et al. (46). In both their studies, atherosclerosis was induced in rabbits by injuring the endothelium with an intraarterial catheter. In each case, the investigators induced a thrombocytopenia by the administration of a specific antiplatelet antiserum. They found that the animals made thrombocytopenic in this manner have no proliferative atherosclerotic lesions, whereas the control animals have extensive lesions.

Using a different approach, Fuster and his colleagues (47) examined the incidence of atherosclerosis in the aortas of swine fed a high-fat, high-cholesterol diet. They were able to study the role of platelets in these swine by trying to induce atherosclerosis with a high-cholesterol diet in a group of swine that were homozygous for von Willebrand's disease compared with a group of normal swine. The swine with severe von Willebrand's disease have essentially no factor VIII—von Willebrand's factor—in their plasma. Normally this factor is required for platelet adherence and release. They showed that the control animals on the high-lipid diet develop extensive proliferative lesions of atherosclerosis, whereas the von Willebrand's swine develop intimal infiltrates of lipid but no smooth-muscle proliferative lesions. In the absence of the von Willebrand's factor, platelet interactions may be inhibited in the hypercholesterolemic von Willebrand swine.

All these studies point to the importance of platelet interactions at the sites of endothelial alterations that precede the formation of experimentally induced proliferative lesions of atherosclerosis, and point to the potential importance of mitogens from platelets like the platelet-derived growth factor.

Lipid Metabolism

Lipids are essential components of all cells; it is not surprising that they are involved in a number of cell functions and metabolic processes, as they represent the principal constituent of all cell membranes. Both the plasma membrane and the internal membranous compartments of all cells, including smooth muscle, are composed of phospholipids, proteins, and cholesterol, principally unesterified cholesterol. Esterified cholesterol is found in smooth muscle only under abnormal conditions. Accumulations of cholesteryl ester in smooth-muscle cells and macrophages lead to the development of foam cells, which are found in the lesions of atherosclerosis. Recent experiments have shown that smooth-muscle cells can acquire cholesterol both by de novo synthesis (48) and from an exogenous source of cholesterol-carrying lipoproteins (49). Such a dual mechanism may help the cell to protect itself against possible deficits in cholesterol.

Smooth-muscle cells and many other cells can also protect themselves against excess cholesterol. The mechanism that has evolved for this purpose is the surface-located, high-affinity LDL receptor (50,51). These receptors bind LDL, and the cell then internalizes the bound LDL by endocytosis and transports it to lysosomes, where the LDL is degraded and free cholesterol is liberated for use by the cell. If the cell is exposed to excess LDL, there is a feedback inhibitory pathway in the cell that inhibits the synthesis of LDL receptors. In addition, the presence of excess cholesterol within the cell inhibits cholesterol synthesis by the rate-limiting intracellular enzyme hydroxymethylglutaryl-coenzyme A reductase (HMG-CoA reductase).

Under normal circumstances, sterol balance in the cell maintains a given level of receptor for LDL at the cell surface. In this way the requirements for extracellular cholesterol are met by concentrations of plasma LDL that are not atherogenic. Increased concentrations of plasma LDL may alter the endothelial barrier and bring large amounts of LDL in direct contact with the smooth-muscle cell, which may ingest much of the LDL by bulk-phase endocytosis, bypassing the high-affinity-receptor mechanism; this leads to the increased esterification and storage of cholesteryl esters and the development of foam cells (Figure 2-3).

LDL has been said to play a mitogenic role for smooth-muscle cells in culture. Wissler and his colleagues (26) have observed that LDL derived from hyperlipemic monkeys is mitogenic in explant cultures of aorta compared with LDL from normolipemic monkeys. The means by which this LDL acts as a mitogen is not clear; however, there do appear to be differences between LDL from normolipemic donors and LDL from hyperlipemic donors in terms of their effects on smooth muscle and endothelium. The elucidation of the effects of hyperlipemic LDL may be important for understanding the basis of the atherogenic effect of hyperlipidemia.

Genetic defects in the cellular metabolism of lipoprotein are relatively common and are undoubtedly important in atherogenesis as well.

Evidence is accumulating in favor of the notion that HDL, in contrast to LDL, is a negative factor in the development of

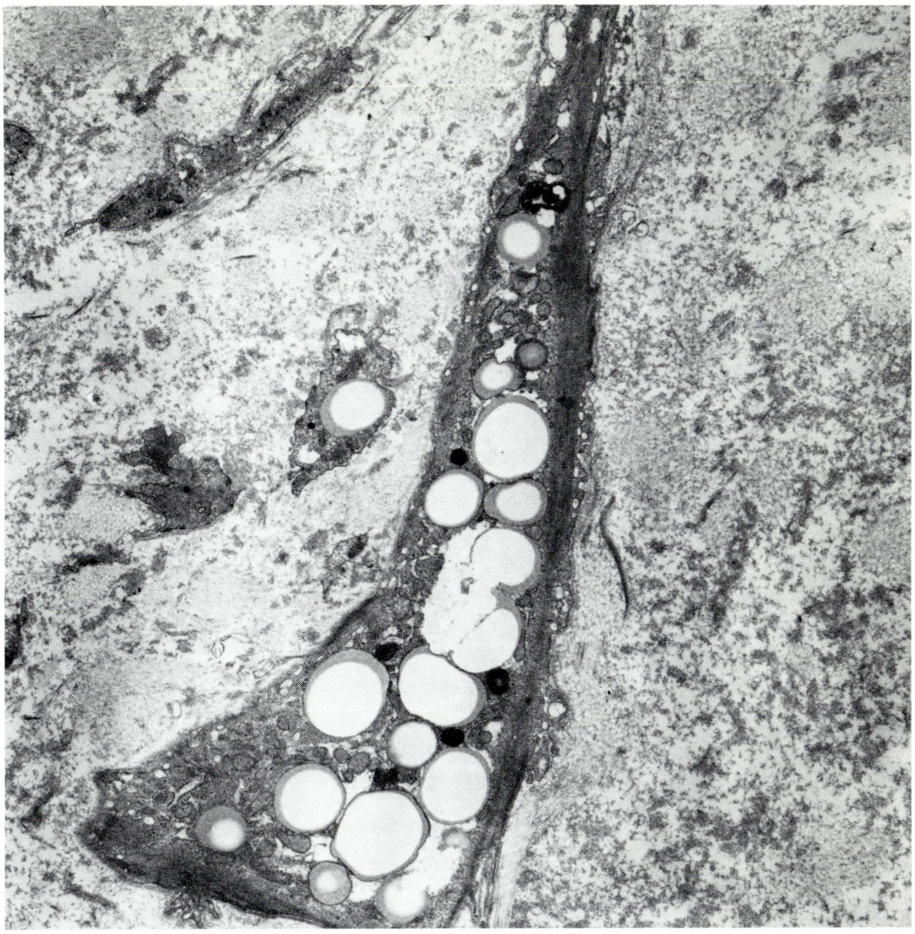

FIGURE 2-3. A transmission electron micrograph of part of an atherosclerotic lesion from the iliac artery of an 8-month-old hypercholesterolemic monkey. The smooth-muscle cell in the center of this micrograph contains numerous lipid droplets and is surrounded by connective tissue.

atherosclerosis. Two hypotheses have been proposed to explain how HDL might be a deterrent against atherosclerosis. The first suggests that HDL augments the removal of cholesterol from cells such as smooth muscle cells. The second mechanism involves the apparent ability of HDL to influence the binding and absorption of LDL by cells such as smooth muscle cells. However, neither of these mechanisms has been shown to be responsible for the control of cellular cholesterol levels.

THE MACROPHAGE

Macrophages are commonly found in early lesions of atherosclerosis as well as in advanced lesions like the fibrous plaque. These cells could conceivably play several roles in lesion progression and possibly in regression as well. In tissue culture, macrophages have been shown to release into the culture medium a mitogen as potent as that derived from platelets (52). Such a growth factor, if formed in vivo, could conceivably be important in lesion progression.

Macrophages have long been known to be largely responsible for tissue debridement. There is increasing evidence in experimental studies and in human beings (23) that some lesions of atherosclerosis are capable of regression. The role of the macrophage in this phenomenon remains to be elucidated.

PLATELETS

The Platelet-Derived Growth Factor

The platelet-derived growth factor is a mitogen that is stored in the alpha granule of the platelets. The factor has been purified to homogeneity. It has a molecular weight of approximately 32,000 and is a highly cationic (pI 9.8), stable disulfide-bonded protein. This growth factor is extremely potent; it causes the proliferation of all susceptible cells in culture at levels of 5 ng/mL of culture medium (equivalent to the addition of 5 percent whole-blood serum). As discussed earlier, in whole-blood serum, platelet-derived growth factor is the principal mitogen to which cells characteristically respond by cell proliferation. When susceptible cells are exposed to this factor, the result is a sequence of events that includes the binding of the molecule to the surface of the cell. This causes the cell to undergo cell-cycle traverse leading to DNA synthesis and cell multiplication.

Upon exposure to smooth-muscle cells, the platelet-derived growth factor stimulates a number of phenomena in addition to DNA synthesis. It causes increases in pinocytosis, protein synthesis, RNA synthesis, and lipid metabolism. Chait et al. (49) have observed that the exposure of arterial smooth-muscle cells to this growth factor results in the increased binding of LDL to the cells because of the formation of an increased number of high-affinity receptors for LDL at the cell surface. This increased binding of LDL permits the cells to more effectively utilize exogenous sources of cholesterol for cell multiplication. Habenicht et al. (48) have demonstrated that this mitogen also stimulates increased cholesterol synthesis by cells if an exogenous source of cholesterol is not available to them. Davies and Ross (53) observed that smooth-muscle cells exposed to the platelet-derived growth factor undergo a marked increase in the rate of endocytosis of tracer molecules. In other words, exposure to this mitogen results in an increase in a number of cellular activities, many of which are associated with cell proliferation and with new protein synthesis, and therefore with connective tissue formation (54). Thus exposure to this factor could trigger the initiation of all the components of a proliferative lesion. The role of functional platelets in inducing experimental atherosclerosis in vivo is unquestioned. The role of the platelet-derived growth factor in stimulating mitogenesis in cell culture is also clear. The question remains whether this factor is active in vivo (Figure 2-4).

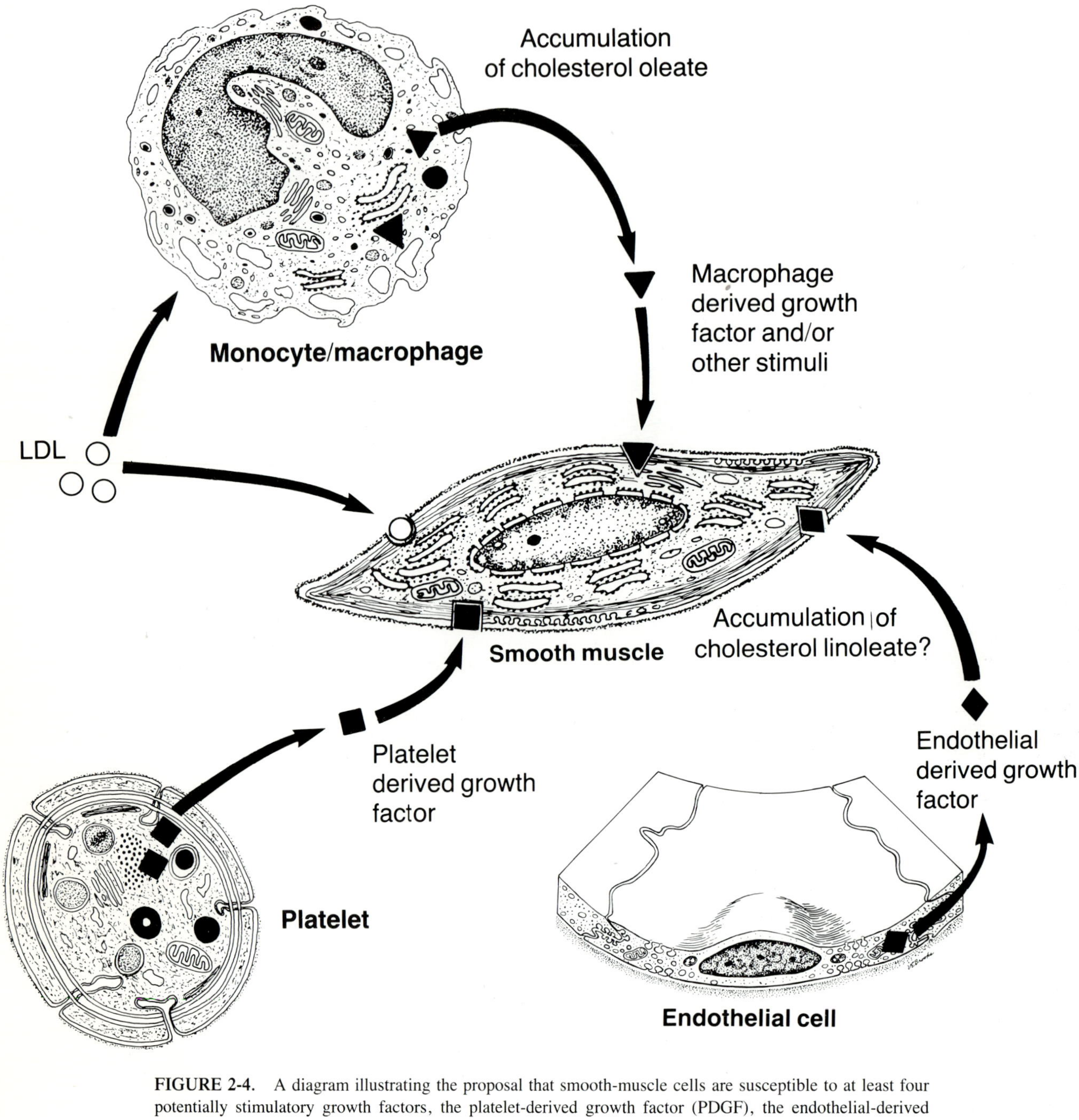

FIGURE 2-4. A diagram illustrating the proposal that smooth-muscle cells are susceptible to at least four potentially stimulatory growth factors, the platelet-derived growth factor (PDGF), the endothelial-derived growth factor (EDGF), the monocyte/macrophage-derived growth factor (MDGF), and LDL. The particular importance of each of these as a cause of smooth-muscle proliferation in the genesis of the lesions of atherosclerosis needs to be better defined for each special set of circumstances, and this provides important opportunities for further research. Reproduced by permission of *Arteriosclerosis*.

PROSTAGLANDINS

A great deal has been learned during the past 10 years about a new category of substances, the prostaglandins, that may play critical roles in the metabolism of platelets, endothelium, and smooth muscle. All three cell types are capable of converting the fatty acid arachidonic acid into prostaglandin endoperoxides. Studies of these endoperoxides identified a number of unstable intermediates in the metabolic pathway of arachidonic acid that leads to the formation of two important end products: thromboxane A_2 (formed by platelets) and PGI_2 (formed by endothelium and smooth muscle). Understanding these two end products has greatly expanded our view of the role played by platelets in thrombosis and by endothelium and smooth muscle in the prevention of thrombosis and atherosclerosis.

Arachidonic acid is derived either from linoleic acid, an essential fatty acid in the membranes of cells, or from the diet. Thromboxane A_2 is a powerful vasoconstrictor and is capable of stimulating smooth-muscle contraction and platelet aggregation. It has a short half-life (30 s) and breaks down spontaneously into a stable substance, thromboxane B_2. A number of inhibitors of thromboxane synthesis markedly reduce platelet aggregation. These include aspirin and indomethacin (55,56).

PGI_2 is the principal product of cycloxygenase activity in the walls of arteries and veins. Endothelium and smooth muscle synthesize PGI_2 from arachidonic acid and may also be able to synthesize this prostaglandin derivative from endoperoxides released from platelets. PGI_2 is unstable and is an extremely potent vasodilator, as well as an inhibitor of platelet aggregation.

It is possible that an imbalance in the relative amounts of thromboxane A_2 and PGI_2 may partly explain the involvement of platelets in cardiovascular diseases. Since platelets contain thromboxane synthetase, the enzyme responsible for the synthesis of thromboxane A_2, and since the inhibition of the activity of this enzyme does not interfere with cycloxygenase activity, it has been speculated that thromboxane synthetase inhibited platelets could donate endoperoxides to endothelial cells, which could then use them as substrates for PGI_2 production. Therefore, attempts are being made to develop specific inhibitors of thromboxane synthesis that do not affect PGI_2 production by cells of the blood vessel wall.

Prostaglandin biosynthesis may be important not only in thrombosis (in terms of platelet adherence and aggregation) but also in the prevention of atherogenesis (by the formation of PGI_2). This had led to the speculation that alterations in the contents of the fatty acids in the diet might offer some protection against the development of atherosclerosis. Populations that consume diets principally composed of marine animals often replace arachidonic acid, the normal substrate for prostaglandin synthesis, with eicosapentaenoic acid. This fatty acid is not completely metabolized by platelets and instead produces a relatively inert form of thromboxane, thromboxane A_3. Eicosapentaenoic acid appears to inhibit the capacity of platelets to metabolize arachidonic acid. When eicosapentaenoic acid is exposed to cells of the blood vessel, they form an analogue of PGI_2, PGI_3. PGI_3 appears to be as effective as PGI_2 in preventing platelet aggregation and in inducing vasodilatation. Thus further studies of the role of this fatty acid derived from marine animals could be important in terms of protecting persons who consume a marine diet against atherogenesis. Clearly, there is much to be learned about prostaglandin metabolism before the agents that have thus far been discovered, and those that are yet undiscovered, can be understood, in relation to both atherogenesis and protection against this disease process.

Future Directions

The field of atherosclerosis research has changed dramatically within the last decade. The emphasis has shifted to probing the fundamental roles of the cells of the artery wall as well as the roles of those in the blood, particularly the platelet and the monocyte. The developments of cell biology, experimental pathology, and immunology have provided tools that should lead to new approaches to diagnosis, intervention, and prevention.

If, for example, it can be demonstrated unequivocally that the platelet-derived growth factor plays a role either in the initiation of the lesions of atherosclerosis or in their progression, or in both, then the development of specific inhibitors of this factor and the development of specific diagnostic tests to measure increased activity would greatly alter present approaches to diagnosis, treatment, and prevention. Future research at the cellular and molecular levels could provide important diagnostic tools that may be of use clinically.

The process of atherogenesis is highly complex, involving many cellular interactions as well as interactions between cells and constituents in the fluid phase of the blood, the plasma. The importance of these interactions is undoubtedly modified by the genetic makeup of each individual. Consequently, from individual to individual, the differences in susceptibility to each of the risk factors, and at the cellular level to the various components considered to be important in atherogenesis, will have to be understood if we are to make further progress, not only in diagnosis and treatment, but ultimately in prevention.

References

1. Ross R, Glomset JA: The pathogenesis of atherosclerosis. N Engl J Med 1976, 295:369.
2. McGill HC Jr: Atherosclerosis: Problems in pathogenesis. Atherosclerosis Rev 1977, 2:27.
3. Bierman EL, Ross R: Aging and atherosclerosis. Atherosclerosis Rev 1977, 2:79.
4. Geer JC, Haust MD: *Monographs on Atherosclerosis.* S Karger, Basel, 1972, vol 2, p 1.
5. "*Arteriosclerosis.* US Dept of Health, Education, and Welfare publication No. (NIH) 72-219. National Heart and Lung Institute Task Force on Arteriosclerosis:" DHEW Publication (NIH) 72-219, vol 2, 1971.

6. DeBakey ME: *Atherosclerosis Reviews*. New York, Raven, 1976, vol 3, p 1.
7. Stemerman MB, Ross R: Experimental atherosclerosis. I. Fibrous plaque formation in primates, an electron microscope study. J Exp Med 1972, 136:769.
8. Bjorkerud S, Bondjers G: Arterial repair and atherosclerosis after mechanical injury. I. Permeability and light microscopic characteristics of endothelium in non-atherosclerotic and atherosclerotic lesions. Atherosclerosis 1971, 13:355.
9. Ross R, Harker L: Hyperlipidemia and atherosclerosis. Science 1976, 193:1094.
10. Harker L, Ross R, Slichter S, Scott C: Homocystine-induced atherosclerosis: The role of endothelial cell injury and platelet response in its genesis. J Clin Invest 1976, 58:731.
11. Minick CR, Murphy GE: Experimental induction of atheroarteriosclerosis by the synergy of allergic injury to arteries and lipid-rich diet. II. Effect of repeatedly injected foreign protein in rabbits fed a lipid-rich, cholesterol-poor diet. Am J Pathol 1973, 73:265.
12. Fabricant CG, Fabricant J, Litrenta MM, and Minick CR: Virus-induced atherosclerosis. J Exp Med 1978, 148:335.
13. Faggiotto A, Ross R, Harker L: Studies of hypercholesterolemia in the nonhuman primate. I. Changes that lead to fatty streak formation. Arteriosclerosis 1984, 4:323.
14. Faggiotto A, Ross R: Studies of hypercholesterolemia in the nonhuman primate. II. Fatty streak conversion to fibrous plaque. Arteriosclerosis 1984, 4:341.
15. Long ER: *Arteriosclerosis. A Survey of the Problem*. New York, Macmillan, 1922, p 19.
16. Virchow R: *Gesammelte Abhandlungen zur wissenschaftlichen Medicin*. Meidinger Sohn, Frankfurt am Main, 1856, p 458.
17. Anitschkow HH: *Cowdry's Arteriosclerosis*. ed 2. New York, Macmillan, 1967, p 21.
18. Duguid JB: Thrombosis as a factor in the pathogenesis of coronary atherosclerosis. J Pathol Bacteriol 1948, 58:207.
19. French JE: Atherosclerosis in relation to the structure and function of the arterial intima, with special reference to the endothelium. Int Rev Exp Pathol 1966, 5:253.
20. Ross R, Glomset J: Atherosclerosis and the arterial smooth muscle cell. Science 1973, 180:1332. (32 references.)
21. Fry DL: *Cerebrovascular Disease*. New York, Raven, 1976, p 77.
22. Moncada S, Higgs HA, Vane JR: Human arterial and venous tissue generate prostacycline, a potent inhibitor of platelet aggregation. Lancet 1977, 2:18.
23. Eissler RW, Vesselinovitch D: Studies of regression of advanced atherosclerosis in experimental animals and man. Ann NY Acad Sci 1976, 275:363.
24. Ross R, Glomset J, Kariya B, Harker LA: A platelet-dependent serum factor that stimulates the proliferation of arterial smooth muscle cells *in vitro*. Proc Natl Acad Sci USA 1974, 71:1207.
25. Geer JC, McGill HC Jr, Strong JP: The fine structure of human atherosclerotic lesions, Am J Pathol 1961, 38:263.
26. Wissler RW: *Biochemistry of Atherosclerosis*. New York, Dekker, 1979, vol 7, p 345 (Extensively referenced.)
27. McGill HC: Risk factors for atherosclerosis. Adv Exp Med Biol 1977, 104:273.
28. Grundy SM: *Nutrition, Lipids, and Coronary Heart Disease*. New York, Raven, 1979, p 89.
29. McGill HC Jr: The relationship of dietary cholesterol to serum cholesterol concentration and to atherosclerosis in man. Am J Clin Nutr 1979, 32(suppl): 2664.
30. Becker CG, Dubin T, Widemann HP: Hypersensitivity to tobacco antigen. Proc Natl Acad Sci 1976, 73:1712.
31. Simionescu N, Simionescu M, Palade GE: Permeability of muscle capillaries to small hemepeptides. Evidence for the existence of patent transendothelial channels. J Cell Biol 1975, 64:586.
32. Renkin EM: Multiple pathways of capillary permeability. Circ Res 1977, 41:735.
33. Stein Y, Stein O: *Biochemistry of Atherosclerosis*. New York, Dekker, 1979, vol 7, p 313.
34. Gimbrone MA Jr: *Progress in Hemostasis and Thrombosis*. New York, Grune & Stratton, 1976, vol 3, p 1.
35. Jaffe EA, Nachman RL, Becker CG, Minick CR: Culture of human endothelial cells derived from umbilical veins. J Clin Invest 1973, 52:2745.
36. Jaffe EA, Adelman B, Minick CR: Synthesis of basement membrane by cultured human endothelial cells, Circulation 1975, 51(suppl 2):11.
37. Moncada S, Higgs EA, Vane JR: Human arterial and venous tissue generate prostacyclin, a potent inhibitor of platelet aggregation. Lancet 1977, 2:18.
38. Jaffe EA, Hoyer LW, Nachman RL: Synthesis of antihemophilic factor antigen by cultured human endothelial cells. J Clin Invest 1973, 52:2757.
39. Gimbrone MA Jr, Alexander RW: Angiotensin II Stimulation of prostaglandin production in cultured human vascular endothelium (abstract). Science 1975, 189:219.
40. Gajdusek C, DiCorleto P, Ross R, Schwartz S: An endothelial cell derived growth factor. J Cell Biol 1980, 85:467.
41. Ross R, Kariya B: *Handbook of Physiology—Circulation, Vascular Smooth Muscle*. Bethesda, Md, American Physiological Society, 1980, p 69.
42. Chamley-Campbell J, Campbell GR, Ross R: The smooth muscle cell in culture. Physiol Rev 1979, 59:1.
43. Kohler N, Lipton A: Platelets as a source of fibroblast growth-promoting activity. Exp Cell Res 1974, 87:297.
44. Heldin C-H, Wasteson A, Westermark B: Partial purification and characterization of platelet factors stimulating the multiplication of normal human glial cells. Exp Cell Res 1974, 87:297.
45. Moore A, Friedman RJ, Singal DP, Gauldie J, Blajchman M: Inhibition of injury induced thromboatherosclerotic lesions by anti-platelet serum in rabbits. Throm Diath Haemorr 1976, 35:70.
46. Friedman RJ, Stemerman MB, Wenz B, Moore S, Gauldie J, Gent M, Tiell ML, Spaet TH: The effect of thrombocytopenia on experimental atherosclerotic lesion formation in rabbits. Smooth muscle cell proliferation and reendothelialization. J Clin Invest 1977, 60:1191.
47. Fuster V, Bowie EJW, Brown AL: Reistance to arteriosclerosis in pigs with von Willebrand's disease. Spontaneous and high cholesterol diet–induced arteriosclerosis. J Clin Invest 1978, 61:722.
48. Habenicht A, Glomset J, Ross R: Relation of cholesterol and mevalonic acid to the cell cycle in smooth muscle and Swiss 3T3 cells stimulated to divide by platelet-derived growth factor. J Biol Chem 1980, 255:5134.
49. Chait A, Ross R, Albers J, Bierman E: Platelet derived growth factor stimulates low density lipoprotein receptor activity. Proc Natl Acad Sci USA 1980, 77:4084.
50. Brown MS, Faust JR, Goldstein JL: Role of the low density lipoprotein receptor in regulating the content of free and esterified cholesterol in human fibroblasts. J Clin Invest 1975, 55:783.
51. Goldstein JL, Brown MS: The low-density lipoprotein pathway and its relation to atherosclerosis. Ann Rev Biochem 1977, 46:879.
52. Leibovich SJ, Ross R: A macrophage-dependent factor that stimulates the proliferation of fibroblasts *in vitro*. Am J Pathol 1976, 84:501.
53. Davies PF, Ross R: Mediation of pinocytosis in cultured arterial smooth muscle and endothelial cells by platelet-derived growth factor. J Cell Biol 1978, 79:663.
54. Burke J, Ross R: *International Review of Connective Tissue Research*. New York, Academic, 1979, vol 8, p 119.
55. Moncada A, Vane JR: Arachidonic acid metabolites and the interactions between platelets and blood-vessel walls. N Engl J Med 1979, 300:1142.
56. Moncada A, Vane JR: Mode of action of aspirin-like drugs. Adv Intern Med 1979, 24:1.

Chapter 3

PATHOPHYSIOLOGY OF HUMAN ATHEROSCLEROSIS

CHRISTOPHER K. ZARINS and SEYMOUR GLAGOV

Atherosclerosis is a degenerative process of the major human elastic and muscular arteries. It is characterized by the formation of intimal plaques consisting of lipid accumulations, smooth-muscle and inflammatory cells, connective tissue fibers, and calcium deposits. Morbidity associated with atherosclerosis arises from plaque enlargement or degeneration. Plaque enlargement may obstruct the lumen, resulting in stenosis and impairment of blood flow. Sudden obstruction of the lumen may result from the dissection of blood from the lumen into or under the plaque or hemorrhage within the plaque from vasa vasorum. Plaque ulceration may result in embolization of plaque elements or thrombus formation on the disrupted intima. Thrombosis may also occlude atherosclerotic vessels without obvious plaque disruption due to local modifications of flow. Finally, atrophy of the media, often associated with atherosclerotic disease, may result in weakening of the artery wall with aneurysmal dilatation, mural thrombosis, and rupture.

Atherosclerosis is a generalized disorder of the arterial tree associated with a number of recognized predisposing risk factors, including altered serum lipid and lipoprotein profiles, hypertension, cigarette smoking, diabetes mellitus, and lifestyle. However, the clinical expression of atherosclerosis tends to be focal with clinical symptoms caused by localized interference with circulation occurring in several critical sites. In addition, the morphologic features underlying morbidity and mortality vary somewhat depending on location. In the coronary arteries, for example, stenosis and thrombosis tend to reduce flow or cause sudden catastrophic occlusion, principally at the site of lesion formation, while at the carotid bifurcation, plaque ulceration and thrombosis often cause characteristic symptoms by embolization to distal cerebral vessels. Extensive disease, often with multiple focal occlusive stenoses, is characteristic of peripheral vascular disease of the lower extremities, while aneurysm formation is a major feature of abdominal aortic disease. While there is a large body of descriptive clinical and experimental knowledge with regard to the general appearance of atherosclerotic lesions, the precise initiating and perpetuating pathogenic mechanisms in human beings remain obscure and the factors which determine human lesion composition, rate of lesion enlargement, lesion organization, and lesion disruption remain to be elucidated.

In this chapter we discuss both the structural features of the artery wall and the hemodynamic factors which may relate to the pathogenesis, localization, and disruption of plaques, and we review the principal features of human lesion composition and configuration. These considerations should help to provide insight into the clinical consequences of differences in plaque localization and composition and serve as a basis for the critical evaluation of currently available methods for the quantitative assessment of human lesions.

Structure of the Artery Wall

The artery wall consists of three concentric layers or zones. From the lumen outward, these are the intima, the media, and the adventitia (Figure 3-1).

INTIMA

The *intima* extends from the luminal endothelial lining to the internal elastic lamina. The *endothelium* is formed by a continuous monolayer of flat, usually elongated, polygonal cells, which tend to be aligned in the direction of blood flow. In areas of slow, reversing, or nonlaminar flow, endothelial cells tend to assume a less clearly oriented configuration (1). Edges of adjacent endothelial cells overlap, with the downstream edges of most endothelial cells overriding their immediate downstream neighbors much like the shingles on a roof. Cytoplasmic bridges, surface ridges, and microvillus projections, as well as interendothelial gaps, stomata, or open junctions between endothelial cells, have been described. These features are, however, largely absent from vessels which have been fixed while distended and which have not been manipulated prior to fixation (2). A protein coating, the glycocalyx, overlies the luminal surface. Immediately beneath the endothelium is a closely associated fibrillar layer, the basal lamina. This structure is thought to form a continuous bond between the endothelial cells and the subendothelial connective tissue matrix. Numerous focal attachments are also present between endothelial cells and the underlying internal elastic lamina (3), while less prominent focal attachments are also formed with other fibers in the intima. The extensive basal lamina provides a supple, pliable junction well adapted to permit

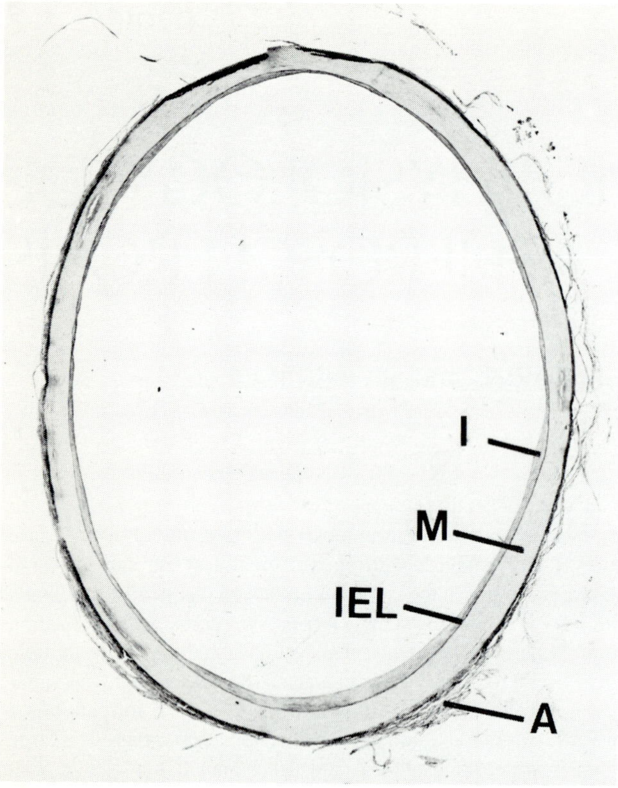

FIGURE 3-1. Transverse section of a normal human superficial femoral artery. Note intima (I), media (M), and adventitia (A). The intima and media are separated by the internal elastic lamella (IEL).

bending and changes in diameter or configuration associated with pulse pressure without disruption or detachment of the endothelium. The focal, tight, relatively rigid junctions may prevent downstream slippage or telescoping which could result from the shear stresses imposed by blood flow. Between the basal lamina and the internal elastic lamina, the intima in most locations normally contains a few scattered macrophages, smooth-muscle cells, and connective tissue fibers.

Since the endothelial cell layer is the immediate interface between the bloodstream and the underlying arterial wall, it is subjected to normal forces exerted by blood pressure and to shearing or drag forces resulting from blood flow. Experimentally imposed shearing stresses in excess of 400 dyn/cm^2 in canine aortas have resulted in morphologic evidences of endothelial injury or disruption and in increased endothelial permeability (4). Other observations have failed to reveal evidences of endothelial injury in areas normally subjected to comparable or higher levels of shear stress (5), suggesting that endothelial cells may withstand relatively high shearing stresses without ill effect in some locations (Figure 3-2).

The endothelial layer has been considered to function as a thrombosis-resistant surface as well as a selective interface for diffusion, convection, and active transport of circulating substances into the underlying artery wall. It would, therefore, be expected to play a critical role in regulating the ingress and egress of lipoproteins and other agents which could determine the subsequent localization of atherosclerotic plaques. Endothelial cells have been shown to participate in an array of metabolic and biosynthetic functions related to thrombosis, prostaglandin formation and smooth-muscle contraction (6). Detachment of endothelial cells with persistence of the basal lamina does not

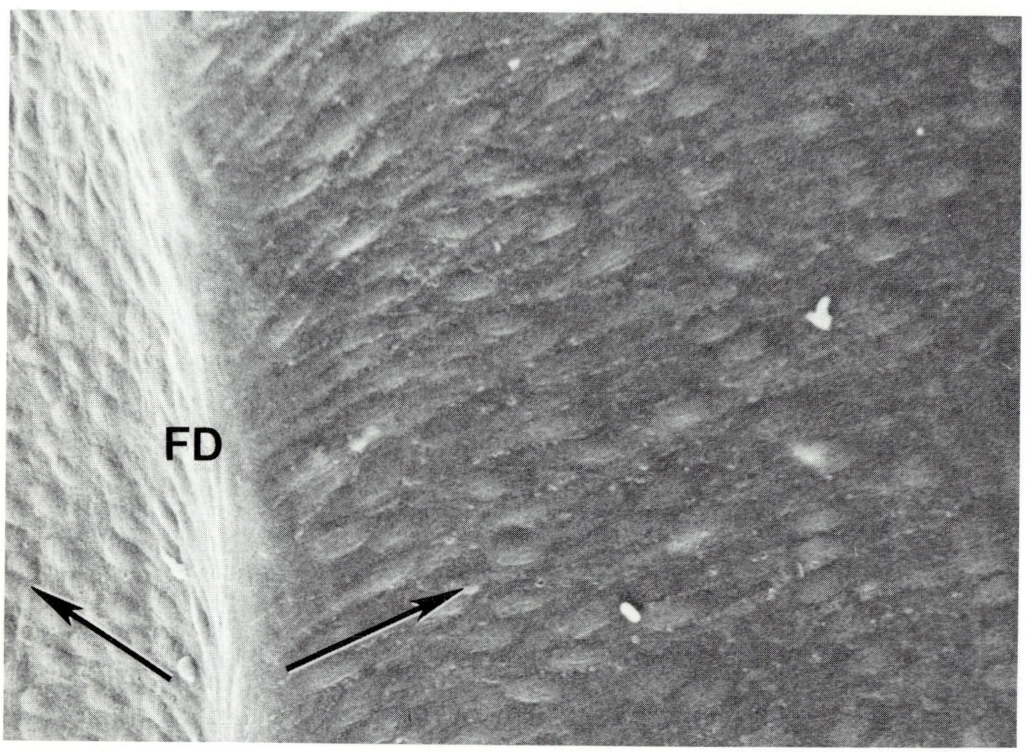

FIGURE 3-2. Scanning electron micrograph of a monkey aortic ostial flow divider (FD). The flow divider is an area subjected to high shear stress. The endothelial cells are intact and elongated in the direction of flow with no disruption. Arrows indicate direction of blood flow.

necessarily result in occlusive thrombus formation. Although a layer of thrombocytes appears to deposit on the denuded basal lamina, large aggregates and fibrin deposits may require the exposure of collagen fibers and other deeper mural components.

MEDIA

The *media* extends from the internal elastic lamina to the adventitia. Although an external elastic lamina demarcates the boundary between media and adventitia in many vessels, a distinct external elastic lamina may not be present, particularly in vessels with a thick and fibrous adventitial layer. The outer limit of the media can nevertheless be distinguished in nearly all intact arteries, for in contrast to the adventitia, the media consists of closely packed layers of smooth-muscle cells in close association with elastin and collagen fibers. Elastic fibers of the media are predominantly wavy or undulating on cross sections of collapsed arteries but appear as relatively straight bands or lamellae in fully distended vessels (Figure 3-3). The smooth-muscle-cell layers are composed of groups of similarly oriented cells, each surrounded by a common basal lamina and a closely associated interlacing basketwork of collagen fibrils which tighten about the cell groups as the media is brought under tension (7). This configuration tends to hold the groups of cells together and prevents excessive stretching or slippage. In addition, each cellular subgroup or fascicle is encompassed by a system of similarly oriented elastic fibers. Focal tight attachment sites between smooth-muscle cells and elastic fibers are normally abundant. In the aorta, the juxtaposition of similarly oriented musculoelastic fascicles results in the appearance on transverse sections of layers of continuous elastic lamellae and intervening smooth-muscle layers. In addition to the pericellular network of fine collagen fibrils, thicker, crimped collagen bundles weave between adjacent lamellae. The elastic fibers are relatively extensible and allow for some degree of compliance; they recoil during the cardiac cycle and tend to distribute mural tensile stresses uniformly. The thick collagen fiber bundles provide much of the tensile strength of the media, and because of their high elastic modulus, limit distension and prevent disruption (Figure 3-4).

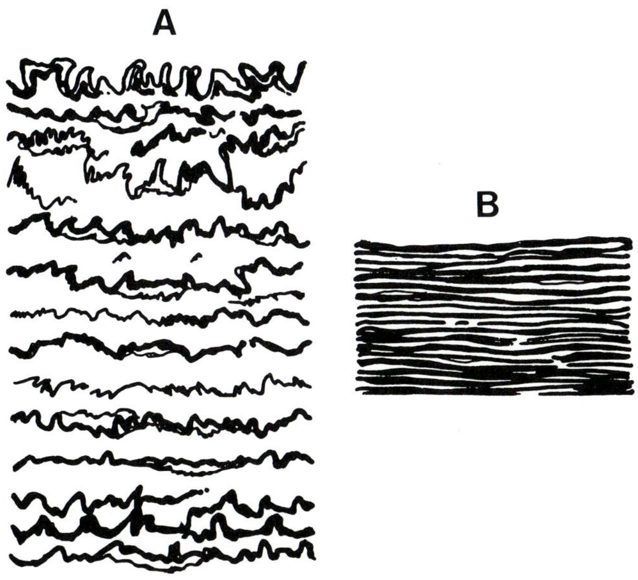

FIGURE 3-3. Tracing of elastic fibers in transverse sections of rabbit aortic media. (*A*) A transverse section of a collapsed aorta demonstrating wavy elastic lamellae and increased thickness of each lamellar unit and increased total thickness of the media. (*B*) A rabbit aorta fixed while distended. Note the straight elastic fibers and thickness of the media.

The aortic elastin lamella and its corresponding smooth-muscle layer has been termed a *lamellar unit*. With increasing mammalian species size, the adult aortic radius increases with a corresponding increase in medial thickness and in the number of transmural lamellar units (Figure 3-5) (8). The total tangential tension exerted on the wall is closely approximated by the product of the distending pressure and the radius (law of Laplace). Since aortic pressure is similar for most adult mammals and individual medial layers tend to be of similar thickness regardless of species, there is a very nearly linear relationship between adult aortic radius and the number of medial fibrocellular lamellar units. On the average, the tangential tension per aortic lamellar unit is close to 2000 dyn/cm.

Smaller *muscular arteries* contain relatively less collagen and elastin and more smooth-muscle cells than the aorta and the proximal, larger *elastic arteries*. The musculoelastic fascicles, which are very prominent in elastic arteries, are also present in muscular arteries and are generally aligned in the direction of the tensile forces (Figure 3-6). However, because of the preponderance of smooth-muscle cells, they are less clearly demarcated and the layering of the media is less distinct (9). Medial thickness and the number of layers is nevertheless closely related to the radius, and the average tension per layer tends to be constant for homologous vessels in mammals (10). In addition, the relative proportion of collagen and elastin varies between muscular and elastic arteries. The media of the proximal aorta and that of the major brachiocephalic elastic arteries contain a larger proportion of elastin and a lower proportion of collagen than the abdominal aorta or the distal peripheral vessels (11). The proximal major vessels are therefore more compliant than the abdominal aorta but also are more friable and prone to tear with suturing.

ADVENTITIA

Although the boundary between media and *adventitia* is usually distinct, even in the absence of a well-defined external elastic lamina, the outer limit of the adventitia may be difficult to identify, for it is often continuous with the surrounding perivascular connective tissues. Although the aorta and pulmonary trunk are normally invested by relatively little adventitial fibrous connective tissue and are closely associated with mediastinal or retroperitoneal adipose tissue and lymph nodes, the adventitia of some of the major arteries, such as the renal and mesenteric branches, are composed of prominent layers of elastic and collagen fibers and may be thicker than the associated media. Compared to the media, cells in the adventitia are relatively sparse and most are fibroblasts. For the normal aorta, removal of the adventitia has little effect on static pressure-volume relationships. In muscular arteries, however, where connective tissue fibers are relatively sparse in the media and smooth muscle contraction may regulate vessel diameter and play a role in maintaining circumferential tensile support, a thick, structured adventitia may serve to provide significant tethering and axial tensile support, prevent excessive dilatation, and dampen the cyclic

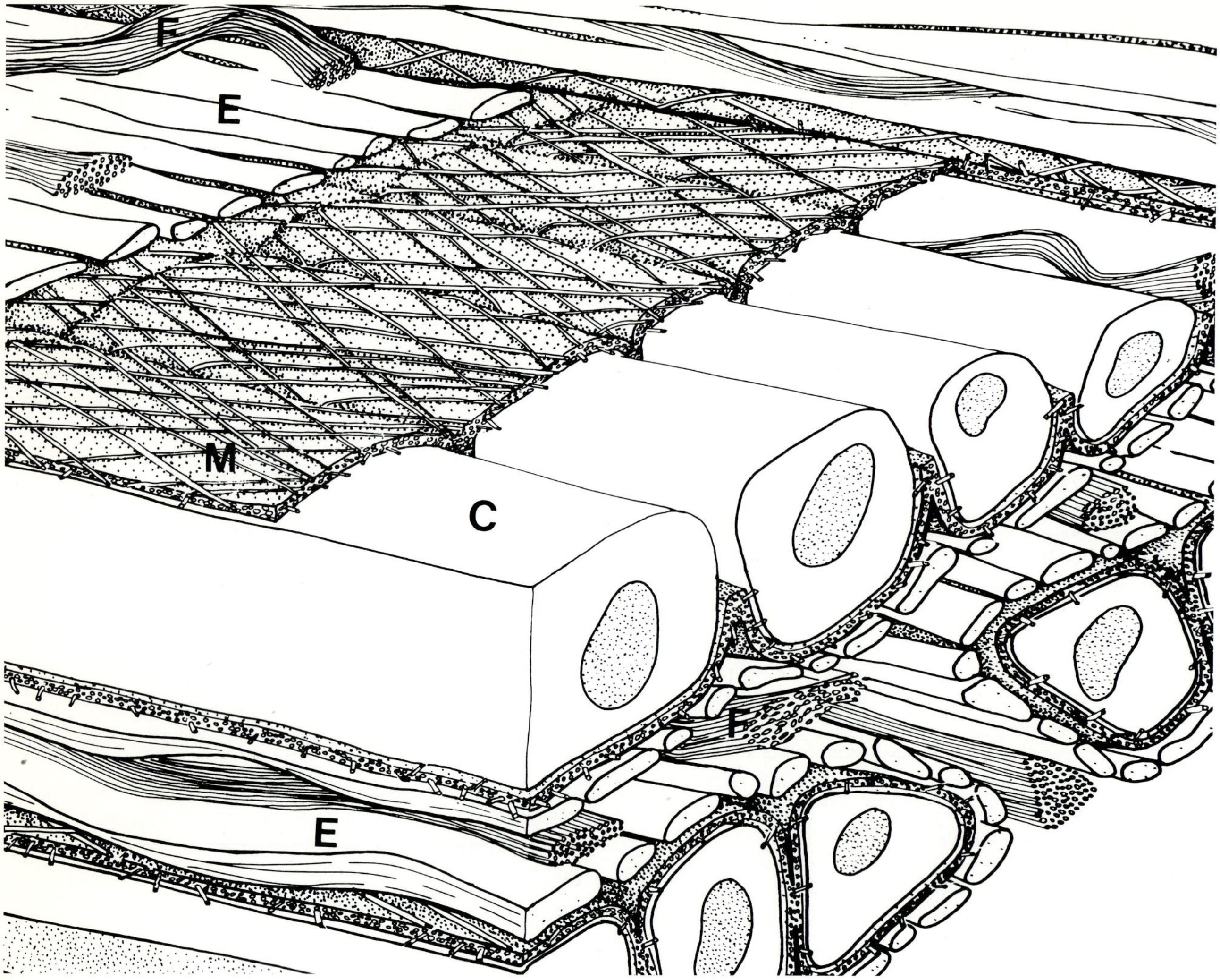

FIGURE 3-4. Diagrammatic representation of the microarchitecture of the media of the aortic wall. The long axes of the smooth muscle cells (C) are oriented circumferentially or perpendicular to the long axis of the artery. Each cell is surrounded by a matrix (M) consisting of basal lamina and a fine meshwork of collagen fibrils. Groups or layers of smooth-muscle cells are surrounded by circumferentially oriented elastic fibers (E), which appear as almost continuous sheets on transverse section of the artery. Wavy collagen bundles (F) course between the successive facing elastic fiber layers. [Adapted with permission from Clark JM, Glagov S: Transmural organization of the arterial media. The lamellar unit revisited. Arteriosclerosis 5:19–34, 1985.]

changes in tangential tension associated with the pulse pressure wave. In instances where a large, intimal atherosclerotic plaque overlies an atrophic media, a thickened adventitia may be the principal mural structural component of the artery wall (see Figure 3-12). During carotid or femoral endarterectomy, the entire intima and extensive portions of remaining media may be removed, leaving only the adventitia to provide support.

Artery Wall Nutrition

The adventitia of all of the major elastic and muscular arteries contains vasa vasorum, i.e., small arteries, arterioles, capillaries, and venous channels which are presumed to participate in nutrition of the artery wall. Except for the aorta, however, precise relationships among vasa supply, vessel location, diameter, wall thickness, and architecture have not been established. The aortic media is nourished directly from the lumen and may also be perfused by means of vasa vasorum from the adventitial side. Passage through the lining endothelium is apparently sufficient to nourish the inner 0.5 mm of the adult mammalian aortic media, which corresponds to approximately 30 medial fibrocellular layers (12). Thus, the aortic media of a small mammal such

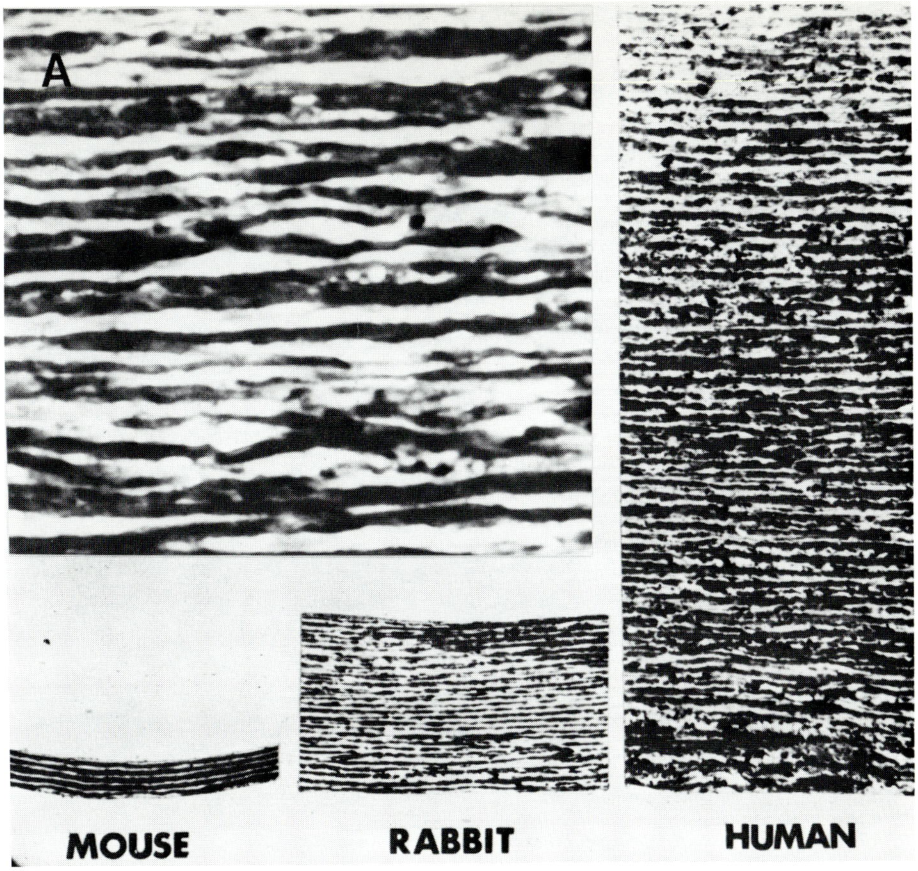

FIGURE 3-5. Aortic lamellar architecture in three mammals. With increasing species size, aortic radius increases. There is a corresponding increase in medial thickness due to an increase in the number of medial lamellar units. (*A*) Higher power of transverse section of media demonstrating lamellar architecture.

as the rat or rabbit, which is less than 0.5 mm thick and has fewer than 30 medial lamellar layers, contains no medial vasa vasorum and is nourished largely from the intimal side. Large mammals such as pigs, sheep, and horses have an aortic media with more than 30 medial lamellar layers. The inner 30 aortic layers in such species are avascular, but the remaining outer medial lamellar units contain vasa vasorum (Figure 3-7). Aortic vasa vasorum arise from major arterial branches close to their origins and usually enter the media at right angles. Within the media, the vasa tend to be oriented axially in several branching levels. The average tension per medial lamellar unit for aortas which contain medial vasa tends to be somewhat higher than for aortas without vasa, suggesting that the presence of nutritive vessels within the media permits each lamellar unit to function at a somewhat higher level of tensile stress. The human abdominal aorta appears to be exceptional when compared to aortas of other mammals, since it is more than 0.5 mm thick but contains fewer than 30 layers (13). It is not furnished with medial vasa vasorum, although the estimated tensile stress per layer is in the range of those aortas with medial vasa (Figure 3-8). The implications of this situation with respect to atherosclerosis and aneurysm formation are discussed below. Although mural stresses and deformations associated with hypertension may impair medial vasal flow (14), the details of aortic media microarchitecture, which permit intramural vasa vasorum to remain open under normal conditions despite the cyclic compressive and shearing stresses within the artery wall, have not been clarified. Vasa vasorum have been identified in atherosclerotic arteries and, in particular, within atherosclerotic plaques. Although vasa vasorum in atherosclerotic plaques have been supposed to underlie disruptive lesion hemorrhages (15), relationships among lesion size, composition, and complications and the presence of vasa vasorum are not clear.

Age-Related Changes in the Artery Wall

Focal intimal thickenings, including cushions or pads at or near branch points, have been observed in infants and fetuses. Many of these tend to be modified and incorporated into the media during growth, and most are therefore likely to represent local

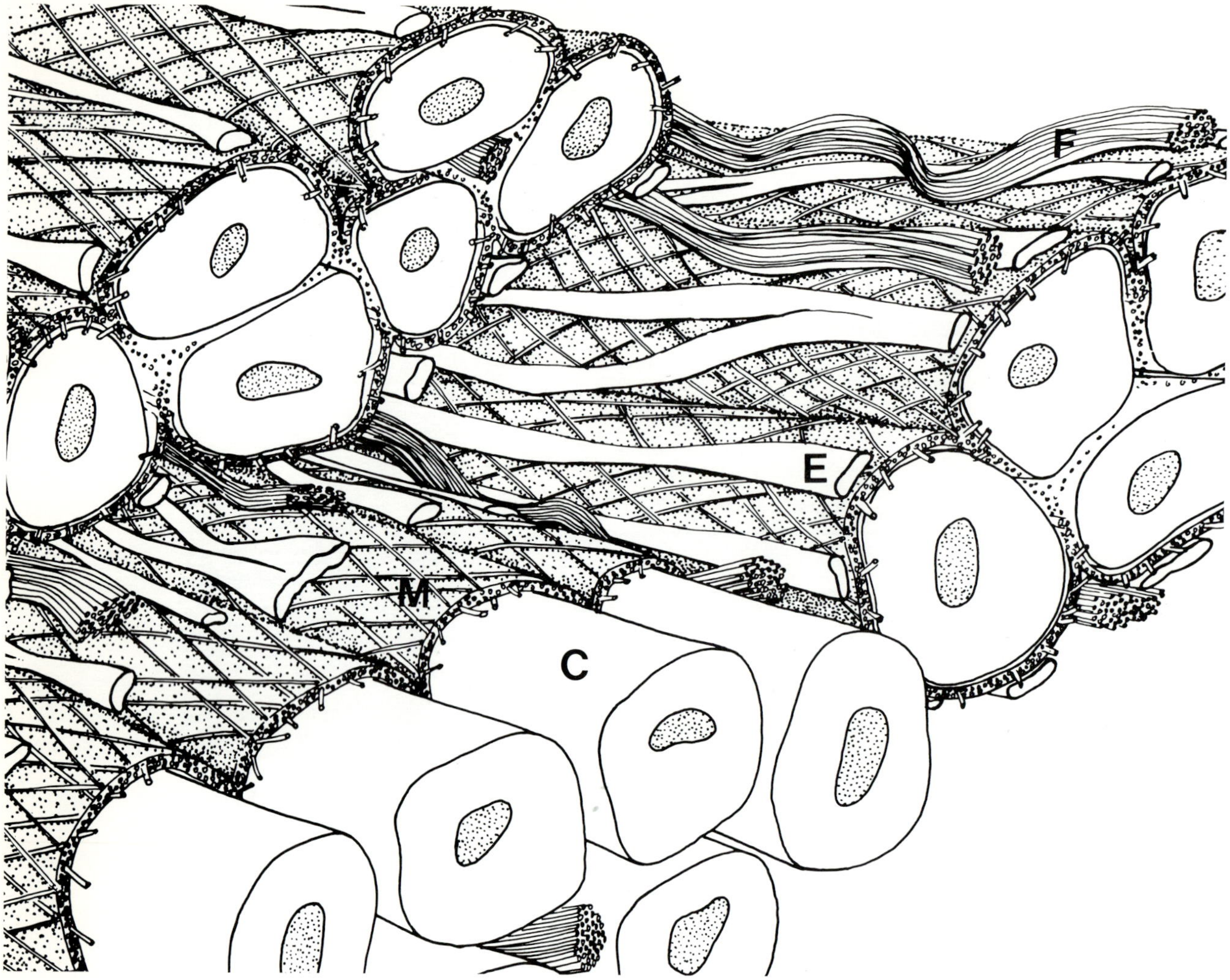

FIGURE 3-6. Diagrammatic representation of microarchitecture of the wall of a muscular artery. The long axes of the smooth muscle cells (C) of the media are oriented circumferentially or perpendicular to the long axis of the artery. Cells are surrounded by a matrix (M) of basal lamina and collagen fibrils. Elastin fiber systems (E) are less prominent. Collagen bundles (F) are interspersed. Compared to elastic arteries (see Figure 3-4), muscular arteries have a greater number of smooth muscle cells and relatively fewer collagen and elastin fibers. [Adapted with permission from Clark JM, Glagov S: Transmural organization of the arterial media: The lamellar unit revisited. Arteriosclerosis 5:19–34, 1985.]

changes in vessel-wall organization related to redistributions of tensile stress associated with developmental changes in diameter, length, and geometric configuration.

Progressive fibrocellular *diffuse intimal thickening,* on the other hand, proceeds from infancy to old age, differing considerably in both extent and degree in different locations in the arterial tree (16,17). This process tends to be more or less uniform about the vessel circumference and is not limited to areas about branch ostia, bifurcations, or the inner aspects of curves. Although the component cells tend to be oriented axially in straight portions of arteries, the organization and composition of thickened intima resemble to some extent that of the underlying media (Figure 3-9). The lumen may not, however, be significantly narrowed by this process, for while the condition may produce an artery wall with an intima thicker than the media, the process tends to be concentric, accumulation of lipid is not a prominent feature, there is no focal stenosis, and the vessel lumen may actually be larger than normal. Diffuse intimal thickening is, nevertheless, especially evident in those vessels which tend to be susceptible to clinically significant atherosclerotic disease (18). There is, however, little evidence to indicate that diffuse intimal thickening is necessarily a precursor of the formation of atherosclerotic lesions. With advancing age, the internal elastic lamina of the aorta and of the large arteries may show gaps, splits, and fragmentation as well as calcium salt deposits. In addition, neoformation of elastin within the thickened intima or in plaques may result in the accumulation of many layers of elastic fibers in the intima.

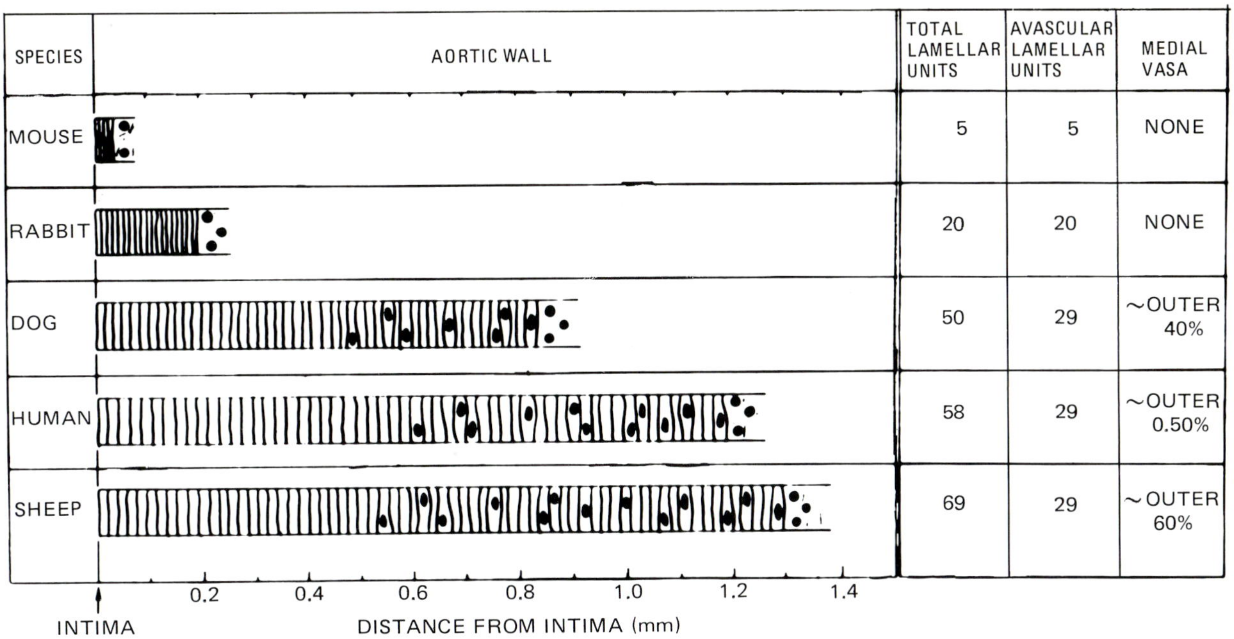

FIGURE 3-7. Relationship between aortic medial lamellar architecture and vasa vasorum blood supply to outer portion of the media in different species. [Reproduced with permission from Glagov S: Hemodynamic risk factors: Mechanical stress, mural architecture, medial nutrition and the vulnerability of arteries to atherosclerosis. In Wissler RW, Geer JC (eds): *The Pathogenesis of Atherosclerosis*. Baltimore, Williams & Wilkins, 1972, pp. 166–199.]

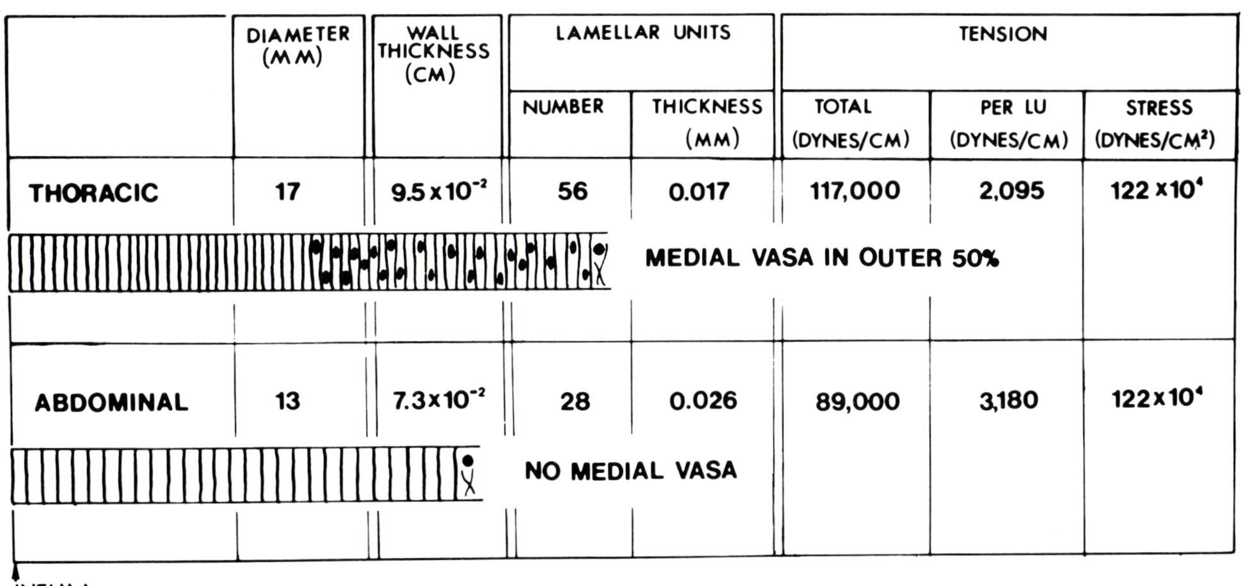

FIGURE 3-8. The human thoracic aorta has medial vasa vasorum in the outer lamellae and each lamellar unit supports approximately 2095 dyn/cm. The human abdominal aorta, however, has 28 lamellar units, has no medial vasa, and each lamellar unit supports about 3180 dyn/cm. This architectural difference may be important in the vulnerability of the abdominal aorta to atherosclerosis and aneurysm formation. [Reproduced with permission from Glagov S: Hemodynamic risk factors: Mechanical stress, mural architecture, medial nutrition and the vulnerability of arteries to atherosclerosis. In Wissler RW, Geer JC (eds): *The Pathogenesis of Atherosclerosis*, Baltimore, Williams & Wilkins, 1972, pp. 166–199.]

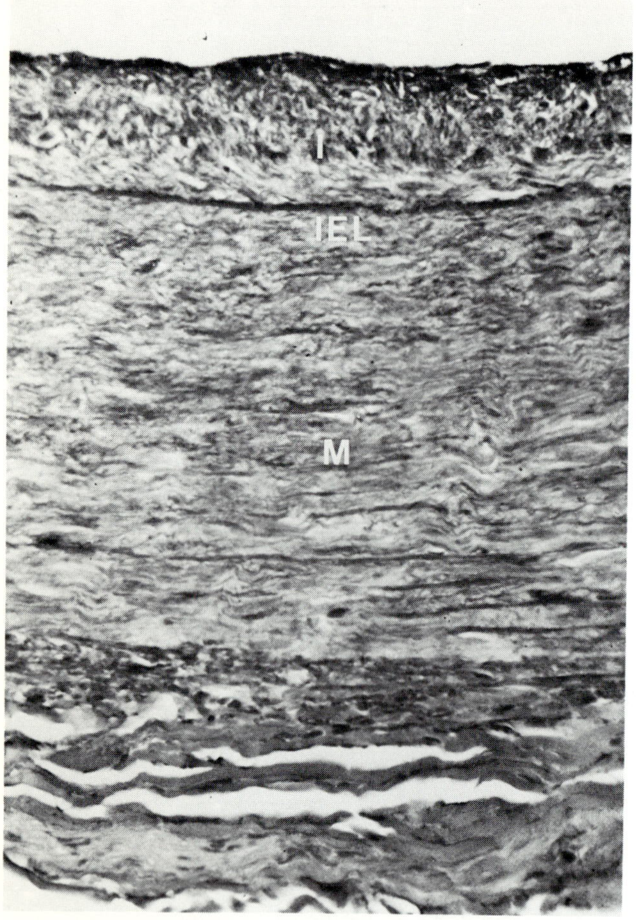

FIGURE 3-9. Transverse section of coronary artery of 18-year-old accident victim demonstrating diffuse intimal thickening (I). Note the organization and composition of the thickened intima resembles the underlying media (M). IEL represents the internal elastic lamina.

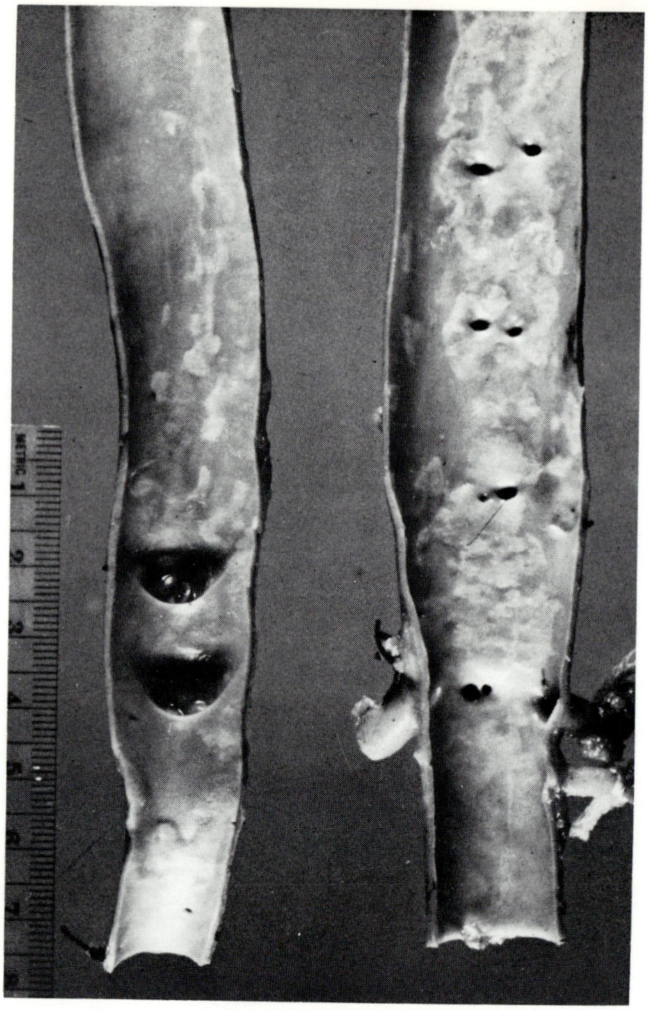

FIGURE 3-10. Fatty streaks in aorta of 45-year-old patient.

In general, arteries tend to increase in diameter, elongate, and become tortuous with age. This diffuse, apparently irreversible enlargement, when marked, is called *ectasia*. The common form of diffuse and extensive ectasia of the aorta and large arteries parallels a relative overall increase in matrix fiber accumulation (19), including an increase in collagen content, a decrease in elastin content, a calcification of the elastic fibers, and a decrease in compliance of the wall. While elongation and tortuosity of the vessel may be quite marked, the diffuse and extensive form of moderate ectasia is not necessarily associated with serious consequences. When complications occur, they are generally attributable to associated atherosclerosis and/or the formation of aneurysms.

Structure of Atherosclerotic Lesions

Atherosclerotic lesions may begin in childhood or adolescence and enlarge progressively over years or decades without associated symptoms. Although intimal plaques are evident in arteries of nearly all adults coming to autopsy in much of the world, little is known concerning the factors which determine individual differences in plaque morphology or govern the gradual or sudden transition from asymptomatic plaques to those which enlarge sufficiently to cause obstruction to flow, ulcerate, or induce occlusive thrombosis or aneurysm formation. On the basis of morphologic appearance and composition, human lesions are usually classified as *fatty streaks* or *fibrous "raised" plaques*. Transitional forms have also been identified. While fatty streaks are not associated with symptoms, raised plaques are more complex and are associated with the alterations which underlie circulatory compromise.

FATTY STREAKS

Fatty streaks are relatively flat, fairly well demarcated patches or minute yellow foci which may appear soon after birth and are seen on the luminal surface of most aortas of individuals over the age of 3 years (Figure 3-10) (20). Fatty streaks are found with increasing frequency between the ages of 8 and 18, becoming most numerous around puberty. These formations are not, however, limited to young persons and may be seen at any age adjacent to or even superimposed upon fibrous plaques. Fatty streaks consist largely of intimal lipid-laden cells (foam cells) and variable quantities of matrix materials beneath an intact endothelium. The extent to which fatty streaks are precursors of subsequent complex fibrous progressive atherosclerotic lesions remains unresolved (21). There is evidence that many human fatty streaks may be evanescent, for the distribution of fatty streaks seen in young individuals does not coincide entirely with the distribution of fibrous plaques seen later in life. It has also been found that cells in human fatty streaks are not monotypic with respect to isoenzyme content (22), but that advanced lesions are composed of cells which contain extensive regions of cellular monotypia (23). These findings have suggested that focal events occurring in some fatty streaks may result in cellular proliferation with the persistence of lesions and the subsequent formation of the more complex fibrous plaques, while other fatty streaks resolve.

FIBROUS PLAQUES

Fibrous plaques do not usually appear until the second decade of life and may not become the predominant lesion type until the fourth decade. The endothelial lining appears to be intact over most uncomplicated lesions, i.e., lesions without evidence of disruption, ulceration, hemorrhage, or thrombus formation. Although plaque composition varies considerably with respect to the relative proportions of the usual lesion components, a predominant mode of composition and organization can be discerned. There is frequently a relatively compact zone of connective tissue fibers and smooth-muscle cells immediately beneath the endothelium known as the *fibrous cap* (Figure 3-11). Deeper in the central portion of the plaque and beneath the fibrous cap is a zone of variable composition and consistency, known as the *necrotic core* or *center*. It contains amorphous debris, lipid-containing cells with morphologic and functional characteristics of either smooth-muscle cells or macrophages (24), extracellular lipids including droplets and cholesterol crystals, calcium salts, and myxoid deposits. In addition, matrix fibers, including elastin, collagen, finer fibrillar material, and structures resembling basal lamina as well as amorphous ground substance are evident. The fibrous cap may become quite thick and form a well-organized fibrocellular, layered structure which may even include a subendothelial elastic lamina. Thrombi formed on lesions as well as fibrin deposits are also incorporated into lesions. Vasa vasorum penetrate from the adventitia or from the lumen to supply the plaque (25) and fibrous cap (Figure 3-12) and to organize thrombotic deposits. There may be thinning and attenuation of the media below the intimal lesion such that the atheromatous deposit and the media bulge outward toward the adventitia. Some advanced lesions, particularly those associated

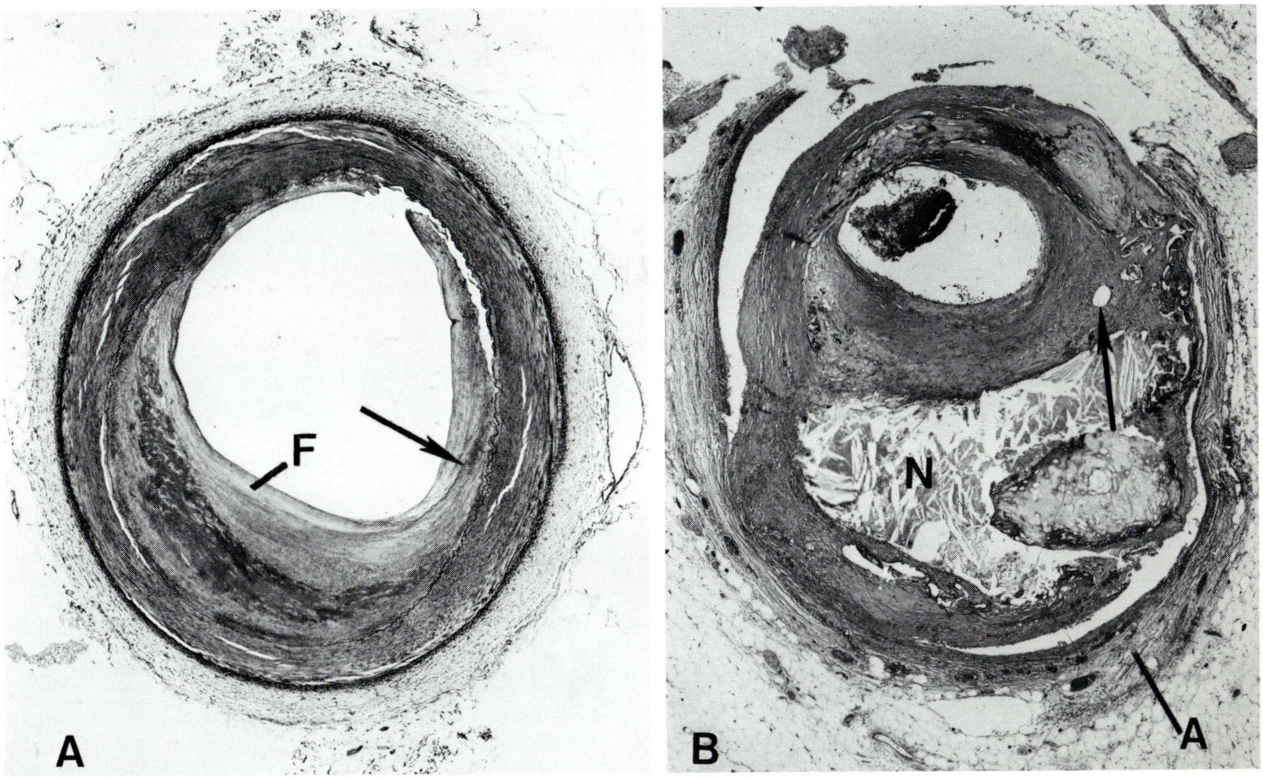

FIGURE 3-11. Transverse section of superficial femoral arteries demonstrating: (***A***) Fibrous plaque with prominent fibrous cap (F). Note thinning of media below the thickest portion of the plaque. Note the formation of a new elastic lamina (*arrow*) near the lumen. (***B***) Plaque with prominent necrotic center (N), medial thinning, and thickened adventitia (A). Note vasa vasorum (*arrow*) penetrating into plaque and fibrous cap.

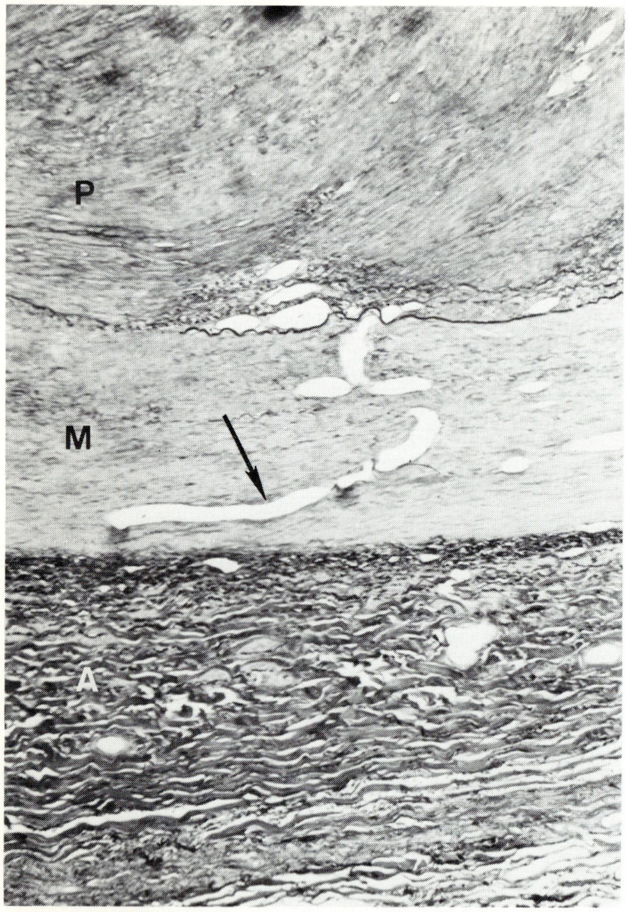

FIGURE 3-12. Transverse section of superficial femoral artery. Note prominent adventitial (A) thickening and vasa vasorum (*arrow*) penetrating through media (M) into plaque (P).

with aneurysms, may appear to be atrophic and relatively acellular, consisting of dense fibrous tissue, prominent calcific deposits, and only minimal evidence of a necrotic center. Calcification is a prominent feature of advanced plaques and may be quite extensive, involving both the superficial and deeper reaches of the plaques. Although there is no consistent relationship between plaque size or complexity and the degree of calcification, calcific deposits are most prominent in plaques of older individuals and in areas, such as the abdominal aortic segment and coronary arteries, where plaques form earliest (26). Advanced lesions are called fibrocalcific, lipid-rich, fibrocellular, necrotic, myxomatous, etc., depending on their morphologic features. The presence of large quantities of lipid, necrotic material, and cells would tend to make a lesion *soft* and friable, in contrast to the *hard* or brittle consistency of a mainly fibrocalcific lesion with an intact and prominent fibrous cap.

LESION COMPLICATIONS

Although it tends to isolate the advanced lesion from the lumen, the fibrous cap may be very thin or virtually absent. It may also be interrupted or disrupted focally, exposing underlying lesion contents to the bloodstream and favoring the formation of thrombi or the penetration of blood from the lumen into the lesion. Since advanced atherosclerotic lesions often contain vasa vasorum, these vessels may rupture and result in hemorrhage into the lesion and degeneration of plaque contents. Degeneration and ulceration of plaques is most common at the sites at greatest risk of advanced lesion formation. Thus, the consequences to the circulation of lesions in those areas derive not only from the tendency to progressive stenosis, but also from the effects of lesion complications leading to rapid or sudden local occlusion or to distal embolization of thrombi or atheromatous fragments. Direct relationships among lesion composition, age of the lesion, lesion complication, and the presence of particular risk factors remain to be demonstrated. Excision of lesions obtained during surgical procedures and at autopsy have revealed complications which may be related spatially and temporally to documented clinical manifestations (27). It should also be noted, however, that lesions studied at autopsy and not associated with known clinical manifestations may show evidences of earlier complications, including hemosiderin deposits from hemorrhages, partially organized thrombi, and inflammatory cells such as macrophages, lymphocytes, plasma cells, and giant cells. These findings indicate that lesions may progress through stages potentially severe enough to induce clinical morbidity but that local tissue reactions may be adequate, at least temporarily, to contain the injury.

Configuration of Lesions

The perception that advanced atherosclerotic lesions protrude or bulge into the arterial lumen is suggested by angiographic or ultrasonic views of arteries in longitudinal projections which reveal narrowing of the lumen. *En face* observations of the luminal surface of arteries opened at operation or autopsy also reveal plaques as projecting elevations, and transverse sections of unopened but undistended atherosclerotic arteries may show narrow, crescentic, or slitlike arterial lumens. These perceptions may be somewhat misleading, for the absence of distending pressure results in partial collapse of the arterial lumen and corresponding deformation of both the artery wall and the plaque. Progressive distension of the normal aorta from zero to diastolic pressure results in a nearly twofold increase in aortic radius, a fourfold increase in lumen cross-sectional area, and a 50 percent reduction in wall thickness (see Figure 3-3) (28). Similar findings are evident for other arteries. Beyond diastolic pressure there is little change in artery wall configuration or lumen diameter in keeping with the mechanical properties related to the connective tissue fiber content and organization of the media as outlined above. Examination of atherosclerotic arteries fixed while distended reveals that the lumen on transverse section is almost always round or oval and only rarely irregular, triangular, or

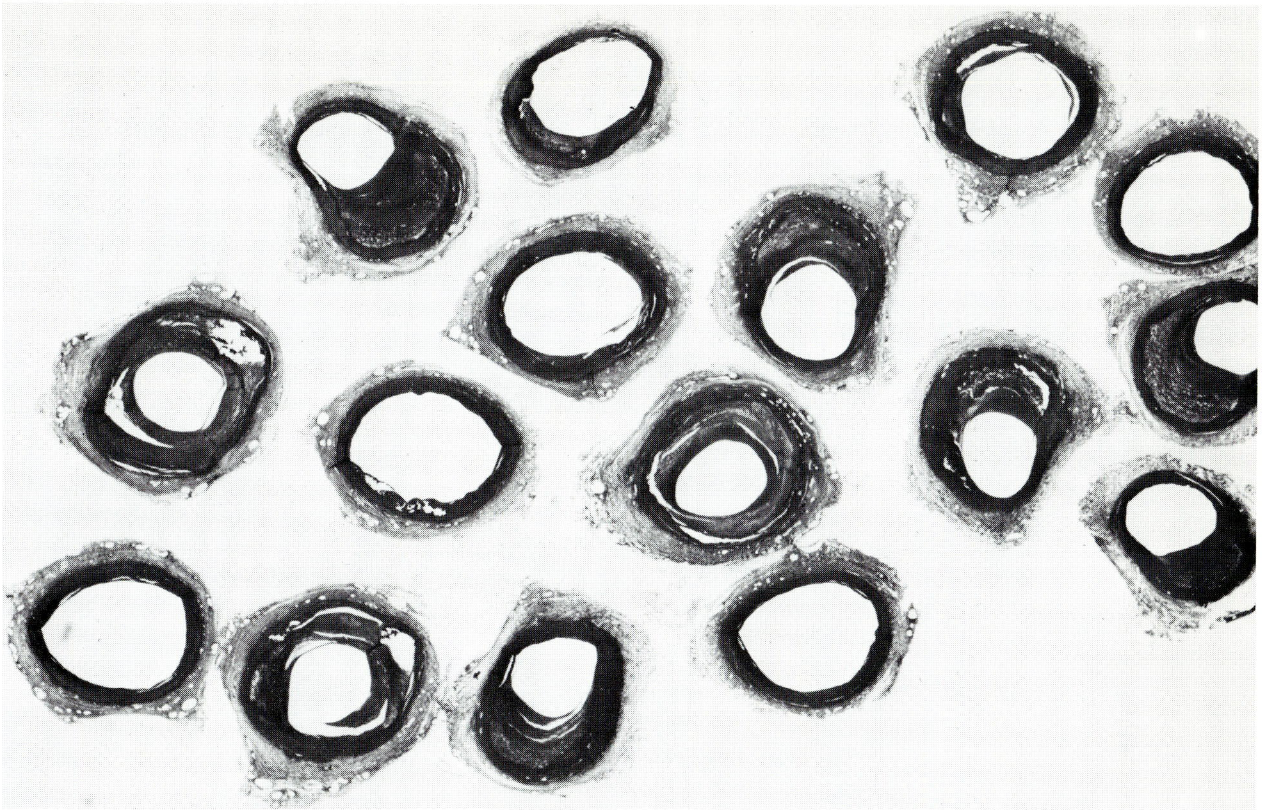

FIGURE 3-13. Multiple transverse sections at 0.5-cm intervals through a 10-cm segment of superficial femoral artery. Despite the presence of large intimal plaques, the lumen remains rounded. The external vessel contour becomes oval as the artery locally dilates to accommodate the enlarging lesion.

slitlike (29). Sequential transverse sections through distended vessels with narrowings on axial projections reveal that the lumen is round even in areas of marked stenosis. In addition, plaques are most often eccentric with respect to the cross section of the artery wall and, under conditions of normal distension, do not usually protrude into the lumen as moundlike projections but tend instead to bulge outward from the lumen. The luminal surface of the fibrous cap is therefore usually concave on transverse section, corresponding to the curvature of the adjacent uninvolved artery wall. As a consequence, the external or outer contour of the artery tends to become oval while the corresponding lumen remains circular (Figure 3-13). As long as the fibrous cap is intact, the necrotic center is effectively sequestered from the lumen and the circular configuration of the lumen is preserved. Thus, while plaques may appear as focal projections into the lumen on angiographic images, cross-sectional views reveal rounded lumen contours and a concave luminal profile of the plaque (30). Circular lumen profiles may also be evident in excised undistended and unopened rigid atherosclerotic arteries when plaques are completely encircling and largely fibrocalcific. Irregular transverse lumen contours on sonograms or distended arteries examined in cross section generally correspond to recent or resolving plaque disruptions, ulcerations, or thrombus deposition.

Studies have indicated that arteries in which lesions are developing tend to dilate (31). Vessel enlargement can occur focally in association with a discrete eccentric plaque or diffusely, resulting in extensive ectasia or arteriomegaly. The mechanism by which atherosclerotic arteries may enlarge and seemingly compensate in some degree for plaque enlargement is unknown. If such a process does indeed occur in human beings, it may follow that failure, inhibition, or exhaustion of the process results in clinically significant stenosis, while an excessive or abnormal response may result in aneurysm formation.

Localization of Atherosclerotic Lesions

Several major arterial sites are particularly prone to the development of advanced atherosclerotic lesions, while others are relatively resistant. The coronary arteries, carotid bifurcation, infrarenal abdominal aorta, and iliofemoral vessels are particularly susceptible, while the mesenteric, renal, intercostal, and mammary arteries tend to be spared (32). The apparently selective localization of plaques which evolve to cause clinical symptoms has been attributed to local differences in vessel wall metabolism, structure, and permeability and to differences in local hemodynamic patterns.

Since many plaques tend to form in relation to branch points and bends where flow profiles have been shown to undergo deviations from unidirectional laminar flow, various flow features related to these changes have been implicated in plaque localization. These include elevated shear stress (4), turbulence (33), flow separation (34), and low shear stress (35). Elevated shear stress has been thought to contribute to plaque initiation by causing endothelial injury. The resulting exposure of intimal connective tissue to the bloodstream would favor platelet deposition and release of platelet growth factor, thereby includng focal intimal thickening by stimulating smooth-muscle-cell proliferation (36). However, evidence that these are major initiating or sustaining mechanisms in human or experimental plaque formation has not been forthcoming. Clinical observations suggest that plaques localize first in areas of low shear stress, such as on the upstream rather than downstream rim of aortic ostia (Figure 3-14). Quantitative correlative studies of flow profiles and early plaque formation in the human carotid bifurcation suggest that flow separation, reduced flow rate, reduced shear stress, and departures from unidirectional laminar flow may be the important hemodynamic factors in plaque pathogenesis (37). At the carotid bifurcation, for example, plaques do not begin in the vicinity of the flow divider where flow velocity is high, laminar, and unidirectional throughout the cardiac cycle. Plaques are formed earliest and are most advanced opposite the flow divider, where flow velocity and shear stress are low (Figure 3-15). Under conditions of pulsatile flow, flow reversal occurs in the same area, particularly during the downstroke of systole (38). These flow properties may be associated with prolonged residence time of atherogenic factors such as lipids or mitogens at geometric sites of predilection. In general, while low flow velocity and stasis promote lesion formation, relatively rapid flow velocity seems to protect. The sparing effect of high flow velocity has also been demonstrated experimentally in stenotic channels (39). Such findings also suggest that an increase in flow velocity and shear in a developing atherosclerotic stenosis could tend to retard further plaque formation. Since the development of complex flow patterns and shear stress reversal occurs during systole, an elevated heart rate may be expected to be associated with the acceleration of plaque formation at sites of predilection, for increased heart rate would prolong the relative time spent in systole. This effect would be expected to be particularly important in the coronary arteries, where systolic flow is biphasic. Experimental studies, as well as clinical epidemiological studies, tend to sup-

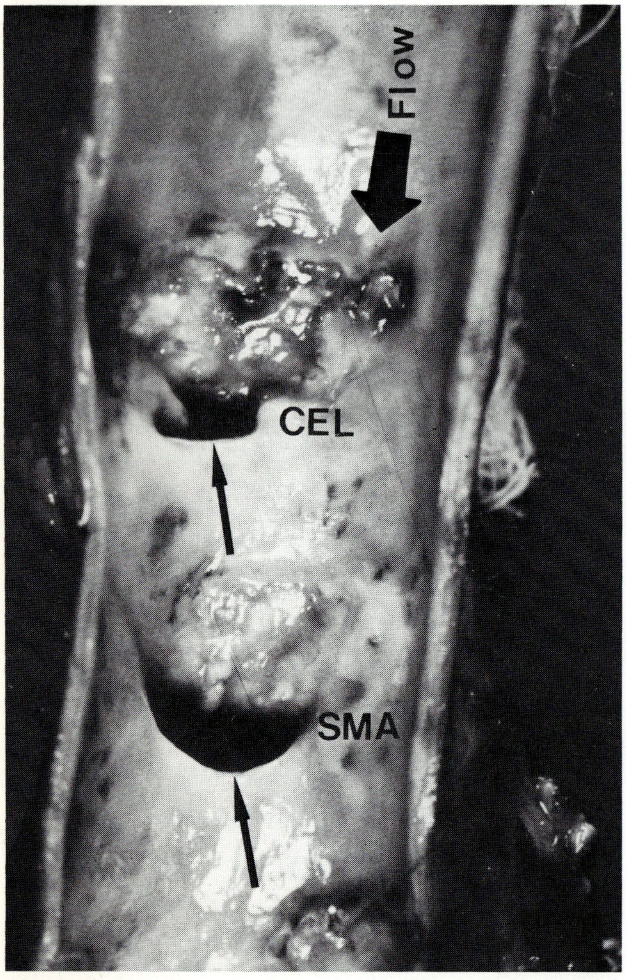

FIGURE 3-14. Celiac (CEL) and superior mesenteric (SMA) ostia of human aorta. Note prominent plaque formation at upstream rim of the ostia with no plaque formation on the flow divider (*arrows*) which is exposed to high shear stress.

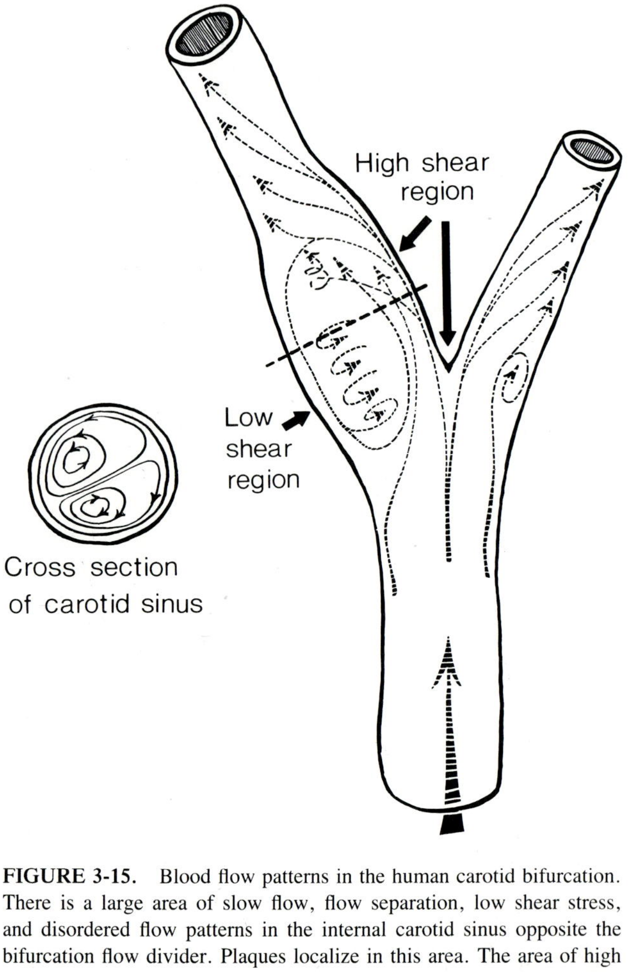

FIGURE 3-15. Blood flow patterns in the human carotid bifurcation. There is a large area of slow flow, flow separation, low shear stress, and disordered flow patterns in the internal carotid sinus opposite the bifurcation flow divider. Plaques localize in this area. The area of high shear stress at the flow divider is relatively spared of plaque formation. [Reproduced with permission from Zarins CK, Giddens DP, Glagov S: Atherosclerotic plaque distribution and flow velocity profiles in the carotid bifurcation. In Bergan JJ, Yao JST (eds): *Cerebrovascular Insufficiency*. New York, Grune & Stratton, Inc., 1983, pp. 19–30.]

port such a relationship (40). Although reduced velocity and shear stress, departures from unidirectional laminar flow, and flow reversal appear to favor plaque formation, turbulence as such does not appear to be a factor. Areas of high turbulence such as occur immediately distal to experimental stenoses are not sites of preferential lesion formation (41).

CAROTID ARTERIES

Intimal thickening is found in the carotid sinus or carotid bulb early in life, and atherosclerotic lesions are common at this site in adults. Although extensive, complex, and complicated plaques may be present in the carotid bifurcation, particularly within the sinus, there is little plaque formation in the immediately proximal common carotid artery or the internal carotid artery immediately distal to the sinus. Within the bony canal in the base of the skull, lesions are unusual, but the basilar artery as well as the proximal segments of the cerebral arteries about the circle of Willis are commonly involved. The distribution of lesions about the bifurcation is probably associated with hemodynamic conditions which derive from the special geometry at this site. The internal carotid sinus is a localized region which has a cross-sectional area twice that of the immediately distal internal carotid segment. This configuration in combination with the branching angle results in a flow profile in which a large area of flow separation is formed along the outer wall of the sinus (Figure 3-15).

Secondary and tertiary flow patterns, vortex formation, and oscillations in the angle of the flow vector occur at the side walls of the sinus. Intimal plaques are deposited early in life in this region. As plaques enlarge at the outer wall, the geometric configuration of the lumen is modified so that other flow patterns may develop which favor plaque formation on the side and inner walls. In its most advanced and stenotic form the disease may involve the entire circumference of the sinus, including the region of the flow divider, but plaques are commonly largest and most complicated at the outer and side walls of the carotid bifurcation (Figure 3-16). The hemodynamic conditions which exist at the carotid bifurcation may also influence the surface characteristics of existing carotid plaques and contribute to their tendency to ulcerate and embolize.

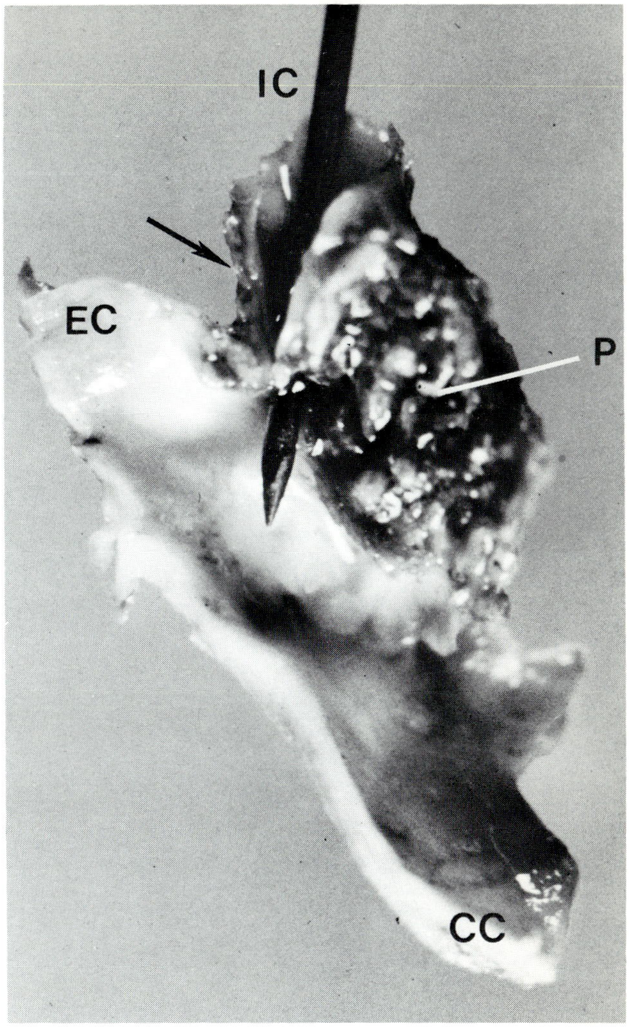

FIGURE 3-16. Longitudinal section of carotid endarterectomy specimen. Note marked plaque formation (P) on outer wall of internal carotid (IC) sinus. This corresponds to the area which is exposed to low flow velocity and low shear stress. The inner wall (*arrow*) has minimal intimal thickening. External carotid (EC), common carotid (CC).

AORTA

Plaques are regularly found in the adult human thoracic aorta, but they are often less abundant, more discrete, less complicated, and less calcific than in the abdominal aortic segment of the same individual. Although plaques tend to deposit about intercostal branch ostia, significant occlusive lesions of the thoracic aorta do not develop and thoracic aorta aneurysms are unusual. The infrarenal abdominal aortic segment, on the other hand, is particularly prone to the early occurrence of plaques and occlusive disease as well as to the development of marked medial atrophy, calcification, and aneurysmal dilatation with mural thrombus formation. Several hypotheses may be invoked to explain the discrepancy between thoracic and abdominal aortic disease. The findings cited above suggest that relatively low flow rates favor atherogenesis. Flow velocity is relatively high in the thoracic aorta, for this segment is the major conduit for the relatively constant elevated levels of flow to the cerebral, upper extremity, and visceral arterial beds, including the delivery of one-quarter of the cardiac output to the renal arteries. By contrast, levels of flow in the infrarenal aorta are largely dependent on muscular activity of the lower extremities. In relation to an increasingly sedentary lifestyle, the abdominal aortic segment is likely to be subjected to relatively reduced flow velocities over the long term. This effect may be further accentuated by the tendency of the aorta to enlarge with age. In addition, as noted above, the perfusion of the human abdominal aortic media may be marginal in relation to its thickness. While the human thoracic aortic media is furnished with intramural vasa vasorum, the abdominal aorta is relatively avascular (13). Thus, reduced and marked variations in luminal flow rate, as well as discrepancies between medial thickness and medial nutrition, may combine to enhance the accumulation of atherogenic substances in the abdominal aortic intima.

ANEURYSM FORMATION

Although 95 percent of aortic aneurysms occur in the infrarenal abdominal segment where atherosclerosis is usually most advanced, the commonly accepted causal relationship between advanced atherosclerosis and abdominal aortic aneurysm has recently been open to question. Theories have been advanced which suggest that a deficiency in copper metabolism (42) produces abnormalities of elastogenesis and eventually affects the mechanical properties of the aortic wall, resulting in the development of abnormal dilatation. It has also been proposed on the basis of chemical analyses that altered collagenase (43) or elastase (44) activity in the media results in weakening of the aortic wall. According to these views, genetic factors acting on matrix fiber formation and maintenance result in inadequate tensile support. However, the striking selective effect on the abdominal aorta may not be consistent with such a mechanism. On the basis of comparisons with other mammalian aortas, and with the human thoracic aorta, the thickness of the abdominal aortic wall should correspond to approximately 40 medial layers and the outer 10 layers should be permeated by vasa vasorum (13). Instead, the human abdominal aorta contains about 29 layers and

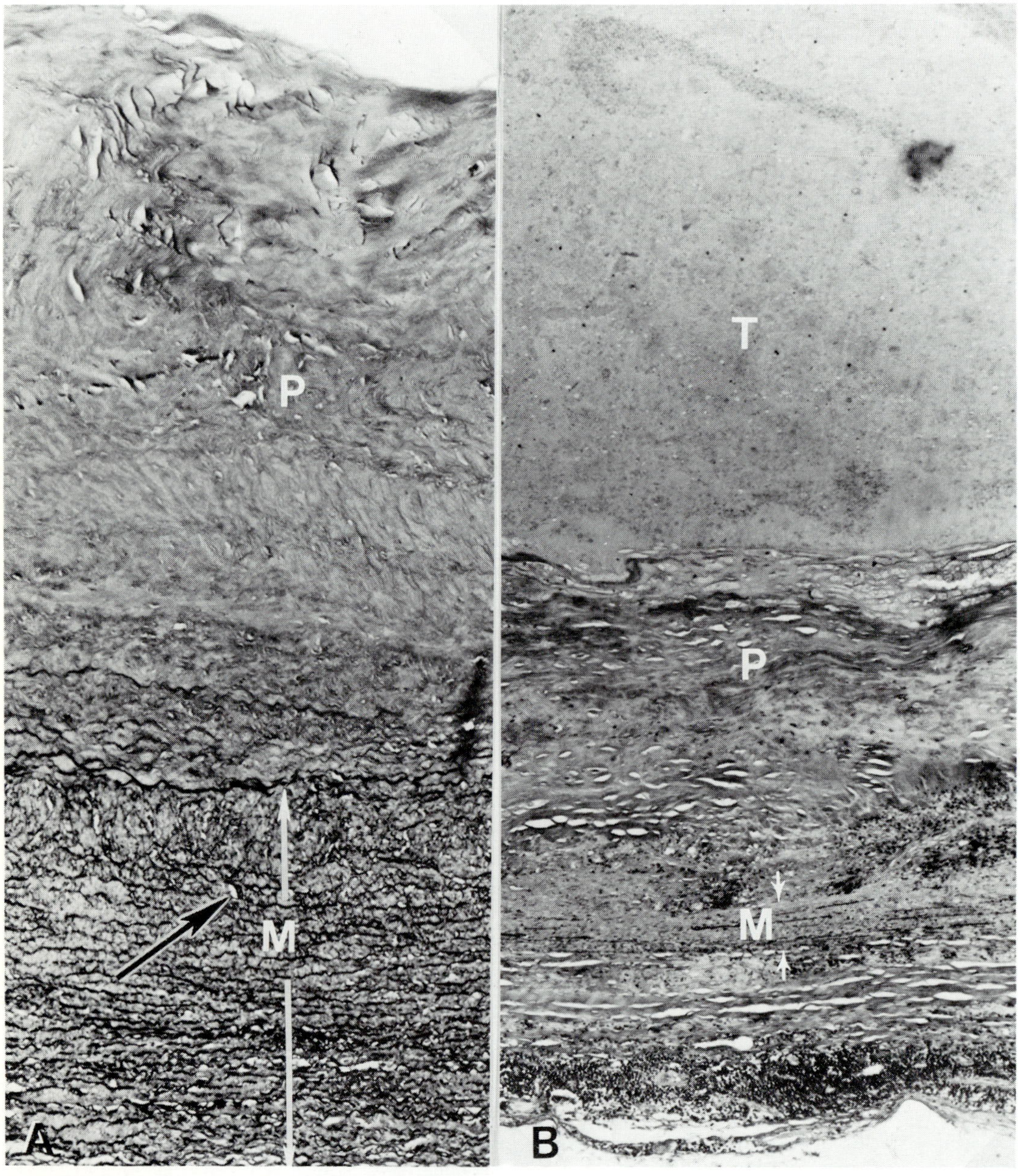

FIGURE 3-17. Transverse section of abdominal aorta demonstrating: (*A*) intimal plaque (P) with preservation of underlying media (M) with its lamellar architecture. Vasa vasorum (*arrow*) are present in the media. (*B*) Aneurysm with marked medial atrophy (M) delineated by arrows, fibrous plaque (P) and large mural thrombus (T).

is devoid of medial vasa (see Figure 3-8). Thus, the average tension per layer is greater than for other mammalian aortas without vasa or for the human thoracic aorta. Presumably, therefore, the human abdominal aortic wall is at a mechanical and nutritional disadvantage. The early advent of intimal thickening and atherosclerosis in this segment may interfere with medial nutrition from the lumen and could be expected to potentiate inborn or acquired metabolic defects which could interfere with normal medial matrix integrity. In general, the media of an aneurysmal aorta is reduced to a dense atrophic fibrous band and the associated intimal atherosclerotic lesions tend to be calcific and bland (Figure 3-17*B*). The lumen contains thrombus in layers of decreasing organization from the media to the lumen. Often the thrombus shows little evidence of organization and is present as a gelatinous mass. These features correspond to a paucity of vasa vasorum in the media or plaque. Occlusive abdominal aortic atherosclerosis on the other hand is usually associated with various degrees of penetration of vasa into the media and the plaque (Figure 3-17*A* and 3-18).

SUPERFICIAL FEMORAL ARTERY

The arteries of the lower extremities are frequently involved by atherosclerotic plaques, while vessels of similar size are spared in the upper extremities. In addition to differences in hydrostatic pressure, the arteries of the lower extremities are subjected to more marked variations in flow rate, depending on the level of physical activity. Similar to the situation which prevails in the abdominal aorta, sedentary lifestyles would tend to favor low flow rates and lead to increased plaque deposition in vessels of the lower extremities. Cigarette smoking and diabetes mellitus are the risk factors most closely associated with atherosclerotic disease of the lower extremities (45). The manner in which these factors and the special hemodynamic conditions are mutually enhancing in the vessels of the lower extremities remains to be elucidated. Of the arteries of the lower extremity, the superficial femoral artery is most commonly the site of multiple stenotic lesions, while the profunda femoris tends to be spared. The superficial femoral artery is a major conduit with relatively few proximal branches, and flow velocity is likely to be relatively slow on the average, varying in relation to activity of the calf

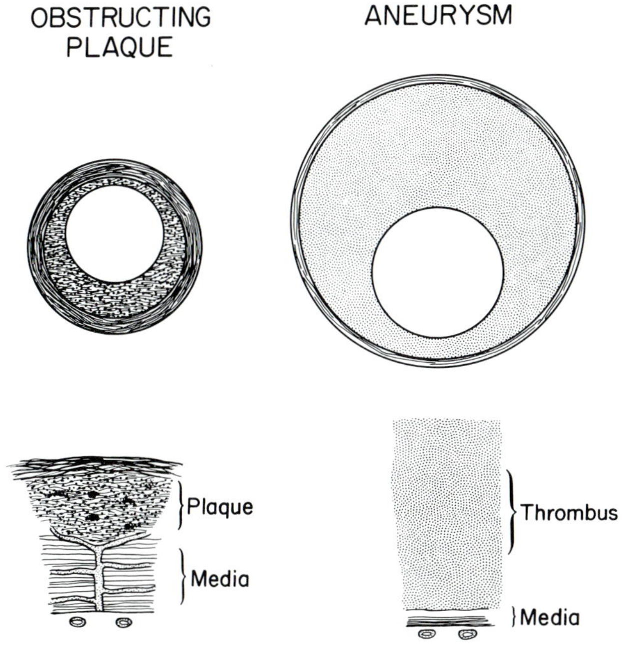

FIGURE 3-18. Obstructing plaques in the abdominal aorta are characterized by ingrowth of vasa vasorum to nourish the media and plaque. Aneurysms are relatively devoid of vasa with atrophy of the aortic wall. A deficiency of medial nutrition may be a factor in aneurysm pathogenesis. [Reproduced with permission from Zarins CK, Glagov S: Aneurysms and obstructive plaques: Differing local responses to atherosclerosis. In Bergan JJ, Yao JST (eds): *Aneurysms: Diagnosis and treatment*. New York, Grune & Stratton, Inc., 1982, pp. 61–82.]

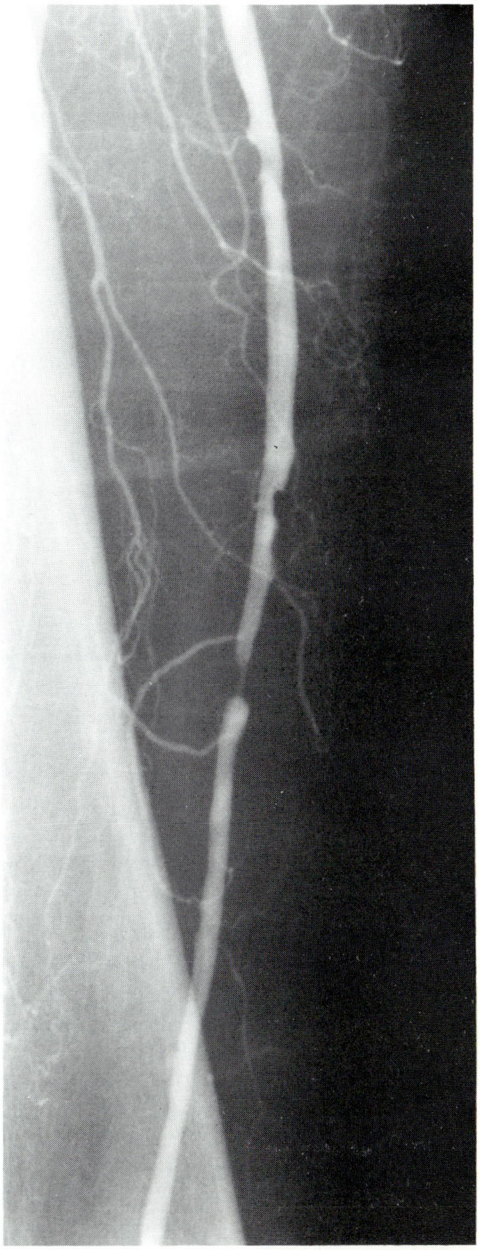

FIGURE 3-19. Focal stenosis of superficial femoral artery at adductor hiatus.

muscles during walking or running. The profunda femoris is a smaller, muscular vessel with many branches to lower extremity muscles; flow velocity is likely to be relatively high under normal conditions. Plaques in the superficial femoral artery have not been shown to occur preferentially at branching sites, but stenotic lesions tend to appear earliest at the adductor hiatus, where the vessel is straight and branches are few (Figure 3-19). Repeated mechanical trauma, limitations on vessel compliance, or enlargement associated with the closely applied adductor magnus tendon may contribute to the selective localization of occlusive disease in this position.

CORONARY ARTERIES

No completely adequate explanation has been furnished for the special propensity of the coronary arteries to develop atherosclerosis or for the discrepancies in severity of involvement between the coronary arteries and the aorta (46). The special hemodynamic features of the coronary circulation, including the marked excursions in flow rate during the cardiac cycle, the geometric configuration of the vessels and their branches, the mechanical torsion and flexions of the vessels associated with cardiac motion, and the special reactivity of coronary artery smooth muscle to vasoactive substances and nervous impulses have been suggested as predisposing factors which could underlie individual differences in lesion distribution. The selective involvement of the left coronary artery opposite the flow divider at the bifurcation of the left circumflex indicates that hemodynamic relationships similar to those which prevail at the carotid bifurcation also occur in the coronary arteries. In addition, compared to other vessels, there are two pulses of flow during systole. Since the oscillatory changes in fluid shear related to the downstroke phase of the systolic pulse (38), an increase in heart rate may exert a greater effect on atherogenesis in the coronary arteries than elsewhere in the arterial tree. Recent studies suggest that reduced heart rate retards the development of experimental, diet-induced plaques (40).

Quantitative Evaluation of Atherosclerosis

Quantitative clinical assessment of atherosclerosis by modern diagnostic methods may include evaluation of several distinct but related aspects of involvement (47). These include the *extent* of the disease process, i.e., the degree to which a given artery segment or arterial bed is involved by the disease and/or the number of distinguishable lesions present in a vessel or group of vessels (Figure 3-20). Irregularities and strictures of lumen contour on angiograms as well as on ultrasonic and axial tomographic images and the presence of calcifications have been considered to be major indicators of *extent* of disease. A second quantifiable feature which bears directly on the consequences to the circulation is the *severity* of the disease, as reflected in the degree of luminal stenosis. Usual estimates are expressed as percent stenosis, based on comparisons between lumen diameter at a definite narrowing and an immediately adjacent segment which appears to be uninvolved. Another discernible index of

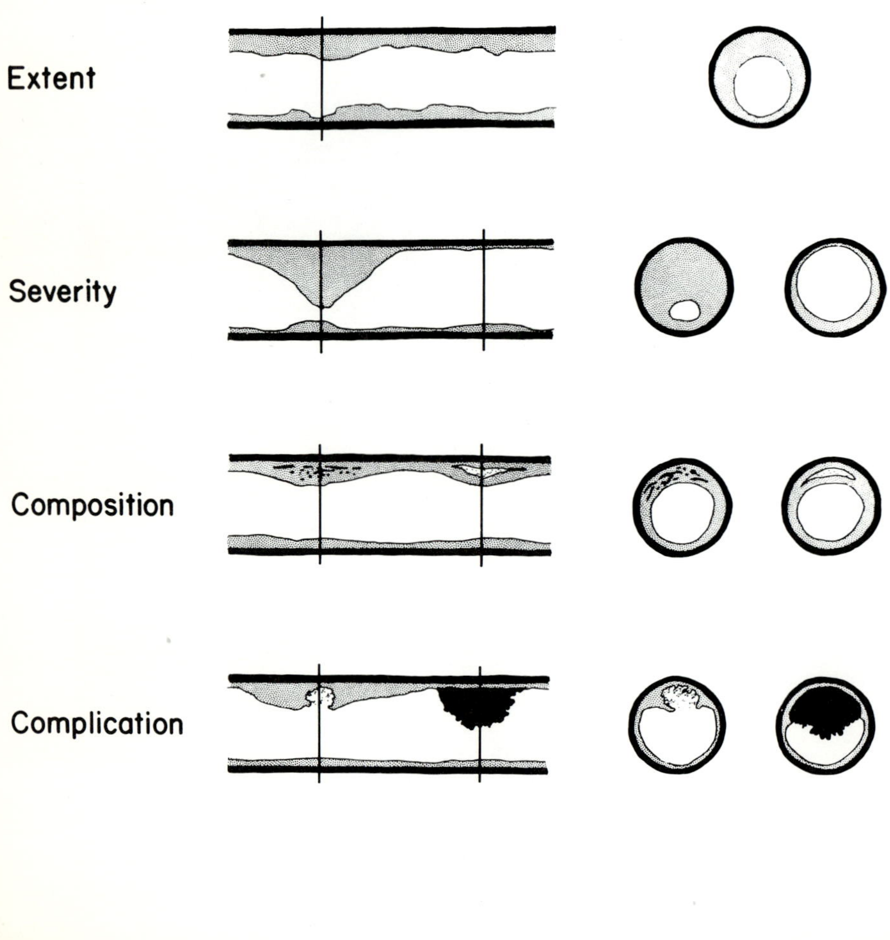

FIGURE 3-20. Quantifiable aspects of atherosclerotic lesions. [Reproduced with permission from Glagov S, Zarins CK: Quantitating atherosclerosis: Problems of definition. In Bond MG, Insull W Jr, Glagov S, Chandler AB, Cornhill JF (eds): *Diagnosis of Atherosclerosis: Quantitative Methods of Evaluation*. New York, Springer-Verlag, 1983, pp. 11–35.]

the atherosclerotic process, independent of both extent of involvement and severity of stenosis, is lesion *complication*. This includes ulceration, necrosis, thrombosis, and plaque hemorrhage. Finally, quantitative information concerning lesion *composition* may be obtained. This includes calcification, frequently revealed by clinical visualization methods and estimates of lipid, cell, and matrix fiber content, usually estimated from histological sections.

Most often, quantitative descriptions of atherosclerosis deal with the severity of disease, or *percent stenosis*, of a lesion imaged by angiography. Since angiography can only demonstrate the opacified artery lumen, the degree of stenosis is calculated by comparing lumen diameter at the narrowest point to an apparently "disease-free" area in the same vessel. In addition to errors in projection, resolution, and magnification, errors may arise if the apparently normal zone is involved by advanced intimal plaques. In comparing sequential angiograms, further errors may result if arteries dilate as atherosclerosis progresses. Such a response to progressing disease has been demonstrated in experimental (31) and human atherosclerosis (30).

Ultrasonic imaging of arteries has the capability of visualizing not only the lumen of the vessel, but also the artery wall (48). Other imaging techniques such as computed tomography and nuclear magnetic resonance have similar potential to visualize the plaque. It is important, however, to recognize the difference in definition of percent stenosis by these imaging techniques compared to angiography (Figure 3-21) when assessing validation studies.

Gross morphologic and histologic examinations of atherosclerotic arteries have the advantage of direct visualization and inspection of the lumen, plaque, and artery wall. However, redistension of the collapsed artery wall during fixation is necessary in order to restore in vivo configuration (30). Failure to do so has led to a misperception that angiography "underestimates" the degree of stenosis when compared to postmortem examination (49). Calculation of percent stenosis from histologic cross sections of arteries is usually performed by comparing the lumen cross-sectional area to the area encompassed by the internal elastic lamina, the presumed lumen size before the plaque developed (Figure 3-21). This difference in definition of percent stenosis may make comparison to other methods difficult. In addition, if vessel enlargement occurred during plaque enlargement, the internal elastic lamina landmark may not accurately represent the "true lumen." Furthermore, accurate quantitative correlation of plaque cross-sectional area as measured on histologic sections with in vivo clinical measurements requires corrections to account for tissue shrinkage during fixation and processing (30).

Although plaques may vary a good deal in *composition*, methods for assessing the distribution of plaque components in vivo are not yet sufficiently sensitive or specific to permit the establishment of criteria for predicting which lesions are likely to enlarge or ulcerate and which lesions will remain relatively stable. Means which provide direct information about actual plaque size and composition are developing rapidly and are likely to gain increased application. These include real-time ultrasound

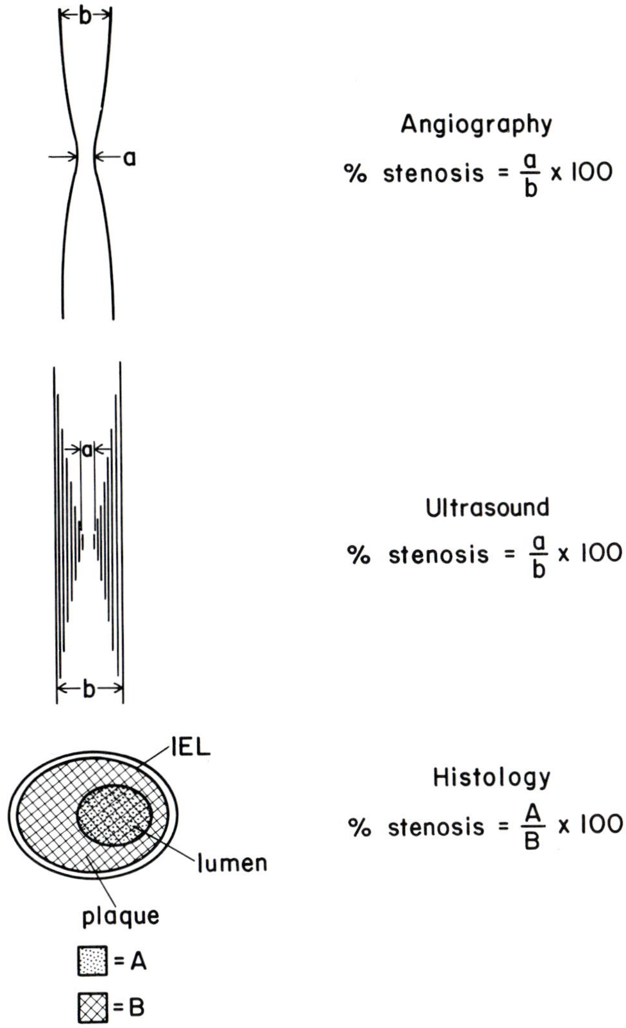

FIGURE 3-21. Different methods of measuring and defining percent stenosis.

imaging, reconstructions from computerized tomography, and nuclear magnetic resonance and positron imaging. Thus, more accurate assessments of the extent of disease may be available in the future, including more quantitative in vivo measurements of lumen diameter, plaque and artery wall thickness, plaque composition, plaque disruption, and thrombosis. For the present, attempts to quantitate atherosclerotic disease in the living patient or from histologic sections in order to evaluate treatment programs dealing with prevention, regression, or early detection must take appropriate account of the features of plaque and vessel morphology outlined above. In particular, the outward sequestration effect, the persistence of a circular lumen which may approximate normal dimensions despite the presence of a large plaque, the association of plaque formation with enlargement of the vessel, and the need for fixation under pressure must be considered.

Acknowledgment

The authors would like to acknowledge Althea B. Zmuidzinas's assistance in the preparation of this manuscript.

References

1. Flaherty JT, Pierce JE, Ferrans VJ, Patel DJ, Tucker WK, Fry DL: Endothelial nuclear patterns in the canine arterial tree with particular reference to hemodynamic events. Circ Res 1972, 30:23.
2. Clark JM, Glagov S: Evaluation and publication of scanning electron micrographs. Science 1976, 192:1360.
3. Ts'Ao CH, Glagov S: Basal endothelial attachments: Tenacity at cytoplasmic dense zone in the rabbit aorta. Lab Invest 1970, 23:520.
4. Fry DL: Acute vascular endothelial changes associated with increased blood velocity gradients. Circ Res 1968, 22:165.
5. Zarins CK, Taylor KE, Bomberger RA, Glagov S: Endothelial integrity at aortic ostial flow dividers. SEM 1980, 3:249.
6. Jaffe EA: *Biology of Endothelial Cells*. Boston, Martinus Nijhoff, 1984.
7. Clark JM, Glagov S: Structural integration of the arterial wall. I. Relationships and attachments of medial smooth muscle cells in normally distended and hyperdistended aortas. Lab Invest 1979, 40:587.
8. Wolinsky H, Glagov S: A lamellar unit of aortic medial structure and function in mammals. Circ Res 1967, 20:99.
9. Clark JM, Glagov S: Transmural organization of the arterial media: The lamellar unit revisited. Arteriosclerosis 1985, 5:19.
10. Glagov S: Hemodynamic risk factors: Mechanical stress, mural architecture, medial nutrition and the vulnerability of arteries to atherosclerosis. In Wissler RW, Geer JC (eds): *The Pathogenesis of Atherosclerosis*. Baltimore, Williams & Wilkins, 1972, pp 164–199.
11. Fischer, GM, Llaurado JG: Collagen and elastin content in canine arteries from functionally different vascular beds. Circ Res 1966, 19:3984.
12. Wolinsky H, Glagov S: Nature of species differences in the medial distribution of aortic vasa vasorum in mammals. Circ Res 1967, 20:409.
13. Wolinsky H, Glagov S: Comparison of abdominal and thoracic aortic medial structure in mammals. Deviation of man from the usual pattern. Circ Res 1969, 25:677.
14. Heistad DD, Marcus ML, Law EG, Armstrong ML, Ehrhardt JC, Abboud FM: Regulation of blood flow to the aortic media in dogs. J Clin Invest 1978, 62:133.
15. Paterson JC: Vascularization and hemorrhage of the intima of arteriosclerotic coronary arteries. Arch Pathol 1936, 22:313.
16. Wilens SL: The nature of diffuse intimal thickening of arteries. Am J Pathol 1951, 27:825.
17. Movat HZ, More TH, Haust MD: The diffuse intimal thickening of the human aorta with aging. Am J Pathol 1958, 34:1023.
18. Tejada C, Strong JP, Montenegro MR, Restrepo C, Solberg LA: Distribution of coronary and aortic atherosclerosis by geographic location, race and sex. Lab Invest 1968, 18:5009.
19. Mendez J, Tejada C: Chemical composition of aortas from Guatemalans and North Americans. Am J Clin Pathol 1969, 51:598.
20. Mitchell JRA, Schwartz CJ: Study of cardiovascular disease at necropsy. In *Arterial Disease*. Oxford, Blackwell Scientific, 1965, pp 377–396.
21. McGill HC Jr: Atherosclerosis: Problems in pathogenesis. In Paoletti R, Gotto AM (eds): *Atherosclerosis Reviews*. New York, Raven, 1977, pp 27–65.
22. Pearson TA, Dillman JM, Solez K, Heptinstall RH: Clonal markers in the study of the origin and growth of human atherosclerotic lesions. Circ Res 1978, 43:10.
23. Benditt EP, Benditt JM: Evidence for a monoclonal origin of human atherosclerotic plaques. Proc Natl Acad Sci 1973, 70:1753.
24. Stary HC: The intimal macrophage in atherosclerosis. Artery 1980, 8:205.
25. Paterson JC: Vascularization and haemorrhage of the intima of arteriosclerotic coronary arteries. Arch Pathol 1936, 22:312.
26. Rifkin RD, Parisi HF, Follard E: Coronary calcification in the diagnosis of coronary artery disease. Am J Cardiol 1979, 44:141.
27. Imparato AM, Riles TS, Mintzer R, Baumann FG: The importance of hemorrhage in the relationship between gross morphologic characteristics and cerebral symptoms in 376 carotid artery plaques. Ann Surg 1983, 197:195.
28. Wolinsky H, Glagov S: Structural basis for the static mechanical properties of the aortic media. Circ Res 1964, 14:400.
29. Glagov S, Zarins CK: Quantitating atherosclerosis: Problems of definition. In Bond MG, Insull W Jr, Glagov S, Chandler AB, Cornhill JF (eds): *Clinical Diagnosis of Atherosclerosis*. New York, Springer-Verlag, 1983, pp 11–35.
30. Zarins CK, Zatina MA, Glagov S: Correlation of postmortem angiography with pathologic anatomy: Quantitation of atherosclerotic lesions. In Bond MG, Insull W Jr, Glagov S, Chandler AB, Cornhill JF (eds): *Clinical Diagnosis of Atherosclerosis*. New York, Springer-Verlag, 1983, pp 283–303.
31. Bond MG, Adams MR, Bullock BC: Complicating factors in evaluating coronary artery atherosclerosis. Artery 1981, 9:21.
32. Roberts JC Jr, Moses C, Wilkins, RH: Autopsy studies in atherosclerosis. I. Distribution and severity of atherosclerosis in patients dying without morphologic evidence of atherosclerotic catastrophe. II. Distribution and severity of atherosclerosis in patients dying with morphologic evidence of atherosclerotic catastrophe. Circulation 1959, 29:511, 520.
33. Stehbens WE: The role of hemodynamics in the pathogenesis of atherosclerosis. Prog Cardiovasc Dis 1975, 18:89.
34. Scharfstein H, Gutstein WH, Lewis L: Changes of boundary layer flow in model systems, implications for initiation of endothelial injury. Circ Res 1963, 18:580.
35. Caro CG, Fitz-Gerald JM, Schroter RD: Atheroma and arterial wall shear: Observation, correlation and proposal of a shear dependent mass transfer mechanism for atherogenesis. Proc R Soc Lond [Biol] 1971, 117:109.
36. Ross R, Harker L: Hyperlipidemia and atherosclerosis. Science 1976, 193:1094.
37. Zarins CK, Giddens DP, Bharadvaj BK, Sottiurai VS, Mabon RF, Glagov S: Carotid bifurcation atherosclerosis: Quantitative correlation of plaque localization with flow velocity profiles and wall shear stress. Circ Res 1983, 53:502.
38. Ku DN, Giddens DP: Pulsatile flow in a model carotid bifurcation. Arteriosclerosis 1983, 3:31.
39. Zarins CK, Bomberger RA, Glagov S: Local effects of stenoses: Increased flow velocity inhibits atherogenesis. Circulation 1981, 64(suppl 2):221.
40. Beere PA, Glagov S, Zarins CK: Retarding effect of lowered heart rate on coronary atherosclerosis. Science 1984, 226:180.
41. Bomberger RA, Zarins CK, Taylor KE, Glagov S: Effect of hypotension on atherogenesis and aortic wall composition. J Surg Res 1980, 28:402.
42. Tilson, MD: Decreased hepatic copper levels: A possible chemical marker for the pathogenesis of aortic aneurysms in man. Arch Surg 1982, 117:1212.
43. Busuttil RW, Abou-Zamzam AM, Machleder HI: Collagenase activity of the human aorta. Arch Surg 1980, 115:1373.
44. Hornebeck W, Adnet JJ, Robert L: Age dependent variation of elastin and elastase in aorta and human breast cancers. Exp Gerontol 1978, 13:293.
45. Gordon T, Kannel WB: Predisposition to atherosclerosis in the head, heart and legs. The Framingham Study. JAMA 1972, 221:661.

46. Glagov S, Rowley DA, Kohut R: Atherosclerosis of human aorta and its coronary and renal arteries. AMA Arch Pathol 1961, 72:558.
47. Strandness DE: Workshop overview. In Bond MG, Insull W Jr, Glagov S, Chandler AB, Cornhill JF (eds): *Clinical Diagnosis of Atherosclerosis*. New York, Springer-Verlag, 1983, pp 1–9.
48. Greene ER, Eldridge MW, Voyles WF, Miranda FG, Davis JG: Quantitative evaluation of atherosclerosis using Doppler ultrasound. In Bond MG, Insull W Jr, Glagov S, Chandler AB, Cornhill JF (eds): *Clinical Diagnosis of Atherosclerosis*. New York, Springer-Verlag, 1983, pp 8–168.
49. Isner JM, Kishel J, Kent KM, Ronan JA Jr, Ross MA, Roberts WC: Accuracy of angiographic determination of left main coronary arterial narrowing. Circulation 1981, 63:1056.

Chapter 4

ARTERITIS AND DYSPLASTIC ARTERIAL LESIONS

BRUCE L. GEWERTZ

The vascular surgeon may occasionally encounter organ or limb ischemia resulting from arteritis or dysplastic lesions distinct from the much more common atherosclerotic process. This chapter discusses these unusual disorders and reviews diagnostic and therapeutic options for the most common lesions.

To aid in clinical differentiation, arteritis is classified by the size of the involved vessel. One such classification is presented in Table 4-1. The most prominent arteritis involving the aorta and its primary branches is Takayasu's arteritis. Other inflammatory disorders involve medium-size and small muscular arteries or the arterioles and capillaries and rarely require operative consideration. Fibrodysplastic lesions will be discussed separately because there is minimal if any inflammatory component to these lesions.

TABLE 4-1. Classification of Arteritis Based on Vessel Size

Large arteries:
Takayasu's arteritis
Medium-sized arteries:
Temporal arteritis (giant cell)
Thromboangiitis obliterans
Polyarteritis (nodosa)
Behçet's disease
Small arteries:
Hypersensitivity vasculitis
Henoch-Schönlein purpura
Mixed cryoglobulinemia

Large-Vessel Lesions

TAKAYASU'S ARTERITIS

Takayasu's arteritis is a dramatic and unusual disorder involving the aorta and its primary branches. Because of its chronic obliterative nature it is also called "pulseless disease" and occlusive thromboaortopathy. Women are much more frequently affected than men (8:1), although the true incidence and distribution of these lesions remains ill-defined. The disease is named for the Japanese ophthalmologist who described associated ocular abnormalities in 1908. Perhaps as a consequence of his early observation, the highest incidence appears to be in the Far East, especially Japan, although more recent reports have contributed large numbers of patients from Mexico and India. In the United States recently, there seems to be an increased recognition of this disorder in Caucasians.

The majority of patients (70 percent) are first affected between 10 and 30 years of age. The precise etiology remains unknown, although infections and autoimmune phenomena have been investigated. The association of this disorder with rheumatoid arthritis, ankylosing spondylitis, and ulcerative colitis appears to reinforce the latter mechanism. Currently, there is no experimental model for this form of aortitis.

Clinical Presentation

The disease process can be broadly divided into two stages: an early phase ("prepulseless") and late phase ("pulseless"). Initial symptoms include generalized malaise and other nonspecific indicators such as skin rash, anorexia, myalgia, weight loss, fatigue, and fever. Laboratory examinations at this time may reflect the general inflammatory process. The erythrocyte sedimentation rate (ESR) is nearly always increased, and mild hypochromic anemia is evident. Elevated alpha 2 and/or gamma globulin fractions are frequently noted.

After a variable period of time from the onset of vague constitutional symptoms, arterial lesions become evident. The vast majority of patients present during the pulseless stage and predictably demonstrate an absence of one or more peripheral pulses. Symptoms at this time reflect the extremity or organ which is rendered ischemic. Light-headedness or vertigo are frequent complaints if the aortic arch or extracranial carotid vessels are involved. Emotional instability, "drop attacks," and headache may also be present, along with more lateralizing signs such as hemiparesis. Ocular symptoms include blurring, diplopia, and progressive blindness. A rare but reported symptom is decreasing vision on physical exertion ("visual claudication"). Such ocular complaints can be associated with retinal atrophy or hemorrhage. Ophthalmoscopic examination may also demonstrate optic atrophy and retinal vein or artery thrombosis.

It has been observed that many of these patients assume a characteristic face-down posturing to prevent neck extension which further compromises carotid or vertebral flow. Extremities with arterial stenoses may manifest exercise-related symptoms; with worsening of occlusive lesions, rest pain or tissue loss may occur. Compromise of the external carotid circulation can result in atrophic facial muscles as well as ulcerations of the palate, nose, or ear. Chronic intestinal or renal ischemia is associated with abdominal aortic involvement.

Noninvasive vascular tests may suggest Takayasu's arteritis if bilateral upper extremity and extracranial occlusive disease are documented in a woman of appropriate age. Arteriography is most useful in confirming the diagnosis and is essential for planning operative therapy. Arteriography also allows classification of Takayasu's arteritis into four main types based on distribution of lesions. *Type 1* is limited to the aortic arch and its primary branches (Figures 4-1 and 4-2); *type 2* includes lesions of the descending thoracic and abdominal aorta; *type 3* extends from the aortic valve to the abdominal aorta (essentially combining types 1 and 2); and *type 4* is defined as pulmonary artery involvement, but it has also been applied to all cases presenting with aneurysms.

Pathology

The classic gross external appearance of the involved blood vessel in Takayasu's arteritis is a "tree-bark" surface not dissimilar to leutic arteritis. Patchy involvement with numerous skip areas is the most common pattern, although some patients present with continuous involvement. Although inflammation is most severe in the adventitia and outer media, Takayasu's arteritis is truly a panarteritis. The media is infiltrated by lymphocytes, plasma cells, and histocytes. Polymorphonuclear and multinucleated giant cells are consistently observed, especially around the vasa vasorum. Elastic and smooth muscular components of the media are gradually eroded by this process, and extensive transmural fibrosis is evident. Additional intimal proliferation may contribute to the occlusive lesion.

Therapy

Unfortunately, corticosteroids are not of proven efficacy in this disorder, although there is still some enthusiasm for this treatment if the disease can be recognized in the prepulseless stage. Other medical therapies have included cytotoxic agents; however, these drugs are also of questionable benefit.

In patients with symptomatic lesions, operative therapy is directed toward bypass of involved and occluded vessels. It is not uncommon for these patients to require bilateral carotid revascularization with grafts originating from the ascending aorta. If possible, it is prudent to delay operation until active signs of the disease have resolved. In patients presenting with cerebrovas-

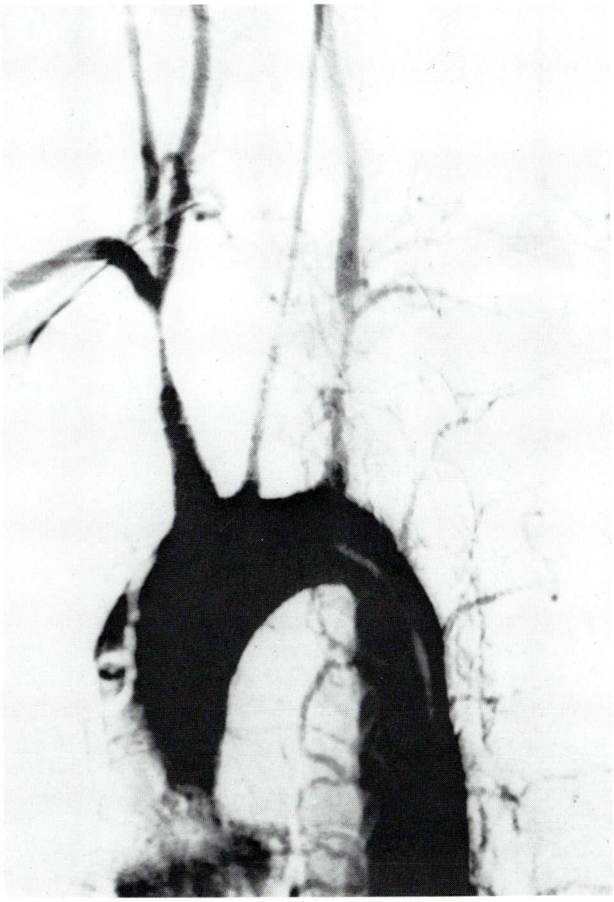

FIGURE 4-1. Typical distribution of lesions in Takayasu's arteritis (type 1) with severe uniform stenoses of brachiocephalic and left common carotid arteries. Patient presented with syncope and dizziness.

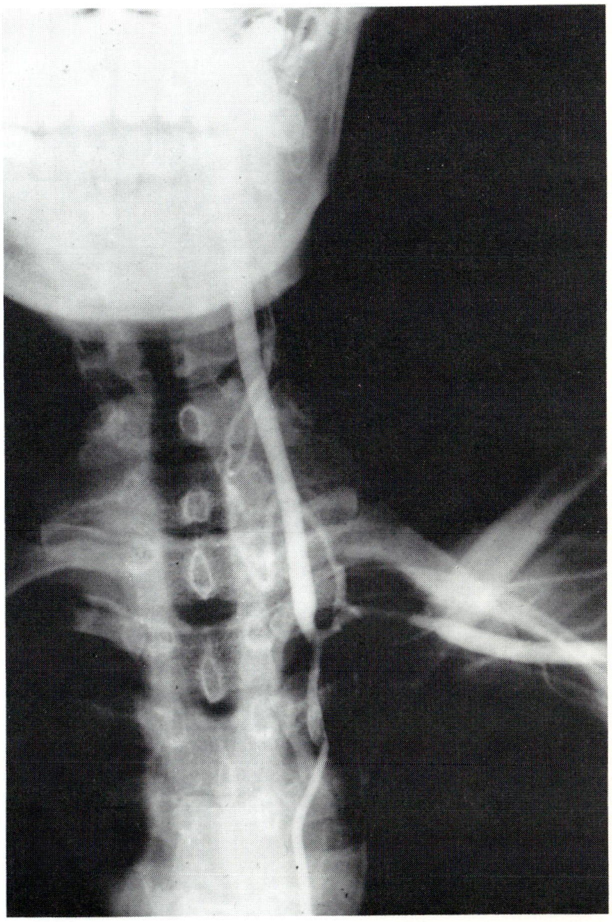

FIGURE 4-2. Selective injection of left subclavian demonstrating poststenotic dilation of patent left vertebral artery. Note restriction of disease to intrathoracic subclavian with normal caliber of left axillary artery.

cular insufficiency, this may be impossible. Indications of quiescence include normalization of markedly elevated ESR and white blood cell counts.

Operative dissection should be confined to the nondiseased portions of the aorta and distal vessels because the inflammatory nature of the arteritis may predispose to injury of adjacent structures. In general, the disease is limited to the more proximal brachiocephalic vessels; carotid bifurcation disease and axillary involvement are minimal. A most versatile procedure is anastomosis of a bifurcated aortic graft to the ascending aorta with limbs to carotid or brachiocephalic vessels. The proximal anastomosis must be tailored obliquely to lie parallel to the ascending aorta to avoid kinking or compression when the sternum is closed (Figure 4-3).

Although endarterectomy has been performed on these lesions, clinical experience strongly favors bypass techniques using prosthetic grafts because of the uncertain strength of the inflamed arterial wall after endarterectomy. Even without endarterectomy, the development of pseudoaneurysms at anastomoses remains a problem. Some surgeons routinely buttress suture lines with pledgets or place interrupted sutures at regular intervals along a continuous suture line.

Medium-Sized Vessel Lesions

TEMPORAL ARTERITIS

Temporal arteritis may be distinguished on clinical grounds from Takayasu's arteritis. It is a far more prevalent disorder and nearly always occurs in patients over the age of 50. While women are affected more commonly than men, the proportion is 2:1 rather than the 8:1 ratio recognized for Takayasu's arteritis. The incidence of temporal arteritis is surprisingly high, especially in the north central regions of the United States. One series documented a prevalence of 133 cases per 100,000 population age 50 and over. Like most vascular inflammatory lesions, autoimmune mechanisms are implicated. This is particularly true in temporal arteritis which is frequently associated with polymyalgia rheumatica.

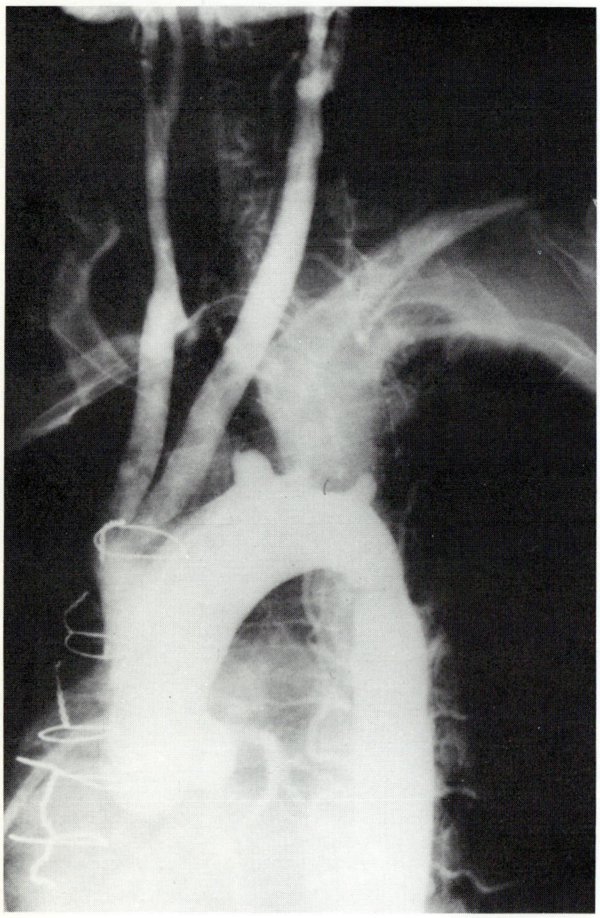

FIGURE 4-3. Bifurcated graft originates from the ascending aorta with distal anastomoses at or below the carotid bifurcations.

Clinical Presentation

In some series, the mean age of onset is as high as 70 years of age. While the onset of ocular symptoms is classically described as abrupt, careful histories will often elicit symptoms present for several months before the diagnosis is established. Fatigue, weight loss, and fever are characteristic of the disorder. Typical presentations also include headache associated with scalp tenderness over the distribution of the temporal artery. The character of the headache is variable, although this manifestation is often severe and may be misdiagnosed as "migraine" headache. The most worrisome presenting symptoms are blindness and diplopia. Fifty percent of patients experience some visual disturbances. While visual loss may be partial or complete, it is generally accepted that once established the deficit is permanent. The mechanism of these visual changes is thought to be ischemia of the retina or optic nerve associated with arteritis of branches of the ophthalmic or posterior ciliary arteries. Ophthalmoscopic examination may occasionally demonstrate central retinal artery occlusion, although this is less common. Before the emphasis on early diagnosis and aggressive treatment with steroids, the incidence of permanent visual loss was as high as 60 percent. More recent series have documented a much lower incidence approximating 10 to 20 percent.

Other specific complaints include difficulty in mastication or swallowing consistent with ischemia of the facial muscles, tongue, and pharynx. Neuropsychiatric symptoms are prevalent and include memory loss, depression, and anxiety. While many patients with temporal arteritis have concomitant atherosclerosis, approximately 10 to 15 percent demonstrate nonatherosclerotic large-artery occlusive lesions similar to those seen in Takayasu's arteritis.

Laboratory examinations reflect the nonspecific inflammatory process. The most common abnormalities include normochromic normocytic anemia associated with decreased albumin and increased fibrinogen, alpha 2 globulins, and gamma globulins. The

ESR usually remains quite high (> 100 mm/h) until successful treatment is initiated. In roughly one-third of patients, liver function tests are abnormal.

The diagnosis should be strongly suspected in any patient over the age of 50 who presents with a new onset of headache, visual symptoms, or hip and shoulder pain compatible with polymyalgia rheumatica. Physical examination may demonstrate scalp tenderness, although this feature can be quite short-lived.

The most definitive diagnostic procedure is biopsy of the temporal artery; adjacent branches of the external carotid can be sampled if other areas of tenderness are elicited. It is important that an adequate length of temporal artery is exposed (at least 2 to 3 cm) and that atraumatic technique is used in removing the specimen. In the few patients with suspected large-artery involvement, arteriography may be indicated. However, such studies are less useful in this disorder in comparison to their central diagnostic role in Takayasu's arteritis. It remains controversial whether all patients with polymyalgia rheumatica should be subjected to temporal artery biopsy even if no other symptoms of temporal arteritis are evident. Such "blind" biopsies yield a 10 to 20 percent incidence of pathologically proven but clinically silent temporal arteritis. In view of this relatively low yield it may be more appropriate to follow patients with polymyalgia rheumatica closely and initiate steroid therapy immediately if scalp tenderness or visual changes are noted.

Pathology

The pathologic lesion is best described as a granulomatous inflammation of the media with varying degrees of fibrocellular intimal proliferation. Mononuclear and polymorphonuclear leukocytes are identified within the media, but lymphocytes and histiocytes predominate. The internal elastic lamina is characteristically necrotic and disrupted. Late in the disease, fibrosis with recanalization of the lumen is often seen. The classic multinucleated or Langhans' giant cells are demonstrated in the majority of cases.

Treatment

Once the diagnosis is made by biopsy, temporal arteritis is best treated nonsurgically. Patients are usually started on 45 to 60 mg of prednisone per day. An equivalent dose of another steroid preparation can also be administered. In patients with active visual symptoms, intravenous steroids are appropriate. Most patients respond to treatment quite rapidly, and visual changes and scalp tenderness subside within 12 to 24 hours. Although some authors have suggested that steroid therapy should be reduced after 1 month, the incidence of early relapse is relatively high (approximately 20 percent), leading many physicians to continue therapy for 1 to 2 years. Despite its lack of specificity, the ESR is the most reliable test to assess activity of the disease during the gradual tapering of the steroid dose.

THROMBOANGIITIS OBLITERANS

Thromboangiitis obliterans, also known as Buerger's disease, involves the medium- and small-size arteries in the distal upper and lower extremities. The prevalence of this disease varies according to the strictness with which the diagnostic criteria are applied. Classic criteria for the disease include (1) most severe involvement in the digital circulation, (2) highest incidence in young males, (3) close association with tobacco dependency, and (4) recurrent episodes of superficial thrombophlebitis. Patients with all four of these components represent a most frustrating, if extremely small, subgroup of those evaluated for finger or toe ischemia. Results of therapy are notoriously poor in these patients and are related to the difficulty in moderating their strong tobacco addiction. Although this disease was originally thought to be limited to those of Jewish descent, additional investigation has revealed a broad incidence across all ethnic groups with a particularly high prevalence in some Asian countries.

Clinical Presentation

Patients present with manifestations of recurrent migratory thrombophlebitis and varying degrees of distal limb ischemia. More than 90 percent of patients are male with a long history of cigarette smoking. It has been suggested by some investigators that tobacco use in Buerger's disease patients may not be excessive, but the disease may reflect a specific hypersensitivity to even small or moderate doses of tobacco. When questioned carefully, patients may describe hand or foot cramping associated with exercise which predates the development of frank ulcerations and other ischemic lesions of the fingers and toes. True claudication of the major muscle mass of the leg occurs only rarely because of the distal distribution of the arterial lesions. Ischemic digits are accompanied by severe pain which often leads to an addictive pattern of analgesic abuse.

Multiple areas of superficial phlebitis may be noted on physical examination. Radial, ulnar, and tibial pulses may be reduced or absent, but popliteal and brachial pulses are generally palpable. Trophic changes of toenails and fingernails may be accompanied by digital clubbing in as many as 50 percent of patients (Figure 4-4). The more proximal areas of the limbs and uninvolved digits are generally normal in character. Because of multiple occlusive lesions in the palmar and plantar arch, cold

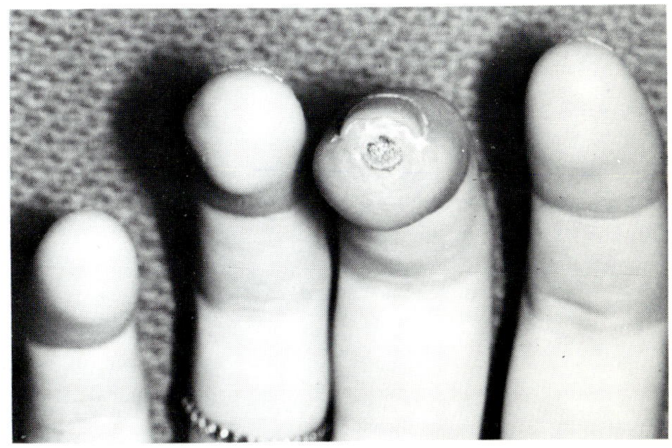

FIGURE 4-4. Distinctive presentation of Buerger's disease with erythema and ulceration of the most distal fingertip. Ulcers are typically unresponsive to local care and severely painful. The general appearance of fingers is "pruned" with a tapered contour caused by wasting of subcutaneous tissue.

sensitivity can be demonstrated in the majority of these patients. (For further discussion of the differential diagnosis of small-artery lesions of the hand, see Chapter 57.)

The noninvasive vascular laboratory may be quite helpful in diagnosis. The Doppler ultrasonic flow detector can be utilized to perform an Allen test to assess patency of the palmar arch. In addition, digital blood flow patterns can be recorded with a pencil probe. The photoplethysmograph allows documentation of digital pressures.

The most confusing differential diagnosis is that of peripheral arterial embolization which may present with "blue toe" or "blue finger" syndromes. Vegetative cardiac lesions and aneurysmal or ulcerative arterial lesions in the axillary, femoral, or popliteal arteries should be investigated. In the absence of ultrasound documentation of intracavitary cardiac thrombi, arteriography may be useful for diagnostic purposes. In Buerger's disease, multiple segmental occlusions are demonstrated in the medium and small arteries of the forearm and hand, leg, and foot. These occlusions and tapered narrowings are not reversible with the intraarterial administration of vasodilators. Many arteriographers have described a corkscrew appearance, which is believed to represent both recanalization of previously occluded arteries and enlargement of periadventitial vessels along thrombosed arterial segments. In some patients, a proximal atherosclerotic lesion may contribute to the distal ischemia.

Pathology

The diagnosis of thromboangiitis obliterans is generally made on a clinical basis supplemented with arteriographic and noninvasive documentation. When arterial specimens have been obtained in active cases, a classic panangiitis is demonstrated. Occasional giant cells, fibroblasts, and lymphocytes are observed within a relatively well preserved arterial wall. Vessels are occluded by chronic thrombus which is highly cellular and composed primarily of fibroblasts. Recanalization of thrombosed arteries and veins is frequently observed. Remarkably, such diseased segments are in direct continuity with normal proximal and distal vessels.

Therapy

Unlike the other forms of arteritis discussed previously in this chapter, steroid therapy has no place in the treatment of thromboangiitis obliterans. The most specific and useful therapy is complete abstinence from tobacco. Unfortunately, results of even the most rigorous behavioral modification programs have been discouraging in this group of patients. Their abuse of cigarettes is a true physiological addiction.

The most crucial surgical therapy is appropriate care of ischemic and gangrenous digits. Cautious applications of tepid soaks and other local therapies are appropriate. Treatment with intravenous antibiotics followed by long-term oral antibiotics is recommended in patients with active ischemic lesions. Although surgical debridement may be associated with poor healing, drainage and removal of infarcted tissue is frequently required. Additional therapies that have been useful include sympathectomy, which is often combined with primary amputation of a single involved digit. The temporary increase in skin blood flow following sympathectomy (lasting 2 to 4 weeks) seems to improve the chances of healing such amputations. Most recent enthusiasm, particularly in Great Britain, has centered on continuous intravenous or intraarterial infusions of prostaglandins including PGE_1 and PGI_2. Although the efficacy of this therapy remains unproven, the rationale is dilation of collateral pathways and an anticoagulation effect in the microcirculation. Other vasodilating agents have *not* been shown to clearly benefit these lesions.

If a proximal atherosclerotic occlusive lesion is demonstrated, bypass or percutaneous angioplasty may be appropriate; unfortunately, such lesions are evident in only a small percentage of patients. Restorative surgery on the microvasculature does not seem to have a role in these patients. Amputation is indicated in instances of secondary infection of gangrenous digits or intractable pain. Even if patients will not permanently restrict their tobacco use, abstinence during the first 7 to 10 days following amputations and other debridement procedures appears to be of some benefit.

BEHÇET'S DISEASE

Behçet's disease is a rare vasculitis with protean manifestations in the systemic arteries and veins as well as the pulmonary circulation. Venous complications include recurrent episodes of deep venous thrombosis which occasionally result in vena cava thrombosis. While arterial symptoms are elicited in only 10 to 20 percent of patients, sudden arterial occlusions and aneurysmal ruptures represent a frequent cause of death in this otherwise benign disease.

Clinical Presentation

First manifestations of Behçet's disease include relapsing iridocyclitis associated with oral and genital ulcerations. Patients may also present with poorly characterized polyarthritis and neurologic deficits compatible with both central lesions and peripheral neuropathies. Involvement of the gastrointestinal tract is unusual but may result in spontaneous ileal and cecal perforations associated with ulcerative enteritis. Abdominal aortic and peripheral aneurysms have been reported, although the frequency of these lesions remains ill-defined.

Diagnosis is based on the history of mucosal ulcerations associated with arterial and venous disease in a young patient. Generally, the disease has a predilection for males, which helps distinguish it from Takayasu's arteritis which has a distinct female predominance.

Physical examination may demonstrate central or peripheral aneurysms and, rarely, absence of peripheral pulses. Ultrasound or computerized tomography (CT) scan can confirm the impression of aneurysmal dilation. Arteriography is occasionally needed to better delineate the pattern of thoracic aortic involvement; however, such studies should generally be reserved for preoperative evaluation (Figure 4-5).

Pathology

The histologic picture is consistent with focal arteriolitis. Lymphocytes and polymorphonuclear leukocytes are widely infiltrated, resulting in fibrinoid necrosis with complete or partial vascular occlusion. This inflammatory process is noted in both the arteries and veins of involved areas.

Aneurysms may appear grossly infected in some patients. While it is impossible to definitively rule out such an infectious etiology, intraoperative cultures are typically negative and graft infections have not been reported following in situ reconstruction. On occasion, however, it may be impossible to differentiate Behçet's disease aneurysms grossly from true infected aneurysms, and extraanatomic reconstruction may be appropriate.

Therapy

Patients frequently are first seen for venous thrombosis. Most authors recommend that patients be maintained indefinitely on both support stockings and anticoagulation with warfarin. The necessity for long-term anticoagulation makes it essential that any complaints of abdominal or back pain be aggressively evaluated because they may herald expansion or rupture of a previously undiagnosed aortic aneurysm.

FIBROMUSCULAR DYSPLASIA

Since the first report of arterial fibrodysplasia in 1938, these lesions have received much attention as a cause of renovascular hypertension. Additional reports have focused on the neurologic manifestations of extracranial dysplastic lesions and the occasional case of mesenteric vascular involvement. Clinically significant fibromuscular dysplasia is most common in women between the ages of 20 and 40 years and can be distinguished from the other lesions discussed previously in this chapter by the absence of any true inflammatory component. The etiology of these lesions remains unknown, although hormonal influences, mechanical stress, and disorders of vascular wall nutrition have been suggested.

Clinical Presentation

The clinical presentation is dependent on the location of the dyplastic lesion. By far the most common site of involvement is the main renal artery and its secondary branches (Figure 4-6). Hemodynamically significant stenoses predictably decrease renal perfusion pressure resulting in hyperrenemia and activation of the angiotensin-aldosterone axis. Dysplastic renal artery lesions must be excluded in any young patient presenting with diastolic hypertension greater than 100 mmHg.

The incidence of renovascular hypertension is bimodal with a first peak at 2 to 4 years of age and a second larger peak at 20 to 40 years. Females predominate 8:1 in the second group, but this sex predilection is less obvious in pediatric patients.

Physical findings other than hypertension are not very specific. Although flank bruits are classically associated with renal artery stenoses, the specificity and sensitivity of this sign are low in most clinical series. Intravenous pyelograms (IVP) may suggest the diagnosis, especially if disparity in renal size, late hyperconcentration of dye, or ureteral notching from collateral vessels

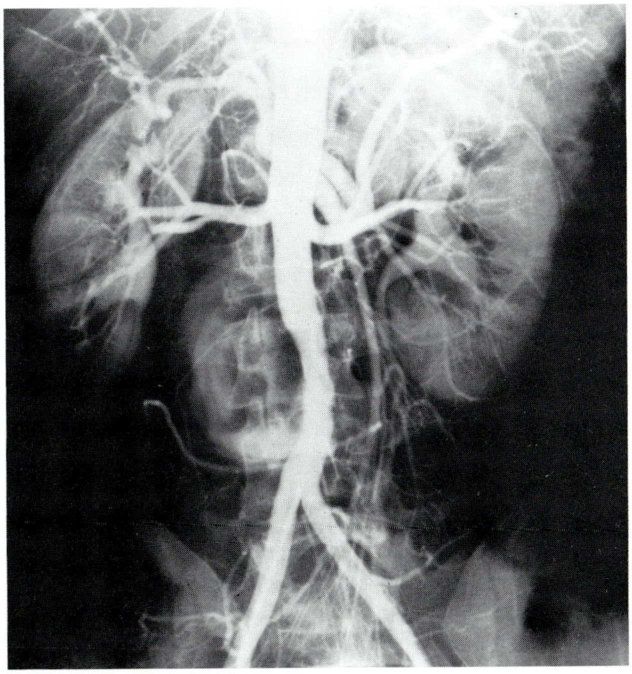

FIGURE 4-5. Preoperative angiogram in a patient with Behçet's disease and abdominal pain demonstrates large infrarenal aneurysm with intraluminal thrombus.

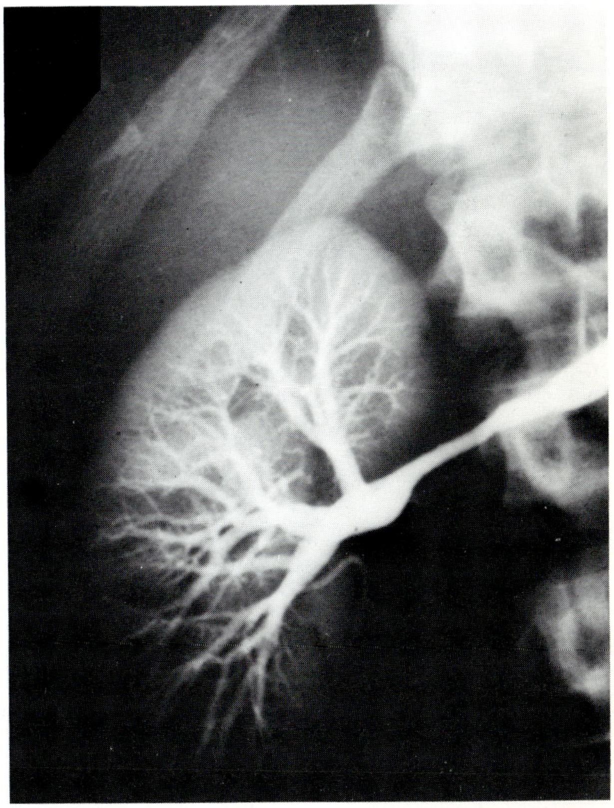

FIGURE 4-6. Tapered fibrodysplastic lesion of right renal artery extends to bifurcation.

is demonstrated. However, the principal function of an IVP is the exclusion of primary renal parenchymal disease.

Specific diagnosis requires arteriography. Intravenous digital angiography can suffice, although it is often more useful to perform direct arterial catheterization by the Seldinger technique, which allows for selective injections and oblique views to obtain better visualization. Fibrodysplastic lesions generally spare the proximal portion of the renal artery but can extend distally to the major branches of the vessel (Figure 4-7).

While renal vein renin ratios and renal systemic renin indices are commonly obtained, the diagnostic reliability of these determinations is compromised by bilateral disease and the multiple medications which are usually required for control of hypertension. Nonetheless, renal systemic renin indices can predict the degree of improvement following successful revascularization. (For further discussion of renovascular disease see Chapter 53.)

Patients with carotid involvement present with intermittent neurologic deficits often corresponding to the middle cerebral artery distribution. Mechanisms for cerebral ischemia include platelet or thrombotic emboli as well as low flow distal to an obstructing lesion. Noninvasive studies such as oculoplethysmography and duplex scanning may detect these lesions; however, arteriography is usually required for full definition of extent of disease. Fibromuscular disease may vary from a localized web at the carotid bifurcation to diffuse involvement of the entire extracranial and intracranial internal carotid artery. These lesions are occasionally associated with subintimal internal carotid artery dissections, distinguished angiographically by irregular arterial walls and "cuffing" as the artery enters the skull. (For further discussion of these carotid lesions see Chapters 49 and 50.)

Pathology

Dysplastic lesions are most conveniently classified into four general types: (1) intimal fibroplasia, (2) medial hyperplasia, (3) medial fibroplasia, and (4) perimedial dysplasia. Of these, medial fibroplasia accounts for more than 85 percent of all lesions (Figure 4-8). Gross examination of excised vessels demonstrates a wide range of morphology from focal stenoses to series of

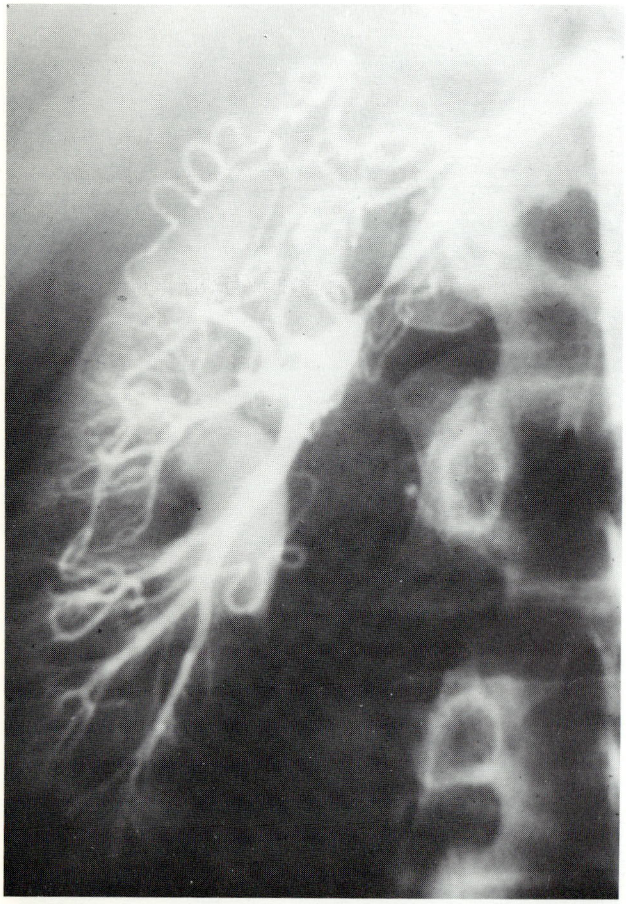

FIGURE 4-7. Severe stenosis of right renal artery associated with extensive network of capsular collaterals from adrenal (*top*) and ureteral (*bottom*) arteries. Presence of these collateral vessels confirms the hemodynamic significance of main renal artery lesion.

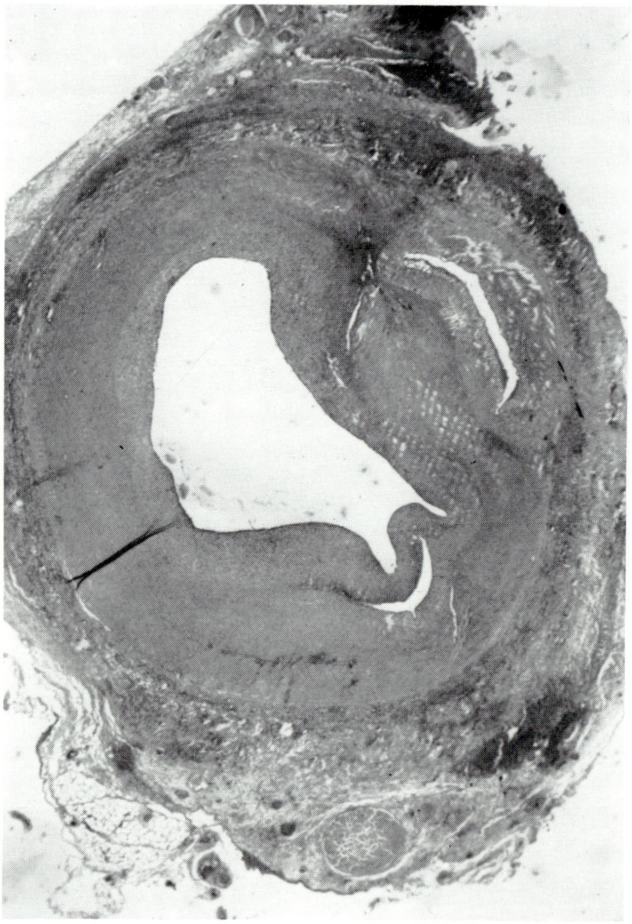

FIGURE 4-8. A spontaneous dissection (*upper right*) compromises the lumen in this renal artery with severe medial fibroplasia. Urgent aortorenal bypass was required.

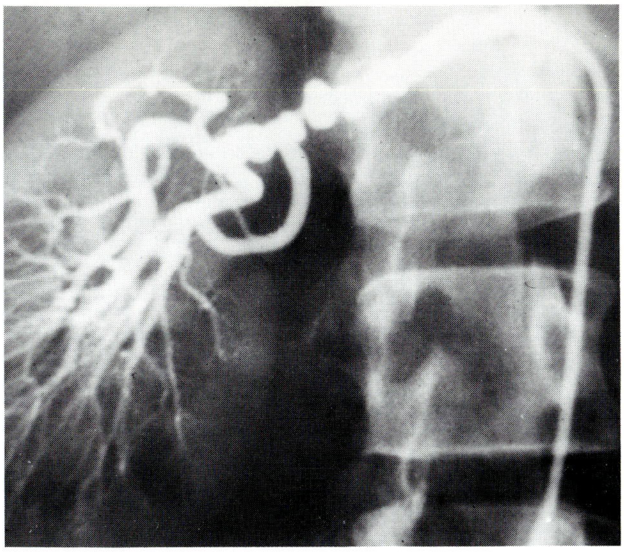

FIGURE 4-9. Classic "chain of lakes" appearance with saccular dilatations and segmental stenoses of this right renal artery.

stenoses with intervening aneurysmal dilatations, the so-called chain of lakes (Figure 4-9).

Histologic examination of medial fibroplasia reveals few intact smooth-muscle cells in the media and a marked increase in collagen and ground substance. Disease may be limited to the outer media or extend throughout the entire media. Although the intima is not primarily involved, in advanced disease the internal elastic lamina may be fractured and some degree of intimal fibrosis can be seen. In the medial and intimal lesions, the adventitia is usually spared completely.

Treatment

Indications for operation in patients with renovascular hypertension include the documentation of an appropriate renal artery lesion in an adult with severe hypertension requiring multiple adrenergic blocking agents for control. Other candidates for surgery in fibrodysplasia include children with severe hypertension and any patient with a documented decrease in renal function.

Renal artery lesions can be treated quite successfully with aortorenal bypass using autologous artery or vein; some surgeons prefer prosthetic graft material, particularly when renal revascularization is combined with aortic reconstruction. In rare instances of distal segmental involvement, ex vivo repair with autotransplantation may be appropriate. Overall, perioperative kidney loss is less than 2 percent and cure or improvement of hypertension can be expected in 90 percent of patients. Percutaneous transluminal angioplasty has demonstrated encouraging early results; however, long-term follow-up is awaited.

Cerebrovascular manifestations of carotid artery disease such as transient ischemic attacks or stroke strongly indicate surgical therapy. Operations have included intraoperative dilation, vein graft bypass, and extracranial-intracranial bypass (EC-IC). Surgery is probably not indicated for carotid artery dissections secondary to fibromuscular dysplasia; the majority of these lesions will resolve with anticoagulant therapy, despite their frightful appearance on angiography. If cerebral ischemia persists, extraanatomic reconstruction with EC-IC may be a more prudent option because distal extension of these lesions into the petrous portion of the carotid artery makes a cervical approach very difficult.

Fibromuscular dysplasia of the mesenteric vessels is quite rare. If acute or chronic intestinal ischemia does result, the operative approach is similar to the treatment of atherosclerotic occlusive lesions. It must be remembered, however, that fibromuscular dysplasia extends more distally along the main mesenteric vessels.

Acknowledgment

The author is indebted to Mrs. Gloria Jones for her preparation of the manuscript.

Bibliography

GENERAL ASPECTS

1. Alarcon-Segovia D: The necrotizing vasculitides. A new pathogenic classification. Med Clin North Am 1977, 61:24–260.
2. Christian CL, Sergent JS: Vasculitis syndromes: Clinical and experimental models. Am J Med 1976, 61:385–392.
3. Fauci AS, Haynes BF, Katz P: The spectrum of vasculitis: Clinical, pathologic, immunologic, and therapeutic considerations. Ann Intern Med 1978, 89(part 1):660–676.

TAKAYASU'S ARTERITIS

1. Alpert HJ: The use of immunosuppressive agents in Takayasu's arteritis. Med Ann DC 1974, 43:69–71.
2. Ask-Upmark E: On the "pulseless disease" outside of Japan. Acta Med Scan 1954, 149:161–178.
3. Bloss RS, Duncan JM, Cooley DA, Leatherman LL, Schnee MJ: Takayasu's arteritis: Surgical considerations. Ann Thorac Surg 1979, 27:574–579.
4. Cipriano P, Silverman J, Perbroth M, Griepp R, Wexler L: Coronary arterial narrowing in Takayasu's arteritis. Am J Cardiol 1977, 39:744–750.
5. Gotsman M, Beck W, Schrine V: Selective angiography in arteritis of the aorta and its major branches. Radiology 1967, 88:232–248.
6. Hachiya J: Current concepts of Takayasu's arteritis. Semin Roentgenol 1970, 5:245–259.
7. Ishikawa KK: Natural history and classification of occlusive thromboaortopathy (Takayasu's disease). Circulation 1978, 57:27–35.

8. Kimoto S: The history and present status of aortic surgery in Japan particularly for aortitis syndrome. J Cardiovasc Surg 1979, 20:107–126.
9. Lande A, Rossi P: The value of total aortography in the diagnosis of Takayasu's arteritis. Radiology 1975, 114:297.
10. Lupi-Herrera E, Sanchey G, Horwitz S, Gutierrey E: Pulmonary artery involvement in Takayasu's arteritis. Chest 1975, 67:69–74.
11. Lupi-Herrera E, Sanchez-Torres G, Marchushamer J, Mispireta J, Horwitz S, Vela JE: Takayasu's arteritis: Clinical study of 107 cases. Am Heart J 1977, 93:94–103.
12. Nakao K, Ikida M, Kimata S: Takayasu's arteritis: Clinical report of eighty-four cases and immunologic studies of seven cases. Circulation 1967, 35:1141–1155.
13. Takayasu M: Case with unusual changes of the vessels in the retina. Acta Soc Ophthalmol 1908, 12:554–563.
14. Young J, Sengupta A, Khaja F: Coronary arterial stenosis, angina pectoris and atypical coarctation of the aorta due to nonspecific arteritis. Am J Cardiol 1973, 32:356–360.

TEMPORAL ARTERITIS

1. Beevers DG, Harpur JE, Turk KAD: Giant cell arteritis: The need for prolonged treatment. J Chronic Dis 1973, 26:571–584.
2. Cochran JW, Fox HJ, Kelly MP: Reversible mental symptoms in temporal arteritis. J Nerv Ment Dis 1978, 6:446–447.
3. Cohen DN, Damaske MM: Temporal arteritis: A spectrum of ophthalmic complications. Ann Ophthalmol 1975, 7:1045–1054.
4. Hamilton CR Jr, Shelley WM, Tumulty PA: Giant cell arteritis and polymyalgia rheumatica. Medicine 1971, 50:1–27.
5. Hunder GG, Allen GL: The relationship between polymyalgia rheumatica and temporal arteritis. Geriatrics 1973, 28:134–142.
6. Hunder GG, Sheps SG, Allen GL, Joyce JW: Daily and alternate day corticosteroid regimens in treatment of giant cell arteritis: Comparison in a prospective study. Ann Intern Med 1975, 82:613–618.
7. Huston KA, Hunder GG, Lie JT, Kennedy RH, Elveback LR: Temporal arteritis: A 25-year epidemiologic, clinical and pathologic study. Ann Intern Med 1978, 88:162–167.
8. Klein RG, Hunder GG, Stanson AW, Sheps SG: Large artery involvement in giant cell (temporal) arteritis. Ann Intern Med 1975, 83:806–812.
9. Mowat AG, Gazleman BL: Polymyalgia rheumatica: A clinical study with particular reference to arterial disease. J Rheumatol 1974, 1:190–202.
10. Ostberg G: Temporal arteritis in a large necropsy series. Ann Rheum Dis 1971, 30:224–235.
11. Pollock M, Blennerhasset JB, Clarke AM: Giant cell arteritis and the subclavian steal syndrome. Neurology 1973, 23:653–657.
12. Seignalet J, Janbon C, Sany J, Janbon J, Bidet JM, Brunel M, Jourdan J, Bussiere JL: HLA in temporal arteritis. Tissue Antigens 1977, 9:69.
13. Stanson AW, Klein RG, Hunder GG: Extracranial angiographic findings in giant cell (temporal) arteritis. AJR 1976, 12:957–963.
14. Wagner HP, Hollenhorst RW: Ocular lesions of temporal arteritis. Am J Ophthalmol 1958, 45:617–630.

BUERGER'S DISEASE

1. Buerger L: *The Circulatory Disturbances of the Extremities, Including Gangrene, Vasomotor and Trophic Disorders*. Philadelphia, Saunders, 1924.
2. McKusick VA, Harris WS, Oltesen OE, Goodman RM, Skelley WM, Bloodwell RD: Buerger's disease: A distinct clinical and pathologic entity. J Am Med Assoc 1962, 181:5.
3. Shionoya S: Pathology of Buerger's disease. Clinico-pathologico-angiographic correlation. Pathol Microbiol 1975, 43:163.
4. Shionoya S, Ban I, Nakata Y, Matsubara J, Hirai M, Miyazaki H, Kawai S: Vascular reconstruction in Buerger's disease. Br J Surg 1976, 63:841.
5. Shionoya S, Ban I, Nakata Y, Matsubara J, Shinjo K, Hirai M, Kawai S, Tsai WH: Diagnosis, pathology, and treatment of Buerger's disease. Surgery 1974, 75:695.

BEHÇET'S DISEASE

1. Behçet H: Uber rezidivierende, aphthose, durch ein Virus verursachte Geschwure am Mund am Auge und an den Genitalien. Dermatol Wochenschr 1937, 105:1152–1157.
2. Chajek T, Fainaru M: Behçet's disease. Report of 41 cases and a review of the literature. Medicine 1975, 54(3):179–196.
3. Enoch BA, Castillo-Olivares JL, Khoo TC, Grainger RG, Henry L: Major vascular complications in Behçet's syndrome. Postgrad Med J 1968, 44:453–459.
4. Haim RS, Reshef R, Peleg E, Riss E: Cardiac involvement and superior vena cava obstruction in Behçet's disease. Thorax 1978, 33:375–377.
5. James DG: Behçet's syndrome: N Engl J Med 1979, 301:431–432.
6. Kansu E, Deglin S, Cantor RI, Burke JF, Cho SY, Cathart RT: The expanding spectrum of Behçet's syndrome. A case with renal involvement. J Am Med Assoc 1977, 237:1855–1856.
7. Ketch LL, Buerk CA, Liechty RD: Surgical implications of Behçet's disease. Arch Surg 1980, 115:759–760.
8. Lebwohl O, Forde KA, Berdon WE, Morrison S, Challop R: Ulcerative esophagitis and colitis in a pediatric patient with Behçet's syndrome. Am J Gastroenterol 1977, 68:550–555.
9. Little AG, Zarins CK: Abdominal aortic aneurysm and Behçet's disease. Surgery 1982, 91(3):359–362.

DYSPLASTIC ARTERIAL LESIONS

1. Ehrenfeld WK, Wylie EJ: Fibromuscular dysplasia of the internal carotid artery: Surgical management. Arch Surg 1974, 109:676–681.
2. Ernst CB, Stanley JC, Marshall FF, Fry WJ: Autogenous saphenous vein aortorenal grafts: A ten-year experience. Arch Surg 1972, 105:855–864.
3. Fry WJ, Ernst CB, Stanley JC, Brink BE: Renovascular hypertension in the pediatric patient. Arch Surg 1973, 107:692–698.
4. Gewertz BL, Stanley JC, Fry WJ: Renal artery dissections. Arch Surg 1977, 112:409–414.
5. Harrison EG, McCormack LJ: Pathologic classification of renal artery disease in renovascular hypertension. Mayo Clinic Proc 1971, 46:161–167.
6. Morris GC Jr, Lechter A, DeBakey ME: Surgical treatment of fibromuscular disease of the carotid arteries. Arch Surg 1968, 96:636–643.
7. Sandok BA, Houser OW, Baker JL, Holley KE: Fibromuscular dysplasia: Neurologic disorders associated with disease involving the great vessels in the neck. Arch Neurol 1971, 24:462–466.
8. Stanley JC, Fry WJ, Seeger JF, Hoffman GL, Gabrielson TO: Extracranial internal carotid and vertebral artery fibrodysplasia. Arch Surg 1974, 109:215–222.
9. Stanley JC, Gewertz BL, Bove EL, Fry WJ: Arterial fibrodysplasia: Histopathologic character and current etiologic concepts. Arch Surg 1975, 110:561–566.
10. Stanley JC, Gewertz BL, Fry WJ: Renal systemic renin indices and renal vein renin ratios as prognostic indicators in remedial renovascular hypertension. J Surg Res 1976, 20:149–155.
11. Wylie EJ, Binkley FM, Palubinskas AJ: Extrarenal fibromuscular hyperplasia. Am J Surg 1966, 112:149–155.

Chapter 5

HEMODYNAMICS OF ABNORMAL BLOOD FLOW

DAVID S. SUMNER

To remain viable and to maintain proper function, all living cells depend on an adequate supply of nutrients and the efficient removal of metabolic products. In all except the most primitive organisms, blood is the vehicle for transporting these substances and the blood vessels are the conduits. Lesions within the human arterial tree produce symptoms and signs only when the integrity of the vessel wall is violated, allowing blood to escape, or when transportation is impaired sufficiently to compromise the viability or function of the tissues. A level of blood flow that suffices under resting conditions may be inadequate under conditions of stress, such as exercise, trauma, or infection. Thus, while the physical dimensions of an obstructing lesion place limitations on the ability of the arteries to transport blood and the strength of the arterial wall determines its resistance to leakage, the needs of the recipient organs ultimately dictate the threshold for the appearance of symptoms.

Like all hydraulic systems, the motion of blood and the behavior of the arterial wall adhere to the laws of physics (1–6). A basic knowledge of the principles of fluid transportation and vessel wall mechanics is, therefore, fundamental to the understanding of arterial disease and to the formulation of a rational approach to treatment.

Basic Hemodynamics

Because blood vessels are not ideal conduits and blood is not a frictionless fluid, the motion of blood from one site to another in the vascular tree involves the dissipation of energy. Consequently, to maintain blood flow, energy must be supplied continuously. Most of this requirement is met by the heart, which transforms chemical energy into mechanical energy. To a lesser degree, some energy is also contributed by the muscles of respiration and locomotion, but for the most part, it is sufficient to focus on the heart as the major source.

Blood leaving the left ventricle is given a potential energy boost in the form of hydraulic pressure and a kinetic energy boost in the form of increased velocity (Figure 5-1). As the blood traverses the intricate network of tubes that make up the circulatory system, potential energy is transformed into kinetic energy and vice versa with each change in velocity and direction. All along the way—but in some regions more than others—energy is converted into heat and is thus "lost." By the time the blood returns to the right atrium, it has given up most of its potential energy but still retains some kinetic energy. Arterial obstruction accelerates the dissipation of energy and interferes with the smooth operation of this system by creating discontinuities in the energy gradient (Figure 5-1).

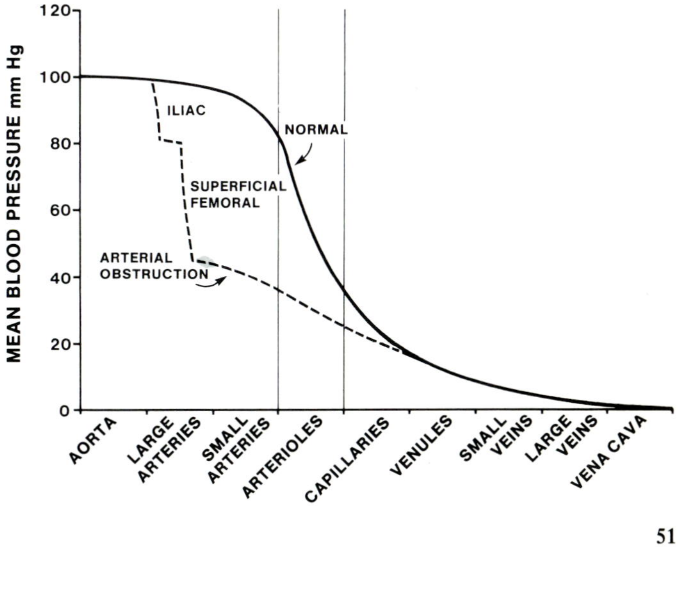

FIGURE 5-1. Potential energy (pressure) gradient from the left ventricle to the right atrium. Normally, the greatest pressure drop is across the arterioles. Note that discontinuities produced by arterial obstructions at the iliac and superficial femoral levels are largely rectified by a reduced gradient across the arterioles.

POTENTIAL ENERGY

In addition to the dynamic pressure P_D produced by the heart, blood is subjected to pressure due to the elastic recoil of the vascular walls and to the effect of gravity (Figure 5-2). Both of these pressures are present even when the circulation is completely static. While they are not ultimately responsible for the motion of blood, they are pertinent to our understanding of vascular physiology.

Although elastic recoil is an important mechanism for storing energy produced during systole for discharge during diastole, the static filling pressure is ordinarily quite small, around 7 mmHg, and can be neglected for most practical purposes. On the other hand, hydrostatic pressure—which represents the weight of a column of blood extending from the right atrium to the point of measurement—may be appreciable. Hydrostatic pressure P_H depends on the density of blood ρ, about 1.056 g/cm^3; the acceleration due to gravity g, 980 cm/s^2; and the distance h from the right atrium:

$$P_H = -\rho g h \qquad (5\text{-}1)$$

At a point 100 cm below the heart, P_H would be 103,488 dyn/cm^2. Since 1.0 mmHg is equal to 1333 dyn/cm^2, the pressure in more familiar terms would be 77.6 mmHg. In general, therefore, hydrostatic pressure in millimeters of mercury can be predicted by multiplying the vertical distance in centimeters from the heart by −0.78. Distances above the heart are given a plus sign, those below, a minus sign.

As shown in Figure 5-3, the total pressure at any point in the arterial tree is the sum of the dynamic and hydrostatic pressures. Below the heart, these pressures are additive, while above the heart, the hydrostatic component acts to reduce the total pressure. In collapsible structures, such as veins or capillaries, intraluminal pressure cannot fall below that of the surrounding tissue (~1 to 5 mmHg); otherwise the lumen would be obliterated and no blood would flow (7).

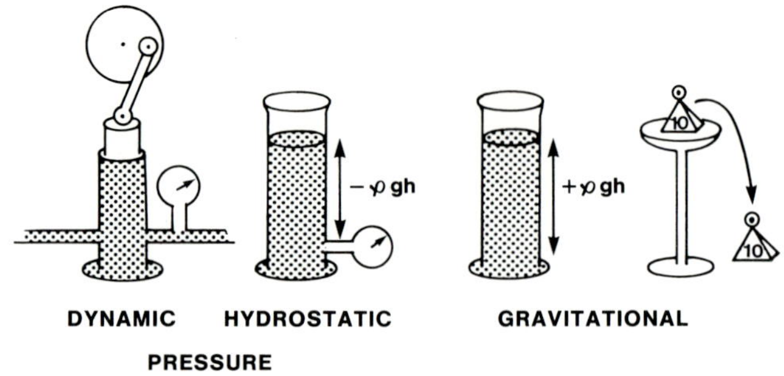

FIGURE 5-2. Forms of potential energy acting on blood. Dynamic pressure is produced by cardiac contraction and is ultimately responsible for the blood circulation. Note that hydrostatic pressure and gravitational potential energy have opposite signs.

In a standing subject, blood flows from a lower pressure in the aortic arch to a higher pressure at the ankle (Figure 5-3). To explain this apparently paradoxical situation requires consideration of gravitational potential energy. Gravitational potential energy is not manifest as pressure but represents the energy that any particle of matter (such as blood) acquires merely because of its distance from the center of the earth (Figure 5-2). A useful artificial convention is to designate the left atrium as the reference point, calling this the point of "zero" gravitational potential energy. Using this convention, the formula for gravitational potential energy E_G is identical with that for hydrostatic pressure but has the opposite sign:

$$E_G = +\rho g h \qquad (5\text{-}2)$$

Therefore, hydrostatic pressure and gravitational potential energy tend to cancel, explaining how blood may move against a pressure gradient but not against an energy gradient.

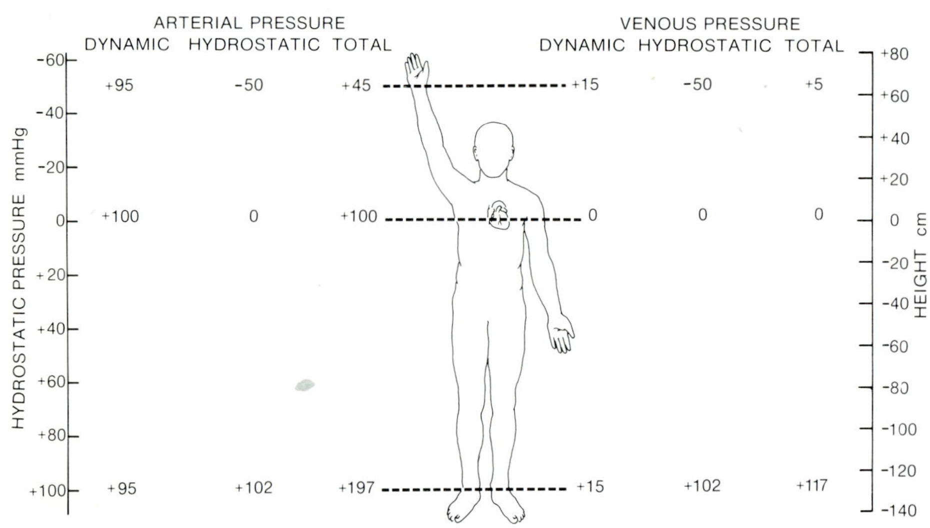

FIGURE 5-3. Effect of hydrostatic pressure on total arterial and venous pressure at various anatomic levels in the standing position. [From Sumner DS: Hemodynamics and pathophysiology of venous disease. In Rutherford RB (ed): *Vascular Surgery*, ed 2. Philadelphia, Saunders, 1984, pp 148–166.]

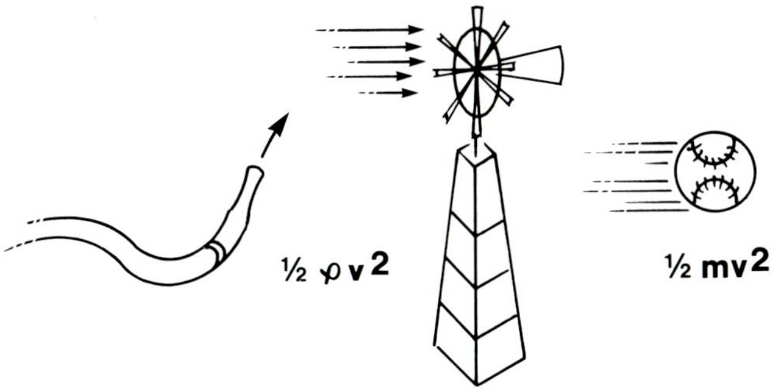

FIGURE 5-4. Blood, like other fluids, gases, or solid bodies in motion, possesses kinetic energy.

KINETIC ENERGY

Like any other matter in motion, blood flowing in the vascular tree possesses kinetic energy (Figure 5-4). In fluid systems, kinetic energy E_K is proportional to the density of the fluid and the square of its velocity v (in centimeters per second):

$$E_K = \tfrac{1}{2}\rho v^2 \tag{5-3}$$

TOTAL FLUID ENERGY

At any point in the vascular system, the total fluid energy E, in ergs per milliliter of blood, is the sum of the potential and kinetic energy:

$$\begin{aligned} E &= P_D + P_H + E_G + E_K \\ &= P_D - \rho gh + \rho gh + \tfrac{1}{2}\rho v^2 \end{aligned} \tag{5-4}$$

Neglecting hydrostatic pressure and gravitational potential energy, most of the energy at the aortic arch is manifested in the form of dynamic pressure, with only a small fraction being kinetic, while in the thoracic venae cavae, most of the energy may be kinetic.

According to Bernoulli's principle, the total energy at one point in a closed system is equal to that at another under ideal conditions of steady flow and no frictional losses. In reality, blood always flows down an energy gradient, since energy is continuously dissipated in the form of heat:

$$\begin{aligned} E_1 &= E_2 + \text{heat} \\ P_1 + \rho g h_1 + \tfrac{1}{2}\rho {v_1}^2 &= P_2 + \rho g h_2 + \tfrac{1}{2}\rho {v_2}^2 + \text{heat} \end{aligned} \tag{5-5}$$

Because the mechanical equivalent of heat is so great, only about 16 cal would be generated per minute in moving 5 L of blood from the left ventricle to the right atrium when the mean pressure differential between these two sites is 100 mmHg. If there were no heat loss to the environment, this would raise the temperature of a 70-kg person only 2.6×10^{-4} °C per minute.

Figure 5-5 illustrates the interchange between one form of energy and another. Fluid flows from a reservoir (1) with a low pressure but high gravitational potential energy to a horizontal tube (2) where the pressure is higher but the gravitational potential energy is lower. In the aneurysmal area (3), velocity is decreased, since flow Q is the product of velocity v and cross-sectional area A:

$$Q = vA \tag{5-6}$$

Conversely, in the stenotic area (4), velocity increases. When velocity decreases, pressure tends to rise as kinetic energy is transformed into potential energy; but when velocity increases, the reverse change occurs—pressure falls as potential energy is converted into kinetic energy. Thus, at several points in the system, fluid may flow against a pressure gradient but never against an energy gradient.

For most practical purposes, total fluid energy can be considered to be roughly equivalent to the dynamic pressure. Neglecting kinetic energy introduces an error that seldom exceeds 2 mmHg and is ordinarily much less; hydrostatic pressure and gravitational potential energy cancel each other out.

ENERGY LOSSES

Viscosity, or the friction between contiguous layers of fluid, accounts for much of the transformation of energy into heat. In an idealized situation (steady, nonpulsatile, laminar flow in a straight cylindrical tube with rigid walls), the energy losses due to viscosity are described by Poiseuille's equation:

$$\Delta P = \bar{v} \cdot \frac{8L\eta}{r^2} = Q \cdot \frac{8L\eta}{\pi r^4} \tag{5-7}$$

where $\bar{v}$ = mean flow velocity, cm^3/s, across a tube with inside radius r, cm
Q = flow, cm^3/s
ΔP = pressure drop, dyn/cm^2, over a length of tube L, cm
η = coefficient of viscosity, P (poise = dyn · s/cm^2)

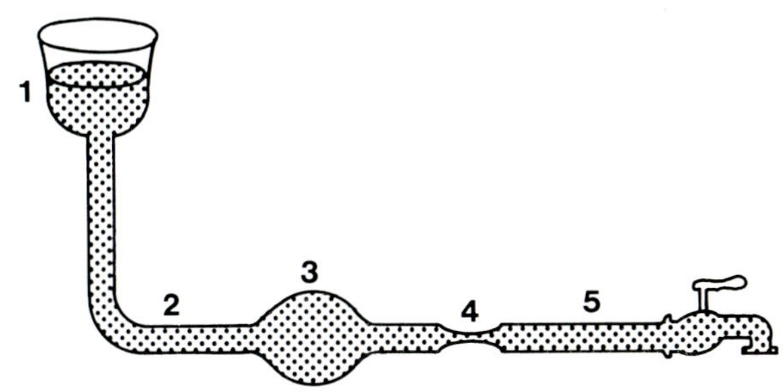

$P_1 < P_2$ $P_2 < P_3$ $P_3 > P_4$ $P_4 < P_5$ $P_2 > P_5$

$K_1 < K_2$ $K_2 > K_3$ $K_3 < K_4$ $K_4 > K_5$ $K_2 = K_5$

$E_1 > E_2 > E_3 > E_4 > E_5$

FIGURE 5-5. Hydraulic model illustrating Bernoulli's principle (Equation 5-5): P, pressure; K, kinetic energy; E, total fluid energy. Although there is a sequential decline in total fluid energy from point 1 to point 5, fluid flows against a pressure gradient in several areas owing to an interchange between pressure and gravitational potential energy or between pressure and kinetic energy.

That ΔP is directly related to flow, length, and viscosity comes as no surprise, but the inverse relationship to the fourth power of the radius is less intuitively evident. As shown in Figure 5-6, diminishing radius has little effect on ΔP until a critical point is reached; thereafter, even small reductions in radius cause a major increase in ΔP. With increasing flow, the point of inflexion occurs at a greater radius, and at any given radius, ΔP is proportional to flow. Large vessels, such as the iliac arteries with diameters of 7 mm, can sustain massive flows of 3000 cm^3/min (50 cm^3/s) over a 10-cm segment with only a 2-mmHg ΔP due to viscous losses. In contrast, the ΔP across a similar length of a 2-mm vessel, such as the posterior tibial artery, would exceed 3 mmHg at a flow of only 30 cm^3/min (0.5 cm^3/s). Diameters of normal vessels are, therefore, consistent with the loads they are expected to carry.

Viscous losses, however, may be overshadowed by those due to inertia. Velocity is a vector quantity; consequently, inertial losses occur any time the speed or direction of blood flow is altered. Because of the pulsatile nature of blood flow, velocity is continuously changing throughout the cardiac cycle and across the vascular lumen (Figure 5-7). Direction changes occur at all branches or bifurcations, in areas of curvature, at the entrance and exit of stenoses or aneurysms, and even during systole and diastole as the vessel wall expands and contracts (Figure 5-8). Turbulence, which creates a multitude of velocity vectors, is a major source of energy loss.

Inertial losses are proportional to the density of blood ρ and to the square of the change in velocity Δv:

$$\Delta P = k\tfrac{1}{2}\rho(\Delta v)^2 \qquad (5\text{-}8)$$

The constant k varies depending upon the nature and rapidity of the velocity change. For example, at the exit from a stenosis, k approaches 1.0 when the orifice is abrupt but is less than 0.2 when the orifice expands gradually at a 6° angle (8). It should be emphasized that Δv may imply a change in "direction" of a blood particle without necessarily a change in its "speed."

As a result of inertial losses, the relationship of pressure gradients and flow in the arterial system never adheres to Poiseuille's law. For a given flow, pressure gradients are always larger than those predicted; likewise, for a given pressure gradient, flows are always less (Figure 5-9). Instead of a linear relationship between pressure gradient and flow, the curve is concave toward the pressure axis and is best described by equations in which flow appears as a squared term. This, of course, would be anticipated from Equation 5-8, since velocity and flow are interdependent. A curve depicting the inertial energy losses for the artery shown in Figure 5-9 could be obtained by subtracting the line representing Poiseuille's equation from the experimentally determined values. The resulting equation ($P = 40Q + 11Q^2$) emphasizes the relationship between inertial losses and flow.

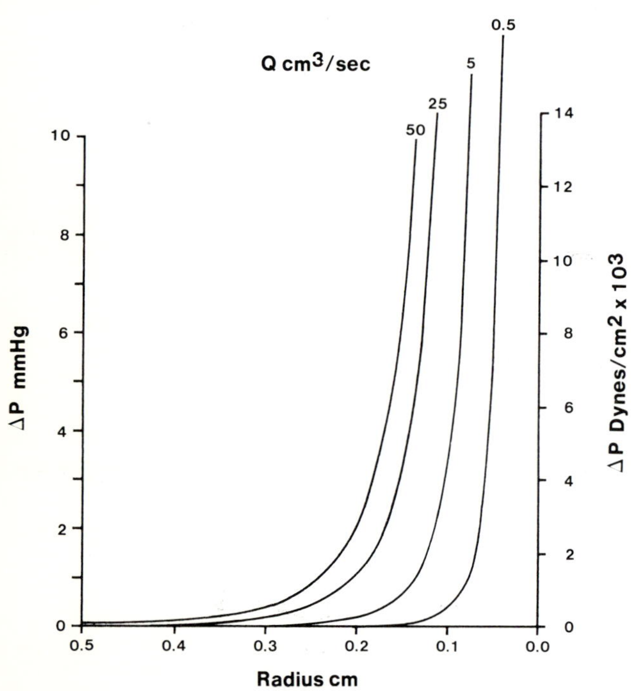

FIGURE 5-6. Curves depicting viscous energy losses ΔP across a 1.0-cm-long tube at various radii and flow rates (Equation 5-7). Viscosity is assumed to be 0.035 P.

Arterial Stenoses

Energy losses caused by stenoses in the arterial system are due to both viscous and inertial factors (9,10). Viscous losses depend on the length of the stenosis and the fourth power of its diameter. According to Poiseuille's law, a reduction in luminal diameter of 50 percent would increase the pressure gradient by a factor of 16, and a reduction of 75 percent would increase ΔP by a factor of 256—provided flow remained constant (Equation 5-7). The diameter of the stenosis, therefore, is far more important than its length (9,11,12).

Energy losses due to inertia occur at the entrance to a stenosis and also at its exit (3,10,11,13,14). Less flow disturbance occurs at the entrance than at the exit, where much of the excess kinetic energy resulting from the increased fluid velocity within the stenosis is dissipated in a turbulent jet. Just beyond the stenosis, areas of flow separation develop near the arterial wall. In these areas, flow may actually reverse.

That inertial losses ordinarily exceed those due to viscous factors is illustrated in Figure 5-10. Viscous factors predominate only at low flow rates or in relatively long stenoses. Because flow disturbances are concentrated at the ends of a stenosis, doubling the length of a stenosis—which affects only the viscous factors—will not double the energy loss.

Based on Poiseuille's law (Equation 5-7) and Equation 5-8, one would predict that narrowing of the arterial lumen would have little effect on the pressure gradient across or the flow through a stenosis until the cross-sectional area is reduced by about 75 percent. These predictions have been substantiated by numerous experimental studies (15,16). As shown in Figure 5-11, in an isolated system with a fixed peripheral resistance and no collateral input, changes in ΔP and flow are mirror images of each other. Flow decreases are commensurate with increases in the pressure gradient. When the peripheral resistance is low and initial flow rates are high, the curves are shifted to the left; in other words, changes in pressure and flow are perceived at a lesser degree of narrowing when initial flow rates are high (15,16). In part, this explains why a lesion that does not appear particularly severe on arteriography may cause no symptoms at rest but causes significant disability during exercise (17).

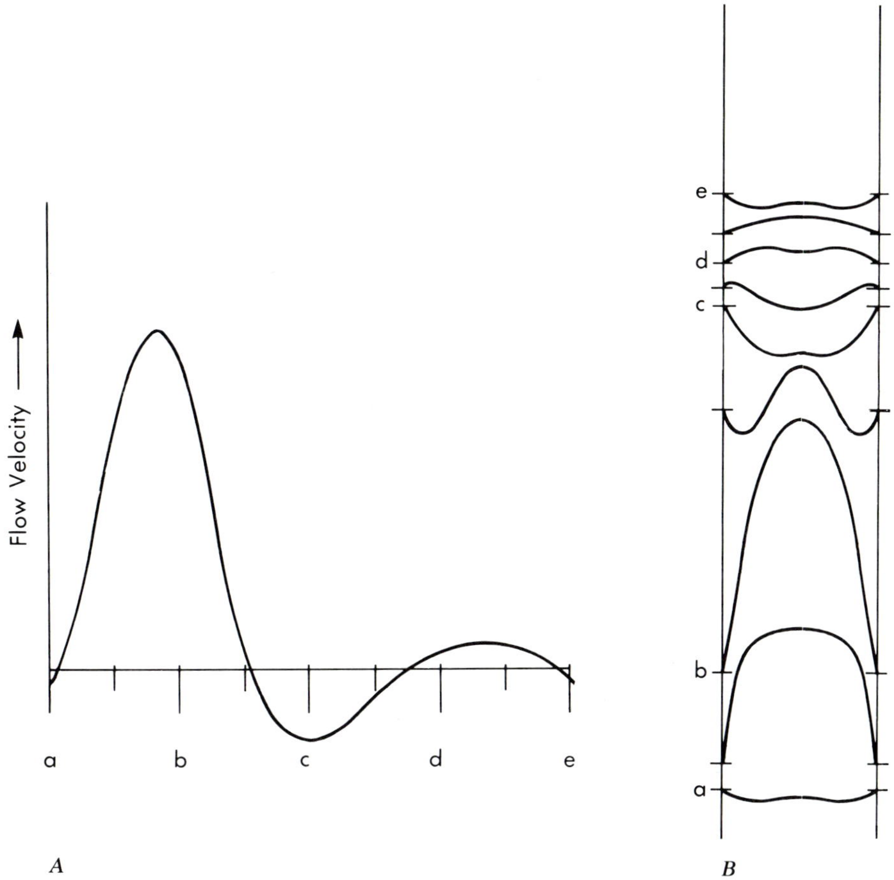

FIGURE 5-7. (*A*) Femoral arterial flow pulse. (*B*) Velocity profiles across the vascular lumen at various phases of the pulse cycle (indicated by lowercase letters). At the wall, velocities are zero. During peak systole *b*, the profile is nearly parabolic; at other times it is quite blunt. When the overall direction of flow is changing rapidly, forward and reverse flow may occur simultaneously. [From Sumner DS: Hemodynamics and pathophysiology of arterial disease. In Rutherford RB (ed): *Vascular Surgery*, ed 2. Philadelphia, Saunders, 1984, pp 19–44.

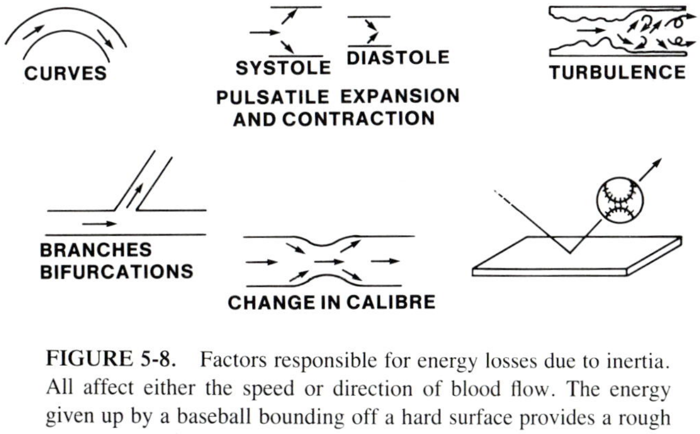

FIGURE 5-8. Factors responsible for energy losses due to inertia. All affect either the speed or direction of blood flow. The energy given up by a baseball bounding off a hard surface provides a rough analogy.

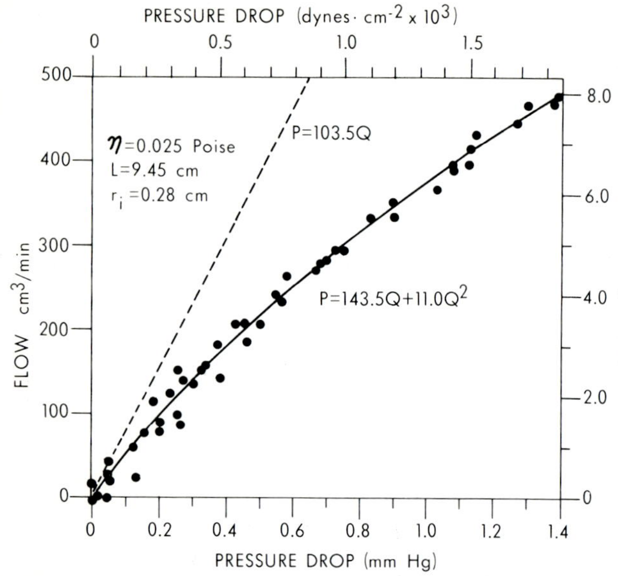

FIGURE 5-9. Flow versus pressure drop across a 9.45-cm length of canine femoral artery. The dashed line represents the pressure-flow curve predicted from Poiseuille's law (Equation 5-7). Note that the formula for the curve that best approximates the experimental data has both a linear and a squared term. [From Sumner DS: Hemodynamics and pathophysiology of arterial disease. In Rutherford RB (ed): *Vascular Surgery*, ed 2. Philadelphia, Saunders, 1984, pp 19–44.]

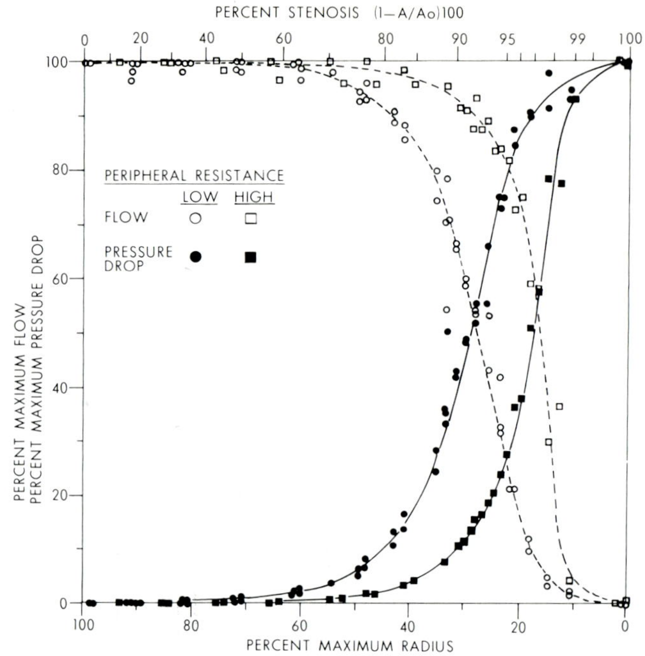

FIGURE 5-11. Effect of increasing stenosis on pressure and flow in isolated segment of canine femoral artery. Peripheral resistance was modified by means of an arteriovenous communication. [From Sumner DS: Hemodynamics and pathophysiology of arterial disease. In Rutherford RB (ed): *Vascular Surgery*, ed 2. Philadelphia, Saunders, 1984, pp 19–44.]

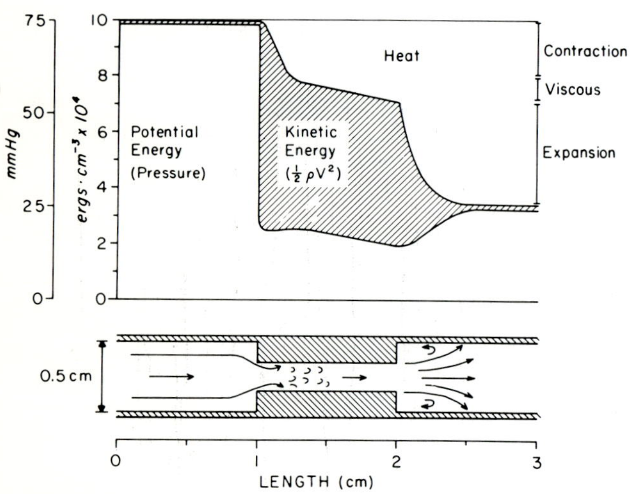

FIGURE 5-10. Calculated energy losses experienced by nonpulsatile blood flow through a 60 percent stenosis. Flow velocity before and after the stenosis is 50 cm/s. Inertial losses are based on Equation 5-8. At the entrance, k is 0.5, and at the exit, 1.0. [From Sumner DS: Hemodynamics and pathophysiology of arterial disease. In Rutherford RB (ed): *Vascular Surgery*, ed 2. Philadelphia, Saunders, 1984, pp 19–44.]

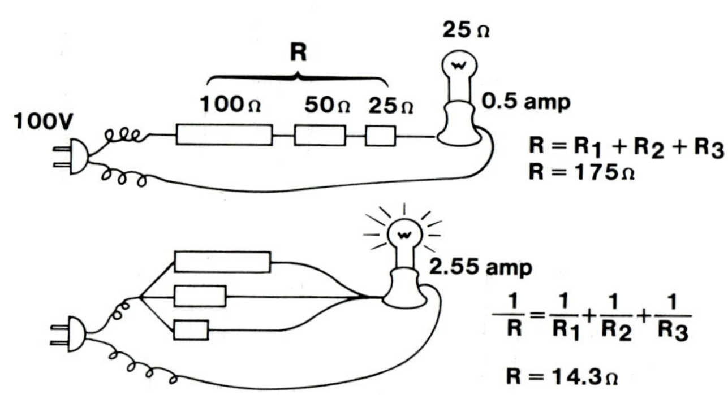

FIGURE 5-12. Electrical analogue showing effect on total resistance R of isolated resistances R_1, R_2, and R_3 arranged in series and in parallel.

When the lesion responsible for a stenosis is axisymmetric, a 75 percent area reduction corresponds to a 50 percent diameter reduction. Stenoses of this magnitude seen on arteriography are frequently labeled "critical" or "hemodynamically significant." While this is a clinically useful concept, permitting the surgeon to predict physiological changes from the arteriographic picture, it must be used cautiously. Because many lesions are not axisymmetric, the arteriographic picture may overestimate or underestimate the degree of stenosis. Moreover, as pointed out above, a lesion may or may not be critical, depending upon the rate of flow.

HEMODYNAMIC RESISTANCE

Hemodynamic resistance (R) is defined as the ratio of the energy gradient between two points along the vessel to the mean blood flow through the vessel:

$$R = \frac{E_1 - E_2}{Q} \sim \frac{P_1 - P_2}{Q} \tag{5-9}$$

For most purposes, R can be roughly approximated by the ratio of ΔP to Q. It must be recognized that the resistance of any vascular segment is not fixed and is not determined exclusively by the diameter of the segment. Because of inertial factors, resistance increases as flow increases. The minimum possible resistance is given by Poiseuille's law*:

$$R_{\min} = \frac{8L\eta}{\pi r^4} \tag{5-10}$$

Analogous to electrical circuitry, resistances in series are roughly additive (Figure 5-12) (18,19). Arranged in parallel, the reciprocal of the total resistance is equal to the sum of the reciprocals of the resistance of each component part (Figure 5-12). The total resistance of vessels in parallel must, therefore, be less than that of the vessel with the least resistance.

*Since blood is a non-Newtonian fluid, its viscosity (η) decreases as its shear rate increases. (Shear rates are directly proportional to velocity and inversely proportional to the vessel diameter). At very low velocities, when blood is practically stagnant, viscosity may be several times higher than that at normal flow velocities; but throughout the wide range of velocities normally present in human arteries, viscosity is nearly constant (3). Therefore, the minimal resistance calculated from Equation 5-10 varies little with changes in flow rate.

Circulatory Effects of Arterial Obstructive Lesions

Stenotic or obstructed arteries are part of a complex hemodynamic circuit which includes the involved artery, a parallel system of collateral arteries, and the peripheral runoff bed (Figure 5-13) (3,20). The parallel resistances of the collaterals R_c and the involved artery R_s constitute a "segmental" resistance R_{seg}, which is in series with the resistance of the runoff bed R_p. Therefore, the total blood flow Q_T to the peripheral tissues is determined by the central arterial pressure P_a, the venous pressure P_v, and the sum of the segmental and runoff resistances:

$$Q_T = \frac{P_a - P_v}{R_{seg} + R_p} \sim \frac{P_a}{R_{seg} + R_p} \tag{5-11}$$

(Because the venous pressure is ordinarily quite low, it can be neglected for the purpose of the following discussion.) To maintain adequate tissue perfusion in the face of a developing stenosis, the body has three options: reduce the segmental resistance, reduce the runoff resistance, or reduce both. The success in accomplishing this task and the mechanisms involved depend not only on the extent and severity of the lesion, but also on its location and the rapidity with which it develops.

Collateral arteries are preexisting pathways consisting of intercommunications between terminal branches of distributing arteries that originate both above and below the obstructing lesion (21). Their recruitment and subsequent enlargement are stimulated by an increased pressure gradient across the involved segment and an increased demand to carry blood flow (22–24). In some areas of the body, the collaterals are sufficiently developed to sustain tissue viability even in the event of an acute obstruction, provided the obstruction does not block the inflow or reentry vessels. In most cases, however, preexisting collaterals are inadequate to prevent ischemia. As a rule, collateral development occurs over a prolonged period; even when they have attained their maximum dimensions, their resistance almost always exceeds that of the major artery whose function they are called upon to supplement or replace. For example, 256 collaterals each with a diameter of 2.5 mm or 10,000 collaterals with a diameter of 1.0 mm would be required to reduce the segmental resistance to that of a major vessel with a diameter of 10 mm (Equation 5-10 and Figure 5-12).

Although the resistance of the collateral bed is relatively fixed, that of the runoff bed is quite variable and acutely responsive to

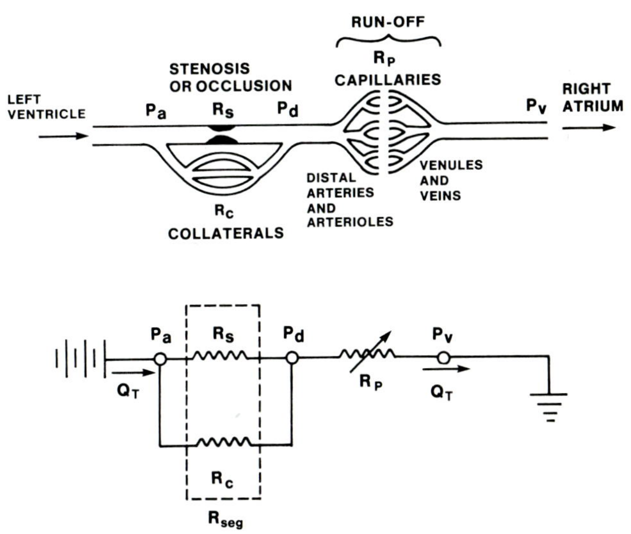

FIGURE 5-13. Diagram illustrating components of a hemodynamic circuit containing an arterial occlusion or stenosis. The lower diagram is an electrical analogue, in which the battery represents the left ventricle and ground potential represents the right atrium.

various exigencies (20,25,26). Most of the resistance is concentrated in the terminal arterioles and precapillary sphincters, which, because of their small diameter and muscular walls, are ideally suited for regulatory functions (Figure 5-1). Their tone is controlled by the sympathetic nervous system, circulating catecholamines, local products of metabolism, and myogenic influences. These vessels have the remarkable ability to autoregulate, dilating in response to a fall in blood pressure and constricting in response to a rise (27,28). By this mechanism, blood flow is maintained within tolerable limits despite wide variations in perfusion pressure. In skeletal muscles, autoregulation ceases when perfusion pressure drops below about 20 to 30 mmHg (28,29). Beyond this point, flow becomes pressure-dependent. When flow drops to the point that ischemia results, metabolic products accumulate. These substances are powerful vasodilators, their influence overcoming the vasoconstrictive effects of sympathetic nerve impulses (30,31).

As the segmental resistance rises, the resistance of the runoff bed falls. At first, the fall in resistance is due to autoregulation; but once blood flow to the periphery is compromised, the products of ischemia play a role. Peripheral vasodilatation, therefore, is immediately available to compensate for an acute elevation of the segmental resistance. With persistence of the obstruction, the collateral arteries dilate, allowing the peripheral resistance to rise. However, peripheral resistance never returns to normal levels as long as arterial obstruction persists.

PRESSURE-FLOW RELATIONSHIPS AT REST

The pressure distal to an arterial obstruction P_d depends on the central arterial pressure P_a and the product of the segmental resistance and the total blood flow (Figure 5-13):

$$P_d = P_a - Q_T R_{seg} \qquad (5\text{-}12)$$

In subjects without arterial disease, R_{seg} is so low that the mean P_d is only a few millimeters of mercury below P_a. Because pulse waves are reflected from the periphery, the systolic pressure distal to the segment may actually be higher than the central systolic pressure; the diastolic pressure, however, will be less (3,32). [This accounts for the observation that systolic blood pressure at the ankle normally exceeds that in the arm (33).]

Segmental resistance becomes appreciable only when the stenosis in the major artery becomes "critical"; and, even then, well-developed collaterals may provide adequate compensation. As the segmental resistance rises, arterioles in the runoff bed dilate, thereby maintaining total blood flow Q_T constant. Because R_{seg} is elevated, the product $Q_T R_{seg}$ increases, and the distal pressure P_d falls (Figure 5-14). Thus, a fall in distal pressure is the earliest objective evidence of arterial obstruction. This explains why blood flow in a limb with well-advanced arterial obstruction is usually normal but the peripheral pressure is reduced (3,33–36).

With increasing disease, poor collateral development, lesions that block collateral inflow or outflow, or multilevel involvement, R_{seg} becomes quite high and the peripheral pressure P_d drops below the limits where autoregulation is possible. Total limb resistance rises; total blood flow Q_T falls, and the peripheral tissues become ischemic at rest (Equation 5-11) (37). Despite the fact that Q_T is decreased, the product $Q_T R_{seg}$ continues to

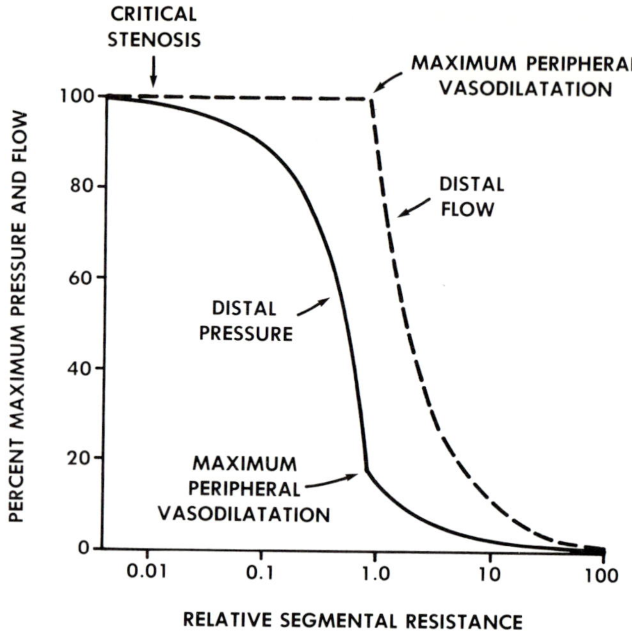

FIGURE 5-14. Relationship between increasing segmental resistance, distal pressure, and distal blood flow. Although flow is maintained at normal levels until maximal peripheral vasodilatation is reached, pressure begins to drop immediately. [From Sumner DS: Correlation of lesion configuration with functional significance. In Bond MC, Insull W Jr., Glagov S, Chandler AB, Cornhill JF (eds): *Clinical Diagnosis of Atherosclerosis: Quantitative Methods of Evaluation*. New York, Springer-Verlag, 1983.]

rise, and the peripheral pressure P_d continues to fall, albeit at a slower rate (Equation 5-12 and Figure 5-14). Noninvasive studies suggest that ischemic signs and symptoms—such as rest pain, ulcers, gangrene, and poor healing—usually become manifest only when the pressure drops below 30 mmHg (38–41).

It is important to recognize that a level of blood flow adequate to maintain tissue viability under normal conditions may not be sufficient to supply the additional nutrients and other blood-borne factors required to heal traumatic wounds or ulcers, especially in the presence of diabetes and infection. Therefore, it is impossible to state precisely what the critical level of tissue perfusion might be in a particular situation.

In most patients with ischemic feet, elevating the legs increases rest pain and impedes healing, while placing the feet in a dependent position often provides relief from pain and may encourage healing. These effects are the result of changes in hydrostatic pressure. Consider a patient who, when lying supine, has an arterial pressure of 25 mmHg and a venous pressure of 10 mmHg in the toes. In this position, the pressure gradient determining blood flow across the arterioles, capillaries, and venules is 15 mmHg. A 20-cm elevation of the feet would decrease the hydrostatic pressure 16 mmHg (Equation 5-1), causing the arterial pressure to fall to 9 mmHg. Since the venous pressure cannot fall below tissue pressure (~1 to 5 mmHg), the gradient across the capillary bed decreases from 15 mmHg to 4 to 8 mmHg; nutritive flow suffers by a like amount; and the patient develops paresthesias or pain in the elevated foot (42). On the other hand, if the patient were to sit up, allowing the feet to rest on the floor, the vertical distance from the heart to the toes would increase by perhaps 80 cm, and the hydrostatic pressure would rise by 62 mmHg. Although both the arterial and the venous pressures increase by the same amount and perfusion pressure across the capillaries remains unchanged (87 mmHg − 72 mmHg = 15 mmHg), the capillary bed dilates in response to the increased intraluminal pressure. This reduces the resistance of the capillaries and venules, thereby augmenting tissue perfusion despite the fact that the transcapillary pressure gradient has not changed (43,44). If the patient contracts the calf muscles and if the venous valves are intact, the venous pressure in the foot will fall from 72 mmHg to some lower value (often to 5 to 10 mmHg). Since arterial pressure is unaffected by calf motion, the pressure gradient across the capillaries will be augmented proportionate to the drop in venous pressure, and tissue perfusion will be similarly enhanced. This explains the somewhat paradoxical observation that ischemic rest pain may be relieved by walking a few steps.

Last, in considering the mechanism if ischemic rest pain, one must not forget that the central pressure P_a also plays a role in determining tissue perfusion (Equation 5-11). Rest pain occurs primarily at night, when the cardiac output falls and arterial pressure decreases. The stimulation of sitting up or moving about usually raises the mean blood prssure, thus augmenting tissue perfusion.

PRESSURE-FLOW RELATIONSHIPS DURING EXERCISE

During exercise, the terminal arterioles supplying the involved muscles dilate, reducing the peripheral resistance R_p. In normal limbs which have a high resting peripheral resistance, exercise produces a marked decrease in total limb resistance and a similarly marked augmentation of limb blood flow (Equation 5-11). Blood flow to the muscles increases commensurate with the vigor of the exercise, often by a factor of five or more (3,36,45,46). Despite the marked increase in blood flow, the product $Q_T R_{seg}$ remains low, and there is little drop in peripheral pressure P_d (Equation 5-12). These relationships are illustrated in Figure 5-15.

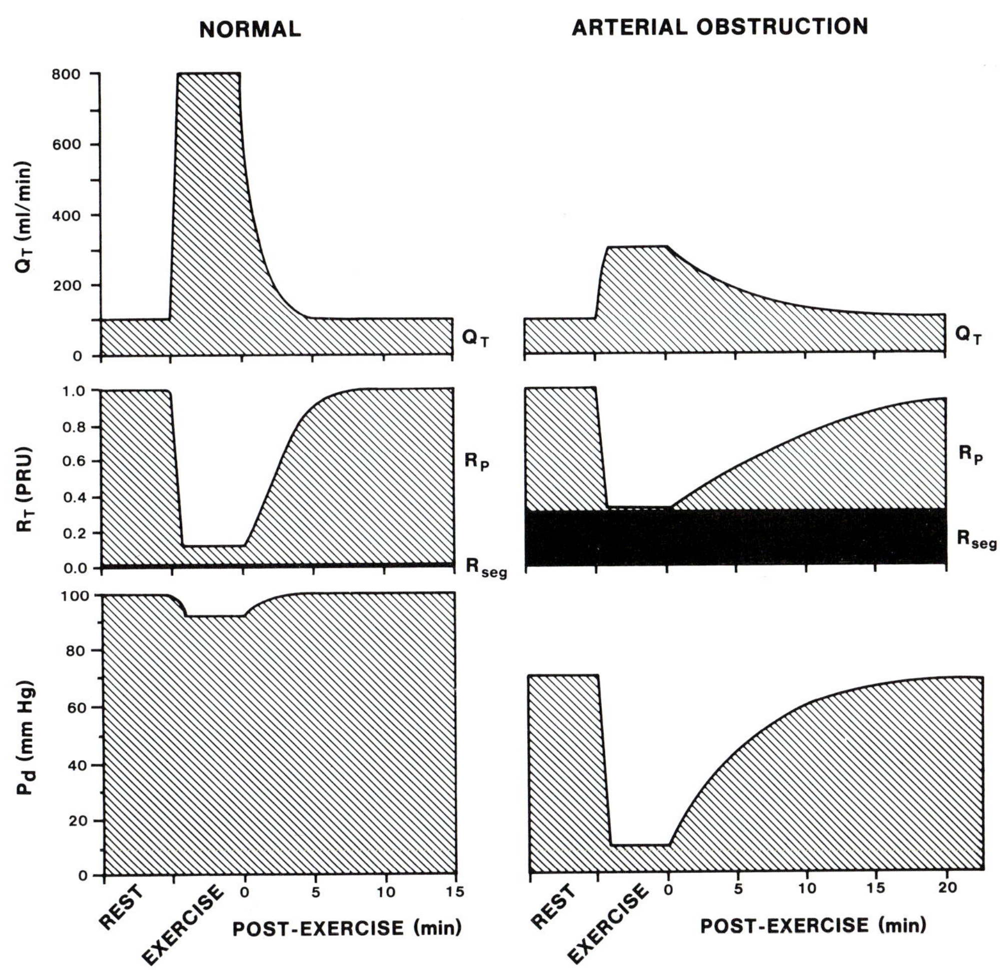

FIGURE 5-15. Relationship between total resistance R_T, segmental resistance R_{seg}, peripheral resistance R_p, blood flow Q_T, and distal blood pressure P_d in normal limbs and limbs with single-level arterial obstruction. Central arterial pressure P_a is 100 mmHg. PRU = mmHg/mL/per minute. (Theoretical curves based on Figure 5-13 and experimental observations.)

In limbs with arterial obstruction, the terminal arterioles—already partially dilated to compensate for the increased segmental resistance—dilate further in response to exercise; but, because of the elevated segmental resistance, the total limb resistance remains relatively high (Figure 5-15). Although exercise induces an increase in blood flow to the muscles, the increase may be inadequate to meet metabolic demands (3,36,44–47). Consequently, the by-products of metabolism accumulate, provoking the symptoms of intermittent claudication. Because blood flow through the elevated segmental resistance increases, peripheral pressure falls (Equation 5-12). This drop in peripheral pressure, usually measured at the ankle level, is one of the most sensitive methods for detecting obstruction of the arteries supplying blood to the legs (33,36,48–50). Even when the resting ankle pressure is imperceptibly reduced, exercise may induce an unequivocal pressure drop, thus establishing the diagnosis (51).

The effects of exercise for a given degree of arterial stenosis are often more severe when the obstruction is located in the proximal arterial segments. A stenosis of the terminal aorta or common iliac artery may impair walking tolerance to a greater degree than a similar stenosis of the superficial femoral artery. Since the iliac artery supplies a much larger muscle mass than that supplied by the superficial femoral artery, the metabolic demands for increased blood flow are correspondingly greater.

The central blood pressure P_a frequently rises during exercise, especially in patients with peripheral vascular disease. This seldom provides much relief from claudication but may disguise small drops in peripheral pressure (Equation 5-12). Consequently, to detect subtle falls in ankle pressure during exercise, one must measure the brachial and ankle pressure simultaneously.

When obstructions involve more than one arterial segment, the hemodynamic situation becomes far more complex (Figure 5-16) (52,53). An arterial segment is composed of a major artery and its collaterals that supply a more or less well-defined peripheral vascular bed. The major artery of a given segment may also constitute the primary inflow source for another more distally located segment. For example, the iliac segment consists of the common and external iliac arteries, which function as major arteries, and the internal iliac system, which make up the collateral channels. These vessels supply not only the buttock and thigh muscles but also provide inflow to the superficial femoral artery, which in turn—with its collaterals—supplies the calf muscle via the popliteal artery. Thus, the leg may be divided into iliac, femoral, calf, and pedal segments.

Walking exercises buttock, thigh, and calf muscles and thus simultaneously involves the iliac, femoral, and calf segments. In a limb with both iliac and superficial femoral disease, exercise provokes increased pressure drops across both segments (Figure 5-17). Because blood flow to the thigh and buttocks increases due to arteriolar vasodilatation, the femoral arterial pressure drops; and the superficial femoral artery and its collaterals will be perfused—not by the central arterial pressure—but by a reduced pressure. Although dilation of the arterioles in the calf muscle decreases the peripheral resistance, the reduction in pressure at the upper end of the femoral segment will further restrict the increase in calf blood flow. Therefore, claudication occurs with less exercise when there is multiple segment disease than when disease is limited to a single segment. In severe cases, the foot and toes, which are at the end of the line, may have virtually no blood flow (33,46,49,54). Thus, in limbs with multilevel obstruction, the proximal segments "steal" blood from those more distally located. This explains why multilevel disease is far more physiologically devastating than disease confined to a

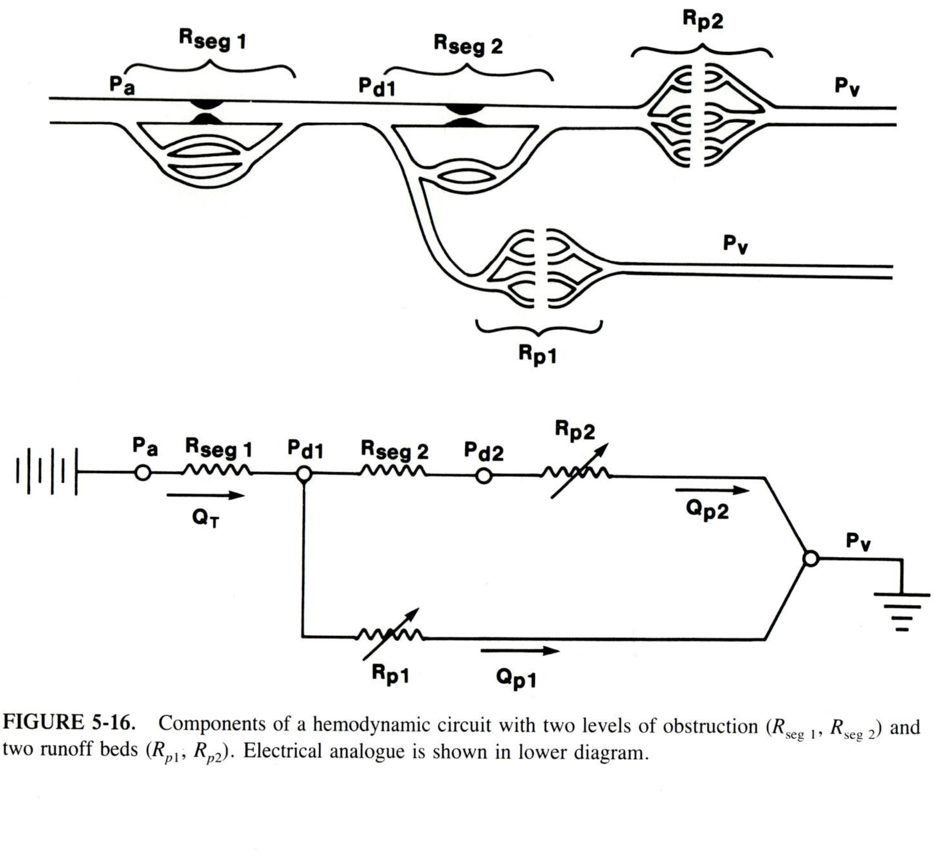

FIGURE 5-16. Components of a hemodynamic circuit with two levels of obstruction ($R_{seg\ 1}$, $R_{seg\ 2}$) and two runoff beds (R_{p1}, R_{p2}). Electrical analogue is shown in lower diagram.

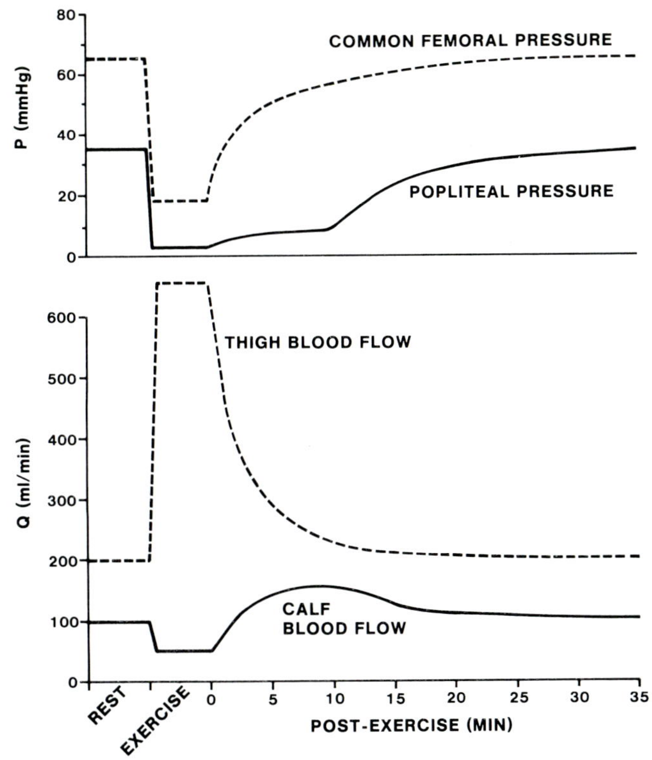

FIGURE 5-17. Relationships between pressure in the common femoral and popliteal arteries and flow in the thigh and calf in a limb with severe occlusive disease of the iliac and superficial femoral segments. Central arterial pressure is 100 mmHg. Note that calf blood flow may drop during exercise and that popliteal pressure remains low for 10 minutes; ankle pressure would be undetectable during this time. (Theoretical curves based on Figure 5-16 and experimental observations.)

single segment. Even with a single obstruction at the iliac level, the proximal muscle compartments may steal blood from the calf, since the superficial femoral artery—though widely patent—is perfused by a reduced common femoral pressure.

Return of blood to the heart is facilitated during walking by the venous pump mechanism. As mentioned earlier, in normal limbs with functioning venous valves, contraction of the calf muscles forces blood cephalad, reduces the effective length of the hydrostatic column, and decreases venous pressure. Since the hydrostatic component of arterial pressure is not affected, the pressure gradient across the capillaries of the exercising muscles is increased and blood flow is augmented. Therefore, one might expect that claudication would occur earlier in limbs with arterial obstruction when chronic venous insufficiency is also present.

PRESSURE-FLOW RELATIONSHIPS AFTER EXERCISE

Following exercise, the greatly increased blood flow in normal limbs rapidly replenishes any nutritional deficiencies that might have developed during muscular contraction and rapidly removes any accumulated products of metabolism. As a result, the dilated arterioles constrict to their resting diameter and blood flow falls to preexercise levels within a few minutes (see Figure 5-15) (3,20,34). Limbs with arterial obstruction, on the other hand, develop a much larger "flow debt" during exercise, the extent of which is roughly proportional to the severity of the obstruction and the duration and magnitude of the muscular work. A prolonged period, therefore, is required to restore the metabolic state to that existing prior to exercise. As a result, postexercise blood flow remains elevated and peripheral pressure remains decreased until the arterioles once again return to their preexercise state (see Figure 5-15) (20,33,34,48–50,52).

In limbs with multilevel disease, repayment of the flow debt of the distal muscular compartments may be delayed until that of the more proximal compartment is satisfied (49,52). For example, in a limb with combined iliac and superficial femoral arterial obstruction, hyperemia of the thigh and buttock muscles must decrease before the femoral pressure can rise (Figure 5-17). As the femoral pressure rises, blood flow to the calf will initially increase and then gradually decrease as the flow debt of the calf muscle is eradicated. Peripheral pressure remains low until calf blood flow begins to fall, returning to preexercise levels only after the hyperemia has subsided.

Recording the ankle pressure after exercise, therefore, provides an excellent method for assessing the severity of arterial obstruction and for predicting the changes occurring in blood flow to the calf and thigh (49). Given an equivalent amount of exercise, one can assume that the greater the decrease in ankle pressure and the longer it remains below preexercise levels, the more severe the obstructive process. An ankle pressure that remains low or undetectable for a prolonged period implies multilevel disease and a diversion of blood flow into the more proximal muscular compartment (Figure 5-17).

Pressure and Flow Pulses

The periodic discharge of blood from the left ventricle into the arterial system during the systolic phase of the cardiac cycle is basically responsible for the pulsatile nature of blood flow. Energy developed during systole is stored within the arterial wall. During diastole, the elastic recoil of the expanded arteries continues to propel blood into the various vascular beds; otherwise, flow would be intermittent and pressure would fall to zero.

Many factors affect the contour of flow and pressure pulses. Among these are resistance to outflow, inertia and viscosity of blood, stiffness of the arterial wall, pulse rate, and wave reflections—all of which are incorporated into the concept of input impedance (3,55). The effect of resistance and wave reflections is perhaps the most easily understood (Figure 5-18). In the normal arterial system, the major site of resistance is in the arterioles. When the surge of blood constituting the flow pulse meets this high resistance, part of the blood is transmitted into the capillaries and part is reflected back up the arterial tree (3,56). The relative magnitude of the reflected wave is therefore a function of the peripheral resistance, being accentuated by vasoconstriction and attenuated by vasodilatation (57).

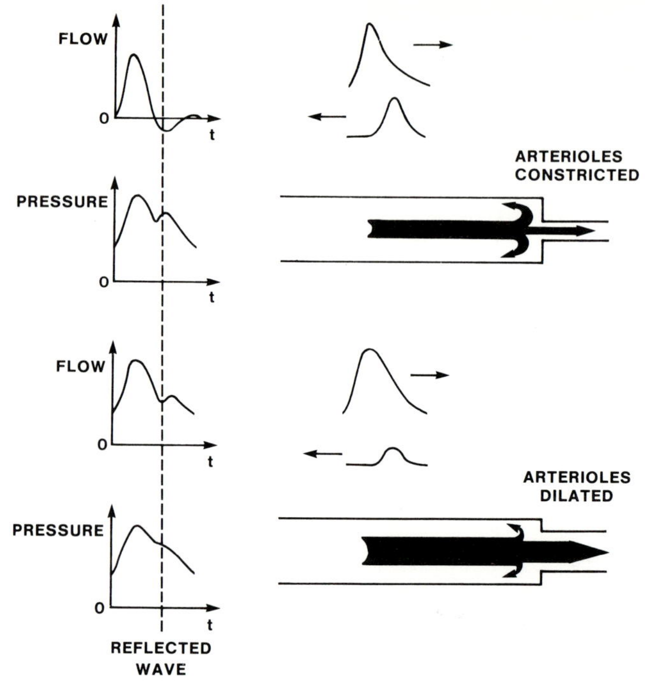

FIGURE 5-18. Effect of reflected waves on the contour of flow and pressure pulses. Reflected waves subtract from forward flow waves but add to pressure waves. Vasoconstriction accentuates the reflected wave, producing flow reversal in diastole and a prominent dicrotic notch in the pressure tracing. Vasodilatation minimizes pulse wave reflection.

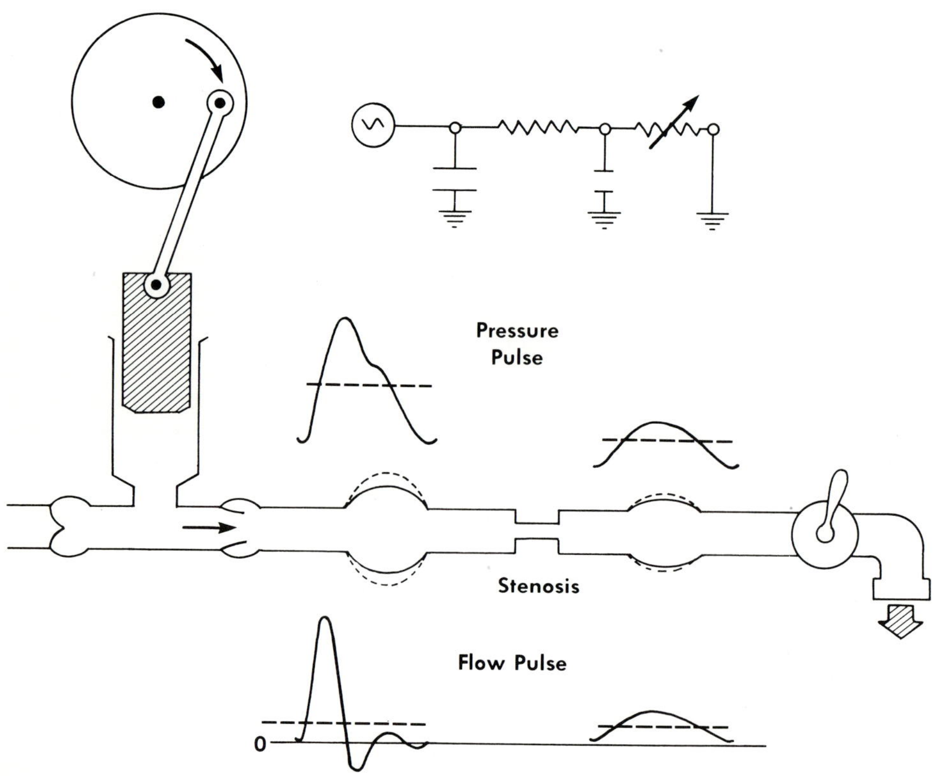

FIGURE 5-19. The combination of a hemodynamically significant stenosis and compliant vessels functions as a "low-pass" filter, attenuating high-frequency components of pulse waves. Arterioles are represented by the faucet and the variable resistance. Mean pressure (*dashed line*) is reduced, but mean flow (*dashed line*) remains unchanged distal to a stenosis. [From Sumner DS: Correlation of lesion configuration with functional significance. In Bond MC, Insull W Jr, Glagov S, Chandler AB, Cornhill JF (eds): *Clinical Diagnosis of Atherosclerosis: Quantitative Methods of Evaluation*. New York, Springer-Verlag, 1983.]

The reflected wave explains the characteristic appearance of the normal flow pulse, which has a large forward flow component in systole, followed by a reversed flow component (representing the reflected wave) in early diastole (Figure 5-18). Finally, another—but much smaller—forward flow wave is often present in late diastole. When the arterioles are dilated, as in exercise, there may be no perceptible reflected wave, and flow is antegrade throughout the cardiac cycle. This configuration is also typical of the pulse in arteries (such as the internal carotid) that supply low resistance vascular beds. The normal pressure pulse has a sharp upslope and a dicrotic wave on the downslope (Figure 5-18). This wave is produced by the return of potential energy reflected from the periphery. Plethysmographic pulses (which represent the interaction of arterial pressure and vessel wall compliance) have contours that are roughly the same as that of the pressure pulse (58,59).

Distal to a critical stenosis, pulse waves are attenuated due to energy losses incurred in the vicinity of the lesion and within the high-resistance collateral pathways (Figure 5-19) (60,61). The combination of high resistance and arterial compliance functions as a low-pass filter. While the lower frequency harmonics are passed with relatively little change, the energy in the higher frequency harmonics is markedly diminished. This produces a characteristic damping of the pulses. The pressure pulse becomes rounded, develops a slow upslope and a downslope that bows away from the baseline, and loses the dicrotic wave. Similarly, the flow pulse displays a slow upslope, a rounded peak, a gradual decline during diastole, and no reversed flow.

Palpation of the peripheral pulse is an essential part of the physical examination in patients with suspected arterial disease. Reduction or absence of palpable arterial pulses distal to an obstruction is the result of both the decrease in mean pressure and the attenuation of the pressure pulse. While gross changes in the flow pulse can be easily recognized with an electromagnetic or Doppler flowmeter, various mathematical manipulations have been introduced to enhance diagnostic accuracy. The simplest of these is the pulsatility index, which is defined as the ratio of the maximum excursion of the velocity pulse wave (from peak systole to the lowest diastolic point) and the mean velocity (62,63). Reduction of the pulsatility index below established normal values indicates proximal stenosis (64,65). Since the accuracy of this test may be compromised by distal obstruction—which also affects the contour of the wave—other more complicated methods, including the use of Laplace transforms, have been devised (66). The relative merits of these calculations have as yet not been established.

Although changes in the envelope of the pulse waves do not become evident until the stenosis reaches critical dimensions, even minor lesions generate turbulent eddies and areas of flow separation (67,68). These disturbances produce a variety of velocity vectors that "broaden" the Doppler frequency spectrum, providing a sensitive method for detecting low-grade stenoses.

Therapy

Improvement of peripheral perfusion is the objective of all methods for treating obstructive arterial disease. When the obstruction is severe and the goal is to eliminate ischemia at rest, a small increase in blood flow may suffice; but when the obstruction is less severe and the goal is to secure relief from claudication, it is necessary to provide a large increase in blood flow during exercise.

To increase blood flow, two basic mechanisms are possible: elevation of perfusion pressure P_a and reduction of hemodynamic resistance (Equation 5-11). While temporary relief of severe ischemia can sometimes be achieved by inducing systemic hypertension, this approach has limited applicability and subjects the patient to additional hazards (69). It follows that eliminating the cause of increased resistance is the most rational approach.

DIRECT ARTERIAL SURGERY

Since the site of increased resistance is the diseased arterial segment and not the peripheral runoff bed (which almost invariably has a decreased resistance), restoration of normal hemodynamics requires removing or bypassing the obstruction. Depending on the nature, extent, and location of the obstructing lesion, it can be removed by embolectomy, thrombectomy, endarterectomy, replacement grafting, or lytic therapy. Bypass grafting is preferred when the lesions are quite extensive or difficult to remove, or when preservation of collateral channels might be jeopardized by attempts to disobliterate the involved artery.

When the obstruction is confined to one arterial segment, it is often possible to return inflow resistance to normal levels and completely restore normal function (70). Peripheral pressures at rest and during and following exercise return to normal levels, and blood flow under the same conditions becomes normal. The same results can be achieved in multisegmental disease when all diseased segments are bypassed. Restricting the operation to one or more segments (usually the more proximal segments), but leaving residual disease, will effect only partial restoration of hemodynamic function. The degree of improvement will depend on the relative reduction in resistance (71). Although peripheral pressures are improved, they continue to be abnormal at rest and to fall during exercise; however, the postexercise decrease in pressure is reduced and recovery time is lessened. Likewise, partial repair is often sufficient to return blood flow to normal levels at rest and to provide sufficient blood flow to prevent claudication during moderate exercise. In cases being operated on for ischemia, it is only necessary to raise the peripheral perfusion pressure to a level that permits autoregulation to occur—about 40 mmHg at the ankle or 30 mmHg at the toe. In cases being operated on for claudication, this degree of improvement would not provide much relief; peripheral pressures need to reach levels that allow some constriction of the intramuscular arterioles at rest. Only then can the arterioles dilate under the influence of exercise to provide the additional flow required to ameliorate claudication.

Even when disease is confined to one segment, the operative procedure may not completely return the resistance of that segment to normal levels. For example, stenosis can occur during closure of an endarterectomy site or at the proximal or distal ends of a bypass graft. Aside from these technical errors, the buildup of pseudointima within a prosthetic graft or the development of fibrodysplastic thickening at the ends of an autogenous graft or within the recipient vessels can narrow the lumen. While these changes may not be clinically evident, they can often be recognized by a less than perfect result in terms of objective hemodynamic data (72,73). Peripheral pressures may not return to normal or, if normal at rest, will show reduction following exercise, and flow disturbances may be detected with a Doppler survey or by the presence of a bruit.

To provide sufficient blood flow at a minimal pressure drop, the diameter of the graft must be selected with its proposed function in mind. Like other blood conduits, the resistance of a graft is directly related to its length and inversely related to the fourth power of its diameter. Thus the minimal resistance of a graft can be estimated from Poiseuille's law (Equation 5-10). This, of course, neglects the inertial energy losses that occur at the graft-host artery junctions—losses that can be appreciable. Table 5-1 lists the minimal pressure gradients that would occur across grafts of various diameters at various flow rates. At flow rates normally observed at rest in a femoropopliteal bypass (about 60 to 150 mL/min), a graft diameter less than 4 mm would be associated with an appreciable pressure drop; the gradient during exercise, when flow rates of 300 to 500 mL/min are required, would be unacceptably high. While a 3-mm femoropopliteal graft might relieve ischemic symptoms, it would provide little benefit in claudicating limbs.

A 7-mm aortofemoral graft having a length of 20 cm would be capable of carrying flows of 3000 mL/min with a pressure drop of only 4.5 mmHg. Due to additional inertial losses, the actual experimental values are considerably higher, about 7 to 20 mmHg at flows of 1200 mL/min (74,75). Nonetheless, grafts of this size should suffice in most circumstances. A 6-mm graft, however, would develop a rather large gradient during exercise and could restrict flow.

Long grafts (80 cm) from the femoral to the tibial regions are ordinarily employed for the treatment of ischemic symptoms. Resting flow rates are not high, and pressure drops of 10 mmHg or more may be acceptable. Still, long segments of such grafts with small diameters (<3 mm) are inefficient blood conduits.

After implantation, prosthetic grafts develop a pseudointima. A thin (0.5-mm) fibrinous layer applied circumferentially to the interior of the graft would reduce the diameter by 1 mm, a reduction that could be of hemodynamic significance if a graft of borderline dimensions had been chosen. On the other hand, if the diameter of the graft is too large, clots tend to form on the inner walls as the flow stream tries to mold itself to the diameter of the recipient vessel. As in the case of aneurysms, this lining has little tensile strength, is loosely attached, and may embolize, causing the graft to fail. A high-flow velocity is conducive to the formation of a tightly adherent pseudointima. Because mean flow velocities are directly related to the flow rate and inversely related to the square of the radius, the velocity in a 7-mm graft would be 1.3 times that in an 8-mm graft and 2.0 times that in a 10-mm graft (Equation 5-6).

TABLE 5-1. Minimal Pressure Gradients across Grafts,* mmHg

Diameter, mm†	Flow, mL/min 300	500	1500	3000
	Aortofemoral, length = 20 cm			
10	0.1	0.2	0.5	1.1
7	0.5	0.7	2.2	4.5
6	0.8	1.4	4.1	8.3
5	1.7	2.9	8.6	17.1
	Femoropopliteal, length = 40 cm			
6	0.3	0.8	1.7	2.8
5	0.6	1.7	3.4	5.7
4	1.4	4.2	8.4	13.9
3	4.4	13.2	26.4	44.0
	Femorotibial, length = 80 cm			
6–4	1.3	2.6	3.9	5.2
5–3	3.5	6.9	10.4	13.8
4–2	13.0	26.0	39.0	52.0

*Based on Equation 5-7, $\eta = 0.035$ P.

†Femorotibial: evenly tapered grafts, largest diameter to smallest.

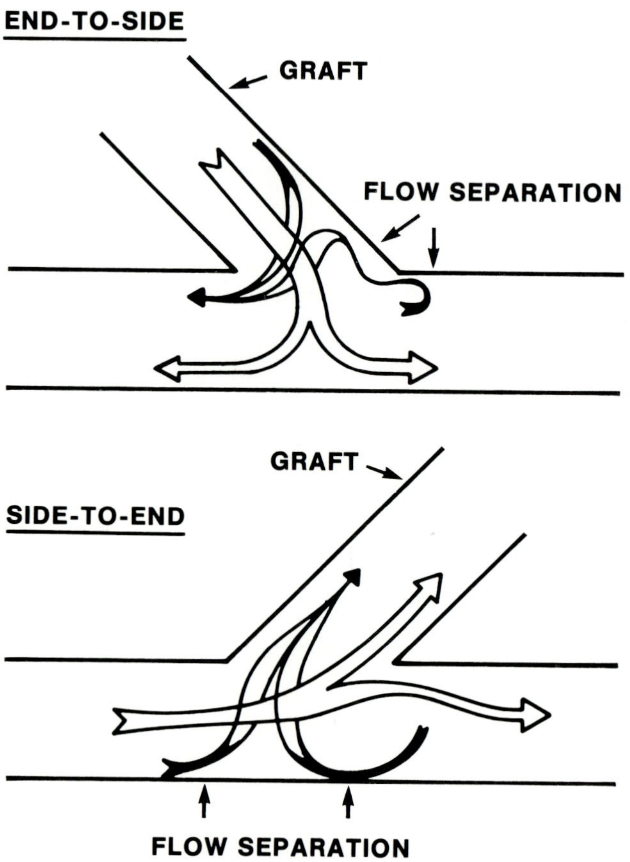

FIGURE 5-20. Flow patterns at end-to-side and side-to-end anastomoses. Note that blood may reverse and travel circumferentially to reach the recipient conduit. Areas where the mainstream flow is separated from that at the wall are prone to neointimal hyperplasia. [Based on studies by LoGerfo FW et al. (76) and Crawshaw HM et al. (77).]

To reduce inertial losses, it is important to make the transition from graft to host vessel as smooth as possible. End-to-end anastomoses, therefore, cause the least flow disturbances (3). End-to-side anastomoses are usually tailored to enter the recipient artery or leave the donor artery at an acute angle. While this diminishes flow disturbances at the entrance to the graft and in the antegrade recipient limb, it accentuates disturbances in the retrograde recipient limb, where the flow vectors are almost completely reversed. No matter what construction is used, there will always be regions of flow separation that contribute to energy losses and, more importantly, to the development of initial thickening or thrombus formation (Figure 5-20) (76,77).

Thus, grafts of all sorts always introduce new hemodynamic problems while they decrease others.

VASODILATORS AND SYMPATHECTOMY

Vasodilators and sympathectomy have little effect on collateral arteries and, therefore, can do little to reduce an elevated segmental resistance. Their function is to dilate the peripheral arterioles, principally in the skin of the more distal parts of the extremity. Since these arterioles are already maximally dilated in ischemic tissues, administration of vasodilators does not enhance blood flow to the critical areas. By dilating arterioles in nonischemic tissues distal to a proximal arterial obstruction, these drugs may actually cause a steal, which, at least theoretically, could be detrimental. Sympathectomy has the advantage of exerting its effect in a more limited area, thus minimizing the likelihood of a steal. Some surgeons feel that sympathectomy hastens demarkation of ischemic tissues, encourages healing of minor skin lesions, and decreases rest pain. The evidence, however, that sympathectomy has a beneficial effect is scant (78–81).

In patients with claudication, sympathectomy and vasodilator drugs do increase blood flow at rest in the nonischemic peripheral tissues. Since resting blood flow is already adequate in these limbs, the only potentially beneficial effect would be to increase the rate of flow through an arterial reconstruction, reducing the chance of thrombosis in the early postoperative period. Exercise itself is the most powerful dilator of intramuscular arterioles (30,79,82,83). Because further dilatation is not possible, these measures are not helpful in the treatment of intermittent claudication (Figure 5-21) (79,84,85).

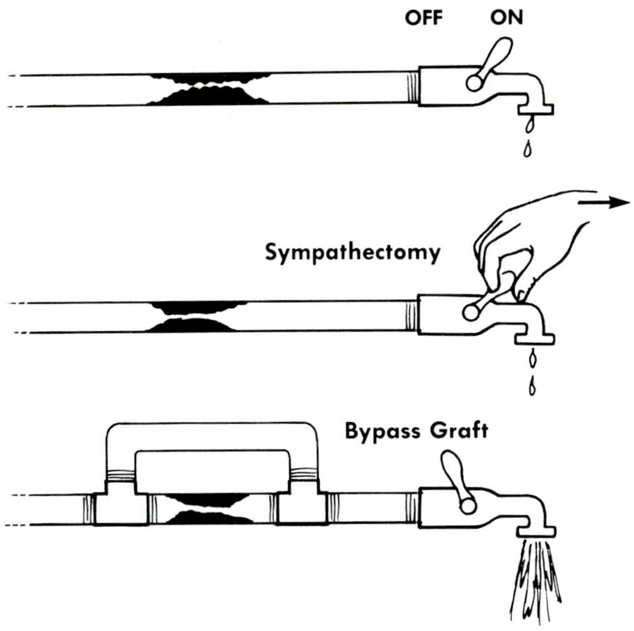

FIGURE 5-21. Contrasting effects of sympathectomy and bypass grafting on blood flow during exercise. Peripheral resistance (represented by the faucet) is maximally decreased during exercise and sympathectomy cannot further reduce resistance. Grafts, bypassing the obstruction, reduce segmental resistance and permit increased blood flow even when there is less peripheral vasodilation. [From Sumner DS: Pathophysiology of arterial occlusive disease. In Hershey FB, Barnes RW, Sumner DS (eds): *Noninvasive Diagnosis of Vascular Disease*. Pasadena, Appleton Davies, 1984, pp 2–15.]

REDUCING VISCOSITY

Blood with a hematocrit of 50 percent is about twice as viscous as that with a hematocrit of 30 percent; consequently, it is possible to augment blood flow somewhat by hemodilution (86–88). Low-molecular-weight dextran, which expands blood volume, raises cardiac output, decreases hematocrit, and reduces erythrocyte aggregtion, has been used for this purpose. The effects, however, are unpredictable, difficult to control, and do not offer a long-term solution to the problems associated with chronic arterial obstructive disease. More recently, pentoxifylline, a drug that increases erythrocyte flexibility, has been shown to increase walking tolerance in claudicants; but again the results are variable (89).

COLLATERAL DILATATION

Collateral development can be stimulated by exercise therapy, thus reducing segmental resistance. Not only are walking times increased appreciably when the patient adheres to an exercise program, but also there may be some improvement in the post-exercise ankle pressure response (69,90–92). Some of the beneficial effects are probably metabolic and not hemodynamic in origin. But this mode of therapy is not applicable to patients with rest pain, and the beneficial effects are variable and are lost when the program is discontinued.

Arteriovenous Fistulas

The components of a typical vascular circuit containing an arteriovenous fistula are illustrated in Figure 5-22. With appropriate modifications, all arteriovenous fistulas, regardless of their complexity, conform to this basic model. Collateral arteries connect the proximal and distal arteries, bypassing the abnormal communication. Similarly, on the venous side, collaterals connect the proximal and distal veins. The critical component of the circuit is the fistula itself, which can be classified as "large"

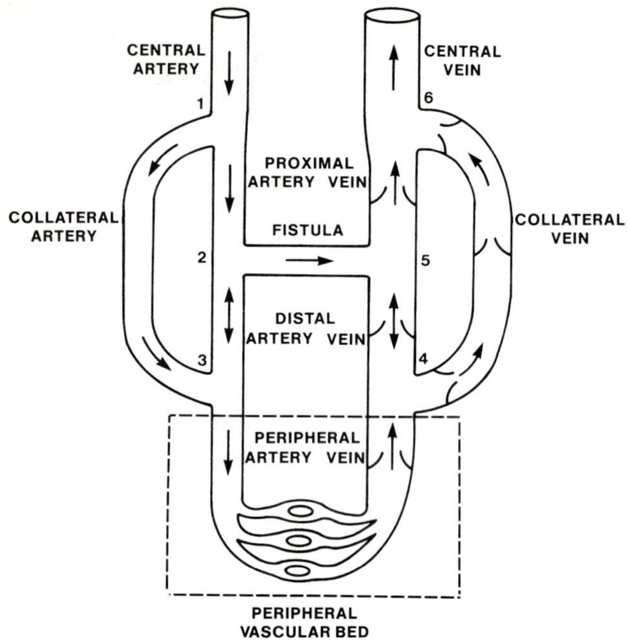

FIGURE 5-22. Diagram of typical H-type or side-to-side arteriovenous fistula.

or "small," depending on its resistance relative to that of the contributing vessels. Fistulas with a narrow diameter or those that are quite long (e.g., a graft between the radial artery and brachial vein) have a high resistance, whereas those with a diameter approaching or exceeding that of the donor artery have a low resistance (3,93).

Blood always traverses the fistula from its arterial to its venous end, the rate of flow being determined by the resistance of the fistula and the arteriovenous pressure gradient (Figure 5-22). Although flow is always directed distally in the proximal artery and proximally in the proximal vein, flow direction varies in the distal artery and vein, depending on the relative resistance of the components of the circuit (3,93–96). When the fistula is "small," a portion of the blood from the proximal artery continues past the fistula, flowing in the normal distal direction in the distal artery, where it joins the collateral inflow to supply the peripheral vascular bed. When the fistula is "large," part of the collateral inflow is diverted into the distal artery, flowing retrograde up the artery to enter the fistula. The peripheral tissues, therefore, are nourished only by input from the collateral arteries. In other words, the fistula "steals" blood from the peripheral vascular bed.

The situation is duplicated on the venous side. Normal flow direction persists in the distal vein when the fistula is small, but the volume of flow is reduced (94). When the fistula is large, there may be no reverse flow in the distal vein if the communication is acute and the valves remain competent. When, however, the fistula is chronic, the distal veins tend to expand; the valves become incompetent; and blood flows retrograde in the distal arteries, returning to the central veins via collateral channels (97,98).

Peripheral arterial pressures (point 3 in Figure 5-22) are always reduced in the presence of an arteriovenous communication, the extent of the pressure reduction increasing as the resistance of the fistula decreases (3,93,99,100). When flow is reversed in the distal artery, the peripheral pressure (point 3) exceeds the pressure at the arterial end of the fistula (point 2) (94). Peripheral venous pressures (point 4) are always elevated, especially when there is reversed flow in the distal veins. The pressure at the venous end of the fistula (point 5) exceeds that at the periphery (point 4) when venous flow is retrograde; otherwise, the normal gradient is maintained (94,99–101).

In summary, all fistulas, regardless of size, tend to impair peripheral perfusion, decrease peripheral arterial pressure, and elevate peripheral venous pressure. Steals associated with "large" fistulas can seriously compromise blood flow to the distal tissues, producing ischemia and venous congestion.

THERAPY

Surgical obliteration of the abnormal communication restores normal hemodynamics and is the optimum form of treatment. Ligation of the proximal artery, a procedure sometimes attempted in the past, is the worst approach (3). This operation ensures that all flow through the fistula will be derived from the collateral arteries; thus an increasing proportion of the collateral input is diverted into the distal artery, further depriving the peripheral tissues of nutrition. On the other hand, quadruple ligation (ligation of all proximal and distal arteries and veins) may be an acceptable compromise. Although this procedure blocks the major inflow arteries and the major outflow veins, it eliminates the devastating effects of the steal. If the fistula is chronic, the collateral arteries and veins are usually well-developed and are capable of sustaining peripheral perfusion. In fact, quadruple ligation usually increases peripheral arterial pressure and reduces peripheral venous pressure (3). These parameters, however, seldom return to normal levels, unless the collateral supply is truly excellent (as it may be when the ulnar artery represents the collateral supply for a radial artery–cephalic vein fistula).

When a significant steal accompanies a side-to-side arteriovenous fistula constructed for vascular access, relief can often be obtained by ligating the distal artery, provided the collateral arteries are well-developed (102). This operation maintains adequate flow through the fistula and ensures that the collateral input will be totally devoted to peripheral perfusion.

Aneurysms

The circumferential stress τ developed within an arterial wall is directly proportional to the transmural pressure p (3,4). Transmural pressure is the difference between the blood pressure within the artery and the surrounding tissue pressure. Wall stress is also directly related to the inside radius r_i of the artery and is inversely proportional to its wall thickness δ:

$$\tau = P\frac{r_i}{\delta} \qquad (5\text{-}13)$$

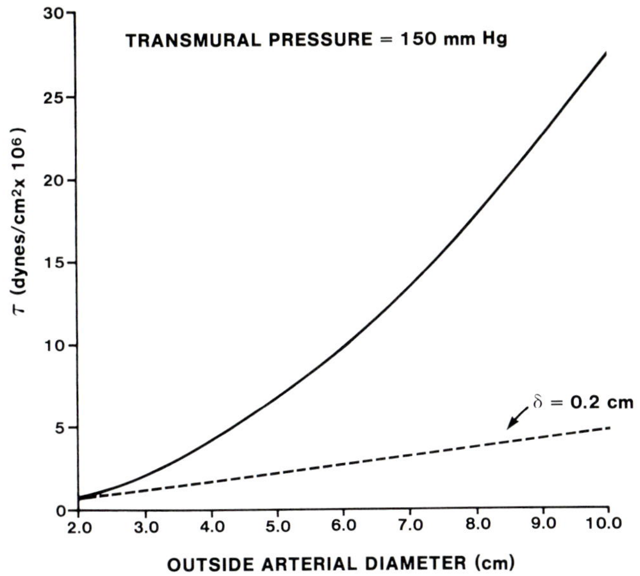

FIGURE 5-23. Effect of increasing arterial diameter on tangential stress τ. Original diameter (2.0 cm) and wall thickness (0.2 cm) correspond to that of a terminal aorta. Solid line assumes that cross-sectional area of the wall remains constant as the artery expands (wall thickness decreases). Broken line assumes constant wall thickness. Aneurysmal rupture occurs when stress exceeds tensile strength.

This explains why large aneurysms are more apt to rupture than small ones and why the risk of rupture is increased in hypertensive patients (Figure 5-23). Rupture is more likely to occur when the wall is thin. Although most aneurysms have thicker walls than normal arteries, the collagen content, which is primarily responsible for tensile strength, is relatively diminished (103). In other words, the functional thickness of an aneurysmal wall may be less than that of a normal artery. It is possible that the thick layer of clot which develops within most aneurysms has some protective effect, but the protection offered is unlikely to be great.

Conclusion

A basic knowledge of hemodynamic principles is necessary to understand the adverse effects that obstructive arterial disease has on the circulation to the multiple organs of the body. Although the factors governing pressure-flow relationships, velocity profiles, blood flow patterns, arterial wall properties, and metabolic interactions are exceedingly complicated and remain a fertile area for investigation, one can work with the knowledge currently on hand to enhance diagnostic accuracy and therapeutic capabilities.

References

1. Burton AC: *Physiology and Biophysics of the Circulation*, ed 2. Chicago, Year Book Medical Publishers, 1972.
2. McDonald DA: *Blood Flow in Arteries*, ed 2. Baltimore, Williams & Wilkins, 1974.
3. Strandness DE Jr, Sumner DS: *Hemodynamics for Surgeons*. New York, Grune & Stratton, 1975.
4. Dobrin PB: Mechanical properties of arteries. Physiol Rev 1978, 58:397.
5. Shephard JT, Vanhoutte PM: *The Human Cardiovascular System, Facts and Concepts*. New York, Raven, 1979.
6. Patel DJ, Vaishnav RN: *Basic Hemodynamics and Its Role in Disease Processes*. Baltimore, University Park Press, 1980.
7. Fry DL, Thomas LJ, Greenfield JC Jr: Flow in collapsible tubes. In Patel DJ, Vaishnav RN (eds): *Basic Hemodynamics and Its Role in Disease Processes*. Baltimore, University Park Press, 1980, pp 407–424.
8. Daugherty HI, Franzini JB: Steady flow of incompressible fluids in pipes. *Fluid Mechanics with Engineering Applications*, ed 6. New York, McGraw-Hill, 1965, pp 191–245.
9. Byar D, Fiddian RV, Quereau M, Hobbs JT, Edwards EA: The fallacy of applying Poiseuille equation to segmented arterial stenosis. Am Heart J 1965, 70:216.
10. Berguer R, Hwang NHC: Critical arterial stenosis: A theoretical and experimental solution. Ann Surg 1974, 180:39.
11. May AG, DeWeese JA, Rob CA: Hemodynamic effects of arterial stenosis. Surgery 1963, 53:513.
12. Kindt GW, Youmans JR: The effect of stricture length on critical arterial stenosis. Surg Gynecol Obstet 1969, 128:729.
13. Young DF, Tsai FY: Flow characteristics of models of arterial stenosis. II. Unsteady flow. J Biomech 1973, 6:547.
14. Anliker M, Stettler JC, Niederer P, Holenstein R: Prediction of shape changes of propagating flow and pressure pulses in human arteries. In Bauer RD, Busse R (eds): *The Arterial System, Dynamics, Control Theory, and Regulation*. Berlin, Springer-Verlag, 1978, pp 15–34.
15. May AG, Van deBerg L, DeWeese JA, Rob CG: Critical arterial stenosis. Surgery 1963, 54:250.
16. Moore WS, Malone JM: Effect of flow rate and vessel calibre on critical arterial stenosis. J Surg Res 1979, 26:1.
17. Moore WS, Hall AD: Unrecognized aorto-iliac stenosis. A physiologic approach to the diagnosis. Arch Surg 1971, 103:633.
18. Flanigan DP, Tullis JP, Streeter VL, Whitehouse WM Jr, Fry WJ, Stanley JC: Multiple subcritical arterial stenoses: Effect on poststenotic pressure and flow. Ann Surg 1977, 186:663.

19. Karayannacos PE, Talukder N, Nerem RM, Roshon S, Vasko JS: The role of multiple noncritical arterial stenoses in the pathogenesis of ischemia. J Thorac Cardiovasc Surg 1977, 73:458.
20. Sumner DS, Strandness DE Jr: The effect of exercise on resistance to blood flow in limbs with an occluded superficial femoral artery. Vasc Surg 1970, 4:229.
21. Longland CJ: The collateral circulation of the limb. Ann R Coll Surg Engl 1953, 13:161.
22. John HT, Warren R: The stimulus to collateral circulation. Surgery 1961, 49:14.
23. Rosenthal SL, Guyton AC: Hemodynamics of collateral vasodilatation following femoral artery occlusion in anesthetized dogs. Circ Res 1968, 23:239.
24. Conrad MC, Anderson JL III, Garrett JB Jr: Chronic collateral growth after femoral artery occlusion in the dog. J Appl Physiol 1971, 31:550.
25. Dornhorst AC, Sharpey-Schafer EP: Collateral resistance in limbs with arterial obstruction: Spontaneous changes and effects of sympathectomy. Clin Sci 1951, 10:371.
26. Ludbrook J: Collateral artery resistance in the human lower limb. J Surg Res 1966, 6:423.
27. Johnson PC: Review of previous studies and current theories of autoregulation. Circ Res 1964, 14:15.
28. Jones RD, Berne RM: Intrinsic regulation of skeletal muscle blood flow. Circ Res 1964, 14:126.
29. Walker JR, Guyton AC: Influence of blood oxygen saturation on pressure-flow curve of dog hind leg. Am J Physiol 1967, 212:506.
30. Remensnyder JP, Mitchell JH, Sarnoff SJ: Functional sympatholysis during muscular activity. Circ Res 1962, 11:370.
31. Kjellmer I: On the competition between metabolic vasodilatation and neurogenic vasoconstriction in skeletal muscle. Acta Physiol Scand 1965, 63:450.
32. Remington JW, Wood EH: Formation of peripheral pulse contour in man. J Appl Physiol 1956, 9:433.
33. Yao ST: Haemodynamic studies in peripheral arterial disease. Br J Surg 1970, 57:761.
34. Shepherd JT: *Physiology of the Circulation in Human Limbs in Health and Disease*. Philadelphia, Saunders, 1963.
35. Carter SA: Clinical measurement of systolic pressures in limbs with arterial occlusive disease. JAMA 1969, 207:1869.
36. Wolf EA Jr, Sumner DS, Strandness DE Jr: Correlation between nutritive blood flow and pressure in limbs of patients with intermittent claudication. Surg Forum 1972, 23:238.
37. Clyne CAC, Ryan J, Webster JHH, Chant ADB: Oxygen tension on the skin of ischemic legs. Am J Surg 1982, 143:315.
38. Carter SA, Lezack JD: Digital systolic pressures in the lower limb in arterial disease. Circulation 1971, 43:905.
39. Holstein P, Noer I, Tønnesen KH, Sager P, Lassen NA: Distal blood pressure in severe arterial insufficiency. Strain-gauge, radioisotopes, and other methods. In Bergan JJ, Yao JST (eds): *Gangrene and Severe Ischemia of the Lower Extremities*. New York, Grune & Stratton, 1978, pp 95–114.
40. Tønnesen KH, Noer I, Paaske W, Sager P: Classification of peripheral occlusive arterial disease based on symptoms, signs, and distal blood pressure measurements. Acta Chir Scand 1980, 146:101.
41. Ramsey DE, Manke DA, Sumner DS: Toe blood pressure—a valuable adjunct to ankle pressure measurement for assessing peripheral arterial disease. J Cardiovasc Surg 1983, 24:43.
42. Matsen FA III, Wyss CR, Robertson CL, Öberg PÅ, Holloway GA: The relationship of transcutaneous PO_2 and laser Doppler measurements in a human model of local arterial insufficiency. Surg Gynecol Obstet 1984, 159:418.
43. Franzeck VK, Talke P, Bernstein EF, Golbranson FL, Fronek A: Transcutaneous PO_2 measurements in health and peripheral arterial occlusive disease. Surgery 1982, 91:156.
44. Hauser CJ, Shoemaker WC: Use of transcutaneous PO_2 regional perfusion index to quantify tissue perfusion in peripheral vascular disease. Ann Surg 1983, 197:337.
45. Pentecost BL: The effect of exercise on the external iliac vein blood flow and local oxygen consumption in normal subjects, and in those with occlusive arterial disease. Clin Sci 1964, 27:437.
46. Lassen NA, Kampp M: Calf muscle blood flow during walking studied by the Xe^{133} method in normals and in patients with intermittent claudication. Scand J Clin Lab Invest 1965, 17:447.
47. Folse R: Alterations in femoral blood flow and resistance during rhythmic exercise and sustained muscular contractions in patients with arteriosclerosis. Surg Gynecol Obstet 1965, 121:767.
48. Strandness DE Jr, Bell JW: An evaluation of the hemodynamic response of the claudicating extremity to exercise. Surg Gynecol Obstet 1964, 119:1237.
49. Sumner DS, Strandness DE Jr: The relationship between calf blood flow and ankle blood pressure in patients with intermittent claudication. Surgery 1969, 65:763.
50. Lewis JD, Papathanaiou C, Yao ST, Eastcott HHG: Simultaneous flow and pressure measurements in intermittent claudication. Br J Surg 1972, 59:418.
51. Carter SA: Response of ankle systolic pressure to leg exercise in mild or questionable arterial disease. N Engl J Med 1972, 287:578.
52. Angelides NS, Nicolaides AN, Needham T, Dudley H: The mechanism of calf claudication: Studies of simultaneous clearance of ^{99m}Tc from the calf and thigh. Br J Surg 1978, 65:204.
53. Angelides NS, Nicolaides AN: Simultaneous isotope clearance from the muscles of the calf and thigh. Br J Surg 1980, 67:220.
54. Allwood MJ: Redistribution of blood flow in limbs with obstruction of a main artery. Clin Sci 1962, 22:279.
55. Farrar DJ, Malindzak GS Jr, Johnson G Jr: Large vessel impedance in peripheral atherosclerosis. Circulation 1977, 56 (suppl II):171.
56. Westerhof N, Sipkema P, Van Den Bos GC, Elzinga G: Forward and backward waves in the arterial system. Cardiovasc Res 1972, 6:648.
57. Rittenhouse EA, Maxiner W, Burr JW, Barnes RW: Directional arterial flow velocity: A sensitive index of changes in peripheral vascular resistance. Surgery 1976, 79:359.
58. Strandness DE Jr, Bell JW: Peripheral vascular disease. Diagnosis and objective evaluation using a mercury strain gauge. Ann Surg 1965, 161 (suppl):1.
59. Darling RC, Raines JK, Brener BJ, Austen WG: Quantitative segmental pulse and volume recorder: A clinical tool. Surgery 1973, 72:873.
60. DeWeese JA, Van de Berg L, May AG, Rob CG: Stenoses of arteries of the lower extremity. Arch Surg 1964, 89:806.
61. Keitzer WF, Fry WJ, Kraft RO, DeWeese MS, Sloan HE: Hemodynamic mechanism for pulse changes seen in occlusive vascular disease. Surgery 1965, 57:163.
62. Woodcock JP, Gosling RG, Fitzgerald DE: A new non-invasive technique for assessment of superficial femoral artery obstruction. Br J Surg 1972, 59:226.
63. Johnston KW, Maruzzo BC, Cobbold RSC: Doppler methods for quantitative measurement and localization of peripheral arterial occlusive disease by analysis of the blood velocity waveform. Ultrasound Med Biol 1978, 4:209.
64. Evans DH, Barrie WW, Asher MJ, Bentley S, Bell PRF: The relationship between ultrasonic pulsatility index and proximal arterial stenoses in a canine model. Circ Res 1980, 46:470.
65. Baird RN, Bird DR, Clifford PC, Lusby RJ, Skidmore R, Woodcock JP: Upstream stenosis, its diagnosis by Doppler signals from the femoral artery. Arch Surg 1980, 115:1316.
66. Skidmore R, Woodcock JP: Physiological interpretation of Doppler-shift waveforms. II. Validation of the Laplace transform method for characterization of the common femoral blood–velocity/

time waveform. Ultrasound Med Biol 1980, 6:219.
67. Blackshear WM Jr, Phillips DJ, Thiele BL, Hirsh JH, Chikos PM, Marinelli MR, Ward KJ, Strandness DE Jr: Detection of carotid occlusive disease by ultrasonic imaging and pulsed Doppler spectrum analysis. Surgery 1979, 86:698.
68. Brown PM, Johnston KW, Kassam M, Cobbold RSC: A critical study of ultrasound Doppler spectral analysis for detecting carotid disease. Ultrasound Med Biol 1982, 8:515.
69. Larsen OA, Lassen NA: Medical treatment of occlusive arterial disease of the legs. Walking exercise and medically induced hypertension. Angiologica 1969, 6:288.
70. Sumner DS, Strandness DE Jr: Hemodynamic studies before and after extended bypass grafts to the tibial and peroneal arteries. Surgery 1979, 86:442.
71. Sumner DS, Strandness DE Jr: Aortoiliac reconstruction in patients with combined iliac and superficial femoral arterial occlusion. Surgery 1978, 84:348.
72. Strandness DE Jr: Abnormal exercise response after successful reconstructive arterial surgery. Surgery 1966, 59:325.
73. O'Mara CS, Flinn WR, Johnson NC, Bergan JJ, Yao JST: Recognition and surgical management of patent but hemodynamically failed arterial grafts. Ann Surg 1981, 193:467.
74. Schultz RD, Hokanson DE, Strandness DE Jr: Pressure-flow relations of the end-side anastomosis. Surgery 1967, 62:319.
75. Sanders RJ, Kempczinski RF, Hammond W, DiClementi D: The significance of graft diameter. Surgery 1980, 88:856.
76. LoGerfo FW, Soncrant T, Teel T, Dewey CF Jr: Boundary layer separation in models of side-to-end arterial anastomoses. Arch Surg 1979, 114:1369.
77. Crawshaw HM, Quist WC, Sarrallach E, Valeri R, LoGerfo FW: Flow disturbance at the distal end-to-side anastomosis. Effect of patency of the proximal outflow segment and angle of anastomosis. Arch Surg 1980, 115:1280.
78. Strandness DE Jr, Bell JW: Critical evaluation of the results of lumbar sympathectomy. Ann Surg 1964, 160:1021.
79. Hoffman DC, Jepson RP: Muscle blood flow and sympathectomy. Surg Gynecol Obstet 1968, 127:12.
80. Carr MJT, Crooks JA, Griffiths PA, Hopkinson BR: Capillary blood flow in ischemic limbs before and after surgery assessed by subcuticular injection of xenon 133. Am J Surg 1977, 133:584.
81. Cronenwett JL, Lindenaur SM: Hemodynamic effects of sympathectomy in ischemic canine hind limbs. Surgery 1980, 87:417.
82. Cousins MJ, Wright CJ: Graft, muscle, skin blood flow after epidural block in vascular surgical procedures. Surg Gynecol Obstet 1971, 133:59.
83. Rutherford RB, Valenta J: Extremity blood flow and distribution: The effects of arterial occlusion, sympathectomy, and exercise. Surgery 1971, 69:332.
84. Coffman JD, Mannick JA: Failure of vasodilator drugs in arteriosclerosis obliterans. Ann Intern Med 1972, 76:35.
85. Weissenhofer W, Schenk WB Jr: Hemodynamic response to vasodilation and exercise in "critical" arterial stenosis. Arch Surg 1974, 108:712.
86. LeVeen HH, Moon I, Ahmed N, Mascardo T, Guinto RB, Falk G, D'Ovidio N: Lowering blood viscosity to overcome vascular resistance. Surg Gynecol Obstet 1980, 150:139.
87. Dormandy JA: Significance of hemorrheology in the management of the ischemic limb. World J Surg 1983, 7:319.
88. Wolfe JHN, Waller DG, Chapman MB, Blackford HN, Prout WG: The effect of hemodilution upon patients with intermittent claudication. Surg Gynecol Obstet 1985, 160:347.
89. Porter JM, Cutler BS, Lee BY, Reich T, Reichle FA, Scogin JT, Strandness DE Jr: Pentoxifylline efficacy in the treatment of intermittent claudication. Am Heart J 1982, 104:66.
90. Skinner JS, Strandness DE Jr: Exercise and intermittent claudication. II. Effect of physical training. Circulation 1967, 36:23.
91. Dahllöf A-G, Holm J, Schersten T, Sivertsson R: Peripheral arterial insufficiency. Effect of physical training on walking tolerance, calf blood flow, and blood flow resistance. Scand J Rehabil Med 1976, 8:19.
92. Snow CJ, Carter SA: Is exercise therapy beneficial in intermittent claudication? Vas Diag Ther Jan/Feb 1984, 5:20.
93. Levigne JE, Mesinna LM, Golding MR, Kerr JC, Hobson RW II, Swan KG: Fistula size and hemodynamic events within and about canine femoral arteriovenous fistulas. J Thorac Cardiovasc Surg 1977, 74:551.
94. Ingebrigtsen R, Wehn PS: Local blood pressure and direction of flow in experimental arteriovenous fistula. Acta Chir Scand 1960, 120:142.
95. Lough FC, Giordano JM, Hobson RW II: Regional hemodynamics of large and small femoral arteriovenous fistulas in dogs. Surgery 1976, 79:346.
96. Anderson CB, Etheredge EE, Harter HR, Graff RJ, Codd JE, Newton WT: Local blood flow characteristics of arteriovenous fistulas in the forearm for dialysis. Surg Gynecol Obstet 1977, 144:531.
97. Hol R, Ingebrigtsen R: Experimental arteriovenous fistulae. Acta Radiol 1961, 55:337.
98. Jamison JP, Wallace WFM: The pattern of venous drainage of surgically created side-to-side arteriovenous fistulae in the human forearm. Clin Sci Mol Med 1976, 50:37.
99. Schenk WB Jr, Bahn RA, Cordell AR, Stephens JG: The regional hemodynamics of experimental acute arteriovenous fistulas. Surg Gynecol Obstet 1957, 105:733.
100. Schenk WB Jr, Martin JW, Leslie MB, Portin BA: The regional hemodynamics of chronic experimental arteriovenous fistulas. Surg Gynecol Obstet 1960, 110:44.
101. Hobson RW II, Wright CB: Peripheral side-to-side arteriovenous fistula. Hemodialysis and application in venous reconstruction. Am J Surg 1973, 126:411.
102. Bussell JA, Abbott JA, Lim RC: A radial steal syndrome with arteriovenous fistula for hemodialysis. Ann Intern Med 1971, 75:387.
103. Sumner DS, Hokanson DE, Strandness DE Jr: Stress-strain characteristics and collagen-elastic content of abdominal aortic aneurysms. Surg Gynecol Obstet 1970, 130:459.

Chapter 6

THE CLINICAL EXAMINATION OF THE VASCULAR SYSTEM

JOHN CONNOR, SAMUEL E. WILSON, and RUSSELL A. WILLIAMS

The value of a complete medical history and physical examination cannot be overstated. They focus attention on the diseased organ system and its likely pathology. To properly apply the sophisticated study techniques of the vascular laboratory it is important to extract maximum information from listening to and examining the patient. Fortunately the vascular system can be very well assessed by the clinical examination, which is the best of all the noninvasive tests, both in terms of information gained and cost effectiveness.

This chapter imparts the general techniques of clinical examination of the vascular system, with illustrative examples. More detailed information on specific diseases is better sought in the appropriate sections of this book.

Clinical Assessment of Arterial Circulation in the Extremities

INSPECTION

The severely ischemic limb has a characteristic atrophic appearance, with muscle wasting, especially in the posterior compartment. The skin is taut, thin, and shiny and hair growth is diminished or absent. With more advanced ischemia the toenails have retarded growth, and the nail plate is thickened and roughened by transverse ridges with claw-shaped nails developing in some patients.

The limb may be white or show varying degrees of pallor, more obvious in the lower parts and the toes. Sometimes the dependent foot has a purple-blue cyanosed appearance which fades to white when the patient lies down and it is elevated. A simple technique to assess the condition of the peripheral arterial circulation is *Buerger's test,* which depends on the change of color occurring on elevation and dependency of the limb. The patient lies on his or her back and lifts both legs to an angle of 45°, keeping the knees straight. Skin with significant impairment of the arterial circulation quickly loses all color and becomes grayish-white, and the veins on the dorsum of the foot empty with "guttering" of the subcutaneous tissue along their course. Slight blanching or loss of color in the extremities is normal on elevation; the feet are then lowered by hanging them, dependent over the edge of the examining table, and a pink flush quickly occurs if the circulation is normal. With significant occlusive disease a brighter red color (reactive hyperemia), later replaced by a cyanotic hue, spreads over the affected foot. These color changes reflect oxygen saturation and blood flow in the capillary venous plexus of the skin that occur because of the loss of the sympathetic reflex vasoconstriction normally found in dependency.

The *venous filling time,* which is the time necessary to fill the superficial veins of the foot after emptying, also gives a measure of peripheral blood flow. This test may be especially valuable in diabetic patients with strong palpable pulses and small-vessel disease. The feet are elevated until the superficial veins collapse, then the feet are allowed to hang over the edge of the table, and the filling time noted. A time greater than 15 s is abnormal. The test is invalid in patients with varicosities or venous obstruction.

The areas of the foot subjected to pressure, heat, or trauma during walking or bed rest will often be the first to show signs of serious trophic changes such as ulceration, so a careful inspection of these areas is made in patients presenting with symptoms of peripheral vascular disease. The diabetic patient with a peripheral neuropathy may have a similarly appearing neuropathic ulcer with or without ischemia.

PALPATION

To accurately assess *skin temperature,* both limbs need to be exposed to the ambient room temperature for at least 5 min. The examiner moves her or his hands over the entire limb to map out warm or cold areas and to find the level at which any abrupt temperature change occurs.

To perform the *capillary refill test* press the nail or pulp of the digit of the affected limb for 2 s. After release of pressure, the color normally returns immediately, and the time taken for the blanched area to turn pink is a crude indication of the blood pressure and flow within the capillaries. The patient should be lying flat with the extremity extended for this test to be useful.

PULSES

Pulses that are usually examined are the radial, femoral, popliteal, dorsalis pedis, posterior tibial, and carotid. Less commonly examined are the other arm pulses (ulnar, brachial, axillary) and the superficial temporal and supraorbital pulses. The popliteal and ulnar peripheral pulses may be difficult to palpate in the normal person. The popliteal pulse is difficult because the popliteal artery does not cross a flat, boney prominence and lies deeply. The ulnar artery is difficult to palpate in the arm as it is a deep structure. The femoral artery lies under the midinguinal point. Differences between the pulses in the groin indicate iliac or femoral artery disease, which is often confirmed by hearing a bruit over the stenosed segment. At times a badly diseased femoral artery may be felt as a solid, pulseless, cylindrical mass along the usual course of the artery, or in contrast very prominent pulses may be found in patients with generalized arterial ectasia or aneurysmal disease.

There are four methods to aid the clinician in palpation of the popliteal pulse, and use of all four may be necessary before deciding the pulse is absent. (1) Flex the knee to approximately 135°, with the heel on the couch and the muscles relaxed. Place the thumbs of both hands on the tibial tuberosity and the fingers on the lower part of the popliteal fossa, then move the fingers from side to side until the pulse is felt. (2) With the leg straight, place one hand around the knee with the finger tips in the midline of the popliteal fossa and hyperextend the knee against this hand with your other hand. (3) With the patient prone, palpate the line of the artery with the fingertips of both hands. This is most reliable if the lower leg is flexed to 90° at the knee with the foot resting on the examiner's brachium. If in doubt about the presence of a pulse, check its rate against your own pulse. (4) The cross-leg test is done while the patient sits with his or her legs crossed; oscillating movements of the foot occur synchronously with the pulse if the popliteal artery is patent. With this test it is useful to continue taking the history to distract the patient's attention from the leg.

One or other of the foot pulses may be absent unilaterally or symmetrically in an asymptomatic patient. To be palpable, the arterial blood pressure in the foot is greater than 90 to 100 mmHg. The dorsalis pedis is the continuation of the anterior tibial artery and extends from a point midway between the malleoli to the base of the first intermetatarsal space. This vessel is most prominent and easily felt on the dorsum of the foot as it lies lateral to the extensor hallucis longus tendon at the ankle joint. The posterior tibial artery pulse is felt behind and a little below the medial malleolus.

The carotid artery pulse is felt with the tips of the examining fingers as it lies on the cervical vertebral transverse processes, moderately deeply in the recess between the esophagus and larynx and the sternocleidomastoid muscle. The carotid siphon may be confused with a lymph node or other tumor or even mistaken for an aneurysm.

The *Allen test* is an excellent check for patency of the ulnar artery. Both the ulnar and radial arteries are compressed, and the patient clenches his or her fist three times. Following release of pressure over the ulnar artery, the palm will be normally perfused if the ulnar artery is patent, but remain blanched if it is occluded. This test can also be used to check for patency of the radial artery.

The *exercise test* is useful when the history is strongly suggestive of arterial occlusion but the pedal pulses are present. The patient is reexamined after exercise such as walking or running which brings on the pain. If the pain is due to arterial insufficiency, then the relevant peripheral pulses will have disappeared or diminished markedly as blood is shunted into the exercised muscles.

One method to record the pulses is to use the scale of 3+ to 0—3+ being easily felt, full and strong; 2+ diminished; 1+ felt with difficulty; and 0 absent. Some surgeons use > 3+ to denote the excessive pulsation of an aneurysm.

Auscultation along the course of all the major arteries in the neck, abdomen, groins, and thighs (using the bell of the stethoscope) may reveal arterial bruits, which denote stenosis. The blood pressure in both arms is measured to detect subclavian or innominate artery disease.

Reactive hyperemia may indicate the severity of arterial ischemia. Inflate a sphygmomanometer around the thigh to 250 mmHg for 3 min and measure the interval between releasing the cuff and the appearance of a red flush in the skin. In normal limbs this interval is 1 to 2 s. In patients with severe arterial disease it is markedly increased.

Chronic Arterial Occlusion

The symptoms of chronic occlusion are intermittent claudication and rest pain. One of the most reliable and easily reproduced symptoms in human disease, *intermittent claudication* is pain which develops with exercise of the muscles, usually in the calf, and is most often described as crampy in nature. The pain occurs only when the muscle is exercised and disappears on resting it. Occasionally the patient will describe his or her leg as feeling "numb" or "going dead" with exercise and often notices paresthesias in the skin of the foot at the time the muscle pain begins. This is caused by shunting blood from the skin to the muscle. He or she also complains of limitation of walking due to pain and the need to modify lifestyle that this imposes.

The physician records as accurately as possible the distance the patient can walk before onset of pain. A particularly useful evaluation is observation of the patient's walking distance in a hospital or office corridor. Pain from other conditions such as arthritis is readily discerned by scrutiny of the gait.

The pain of claudication may begin suddenly or insidiously, the latter being the more common. The claudication distance gradually shortens over a few months and then becomes static. Sometimes the distance begins to increase again, corresponding with development of collaterals. The limb of the patient with intermittent claudication may show changes due to poor nutrition with decreased hair growth, shiny skin, and coolness of the extremity to the touch. The pulses immediately above the involved muscle will be diminished or absent and there may be a bruit.

Rest pain describes the continuous pain caused by severe ischemia. It is of far graver significance than intermittent claudication as gangrene is never far away. The pain is described as a continuous, severe, aching pain that prevents the patient from sleeping or walking on the limb. It usually occurs in the feet, often at the metatarsal heads, and worsens at night as the foot becomes warm beneath the bedclothes, thus increasing oxygen demand. The patient seeks relief by hanging the leg over the side of the bed or standing on a cold floor, and swelling of the extremity with worsening of perfusion results. Sometimes the pain is so severe that the patient elects to sleep in a chair. Patients' lives are made so miserable from the severe rest pain that they frequently require narcotics for relief and may request an amputation. A trophic ulcer in a patient with rest pain is often a precursor of gangrene.

Gangrene of the limb refers to necrotic tissue which is black or brown, and contracts into a crinkled, withered, hard mass. The dead tissue is senseless, and the junction between dead and living tissue becomes distinct and is known as the line of demarcation. The dead tissue may eventually separate and fall off (autoamputation). The living tissue on the proximal side of the line of demarcation is likely to be ischemic and is often painful and tender and may give rise to rest pain. The most distal parts of the limb, i.e., the tips of the toes and the pressure areas, are the most likely to become gangrenous (Figure 6-1).

If the dead tissue becomes infected, it is soft and boggy and pus appears at the line of demarcation. When the gangrenous tissue is hard and not infected, it is known as dry gangrene and when infected it is known as wet gangrene.

Ischemic ulceration is ulceration caused by inadequate blood supply; ischemic ulcers are usually very painful and may be accompanied by rest pain. Although the ulcer bleeds very little, it may discharge a thin serous exudate. The patient may remember some minor trauma to the site which did not heal despite care and attention and indeed will often have become deeper and larger. The causes of ischemic ulcers are atherosclerosis, embolism, renal disease, scleroderma, Buerger's disease, diabetes, and physical agents such as pressure necrosis, radiation, trauma, and electrical burns. The patients often give a history of long-standing, generalized vascular disease. On examination, the ischemic ulcers associated with vascular disease are usually found on the tips of the toes or fingers and over the pressure areas, and occasionally between the toes and the ulcer and surrounding tissues are usually very tender. Removing a dressing can cause severe exacerbation of the pain. The surrounding tissues are usually cold because they are ischemic; warm, healthy tissues suggest the ulcer is due to another cause.

Ischemic ulcers can be any size, from small, deep lesions to large, flat ulcers, and the edge of the ulcer is punched out because there is no attempt at healing by surrounding tissues. The skin at the edge of the ulcer is usually a blue-gray color. The base may contain gray-yellow sloughing tissue and may be infected. The tissue forming the base has a deficient blood supply inadequate to support growth of granulation tissue.

Ischemic ulcers may be very deep, penetrating down to bone and into the underlying joints, and it is not uncommon to see bare bone, ligaments, and tendons exposed in the base. The discharge from an ulcer is either clear fluid or pus, but rarely blood-stained. The surrounding tissue shows signs of ischemia, the pulses are absent, and there may be loss of superficial and deep sensation, weakness of muscles, and loss of reflexes. It is important to examine the peripheral nervous system of patients presenting with what is thought to be an ischemic ulcer, as sensory neuropathy may be the cause of the ulcer.

The *Leriche syndrome* occurs in relatively young patients who complain of intermittent claudication mainly in the thigh or buttocks, characteristically affecting both lower extremities. In men there is diminishing and later disappearance of penile erection. The physical signs in the legs are pallor, wasting, and absence of femoral arterial pulse. Thrombosis starts in an iliac artery and propagates superiorly into the bifurcation of the aorta.

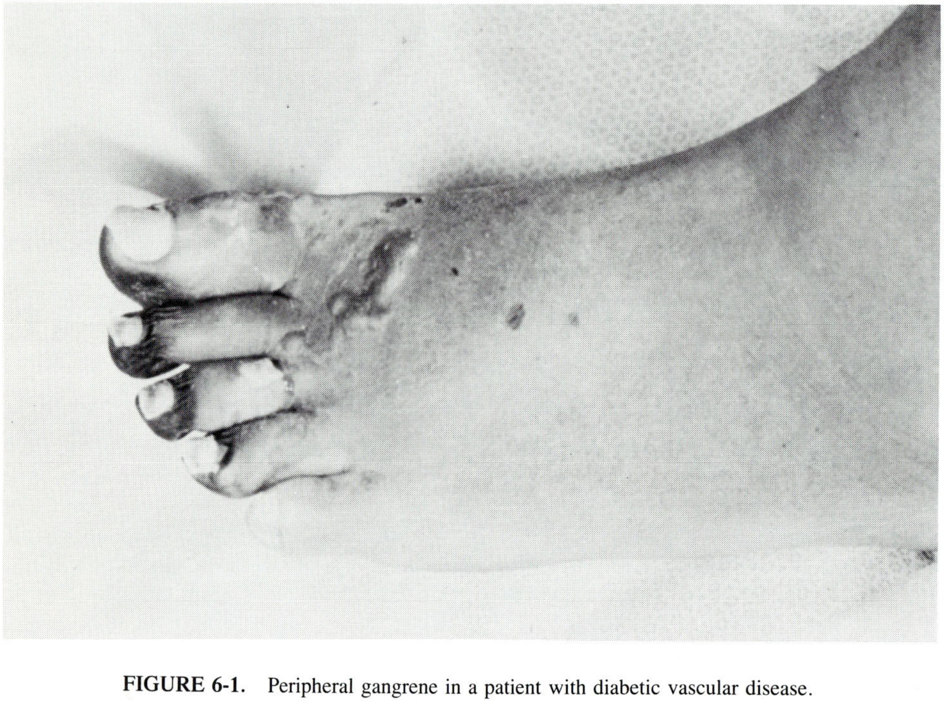

FIGURE 6-1. Peripheral gangrene in a patient with diabetic vascular disease.

SPECIAL VARIETIES OF OCCLUSIVE PERIPHERAL VASCULAR DISEASE

Thromboangiitis Obliterans, or Buerger's Disease

This condition gives rise to symptoms in men under 40 years of age and is virtually unknown in women. The patient is always a heavy smoker, and indeed the disease may be ameliorated by cessation of smoking. Signs of arterial insufficiency usually appear first in the lower extremities, but the hands are also involved, and intermittent claudication of the feet and hands is often a leading symptom, along with coldness and color changes in both lower extremities. Distal pulses are diminished or absent, and ulcerations of the fingertips are common. Usually the episodic nature of the disease allows an adequate collateral circulation to develop in response to successive vessel occlusion, but this condition may present with acute thrombosis and cause loss of all four limbs in a very short time.

Superficial Migratory Thrombophlebitis

This condition typically appears first in the veins of the lower leg, occurs in the majority of patients with Buerger's disease, and indeed may precede the onset of the arterial symptoms.

Acrocyanosis

Acrocyanosis is the condition in which the hands and feet are persistently blue and cold. The color of the skin does not alter with changes in temperature as it does in Raynaud's phenomenon, but the blueness may come and go, leaving the hands pink and normal between attacks. The condition occurs in youth and is much more common in females.

Erythromelalgia (Erythermalgia)

This condition leads to complaints of severe burning pain in the palms or soles which is precipitated by exposure to heat. During an attack, the feet are flushed, the veins prominent, the skin temperature is slightly raised, and the skin surface is hyperesthetic and very tender. Even the warmth of bedclothes may be enough to precipitate an attack.

Raynaud's Syndrome

Raynaud's syndrome is comparatively rare and occurs almost exclusively in females with its onset between the ages of 25 to 45, usually as a unilateral affliction. Patients complain of severe pain in the fingers on exposure to cold and with time the attacks become more frequent, bilateral, and last longer. Often the tip of one finger remains numb after the rest of the digits have regained an adequate circulation. The syndrome is produced by spasm of the digital arteries and in the severe form may produce gangrene of the fingertips. In an attack the skin first turns white and becomes cold and numb. It next turns blue, but remains cold and numb, and last it turns red, hot, and painful. As the disease progresses, there is atrophy of the terminal pulp of the finger or fingers affected. This gives a tapering appearance to the nails, which become ridged and brittle. Small, pitlike scars appear following necrosis of areas of the fingertips, and sometimes small painful ulcers develop on the fingertips (Figure 6-2). The disease may progress so the patient has rest pain and gangrene.

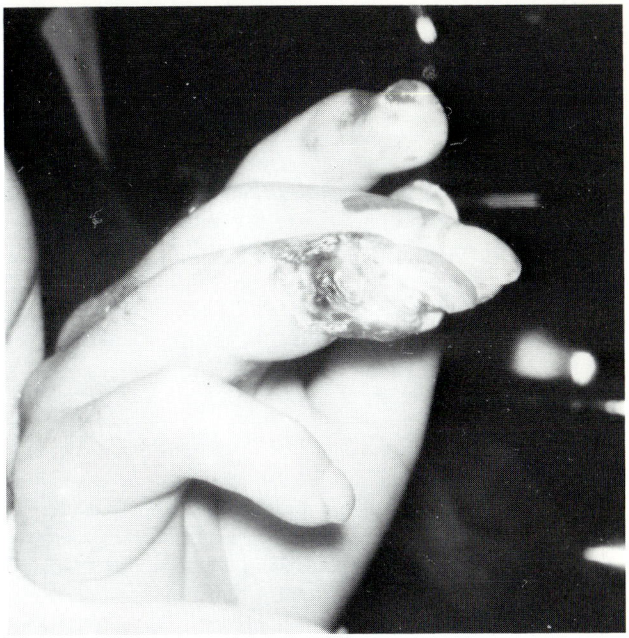

FIGURE 6-2. Advanced Raynaud's disease.

Livedo Reticularis

The most common finding in this condition is a diffuse, meshlike pattern of bluish, intradermal vessels of the limbs and occasionally the trunk. Primary livedo reticularis usually appears after puberty and is a permanent discoloration, although the intensity of cyanosis may increase with cold or emotional stimuli. The findings are usually symmetric, are more marked distally, and may involve the trunk. The distribution of secondary livedo reticularis is more patchy and asymmetric, and occasionally some of the more prominent lesions may ulcerate.

Acute Arterial Occlusion

Acute arterial occlusion results from arterial thrombosis, embolism, or trauma.

ACUTE ARTERIAL THROMBOSIS

The most common site for acute arterial thrombosis is the lower end of the femoral artery where it leaves the subsartorial canal. Thrombosis at this site produces acute ischemia and is very difficult to differentiate from an embolus. The patient will typically give a history of intermittent claudication with this, and when there is no obvious source for an embolus, thrombosis is the likely diagnosis. Ischemia is limited by the collaterals that usually have developed around a chronically narrowed artery.

In the early stages the limb is painful and pale with loss of sensation and muscle power. In addition, pulses will not be palpable. Although with underlying chronic atherosclerosis these may not have been palpable prior to the acute thrombosis, presence of the pulse at the corresponding site on the other limb is suggestive that the pulse in question was obliterated. (Atherosclerosis tends to progress symmetrically.)

The ischemic limb then swells, remains waxen and cyanotic, developing watery skin blisters which rupture, leaving superficially denuded areas of tissue. Eventually the dead tissue mummifies or becomes infected. The signs and symptoms of arterial thrombosis will vary with the anatomical site, e.g., infrarenal aortic thrombosis, subclavian artery thrombosis. (Figure 6-3).

EMBOLISM

It is important to seek out a source for an embolus such as a mural thrombus from the heart in a patient with atrial fibrillation, a recent myocardial infarction, an aortic aneurysm, or a peripheral aneurysm. Pain is present in 95 percent of cases and is usually abrupt in onset and excruciating. There is also weakness and numbness in the affected limb. Color change is normally limited to the distal part of the limb, which assumes a cadaveric pallor and about 1 to 2 hours later becomes cyanosed distally and mottled proximally. The level of ischemia begins some distance distally to the site of embolus; for example, a popliteal embolus will manifest ischemic signs beginning in the lower third of the leg. There are no pulses beyond the occlusion, and the distal extremity is cold. The embolus commonly impacts proximal to the bifurcation of a major artery. To determine the site of impaction a sphygmomanometer cuff is inflated around the affected limb and a stethoscope is applied progressively along the course of the artery. As the pressure is released, a booming sound signals returning arterial flow which is heard until the embolus is reached, when there is an abrupt end to the sound (Figure 6-4).

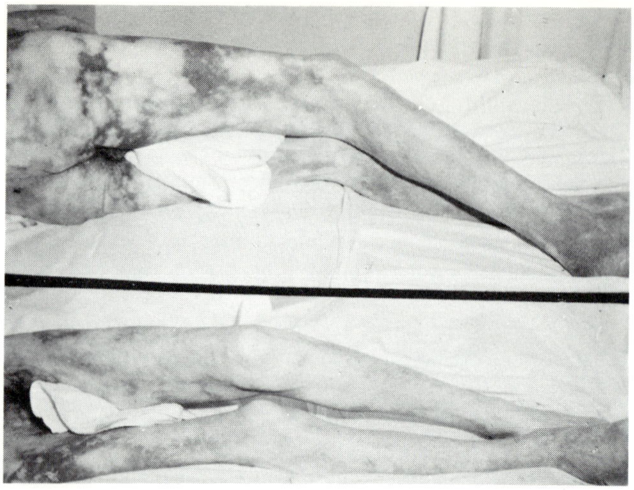

FIGURE 6-3. Aortic thrombosis showing reticular marbled appearance of severe ischemia.

TRAUMA

Arterial occlusions following blunt trauma may occur as a result of injury by bony fragments, pressure on an artery by an angulated bone end, or intimal rupture of an artery due to a fracture or dislocation or the compartment syndrome.

The following fractures and dislocations are the most often implicated in arterial injury: supracondylar fracture of the shaft of the humerus, dislocation of the shoulder, supracondylar or shaft fracture of the femur, dislocation of the elbow, and dislocation of the knee. Besides the symptoms and signs of the bony injury, the clinical presentation of traumatic occlusion of an artery is the same as for embolism.

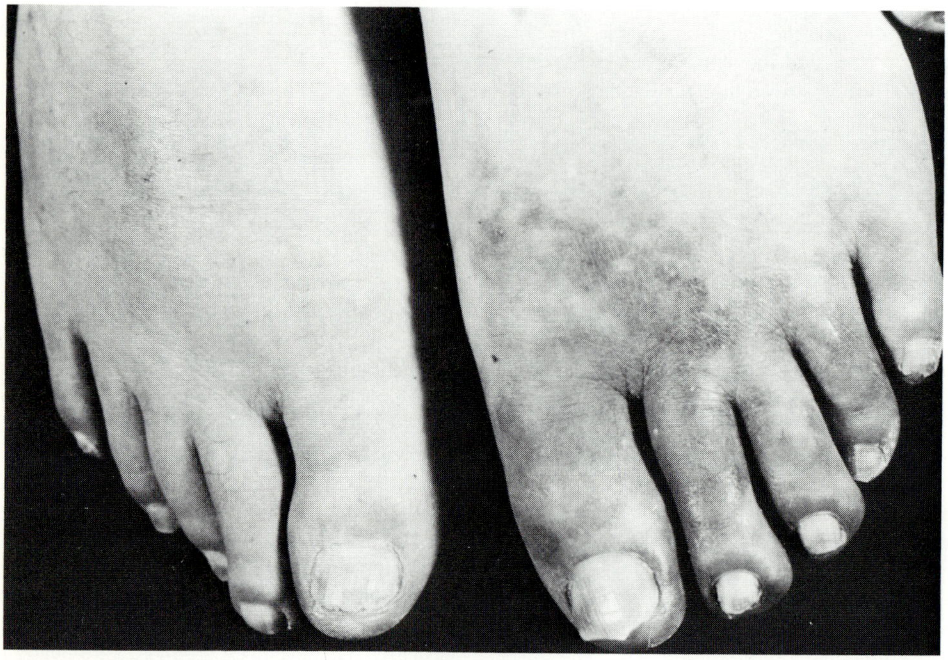

FIGURE 6-4. Emboli to foot following aorto-bifemoral reconstruction (''trash foot'').

Aneurysmal Disease

An *aneurysm* is an abnormal dilatation of the whole or part of the circumference of a length of artery. The most frequent *congenital aneurysm* is a Berry aneurysm of the cerebral arteries or less commonly arterial dilatation associated with an arteriovenous fistula. *Acquired aneurysms* are due to trauma, infection, and degenerative diseases. False aneurysms occur after an injury to an artery. The most common locations for atherosclerotic aneurysms are the abdominal aorta and the common femoral and popliteal arteries. Syphilitic aneurysms affect the thoracic aorta.

Atherosclerotic aneurysms are rarely found in patients below the age of 50 years, and men are affected 10 times more often than women. The most common symptom is a dull, aching pain, and with an abdominal aortic aneurysm, this is felt in the abdomen and often radiates through to the back. The pain is caused by stretching of the arterial wall. Acute pain occurs if the vessel suddenly stretches and begins to tear, and severe pain, bursting in nature, referred to the back is the most common symptom of a ruptured abdominal aneurysm. Referred pain due to pressure on a nerve by the aneurysm is not uncommon, and indeed some patients do present with sciatica. It is not unusual for patients to notice a pulsatile mass in their abdomen.

Patients may present with severe ischemia of the lower limb due to thrombosis of the aneurysm. This is unusual with aortic and femoral aneurysms but is a common occurrence with a popliteal aneurysm. Aneurysms may also be the source of emboli, the patient presenting with small areas of acute ischemia. At times aneurysms cause thrombosis in veins that are closely related to them—the patient will then present with a swollen blue and painful limb. Before examining the patient with an aneurysm it should be borne in mind that aneurysms tend to be progressive and multiple. With an abdominal aortic aneurysm the examiner has a 5 to 10 percent chance of finding an additional aneurysm in the limb. When a popliteal aneurysm presents, there is about a 50 percent chance of finding a similar contralateral lesion and a 30 to 40 percent chance of finding an aneurysm in the aorta or its branches.

An abdominal aneurysm is felt as a large, expansile, pulsating mass in the abdomen, particularly to the left of the midline. If the fingers are placed on the swelling in a fanlike manner, they are not only lifted but also separated. This is differentiated from a transmitted pulsation, in which the fingers are simply lifted upward. Lateral pulsation signifies an aneurysm. The aneurysm may be tender and is firm and not compressible. Peripheral pulses are usually present in patients with an abdominal aortic aneurysm, unless in the rare case where it is thrombosed or more likely the iliac arteries are diseased. The aneurysm is best felt by fairly light palpation as deep palpation may be misleading, and if the examiner's fingers cannot be insinuated between the dome of the aneurysm and the left costal margin, a suprarenal aneurysm is in all likelihood present.

Beware of the tortuous aorta and a prominent aortic pulsation, which are particularly well felt in a thin patient or one with scoliosis, leading to misdiagnosis of an aneurysm. Before proceeding to palpation careful observation of the patient's abdomen may reveal the visible pulsation.

Femoral aneurysms are usually found in the common femoral artery just below the inguinal ligament (Figure 6-5). They are very easy to palpate, but it should be confirmed that the pulsation is expansile and not transmitted. The distal pulses of the limb may be absent due to embolization or there may be an associated popliteal aneurysm. The limb is carefully examined for evidence of arterial insufficiency or venous obstruction, and auscultation over both of the femoral arteries and the abdomen may reveal a bruit.

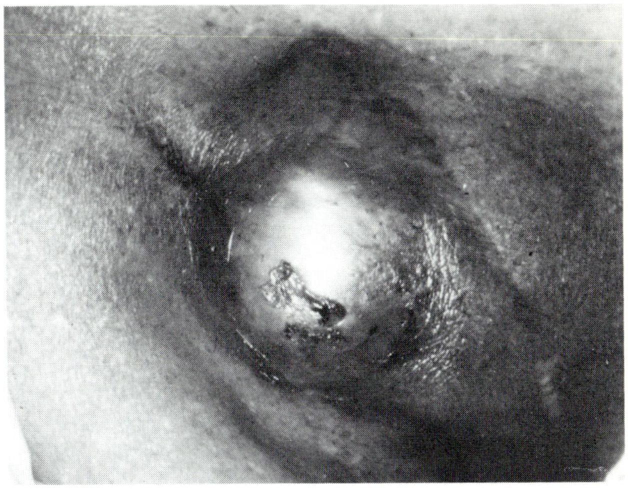

FIGURE 6-5. Femoral artery aneurysm with ulceration of the skin overlying it.

The classic sign of the *popliteal artery aneurysm* is an expansile pulsation in the popliteal fossa—if the popliteal pulses are too readily palpated, suspect an aneurysm. A palpable thrill may be present, and accompanying it, on auscultation, a systolic bruit is heard. Patients may complain of pain radiating toward the distal portion of the extremity due to pressure on the sensory nerves adjacent to the aneurysm.

There is a high incidence of thrombosis and embolization with distal ischemia ensuing in patients with popliteal artery aneurysms; early recognition and surgery are important to prevent loss of the limb. The thrombosed popliteal aneurysm may be difficult to diagnose and confused with a Baker's cyst or a semimembranosis bursa. It is solid, dull to percussion, does not fluctuate, and its size is unchanged when the knee is flexed as opposed to the Baker's cyst or semimembranosis bursa. Ankle pulses are not palpable if the aneurysm is thrombosed and are often not palpable even though the aneurysm is pulsatile, because concomitant occlusive disease or emboli have blocked the popliteal bifurcation. There is a high incidence of popliteal vein thrombosis in association with popliteal aneurysm, so evidence of venous obstruction may be found.

A *false aneurysm* originates from an organized hematoma, the center of which still contains blood that directly communicates with the mainstream in the lumen of the vessel. This is secondary to trauma, and the commonest causes are an iatrogenic vascular puncture or a stab wound. The signs, symptoms, and complications of false aneurysms are the same as those of true aneurysms except for a history of trauma or sudden appearance after the trauma and location of the aneurysm in an unusual site such as the wrist or ankle.

Cerebral Vascular Insufficiency

Cerebral vascular insufficiency may present with transient neurologic deficits or transient ischemic attacks, and there may be ipsilateral loss of vision. This transient loss of vision is called *amaurosis fugax,* which the patient describes as the "closing of a curtain or shade" in the eye, not just a sudden loss of vision. Contralateral sensory or motor deficits involving the limbs often accompany the eye symptoms.

Vertebrobasilar insufficiency presents with the somewhat less discrete complaints of dizziness, vertigo, and blurred vision. Either set of symptoms results from a stenotic mass lesion causing decreased cerebral blood flow or an ulcerated atheromatous plaque in the extracranial vessels from which microemboli detach to the retina or cerebrum.

On *physical examination* the subclavian pulse is felt by digital compression in the neck, superior to the center of the clavicle; the common carotid arteries are easily palpated in the neck by gentle compression against the vertebrae. Auscultation over these vessels for bruits detects stenotic arterial lesions in the neck and is a routine part of the general examination of the vascular system. An innominate artery stenosis produces bruits in both the subclavian and carotid arteries and is differentiated from the bruit of aortic stenosis, which decreases in intensity as one ascends the carotid artery. A vertebral artery stenosis may be very faint and is heard best over the tip of the shoulder.

Severe stenosis of the innominate or subclavian artery may stimulate the development of sufficient collaterals to maintain a weak brachial or radial pulse, but the blood pressure in the affected limb will be decreased, hence the importance of measuring blood pressure in both arms. The most common cause of cerebral vascular insufficiency is arteriosclerosis, much less common is fibromuscular hyperplasia of the internal carotid, and a rare cause is Takayasu's arteritis.

Gastrointestinal Ischemia

Patients complain of very severe abdominal pain, 15 to 30 minutes after eating, which is called "abdominal angina." This is most commonly in the epigastrium but may occur anywhere in the abdomen. Patients often lose a large amount of weight as they are frightened to eat because of the ensuing pain.

Palpation of the abdomen is unhelpful, and the most useful part of the physical exam is auscultation. Many patients have a bruit in the midline between the umbilicus and the xiphoid process due to stenosis of either (or both) the celiac or superior mesenteric arteries. Diagnosis is confirmed by arteriography. Without surgical intervention chronic visceral ischemia may progress to acute intestinal infarction.

Subclavian Steal Syndrome

With obstruction of the proximal subclavian artery, use of the arm on the affected side may lead to a reversal of blood flow in the ipsilateral vertebral artery, which results in brainstem ischemia. Dizziness and a murmur are noted; the murmur is systolic and in the lower neck.

Compression of the common carotid artery in the neck of the affected side leads to a decrease in the retrograde vertebral flow (the circle of Willis anastomosis being reduced), which in turn diminishes the radial pulse—this sign was described by Javid. In this syndrome the blood pressure in the affected arm is lower (usually greater than 50 mmHg difference to be symptomatic) than that of the normal side.

Costoclavicular Syndrome

This syndrome is seen less frequently than the cervical rib syndrome, and it occurs in older individuals, in whom the muscles normally responsible for holding the clavicle away from the rib, i.e., the sternocleidomastoid, trapezius, and levator scapulae, have atrophied and weakened and the subclavian artery is then compressed between the clavicle and the first rib. This is especially common if there is already a congenital narrowing of the interval between the first rib and the clavicle. To test for this syndrome the patient stands up with the arm by the side, and the volume of the pulse is noted. He or she abducts the arm to a right angle and then raises it above the head. With the costoclavicular syndrome the pulse weakens.

Cervical Rib Syndrome

Approximately 0.4 percent of the population has a cervical rib and in 7 percent of those affected this is bilateral. Usually these ribs are asymptomatic. However, the vascular symptoms of the cervical rib include pallor, coldness, and cyanosis of the hands and fingers. In severe cases, partial (mural) thrombosis of the subclavian artery occurs, and small emboli cause peripheral gangrene, particularly of the index finger tip.

The symptoms from a cervical rib are usually unilateral, tend to come on toward the end of the day, and are often improved by raising the arm. The radial pulse may become considerably weaker when the arms are forcibly depressed by traction in a downward direction. Obliteration of the pulse may occur with tensing of the scalenus anterior muscle. There may be a subclavian artery murmur.

To examine the region of the thoracic outlet first look and feel in the supraclavicular fossa for an abnormally elevated subclavian artery. Pressure on this artery may reproduce the symptoms, and a well-formed, easily palpable cervical rib may rarely be found. As a rule palpation is unhelpful because the ribs are either very small or represented by a fibrous band.

Veins

VENOUS THROMBOSIS

Thrombosis can develop within the superficial or deep venous systems. Only 25 to 40 percent of deep venous thromboses cause signs and symptoms. However, it is most important to detect deep venous thrombosis early to avoid pulmonary embolism and the postthrombotic syndrome. High-risk patients are identified and examined daily. These include patients who are greater than 40 years of age, are obese, have an unexplained fever, have organic heart disease, and have undergone recent abdominal or pelvic surgery, especially prostatectomy, cholecystectomy, or abdominal hysterectomy, or nailing of a fractured femur. They may complain of pain and swelling in the calf or leg but more often there are no symptoms. The clinical examination exposes the patient to a small risk of dislodging a clot, so it is undertaken gently and slowly. With the patient supine and both limbs fully exposed, the physician looks for inequality of leg girth, noting the relative prominence of the veins on the dorsum of the feet and any visible veins over the upper third of the tibia on the suspected side. The instep and the sulcus beneath the medial malleolus are examined for pitting edema. Dorsiflexion of the foot exerts traction on the posterior tibial vein, which if involved causes pain in the calf. This is known as Homans' sign, but it is well known to be frequently falsely positive, especially among females who wear high-heeled shoes, and it risks dislodging a clot.

The calf is examined gently, and the patient is asked to flex the knee. Starting at the Achilles tendon the calf is grasped and, while retracting it from the tibia, is gently squeezed. This is continued upward until the main calf muscle belly is reached, to ascertain if the soleus is tender, as the veins in the soleus muscle are a common site for thrombosis. Next the main muscle belly anteriorly is compressed; tenderness elicited here is suggestive of thrombosis in the posterior tibial vein. Always compare limbs.

Proceeding up the limb, the popliteal space is examined for tenderness, and at this stage the patient can rest his or her legs on the bed. The medial aspect of the thigh, from the saphenous opening below the inguinal ligament to the knee, is examined to detect femoral vein thrombosis. Early edema, if present, is detected by pinching the skin; this is difficult, due to thickening of the dermis and subcutaneous tissue. After palpating the entire leg, calf, and thigh, girths of both limbs are measured at standard distances from bony points and compared.

ACUTE VENOUS THROMBOSIS

Phlegmasia alba dolens (white leg, milk leg) is due to ileofemoral venous thrombosis. Rarely this arises spontaneously; more commonly it follows immobilization postoperatively or postpartum. The process often starts in the veins of the soleus muscle and proceeds upward, or begins at a valve in the femoral vein or the pelvic veins. The patient has an elevated temperature without any obvious cause, and there is pain in the groin and medial thigh. During the next 12 hours the limb becomes swollen with pitting edema and is pale, with considerable tenderness along the course of the femoral vein and into the iliac fossa. The foot becomes cool, and enlargement of the groin lymph nodes is common. The acute phase lasts 2 to 6 weeks and is followed by a chronic phase, characterized by a swollen, edematous, and cool and aching limb. There may be a venous ulcer present.

Phlegmasia cerulea dolens is due to massive thrombosis of the ileofemoral venous segment. It starts with tingling and numbness in the extremity and is followed by a sudden onset of crampy pain in the limb, which quickly becomes deeply cyanotic and hugely swollen, especially inferior to the knee. The pain is severe; the limb feels tense, firm, and rubbery, and there is little pitting on pressure. The patient can be in shock; the limb is cool, and venous gangrene may appear quickly. The pulses are difficult to palpate due to the swelling initially, and later disappear due to compression. The differential diagnosis between an arterial and venous occlusion is difficult. Treatment must be started immediately for the limb to be salvaged.

With *superficial thrombophlebitis* the vein wall is always inflamed, and this may actually be the cause of the thrombosis. Superficial thrombophlebitis may occur in varicose veins or in patients with an occult carcinoma, especially of the bronchus, pancreas, stomach, or kidney, lymphoma, or in those with Buerger's disease, polycythemia, polyarthritis, or be idiopathic. It is not uncommon for it to occur secondarily to intravenous site infiltration.

The patient complains of a sudden appearance of a painful lump on the arm or leg, there may be a slight fever, and the surrounding skin may feel warm. Examination reveals a lump in the subcutaneous tissue which has an elongated pipelike shape. The mass is tender, and the overlying skin is warm, edematous, and may be stained with a pale brown pigment. Local nodes are usually not involved early.

Thrombophlebitis migrans appears in previously healthy veins in patients who appear to be in good health and develops in different veins over varying periods of time. It is a sinister sign that should alert the physician to search for an occult malignancy. The association of superficial migratory thrombophlebitis with an occult carcinoma is known as Trousseau's sign. This may also be the presenting sign of Buerger's disease.

Mondor's disease, also known as string phlebitis, is a rare, self-limiting thrombophlebitis of the veins overlying the chest wall. It is more common in females where veins overlying the breast may be affected and can be mistaken for carcinoma.

Axillary or subclavian vein thrombosis may follow trauma to, or excessive use of, the arm. Typically the patient is an active young to middle-aged man. He complains of discomfort in the arm, and the upper arm, forearm, and hand swell, with pain on the medial side of the upper arm and in the axilla. The arm may feel hot, and its range of movement may be limited.

The whole arm is swollen, sometimes congested and blue; the superficial veins, particularly those around the shoulder, are distended and do not collapse if the arm is raised above the level of the heart. The axillary vein may be palpable in the axilla and is very tender. Examination should include the head and neck, breasts, and abdomen to detect diseases that can cause enlarged deep cervical, axillary, supraclavicular, or mediastinal lymph nodes.

CONGENITAL VENOUS ABNORMALITIES

The *Klippel-Trénaunay syndrome* is a rare vascular malformation that can be confused with varicose veins. Dilated veins have been present since birth, usually on the outer side of the leg, in contrast to varicose veins, which are commonly on the inner aspect of the leg. The affected limb is often larger than the normal side, and there may be cutaneous angiomas (port-wine stain). There are no associated arterial abnormalities or arteriovenous fistulas with this syndrome.

Congenital arteriovenous fistula is found most commonly in the leg. The fistula usually presents in youth with the following signs: a leg ulcer that is often very painful, surrounded by warm skin, and varicose veins together with cutaneous angiomas are often present. The affected limb may be longer and have a greater girth than the normal side and is warmer and moister than the normal side. There is a positive Branham's sign, elicited by digital occlusion of the fistula, which increases peripheral resistance causing a prompt slowing of the pulse due to decreased cardiac output. A machinery murmur with systolic accentuation is usually heard.

An arteriovenous fistula may be acquired as a result of penetrating trauma, particularly in the groin between the femoral vessels, or, unusually, as a complication of lumbar disk surgery when the fistula may form between the common iliac artery and veins.

VARICOSE VEINS

Varicose veins are the most common of all peripheral vascular diseases. They are dilated, tortuous, and lengthened, with incompetent valves, and usually they involve the long or short saphenous vein or the tributaries, the long saphenous vein being the most commonly involved. The superficial and deep venous system are connected by perforating veins which pierce the deep fascia. The long saphenous vein has three sets of perforators, one related to the subsartorial canal, a second related to the calf muscles, and the third set just above the ankle joint. If the lowest set has incompetent valves, contraction of the calf muscles causes reversed flow, giving the "flare sign" of venules radiating out in all directions from the perforator above the ankle joint.

Varicose veins affect all ages but are most common in young and middle-aged females; in children they are almost always due to a congenital abnormality. Women are affected 10 times more often than men. The patient's employment quite commonly involves standing for long periods, which, while not causing varicose veins, certainly exacerbates the symptoms. She or he often complains of a dull ache in the calves and lower leg which gets worse toward the evening, especially while standing, and which is relieved by lying down. Patients often complain of night cramps.

Some patients may be pain-free but present because they have noted dilated veins, venous stars, pigmentation, eczema, and ulceration. There may also be mild swelling of the ankle at the end of the day. Pregnancy often exacerbates the disease, and in other cases, symptoms or signs that might indicate a pelvic tumor are sought.

With the patient standing, inspect the lower limbs from umbilicus to toes, remembering to inspect the back of the legs for varicosities along the short saphenous veins, noting large visible veins, their extent and size, looking for evidence of chronic venous hypertension such as brown pigmentation, eczema, and ulceration, especially above the medial malleolus. Also examine the lower abdomen and pelvis.

Palpation over the course of the long and short saphenous veins detects varicosities that are not visible, especially along the proximal portions of both veins, which may be covered by a thicker layer of subcutaneous fat.

The *cough impulse test* assesses the competence of the valves in the long saphenous vein. The fingers are placed on the thigh just below the saphenous opening in such a way that the distal phalanx of the middle finger rests on the vein, and the patient coughs. If the valve at the saphenofemoral junction is incompetent, a fluid thrill is felt.

Trendelenburg's test is done with the patient lying down and the limb raised to drain the blood from the veins. The fingers are placed over the saphenous opening, and firm pressure is maintained over this point while the limb is lowered by the patient standing. If removal of the fingers from the saphenous opening is followed by filling of the veins immediately, the valves in the saphenous vein are incompetent.

The *tourniquet test* will reveal the presence and site of incompetent valves, especially the valves connecting the deep to superficial veins. The patient lies down, elevates the leg to allow the superficial veins to empty, and a tourniquet is placed around the upper third of the thigh tightly enough to occlude the superficial veins, and the patient then stands. If the veins above the tourniquet fill while those below it remain collapsed, there is an incompetent communicating vein above the tourniquet. If the veins below the tourniquet fill rapidly, there is an incompetent communicating vein below the tourniquet. This test is repeated progressing down the limb to map out the location of the incompetent communicating veins.

In *Fegan's method* the initial step to locate the site of perforators is marking the varicosities with a skin pen while the patient stands; he or she then lies down, and the affected limb is raised, resting its heel against the examiner's chest. The line of the varicosities is felt for gaps in the deep fascia through which the perforating veins pass; these are circular openings with sharp margins, and they are marked with an X. To confirm filling of the superficial veins via the perforating vein the Trendelenburg or tourniquet test may be applied, or more simply, finger pressure is maintained over the perforator site and the patient restands to determine if this provides "control" of the perforator.

Percussion of the veins when they are full transmits a percussion wave; the longer the vein and the fewer its valves, the better this wave will be transmitted. The fingers of one hand are placed on the lower limit of the visible vein, which is tapped at its upper limits, and a palpable percussion impulse implies a dilated vein with incompetent valves between the sites of palpation and percussion.

Auscultation over clusters of veins is a simple but sometimes forgotten means to diagnose an arteriovenous fistula.

The abdomen is carefully examined, including a rectal and vaginal exam, to exclude a pelvic or abdominal cause for the varicose veins. In males the testes are examined carefully, as metastases from testicular tumors cause enlargement of the abdominal lymph nodes which may obstruct the inferior vena cava.

The *postphlebitic syndrome* develops secondarily to valvular incompetence of the deep veins in the legs after deep vein thrombosis and includes characteristic changes of ulceration, which are common, along with a brawny edema of the leg most marked at the ankle, and a brownish pigmentation and eczema. There may be associated secondary varicosities. Occasionally a dusky cyanosis of the lower leg with purplish mottling is seen, but usually the only skin color change is to a brownish pigmentation due to hemosiderin deposition. The changed shape of the leg has been likened to an inverted champagne bottle.

Venous ulceration usually occurs after many years of venous disease, so most patients with ulcers are in the sixth or seventh decade; women are more commonly affected. Patients complain of pain, especially when dressing the ulcer and on slight trauma. Ulcers are commonly in the lower one-third of the leg on its medial side, but they can occur elsewhere, even on the foot, though almost never above the junction of the middle and upper third of the lower leg. The ulcers may be any shape or size, with a sloping edge and a pale purplish blue color. The base of a venous ulcer is usually covered with pink granulation tissue, but areas of white fibrous tissue may be seen. In severe cases tendons and bone may be exposed. The ulcers are, however, usually shallow and flat, and the surrounding tissues are usually indurated and pigmented.

Squamous cell carcinoma can arise in a chronic benign ulcer, and if the ulcer has a raised edge, is thickened, or is in any way different from a typical venous ulcer, suspicion of malignant change should be raised. Malignant change in a chronic ulcer is known as a *Marjolin's ulcer*.

OBSTRUCTION OF THE VENA CAVA

Superior vena cava obstruction presents with engorgement of the veins in the neck, anterior chest, upper arms, and face and may be due to external compression or intrinsic thrombosis or both. The onset may be gradual or acute. If it is acute, the patient has marked suffusion and edema of the face and neck; particularly notable are the bulging, edematous, bloodshot eyes. In chronic occlusion venous stars appear over the chest (Figure 6-6).

The most common causes are primary or secondary mediastinal malignancy and thyroid malignancy. Other causes are tuberculous lymph nodes, sarcoidosis, aneurysm of the aortic arch, idiopathic mediastinitis, substernal goiter, and iatrogenic reasons associated with indwelling catheters.

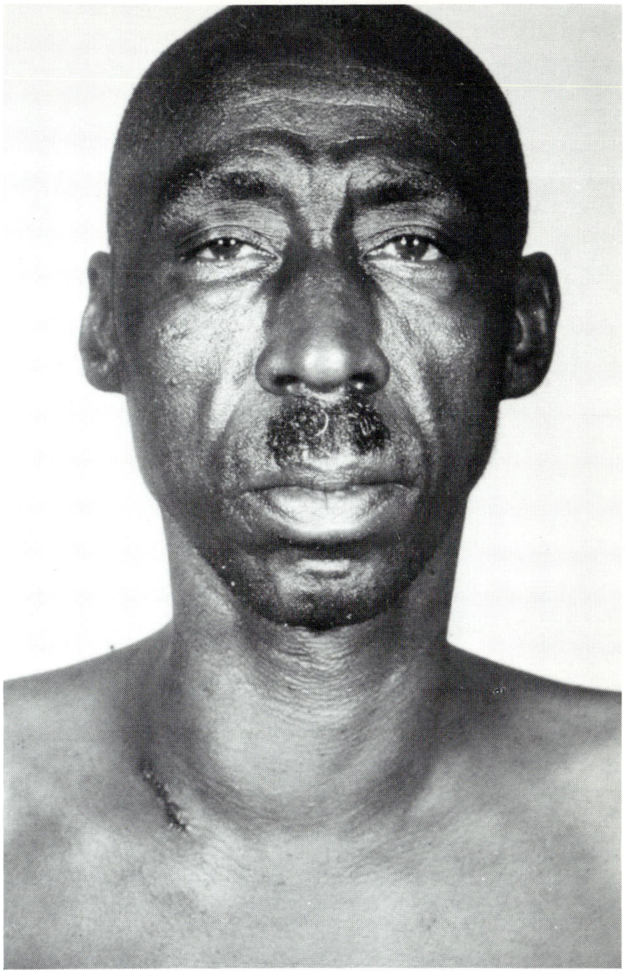

FIGURE 6-6. Cyanosis of head and neck in a patient with superior vena caval occlusion.

Obstruction of the inferior vena cava may also be gradual or acute in onset, and the development of collaterals that occurs with time dictates the degree of venous congestion and distal edema. There are often stasis changes of the skin on the legs, and venous collaterals may be seen about the hips and abdomen. It may be difficult to differentiate between inferior vena cava obstruction and portal vein obstruction as both systems use the same superficial collateral vessels. To try to differentiate between these two syndromes, an empty superficial collateral vein is isolated between two fingers, one of which is released alternately. If the flow is cephalad, caval obstruction is more likely, and if distally the portal system is implicated. But this is not a very reliable sign as both systems may be involved simultaneously.

Inferior vena cava obstruction is caused by intraabdominal malignancy in about 50 to 60 percent of cases. Other causes include retroperitoneal fibrosis, extension of ileofemoral venous thrombosis, extensive lymphadenopathy, pelvic lipomatosis, and aneurysm of the abdominal aorta. The patient's abdomen is commonly covered with dilated superficial veins, and there may be considerable peripheral edema.

Chapter 7

RADIOISOTOPES AND THEIR APPLICATION TO THE STUDY OF PERIPHERAL VASCULAR DISEASE

MARTIN A. WINSTON

Radioisotope techniques have been devised to study both anatomic and functional characteristics of the peripheral circulation. Broadly speaking, depending on the tracer used, one can study its rate of delivery to the tissues, eventual tissue concentration, or rate of clearance (washout) from the tissues. Vascular channels can be visualized in a manner similar to, but with less spatial resolution than, that of a contrast angiogram.

The Tracers

Historically, the first isotope studies employed intravenously injected sodium 24 and detected the initial arrival of the radioactive bolus with Geiger probes. In such studies the circulation time of course depends not only on the local blood flow but also on the cardiac status and blood volume (1).

Nondiffusible or slowly diffusible tracers which remain within the vasculature for at least one circulation time may be injected intravenously, and a rapid sequence of images, i.e., every 1 to 4 s, may be obtained to demonstrate the local vasculature. Typically technetium 99m is employed either in its native form as pertechnetate, which is slowly diffusible, or complexed to serum albumin or erythrocytes (nondiffusible).

The results are not quantitative but can give quick qualitative comparison of right/left symmetry. This has been most widely used in studies of cerebral blood flow, but is equally applicable to paired organs such as kidneys or extremities (so long as the injection is remote from the extremity to be studied).

In a semiquantitative method, ^{131}I-labeled serum albumin is injected intravenously while a cuff occludes the circulation to a lower extremity; during the reactive hyperemia following the release of the cuff, the arrival time and buildup rate of activity in the foot are monitored by a rapidly responding probe. A delay in the arrival of the tracer indicates a reduced blood velocity, while the time from the initial arrival to reach 50 percent of the eventual peak activity depends on the blood flow and the volume of blood in the monitored vascular bed (2).

Radioisotopically labeled particulate matter of sufficient size is trapped in the first capillary bed encountered, providing a more permanent record of perfusion at the time of injection (limited only by the physical decay of the tracer and the metabolism, if any, of carrier). This is the basis of the familiar lung scan and represents 100 percent clearance of the tracer from the blood during the first passage. The obvious disadvantage is that for any other organ to be studied, an intraarterial injection is required (3,4).

A freely diffusible tracer such as xenon 133 is used to quantitate the blood flow per unit of tissue. When it is dissolved in saline and injected directly into the muscle or skin being studied, its rate of washout (clearance) directly depends on tissue perfusion and the relative solubility of xenon in tissue and blood (partition coefficient). Even at higher rates of blood flow, the diffusion of the isotope is so rapid that blood flow is the only limiting factor in the rate of removal of the isotope. One of the few other materials with this characteristic is ^{131}I- or ^{125}I-labeled iodoantipyrene. As the partition coefficient (λ) of these compounds is known, perfusion can be directly calculated. Thus radioxenon can be used to study maneuvers designed to maximize perfusion such as a change in position, reactive hyperemia following occlusion and/or exercise, and pharmacologic interventions. Recirculation does not occur because the tracer is nearly 100 percent cleared by passage through the lungs because of its decidedly greater solubility in air than in tissue or blood.

The rate of flow for freely diffusible tracers in milliliters per 100 g of tissue per minute $= (\ln 2/T_{\frac{1}{2}}) \times \lambda \times 100$, where $T_{\frac{1}{2}}$ is the time required for the activity to diminish by 50 percent.

Radioxenon has been used to study the perfusion of cardiac muscle, bowel, kidneys, and brain, in addition to skeletal muscle. Indeed its application is limited only by the ingenuity required to deliver it to a particular organ (5–7).

Krypton 81m is an inert gas with physical properties similar to those of xenon but with a much shorter half-life. When it is delivered by a continuous intraarterial infusion, its concentration in a given area is proportional to regional blood flow (8).

Thallium 201 is representative of a class of agents concentrated within muscular tissue presumably because of the resemblance of the atomic structure to that of potassium. Potassium itself and rubidium are other elements which have been explored, but their isotopes (potassium 43 and rubidium 86) are less suitable for use as tracers because of either an excessively long half-life and therefore radiation dose, or the excessively high energy of the gamma radiation.

Although the isotope is freely diffusible, nearly 100 percent of thallium 201 is trapped during its first passage through muscular tissue, so its regional activity is proportional to the regional tissue perfusion at the time of the injection. The situation is thus analogous to that described earlier for particulates, but radioactive thallium has the advantage that it can be administered intravenously and given during exercise stress. Release from the tissue and recirculation do occur but are slow enough (1 or more hours) for studies to be obtained showing the perfusion pattern during exercises before significant redistribution occurs. This is the basis for regional myocardial perfusion scans, but application in peripheral musculature has now been widely reported as well (9–12).

Application

Radioactive tracers provide physiological information about the level and distribution of perfusion to the tissues, in contrast to the anatomic delineation of the larger vessels provided by angiography. These data may well be complementary, and the data from tracer experiments can be used to determine the physiological significance of mild to moderate stenosis seen on angiography, or the viability of the tissue distal to a severe stenosis.

PERIPHERAL VASCULAR DISEASE

If a relatively large dose of nonparticulate material such as ^{99m}Tc-labeled diethylenetetramine pentaacetic acid (^{99m}Tc DTPA) or ^{99m}Tc-labeled albumin is rapidly injected intravenously and a sequence of images is obtained at short intervals, e.g., every 1 to 4 s, the bolus may be followed through large and medium-sized vessels, thus supplying a low-resolution angiogram. Aneurysms or arterial injuries may be delineated. Vascular-graft patency is particularly well evaluated in this way. Time-versus-activity curves may be obtained from areas of interest in paired organs, e.g., kidneys or cerebral hemispheres. The curves are contributed to both by the transit time of the material from the point of injection through the organ and the blood volume within the selected areas of interest. A comparison of the flow in paired structures is thus possible, but a calculation of the flow rate is not (13–17). (See Figure 7-1.)

In the work-up of peripheral vascular disease, the intraarterial injection of macroaggregates or the intravenous administration of thallium 201 has been applied, both to estimate the level of the disease and to determine the physiological significance of angiographically visible lesions. Thallium 201 provides images of the tissue perfusion at the time of the injection, and the injection may be timed to coincide with maneuvers (such as treadmill exercise) designed to maximally increase perfusion (see Figure 7-2).

These materials have been employed to predict the healing of ischemic ulcers. If reactive hyperemia can be demonstrated in their neighborhood, the ulcers are far more likely to heal. Criteria based on studies with both intraarterial macroaggregates and intravenous thallium 201 are more accurate than the previous criteria of palpable pulses or the presence of runoff vessels seen on arteriograms (18).

A theoretical objection exists to the use of thallium 201 in the case of ulcers in nonmuscular areas, e.g., the feet, since it is concentrated only in muscular tissue.

Xenon 133 injected intracutaneously has been employed to predict the healing of both ulcers and amputation sites. Since cutaneous flow largely determines whether an amputation will successfully heal, a very small volume of xenon 133 is injected intradermally at various sites of potential tissue breakdown, and the rate of flow is determined from the rate of clearance. By this means, a flow of 2.4 mL/100 g per minute has been found to virtually guarantee healing, although healing may occur with a flow as little as 0.8 mL/100 g per minute (5).

Reduced xenon clearance from muscle during stress-induced hyperemia may provide early indications of small-vessel disease not angiographically visible (19).

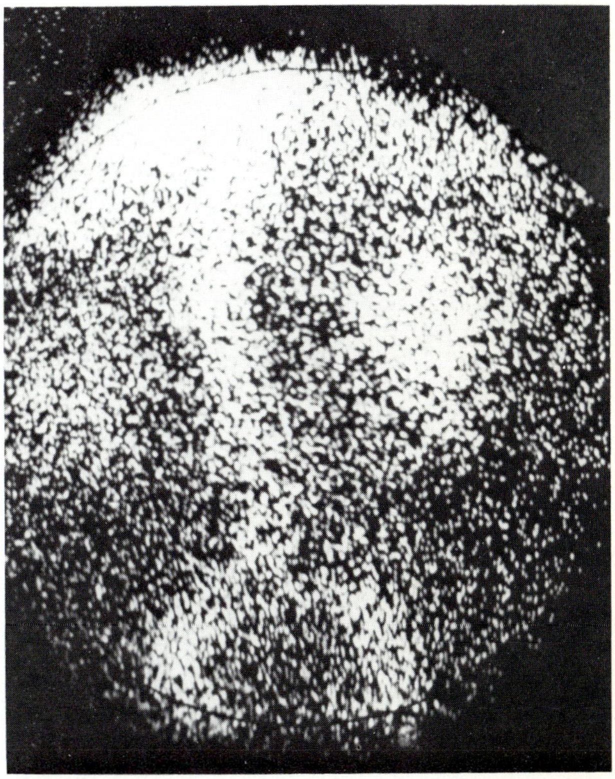

FIGURE 7-1. A dynamic scintiphoto study of the aortoiliac region obtained after the rapid intravenous injection of 20 mCi of ^{99m}Tc DTPA. Note also the symmetrical perfusion of the kidneys.

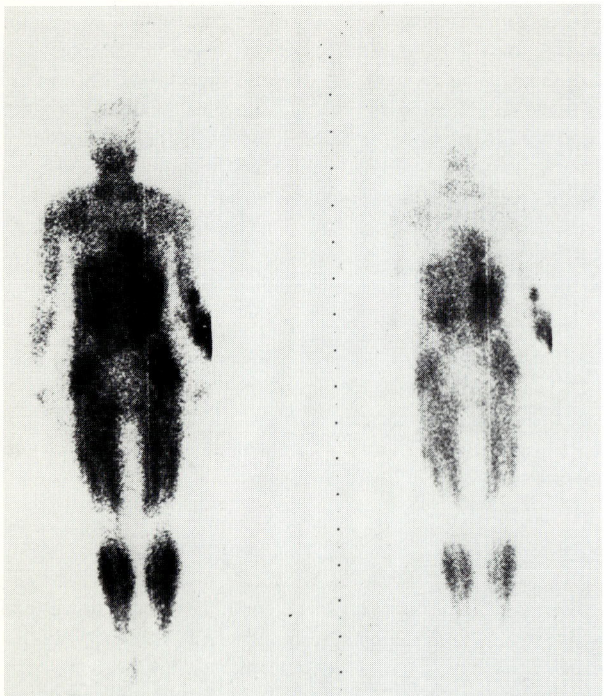

FIGURE 7-2. A normal whole-body scan with 2 mCi of thallium 201. Note the symmetrical thigh and calf activity in contrast to the greatly reduced activity in the knees and the ankles. (Courtesy Dr. E. Glass, St. John's Hospital, Santa Monica, Calif.)

CEREBROVASCULAR DISEASE

The assessment of cerebral perfusion by isotope techniques is currently receiving extensive clinical investigation. Sequential images of the passage of a tracer bolus through the carotid arteries and cerebral hemispheres provide a gross comparison of flow in the two sides. Such perfusion studies may be done preliminary to brain scintiscanning; major differences in perfusion are detectable, but it is not always clear whether these differences are due to vascular obstruction on one side or to hyperemia on the other, such as occurs during the phase of luxury perfusion following infarct, or as a response to status epilepticus.

The delivery of xenon 133 to the cerebrum can be accomplished either by intraarterial injection or by a period of rebreathing. The washout rate may then be monitored from multiple sites by means of an array of probes, and thus regional perfusion rates may be established. If the rebreathing method is chosen, the exhaled air must be monitored during the washout period to account for recirculation. Activity in the scalp and skull also needs accounting for but can be detected by its slower rate of washout (20).

A number of other materials and procedures, not yet widely applied, are available for special applications.

Platelets may be separated from blood, radiolabeled with indium-111 which is carried into the cell by 8-hydroxyquinoline (oxine), and then readministered. They will localize along areas of active thrombus formation or endothelial damage either in arteries or veins (21,22).

^{99m}Tc-labeled macroaggregates or microspheres, when injected into the common carotid artery, can be used to demonstrate the intracerebral perfusion pattern. This is a useful technique for demonstrating the patency of superficial temporal–middle cerebral artery transcranial anastomosis (21,23).

Ultrashort-lived isotopes, most notably krypton 81m, when infused intraarterially, allow visualization of regional perfusion in a manner analogous to that described for macroaggregates or thallium 201. Most interesting, however, is krypton's ability to demonstrate a constantly shifting pattern as perfusion changes, for example, in response to a pharmaceutical agent (6).

Gold 195m, eluted from a mercury 195m generator, has only a 30-s half-life, but because it is not eliminated in the lungs as krypton 81m is, it can be continuously infused intravenously and can provide excellent angiograms (24).

The pulsation of the arterial wall in response to the heartbeat has been studied utilizing ^{99m}Tc-labeled autologous erythrocytes which remain within the circulation. Images of the carotid vessels were obtained in conjunction with ECG gating, i.e., a series of images was obtained from different points in the cardiac cycle. A changing activity level at each point along the vessel during the heartbeat indicates that pulsation is occurring; such evidence of pulsation is diminished or lost distal to stenosis of 50 percent or greater reduction in the lumen (25).

Finally, newer tracers are facilitating the study of tissue metabolism and its correlation to blood flow. An example of such a tracer is oxygen 15, a short-lived (half-life = 2.1 minutes) cyclotron product and positron emitter. When inhaled or infused into the circulation, it is carried by hemoglobin to the tissues, where it is extracted. At equilibrium, its concentration is proportional to the local aerobic metabolic rate.

If the oxygen is inhaled in the form of $C^{15}O_2$, which is rapidly metabolized to bicarbonate, and thence by exchange to $H_2{}^{15}O$, the labeled water is deposited in tissues in direct proportion to the blood flow.

Ischemic tissues at rest continue to metabolize oxygen despite a reduced flow, largely through increased oxygen extraction (26). When methods of quantification, using positron tomographic imaging devices (PETT) are perfected, it is expected that such questions as the need for limb salvage, or the effects of drugs and surgery, may ultimately be decided on the basis of tissue function by an accurate evaluation of metabolic activity.

References

1. Smith BC, Quimby EA: Use of radioactive sodium in studies of circulation in patients with peripheral vascular disease: Preliminary report. Surg Gynecol Obstet 1944, 79:142–147.
2. Cuypers Y, Steels P: Clinical significance of the radioisotope test using I-131 labelled serum albumin for evaluating the peripheral circulation in the foot during a period of reactive hyperemia. Angiology 1983, 34:91–101.
3. Siegel ME, Wagner HN: Radioactive tracers in peripheral vascular disease. Semin Nucl Med 1976, 6:253–278.
4. Giargiana FA Jr, Siegel ME, James AE Jr, et al: A preliminary

report on the complementary roles of arteriography and perfusion scanning in assessment of peripheral vascular disease. Radiology 1973, 108:619–622.

5. Silberstein EB, Thomas S, Cline J, et al: Predictive value of intracutaneous xenon clearance for healing of amputation and cutaneous ulcer sites. Radiology 1983, 147:227–229..
6. Moore WS: Determination of amputation level. Arch Surg 1973, 107:798–802.
7. Hinsenkamp M, d'Hollander A, Coussaert E, et al: Measurement of blood flow in peripheral muscles using Xe-133. Angiology 1980, 31:50–65.
8. Gerritsen HA, Perquin JW, de Smet HL, et al: Continuous imaging of regional blood flow in peripheral vascular disease using krypton-81m: Effect of Ketanserin, a new selective serotonin antagonist. Diagn Imaging 1983, 52:85–92.
9. Siegel ME, Stewart CA: Thallium-201 peripheral perfusion scans: Feasibility of single dose, single day, rest and stress study. AJR 1981, 136:1179–1183.
10. Christenson J, Larsson I, Svensson SE, et al: Distribution of intravenously injected thallium-201 in the legs during walking. Eur J Nucl Med 1977, 2:85–88.
11. Seder JS, Botvinick EH, Rahimtoola SH, et al: Detecting and localizing peripheral arterial disease. Assessment of Tl-201 scintigraphy. AJR 1981, 132:373–380.
12. Siegel ME, Stewart CA, Kwong P, et al: Tl-201 perfusion study of ischemic ulcers of the leg: Prognostic ability compared with Doppler ultrasound. Radiology 1982, 143:233–235.
13. Barnes RW: Noninvasive diagnostic techniques in peripheral vascular disease. Am Heart J 1979, 97:241–258.
14. Diamond AB, Meng CH, Wolanski AC, et al: Radionuclide demonstration of traumatic arterial injury. Radiology 1973, 109:623–626.
15. Klingensmith WC: Regional blood flow with first circulation time-indicator curves. A simplified physiologic method of interpretation. Radiology 1983, 149:281–286.
16. Oshima M, Koh Y, Kobayashi M, et al: Radioisotopic dynamic study of the assessment of peripheral arterial disease (abstract). J Nucl Med 1981, 22:P48.
17. Moss CM, Rudavsky AV, Veith FJ: Isotope angiography: Technique, validation, and value in assessment of arterial reconstruction. Ann Surg 1976, 184:116–121.
18. Siegel ME, Williams CM, Giargiana FA, et al: An objective useful criterion for determining the healing potential of an ischemic ulcer. J Nucl Med 1975, 16:993–995.
19. Steinbach JJ, Pendergast D, Blau M: Muscle blood flow in insulin dependent patients with diabetes mellitus using small solid state CdTe detectors and xenon-133 (abstract). J Nucl Med 1981, 22:P48.
20. Obrist WD, Thompson HR Jr, Wang HS, et al: Regional cerebral blood flow estimated by xenon-133 inhalation. Stroke 1975, 6:245–256.
21. Davis HH, Heaton WA, Siegel BA, et al: Scintigraphic detection of atherosclerotic lesions and venous thrombi in man by indium-111 labelled autologous platelets. Lancet 1978, 1:1185–1187.
22. Goodwin DA, Bushberg JT, Doherty PW, et al: Indium-111 labelled autologous platelets for location of vascular thrombi in humans. J Nucl Med 1978, 19:626–634.
23. Etani H, Kimura K, Iwata Y, et al: Internal carotid occlusion assessment, by Tc-99m-tagged microspheres, of bypass from superficial temporal to middle cerebral artery. J Nucl Med 1981, 22:856–860.
24. Brihaye C, Guillaume M, Lavi N, et al: Development of a reliable Hg-195m–Au-195m generator for the production of Au-195m, a short-lived nuclide for vascular imaging. J Nucl Med 1982, 23:1114–1120.
25. Winston MA, Cohen SN: ECG-gated blood-pool study of carotid arterial pulsation as a sign of stenosis. J Nucl Med 1983, 24:470–474.
26. Clyne CA, Jones T, Moss S, et al: The use of radioactive oxygen to study muscle function in peripheral vascular disease. Surg Gynecol Obstet 1979, 149:225–228.

Chapter 8

NONINVASIVE STUDIES OF PERIPHERAL VASCULAR DISEASE

JAMES S. T. YAO

Plethysmography

Plethysmography probably is the oldest method for measuring blood flow. In this method, measurements are made of changes in volume of an organ or region of tissue. The word "plethysmography" was derived from the Greek and literally means "the recording of increase." Swammerdam, in 1737, is credited with being the first to introduce this principle. It was not until the introduction of venous occlusion plethysmography, however, that measurements were made on a qualitative basis dependent on the alteration of pulse waveforms.

In the modern practice of vascular surgery, the use of plethysmography has been expanded to include detection of not only arterial occlusive disease but also carotid artery disease and venous problems. The use of oculoplethysmography and impedance plethysmography will be discussed in Chapters 10 and 11, respectively, and hence will not be discussed here. In addition to clinical application, plethysmography has been shown to provide valuable information on both arterial and venous physiology.

Several types of plethysmographs are now available for clinical use in the evaluation of arterial occlusions. These are volume, strain-gauge, and photoelectric plethysmographs. The water-filled volume recorder, popular in the early use of plethysmography, is now obsolete and has been replaced by the air-filled volume plethysmograph, notably, the pulse-volume recorder developed by Raines (1). For clinical application, the newer plethysmographs, such as the strain-gauge, photoplethysmograph, and pulse-volume recorder, are now standard equipment in many vascular laboratories.

INSTRUMENTATION

Strain-Gauge Plethysmograph

Strain-gauge plethysmographs use fine-bore silicone rubber tubes filled with mercury or a liquid-metal alloy that makes contact with copper electrodes at either end. The gauge is wrapped around the part being studied. As the part (calf or forearm) expands or contracts, the length of the gauge increases or decreases by a corresponding amount. The changes in length of the gauge reflect changes in the circumference of the part and are interpreted as volume changes. Because the resistance of the liquid-metal column varies with its length, changes in voltage across the gauge, when amplified, can be calibrated to reflect changes in circumference (volume) of the circumscribed part.

Changes in strain-gauge length can be calibrated mechanically to reflect volume flow, or electrical calibration by a bridge circuit can be used to measure voltage drop across the gauge.

Photoelectric Plethysmograph

The term *photoelectric plethysmograph* was first introduced by Hertzmann (2), who used it to measure blood volume changes induced in the skin by exercise in normal individuals and in patients with peripheral arterial disease. Early instrumentation included the use of a photo cell for pulse recording by means of alternating current (ac) signals. Recently, an infrared sensor has been used in the newer generation of photoelectric plethysmographs. In this newer instrument, a direct current (dc) coupling technique is also provided. The dc signal is not related to the pulse, is slow to change, and depends on changes in the total blood volume in the skin. With refinement in probe design, the photoplethysmograph has become a standard instrument for the study of venous problems and for the recording of pulse waveforms in most laboratories. The use of the dc mode to detect volume changes is helpful in recording finger or toe pressure.

Air-Filled Plethysmograph

One of the popular instruments used in the noninvasive laboratory is the pulse-volume recorder. In essence, this is an air-filled, segmental plethysmograph designed to measure segments of the leg. The air-filled plethysmograph uses a pneumatic cuff placed around the part being examined, often at several levels. By injecting a known volume of air into the cuff bladder, instantaneous volume changes in the limb segment beneath the cuff can be calibrated and recorded with a sensitive pressure transducer to provide pulsatile flow tracings. Changes in the configuration of such pulse-volume tracings indicate proximal arterial occlusion. By visual inspection, the pulse waveforms can be related to different degrees of ischemia (Figure 8-1).

In addition to recording arterial pulse-volume waveforms, the pulse-volume recorder can be converted for recording venous outflow and capacitance using the dc mode. Also, the instrument is useful to record penile pulse waveforms and to record ophthalmic

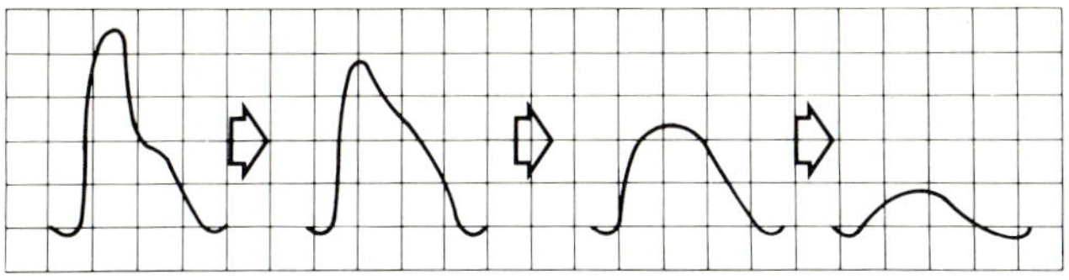

FIGURE 8-1. Changes in waveforms recorded by the pulse-volume recorder with progressive arterial disease. Severe ischemia is manifested by marked damping of the waveform. [From Kempczinski RF: Segmental volume plethysmography: The pulse volume recorder. In Kempczinski RF, Yao JST (eds): *Practical Noninvasive Vascular Diagnosis*. Chicago, Year Book Medical Publishers, 1982, pp 105–117.]

artery pressure by methodology similar to the Gee-OPG technique. (See Chapter 10.)

CLINICAL APPLICATIONS

Clinical use of plethysmography includes (1) determination of segmental systolic arterial pressures in the upper or lower limb, including the digits, (2) determination of limb blood flow (volume) expressed in milliliters per minute per 100 g of tissue, (3) pulse registration of the fingers or toes, (4) penile waveform analysis, and (5) testing for the thoracic outlet syndrome.

Systolic Pressure Recording in Limbs

Although Doppler ultrasound methods have largely replaced the use of the plethysmograph for indirect measurement of limb or digital systolic arterial pressure, there are applications when recordings of toe pressure or finger pressure are required. The plethysmograph (strain-gauge or photoelectric) in a dc mode is of particular use to record finger or toe pressures because signals may be inaudible by Doppler in a low flow state. The dc mode is designed to detect instantaneous changes of volume by a shift of the baseline in the recorder. Such a shift is often used as the end point for systolic pressure determination during inflation of the pressure cuff. This technique is also useful to study finger pressure and its response to cold stimulation (3).

Limb Blood Flow

Recording of limb blood flow requires the use of the venous occlusion technique introduced by Brodie and Russell in 1903 (4). Since then, numerous studies have appeared on measurement of quantitative blood flow using this principle. In 1949, Whitney (5) first introduced the mercury-in-rubber strain-gauge for venous occlusive plethysmography, and this simple method has emerged as a standard plethysmographic technique for recording limb blood flow.

Limb volume changes instantaneously with the rate of arterial inflow and venous outflow. If a blood pressure cuff is placed around the thigh and then inflated to a suitable pressure, the venous outflow from the limb will be stopped without altering the rate of arterial inflow. The resulting increase in limb volume distal to the cuff is caused by a similar increase in blood volume. Initially, the rate of increase in venous blood volume is equal to the rate of arterial inflow. The limb volume change per minute is expressed as a percentage increase, or milliliters per 100 mL per minute.

In principle, the segment to be measured is encircled by a fine elastic tube filled with mercury, which is connected to an electrical resistance-measuring circuit. The measuring circuit detects change in the length of the gauge. According to the formula of Whitney (5), changes in the volume of the segment are derived from changes in its circumference. With no significant tissue compression beneath the gauge, the percentage change in gauge length per minute is equal to a similar change in the segment circumference. Assuming that the segment length (length of the limb) is constant, the percentage change in cross-sectional area per minute is equal to a similar percentage change in volume per minute (milliliters per 100 mL per minute). With the use of a Wheatstone bridge, the changes in strain-gauge length are represented as changes in electrical resistance that can, in turn, be graphically displayed on any standard recorder.

Calibration of the strain-gauge is done by a mechanical method (6). The gauge is calibrated by changing the length by a known amount with the adjustment screw and noting the resulting recorder deflection (X mm). The calibration deflection (X mm) is compared with the flow deflection (Y mm) to give actual changes in gauge length per minute following proximal venous occlusion. This is compared with the original gauge length and expressed as a percentage change in circumference per minute (equivalent to one-half the percentage change in segment volume per minute). Other investigators prefer electrical calibration, which allows "on limb" calibration to be carried out at any time during a period of flow measurement without handling the gauge.

Both calf and foot blood flow can be measured simultaneously by placing the gauge around the calf and the foot. Because of the makeup of tissue in the calf, composed largely of muscle, it is generally thought that calf blood flow is a representation of muscle blood flow. Similarly, the relative lack of muscle in the foot means that flow recorded there is representative of the skin blood flow.

Recording of the volume flow using milliliters per 100 g of tissue per minute obtained at the calf (muscle) or foot (skin) has long been of interest to physiologists studying vasomotor tone of the lower extremity in both health and disease states. For the study of the upper extremity, both forearm and digital flow may be recorded by a similar technique. In addition to resting flow, measurement of reactive hyperemic flow may be accomplished using a pressure cuff inflated above the systolic pressure for 3 to 5 minutes. Reactive hyperemic flow is designed primarily to evaluate the status of the vascular bed distal to the site of examination. Both resting and reactive hyperemic flows are of value in the study of vasomotor tone and the effect of vasodilating agents in the forearm or digits (fingers or toes). For occlusive arterial disease of the lower limb, however, resting flow has neither diagnostic nor prognostic value (7). Conversely, reactive hyperemic flow provides better information. Storen (8) as well as others (9,10) have shown the extent of hyperemic flow to be of diagnostic value in patients with occlusive arterial disease. Strandness and Bell (11) and Myers and Irvine (12) have shown a significant correlation between an increase ($>$ 50 percent) in pulse amplitude or volume flow during hyperemia and beneficial effects of lumbar sympathectomy.

In the clinical practice of vascular surgery, the use of calf (muscle) or skin (foot) flow is of limited value. Flow measurement may be useful in the evaluation of the acute effect of various pharmacologic agents.

Pulse Registration of Fingers or Toes

Strain-gauge, air-filled volume- and photoplethysmographs are useful to record the pulse volume of fingers or toes or a segment of the limb as an organ. Because the contour and volume of these pulses have diagnostic significance, this qualitative information has been used to supplement diagnostic information from indirect pressure determinations. Normal waveforms have a sharp upstroke and a distinct dicrotic notch (Figure 8-2). In the presence of occlusive arterial disease, pulse waveforms recorded distal to the occlusive process become rounded, with slow acceleration and loss of the dicrotic notch (Figure 8-2). In the fingers, a special configuration of a so-called peaked pulse (Figure 8-2*A*) may be seen in patients with small-vessel involvement, such as with collagen disease, Buerger's disease, frostbite, and traumatic arteritis (13). This peaked pulse has a fairly rapid upswing, an anacrotic notch or bend, and a dicrotic wave located high on the downslope. In addition to visual inspection of pulse contour, the ability of the peripheral arterioles to dilate can be assessed by a change of contour following reactive hyperemia. This is done by placing a pneumatic cuff around the finger proximal to the gauge and inflating the cuff to a pressure above the brachial systolic pressure. After a 5-minute period of ischemic arrest, the cuff is suddenly deflated, and the pulses are continuously recorded until maximal hyperemia is reached. In normal individuals, an increase of pulse contour (flow acceleration) is observed. In the presence of obstruction proximal to the digits, peak volume will be delayed.

Failure of the pulse volume to increase indicates the presence of fixed resistance either due to stiff arterioles or because maximal hyperemia has already occurred. In either case, vasodilatation or surgical sympathectomy would not be effective in these patients. In multilevel occlusive disease, the reactive hyperemic response may show a decrease of pulse volume, and this finding indicates the presence of severe ischemia.

Digital pulse recording may also be of use to assess sympathetic activity in patients with vasospastic disorders. This is done by observing the change of pulse contours during deep breathing, with ice placed on the forehead, or while the patient performs mental arithmetic. An increase of pulse volume suggests the presence of sympathetic activity. For quantitative analysis, pulse contour may be subjected to Fourier analysis (14).

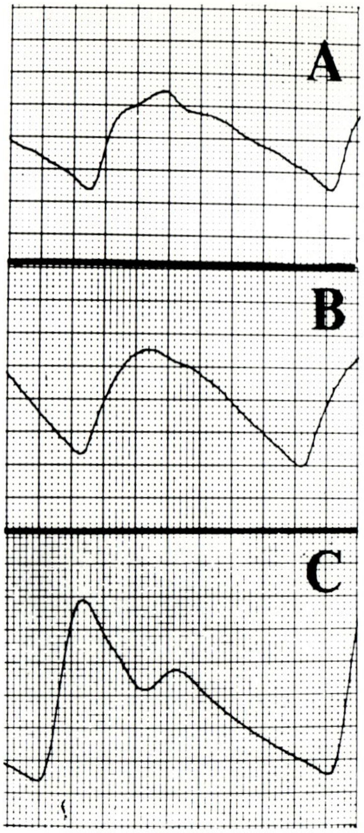

FIGURE 8-2. Finger pulse contour. *(A)* Peaked, *(B)* obstructive, *(C)* normal. (From Summer DS, Strandness DE: An abnormal finger pulse associated with cold sensitivity. Ann Surg 1972, 175:294–298.)

Penile Waveform Analysis

The use of the pulse-volume recorder or impedance plethysmograph to register penile pulse waveforms has been reported to be of value in the diagnosis of vasculogenic impotence (15,16).

Thoracic Outlet Testing

The photoplethysmograph sensor is a convenient tool to evaluate arterial thoracic outlet compression. The sensor is placed on the digits, and a change of pulse contour during various thoracic outlet maneuvers indicates the presence of thoracic outlet compression.

Doppler Segmental Pressure Determination in the Limbs

Since the introduction of the Doppler technique, recording of systolic pressure using a plethysmograph has received less attention. The Doppler technique is ideal for bedside, office, and intensive care monitoring. Although the technique of recording systolic pressure with the Doppler method is simple, the principles of measuring blood pressure must be observed in order to obtain accurate readings.

EQUIPMENT AND TECHNIQUE

Proper blood pressure cuffs, manometers, and control valves are prerequisites for accurate blood pressure recording. Regardless of the type of instrument used, the cuff size applied to the limb is of paramount importance in achieving accurate readings. An inflatable bladder is surrounded by an unyielding cover, called the cuff. The width of the bladder is critical. If it is too narrow (undercuffing), the blood pressure reading will be erroneously high, and if it is too wide (overcuffing), the reading may be too low. The American Heart Association (AHA) now recommends that the cuff size be based on limb circumference (17). It is recommended that the width of the inflatable bladder be 40 percent of the circumference of the midpoint of the limb, or 20 percent wider than the diameter. The length of the bladder should be twice its width (bladder length equal to 80 percent of the arm circumference). Table 8-1 lists the recommendations for blood pressure cuff bladder dimensions made by the AHA in 1980 (17).

Since the recording of ankle pressure closely parallels the recording of brachial pressure, the bladder dimension and ankle circumference must be taken into consideration for accurate measurement. For measurement of ankle blood pressure, the conventional arm cuff is sufficient. Standard adult arm cuffs used in clinical medicine at the present time contain an air-inflatable rubber bladder that is 23 cm long and 12 to 12.5 cm wide, which should be sufficient for use at the ankle level. Measurements using cuffs of this size yield values that agree with intraarterial measurements.

The size of the thigh cuff is important. It should be 18 to 20 cm wide. For recording pressure of the lower thigh, we have found that a 19-cm cuff is useful. Barnes (18) has suggested a narrow cuff (11 cm) for upper thigh pressure measurement. In obese patients, a wider cuff may be more appropriate because of the large size of the thigh.

Digital cuffs for recording finger or toe pressures may be constructed of a bladder made of Penrose drain on a backing of nylon Velcro strip. Digital cuff width varies from finger to toe. The proper width for a finger is 2 to 2.5 cm and for the toe, 2.5 to 3 cm. Table 8-2 summarizes the different sizes of cuffs that should be used for recording lower limb pressure.

Two types of pressure registering systems are in general use: the mercury gravity and the aneroid manometer. Both give accurate and reproducible results when working properly. The aneroid manometer is probably more versatile for bedside or laboratory use. If an aneroid manometer is used, the instrument should be calibrated yearly by interposing a Y-connector in the tube from the cuff to a mercury manometer and attaching the sphygmomanometer to be tested to the free end of the connector.

All measurements are made with the patient in the supine position after a 10- to 15-minute period of rest. Brachial pressure is recorded with the Doppler method or with a conventional stethoscope before lower limb pressure measurement.

Ankle Systolic Pressure

The arm pressure cuff is applied snugly above the malleolus. The cuff is then inflated above the brachial systolic pressure (about 20 to 30 mmHg). The end point of systolic pressure is determined by the reappearance of the pulse (an audible sound by Doppler method or pulse waveform by plethysmography). Two or three measurements should be made on each limb.

TABLE 8-1. Recommended Bladder Dimensions for Blood Pressure Cuffs

Arm Circumference at Midpoint,* cm	Cuff Name	Bladder Width, cm	Bladder Length, cm
5–7.5	Newborn	3	5
7.5–13	Infant	5	8
13–20	Child	8	13
17–26	Small adult	11	17
24–32	Adult	13	24
32–42	Large adult	17	32
42–50†	Thigh	20	42

*Midpoint of arm is defined as half the distance from the acromion to the olecranon.

†In persons with very large limbs, the indirect blood pressure should be measured in the leg or forearm.

SOURCE: From Kirkendall et al. (17). Used by permission of the American Heart Association, Inc.

TABLE 8-2. Recommended Cuff Size for Lower Limb Pressure Measurement

Location	Cuff Width, cm
Adult upper thigh	11
Adult lower thigh	19
Adult thigh (contour-type cuff)	22
Adult ankle	12
Adult finger	2–2.5
Adult toe	2.5–3

SOURCE: Reproduced by permission from Yao JST: Noninvasive techniques of measuring lower limb arterial pressures. In Bernstein EF (ed): *Noninvasive Diagnostic Techniques in Vascular Disease,* 3d ed, St Louis, Mosby, 1985, pp 1–24.

Upper Thigh Pressure

A narrow cuff (11 cm) is placed just below the inguinal ligament, and the Doppler probe is placed over the popliteal artery for end point determination.

Lower Thigh Pressure

The thigh cuff is applied just above the knee. If the Doppler technique is used, the sound probe is placed over the popliteal artery to detect sound signals. It has been shown that placing the sensor close to the pressure cuff is critical to obtain accurate thigh pressure measurement, especially in patients with multiple-level occlusions (19). If plethysmography is used, pulse registration is normally done on the big toe. The end point of the systolic pressure is determined by the same maneuver used to obtain the ankle pressure.

Toe Pressure

A strain-gauge or photosensor is placed on the big toe to record pulse or volume changes (dc mode), and the cuff is placed at the base of the toe.

Postexercise Measurements

Ankle pressure can be measured after exercise in a similar manner. Standard treadmill walking is used. Immediately after termination of the treadmill exercise, the patient resumes the supine position, and ankle pressure is recorded at 1-minute intervals until the pressure reaches the preexercise level. Exercise testing is not advisable if the patient has angina or a severe arrhythmia. When indicated, monitoring of cardiac rhythm during treadmill exercise is needed to ensure safety of the procedure.

Postischemic Measurements (Reactive Hyperemia)

To simulate the reactive hyperemia induced by exercise, a pressure cuff applied to the thigh may be used to induce distal ischemia. The cuff is inflated to a level of 50 mmHg above the systolic pressure for a period of 3 to 5 minutes and then abruptly deflated. Reactive hyperemia will follow immediately. Ankle systolic pressure is then recorded at 1-minute intervals until it returns to the resting pressure level.

CLINICAL APPLICATIONS

Segmental pressure measurements in the lower extremity include those at the high and low thigh, calf, and ankle levels. Also, toe pressure recorded by either the Doppler or photoplethysmograph may offer further hemodynamic information. Table 8-3 shows the normal values of systolic pressures commonly used in many vascular laboratories. Similar to all physiological measurements, ankle pressure is subject to variability, and this variation must be considered when evaluating the results of a longitudinal study. In our laboratory (20) as well as others (21), a change in the ankle pressure index of 0.15 is considered to be significant, but any change less than 0.15 is considered a result of measurement variation. Each laboratory must establish its own variability in this regard.

TABLE 8-3. Normal Values for Doppler Arterial Examination

Ankle systolic pressure	>Brachial systolic pressure (< 40 mmHg = limb-threatening ischemia)
Ankle pressure index (ankle-brachial ratio)	> 1.0
Thigh systolic pressure:	
High (narrow cuff)	30–40 mmHg > brachial systolic pressure
Low (wide cuff)	20–30 mmHg > brachial systolic pressure
Thigh pressure index	> 1.1
Pressure gradients	< 30 mmHg between adjacent sites
Toe systolic pressure	= to or 70% of brachial systolic pressure (< 30 mmHg = severe ischemia)
Toe systolic pressure index	0.7 ± 0.19 (0.35 ± 0.15 = claudication) (0.11 ± 0.10 = rest pain)
Penile pressure index	> 0.75 (0.60 ≐ vascular impotence)
Finger systolic pressure index	> 0.95
Treadmill exercise test (2 mph, 12% grade)	Elevated or no decrease of ankle pressure after 5 min walking time

SOURCE: Modified from Pearce WH, Yao JST, Bergan JJ: Noninvasive vascular diagnostic testing. Curr Probl Surg 1983, 20(no 8). Used by permission of Year Book Medical Publishers, Inc., Chicago, pp 460–538.

Diagnostic Use

The absence of a palpable pedal pulse often leads to the diagnosis of occlusive arterial disease. In borderline situations, such as in the presence of ankle edema or obesity, which make palpation of the pedal pulse difficult, the level of ankle pressure recorded by the Doppler technique often refutes or confirms the diagnosis instantly. In patients with occlusive arterial disease in whom the pedal pulses are not palpable, the Doppler flow velocity detector is able to detect flow signals from either the posterior tibial or dorsalis pedis artery. These flow signals represent the supply by collateral flow pathways, which could be used for registration of the systolic pressure end point by the indirect cuff technique.

Pressures measured at the thigh, calf, and ankle may aid in establishing the site or sites of occlusion. In the presence of iliac artery or common femoral artery occlusion alone, pressure recorded at these sites gives similar information, i.e., there is no pressure gradient. In contrast, a pressure gradient is noted between thigh and ankle levels when there is occlusion affecting the femoropopliteal segment. In multiple occlusions affecting the aortoiliac and femoropopliteal segments, different pressure gradients in the thigh and ankle are seen, with the ankle pressure being much lower than in patients with single occlusions.

In addition to establishing the diagnosis of arterial occlusive disease, recording of the ankle systolic pressure may help in detection of the popliteal artery entrapment syndrome. A marked decrease in ankle systolic pressure when the leg is placed in passive dorsiflexion and hyperextension suggests the presence of an entrapment syndrome. Also, when a steal phenomenon with an arteriovenous fistula is suspected, measurement of the ankle systolic pressure and observation of its change after compression of the fistula may help to confirm the diagnosis. An increase in systolic pressure with the arteriovenous fistula (proximal to the site of measurement) closed indicates a significant hemodiversion causing distal ischemia. With increasing use of the in situ vein graft, this diagnostic maneuver may help to determine the significance of an abnormal arteriovenous communication.

Degree of Ischemia

Ankle systolic pressure, when compared with the brachial systolic pressure, gives an index of ischemia. Such a pressure index, as suggested by Winsor (22), has been shown to correlate significantly with initial clinical symptoms and with angiographic findings (23). The majority of patients with claudication have a pressure index of 0.59 ± 0.15. A low pressure index (0.26 ± 0.13) is often seen in patients with rest pain. In patients with impending gangrene, the pressure index is often extremely low (0.05 ± 0.08) or unrecordable (23). In multiple-level disease, the ankle systolic pressure is usually much lower than with a single-segment occlusion.

The absolute level of ankle systolic pressure and the pressure index are useful to express hemodynamic data. The pressure index helps distinguish normal from abnormal limbs, whereas the absolute pressure level helps in determining limb viability. Figure 8-3 illustrates the receiver operating characteristic (ROC) curves reported by Ouriel and Zarins (24) for these two parameters in the diagnosis of arterial occlusive disease. Ankle-brachial pressure index was a better predictor of pressure or absence of disease than absolute ankle pressure. Ankle systolic pressure, however, is more useful to determine limb viability. Ankle systolic pressure less than 40 mmHg is indicative of limb-threatening ischemia, and such a level has been recommended as an objective hemodynamic criterion for defining critical ischemia (25). However, this parameter alone should not mandate interventional treatment since some patients can tolerate such pressures for protracted periods without difficulty.

In patients with symptoms of limb-threatening ischemia, recording of the toe pressure is necessary when the ankle pressure exceeds 40 mmHg. Carter and Lezack (26) have found that

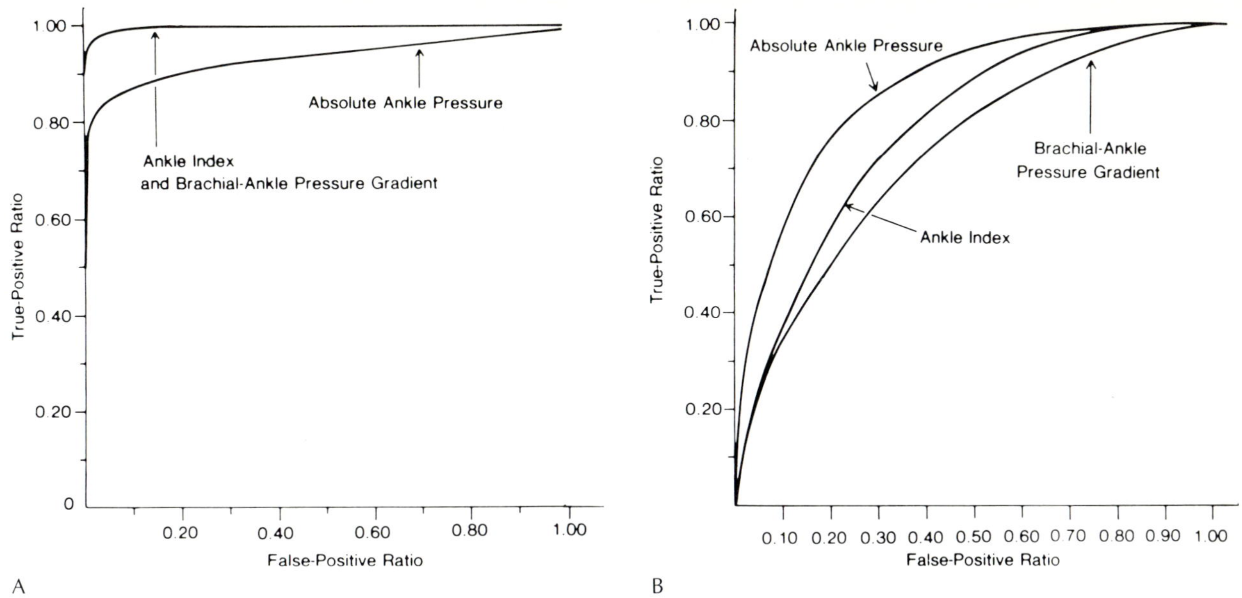

FIGURE 8-3. Receiver operator characteristic (ROC) curves illustrating the ability of absolute ankle pressure and ankle index to discriminate between normal and arteriographically diseased limbs *(A)*, and between viable and nonviable limbs *(B)*. (From Ouriel K, Zarins CK: Arch Surg 117:1297–1300, 1982. Copyright 1982, American Medical Association.)

systolic pressure in the toe was below 20 mmHg in 85 to 90 percent of limbs with rest pain, and below 40 mmHg in 100 percent. There was no difference between diabetics and nondiabetics. When arterial occlusion involves the plantar arteries, the toe pressure is a better index to establish the presence of severe ischemia. Also, toe pressure measurement is helpful in diabetic patients when an abnormally high ankle pressure is recorded. Toe pressure measurements may be subject to wide variation, however, and duplicate measurements may be needed for a reliable study (27).

The main objective in using the pressure index or critical level of ankle or toe systolic pressure is confirmation of the presence of severe ischemia. Although diagnosis of ischemic pain is not often difficult, the confirmatory finding of a low systolic pressure is rewarding, and it may help to differentiate ischemic pain from that of neurogenic origin, especially in patients with diabetic neuropathy. In high-risk patients, the decision to proceed with a limb salvage operation without objective documentation of severe ischemia may subject the patient to an unnecessary procedure.

Evaluation of Intermittent Claudication

Measurement of ankle pressure and observation of its change after standard treadmill exercise provide a simple test for the diagnosis of claudication of vascular origin. This is particularly true in patients initially having intermittent claudication who are found to have pedal pulses. These pulses, derived from collateral flow, often are associated with a decreased ankle pressure and often disappear after exercise. This "pulse-disappearing phenomenon" can be verified simply by recording the ankle pressure after exercise. When there is a significant drop in ankle pressure after exercise, the relationship between disability and arterial occlusion can be safely established. The relationship between postexercise ankle pressure and calf blood flow has been studied by plethysmographic and isotope techniques (28,29). A good correlation between flow and ankle pressure changes has been demonstrated. Since ankle pressure is easy to use, measurement of the ankle pressure response to exercise is now a standard laboratory test.

After treadmill exercise, the degree of ankle pressure drop and the time for the pressure to return to the preexercise level are the two important components that offer hemodynamic information. The degree of ankle pressure drop immediately after termination of exercise reflects the degree of inflow obstruction, whereas the recovery time denotes the adequacy of collateral pathways. In the presence of superficial femoral or femoropopliteal artery occlusion, the pressure drop is often to 50 percent of the preexercise level. In contrast, patients with iliac artery occlusion will have a greater drop in ankle pressure (70 to 90 percent) immediately after exercise because of shunting of blood to the thigh muscle group. The return of pressure to the preexercise level often occurs within 5 to 7 minutes because of the adequacy of collateral pathways in these patients. When two levels of occlusion are present, the picture becomes more complex. Following exercise, blood flow must traverse two collateral networks. A profound drop of ankle systolic pressure, often to an unrecordable level, results. Likewise, the recovery time is prolonged because of multiple levels of occlusion. An understanding of these hemodynamic changes helps determine the type of surgical corrective procedure to be used in these patients.

Treadmill exercise testing also helps to evaluate claudicants with an occult angiographic stenotic lesion or an inapparent stenosis on the anteroposterior (AP) view of the arteriogram. In this circumstance, treadmill exercise establishes the hemodynamic significance of the iliac artery lesion.

Treadmill exercise is helpful in differentiating between atypical claudication and neurogenic claudication. A normal exercise response in a patient with exercise intolerance virtually eliminates a vascular etiology. In patients with coexisting neurospinal compression and arterial occlusive disease, a decision regarding appropriate therapy may be based upon the results of exercise testing (30).

Because of the nature of atherosclerotic disease, it is not surprising to find that patients with claudication may also have asymptomatic ischemic heart disease. The latter may assume clinical significance during stress testing. With the increasing use of the treadmill for assessing claudicants, the necessity for cardiac monitoring in these patients has become apparent. In a series of 100 consecutive claudicants who did not have any cardiac symptoms, the electrocardiogram was recorded at rest and during treadmill exercise. Evidence of ischemic heart disease was present in 56 percent of these patients at rest, and gross ischemic changes (for example, a 4-mm ST-segment depression), including arrhythmias, developed in 20 percent during exercise (31). A significant increase in cardiac arrhythmias in patients undergoing treadmill testing for claudication has been reported by others (32). In one study of 16 patients who developed abnormal ECG findings during exercise, 6 suffered a myocardial infarction after vascular reconstructive surgery (33). Although complications of the treadmill test are rare, the sequelae are potentially serious. To ensure safety and guard against litigation, treadmill exercise testing is best avoided in claudicants with overt cardiac abnormalities. Moreover, treadmill testing in claudicants should be done with cardiac monitoring and with resuscitation equipment and medical personnel trained in its use present in the laboratory.

The reproducibility of the standard treadmill test has been investigated in a series of 117 patients with stable claudication (34). Paired treadmill tests were done 1 week apart. The Doppler pressures were reproducible for the group as a whole, but there was a marked individual variation. The coefficient of variation was 15 percent for the pressures in the better leg and 24 percent in the more symptomatic leg. In the recent report by Ouriel and Zarins (24), a relative standard deviation of 15.6 percent for treadmill exercise and 14.7 percent for postocclusive reactive hyperemia was described. It was also found that brachial pressure after exercise was, on the average, 20 mmHg higher than the preexercise level (35). Failure of the brachial pressure to increase in response to exercise, or the finding of a decrease, is suggestive of poor myocardial performance.

Evaluation of Inflow (Aortoiliac Segment)

The importance of recognizing iliac artery stenosis before superficial femoral artery reconstruction has been stressed by many authors (see Chapter 28). Failure to correct a significant inflow lesion often results in occlusion of a femorodistal bypass or failure to improve hemodynamic status. When there is angiographic evidence of stenotic lesions affecting both the iliac and superficial femoral arteries, the crucial lesion producing the ischemic symptoms must be identified. Evaluation of inflow can be assisted by (1) common femoral artery waveform analysis, (2) thigh pressure measurement, (3) thigh-ankle pressure gradient, and (4) ankle pressure response to exercise. However, all these data must be correlated with clinical and arteriographic findings, and some groups find these noninvasive tests to be of little value in assessing combined segment disease (see Chapter 28). For claudicants, the use of treadmill testing offers more conclusive information.

To identify iliac artery stenosis, Bone et al. (36) have recommended the use of a narrow cuff to record upper thigh pressure. In our laboratory, as well as others (37), it has been found that the upper thigh pressure measurement adds little information on the status of inflow. The presence of a superficial femoral artery occlusion alters the result of upper thigh pressure recordings. Whereas a normal upper thigh pressure is generally reliable in ruling out hemodynamically significant aortiliac occlusive disease, an abnormal pressure does not differentiate between aortoiliac and superficial femoral artery disease. In the study by Flanigan et al. (37), it was found that the upper thigh pressure could not identify a significant iliac lesion when there was an associated femoropopliteal artery occlusion. Inconclusive thigh pressure readings may also be caused by artifacts of the thigh cuff (38) or the presence of a calcified superficial femoral artery. If there is difficulty in determining which lesion is hemodynamically significant, some authors have recommended intraoperative pressure measurement with pharmacologic vasodilatation (39,40).

Using the ankle pressure measurement and flow waveform recordings from the common femoral artery, the hemodynamic significance of anatomic disease in the iliac artery can be estimated. The presence of a monophasic common femoral artery waveform and the absence of a significant thigh-ankle pressure gradient indicate a significant inflow lesion. On the contrary, a segmental pressure measurement that shows a significant pressure gradient (greater than 30 mmHg) between thigh and ankle levels and a triphasic femoral waveform signify that the occlusion of the femoropopliteal segment is of hemodynamic significance. The degree of ankle pressure drop following treadmill exercise is also helpful in the evaluation of proximal arterial lesions. Since there is only minor shunting of blood to the thigh muscles, patients with femoropopliteal disease alone have only moderate reduction in postexercise ankle pressure. Conversely, inflow disease of the aortoiliac segment produces more profound drops in ankle pressure. When functionally significant disease is present in both arterial segments, ankle pressures often fall to zero following exercise and remain depressed for a prolonged period. Correction of the aortoiliac arterial occlusion often reverts the postexercise pattern to that of a single anatomic occlusion.

Obviously, the hemodynamic data must be correlated with presenting symptoms. For claudication, the use of exercise testing or reactive hyperemia is needed to achieve an adequate assessment. When a femorofemoral graft is considered, the adequacy of the donor artery inflow must be evaluated by treadmill exercise. A decrease in ankle pressure in the donor limb after exercise is ominous. In our analysis of 44 patients who underwent femorofemoral grafting for claudication, 20 (45 percent) of the patients had deterioration of donor limb hemodynamics after surgery. Seven of 14 patients who had abnormal treadmill exercise testing preoperatively had worsening of the ankle pressure response to exercise of the donor limb. On the other hand, a femorofemoral graft may remain functional and effective even when there is less than perfect inflow, especially if the procedure is done for limb salvage. It would appear that strict patient selection criteria are needed when femorofemoral grafting is done for claudication.

Selection of Patients for Femorodistal Bypass

A low ankle pressure or unrecordable pressure does not indicate an unsalvageable situation. Several studies have now shown that the level of ankle pressure bears little relation to the prognosis of a femorodistal bypass (41,42). However, ankle pressure recording prior to reconstructive surgery below the inguinal ligament may be helpful (1) to supplement arteriographic findings and (2) to determine the exact site of distal anastomosis.

In the absence of acute occlusion, a low or unrecordable ankle pressure in patients with chronic ischemia caused by a femoropopliteal occlusion suggests the presence of severe occlusive disease distal to the popliteal trifurcation. Therefore, arteriographic examination must include the arteries in the calf and ankle region. In our recent analysis (43), the level of ankle pressure or the pressure index correlated well with the status of popliteal artery run-off in patients with normal aortoiliac inflow. In the presence of severe popliteal occlusive disease with involvement of the tibial or peroneal artery, the pressure index was often much lower (0.22 ± 0.13) than in patients with patent vessels distal to the popliteal trifurcation (0.55 ± 0.09). Also, the pressure gradient between the thigh and ankle helps to determine the severity of popliteal disease with tibial vessel involvement. When severe trifurcation disease is present, a large pressure gradient may develop between the lower thigh and ankle levels. In this situation, a reconstruction with the anastomosis placed into a tibial vessel to bypass the segments having the pressure gradient is desirable. A bypass graft to the popliteal artery proximal to diseased tibial and peroneal arteries is frequently associated with thrombosis (44), although this may not always be the case (see Chapter 26). In chronic ischemia, therefore, very low ankle pressure mandates complete arteriography including examination below the popliteal trifurcation.

The ankle pressure is helpful to supplement arteriographic findings when there is nonvisualization of arteries distal to the popliteal trifurcation on the preoperative arteriogram, especially the translumbar aortogram. The presence of a recordable pressure invariably indicates an operable situation (45), and nonvisualization by arteriography should not be an indication for amputation. Also, the difference between pressure recorded from the dorsalis pedis and posterior tibial arteries may help to determine the exact site of distal anastomosis. This is especially true in patients with inadequate visualization of distal arteries on preoperative arteriography.

Determination of Response to Sympathetic Ablation

The use of pressure studies to determine the response to sympathetic ablation will be discussed in Chapter 32, and hence, will not be repeated here. The importance of pressure measurements in relation to sympathectomy lies in the selection of patients who will certainly not respond to the procedure. Unless there is adequate distal perfusion (> 30 mmHg), lumbar sympathectomy is seldom effective. These patients, when identified preoperatively, will be spared an unnecessary operation (see Chapters 26 and 32 for even more restrictive views regarding sympathectomy).

Selection of Amputation Level and Prediction of Wound Healing after Minor Amputation

Determining the level of amputation for severe, uncorrectable ischemia remains a challenging problem, particularly after failed femoropopliteal or femorotibial grafting. A major objective of noninvasive technology has been to predict the most distal amputation that would heal primarily. Doppler segmental pressure measurement is a simple method to obtain helpful information. In a series of 66 patients who had major amputations, we used the ankle systolic pressure; the waveforms recorded from the posterior tibial, anterior tibial, and dorsalis pedis arteries; and the pressure in the lower thigh to determine the level of amputation (46). Our data suggest that, when there is no detectable flow in the popliteal artery, an above-knee amputation is advisable. On the other hand, detectable flow in the popliteal artery allows the recording of thigh pressure, and if the thigh pressure exceeds 50 mmHg, a below-knee amputation should be attempted because the chance for success is high. This has also been suggested by other authors (47,48). All patients who had audible signals at the posterior tibial or dorsalis pedis artery had a successful below-knee amputation. Of course, the use of pressure level alone may be fallacious, because the presence of infection and the operative technique strongly influence the surgical result. Nicholas (49), using a calf systolic pressure greater than 70 torr and an ankle pressure greater than 30 torr as an index that below-knee amputation would heal, found that this could not be achieved in 32 and 40 percent of cases, respectively.

Measurement of ankle pressure alone may not be sufficient to determine the success of minor amputation, including digit or forefoot amputation, and the use of toe pressure is needed to predict wound healing. Carter has stated that the chance of healing was nearly 100 percent in nondiabetic patients if digital pressure exceeded 30 mmHg (50). In diabetics, healing occurred in 75 percent of limbs with a pressure of 30 to 55 mmHg, and in 95 percent with higher pressures. A similar result has been reported by others, especially by Scandinavian investigators (51,52).

Photoplethysmography (PPG) may be used instead of Doppler ultrasound or strain-gauge recording. Using a PPG end point of 20 mmHg, Schwartz et al. (53) and Barnes et al. (54) observed uniform healing in all minor forefoot and digital amputations. Forefoot pulse-volume recording waveforms of only 4 mm or less have also been used to indicate that a toe or partial foot amputation will not heal (see Chapter 26).

Similar to selection of patients for lumbar sympathectomy, the purpose of pressure measurements to determine the level of amputation is to avoid an unnecessary amputation at a level where healing cannot occur.

Determination of Graft Patency and Graft Limb Occlusion after Reconstructive Surgery

The return of a pedal pulse usually indicates successful surgery, but the variability in palpation of pulses by different observers, especially in borderline cases and in the presence of postoperative edema, often makes this method unreliable. Doppler ankle pressure measurement offers a simple and reliable method of assessing the patency of arterial reconstructions. Determination of ankle systolic pressure can be made as often as required and is of particular value in patients in whom a residual lesion is present, making the return of a palpable pedal pulse unlikely. This situation is often encountered in patients with occlusions affecting both the aortoiliac and superficial femoral arteries, where reconstruction is done only at the aortoiliac level. It may also be seen in patients with occlusion of the femoropopliteal artery and severe disease below the trifurcation of the popliteal artery. In deep femoral artery reconstruction, where there is a concomitant occlusion of the femoropopliteal segment, ankle systolic pressure recording is probably the only reliable, objective method to ascertain the result of operation.

Successful arterial reconstruction in single-segment disease (aortoiliac or superficial femoral) is always followed by an immediate increase in ankle pressure to a level close to a pressure index of 1.0 at the termination of the surgical procedure or within 6 hours postoperatively. On occasion, despite the absence of palpable pedal pulses immediately following the procedure, a delayed return of ankle pressure may be observed, especially with vein grafts. As long as the ankle pressure is not less than the preoperative level, continuous monitoring of pressure at hourly intervals will help to determine graft patency. Infrequently, the return of ankle pressure is delayed after aortoiliac reconstructions because of prolonged clamping of the aorta or excessive blood loss. In these cases, low thigh pressure recording is helpful to determine the success of the operation. Usually, after the effects of all anesthetic agents are dissipated 6 hours or more after surgery, ankle pressure returns to a higher level than before surgery. The use of thigh pressure is also helpful in composite-sequential bypasses, demonstrating the patency of the proximal bypass even when the ankle pressure is not improved after the procedure.

Ankle pressure recording is a simple method to monitor patency of arterial reconstructions. Perhaps the greatest value of this technique is in detection of failure when success has been assumed. Failure of a reconstruction is indicated by a steady drop in ankle pressure or ankle pressure index in the immediate postoperative period, or by failure of ankle pressure to improve to higher than the preoperative level in a 6- to 12-hour observation period. Early return to the operating room for correction of technical error often converts failure to success. The simplicity of ankle pressure measurement allows nursing personnel to perform hourly determinations in the recovery room and intensive care unit. Such measurements should be made routinely in addition to palpation of pedal pulses in all hospitals dealing with vascular reconstructive procedures.

Evaluation of New Treatment Modalities and Follow-up of Bypass Grafts

The use of noninvasive tests is essential in epidemiological settings for the diagnosis of atherosclerotic peripheral arterial disease and for recording the progress of the disease process. In an epidemiological study, Marinelli et al. (55) have found clinical examination of pulses to be totally unreliable. One-fifth of the patients with normal physical examination results were found to have abnormal results by ankle pressure determination. Recently, the American Heart Association Council on Epidemiology has recommended the use of Doppler ultrasound to record the ankle-arm pressure index before and after standard treadmill exercise as a diagnostic tool for field studies (56). The ankle pressure index can serve as baseline data to follow the natural history of the disease.

New therapeutic procedures are always being introduced as alternative treatments to surgery, and Doppler ultrasound examination provides an objective means to evaluate these procedures. The efficacy of transluminal balloon dilatation or thrombolytic therapy, for example, needs to be verified objectively. Several studies (57,58) have demonstrated that the results of balloon dilatation, when assessed by hemodynamic measurement, are inferior to those obtained by assessment of symptomatic improvement alone. The role of vasodilating agents in the treatment of claudication remains unclear. Evaluation of such vasodilator treatment can be obtained, since resting and exercise ankle systolic pressures provide objective tests to determine the efficacy of this pharmacologic approach (59). More importantly, assessment of the result of any type of reconstructive surgery by an objective technique is essential to establish the effectiveness of the procedure. For instance, we have found that the femorofemoral graft is effective in limb salvage situations, but that the procedure gives less than optimal results in patients with claudication (60). There has been concern about the effect of knee flexion on limb hemodynamics when prosthetic grafts are used, but ankle pressure measurement has demonstrated no ill effect during knee flexion (61).

In later follow-up, ankle pressure measurement has, in our hands, been the single most useful method to detect graft stenosis (62) and to confirm graft occlusion. A steady decrease in ankle pressure is indicative of progression of the disease distal to the bypass or of graft stenosis. The latter is frequently observed in patients with saphenous vein grafts.

A patent bypass graft by arteriography has been considered the hallmark of success of reconstructive arterial surgery. In contrast to this belief, a bypass graft may be patent by arteriography yet provide no functional improvement. This patent, but hemodynamically failed, graft can be detected by serial Doppler ultrasound examinations. A decrease in ankle pressure of 0.15 is considered to be hemodynamically significant and calls for repeat arteriography. A hemodynamically failed graft, if recognized early, may be corrected by surgery before graft thrombosis occurs (63). The frequent use of Doppler ankle pressure recording during the follow-up period should be routine in the assessment of the results of reconstructive arterial surgery.

Finally, postoperative or follow-up study by noninvasive techniques can determine whether an additional reconstructive procedure is necessary to achieve the desired result. The need for a further bypass procedure is often seen in patients who have multiple-level disease and in whom a proximal reconstruction is performed in the presence of a distal occlusion. If there is no improvement in the ankle pressure after aortoiliac or deep femoral artery reconstruction, a distal bypass graft to relieve symptoms is often warranted.

LIMITATIONS OF DOPPLER SEGMENTAL PRESSURE MEASUREMENT

In diabetics or in azotemic patients, it is not uncommon to find an abnormally elevated pressure because of calcification of the arterial wall. Systolic pressure may exceed 300 mmHg if there is an incompressible artery caused by circumferential calcification. Under this circumstance, recording pulse waveforms from the pedal arteries or toe pressure measurement will help to determine the status of ischemia. False-elevated systolic pressure is a limitation of indirect pressure measurement. On the other hand, the presence of a pressure > 300 mmHg invariably indicates arterial wall calcification.

Acknowledgments

This work was supported in part by the Conrad Jobst Foundation, the Seabury Foundation, and the Northwestern Vascular Foundation.

References

1. Raines JK, Darling RC, Buth J, Brewster DC, Austin WG: Vascular laboratory criteria for the management of peripheral vascular disease of the lower extremities. Surgery 1976, 79:21–29.
2. Hertzmann AB: The blood supply of various skin areas as estimated by the photoelectric plethysmograph. Am J Physiol 1938, 124:328.
3. Nielsen PE, Bell G, Lassen NA: The measurement of digital systolic blood pressure by strain-gauge technique. Scand J Clin Lab Invest 1972, 29:371.
4. Brodie TG, Russell AE: On the determination of rate of blood flow through an organ. J Physiol 1905, 32:47.
5. Whitney RJ: The measurement of volume changes in human limbs. J Physiol 1953, 121:1.
6. Needham TN: The measurement of blood flow: Strain gauge plethysmography. Bio-Med Engineering, July, 1972, pp 266–269.
7. Yao JST, Needham TN, Gourmos C, Irvine WT: A comparative study of strain-gauge plethysmography and Doppler ultrasound in the assessment of occlusive arterial disease of the lower extremities. Surgery 1972, 71:4–9.
8. Støren G: Postischemic calf volume recording in functional evaluation of patients with intermittent claudication. Scand J Clin Lab Invest 1969, 23:339.
9. Shepherd JC: The blood flow through the calf after exercise in subjects with arteriosclerosis and claudication. Clin Sci 1950, 9:49.
10. Jacobs S, Reich T: Calf blood flow in intermittent claudication. Arch Surg 1975, 110:1465.
11. Strandness DE Jr, Bell JW: Peripheral vascular disease: Diagnosis and objective evaluation using a mercury strain gauge. Ann Surg 1965, 161(suppl):1–35.
12. Myers KA, Irvine WT: An objective study of lumbar sympathectomy. I. Intermittent claudication. Br Med J 1966, 52:879.
13. Sumner DS, Lambeth A, Russell JB: Diagnosis of upper extremity obstructive and vasospastic syndromes by Doppler ultrasound, plethysmography, and temperature profiles. In Puel P, Boccalon H, Enjalbert A (eds): *Hemodynamics of the Limbs I*. Toulouse, France, GEPESC, 1979, pp 365–373.
14. Strandness DE Jr, Sumner DS: *Hemodynamics for Surgeons*. New York, Grune & Stratton, 1975.
15. Kempczinski RF: Role of the vascular diagnostic laboratory in the evaluation of male impotence. Am J Surg 1979, 138:278–282.
16. DePalma RG, Kedia K, Persky L: Vascular operations for preservation of sexual function. In Bergan JJ, Yao JST (ed): *Surgery of the Aorta and Its Body Branches*. New York, Grune & Stratton, 1979, pp 277–296.
17. Kirkendall WM, Feinleib M, Freis ED, Mark AL: Recommendations for human blood pressure determination by sphygmomanometers. Subcommittee of the AHA Postgraduate Education Committee. Circulation 1980, 62:1146A–1155A.
18. Bridges RA, Barnes RW: Segmental limb pressures. In Kempczinski RF, Yao JST (ed): *Practical Noninvasive Vascular Diagnosis*. Chicago, Year Book Medical Publishers, 1982, pp 79–92.
19. Franzeck UK, Bernstein EF, Fronek A: The effect of sensing site on the limb segmental blood pressure determination. Arch Surg 1981, 116:912.
20. Yao JST: Discussion of Baker JD, Dix D: Surgery 1981, 89:137.
21. Baker JD, Dix D: Variability of Doppler ankle pressures with arterial occlusive disease: An evaluation of ankle index and brachial-ankle pressure gradient. Surgery 1981, 89:134–137.
22. Winsor T: Influence of arterial disease on the systolic blood pressure gradients of the extremity. Am J Med Sci 1950, 220:117.
23. Yao JST, Hobbs JT, Irvine WT: Ankle systolic pressure measurement in arterial disease affecting the lower extremities. Br J Surg 1969, 56:676.
24. Ouriel K, Zarins CK: Doppler ankle pressure. An evaluation of three methods of expression. Arch Surg 1982, 117:1297–1300.
25. Jamieson CW: Editorial. The definition of critical ischaemia of a limb. Br J Surg 1982, 69(suppl):S-2.
26. Carter SA, Lezack JD: Digital systolic pressures in the lower limb in arterial disease. Circulation 1971, 43:905–914.
27. Sondergroth TR, Salles-Cunha SX, Vollrath KD, Towne JB: Variability of toe pressure measurements. Bruit 1982, 6:14–16.
28. Lewis JD, Papathanasiou C, Yao JST, Eastcott HHG: Simultaneous flow and pressure measurements in intermittent claudication. Br J Surg 1972, 59:418–423.
29. Sumner DS, Strandness DE: The relationship between calf blood flow and ankle blood pressure in patients with intermittent claudication. Surgery 1969, 65:763–771.
30. Goodreau JJ, Creasy JK, Flanigan DP, Burnham SJ, Kudrna JC, Schafer MF, Bergan JJ, Yao JST: Rational approach to the differentiation of vascular and neurogenic claudication. Surgery 1978, 84:749–757.
31. Kovamees SA, Brundin T: Continuous electrocardiography recording and examination of walking capacity in patients with intermittent claudication. J Cardiovasc Surg 1976, 17:509–513.
32. Carroll RM, Rose HB, Vyden J: Cardiac arrhythmias associated with treadmill claudication testing. Surgery 1978, 83:284–287.
33. Cutler B, Wheeler HB, Panaskos JA, Cardullo PA: Assessment of operative risk with electrocardiographic exercise testing in patients with peripheral vascular disease. Am J Surg 1979, 137:484–490.
34. Clyne CN, Tripolitis A, Jamieson CW: The reproducibility of the treadmill walking test for claudication. Surg Gynecol Obstet 1979, 149:727–731.
35. Yao JST, O'Mara CS, Flinn WR, Blackburn D, Bergan JJ: Postoperative evaluation of graft failure. In Bernhard VM, Towne JB (eds): *Complications in Vascular Surgery*. New York, Grune & Stratton, 1980, pp 1–19.
36. Bone GE, Hayes AC, Slaymaker EE, Barnes RW: Value of segmental limb pressures in predicting results of aorto-femoral bypass. Am J Surg 1976, 132:733–738.
37. Flanigan DP, Gray B, Schuler JJ, Schwartz JA, O'Connor RJA, Williams LR: Utility of wide and narrow blood pressure cuffs in the hemodynamic assessment of aortoiliac occlusive disease. Surgery 1982, 92:16–20.
38. Bernstein EF, Witzel TH, Stotts JS, Fronek A: Thigh pressure artifacts with noninvasive techniques in an experimental model. Surgery 1981, 89:319–323.
39. Flanigan DP, Ryan TJ, Williams LR, Schwartz JA, Gray B, Schuler JJ: Aortofemoral or femoropopliteal revascularization? A pro-

spective evaluation of the papaverine test. J Vasc Surg 1984, 1:215–223.

40. Archie JP Jr, Feldtman RW: Intraoperative assessment of the hemodynamic significance of iliac and profunda femoris artery stenosis. Surgery 1981, 90:876–880.
41. Corson JD, Johnson WC, LoGerfo FW, Bush HL Jr, Menzoian JO, Kumaki DJ, Nabseth DC: Doppler ankle systolic blood pressure: Prognostic value in vein bypass grafts of the lower extremity. Arch Surg 1978, 113:932–935.
42. Williams LR, Flanigan DP, Schuler JJ, O'Connor RJA, Castronuovo JJ: Prediction of improvement in ankle blood pressure following arterial bypass. J Surg Res 1984, 37:175–179.
43. Yao JST, Nicolaides AN: Transcutaneous Doppler ultrasound in the management of lower limb ischemia. In Nicolaides AN, Yao JST (eds): *Investigation of Vascular Disorders*. London, Churchill Livingstone, 1981, pp 249–273.
44. Dean RH, Yao JST, Stanton PE, Bergan JJ: Prognostic indicators in femoro-popliteal reconstructions. Arch Surg 1975, 110:1287–1293.
45. Ricco JB, Pearce WH, Yao JST, Flinn WR: The use of operative pre-bypass arteriography and Doppler ultrasound recordings to select patients for extended femoro-distal bypass. Ann Surg 1983, 198:646–653.
46. Dean RH, Yao JST, Thompson RG, Bergan JJ: Predictive value of ultrasonically derived arterial pressure in determination of amputation level. Am Surg 1975, 41:731–737.
47. Barnes RW, Shanik GD, Slaymaker EE: An index of healing below the knee amputations using leg blood pressure by Doppler ultrasound. Surgery 1976, 79:13–20.
48. Lee BY, Trainer FS, Kavner D: Noninvasive hemodynamic evaluation in selection of amputation level. Surg Gynecol Obstet 1979, 149:241–244.
49. Nicholas GG, Myers JL, DeMuth W: The role of the vascular laboratory. Criteria in the selection of patients for lower extremity amputation. Ann Surg 1982, 195:469–473.
50. Carter SA: Role of pressure measurements in vascular disease. In Bernstein EF (ed): *Noninvasive Diagnostic Techniques in Vascular Disease*, 2d ed. St Louis, Mosby, 1982, pp 317–343.
51. Tønnesen KH, Noer I, Paaske W, Sager P: Classification of peripheral occlusive arterial diseases based on symptoms, signs, and distal blood pressure measurements. Acta Chir Scand 1980, 146:101–104.
52. Paaske WP, Tønnesen KH: Prognostic significance of distal blood pressure measurements in patients with severe ischaemia. Scan J Thorac Cardiovasc Surg 1980, 14:105–108.
53. Schwartz JA, Schuler JJ, O'Connor RJA, Flanigan DP: Predictive value of distal perfusion pressure in the healing of the digits and the forefoot. Surg Gynecol Obstet 1982, 154:865–869.
54. Barnes RW, Thornhill B, Nix L, Rittgers SE, Turley G: Prediction of amputation wound healing. The roles of Doppler ultrasound and digit photoplethysmography. Arch Surg 1981, 116:80–83.
55. Marinelli MR, Beach KW, Glass MJ, Primozich JF, Strandness DE Jr: Noninvasive testing vs. clinical evaluation of arterial disease. A prospective study. JAMA 1979, 241:2031–2034.
56. Prineas RJ, Harland WR, Janzon L, Kannel W: Recommendations for use of non-invasive methods to detect atherosclerotic peripheral arterial disease—in population studies. American Heart Association Council on Epidemiology. Circulation 1982, 65:1561A–1566A.
57. O'Mara CS, Neiman HL, Flinn WR, Herman RJ, Yao JST, Bergan JJ: Hemodynamic assessment of transluminal angioplasty for lower extremity ischaemia, Surgery 1981, 89:106–117.
58. Flanigan DP, Schuler JJ, Spigos DG, Lim LT: Anatomic and hemodynamic evaluation of percutaneous transluminal angioplasty. Surg Gynecol Obstet 1982, 154:181–185.
59. Porter JM, Baur GM: Pharmacologic treatment of intermittent claudication. Surgery 1982, 92:966–971.
60. Harris JP, Flinn WR, Rudo ND, Bergan JJ, Yao JST: Assessment of donor limb hemodynamics in femorofemoral bypass for claudication. Surgery 1981, 90:764–773.
61. Burnham SJ, Flanigan DP, Goodreau JJ, Yao JST, Bergan JJ: Nonvein bypass in below-knee reoperation for lower limb ischemia. Surgery 1978, 84:417–424.
62. Pearce WH, Yao JST, Bergan JJ: Noninvasive vascular diagnostic testing. Curr Prob Surg 1983, 20(8):460–538.
63. O'Mara CS, Flinn WR, Johnson ND, Bergan JJ, Yao JST: Recognition and surgical management of patent but hemodynamically failed arterial grafts. Ann Surg 1981, 193:467–476.

Chapter 9

ULTRASOUND AND COMPUTERIZED TOMOGRAPHY IN THE EVALUATION OF ARTERIAL ANEURYSMS

EUGENE F. BERNSTEIN and RONALD D. HARRIS

Aneurysms of the arterial tree are common and dangerous lesions which represent a threat to life because they frequently rupture (1,2). In the thoracic aorta they may be due to Marfan's syndrome, dissection, trauma, lues, or atherosclerosis. Below the diaphragm they are almost invariably due to atherosclerosis, although there are exceptional cases associated with mycotic infections and other unusual entities. Because of their threat to life, it is critical to be able to confirm the diagnosis in a reliable fashion. In addition, it is often useful to obtain information about the size of the aneurysm in three dimensions and also to learn about the anatomy of other structures in relation to it.

A clinical diagnosis of aneurysm may be made on the basis of the physical examination, particularly for the abdominal aorta and the femoral and popliteal arteries. However, sometimes these physical findings can be unreliable, since aortic aneurysms can be missed in obese patients and since overlying retroperitoneal and other visceral masses may simulate aneurysms in the abdomen, especially in thin patients with easily transmitted aortic pulsations. Moreover, a tortuous aorta or iliac arteries may mimic an aneurysm. Thus to avoid unnecessary surgery, it is critical to obtain independent and objective confirmation of the diagnosis. In addition, more detailed information concerning the size and configuration of abdominal aneurysms increases the data base from which a decision for surgery may be made, particularly in poor-risk patients with small, asymptomatic aneurysms.

Conventional contrast, digital subtraction, and isotope angiograms have been advocated for the diagnosis and characterization of abdominal aortic aneurysms (3–8). However, all angiographic studies define only the inner lumen of the aneurysm and may provide grossly inaccurate data regarding the overall aneurysmal size. Further, conventional contrast angiography is invasive and expensive and has a small but definite complication rate (9). Therefore, angiography should not be performed as a primary diagnostic procedure for most aneurysms, but rather as a preoperative investigation, when indicated, after surgery has definitely been decided upon. The purpose of the angiogram is to further delineate the anatomy of paraaneurysmal structures, with particular emphasis on renal artery and visceral vessel lesions, the presence of iliac aneurysms, and the distribution of iliofemoral occlusive disease.

Role of Ultrasound and Computerized Tomography

Ultrasonic techniques first became available for the diagnosis of abdominal aortic aneurysms in 1966 with the publications by Goldberg (10) and Segal (11), and achieved widespread clinical use for this purpose by the early 1970s (12–21). In 1976, with the introduction of CT body scanning, this technique was also rapidly recognized as a valuable radiodiagnostic tool (22–24). Both ultrasound and CT scanning are excellent imaging modalities for the study of arterial aneurysms. Both permit the routine documentation of the presence or absence of an aneurysm and accurately depict its configuration, location, and size. The two methods appear to be equally accurate in properly diagnosing conditions in which aortic ectasia, tortuosity, an overlying abdominal mass, or a normal aorta in an asthenic person has mimicked an aneurysm sufficiently to cause a clinical suspicion of aneurysm. Both techniques are safe, fast, noninvasive, and easily performed on an outpatient basis. In addition, their fine detail also provides added information about other structures important to the surgeon at the time of the operation.

Accuracy of Ultrasound Techniques

A beam of ultrasound moving in the transducer plane of section is reflected from various tissues, and those echoes can be detected to produce images on a video screen in accordance with the transducer position and the echo characteristics of the tissue, thus providing a two-dimensional impression of the interior of the body. In this procedure, referred to as B-mode scanning or

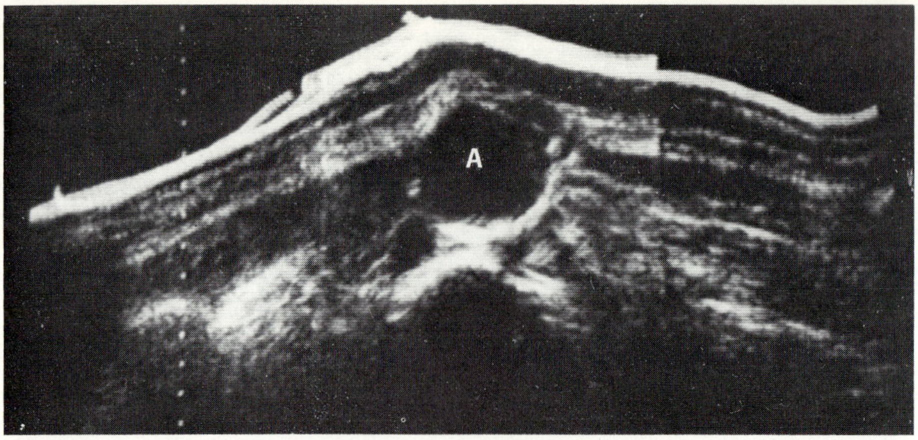

FIGURE 9-1. A B-scan echogram in the transverse plane, demonstrating an abdominal aortic aneurysm (A). (From Bernstein EF: *Noninvasive Diagnostic Techniques in Vascular Disease*, ed 2. St Louis, Mosby, 1982, p 419. With permission of the CV Mosby Co.)

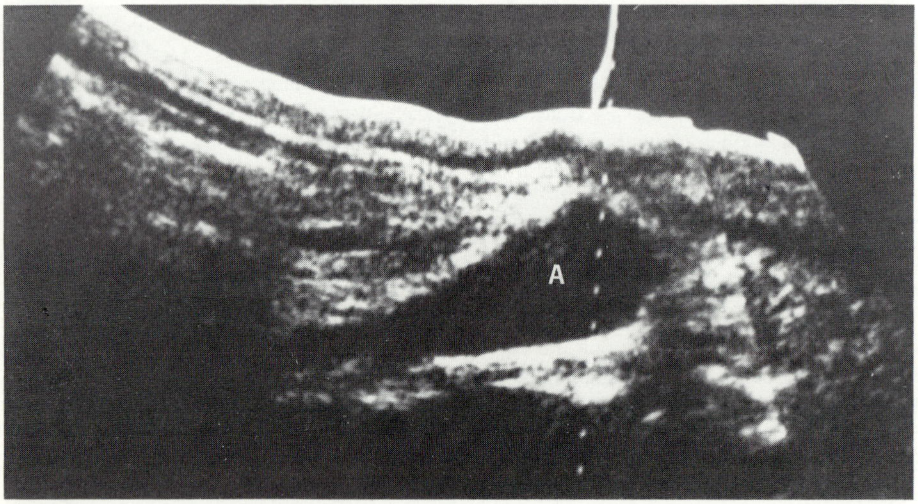

FIGURE 9-2. A sagittal-plane B-scan echo through an abdominal aortic aneurysm (A) with a sizing scale. (From Bernstein EF: *Noninvasive Diagnostic Techniques in Vascular Disease*, ed 2. St Louis, Mosby, 1982, p 420. With permission of the CV Mosby Co.)

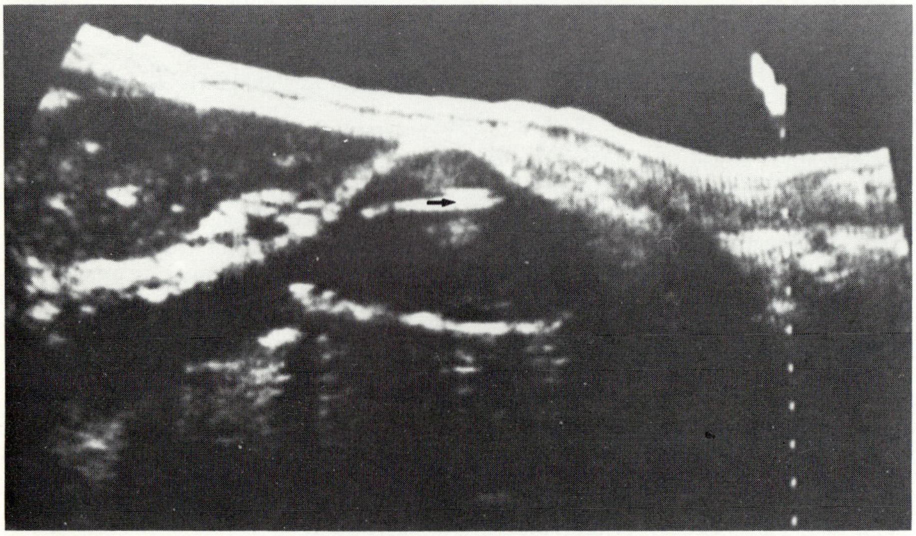

FIGURE 9-3. A sagittal-plane demonstration of a large abdominal aortic aneurysm with a thrombus (*arrow*) within the lumen. (From Bernstein EF: *Noninvasive Diagnostic Techniques in Vascular Disease*, ed 2. St Louis, Mosby, 1982, p 420. With permission of the CV Mosby Co.)

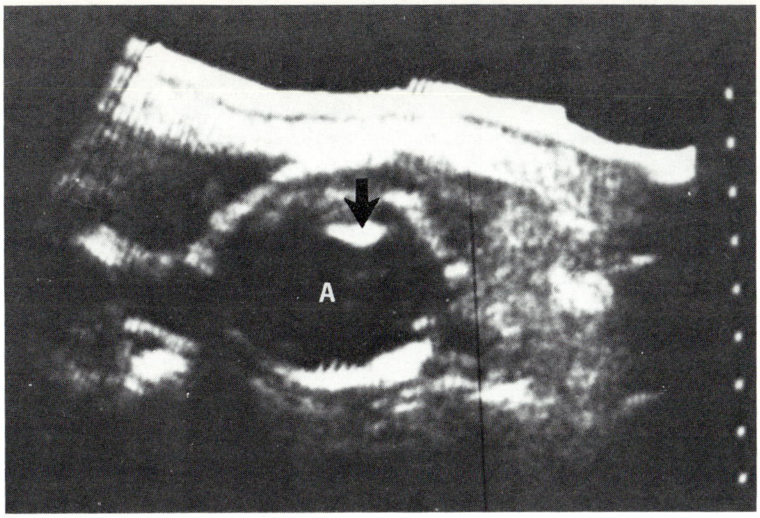

FIGURE 9-4. A transverse B-scan echogram of an abdominal aneurysm (A) with a thrombus (*arrow*) of varying acoustic density in the anterior portion of the lumen. (From Bernstein EF: *Noninvasive Diagnostic Techniques in Vascular Disease,* ed 2. St Louis, Mosby, 1982, p 421. With permission of the CV Mosby Co.)

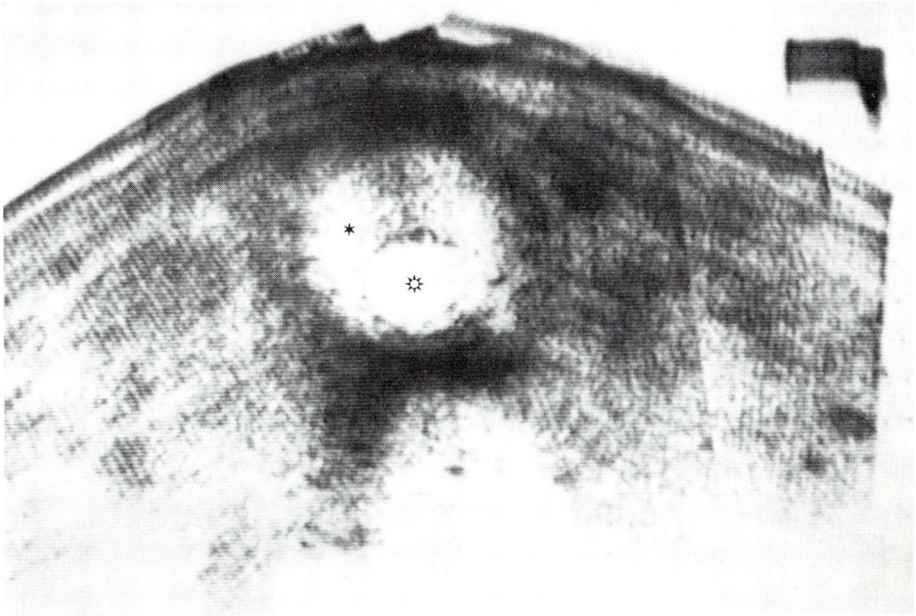

FIGURE 9-5. A transverse section of a large abdominal aneurysm in which the intraluminal thrombus (*) is circumferential and the lumen (✲) is of normal size. Such a lesion might appear normal on aortography. (From Bernstein EF: *Noninvasive Diagnostic Techniques in Vascular Disease,* ed 2. St Louis, Mosby, 1982, p 422. With permission of the CV Mosby Co.)

ultrasonic scanning, the transducer may be moved in any plane or section to provide a two-dimensional echo image. The use of this technique began at the University of California, San Diego, in 1968 (15) and our experience currently exceeds 700 cases (25). The accuracy of this approach in confirming the diagnosis of abdominal aortic aneurysms has been confirmed in several publications. In 1971, Nusbaum reported the accurate diagnosis of 79 cases out of 80 when abdominal aneurysms were tested with B-mode scanning; there was one false-positive diagnosis in a patient with paraaortic lymph node enlargement (20). Current equipment would easily detect this error (26). Studies by Maloney at the Mayo Clinic (27) and Hertzer at the Cleveland Clinic (28) demonstrated that B-mode ultrasound images were within a few millimeters of operating room measurements of aneurysm size in essentially all cases. In the Cleveland Clinic study, the measurements were identical in 34 percent of the patients and within 0.5 cm in 75 percent. (See Figures 9-1 to 9-5.)

The reproducibility of B-mode ultrasound techniques has also been demonstrated in our own experience, in which several hundred patients with abdominal aneurysms have been examined and followed with repeated studies for up to 6 years, because they were poor-risk patients with small, asymptomatic lesions.

The results of studies performed at 3-month intervals in these patients rarely varied by more than 2 or 3 mm; such consistent data permitted aneurysm expansion rates to be accurately defined.

Other important advantages of ultrasound imaging include the ability to perform longitudinal reconstructions, which are very helpful in differentiating tortuous aortas from those with small aneurysms, and the ability to measure the anteroposterior (AP) diameter. In addition, the ability of real-time B-mode scanning to identify areas of aortic pulsation which are particularly prominent may permit the selection of those lesions with an area of localized weakness that may be prone to early rupture. However, data proving this possibility are not yet available.

Abdominal Aneurysm Expansion Rates

Serial ultrasound studies have been done in 110 poor-risk patients with asymptomatic abdominal aortic aneurysms initially measuring 3.0 cm or greater in the largest transverse diameter. The expansion rates of the aneurysms in these patients averaged 0.4 cm/year, and this mean is a useful general guideline in predicting the potential of any aneurysm to increase in size and to rupture (29–31). Although individual expansion rates of abdominal aneurysms may vary substantially from this mean expansion rate, and although sudden expansion and rupture is always possible, these data have permitted us to observe without operation a group of poor-risk patients with small, asymptomatic abdominal aneurysms. The overall mortality in this group of patients has been low.

The outcome in these 110 patients may be summarized as follows. A total of 46 patients underwent elective resection because the aneurysms increased in size to 6 cm or more in diameter, or because symptoms developed; 36 died from causes unrelated to their unoperated aneurysms; and 22 were still alive without surgery at the time of their most recent follow-up visit. Only 6 patients suffered aneurysm rupture, and of these, 3 had not been operated on electively, even though their aneurysms had been larger than 6 cm, because of major contraindications, such as residual hemiplegia and aphasia after a stroke. Of the 6 patients whose aneurysms ruptured, 2 had failed to continue the serial 3-month examinations and had not been studied for at least 18 months before the rupture. Therefore, only 4 of the 110 patients ruptured without warning while under this surveillance. The total mortality in the 110 patients due to aneurysm rupture or surgery was 8 patients, or 7.3 percent. It appears that using serial ultrasonic examinations to evaluate and follow poor-risk patients with small and asymptomatic abdominal aneurysms permits the surgeon to identify those in whom rupture is likely to occur. This identification, which is based either on the development of symptoms or on an increase in aneurysm size to 6 cm, permits elective surgery to be done selectively in those patients. On the other hand, over half the patients, those who remain symptom-free and whose aneurysms remain less than 6 cm in diameter, can be managed without surgery.

Computerized Tomography

With CT, an array of highly sensitive x-ray detectors are placed in precise alignment with an x-ray tube. The x-ray beam is tightly collimated into a shape that matches the configuration of the detectors. The tube and detectors are then rotated through 360°. The intensity of the beam in each radial is altered by tissue absorption in the beam's path, and the detectors convert this information into electric signals which are precisely digitized and manipulated by a computer to produce a two-dimensional cross-sectional image. This image is displayed on a video system and can be manipulated to provide optimal information. With the newest generation of scanners, a complete scan can be performed in 2 to 5 s with a skin-surface radiation dose as low as 0.1 rad per section. In our institution, these studies are specifically tailored to the individual needs of the patient, so a limited abdominal scan for aneurysm diagnosis and size is performed. In our standard approach, the scan is performed from 3 cm above to 3 cm below the maximal abdominal mass as detected by clinical palpation. Then the patient who has no contraindications to the use of contrast material is given an intravenous bolus or infusion of radiographic contrast material, generally consisting of 50 to 100 mL of diatrizoate (Renografin-76) or 300 mL of 30 percent diatrizoate (Reno-N-Dip), and the scans are then repeated. This allows the definition of liquid blood and clot within the aneurysm. It also provides information about the patient's renal status by identifying problems in dye excretion and outflow obstruction.(See Figures 9-6 to 9-8.)

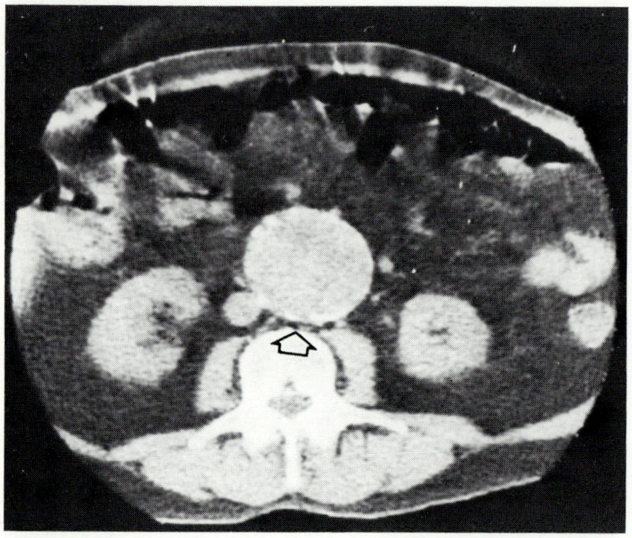

FIGURE 9-6. A CT scan from a patient with a large amount of body fat shows how the fat acts as a contrast substance against which the organs stand out. The arrow points to an aortic aneurysm. (From Bernstein EF: *Noninvasive Diagnostic Techniques in Vascular Disease,* ed 2. St Louis, Mosby, 1982, p 424. With permission of the CV Mosby Co.)

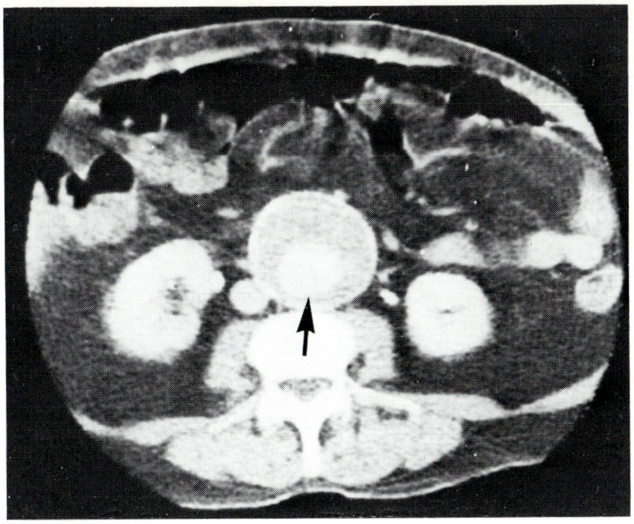

FIGURE 9-7. After the intravenous administration of contrast material in this CT scan, the lumen of the aorta is enhanced by flowing blood (*arrow*). The thrombus is easily differentiated and is typically located anterior and lateral to the lumen. (From Bernstein EF: *Noninvasive Diagnostic Techniques in Vascular Disease,* ed 2. St Louis, Mosby, 1982, p 424. With permission of the CV Mosby Co.)

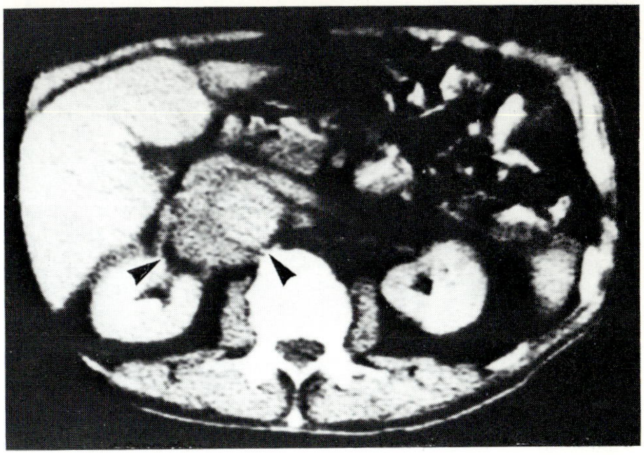

FIGURE 9-8. This contrast-enhanced CT scan demonstrates the amount of tortuosity that can occur in a dilated aorta. Here the aorta is seen far to the right (*arrowheads*). The inferior vena cava is anterior to the aorta, with the renal veins stretched to gain access to it. (From Bernstein EF: *Noninvasive Diagnostic Techniques in Vascular Disease,* ed 2. St Louis, Mosby, 1982, p 423. With permission of the CV Mosby Co.)

CT scans not only demonstrate the wall of the abdominal aneurysm in two dimensions with 2- to 3-mm accuracy, but also identify other intraabdominal and retroperitoneal masses, vertebral body erosion (Figure 9-9), leaks or hematomas in the perianeurysmal area, perianeurysmal fibrosis or inflammation (Figure 9-10), and aneurysmal dilatation of the iliac arteries (Figure 9-11) (23,32–37).

CT scanning is of particular value in obese patients or those with barium retention or excessive intestinal gas, because all these conditions may interfere with ultrasound examination. Obese patients are more readily studied by CT scans because fat acts as a contrast material against which other organs stand out quite clearly (Figure 9-6). One source of CT artifact is the presence of metallic foreign bodies, including surgical clips, which obscure the surrounding area, especially if there is associated clip motion.

The use of intravenous radiographic contrast material has improved the CT evaluation of abdominal aneurysms considerably. The contrast material has permitted the delineation of lumen position and size. Clot close to the lumen is less dense than older clot close to the outer wall. In most instances the lumen is located posteriorly and is symmetrically situated within the aneurysm (Figure 9-7). However, in some cases the lumen is clearly asymmetrical and anterior, and these conditions may be more

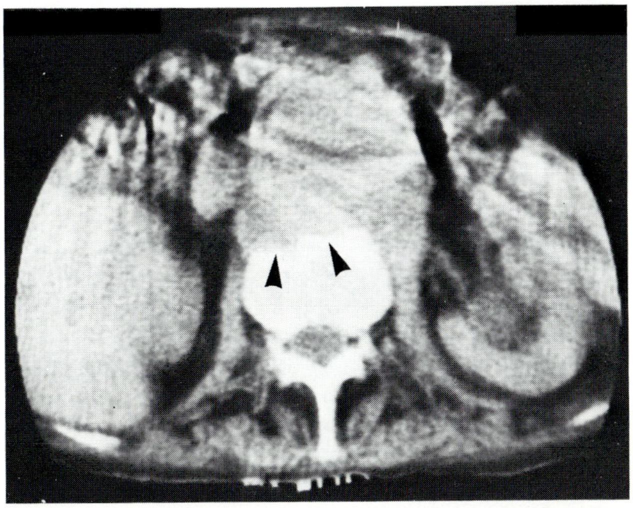

A

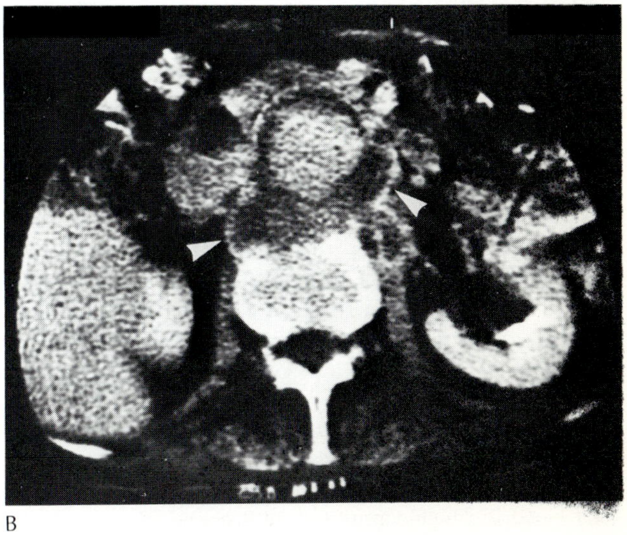

B

FIGURE 9-9. A retroperitoneal hematoma surrounds a leaking aortic prosthesis. ***(A)*** The high-density blood obscures the normal anatomic configurations of the aorta and anterior psoas muscle margins. Vertebral body erosions are also noted (*arrowheads*). The bleeding was due to an aortoprosthetic graft disruption. ***(B)*** Contrast enhancement clearly delineates the aortic lumen and the limits of the periprosthetic hematoma (*arrowheads*). (From Bernstein EF: *Noninvasive Diagnostic Techniques in Vascular Disease,* ed 2. St Louis, Mosby, 1982, p 425. With permission of the CV Mosby Co.)

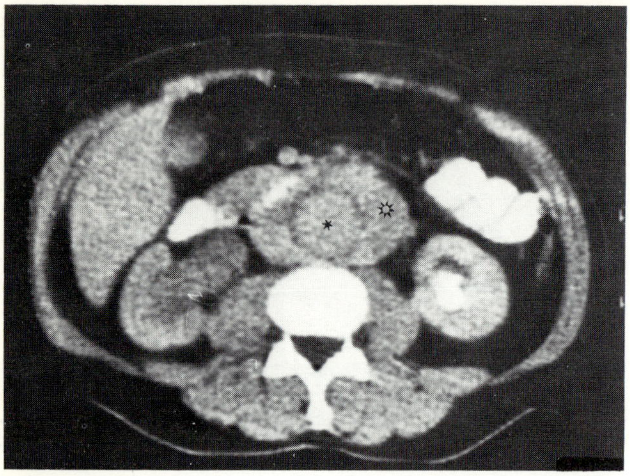

FIGURE 9-10. An inflammatory aneurysm is clearly demonstrated, with a thick mantle of tissue (✲) lateral to the aneurysm lumen (*). Bilateral hydronephrosis is also present, presumably due to perianeurysmal fibrosis.

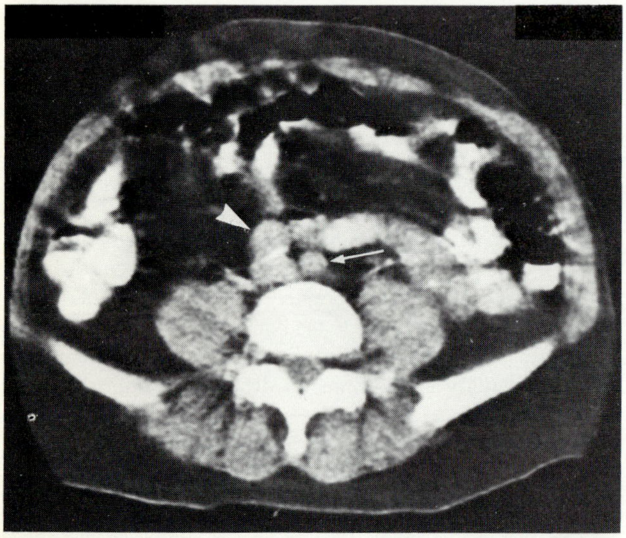

FIGURE 9-11. This CT scan obtained below the aortic bifurcation shows an aneurysm of the right common iliac artery (*arrowhead*) next to a normal left common iliac artery (*small arrow*). (From Bernstein EF: *Noninvasive Diagnostic Techniques in Vascular Disease,* ed 2. St Louis, Mosby, 1982, p 423. With permission of the CV Mosby Co.)

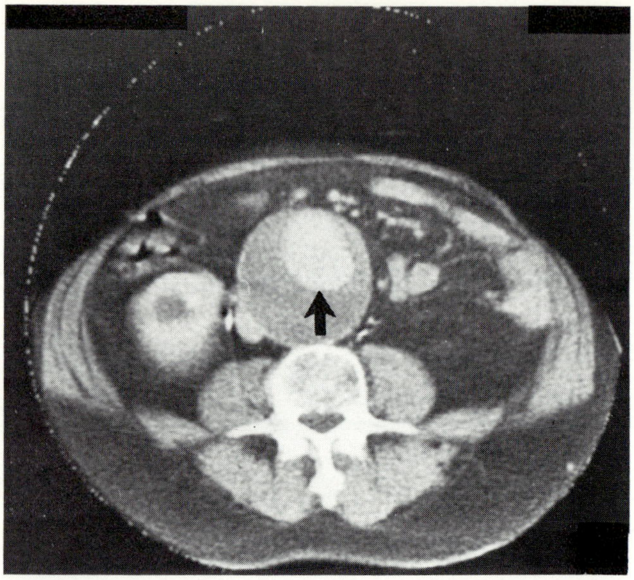

FIGURE 9-12. In this contrast-enhanced CT scan, the lumen of the abdominal aortic aneurysm is eccentric (*arrow*), suggesting clot dissection.

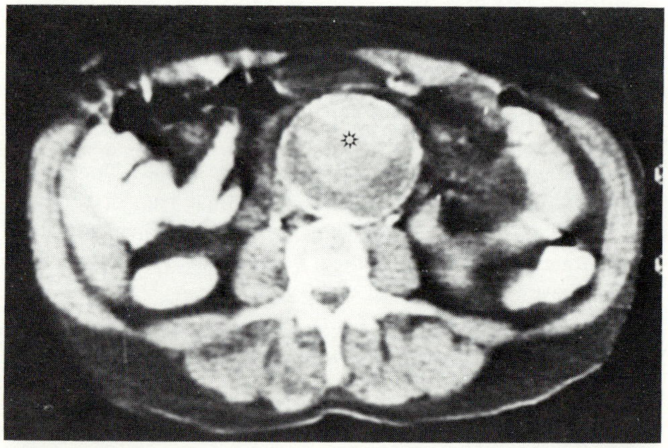

FIGURE 9-13. The anterior lumen of an aortic aneurysm (✲) with no thrombus between the aneurysm wall and lumen suggests the possibility of early wall disruption.

likely to be associated with early rupture, particularly if localized wall asymmetry is present. Clot liquefaction or dissection can also be identified in the presence of an eccentric lumen (Figures 9-12 and 9-13), often with a tail of contrast material seen close to the lateral wall, indicating the separation of clot from the wall (Figure 9-14).

The presence of actual or impending rupture or leakage of an aneurysm may be rapidly assessed by CT, particularly with contrast-enhanced scans (Figures 9-9 and 9-12 to 9-15.) Extravascular blood is a high-density CT substance which can be seen to disrupt the normal anatomic configuration of the aortic wall and the retroperitoneum. After the injection of contrast material, the clot takes on a characteristic lower density than surrounding structures, which normally enhance with contrast material. In addition, a hematoma may have some rim enhancement because of an inflammatory response to the hematoma (Figure 9-9*B*).

CT scanning has been particularly important in the postoperative evaluation of patients after aneurysmectomy or other abdominal aortic surgery when there is a question of recurrence of pseudoaneurysm or, particularly, graft infection (38). Repeated scans can follow the resolution of periprosthetic hematomas. Both aortic prosthesis disruption and false-aneurysm formation may be diagnosed. The identification of small pockets of gas caused by pyogenic organisms is pathognomonic for aortic prosthetic infection when the gas is located posterior to the lumen of the graft and persists more than 2 weeks after surgery (Figure 9-16). It is normal to see some gas as a single collection anteriorly for up to 10 days after operation. Inflammatory rim enhancement surrounding an abscess involving an aortic or iliac graft is also pathognomonic for graft infection, but requires contrast injection.

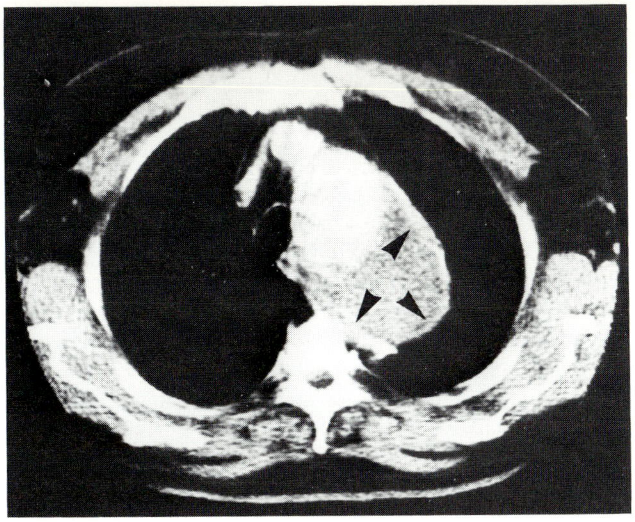

FIGURE 9-14. In this thoracic aneurysm, contrast material is seen around the edge of the thrombus just beneath the wall of the aorta (*arrowheads*). This is a sign of clot liquefaction and dihiscence. (From Bernstein EF: *Noninvasive Diagnostic Techniques in Vascular Disease*, ed 2. St Louis, Mosby, 1982, p 425. With permission of the CV Mosby Co.)

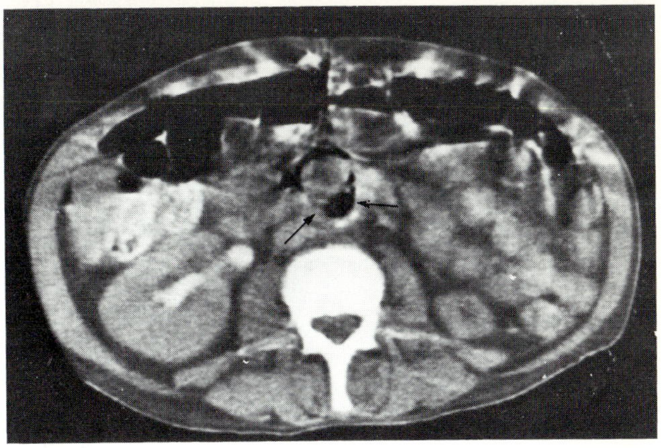

FIGURE 9-16. This patient became febrile after aortic graft surgery. The scan shows collections of gas, which appear as black areas posterior to the lumen of the aorta (*arrows*). When present long after aortic graft implantation, these gas pockets are pathognomonic for a pyogenic infection. (From Bernstein EF: *Noninvasive Diagnostic Techniques in Vascular Disease*, ed 2. St Louis, Mosby, 1982, p 426. With permission of the CV Mosby Co.)

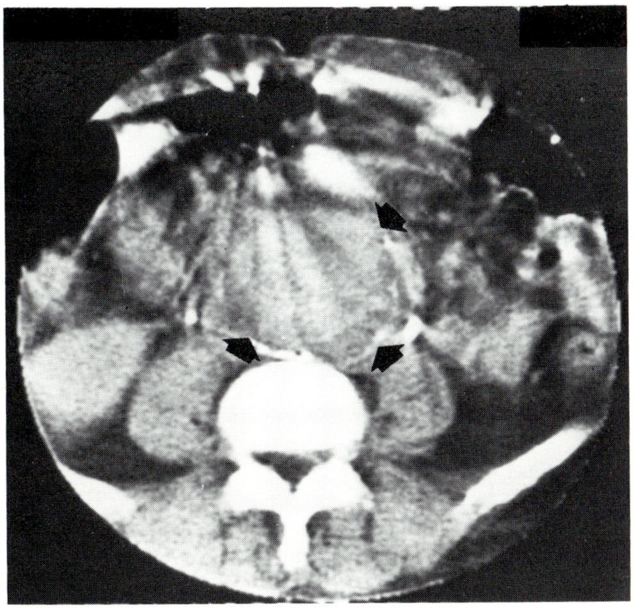

FIGURE 9-15. A ruptured aneurysm of the abdominal aorta. Note the obscure boundaries of the anterior aortic wall (*arrows*).

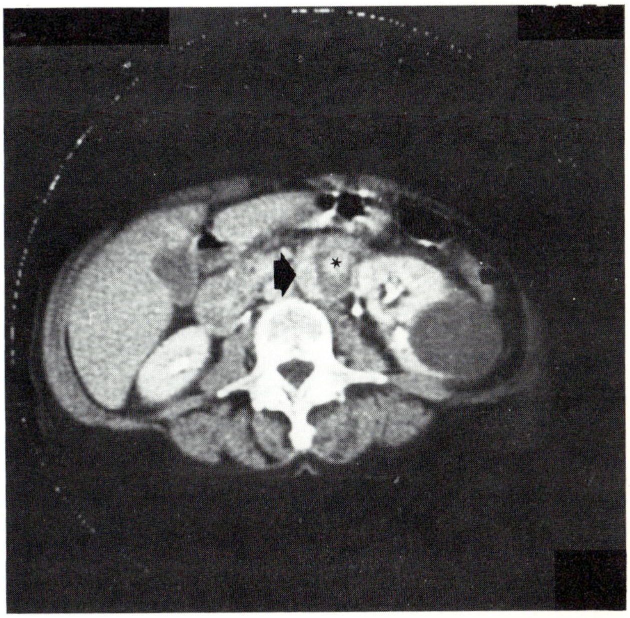

FIGURE 9-17. A dissecting aneurysm of the aorta; the two lumens (*white*) are demonstrated by the star (*) and the arrow and are separated by the dissected aortic wall layer. A left renal cyst is also present.

Comparative Roles of Ultrasound and CT Scanning in the Evaluation of Abdominal Aortic Aneurysms

Both echography and CT scanning are close to 100 percent accurate in diagnosing abdominal aortic aneurysms, and both provide size measurements which are generally within 3 mm of the actual measured size of the aneurysm at surgery (39). However, errors in diagnosis and size estimation are more common with B-mode scanning, which is more dependent on both the skills of the technician and the radiographic interpretation. With echography, errors may also be caused by tortuous arteries and because of increased wall thickness and old organized thrombus which may make it difficult to acoustically separate the aortic wall from surrounding tissue. Echography has limitations in patients in whom there are large amounts of intestinal gas, particularly those with paralytic ileus, as in the postoperative state. In addition, radiodense contrast material such as barium in the intestine, or massive obesity, may limit the penetration of the sound beam and thereby preclude an accurate anatomic examination. On the positive side, ultrasonography is extremely fast, simple, cheap, and usually effective in making the diagnosis. Scans in both a transverse and a longitudinal plane are routine, and the likelihood of confusing a tortuous aorta with a small aneurysm is extremely small. Contrast injections are not necessary, avoiding the small but real risks of contrast reactions and toxicity. The longitudinal scan serves as a check on the transverse measurements and helps identify tortuous aortic segments which may mimic aneurysms. In addition, real-time ultrasonography offers an opportunity to study aortic wall motion and may permit the identification of localized rupture-prone sites.

The rapid evolution of newer and faster CT scanning techniques that require less radiation, coupled with the willingness of some radiologists to perform limited CT scans of the abdominal aorta, which are competitive in price with ultrasonography, has made this technique the modality of choice in our institution, both for making the initial diagnosis of abdominal aortic aneurysm and for investigating patients who have postoperative problems. The radiation dosage is no longer a drawback, even in serial studies, since the skin dose is now reduced to 0.1 rad per section studied. In addition, the newer CT software packages permit longitudinal and coronal reconstructions of abdominal aortic images. One of the important residual limitations of CT scanning is its sensitivity to the presence of intraabdominal metallic foreign bodies such as hemostatic surgical clips. Because such clips scatter the x-ray beam and destroy the image of surrounding tissues, many neurosurgeons have ceased using clips for hemostasis, or have replaced metallic clips with nonmetallic ones. Abdominal and vascular surgeons may find a similar tactic essential if CT scanning becomes as important a postoperative diagnostic tool as now seems likely.

Current advances in the technology of both the ultrasound and CT scanning should permit the risk-free accurate diagnosis of abdominal aortic aneurysms on a routine basis in an outpatient setting. The identification of patients with aortic ectasia or tortuosity saves such patients from unnecessary angiography and laparotomy. The clear detection of unsuspected aneurysms and their differentiation from other intraabdominal and retroperitoneal masses permits early elective aneurysm resection in good-risk patients and should eventually decrease the mortality from this disease. In addition, the anatomic delineation of small details which appears possible with both these techniques may permit the localization of paraaneurysmal structures including renal artery lesions, anomalous venous conditions, and other anatomic items of importance to the vascular surgeon. The increasing trend toward the mass screening of patients for asymptomatic cardiovascular disease may lead to the use of routine ultrasound or CT screening for aneurysmal disease in elderly patients, particularly those with a significant cardiovascular history. Both ultrasound and CT scanning appear to be excellent modalities for these purposes. The rapid development of faster and cheaper CT procedures, which provide additional anatomic detail, have few limitations or contraindications, and are competitively priced with ultrasound techniques, appears to make CT scanning somewhat superior at the present time.

Thoracic Aortic Aneurysms

In the thoracic area, ultrasonography is rarely of value because of ultrasound's attenuation by the air-containing lungs. Thus CT scanning (Figure 9-17) and digital subtraction angiography (DSA) have become the only relatively noninvasive modalities capable of identifying thoracic aortic aneurysms (40,41). However, in this area of the body, preoperative standard angiography is considered mandatory to define the lesion and its relationship to other critical vessels. Further, since there are few or no data regarding the relationship of thoracic aneurysm size and the likelihood of rupture, measurements of thoracic aneurysms have not achieved the widespread clinical significance that measurements have in the abdomen.

Femoral and Popliteal Arterial Aneurysms

Both ultrasound and CT scanning are equally effective diagnostic tools in the femoral and popliteal areas (42–44,7). However, echography has achieved far greater popularity in these anatomic areas, both because of the ease of such scanning and because the images are usually of very high quality, since higher-frequency probes which yield finer sensitivity can be used in these relatively superficial applications. Since the presence of aneurysms in these locations is often an indication for surgery, details regarding size, shape, and neighboring structures are relatively unimportant.

The Place of Digital Subtraction Angiography

The recent development of DSA provides the physician with a means to obtain anatomic information regarding vascular structures which may be of interest to the surgeon; the method uses an intravenous injection of radiographic contrast material and thus avoids the risks of arterial puncture (7). DSA may sometimes replace direct contrast angiography for providing this anatomic information but should not be used as a primary diagnostic technique for aneurysms, or as one to evaluate aneurysm size. It has the same limitations as any other angiographic method, i.e., it demonstrates the aneurysm lumen and provides no information about the thickness of the clot or the true outer dimensions of the aneurysm, both of which are more important in determining the risk of rupture, at least for the abdominal aorta. In addition, DSA is more expensive than either CT or ultrasound techniques, and carries some risk of contrast medium toxicity.

Summary

Both ultrasound and CT scanning are safe, noninvasive methods with a high reliability in diagnosing abdominal aortic aneurysms. Both approaches appear to be capable of determining aneurysm size within 3 or 4 mm. The usefulness of echography is somewhat limited in the presence of large amounts of intestinal gas, retained abdominal barium, and marked obesity. However, these limitations are offset by the ease of obtaining longitudinal as well as transverse scans in the absence of ionizing radiation. The drawbacks of CT scanning include its limited usefulness in the presence of metallic objects, the radiation dose, and the cost. However, the excellent intraluminal definition which is possible, as well as the detailed anatomic delineation of other retroperitoneal structures, appears to make CT the preferred method for diagnosing abdominal aortic aneurysms at present. Long-term reductions in cost may permit the application of either of these techniques to the screening of asymptomatic patients as well as to the observation of the asymptomatic patient with a small aneurysm who is too high a risk for early surgery.

References

1. Bernstein EF: The natural history of abdominal aortic aneurysms. In Najarian JS, Delaney JB (eds): *Vascular Surgery*. Miami, Symposia Specialists, 1978, pp 441–452.
2. Gore J, Hirst AJ: Arteriosclerotic aneurysms of the abdominal aorta: A review. Prog Cardiovasc Dis 1973, 16:113–149.
3. Birnholtz JC: Alternatives in the diagnosis of abdominal aortic aneurysm: Combined use of isotope aortography and ultrasonography.AJR 1973, 111:809–813.
4. Brewster DC, Retana A, Waltman AC, Darling RC: Angiography in the management of aneurysms of the abdominal aorta. N Engl J Med 1975, 292:822–825.
5. Brewster DC, Darling RC, O'Donnell TF, Raines JF, Sarno R, Athanasoulis C: Assessment of abdominal aortic aneurysm size. Circulation 1977, 56(suppl II):164–169.
6. Robicsek F, Daugherty HK, Mullen DC, Tam W, Scott WP: The value of angiography in the diagnosis of unruptured aneurysms of the abdominal aorta. Ann Thorac Surg 1971, 11:538–550.
7. Turnipseed WD, Acher SW, Detmer DE, Berkoff HA, Myerowitz PD, Crummy AB, Belzer FO: Digital subtraction angiography and B-mode ultrasonography for abdominal and peripheral aneurysms. Surgery 1982, 92:619–626.
8. Wheeler WE, Beachley MC, Ranniger K: Angiography and ultrasonography. AJR 1976, 126:95–100.
9. Nuno IN, Collins GM, Bardin JA, Bernstein EF: Should aortography be used routinely in the elective management of abdominal aortic aneurysm? Am J Surg 1982, 144:54–57.
10. Goldberg BB, Ostrum BJ, Isard HJ: Ultrasonic aortography, JAMA 1966, 198:353–358.
11. Segal BL, Likoff W, Asperger Z, Kingsley B: Ultrasound diagnosis of an abdominal aortic aneurysm. Am J Cardiol 1966, 17:101–103.
12. Evans GC, Lehman JS Sr, Segal BL, Likoff W, Ziskin M, Kingsley B: Echo-aortography. Am J Cardiol 1967, 19:91–96.
13. Goldberg BB, Lehman JS: Aortosonography, ultrasound measurement of the abdominal and thoracic aorta. Arch Surg 1970, 100:652–655.
14. Goldberg BB: Suprasternal aortosonography. JAMA 1971, 215:245–250.
15. Leopold GR: Ultrasonic abdominal aortography. Radiology 1970, 96:9–14.
16. Leopold GR, Goldberger LE, Bernstein EF: Ultrasonic detection and evaluation of abdominal aortic aneurysm. Surgery 1972, 72:939–945.
17. McGregor JC, Pollock JG, Anton HC: The value of ultrasonography in the diagnosis of abdominal aortic aneurysm. Scott Med J 1975, 20:133–141.
18. McGregor JC, Pollock JG, Anton HC: The diagnosis and assessment of abdominal aortic aneurysms by ultrasonography. Ann R Coll Surg, Engl 1976, 58:388–392.
19. Mulder DS, Winsberg F, Cole CM, Blundell PE, Scott HJ: Ultrasonic "B" scanning of abdominal aneurysms. Ann Thorac Surg 1973, 16:361–367.
20. Nusbaum JW, Fremanis AK, Thomford NR: Echography in the diagnosis of abdominal aortic aneurysm. Arch Surg 1971, 102:385–388.
21. Winsberg F, Cole-Beuflet C, Mulder DS: Continuosu ultrasound "B" scanning of abdominal aortic aneurysms. AJR 1974, 121:626–633.
22. Axelbaum SP, Schellinger D, Gomes MN, Ferris RA, Hakkal HG: A computed tomographic evaluation of aortic aneurysms. AJR 1976, 127:75–78.
23. Gomes MN: ACTA scanning in the diagnosis of abdominal aortic aneurysms. Comput Tomogr 1977, 1:51–61.
24. Schellinger D: CT of abdominal aortic aneurysms. Society of Computerized Tomography, postgraduate course, San Diego, Feb 24–Mar 1, 1979.
25. Gosink B: Natural history of unresected abdominal aortic aneurysms: 12 years of experience. Unpublished data.
26. Leopold GR: Gray scale ultrasonic angiography of the upper abdomen. Radiology 1975, 117:665–671.
27. Maloney JD, Pairolero PC, Smith BF Jr, Hattery RR, Brakke DM, Spittell JA Jr: Ultrasound evaluation of abdominl aortic aneurysms. Circulation 1977, 56(suppl II):80–85.
28. Hertzer NR, Beven EG: Ultrasound measurement and elective aneurysmectomy. JAMA 1978, 240:1966–1968.
29. Bernstein EF: Considerations in the management of poor-risk patients with small asymptomatic abdominal aortic aneurysms. In Varco RL, Delaney JP (eds): *Controversy in Surgery*. Philadelphia, Saunders, 1976, pp 267–276.
30. Bernstein EF, Harris RD, Leopold GR: Noninvasive evaluation of abdominal aortic aneurysms by ultrasonic imaging and computed tomography scanning. In Bernstein EF (ed): *Noninvasive Diagnostic Techniques in Vascular Disease*. St. Louis, Mosby, 1985, pp 652–665.
31. Bernstein EF, Dilley RB, Goldberger LE, Gosink BB, Leopold GR: Growth rates of small abdominal aortic aneurysms. Surgery 1976, 80:765–773.
32. Carter BL, Wechsler RJ: Computed tomography of the retroperitoneum and abdominal wall. Semin Roentgenol 1978, 13:201–211.
33. Gomes MN, Hakkal HG, Schellinger D: Ultrasonography and CT scanning: A comparative study of abdominal aortic aneurysms. Comput Tomogr 1978, 2:99–110.

34. Gomes MN, Schellinger D, Hufnagel CA: Abdominal aortic aneurysms: Diagnostic review and new technique. Am Thorac Surg 1978, 27:479–488.

35. Haaga J, Reich NE: *Computed Tomography of Abdominal Abnormalities*. St. Louis, Mosby, 1978, pp 163–169.

36. Pond GD, Hillman B: Evaluation of aneurysms by computed tomography. Surgery 1981, 89:216–223.

37. Ramirez AA, Riles TS, Imparato AM, Hegibown AH: CAT scans of inflammatory aneurysms: A new technique for preoperative diagnosis. Surgery 1982, 91:390–393.

38. Haaga Jr, Baldwin GN, Reich NE, Bevan E, Kramer A, Weinstein A, Harsilla TR, Seidelmann FE, Namba AH, Parrish CM: CT detection of infected synthetic grafts: Preliminary report of a new sign. AJR 1981, 131:317–320.

39. Raskin MM, Cunningham JB: Comparison of computed tomography and ultrasound for abdominal aortic aneurysms: Preliminary study. J Comput Assist Tomogr 1978, 2:21–30.

40. Harris RD, Hougen ML: Early diagnosis of tuberculous thoracic aortic aneurysm by computerized axial tomography. Comput Tomogr 1978, 2:49–53.

41. Harris RD, Usselman JA, Vint V, Warmath M: Computerized tomography of an aneurysm of the thoracic aorta. Comput Tomog 1979, 3:81–86.

42. Davis RP, Neiman HL, Yao JST, Bergan JJ: Ultrasound scan in diagnosis of peripheral aneurysms. Arch Surg 1977, 1112:55–58.

43. Dent TL, Lindenauer SM, Ernst CB, Fry WJ: Multiple arteriosclerotic arterial aneurysms. Arch Surg 1972, 105:338–344.

44. Graham LM, Zelenock GB, Whitehouse WM Jr, Erlandson EE, Dent TL, Lindenauer SM, Stanley JC: Clinical significance of arteriosclerotic femoral artery aneurysms. Arch Surg 1980, 115:502–506.

Chapter 10

NONINVASIVE CEREBROVASCULAR DIAGNOSTIC TECHNIQUES

THOMAS G. LYNCH and ROBERT W. HOBSON II

Hemodynamic changes associated with internal carotid artery stenosis and occlusion provide the basis for a wide range of noninvasive cerebrovascular diagnostic techniques. Because of this relationship, any review of the development and application of these techniques must also include a discussion of the carotid arterial circulation and the alterations and collateral pathways that develop following stenosis or occlusion.

Cerebrovascular Doppler examination (CDE), supraorbital photoplethysmography (SOPPG), oculoplethysmography (OPG-K), and ocular pneumoplethysmography (OPG-G) are sensitive to abnormal patterns of collateral circulation, ocular pulse delay, or a decrease in the end-ophthalmic (distal internal carotid) artery pressure and provide indirect evidence of carotid arterial obstruction. These indirect techniques, however, cannot quantitate the degree of stenosis or distinguish between stenosis and occlusion, and they are unable to detect nonstenotic ulcerative disease. Techniques which directly assess the cervical carotid artery, such as Doppler ultrasonic scanning, spectral analysis, and real-time B-mode ultrasonography, provide additional information relative to the morphology and degree of the obstruction.

Noninvasive studies have become an effective means with which to screen asymptomatic individuals for atherosclerotic involvement of the cervical carotid artery. Such patients include those with asymptomatic cervical bruits; those with symptoms of posterior circulation or vertebrobasilar insufficiency; those who are candidates for major vascular reconstructive procedures; and those patients with risk factors associated with atherosclerotic occlusive disease. In patients with anterior circulation or lateralizing symptoms, however, contrast arteriography is still a requisite study. Under these circumstances, noninvasive techniques are useful for purposes of registration and baseline measurements. Both indirect and direct techniques have also been employed intraoperatively and postoperatively to evaluate the adequacy and continued patency of carotid reconstructions.

Arteriography is the standard against which all noninvasive studies are compared. The percentage of stenosis, when present, is determined by comparing the least transverse diameter of the internal carotid artery at the stenosis with the diameter of the distal uninvolved artery (Figure 10-1). This percentage may be expressed as a function of the diameter or the cross-sectional area. Brown and Johnston (1), however, have suggested that the minimum residual lumen diameter (MRLD), defined as the least transverse diameter seen in either the anteroposterior or lateral view, should be the preferred method for quantifying carotid stenosis (Figure 10-1). The authors conclude that the MRLD is reproducible and more accurately reflects the extent of disease. They do admit, however, that the percentage of stenosis has been used more commonly, facilitating comparisons with previously published data. While arteriography is the only practical standard at present, it is not a perfect standard. Since arteriography yields a two-dimensional image of a three-dimensional process, the extent of disease may be over- or underestimated, depending upon which plane or planes of the artery are transected (Figure 10-2*A* and *B*).

Sensitivity and specificity are frequently used to express the accuracy of a technique relative to a standard, in this case arteriography. The sensitivity of a technique is defined as the percentage of those arteries with disease demonstrated arteriographically, that are correctly identified noninvasively. Specificity is defined as the percentage of those arteries without arteriographically demonstrated disease, that are correctly identified noninvasively (Table 10-1). In reviewing the literature it is important to be aware that the extent of disease, expressed as a percentage stenosis or an MRLD, upon which the sensitivity and specificity are based may vary between reported series and that calculations may be made on a per artery or a per patient basis.

Positive and negative predictive values (Table 10-1) have also been used to characterize the value of a technique. The positive predictive value represents the percentage of noninvasively abnormal studies which were also abnormal by contrast arteriography, while the negative predictive value represents the percentage of negative noninvasive studies which were associated with normal arteriograms. Unlike sensitivity and specificity, which characterize the percentage of arteriographic studies that are correctly identified noninvasively, the positive and negative predictive values yield the percentage of noninvasive studies that are in agreement with arteriography. Thus the predictive value represents the probability that a given noninvasive test result will accurately reflect the arteriographic findings.

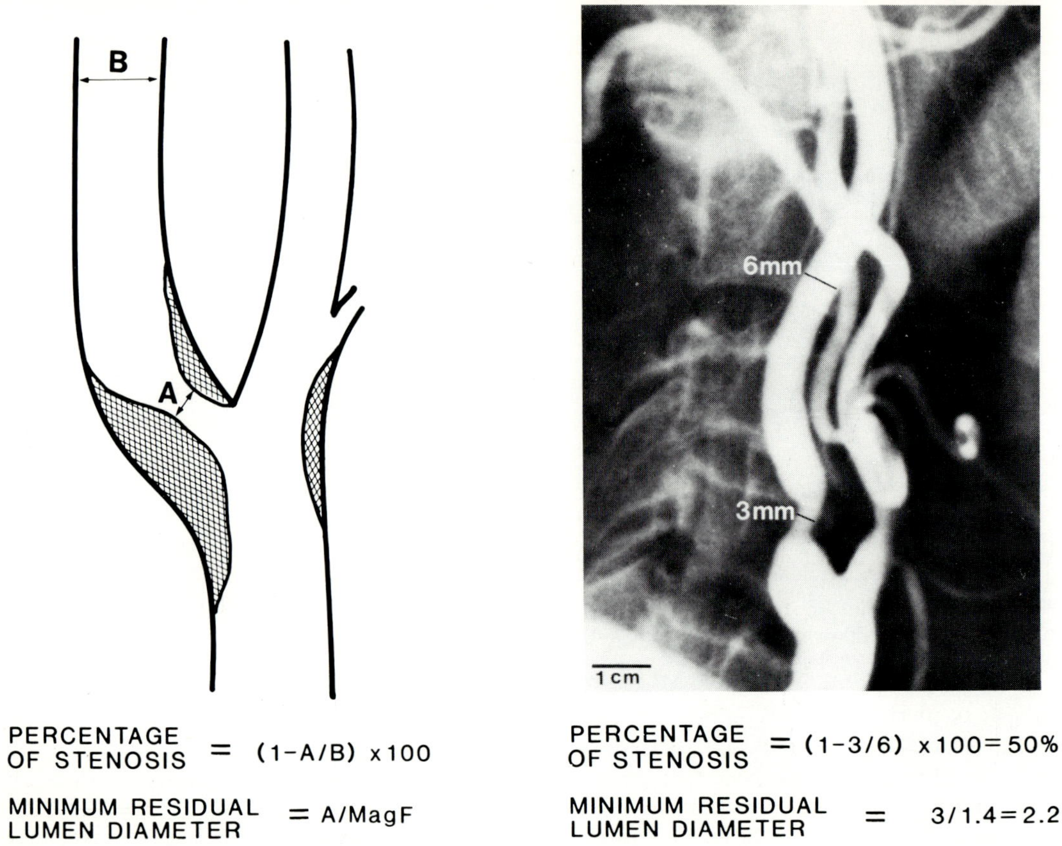

FIGURE 10-1. The percentage of stenosis is calculated by dividing the least transverse diameter of the internal carotid artery at the stenosis (A), by the diameter of the distal, uninvolved artery (B). The minimum residual lumen diameter is equivalent to the least transverse diameter (A) divided by the magnification factor (MagF) of the arteriogram. The example (*right*) illustrates a 50 percent stenosis, by diameter, and a minimum residual lumen diameter of 2.2 mm.

TABLE 10-1. Statistical Calculations Used in the Evaluation of Noninvasive Cerebrovascular Diagnostic Techniques

		Noninvasive Examination	
Carotid Arteriography		Abnormal	Normal
Positive (stenosis or occlusion)		A	B
Negative		C	D
Sensitivity	A/A + B		
Specificity	D/C + D		
Positive predictive value	A/A + C		
Negative predictive value	D/B + D		
Accuracy	A + D/A + B + C + D		

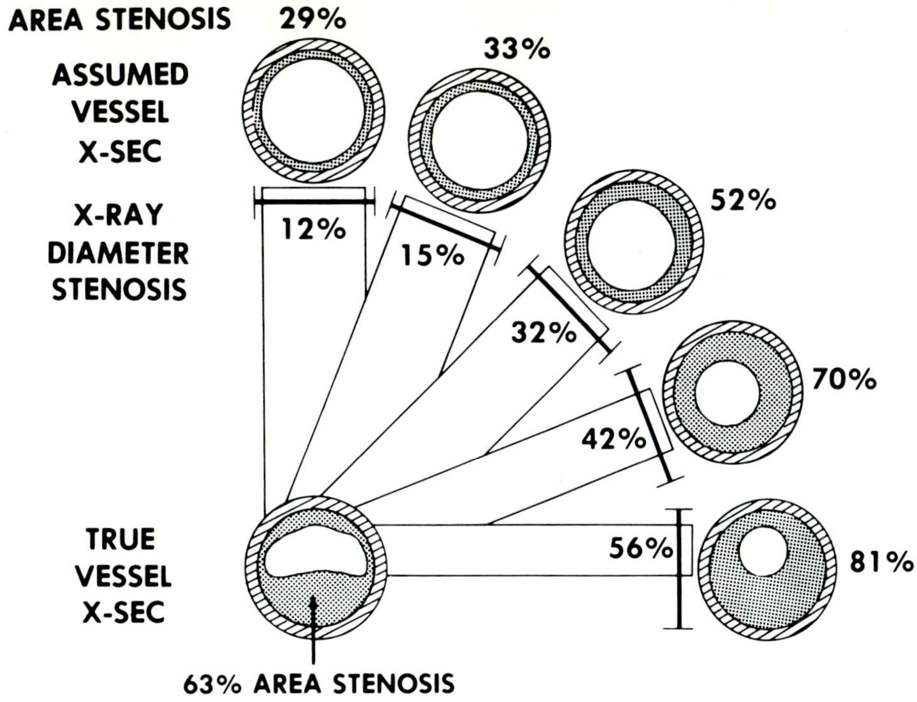

A

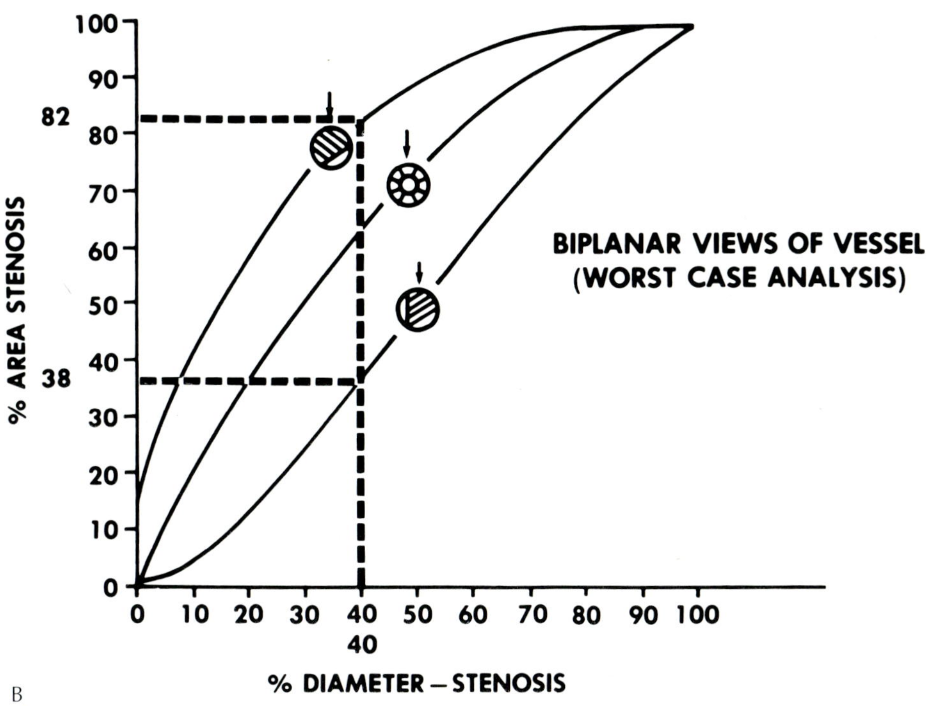

B

FIGURE 10-2. *(A)* The assumed, or apparent, degrees of diameter and area stenosis when an asymmetrical lesion is visualized in different projections. [Sumner DS, Russell JB, Miles RD: Pulsed Doppler arteriography and computer assisted imaging of the carotid bifurcation. In Bergan JJ, Yao JST (eds): *Cerebrovascular Insufficiency*. New York, Grune & Stratton, 1983, pp 115–135. Reproduced by permission of Grune & Stratton, Inc.] ***(B)*** The relationship between area stenosis and diameter stenosis when the artery is asymmetrically narrowed (*top* and *bottom* lines) and when it is symmetrically narrowed (*middle* line). Arrows indicate the direction of the x-ray beam in the projection that shows the greatest degree of narrowing. If the stenosis is asymmetrical and if two orthogonal views are assumed, the actual area stenosis for any given diameter stenosis must lie between the upper and lower lines. Only if the stenosis is symmetrical can a precise estimate of area be obtained. [Sumner DS, Russell JB, Miles RD: Pulsed Doppler arteriography and computer assisted imaging of the carotid bifurcation. In Bergan JJ, Yao JST (eds): *Cerebrovascular Insufficiency*. New York, Grune & Stratton, 1983, pp 115–135. Reproduced by permission of Grune & Stratton, Inc.]

The Cerebrovascular Doppler Examination (CDE)

The early noninvasive cerebrovascular diagnostic techniques developed from an understanding of the carotid circulation and its potential collateral pathways (Figure 10-3*A* and *B*). The ophthalmic artery is the first branch of the internal carotid artery. It divides into the frontal, supraorbital, and nasal arteries, which pass onto the anterior face and forehead and communicate through collateral channels with the superficial temporal, facial, and infraorbital branches of the external carotid artery. In the absence of an obstruction, flow passes through the internal carotid artery and out of the orbit via the ophthalmic artery and its branches.

May et al. (2) have shown experimentally that the cross-sectional area of the internal carotid artery must be reduced by 75

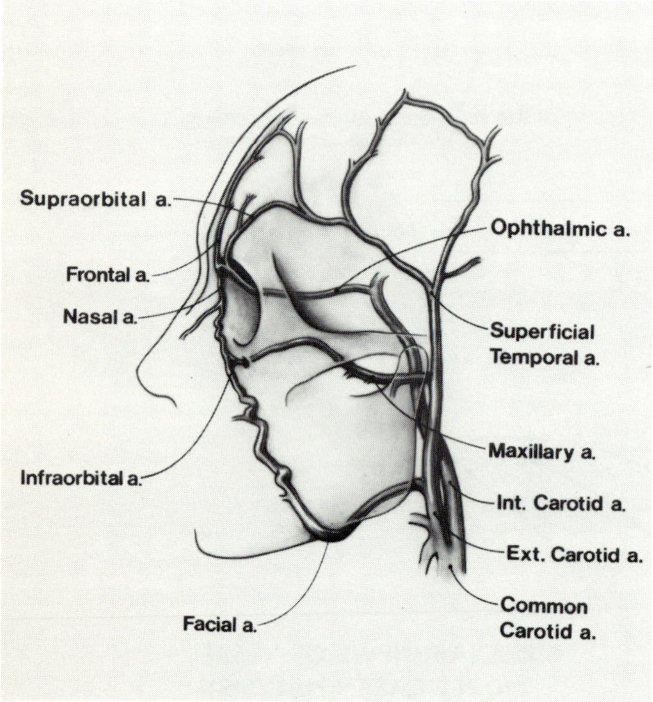

A

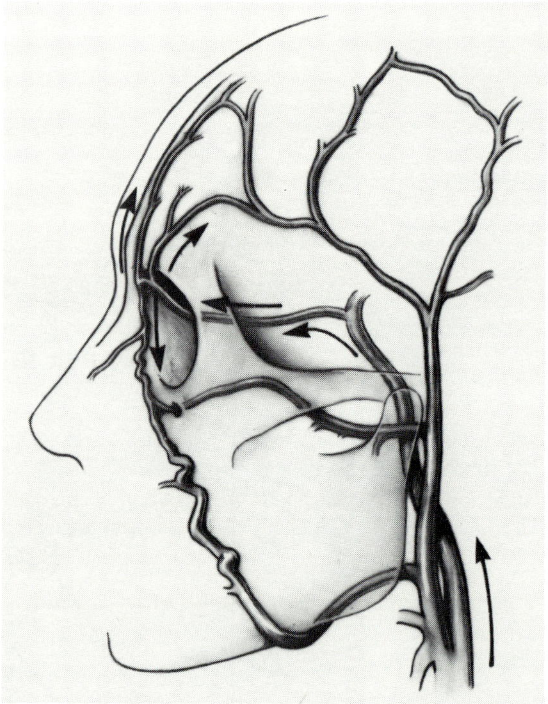

B

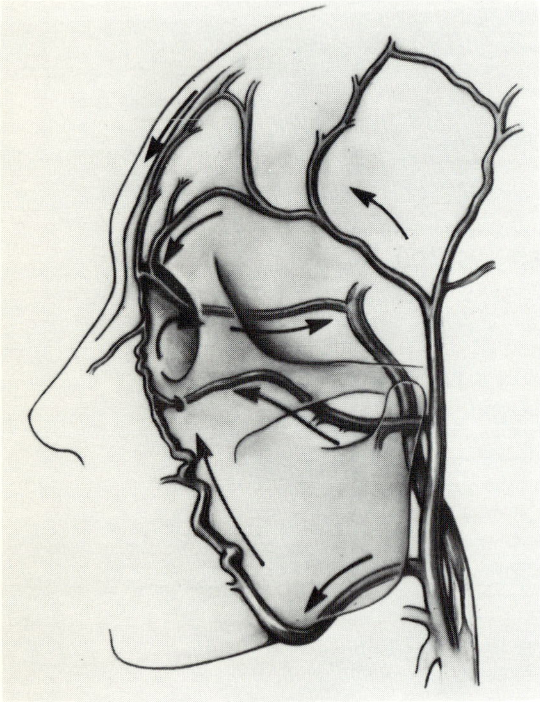

C

FIGURE 10-3. *(A)* The common carotid artery and its bifurcation demonstrating the branches of the internal and external carotid arteries. The direction of flow is indicated in the absence ***(B)*** and presence ***(C)*** of a hemodynamically significant stenosis.

percent before flow is decreased distal to an obstruction. This is equivalent to a 50 percent reduction in diameter as seen arteriographically. In the presence of a hemodynamically significant internal carotid artery stenosis or occlusion, flow in the distal artery is augmented by collateral circulation through the superficial temporal, facial, and infraorbital branches of the external carotid artery. This flow passes into the orbit via the nasal, frontal, and supraorbital branches of the ophthalmic artery (Figure 10-3*C*).

Early experience with a cerebrovascular Doppler examination was reported by Brisman et al. (3). They observed that stenosis or occlusion of the internal carotid artery was associated with a reduction in the amplitude and velocity of common carotid artery flow. Maroon et al. (4) employed Doppler ultrasonography to assess ophthalmic artery flow velocity in a transorbital fashion (Figure 10-4), while Muller (5) reported the use of a directional Doppler velocimeter to evaluate flow in the frontal artery (Figure 10-5). Brockenbrough (6) described the use of superficial temporal and common carotid artery compression maneuvers in 1969. Combining these techniques with directional flow assessment in the periorbital arteries, he was able to describe five dominant collateral patterns (7).

Maroon et al. (4) were able to predict the presence of an internal carotid artery occlusion or a significant stenosis by evaluating the amplitude and velocity of ophthalmic artery flow; however, their accuracy decreased when there was adequate collateral circulation through the branches of the external carotid artery. Evidence of this collateral circulation was demonstrated by Muller (5). Using a directional Doppler velocimeter, he observed that an internal carotid artery stenosis or occlusion was associated with flow reversal in the frontal and ophthalmic arteries. Normally flow in the frontal artery is out of the orbit, while collateral circulation from branches of the external carotid artery results in a reversal of flow into the orbit (Figure 10-3*B* and *C*). Muller reported no falsely positive studies in 50 normal subjects. Fourteen of fifteen carotid occlusions and six of twelve high-grade stenoses were identified for a sensitivity of 74 percent.

Brockenbrough (6) described the addition of ipsilateral temporal and common carotid artery compression maneuvers in 1969. As subsequently refined by Bone and Barnes (8) and Barnes et al. (9,10), the CDE is performed using a 10-MHz directional Doppler. The supraorbital and/or frontal arteries are identified, and the direction of flow is determined. The response to superficial temporal, facial, infraorbital, and common carotid artery compression is then determined. The study is abnormal if the direction of flow is reversed in either or both arteries or if flow decreases with external carotid branch compression. Flow normally decreases with ipsilateral common carotid artery compression and is abnormal if it does not decrease with ipsilateral compression or if it decreases with contralateral common carotid artery compression.

Greater than 90 percent of the collateral patterns involve the ipsilateral external carotid artery and its branches and can be detected by these compression maneuvers (9). In the presence of a common carotid artery occlusion, collateralization will be from the contralateral carotid artery. Thus, if the right common carotid artery is occluded, flow in the right supraorbital or frontal

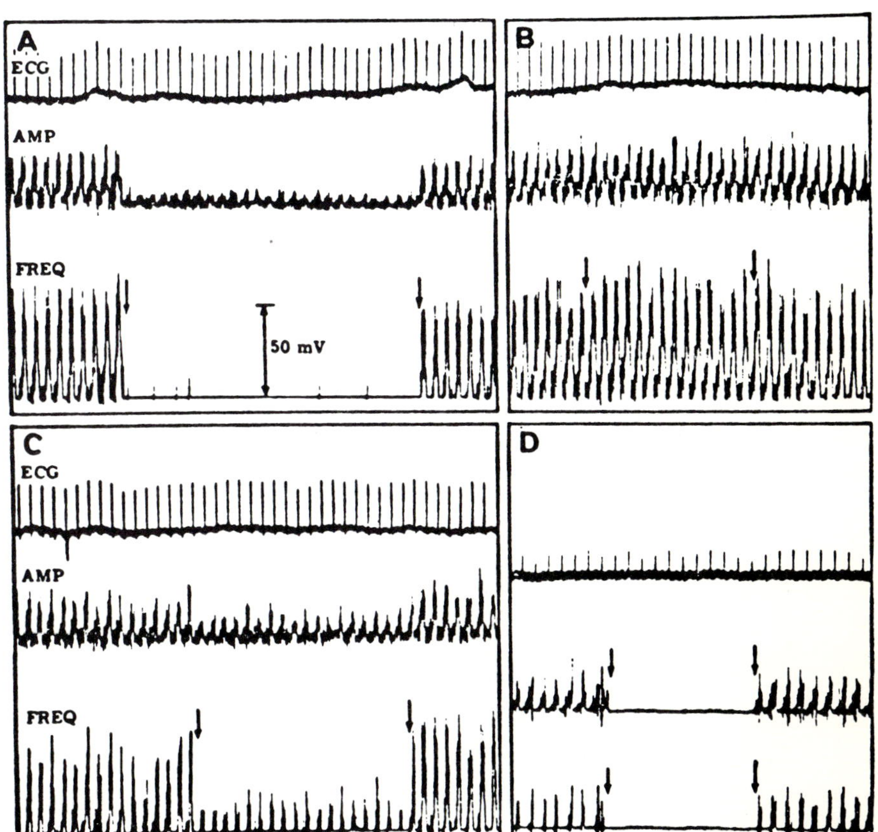

FIGURE 10-4. Experimental data obtained from the monkey (*Macaca speciosa*) demonstrating the source of the transorbital Doppler signal. Illustrated is a continuous recording of the electrocardiogram (ECG), mean amplitude (AMP), and frequency (FREQ) of the ophthalmic artery Doppler signal. There is a marked decrease in the amplitude and frequency of the Doppler signal with common carotid (*A*), internal carotid (*C*), and ophthalmic artery (*D*) compression (*between the arrows*). There were no changes with external carotid artery compression. [From Maroon JC, Piero DW, Campbell RL (4).]

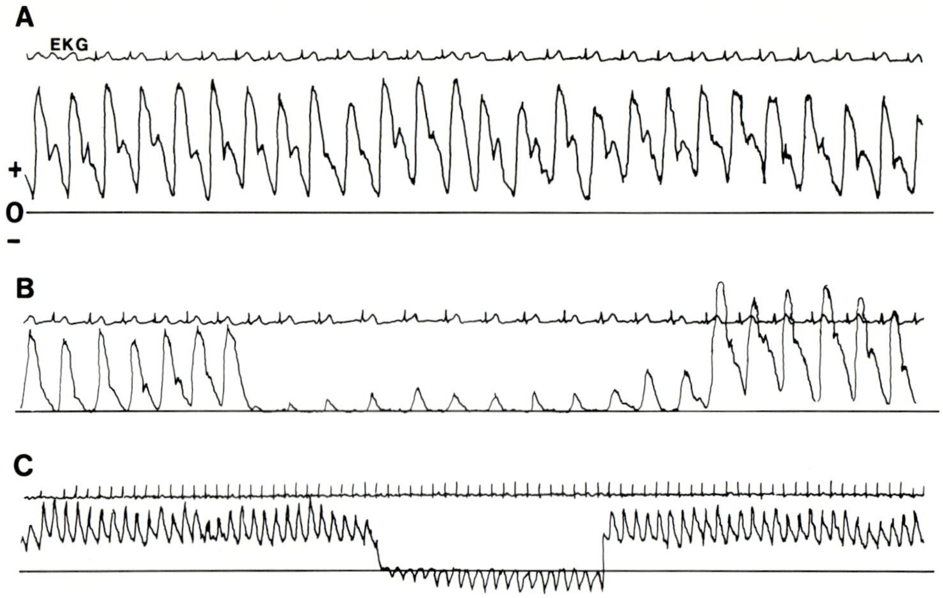

FIGURE 10-5. *(A)* Normal ophthalmic artery Doppler tracing demonstrating forward (+) flow. *(B)* Common carotid artery compression results in a decrease in forward flow, and *(C)* intraoperative clamping of the internal carotid artery results in flow reversal. [From HR Muller (5).]

artery will decrease when the left common carotid artery is compressed. Occasionally, collateral pathways may involve the internal maxillary or vertebral arteries. The CDE is insensitive to these variations, however.

Since Brockenbrough's description, the use of Doppler ultrasonography in cerebrovascular noninvasive testing has been extensively reported. The results, however, have been inconsistent, and the accuracy influenced by the technique employed, the definition of hemodynamically significant disease, and the relative distribution within the study population of stenotic and occluded vessels.

LoGerfo and Mason (11) assessed supraorbital artery flow direction alone and reported an unacceptable rate of falsely negative studies. Lye et al. (12) evaluated supraorbital artery flow direction and temporal artery compression, with an overall accuracy rate of 89 percent and a 22 percent incidence of falsely negative studies. They reported their greatest incidence of error in patients with stenosis or occlusion of the common carotid artery and in those patients with coexistent internal and external carotid artery stenoses. In such cases flow is reduced equally in the internal and external carotid arteries, so there is no pressure gradient between these circulations to promote flow reversal and collateralization.

Assessing flow direction in the supraorbital and/or frontal arteries, as well as the response to superficial temporal, facial, infraorbital, and common carotid artery compression, Bone and Barnes (8), Barnes et al. (9,10), and Duke et al. (13) reported an overall accuracy rate in excess of 90 percent, with a sensitivity which varied from 87 to 95 percent. McDonald et al. (14), however, reported a sensitivity of only 55 percent and an 81 percent accuracy using a similar technique, except that common carotid artery compression maneuvers were not employed. Evaluating 320 carotid arteries in our own series (15), the CDE had an accuracy of 87 percent, with a sensitivity of 84 percent and a specificity of 88 percent. There was a 50 percent sensitivity to the 50 to 59 percent stenosis, 71 percent to the 60 to 70 percent stenosis, 93 percent to the 71 to 99 percent stenosis, and a 94 percent sensitivity to carotid occlusion.

If the distribution of falsely negative studies is analyzed, the CDE is most sensitive to tightly stenotic or occluded arteries. Duke et al. (13) and Kempczinski (16) reported no falsely negative studies in those patients with carotid artery occlusion. Towne et al. (17) noted that two-thirds of his falsely negative studies were in those arteries with 50 to 99 percent stenoses. In our own series (15) there was a 95 percent sensitivity to carotid occlusion compared to a 78 percent sensitivity to the 50 to 99 percent stenosis ($p < 0.01$). Further, there was a 50 percent sensitivity to the 50 to 59 percent stenosis and an 85 percent sensitivity to the 60 to 99 percent stenosis ($p < 0.01$).

While the directional Doppler velocimeter used in the CDE is relatively inexpensive and there are no contraindications to the technique, it is highly technician- or operator-dependent. As a result, its reported accuracy has been variable, and the technique is no longer employed commonly. It remains valuable, however, as a framework upon which to discuss the anatomy and hemodynamics of the carotid arterial circulation and the collateral pathways that are associated with stenosis or occlusion of the internal carotid artery.

Supraorbital Photoplethysmography (SOPPG)

Supraorbital photoplethysmography employs an infrared light-emitting diode and an adjacent phototransistor to detect backscattered light. The amount of reflectance varies with the tissue microcirculation and thus can be used to detect a change in overall flow (18).

Unlike the directional Doppler, the SOPPG cannot determine

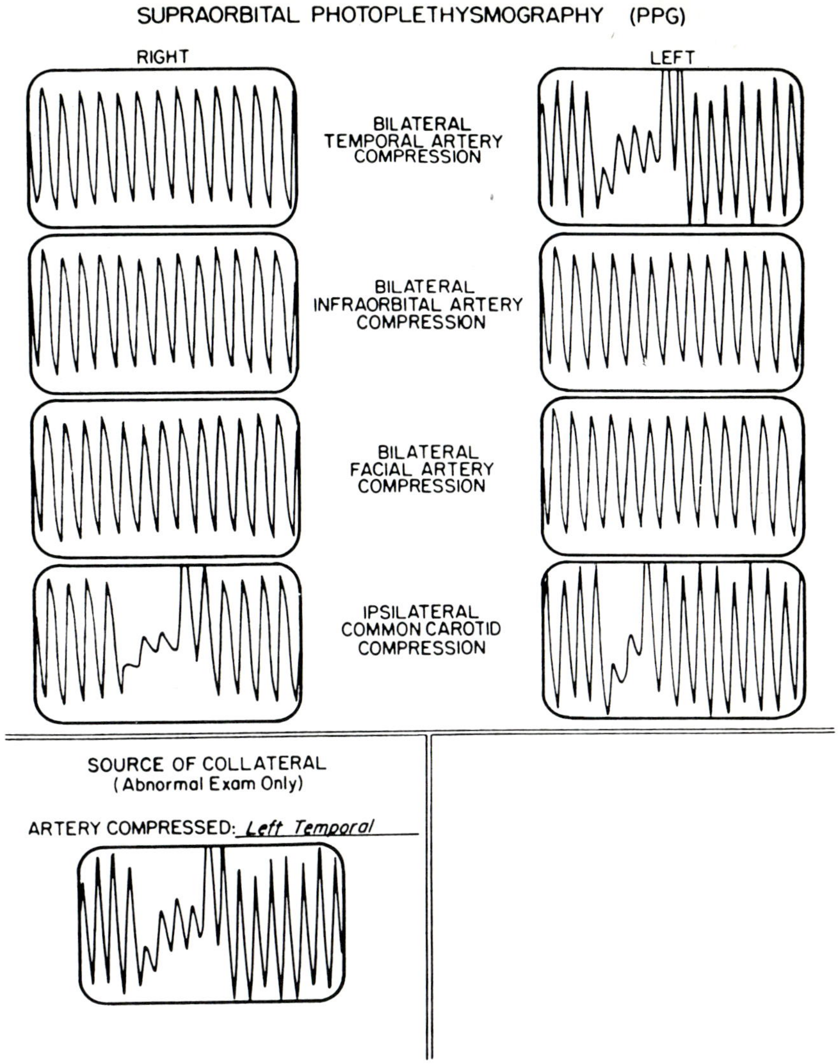

FIGURE 10-6. An abnormal supraorbital photoplethysmographic study demonstrating a decrease in left supraorbital flow with bilateral temporal artery compression (*upper right*) and with compression of the left superficial temporal artery (*lower left*). Flow is normally decreased with ipsilateral common carotid compression. This study is consistent with a hemodynamically significant obstruction of the left internal carotid artery, with collateral flow through the left external carotid and superficial temporal arteries.

the direction of flow. It can, however, detect a change in the amplitude of flow in response to common carotid and external carotid artery branch compression. The diode-sensor is placed over the eyebrow in the vascular watershed of the supraorbital and frontal arteries and is connected to an analogue recorder. The response to the compression maneuvers is then observed. A 15 percent decrease in amplitude with facial or infraorbital artery compression and/or a 33 percent decrease with superficial temporal artery compression correlates with a hemodynamically significant internal carotid artery obstruction (Figure 10-6).

The SOPPG was overly sensitive and had an 85 percent specificity (10,13). However, if the CDE and SOPPG were performed in combination and if the results were concordant, the presence or absence of a hemodynamically significant lesion was predicted in 98 percent of cases.

Oculoplethysmography

Oculoplethysmography (OPG-K), first described by Kartchner and McRae (19), employs a fluid medium for the transmission and recording of phasic changes in ocular volume. Since venous outflow from the eye is relatively constant, the cyclic variation in net ocular volume is a direct function of pulsatile arterial flow. The ascending, or anacrotic, limb of the ocular pulse volume wave begins when arterial inflow exceeds venous outflow and continues until the arterial flow is once again less than venous outflow. At this point the pulse wave peaks and begins the descending, or dicrotic, limb (Figure 10-7). Obstruction of the common or proximal internal carotid artery reduces flow to the ophthalmic artery and alters the pulse volume wave. Minimal stenoses decrease the slope of the ascending limb, resulting in a delayed peak, while increasing degrees of proximal arterial obstruction delay the onset of the ascending limb. Severe proximal stenosis, with poor collateralization, may also result in a decreased pulse amplitude (Figure 10-8). Alterations in the descending, or dicrotic limb, are generally the result of venous pathology.

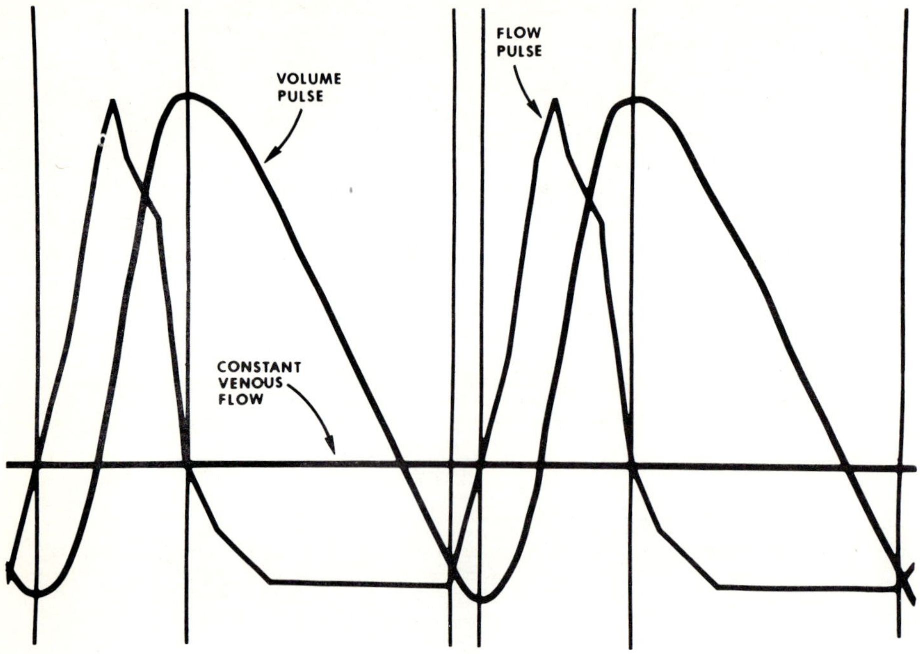

FIGURE 10-7. The relationship between the arterial flow pulse and the ocular pulse volume wave. [Reproduced with permission from McRae LP, Kartchner MM: Oculoplethysmography. In Kempczinski RF, Yao JST (eds): *Practical Noninvasive Vascular Diagnosis*. Chicago, Year Book Medical Publishers, 1983, pp 181–202. Copyright © 1982 by Year Book Medical Publishers, Inc., Chicago.]

Defining a hemodynamically significant stenosis as one which reduced the arterial diameter by 40 percent or more and resulted in a 0.01-s delay in the onset of the ocular pulse volume wave, Kartchner and McRae (19) initially reported an overall accuracy for the technique of 91 percent compared with arteriography. The specificity was 97 percent and the sensitivity 76 percent. The presence of bilateral carotid artery occlusions or a contralateral carotid artery stenosis or occlusion accounted for 62 percent of the falsely negative studies.

In order to reduce the number of falsely negative studies, carotid phonoangiography and, later, earlobe photoplethysmography were incorporated as adjuncts to the OPG-K. Phonoangiography permits the visual analysis of carotid bruits, employing a handheld microphone to allow auscultation of the cervical carotid artery in the low, mid-, and high neck. The results are displayed on an oscilloscope. The source of a bruit may thus be localized and its duration evaluated with respect to the first and second heart sounds. Bruits localized to the low neck are generally transmitted thoracic murmurs, while those in the mid- and high neck are generally carotid in origin (Figure 10-9). The pitch and duration of the bruit increase directly with the percentage of stenosis; and, while the bruit is primarily a systolic phenomenon, it may extend into diastole when the stenosis exceeds 70 percent. As the obstruction approaches 80 to 90 percent, however, flow decreases and the bruit may disappear (Figure 10-10). Because this technique is unable to consistently identify high-grade stenoses, phonoangiography alone has an unacceptably high incidence of falsely negative studies, 31 percent (19).

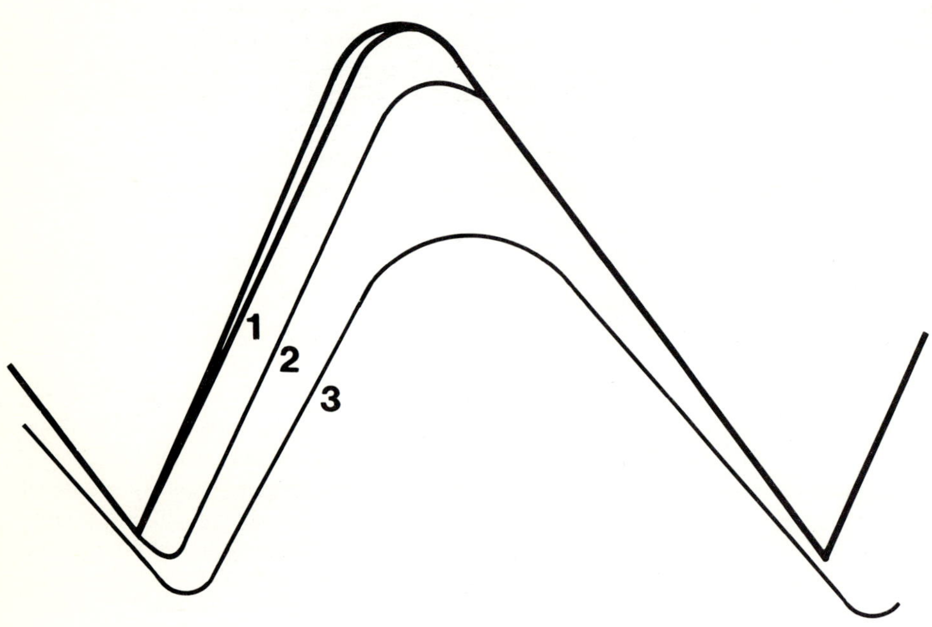

FIGURE 10-8. Minimal stenoses alter the slope of the ascending limb of the ocular pulse volume wave resulting in a delayed peak (1), while moderate to severe stenoses delay the onset of the ascending limb (2) and/or result in a decreased pulse amplitude (3). [Modified from Kartchner MM, McRae LP (25).]

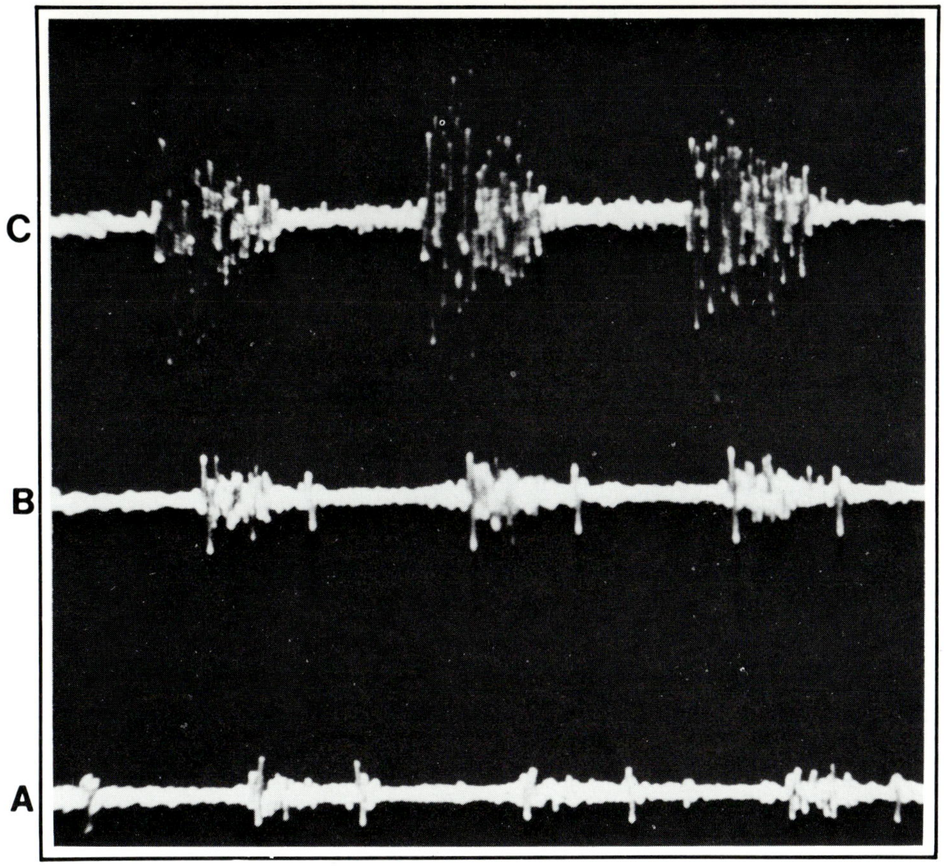

FIGURE 10-9. Carotid phonoangiograms from the *(A)* low, *(B)* mid, and *(C)* high neck demonstrating a bruit of probable carotid origin, which begins in the midneck and radiates upward.

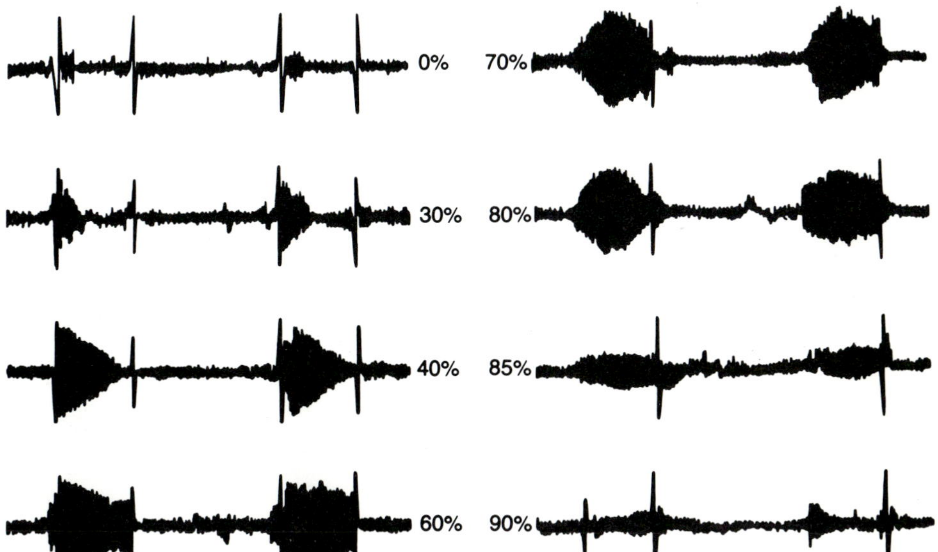

FIGURE 10-10. The relationship between carotid artery stenoses and their representative carotid bruits. [From Kartchner MM, McRae LP (25).]

However, in combination with oculoplethysmography, it increases the sensitivity to bilaterally symmetrical disease and lesser stenoses associated with a minimal reduction in flow. In addition, Kartchner et al. (20) have suggested that a decrease in the intensity of a significant bruit may indicate progression of a stenosis toward occlusion in the patient with a markedly positive OPG-K.

Photoplethysmography employs a photosensor attached to the earlobe to detect flow from branches of the external carotid artery. This was initially employed to establish a reference baseline for measuring bilateral ocular pulse wave delays in the patient with severe bilateral internal carotid artery stenosis or occlusion. It has subsequently been used to detect severe external carotid artery stenosis as a source of cervical bruits (20). Using phonoangiography and earlobe photoplethysmography to supplement the oculoplethysmographic data, Kartchner et al. (20) reported an accuracy approaching 90 percent, with a specificity of 92 percent and a sensitivity of 88 percent. Gross et al. (21) also reported an overall accuracy of 90 percent, with an 87 percent specificity and a 91 percent sensitivity.

Despite these reports, however, Blackshear et al. (22) have suggested that the bilateral presence of hemodynamically significant disease still adversely affects the accuracy of the OPG-K. In their original report Kartchner et al. (19) noted a sensitivity of 76 percent when the technique was used without adjunctive carotid phonoangiography. Of the 24 falsely negative studies, 15 were associated with significant contralateral disease. In our own series (23), 132 arteries in 66 patients were examined prospectively with the OPG-K. The sensitivity was 70 percent, while the specificity was 83 percent. Analysis of the 17 falsely negative studies demonstrated that 10 of 28 (36 percent) significant lesions were misdiagnosed in 6 of 14 patients. The remaining falsely negative studies were in patients with unilateral lesions. In a subsequent report, Kartchner et al. (20) obtained an 88 percent sensitivity using carotid phonoangiography and earlobe photoplethysmography as adjuncts. However, these data were interpreted on a per patient, rather than a per artery, basis. Thus if only one of two bilaterally significant stenoses were identified, the study would be correct on a per patient basis. In addition, even though Gross et al. (21) reported a 91 percent sensitivity, all of their falsely negative studies occurred in patients with bilateral disease.

Blackshear et al. (22) observed bilateral disease in 27 of 54 patients, with hemodynamically significant lesions bilaterally in 14. Three of these patients had positive studies bilaterally, while results were negative bilaterally in four patients and positive on one side only in seven. They further observed that phonoangiography demonstrated significant bruits in only 14 of 41 arteries with greater than 50 percent stenosis by arteriography. Six of ten occluded internal carotid arteries were associated with a bruit in the high neck.

Kartchner and McRae (24,25) also reported that they have electronically extracted a differential waveform (Diff) from the two ocular pulse waves by continuously subtracting the amplitude of the left pulse wave (L) from that of the right (R):

$$\mathrm{Diff}(t) = 2[R(t) - L(t)]$$

Correlating these data with operative flow measurements, they have defined five grades of stenosis. If the bruit does not extend through systole and if there is no delay in the ocular pulses or if the deflection of the differential from baseline is less than 10 percent of the ocular pulse amplitude, the stenosis is less than 40 percent and the mean flow reduction is less than 20 percent. A 40 to 60 percent stenosis is associated with a 20 to 30 percent mean flow reduction and is characterized by a bruit extending through systole and a deflection of the differential from the baseline of between 10 and 20 percent of the ocular pulse amplitude. If the deflection of the differential is accompanied by a slight or inconsistent visible delay in the ocular pulse, the stenosis is between 60 and 70 percent and the mean flow reduction between 30 and 40 percent. A 70 to 85 percent stenosis, and a mean flow reduction exceeding 40 percent is accompanied by a pansystolic bruit, possibly extending into diastole and consistent, visible delays in the ocular pulse wave at its peak and possibly at the onset of the anacrotic limb. The difference between a severe stenosis and an occlusion is determined by carotid phonoangiography. An occlusion is characterized by the absence of a bruit and OPG-K findings similar to those for a 70 to 85 percent stenosis.

In addition to screening for the presence of hemodynamically significant carotid artery obstruction, attempts have been made to correlate an abnormal OPG-K with a higher incidence of ischemic cerebrovascular events. Kartchner and McRae (24) reported a 12 percent stroke rate, after 2 years, in a group of asymptomatic patients with hemodynamically significant stenoses identified by OPG-K and carotid phonoangiography. Forty-one percent of the strokes, however, were unrelated to the stenotic lesion, and a large number of the patients were nonrandomly selected for prophylactic carotid endarterectomy. In a subsequent study (26), the same authors evaluated 234 patients with the OPG-K prior to planned cardiovascular surgical procedures and reported a 1 percent stroke rate in patients with a normal OPG-K and a 17 percent incidence in those with an abnormal OPG-K. Only 47 percent of the patients were asymptomatic, however, while 27 percent had had nonlateralizing symptoms, 18 percent transient ischemic attacks (TIAs), and 8 percent a previous stroke.

Ocular Pneumoplethysmography

Ocular pneumoplethysmography (OPG-G) employs an air-filled system which, like the fluid medium of the OPG-K, provides a means to record the phasic variations in ocular volume. Unlike the OPG-K, it incorporates a system of induced and controlled ocular hypertension to measure ophthalmic artery pressure. The pulse volume changes are recorded via hemispherical suction cups (12 mm in diameter) applied to the sclera of each eye and held in place by a vacuum. As the vacuum is increased, the intraocular geometry is distorted and the intraocular pressure increased. The amount of vacuum applied has been correlated with the intraocular pressure, and thus it is possible to determine that pressure at which ophthalmic artery flow ceases—that is, the ophthalmic artery systolic pressure (OAP). As initially conceived, measurement of the ophthalmic artery pressure was combined with ipsilateral common carotid artery compression as a means of measuring collateral cerebral blood flow (27). When the noninvasively determined pressure was compared with the operatively measured internal carotid artery back pressure, only 3 of 81 patients showed a difference of 5 mmHg or more between the noninvasively predicted and operatively measured values (28).

Initial reports stressed the value of this technique in assessing the adequacy of collateral cerebral circulation. Martinez et al. (29) evaluated 11 patients with head and neck cancers, who potentially might have required resection of the carotid artery at the time of tumor dissection. Citing a 64 percent mortality rate associated with acute disruption of the carotid artery, compared with a 14 percent mortality rate following elective resection, the authors employed the OPG-G to predict tolerance of elective carotid artery resection. Of the 11 patients, 4 subsequently underwent carotid artery resection. The noninvasively measured common carotid artery back pressures varied from 52 to 82 mmHg, and there were no neurologic complications. The authors concluded that 50 mmHg was the critical value for determining resectability of the internal carotid artery, basing this estimate on previous experience with temporary carotid artery occlusion during endarterectomy. In a subsequent report, Nolph and associates (30) examined results in nine patients who underwent carotid artery resection or ligation. A pressure of 60 mmHg was the discriminate value in this study. One patient had hemiparesis, attributed to systemic hypotension, in the immediate postligation period.

In 1977, Gee and associates (31) first reported use of the OPG-G as a screening device to determine the presence of hemodynamically significant carotid stenoses. The following four criteria were considered diagnostic of a significant carotid stenosis: (1) if the systemic systolic blood pressure (brachial systolic pressure, BSP) was 142 mmHg or less and the OAP/BSP ratio was less than 0.77; (2) if the BSP was greater than 142 mmHg and the OAP was 110 mmHg or less; (3) if the difference between OAPs was 5 mmHg or more; and/or (4) if the OAP was greater than 110 mmHg and there was a difference in pulse amplitude at any point in the tracing. Defining a hemodynamically significant obstruction as a 75 percent stenosis or greater, they reported a 95 percent accuracy, with a sensitivity of 95 percent and a specificity of 95 percent. McDonald et al. (32) modified criteria 1 and 3, suggesting that the OAP/BSP index should be 0.66 or less and not "less than 0.77" and that pulse amplitude differences should be 2 mm or greater at 110 mmHg rather than "a difference in pulse amplitude at any point in the tracing" (Figure 10-11*A* to *D*). Using these modified criteria, they reported a 92 percent accuracy, with a specificity of 100 percent and a sensitivity of 87 percent.

Initially the OPG-G could generate a maximum vacuum of only 300 mmHg. The maximum intraocular pressure achieved with a 300-mmHg vacuum was 110 mmHg. Twenty-seven of the sixty-three patients reported by McDonald et al. (32) were hypertensive, and eight had positive studies. Of these eight, four had an OAP on the affected side which was less than 110 mmHg and four had an OAP which was greater than 110 mmHg with pulse amplitude differences present. Because the ophthalmic artery systolic pressure in hypertensive patients often exceeds 110 mmHg, a modification was introduced which permitted the generation of a 500-mmHg vacuum (Figure 10-12). This produced a maximum intraocular pressure of 144 mmHg. Employing this modification, Gee (33) reported his results for 1534 arteries. The sensitivity was 96 percent, the specificity 98 percent, and the overall accuracy 97 percent. As reported previously, the study was abnormal if the difference between ophthalmic artery systolic pressures was 5 mmHg or greater. However, the author modified the simple ratio used to compare the ophthalmic and brachial artery systolic pressures. Instead of the previous index of 0.77 reported by Gee et al. (31) or 0.66 reported by McDonald and associates (32), the linear regression, OAP = 0.43 BSP + 39, had been substituted. Data from this series indicated that, unlike the OPG-K, the OPG-G was more accurate in the diagnosis of bilateral disease. Of 31 patients with bilateral carotid occlusions or with a unilateral occlusion opposite to a hemodynamically significant stenosis, the OPG-G correctly diagnosed 57 of 62 (92 percent) obstructions.

While the OPG-G can neither distinguish between stenosis or occlusion nor quantitate the degree of stenosis, the ophthalmic artery pressure gradient does increase in relation to the type of obstruction and the sensitivity is a direct function of the percentage of stenosis. Of the 208 patients studied by Gee (33) with a hemodynamically significant stenosis opposite to an undiseased artery, the gradient between ophthalmic artery pressures was 5 to 9 mmHg in 50 percent, 10 to 14 mmHg in 26 percent, and >14 mmHg in 24 percent. This distribution was shifted in the 111 patients with an occlusion opposite to an undiseased artery. In these patients the gradient was 5 to 9 mmHg in 18 percent, 10 to 14 mmHg in 25 percent, and >14 mmHg in 57 percent. Of the 111 patients with a unilateral occlusion, 35 (32 percent) had a normal OAP/BSP ratio, suggesting adequate collateral circulation. In our own series (15) the OPG-G had an accuracy of 90 percent, with a 93 percent specificity and an 85 percent sensitivity. Only 287 of 320 arteries could be studied with the OPG-G. Exclusions were made on the basis of specific medical contraindications including conjunctivitis, untreated glaucoma, a history of spontaneous retinal detachment, or recent trauma. The sensitivity of the technique was directly related to the degree of stenosis. There was a 53 percent sensitivity to 50 to 59 percent stenoses, a 79 percent sensitivity to 60 to 70 percent stenoses, an 86 percent sensitivity to 71 to 99 percent stenoses, and a 96 percent sensitivity to carotid occlusion (Table 10-2).

The OPG-G has also been used to document the increase in distal carotid artery pressure following carotid endarterectomy, as well as to confirm patency of the endarterectomy following surgery. In 14 of 15 patients (34) with a hemodynamically significant stenosis and a contralateral occlusion, endarterectomy of the stenotic artery resulted in hemodynamic improvement on the ipsilateral side, with an average increase in the OAP of 17 mmHg. In addition, 12 of 15 patients also demonstrated improvement on the contralateral side, with an average increase in the OAP of 12 mmHg (34). During late follow-up, the OPG-G has also been useful in identifying recurrent stenosis. While the incidence of symptomatic carotid restenosis is low, Kremen et al. (35) used the OPG-G to demonstrate a 9.8 percent incidence of recurrent stenosis following 172 endarterectomies. Only 2 percent were symptomatic.

The technique can also yield physiologic data. Gee et al. (36) have calculated ocular blood flow from the pulse rate and amplitude, demonstrating a significant decrease in flow in patients

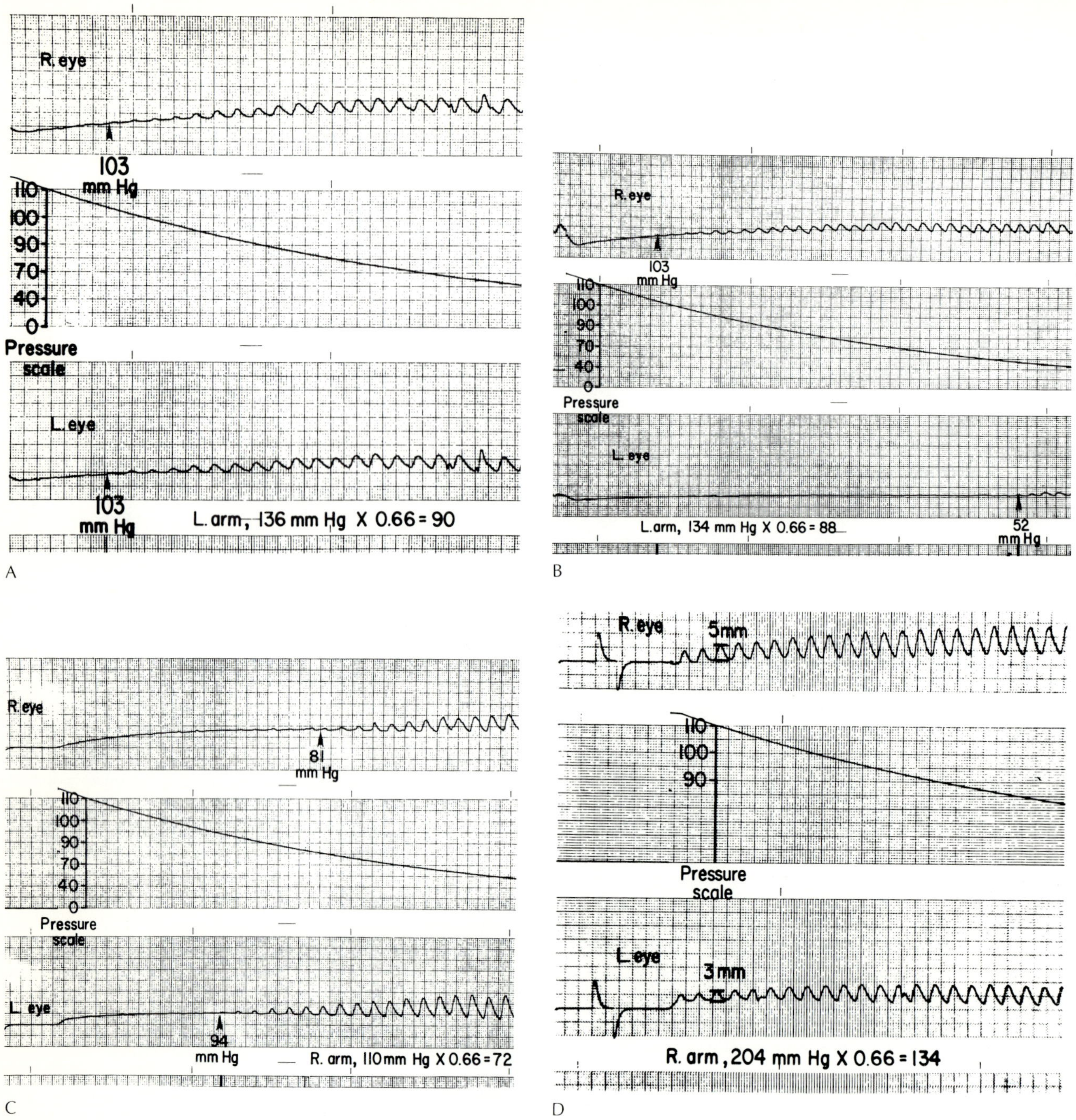

FIGURE 10-11. Studies obtained using the OPG-G. *(A)* The normal tracing demonstrates the simultaneous return of pulsatile flow in the right (*top scale*) and left (*bottom scale*) eyes. The ophthalmic artery pressures (103 mmHg) are determined using the center scale and exceed two-thirds (0.66) of the brachial systolic pressure (left arm, 136 mmHg). (From Lynch TG, Wright CB, Miller EV: Oculopneumoplethysmography, Doppler examination and supraorbital photoplethysmography. A comparison of hemodynamic techniques in assessing cerebrovascular occlusive disease. Ann Surg 1981, 194:731–736.) ***(B)*** The left ophthalmic artery pressure (52 mmHg) is less than two-thirds of the brachial systolic pressure (left arm, 134 mmHg × 0.66 = 88), indicating a hemodynamically significant obstruction of the left common or internal carotid artery. ***(C)*** Both ophthalmic artery pressures (right eye, 81 mmHg; left eye, 94 mmHg) are greater than two-thirds of the brachial systolic pressure (right arm, 110 mmHg × 0.66 = 73); however, the right ophthalmic artery pressure is 13 mmHg less than that on the left. This indicates a hemodynamically significant obstruction of the right common or internal carotid artery. ***(D)*** The hypertensive individual in this study had ophthalmic artery pressures which exceeded 110 mmHg. The difference in pulse wave amplitudes (right eye, 5 mm; left eye, 3 mm), measured at an ophthalmic artery pressure of 110 mmHg, was 2 mm, however, indicating a hemodynamically significant obstruction of the left common or internal carotid artery.

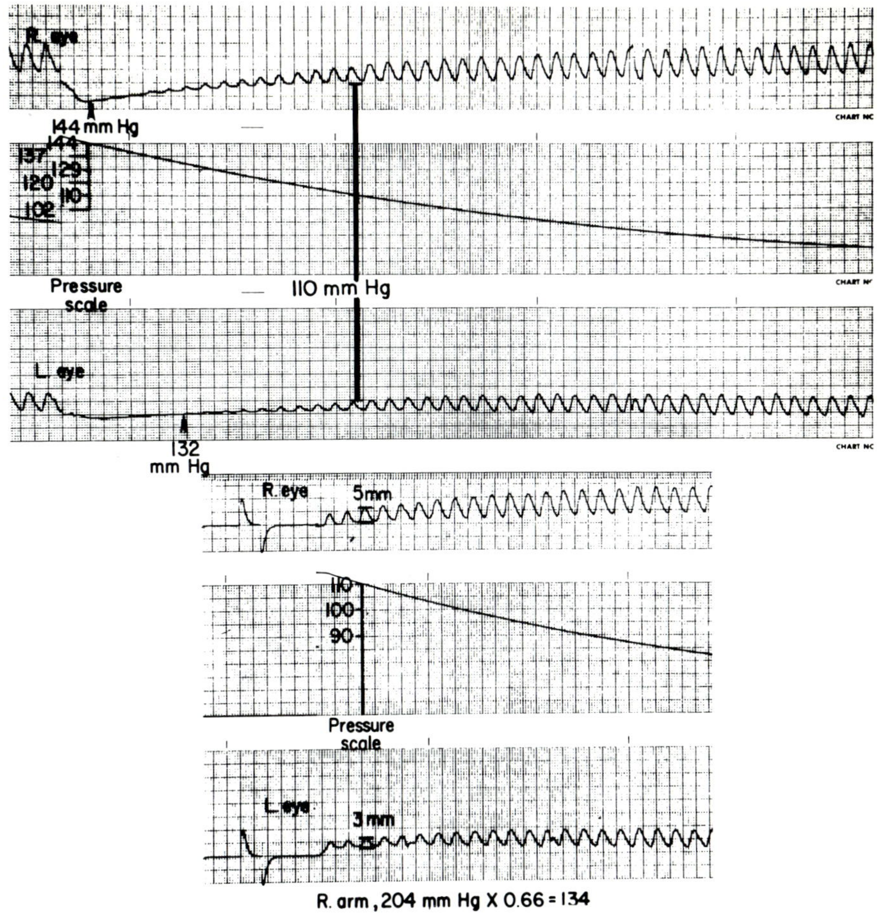

FIGURE 10-12. The tracing from Figure 10-11D (*below*) is compared with a tracing, from the same patient, obtained using an OPG-G with a 500-mmHg vacuum (*above*). The latter device is capable of generating an intraocular pressure of 144 mmHg and demonstrates the difference between ophthalmic artery pressures (right eye, 144 mmHg; left eye, 132 mmHg) characteristic of a hemodynamically significant obstruction of the left common or internal carotid artery.

with hemodynamically significant obstruction. Further, the pulse wave morphology provides a noninvasive correlate of intracranial pressure (37). Morphologically, the normal pulse wave obtained using the OPG-G lacks a dicrotic notch, reflecting the low resistance of the intracranial circulation and the damping effect of the carotid siphon. In a study of 81 head-injured patients (37), Gee observed a consistent relationship between increased intracranial pressure measurements and the presence of a dicrotic notch (Figure 10-13). There was, in addition, a significant decrease in ocular blood flow in these patients, which could be correlated with subsequent mortality.

Similar to studies done using the OPG-K, attempts have also been made to correlate an abnormal OPG-G with subsequent ischemic cerebrovascular events. Cullen et al. (38) using the OPG-G to characterize 106 patients with asymptomatic carotid bruits, identified 77 patients with hemodynamically insignificant

TABLE 10-2. The Accuracy of Ocular Pneumoplethysmography (OPG-G)

Accuracy = 90% | Specificity = 93% | Sensitivity = 85%

Carotid Arteriogram (Arteries)		OPG-G Examination: Normal	OPG-G Examination: Abnormal	Accuracy, %
Occlusion	(47)	2	45	96
71–99% stenosis	(37)	5	32	86
60–70% stenosis	(24)	5	19	79
50–59% stenosis	(15)	7	8	53
<50% stenosis	(164)	153	11	93

Note: Statistical comparisons using chi-square analysis and Bonferroni's inequality equation for multiple comparisons ($p < 0.0167$ for 95% confidence): 50–99% vs. 100%; 50–59% vs. 60–99%; 50–71% vs. 71–99%; $p = 0.0312$; $p = 0.135$.

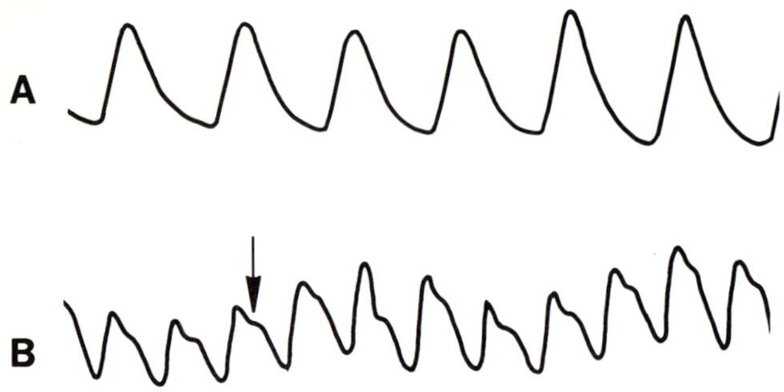

FIGURE 10-13. Two tracings obtained with the OPG-G illustrating *(A)* a normal pulse wave contour and *(B)* one with catacrotic or dicrotic notching (*arrow*).

carotid stenoses and 29 with hemodynamically significant stenoses. Follow-up at 18 months demonstrated that 11 percent of those without significant stenoses had become symptomatic compared to 24 percent of the group with significant stenoses. The relative percentage of strokes and TIAs was not reported, but this series does demonstrate a higher percentage of cerebral ischemic events occurring in patients with hemodynamically significant carotid stenoses. Busuttil et al. (39) also reported an increase in the incidence of strokes (6.6 percent) and a significant increase in the incidence of TIAs (29 percent) in 45 patients with asymptomatic and hemodynamically significant carotid stenoses followed for an average of 19 months. In 28 patients with asymptomatic and hemodynamically insignificant bruits, there were no strokes and a 7.1 percent incidence of TIAs.

Ultrasound

The early noninvasive, cerebrovascular diagnostic techniques were dependent upon Doppler ultrasound. With the exception of plethysmographic techniques such as the OPG-K and the OPG-G, subsequent procedures have also depended heavily on ultrasound. In theory, when transmitted ultrasound strikes a moving interface, the frequency of the reflected wave is shifted in proportion to the velocity of that interface. Conversely, when transmitted ultrasound strikes a stationary interface, it is reflected, unchanged, in proportion to the density of the interface. The Doppler ultrasonic velocimeter is the practical application of the former physical principle, while B-mode (brightness modulation) ultrasonic imaging results from the latter.

The Doppler transducer, a polarized, synthetic, ceramic crystal with piezoelectric properties, emits a high-frequency, ultrasonic pressure wave with the application of an electrical field (40–42). When the transmitted ultrasonic waves are reflected from moving red blood cells, the frequency of the ultrasound is altered, or shifted, in proportion to the velocity of the blood cells. The reflected ultrasonic wave then strikes the same, or a second, piezoelectric crystal, producing a voltage which is proportional to the frequency of the wave. The resulting frequency shift, relative to the transmitted frequency, may then be interpreted as an audible signal or an analogue record.

The Doppler effect is used to explain the frequency shift which occurs when transmitted ultrasound is reflected from a moving interface, such as red blood cells. The velocity V of blood flow can then be determined from the following relationship:

$$V = \frac{\Delta F \mu}{2 \cos \theta f_0}$$

where ΔF is the frequency shift, μ the speed of sound through blood, θ the probe angle relative to the longitudinal axis of the blood vessel, and f_0 the transmitted frequency.

If the above relationship is rewritten, it is evident that the magnitude of the frequency shift is related not only to the velocity of blood flow, but also to the transmitted frequency f_0 and the probe angle θ:

$$\Delta F = \frac{2 \cos \theta V f_0}{\mu}$$

While the magnitude of the frequency shift is directly related to the transmitted frequency f_0, absorption of the ultrasound by tissue is proportional to the square of the transmitted frequency f_0^2. Thus greater tissue penetration is achieved at lower transmitting frequencies, but at the expense of a decrease in the magnitude of the frequency shift (41,42). The optimum frequency f_{opt} is related to the depth d in centimeters by the following relationship (43):

$$f_{opt} = \frac{9}{d}$$

The Doppler transducer can be modified to permit continuous or pulsed (gated) sampling of the reflected ultrasound. The continuous-wave Doppler transducer (Figure 10-14*A*) has two piezoelectric crystals, one of which transmits ultrasound while the other continuously receives the reflected, Doppler-shifted signal. The ultrasound is reflected from red blood cells across the diameter of the vessel, so that the reflected and Doppler-shifted frequencies represent a range of red cell velocities in the plane of insonation. The pulsed Doppler transducer (Figure 10-14*B*) has a single crystal, which alternately transmits and receives ultrasound. The timing of the receiving mode relative to the preceding transmission determines the depth, or distance from the probe, at which the reflected ultrasound is sampled. This permits flow velocity measurements within a discrete sampling area, such as the midstream of an artery.

While the magnitude of the frequency shift is directly related to flow velocity, the direction of the frequency shift is a function of the direction of flow. Flow toward the transducer results in a Doppler-shifted frequency which is greater than the transmitted frequency, while flow away from the transducer results in a decrease in the transmitted frequency. A continuous-wave directional Doppler velocimeter is employed in the cerebrovascular Doppler examination (CDE) to determine the direction and amplitude of periorbital blood flow. With the addition of a position-sensing arm, both continuous-wave and pulsed Doppler transducers have been used to generate a flow-dependent map of the carotid artery and its branches (ultrasonic arteriography or Doppler ultrasonic imaging).

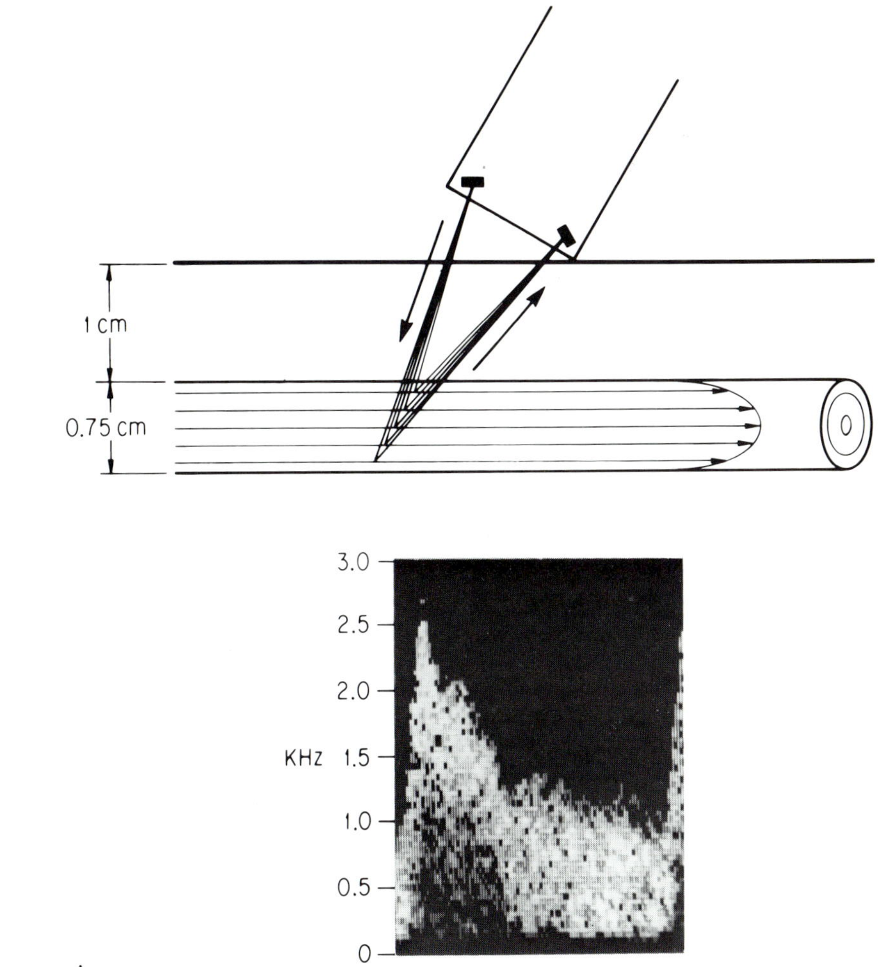

A

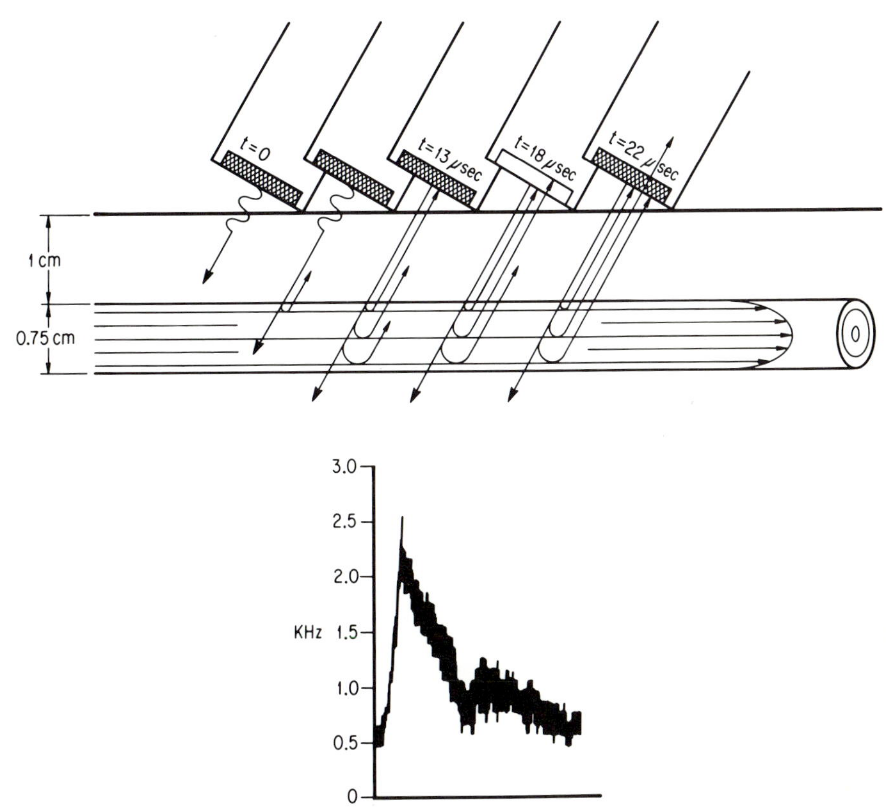

B

FIGURE 10-14. (***A***, *top*) The sampling range of a continuous-wave Doppler velocimeter encompasses the entire diameter of the insonated vessel. (***B***, *top*) The range of the pulsed Doppler velocimeter, however, is limited to a small sample volume, the relative position of which is dependent upon the time relationship between the transmitting and the receiving modes of the single piezoelectric crystal. In the example, an ultrasonic wave is emitted at time $t = 0$; only at time $t = 18$ μs does the crystal receives a wave, which was reflected from the midstream of the vessel.

A parabolic profile characterizes laminar flow at peak systole. The midstream spectral profile obtained with a pulsed instrument (***B***, *bottom*) reflects the well-defined spectral envelope and window, which are characteristic of midstream flow velocity. The spectral profile obtained with a continuous-wave instrument (***A***, *bottom*), however, is characterized by a relative spectral broadening. Because the continuous-wave velocimeter reflects the velocity profile across the entire diameter of the vessel, the spectral envelope is more divergent and the window less well defined.

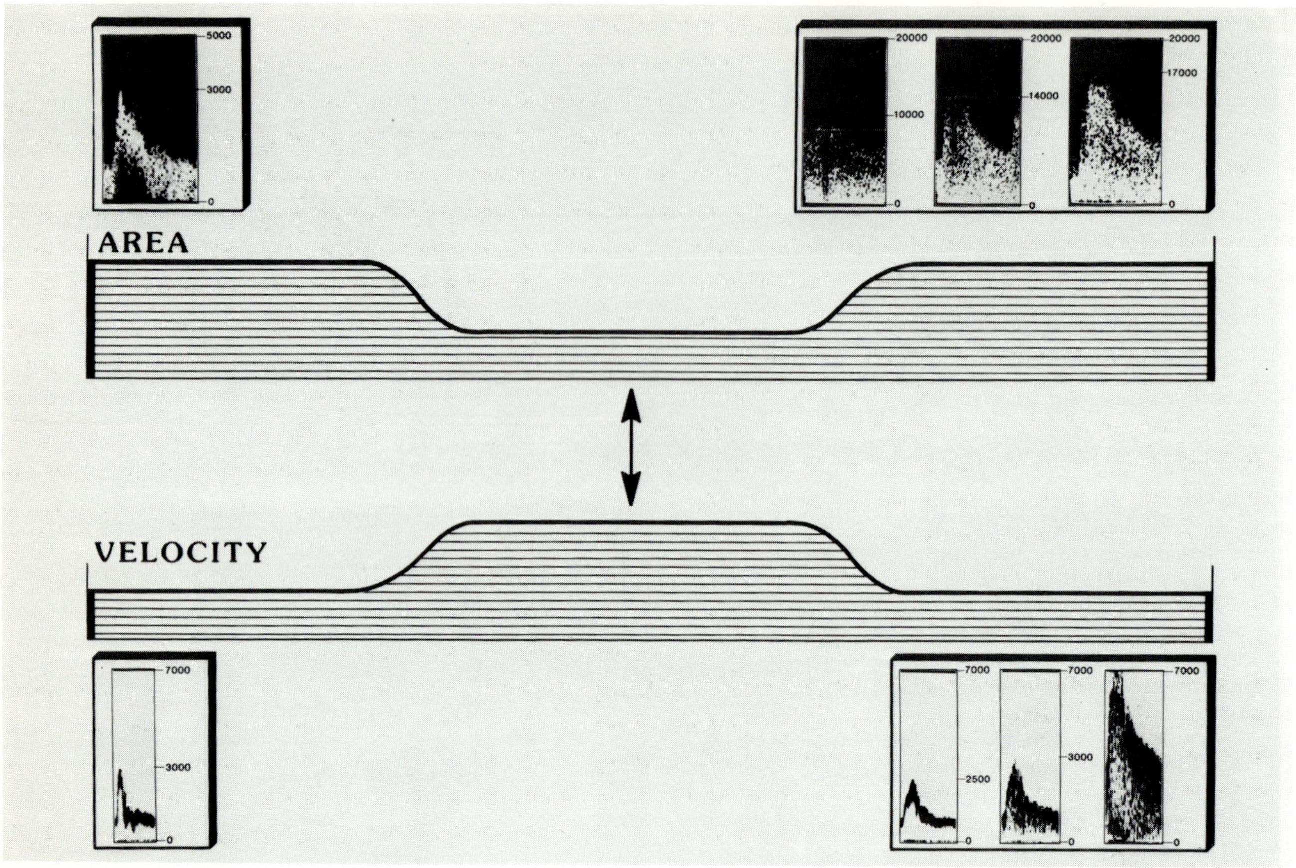

FIGURE 10-15. The figure illustrates the inverse relationship between the cross-sectional area of an artery (area) and flow velocity (velocity). Also illustrated are normal spectral profiles characteristic of the continuous-wave (*top left*) and pulsed Doppler velocimeter (*bottom left*), and profiles demonstrating the changes that occur with progressive stenoses (*top right* and *bottom right*, respectively). [Bottom right and left from Zierler RE, Roederer GO, Strandness DE: The use of frequency spectral analysis in carotid artery surgery. In Bergan JJ, Yao JST (eds): *Cerebrovascular Insufficiency*. New York, Grune & Stratton, 1983, pp 137–163. Reproduced by permission of Grune & Stratton, Inc.]

In addition, both continuous-wave and pulsed Doppler velocimeters have been used in an attempt to quantitate, noninvasively, the degree of stenosis (spectral analysis). Since flow Q is a function of velocity V and cross-sectional area A,

$$Q = VA$$

Velocity is directly related to flow and indirectly related to cross-sectional area:

$$V = \frac{Q}{A}$$

If the flow is constant, then the velocity of flow must increase as the cross-sectional area of the artery is reduced by stenosis. This increased flow velocity is reflected in an increased peak systolic frequency (Figure 10-15). Using spectral analytic techniques, the arterial flow velocity profile can be characterized using the Doppler-shifted frequency output of continuous-wave and pulsed Doppler velocimeters.

Depending upon the electronic processing, ultrasound may be used not only to determine the direction and velocity of a moving interface, but also to sense the depth and amplitude of signals reflected from a stationary interface, thus creating a visual image of the subjacent structures. The amplitude of the reflected signal is proportional to the difference in density of the two media at the interface. B-mode (brightness modulation) ultrasonic imaging employs time relationships to sense the depth of these interfaces and brightness variations to express differences in amplitude. If the changes in the reflected ultrasound can be displayed at a sufficient rate (greater than 15 frames per second), then a real-time image can be obtained, providing information about physiologic movement (real-time B-mode ultrasonography).

Doppler Ultrasonic Imaging

Using a position sensing arm and a storage oscilloscope, continuous-wave or pulsed Doppler imaging systems can be used to generate a flow-dependent image of the carotid artery and its branches. The continuous-wave image is relative and cannot be used to determine the vessel size or to visualize and measure stenotic lesions (Figure 10-16). Diagnostic implications are drawn from the Doppler audio signals recorded at various points along the imaged artery (44). In addition, initial evaluations of continuous-wave Doppler imaging also employed the CDE as an adjunct. Spencer et al. (45) reported an accuracy of 84 percent, but did not calculate the sensitivity or specificity. Thomas et al. (46) reported an accuracy of 89 percent, with 6 of 13 incorrect studies being falsely positive. Using data reported by Blackwell et al. (47), a sensitivity of 81 percent and a specificity of 78 percent were calculated. There was, however, a 100 percent correlation with total occlusion.

While some authors (48) have measured the percentage stenosis directly from a pulsed Doppler image, this has generally proved to be unsatisfactory because of calcification and shadowing (Figure 10-17*A* and *B*). The densely calcific plaque prevents the further transmission of ultrasound, resulting in subjacent shadows or echo-free areas which obscure portions of the arterial lumen and make precise diagnosis difficult. In a series reported by Wasserman et al. (23), 33 percent of patients with stenoses, determined angiographically to exceed 50 percent, had calcification and resulting echo-free areas which interfered with determination of the percentage stenosis. While 22 of 26 (85 percent) internal carotid artery occlusions were correctly predicted, it was not possible to quantify the degree of stenosis accurately. Only 54 percent of stenoses less than 50 percent and 73 percent of stenoses greater than 50 percent were accurately quantified. Barnes et al. (49) reported a high diagnostic accuracy using pulsed Doppler imaging; however, spectral analysis of the Doppler audio output was necessary to accurately predict the percentage stenosis.

Sumner et al. (48) reported the results of pulsed Doppler imaging in 200 carotid arteries. The percentage of stenosis was determined from the ultrasonic image, obtaining measurements, to the nearest millimeter, at the point of maximum stenosis and from the internal carotid image distal to the stenosis. When the image was difficult to measure, however, "the audible Doppler signal was used to supplement the visual data in estimating the degree of stenosis." When the noninvasively estimated stenosis was compared with the angiographically determined standard, the correlation coefficient was 0.75. Noninvasive estimates and angiographic stenoses agreed within limits of ± 20 percent in 81 percent of the studies. If a 40 percent stenosis (by diameter) was considered hemodynamically significant, the sensitivity of the technique was 86 percent and the specificity 90 percent. In a subsequent report by Moore et al. (50), the components of this technique were evaluated to determine their relative contribution to overall accuracy. Knowledge of the technician's subjective impressions regarding signal quality and the etiology of echo-free areas significantly improved the accuracy of image interpretation alone. Spectral analysis was significantly more accurate than image interpretation alone and was equivalent to image interpretation with knowledge of the technician's impressions.

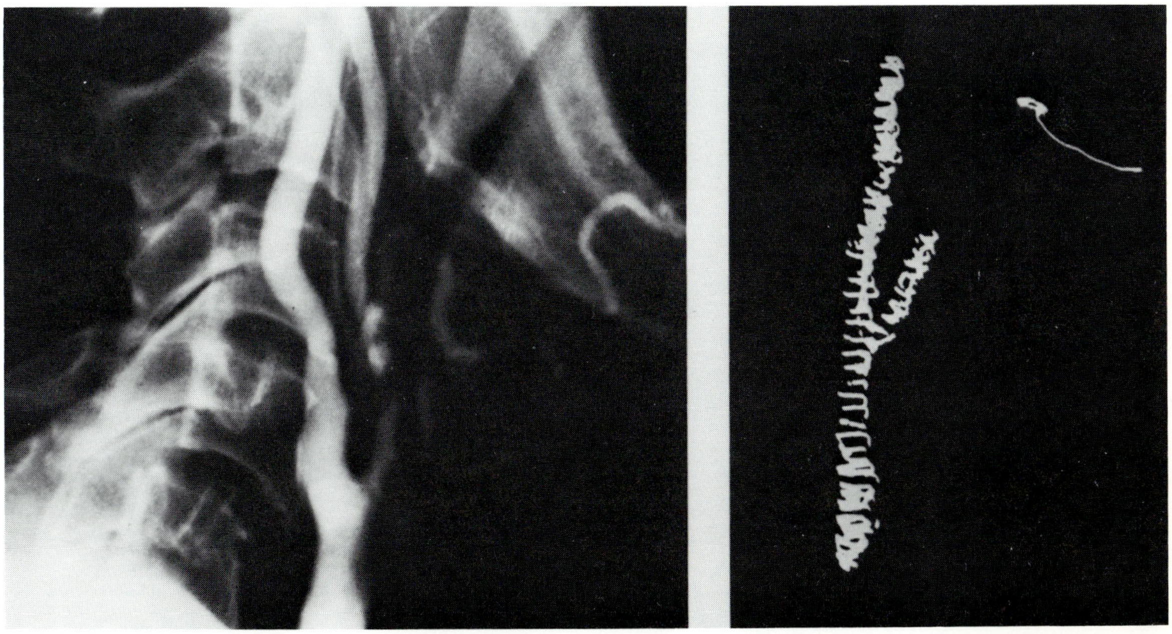

FIGURE 10-16. A continuous-wave Doppler image (*right*) of a normal carotid artery bifurcation (*left*). The image is relative and is not useful in quantitating the degree of stenosis. Diagnostic implications are drawn from an analysis of the spectral profile (see Figures 10-15 and 10-18).

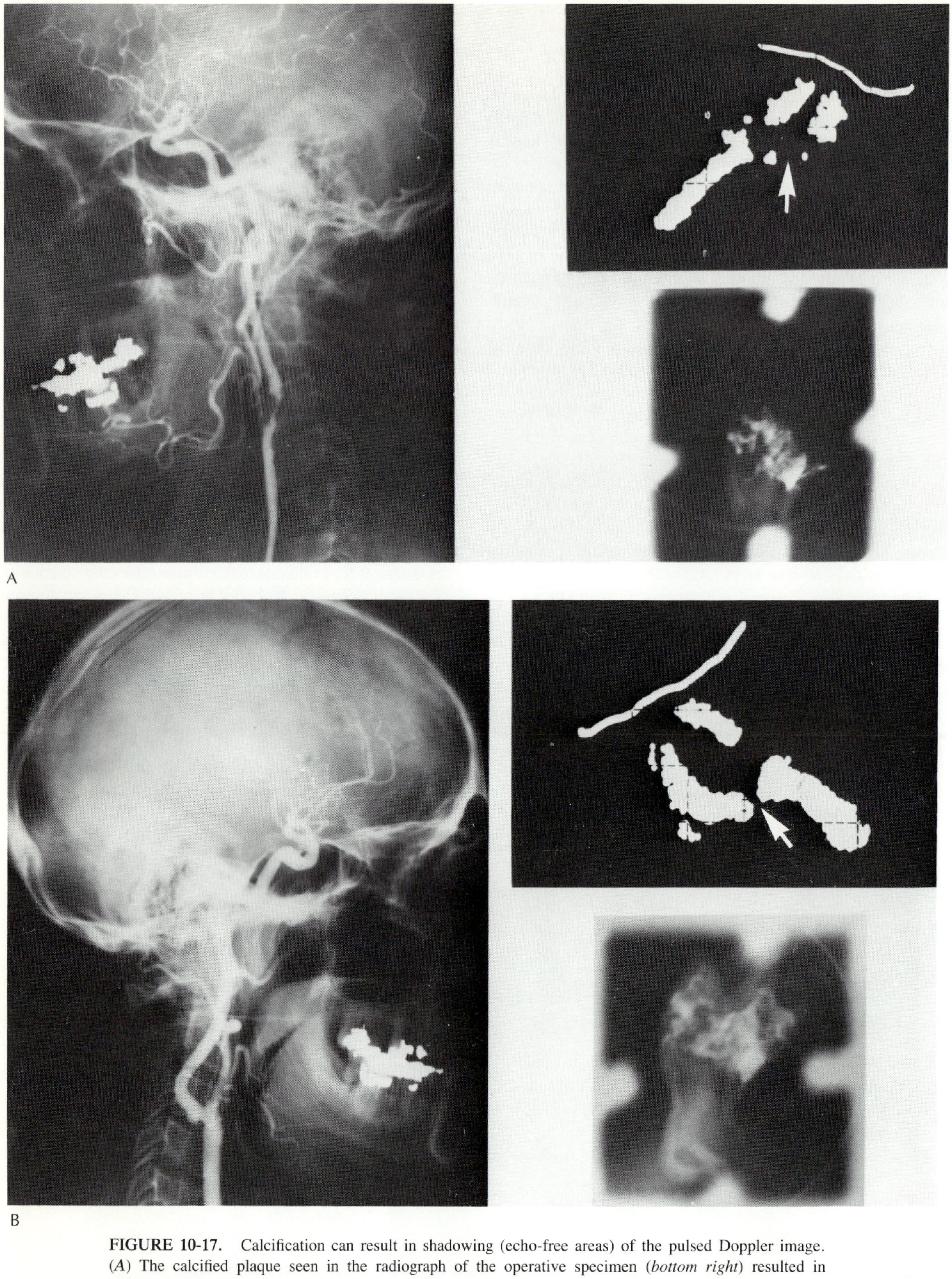

FIGURE 10-17. Calcification can result in shadowing (echo-free areas) of the pulsed Doppler image. (*A*) The calcified plaque seen in the radiograph of the operative specimen (*bottom right*) resulted in shadowing (*arrow*) at the origin of the internal carotid artery on the pulsed Doppler image (*top right*) and prevented accurate quantification of the angiographically documented stenosis (*left*). [From Berry SM, O'Donnell JA, Hobson RW: Capabilities and limitations of pulsed Doppler sonography in carotid imaging. J Clin Ultrasound 1980, 8:405–412.] ***(B)*** The calcified plaque (*bottom right*) resulted in shadowing (*top right*). In this example, however, the shadowing was associated with a nonstenotic ulcer (*left*) and not a stenosis.

Spectral Analysis

Because changes in the Doppler-shifted frequency profile are pivotal to the interpretation of continuous-wave imaging data and because calcification and echo-free areas interfere with direct interpretation of the pulsed Doppler image, spectral analysis has become increasingly important in the effort to quantify the magnitude of the Doppler frequency shift and, indirectly, the degree of stenosis. The normal internal carotid artery has a peak systolic frequency of 2 to 4 kHz, with a prominent diastolic flow component. The frequency profile reflects the laminar flow pattern and is tightly distributed about the peak midstream frequency. The normal external carotid artery flow signal is systolic in character and may occasionally have a peak frequency greater than 4 kHz. There is little diastolic flow because of distal, high-resistance runoff. The common carotid artery flow pattern is intermediate between that of the internal and external carotid arteries and has both systolic and diastolic components (44,51) (Figure 10-18*A* and *B*).

The peak systolic frequency, the relative distribution of the frequency profile, and the end-diastolic frequency have each been used in an attempt to characterize the extent of stenosis. The shift, or abnormal distribution of frequencies, associated with increasing stenosis is also referred to as spectral broadening. In the absence of poststenotic turbulence, laminar flow results in a frequency profile which is tightly distributed about the peak, or midstream, frequency. This results in an open area, or "window," beneath the peak systolic envelope. In addition to the increase in peak systolic frequency which occurs with increasing stenosis, there is also poststenotic turbulence. This loss of a laminar flow profile results in disordered, low-velocity flow patterns. These are reflected in a shift in the frequency distribution, with more low-frequency components and an opacification of the "window" (spectral broadening) (Figure 10-15).

When interpreting the spectral profile, differences between pulsed and continuous-wave Doppler velocimeters must be considered. Because of the physical principles involved, the pulsed Doppler will only detect a Doppler-shifted frequency which does not exceed 5 to 8 kHz, depending on the instrumentation. Within the range of the pulsed Doppler, the peak systolic frequency will not differ significantly from that measured with a continuous-wave Doppler. However, the peak frequency resulting from a tightly stenotic lesion which exceeds 5 to 8 kHz will only be detected by a continuous-wave Doppler velocimeter. While the continuous-wave Doppler may reflect peak frequency with a greater accuracy than the pulsed Doppler, the latter is more sensitive to changes in frequency distribution. The continuous-wave Doppler reflects the velocity profile across the entire diameter of the artery. Because the normal, laminar flow profile is parabolic, low-velocity flow at the periphery is insonated along with midstream high-velocity flow, resulting in spectral broadening. The pulsed Doppler, on the other hand, reflects the velocity profile within a discrete sample area. Thus the midstream profile demonstrates a discrete spectral envelope without significant spectral broadening (see Figure 10-14).

The relationship between the peak systolic frequency and the percentage of stenosis (or the reduction in cross-sectional area) is nonlinear or curvilinear. The slope of this relationship is more gradual than that predicted by a straight-line regression (Figure 10-19) when subcritical stenoses reduce the cross-sectional area by 5 to 50 percent. Conversely, the slope is much steeper than might be expected from a straight-line relationship when the reduction in cross-sectional area exceeds 80 percent (52). Clinically, Spencer and Reid (53), as well as Zwiebel and associates (54), have demonstrated this nonlinear, exponential relationship between the Doppler-shifted peak systolic frequency and the percentage of stenosis. Spencer and Reid observed that the actual frequency range recorded from a given stenosis was in reality much less than that predicted theoretically and suggested that turbulence limited the peak frequencies attained.

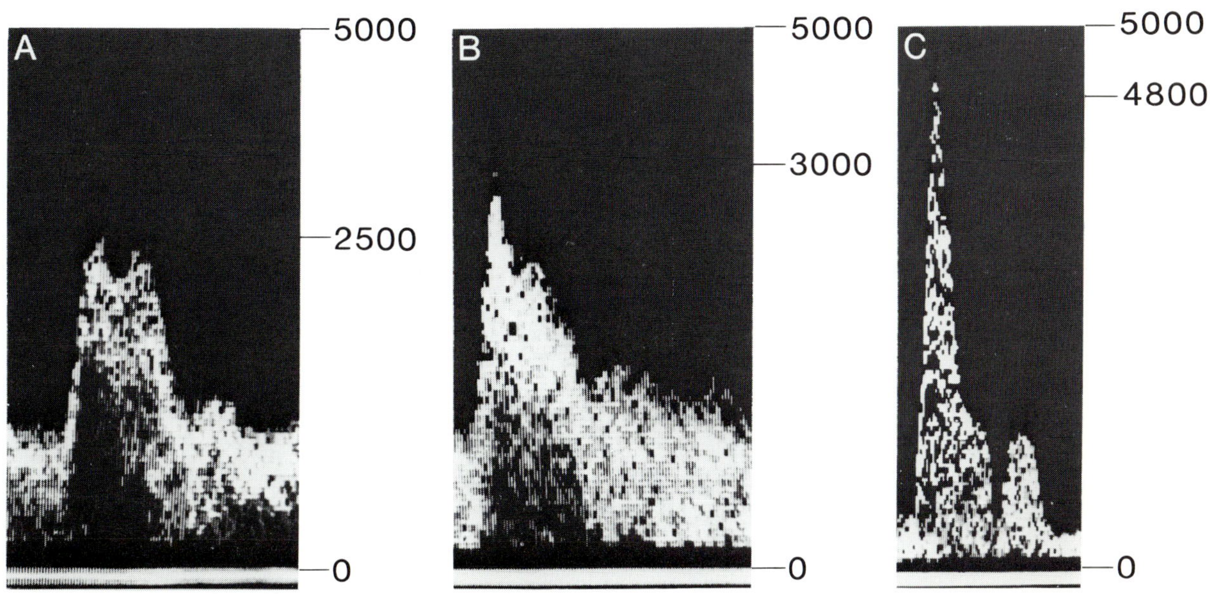

FIGURE 10-18. Normal spectral profiles from the *(A)* common, *(B)* internal, and *(C)* external carotid arteries.

Since flow is a function of cardiac output, it is reasonable to assume that the components of cardiac output, stroke volume and pulse rate, also influence flow and flow velocity across a stenosis. Using a microprocessor controlled in vitro flow loop (52), we have demonstrated in recent experimental studies that the elevation, or *y* intercept, of the relationship between peak systolic frequency (PSF) and reduction in cross-sectional area is directly related to pulse rate (Figure 10-20). Thus the peak systolic frequency is greater at a pulse rate of 90 cycles per minute (cpm) than it is at 60 cpm. Variations in the clinically observed

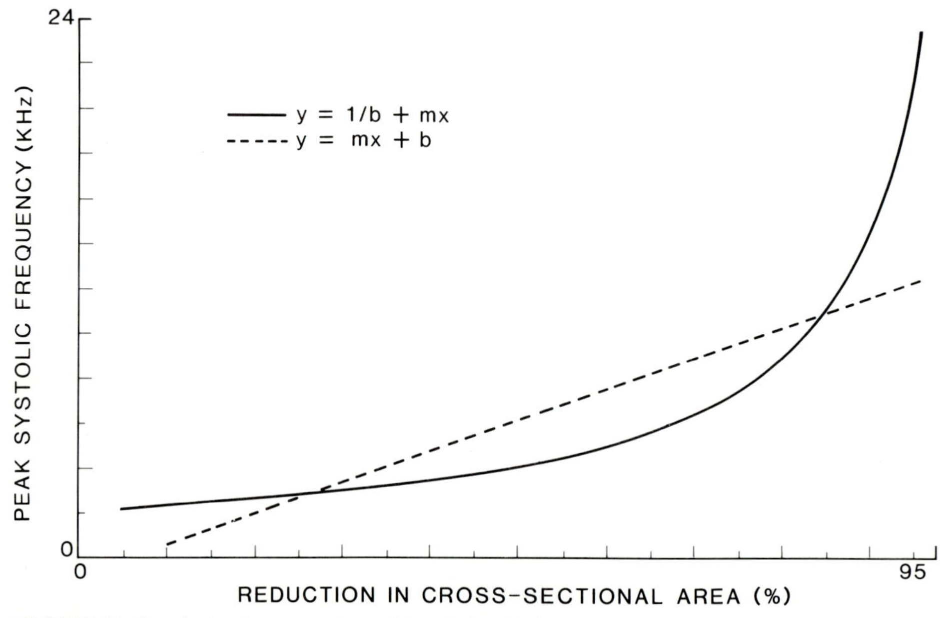

FIGURE 10-19. An in vitro comparison of the relationship between peak systolic frequency and reduction in cross-sectional area represented by linear [$Y = MX + B$; r value $= 0.87$] and nonlinear [$y = 1/(b + mx)$; r value $= 0.98$] regression lines at a pulse rate of 60 cpm and at one diameter distal to the stenosis.

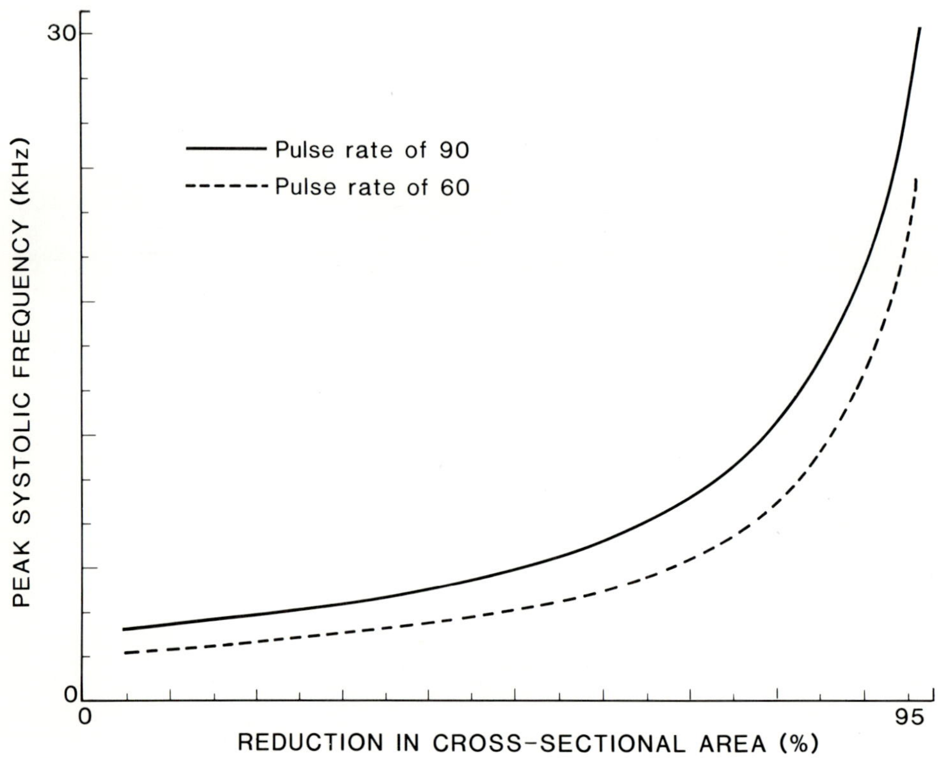

FIGURE 10-20. An in vitro comparison of the relationship between peak systolic frequency and reduction in cross-sectional area of pulse rates of 60 and 90 cpm.

peak systolic frequency may also be a function of the relative point of insonation. Experimentally there is no significant difference between observations obtained within two diameters of the stenosis. Beyond two diameters, however, there is a progressive decrease in the peak systolic frequency as the point of insonation is moved distally (Figure 10-21). Further, these differences are directly related to the percentage reduction in cross-sectional area.

Clinically, Rittgers et al. (55) have demonstrated a wide range in the PSFs recorded from a given percentage stenosis. In addition, Zwiebel et al. (54) were led to conclude that it was a range of frequencies, from 5 to 8 kHz, which was associated with 50 to 75 percent stenoses and a range from 8 to 12 kHz which was associated with 75 to 90 percent stenoses. While pulse rate and distance from the stenosis may not be the only variables influencing poststenotic flow velocity changes, they do offer an explanation for the variations in PSF which are observed clinically. Additionally, variables such as arterial diameter and compliance, the geometry of the stenosis, distal resistance, and the influence of collateral circulation must also be considered.

Using pulsed Doppler ultrasonography Blackshear et al. (56) examined the relationship between spectral broadening and the percentage of stenosis. In a normal artery, the midstream spectral profile shows no opacification of the peak systolic window (see Figure 10-15, bottom left). There were lesser degrees of spectral broadening, but no increase in peak frequency, when the stenoses ranged from 10 to 49 percent. Total opacification of the spectral window and an increase in PSF were associated with 50 to 99 percent stenoses (see Figure 10-15, bottom right). Using these criteria, they correctly identified 88 percent ($n = 8$) of normal arteries, 78 percent ($n = 23$) of those arteries with 10 to 49 percent stenoses, and 100 percent ($n = 22$) of those with 50 to 99 percent stenosis.

In an attempt to characterize more precisely those stenoses from 50 to 99 percent, Roederer et al. (57) used pulsed Doppler ultrasound and measured the end-diastolic frequency. Using 4.5 kHz as a cutoff, they correctly identified 88 percent of stenoses less than 80 percent and 84 percent of those greater than 80 percent.

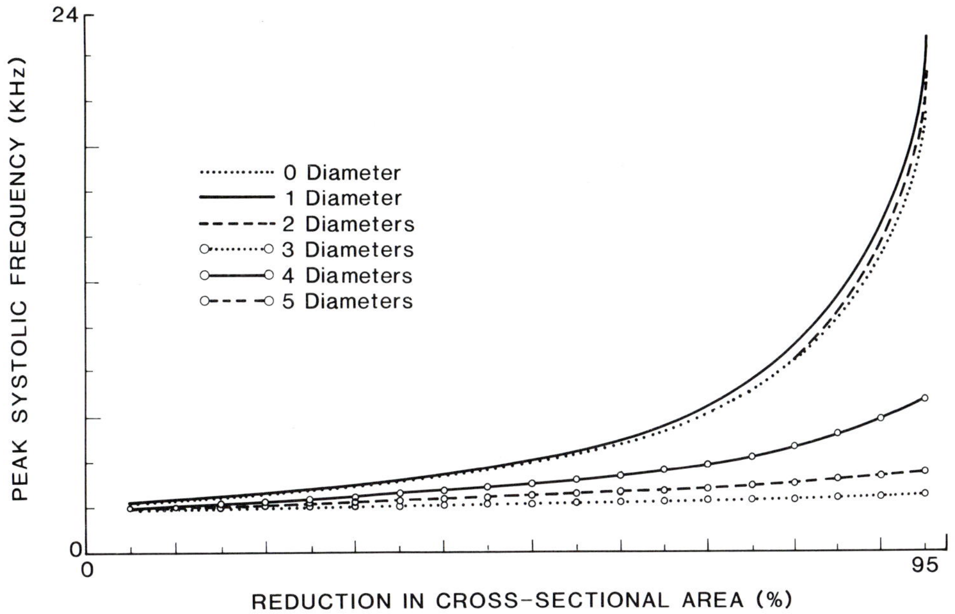

FIGURE 10-21. A comparison of the relationship between peak systolic frequency and the reduction in cross-sectional area at the stenosis and at 1, 2, 3, 4, and 5 diameters distal to the stenosis.

Real-Time B-Mode Ultrasonography

The capabilities and limitations of real-time B-mode ultrasonography are best demonstrated by illustrative examples of the technique. Patients are routinely examined in a supine position with the neck slightly extended and the head rotated away from the side of the examination. Two longitudinal scans are obtained in planes lateral and posterior to the carotid artery. The transducer is then rotated 180° for cross-sectional visualization. Figure 10-22 is representative of a normal carotid bifurcation, seen in longitudinal and cross-sectional views. In the longitudinal plane, the sternomastoid muscle and jugular vein are superficial to the artery. On cross section, identification of the medially placed thyroid gland will facilitate identification of the internal and external carotid arteries. Carotid visualization and interpretation are also dependent upon the relationship of the transducer to the carotid artery. When the transducer can be positioned so that the scanning plane includes the internal and external carotid arteries, an image demonstrating the bifurcation and its branches is obtained. In 70 percent of cases, however, the probe must be moved laterally from the bifurcation to visualize the internal carotid artery or medially toward the thyroid gland to visualize

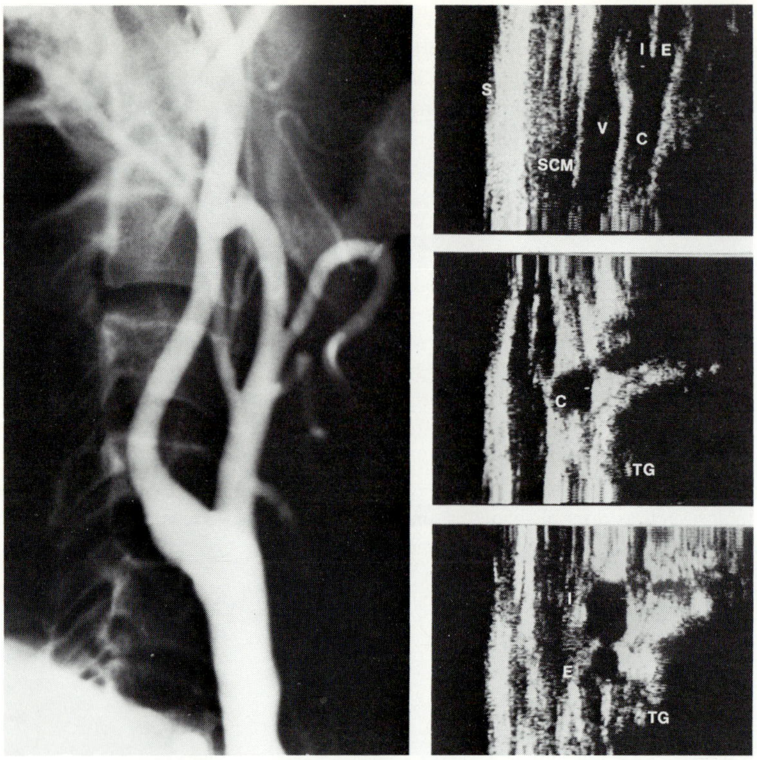

FIGURE 10-22. Normal arteriogram (*left*) with corresponding longitudinal (*top right*) and cross-sectional (*middle* and *bottom right*) images. Skin (S), sternocleidomastoid muscle (SCM), and jugular vein (JV) are seen anterior to the carotid artery. The common carotid (C), internal carotid (I), and external carotid (E) arteries are demonstrated. Location of the thyroid gland (TG) is indicated.

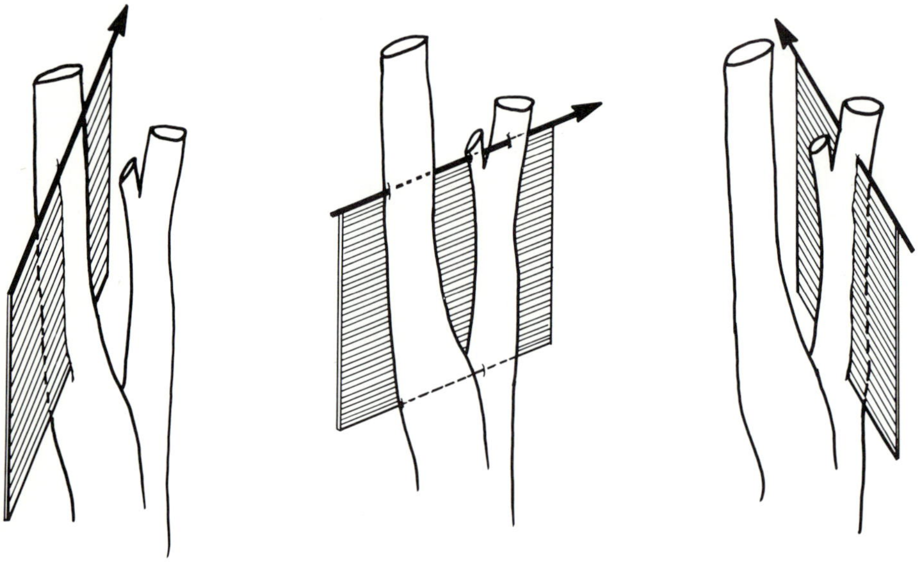

FIGURE 10-23. Spatial relationships are relevant to the appearance of real-time images. An artist's conception of various anatomical examples. [From RW Hobson et al. (51). Reproduced by permission of Grune & Stratton, Inc.]

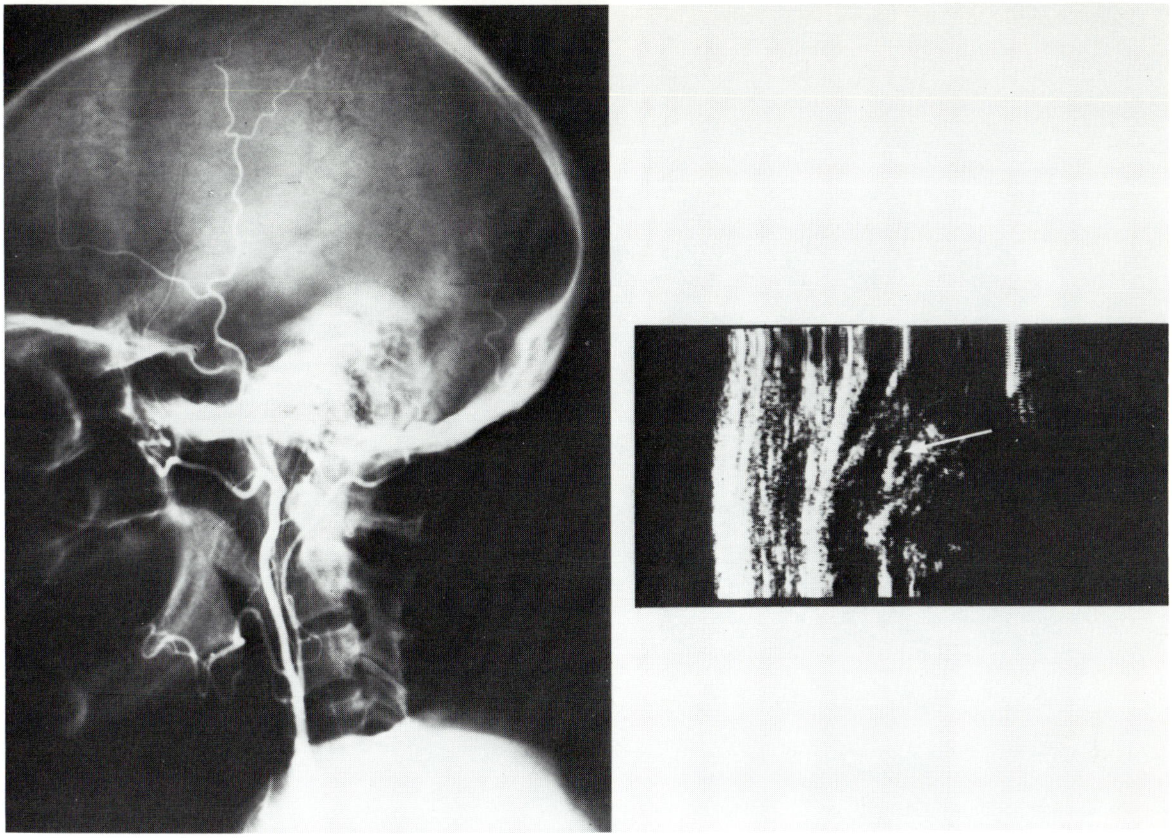

FIGURE 10-24. The arteriogram (*left*) demonstrates occlusion of the internal carotid artery. Multiple reflective densities (*arrow*) within the proximal internal carotid artery of the corresponding image (*right*) suggest occlusion of the internal carotid artery.

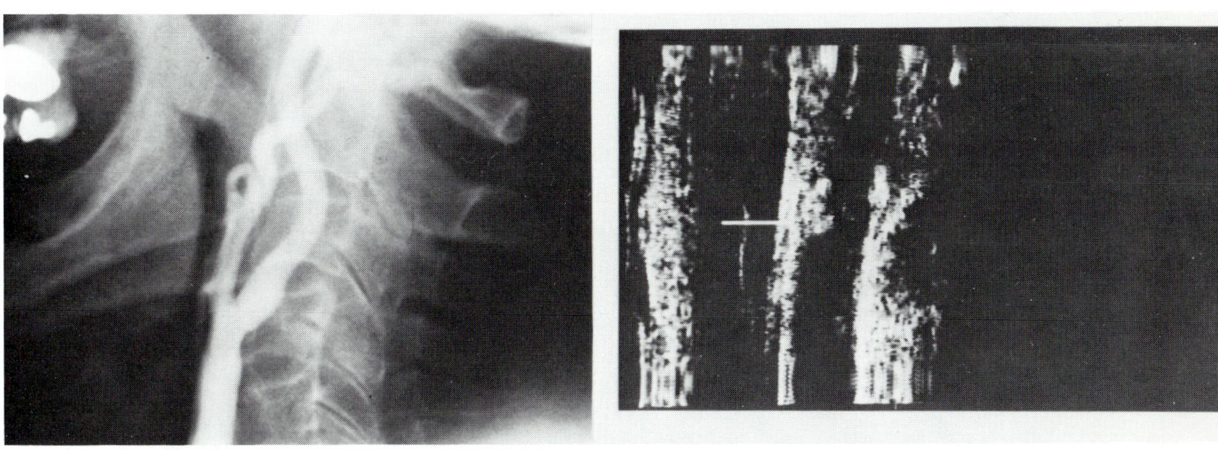

FIGURE 10-25. Normal contrast arteriogram (*left*) and accompanying scan (*right*) demonstrating an ulcerative lesion.

the external carotid artery. The spatial relationship of the bifurcation to the external and internal carotid arteries is illustrated in Figure 10-23.

Figure 10-24 illustrates characteristics of internal carotid artery occlusion. While the presence of intraluminal reflectivity and the absence of arterial pulsatility are consistent with internal carotid artery occlusion, a recent thrombosis may not be sufficiently organized to confirm the diagnosis without the use of flow-detecting Doppler circuitry.

Minimal atherosclerotic changes are demonstrated in Figures 10-25 and 10-26. The appearance of intimal thickening (Figure 10-27) is the first ultrasonic evidence of early atherosclerotic change. Smaller ulcerative lesions can occasionally be associated with normal contrast arteriography (see Figure 10-25).

The identification of highly stenotic lesions may be complicated by the presence of calcification which results in "shadowing" (Figure 10-28). Nonetheless, the technique is often of value in the diagnosis of moderate and severe stenosis (Figure

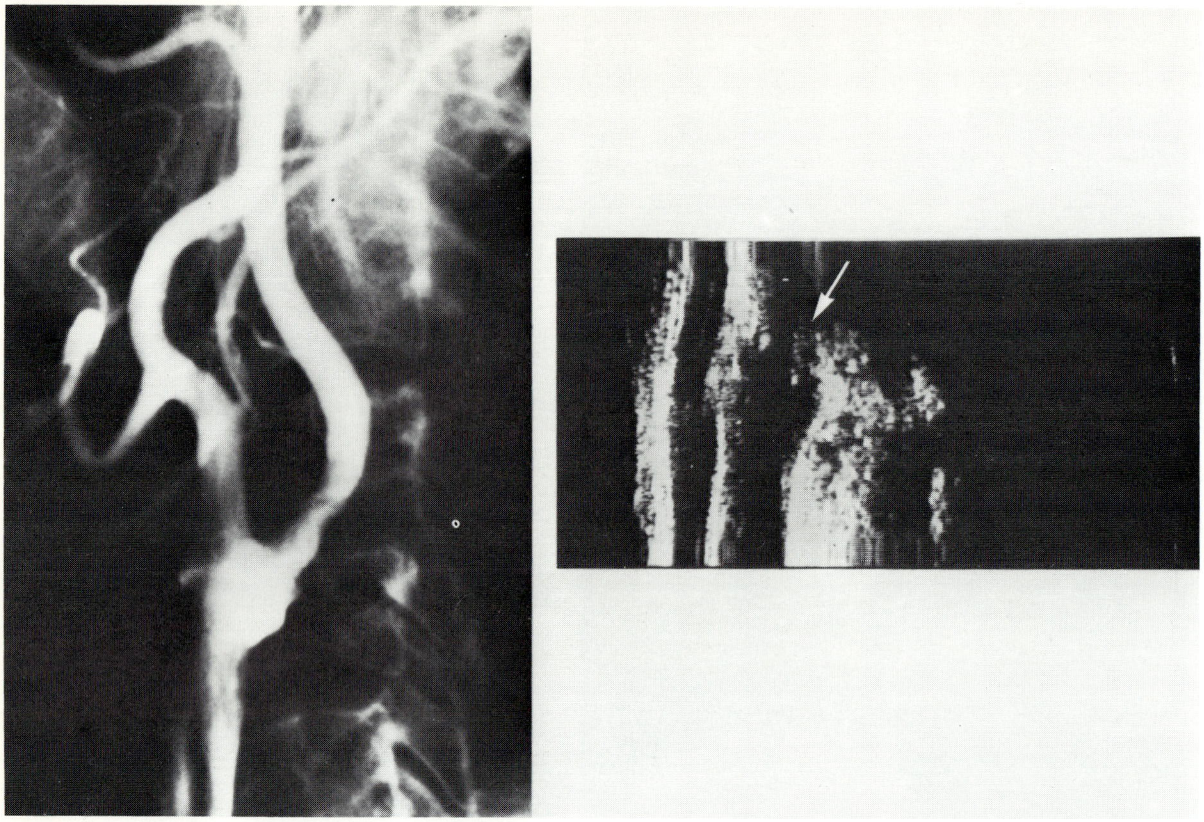

FIGURE 10-26. Contrast arteriogram (*left*) demonstrating an ulcerative plaque involving the common carotid bifurcation and the proximal internal carotid artery. The arrow demonstrates the ultrasonic appearance in the accompanying scan (*right*).

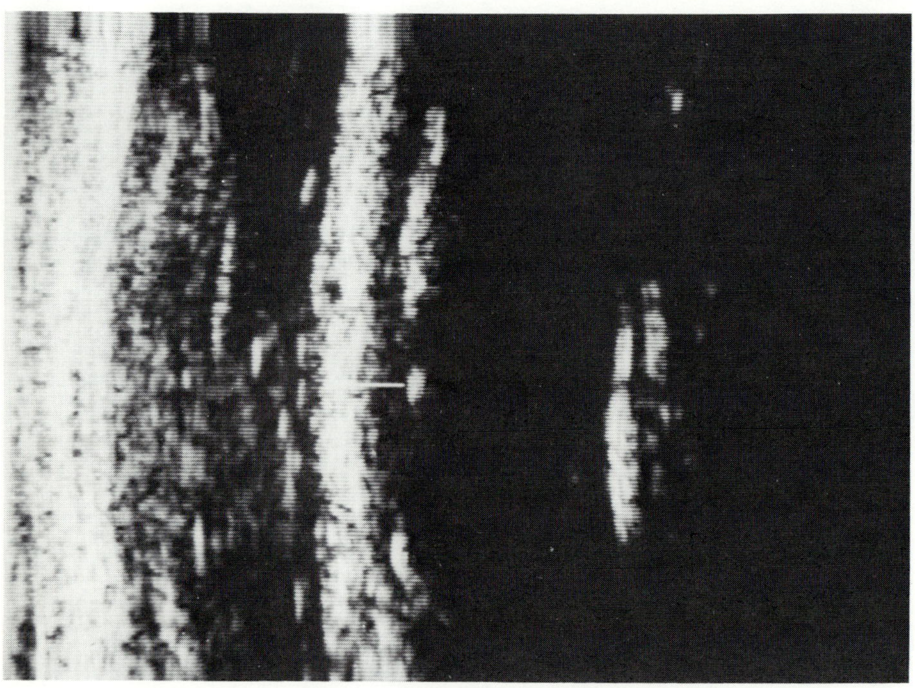

FIGURE 10-27. Image demonstrating intimal thickening (*arrow*) along the arterial wall. [From TG Lynch et al. (61).]

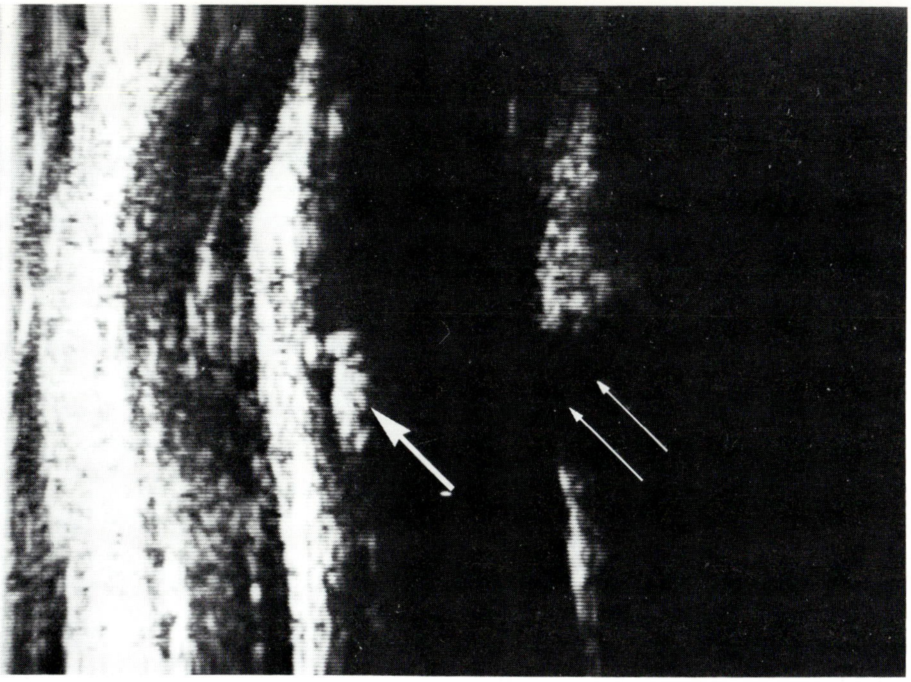

FIGURE 10-28. A calcified plaque (*single arrow*) is seen on the anterior wall of the bifurcation, with shadowing (*double arrow*) obscuring the posterior portion of the scan. [From TG Lynch et al. (61).]

10-29*A*,*B*, and *C*). The common carotid stenosis seen in Figure 10-29*A* demonstrates the relationship between the variable densities within an atherosclerotic plaque and the arterial wall.

Early data published by Hobson and associates (58) demonstrated an 89 percent specificity for hemodynamically insignificant stenoses or normal arteries. There was a 58 percent sensitivity to the presence of stenoses exceeding 50 percent and only an 18 percent sensitivity to carotid occlusion. In this early study, B-mode imaging was particularly useful in excluding disease in those patients with normal arteries and in characterizing hemodynamically insignificant stenoses. The real-time instrument provides images of high resolution which define the relationship between the arterial wall and the atherosclerotic plaque, characterizing as well the size and ultrasonic morphology of the plaque. The presence of calcification and shadowing, as well as the degree of organization, interferes with the characterization of significant stenoses or carotid occlusion.

Data from that same series (58), however, demonstrated that pulsed Doppler ultrasonic imaging had a 100 percent sensitivity to carotid occlusion in these same patients. These results can be explained by the differences in the approach to vascular imaging. A technique such as pulsed Doppler imaging, which is based upon flow detection, might reasonably be expected to detect occlusion or absence of flow with a high degree of accuracy. However, images produced by real-time B-mode ultrasonography, which define anatomical relationships rather than hemodynamics, might not be as accurate.

The use of duplex scanning equipment has provided the technology to image arteries in real time, as well as to assess the Doppler velocity profile. Comerota et al. (59) employed a real-time B-mode imager, with pulsed Doppler circuitry, in a multicenter trial. They demonstrated the expected specificity of 87 percent for arteries with 0 to 39 percent stenoses, and also showed a 74 percent sensitivity to carotid occlusion during the last 2 years of the study. The sensitivity to 40 to 69 percent and 70 to 99 percent stenoses was 72 percent and 66 percent, respectively, and was directly related to the quality of the scan.

Of additional significance is the application of B-mode ultrasonography during the operative and postoperative management of vascular surgical procedures. Sigel and colleagues (60) have recommended operative use of B-mode imaging to evaluate the adequacy of carotid endarterectomy and to assess the presence of unsuspected technical errors (Figure 10-30). Lynch and associates (61) have utilized B-mode imaging and ocular pneumoplethysmography in a clinical follow-up of 41 patients (54 arteries) after carotid endarterectomy. Recurrent stenosis was observed in three (6 percent), occlusion in three (6 percent), and external carotid occlusion in one patient, the latter resulting in lateralizing neurological symptoms secondary to atheroembolism. Only two of these patients were symptomatic, and three of the seven had hemodynamically insignificant stenoses. B-mode ultrasonography also permitted the identification of several additional postoperative findings. An intimal shelf was observed frequently at the proximal limit of the endarterectomy, and thickening of the arterial wall was observed in 74 percent of cases.

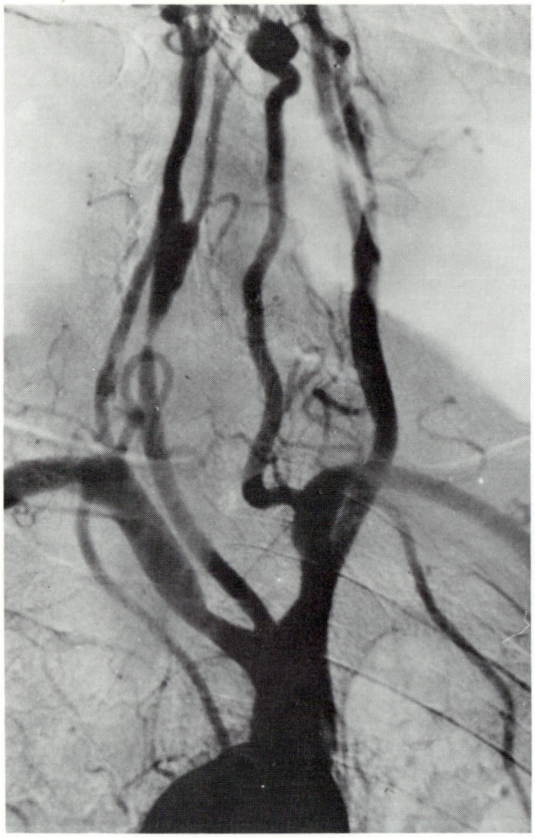

A

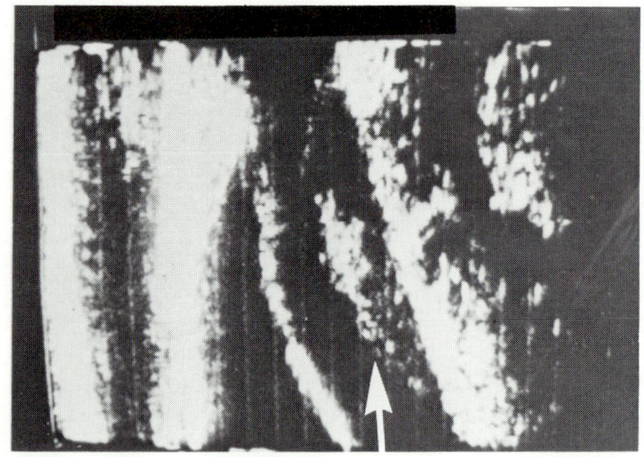

FIGURE 10-29. *(A)* The arch arteriogram (*left*) demonstrates a significant common carotid artery stenosis proximal to the carotid bifurcation. The accompanying B-mode image (*right*) demonstrates the ultrasonic morphology of the plaque (*arrow*) within the common carotid artery. [From RW Hobson et al. (58).]

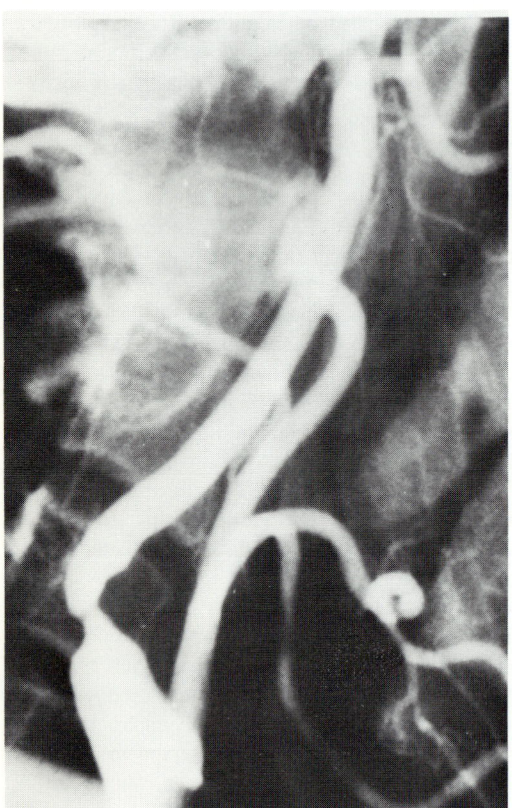

B

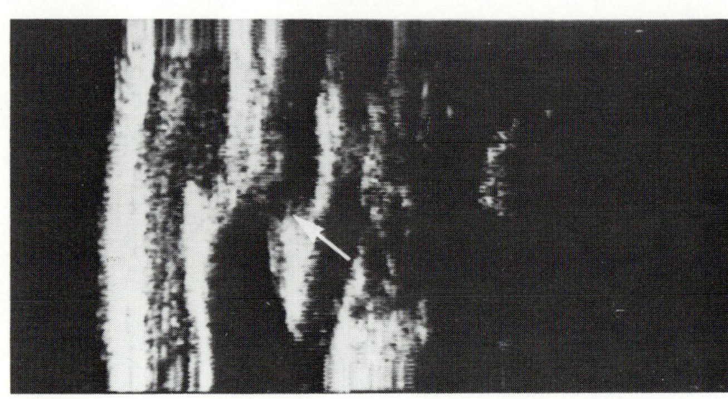

FIGURE 10-29 (continued). (*B*) Comparison of the arteriographic and ultrasonic appearance of a 50% stenosis of the proximal internal carotid artery.

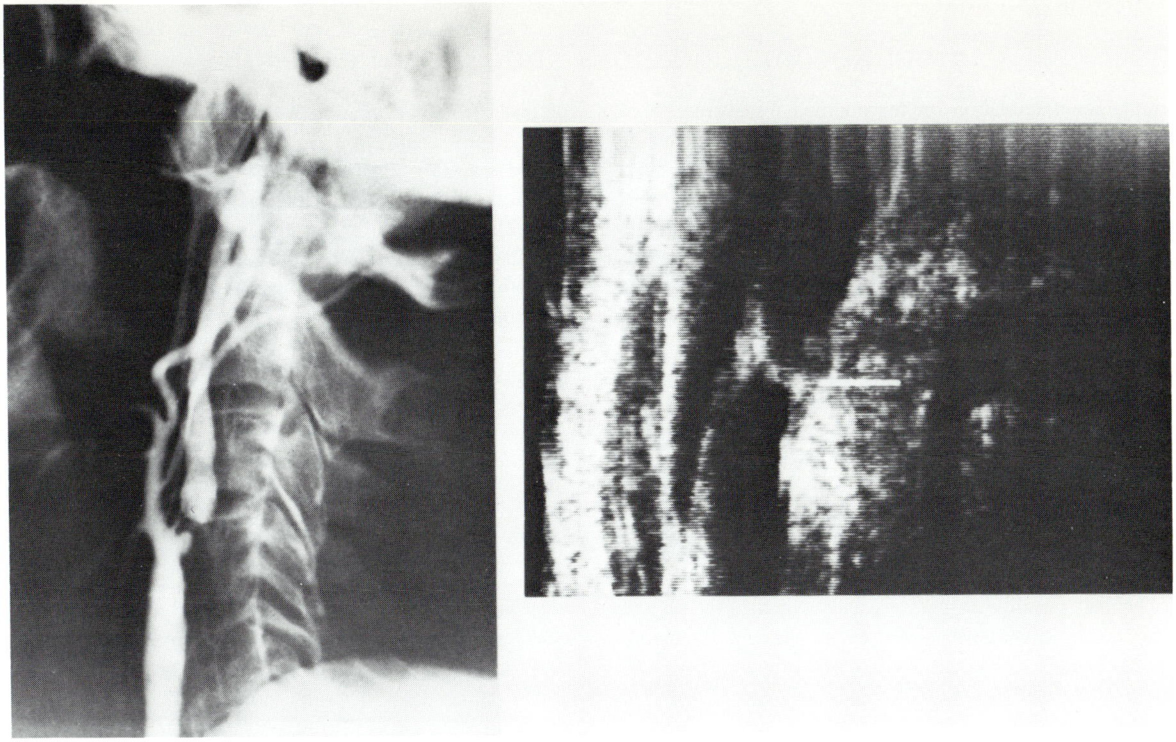

C

FIGURE 10-29 (continued). (*C*) Comparison of the arteriographic and ultrasonic appearance of a 99 percent stenosis of the proximal internal carotid artery.

FIGURE 10-30. A normal completion arteriogram (*top*) obtained following carotid endarterectomy and the corresponding intraoperative real-time B-mode image (*bottom*). The common carotid artery (C), the area of the bulb (B), and the distal internal carotid artery (I) are indicated. The arrow indicates a shelf or step-off characteristic of the proximal limits of the endarterectomy.

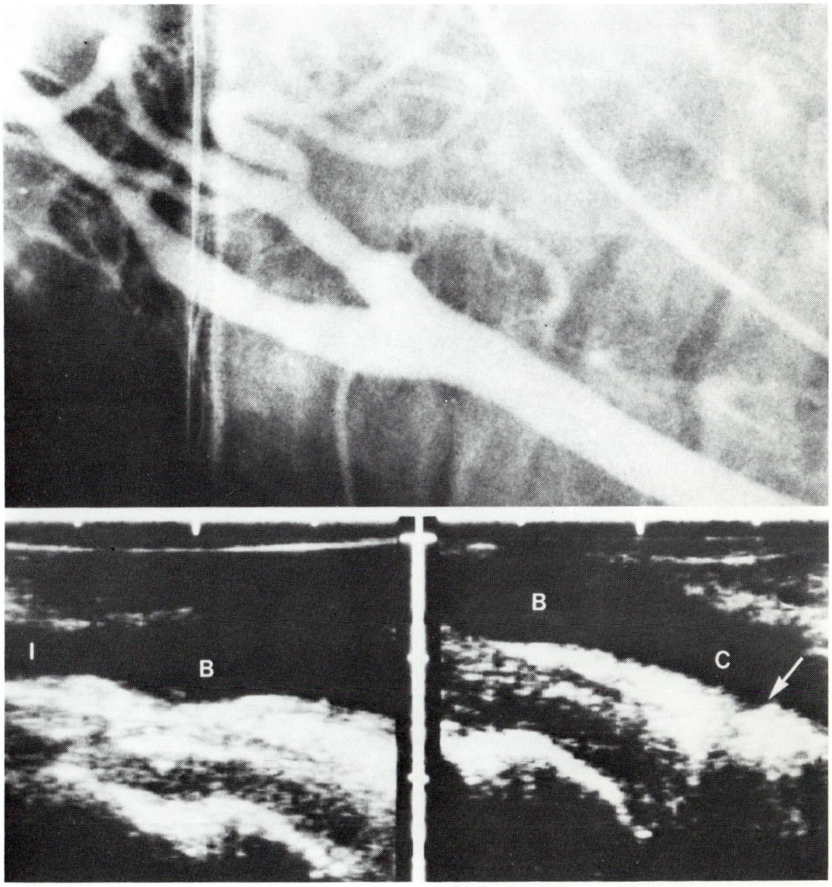

Current Recommendations and Future Perspectives

Our current recommendation for the noninvasive evaluation of carotid occlusive disease is a combination approach using the OPG-G, spectral analysis, and real-time B-mode ultrasonography. The OPG-G with a sensitivity of 85 to 96 percent (15,33) is used as the primary screening tool to identify hemodynamically significant disease in asymptomatic patients. Spectral analysis and B-mode ultrasonography are then used to quantify the degree of stenosis and its morphologic characteristics, as well as to confirm patency of the artery. Thus, the combination of direct and indirect techniques provides an accurate anatomic and physiologic assessment of the hemodynamic significance of a lesion. These methods enable easy, reproducible screening of patients and can also be used to quantify the degree of stenosis and follow the progression of disease. In symptomatic individuals real-time B-mode ultrasonography may be used to characterize nonstenotic ulcerative plaques, prior to angiography, in patients with a normal OPG-G and hemodynamically insignificant disease.

As it becomes possible to noninvasively quantify the degree of stenosis and to distinguish between stenosis and occlusion, future research must ultimately focus on the noninvasive characterization of plaque morphology. Although a great deal of research has been directed toward the identification and quantification of stenotic lesions (61,62), the number of studies evaluating the relationship between plaque morphology and the transcutaneous sonographic image have been limited. Real-time B-mode ultrasonography, alone or in combination with indirect tests of hemodynamic significance, has become an accepted method with which to characterize the extent of carotid atherosclerosis. It is apparent, however that certain atherogenic patterns are associated with the development of TIAs and stroke. Imparato et al. (63) reported a relationship between the presence of intraplaque hemorrhage and focal neurologic symptoms. In addition, he further noted that atherosclerotic morphology tended to be symmetrical, observing that the pathologic characteristics of one carotid bifurcation were not dissimilar to those of the contralateral bifurcation. Persson and colleagues (64) also reported that 33 of 34 (97 percent) symptomatic patients had intraplaque hemorrhage, while asymptomatic patients demonstrated similar pathologic findings in only 11 of 21 (52 percent) patients. Lusby et al. (65) subsequently published a prospective study of carotid endarterectomy speciments. Acute or recent intraplaque hemorrhage was present in 49 of 53 (92 percent) symptomatic patients, but only 7 of 26 (27 percent) asymptomatic patients. Luminal stenoses exceeding 50 percent of the arterial diameter were present in 46 of 53 symptomatic patients, of whom 43 had evidence of intraplaque hemorrhage. Unfortunately, the number of studies designed to establish the relationship between noninvasively defined morphology and the actual pathologic morphology are few. Katz et al. (62) were unable to consistently identify ulcerative plaques using real-time B-mode ultrasonography. These investigators reported a 33 percent sensitivity to ulcerations of less than 2 mm, while the sensitivity was 58 percent for ulcerations of greater than 2 mm. Interestingly, however, arteriography had corresponding sensitivities of only 58 and 74 percent, respectively. Conversely, O'Donnell et al. (66) reported an 89 percent sensitivity to ulcerative carotid plaques. Of additional significance, Reilly and associates (67) ascribed a greater risk to those plaques which had a heterogeneous character when visualized with B-mode ultrasonography.

If plaque morphology could be determined noninvasively using real-time B-mode ultrasonography, these findings might contribute significantly to the management of patients with atherosclerotic involvement of the carotid bifurcation. Specifically, asymptomatic patients with high-risk plaque morphology could be identified and considered for endarterectomy, while other patients could be observed. Prospective longitudinal studies of atherogenic risk factors could also be interpreted relative to actual pathologic abnormalities.

References

1. Brown PM, Johnston KW: The difficulty of quantifying the severity of carotid stenosis. Surgery 1982, 92:468–473.
2. May AG, VandeBerg L, DeWeese JA, Rob CG: Critical arterial stenosis. Surgery 1963, 54:250–257.
3. Brisman R, Grossman RL, Correll JW: Accuracy of transcutaneous Doppler ultrasonics in evaluating extracranial vascular disease. J Neurosurg 1970, 32:529–533.
4. Maroon JC, Pieroni DW, Campbell RL: Ophthalmosonometry: An ultrasonic method for assessing carotid blood flow. J Neurosurg 1969, 30:238–246.
5. Muller HR: The diagnosis of internal carotid artery occlusion by directional Doppler sonography of the ophthalmic artery. Neurology 1972, 22:816–823.
6. Brockenbrough EC: Screening for the prevention of stroke: Use of the Doppler flowmeter. Washington/Alaska Regional Medical Program Brochure, 1970.
7. Brockenbrough EC: Periorbital Doppler velocity evaluation of carotid obstruction. In Bernstein EF (ed): *Noninvasive Diagnostic Techniques in Vascular Disease*. St Louis, CV Mosby Co, 1982, pp 231–238.
8. Bone GE, Barnes RW: Clinical implications of the Doppler cerebrovascular examination: A correlation with angiography. Stroke 1976, 7:271–274.
9. Barnes RW, Russell HE, Bone GE, Slaymaker EE: Doppler cerebrovascular examination: Improved results with refinement in technique. Stroke 1977, 8:468–471.
10. Barnes RW, Garrett WV, Slaymaker EE, Reinertson JE: Doppler ultrasound and supraorbital photoplethysmography for noninvasive screening of carotid occlusive disease. Am J Surg 1977, 134:183–186.
11. LoGerfo FW, Mason GR: Directional Doppler studies of supraorbital artery flow in internal carotid stenosis and occlusion. Surgery 1974, 76:723–728.
12. Lye CR, Sumner DS, Strandness DE: The accuracy of the supraorbital Doppler examination in the diagnosis of hemodynamically significant carotid occlusive disease. Surgery 1976, 79:42–45.
13. Duke LJ, Slaymaker EE, Lamberth WC, Wright CB: Results of ophthalmosonometry and supraorbital photoplethysmography in evaluating carotid arterial stenoses. Circulation 1979, 60(suppl I):127–131.

14. McDonald PT, Rich NM, Collins GJ, Anderson CA, Kozloff L: Doppler cerebrovascular examination, oculoplethysmography, and ocular pneumoplethysmography. Arch Surg 1978, 113:1341–1349.
15. Lynch TG, Wright CB, Miller EV, Slaymaker EE: Evaluation of cerebrovascular Doppler examination and oculopneumoplethysmography in a clinical perspective. Stroke 1981, 12:325–330.
16. Kempczinski RF: A combined approach to the noninvasive diagnosis of carotid artery occlusive disease. Surgery 1979, 85:689–694.
17. Towne JB, Bernhard VM, Salles-Cunha S, Ray LI: Supraorbital Doppler evaluation in vascular surgery. Med Instrum 1979, 13:92–94.
18. Barnes RW, Clayton JM, Bone GE, Slaymaker EE, Reinertson J: Supraorbital photoplethysmography: Simple, accurate screening for carotid occlusive disease. J Surg Res 1977, 22:319–327.
19. Kartchner MM, McRae LP, Morrison FD: Noninvasive detection and evaluation of carotid occlusive disease. Arch Surg 1973, 106:528–535.
20. Kartchner MM, McRae LP, Crain V, Whitaker B: Oculoplethysmography: An adjunct to arteriography in the diagnosis of extracranial carotid occlusive disease. Am J Surg 1976, 132:728–732.
21. Gross WS, Verta MJ, van Bellen B, Bergan JJ, Yao JST: Comparison of noninvasive diagnostic techniques in carotid artery occlusive disease. Surgery 1977, 82:271–278.
22. Blackshear WM, Thiele BL, Harley JD, Chikos PM, Strandness DE: A prospective evaluation of oculoplethysmography and carotid phonoangiography. Surg Gynecol Obstet 1979, 148:201–205.
23. Wasserman DH, Hobson RW, Lynch TG, Berry SM, Jamil Z: Ultrasonic imaging and oculoplethysmography in diagnosis of carotid occlusive disease. Arch Surg 1983, 118:1161–1163.
24. Kartchner MM, McRae LP: Noninvasive evaluation and management of the "asymptomatic" carotid bruit. Surgery 1977, 82:840–847.
25. Kartchner MM, McRae LP: Carotid phonoangiography and oculoplethysmography. In Nicolaides AN, Yao JST (eds): *Investigations of Vascular Disorders*. New York, Churchill Livingstone, 1981, pp 91–120.
26. Kartchner MM, McRae LP: Carotid occlusive disease as a risk factor in major cardiovascular surgery. Arch Surg 1982, 117:1086–1088.
27. Gee W, Smith CA, Hinsen CE, Wylie EJ: Ocular pneumoplethysmography in carotid artery disease. Med Instrum 1974, 8:244–248.
28. Gee W, Mehigan JT, Wylie EJ: Measurement of collateral cerebral hemispheric blood pressure by ocular pneumoplethysmography. Am J Surg 1975, 130:121–127.
29. Martinez SA, Oller DW, Gee W, deFies HO: Elective carotid artery resection. Arch Otolaryngol 1975, 101:744–747.
30. Nolph MB, Martinez SA, Gee W, deFries HO: Ophthalmoplethysmography in head and neck surgery. Arch Otolaryngol 1979, 105:492–495.
31. Gee W, Oller DW, Amundsen DG, Goodreau JJ: The asymptomatic carotid bruit and the ocular pneumoplethysmography. Arch Surg 1977, 112:1381–1388.
32. McDonald PT, Rich NM, Collins GJ, Kozloff L, Andersen CA: Ocular pneumoplethysmography: Detection of carotid occlusive disease. Ann Surg 1979, 189:44–48.
33. Gee W: Carotid physiology with ocular pneumoplethysmography. Stroke 1982, 13:666–673.
34. Gee W, McDonald KM, Kaupp HA, Celani VJ, Bast RG: Carotid stenosis plus occlusion: Endarterectomy or bypass? Arch Surg 1980, 115:183–187.
35. Kremen JE, Gee W, Kaupp HA, McDonald KM: Restenosis or occlusion after carotid endarterectomy: A survey with ocular pneumoplethysmography. Arch Surg 1979, 114:608–610.
36. Gee W, Morrow RA, Stephens HW, Lin FZ: Ocular pneumoplethysmography in carotid-cavernous sinus fistula. J Neurosurg 1983, 59:40–45.
37. Gee W, Rhodes M, Denstman FJ, Jaeger RM, Tilly DA, Stephens HW, Morrow RA, Lin FZ: Ocular pneumoplethysmography in head-injured patients. J Neurosurg 1983, 59:46–50.
38. Cullen SJ, Correa MC, Calderon-Ortiz M, Walburn FJ, Raines J: Clinical sequelae in patients with asymptomatic carotid bruits. Circulation 1983, 68(suppl II):83–87.
39. Busuttil RW, Baker JD, Davidson RK, Machleder HI: Carotid artery stenosis—Hemodynamic significance and clinical course. JAMA 1981, 245:1438–1441.
40. Geddes LA, Baker LE: *Principles of Applied Biomedical Instrumentation*. New York, Wiley, 1968.
41. Leopold GR: Pulse echo ultrasonography for the noninvasive imaging of vascular anatomy. In Bernstein EF (ed): *Noninvasive Diagnostic Techniques in Vascular Disease*. St Louis, CV Mosby Co, 1982, pp 174–179.
42. Sumner DS: Ultrasound. In Kempczinski RF, Yao JST (eds): *Practical Noninvasive Vascular Diagnosis*. Chicago, Year Book Medical Publishers, 1983, pp 21–47.
43. Johnston KW: Doppler signal processing and waveform analysis: Problems and solutions. In Bernstein EF (ed): *Noninvasive Diagnostic Techniques in Vascular Disease*. St Louis, CV Mosby Co, 1982, pp 28–43.
44. Lynch TG, Wright CB, Miller EV, Slaymaker EE: Comparison of continuous-wave Doppler imaging, oculopneumoplethysmography, and the cerebrovascular Doppler examination. Circulation 1982, 66(suppl I):106–110.
45. Spencer MP, Reid JM, Davis DL, Paulson PS: Cervical carotid imaging with a continuous-wave Doppler flowmeter. Stroke 1974, 5:145–154.
46. Thomas GI, Spencer MP, Jones TW, Edmark KW, Stavney LS: Noninvasive carotid bifurcation mapping. Its relation to carotid surgery. Am J Surg 1974, 128:168–174.
47. Blackwell E, Merory J, Toole JF, McKinney W: Doppler ultrasound scanning of the carotid bifurcation. Arch Neurol 1977, 34:145–148.
48. Sumner DS, Russell JB, Ramsey DE, Hajjar WM, Miles RD. Noninvasive diagnosis of extracranial carotid arterial disease. Arch Surg 1979, 114:1222–1229.
49. Barnes RW, Bone GE, Reinertson J, Slaymaker EE, Hokanson DE, Strandness DE: Noninvasive ultrasonic carotid angiography: Prospective validation by contrast arteriography. Surgery 1976, 80:328–335.
50. Moore DJ, Miles RD, Ohgi S, Landholt G, Call PJ, Sumner DS: An analysis of factors influencing non-invasive carotid diagnosis. San Diego Symposium on Noninvasive Diagnostic Techniques in Vascular Disease, 1985, p 82.
51. Hobson RW, Berry SM, Lynch TG: Applications of B-mode ultrasonography and ocular pneumoplethysmography in the diagnosis of carotid occlusive disease. In Bergan JJ, Yao JST (eds): *Cerebrovascular Insufficiency*. New York, Grune & Stratton, 1983, pp 165–177.
52. Lynch TG, Hobson RW, Pawel HE: Microprocessor-controlled pulsatile flow loop for hemodynamic studies. J Surg Res (in press).
53. Spencer MP, Reid JM: Quantitation of carotid stenosis with continuous-wave (C-W) Doppler ultrasound. Stroke 1979, 10:326–330.
54. Zwiebel WJ, Zagzebski JA, Crummy AB, Hirscher M: Correlation of peak Doppler frequency with lumen narrowing in carotid stenosis. Stroke 1982, 13:386–391.
55. Rittgers SE, Thornhill BM, Barnes RW: Quantitative analysis of carotid artery Doppler spectral waveforms: Diagnostic value of parameters. Ultrasound Med Biol 1983, 9:255–264.
56. Blackshear WM, Phillips DJ, Thiele BL, Hirsch JH, Chikos PM, Marinelli MR, Ward KJ, Strandness DE: Detection of carotid occlusive disease by ultrasonic imaging and pulsed Doppler spectrum analysis. Surgery 1979, 86:698–706.
57. Roederer GO, Langlois YE, Jager MD, Lawrence BS, Primozich JF, Phillips DJ, Strandness DE: A simple spectral parameter for

accurate classification of severe carotid disease. Bruit 1984, 8:174–178.
58. Hobson RW, Berry SM, Katocs AD, O'Donnell JA, Jamil Z, Savitsky JP: Camparison of pulsed Doppler and real-time B-mode echo arteriography for noninvasive imaging of the extracranial carotid arteries. Surgery 1980, 87:286–293.
59. Comerota AJ, Cranley JJ, Katz ML, Cook SE, Sippel PJ, Hayden WG, Fogarty TJ, Tyson RR: Real-time B-mode carotid imaging. A three-year multicenter experience. J Vasc Surg 1984, 1:84–95.
60. Sigel B, Coelho JCU, Flanigan DP, Schuler JJ, Machi J, Beitler JC: Detection of vascular defects during operation by imaging ultrasound. Ann Surg 1982, 196:473–480.
61. Lynch TG, Hobson RW, Berry SM: The role of real-time B-mode ultrasonography and ocular pneumoplethysmography following carotid endarterectomy. Am Surg 1983, 49:31–36.
62. Katz ML, Johnson M, Pomajzl, Comerota AJ, Ahrensfeld D, Mandel L, Hayden W, Fogarty T: The sensitivity of real-time B-mode carotid imaging in the detection of ulcerated plaques. Bruit 1983, 8(Sept):13–16.
63. Imparato A, Riles T, Mintzer R: The importance of hemorrhage in the relationship between gross morphologic characteristics and cerebral symptoms in 376 carotid artery plaques. Ann Surg 1983, 197:195–203.
64. Persson AV, Robichaux WT, Silverman M: The natural history of carotid plaque development. Arch Surg 1983, 118:1048–1052.
65. Lusby RJ, Ferrell LD, Ehrenfeld WK: Carotid plaque hemorrhage. Arch Surg 1982, 117:1479–1487.
66. O'Donnell TF, Erdoes L, Mackey WC, McCullough J, Shepard A, Heggerick P, Isner J, Callow AD: Correlation of B-mode ultrasound imaging and arteriography with pathologic findings at carotid endarterectomy. Arch Surg 1985, 120:443–449.
67. Reilly LM, Lusby RJ, Hughes L: Carotid plaque histology using real-time ultrasonography: Clinical and therapeutic implications. Am J Surg 1983, 146:188–193.

Chapter 11

NONINVASIVE DIAGNOSIS OF VENOUS OBSTRUCTION AND INSUFFICIENCY

GEORGE J. COLLINS, JR., J. LEONEL VILLAVICENCIO, CREIGHTON B. WRIGHT, NORMAN M. RICH, and JAMES M. SALANDER

It has been estimated that each year nearly 200,000 people in the United States die from complications of lower extremity venous thrombosis (12). The figures from Great Britain are no less impressive with an estimated annual mortality rate of 21,000 (32). Lower extremity venous thrombosis frequently accompanies other disease processes, and several conditions predispose to its development (Table 11-1). Innovations such as transjugular and transsubclavian monitoring and infusion lines, transvenous pacemaker insertions, and intravenous hyperalimentation have led to a remarkable increase in the incidence of brachiocephalic and upper extremity venous thrombosis. This is superimposed on a generally low, but potentially devastating, incidence of upper extremity venous thrombosis associated with thoracic outlet syndrome. While it was formerly believed that pulmonary embolism rarely occurred in patients with brachiocephalic or upper extremity venous thrombosis, an incidence of pulmonary embolism of 12 percent has now been documented (2,10).

Despite a great deal of experience with lower extremity venous thrombosis, uncertainty continues regarding optimum treatment during the acute stages and optimum methods of long-term management. However, there has been significant progress over the last several years in the development of noninvasive techniques for diagnosing both venous obstruction and venous insufficiency. As will be discussed in subsequent sections, these techniques have significant advantages over contrast phlebography, and they have been shown to have comparable cost effectiveness (28).

The purpose of this chapter is to acquaint the reader with recent developments in this field. First, the salient clinical features of venous disease are reviewed. The discussion is almost exclusively confined to lower extremity problems because they are more common and frequently more perplexing than those of the upper extremity.

TABLE 11-1. Conditions Associated with or Predisposing to Development of Venous Thrombosis

1. Cardiovascular disease
2. Coagulopathies (including the use of birth control pills)
3. Malignancy
4. Immobility
5. Obesity
6. Old age
7. Operations
8. Pregnancy
9. Previous deep venous thrombosis
10. Sepsis
11. Thrombocytosis
12. Trauma
13. Varicose veins

Clinical Features of Lower Extremity Venous Thrombosis

The most common symptom reported by patients with lower extremity venous thrombosis is pain. The pain may be mild and insidious in patients with thrombosis of one of the calf veins, or it may be acute and excruciating in patients with iliofemoral thrombosis. Most commonly, it is described as a dull ache, throbbing sensation, feeling of tightness, or a feeling that the leg is about to burst. These symptoms are present at rest and may be aggravated by walking. Unfortunately, many patients, and particularly those who are postoperative or critically ill from other diseases, have no symptoms related to the leg, and their first manifestation of venous thrombosis is a pulmonary embolus.

When signs of toxicity such as extreme temperature elevation or extreme tachycardia are present, septic thrombophlebitis or massive iliofemoral venous thrombosis should be suspected. The presence or absence of these signs of inflammation was previously thought to be quite important, and distinctions were made between phlebothrombosis, in which there was little or no inflammation of the vein, and thrombophlebitis, in which inflammation of the vein was prominent (38). Patients with phlebothrombosis were thought to be at much greater risk of pulmonary embolism than those with thrombophlebitis. While these distinctions may have enhanced our understanding of the basic disease, the categorizations are almost impossible to make on the basis of clinical findings. The term phlebothrombosis is rarely used nowadays, and all patients with venous thrombosis should be considered to be at significant risk of pulmonary embolism.

Some patients seek medical care only after the onset of leg swelling. Leg swelling and edema may also be a subtle clue to the onset of venous thrombosis in bedridden patients. As illustrated in Figure 11-1, edema fluid may collect behind the malleoli before it becomes more diffuse. This subtle finding of ret-

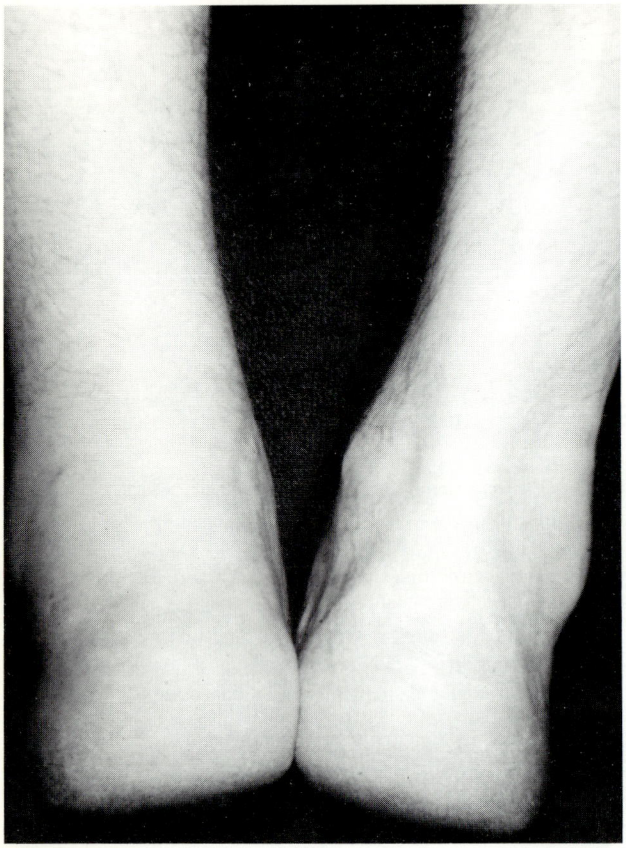

FIGURE 11-1. Retromalleolar edema may be a subtle clue to the development of deep venous thrombosis, particularly in bedridden patients.

romalleolar edema in bedridden patients should alert one to the possibility of deep vein thrombosis (20). In searching for leg swelling and edema, one should remember that there is normally some discrepancy between the sizes of the two lower extremities. However, size discrepancies greater than 1 cm are considered significant (14). In comparing sizes between the two extremities, it is helpful to use fixed landmarks (medial malleolus, midpoint of patella, and anterior superior iliac spine) as refererence points and to make sequential measurements at the same distance from these fixed reference points.

Local heat and erythema are common in superficial thrombophlebitis, but not in thrombosis of the deep veins. Superficial tenderness and the presence of a palpable cord are also common in superficial thrombophlebitis. The tetrad of local heat, erythema, superficial tenderness, and palpable cord should help to distinguish superficial thrombophlebitis from deep venous thrombosis.

The principal physical findings in deep venous thrombosis are leg swelling, edema, dilatation of superficial veins, and tenderness. In iliofemoral thrombosis, the area of maximum tenderness is generally in the thigh or groin. At times, however, it may be in the lower abdominal quadrants and may mimic the tenderness elicited in conditions such as appendicitis and diverticulitis.

When calf tenderness is present, one must try to determine whether it arises from the underlying muscles or veins. Tenderness due to a partial tear of the gastrocnemius muscle or rupture of the plantaris tendon is usually elicited by side-to-side compression of the muscle bellies, and ecchymosis over the calf is common. A history of recent participation in athletics provides a further clue to the diagnosis of these acute muscular disorders. Calf tenderness due to venous thrombosis is usually elicited by compression of the muscle bellies directly forward against the tibia. Homans' sign refers to pain in the calf produced by dorsiflexion of the foot with the knee slightly flexed. It increases one's index of suspicion, when present, but similar findings occur in patients with heel cord tightness, discogenic pain, and primary muscle disorders.

Clinical Features of Venous Insufficiency

The predominant and most easily recognized feature of venous insufficiency is varicose veins. The external manifestations of disease are reflected in the serpiginous greater and lesser saphenous veins and their connecting tributaries. However, these findings are frequently indicative of incompetence in the underlying deep veins and perforating veins. Incompetence in any of these three sets of veins (deep veins, perforating veins, superficial veins) can lead to the same end results of edema, eczema, hyperpigmentation, and finally skin breakdown with poor healing and ulceration (Figures 11-2 and 11-3).

As shown in Table 11-2, a functional classification aids in understanding the pathophysiology of venous insufficiency and further aids in selection of proper treatment (18). Veins that are incompetent on the basis of congenitally defective valves are referred to as primary, or familial, varicose veins. They can be further subdivided into varicosities of the greater (long) saphenous vein, varicosities of the lesser (short) saphenous vein, and varicosities related to primary incompetence of ankle perforators (33).

Secondary varicosities are caused by deep venous obstruction. This is usually related to thrombosis, but other causes such as tumor ingrowth or external compression by tumor may also lead to venous obstruction. Secondary varicosities can be further subdivided into three major types. The first type is due to generalized venous hypertension following permanent blockage of a major iliac vein as often occurs after iliofemoral thrombosis. In this type, venous hypertension causes gradual dilatation of small venules, particularly in the leg, ankle, and foot. There is usually no dilatation of the main saphenous veins. The second type is due to destruction of the valves in the ankle perforating veins and is common after deep venous thrombosis. Valve destruction at the mouth of the short and/or long saphenous vein may also occur, resulting in varicosities of either or both veins. The third type of secondary varicosities are those about the pubis and lower abdomen. Pudendal varicose veins occur as a postpregnancy phenomenon related to uterine pressure.

Rarely, varicose veins may be associated with either congenital or acquired arteriovenous fistulas. In the Klippel-Trénaunay syndrome (lateral venous anomaly) varicose remnants of the sciatic venous system persist on the lateral aspect of the leg (18). This syndrome is characterized by varicosities, hemangiomas, and limb hypertrophy. Arteriovenous fistulas are present in some cases (21).

Diagnosis of Venous Diseases

In superficial thrombophlebitis, septic thrombophlebitis of the lower extremities, phlegmasia alba dolens, and phlegmasia cerulea dolens, diagnosis based solely on symptoms and physical findings should be relatively easy. The diagnosis of varicose veins is also straightforward, but additional studies are needed to define the pathophysiology.

In superficial thrombophlebitis, in particular, the diagnosis can usually be made with a high degree of accuracy on clinical grounds, and special diagnostic tests are not needed. The diagnosis is rarely confused, but conditions such as acute gout, bacterial cellulitis, lymphangitis, fat necrosis, and vasculitis must be ruled out.

Phlegmasia alba dolens refers to severe iliofemoral thrombosis in which there is marked pain and swelling of the involved extremity. Color ranges from white to deeply cyanotic. Despite the ominous appearance, there is no immediate threat of limb loss. In phlegmasia cerulea dolens, the entire venous outflow from the leg becomes blocked by the thrombotic process, and the leg becomes massively swollen and violaceous (Figure 11-4). Arterial pulsations are initially present but are later lost as the outflow resistance increases. Cutaneous blebs and bullae may develop. As the process worsens, cardiovascular collapse due to sequestration of fluid in the lower extremity (or extremities) may occur, and gangrene will occur unless some degree of venous outflow can be established (16). Because of the massive involvement, the diagnosis is seldom in question in either phlegmasia alba dolens or phlegmasia cerulea dolens.

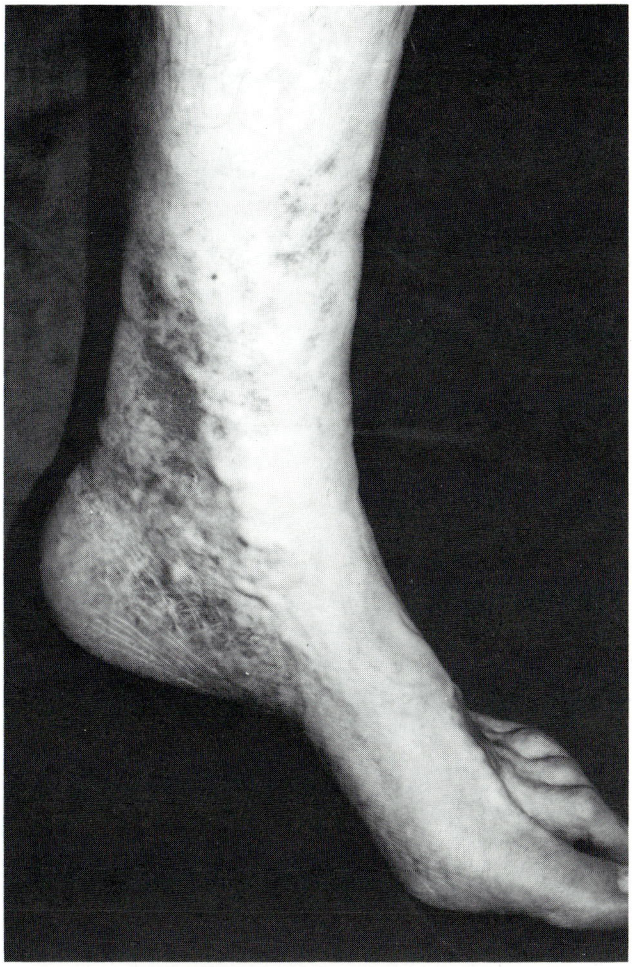

FIGURE 11-2. Secondary varicose veins, eczema, and hyperpigmentation occur relatively early in the postphlebitic limb.

In the less dramatic but more common variants of deep venous thrombosis, diagnosis is often difficult because of the vague signs and symptoms. Clinical diagnosis is in error in at least 50 percent of cases (14). Venous thrombosis should be suspected and ruled in or out in any patient with lower extremity pain if no other obvious cause is present. Even in the absence of pain or discomfort, it should also be suspected in bedridden patients who develop lower extremity edema. Although unilateral edema makes one more suspicious, the presence of bilateral edema does not rule out the diagnosis.

The postphlebitic limb poses special problems for the clinician because of the combined problems of venous obstruction and venous insufficiency. Important distinctions must be made between primary and secondary varicosities. Also, the chronic leg edema must be distinguished from that of lymphedema or, in the case of bilaterality, from that of congestive heart failure and/or anasarca from other causes.

Because of the high rate of inaccuracy of clinical diagnosis in both acute and chronic conditions, physicians initially turned to phlebography as the gold standard for diagnosis of venous thrombosis. Important aspects of phlebography will be discussed in the ensuing paragraphs.

PHLEBOGRAPHY

Several techniques of performing phlebography have been described (4,34,36,43). Excellent phlebograms are obtained using the technique outlined by Rabinov and Paulin (39), and it is regarded as one of the preferred techniques. In this technique, the extremity to be examined is unweighted, the patient is semi-upright, and no tourniquet is used.

The more common radiographic signs of venous thrombosis are outlined in Table 11-3. Generally speaking, phlebography is a safe procedure which can even be done on an outpatient basis. However, it does have some inherent drawbacks in that it causes discomfort and is hazardous in patients with a sensitivity to iodine. Chemical thrombophlebitis in reaction to the contrast medium may also develop as a result of the procedure in a small percentage of cases. Clinically manifest postvenogram chemical phlebitis has been reported to occur in roughly 2.0 percent of cases, while the incidence of subclinical chemical phlebitis may be as high as 33 percent (3). Because of the drawbacks

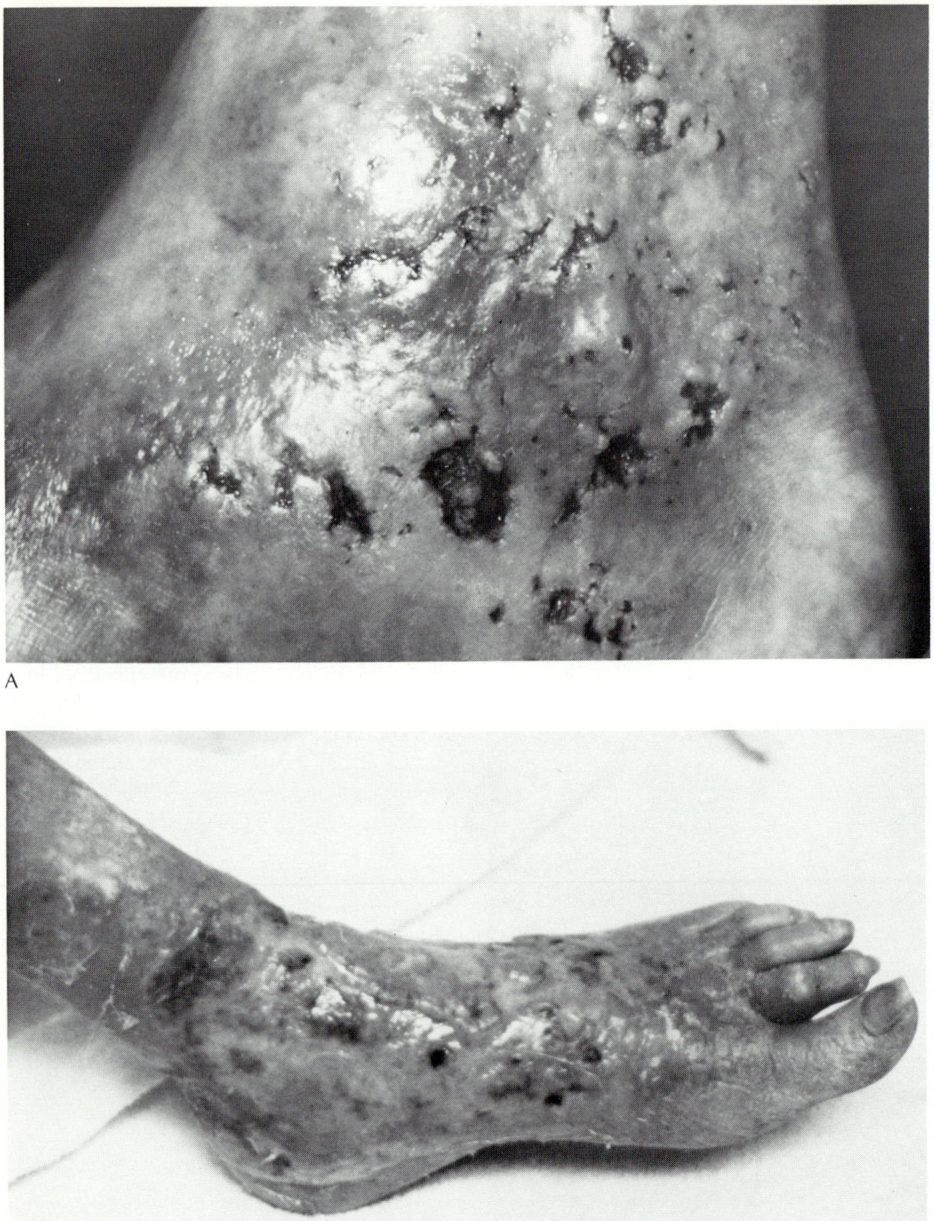

A B

FIGURE 11-3. (*A*) Skin ulceration and (*B*) even massive tissue necrosis may occur as late manifestations of the postphlebitic syndrome.

TABLE 11-2. Functional Classification of Venous Insufficiency

I.	Primary, or familial, varicose veins
	a. Greater saphenous incompetence
	b. Lesser saphenous incompetence
	c. Perforator vein incompetence
II.	Secondary varicosities
	a. Postphlebitic syndrome with severe varicosities
III.	Varicosities of pregnancy
IV.	Miscellaneous causes of varicosities
	a. Congenital arteriovenous malformations
	b. Acquired arteriovenous fistulas
	c. Klippel-Trénaunay syndrome

associated with contrast phlebography and technological developments leading to the capability of arriving at an accurate diagnosis noninvasively, there has been a decline over the past several years in the number of phlebograms performed in many major institutions. Related techniques which require minor invasiveness but little discomfort or risk include several radioisotope techniques which will be discussed in the next section.

RADIOISOTOPE TECHNIQUES

Radionuclide phlebography refers to a technique in which a radioactive substance is injected into a pedal vein. Dynamic

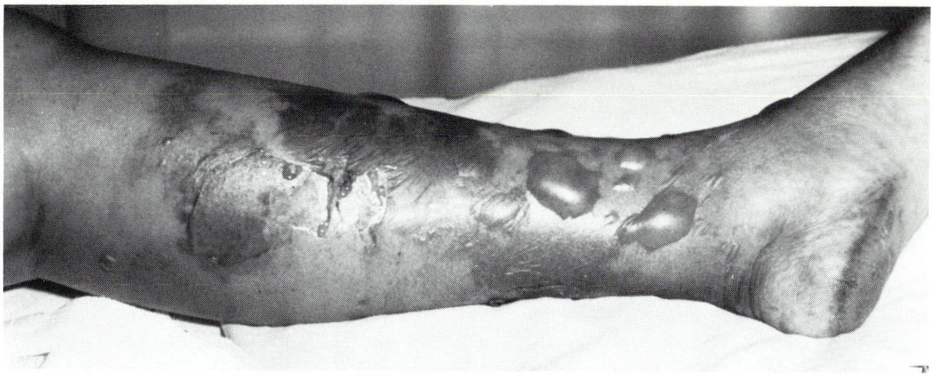

A

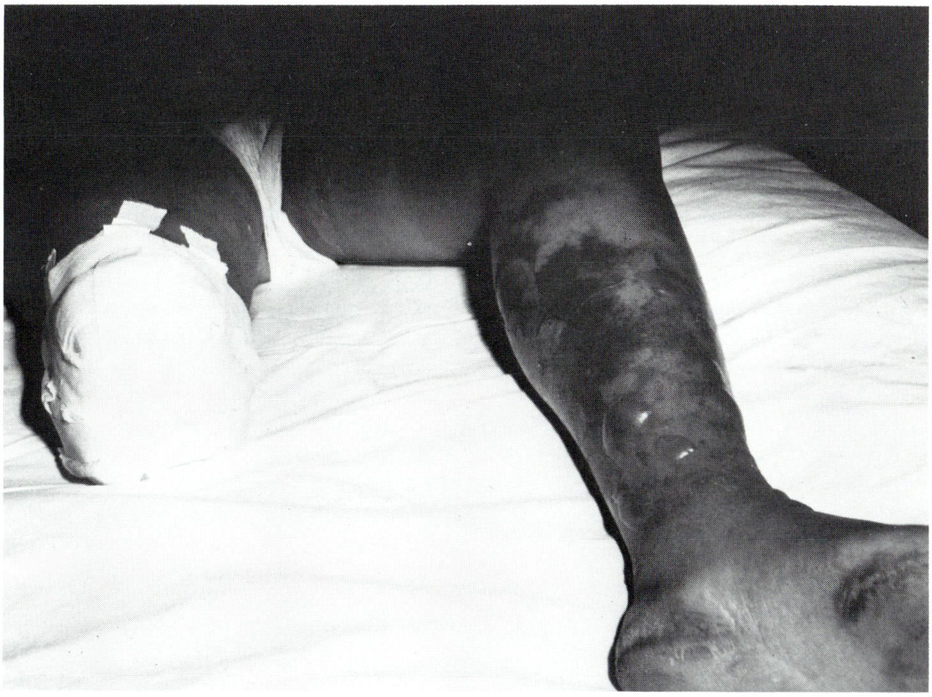

B

FIGURE 11-4. (*A*) Phlegmasia cerulea dolens represents near total obstruction of venous outflow resulting in massive swelling and violaceous discoloration. Cutaneous blebs and bullae may develop. (*B*) As shown, limb loss occurs if some degree of venous outflow cannot be established.

imaging using a scintillation camera is then done over the extremity veins, iliac veins, and inferior vena cava. Some of the substances that have been used are ^{99m}Tc macroaggregated albumin, ^{99m}Tc macroaggregated fibrinogen, and ^{99m}Tc human albumin microspheres (HAM). The basis for the test is that, in the presence of venous thrombosis, a portion of intravenously injected macroaggregated albumin particles will become adherent to thrombus. Thrombi are identified by recognition of delayed clearance of radioactivity from the extremity after intravenous injection of radiolabeled particles.

Compared with contrast phlebography, radioisotope imaging techniques have yielded accuracy rates ranging from 89 to 96 percent (26,41). They have a great deal of appeal, because of a high degree of patient acceptance and the ability to perform a lung scan using the same injection of radioactive substance (40). However, they also have some drawbacks. In the early studies, the contralateral extremity was used as a reference. Thus, results were difficult to interpret when there was bilateral lower extremity involvement. Furthermore, sluggish flow of blood through the popliteal space may lead to false-positive results. Further studies of these types of imaging techniques are warranted in view of their low risk and potential application.

Another radioisotope technique involves trapping of radiolabeled fibrinogen in developing thrombus. Serial counts are

TABLE 11-3. Radiographic Signs of Deep Venous Thrombosis

1. Constant, well-delineated filling defects
2. Abrupt termination of contrast medium at a constant site above or below obstruction
3. Nonfilling of the entire deep system or portions thereof, providing proper technique was used
4. Diversion of flow through collaterals

obtained over the extremity, but no images are obtained. These techniques were made possible by the recognition that radiolabeled fibrinogen could be incorporated into developing thrombi in sufficient quantity to make it detectable by scintillation counting (27). ^{131}I was used in the early studies, but a major shortcoming of the technique related to the short half-life of this isotope (5,27). This was overcome when it was found that the more stable isotope, ^{125}I, gave similar results (31). Incorporation of ^{125}I-labeled fibrinogen into a developing thrombus now forms the basis of the *fibrinogen uptake test*. Many of the early studies of the fibrinogen uptake test were done in surgical patients. It was found that in some cases in which venous thrombosis became apparent later in the postoperative period, the clotting process actually began before or during operation or as early as the first postoperative day (25).

To perform the fibrinogen uptake test, thyroid uptake of iodine is blocked with 100 mg of sodium iodide, which can be given orally or intravenously, and a 100-Ci dose of ^{125}I-labeled fibrinogen is given intravenously. Radioactivity counts are then taken at various points over each extremity and expressed as a percentage of reference counts made over the precordium. Based on phlebographic comparisons, accuracy rates ranging from 80 to 93 percent have been reported (8,24,31,32). However, the fibrinogen uptake test is not useful in traumatized extremities or recently operated upon extremities, and it has a low degree of accuracy in the iliofemoral venous segment. Its greatest usefulness has been as a screening technique in trials comparing various methods for preventing postoperative venous thrombosis. Development of this test also contributed greatly to identification of categories of patients who are at high risk of developing postoperative venous thrombosis.

Thus far, neither phlebography nor radioisotope techniques have provided the degree of clinical utility needed for the rapid, safe, and accurate diagnosis of deep venous thrombosis. Thus, noninvasive tests have gained in popularity and are now widely used as the first test in patients with suspected lower extremity venous thrombosis. The Doppler test, which will be discussed further, can also be used to evaluate suspected upper extremity venous thrombosis (42).

Noninvasive Techniques

A number of totally noninvasive techniques for diagnosing venous obstruction and/or venous insufficiency are available. As these techniques have improved, they have begun to supplant contrast phlebography, which is now being used in several institutions only when the diagnosis remains in question after noninvasive testing. The most commonly used techniques will be discussed in the ensuing paragraphs.

IMPEDANCE PLETHYSMOGRAPHY

Impedance plethysmography was one of the earliest noninvasive tests to be developed. It is based on the principle that during respiration there are cyclic variations in venous volumes and pressures in the lower extremities (35,45). Volume changes cause variations in electrical impedance, with the two being inversely related. Normally, with deep inspiration the volume of the extremity increases and the electrical impedance decreases. During expiration the opposite takes place. This is in accordance with Ohm's law (voltage = current × resistance). The difference between the lowest impedance achieved during inspiration and the highest impedance achieved during expiration is called the "maximum respiratory impedance excursion." In patients with obstructed venous outflow, "maximum respiratory impedance excursion" is less than in normal controls. In early studies of normal extremities it almost invariably exceeded 0.2 percent of baseline impedance, while in extremities with thrombophlebitis it rarely achieved that value (45). Early on, impedance plethysmography was shown to be highly useful as a rapid screening test. However, it was criticized as being of little value in detecting below-knee thrombi, with accuracy rates as low as 60 percent (23).

The accuracy of impedance plethysmography was greatly increased by the introduction of the cuff occlusion technique (24). This technique has been described in detail by several workers (29,30,44,45). To perform it, an occlusion cuff is placed around the thigh and inflated to a level greater than venous pressure but less than arterial pressure. Pressures in the range of 50 to 60 mmHg are usually satisfactory. In normal extremities, cuff inflation causes a rapid increase in calf blood volume and a concomitant rise in the baseline of the impedance tracing. Rapid cuff deflation causes a rapid return to baseline calf blood volume. Obstruction caused by deep venous thrombosis impedes outflow and causes a slow return to baseline. By calculating the percentage of trapped venous blood that leaves the calf in the first 2 seconds after cuff release, the rate of venous outflow can be quickly obtained. Using venous occlusion impedance plethysmography, accuracy rates as high as 98 to 100 percent for proximal venous thrombi have been obtained (29,45).

SEGMENTAL PLETHYSMOGRAPHY (AIR AND STRAIN GAUGE)

Segmental air plethysmography and strain-gauge plethysmography are similar in principle to cuff occlusion impedance plethysmography. In this technique, however, changes in limb volume and pressure are detected by pneumatic bladders or mercury strain gauges which encircle the leg at one or more points. When a proximal occlusion cuff is inflated to a level between arterial and venous pressure (50 to 60 mmHg), limb volume increases and the baseline of the tracing rises. With cuff release, a rapid return toward baseline occurs in normal extremities. The rate of venous emptying in the presence of venous obstruction is retarded. By dividing the fall occurring in the first 1 to 2 seconds after release by the total rise, a ratio can be established which will separate extremities with normal venous emptying from those with abnormal venous emptying (Figure 11-5). In most normal extremities, 50 percent of venous emptying occurs during the first 2 seconds after cuff release (37). Overall accuracy is in the range of 80 percent. False positives are not common for major obstructing thrombi and have been reported at less than 3.0

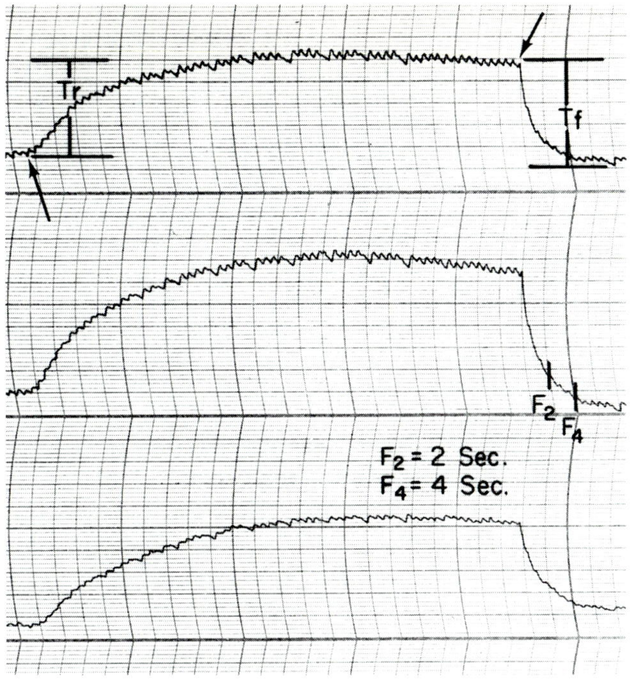

A

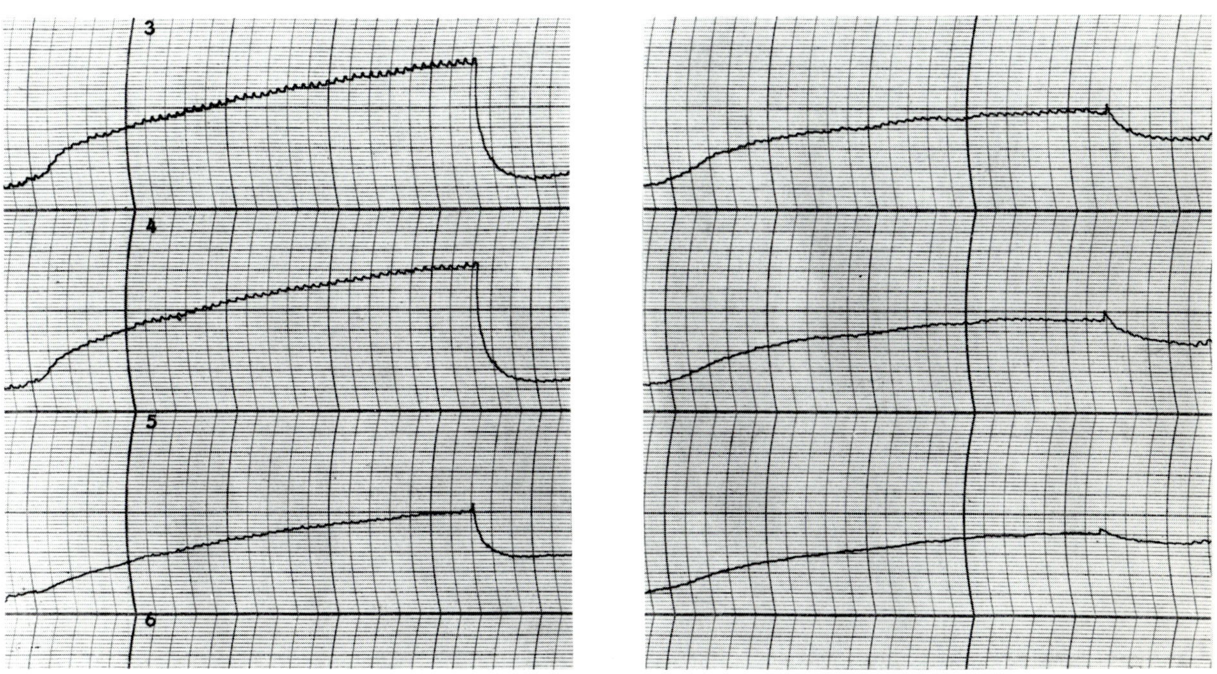

B

FIGURE 11-5. (*A*) In segmental venous occlusion plethysmography, the baseline begins to rise when the occluding cuff is inflated to greater than venous pressure (*arrow*). When the capacitance bed is filled, the tracing stabilizes at a higher level (Tr). When the cuff is released (*arrow*), the tracing returns to baseline. Venous outflow is calculated by dividing the fall at 2 s (F_2) by the total rise (Tr). (***B***) Outflow tracing from the normal (*left*) and abnormal (*right*) lower extremities in a patient with acute deep venous thrombosis.

percent (37). There are significant drawbacks, however, to segmental plethysmography. False-positive results are obtained in a high percentage of patients if the leg is improperly positioned. This is usually related to having the knee straight rather than slightly bent. The recent finding of a sensitivity of only 77.3 percent and a specificity of 62.4 percent has led to a discontinuation of routine usage of segmental air plethysmography at Massachusetts General Hospital where it was developed (22).

PHLEBORHEOGRAPHY

Phleborheography is a highly useful technique which will detect thrombi in both above-knee and below-knee veins (13,15). In the initial description of the technique, only three false-negative and four false-positive results were reported from the examination of 304 extremities (13). Accuracy was determined by comparison to phlebograms. In a later report involving 133 extremities, the accuracy compared with phlebography was 100 percent (15). Others have reported lower levels of accuracy (85 percent) (9), but the incidence of false positives is low, and one is justified in instituting treatment in patients with positive results.

Phleborheography is a highly useful technique for screening patients with suspected deep venous thrombosis. In a series involving 328 extremities, useful information was obtained in over 98 percent (11). In 64 extremities, phlebograms were also done, and the overall accuracy for detecting venous obstruction was 95.3 percent.

To perform the test, pneumatic cuffs connected to low pressure transducers are placed on the foot; the lower, middle, and upper calf; and the thorax. The thoracic cuff is used to monitor respiration, and the foot and lowermost calf cuffs are used interchangeably as compression and recording cuffs. In a normal tracing, good respiratory waves are transmitted throughout the lower extremity, and there is no rise in baseline with three short bursts of 50 mmHg delivered to the calf cuff or 100 mmHg delivered to the foot cuff. In extremities with acute venous obstruction, respiratory waves are diminished or absent and there

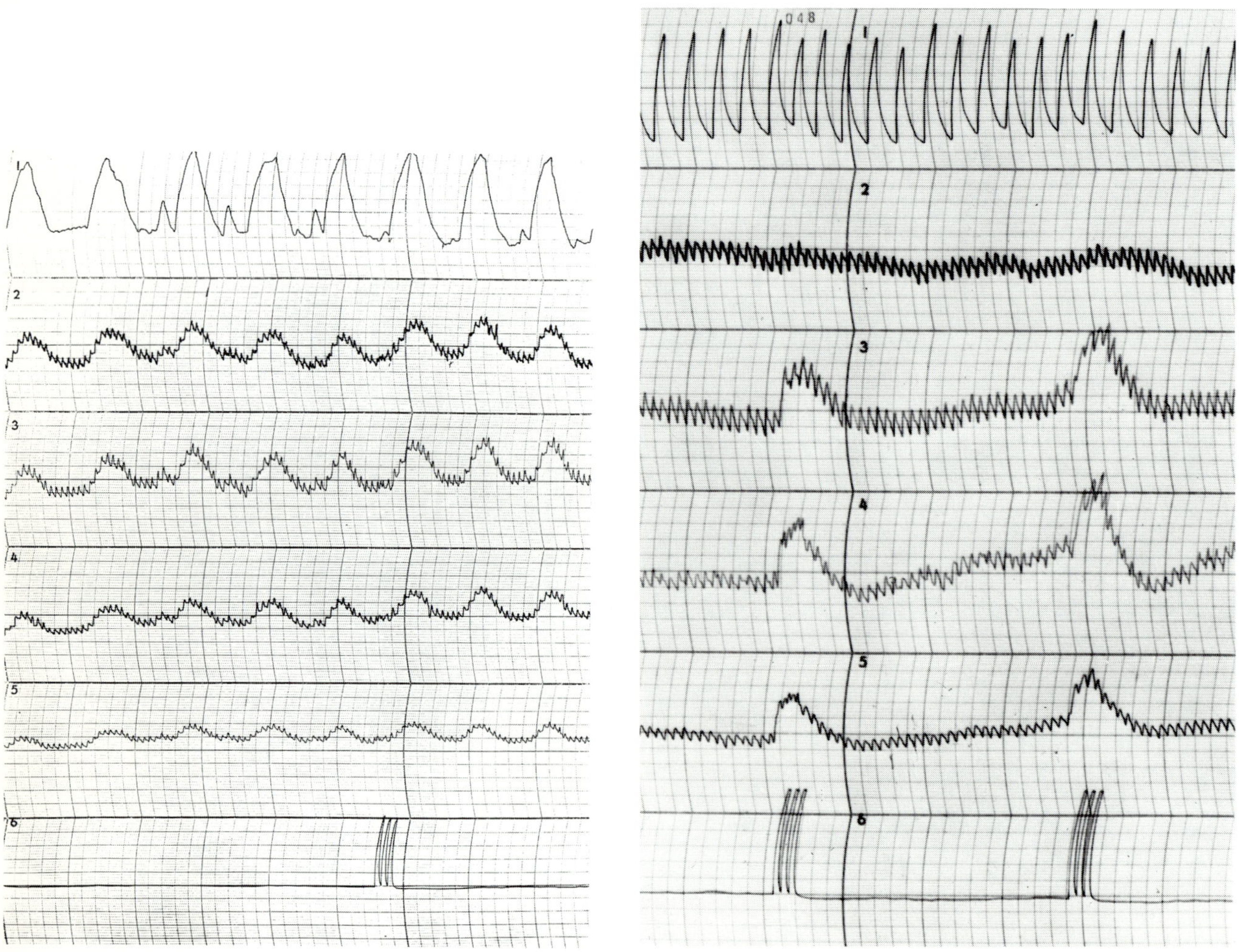

A B

FIGURE 11-6. (*A*) The normal phleborheogram is characterized by good transmission of respiratory waves and no change in baseline with distal compression. Tracings from top to bottom are from the thorax; thigh; upper, middle, and lower calf; and foot. The foot cuff is being used for distal compression. (***B***) In acute deep venous thrombosis, respiratory waves (tracing 1) are not transmitted (tracings 2–5). There is also a rise in baseline (tracings 3–5) when distal compression is applied.

is a rise in baseline with distal compression. In patients with chronic venous obstruction and those with subacute obstruction with recanalization or collaterization, respiratory waves are present or even exaggerated, but there is a rise in baseline with distal compression. Representative tracings are illustrated in Figure 11-6.

Like other noninvasive techniques, phleborheography does not detect thrombi in superficial veins, the profunda femoris veins, or muscular veins. It also requires a short period of special training in both test performance and tracing interpretation. Nonetheless, properly used it is one of the most accurate of the noninvasive tests for the detection of lower extremity venous obstruction. There are limited data on the use of phleborheography in diagnosing upper extremity venous obstruction. However, the positive predictive value of 94 percent reported in a recent study suggests that it might be of use in the upper as well as the lower extremity (42).

ULTRASOUND TECHNIQUES

Doppler ultrasound techniques have been used extensively to detect both venous obstruction and venous insufficiency. The detection of venous obstruction is based on impedance of forward flow and a consequent reduction in transmitted venous flow sounds. Using a bidirectional flow probe, forward flow is recorded as flow away from the probe (Figure 11-7). Contrarily, certain maneuvers used to elicit valvular incompetence will augment flow toward the probe with a bidirectional unit. For simplicity and ease of application, however, both obstruction and insufficiency can be detected using a unidirectional probe. With a trained ear, one can rapidly assess the lower extremity veins using the Doppler. Recording of tracings is not entirely necessary but is highly useful for documentation of findings, for physician interpretation of technician's findings, and for providing a permanent record. Representative tracings are shown in Figure 11-8. In performing the Doppler examination, one needs to assess five elements of the venous Doppler signal: spontaneity, phasicity, augmentation, competence, and pulsatility. Each is discussed in greater detail below. Excellent descriptions are also available in basic texts (6).

Spontaneity. Normally, there are spontaneous venous flow sounds that can be recorded from all the major veins. In vasoconstricted extremities, these sounds may be greatly attenuated or absent over the posterior tibial veins or superficial veins but are still present over the deep veins in the popliteal space and thigh. Absence of a spontaneous venous flow signal thus represents an abnormal finding and is one of the early signs of venous obstruction.

Phasicity. This refers to the normal waxing and waning of the venous flow signal with respiration. During descent of the diaphragm during inspiration, venous flow is greatly diminished or totally interrupted. The flow signal then increases maximally during expiration. In the presence of proximal venous obstruction, the venous flow signal becomes more continuous and respiratory variation becomes markedly diminished.

Augmentation. The venous flow signal is normally increased by compression of the limb distal to the probe or by release of compression proximal to the probe. Such augmentation is diminished or absent in the face of venous obstruction.

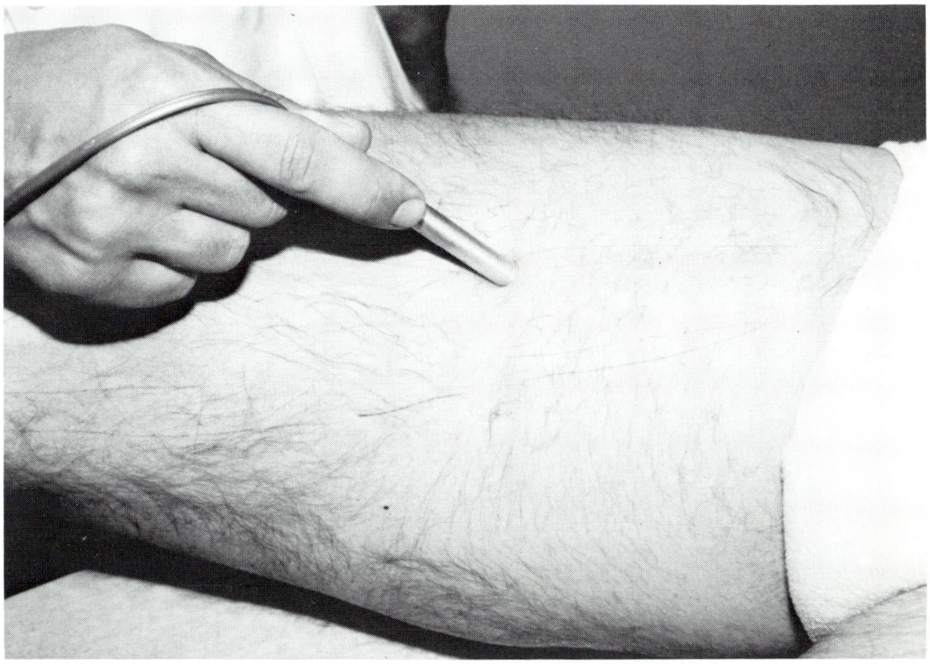

FIGURE 11-7. With the bidirectional probe at a 45° angle to the skin and directed toward the heart, forward flow is recorded as flow *away* from the probe. If reflux occurs with a Valsalva maneuver, there is augmentation of flow *toward* the probe. This photograph shows the proper orientation of the probe.

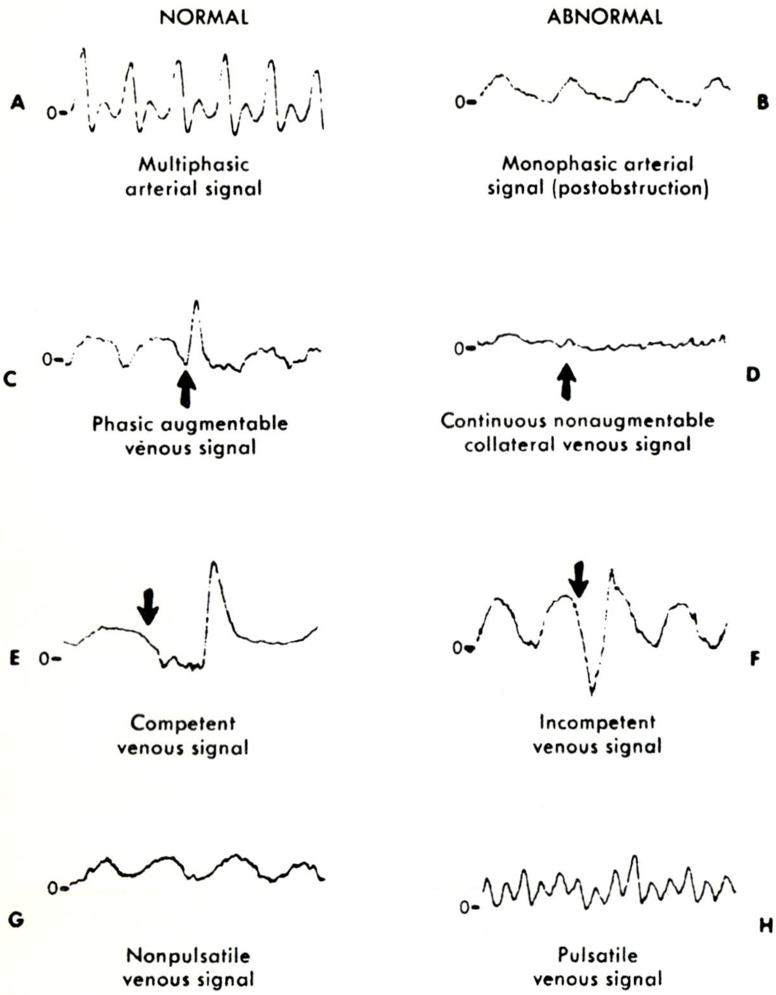

FIGURE 11-8. Normally, venous flow is nonpulsatile and phasic as shown in (*C*) and valvular competence prevents a venous flow signal during proximal compression as shown in (*E*). When venous obstruction is present, the venous flow signal may be continuous due to flow through collaterals (*D*), and proximal limb compression causes an augmented retrograde flow signal due to valvular incompetence (*F*). The venous flow signal may also take on a pulsatile arterial quality when venous pressure is elevated as shown in (*H*). [From Barnes (6).]

Competence. Competent venous valves prevent reflux flow of blood. In cases of congenitally incompetent or absent valves and in cases of valvular destruction, there will be retrograde flow of blood during compression of the limb proximal to the flow probe. Also, when venous valves are competent, a Valsalva maneuver causes prompt cessation of flow. Contrarily, in the face of valvular incompetence, the Valsalva maneuver augments retrograde flow.

Pulsatility. Venous signals are normally nonpulsatile and vary in intensity with respiration but not with the heart beat. When venous pressure is elevated, such as in congestive heart failure, venous sounds may be difficult to distinguish from arterial sounds. However, limb compression maneuvers and the Valsalva maneuver continue to alter venous flow sounds. These maneuvers have no effect on arterial flow sounds.

To perform the Doppler examination, the patient should be positioned supine in a comfortable position with the head of the bed or examining table slightly elevated to increase venous pooling. The legs should be in a comfortable, relaxed position with the hips externally rotated and the knees slightly flexed. Examination of the popliteal veins is best accomplished with the patient in the prone position.

One should routinely examine the posterior tibial vein, the popliteal vein, the superficial femoral vein, and the common femoral vein. Close attention should be paid to the presence of spontaneous venous flow sounds and to the influence of proximal and distal compression.

The superficial venous system, especially the greater saphenous vein, can also be tested for incompetence using the Doppler instrument. As mentioned earlier, the Doppler can also be used to detect upper extremity venous obstruction (42).

The accuracy of the venous Doppler examination is observer-dependent, and the test requires time, experience, and practice to learn. However, a competent observer should be able to obtain an accuracy on the order of 90 percent. Sources of error, in addition to observer inexperience, include nonobstructive thrombi, thrombi in parallel (duplicated) veins, and thrombi in veins that are not in the axial stream. Examples include thrombi in muscular veins, veins of the soleal plexus, and the profunda femoris veins. All the previously mentioned noninvasive tests are subject to these same limitations.

A promising recent development is use of the continuous wave Doppler to perform B-mode images of the veins. With this technique intraluminal images are obtained, and both acute and chronic thrombi can be seen. It can be used for upper extremity and

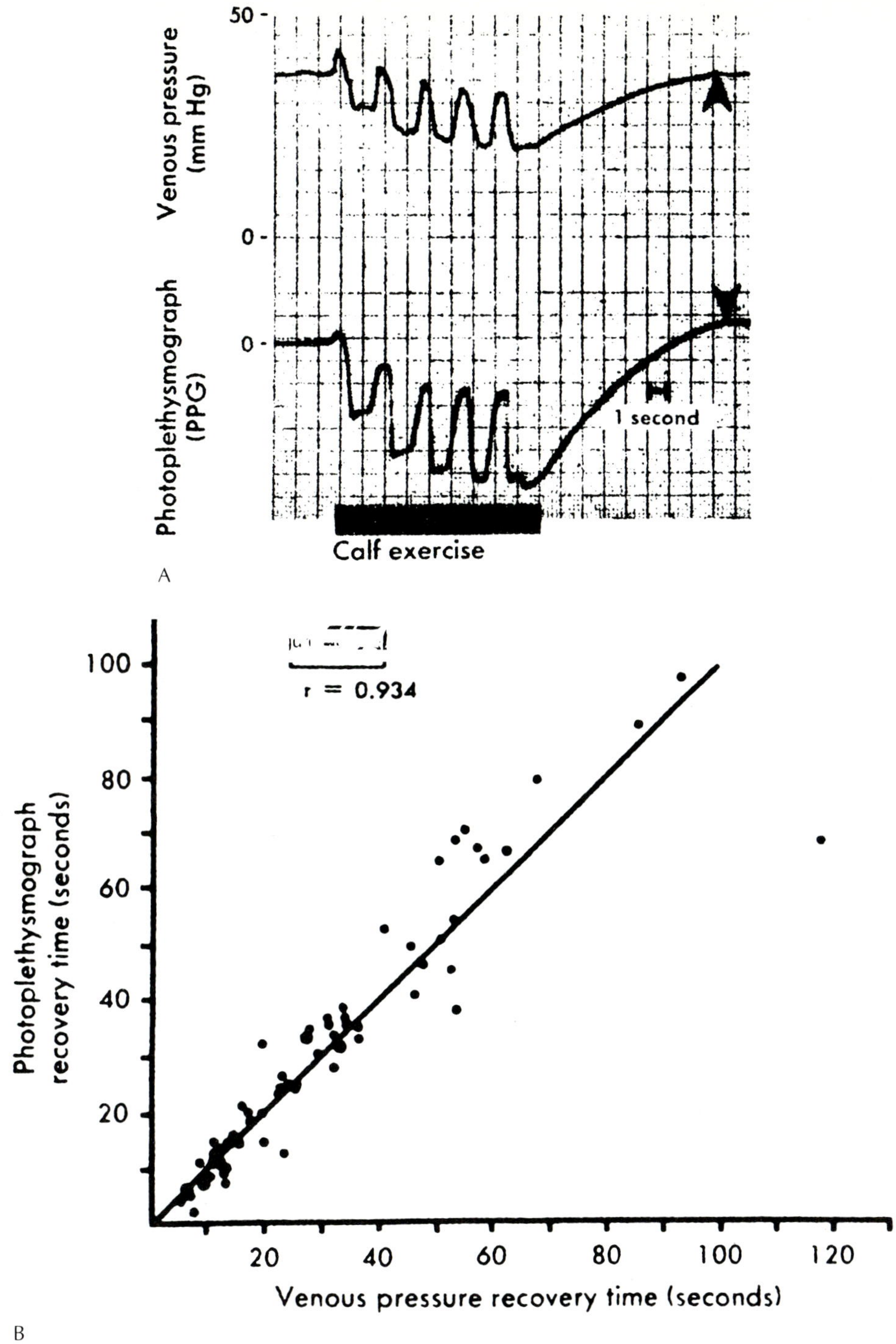

FIGURE 11-9. (*A*) Photoplethysmographic and venous pressure tracings have similar contours, and as shown in (*B*) there is a high degree of correlation between the two. [From Abramowitz (1).]

neck veins. However, the iliac veins cannot be reliably imaged. Venographic comparisons have indicated a positive predictive value of 92 percent and a negative predictive value of 96 percent in the lower extremities (19). Because this test is totally noninvasive, it can be repeated to follow the progression of known thrombi. Thus it may yield important information related to response to therapy. Also, the test results may influence therapy as in the case of free-floating thrombi.

PHOTOPLETHYSMOGRAPHY

Among recent developments in noninvasive vascular diagnosis, photoplethysmography, as applied to the diagnosis of chronic venous insufficiency, is one of the most useful. It has been shown to correlate very well with direct pressure measurements (Figure 11-9) (1). Thus, it has essentially replaced the need to make such measurements. This technological advance was made possible by direct current (dc) coupling of the voltage output of an infrared photoplethysmograph (PPG) to permit continuous recording of the relative amount of blood in the cutaneous microcirculation (7).

The PPG transducer contains an infrared light-emitting diode and an adjacent phototransistor to receive back-scattered light reflected from the superficial layers of the skin. The amount of reflected light varies with the number of red blood cells in the microcirculation. Arterial waveforms can be recorded in the alternating current (ac) mode. In the dc mode, the voltage output is filtered to provide a longer time constant, permitting a record of relative changes in skin blood content over the course of time. The dc mode is used for venous studies.

The examination is performed with the patient in the sitting position with both feet on the floor. The transducer is fixed to the skin above the medial malleolus, using double-faced clear plastic tape. Comparison tracings are obtained by examining both extremities at the same time.

When stable baselines are achieved, the patient is instructed to actively contract the muscles of each calf by alternately plantar flexing the foot five times in succession. The recording is continued until the PPG tracing returns to baseline. The function of the deep and perforating veins can be tested by serially occluding the subcutaneous veins with tourniquets. The exercise test is then repeated with the tourniquets in place.

Since the PPG output cannot be calibrated, the quantitative end points for this study are related to the recovery time of the baseline skin blood content after active leg muscle exercise. Recovery time is recorded as the total number of seconds required for the recording to return to the preexercise baseline level or to one-half of the preexercise baseline level ($t_{\frac{1}{2}}$) as shown in Figure 11-10.

Normally, skin blood content decreases in response to active or passive calf muscle exercise due to venous emptying. The recovery time is usually greater than 20 seconds, and it is not affected by application of a tourniquet. In chronic venous insufficiency, three patterns may be observed: (1) In the decompressive pattern, skin blood content decreases initially, as in normal extremities, but the recovery time is short, usually less than 10 seconds. (2) In the static pattern, there is no significant change in the amount of blood in the skin after muscle exercise. (3) In the congestive pattern, an increase in blood content in the skin is noted immediately after exercise.

In patients with secondary varicose veins, application of leg tourniquets does not change the abnormal pattern of venous reflux. On the contrary, in patients with primary varicosities, there is a restoration of $t_{\frac{1}{2}}$ toward normal (Figure 11-11).

The decompressive pattern of venous reflux appears more commonly in patients with stasis dermatitis but no ulceration, while static and decompressive patterns are observed more commonly in patients with ulceration. The congestive pattern also appears more often in patients with ulcers of long duration.

A normal study does not rule out the presence of deep venous disease, because the PPG test does not directly assess venous outflow obstruction. The test is abnormal only if there are incompetent superficial or perforating veins.

Limitations of the technique include its qualitative nature, although the measurement of recovery times permits some degree of quantification of altered venous hemodynamics. The test may be falsely positive with rapid recovery times in areas of acute inflammation or infection. All in all, venous phase PPG is an excellent test in patients with primary or secondary varicose veins, stasis dermatitis, and postphlebitic stasis ulceration. It is rapidly becoming the state of the art in most venous laboratories.

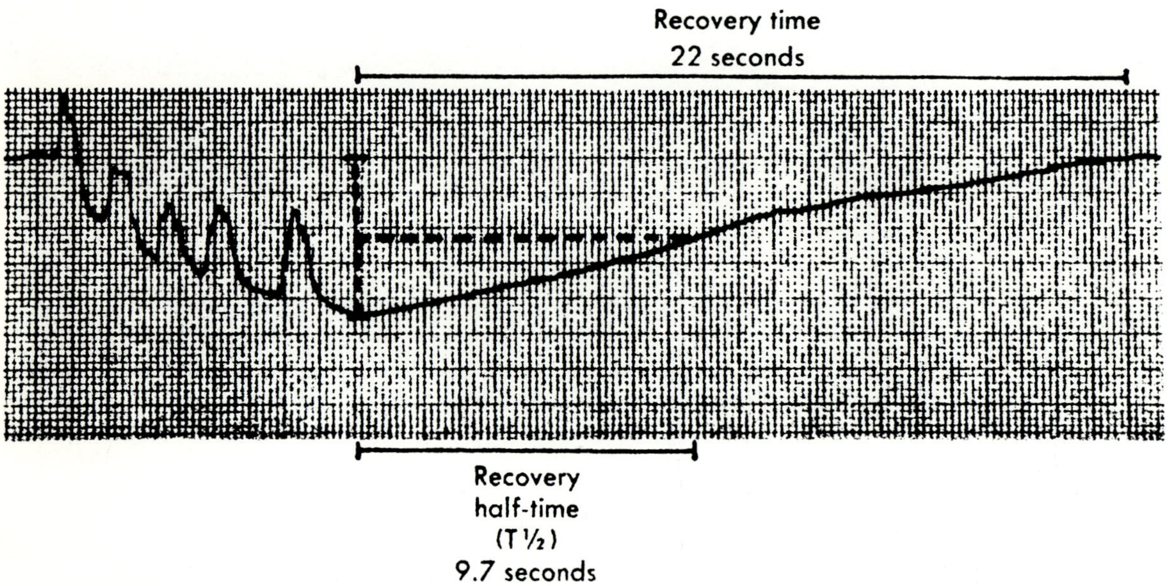

FIGURE 11-10. Photoplethysmography is not strictly quantitative, but measurement of the recovery half-time allows one to distinguish between extremities with normal hemodynamics and those with venous insufficiency with a high degree of accuracy. [From Barnes (7).]

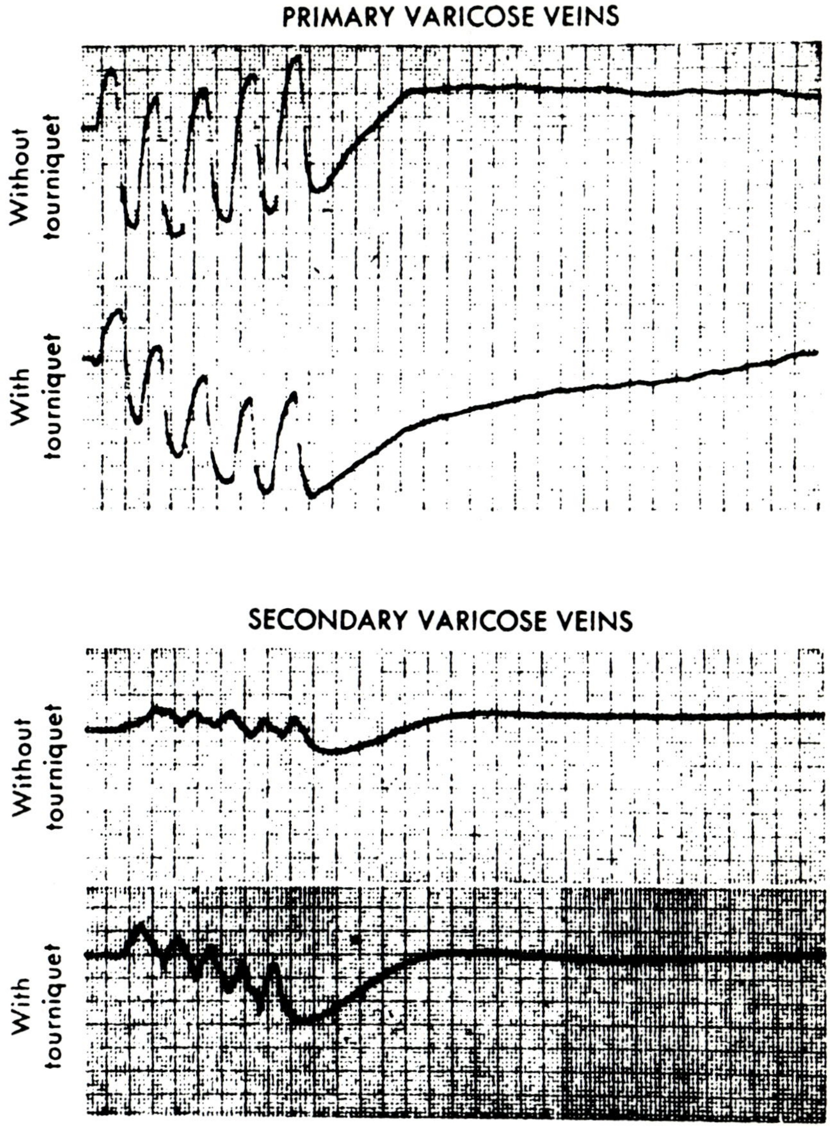

FIGURE 11-11. The application of tourniquets does not alter the abdominal PPG in patients with secondary varicose veins. However, in patients with primary varicosities the recovery half-time $t_{1/2}$ returns toward normal with the application of tourniquets [From Barnes (6).]

References

1. Abramowitz HB, Queral LA, Flinn WR, Nora PF Jr, Peterson LK, Bergan JJ, Yao JST: The use of photoplethysmography in the assessment of venous insufficiency: A comparison to venous pressure measurements. Surgery 1979, 86:434.
2. Adams JT, McEvory RK, DeWeese JA: Primary deep venous thrombosis of upper extremities. Arch Surg 1965, 91:27.
3. Albrechtsson J, Olsen CG: Thrombotic side effects of lower limb phlebography. Lancet 1976, 1:723.
4. Athanasoulis CA: Phlebography for the diagnosis of deep vein thrombosis. In *Prophylactic Therapy of Deep Vein Thrombosis and Pulmonary Embolism*. DHEW Publication No. (NIH) 76:860, 1975.
5. Atkins P, Hawkins LA: Detection of venous thrombosis in the legs. Lancet 1965, 2:1217.
6. Barnes RW: Doppler ultrasonic diagnosis of venous disease. In Bernstein EF (ed): *Noninvasive Diagnostic Techniques in Vascular Disease*. St Louis, CV Mosby Co, 1982, pp 452–457.
7. Barnes RW, Yao JST: Photoplethysmography in chronic venous insufficiency. In Bernstein EF (ed): *Nonvasive Diagnostic Techniques in Vascular Disease*. St Louis, CV Mosby Co, pp 514–521.
8. Browse NL: The ^{125}I fibrinogen uptake test. Arch Surg 1972, 104:160.
9. Bynum LJ, Wilson JE III, Crotty CM, Curry TS III, Smitson HL: Noninvasive diagnosis of deep venous thrombosis by pleborheography. Ann Intern Med 1978, 89:162.
10. Campbell CB, Chandler JG, Tectmeyer CJ, Bernstein EF: Axillary, subclavian, and brachiocephalic vein obstruction. Surgery 1977, 82:816.
11. Collins GJ Jr, Rich NM, Andersen CA, McDonald PT, Kozloff L: Phleborheographic diagnosis of venous obstruction. Ann Surg 1979, 189:25.
12. Coon WW: Epidemiology of venous thromboembolism. Ann Surg 1977, 186:149.

13. Cranley JJ, Canos AJ, Sull WJ, Grass AM: Phleborheographic technique for diagnosing deep venous thrombosis of the lower extremities. Surg Gynecol Obstet 1975, 141:331.
14. Cranley JJ, Canos AJ, Sull WJ: The diagnosis of deep venous thrombosis, fallibility of clinical symptoms and signs. Arch Surg 1976, 111:34.
15. Cranley JJ, Gay AY, Grass AM, Simeone FA: Plethysmographic technique for the diagnosis of deep venous thrombosis of the lower extremities. Surg Gynecol Obstet 1973, 136:385.
16. DeBakey M, Ochsner A: Phlegmasia cerulea dolens and gangrene associated with thrombophlebitis. Surgery 1949, 26:16.
17. DeWeese JA, Rogoff SM: Clinical uses of functional ascending phlebography of the lower extremity. Angiology 1958, 9:268.
18. Dodd H, Cockett HB: Diagnosis of varicose veins. In *The Pathology and Surgery of the Veins of the Lower Limb*. Edinburgh, Churchill Livingstone, pp 74–98.
19. Flanagan LD, Sullivan ED, Cranley JJ: Venous imaging of the extremities using real time B-mode ultrasound. In Bergan JJ, Yao JST (eds): *Surgery of the Veins*. New York, Grune and Stratton, 1985, pp. 89–98.
20. Gibbs NM: Venous thrombosis of the lower limbs with particular reference to bed rest. Br J Surg 1957, 45:209.
21. Gloviczki P, Hollier LH, Telander RL, Kaufman B, Bianco AJ, Stickler GB: Surgical implications of Klippel-Trenaunay syndrome. Ann Surg 1983, 197:353.
22. Hanel KC, Abbott WM, Reidy NC, Fulchino D, Miller A, Brester DC, Athanasoulis CA: The role of two noninvasive tests in deep venous thrombosis. Ann Surg 1981, 194:725.
23. Harris WH, Sara SM, Salzman EW, DeSanctis RW, Waltman AC, Athanasoulis S: Impedance phlebography: A correlation with lower limb venography in the diagnosis of deep vein thrombosis. Surgery 1973, 74:385.
24. Harris WH, Athanasoulis C, Waltman AC, Salzman EW: Cuff-impedance phlebography and ^{125}I fibrinogen scanning versus roentgenographic phlebography for diagnosis of thrombophlebitis following hip surgery. J Bone Joint Surg 1976, 58A:939.
25. Heatley RV, Morgan A, Hughes LE, Okwonga W: Preoperative or postoperative deep-vein thrombosis? Lancet 1976, 1:437.
26. Henkin RE, Quinn JL: Nuclear medicine techniques in the diagnosis of deep vein thrombosis. Surg Clin North Am 1974, 54:57.
27. Hobbs JT, Davies JWL: Detection of venous thrombosis with ^{131}I-labelled fibrinogen in the rabbit. Lancet 1960, 2:134.
28. Hull R, Hirsch J, Sackett DL, Stoddart G: Cost effectiveness of clinical diagnosis, venography, and noninvasive testing in patients with symptomatic deep-vein thrombosis. N Engl J Med 1981, 304:1561.
29. Johnston KW, Kakkar VV: Plethysmographic diagnosis of deep vein thrombosis. Surg Gynecol Obstet 1974, 139:41.
30. Johnston KW, Kakkar VV, Spindler JJ, Corrigan TP, Fossard DP: A simple method for detecting deep vein thrombosis: An improved electrical impedance technique. Am J Surg 1974, 349.
31. Kakkar V: The diagnosis of deep vein thrombosis using ^{125}I-fibrinogen test. Arch Surg 1972, 104:152.
32. Kakkar V: Deep vein thrombosis, detection and prevention. Circulation 1975, 51:8.
33. Kistner RL: Primary venous incompetence of the leg. Am J Surg 1980, 140:218.
34. Lockhart-Mummery HE, Smitham JH: Varicose ulcer—A study of the deep veins with special reference to retrograde venography. Br J Surg 1951, 38:284.
35. Mullick SC, Wheeler HB, Songster GF: Diagnosis of deep venous thrombosis by measurement of electrical impedance. Am J Surg 1970, 119:417.
36. Nicolaides AN, Kakkar VV, Field ES, Renney JTG: The origin of deep vein thrombosis: A venographic study. Br J Radiol 1971, 44:653.
37. Nicholas GG, Miller FJ Jr, Demuth WE Jr, Waldhausen JA: Clinical vascular laboratory diagnosis of deep venous thrombosis. Ann Surg 1977, 186:213.
38. Ochsner A, Ochsner JL: Prevention of pulmonary embolism. Milit Med 1971, 136:829.
39. Rabinov K, Paulin S: Roentgen diagnosis of venous thrombosis in the leg. Arch Surg 1972, 104:134.
40. Rosenthall L: Combined inferior vena cavography, iliac venography, and lung imaging with ^{99m}Tc albumin macroaggregates. Radiology 1971, 98:623.
41. Ryo UY, Qazi M, Srikantaswamy S, Pinsky S: Radionuclide venography: Correlation with contrast venography. J Nucl Med 1977, 18:11.
42. Sottiurai VS, Towner K, McDonnell AE, Zarins CK: Diagnosis of upper extremity deep venous thrombosis using noninvasive technique. Surgery 1982, 91:582.
43. Thomas ML: Phlebography. Arch Surg 1972, 104:145.
44. Wheeler HB, Mullick SC, Anderson JN, Pearson D: Diagnosis of occult deep vein thrombosis by a noninvasive bedside technique. Surgery 1971, 70:20.
45. Wheeler HB, O'Donnell JA, Anderson FA, Benedict K: Occlusive impedance phlebography: A diagnostic procedure for venous thrombosis and pulmonary embolism. Prog Cardiovasc Dis 1974, 17:199.

Chapter 12

TRANSCUTANEOUS OXIMETRY IN VASCULAR SURGERY

CARL J. HAUSER and WILLIAM C. SHOEMAKER

History of Transcutaneous Gas Tension Monitoring

Oxygen transport through the skin was first reported by von Gerlack in 1851 (1); he varnished a shaved area of skin in animals and then analyzed gases in the bubbles formed under the varnish. Shaw et al. (2) later demonstrated that increasing temperature accelerates the rate of gas transport through skin. In 1951 Baumberger and Goodfriend (3) observed that immersing a finger in a 45°C electrolyte solution results in equilibration of the oxygen tension (P_{O_2}) of the solution and arterial oxygen tension (Pa_{O_2}). Direct measurements, however, on unheated skin revealed very low P_{O_2} values (4). Drug-induced hyperemia was noted to increase the skin surface P_{O_2} transiently, but it was not until the miniaturized heated Clark (5) P_{O_2} electrodes were developed by Huch et al. (6,7) and Eberhard et al. (8,9) that monitoring of skin oxygen tension became a practical reality.

Transcutaneous oxygen tension (Ptc_{O_2}) monitoring with such electrodes was originally studied and developed as a noninvasive method for tracking Pa_{O_2} in neonates. Numerous early reports (9–11) in the pediatric literature documented high correlation coefficients between the Ptc_{O_2} and the Pa_{O_2}, and so the idea that the Ptc_{O_2} is equivalent to the Pa_{O_2} became firmly entrenched. Subsequently, it became clear that although the Ptc_{O_2} reflects the Pa_{O_2} in the hemodynamically stable neonate, the Ptc_{O_2} is often much lower than the Pa_{O_2} in the seriously ill neonate. When the Pa_{O_2} and the Ptc_{O_2} differed, however, it was tacitly assumed the Ptc_{O_2} sensor was somehow at fault.

In adults, the Ptc_{O_2} is almost always considerably lower than the Pa_{O_2}. In part, this is because the thicker adult skin acts as a barrier to oxygen diffusion. Nonetheless, the incorrect assumption that the Ptc_{O_2} had to equal the Pa_{O_2} led to the erroneous conclusion that the Ptc_{O_2} was inaccurate in adults. Later studies (12,13), however, demonstrated that the Ptc_{O_2} in the adult is indeed a valid measure of the oxygenation of the skin. Thus the Ptc_{O_2} measured on the chest became accepted as a measure of the adequacy of the systemic oxygen delivery ($\dot{D}_{O_2}$). More recently, it has become apparent that when the Ptc_{O_2} is measured on a limb, the Ptc_{O_2} may also vary with the vascular status of the limb (14–16); it has also been found that the relationship of limb Ptc_{O_2} to chest Ptc_{O_2} assesses the adequacy of oxygen delivery to the limb in a variety of functional conditions (17).

Ptc_{O_2} Monitoring of Arterial Oxygenation

Heating skin liquifies the crystalline lipid structure of the stratum corneum (Figure 12-1), facilitating oxygen diffusion to the sensor; it heats the tissue and blood, decreasing the oxygen solubility and shifting the oxyhemoglobin dissociation curve to the right; and it dilates the local metarterioles and capillaries, thereby hyperperfusing the skin. This last effect, which has unfortunately become known as "arterialization," is subject to limitation by the body's hemodynamic status. These temperature-related increases in tissue P_{O_2} tend to obviate the oxygen diffusion gradient from capillary to electrode and the temperature-dependent increases in oxygen consumption by dermal and epidermal cells. Electrode temperatures of 44 to 45°C produce approximate compensation of these opposing effects, allowing the Ptc_{O_2} to approach the Pa_{O_2} in hemodynamically stable subjects, i.e., the Ptc_{O_2} approximates the Pa_{O_2} for neonates and is about 80 percent of the Pa_{O_2} in adults (18). As long as the cardiac output and the hematocrit are stable, this relationship is stable. The Pa_{O_2} can therefore be estimated continuously from the Ptc_{O_2} without multiple arterial punctures (Figure 12-2). This method is of great value when rapid changes in the Pa_{O_2} are expected. A direct Pa_{O_2} measurement should be performed and a stable relationship with the Ptc_{O_2} should be corroborated whenever a significant Ptc_{O_2} change occurs, or when the sensor site is changed.

HEMODYNAMIC ASSESSMENT BY Ptc_{O_2}

The skin is an ideal location to monitor oxygenation for early warning of incipient circulatory problems, because the cutaneous circulation is exquisitely susceptible to vasoconstriction during acute circulatory failure, whereas the circulations to the heart, brain, and other vital organs are preferentially preserved. Therefore, the Ptc_{O_2} has been found to be a useful variable for monitoring the acutely disturbed systemic circulation. Comparative

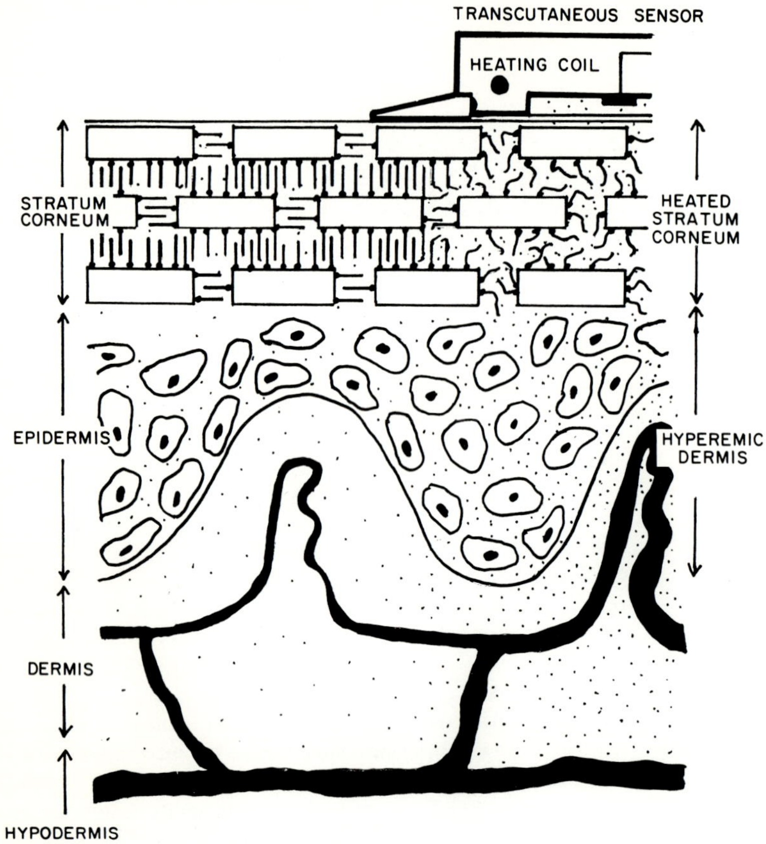

FIGURE 12-1. A schematic cross section of the electrode and skin including the stratum corneum, epidermis, dermis, and hypodermis. The irregular structure of the stratum corneum beneath the heated electrode represents the melted lipid. The small dots represent oxygen. Note the dilated dermal capillaries and the increased oxygen concentration under the heated electrode. The higher oxygen concentration is due to the greater blood flow and the greater oxygen release by the right-shifted oxyhemoglobin dissociation curve. (From Tremper KK, Waxman K, and Shoemaker WC. Crit Care Med 1979, 7:526.)

intraoperative and intensive care unit clinical studies indicate that the Ptc_{O_2} is, in some ways, a more sensitive indicator of circulatory insufficiency than conventional monitoring variables such as arterial pressure, heart rate, central venous pressure (CVP), ECG, and urine output (13).

Transcutaneous oxygen values depend on both the flow and the Pa_{O_2} (18,19). When the flow is adequate, the Ptc_{O_2} follows the Pa_{O_2}; when the flow is compromised but the Pa_{O_2} is adequate, the Ptc_{O_2} tracks the flow. In either case, the Ptc_{O_2} follows the D_{O_2}, which is defined as the product of the arterial oxygen content (which varies acutely with the Pa_{O_2}) and the cardiac output. Thus when the normovolemic patient goes into or out of respiratory failure, the Ptc_{O_2} follows the Pa_{O_2}; but as soon as the patient develops circulatory problems with low cardiac output, the Ptc_{O_2} and the Pa_{O_2} diverge (Figure 12-3).

In a large clinical series, the Pa_{O_2} and Ptc_{O_2} values from 106 adult patients were analyzed according to their cardiac index (CI). The patients were divided into three groups: (1) those with

TABLE 12-1. Ptc_{O_2} vs. Pa_{O_2} Linear Regression Values and Ptc_{O_2} Index Values for Patients in Three Ranges of CI

	Group 1 (Stable) CI >2.2	Group 2 (Moderate Shock) 2.2 >CI >1.5	Group 3 (Severe Shock) CI <1.5
No. data sets/no. patients	934/92	74/5	65/9
CI, L/min per square meter	4.1 ± 1.0	2.0 ± 0.2	0.9 ± 0.2
MAP, mmHg	96 ± 17	94 ± 18	39 ± 21
Ptc_{O_2} vs. Pa_{O_2}:			
Linear regression, *r* value	0.89	0.78	0.06
Slope	0.78	0.5	
Intercept	4.1	6	
Ptc_{O_2} index	0.79 ± 0.12	0.48 ± 0.07	0.12 ± 0.12
Ptc_{O_2} index vs. CI:			
Linear regression, *r* value			0.86

CI, Cardiac index; MAP, mean altered pressure.
SOURCE: Tremper KK, Shoemaker WC. Crit Care Med 1981, 9:706.

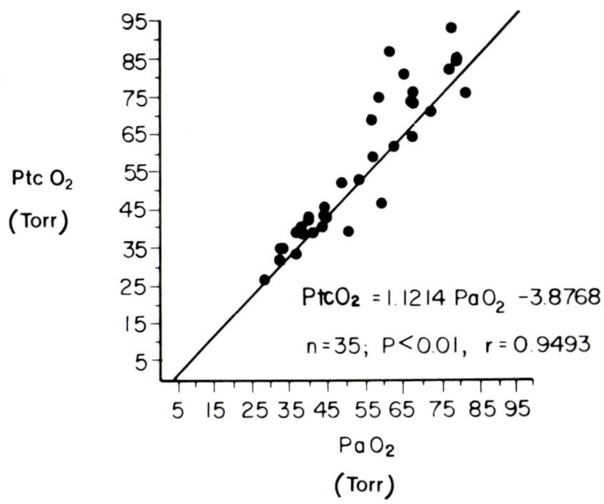

FIGURE 12-2. The relationship between the Ptc_{O_2} and the Pa_{O_2} in infants. (From Venus B, Patel KC, Pratap KS, Konchigeri H, Vidipsagar B. Crit Care Med 1981, 9:714.)

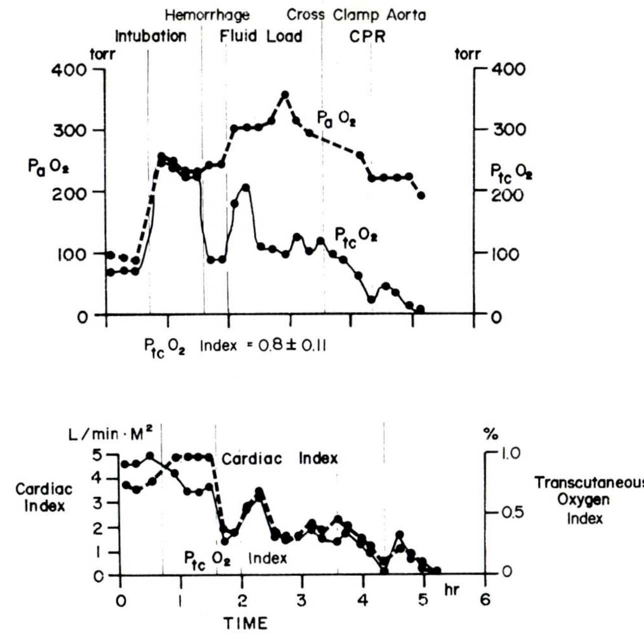

FIGURE 12-3. The relationships of the Ptc_{O_2}, Pa_{O_2}, cardiac index, and Ptc_{O_2} index (Ptc_{O_2}/Pa_{O_2}) in a patient who bled massively and subsequently suffered a cardiac arrest during an emergency portacaval shunt. The Ptc_{O_2} is related to the Pa_{O_2} while the patient is stable. When the CI decreases, the Pa_{O_2} becomes flow-dependent. The Ptc_{O_2} index is highly correlated ($r = 0.90$) to the flow. (From Tremper KK and Shoemaker WC. Crit Care Med 1981, 9:706.)

a relatively normal flow, CI > 2.2 L/min per square meter; (2) those with a moderately low flow, 2.2 > CI > 1.5 L/min per square meter; and (3) those with a severely low flow, CI < 1.5 L/min per square meter. The transcutaneous values were indexed to their corresponding arterial value by the formula: Ptc_{O_2} index $= Ptc_{O_2}/Pa_{O_2}$. This index determines if the Ptc_{O_2} values are in the normal range for Pa_{O_2} dependence (1.0 to 0.6) or in a flow-dependent range (<0.5). The Ptc_{O_2} accurately reflects the Pa_{O_2} in hemodynamically stable patients who are not in shock (Table 12-1, group 1). The correlation is poorer in patients with moderate shock (Table 12-1, group 2) and is nonexistent in patients with severe shock (Table 12-1, group 3) (18).

From the clinical point of view, this relationship between the Ptc_{O_2} and the Pa_{O_2} constitutes a highly significant noninvasive estimate of the hemodynamic status and the tissue perfusion. After control measurements of the Ptc_{O_2} and the Pa_{O_2} document this relationship, a patient may be monitored continuously through a life-threatening episode in the operating room or intensive care unit. When the Ptc_{O_2} drops, the Pa_{O_2} is measured; if the Pa_{O_2} has fallen, the patient has respiratory impairment; if the Pa_{O_2} and hemoglobin values are constant, the Ptc_{O_2} drop reflects a fall in the cardiac output.

Transcutaneous CO_2 Monitoring

With the development of the Stowe-Severinghaus CO_2 electrode, Ptc_{CO_2} monitoring was first used to measure the Pa_{CO_2} in neonates (20–22). It was originally hoped that the Ptc_{CO_2} would approximate the Pa_{CO_2}, but the Ptc_{CO_2} is consistently higher than the Pa_{CO_2} in neonates as well as adults. This situation is analogous to that in transcutaneous oxygen sensing, with the exception that oxygen is consumed by the tissues and the P_{O_2} gradient is from the capillary to the skin, whereas CO_2 is produced in the tissues and diffuses to the capillaries, where it is cleared. Thus we would expect the Ptc_{CO_2} to be higher than the venous P_{CO_2} and certainly higher than the Pa_{CO_2}. This is, in fact, just what is observed (12,13). Also, just as oxygen delivery to the skin is flow-dependent, CO_2 clearance from the skin is flow-dependent. The Ptc_{CO_2} is consistently correlated with the Pa_{CO_2} as long as the flow is constant, but when the flow decreases, the ratio of Ptc_{CO_2} to Pa_{CO_2} rises; conversely, an observed rise in this ratio indicates a decrease in the cardiac output.

Summary

Transcutaneous P_{O_2} and P_{CO_2} monitoring methods are useful in the noninvasive estimation of arterial blood gases when frequent arterial sampling would otherwise be necessary. Poor cutaneous perfusion, however, results in a divergence of the arterial and transcutaneous gas tensions. This effect makes transcutaneous monitoring a useful variable to assess the overall cardiorespiratory status of patients at risk for respiratory and circulatory failure. Such properties have important applications to the care of the surgical patient, including the titration of ventilatory and circulatory support systems, the assessment of the adequacy of resuscitation, and the on-line continuous monitoring of high-risk patients both inside and outside intensive care settings. This same property of assessing cutaneous perfusion allows transcutaneous monitoring to be applied to the evaluation of peripheral vascular disease.

Regional Transcutaneous Oximetry in Vascular Disease

The assessment of limb perfusion by transcutaneous oximetry is dependent upon the relationships which exist between the oxygen supply ($\dot{D}_{O_2}$), oxygen demand ($\dot{V}_{O_2}$), and oxygen tension (P_{O_2}) in the skin. Warming the skin is necessary to allow sensors on the skin surface to measure the P_{O_2} through the otherwise impervious stratum corneum. Such warming, however, causes significant artifactual changes in local oxygen transport. These include, on the one hand, local hyperemia (increased $\dot{D}_{O_2}$) and enhanced oxyhemoglobin dissociation, which raise the tissue P_{O_2}, and on the other hand, increased tissue $\dot{V}_{O_2}$, which tends to lower the tissue P_{O_2}. As long as the regional blood flow is adequate, the hyperemia and enhanced oxygen dissociation caused by the sensor predominate, and the local $\dot{D}_{O_2}$ is increased relative to the $\dot{V}_{O_2}$. Under these circumstances, the mean tissue P_{O_2} is close to the Pa_{O_2}. It is this mean tissue P_{O_2} which creates the gradient down which oxygen flows, across the stratum corneum, to the Ptc_{O_2} sensor, and, indeed, when the regional perfusion is adequate, the Ptc_{O_2} on the chest is about 80 percent of the Pa_{O_2} in adults. This situation is clearly distinct from that which exists under the nonheated sensors, such as conjunctival P_{O_2} electrodes or tissue fluid chambers, where the $\dot{D}_{O_2}$ and the $\dot{V}_{O_2}$ are unchanged and the mean tissue P_{O_2} assessed by the sensor tends to reflect end capillary or venular P_{O_2}.

When regional $\dot{D}_{O_2}$ decreases below critical values, the hyperemia achieved under the warmed sensor appears to be inadequate to maintain the close relationship between the Ptc_{O_2} and the Pa_{O_2}, and the Ptc_{O_2} falls away from the Pa_{O_2}. Decreases in systemic $\dot{D}_{O_2}$, whether caused by low cardiac output states or a decreased arterial oxygen content (Ca_{O_2}), result in proportional decreases in the systemic Ptc_{O_2} (Table 12-1). Such generalized Ptc_{O_2} decreases are seen with advancing age (16,17) and with cardiorespiratory diseases (Figure 12-4). Symmetrical peripheral Ptc_{O_2} decreases may occasionally result from peripheral vaso-

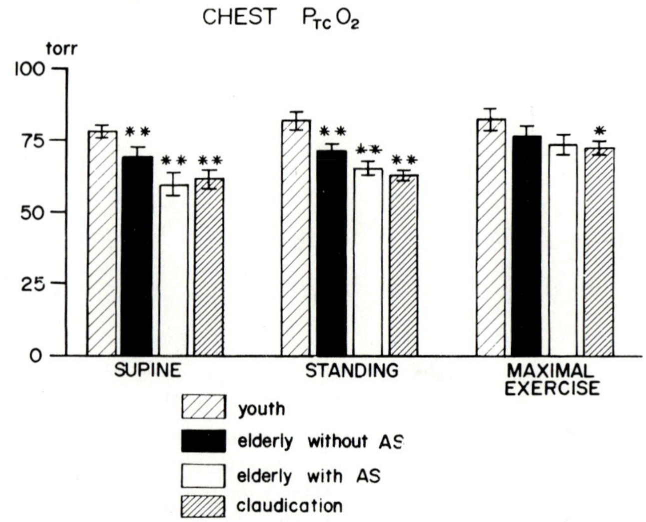

FIGURE 12.4 The chest Ptc_{O_2} in young volunteers, elderly volunteers with and without atherosclerosis AS, and patients with intermittent claudication. Age and cardiovascular disease decrease the resting chest Ptc_{O_2} significantly (*$P < 0.05$, **$P < 0.01$) by Student's *t*-test. Exercise increases the chest Ptc_{O_2} to near-normal levels unless limited by claudication. (From Hauser CJ, Shoemaker WC. Ann Surg 1983, 197:337–343.)

constriction in hemodynamically unstable subjects or in patients with vasospastic disorders. Except in these unusual circumstances, however, experience has shown that *a limb-chest Ptc_{O_2} ratio, or regional perfusion index (RPI), of significantly less than 1.0 (or 100 percent) always indicates localized tissue ischemia* (17,23).

Classification of Peripheral Vascular Disease by Transcutaneous Oximetry

The clinical signs and symptoms which define vascular insufficiency syndromes reflect the relative supply of and demand for oxygen in the limb. No ischemic symptoms are present when the oxygen supply is adequate under all conditions. When limb $\dot{D}_{O_2}$ is adequate in the resting state but exercise $\dot{V}_{O_2}$ cannot be met because of arterial obstruction, we expect exercise ischemia, i.e., claudication. Rest pain implies significant continuous ischemia. Ischemic "dry" gangrene occurs when the $\dot{D}_{O_2}$ is inadequate to support the basic oxidative requirements of the tissue. Before this end stage is reached, though, lesser degrees of ischemia compromise both tissue repair and the resistance to bacteria. Thus invasive infection frequently follows an otherwise minimal trauma, and "wet" gangrene, which is to say necrolizing infection, results. Because our understanding of the natural history of peripheral vascular disease (PVD) is predicated upon the conditions of oxygen supply and demand implied by the vascular insufficiency syndromes, accurate classification is the key to developing valid indications for therapeutic intervention. Unfortunately, the subjectivity of symptoms and the frequent coexistence of neurologic and orthopedic disease, can make accurate classification difficult on clinical grounds alone.

One of the primary purposes of noninvasive vascular testing is to assist in such classification. Transcutaneous oximetry would be expected to be of special value in this task since, alone among noninvasive modalities, it reflects precisely those oxygen supply-demand relationships which are the pathophysiological basis of the vascular insufficiency syndromes (23). In fact, the primary significance of transcutaneous oximetry in vascular surgery is that the Ptc_{O_2} (or, more exactly, the RPI) provides *a semiquantitative assessment of the adequacy of oxygenation in the area of the limb studied under the conditions prevailing during the study.*

Limb classification by Ptc_{O_2} should be based upon results from the most distal available sensor site, usually the dorsum of the foot, since the most distal location reveals the greatest extent of hypoxia. On this basis, limbs may be categorized into (1) normal limbs, which manifest no evidence of hypoxia under any physiological conditions, (2) limbs which manifest hypoxia all or nearly all the time, and (3) limbs which manifest hypoxia only under specified conditions. In the third group, significant limb hypoxia must be elicited by provocative testing, and the ease of difficulty of provoking RPI decreases is indicative of the extent of disease.

UNPROVOKED HYPOXIA

In control subjects without vascular disease limb Ptc_{O_2} is very close to the chest Ptc_{O_2}; the pedal RPI in this group is 91 ± 7 (SD) percent in the supine position. This control group comprised a mixture of youthful, as well as elderly and elderly smoking, subjects who were free of clinical peripheral vascular disease. In fact, though, some of those elderly controls may have had subclinical circulatory disease since the supine pedal RPI in 25- to 35-year-old controls is somewhat higher (16,17). Nonetheless, 98 percent of such unselected normal subjects have supine pedal RPI values greater than 75 percent. Values lower than 75 percent, therefore, indicate significant ischemia at rest (Table 12-2). This degree of supine ischemia is not necessarily enough to cause symptoms at rest, since the majority of limbs with a supine pedal RPI between 50 and 75 percent manifest only claudication. At the lower end of this RPI spectrum, however, patients who present with claudication, if closely questioned, usually describe some rest symptoms, such as night pain, numbness, or tingling. At supine pedal RPI values less than 50 percent, almost all patients who have sensation in the foot have rest pain. Supine pedal RPI values less than 25 percent are almost always associated with gangrenous skin changes, either with or without infection (23–25). The occasional patient with a very low pedal RPI who has escaped trivial injury and subsequent infection may present with a precadaveric "mummified" foot.

PROVOKED HYPOXIA

In limbs which have normal or near normal pedal RPI values in the supine position, definitive evidence of ischemia may be obtained either by increasing the limb $\dot{V}_{O_2}$ (by exercise) or decreasing the limb $\dot{D}_{O_2}$ by decreasing the arterial inflow. In either case, it is the *vascular reserve* of the limb which is tested, the principle being that in normal limbs the $\dot{D}_{O_2}$ remains matched to the $\dot{V}_{O_2}$ and the RPI remains relatively constant in spite of the challenge, whereas limbs with significant vascular disease cannot maintain compensation, and the RPI falls.

TABLE 12-2. Classification of Limb Perfusion Regional Transcutaneous Oximetry

Oximetry Class	Equivalent Clinical Class	Limb RPI Value, %			Perfusion
		Standing	Supine	Elevated 30°	
0	Normal	103 ± 14 (2 SD)	91 ± 15 (2 SD)	85 ± 14 (2 SD)	Adequate reserve
I	Minimal impairment	> 85	> 75	> 60	Reserve adequate under most conditions
II	Intermittent claudication	> 75	> 50	< 50	Adequate at rest; inadequate reserve
IIIA	Night pain	> 75	< 50	< 25	Inadequate supine; good dependent augmentation
IIIB	Rest pain	< 75	< 50	< 25	Poor dependent augmentation
IV	Impending gangrene	< 50	< 25	< 25	Inadequate for tissue survival

Exercise Oximetry

The diagnosis of claudication and the assessment of functional impairment which is actually due to exercise ischemia may occasionally present significant problems. Vascular, neurologic, and orthopedic disease often coexist, and vascular reconstruction is of little benefit to the patient whose exercise tolerance is otherwise limited. Thus, the finding by Doppler or angiographic criteria that a patient has significant vascular disease does not always predict that successful reconstruction will lead to symptomatic relief.

On the contrary, decreases in limb RPI during treadmill exercise are a specific correlate of ischemic claudication. In our experience, patients without arterial occlusion maintain a stable limb RPI under almost any workload (17). In contrast, patients with vascular disease demonstrate significant decreases in the limb RPI *at the same time as or shortly after* they develop symptoms (Figure 12-5). Exercise changes in the RPI are best measured at the thigh and calf, where, presumably, muscle ischemia leads to the diversion of the blood flow away from the skin. RPI decreases larger than 15 to 20 percent from the standing control value are highly significant, but the magnitude of the oximetry changes observed per se do not correlate well with the severity of disease. In fact, patients with rest pain who can walk demonstrate RPI decreases similar to those seen in claudicants, but need to walk considerably less distance to elicit them. This seems to occur because as they walk, most patients with PVD begin to have pain when the RPI falls below 75 percent, and they cease to walk very soon thereafter. The RPI only assesses the cutaneous ischemia, however, and under these circumstances, the muscle ischemia is probably much more profound. Thus the development of significant skin hypoxia and its temporal correlation with the onset of symptoms make the diagnosis of ischemic claudication certain. The degree of functional impairment is better correlated with the amount of work necessary to incur significant limb hypoxia.

Alone among noninvasive vascular tests, oximetry can be used *during* exercise. Also, however, as with Doppler testing, the rapidity of the reflow after exercise may be used as a measure of the vascular integrity (17). As PVD increases in severity, more time is required for the limb RPI to return toward normal levels. We have used the standing position to measure the half-life of RPI recovery (Figure 12-5), but allowing recovery in the supine position would be expected to lengthen the recovery time. This maneuver might make it easier to classify patients by the RPI recovery time but would also make the test more cumbersome.

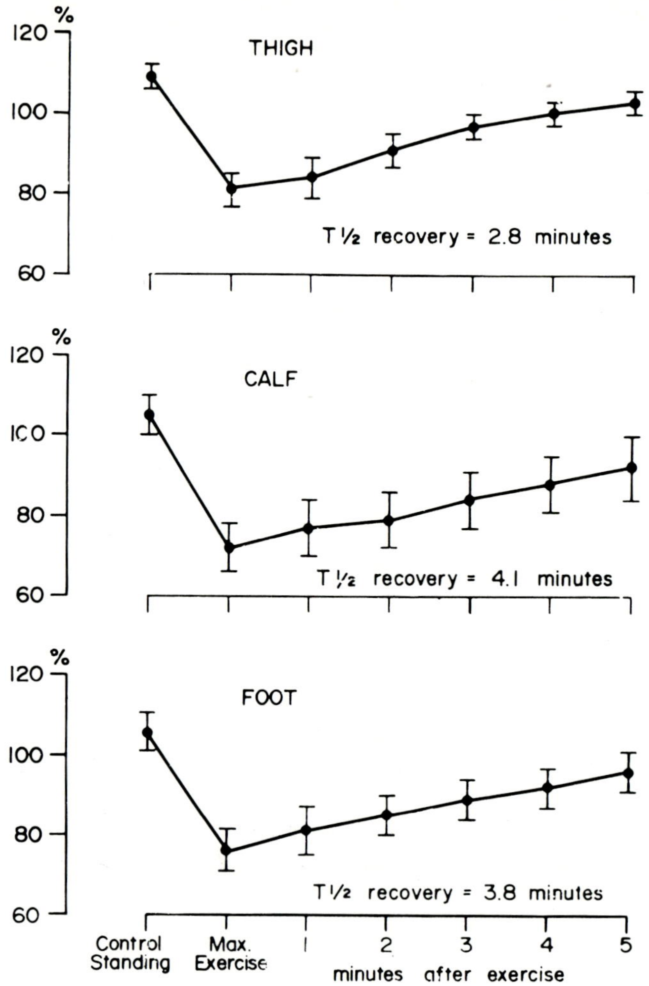

FIGURE 12-5. The effect of treadmill exercise on RPI in claudicant limbs. The $T_{1/2}$ recovery is the time required to recover half the RPI decrease caused by exercise. (From Hauser CJ, Shoemaker WC. Ann Surg 1983, 97:337–343.)

Positional Oximetry

Treadmill oximetry is a very sensitive test for PVD, but it is relatively cumbersome and by nature entails some discomfort to the patient. Electrocardiographic monitoring is necessary in patients with cardiac disease. Moreover, many patients with far-advanced PVD cannot walk well enough to use a treadmill.

We have found (23) that simple positional changes of the limbs in such patients yield distinctive Ptc_{O_2} and RPI variations. Positional oximetry works by varying the arterial inflow ($\dot{D}_{O_2}$) into the limb while the $\dot{V}_{O_2}$ remains fixed. The positions used are standing, supine, and supine with 30° limb elevation. In subjects free from vascular occlusions, the limb perfusion is relatively independent of the position. Such subjects show only small variations in the RPI with position changes (Table 12-2); this may reflect positional changes in capillary recruitment. Patients with arterial occlusions demonstrate marked positional variation in the limb Ptc_{O_2} and RPI.

POSITIONAL CHANGES IN CLAUDICATION

Claudicant limbs (Figure 12-6) demonstrate modest but significant decreases in the supine RPI, especially at the calf and foot, when compared with normal limbs. Standing (or sitting) raises the RPI values of claudicant limbs 20 to 25 percent, and normal values are achieved in this position. With 30° elevation, the pedal RPI in the claudicant limb falls to below 50 percent, whereas 98 percent of normal limbs show an RPI greater than 70 percent in this position.

Clearly, simple limb elevation distinguishes the claudicant limb, and the positional oximetry changes observed clearly reflect the characteristic pathophysiology of this class of patient. Decreased intraarterial pressure distal to obstructive lesions causes the limb $\dot{D}_{O_2}$ to be decreased at rest when the patient is supine; this decrease is enough to decrease the RPI modestly, but not

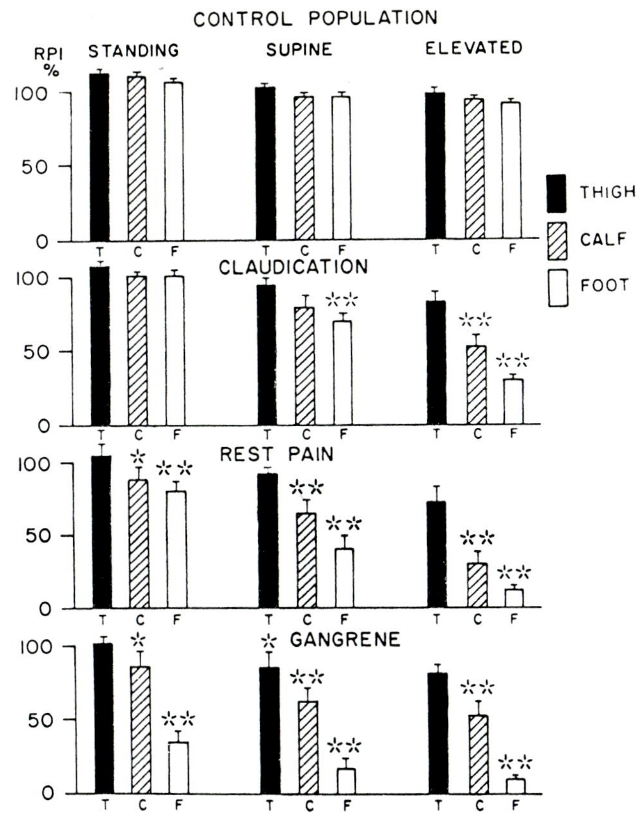

FIGURE 12-6. RPI values in the standing, supine, and leg elevated 30° positions in control patients and patients with claudication, rest pain, and gangrene. (From Hauser CJ, Appel P, Shoemaker WC. Surgery, in press.)

enough to cause symptoms. When the perfusion pressure is further decreased by limb elevation, gross oxygen supply-demand inequality occurs. The resultant RPI drop is especially obvious at the foot and calf sensor sites, where the elevation is greatest and the perfusion pressure is most decreased. Analogously, standing upright tends to increase the pressure and improve the flow distal to the obstructive sites, resulting in normalized $\dot{D}_{O_2}$ and RPI values.

POSITIONAL CHANGES IN REST PAIN

Limbs manifesting ischemic rest pain (Figure 12-6) have RPI values below 50 percent when the patient is supine. Limb elevation diminishes the RPI to 25 percent or below. Standing values, however, tend to segregate into two groups. Persons who have good dependent flow augmentation have standing RPI values in the 75 percent range, similar to the supine foot RPI in claudicants. These patients' pain is relieved upon standing, thus really putting them in a night pain rather than a continuous rest pain category. Limbs which fail to achieve a pedal RPI >50 percent on standing have little pain relief. This distinction has considerable practical importance, since limbs with continuous hypoxia are physiologically similar to limbs with gangrene and are therefore likely to be at risk for an early onset of complications.

POSITIONAL CHANGES IN LIMBS WITH GANGRENE

Limbs with ischemic gangrene are observed to have RPI values below 50 percent in all positions and usually below 25 percent when the patient is supine (Figure 12-6). Limb elevation causes little decrease since the RPI is already so low. Not all limbs having such poor pedal oxygenation have gangrene, but since the oxygenation is inadequate for tissue repair, all are at very high risk to develop gangrene subsequent to minor trauma unless reconstruction is achieved. Investigation of limbs which fit these criteria for potential revascularization should therefore proceed rapidly, since they are at continual risk for the development of complications, especially infections, which will further compromise the limb and the patient, and may potentially limit therapeutic options.

Transcutaneous Oximetry in Diabetes

Noninvasive vascular diagnosis presents a particular challenge in diabetes. The medial calcification which characterizes the large and medium-sized arteries of diabetics causes spurious elevations of limb blood pressure as measured by Doppler techniques. Also, decreased compliance of the vascular bed results in plethysmographic findings which may or may not coincide with limb ischemia. Lastly, cutaneous ischemia caused by arteriolar disease or the obliteration of capillaries is not detectable by any of these means.

Transcutaneous oximetry, by the direct assessment of skin hypoxia, avoids many of these pitfalls. In our experience (24,25), diabetic limbs show the same positional criteria for classification as nondiabetic limbs. In contrast, Doppler limb assessment in these patients has a very high false-negative test rate, because of artifactual hypertension. RPI measurement on the dorsal foot clearly demonstrates diagnostic accuracy superior to that of Doppler pressure measurements in diabetics. Also, we have not encountered any situations in which meaningful Ptc_{O_2} measurements cannot be made, whereas in many patients, Doppler pressures, pulse volumes, and reappearance times cannot be measured because of the presence of ulcers, or the absence or noncompressibility of foot and toe pulses (25).

We noted that a subset of diabetic patients with gangrene had RPI values which, though clearly hypoxic, were above 50 percent in the supine position. We feel that these values represent instances in which the primary event leading to tissue loss is invasive infection superimposed upon otherwise moderate ischemia. Because of the difficulty in retrospectively assessing the relative contributions of hypoxia and infection to the gangrene, all the patients were considered as one group for the purposes of those studies. The relationship, however, between the adequacy of pedal oxygenation and the nature of infection in the diabetic foot is currently being prospectively analyzed.

Oximetry and Arteriography

INDICATIONS FOR ARTERIOGRAPHY

Contrast angiography is usually regarded as the gold standard for the anatomic assessment of vascular disease. The importance of preoperative angiography in planning operative strategy is such that very few, if any, patients undergo reconstructive surgery without it. The primary importance of noninvasive studies is therefore to function as a triage step in which patients are selected for invasive angiographic study. Doppler blood pressure measurements, however, only serve to corroborate clinical indications for angiography and should not, in and of themselves, determine the need for arteriography. This is because limb blood pressure frequently does not parallel limb perfusion. Patients may therefore be denied an angiographic work-up on the basis of false-negative noninvasive tests, especially when the patients are primarily managed by clinicians unfamiliar with these problems. Conversely, experienced clinicians occasionally proceed to low-yield angiography despite normal noninvasive studies to rule out a correctable lesion. In either case, however, unnecessary morbidity may result.

Since regional oximetry directly assesses limb hypoxia, and limb hypoxia is almost always due to arterial occlusion, we feel that RPI measurements can markedly clarify the indications for angiography. Simply put, the demonstration of significant hypoxia (RPI <50 percent supine or <25 percent elevated) in any potentially salvageable limb indicates prompt arteriography. To date, all limbs studied on such oximetric indications have had positive angiograms.

In limbs with a supine foot RPI greater than 75 percent, pain or ulceration is not primarily due to hypoxia, and angiography is not usually warranted. Intermediate limbs (supine pedal RPI >50 percent but <75 percent) have significant hypoxia but not of such magnitude that it is immediately limb-threatening. Many patients in this group present with claudication. These patients should not undergo angiography unless intervention is clinically indicated because of functional impairment, or progressive deterioration of limb perfusion, as can be objectively assessed by treadmill oximetry (17). Angiography may be undertaken electively in this group.

FUNCTIONAL ASSESSMENT OF ANGIOGRAPHIC FINDINGS

Although angiograms are usually successful in localizing and describing arterial lesions, they are relatively poor at the assessment of the functional significance of the lesions. This is because angiograms yield only qualitative information about the flow restrictions imposed by axial vascular lesions and provide little information about the adequacy of collateralization. When a functional assessment of the lesions is important, transcutaneous oximetry appears to be of great use, providing the physiological correlates of anatomic arteriographic data (17,23–25).

In order to measure the oxygen-transport effects of anatomic lesions in specific areas of the leg, we have used a system of *segmental oximetry*, by which the limb can be mapped for the Ptc_{O_2}, and changes in the oxygenation can be correlated with specific vascular lesions. We have found that measurements performed at four peripheral sensor sites (the hip, the distal medial thigh, the proximal medial calf, and the dorsum of the foot) are adequate for the functional assessment of most angiographic lesions (26). The Ptc_{O_2} drop offs between the chest and the hip and thigh sites usually reflect severe aortoiliac disease, but diminution of the thigh Ptc_{O_2} may also occur secondary to high-grade disease in the thigh vessels without disease above the inguinal ligament. When the calf-thigh Ptc_{O_2} ratio falls, this reflects severe femoropopliteal disease; similarly, decreases in the foot-calf Ptc_{O_2} ratio reflect the severity of calf disease. The interpretation of multilevel disease must be undertaken cautiously, however, since proximal lesions may cause *progressive* decreases in the Ptc_{O_2} down the leg. This is especially true when limb elevation is used to elucidate marginal ischemia, since the effect of elevation on the limb Ptc_{O_2} is greatest distally. At our present level of experience, therefore, sequential Ptc_{O_2} drops can generally be used only to demonstrate the highest level of significant vascular obstruction. It is possible that with increasing experience, the magnitude of segmental Ptc_{O_2} decreases may be helpful in elucidating the relative metabolic significance of lesions in multilevel disease.

Assessment of Wound Healing

No single element is as vital to the process of wound healing as the adequate perfusion and oxygenation of healing tissues. Direct measurements of tissue oxygenation in the region of the wound might, therefore, be expected to provide information of vital importance in the prediction of wound healing. The accurate prediction of wound healing might lead to a more accurate selection of patients for conservative or nonconservative management, thus shortening hospitalization and decreasing morbidity and mortality. We have found that regional Ptc_{O_2} measurements are frequently of great help under such circumstances, but that the relationship between the Ptc_{O_2} and wound healing appears not to be entirely direct. If this is so, it is probably because the relationship of tissue oxygenation to tissue oxygen metabolism is not entirely direct.

The vast majority of oxygen delivered to most tissues is consumed by oxidative phosphorylation, thus producing adenosine triphosphate (ATP) for cellular metabolic requirements. However, the Michaelis constant (K_m) of cytochrome oxidase for molecular oxygen is much less than 1 torr, so the $\dot{D}_{O_2}$ and the mean tissue P_{O_2} must be markedly depressed before the $\dot{V}_{O_2}$ falls, marking the onset of anaerobic metabolism in the tissue regions most distant from perfusion. Certainly, wounds in tissues with minimal perfusion would not be expected to heal, since energy is unavailable even for much more basic tissue functions. Experience to date suggests that wounds in areas with very low Ptc_{O_2} (<25 torr) and RPI values (<50 percent) will not heal, whereas wounds on limbs with nearly normal perfusion and Ptc_{O_2} values will heal normally (14,16,25,27). The middle ground, however, is very wide and may reflect the status of other processes crucial to wound healing which are affected by the smaller variations in the tissue P_{O_2} produced by moderate decreases in the $\dot{D}_{O_2}$. These processes include collagen cross-linking and oxygen-dependent bacterial killing. The interreactions of such factors and, no doubt, many others, have made the assignment of firm Ptc_{O_2} cut-off values for wound healing in specific locations very difficult. Also, the circulatory status of the area in question may change over time, making it necessary to repeat Ptc_{O_2} measurements to obtain updated information on wound oxygenation. Studies continue, however, to try to assign confidence limits at specific locations to the healing of lesions at specific RPIs. At the present, the majority of the information we present should be considered anecdotal.

ULCER HEALING

Foot ulcers fall into three general categories. Vascular ulcers may be arterial or venous, or due to a combined disease. All arterial ulcers studied to date have occurred in hypoxic areas, with the surrounding skin demonstrating RPI values less than 50 percent (23–25). We have not seen such an ulcer heal spontaneously without vascular reconstruction which improved the RPI to >75 percent. Venous ulcers, in our small experience, have been somewhat hypoxic, but it is unclear at this time whether this represents coexisting arterial disease or the direct effects of venous hypertension upon the perfusion and oxygenation of the skin.

Neuropathic ulceration of the foot occurs most frequently in diabetics when a loss of protective sensation allows repetitive injury and tissue loss, with or without infection, to ensue. Coexistent ischemia frequently plays a permissive role in the development of neuropathic ulcers, but ischemia is, by definition, not a prerequisite. Irrespective of the original pathophysiology, however, in the presence of a significantly decreased Ptc_{O_2}, such neuropathic ulcers do not heal spontaneously. RPI values above 75 percent suggest that with adequate protection of the ulcer and control of infection, healing is possible. We are presently conducting prospective trials to ascertain the likelihood of healing at different Ptc_{O_2} levels.

The third group of ulcers we have studied occurs in the presence of skin diseases, most notably the vasculitides. Our experience with dermal vasculitis due to immunologic lesions, radiation therapy, and old thermal injury, and miscellaneous lesions such as heroin-induced vasculitis, has all been quite consistent; whatever the inciting event, ulceration only occurs in the presence of ischemia and hypoxia (27). This information has two important clinical correlates. First, skin grafts will not take on a hypoxic ulcer, and any attempt to excise and close the ulcer will be unsuccessful if the wound closure uses skin which is involved by the hypoxic process. A surgical closure of such defects will be successful only when accomplished with adequately perfused tissue. This sometimes will entail reconstruction with pedicle, myocutaneous, or vascularized free flaps. Second, when the underlying disease process is being treated pharmacologically, we would expect that the resolution of the hypoxia would be a marker for the therapeutic effect and a requisite for ulcer healing, just as it would be after revascularization.

AMPUTATION HEALING

The accurate prediction of amputation healing would enable the surgeon to choose a site where the conservation of tissue would be maximal while minimizing the chances of amputation failure. Early experience in this laboratory indicated that Ptc_{O_2} values above 40 torr on the calf suggest that perfusion is adequate to perform a below-knee amputation (14). Other investigators have suggested that a Ptc_{O_2} above 35 torr is adequate (16). It is likely, however, that a confident prediction of amputation healing at certain levels will not be possible on the basis of an isolated Ptc_{O_2} or RPI value at that level. Using preamputation RPI mapping of the calf, we have found significant variations in the perfusion of the skin of various quadrants of the calf. For example, pretibial skin generally has a lower RPI than the skin over the gastrocnemius muscles. At present, we are mapping the margins of a standard below-knee amputation incision (10 cm distal to the tibial tubercle anterior and bilaterally, and 20 cm distal posteriorly) and are prospectively assessing the relationship of the RPI in these areas to healing. Our preliminary impression is that in below-knee amputation, the posterior-flap RPI is more crucial than the RPI on pretibial skin. We do not have enough data at this time to assess other amputation sites.

Future Applications

The establishment of surface oximetry as a valid correlate of tissue perfusion opens the way to the noninvasive assessment of perfusion in a wide variety of situations. Specifically, oximetry can assess the vascular class and the need for reconstruction in peripheral vascular disease. Intraoperatively, this technique generates continuous data that quantify limb perfusion and thus immediately evaluate the functional adequacy of revascularization. In the postoperative period, oximetry can be used to monitor reconstructed limbs for early, potentially correctable, graft failure (28–30) without the discomfort and graft compression necessitated by cuff occlusion.

In such prolonged use of settings, it must be remembered that Ptc_{O_2} sensors can cause burns if left turned on in the same location for more than 4 to 6 hours. This is especially true when the limb perfusion is very poor and thus heat is poorly dissipated from the sensor site.

New evidence suggests that Ptc_{O_2} data may be of value in the diagnosis of arterial trauma. Clearly, when axial vessel obstruction occurs, the distal Ptc_{O_2} and RPI are markedly decreased, but evidence suggests that traumatized limbs with nonocclusive arterial injuries, such as lacerations or intimal flaps, show a decreased Ptc_{O_2} when compared with the contralateral limb (31,32). In contrast, limbs suffering penetrating trauma without arterial injury appear to show a slight *increase* in the Ptc_{O_2} relative to the contralateral limb. If the phenomenon is confirmed, it would seem that it must reflect differences in the local neural and humoral responses to injury, rather than anatomic factors. Care must be used in extending these findings to the setting of blunt trauma, where we have observed that venous obstruction or edema may lead to a marked depression of the distal Ptc_{O_2} in the presence of excellent arterial inflow.

The development of sterile nonheated electrodes will add a new dimension to surface oximetry, enabling the direct assessment of the metabolic status of ulcer bases, and transsected muscle bellies during amputation, and the intraoperative assessment of the perfusion of viscera such as the bowel. Thus in addition to its importance in noninvasive vascular diagnosis, surface oximetry promises to be an important investigational tool in vascular surgery, as well as in other disciplines, when the optimization of organ perfusion is a primary goal.

Key Points

1. Transcutaneous oximetry assesses the oxygenation of the skin. The relationship of the peripheral to the central Ptc_{O_2} (RPI) assesses relative local perfusion.

2. A progressive RPI diminution at rest reflects a progressive metabolic impairment of the area in question.

3. The provocation of an oxygen supply-demand imbalance may be used to create a functional categorization of vascular insufficiency syndromes.

4. Limbs demonstrating severe resting hypoxia require urgent investigation and, if possible, vascular reconstruction.

5. Healing is primarily P_{O_2}-dependent.

References

1. von Gerlack A: Über das Hautatmen. Arch Anat Physiol, Leipzig, 1851, 431–479.
2. Shaw LA, Messer AC, Weiss M: Cutaneous respiration in man. I: Factors affecting the rate of carbon dioxide elimination and oxygen absorption. Am J Physiol 1929, 90:107–118.
3. Baumberger JP, Goodfriend RB: Determination of arterial oxygen tension in man may be equilibration through intact skin. Fed Proc Am Soc Exp Biol 1951, 10:10–11.
4. Rooth G, Sjostedt S, Caligara F: Bloodless determination of arterial oxygen tension by polarography. Science Tools, LKW Instrument J 1957, 4:37.
5. Clark LC Jr: Monitor and control of blood tissue oxygen tensions. Trans Am Soc Artif Intern Organs 1956, 2:41–46.
6. Huch A, Huch R, Lubbers DW: Quantitative polarographische Sauerstoff-Druckmessung aut der Lopthaut des Neugeborenen. Arch Gynecol 207:443, 1969.
7. Huch A, Huch R, Meinzer K, et al: Eine schnelle, behizte Pt Oberflächen-Elektrode zur kontinuierlichen Überwachung des P_{O_2} beim Menschen. Elektrodenaufbau und Eigenschaften. Stuttgart, Proc Medizin-Technik, 1972, p 26.
8. Eberhard P, Hammacher K, Mindt W: *Perkutane Messung des Sauerstoff-Partialdruckes. Methodik und Anwendungen*. Stuttgart, Proc Medizin-Technik, 1972, p 26.
9. Eberhard P, Mindt W: Skin sensors for continuous oxygen monitoring of newborns. Biotelemetry 1977, 4:48–51.
10. Huch A, Huch A, Albani M, et al: Transcutaneous P_{O_2} monitoring in routine management of infants and children with cardiorespiratory problems. Pediatrics 1976, 57:681–687.
11. Horbor JD, Clark JT, Lucey JF: The newborn oxygram: Automated processing of transcutaneous oxygen data. Pediatrics 1980, 66:84–51.
12. Shoemaker WC, Vidyasagar D: Physiologic and clinical significance of Ptc_{O_2} and Ptc_{CO_2} measurements. Crit Care Med 1981, 9:689–690.
13. Nolan LS, Shoemaker WC: Transcutaneous O_2 and CO_2 monitoring of high risk surgical patients during the perioperative period. Crit Care Med 1982, 10:762–764.
14. White RA, Nolan L, Harley D, et al: Noninvasive evaluation of peripheral vascular disease using transcutaneous oxygen tension. Am J Surg 1982, 144:68–75.
15. Franzeck UK, Talke P, Bernstein EF, Golbranson FL, Fronek A: Transcutaneous P_{O_2} measurements in health and in peripheral arterial occlusive disease. Surgery 1982, 91:156–163.
16. Mustapha NM, Redhead RG, Jain SK, Wielogorski JWJ: Transcutaneous partial oxygen pressure assessment of the ischemic lower limb. Surg Gynecol Obstet 1983, 156:582–584.
17. Hauser CJ, Shoemaker WC: Use of a transcutaneous P_{O_2} regional perfusion index to quantify tissue perfusion in peripheral vascular disease. Ann Surg 1983, 197:337–343.
18. Tremper KK, Shoemaker WC: Transcutaneous oxygen monitoring of critically ill adults with and without low flow shock. Crit Care Med 1981, 9:706–709.
19. Tremper KK, Waxman K, Shoemaker WC: Effects of hypoxia and shock on transcutaneous P_{O_2} values in dogs. Crit Care Med 1979, 7:526–531.
20. Hansen TN, Tooley WH: Skin surface carbon dioxide in sick infants. Pediatrics 1979, 64:942–944.
21. Severinghaus JS, Stafford M, Bradley AF: Ptc_{CO_2} electrode design, calibration and temperature gradient problems. Acta Anaesth Scand 1978, 68:118–122.
22. Beran AV, Shigezawa GY, Yeung HN, Huxtable RF: An improved sensor and a method for transcutaneous CO_2 monitoring. Acta Anaesthesio Scand 1978, 68:118–121.
23. Hauser CJ, Appel P, Shoemaker WC: Pathophysiologic classification of peripheral vascular disease by positional changes in regional transcutaneous P_{O_2}. Surgery 1984, 95:689–693.
24. Hauser CJ, Klein SR, Mehringer CM, Appel P, Shoemaker WC: Assessment of perfusion in the diabetic foot by regional transcutaneous oximetry. Diabetes 1984, 33:527–532.
25. Hauser CJ, Klein SR, Mehringer CM, Appel P, Shoemaker WC: Superiority of regional transcutaneous oximetry in non-invasive vascular diagnosis in patients with diabetes. Arch Surg 1984, 119:690–695.
26. Hauser CJ, Mehringer CM, Appel P, Shoemaker WC: Diagnosis and assessment of aorto-iliac occlusion by segmental transcutaneous oximetry. Unpublished data.
27. Hauser CJ, Shoemaker WC: Estimation of the healing potential of ulcerating skin lesions by transcutaneous oximetry. Unpublished data.
28. Kram HB, Shoemaker WC: Use of transcutaneous oxygen monitoring in the intraoperative management of severe peripheral vascular disease. Crit Care Med 1983, 11:482–483.
29. Bratanow N, Klein SR, Hauser CJ, Kram HB, Wright JF, Appel P, Shoemaker WC, White RA: Transcutaneous oximetry: Continuous intraoperative multilevel assessment of limb perfusion in distal reconstruction. Arch Surg, in press.

30. Kram HB, Appel PL, White RA, Shoemaker WC: Assessment of peripheral vascular disease by postocclusive transcutaneous oxygen recovery time. J Vasc Surg 1984, 1:628–634.
31. Kram HB, Wright J, Shoemaker WC, Klein S: Perioperative transcutaneous O_2 monitoring in the management of major peripheral arterial trauma. J. Trauma 1984, 147:776–780.
32. Kram HB, Shoemaker WC: Diagnosis of major peripheral arterial trauma by transcutaneous monitoring. Am J Surg 1984, 147:628–634.

Chapter 13

ANGIOGRAPHY

VERITY S. GRINNELL, C. MARK MEHRINGER, and GRANT B. HIESHIMA

The history of angiography is short, with its centennial approaching. A very brief review of milestones begins with the discovery of x-rays in 1895 by Roentgen. Only a few months later contrast agents too toxic for human use were being injected into cadavers, severed limbs, and animals. The next major developments came in the late 1920s when percutaneous translumbar aortography and cerebral angiography were described by the Portuguese surgeons Dos Santos and Moniz, respectively. Contrast agents were now less toxic, and clinically useful angiography was a reality. In 1953 Seldinger described his technique for percutaneous vascular catheterization (1) which formed the basis of many catheterization techniques to follow. In the 1970s the development of less invasive diagnostic methods such as computed tomography and diagnostic ultrasound decreased the indications for angiography, but newer interventional techniques such as embolization therapy and angioplasty have taken up the slack.

Angiography remains the most important way to demonstrate vascular diseases graphically. Specific techniques such as angioplasty and digital subtraction angiography will be dealt with in other chapters. We hope to provide an overview of major areas of angiographic utilization. The basic techniques of arterial puncture and catheterization have been well described elsewhere (2–4).

Contrast Agents

The contrast agents most widely used for angiography in the United States are iodinated benzoic acid salts with diatrizoate or iothalamate as their cationic component and sodium and methylglucamine as their anionic component. In concentration ranges which allow satisfactory contrast, they are hypertonic and have some myocardial depressant effect. This must be taken into consideration in patients with heart failure. The agents are vasodilators and mild anticoagulants.

Arrythmias may occur when a contrast agent is injected into the heart or ascending aorta. This is more likely if the sodium concentration of the contrast agent is too high or too low. Contrast agents with methylglucamine and physiologic sodium levels should be employed in cardiac work (5). Pure methylglucamine salts, however, are better tolerated in the cerebral vascular bed (6). The agents are cleared by glomerular filtration with minor contributions to excretion by the liver and small bowel. A few patients, especially those with multiple myeloma or diabetes (7), may show impaired renal function after contrast agent administration. This is usually a self-limited state similar to acute tubular necrosis, but in some cases permanent renal impairment can occur. The contrast agent may cause sickling in patients with hemoglobin S. Limiting the contrast agent dose as much as possible and keeping the patient well hydrated are the best preventions.

Non-dose-related idiosyncratic or allergic reactions to a contrast agent are manifested by symptoms ranging from urticaria to bronchospasm and cardiovascular collapse. Previous episodes of nausea and vomiting or feelings of warmth during contrast agent administration are usually direct irritant effects and do not mean that the patient is allergic.

Pretesting for allergy is of no predictive value and should be abandoned (8). Patients with a history of previous reaction have approximately a 15 percent chance of having another reaction. This should be weighed against the benefit to be derived and premedication with steroids and anesthesia standby employed if the study is to be performed. The mortality rate related to contrast agent reaction in one large series of 300,000 patients was 1:75,000 (9). Newer, nonionic contrast agents coming on the market promise fewer toxic effects, but their acceptance is currently hampered by high cost.

Angiographic Catheters

Angiographic catheters are most commonly made of polyethylene, polyurethane, Teflon, or woven Dacron. Polyethylene is the most widely used. It can be formed in hot water or steam to a desired shape which it retains after cooling. Polyurethane has a similar characteristic. Teflon can hold higher injection pressures and therefore deliver higher flow rates but requires extreme heat to modify its shape. It is also stiffer than the other materials. The torque control of a catheter is a function of its stiffness, which in turn relates to size, wall thickness, and composition. Stiffer catheters are easier to use but can more easily dislodge plaques or injure the vessel wall. It has been said that the stiffness and size of catheters are inversely related to the skill of the angiographer. Of course, larger catheters may be necessary to deliver high rates of flow. Increasing emphasis on outpatient studies will speed the acceptance of smaller diameter catheters.

Thoracic Aortography

Percutaneous femoral puncture is the most widely used approach to the aorta and its branches. This technique is most comfortable for the patient, is associated with the lowest rate of puncture complications, and allows easiest manipulation of the catheter into the desired position including small aortic branches. Mani (10) cites a rate of 0.1 percent of damage to the femoral artery in a large series, and we have had only three complications serious enough to require surgery in approximately 3000 recent femoral punctures at the Harbor-UCLA Medical Center. Dissection of the intima or laceration of the whole arterial wall is the most common danger with resulting thrombosis, embolism, false aneurysm, or uncontrollable hemorrhage. This results from extraluminal placement of the needle, guide wire, or catheter and may be detected on test injections. An arteriovenous fistula may also develop if the vein is concomitantly punctured. The incidence of these complications clearly increases with the size of the catheter used (10) and is higher with the inexperienced angiographer. Thoracic aortography requires a large catheter, such as a no. 7 French outer diameter or larger, since a contrast agent flow approaching 40 mL/s of standard concentrations is usually needed to opacify this large vessel. Smaller catheters may be used if only branch selection is required, reducing the risk at the puncture site. Other very uncommon risks are infection at the puncture (none in Mani's series or ours) and breakage of the catheter or guide wire, necessitating surgical removal.

If the femoral artery is not available, we select the axillary artery, which is smaller and deeper and therefore carries a higher risk of local damage than a comparable femoral catheter placement (10,11). In addition, the musculature in the axilla makes postangiographic control by compression more difficult, and axillary hematoma may result in nerve damage to the brachial plexus. This may be avoided by careful postangiogram observation and urgent surgical evacuation of any significant hematoma. Because the brachial and radial arteries are even smaller, we do not use these routes, although aortic catheterization via cutdown on the brachial artery is popular among cardiologists (12). Damage to the brachial artery with this approach is not uncommon but usually insignificant clinically.

If neither axillary nor femoral sites are available, retrograde carotid puncture may be used. We have done repeated retrograde carotid punctures in a multiple amputee without difficulty and under local anesthesia with a no. 6 French catheter in a case where branch selection was mandatory. This is clearly an approach of last resort since damage at the puncture site would carry the risk of stroke which would not be present with other vessels.

In cases where a prosthetic graft is in place, puncture is accomplished easily by routine transfemoral technique, and in our experience, as long as the graft is mature enough to have a firm neointima, no complications have occurred. The safety of this procedure has been confirmed in some reports (13) and denied in others (14).

Risks other than those associated with the puncture are uncommon and include cerebral embolus and seizures from injection proximal to the brachiocephalic vessels and dissections from improper placement of the catheter, such as into a coronary artery orifice or injection recoil into a carotid. Arrhythmias, hypotension, and contrast agent–induced renal failure also occur. An exact incidence of complications from thoracic aortography is uncertain, but a recent large series of angiography complications, which include a high proportion of aortograms, cited a mortality rate of 0.032 percent and a complications rate of 1.7 to 3.3 percent, depending on the puncture site (11).

Aneurysms

The most common etiology of thoracic aneurysms is arteriosclerosis; 81.6 percent of aneurysms in DeBakey's surgical series of 500 descending aortic aneurysms were arteriosclerotic (15). These aneurysms are usually fusiform but may be saccular and even multiple. They may extend into the brachiocephalic vessels and into the abdominal aorta; they are frequently calcified. Other etiologies of thoracic aneurysms are syphilis, bacterial infection, trauma, and aneurysms associated with congenital malformations. Luetic and mycotic aneurysms are usually saccular and more commonly found in the ascending aorta; mycotic aneurysms rarely calcify (16). Since arteriosclerotic aneurysms may mimic these patterns, the precise etiology of the aneurysms is often not evident on aortogram. Aneurysms appear as mediastinal masses on plain chest x-rays and have a diagnostic appearance on computed tomography.

Traumatic false aneurysms are the second most common thoracic aneurysms and have a characteristic appearance (Figure 13-1). Although large autopsy series (17) show that only 45 percent of these aneurysms occur at the site of the ligamentum arteriosum, 95 percent of radiologically demonstrated aneurysms occur here. As many as 22 percent of aortic ruptures described on postmortem examination are in the ascending aorta, but there are only isolated reports (18) of aneurysms in this area diagnosed by angiography. This discrepancy is ascribed to the much higher mortality rate of aortic root ruptures from associated cardiac injury and hemorrhage into the pericardium causing tamponade, whereas 15 to 20 percent of isthmus injuries survive hours to days to allow diagnosis (17).

Plain chest x-ray findings suggesting the diagnosis of aortic rupture include widened mediastinum, present in the majority of

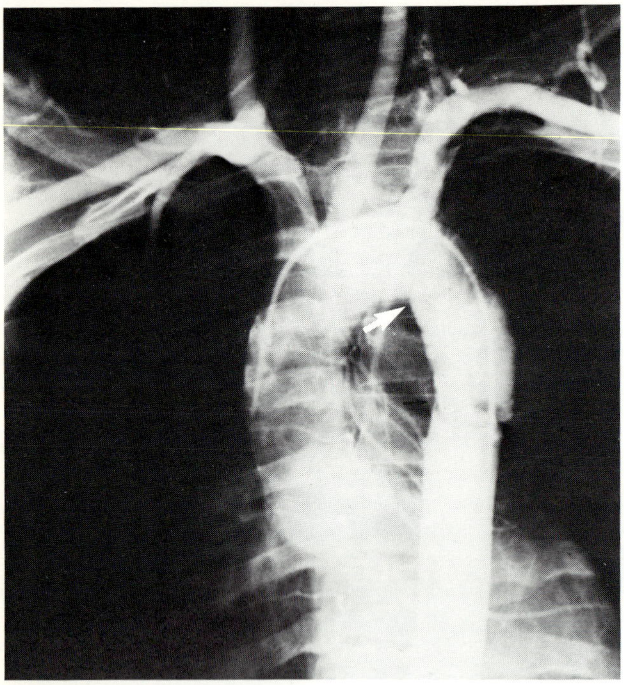

FIGURE 13-1. Traumatic aortic rupture demonstrated on arch aortogram. Irregularity and/or a step-off in the contrast column indicates transection with false aneurysm formation at the level between the two arrows.

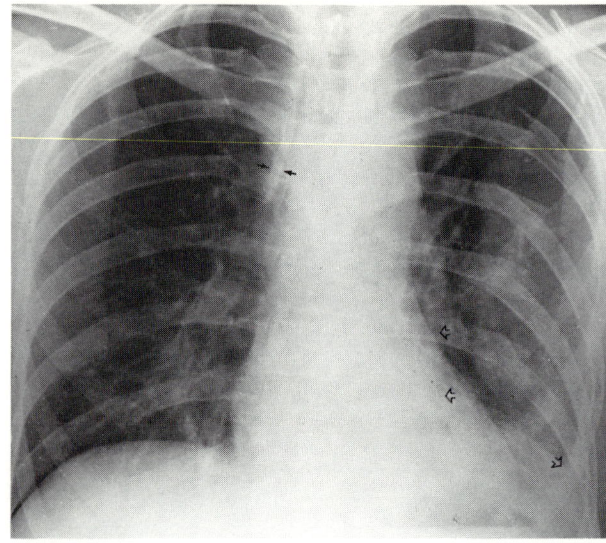

FIGURE 13-2. Chest x-ray showing signs of major vessel injury. The trachea is displaced to the right; the aortic knob is enlarged; there is left pleural fluid (*open arrows*). The right paratracheal stripe is wider than the normal 5 mm (*black arrows*). Multiple rib fractures are also seen.

cases of aortic rupture (also 25 percent of other matched patients and therefore nonspecific) (19); depression of the left main stem bronchus; tracheal and nasogastric tube deviation to the right; pleural fluid; and obliteration of the normal contour of the aortic knob. A widening of the right paratracheal stripe that exceeds 5 mm (Figure 13-2) has recently been reported as a reliable sign of mediastinal hematoma (20). Some have advocated routine aortography in patients with fractures of the first rib because of the presumed correlation with a high incidence of aortic and brachiocephalic artery injuries (21). Recent series (22,23), however, have demonstrated a low correlation of rib fractures and vascular injuries, which concurs with our experience (24).

Dissecting Aneurysm

Aortic dissections arise in the thorax unless they are induced by abdominal surgery or trauma. The chest x-ray, along with the typical history of chest pain and findings of pulse deficits, provides important diagnostic information. Progressive mediastinal widening and haziness or a knobby appearance of the aortic arch or descending aorta are suggestive of dissection. A more specific sign is separation of a calcified intimal plaque from the outer wall of the aorta by 6 mm or more. However, this sign is present in a minority of cases and if present may not be diagnostic; separation of up to 10 mm in arteriosclerosis without dissection has been seen (25).

In patients with suspected dissection we approach the aortogram from the femoral route because we have found that false lumen entry is just as likely from the axilla. A guide wire with a very flexible tip is carefully advanced before the catheter, and small test injections are used to avoid high-pressure injections into the false lumen. In this way we have been able to demonstrate both true and false lumens without extending the dissection (Figure 13-3).

Signs of dissection on aortogram include narrowing and distortion of the intraluminal contrast agent along with a section of unopacified lumen that may be seen as a linear soft tissue density paralleling the contrast column (Figure 13-4), nonfilling of aortic branches, and associated aortic insufficiency. In other cases, the true and false lumens may both fill and empty at slightly different times. If the tear is widely patent and the lumens fill and empty simultaneously, the wall between them may be seen as a thin, linear filling defect in the contrast agent (Figure 13-3). This may be difficult to demonstrate because not only does this dissected wall assume a spiral configuration but also it may flap quite violently with the heartbeat and appear and disappear on sequential films.

Dissections arising at the aortic root and extending into the descending aorta (DeBakey type I) or limited to the ascending aorta (DeBakey type II) are considered most common (26). In our experience and that of Earnest (27), type III have been more frequent; that is, the tear arises near the left subclavian and dissects distally and often proximally as well. Whenever possible, the angiography should demonstrate the site of the tear by sequential visualization of filling of the uncatheterized lumen (Figure 13-3); however, the filling may be too fast to see this or there may be reentry tears at multiple sites. Abrams has been able to demonstrate the site in only 50 percent of cases (28).

High-resolution computerized tomography (CT) is a valuable

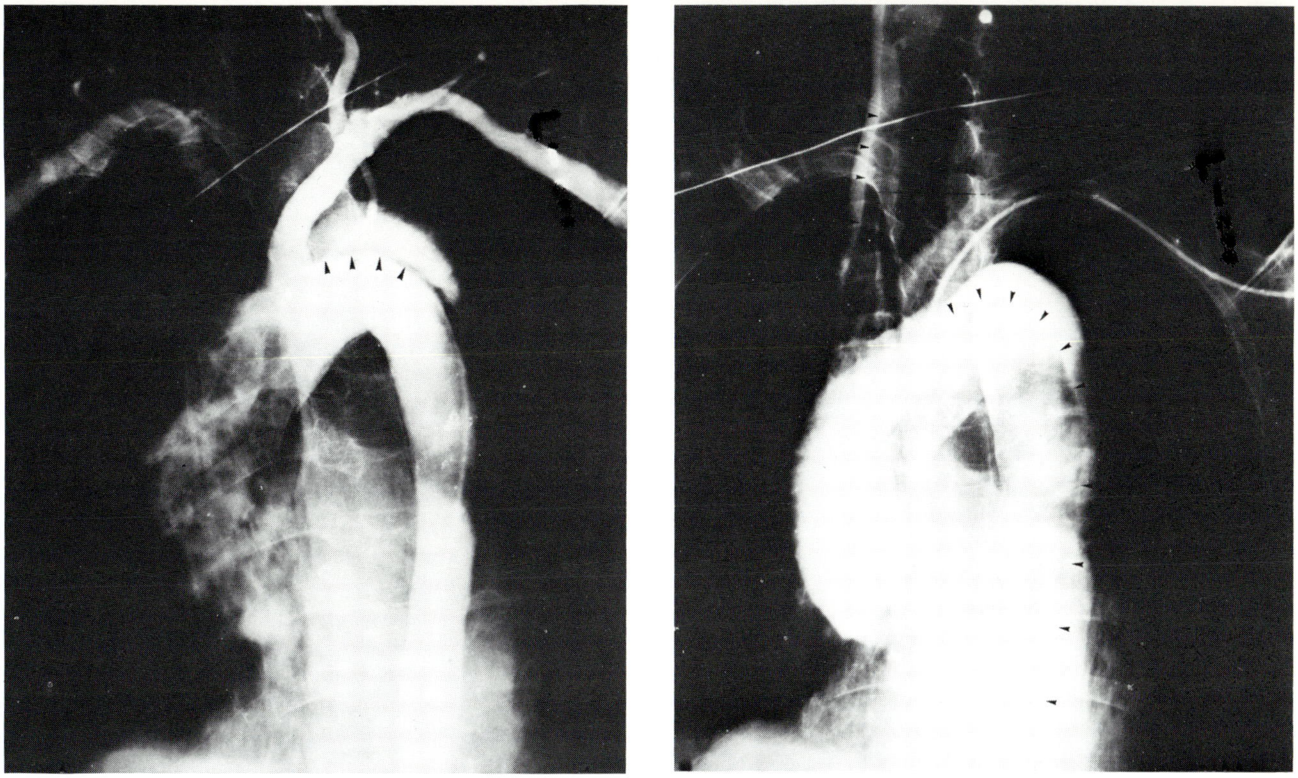

A B

FIGURE 13-3. (*A*) Type-3 dissection with retrograde extension demonstrated by transfemoral aortogram. The catheter is in the true lumen, which fills the left subclavian. Early filling of the false lumen at site of tear is indicated by arrowheads. (*B*) The false lumen is demonstrated via left subclavian; true lumen appears as a filling defect (*arrowheads*).

tool for diagnosis of dissection. Although the exact anatomy of the tears or extension into small branches still necessitates angiography, CT is accurate in ruling out the diagnosis if questionable and in follow-up of old dissections, particularly after surgery where persistence of the false lumen is often seen (29).

Occlusive disease of the aorta and brachiocephalic vessels, such as arteriosclerosis (Figure 13-5), arteritis, and congenital coarctation (Figure 13-6), is a common indication for arch aortography. Arteriosclerotic plaques of the carotid bifurcation are best demonstrated by selective injection; aortography of the upper thorax demonstrates proximal stenoses and any areas of collateral or retrograde flow. The most common example of the latter is filling of the distal portion of an occluded subclavian artery by retrograde flow down the vertebral artery, so-called subclavian steal (Figure 13-7). Retrograde filling of the right carotid may similarly fill an occluded right subclavian artery.

Takayasu's arteritis occurs in females who typically have pulse deficits and is visualized as long or short segments of smooth stenosis in the aorta itself or any of its branches. Atypically it may cause aneurysms, usually in old people, and in advanced cases superimposed arteriosclerosis may mask the diagnosis of arteritis. Most other types of arteritis cause dilatation and irregularity of the aorta and do not have a diagnostic radiologic picture. Examples include giant-cell arteritis, which may also cause stenosis, and arteritis associated with syphilis, rheumatic fever, rheumatoid arthritis, ankylosing spondylitis, and Reiter's syndrome (30).

Congenital coarctation appears in one of three patterns: (1) a short segment stenosis in the high thoracic aorta not far from the origin of the left subclavian artery (Figure 13-6), which is most common; (2) distal thoracic segmental narrowing, which is probably a form of Takayasu's arteritis (21); and (3) complete interruption of the aortic arch (Figure 13-8) or hypoplasia over a long segment involving the brachiocephalic origins.

Pulmonary Angiography

The two most common approaches to the pulmonary artery are percutaneous femoral or brachial vein puncture using the Seldinger technique similar to that used in an artery. Because the right heart and pulmonary arteries are relatively thin walled and delicate compared to major systemic arteries, the catheters generally in use have either a pigtail shape or a round, smooth end with no end hole to reduce the risk of cardiac or vessel puncture. Multiple side holes help to prevent recoil on injection and further protect against puncture or injection at intended sites. The catheters must be large, nos. 7 or 8 French, to allow an injection

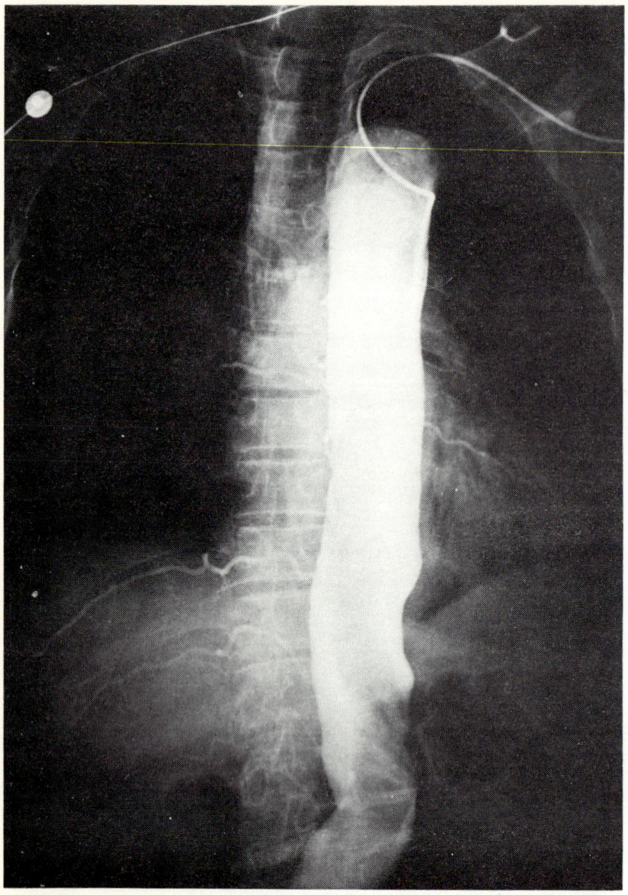

FIGURE 13-4. Aortic dissection: A descending aortogram via the left subclavian opacifies the false lumen. The true lumen appears as a filling defect.

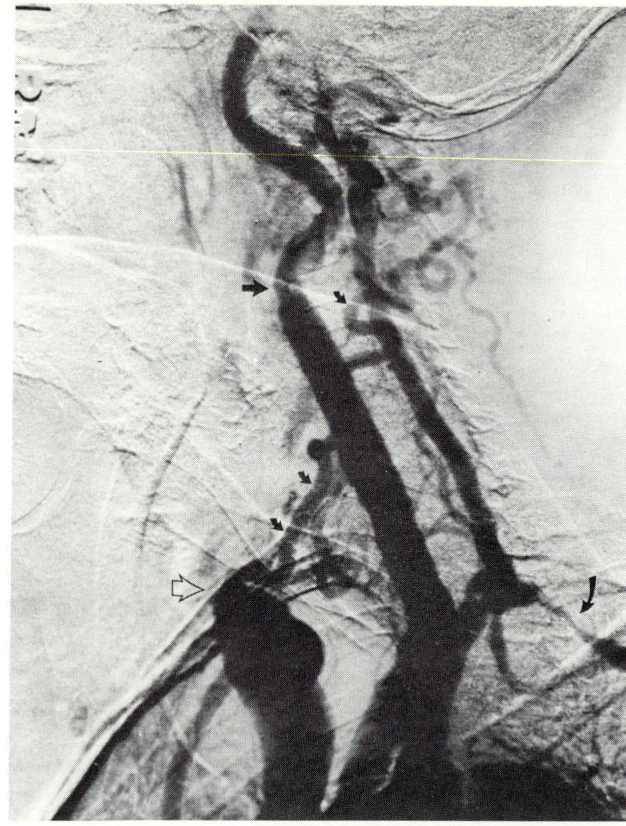

FIGURE 13-5. Severe arteriosclerotic occlusive disease in an asymptomatic patient. The right innominate artery is occluded (*open arrow*) so the carotid and vertebral do not fill, but a large muscular collateral arises off the innominate stump (*small curved arrow*). The left carotid has a stenosis at its bifurcation (*straight arrow*) and the left subclavian is almost completely occluded (*large curved arrow*).

rate of 30 to 40 mL/s, which is necessary to opacify the entire pulmonary vasculature. A preformed pigtail catheter designed to pass easily through the heart and select the pulmonary artery and major branches is our choice (31). The usual alternative is a straighter catheter with a closed end, "the NIH catheter," which is looped in the right atrium to get through the tricuspid valve and requires a tip deflector for subselective injections.

Two major risks complicate pulmonary arteriography. The first is arrhythmia induced by passage of the catheter through the tricuspid valve. Close monitoring of the electrocardiogram is therefore mandatory. Fortunately arrhythmias usually resolve when the catheter is withdrawn into the right atrium. In Mills's series of 1350 pulmonary arteriograms (32) 11 serious arrhythmias and 5 cardiac arrests occurred. Thus, defibrillation apparatus and antiarrhythmic drugs should be readily available. The second danger is that of acute right heart failure from contrast agent injection in patients with preexisting pulmonary hypertension. Pulmonary artery pressures must therefore be obtained through the catheter before contrast agent injection. In Mills's report all three patients who died had pulmonary artery pressures of 75/28 mmHg or above. A right ventricular diastolic pressure of 20 or above should be considered a danger sign. Our guidelines are that a systolic pulmonary artery pressure above 60 mmHg is a contraindication to continuing the study. If the pressure is between 40 and 60 mmHg, we proceed carefully with

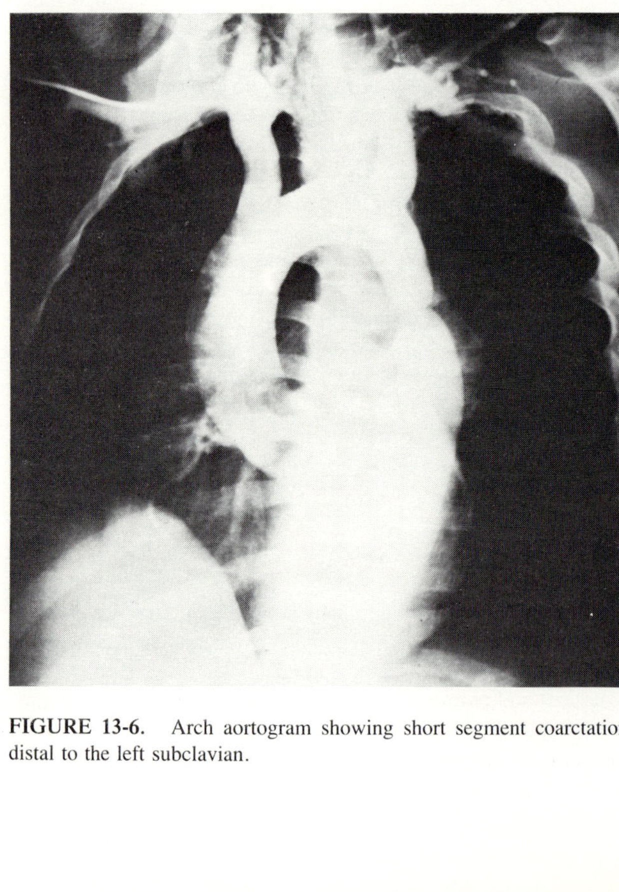

FIGURE 13-6. Arch aortogram showing short segment coarctation distal to the left subclavian.

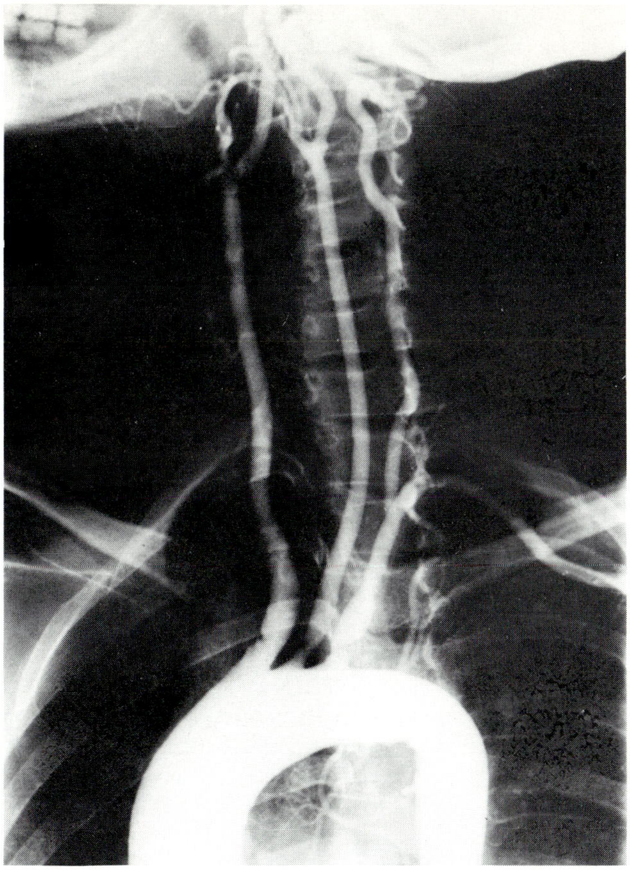

A

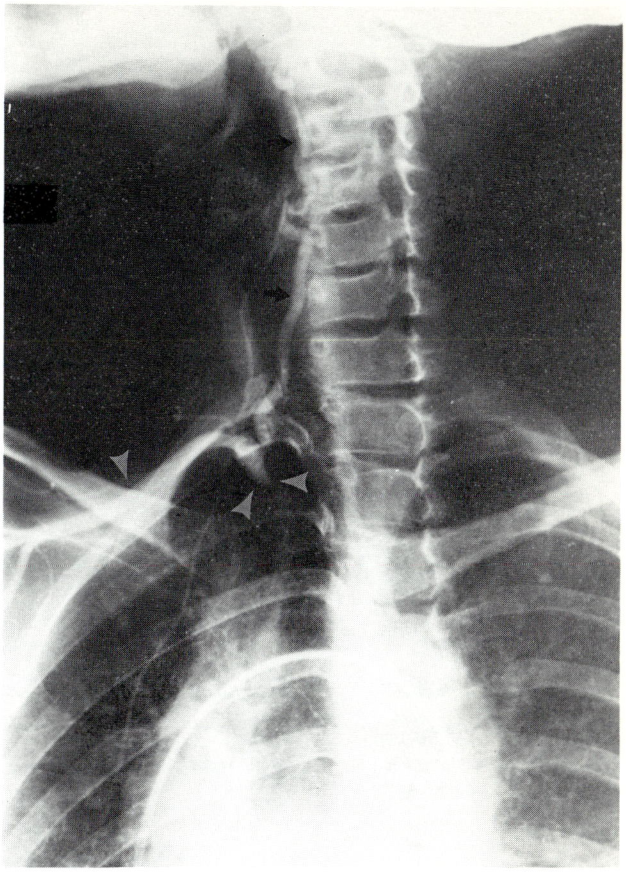

B

FIGURE 13-7. (*A*) Arch aortogram showing nonfilling of the right subclavian and right vertebral arteries, as well as stenoses at the origins of all the other brachiocephalic vessels. (*B*) Delayed film shows retrograde filling of the right vertebral (*arrows*) which fills the subclavian (*arrowheads*) ''subclavian steal''.

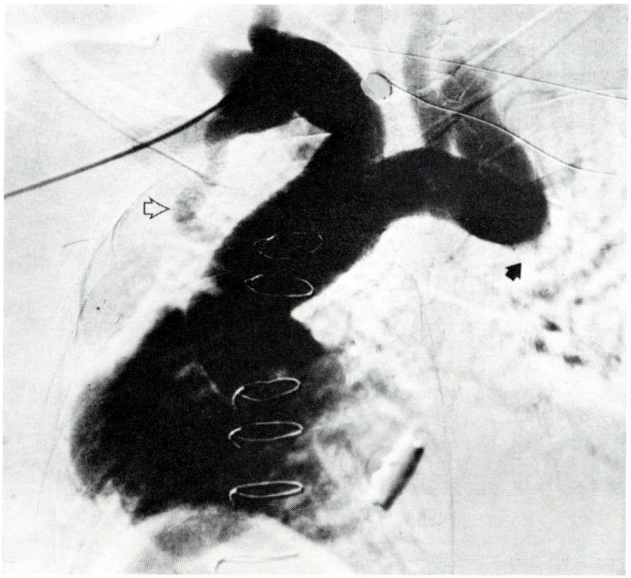

FIGURE 13-8. Arch aortogram showing complete interruption of the aorta (*black arrow*) just distal to the left subclavian. All the brachiocephalic branches are massively dilated to provide collaterals; an enlarged internal mammary artery on the right is seen (*open arrow*). The patient has a prosthetic aortic valve, and postoperative leakage into the right atrium is also demonstrated.

subselective injections in the areas of highest suspicion for pathology, continuing if the first injections are well tolerated.

Cardiac perforation has been reported as a complication (23) of pulmonary angiography, usually in association with whipping or recoil of the catheter during the injection or overly forceful handling of the wire or catheter. Perforation has not been reported with the pulmonary pigtail modification. Perforation or subintimal injection was noted by Mills in 14 patients, but none of these patients had any serious sequelae. It is wise to bear in mind the theoretical danger of dislodging and advancing emboli either from the cava or right atrium while advancing the catheter or from the proximal pulmonary arteries during injection. We minimize this risk by gentle catheter advancement with frequent test injections.

A balloon-tipped, flow-directed pulmonary catheter that may be used at the bedside and advanced into pulmonary branches is also available (33). Emboli could theoretically be visualized with portable filming in a patient too unstable to move. In practice, however, the rate limitations of contrast agent injection imposed by a double-lumen catheter have resulted in flow defects and sampling errors leading to a high incidence of false positives (33).

The most common indication for pulmonary arteriography is documentation of pulmonary emboli. A negative isotope perfusion defect in areas that are well ventilated by inhalation isotope scan is strong evidence for emboli and sufficient indication

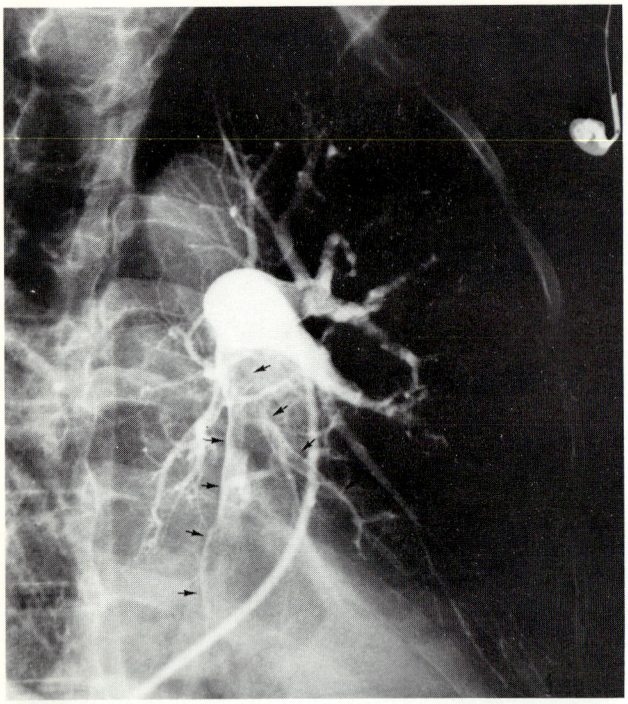

FIGURE 13-9. Left pulmonary arteriogram showing branching filling defect along multiple lower lobe segmental arteries (*arrows*) indicating a large pulmonary embolus.

for anticoagulation. If, however, the defects are matched on perfusion and ventilation scans, then scanning does not help and the definitive study is arteriography. Undue delay may result in missing the diagnosis because lysis of clots has been documented in 2 days, although most persist longer (34). The diagnosis is made by the demonstration of an intraluminal filling defect in one of the pulmonary arteries (Figure 13-9). Amputated vessels and avascular areas may be seen, but these also occur in pneumonia, emphysematous bullae, tumors, and other conditions. Often selective injections into second- or third-order pulmonary arteries with magnification or oblique projections is necessary to distinguish emboli from these other types of occlusions.

Congenital or acquired arteriovenous fistulas (Figures 13-10 and 13-11) are an indication for pulmonary arteriography. Any associated false aneurysms should be identified since these may rupture. The lobe containing the fistula may be resected, or the fistulas may be closed by detachable balloon embolization (35). Small fistulas may be closed by a balloon alone, but balloon closure of a fistula over 6 to 8 mm in diameter incurs the high risk of balloon passage into the systemic arteries. The "spider" or Amplatz vascular occluding device is used to anchor the balloons in fistulas of up to 11 mm (Figure 13-10).

Other anomalies of the pulmonary vasculature that may be demonstrated on angiogram include pulmonary artery atresia, aneurysm or venous varix, or anomalous pulmonary drainage. Displacement and encasement of pulmonary arteries may be caused by a tumor, but tumor vascularity of both primary and metastatic lung cancers is supplied by systemic vessels (36).

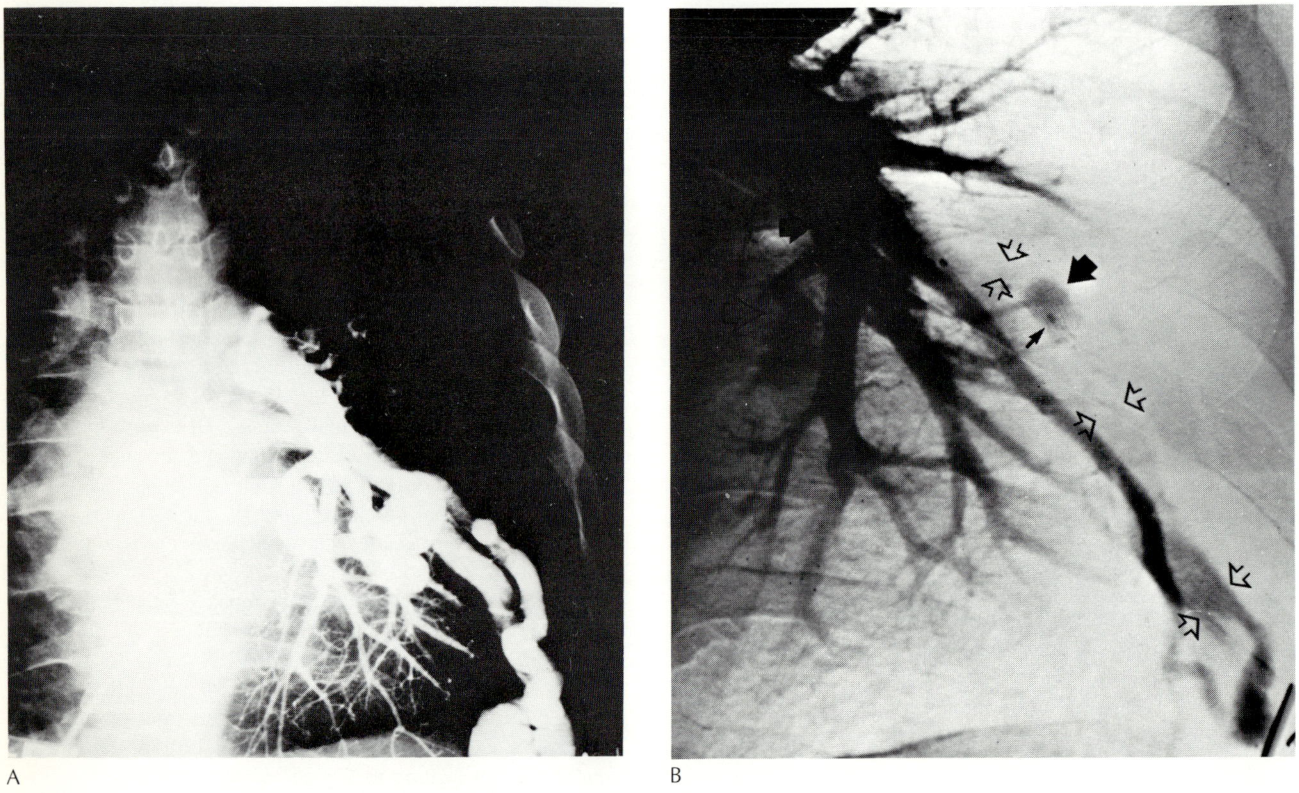

FIGURE 13-10. (*A*) Multiple AV fistulas in the left lower lobe associated with large venous varices shown by left pulmonary arteriogram. (*B*) Postembolization arteriogram. Two detachable balloons were placed at the sites of the large arrows. The most lateral feeding vessel (*open arrows*) has now thrombosed. Slow filling of the most medial varix persists. The balloons were anchored by "spiders" (Amplatz Vascular Obstructing Device, Cook, Inc.) to prevent migration through the fistulas.

Mesenteric Venography

The portal vein and its tributaries are usually well visualized 8 to 12 seconds after selective injection of either the celiac or the superior mesenteric artery. An injection of 50 mL over 6 to 7 seconds is our routine dose, but we have safely used injections of up to 100 mL in large arteries to increase the venous contrast; this is particularly useful in cases of gross splenomegaly for dense opacification of the splenic vein. Venous contrast can be further enhanced by injecting 25 to 50 mg of tolazoline (Priscoline) through the catheter immediately prior to the contrast injection. We have rarely found it necessary to inject the mesenteric veins directly, but this may be done by three approaches.

SPLENOPORTOGRAPHY

Mesenteric venography may be approached directly for selected indications. Splenoportography is the oldest direct technique. During inspiration the spleen is punctured with a long needle surrounded by a closely fitting Teflon sheath. The needle is withdrawn, and the contrast agent is injected into the splenic pulp through the sheath. Portal venous pressure may be accurately measured through this catheter. The splenic and portal veins are more densely opacified by this method than by the arterial route, as are systemic collaterals including esophageal varices. In cases of very high portal hypertension, however, the splenic vein fills in a retrograde manner, emptying into these collaterals; therefore, in this instance visualization of the portal system will not occur from a splenic injection. The main complication of splenoportography is bleeding at the puncture site, and the study is therefore contraindicated in patients with impaired clotting and relatively contraindicated in patients with ascites, both common occurrences in patients with portal hypertension secondary to cirrhosis.

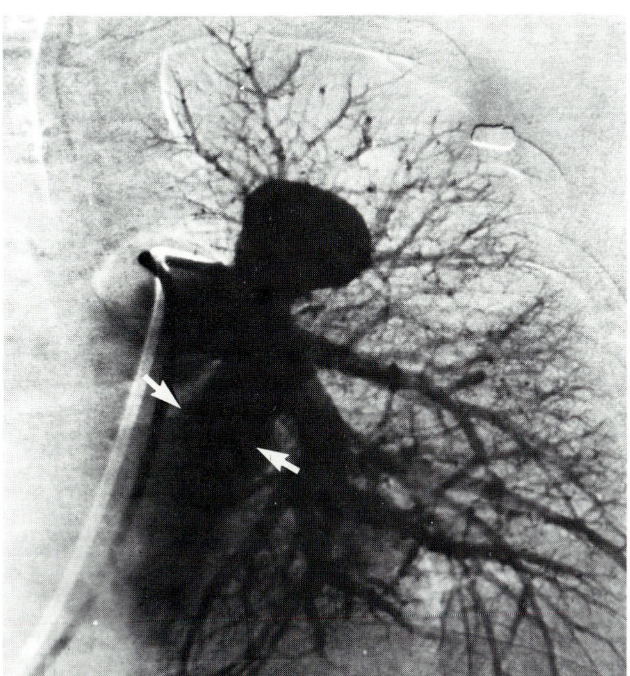

FIGURE 13-11. Subtraction left pulmonary arteriogram showing post-traumatic false aneurysm at site of a gunshot wound a year before. Contrast jet into left atrium (*arrows*) indicates an AV fistula is also present.

TRANSHEPATIC PUNCTURE

The most commonly used direct approach at present is the transhepatic puncture, which is performed with a Chiba needle and sheath inserted in the right midaxillary line. The needle's stylet is then removed and the needle and sheath slowly withdrawn until blood is aspirated. If a test injection of contrast agent demonstrates portal vein filling, the needle is removed and a guide wire advanced into the portal lumen. The sheath may then be advanced over the wire or may be exchanged for any other suitable catheter allowing selective injection of the portal tributaries. Excellent opacification may be obtained; variceal embolization may also be performed (which is not possible via splenic puncture) (Figure 13-12). Complications of transhepatic puncture include hemorrhage and puncture of adjacent organs. The complication rate in most series is low. Impaired clotting and ascites are again contraindications. In Widrich's series of 89 transhepatics only 2 serious complications occurred, even though the gut was punctured in 4 patients and the bile ducts in 30 (37).

Transhepatic variceal embolization, described by Lunderquist in 1974, has been effective in controlling life-threatening bleeding in the short term (38). The incidence of rebleeding, however, is high (39). Multiple sorts of emboli have been utilized including Gelfoam, Ivalon, sclerosing agents, balloons, coils, and cyanoacrylate. Cyanoacrylate embolization results in a high incidence of portal vein thrombosis; in a series of 43 patients embolized by the group that originated the procedure, 13 rebled and there were 7 deaths attributed to the embolization procedure (40). Other complications of embolization reported in other series are aberrant emboli, both pulmonary and systemic. The systemic emboli arise from spontaneous portal-to-pulmonary-vein shunts, which have been well demonstrated pathologically but only twice in living patients (41,42).

UMBILICAL VEIN CUTDOWN

Umbilical vein catheterization by surgical cutdown is the third direct approach and allows embolization. Portal cannulation was described in 1959 (43) in children; high rates of unsuccessful cannulation have occurred until recently, when Spigos (44) reported successful cannulation and embolization in seven of seven patients through a small midline incision. Few other reports have appeared, but the approach seems promising.

Indications for mesenteric venography include most cases of portal hypertension being considered for surgical or embolic therapy. As well as giving the surgeon a "road map" of the veins available and their calibers, it will demonstrate the venous dynamics; hepatofugal flow in advanced cirrhoses is shown by retrograde flow down a portal tributary from an organ whose artery was not injected, i.e., superior mesenteric or inferior mesenteric vein filling on a celiac injection, or splenic or inferior mesenteric vein filling from the superior mesenteric arteriogram

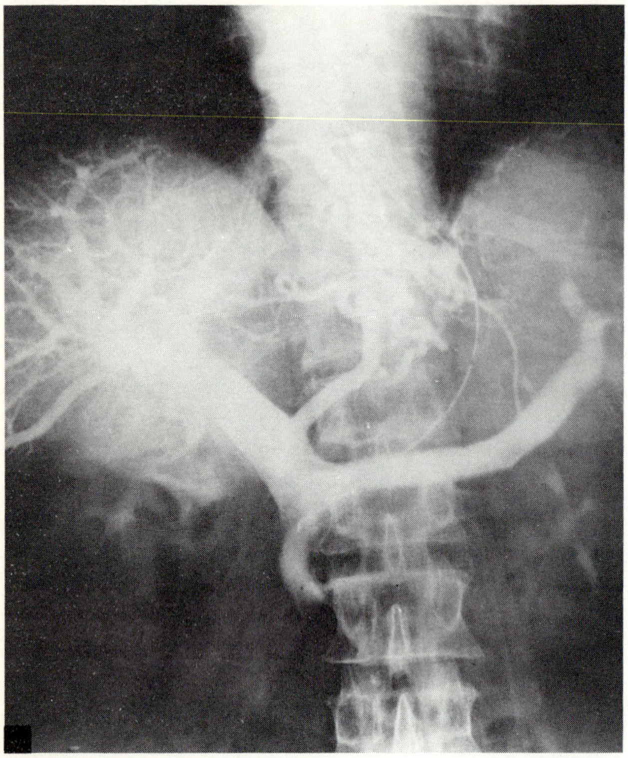

A

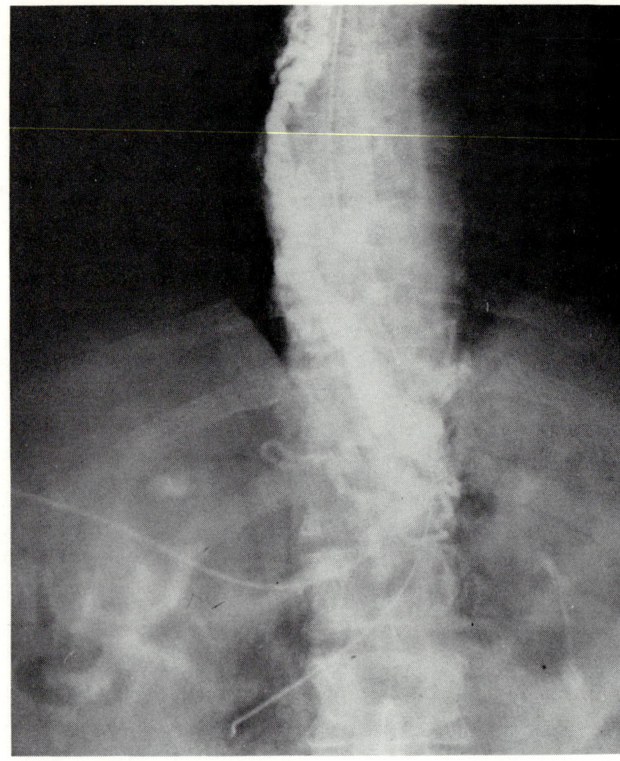

B

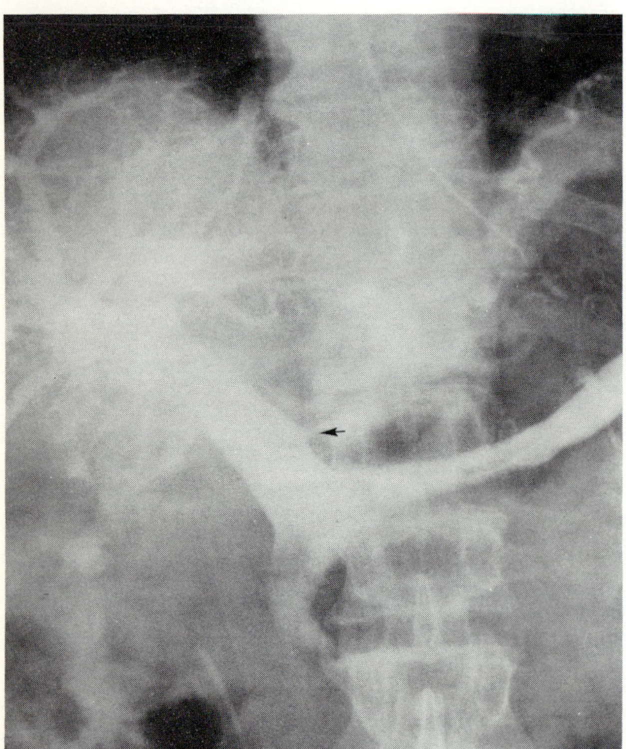

C

FIGURE 13-12. (*A*) transhepatic portogram showing large esophageal varices. (*B*) Selective catheterization of the coronary vein for variceal embolization. (*C*) Postembolization portogram showing occluded coronary vein (*arrow*). Courtesy of Dr. Robert Conroy, Long Beach Veterans Administration Hospital.

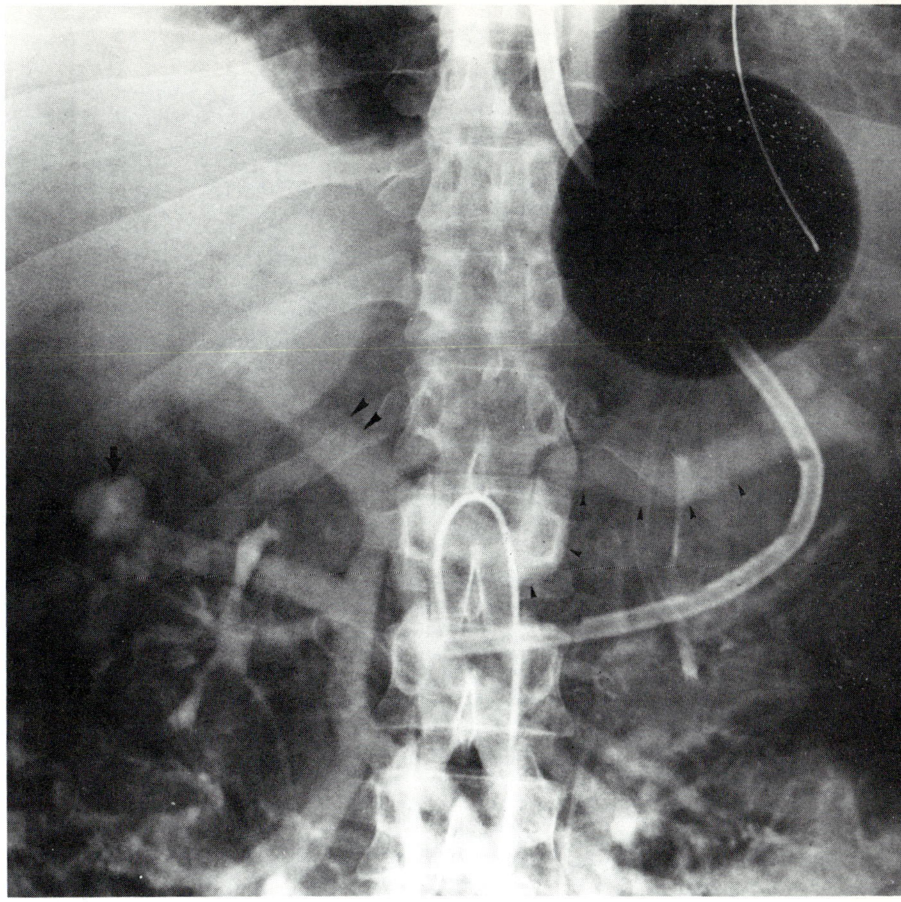

FIGURE 13-13. Hepatofugal flow demonstrated on venous phase of superior mesenteric arteriogram. Splenic vein fills retrograde (*small arrowheads*). Right colonic vein fills colonic varix (*arrows*). Portal vein (*large arrowheads*) does not fill hepatic branches.

(Figure 13-13). Also varices at unsuspected sites such as the ileum (Figure 13-14) or colon (Figure 13-15) will be seen; these may be sites of gastrointestinal bleeding not visible on barium studies. Portal vein thrombosis, sometimes an unsuspected etiology of variceal bleeding, will be revealed (Figure 13-16). In addition, patients with previous surgical portal-systemic shunts may be evaluated for shunt patency (Figures 13-17 and 13-18). Finally invasion of the portal vein by hepatic tumors, a grave prognostic sign and usually a contraindication to resection, is best shown by this technique.

Hemodynamic information about the portal system can also be obtained by hepatic venography. A wedge pressure may be taken by advancing a catheter from the inferior vena cava far into a hepatic vein until it blocks a small hepatic branch. Pressure measurements then accurately reflect the sinusoidal pressure and also the portal pressure in cases of postsinusoidal portal hypertension, as in most cases of alcoholic cirrhosis. Injection of contrast agent will demonstrate distorted hepatic venules in cases of cirrhosis and even portal radicle filling if cirrhosis has advanced to stage III where the flow in the portal vein is reversed (hepatofugal).

In cases of presinusoidal portal hypertension, such as portal vein thrombosis or schistosomiasis, the wedge study will be normal. However, in cases of Budd-Chiari syndrome or hepatic vein thrombosis, if a hepatic vein can be catheterized, contrast agent injection reveals a typical ''spiderweb'' pattern of hepatic vein collaterals (Figure 13-19). A more detailed discussion of all forms of mesenteric venous pathology may be found in Reuter and Redman's text (45).

Mesenteric Arteriography

The mesenteric vessels may be approached by the femoral or axillary routes for selective catheterization. Stenosis of the origins of these vessels is best appreciated on the lateral aortogram (see Figures 13-25 and 13-26). Risks of mesenteric arteriography are small; beyond problems with femoral puncture, the most common complications are intimal damage by the catheter or guide wire. This is easily detected on the arteriogram and is not rare; Sigstedt and Lunderquist (46) reported 37 subintimal injections in 1804 mesenteric arteriograms; this may lead to occlusion, stenosis, or aneurysm formation, but very few patients have symptomatic sequelae (46,47) because of the excellent collateral circulation to these vessels. The aneurysms are usually small and thrombose spontaneously.

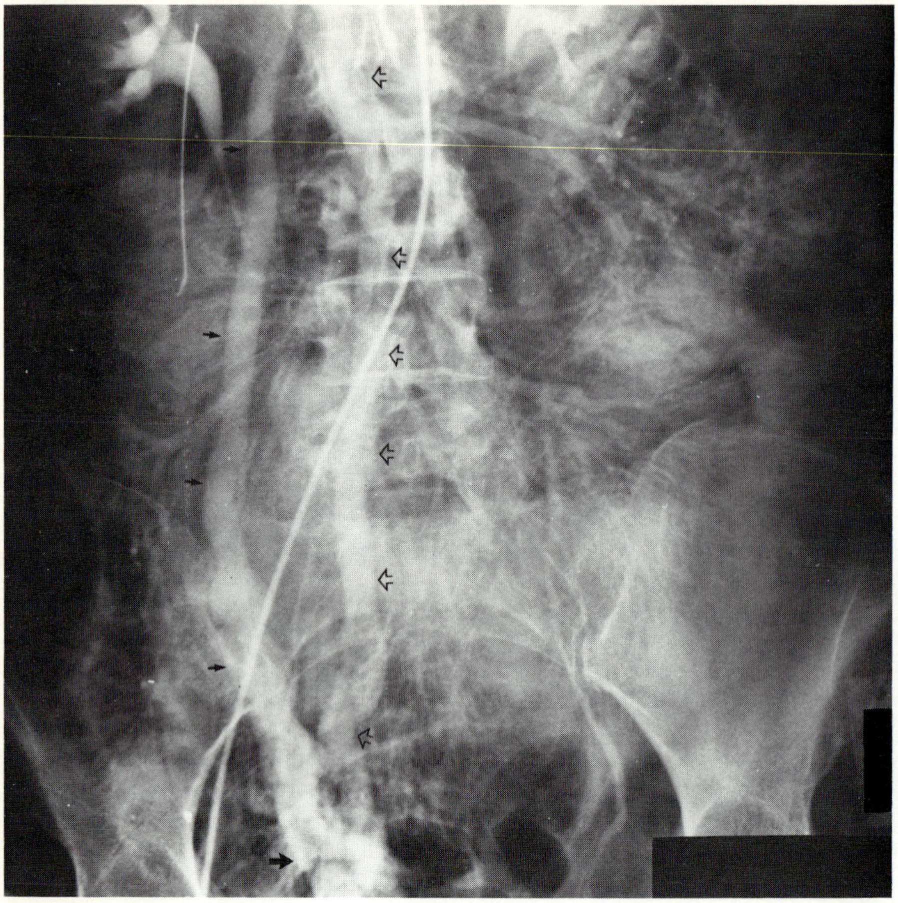

FIGURE 13-14. Ileal varix demonstrated on venous phase of superior mesenteric arteriogram. The superior mesenteric vein fills retrograde (*open arrows*) down to varix (*large arrow*) and up the left ovarian vein (*arrows*) to inferior vena cava.

Trauma

Suspected injury to the liver or spleen from blunt trauma is a common indication for celiac arteriography. Areas of high-flow bleeding may be visualized on aortogram, but a selective injection is necessary to rule out a laceration. Signs of vascular injury are similar in the liver and spleen and include areas of extravasation or puddling of contrast agent (Figure 13-20); filling of false aneurysms (Figure 13-21); avascular clefts; arteriovenous shunting; and displacement of the parenchymal blush away from the body wall, which is a sign of subcapsular hematoma. Care must be taken, however, in interpreting the splenic angiogram because congenital lobulations and accessory spleens occur commonly and may simulate splenic rupture (Figure 13-22). Most accessory spleens lie near the hilus, but those below the lower pole can be confusing. Oblique projections and CT are helpful in making the distinction.

Although it has been shown experimentally that a splenic hematoma is isodense with normal splenic tissue, fast, high-resolution CT scans using infusion are highly accurate in diagnosing splenic injury; for example, 96 percent was demonstrable by CT in Jeffrey's series of 22 surgically proven lacerations (48). The mistakes occurred in children whose scans had movement artifact. A good scan is therefore an excellent screening study. Accurate diagnosis of liver injury has not been so well documented but may be substantiated when large series of patients studied with higher resolution scans are available. CT has the additional advantage of demonstrating associated injuries that may have been previously unsuspected.

Gastrointestinal Bleeding

Bleeding into the gut is reliably demonstrated by selective mesenteric arteriography if the patient is bleeding at a rate of at least 0.5 to 1.0 mL/min at the moment of contrast agent injection. The diagnosis is made by demonstration of extravasation or puddling of contrast agent which persists beyond the phase of venous emptying (Figure 13-23). The major problem with arteriographic diagnosis is that bleeding is often intermittent and may have stopped at the time of injection. Endoscopy immediately prior to the angiogram helps to localize the site and limits the number of vessels to be injected. This avoids the dangerously long catheter time and high contrast agent load often required to select all possible gut vessels. Recent barium studies preclude arteri-

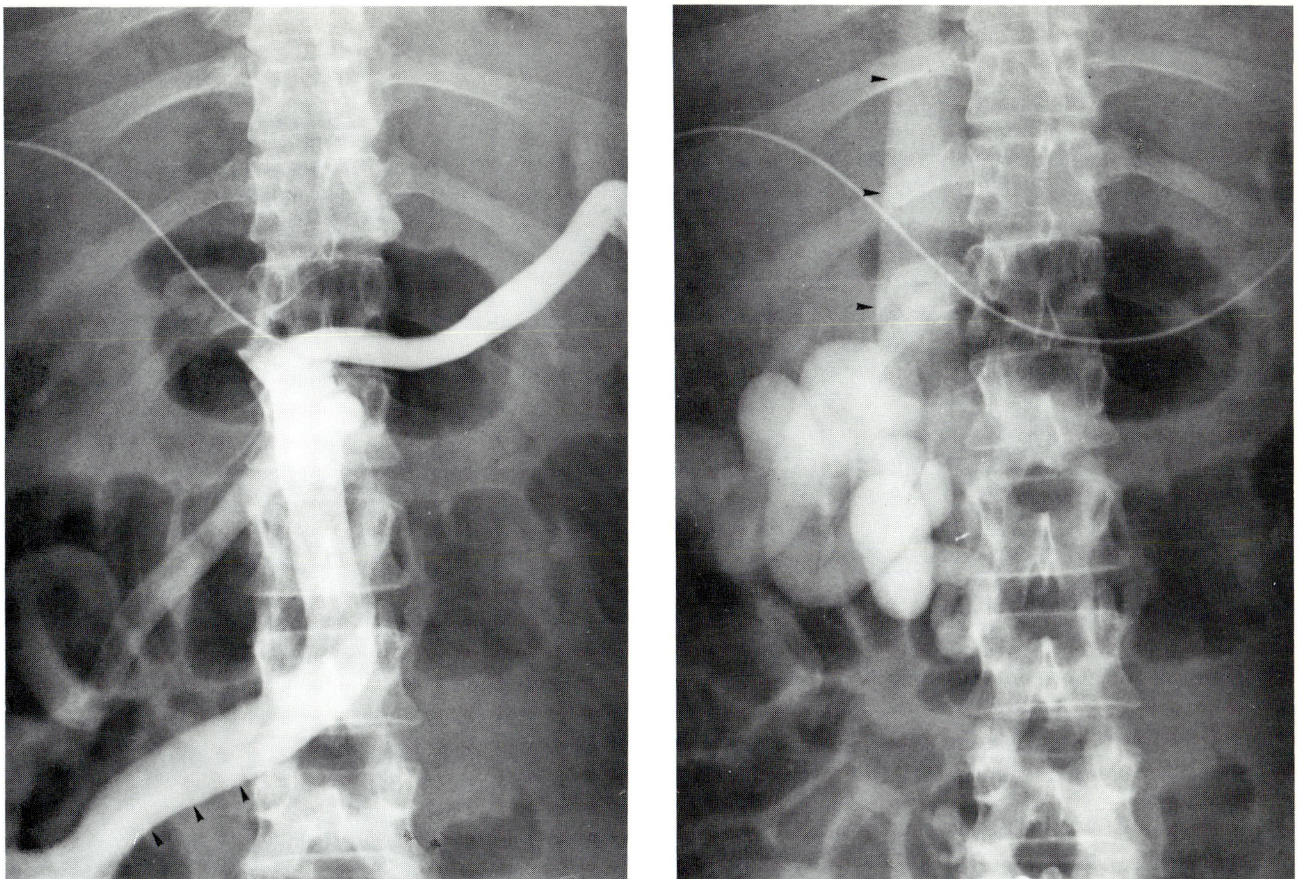

A B

FIGURE 13-15. (*A*) Transhepatic injection of the splenic vein showing retrograde (hepatofugal) flow down the superior mesenteric vein (*arrowheads*). (*B*) Later film of transhepatic splenic venogram showing filling of large colonic varix and drainage into inferior vena cava (*arrowheads*). Courtesy of Dr. Robert Conroy, Long Beach Veterans Administration Hospital.

FIGURE 13-16. Portal vein thrombosis with ''cavernous transformation'' of the portal vein (*curved arrows*) demonstrated on the venous phase of a splenic artery injection. The splenic vein (*arrow*) and coronary vein (*open arrow*) are normal, but retrograde filling of mesenteric collaterals (*arrowheads*) indicates portal hypertension.

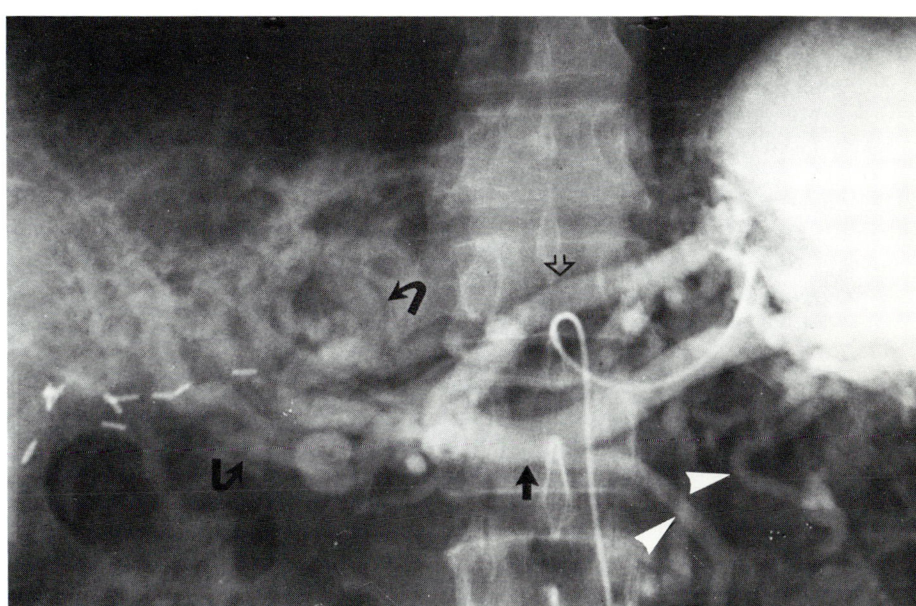

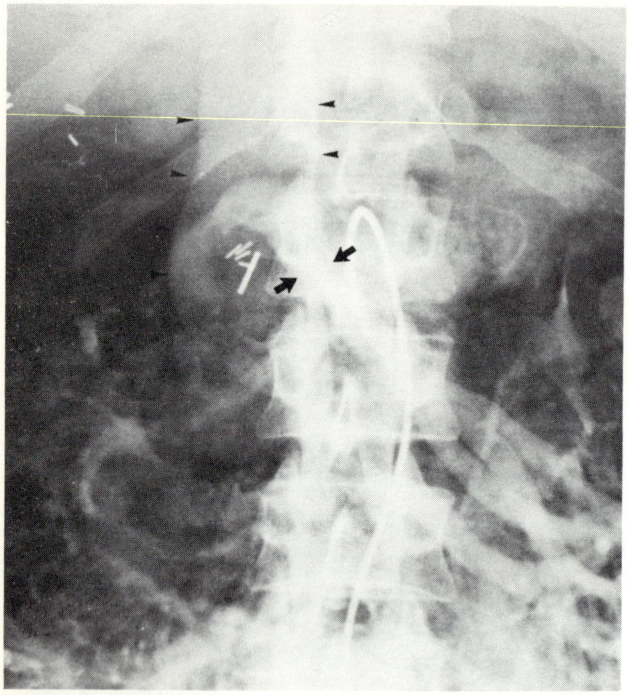

FIGURE 13-17. Patent portocaval shunt demonstrated on venous phase of superior mesenteric arteriogram. The portal vein is indicated by arrows; the inferior vena cava by arrowheads.

ography because the residual barium masks extravasation. Several intravenous isotope studies are available which are more sensitive than the arteriogram to low rates or intermittent bleeding. Extravasation at 0.1 mL/min may be visible on scan after injection of ^{99m}Tc-labeled sulfur colloid (49) or ^{99m}Tc-labeled red blood cells (50). Bleeding under the liver is obscured in the sulfur colloid scan, and in areas where segments of upper and lower bowel are superimposed, it may be difficult to tell which segment is bleeding.

Gastrointestinal bleeding can be controlled by transcatheter therapy with vasopressin (Pitressin) infusion or embolization in a high percentage of patients. In general vasopressin infusion is easier because catheter placement is not so critical and the risk of bowel infarction is negligible; however, the prolonged presence of the catheter in the femoral artery carries a risk of thrombus formation and embolization in the leg that increases with the size of the catheter and the duration of infusion. In the stomach, embolization is an attractive choice since the left gastric artery can usually be catheterized without difficulty and the risk of stomach infarction is exceedingly low. Control of gastric bleeding by vasopressin has been reported at approximately 80 percent in multiple series (51). Pyloroduodenal bleeding is more difficult because of the double blood supply from the pancreaticoduodenal arcade, and the success of vasopressin is correspondingly lower at 40 percent or less (51). For better control, selection of the gastroduodenal artery for embolization is desirable but often difficult. Even after gastroduodenal embolization, bleeding may persist from superior mesenteric artery (SMA) collaterals. Selective embolization can control the bleeding in

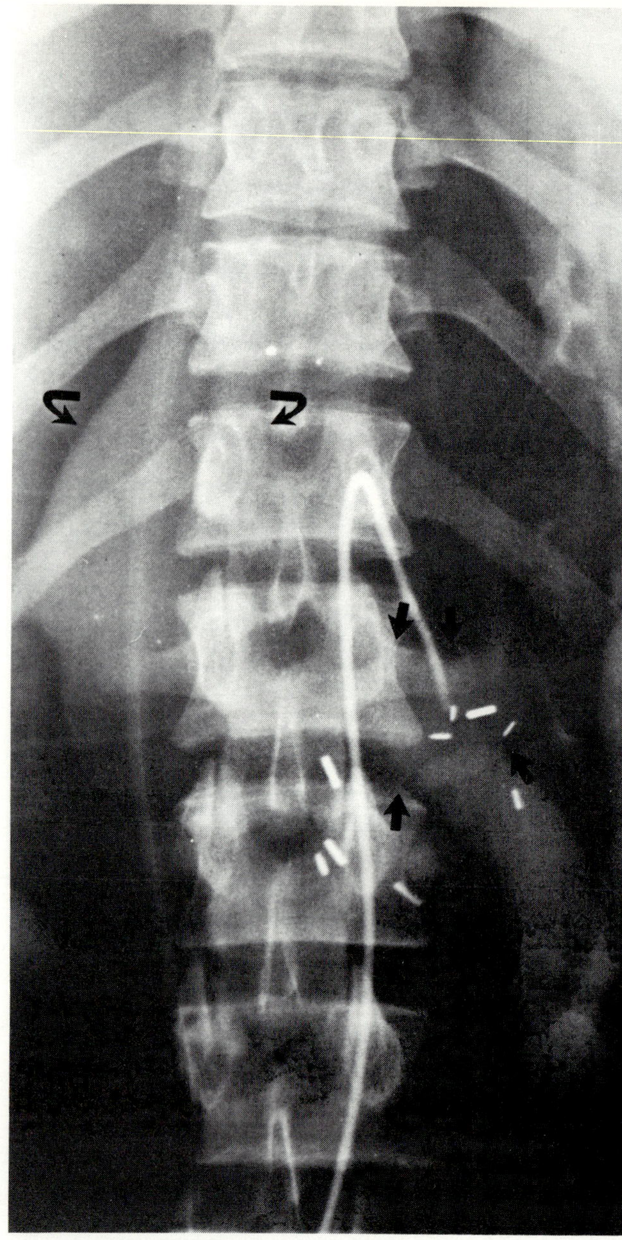

FIGURE 13-18. Patent Warren shunt demonstrated on venous phase of high volume splenic arteriogram. Straight arrows outline renal vein; curved arrows the inferior vena cava.

65 to 70 percent of cases (51). Experience with small bowel embolization is limited; we were successful in one case, but bowel infarction has been reported elsewhere. Colon infarcts after embolization are known to occur in approximately 12 percent of patients (52) so that in the lower bowel, infusion is the treatment of choice, achieving success in 80 to 90 percent of cases (53) (Figure 13-23).

Although intraarterial infusion of vasopressin into the SMA reduces splanchnic blood flow, it has been demonstrated that intravenous infusion is just as effective at controlling variceal bleeding (54); we have therefore abandoned intraarterial therapy in these cases.

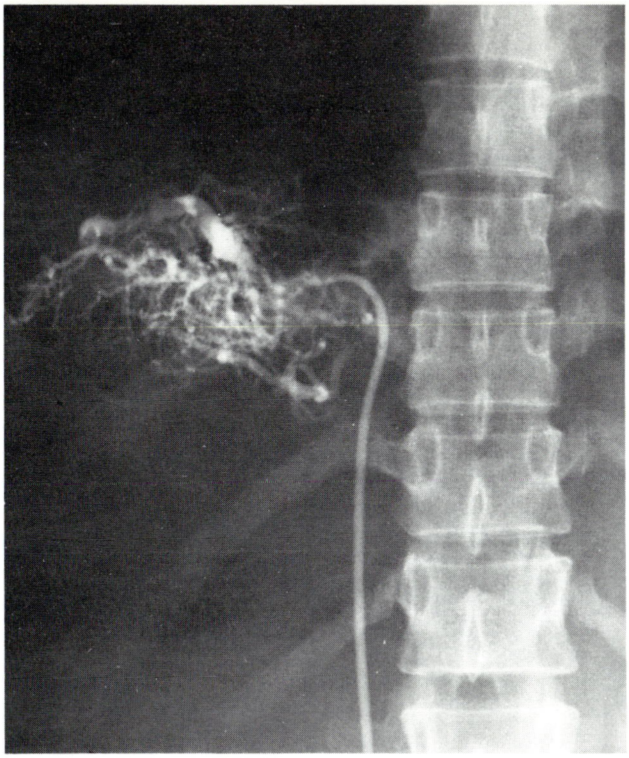

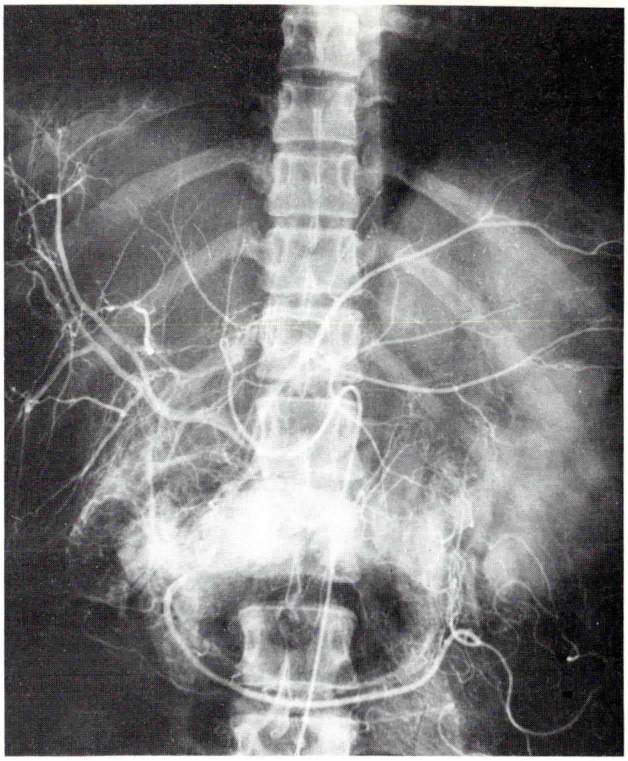

A B

FIGURE 13-19. (*A*) Wedged hepatic venogram in patient with Budd-Chiari syndrome, showing typical pattern of tortuous hepatic venous collaterals. (*B*) Late arterial phase of celiac arteriogram showing stretching of hepatic branches from diffuse central mass effect in both left and right lobes characteristic of Budd-Chiari syndrome.

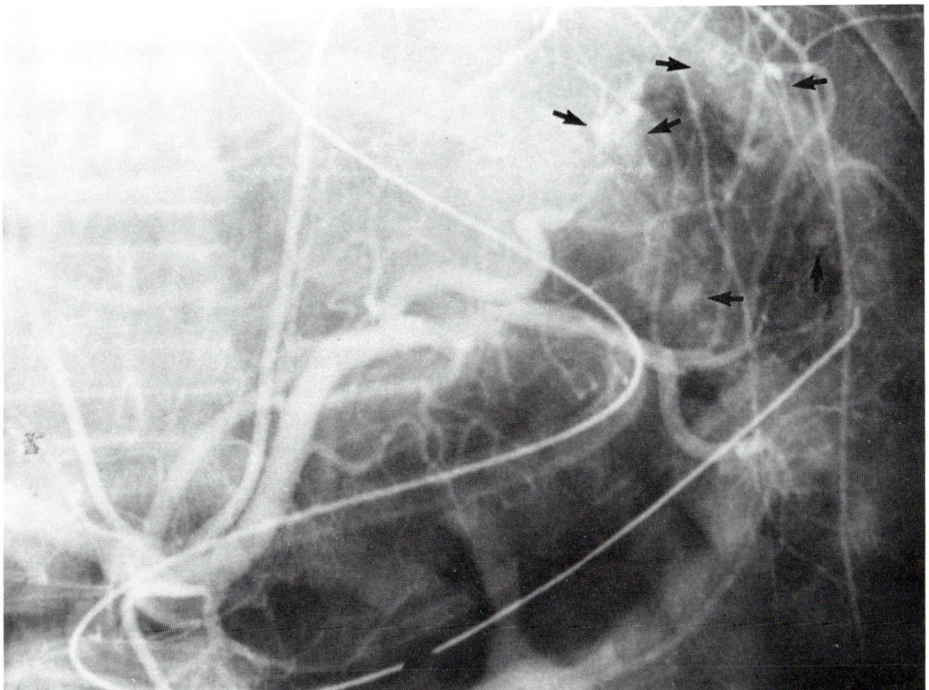

FIGURE 13-20. Celiac arteriogram showing evidence of splenic injury: sharp attentuation of multiple intrasplenic branches with areas of puddling of contrast (*arrows*).

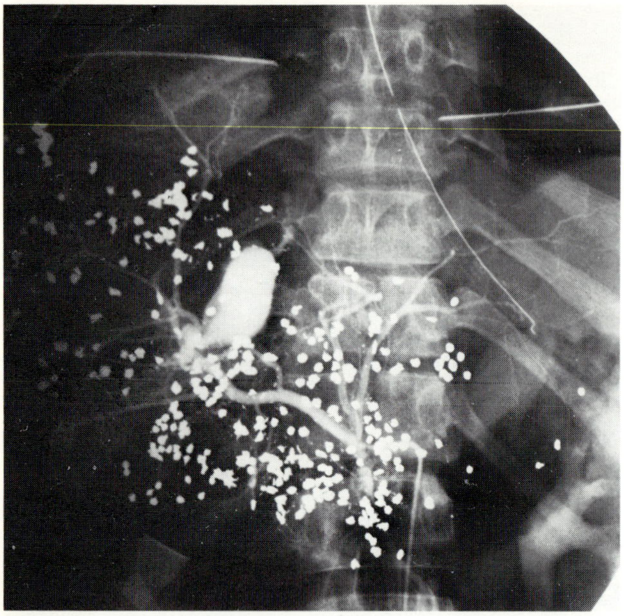

A

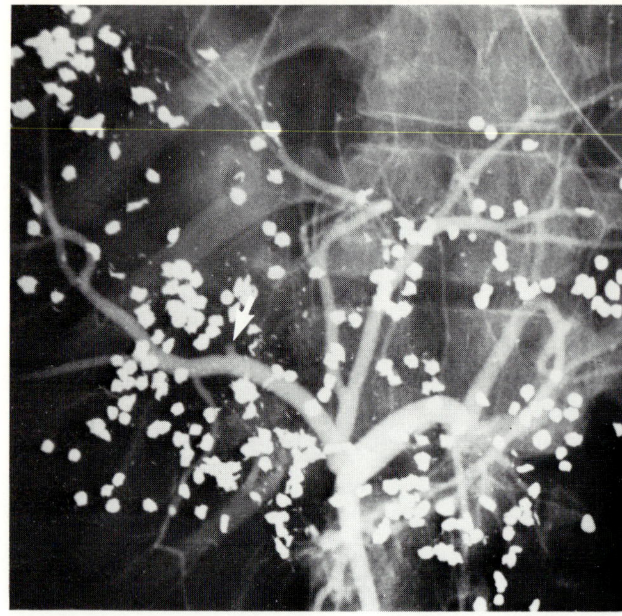

B

FIGURE 13-21. (*A*) Selective proper hepatic arteriogram showing large hepatic false aneurysm secondary to shotgun wound. (*B*) Close-up of right hepatic branch postparticulate embolization shows stump of occluded vessel at site of aneurysm (*arrow*).

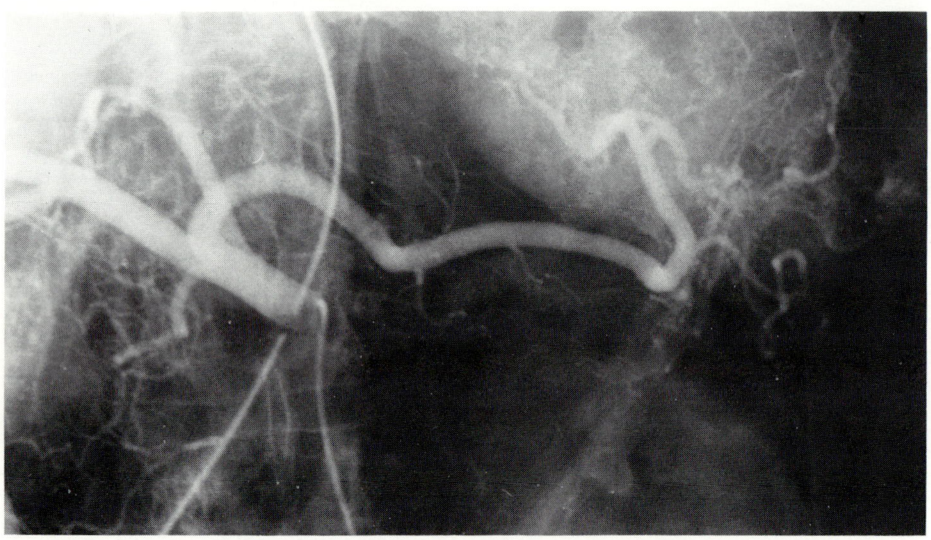

FIGURE 13-22. Celiac arteriogram showing an accessory spleen mimicking splenic rupture.

Mesenteric Ischemia

CHRONIC ISCHEMIA

Angiography is not a precise diagnostic tool in many cases of suspected chronic mesenteric ischemia, because stenoses and occlusions correlate very poorly with ischemic symptoms or bowel infarcts in radiological or pathological series. It is not rare to see proximal stenoses or occlusions of all three mesenteric vessels in asymptomatic patients (55). The rich collateral supply of the gut often compensates adequately in slowly progressive stenoses.

Proximal occlusions are seen best on the lateral aortogram, while the anterior projection demonstrates the anatomy of collaterals. Collateral flow between the SMA and the inferior mesenteric artery (IMA) develops along the left colic to middle colic anastomoses, along the marginal artery of Drummond (the "functional artery" of the colon) in the mesenteric edge of the descending colon, and along the arc of Riolan between the proximal IMA and SMA (Figure 13-24). Enlarged pancreaticoduodenal arteries are the most commonly seen collaterals between the SMA and celiac artery, although routes around the stomach

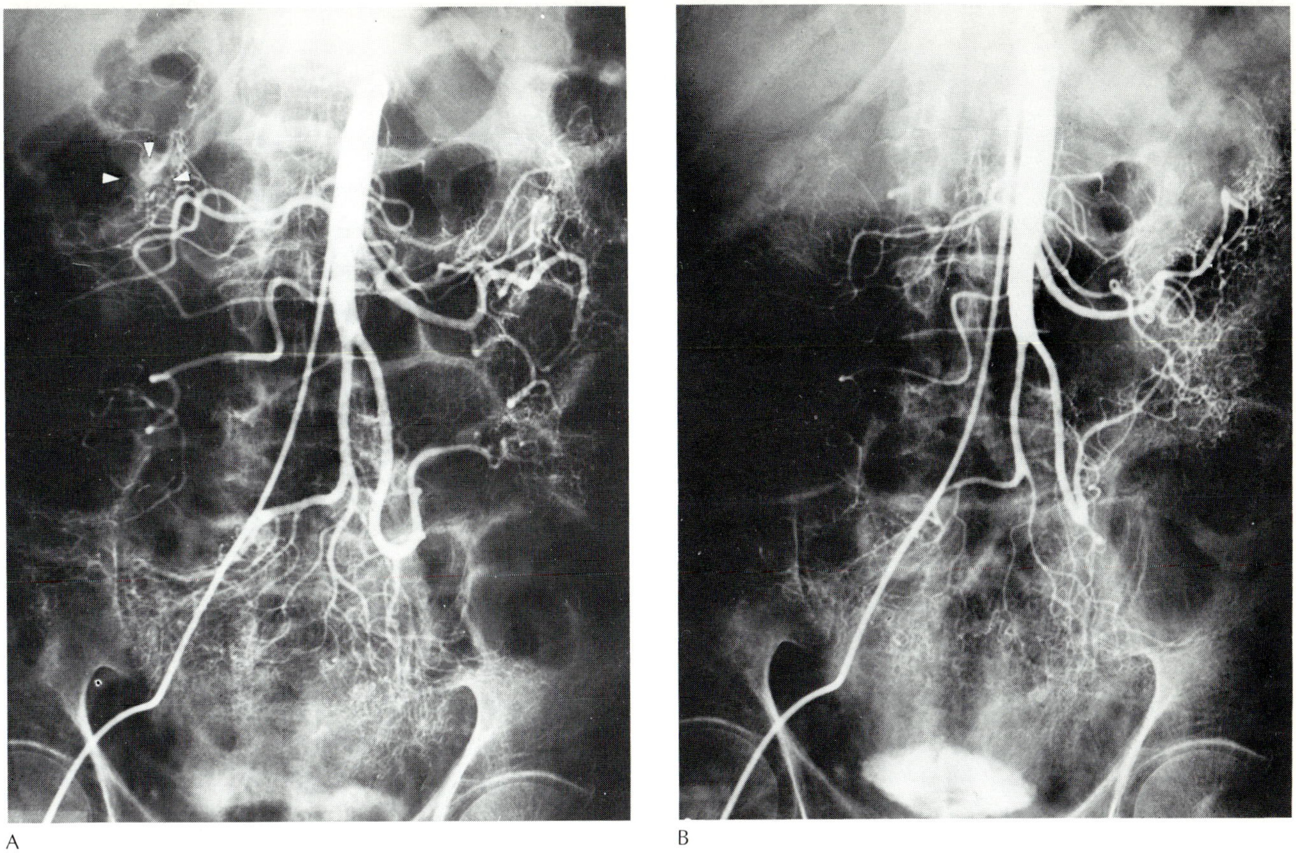

FIGURE 13-23. (*A*) Superior mesenteric arteriogram showing extravasation (*arrowheads*) of contrast from a branch of the middle colic artery, indicating an active bleeding site at the hepatic flexure. (***B***) Repeat injection of superior mesenteric artery after a trial of pitressin infusion. The caliber of all the branches is reduced, and the extravasation is no longer seen.

are available. Arteriosclerosis is the most common etiology for stenoses; the most frequently affected vessel is the IMA. Other etiologies include Takayasu's arteritis, dissecting aneurysm, fibromuscular dysplasia, and the controversial median arcuate ligament syndrome (Figure 13-25).

ACUTE MESENTERIC ISCHEMIA

Angiography is indicated in cases of acute mesenteric ischemia to delineate an obstructive lesion and differentiate obstruction from nonocclusive ischemia; in some cases of nonocclusive ischemia transcatheter therapy is indicated. Obstructive ischemia is usually caused by either thrombus or embolus, or occasionally by an acute aortic dissection (Figure 13-26). Emboli appear as rounded filling defects in the artery; thrombi are usually associated with arteriosclerotic stenoses that are often evident in other vessels as well. Radiological differentiation between thrombi and emboli may not be possible.

Nonocclusive ischemia is caused by mesenteric vasoconstriction, which appears on the angiogram as diffusely decreased caliber of the mesenteric arteries, impaired filling of distal branches, giving a "pruned" appearance, and a series of segmental stenoses forming a "string of sausages" configuration. The constriction may be precipitated by a variety of insults including hypotension, transient SMA occlusion, pressor agents, or decreased cardiac output, but it may persist after correction of the initial event. Infusion of vasodilators, either papaverine or tolazoline (56,57), has been successful in relieving symptoms and avoiding bowel resection. Papaverine has been used successfully after demonstrating a clot (57) in a few patients.

Acute venous thrombosis is an infrequent cause of bowel infarction and often is not visible on angiography. Nonvisualization of the portal vein or tributaries and delayed washout of the small vessels and mucosal blush are seen with an extensive thrombosis.

Renal Arteriography

Either selective renal artery injections or abdominal aortography can be used to evaluate the renal vasculature. The best images result from selective injections; however, when disease is suspected at the renal artery origin, aortography may be used first in lieu of renal artery catheterization. A slight right posterior oblique projection shows the renal artery orifice optimally in

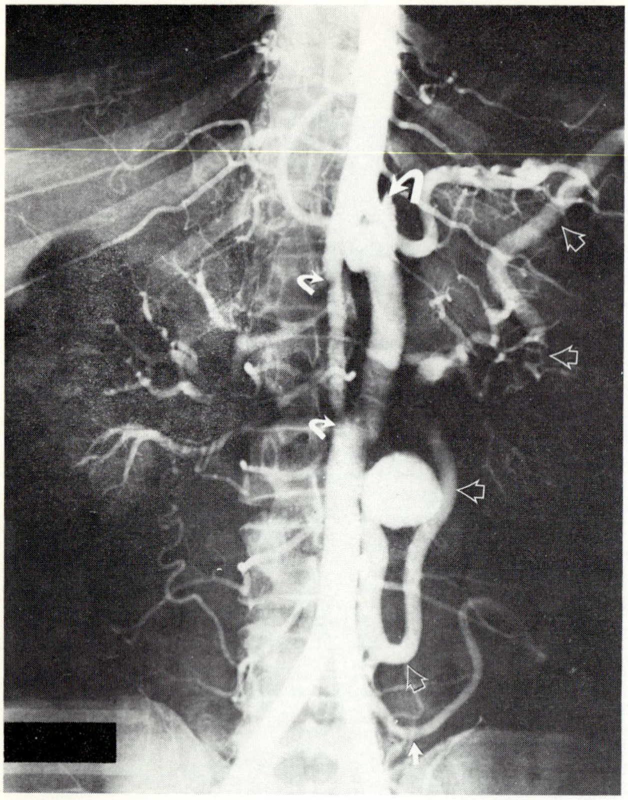

A

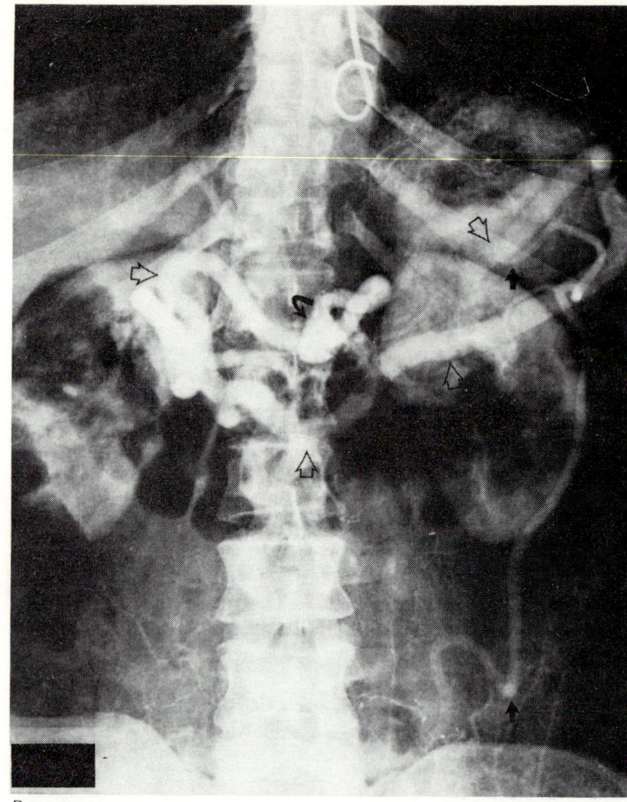

B

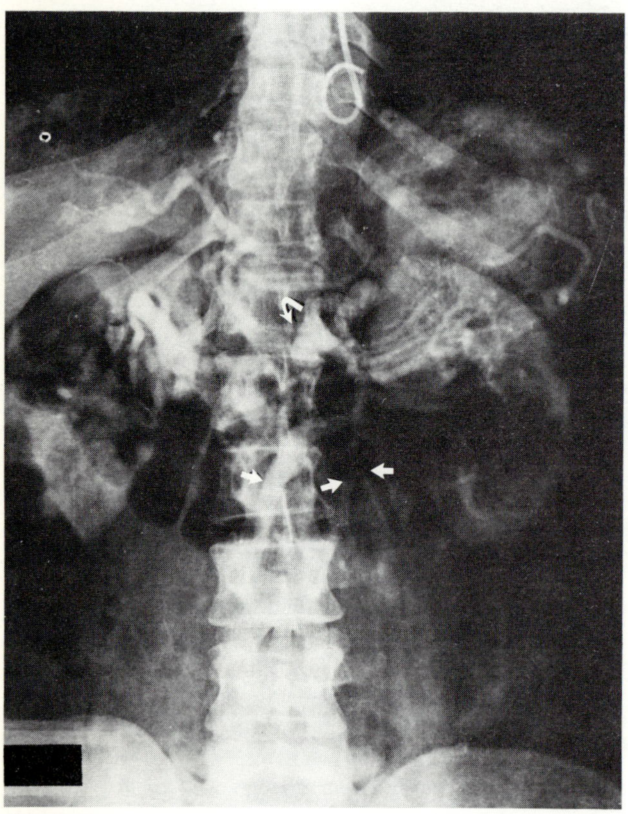

C

FIGURE 13-24 (*A*) Abdominal aortogram in a patient with a long abdominal coarctation (*small curved arrows*) which has been bypassed. There is a false aneurysm at the origin of the graft (*large curved arrow*) and a true aneurysm at the origin of an enlarged inferior mesenteric artery, the only gut artery filling. Collateral pathways are demonstrated including the Arc of Riolan (*open arrow*) and the marginal artery (*straight arrow*). (*B*) Later phase showing filling back to the origin of the superior mesenteric (*curved arrow*) via a large middle colic (*open arrows*). (*C*) Even later phase showing antegrade filling of superior mesenteric (*small arrows*) and filling of the hepatic artery via the gastroduodenal.

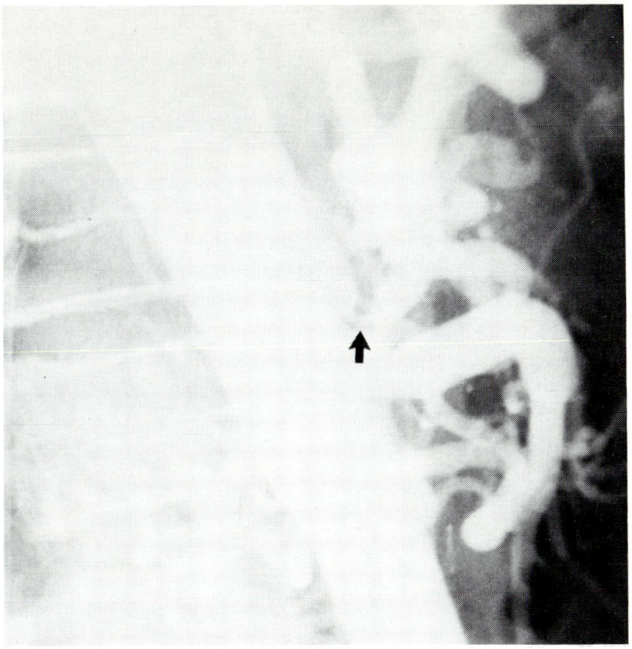

A

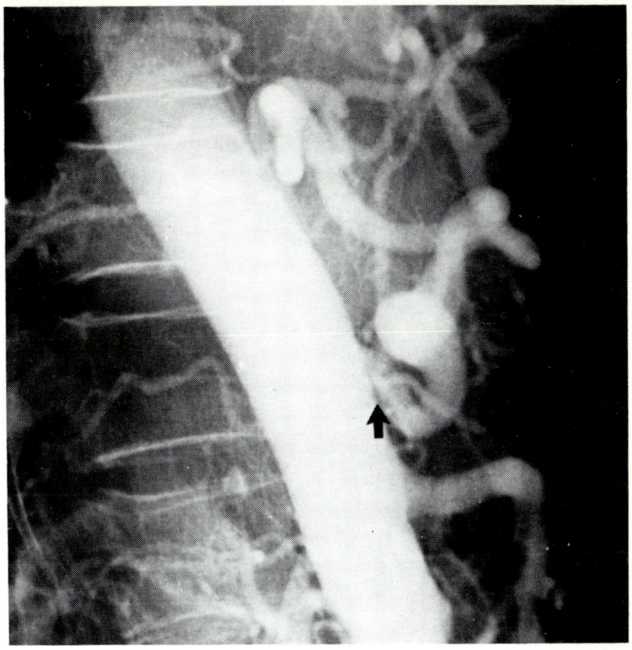

B

FIGURE 13-25. (*A*) Lateral aortogram in expiration showing narrowing at the origin of celiac axis typical of median arcuate ligament syndrome. (*B*) Aortogram in inspiration. The stenosis has disappeared.

most patients (Figure 13-27). Aortography may also be preferred in cases of renal trauma, for large renal tumors with parasitized blood supply, and for evaluating renal donors. Aortography provides an anatomical overview which is useful in demonstrating multiplicity of renal arteries, which is present in 20 to 30 percent of cases (58).

Selective catheterization of the renal artery is usually straightforward; however, an acute takeoff from the aorta may make a recurved catheter shape or an approach from the axillary artery necessary. Injection of epinephrine into the renal artery immediately prior to filming has been recommended in cases of suspected renal tumor (59). Normal vessels respond by constricting. Neovascularity does not respond as much and is thereby rendered more prominent. This form of pharmacoangiography does enhance visualization of tumor vessels but has in our experience seldom made a diagnosis which was not already possible from routine films.

In our practice, the greatest usage of renal angiography currently is for renal masses and vascular lesions, such as renal artery stenosis, renal arteriovenous fistula or malformation, renal artery aneurysm, fibromuscular dysplasia, and arteritis. When lesions are not primarily vascular in nature, less invasive tests such as intravenous pyelography, ultrasound, CT, and isotope studies almost always precede angiography. If less invasive procedures are not diagnostic, however, angiography may demonstrate an etiology in some cases of oliguria, hypertension, hematuria, or hydronephrosis, and it may elucidate the extent of renal tumor spread in cases of renal carcinoma.

Atherosclerotic narrowing is the most common renal vascular lesion. Atherosclerosis usually involves the proximal third of the renal artery and is seldom present without associated abdominal aortic disease. Since only a small percentage of hypertension is renovascular and patients with renal artery stenosis may be normotensive, the presence of renal artery narrowing alone is rarely appropriate as the sole determinant for surgery or angioplasty. A narrowing of 80 percent or more, however, is usually significant (60).

Renal artery aneurysms have been incriminated as a cause of pain, hematoma, and hypertension. They may rupture, and an increased incidence of rupture during pregnancy has been described (61). Selected patients can be treated by embolization (Figure 13-28).

Renal arteriovenous fistulas are usually associated with congenital arteriovenous malformations or penetrating trauma or are iatrogenically induced. The most common cause overall is percutaneous needle biopsy. Most postbiopsy fistulas resolve with time, but a few go on to severe hypertension or heart failure. Arteriovenous fistulas and malformations may also be treated by embolization techniques (62) (Figure 13-29).

Renal artery dysplasia or fibromuscular dysplasia occurs most frequently in women in the middle decades of life. Other visceral and cerebral vessels may be involved. Renal artery dysplasia can be associated with spontaneous renal artery dissection, aneurysms, and hypertension. The proximal third of the main renal artery is usually spared, unlike with atherosclerotic involvement. A number of classification systems based on location and type of arterial involvement have been described (63). In some instances, dysplasia may be difficult to differentiate from arteritis.

Arteritis of the renal vasculature causes changes which are not specific for different etiologies. Vessel irregularities, stenoses, occlusions, and aneurysms may be seen. Small aneurysms of medium- and smaller-sized renal artery branches are suggestive of periarteritis nodosa (Figure 13-30), but other necrotizing vasculitides may cause similar aneurysms.

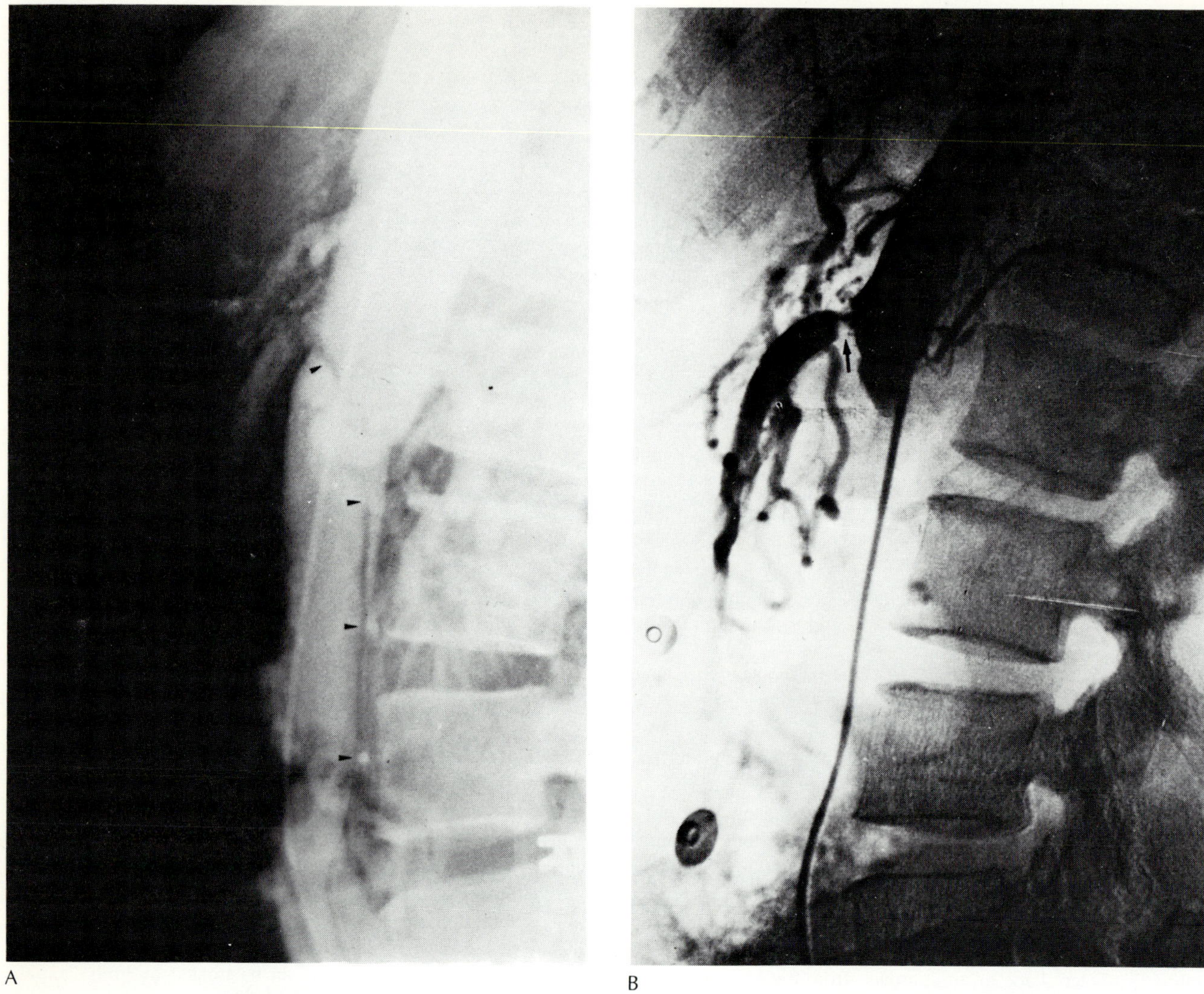

FIGURE 13-26. (*A*) Extension of a thoracic aortic dissection causing acute mesenteric ischemia shown on lateral aortogram. The septum is indicated by arrowheads. There is a tight stenosis of the superior mesenteric and no celiac filling. (*B*) Subtraction of true lumen arteriogram showing superior mesenteric stenosis (*arrow*) and hepatic artery filling via collaterals. (*C*) Lower portion of severely narrowed true lumen giving rise to normal lumbar arteries.

Abdominal Aortic and Lower Extremity Arteriography

We prefer the femoral approach to arteriography of the abdominal aorta and lower extremity. The femoral artery on the least symptomatic side is usually employed. When a femoral pulse cannot be palpated or grafts have been placed in the femoral area, we utilize the axillary artery as the next approach. The translumbar aortic approach can also be employed, and some angiographers prefer this route.

The translumbar technique, originally described by Dos Santos in 1929 (64), has been modified by the use of guide wires and replacement of the needle with a Teflon sheath or catheter after the aortic puncture. Severe hypertension or coagulopathy are firmer contraindications to the use of translumbar aortography than to angiography using peripheral access sites, because the inability to compress the puncture site following catheter withdrawal or to visualize the site makes bleeding more problematic. Thousands of aortograms have been performed using the translumbar approach with a surprisingly low complication rate, but the approach is lacking in flexibility in that selective catheterizations and interventional techniques such as angioplasty or thrombolytic therapy are not easily performed by this route.

It is possible to catheterize mature grafts with a low complication rate, but the tough scar and graft material may make catheter passage difficult. Even if the incidence of complications is similar, the gravity of a complication such as infection is much greater with a prosthesis. We therefore reserve a graft as our last choice of approach, unless it offers a special advantage such as the direct visualization of an axillofemoral graft and its runoff.

The amount, rate, and location of contrast agent injection and the sequence and centering of filming vary depending upon the

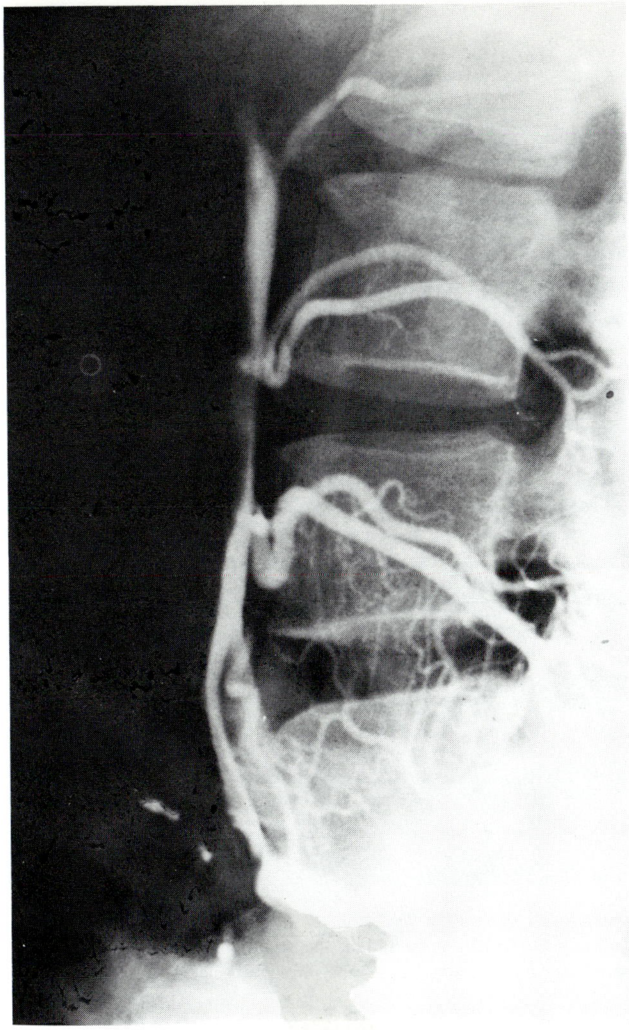

C

FIGURE 13-26. *(continued.)*

suspected pathology. For example, an arteriovenous fistula would require rapid injection and filming, while the slowed, turbulent flow of an aneurysm would be better demonstrated by slower rates of injection and filming. Atherosclerotic occlusive disease of the lower extremity is one of the most common indications for angiography in our practice, and when performed for that indication, the study is accomplished by placing a no. 5 French pigtail catheter at the level of the renal arteries. At the rate of 15 mL/s, 75 mL of contrast agent is injected, and films are exposed at intervals for up to 30 s from the beginning of the injection. Because of the generalized nature of atherosclerosis, the aorta is included in the films even when symptoms suggest disease limited to the lower extremity. Films extend at least down to the ankle. Long films which cover the entire lower extremity or a programmed moving table top are invaluable for obtaining films which show all vessels maximally opacified and for minimizing the need to repeat injections. Biplane angiography is advantageous for showing areas which are often obscured by superimposition in the frontal projection, such as the profunda femoris origin, or posteriorly located plaques. It also minimizes the need for repeat injections. It is desirable to keep the contrast agent load within limits so as not to impair renal function. Injection of contrast agent is also uncomfortable for the patient, especially in the extremities. Some authors have advocated intraarterial injection of lidocaine to alleviate pain, but results are conflicting (65,66) and we are not using the technique currently. Nonionic contrast agents coming on the market now may be less painful than ionic agents. A diluted, less hypertonic contrast agent is definitely less painful than the standard dilutions but offers less opacification. When aortography is performed to examine the abdominal aorta alone, smaller amounts of contrast agent are employed; 25 to 40 mL injected over 2 s is usually sufficient.

Atherosclerotic occlusive disease is seldom a diagnostic dilemma per se because the vessel irregularities, stenoses, and occlusions are easily diagnosed. Performance of the examination may be the most challenging aspect of the study. Vascular access may be limited, and plaques which compromise the lumen increase the chance of subintimal passage of the guide wire. Distal emboli in the form of dislodged plaque fragments or showers of cholesterol emboli may complicate the procedure. For these reasons we prefer small, soft catheters and soft guide wires such as the 0.32-inch Bentson guide* as our standard equipment.

Certain patterns of atherosclerotic occlusion occur with predictable frequency. The most frequently involved area is the distal superficial femoral artery at the adductor canal, presumably because of repeated trauma as the artery enters the canal. The calf vessels and popliteal artery are involved in order of decreasing frequency after the superficial femoral artery. Profunda femoris occlusion is uncommon, although there may be stenoses at its origin. This is fortunate because it is the collateral for sparing superficial femoral disease. The patterns of occlusive disease have been well described for the lower extremity (67,68) as well as the abdominal aorta and pelvic vessels (69–71).

Pathways of collateralization in chronic distal aortic and iliac disease are testimony to the body's ability to adapt to adversity. If unsuspected or incompletely defined, they can lead to unpleasant surprises, as indicated by the story of the surgeon who performs a bowel resection only to face lower limb ischemia. When the aorta is occluded, both parietal and visceral collateral networks may form. The visceral network involves connections between branches of the superior mesenteric to inferior mesenteric to internal iliac to profunda femoris systems. The level of obstruction will determine which portion of the network develops. The parietal network involves aortic branches such as the intercostal, subcostal, lumbar and middle sacral arteries, anastomosing with external iliac, internal iliac, and profunda femoris branches. The epigastric arteries may be important collaterals in the form of Winslow's pathway, which is a superior epigastric to inferior epigastric connection linking the internal mammary and intercostal arteries to the internal iliac artery. This pathway should be remembered because it is not evaluated by standard injections in the abdominal aorta.

Vascular trauma is the second most frequent indication for lower extremity angiography in our practice. The injury patterns include vasospasm, intimal flap, occlusion, laceration, complete transection, arteriovenous fistula, pseudoaneurysm, and combinations of these. When an intimal flap, fistula, or pseudoaneurysm is seen, the diagnosis is straightforward, but an angiogram

*Cook, Inc., Bloomington, Indiana.

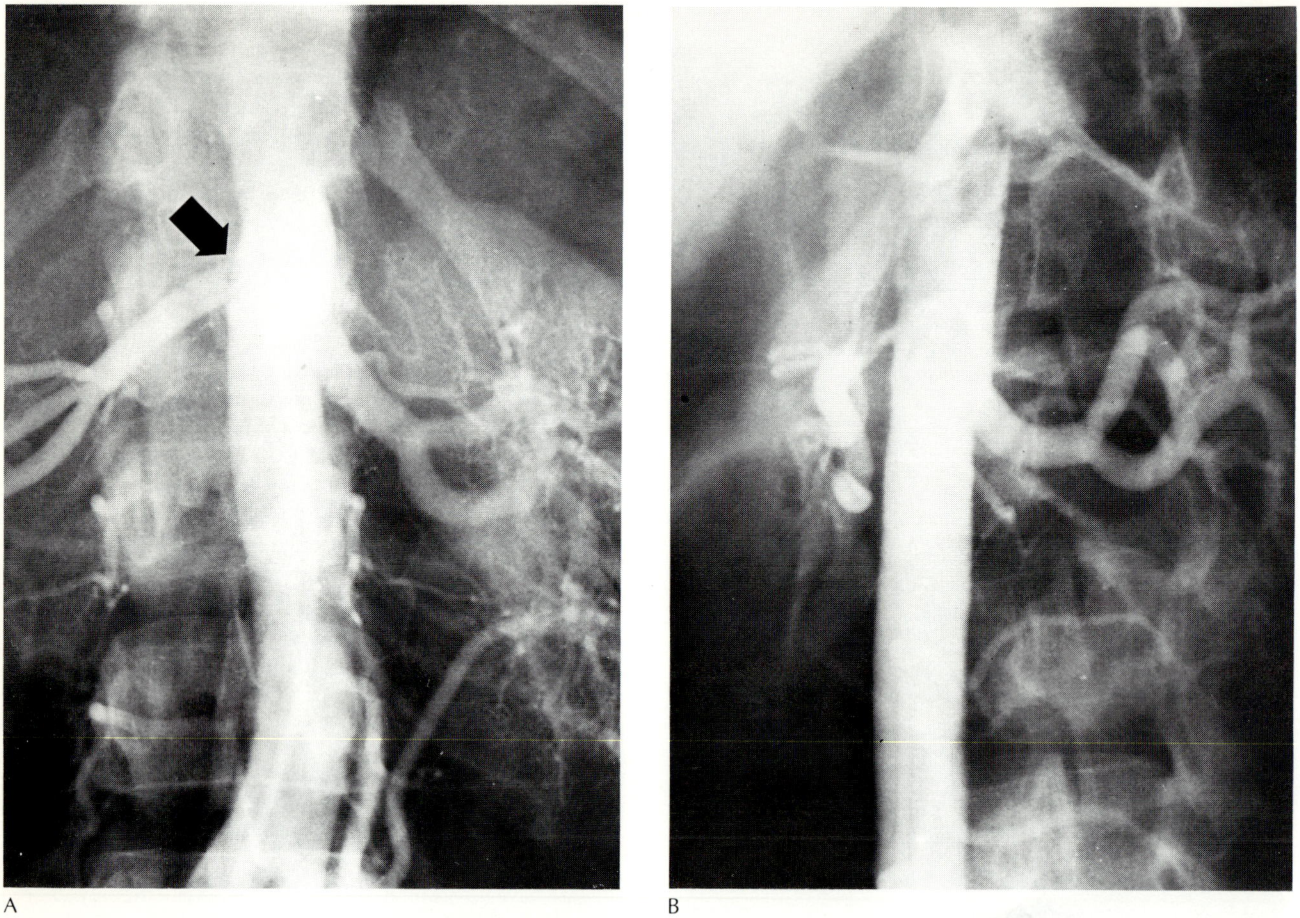

FIGURE 13-27. (*A*) The proximal right renal artery origin is partially obscured in the straight AP projection (*arrow*). (*B*) A right posterior oblique projection more clearly demonstrates the proximal renal artery stenosis.

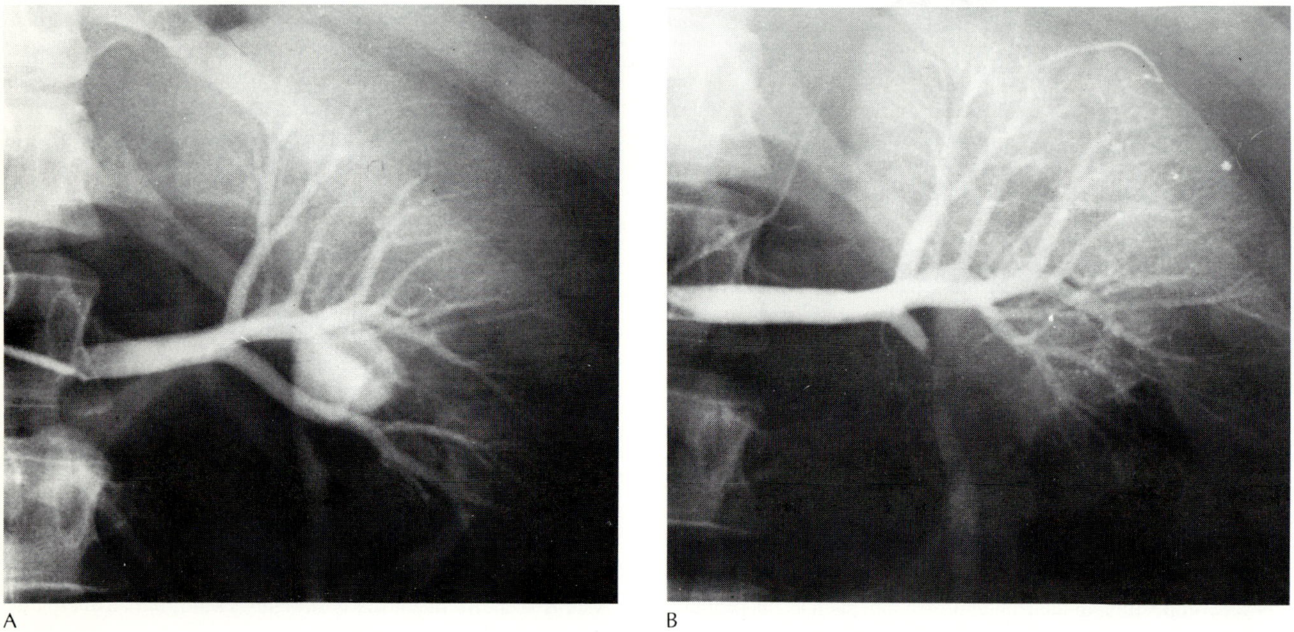

FIGURE 13-28. Traumatic renal artery aneurysm arising from the lower pole artery before (*A*) and after (*B*) embolization.

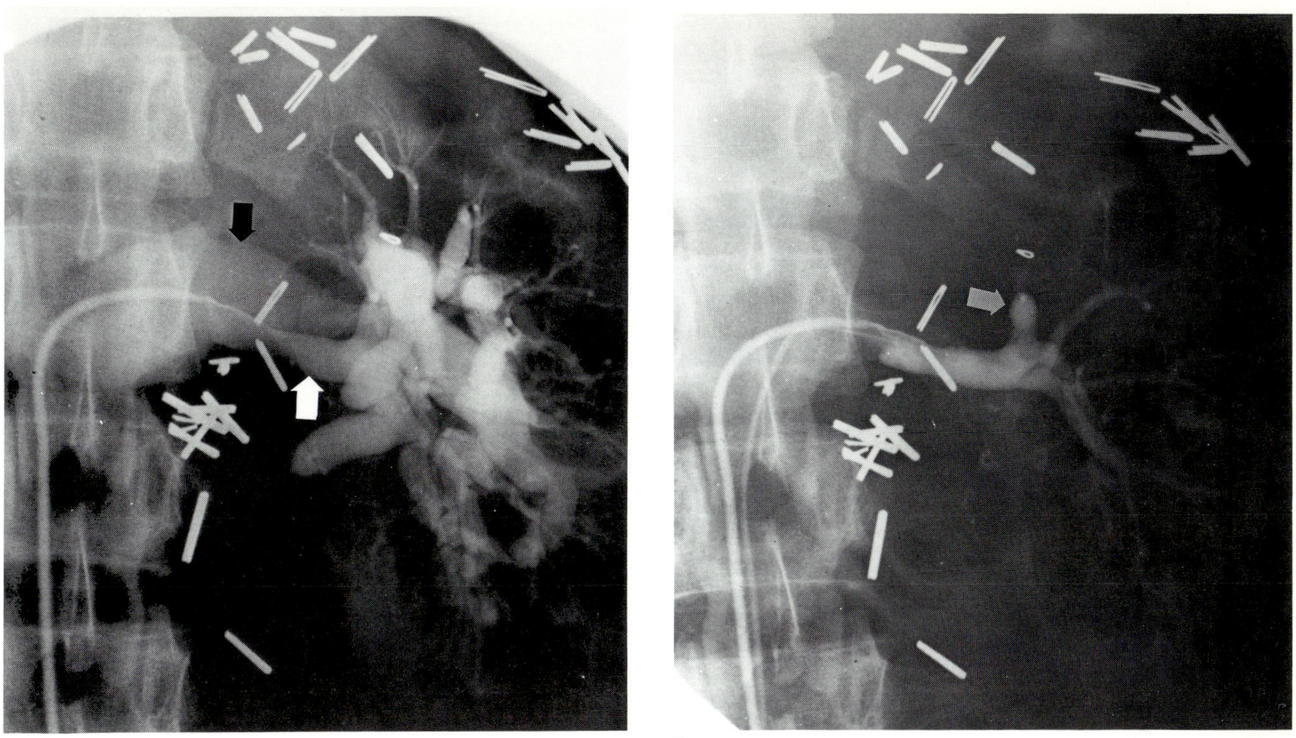

A B

FIGURE 13-29. (*A*) Traumatic renal AV fistula, unsuccessfully treated by surgery. Arrow shows venous shunting (*light arrow*, renal artery). (*B*) A single detachable balloon (*arrow*) occludes the fistula with almost immediate cessation of pain and hypertension.

may not be able to differentiate the others. It is possible to have a complete arterial transection with intact flow. Angiography generally underestimates the severity of injury. Penetrating wounds cause the majority of injuries and more commonly cause lacerations and transections. Blunt trauma is more commonly associated with intimal flaps (72,73). The mainstays of diagnostic testing in peripheral vascular trauma are angiography and Doppler ultrasound. Intravascular embolization therapy is useful in arteriovenous fistula, hemorrhage, and some false aneurysms. It is especially useful in traumatic pelvic bleeding, which may be difficult to control surgically.

Abdominal aortic aneurysms are usually arteriosclerotic in origin. Thoracic aortic dissection may extend into the abdomen, but a dissecting aneurysm originating in the abdominal aorta is rare (Figure 13-31). Traumatic, mycotic, and arteritic aneurysms are also rare. Most abdominal aortic aneurysms are fusiform, some are saccular. Angiography allows precise definition of which aortic branches are involved. Extension into renal and iliac arteries can be demonstrated. Angiography may fail to demonstrate the full size because of thrombus in the lumen (Figure 13-32). The accuracy of ultrasound may be as high as 98 percent, and it offers a noninvasive way to serially assess the size, which is of prognostic importance. CT scanning gives similar data but costs more and involves radiation. It is more useful in evaluating thoracic aneurysms where ultrasound is less accurate.

Lower Extremity Venography

Many different techniques for performing lower extremity venography have been described. The choice of technique will depend in part upon the equipment available, the patient's clinical status, and the personal preference of the radiologist.

We perform venography of the lower extremity using the following technique. A superficial vein on the dorsum of the foot is cannulated with a butterfly needle. Fifty milliliters of contrast agent is then injected by hand with tourniquets in place at the ankle and above the knee to force flow into the deep venous system. The deep venous system will fill best in an erect or semierect, non-weight-bearing position. Tourniquets are removed just before the final films to better demonstrate superficial, soleal, and gastrocnemius veins. When the examination is performed on a tilting table, the iliac veins and inferior vena cava may be better filled immediately after tilting the patient head down. The use of larger volumes of contrast agent and no tourniquets is advocated by some (74). Diluting the contrast agent, using a heparin flush, or using a nonionic contrast agent may decrease complications. We do not employ these methods but do flush the veins with normal saline immediately following filming.

Major complications of the procedure include contrast agent reaction, reactivation or causation of thrombophlebitis, and skin slough secondary to extravasation at the injection site. Skin slough is rare and usually occurs when skin viability is already compromised by chronic venous or arterial disease. Thrombophle-

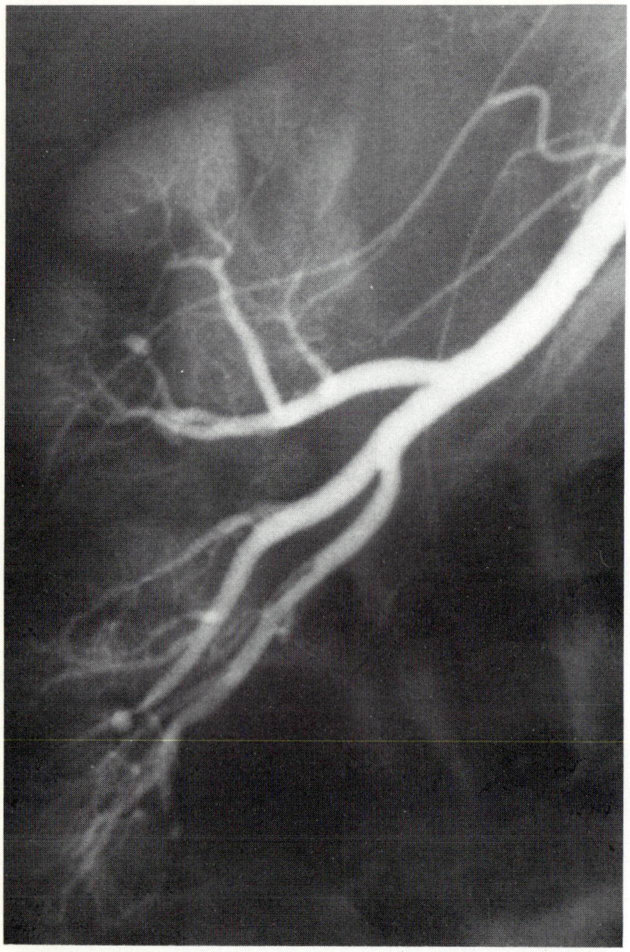

FIGURE 13-30. Multiple small aneurysms and renal infarcts in polyarteritis nodosa.

bitis related to the procedure is usually a mild, self-limited phenomenon. The risk of dislodging thrombi by using the technique described here is negligible, but if catheter technique is employed, the risk is higher. Overall, the risks of lower extremity venography are quite low (75).

The most accurate venographic sign of thrombosis is direct demonstration of thrombus as an intraluminal filling defect with a thin layer of contrast agent surrounding the clot (Figure 13-33). Visualization of collaterals and nonfilling of veins are less direct, less accurate signs of thrombosis. In cases of chronic venous occlusive disease, collateral pathways, irregular vessel walls, and a loss of valvular detail may be seen.

Contrast venography is the most invasive of the techniques employed in diagnosing deep vein thrombosis, but it is the standard by which other methods are judged. It is 95 percent accurate and can be performed quickly in a standard fluoroscopy suite. The labeled fibrinogen test may be more sensitive for acute thrombi in the calf, but it is not widely available, takes more time to complete, and is of less use in chronic thrombosis. Noninvasive testing using Doppler ultrasound, impedance plethysmography, or ^{99m}Tc radionuclide venography has an accuracy which approaches 90 percent in the iliofemoralpopliteal venous pathways, but these methods are less accurate in the calf and lack specificity for thrombosis compared to contrast venography (76,77).

The use of venography in varicose veins is moot. Most authors feel that it is of value. Venography can demonstrate incompetent perforators, although they may not all be opacified. The status of the deep venous system can be demonstrated and varicosities themselves may be opacified. The technique is utilized when such data are judged useful for management.

It is our opinion that there is a tendency to overutilize lower extremity venography. This may be understandable in view of the nonspecificity of clinical signs and symptoms (78). More patients could probably be diagnosed solely on the basis of noninvasive testing, but because of its higher accuracy rate, venography remains the diagnostic gold standard.

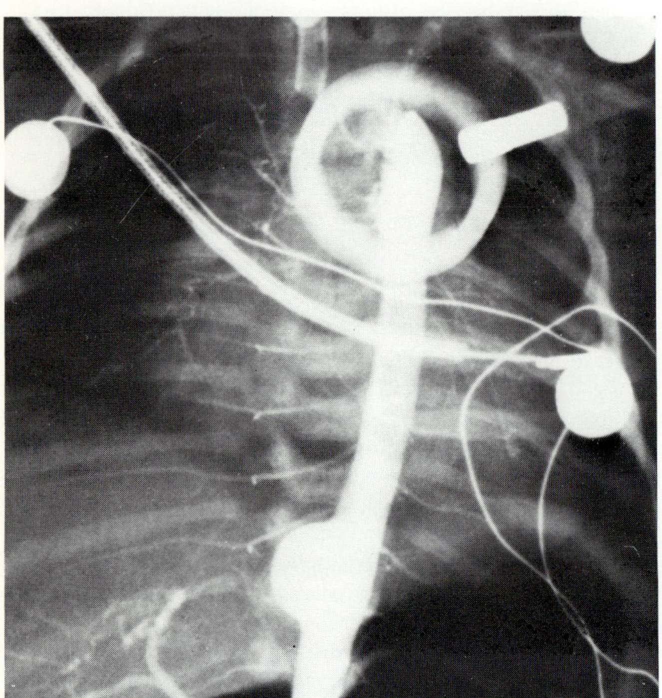

FIGURE 13-31. Mycotic aneurysm of the high abdominal and low thoracic aorta in a neonate at the site of a previous umbilical catheter tip. Previous aortogram through the umbilical catheter was normal.

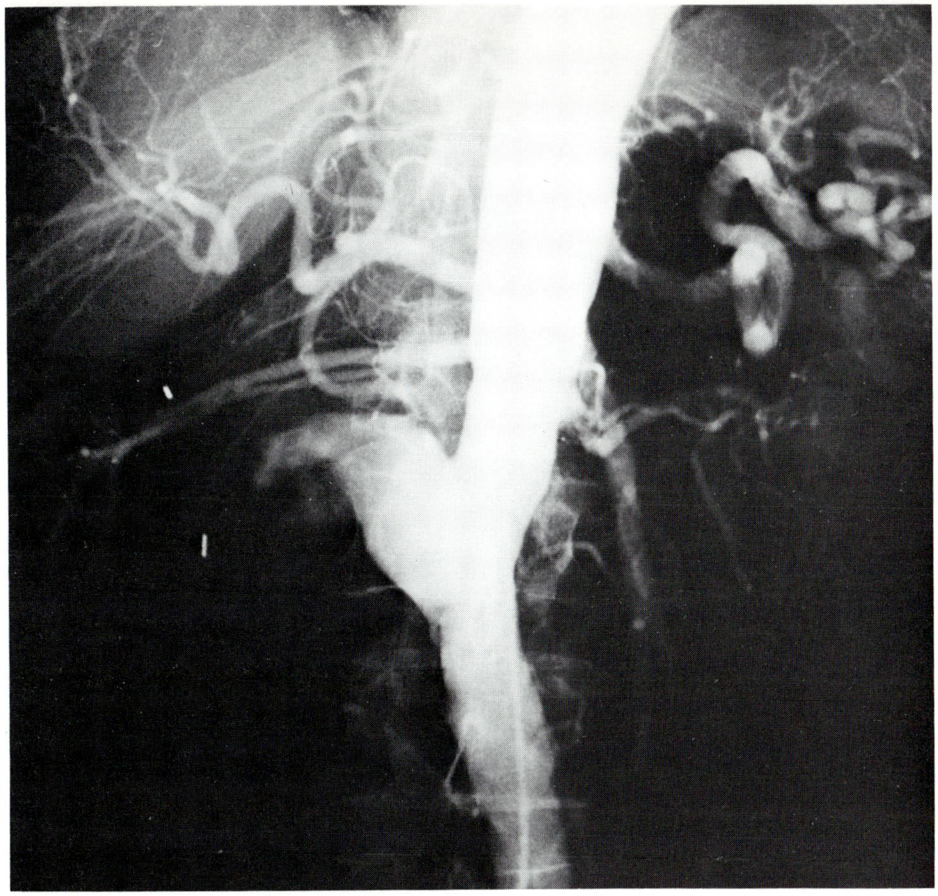

FIGURE 13-32. Saccular abdominal aortic aneurysm. Most of the aneurysm is filled with thrombus.

Upper Extremity Arteriography

Arteriography of the upper extremity is performed in most cases via retrograde catheterization from the femoral artery. Antegrade puncture of the brachial artery may be utilized when embolization therapy of lesions in the forearm or hand is performed. We do not use the brachial approach for diagnostic studies. Upper extremity angiography is most often performed for evaluation of traumatic injuries, arteriovenous malformations and fistulas, vasospastic and vasoocclusive phenomena, and thoracic outlet syndrome.

Acute traumatic injuries show a gamut of findings similar to vascular injuries elsewhere. Delayed or chronic traumatic effects are most often manifested by signs of ischemia when there is vessel occlusion, an enlarging mass in cases of false aneurysm, and a thrill or bruit in an acquired arteriovenous fistula (Figure 13-34). An arteriovenous fistula may also cause local ischemia, cardiac failure, and swelling related to venous engorgement. Congenital arteriovenous malformations of the upper extremity may become very large and present with pain, ulceration, and hemorrhage. They may be management problems, and when they are so extensive that they cannot be resected with limb salvage, embolization therapy may be able to palliate symptoms or make surgery possible.

Evaluation of vasospastic and vasoocclusive disease in the hand can be frustrating in so far as defining a specific etiology. If vasospasm is severe, thrombosis may occur, and conversely some component of vasospasm may accompany occlusive disease or be caused by the angiogram itself. Injection of an intraarterial vasodilator (e.g., tolazoline, 75 mg) may help to differentiate vasospasm from occlusive disease. An overview of the manifold causes of upper extremity and digital ischemia has been presented by Yao et al. (79).

Thoracic outlet syndrome is an important cause of neurovascular compression in the upper extremity, but the symptoms are usually not due to arterial compression. Arteriography is probably best limited to patients with a pulse deficit or a bruit in the neutral position or when a subclavian aneurysm or peripheral emboli are suspected. Demonstrating a vascular compression does not prove that it is the cause of symptoms. Many normal, asymptomatic patients may show compression in certain positions of stress, and patients with severe outlet syndrome may have a normal arteriogram. When evaluating for thoracic outlet syndrome, we inject in the subclavian artery in the neutral position and in the position which recreates symptoms if such can be elicited (Figure 13-35). A more extensive technique is advocated by Lang (80) who also recommends radionuclide flow studies to decrease false-positive results.

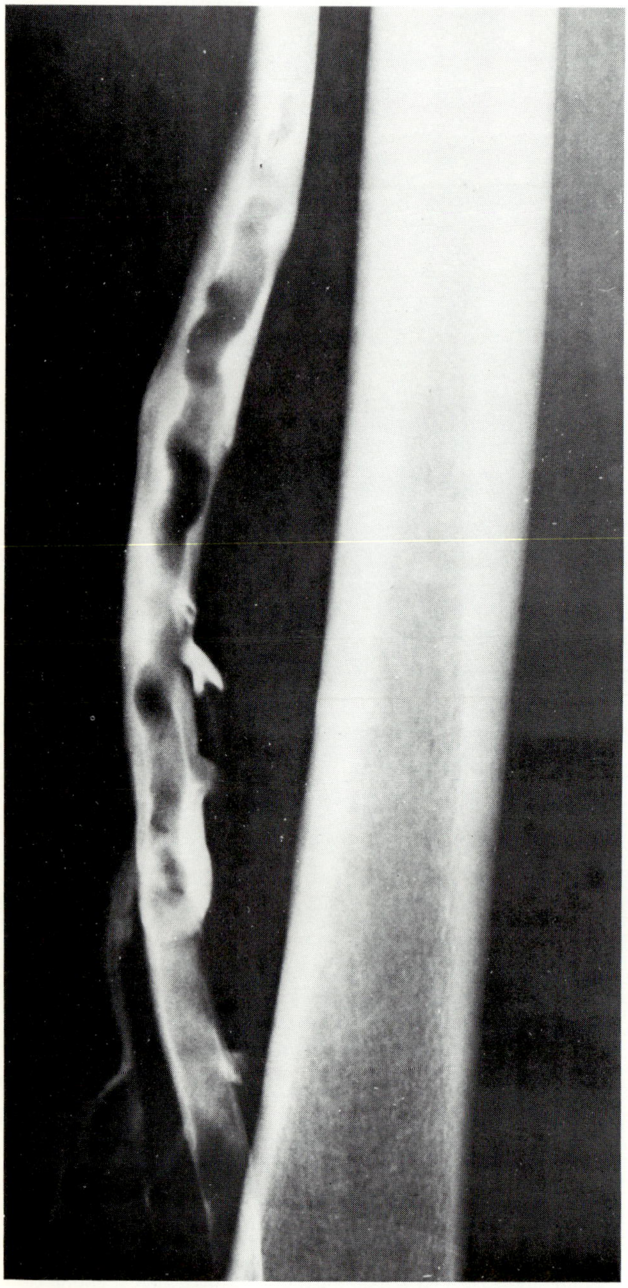

FIGURE 13-33. Clot causing a serpiginous intraluminal filling defect in the femoral vein in a patient with recent thrombophlebitis.

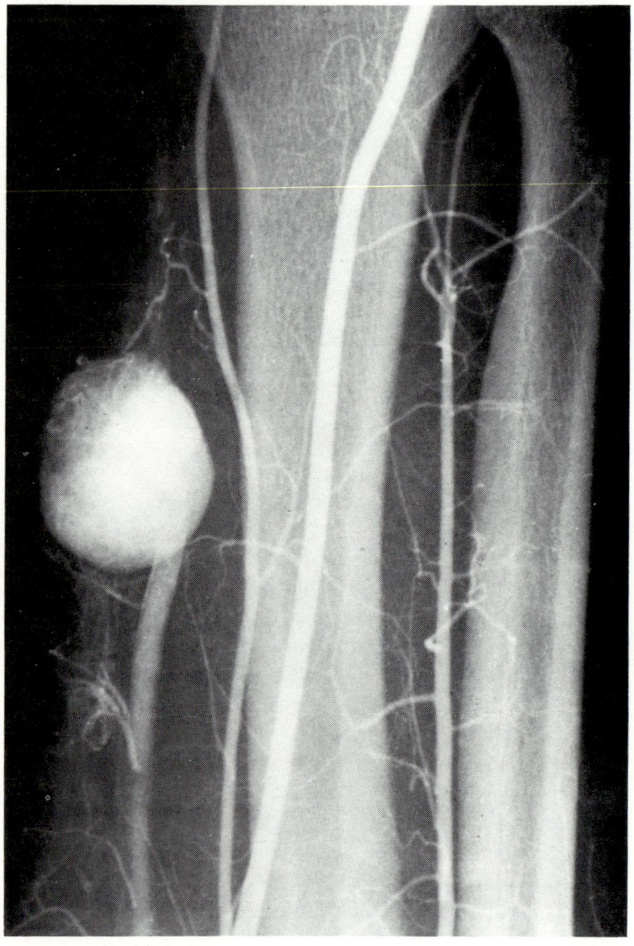

FIGURE 13-34. Traumatic false aneurysm of the radial artery presented with enlarging pulsatile mass.

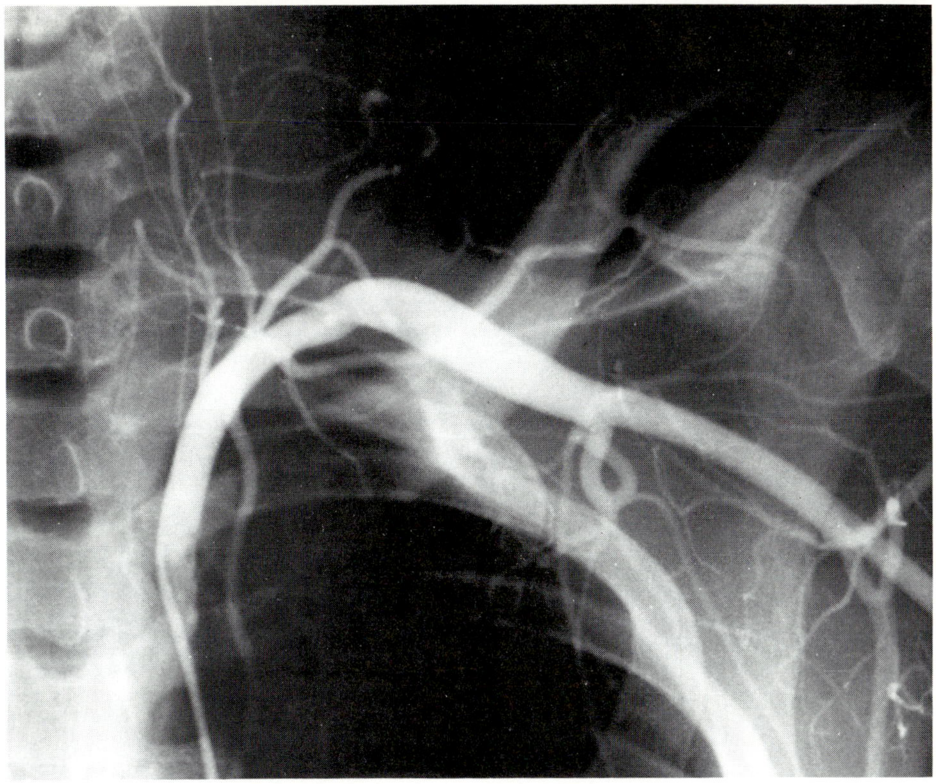

A

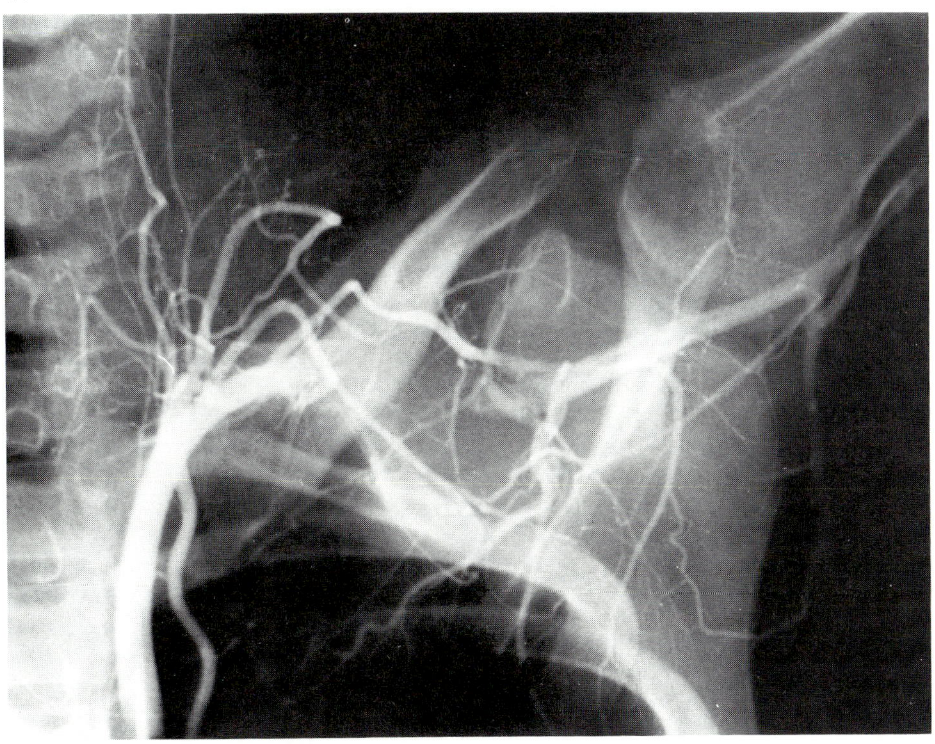

B

FIGURE 13-35. Thoracic outlet syndrome. Vascular compression related to an anomalous 1st rib with a pseudarthrosis. There is slight poststenotic dilatation with the arm in neutral (*A*) but marked compression when elevated (*B*).

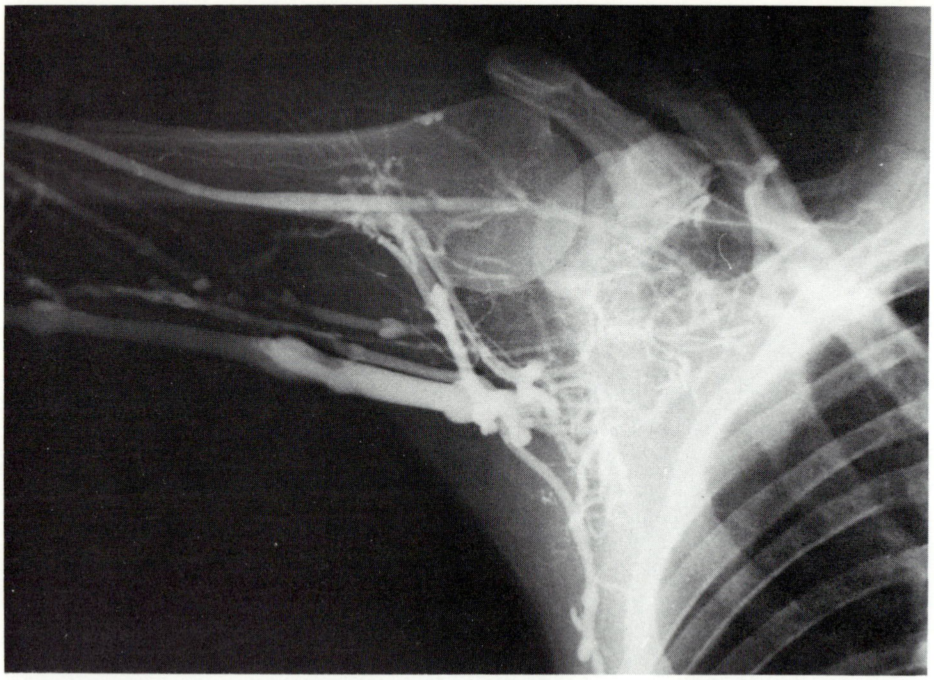

FIGURE 13-36. Exertional thrombosis of the axillary vein in a young manual laborer.

Venography of the Upper Extremity and Superior Vena Cava

The technique of upper extremity venography is simple. A vein distal to the suspected site of occlusion is cannulated with a butterfly needle, and 50 mL of contrast agent is injected by hand. Tourniquets are not employed during injection. Elevation of the arm prior to the final films may give better opacification of the subclavian vein and superior vena cava. Manual compression of the jugular vein during filming may avoid confusing filling defects in the subclavian vein due to inflow of unopacified jugular blood. When visualization of the superior vena cava is desired, both upper extremities are simultaneously injected. Although it is seldom necessary to do so, the superior vena cava and upper extremity veins can be visualized by retrograde or antegrade catheterization. When the study is performed for evaluation of the axillary and subclavian veins and the initial films in a neutral position are negative, it may be advisable to perform a second injection with the arm above the head to evaluate for positional compression by muscle or fibrous bands or the first rib.

In some cases of superior vena caval and arm vein obstruction, CT with contrast agent infusion is a useful adjunct because it can image masses which are responsible for venous occlusion. It may also show filling of collateral channels which implies occlusion; however, it does not show intraluminal clot as well as venography. Symptoms of upper extremity venous thrombosis are usually less severe and more self-limited than in most cases of venous thrombosis of the lower extremity. This may explain the less frequent utilization of venography in the upper extremity. Etiologic factors which we have seen include exertion, penetrating trauma, intravenous drug abuse, congenital venous web, central venous catheter placement, and hypercoagulable states (Figure 13-36). Significant pulmonary embolism is thought to be uncommon from the upper extremity, but in our experience the incidence has been underrated (81).

Cerebral Angiography

Techniques of cerebral angiography have evolved from direct percutaneous puncture of the carotid and vertebral arteries and retrograde brachial artery injection to the almost exclusive use of femoral or axillary catheter techniques. We prefer small (no. 5 French), soft, polyethylene catheters with simple, atraumatic curves for selective carotid injections. If the vessels are tortuous, stiffer catheters with more complex shapes such as "head-hunter" or recurved Simmons types may be necessary. Visualization of at least the proximal intracranial vessels is desirable when evaluating for extracranial occlusive disease. The presence of unsuspected distal lesions may alter a treatment plan based on knowledge limited to the extracranial vasculature alone. Our technique includes two views of the neck with a field of view from above the supraclinoid carotid to below the carotid bifurcation while injecting in the common carotid artery. If more of the intracranial vasculature or superficial temporal artery needs to be demonstrated, a second series of films can be performed centered over the head. The small catheter is then replaced with

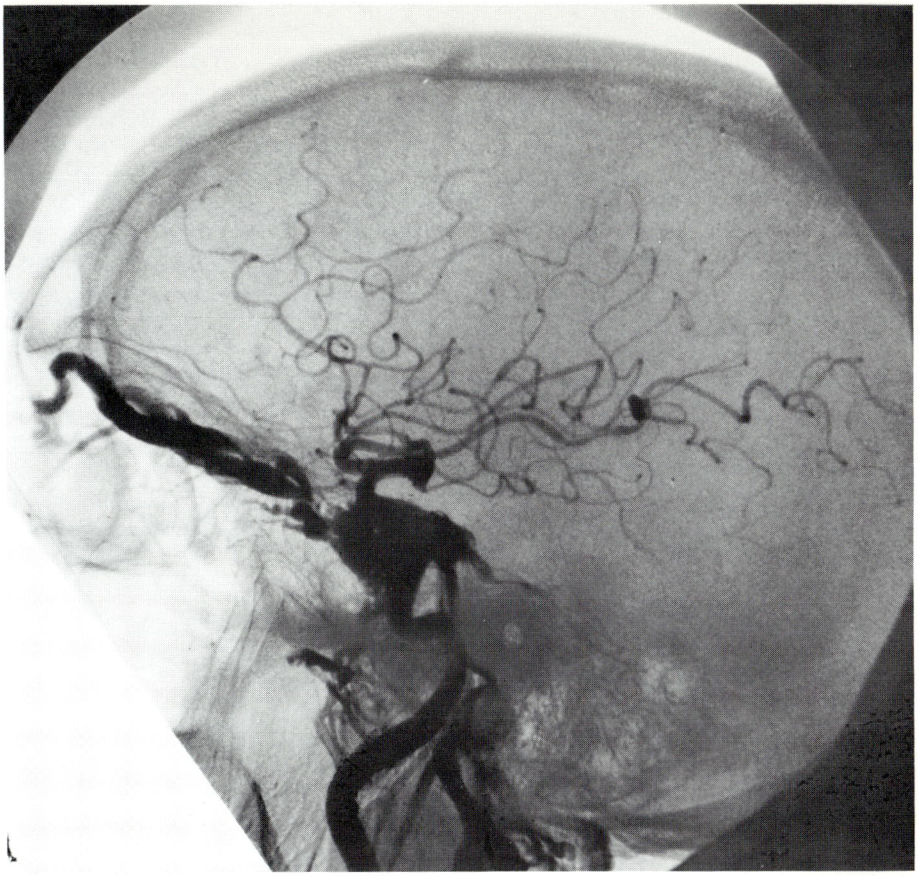

A

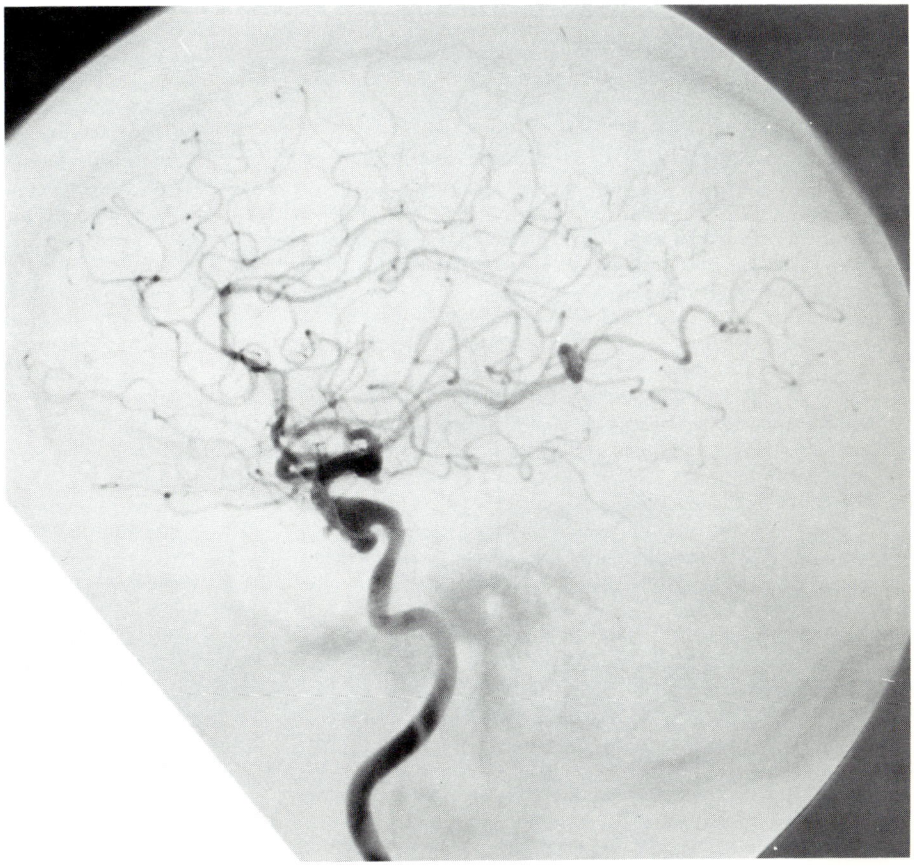

B

FIGURE 13-37. Traumatic carotid cavernous fistula before (***A***) and after (***B***) treatment with a detachable balloon. A small false aneurysm remains.

a larger (no. 6 or 7 French) catheter, which is placed with its tip above the aortic root. A right posterior oblique (with respect to the table top) view of the aortic arch is then obtained. This shows the origin of the vessels off the arch adequately in most cases, although the right common carotid or subclavian artery origins may be superimposed. If necessary a left posterior oblique view can be obtained. When digital subtraction angiography is available, the aortic injection may be performed through a small catheter and may precede attempts at more selective injections rather than follow them. Contrast agent volumes can also be kept at a lower level. Selective injection into the internal carotid artery yields the best visualization of intracranial vessels and is preferred in cases of intracranial disease so long as there is no pathology in the common or cervical internal carotid artery which makes catheter placement in the internal carotid hazardous. Digital subtraction technique provides adequate resolution in most cases. On occasion the higher resolution of small focal spot magnified cut film angiography is useful. This is especially true in intracranial disease where, for example, the question of a vessel turn or infundibulum versus aneurysm may call for images with the maximum spatial resolution.

Noninvasive vascular imaging is a useful screening technique for extracranial occlusive disease, especially when a battery of tests are employed, but it is not as accurate as angiography. Doppler oculoplethysmography, carotid phonoangiography, and small parts ultrasound are prevalent methods in use. Magnetic resonance imaging may play a role in the future (82).

Vascular trauma is being recognized with increasing frequency as angiography is utilized more often to evaluate trauma patients. The usefulness of angiography in trauma is shown by one study where 42 percent of patients with clinical evidence of carotid injury had normal angiograms and 20 percent of those with no cranial signs subsequently had positive studies (83). Cranial CT is useful to rule out intra- and extraaxial hematomas as a cause of neurologic findings but of course does not rule out associated vascular injury, and unfortunately CT seldom demonstrates infarcts in the first few hours. Injury patterns in the head and neck are the same as elsewhere, but clinical presentation may differ. Blunt trauma to the neck may result in delayed carotid occlusion with a lucid interval of 1 to 24 hours before symptoms develop. The postulated mechanism is stretching of the vessel with intimal disruption or disruption of a preexisting atheromatous plaque. A wall hematoma or intimal flap then forms with resultant occlusion or stenosis (84). The carotid bifurcation and proximal internal carotid are most frequently involved. The vertebral artery is less commonly involved in trauma than the carotid, presumably because it is encased in a bony canal for most of its course. Arteriovenous fistulas in the head and neck offer a challenge to the interventional neuroradiologist, especially when they are located in surgically difficult areas such as the cavernous sinus, vertebral canal, and high cervical carotid regions (85) (Figure 13-37).

References

1. Seldinger SI: catheter replacement of needle in percutaneous arteriography: New technique. Acta Radiol (Stockh) 1953, 39:368.
2. Neiman HL, Yao JST: *Angiography of Vascular Disease*. New York, Churchill Livingstone, 1985.
3. White RI: *Fundamentals of Vascular Radiology*. Philadelphia, Lea & Febiger, 1976.
4. Gerlock AJ Jr, Mirfakhraee M: *Essentials of Diagnostic & Interventional Angiographic Techniques*. Philadelphia, Saunders, 1985.
5. Snyder C, Cramer R, Amplatz K: Isolation of sodium as a cause of ventricular fibrillation. Invest Radiol. 1971, 6:245–248.
6. Hilal SK: Hemodynamic responses in the cerebral vessel to angiographic contrast media. Acta Radiol [Diagn] (Stockh) 1966, 5:211–231.
7. Pillay UKG, Robbins PC, Schwartz FP, Kark RM: Acute renal failure following intravenous urography on patients with longstanding diabetes mellitis and azotemia. Radiology 1970, 95:633–636.
8. Shehadi WH: Contrast media adverse reactions: Occurrence, recurrence, and distribution patterns. Radiology 1982, 143:11–17.
9. Hartman GW, Hattery RR, Wilton DW, Williamson B: Mortality during excretory urography: The Mayo Clinic experience. AJR 1982, 139:919–922.
10. Mani RL, Eisenberg RL, McDonald EJ Jr: Complications of catheter cerebral ateriography: Analysis of 5,000 procedures. I. Criteria and incidence. AJR 1978, 131:861.
11. Hessel SJ, Adams DF, Abrams HL: Complications of angiography. Radiology 1981, 138:273.
12. Braunwald E: *Heart Disease*. Philadelphia, Saunders, 1980.
13. Wade GL, Smith DC, Mohr LL: Follow-up of 50 consecutive angiograms obtained utilizing puncture of prosthetic vascular grafts. Radiology 1983, 146:663.
14. Weinshelbaum A, Carson SN: Separation of angiographic catheter during arteriography through vascular graft. AJR 1980, 134:583.
15. DeBakey ME, McCollum CH, Graham JM: Surgical treatment of aneurysms of the descending thoracic aorta: Long-term results in 500 patients. J Cardiovasc Surg (Torino) 1978, 19:571.
16. Randal PA, Tarmolowski CR: Aneurysms of the thoracic aorta. In Abrams HL (ed): *Abrams Angiography*. Boston, Little, Brown 1983, p. 417.
17. Parmley LF, Mattingly TW, Manion WC, Jahnke EJ Jr: Nonpenetrating traumatic injury of the aorta. Circulation 1958, 17:1086.
18. Daniels DL, Maddison FE: Ascending aortic injury: Angiographic diagnosis. AJR 1981, 136:812.
19. Seltzer SE, D'Orsi CJ, Kirshner R, DeWeese JA: Traumatic aortic rupture: Plain radiographic findings. AJR 1981, 137(2):1011.
20. Woodring JH, Pulmano CM, Stevens RK: Right paratracheal stripe in blunt chest trauma. Radiology 1982, 143:605.
21. Richardson JD, McElvin RB, Trunkle JK: First rib fracture: A hallmark of severe trauma. Ann Surg 1975, 181:251.
22. Fisher RG, Ward RE, Ben-Menachem Y, Mattox KL, Flynn TC: Arteriography and fractured first rib: Too much for too little? AJR 1982, 138(2):1059.
23. Woodring JH, Fried AM, Hatfield DR: Fractures of first and second ribs: Predictive value for arterial and bronchial injury. AJR 1982, 138:211.
24. Lazro S, Harley DP, Grinnell VS, White RA, Nelson RJ: Should all patients with first rib fracture undergo arteriography? J Thorac Cardiovasc Surg 1982, 83:532.
25. Abrams HL: Dissecting aortic aneurysm. In Abrams HL (ed): *Abrams Angiography*. Boston, Little, Brown, 1983, p 457.
26. Lindsay J Jr, Hurst JW: Clinical features and prognosis in dissecting aneurysms of the aorta. Circulation 1967, 35:880.

27. Earnest FE IV, Muhm JR, Sheedy FP II: Roentgenographic finding in thoracic aortic dissection. May Clin Proc 1979, 54:43.
28. Abrams HL: Dissecting aortic aneurysm. In Abrams HL (ed): *Abrams Angiography*. Boston, Little, Brown, 1983, p 455.
29. Godwin JP, Turley K, Herfkens RJ, Lipton MJ: Computed tomography for follow-up of chronic aortic dissections. Radiology 1981, 139:655.
30. Lande A, Berkmen YM: Aortitis: Pathologic, clinical and arteriographic review. Radiol Clin North Am 1976, 14:219.
31. Grollman JH, Renner JW: Transfemoral pulmonary angiography: Update on technique. AJR 1981. 136:624.
32. Mills SR, Jackson DC, Older RA, Heaston DK, Moore AV: Incidence, etiologies and avoidance of complications of pulmonary angiography in a large series. Radiology 1975, 136:295.
33. Loop JW, Archer G, Northrop CH: Bedside pulmonary arteriography. Radiology 1975, 114:469.
34. Mathur VS, Dalen JE, Evans H, Haynes FW, Pur-Shahriari AA, Stein PD, Dexter L: Pulmonary angiography one to seven days after experimental pulmonary embolism. Invest Radiol 1967, 2:304.
35. Wildrich WC, Robbins AH, Nabseth DC, Johnson WC, Goldstein SA: Pitfalls of transhepatic portal venography and therapeutic coronary vein occlusion. AJR 1978, 131(2):637.
36. Hoiseth A, Amundsen P: Pulmonary angiography in lung and mediastinal tumor. In Abrams HL (ed): *Abrams Angiography*. Boston, Little, Brown, 1983, p 817.
37. Widrich WC, Robbins AH, Nabseth DC, Johnson WC, Goldstein SA: Pitfalls of transhepatic portal venography and therapeutic coronary vein occlusion AJR 1978, 131:637.
38. Lunderquist A, Vang J: Transhepatic catheterization and obliteration of the coronary vein in patients with portal hypertension and esophageal varices. N Engl J Med 1974, 291:646.
39. Keller FS, Rosch J, Dotter CT: Transhepatic obliteration of gastroesophageal varices with absolute ethanol. Radiology 1983, 146:615.
40. Bengmarks S, Borjesson B, Hoevals J, Joelsson B, Lunderquist A, Owman T: Obliteration of esophageal varices by PTP: Follow-up of 43 patients. Ann Surg 1979, 190:549.
41. Ellman BA, Curry TS III, Glotzbach RE, Simpson PR: Systemic embolization as a complication of transhepatic venography. Radiology 1981, 141:67.
42. Sano A, Yasumasa K, Funinori M, Takahashi Y, Koizumi S, Kimura S, Okuda K: Porto-pulmonary venous anastomosis in portal hypertension demonstrated by percutaneous transhepatic cineportography. Radiology 1982, 144:479.
43. Gonzalez: Portography: A preliminary report of a new technique via the umbilical vein. Clin Proc Child Hosp DC 1959, 15:120.
44. Spigos DG, Tauber JW, Tan W, Mulligan BD, Espinoza GA: Work in progress: Umbilical venous cannulation: A new approach for embolization of esophageal varices. Radiology 1983, 146:53.
45. Reuter SR, Redman HC: *Gastrointestinal Angiography*. Philadelphia, Saunders, 1977.
46. Sigstedt B, Lunderquist A: Complications of angiographic examinations. AJR 1978, 130:455.
47. Soo C-S, Wallace S, Chaung VP, Charnsangavej C, Bowers TA: Injury to the intima of the hepatic artery. Radiology 1982, 143:373.
48. Jeffrey RB, Laing FC, Federle MP, Goodman PC: Computed tomography of splenic trauma. Radiology 1981, 141:729.
49. Alavi A, Ring EJ: Localization of gastrointestinal bleeding: Superiority of ^{99m}Tc sulfur colloid compared with angiography. AJR 1981, 137:741.
50. Winzelberg GG, Froelich JW, McKusick KA, Waltman AC, Greenfield AJ, Athanasoulis CA, Strauss HW: Radionuclide localization of lower gastrointestinal hemorrhage. Radiology 1981, 139:465.
51. Athanosoulis CA: Upper gastrointestinal bleeding of artero-capillary origin. In Athanosoulis CA, Pfister RC, Greene RE, Roberson GH (eds): *Interventional Radiology*. Philadelphia, Saunders, 1982, p 81.
52. Rosenkrantz H, Bookstein JJ, Rosen RJ, Goff WB II, Healy JF: Postembolic colon infarction. Radiology 1982, 142:47.
53. Baum S: Arteriographic diagnosis and treatment of gastrointestinal bleeding. In Abrams HL (ed): *Abrams Angiography*. Boston, Little, Brown, 1983, p 1689.
54. Johnson WC, Widrich WC, Ansell JE, Robbins AH, Nabseth DC: Control of bleeding varices by vasopressin: A prospective randomized study. Ann Surg 1977, 186:369.
55. Reuter SR, Redman HC: *Gastrointestinal Angiography*. Philadelphia, Saunders, 1977, p 88.
56. Boley SJ, Brandt LJ, Verth FJ: Ischemic disorders of the intestines. Curr Prob Surg 1978, 15(4):1.
57. Boley SJ, Sprayregan S, Siegelman SS, Verth FJ: Initial results from an aggressive roentgenological and surgical approach to acute mesenteric ischemia. Surgery 1977, 82:848.
58. Boijsen E: Angiographic studies of the anatomy of single and multiple renal arteries. Acta Radiol 1959, (suppl)183.
59. Bosniak MA, Ambos MA, Madayag MA, Lefleur RS, Casarella WJ: Epinephrine enhanced renal angiography in renal mass lesions: Is it worth performing? AJR 1977, 129(2):647.
60. Bookstein JJ: Appraisal of arteriography in estimating the hemodynamic significance of renal artery stenoses. Invest Radiol 1966, 1:281.
61. Burt RL, Johnston FR, Silverthorne RG, Lock FR, Dickerson AJ: Ruptured renal artery aneurysm report of a case with survival. Obstet Gynecol 1956, 7:229.
62. Grinnell VS, Hieshima SB, Mehringer CM, Tsai F, Shaw S, Irwin RJ: Therapeutic renal artery occlusion with a detachable balloon J Urol 1981, 126:233–237.
63. Abrams HL: Renal arteriography in hypertension. In Abrams HL (ed): *Abrams Angiography*. Boston, Little, Brown, 1983, pp 1255–1257.
64. Dos Santos R, Lamas AC, Pereira-Caldas J: Arteriografiada aorta e dos vosos abdominais. Med Contemp 1929, 47:93.
65. Gordon IJ, Wescott JL: Intraarterial lidocaine. An effective analgesic for peripheral angiography. Radiology 1977, 124:43.
66. Eisenberg RL, Mani RL, Hedgicock MW: Pain associated with peripheral angiography: Is lidocaine effective? Radiology 1978, 127:109.
67. Haimavia H, Shapiro JH, Jacobson HG: Serial femoral arteriography in occlusive disease: Clinical roentgenologic considerations with a new classification of occlusive patterns AJR 1960, 83:1042.
68. Lindblom A: Arterosclerosis and arterial thrombosis in the lower limb: A roentgenological study. Acta Radiol (Stockh) 1950, 80(suppl):1.
69. Edwards EA, LeMoy M: Occlusion pattern and collateral in arteriosclerosis of the lower aorta and iliac arteries. Surgery 1955, 38:950.
70. Lipchik EO, Rogoff SM: The abnormal abdominal aorta: Arteriosclerosis and other diseases. In Abrams HL (ed): *Abrams Angiography*. Boston, Little, Brown, 1983, pp 1069–1076.
71. Chart A, Maltz A, Wilson JH: The collateral arterial circulation in the pelvis: An angiographic study. AJR 1968, 102:392.
72. Draponos T, Hewit RL, Weichert RF III, Smith AD: Civilian vascular injuries: A critical appraisal of three decades of management. Ann Surg 1970, 172:351–360.
73. Hardin WD Jr Mattox KL, Feliciano AV, DeBakey ME: Vascular injuries of the axilla. Ann Surg 1982, 195:232–238.
74. Rabinov K, Paulin K: Venography of the lower extremities. In Abrams HL (ed): *Abrams Angiography*. Boston, Little, Brown, 1983, p 1877.
75. Grollman JH, Weber MW, Soms AS: Phlebography and radionuclide clot localization in the lower extremities. Radiol Clin North Am 1976, 14:309.

76. Browse W: Diagnosis of deep vein thrombosis. Med Bull 1978, 34:163–167.
77. Lisbona R, Stern J, Derbekyan V: ^{99m}Tc red blood cell venography in deep vein thrombosis of the leg: A correlation with contrast venography. Radiology 1982, 143:771–773.
78. Cranley JJ, Canos AJ, Sull WS: The diagnosis of deep venous thrombosis. Arch Surg 1976, 111:34–36.
79. Yao STY, Bergan JJ, Neiman HL: *Angiography of Vascular Disease*. New York, Churchill Livingstone, 1985, pp 353–391.
80. Lang EK: Arteriography of thoracic outlet syndrome. In Abrams HL (ed): *Abrams Angiography*. Boston, Little Brown, 1983, pp 1001–1015.
81. Harley DP, White PA, Nelson RJ, Mehringer CM: Pulmonary embolism secondary to venous thrombosis of the arm. Am J Surg 1984, 147:221–224.
82. Herfkens RJ, Higgins CB, Hricak H, Lipton MJ, Crooks LE, Sheldon PE, Kaufman L: Nuclear magnetic resonance imaging of atherosclerotic disease. Radiology 1983, 148:161.
83. McCormack TM, Burch BH: Routine angiographic evaluation of neck and extremity injuries. *J Trauma* 1979, 19:384–387.
84. Yamada S, Kindt GW, Youmans JR: Carotid artery occlusion due to non-penetrating trauma. J Trauma 1967, 7:333–342.
85. Mehringer CM, Grinnell VS, Hieshima GB: Therapeutic embolization of trauma to the head and neck. AJNR 1983, 4:137–142.

Chapter 14

DIGITAL SUBTRACTION ANGIOGRAPHY: ITS USE IN THE DIAGNOSIS AND MANAGEMENT OF VASCULAR DISEASE

WILLIAM D. TURNIPSEED

Since the pioneering work of Moniz and Dos Santos, standard angiography has played an essential role in the diagnosis and management of vascular disease. Arterial imaging made it possible to accurately define the anatomic characteristics of occlusive and aneurysmal disease within the arterial circulation. This ability to precisely define the location and severity of arterial lesions combined with new surgical techniques made vascular reconstructive surgery a reality. Although angiography was originally used to diagnose patients suspected of having vascular occlusive disease, physicians soon became aware of the risks and costs that were involved in using angiography for diagnostic screening. The need for hospitalization and arterial catheterization combined with rather poor patient acceptance restricted the use of standard angiography. Standard arteriography is generally used to provide an anatomic display of vascular disease in symptomatic patients who are considered candidates for vascular reconstructive surgery.

Because of the arteriography's limited practical use, the development of noninvasive techniques has flourished. These tests have enabled clinicians to more accurately evaluate persons at risk for vascular disease and to more objectively define the hemodynamic and physiological significance of known or suspected vascular lesions. Most of these tests were designed to identify the presence of hemodynamically significant occlusive disease in isolated vascular segments and require the expertise and interpretative skills of trained personnel. They cannot accurately define the vascular anatomy in remote areas of the circulation (intrathoracic, intraabdominal, intracranial segments) and easily miss minor stenoses, ulcerated plaques, or aneurysmal lesions. Although noninvasive testing has improved our ability to identify potentially threatening vascular diseases and to more objectively define the functional consequences of known arterial lesions, it has not eliminated the need for the anatomic information provided by angiography (1–7).

Recent developments in the area of computerized image enhancement have made it possible to visualize the arterial circulation by the intravenous injection of a contrast agent. This technique has been referred to by a variety of terms including digital video angiography (DVA), digital video imaging (DVI), or digital subtraction angiography (DSA). These terms are interchangeably used to describe a process of arterial imaging made possible by computerized fluoroscopy (8–12). DSA has generated interest among physicians because of its ability to combine many of the safety features of noninvasive testing with the anatomic information provided by standard angiography. Intravenous DSA significantly reduces the risk of hemorrhage and thrombosis by avoiding arterial catheterization and lowers the potential costs by reducing the need for hospitalization. The patient acceptance is better because there is less discomfort and because the time required to perform the procedure is significantly shorter. However, in order to determine the appropriate clinical applications of DSA, one must look critically not only at its strengths, but at its weaknesses as well.

Technique

Although DSA can be performed by the intravenous or intraarterial injection of contrast medium, initial interest was focused on the intravenous technique. Arterial imaging is obtained by power-injecting a bolus of standard contrast medium (40 to 60 mL) into the peripheral venous circulation at a rate of 11 to 15 mL/s. Although contrast material can be injected through a short catheter placed in an antecubital vein, experience suggests that better results can be obtained by using a long no. 5F catheter which is threaded retrograde through a vein in the antecubital fossa into the subclavian vein or superior vena cava. If upper-extremity venous access is not available, contrast medium can be injected through a catheter placed retrograde from the femoral vein into the iliac or inferior vena cava. The central placement of the catheter and the use of power injection ensure a crisp delivery of the contrast bolus to the right side of the heart and reduce the possibility of the extravasation or perforation of the vein. Immediately after the contrast medium is injected, a fluoroscopic mask image is taken of the area of anatomic interest. This image is stored in one of two memory units within the digital videoprocessor and is referred to as the mask image. The mask image stores bone and soft densities before the arrival of the contrast medium in the peripheral vessels. As the contrast agent is pumped from the heart into the peripheral circulation, it is identified under fluoroscopy, and then a sequence of 6 to 10 serial images are taken at 1-s intervals. These sequential images are stored in the second, parallel memory unit, where contrast densities are summated and then subtracted from the video mask. This gives an enhanced arterial image which is displayed on a television screen and which can be converted to hard-copy angiograms by a multiformat camera. Image reprocessing can be performed by using later serial images as a video mask to refine the image quality and is of particular value in cases in which image distortion has occurred because of patient movement.

When compared with standard angiography, intravenous DSA (IVDSA) has some obvious advantages. It is safer because arterial catheterization and its complications can be avoided. It is also cheaper because studies can be performed on an outpatient basis. An outpatient IVDSA exam costs approximately 450 dollars, while a standard arteriogram costs about 1500 dollars (including interpretation fees and hospitalization costs). Despite these apparent advantages, IVDSA has some shortcomings as well. The limitations intrinsic to IVDSA include a small image-field size (9 in = 22.9 cm), an image-quality degradation associated with motion, a limited spatial resolution, and a restriction to single-plane imaging. The small field size and the restriction to single-plane imaging mean that multiple injections of contrast material are necessary for complete peripheral vascular imaging. The amount of contrast material required has been significantly reduced by using new-generation image intensifiers which have a 14-in field (35.6 cm). Limited spatial resolution is another problem. The focal spot is about 0.6 mm, which means that the fine detail in small vessels cannot be accurately seen and that web stenosis and small ulcerations can be easily missed. IVDSA increases the contrast opacification but at a sacrifice of spatial detail. The resolution of a digital angiogram with a 512 × 512 pixilformat is in the range of 2 line pairs per millimeter, whereas standard angiography provides resolution of 6 to 10 line pairs per millimeter (8–14). Biplane imaging with IVDSA is not feasible because a costly duplication of hardware is necessary. As a consequence additional contrast injections are required if more than one arterial projection is needed. The risk for renal complications increases significantly when more than 200 mL of contrast medium is used in patients who have altered kidney function or insulin-dependent diabetes.

Any motion on the part of the patient, be it voluntary or involuntary, causes image distortion and detracts from the clinical value of the study. Involuntary motion is most commonly encountered because of a hot, painful sensation when the contrast agent is injected into the vascular system. Patient discomfort can be significantly reduced by mixing lidocaine with the ionic contrast medium (1 mL per 10 mL of contrast medium). Nonionic contrast agents are currently being tested, and the initial results suggest that these agents are safer for patients who are sensitive to the ionic contrast agents and that they reduce the problem of patient motion because there is less discomfort when they are injected (15). The high cost of these agents at present precludes their routine clinical use, however. Involuntary motion is also a problem when the abdominal vessels are imaged. Peristalsis of the gastrointestinal tract can cause artifacts which impair image quality. Intravenous glucagon has proved to be useful in suppressing gut activity during these DSA studies (16). Although it is possible to minimize the image distortion from involuntary patient movement, it is obvious that complete patient cooperation is necessary in order to obtain an adequate clinical study. Therefore, patient selection is important. Persons who cannot follow verbal commands, patients in cardiorespiratory distress, and victims of massive soft tissue injury are poor candidates for IVDSA because of the high probability of artifact imaging.

Although the initial focus of interest was on IVDSA, there has been a growing awareness that computer techniques can significantly enhance the safety and quality of imaging obtained by standard intraarterial methods. The advantages of intraarterial (IA)DSA include an increased contrast resolution, reduced contrast-volume requirements, and the use of smaller arterial catheters. The direct injection of contrast medium into the arterial system means that better opacification of the contrast medium can be obtained and that fine detail in the smaller vessels of the distal peripheral circulation can be expected (17). In addition, IADSA can reduce the absolute volume and concentration of the contrast agents used for arterial imaging. This means that the risk for renal failure, particularly in insulin-dependent diabetics and in patients with altered renal function, can be significantly reduced. It also means that diagnostic angiography can be performed in the neonatal and pediatric age groups in a much safer fashion. Clinicians are just now becoming aware of the important ways that DSA can be used to improve the accuracy and safety of intraarterial imaging. The smaller catheters and the smaller volumes of the contrast agent required for imaging should make it feasible to perform outpatient intraarterial imaging. The improved contrast opacification makes it possible to more precisely define the true anatomic condition of distal tibial vessels in ischemic lower extremities, which are often poorly visualized by standard injection techniques. IADSA makes it possible to avoid many of the technical errors which make clinical interpretation difficult and which may adversely affect management decisions. IADSA techniques can also be used during routine standard angiography as a means of screening for main stem in situ coronary occlusive disease and to determine the anatomic significance of suspected carotid lesions.

Clinical Applications of IVDSA

The most common application of IVDSA has been in the evaluation of the cerebral vascular system. This technique has been very attractive as a means of diagnostic screening because it provides anatomic information about the brachiocephalic circulation without the risks of standard angiography. Although IVDSA has played an increasingly important role in the assessment of patients suspected of being at risk for stroke, its exact role in the diagnosis and management of cerebral vascular disease has not been completely defined. The proper utilization of DSA can be clinically rewarding, but its inappropriate use can be frustrating and oftentimes misleading. Numerous studies have clearly demonstrated that IVDSA is very effective in identifying occlusive and severely stenotic lesions in the brachiocephalic and extracranial arterial circulation (18–24). Interestingly enough, the same group of hemodynamically significant lesions can be accurately detected by a number of noninvasive techniques including oculoplethysmography (Karchner/Gee), phonoangiography, duplex scanning, and Doppler spectral frequency analysis. The general trend of experience thus far suggests that for hemodynamically significant lesions (stenoses with diameter reductions exceeding 50 percent), there is little difference in diagnostic accuracy between IVDSA and noninvasive testing (25–27). The sensitivity, defined as the proportion of positive DSA or noninvasive tests in arteries with positive conventional angiograms, and the specificity, defined as the proportion of negative DSA or noninvasive tests in comparison with negative conventional angiograms, are nearly identical as measured by either technique. However, IVDSA is more dependable than noninvasive testing for the detection of complete internal carotid occlusion (25–28).

It is important to consider the risk and cost of diagnostic screening. Although IVDSA is safer than standard angiography, it remains an invasive technique with identifiable risks (contrast hypersensitivity, renal failure, etc.). Noninvasive tests are almost free of complications. DSA is more expensive than noninvasive tests. A noninvasive diagnostic study costs between 115 and 240 dollars, whereas an outpatient digital angiogram costs about 450 dollars. This suggests that noninvasive testing is appropriate for the evaluation of patients with asymptomatic cervical bruits (25,27). The hemodynamically significant carotid bifurcation lesions can be accurately determined in this manner, and on the basis of these preliminary screening tests, specific anatomic information can be obtained by digital or standard angiography if so desired.

The anatomic definition of disease becomes more important in patients who have symptoms of cerebral vascular insufficiency (Figure 14-1). Transient or permanent neurologic deficits that can be localized to one hemisphere suggest carotid-origin ischemia. Before the advent of DSA, most patients with transient or stabilized symptoms of cerebral insufficiency were evaluated by standard arteriograms. Noninvasive testing in these symptomatic patients was not as important because management was based on the anatomy of carotid disease shown by arteriography. In many ways, the development of DSA has enhanced the role of noninvasive testing in symptomatic patients. The hemodynamic classification of disease by noninvasive tests makes it

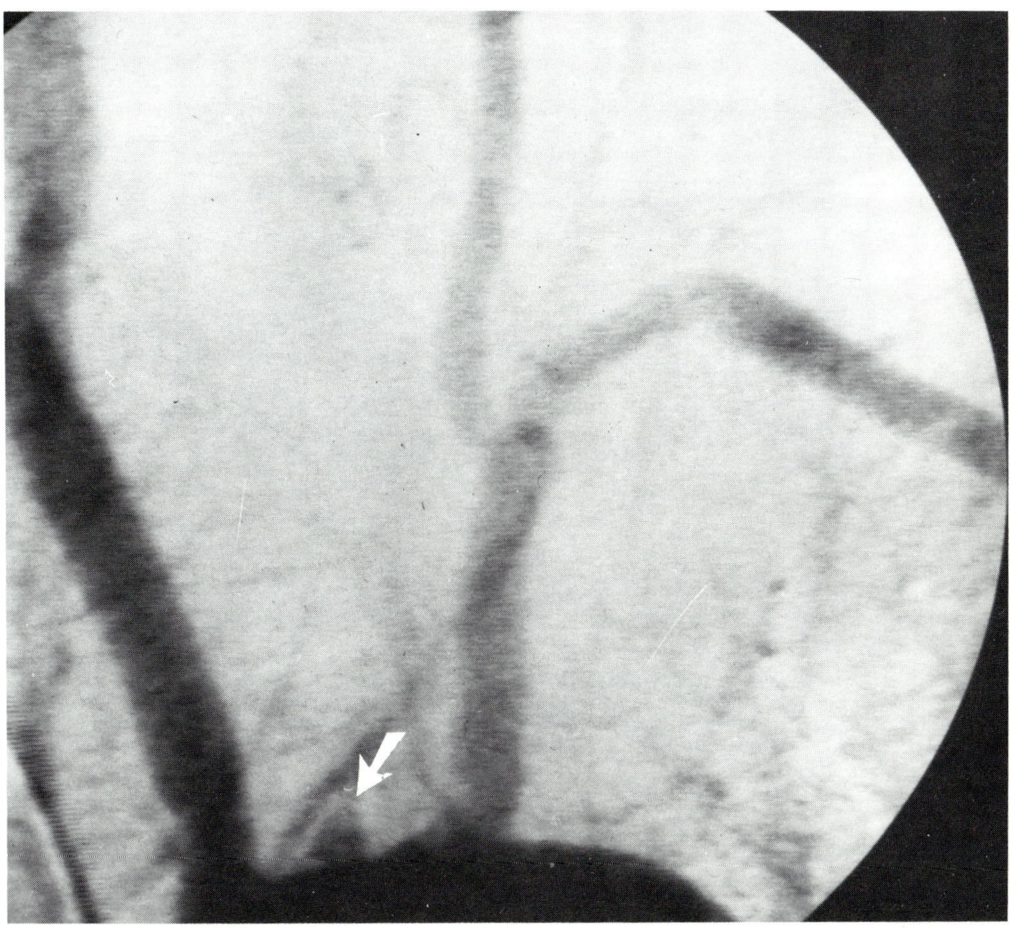

FIGURE 14-1. This intravenous digital arteriogram of the aortic arch demonstrates complete occlusion of the left common carotid artery (*arrow*). Arch views are suggested in all symptomatic patients in order to rule out stenotic or occlusive lesions at the origin of the brachiocephalic vessels.

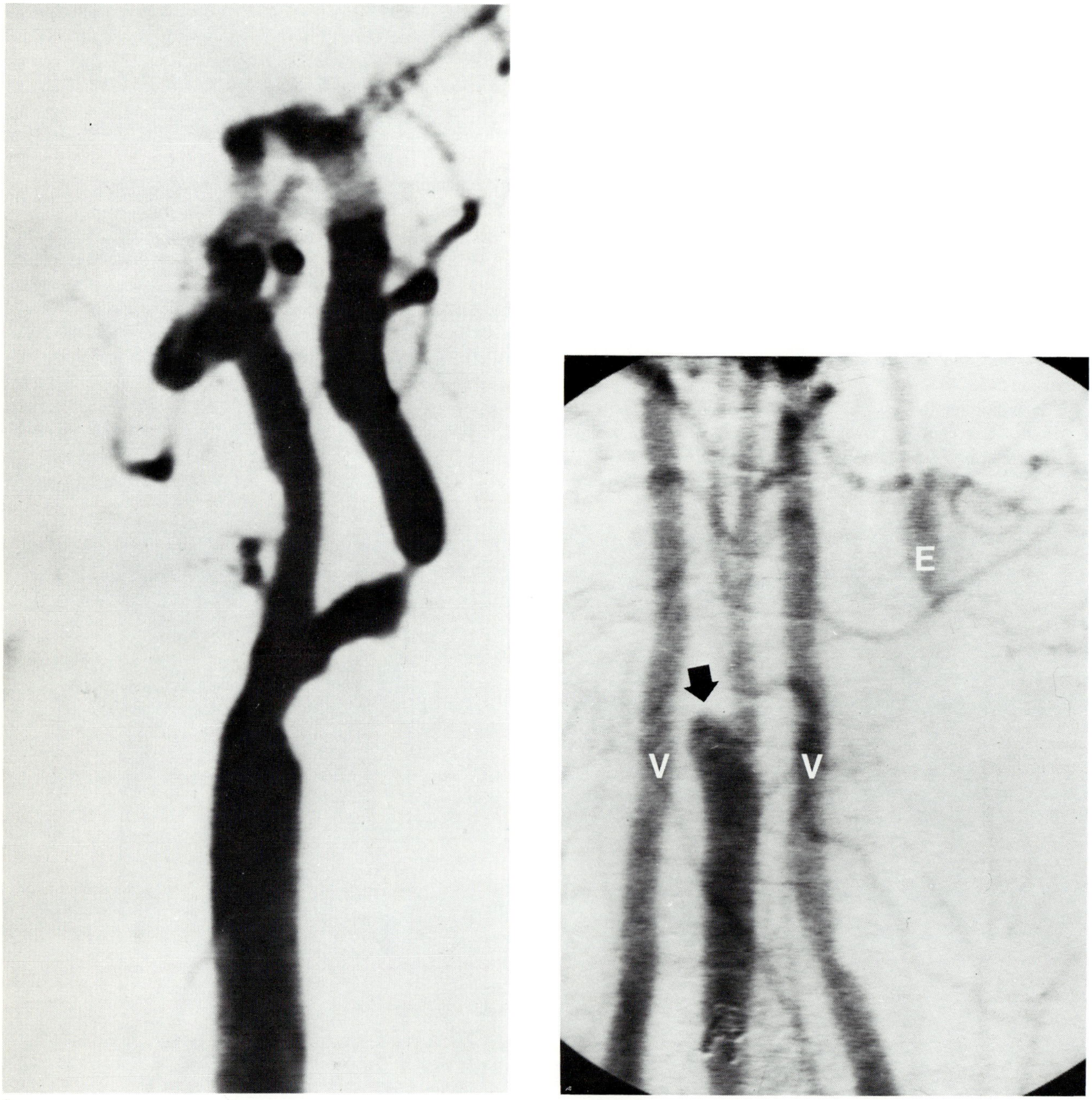

A B

FIGURE 14-2. (*A*) This IVDSA demonstrates a hemodynamically significant stenosis of the internal carotid branch. IVDSA is most accurate in identifying lesions of hemodynamic significance in the carotid bifurcation. (*B*) This intravenous digital arteriogram demonstrates large vertebral arteries V bordering the common carotid artery and occluded internal branch (*arrow*). The left common carotid artery is completely obstructed, and the external branch E is reconstituted by a collateral branch from the right external carotid artery.

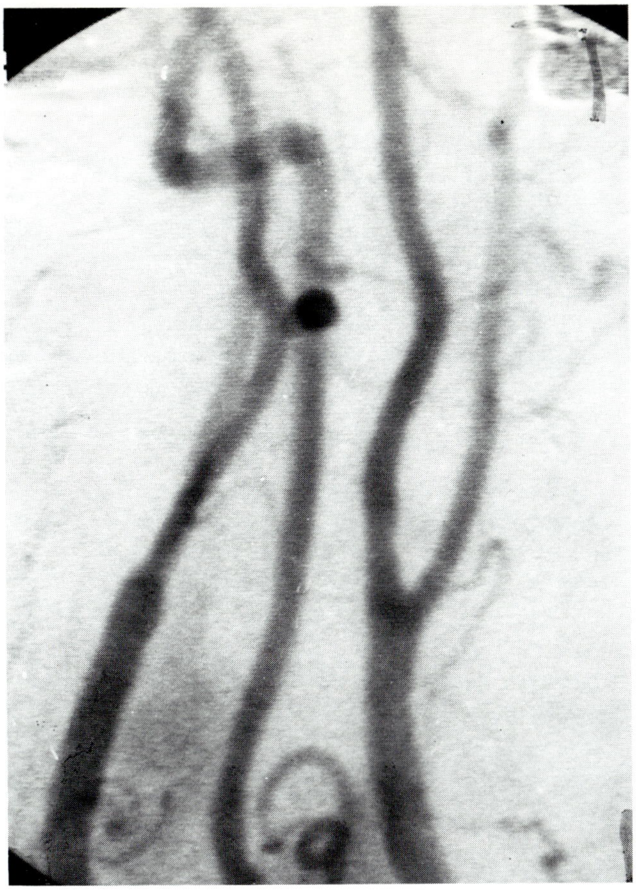

FIGURE 14-3. This IVDSA study performed in the left oblique projection demonstrates a normal left carotid bifurcation. Another injection in the right oblique position is necessary in order to profile the obscured right carotid bifurcation. Failure to profile both carotid bifurcations may result in a false-negative study.

possible to more appropriately select the most productive form of diagnostic arterial imaging (7,18,19, 24–29). In patients who show focal symptoms of cerebral insufficiency, IVDSA is the safest, cheapest, and most accurate method of determining the anatomy of carotid disease when noninvasive tests show severe occlusive disease to be present (>75 percent reduction in the transverse diameter). In symptomatic patients 96 percent of the severe carotid lesions can be identified by IVDSA (25,26) (Figure 14-2). Failure to identify a critical stenosis usually results from a technically inadequate study due to a motion artifact, poor positioning, a failure to profile the carotid bifurcation, decreased cardiac output and prolonged circulation time, or resolution limitations of the technique (Figure 14-3). Failure to identify a suspected critical lesion occurs in about 4 percent of the cases and mandates intraarterial angiography (25,27).

In patients with focal cerebral ischemic symptoms who are found by noninvasive testing to have noncritical, but hemodynamically significant, disease (50 to 75 percent reduction in the diameter of the transverse lumen), the accuracy of IVDSA is less predictable. The sensitivity for detecting disease is about 88 percent, and the specificity for ruling out disease is about 86 percent. Clinically inadequate studies occur in about 5 percent of all symptomatic carotids that have hemodynamic lesions of moderate severity (25,27–29).

Comparative studies suggest that IVDSA is more accurate than noninvasive testing in the evaluation of hemodynamically insignificant disease (<50 percent reduction in the diameter of the transverse lumen) (25–29). With the exception of real-time imaging, most noninvasive tests are incapable of identifying ulcerative lesions in the carotid circulation. IVDSA is capable of demonstrating the larger ulcerations commonly associated with stenosis, but misses minor ulcerations because of limitations in spatial resolution (Figure 14-4). IVDSA identifies approximately 33 percent of all ulcerated lesions that can be identified by standard imaging techniques (25,27). These data suggest that patients presenting with focal symptoms of cerebral ischemia who are found by noninvasive testing to have hemodynamically insignificant disease should have intraarterial angiography (standard or DSA). The intraarterial angiography is better than IVDSA for identifying minor grades of stenosis and ulceration in the carotid bifurcations and for visualizing small vessels in the intracranial circulation (Figure 14-5). The technique of intraarterial imaging can be tailored to the needs of the patient. IADSA has significant advantages over standard angiography. Smaller catheters can be used, and selective catheterization is less commonly necessary. The spatial resolution is nearly equivalent to that of standard angiography, and the contrast opacification is actually improved when one considers that the volume of the contrast medium can be reduced by 30 percent and that the concentration of the contrast medium can be reduced by almost 75 percent. Therefore, diagnostic radiography can be performed more safely in neonatal and pediatric patients, and the risks for renal failure can be reduced in patients with diabetes or altered renal function. IADSA or intraarterial standard angiography is preferred over IVDSA for diagnosing intracranial aneurysms, occlusions, arterial venous malformations, and tumors (Figure 14-6). Although IVDSA can detect major stenoses or aneurysms of the carotid siphon, the small-vessel detail is inadequate (Figure 14-7). The use of standard angiography will undoubtedly be reduced as IADSA techniques are learned (19,28).

Noninvasive testing and DSA also play an important role in the postoperative assessment of patients after carotid endarterectomy or intracranial vascular reconstructive surgery (30). Noninvasive tests are the cheapest and most effective way of following patients who remain asymptomatic after carotid endarterectomy. The noninvasive tests are very accurate in identifying hemodynamically significant occlusive disease and can be used to identify recurrent stenosis at postoperative sites and to monitor the progression of disease in the unoperated carotids. IVDSA should be performed only on patients who have recurrent symptoms of cerebral insufficiency or severe recurrent stenosis after carotid endarterectomy (20,21,26) (Figure 14-8). Noninvasive tests are less likely to be of value in the assessment of intracranial vascular reconstructive procedures. Although IVDSA can identify patent intracranial grafts, the fine vascular detail is better displayed by intraarterial DSA or by standard angiography (28).

In summary, standard arteriograms are more accurate than IVDSA or noninvasive tests in identifying minor carotid stenoses and ulcerated plaques. IVDSA is almost as accurate as standard arteriography or noninvasive testing in the identification of hemodynamically significant stenoses and complete internal carotid

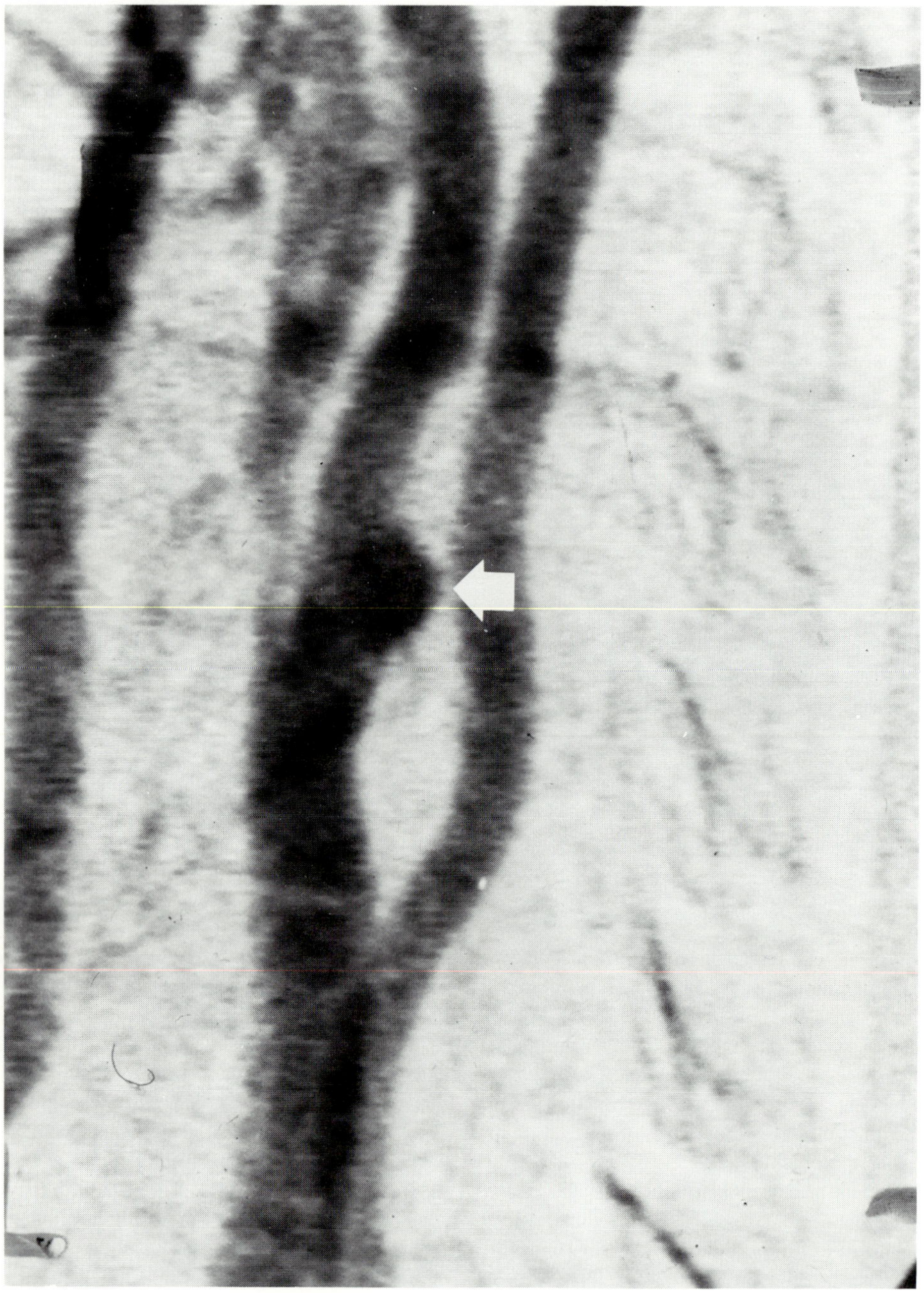

FIGURE 14-4. This IVDSA study shows a large ulceration in the carotid bifurcation area (*arrow*). Although IVDSA can demonstrate larger ulcerations, it misses small ulcerative lesions or web stenoses because of limited spatial resolution. Intraarterial studies (standard or digital) should be done in symptomatic patients when noninvasive tests suggest insignificant disease or when IVDSA studies appear normal.

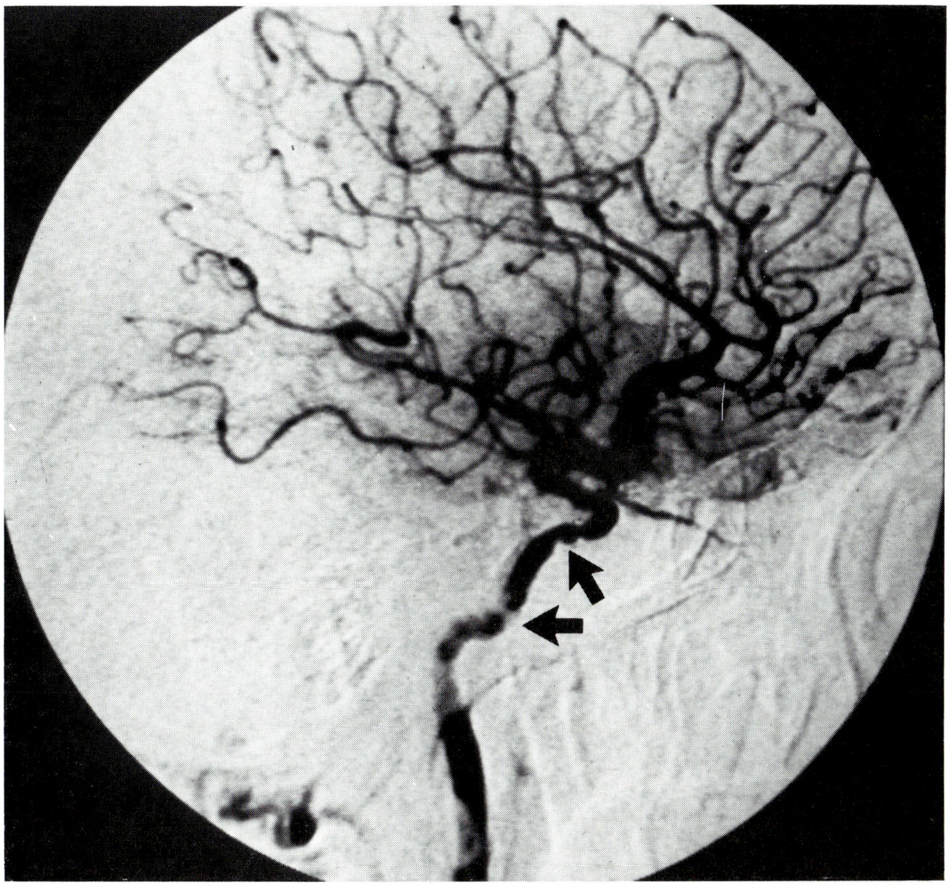

FIGURE 14-5. This IADSA digital arteriogram (performed by injecting 1 mL of contrast material into the common carotid artery) has spatial resolution and fine-vessel detail nearly equivalent to that of standard angiography. Note the stenotic lesion in the siphon (*arrows*) and the small-vessel detail in the peripheral branches.

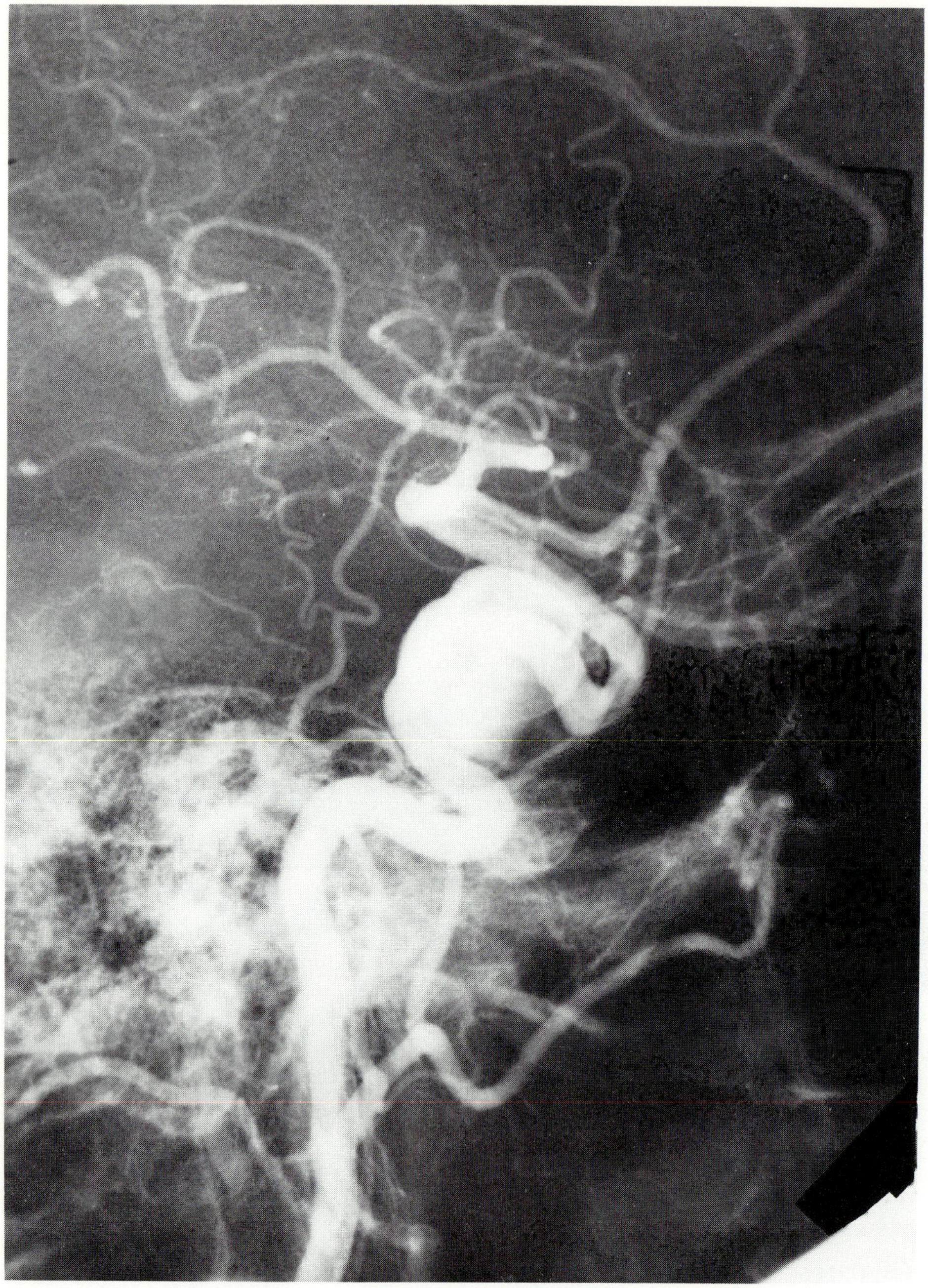

A

FIGURE 14-6. (*A*) This standard arteriogram (obtained by injecting 10 mL of contrast material into the right common carotid artery) demonstrates a large intracerebral aneurysm involving the carotid siphon.

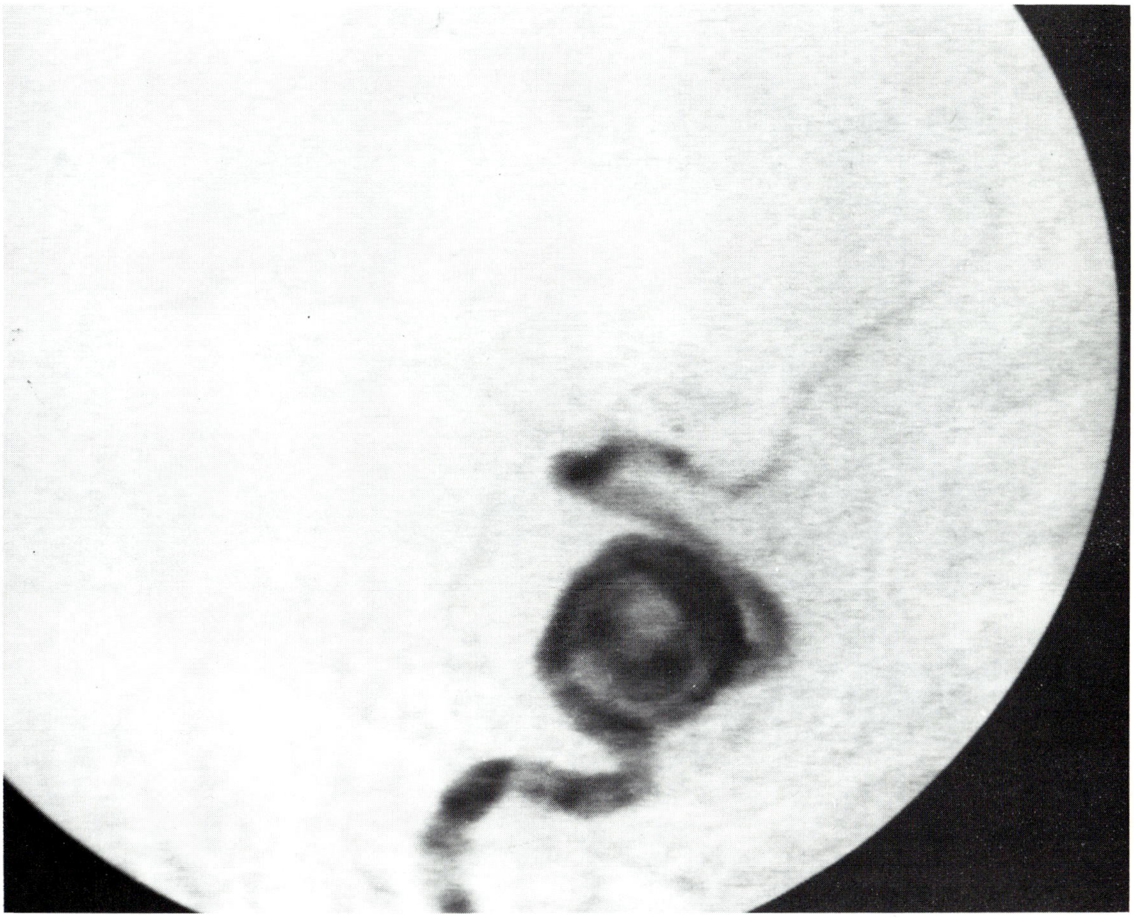

B

FIGURE 14-6 (*continued*). (***B***) An IADSA obtained by injecting 1 mL of contrast material demonstrates the same intracranial aneurysm.

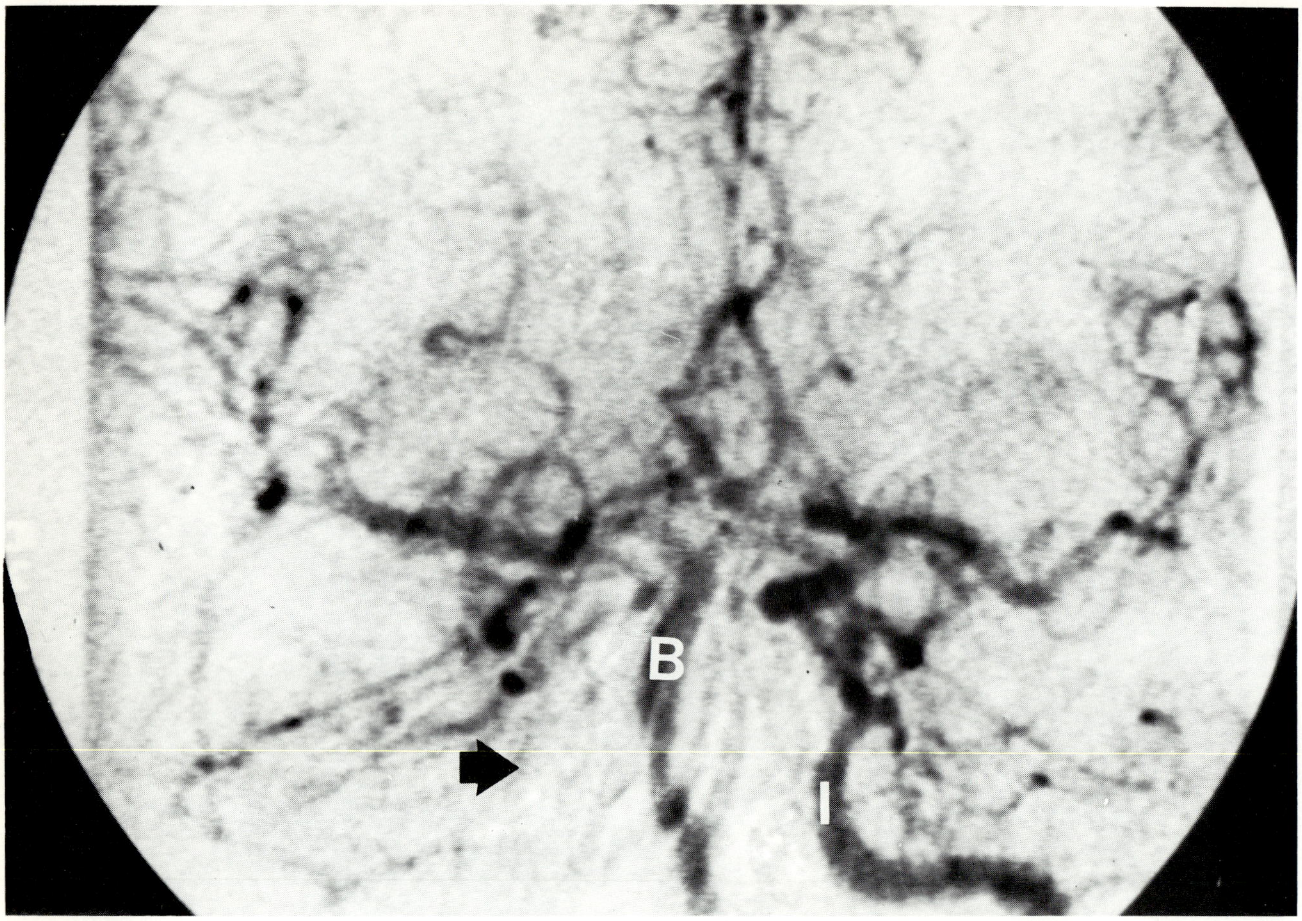

FIGURE 14-7. This IVDSA demonstrates complete occlusion of the right internal carotid artery siphon (*arrow*). Collateral perfusion of the right hemisphere is derived from the contralateral internal carotid I and from the basilar artery B posteriorly. IVDSA can be used to identify major occlusions or large aneurysms in proximal vessels of the circle of Willis. It is unacceptable as a means of evaluating small-vessel disease in the peripheral intracranial vessels.

artery occlusions. Although IVDSA can be used to identify major occlusions and large aneurysms (in the carotid siphons) and to screen for cortical arterial venous malformations, intraarterial studies (digital or standard) are more appropriate in evaluating patients suspected of having intracranial disease. Digital enhancement methods can be safely combined with standard coronary or peripheral angiography to obtain additional anatomic information about the carotid arteries. It is apparent that DSA (intravenous and intraarterial) will expand the role of arterial imaging and alter our use of noninvasive testing in the evaluation of patients with known or suspected cerebral vascular problems (8).

Thoracic and Cardiopulmonary Vascular Disease

IVDSA is useful in diagnosing congenital or acquired lesions of the thoracic aorta. Coarctation, right aortic arch, duplication of the aortic arch, dissection, and aneurysm of the thoracic aorta have all been confirmed by IVDSA (Figure 14-9). This technique also serves as a rapid means for identifying major blunt or penetration injuries to the thoracic aorta in trauma patients whose chest x-rays show mediastinal widening (31–33).

However, the static digital technique (mask-mode radiography) used for imaging the thoracic aorta is inadequate for the dynamic evaluation of cardiac function. Mask-mode fluoroscopy, a method of real-time evaluation in which the mask image is subtracted from a succession of fluoroscopic images at a rate of up to 60 frames per second, makes the dynamic assessment of the contractile heart possible and can be used for performing ventriculography. The image quality is comparable to that of standard angiographic methods. Digital fluoroscopy can be used to calculate ejection fractions by a method of videodensitometry. This technique quantitates the relative volume of iodine in the ventricle during systole and diastole by using a light gun to trace volume changes during the systolic and diastolic motion of the

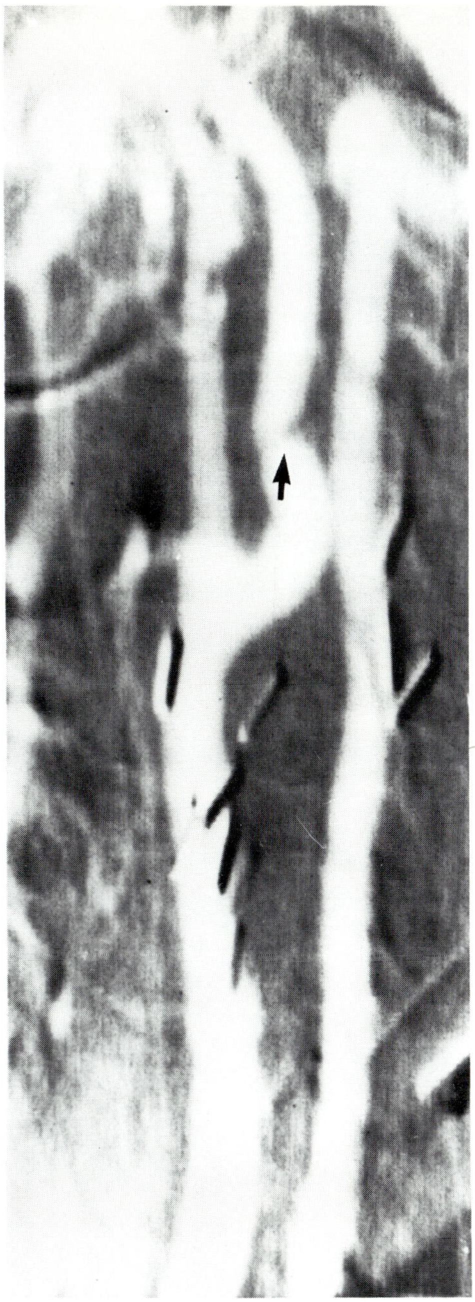

FIGURE 14-8. This asymptomatic patient has a recurrent stenosis of the carotid artery following endarterectomy (*arrow*). A hemodynamically severe lesion was identified by noninvasive testing and confirmed by IVDSA.

left ventricle. These window tracings are stored in the videoprocessor, the image sequences are again played, and a ventricular-volume curve for multiple beats is constructed. The ejection fraction (EF) is calculated by the formula:

$$EF = \frac{(d - d_0) - (s - s_0)}{d - d_0}$$

where d_0 and s_0 are baseline corrections for endiastolic (d) and endsystolic (s) volumes. The ejections figures obtained in this manner compare favorably with those obtained by area length determinations (33,34).

IVDSA can also determine the patency of coronary artery bypass grafts and has potential as a means of diagnostic screening for graft occlusion in patients who have recurrent symptoms of angina or chest pain following coronary bypass procedures (Figure 14-10). IVDSA is of no value in planning reconstructive coronary surgery, however, because of the limitations in spatial resolution, the overlapping contrast material in the chambers of the heart, and the continuous motion of the heart. These factors make it impossible to clearly define the anatomic status of proximal or distal coronary artery bypass anastomoses and make it impossible to accurately determine the severity and distribution of atherosclerotic lesions within the in situ coronary system (31–33).

Recent experimental and clinical evidence clearly demonstrate that in situ coronary arteries can be accurately displayed by injecting small volumes of contrast medium into the root of the aortic arch at the level of the coronary ostia and using digital enhancement methods. Occlusive, stenotic, and aneurysmal lesions of the proximal coronaries can be identified, and the anatomic status of aortocoronary bypass grafts can be more precisely defined. Although the utilization of intraarterial digital coronary imaging has been limited, there is great potential for its development. The major advantage of this technique is that critical occlusive lesions in the proximal right or left in situ coronary artery system can be identified during peripheral angiography in patients with symptomatic cerebral or peripheral vascular disease. In addition, the patency and anatomic status of coronary bypass grafts can be precisely defined (33). Standard coronary artery catheterization is recommended for all patients who on DSA are suspected of having major occlusive lesions in the proximal right or left main stem and main stem equivalent distribution of the coronary circulation, and in patients with occlusion or stenosis of coronary artery bypass grafts. These patients appear to be at increased risk of postoperative cardiac problems following elective peripheral vascular reconstruction. DSA is safe because selective coronary catheterization is unnecessary and because relatively small volumes of contrast medium are needed. The information derived from this simple addition to standard peripheral angiography can be of importance in determining the perioperative risks associated with elective vascular surgery. Although there is great potential for the use of digital techniques in evaluating the coronary circulation and the ventricular dynamics of cardiovascular function, clinical experience in this area remains limited (Figure 14-10).

The ability of IVDSA to visualize the heart and the pulmonary vessels suggests that it might be a useful method for diagnosing pulmonary emboli. Clinical experience, however, has shown that although it is possible to visualize pulmonary emboli with IVDSA, standard arteriographic methods are more accurate. The resolution limitations of the intravenous technique make it very difficult to get good detail of the peripheral branches in the pulmonary artery system. This means that small pulmonary emboli can be missed entirely by the digital method. Another problem is that respiratory motion degrades image clarity. The probability of getting a good study in an acutely ill patient who is air-hungry and breathing rapidly is quite small. Although large proximal emboli can be visualized by IVDSA, the results of

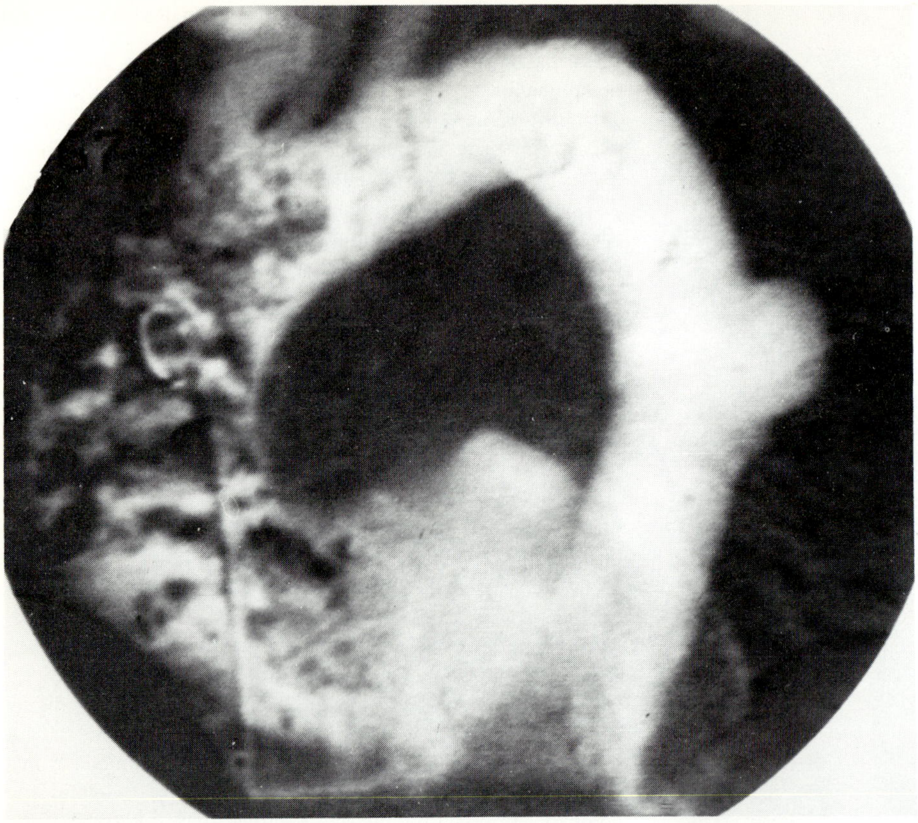

FIGURE 14-9. This IVDSA digital arteriogram shows a traumatic aneurysm of the thoracic aorta. DSA is accurate in diagnosing congenital and acquired lesions of the thoracic aorta.

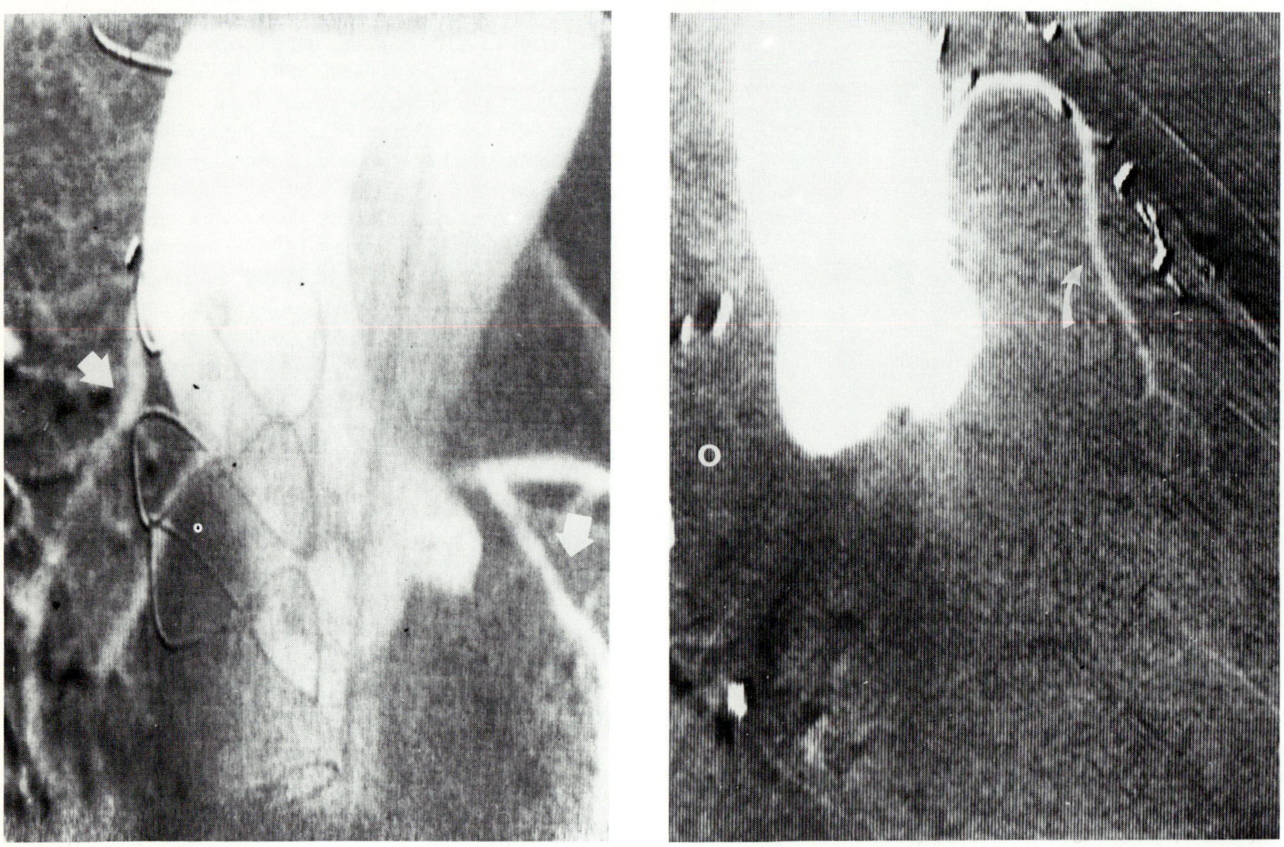

A B

FIGURE 14-10. (*A*) This IVDSA study demonstrates the patency of aortocoronary bypass grafts (*arrows*). The intravenous technique cannot adequately evaluate distal anastomoses or in situ coronary vessels because of limited spatial resolution, and motion artifacts. (***B***) This IADSA study demonstrates the occlusion of a right aortocoronary graft, and a patent left graft with good distal runoff (*arrow*). Intraarterial DSA makes it safer to screen for proximal in situ disease and to determine coronary graft patency during peripheral angiography.

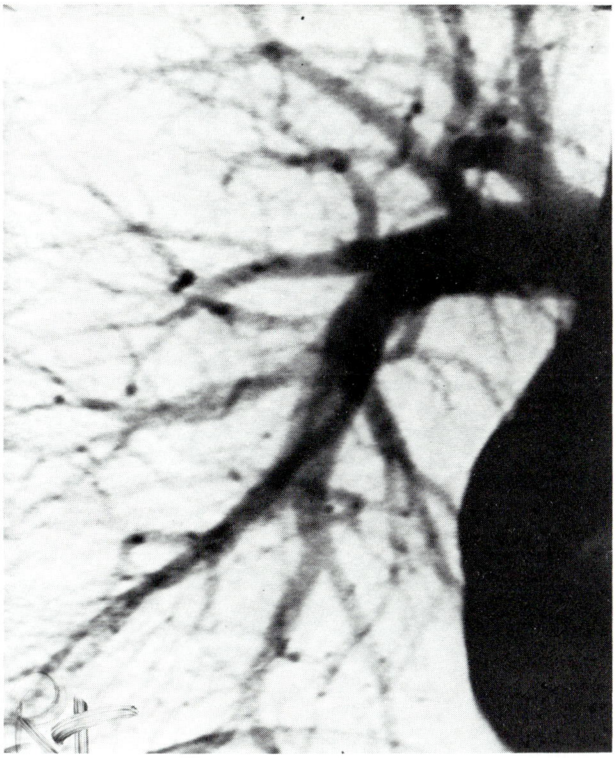

A

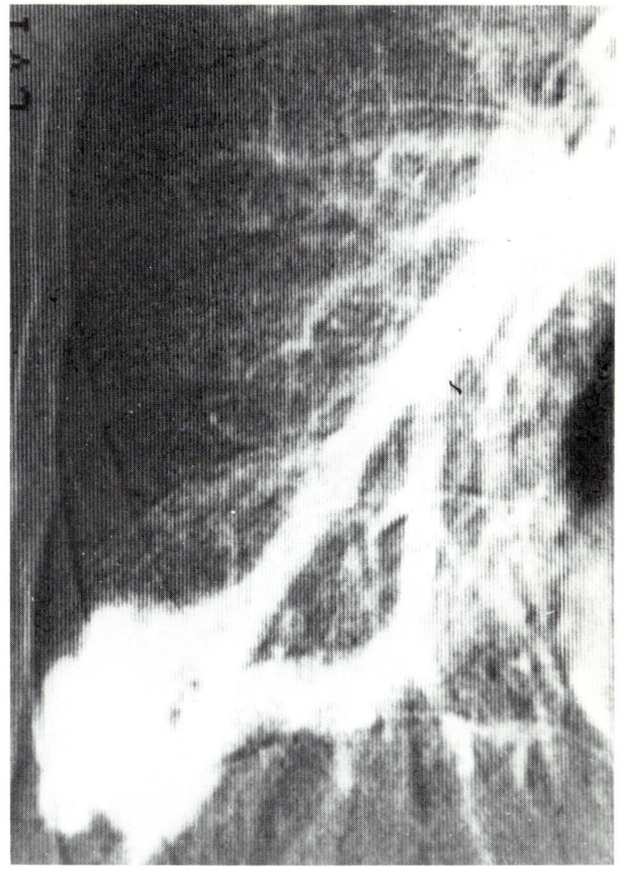

FIGURE 14-11. (*A*) This pulmonary angiogram was obtained with IVDSA. Good detail of the proximal artery and its major branches can be observed. This technique is capable of identifying large pulmonary emboli in the proximal branches of the artery. The technique is less suitable for identifying small peripheral emboli because of spatial-resolution problems and because the imaging detail may be severely obscured if the patient is air-hungry and breaths during the filming sequence. (*B*) IVDSA is an acceptable method for identifying congenital pulmonary lesions such as AV fistulas.

standard pulmonary angiography have been much more dependable (8,31,32). Intravenous angiography can, however, be used as a means of identifying congenital or acquired pulmonary arteriovenous fistulas (Figure 14-11).

Abdominal and Lower-Extremity Vascular Disease

IVDSA can be used to diagnose a number of intraabdominal vascular problems. This technique has been used to screen for renal vascular hypertension. The number, location, and anatomic status of renal arteries can be determined by IVDSA, along with physiological information about the excretory function of the kidney. IVDSA is most accurate in identifying critical stenoses and occlusions at the origin or midportion of the renal artery. Larger atherosclerotic aneurysms can be identified (Figure 14-12). IVDSA is not adequate in the evaluation of patients suspected of having fibromuscular disease because Web stenoses and pathology in the hilar vessels can easily be missed. Consequently, IVDSA should be performed only when atheroocclusive disease is suspected in the elderly hypertensive patient. Intraarterial angiography (standard or digital) is more appropriate in the evaluation of hypertensive young females who are likely to have fibromuscular renal disease (Figure 14-13). In general, whenever IVDSA is done in order to rule out renal vascular hypertension, the percutaneous retrograde femoral vein approach should be used. Selective renal vein reins can be obtained before the injection of the contrast medium. Timed exposures using standard imaging techniques can be utilized to evaluate the excretory function of the kidney.

IVDSA is also useful in evaluating patients who are suspected of having trauma to the kidneys, and it is recommended for patients who have hematuria following blunt abdominal injury. Complete occlusion of the renal artery can be quickly and accurately diagnosed in this fashion.

IVDSA can also be used to visualize the celiac axis and the mesenteric arteries. Lateral projections of the aorta provide adequate definition of the celiac and superior mesenteric artery origins and make it possible to rule out major occlusive lesions in these vessels. IVDSA is most appropriate in evaluating patients with chronic intestinal ischemia because the disease is most commonly localized at the origin of the celiac or superior mesenteric arteries. Patients with clinical evidence of acute intestinal ischemia are probably better evaluated by intraarterial imaging

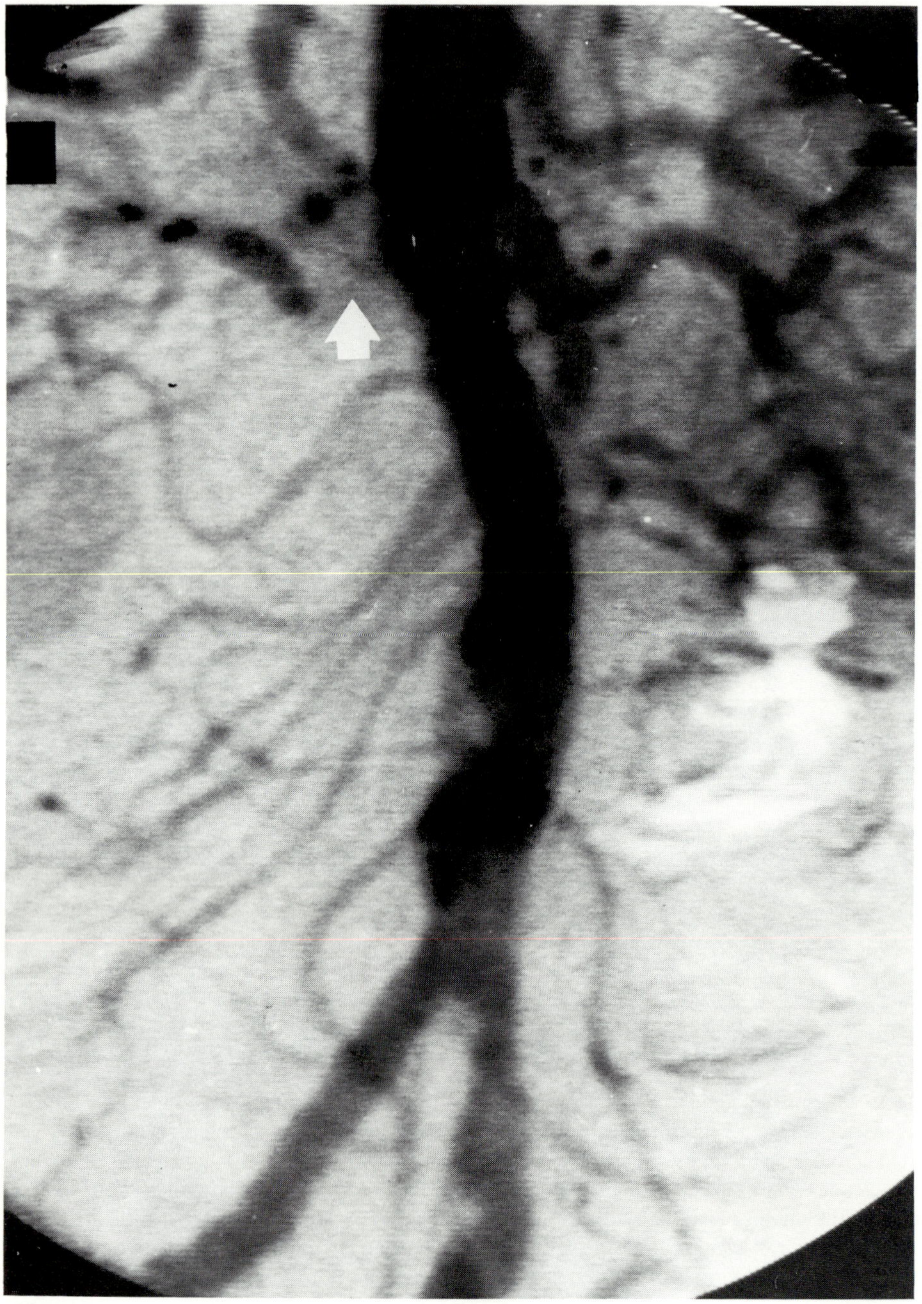

FIGURE 14-12. IVDSA can be used as a method of screening for renal vascular hypertension. IVDSA is most effective in screening for atheroocclusive lesions involving the origin or midportions of the renal artery (*arrow*).

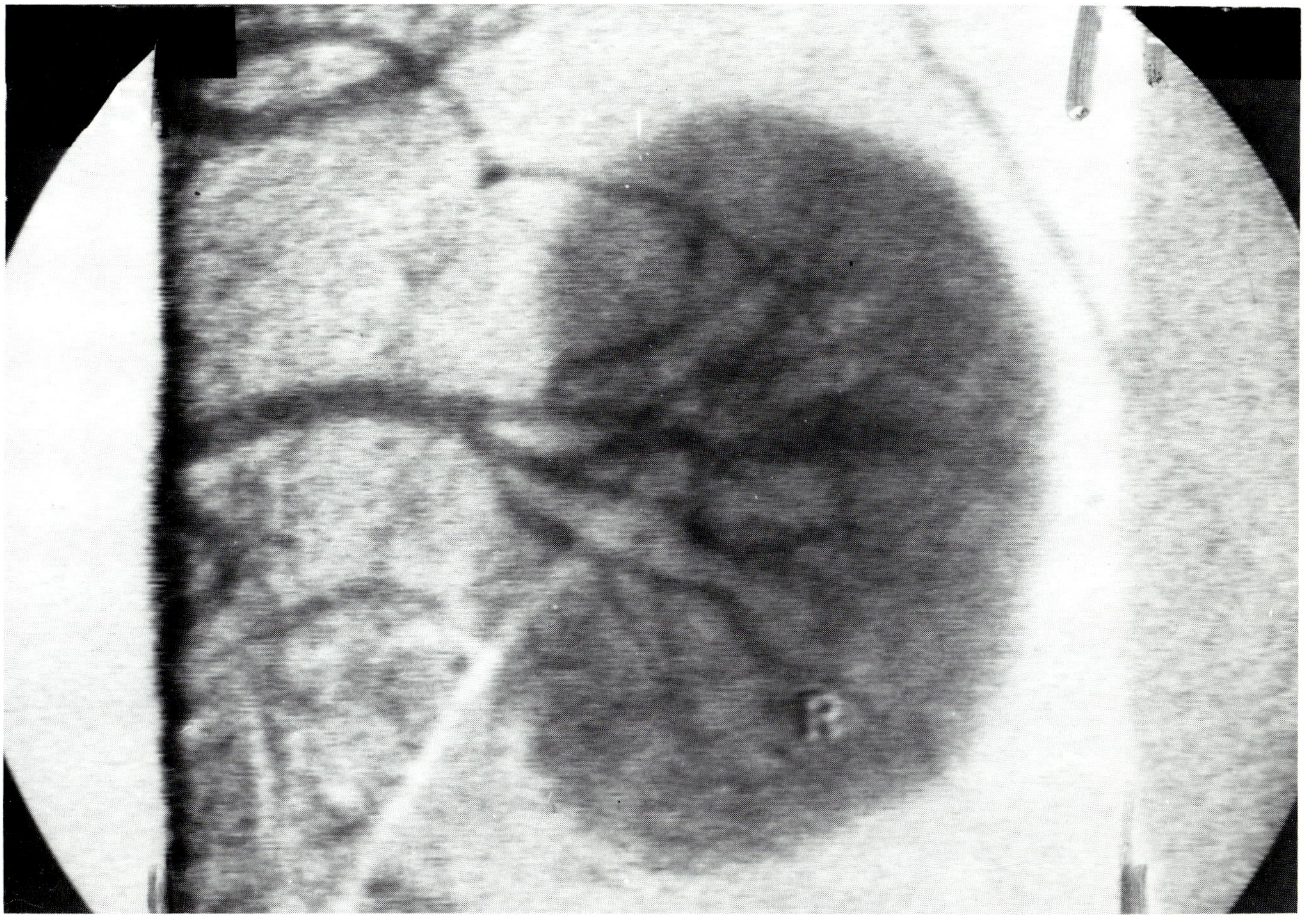

A

FIGURE 14-13. (*A*) IVDSA can visualize the hilar branches of the renal vessels, but does not provide the detail that IADSA studies afford.

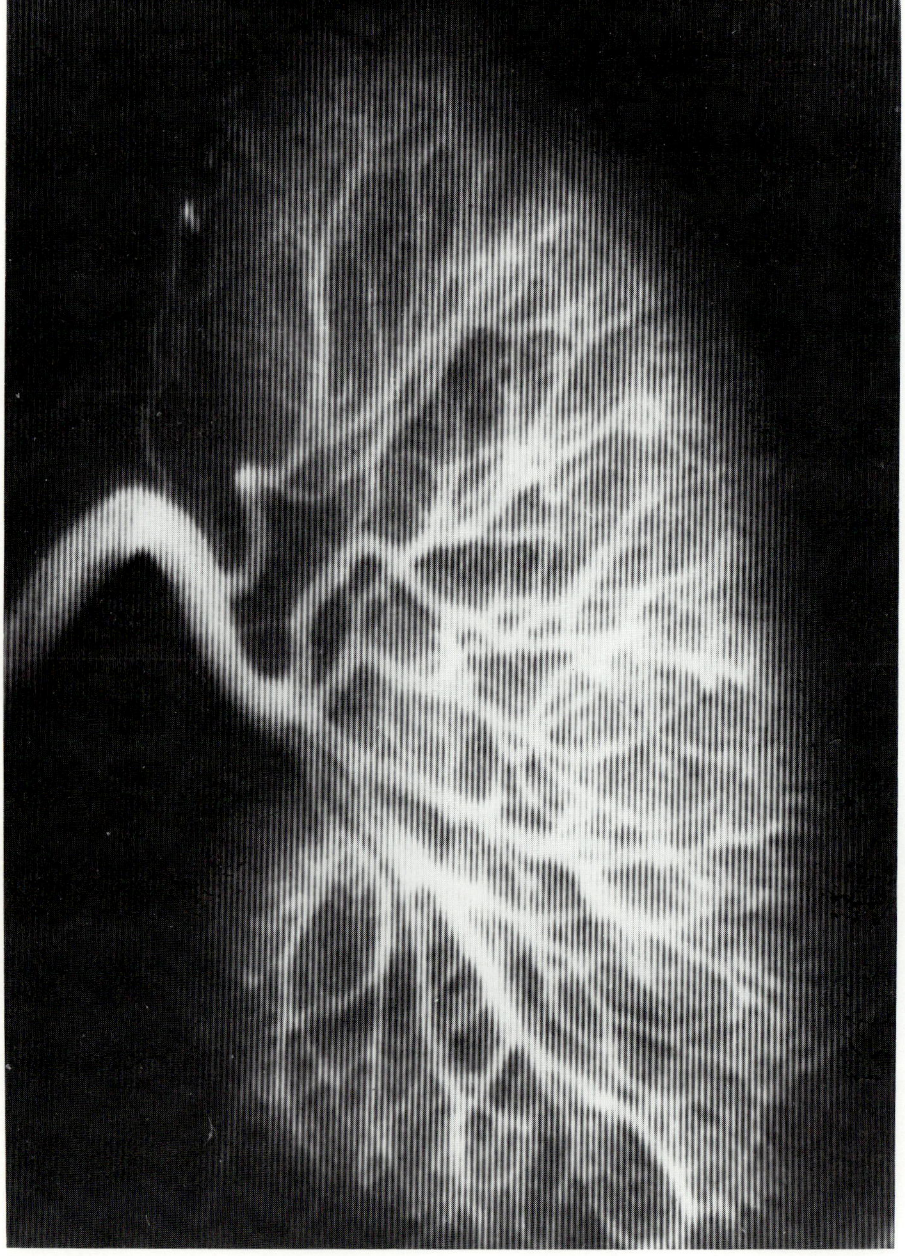

B

FIGURE 14-13 (*continued*). (*B*) IADSA provides increased small-vessel resolution with smaller injections of the contrast medium.

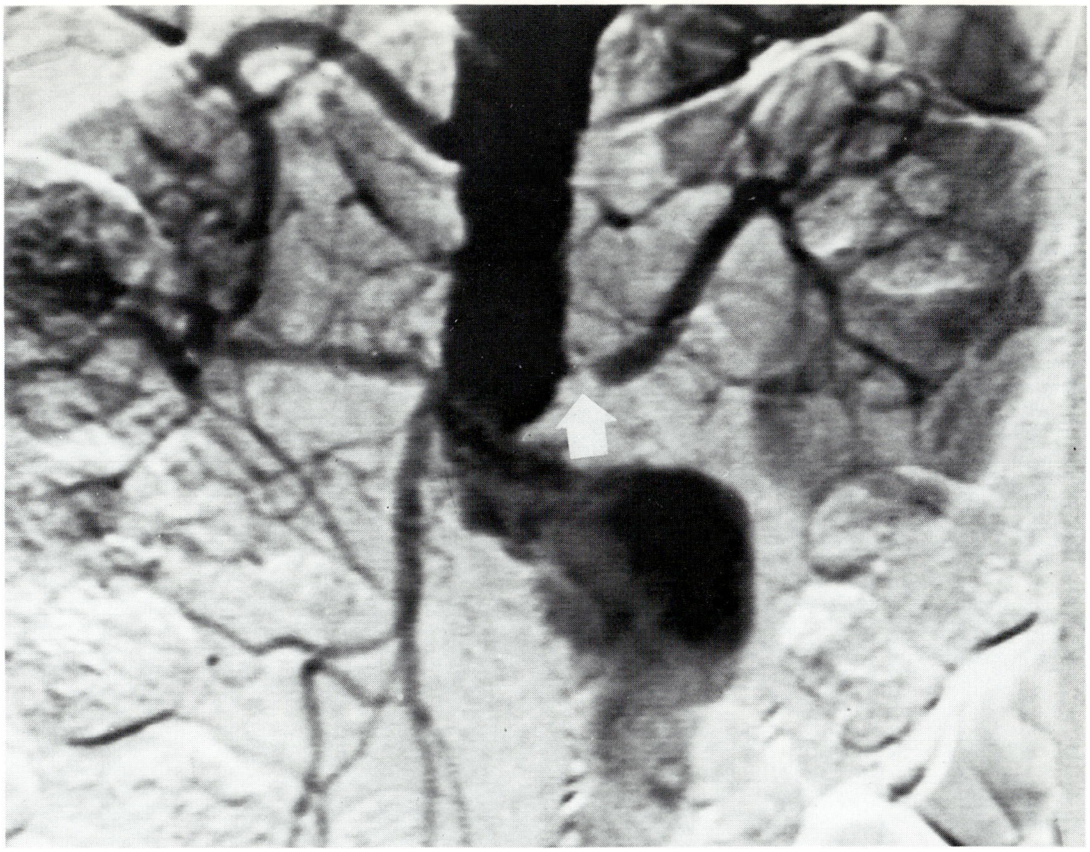

A

FIGURE 14-14. (*A*) IVDSA is useful in the preoperative evaluation of patients with intraabdominal aneurysms when renal vascular hypertension, claudication, or multiple peripheral aneurysms are clinically suspected. This intravenous angiogram shows a severe stenosis at the origin of the left renal artery (*arrow*).

techniques because fine detail in the mesenteric arcades cannot be obtained by intravenous methods. The chances of missing smaller emboli in the distal branches of the mesenteric celiac vessels are so great that the use of IVDSA does not seem justified. For the same reason, IVDSA has proved to be an inaccurate and disappointing method for identifying the location of gastrointestinal bleeding (8,33).

At present, there is no consistent opinion about whether standard arteriography is essential for the diagnosis and management of abdominal aneurysms. These lesions can usually be diagnosed by physical examination, and their size can usually be accurately defined by B-mode ultrasonography or CT scan. In the otherwise asymptomatic patient, standard arteriography may have greater risks than diagnostic value since most of the anatomic information needed for surgical management can be determined at the time of the operative procedure. Standard arterial imaging in these patients is frequently of poor quality because of reduced contrast opacification caused by dissolution and slow flow through the aneurysmal vessels. IVDSA makes it possible to improve arterial imaging because contrast opacification is better and to reduce the risks by avoiding the catheterization of thin-walled or clot-filled aneurysms (35). Patients suspected of having multiple or suprarenal aneurysms, or aneurysms with coexistent peripheral vascular disease manifest by hypertension or lower-extremity claudication, should be evaluated by IVDSA. The number, status, and anatomic location of renal vessels and their relationship to the aneurysm neck, and the presence of occlusive or aneurysmal changes in the iliac arteries, can be adequately determined in this manner (Figure 14-14).

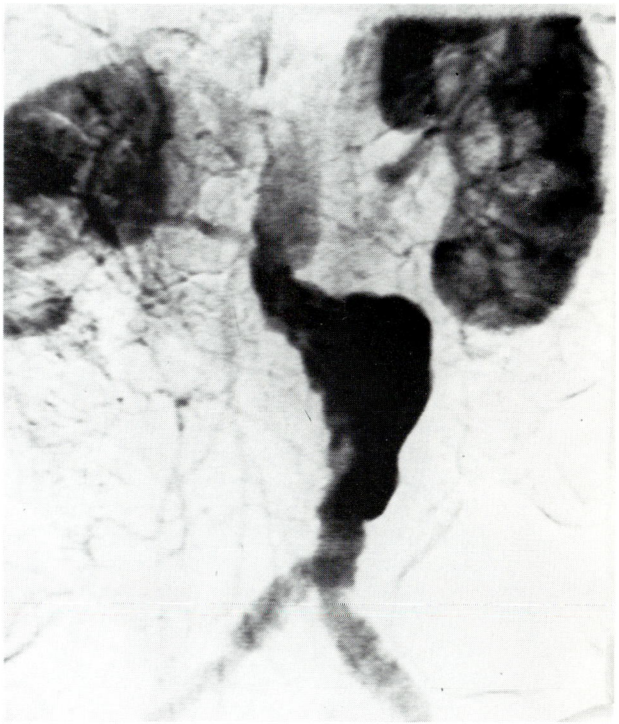

B

FIGURE 14-14 (*continued*). (*B*) This aortic aneurysm extends to the bifurcation and involves the proximal common iliac arteries.

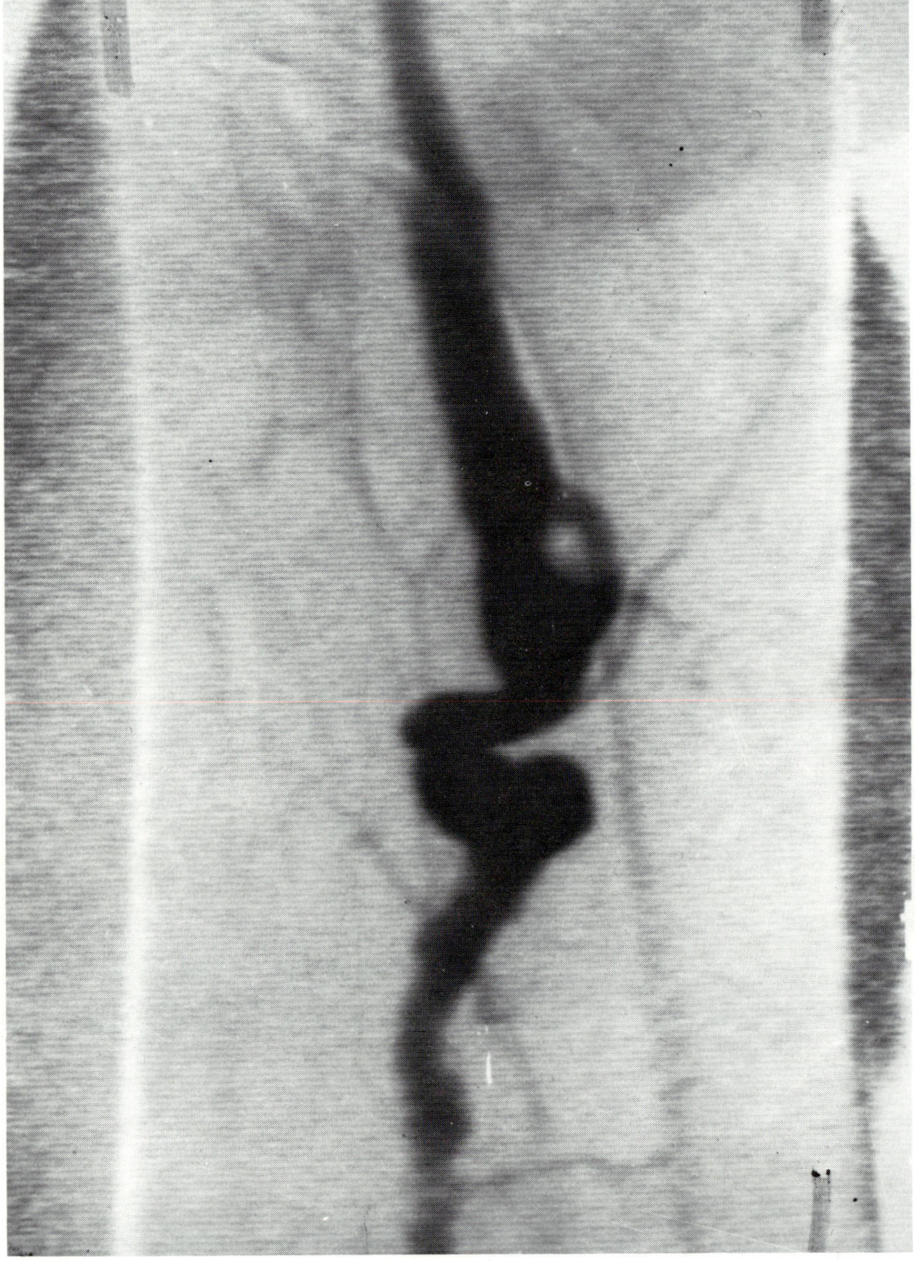

FIGURE 14-15. This IVDSA shows an aneurysm of the popliteal artery. IVDSA is ideally suited for evaluating isolated segments of the peripheral circulation. In this case, the anatomic condition of vessels proximal and distal to the aneurysm are clearly defined.

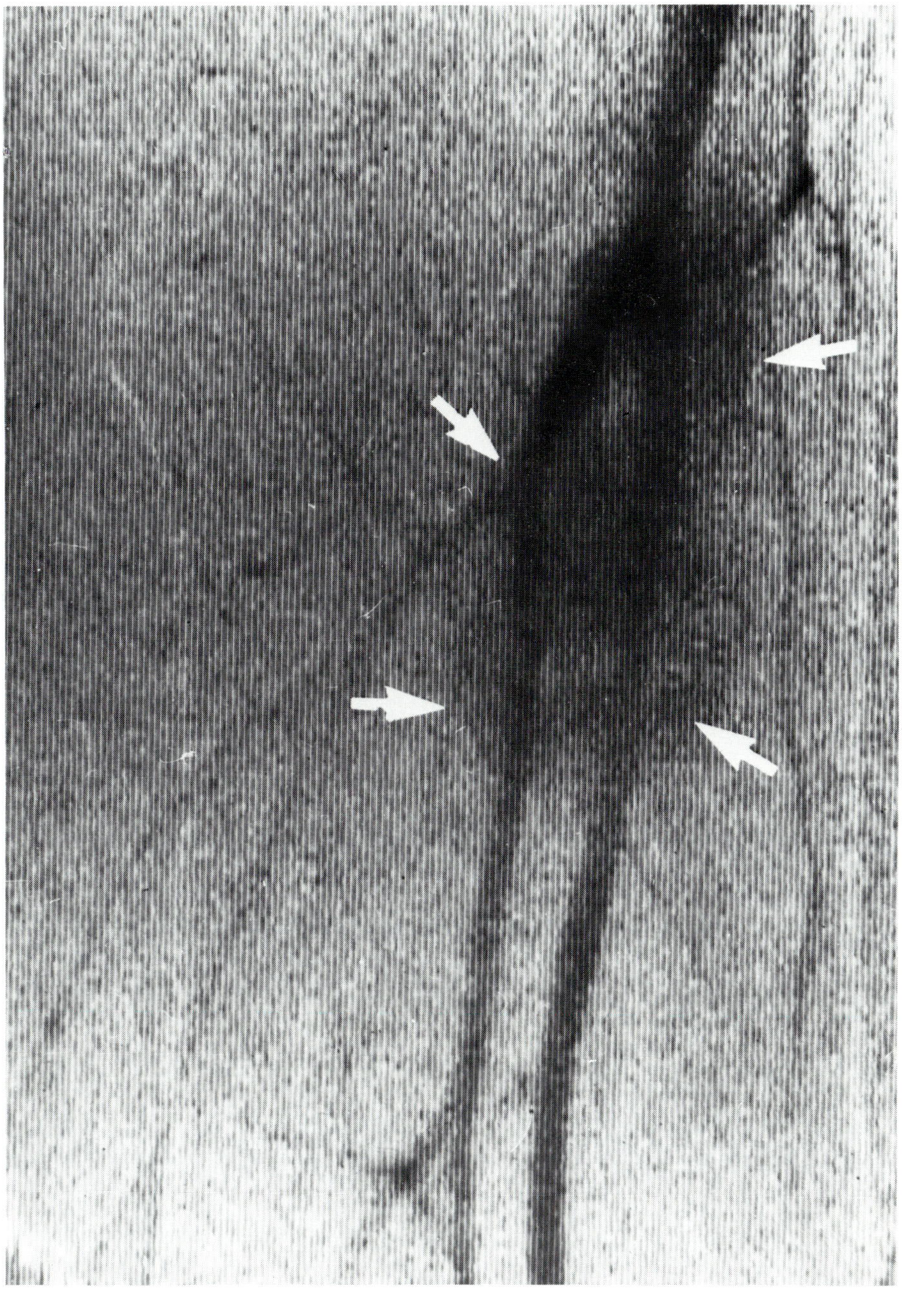

FIGURE 14-16. IVDSA is a rapid and effective method of identifying penetrating or blunt arterial trauma in the stabilized patient. This study demonstrates a pseudoaneurysm (*arrows*) resulting from a stab wound to the right groin.

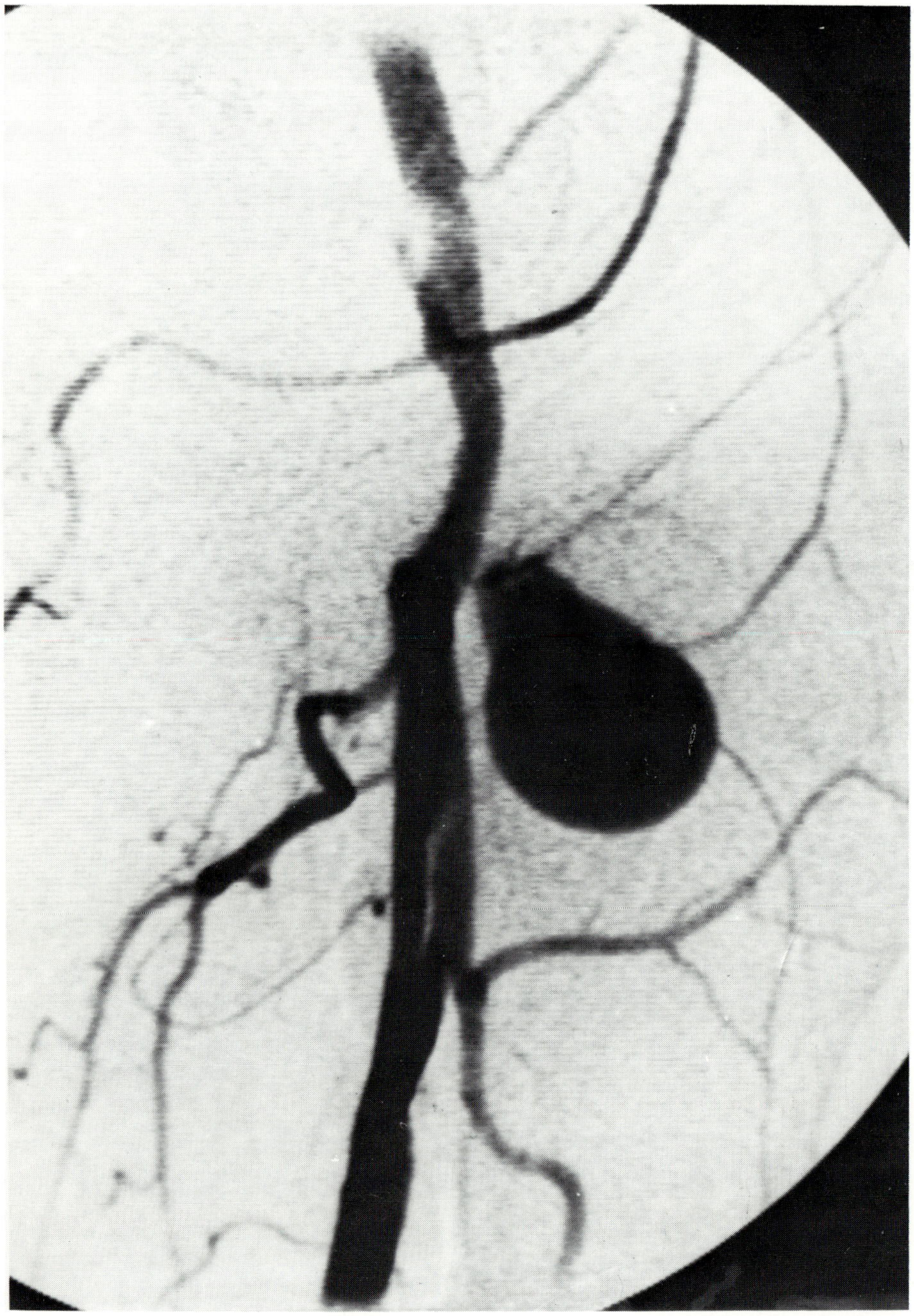

FIGURE 14-17. This IVDSA study shows a pseudoaneurysm of the common femoral artery which developed following percutaneous transluminal angioplasty. IVDSA is ideal for evaluating iatrogenic vascular trauma that occurs during standard cardiac or peripheral artery catheterization.

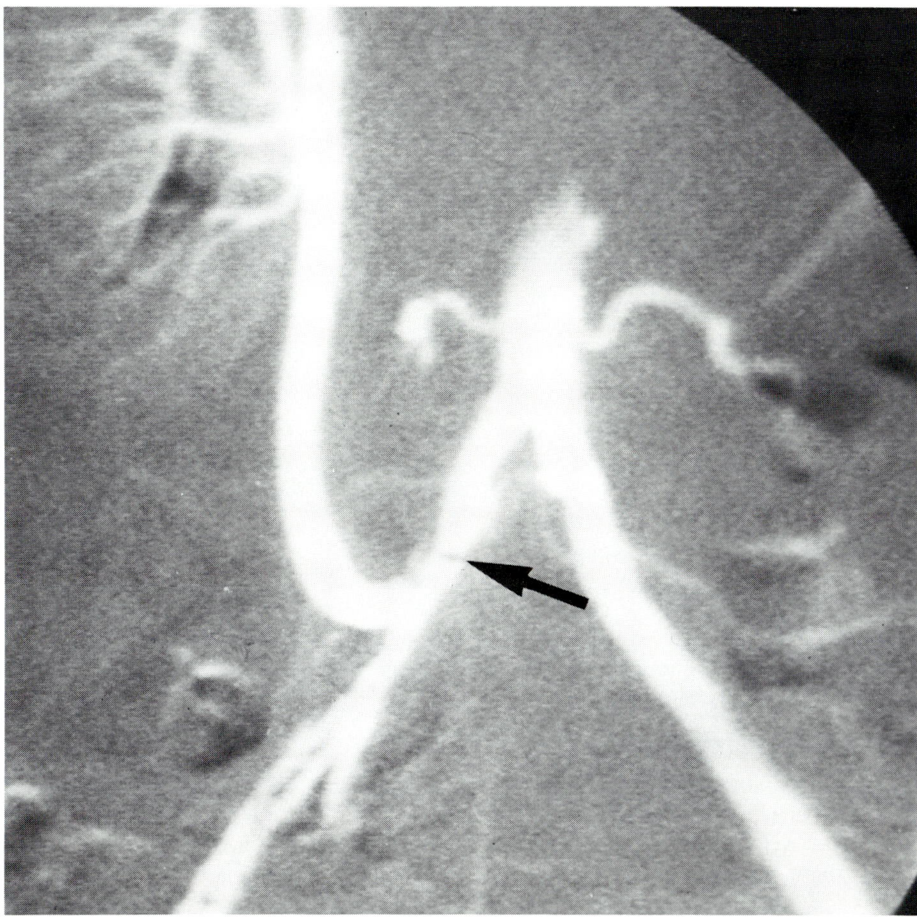

FIGURE 14-18. IVDSA is a useful method in evaluating intraabdominal vascular anastomoses. This patient had a renal transplant and developed hypertension 3 years postoperatively. A significant stenosis is identified in the iliac artery proximal to the graft anastomosis (*arrow*).

The role of DSA in the evaluation of lower-extremity claudication has been limited because of the small image-field size, the inability to perform biplane imaging, and the limited spatial resolution. These intrinsic limitations have made it difficult to obtain detailed anatomic information about the entire peripheral vascular system without using excessive volumes of contrast medium. This excessive contrast medium invites a greater risk for renal failure, particularly in the insulin-dependent diabetic and in patients who have a chronic impairment of renal function or renal transplants. For this reason, IVDSA has most commonly been employed to evaluate local segments of the peripheral vasculature. It has proved useful in the diagnosis of femoral and popliteal aneurysms, in the assessment of suspected blunt or penetrating arterial injuries, and in the postoperative assessment of bypass grafts and balloon angioplasty (31,36,37).

IVDSA used in conjunction with B-mode ultrasonography is adequate for diagnosing and treating most peripheral aneurysms. These lesions are potentially dangerous, tend to be multiple, and are easily missed on physical examination. Diagnostic screening with ultrasonography is indicated in patients with aortoiliac aneurysms and in patients with embolic infarcts in the toes. IVDSA should be performed when ultrasonographic findings are positive. The extent of the aneurysm and the anatomic status of the proximal and distal vessels can be determined while avoiding the potential complications of standard catheterization (Figure 14-15).

IVDSA can be used for diagnostic screening in stabilized patients with suspected blunt or penetrating arterial trauma. Pseudoaneurysms, arteriovenous fistulas, and occlusions can be easily identified (Figure 14-16). The major advantage is the speed and safety with which the studies can be performed. Intravenous access is usually available, and arterial catheterization is unnecessary. IVDSA is contraindicated when cardiac tamponade, uncontrolled hemorrhage, or massive soft tissue injury is present. Reduced cardiac output in hemodynamically unstable patients with tamponade adversely affects the contrast delivery and image quality. Likewise, major soft tissue injury causes misregistration with the video mask, and this destroys the image quality. Incoherent patients and persons unable to hold still or obey verbal commands are poor candidates for intravenous arterial screening because motion artifacts seriously alter the clinical value of the study. IVDSA is ideally suited for evaluating patients with iatrogenic vascular injury following standard angiography, cardiac catheterization, or the placement of subclavian lines. Important clinical information can be obtained without submitting the patient to the risk of further arterial injury (Figure 14-17).

IVDSA should be selectively used in postoperative assessment. It is preferred for evaluating intraabdominal vascular procedures involving renal or visceral artery branches (Figure 14-18). Postoperative surveillance of the lower extremity should combine safety and cost efficiency. Because DSA is an invasive technique with some attendant risk, noninvasive tests are safer and just as accurate in screening for hemodynamically significant stenoses. Noninvasive tests are recommended before patient discharge because they provide an objective physiological baseline against which to compare clinical changes following bypass grafts or percutaneous transluminal angioplasty. These tests repeated 6 to 8 weeks later help identify occult surgical errors. Additional testing at 6 months and at yearly intervals helps screen for late-developing suture-line stenoses or significant progression of the disease in host vessels. IVDSA is recommended whenever segmental pressure indices drop more than 15 percent, when recurrent symptoms of ischemia occur, or at yearly intervals. The patency, the anastomotic integrity, and the distinction between the graft and host-vessel progression of stenosis can be determined (Figure 14-19). This combination of surveillance techniques maximizes safety and cost efficiency and accurately identifies recurrent or progressive disease. The early identification of technical problems after reconstructive procedures and the identification of clinically occult lesions in the peripheral circulation make it possible to extend graft patency rates by correcting these problems before graft thrombosis occurs.

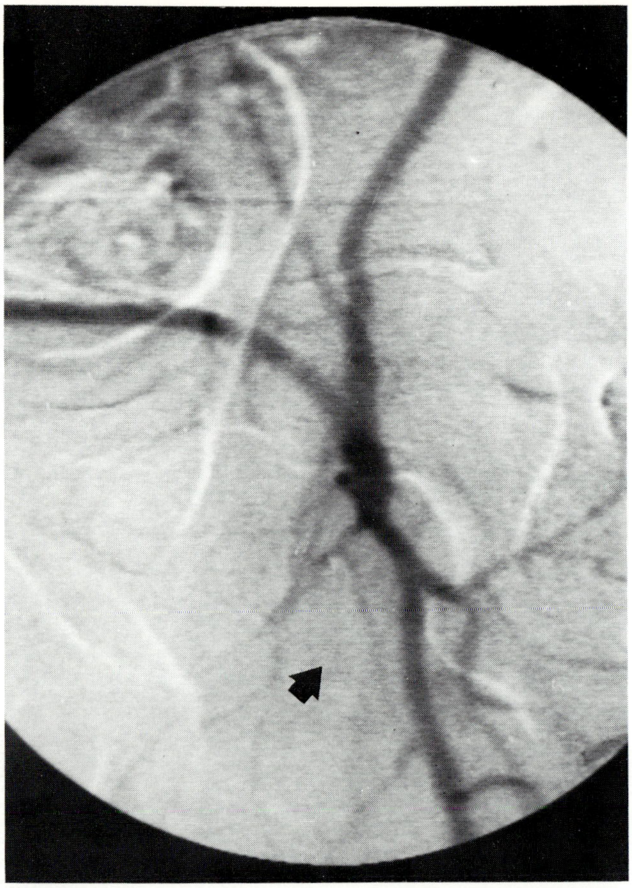

A

FIGURE 14-19. IVDSA is effective as a means of postoperative follow-up in patients with recurrent symptoms of ischemia, or noninvasive evidence of progression. (*A*) A patent axillofemorofemoral bypass. This patient complained of recurrent claudication and had a drop in segmental Doppler pressures in that leg. DSA demonstrates a patent graft and recent occlusion of the superficial femoral artery (*arrow*).

IADSA is effective in the evaluation of ischemic claudication when the complete display of the abdominal and extremity vasculature is necessary. The advantages include the increased contrast opacification, the reduced contrast-volume requirement, and the improved spatial resolution. The direct injection of contrast material into the arterial system allows better opacification and more precise detail in smaller vessels of the peripheral

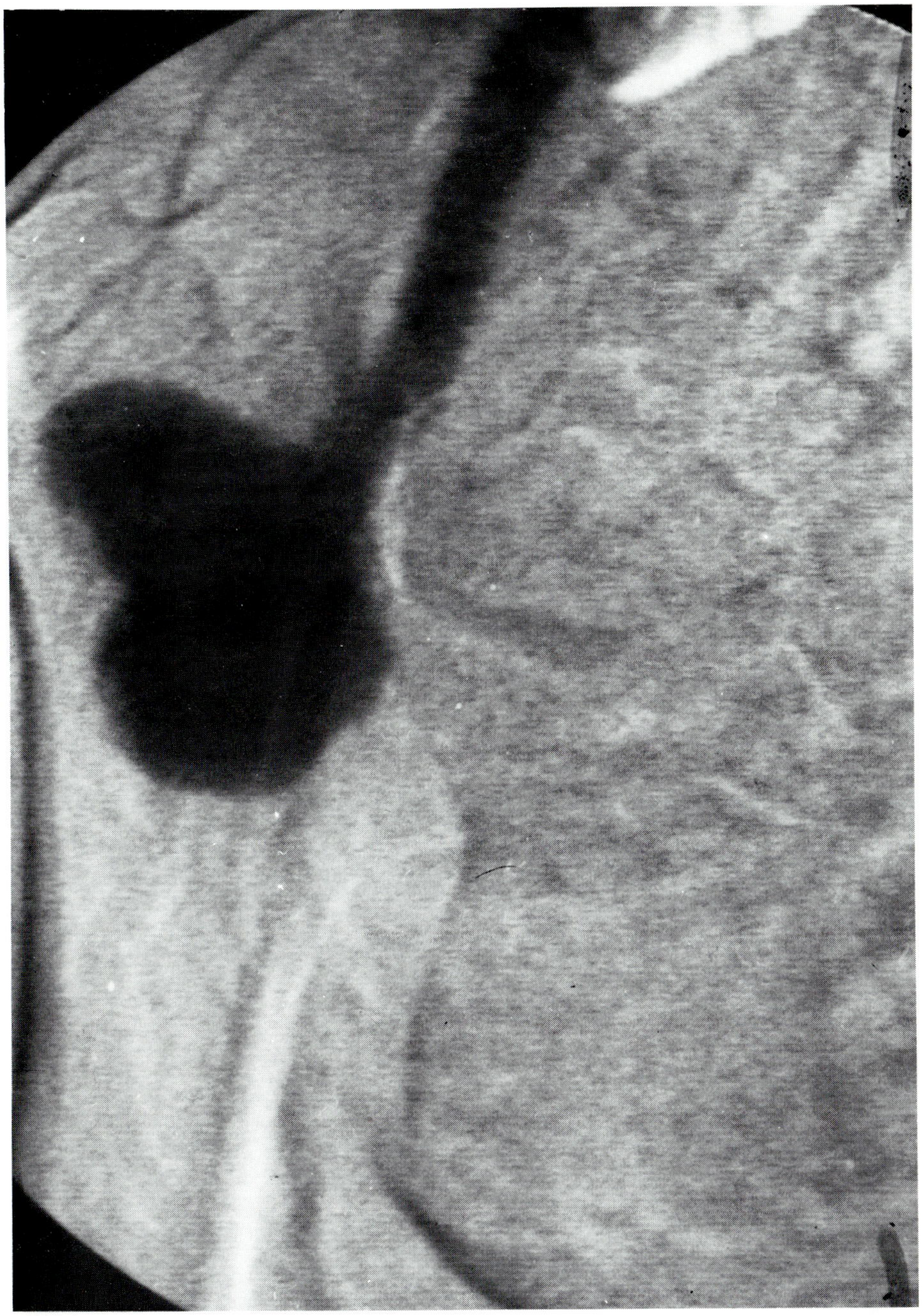

B

FIGURE 14-19 (*continued*). (*B*) A large pseudoaneurysm at the diatal anastomosis of an aortofemoral bypass graft is demonstrated IVDSA.

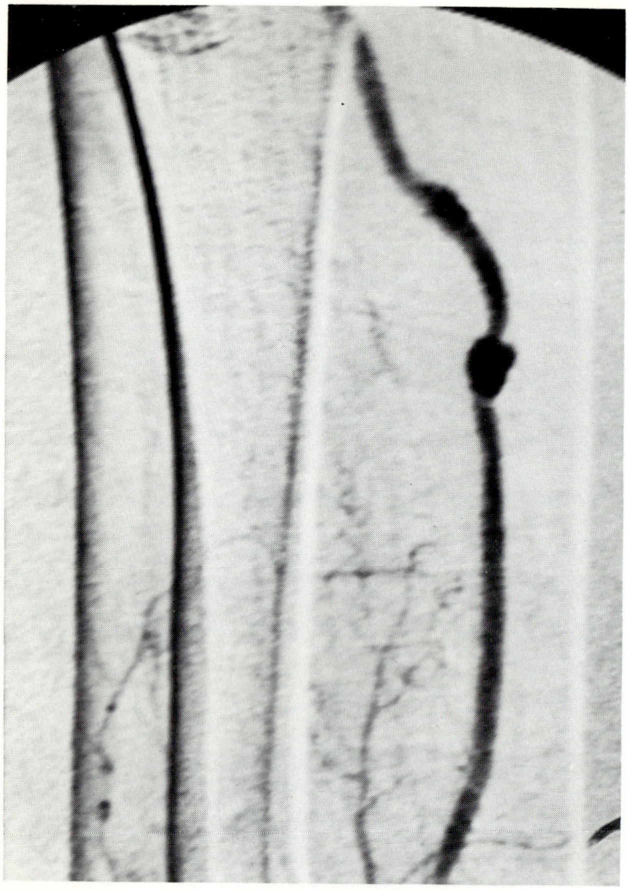

C

FIGURE 14-19 (*continued*). (*C*) IVDSA shows aneurysmal and stenotic degenerative changes in a saphenous femoropopliteal bypass. Segmental Doppler pressures fell progressively during several months of observation. DSA identified the anatomic cause for this change. The lesion was surgically excised and graft patency maintained.

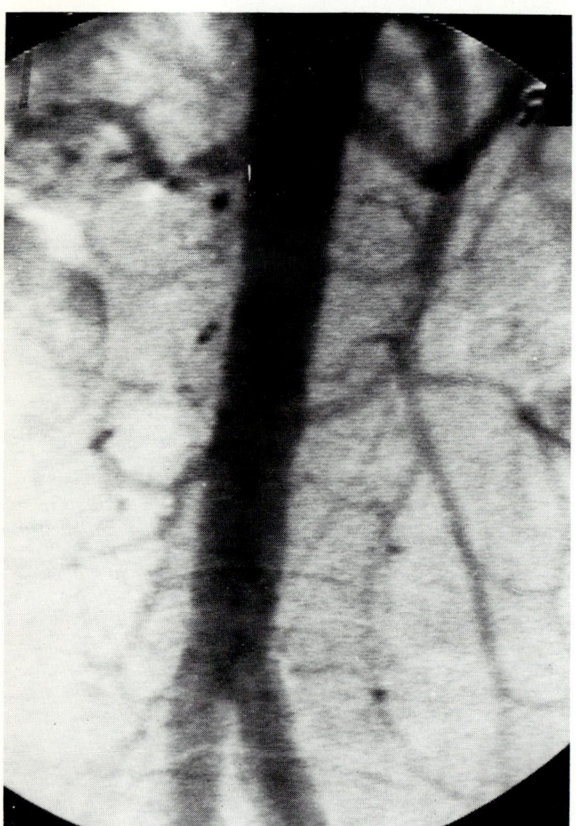

A

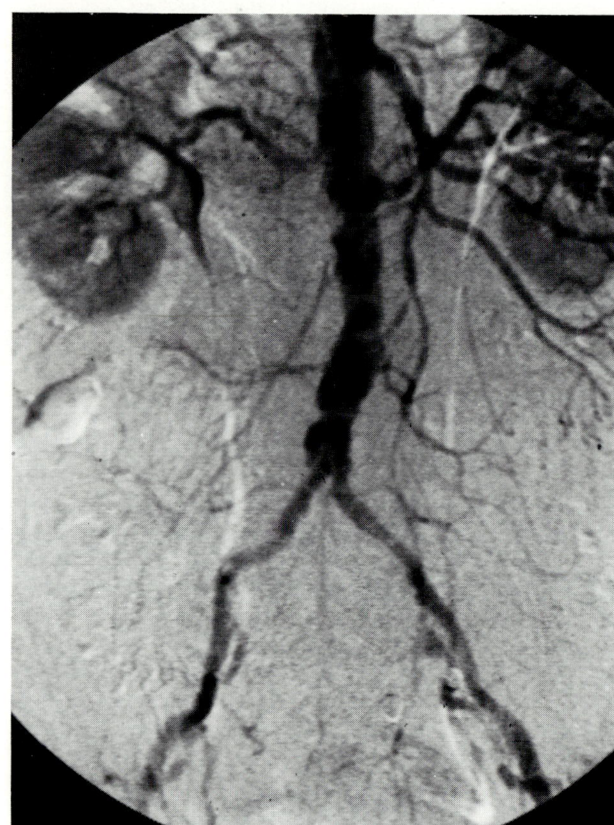

B

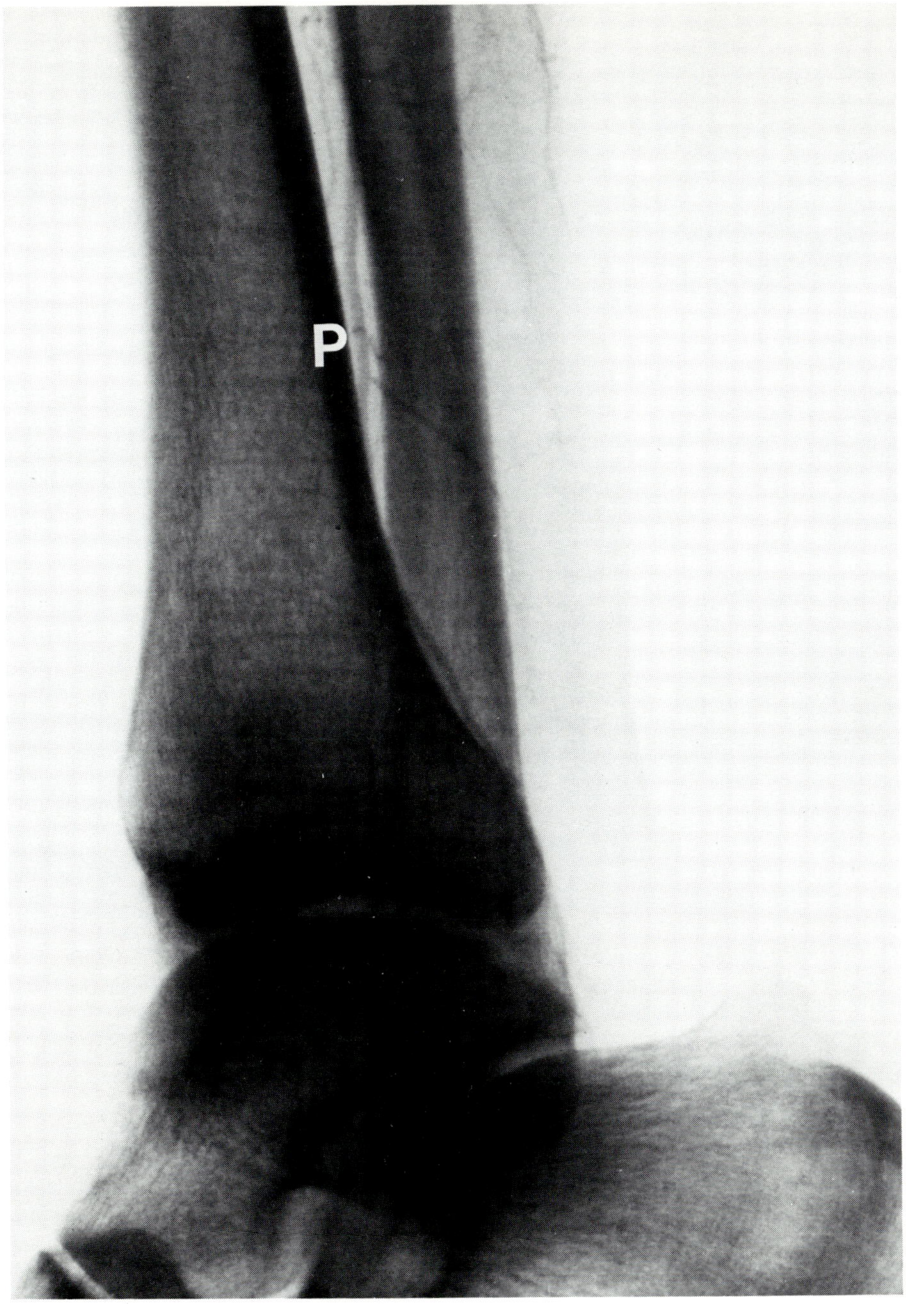

A

FIGURE 14-21. (*A*) This standard angiogram shows faint visualization of the peroneal artery P. No communication with the pedal arch is demonstrated.

FIGURE 14-20. (*A*) This IVDSA study demonstrates the field-size restriction of a 9-in fluoroscope. (*B*) More extensive vascular anatomy can be displayed with a single injection of contrast material using the 14-in fluoroscope. The larger fluoroscope makes it possible to reduce the volume of contrast material required for both intravenous and intraarterial digital angiography.

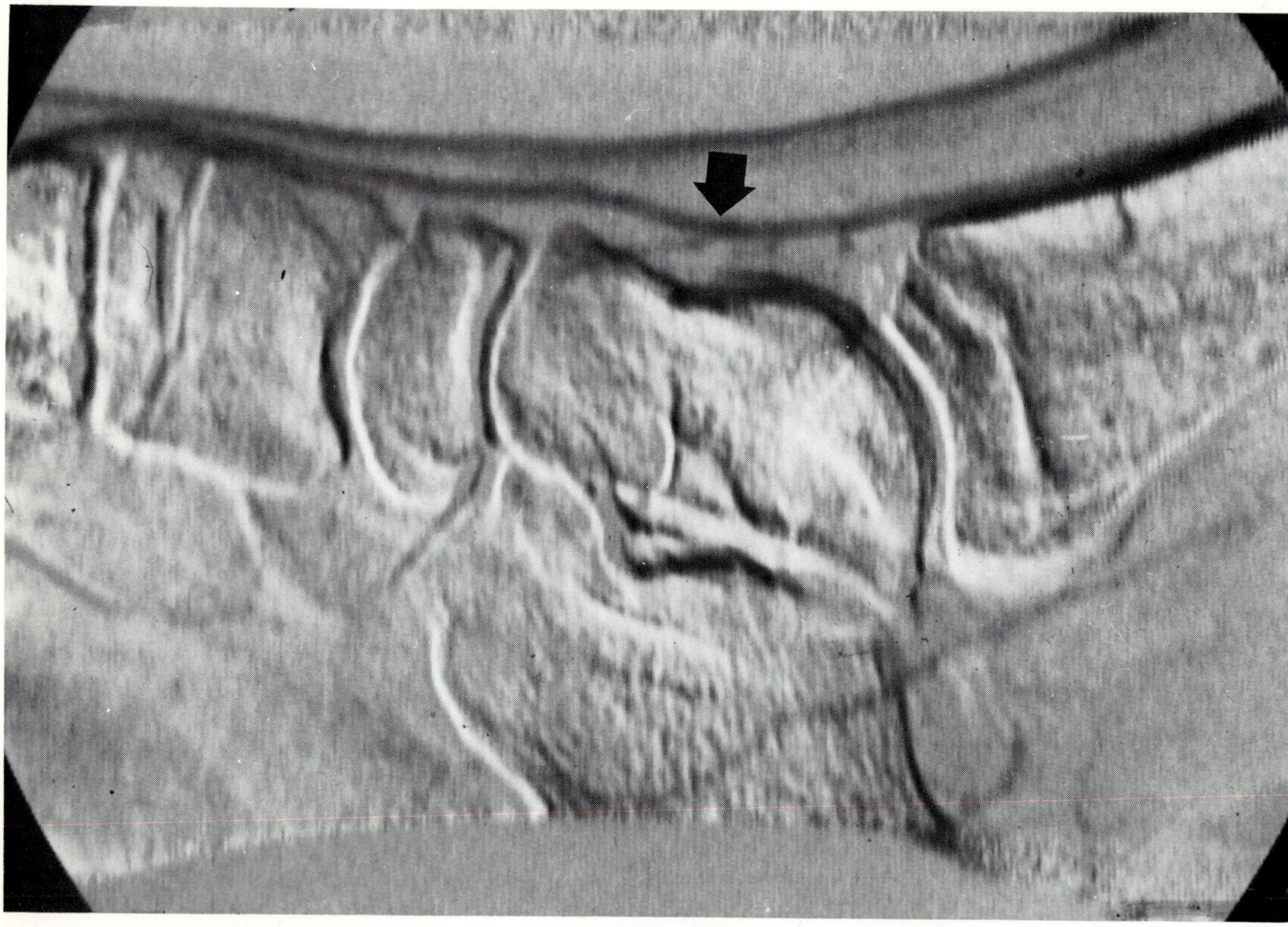

B

FIGURE 14-21 (*continued*). (*B*) IADSA performed after 7 minutes of reactive hyperemia demonstrates a patent anterior tibial artery which extends into the arcade of the foot (*arrow*). Intraarterial digital techniques improve the preoperative selection of patients for limb-salvage distal vascular reconstructions.

circulation and significantly reduces the absolute volume and the concentration of the contrast agents used. These advantages and the recent availability of a 14-in image intensifier make complete diagnostic angiography of the abdominal and lower-extremity circulation safer and more practical (Figure 14-20). IADSA is recommended for all patients with insulin-dependent diabetes and for persons who have kidney transplants or altered renal function (17,31). IADSA combined with reactive cuff hyperemia is also valuable in the assessment of patients with limb-threatening ischemia who are found on standard angiography to have poorly visualized distal vascular segments. The failure to image the distal circulation may be due to severe occlusive disease but frequently results from technical errors, such as the improper timing of the film exposure and inadequate injection contrast medium rates. IADSA is performed by inflating a thigh pressure cuff to slightly above systolic pressure and restricting arterial flow to the limb for 7 minutes. Just before the cuff is released, the fluoroscopic mask image is taken, and then 60 to 80 mL of contrast medium is intraarterially injected at 10 mL/s. Arterial exposures are taken at 1-s intervals for 60 s. The reduction in peripheral resistance caused by the hyperemia improves the delivery of contrast material to the limb, and digital amplification enhances the contrast opacification, thus improving the anatomic display of the popliteal artery runoff and tibial vessel communications with the pedal arch (Figure 14-21). The information derived from this method of arteriography makes it possible for the vascular surgeons to more accurately plan vascular reconstruction and to prevent untimely amputation (36).

The need for arterial catheterization has been the major impediment to the widespread use of angiography in the diagnosis and management of vascular disease. DSA effectively reduces the dangers associated with arterial catheterization and as a result will undoubtedly expand the application of and liberalize the indications for arteriographic imaging. It is unlikely that IVDSA will eliminate the need for intraarterial imaging or for noninvasive testing, but in all likelihood IVDSA will alter the way in which these techniques will be used. It is clear that digital subtraction techniques, when combined with current methods of regional noninvasive assessment, should provide objective information which will result in better health care.

References

1. Barnes RW: Non-invasive techniques in peripheral vascular disease. Am Heart J 1979, 79:241.
2. Bone GE, Slaymaker EG, Barnes RW: Noninvasive assessment of collateral blood flow of the cerebral hemisphere by Doppler ultrasound. Surg Gynecol Obstet 1977, 145:873.
3. Kempczinski RF, Rutherford RB: Current status of the vascular laboratory. Adv Surg 1978, 12:1.
4. Mulder DS, Winsberg F, Cole CM, Blundell PE, Scott HJ: Ultrasonic "B" scanning of abdominal aneurysms. Ann Thorac Surg 1973, 16:361.
5. Pond GD, Hillman B: Evaluation of aneurysms by computed tomography. Surgery 1981, 89:216.
6. Winsberg F, Cole-Beuglet C, Mulder DS: Continuous ultrasound "B" scanning of abdominal aortic aneurysms. Am J Roentgenol 1974, 121:626.
7. Crummy AB, Zweibel WJ, Barriga P: Doppler evaluation of extracranial cerebrovascular disease. Am J Radiol 1979, 132:91.
8. Mistretta CA, Crummy AB, Strother CM, Sackett JF: *Digital Subtraction Arteriography: An Application of Computerized Fluoroscopy*. Chicago, Year Book, 1982.
9. Ergun DC, Mistretta CA, Kruger RA, Riederer SJ, Shaw CG: A hybrid computerized fluoroscopy technique for noninvasive cardiovascular imaging. Radiology 1979, 132:739.
10. Kruger RA, Mistretta CA, Hauk TL, Kubal W, Riederer SJ, Ergun DC, Sharo CG, Lancaster JC, Rowe CG: Computerized fluoroscopy techniques for intravenous study of cardiochamber dynamics. Invest Radiol 1979, 14:279.
11. Kruger RA, Mistretta CA, Hauk TL, Riederer SJ, Shaw CG, Goodsitt MM, Crummy AB, Zweibel WJ, Lancaster JC, Rowe CG, Flemming D: Computerized fluoroscopy in real time for non-invasive visualization of the cardiovascular system—Preliminary studies. Radiology 1979, 130:49.
12. Kruger RA, Mistretta CA, Lancaster J, Houk TL, Goodsitt MM, Shaw CG, Riederer SJ, Hicks J, Sackett JF, Crummy AB, Flemming D: A digital video image processor for real time x-ray subtraction imaging. Optic Eng 1978, 17:652.
13. Ovitt T, Capp MP, Christenson P: Development of a digital video subtraction system for intravenous angiography. SPIE 1979, 206:73.
14. Meany TF, Weinstein MA, Buonocou P: Digital subtraction angiography of the human cardiovascular septum. SPIE 1980, 233:272.
15. Sackett JF, Mann FA: Contrast media for digital subtraction angiography. In Mistretta CA, Crummy AB, Strother CM, Sackett JF (eds): *Digital Subtraction Arteriography: An Application of Computerized Fluoroscopy*. Chicago, Year Book, 1982.
16. Crummy AB, Strother CM, Lieberman RP: Digital subtraction angiography for evaluation of peripheral vascular disease. Radiology 1981, 141:33.
17. Turnipseed WD, Detmer DE, Berkoff HA, Acher CW, Crummy AB, Belzer FO: Intraarterial angiography: A new diagnostic method for determining limb salvage bypass candidates. Surgery 1982, 92:322.
18. Turnipseed WD: The diagnosis of carotid artery stenosis by digital subtraction angiography. In Bergan JJ, Yao JS (eds): *Cerebrovascular Insufficiency*. New York, Grune & Stratton, 1983.
19. Strother CM, Sackett JF, Crummy AB: Clinical application of computerized fluoroscopy: The extracranial carotid artery. Radiology 1980, 136(2):781.
20. Hertzer NR, Modic MT: Digital subtraction angiography after extracranial carotid reconstruction. In Bergan JJ, Yao JS (eds): *Cerebrovascular Insufficiency*. New York, Grune & Stratton, 1983.
21. Chilcote WA, Modie MT, Pavlicek WA: Digital subtraction angiography of the carotid arteries: A comparative study in 100 patients. Radiology 1981, 139:287.
22. Modic MT, Weinstein MA, Chilcote WA: Digital subtraction angiography of the intracranial septum: A comparative study in 55 patients. AJNR 1981, 2:527.
23. Hertzer NR, Beven EG, Modic MT: Early patency rates of the carotid artery following endarterectomy. Digital subtraction angiography after 262 operations. Surgery 1983, 92:1049.
24. Turnipseed WD, Sackett JF, Strother CM, Crummy AB, Mistretta CA, Kruger RA: Computerized arteriography of the cerebrovascular system. Arch Surg 1981, 116:470.
25. Turnipseed WD, Sackett JF, Strother CM, Crummy AB, Mistretta CA: A comparison of standard cerebral arteriography with an invasive Doppler imaging and intravenous angiography. Arch Surg 1982, 117:419.
26. Acher CW, Turnipseed WD, Sackett JF, Strother CM, Mistretta CA: Digital subtraction angiography and continuous-wave Doppler studies. Arch Surg 1983, 118:462.
27. Russell JB, Watson TM, Madi JR, Lambeth A, Sumner DS: Digital subtraction angiography for evaluation of intracranial carotid occlusive disease: Comparison with conventional arteriography. Surgery 1983, 94:604.
28. Earnest F, Houser DW, Forbes GS, Kispert DB, Folger NN, Sundt TM: The accuracy and limitations of intravenous digital subtraction angiography in evaluation of atherosclerotic cerebrovascular disease: Angiographic and surgical correlations. Mayo Clinic Proc 1983, 58:735.
29. Eikelboom BC, Acherstaff AA, Ludwig JW, Moll FL, Vries AR, Vermulen FE: Digital video subtraction angiography and duplex scanning in assessment of carotid artery disease: Comparison with conventional angiography. Surgery 1983, 94:821.
30. Turnipseed WD, Berkoff WD, Crummy AB: Postoperative occlusion after carotid endarterectomy. Arch Surg 1979, 115:573.
31. Turnipseed WD: Potential clinical applications of digital subtraction angiography. Vasc Diagn Ther 1982 3(4):17.
32. Myerowitz PD, Turnipseed WD, Shaw GG, Swanson D, Chopra PJ, Berkoff HA, Kroncke GM, Dhanani SP, Rowe GG, VanLysel M, Crummy AB: Computerized fluoroscopy: J Thorac Cardiovasc Surg 1982, 83:65.
33. Myerowitz PD, Turnipseed WD, Swanson D, VanLysel M, Peppler W, Mistretta CA, Kroncke GG, Hasegawa B, Steighorst M, Turski P, Crummy AB: Digital subtraction angiography as a method of screening for coronary artery disease during peripheral vascular angiography. Surgery 1982, 92:1042.
34. Myerowitz PD, Swanson D, Turnipseed WD, Mistretta CA: The role of digital subtraction angiography in the evaluation and management of patients with coronary artery disease. In Roberts AJ (ed): *Coronary Artery Surgery: Applications of New Technologies*. Chicago, Year Book, 1983.
35. Turnipseed WD, Acher CW, Detmer DE, Berkoff HA, Myerowitz PD, Crummy AB, Belzer FO: Digital subtraction angiography and B-mode ultrasonography for abdominal and peripheral aneurysms. Surgery 1982, 92:619.
36. Turnipseed WD, Crummy AB, Sackett JF, Ergen D, Shaw C, Kruger R, Mistretta CA, Liberman RP, Belzer FO: Computerized intravenous arteriography: A technique for visualizing the peripheral vascular system. Surgery 1981, 89:118.
37. Crummy AB, Strother CM, Lieberman RP, Stighrost MF, Sackett JF, Woutowycz MM, Kruger RA, Turnipseed WD, Ergun DL, Shaw CG, Mistretta CA, Ruzicka FF: Digital video subtraction angiography for evaluation of peripheral vascular disease. Radiology 1981, 141:33.

PART TWO

Medical Treatment

Chapter 15

MEDICAL MANAGEMENT OF ATHEROSCLEROTIC VASCULAR DISEASE

RALPH G. DePALMA

Atherosclerosis is the most important disease treated by the vascular surgeon. It is also the most common serious disease of modern western society, though within the last two decades, cardiovascular mortality in the United States has decreased (1). Since the pioneering surgical efforts of the 1950s, there has been remarkable progress in relieving the morbidity and mortality of atherosclerosis, particularly the lethal consequences of aortic aneurysms and left main coronary artery and carotid bifurcation plaques. The recognition by surgeons that the complications of atherosclerosis relate to segmental arterial involvement was critical in developing techniques to treat this disease (2,3). Vascular surgical interventions remain the most effective means of ameliorating the complications of the atherosclerotic process. However, atherosclerosis is also a systemic disease which remains dormant in arteries until a complication signals its presence.

Recently, there has been intense interest in medical treatment to control, or at least arrest, atherosclerotic lesions sufficiently to improve the outcome in this disease. Although there is general agreement about the epidemiology of risk factors which predispose to atherosclerosis (4), the medical control of established atherosclerosis remains controversial (5,6). To understand this discrepancy, the dynamics of atherosclerotic plaques and limitations in detecting change in the disease process must be understood. There is little doubt about the feasibility of inducing plaque regression or arrest in experimental animals by drastically reducing low-density lipoprotein (LDL) cholesterol levels in the blood (7–13). These experiments reduce the usual single risk factor used to cause experimental disease. Whether human atherosclerosis has the same potential for regression or arrest is debated (14). This chapter discusses the medical management of atherosclerotic vascular disease for surgeons, who are often required to choose medical and surgical alternatives before and after operation. Concepts about the dynamics of the atheroma, lesion quantification, and risk-factor interventions are reviewed. It will be seen that indirect interventions might be applicable to certain atherosclerotic lesions, while surgical intervention is required for many other arterial lesions.

The Atheroma

The first events provoking atheroma formation and localization are incompletely understood. The initial process may be increased endothelial permeability resulting from altered endothelial cell function or possibly from actual endothelial injury (15,16). The first lesion of atherosclerosis, considered to be the progenitor of the more advanced lesions, occurs because of the entry of LDL through the intima into the arterial wall. The lipids of plasma are similar to those of the early plaque (17). This LDL entry stimulates arterial smooth muscle to form foam cells; a significant fraction of the foam cells are believed to be derived also from macrophages. Early fatty streaks appear grossly as minimally raised yellow lesions and are found commonly in younger people, i.e., in the first through the third decades of life. The fatty streak contains intracellular lipid in macrophages and smooth-muscle cells; the bulk of the lipid occurs intracellularly. When lipid escapes from the cell, extracellular cholesterol esters are intensely irritating to the arterial wall (18). It is believed that some, but not all, fatty lesions evolve into more advanced lesions, or fibrous plaques (19). As the disease advances, these plaques intrude into the arterial lumen. Fibrous plaques are composed of large numbers of smooth-muscle cells and connective tissue, forming a fibrous cap over an inner core containing mainly cholesterol esters. In the early fatty streaks, the cholesterol esters appear as ordered crystalline arrays, i.e., in the form of liquid crystals, while in the advanced plaques, the lipid appears in isotropic and in extracellular sites (18,20). These lipid deposits in advanced plaques may be more difficult to reabsorb, possibly limiting lesion arrest or regression (21). Whether all fibrous plaques characteristic of advanced atherosclerosis evolve through a fatty streak stage is uncertain (22). However, fibrous plaques often appear chronologically after fatty streaks, often in the same anatomic locations, and characterize clinically apparent atherosclerosis (23,24).

Contrary to a traditional definition of atherosclerosis as "a variable combination of changes in *the intima* [sic.] of arteries consisting of focal accumulation of lipids, complex carbohydrates, blood and blood products, fibrous tissue and calcium deposits" (25), the advanced atheroma often invades the media. In its early stages it can produce a beadlike appearance of smaller arteries. It is also associated with varying degrees of periarterial

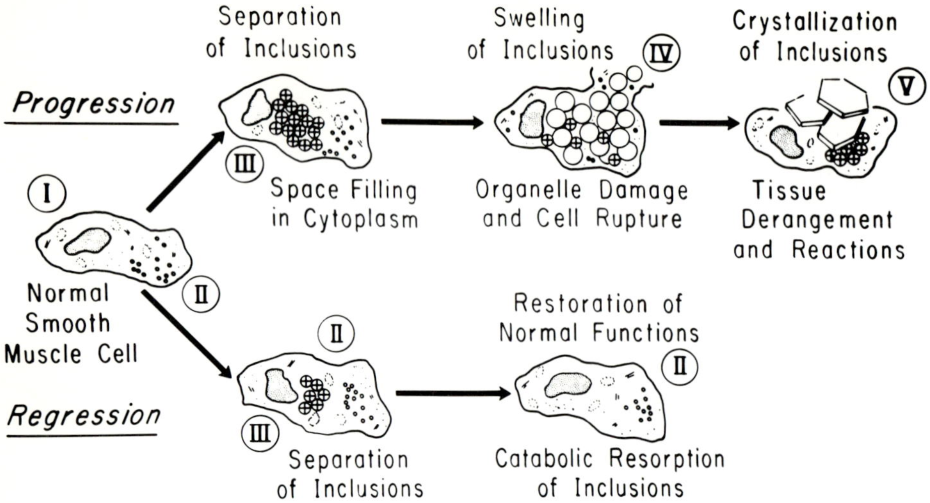

FIGURE 15-1. Possible role of lipid inclusions in atherogenesis and regression, after Hata (20). (I) Structure-bound lipids in a normal smooth-muscle cell, e.g., mainly in cell membranes; (II) lipoprotein in lipid forms; (III) anisotropic lipid inclusions in early stage; (IV) isotropic lipid inclusions and cell rupture; (V) solid crystals. Note that during regression intracellular anisotropic lipids may resorb. [*Reprinted from DePalma RG, Clowes AW (64).*]

inflammation. Figure 15-1 illustrates the key role of lipid inclusions in human atherosclerosis. During atherosclerotic progression, liquid lipids crystallize, probably causing tissue derangements and the inflammatory reaction of atherosclerosis. During regression, both lipoprotein lipids and anisotropic lipid inclusion bodies are resorbed, and this results in the restoration of normal smooth-muscle cell function. These sequences are important in evaluating the possibilities as well as the constraints of medical therapy.

Complicated plaques—fibrous plaques which have become calcified, ulcerated, or necrotic—constitute end-stage atherosclerosis and cause clinical symptoms. Because of their friability, they can dissect from the arterial wall to cause sudden occlusion. Catastrophic events, such as sudden expansion or overlying thrombosis, within the plaque result in sudden death, limb loss, or stroke. Carotid plaques are particularly unstable entities in the arterial wall. Hemorrhage from neovascularization within the plaque can produce rapid lesion expansion, and this raises serious questions about therapies which might predispose to bleeding in plaques (26). Ulcerated carotid plaques may also suddenly dissect, and porridgelike material within them may rupture into the lumen, embolizing distally to the brain and retina. Imparato (27) has long emphasized these mechanisms. A means of stabilizing the fibrous or complicated plaque would prevent these clinical catastrophes; this would involve much more than anticoagulation, or a modest reduction in the plasma lipid levels.

Unstable plaque components, related to connective tissues, can cause capricious behavior. Unpredictable events in atherosclerotic plaques often account for the protean manifestations of the disease. The many variants of atherosclerotic disease and its polypathogenic nature (28) make its prognosis and control an enormous problem. The classification of certain types of lesions and their rates of progression within particular arterial beds provide a useful tool for prognosis (29). It is obvious, but usually overlooked, that any treatment intended to improve the outcome must have a beneficial effect on the lesions within the arterial wall itself. Clinical treatment trials to reduce morbidity and mortality often yield blurred results; the cause of this is discussed in some detail in a later section. To date, there remain problems in quantifying the severity of atherosclerotic lesions and the involvement of arterial walls. When these problems are solved, the efficacy of medical management might be better assessed.

Although atherosclerosis is a segmental disease involving mainly the arteries of the head, heart, and lower extremities, it is also a systemic problem. Some atheromatous involvements are associated; for example, a high incidence of coronary lesions is found in patients with aortic (30), carotid (31,32), and peripheral atherosclerosis (4). The reverse is not necessarily true; patients often have coronary disease in the absence of significant peripheral atherosclerosis. Bodily patterns of peripheral atherosclerosis suggest that particular arterial beds are affected by particular risk factors (33). The challenge is to identify asymptomatic early lesions which may be amenable to regression or arrest.

Lesion Detection and Quantification

Ideally, we should be able to detect asymptomatic lesions. These lesions will probably not be found by conventional noninvasive flow studies. The asymptomatic nonhemodynamically significant lesions will be found only by scans which delineate arterial wall abnormalities. Once the clinician identifies wall involvement and early luminal intrusion, he or she might choose the best clinical treatment. The beneficial effects of intervention would result in less luminal intrusion or arterial wall involvement. Although this technology is still not routinely available, there has been important progress in attempts to detect and to quantify lesions (34–36). For this purpose, serial angiography and ultrasound imaging are being used.

It is important for the surgeon to examine gross morphologic characteristics for clues about the activity of the disease process.

TABLE 15-1. **Atherosclerosis**

	Active	Nonactive
Adventitia	Inflammatory reaction Yellow beadlike bulges	Fibrosis White scar
Media	Friable Necrotic central lesions	Tough Calcified
Intima	Grumous ulcers Intima-media poorly attached Many yellow plaques	Ulcers: calcified base Pearly elevated scars Many white plaques
Lumen	Porridgelike debris Loose clot	Fibrotic stenosis Adherent clot

Table 15-1 outlines the findings in active and nonactive phases of the disease; intermediate stages also exist. *Atheroma* comes from the Greek word for "porridge," and *sclerosis* signifies "induration" or "hardening." When the surgeon encounters friable atheromas in younger patients, e.g., those in the fourth decade, he or she should note the nature and intensity of the risk factors pertaining to that patient. In my experience, one can almost always identify heavy cigarette smoking or a metabolic disorder in these cases. If the problem is mainly dilating or aneurysmal disease, this too should be recorded, since the only treatment for inexorably progressive dilating or aneurysmal disease is surgical.

Experimental plaque regression relates mainly to the reduction of plaque bulk by lipid absorption (5,12,37); connective tissue accumulations can also regress slowly (38). Experiments show that it is possible to lessen luminal intrusion and plaque bulk by drastically reducing serum cholesterol (39). There appears, moreover, to be a critical serum lipid threshold above which lesions continue to progress in an inevitable fashion (40–42). Based on experimental data, this threshold probably approximates a total serum cholesterol concentration of 150 to 170 mg/dL. In humans, the regression of early lesions with lipid and other interventions can be documented by using serial angiograms, which show less luminal (34,43) intrusion. To date, angiography has been the main method applied to quantitate lesion regression clinically (44,45).

Possibly critical to the fate of plaques are the particular fibrous-protein responses elicited in the artery wall by the disease process. The collagen which forms in atherosclerotic lesions is not the normal type III arterial collagen; it is a type I scar collagen elaborated by transformed medial cells (46). The friability of the intima and media of atherosclerotic arteries is familiar to all surgeons who suture these vessels. The thin and uninvolved outer arterial layer often holds sutures well. The behavior of the complex lesions, lipid core, smooth muscle, and collagen mass might be determined mainly by the quality of the fibrous protein strength. The atheroma is also an inflammatory lesion and can be regarded as a form of continually sustained injury, as reviewed by Ross and Glomset (15). Although it appears logical to ameliorate the factors continuing to initiate arterial injury, no other *specific* medical therapy exists. In animal models, plaques regress within certain limits of individual variability, depending upon the rate and degree of elevation of the serum cholesterol level or its reduction below the threshold for regression or arrest. However, the ultimate fate of advanced human plaques may also be a function of connective tissue, hemodynamic, and coagulation responses, in turn related to the multiple risk factors promoting this disease (see Chapter 2).

In spite of these caveats related to connective tissue, hemodynamic and coagulative responses over which we have little control, having the ability to detect atherosclerotic plaques and to document changes in luminal intrusion serially is a valid goal. Both the advantages and the limitations of angiography can be determined in animal experiments (47). Our experiments in rhesus monkeys, using serial angiography as a tool to estimate disease severity, were instructive. Luminal changes in fatty fibrous plaques were documented angiographically and confirmed morphologically, a procedure that can only be done in animal models. Angiography showed that the progression of luminal intrusion is related to a degree of hypercholesterolemia. We found that the most effective diet for producing disease in monkeys is one in which sugar and egg yolk are combined and which does not contain as much cholesterol as regimens that produce less disease. The regressive effects of lowered serum cholesterol levels induced by diet, internal biliary diversion, and bile acid sequestrant are directly related to the degree of serum lipid reduction.

Angiography is a specific method to detect advanced plaques. However, its sensitivity for early lesion detection is limited and differs from site to site. The sensitivity for the detection of rhesus monkey lesions of the internal carotid artery was .45; for the inferior mesenteric artery, .73; for the lumbar aorta, .54; and for the spermatic artery, .58 in 146 observations in which specimens were examined soon after the angiograms. Angiography did not yield information about changes in wall thickness or show the external bulging of the arterial wall often produced by fatty plaques. These are important limitations for the clinician to consider when using angiography to estimate the extent of atherosclerotic involvement. The detection of a change in wall thickness is critical if treatment is to be started in early stages of the disease. Refined B-mode imaging and computerized axial tomography are now important tools for the examination of the arterial wall. It is worth reemphasizing that the detection of dilating or aneurysmal disease by angiograms alone can be deceptive if the arterial lumen is filled with laminated clot.

Luminal-plaque encroachment has been quantified by computerized methods by Blankenhorn and associates (34–36). This method has been applied to the femoral artery, which can be conveniently imaged by serial angiography in humans. Numerical estimates of atherosclerotic change can be provided with an orderly review of morphometric data, and responses to particular therapeutic interventions can be determined. Plaque regression in humans occurs in instances where the disease causes minimal intrusion into the arterial lumen. Such lesions are rarely hemodynamically significant, and plaque regression, overall, is a rare clinical response. Malinow (14) documented 32 such instances in 143 serial angiograms. The reasons for this include a lack of control of multiple risk factors and even a failure to achieve threshold lipid reductions such as can be done in animals in a laboratory.

Human atherosclerotic disease, by and large, has progressed for three or more decades before it is detected. Regression of human arterial lesions may require a longer time than that of the studies so far done. Experimental interventions use quantitative methods to measure the components of the arterial wall and to take into account the effects of arterial pressure. The surgeon should attempt to estimate the degree of lesion severity, recognizing limitations in his or her perceptual ability in an open vessel. A better quantitative grasp of this disease results from repeated clinical correlations between the plaque morphology, angiograms, and arterial wall scans. Ultimately, such correlated morphometric observations will permit a more objective evaluation of treatment.

Risk Factors as Etiologic Factors

It is useful, but not necessarily absolutely rigorous to consider epidemiologically defined risk factors as etiologic factors. When these factors are considered together with pathological factors, human atherosclerosis can be seen as a family of closely related vascular lesions (28,29). Its etiology is multifactorial. From a practical standpoint, the clinician often detects four major risk factors which interact in varying degrees. These are diabetes mellitus, hyperlipidemia, cigarette smoking, and hypertension. In some cases none of these are present when the patient presents. Nonetheless, epidemiologic studies done by the Framingham group (4) relate quantitatively the intensity and duration of these risk factors to the frequency of clinical disorders signaling atherosclerotic disease.

It is useful to examine each risk factor as it relates to lesion pathogenesis. When diabetes is the only risk factor present, it causes diffuse involvement of the infrageniculate arteries with relative sparing of the aortoiliac segments (33). It is also associated with an increased risk of disease in other vessels. An experienced observer can often identify diabetes-caused atherosclerosis from arteriograms of the tibial vessels. We still do not know whether the meticulous control of diabetes influences atherosclerosis in general. However, the addition of cigarette smoking to diabetes portends disaster, especially for patients with distal disease. Current emphasis among diabetologists is on the rigorous control of blood glucose levels without the use of oral agents, which are possibly associated with a higher incidence of atherosclerotic complications (48). The pathogenic mechanisms by which diabetes promotes atherosclerosis are poorly understood. Some fragments of information exist. It has been shown that insulin therapy controls hyperlipidemia and decreases total cholesterol synthesis (49). Studies in wound healing demonstrate that insulin treatment restores impaired collagen formation in laboratory animals (50). Hyperlipidemia is a complex subject because there are uncertainties in the role of each plasma protein fraction as related to actual pathological changes in the arterial wall (51).

Although a high level of LDL cholesterol is a major etiologic factor, a high level of high-density lipoprotein (HDL) is a negative risk factor. At all ages in the United States the total cholesterol level mirrors the LDL level (52); measurements of LDL cholesterol and HDL cholesterol provide refinements. Estimates of abnormally elevated cholesterol levels are changing. In general cross-sectional data in middle-aged men, total cholesterol levels of 185 mg/dL with an LDL level of 140 mg/dL or lower and an HDL level of over 45 mg/dL are favorable. Whether or not the lipid will enter the arterial wall is believed to depend on the apoprotein moiety, or the protein constituent of the lipoprotein molecule. Apoprotein B is associated with LDL and the tendency to enter the arterial wall, while apoprotein A is the main constituent of HDL (''helper'' lipoprotein). Hyperapobetalipoproteinemia identifies hypertriglyceridemic patients prone to atherosclerotic disease (53). It is possible that measurements of apoprotein B alone will be used in the future to identify risk for atherosclerotic disease.

A worrisome relationship between low plasma cholesterol levels, noncardiovascular mortality, and cancer of the colon has been suggested (54). Increased mortality from cancers occurs in groups with levels of total cholesterol below 195 mg/dL. What does this imply for lipid-risk-factor interventions? This issue has been reviewed by Levy (55), who noted that the cholesterol-cancer relationship has been inconsistent and mainly apparent in males. A panel sponsored by the National Heart, Lung, and Blood Institute (NHLBI) concluded that ''the data did not preclude, countermand, or contradict the current public health message which recommends that those with elevated cholesterol levels seek to lower them. . . .'' One suggestion is that the lower cholesterol level in colon cancer patients is a biological marker, possibly genetic in origin. Another (56) is that the ideal cholesterol level is somewhat below the average U.S. level, but not at very low levels.

Cigarette smoking is the most prevalent and ominous risk factor in the atherosclerotic patient. It is associated with the progression of peripheral atherosclerotic disease to amputation (56), a high mortality from ischemic heart disease (57), and late failures of aortic reconstruction (58,59). The exact mechanisms by which smoking promotes atherosclerosis are incompletely understood. Intermittent carbon monoxidemia possibly predisposes to endothelial injury (60), leading to increased plasma flux into the arterial wall. Cigarette smoking causes increased platelet reactivity, promotes peripheral vasoconstriction, and is associated with reduced levels of HDL (61).

Hypertension is a potent risk factor; atherosclerosis due to hyperlipidemia is accelerated by chronic hypertension in the experimental animal (62), and hypertension probably has the same effect in humans. It causes vascular complications such as cerebral hemorrhage and renal failure, and its control prolongs life (63). Certain populations in the orient and in the Caribbean exhibit hypertension with a relative absence of atherosclerotic disease when other risk factors promoting atherocslerosis are absent. Hypertension predisposes to more continued arterial injury hemodynamically, probably accelerating plaque complications.

Trauma-induced local risk factors predisposing to plaque development have been reviewed (64). These risk factors include procedures that involve damage to the arterial wall, such as clamping, balloon embolectomy, and radiation therapy. The local damage particulary predisposes to the development of plaques in muscular arteries, even when other risk factors are reduced. This effect should be anticipated in patients after arterial injury and radiation therapy. Males receiving estrogen therapy for carcinoma of the prostate are more liable to the thrombotic complications of atherosclerosis. Finally, a higher incidence of coronary artery disease has been reported with a combination of birth control pills and cigarette smoking in young women (65).

Interventions

The surgeon needs to document risk factors that exist in individual patients. Risk-factor intervention assumes that altering or abolishing a risk factor will result in a clinical benefit. The evidence for this belief will be reviewed later. The postoperative maintenance of graft patency and the prevention of the progression of disease in other native arteries are the goals of intervention. Because of the dramatic beneficial results of surgery, the operating surgeon often exerts considerable influence over the patient's motivation to follow a program of risk-factor reduction. The surgeon's advice must be tailored to individual patient needs and realistically based on alterable risk factors. In many cases, this advice essentially amounts to two practical recommendations: the cessation of smoking and the treatment of hyperlipidemia.

CIGARETTE SMOKING

Cigarette smoking is the most pervasive risk factor predisposing to postoperative reconstructive failures. The patient must be induced to relinquish this habit before surgery. This is best done during admission for preoperative studies and during postoperative care. Compliance with the advice given can be assessed by measurement of the blood thiocyanate (66) or carboxyhemoglobin levels (67). The surgeon must constantly reinforce the advice about the cessation of cigarette smoking. Patients who change to cigar or pipe smoking also inhale and should not resume smoking until the habit of smoke inhalation is completely under control. The biochemical tests will detect whether the patient has adopted a pattern of inhaling tobacco smoke from a pipe or cigar. An alteration of smoking habits does not compete with measures to lower lipid levels, nor should smoking habits and dietary measures become bargaining chips between the patient and the physician. In a study of biochemical factors after reconstruction, Greenhalgh (68) concluded that little evidence exists to warrant dietary advice at all. This recommendation relates to graft patency and is consonant with my experience. It does appear logical, however, to control hyperlipidemia to prevent disease progression.

LIPID REDUCTION

Diet

Many patients who present for peripheral reconstruction have no lipid abnormality detectable by current methods (33). In these circumstances, it is irrational to recommend dietary alterations or drug treatment. When patients exhibit hypercholesterolemia or hypertriglyceridemia, I have recommended the following diet since 1970 (69).

Meat. Three meals a week may contain lean beef or lamb. Meat should be trimmed of visible fat. Fatty meats, such as hot dogs, canned processed meats, cold cuts, and sausages, should be eliminated completely.

Chicken, veal, turkey, and fish are permitted in any amount. Shellfish of all kinds (shrimp, lobster, crab, etc.) are allowed. Even though shellfish are high in cholesterol, some authorities believe that they do not elevate blood cholesterol levels.

Carbohydrates. Foods such as rice, potatoes, pasta, bread, and popcorn are allowed in moderation. The major concern with these is weight gain. There are two restrictions: (1) Bread should have as high a fiber content as possible, thereby eliminating most commercial brands; (2) popcorn should be made at home with margarine flavoring; that made at the movies is not allowed, since it usually is made with peanut or coconut oils, which are intensely irritating to the arteries.

Vegetables. A liberal intake of all kinds of vegetables is encouraged.

Dairy Products. No butter, eggs, or whole milk is recommended.

Margarine and skim milk are allowed. Cheeses are limited to skim milk products such as cottage, ricotta, or Greek cheese.

Sugar. Sucrose should be eliminated from the diet as much as possible. No desserts, candy, or soft drinks which contain this sugar are allowed.

Fruit. Whole natural fruits are used as a substitute for desserts with a high sugar content. Fruits which have been canned in sugar syrup are not permitted.

Beverages. Coffee is permitted in moderation, as are tea and alcohol; wine is allowed with meals.

Cooking Oil. Oils such as olive, corn, or safflower are to be used for salad dressings and for cooking, instead of shortening.

Vitamin Supplements. A daily vitamin supplement containing 300 mg of ascorbic acid, 5000 U.S.P. units of vitamin A, and vitamin B complex are advised during dietary alteration.

There is enormous popular interest in intensive dietary and exercise programs to treat ischemic heart disease. The Pritikin program (70) consists of a 10 percent fat diet which rigorously excludes salt, sugar, alcohol, and caffeine. Dietary protein is derived primarily from plant sources, with the addition of skim milk and small amounts of fish or fowl. This diet minimizes fat consumption to 10 percent or less of the calories and is often taught in a center. Smoking is not allowed. Falls in average serum cholesterol levels from 236 ± 9 to 179 ± 6 mg/dL have been obtained with increased maximal work capacity. Combined with intensive medically supervised exercise programs, this program also has a favorable effect on non-insulin-dependent diabetes (71). The long-term effects of aggressive dietary intervention on survival, and its effects of such intervention on the arterial wall itself, need evaluation. It is my belief that the diets outlined above do reduce serum lipid levels to threshold levels consistent with the regression or arrest of early lesions. The problems are patient acceptance and compliance.

Drugs for Hyperlipidemia

Drugs are used when dietary therapy has not reduced lipid levels to normal and after the hyperlipidemia has been classified. As pointed out in a recent review by LaRosa (72) hyperlipidemia should be considered to have a sufficiently high risk that the physician should consider prescribing drugs for hyperlipidemic patients for an indefinite period. For patients with elevated LDL (type II hyperlipoproteinemia), a bile acid sequenstrant, cholestyramine, and a similar agent, colestipol, are mainstays of treatment. These agents interrupt the enterohepatic circulation of bile and cause increased bile acid excretion in the stool, thus lowering serum cholesterol levels. The major side effect of cholestyramine is constipation, which requires stool softeners or Metamucil. These drugs must be taken as powders in juice or water, and this dosage form plus their constipating side effects may lead to poor compliance. Experimentally, in monkeys, cholestyramine produced plaque regression or arrest (41,42).

For patients with elevated very-low-density lipoprotein (VLDL; triglyceride) levels, gemfibrozil, an agent related to clofibrate, is effective. It has an advantage over clofibrate in that it elevates HDL levels in addition to lowering VLDL levels. Nicotinic acid is effective in all types of hyperlipoproteinemia and can be particularly useful when combined with bile acid sequestrants. It is limited by the side effects pruritis and flushing; these two complaints may limit compliance.

Metabolic Surgical Interventions

An important alternative for certain patients with elevated LDL cholesterol levels, based on either genetic or acquired factors, is the ileal bypass described by Buchwald, Moore, and Varco (73). The most recent results from Buchwald's group (74) show a reduction of LDL cholesterol levels from 182.3 ± 35 mg/dL before operation to a range of 95.8 to 109.8 mg/dL 3 months to 4 years after the ileal bypass. The mean total plasma cholesterol level fell from 255 mg/dL to a range of 167 to 185.3 mg/dL over the same intervals. This unifactorial secondary-intervention trial on survivors of myocardial infarction aims to document the changes in coronary atherosclerotic plaques. The results will be important in asssesing the effect of an obligatory single risk-factor reduction in patients with coronary heart disease (CHD). The study is designed deliberately not to alter smoking behavior.

Portacaval shunts (75,76) have been suggested for patients with type II familial hyperlipoproteinemias, which are associated with LDL elevations of extreme degree. In these rare patients, LDL receptors are lacking (77,78); the patients cannot metabolize LDL or regulate endogenous cholesterol synthesis (79), and untreated homozygotes usually die in their teens or twenties of coronary atherosclerosis. Because their prognosis is exceedingly poor, end-to-side portacaval shunts have been done for a few of these patients. The patients are identified by their family history. A biopsy of the proband's connective tissue cells can be processed to identify a lack of LDL receptors. Since the initial reports (75,76), there has been cautious study of this procedure in these patients. The shunt causes a decreased synthesis of hepatic lipoprotein, an increased degradation of lipoprotein, and decreased plasma LDL levels (80).

CONTROVERSY IN RISK-FACTOR INTERVENTIONS

If risk-factor intervention is advised, we must also consider the results achieved in multiple-risk-factor-intervention trials. A 7-year trial was designed to test the effects of multiple-risk-factor interventions on the outcome of CHD in 12,866 high-risk men, aged 35 to 57 years (81). Half these men were randomly assigned to a special intervention (SI) program consisting of the treatment of hypertension, counseling about cigarette smoking, and dietary advice about lowering serum cholesterol levels. The other half, called the usual-care (UC) group, were referred to the usual sources of health care in the community. Serum cholesterol levels fell from an average of 255 mg/dL in both groups to approximately 235 mg/dL in the SI group and 240 mg/dL in the UC group. Thiocyanate-adjusted cigarette smoking fell from about 65 percent in both groups to 35 percent in the SI group and 45 percent in the UC group. These differences are very small. Based on what is known experimentally, these changes would not be expected to cause arterial wall changes. In fact, the total mortality and the CHD rates were identical for the two groups. However, among the UC group based on assumptions about risk-factor and the Framingham risk functions, 442 deaths, including 187 from CHD, were expected by the end of the study. Only 219 deaths occurred, including 104 from CHD. It is possible that the UC group did, in fact, do something about their own risk factors. Two other explanations for why the SI program did not affect CHD mortality were offered: (1) the intervention affected CHD mortality, but this effect was not observed in this 7-year trial in which the UC group had a lower-than-expected mortality and a considerable risk-factor change; or (2) measures to reduce cigarette smoking and lower blood cholesterol levels reduced the CHD mortality within some groups of the SI cohort, but an unfavorable response to antihypertensive drug therapy occurred in certain of the hypertensive subjects. On the surface, these results appear discouraging for risk-factor interventions. A Norwegian single-center two-factor CHD-prevention trial (82) did significantly reduce the incidence of total cardiovascular and CHD end points. This study excluded hypertensive subjects. With two-factor interventions—reducing smoking and lowering lipid levels—the single-center study achieved a significant reduction in CHD.

These data underscore the difficulty of analyzing lifestyle alterations in large groups. Physicians and surgeons following individuals with established disease have a better opportunity to define actual alterations in individual risk factors. To quote Gertrude Stein: "A difference to be a difference must make a difference." In undertaking a risk-factor alteration, the clincian must comprehend the magnitude of this task in practice. Barmeyer and associates (83), in spite of frequent counseling, noted that the risk factors cigarette smoking and hyperlipidemia were poorly controlled. Their serial angiographic studies revealed progression in all cases, as did the angiographic studies of Kuthan et al. (84). In other instances, partial regression of lesions with diet and exercise were documented with serial angiography, but only in *nonsmokers* (85). The blurred effect in large trials could be clarified by following single patients using objective methods to quantify arterial wall changes.

ANTIPLATELET THERAPY

Aspirin, dipyridamole, and other antiplatelet agents are now used commonly to treat or prevent the thrombotic or thromboembolic complications of atherosclerosis. Prostaglandin inhibitors have been shown to reduce platelet adherence to grafts (86–89). Experimentally, they may inhibit anastomotic intimal hyperplasia (86,87,90). However, in addition to the potential beneficial effects on platelet-induced thrombosis resulting from the inhibition of thromboxane A_2 production, they also inhibit the endothelial cell production of prostacyclin, which is believed to protect the intima by preventing platelet adherence. Antiplatelet therapy could be a two-edged sword. In an experiment using serial angiography and arterial biopsy in rhesus monkeys, we noted deleterious effects of aspirin and dipyridamole on diet-induced atherosclerosis (91,92). During 1 year of treatment, antiplatelet therapy accelerated the disease and caused plaque calcification which was absent in untreated animals. We also observed that aspirin and dipyridamole, in dosages of 13.5 mg/kg per day of aspirin and 15 mg/kg per day of dipyridamole, inhibit the rate of endothelial regrowth in balloon-injured rabbit arteries (93). Recent work from our laboratory showed an overall 66 percent increased thickening of the more slowly growing endothelium in the antiplatelet-treated animals (94). Carson et al. (95) reported that antiplatelet treatment in humans results in more emergency surgical interventions for carotid atheromas. Aspirin and dipyridamole do not alter ^{111}In-labeled platelet adherence in recently thrombectomized carotid artery segments (96). All these experimental data indicate problems in current choices and dosages of antiplatelet agents.

Thus the physician considering antiplatelet therapy faces a dilemma. Although antiplatelet agents are beneficial after coronary vein bypass operations (97), their experimental effects on indigenous arteries and regrowing areas of endothelium are troubling. The negative effect of these agents on endothelial prostacyclin production is an important problem. Antiplatelet therapy could be indicated after certain types of reconstruction, but perhaps not for the general management of atherosclerosis. Pending further study, I am not using combination antiplatelet agents routinely before or after carotid endarterectomy. Although the interactions of platelets, endothelial regrowth, and plaque development present challenging research prospects, current antiplatelet therapy should not be accepted uncritically as an alternative treatment. For symptomatic carotid disease, I believe that carotid endarterectomy is safer than the use of antiplatelet agents and that antiplatelet agents should not be used postoperatively without specific indications.

HYPERTENSION

A general decrease in cerebrovascular disease mortality has occurred (98). Although stroke is related to the risk factors of atherosclerosis, its intimate association with hypertension is strongly established. A considerable reduction in the risk of stroke results from the treatment of hypertension. It has been suggested that the reduced cerebrovascular disease mortality might be attributed to the use of modern antihypertensive agents, especially beta-adrenergic blocking agents. The worrisome negative effect of antihypertensive treatment in the multiple-risk-factor-intervention trial (81) has been postulated to relate to diuretics rather than to the newer beta blockers. Although hypertension alone does not necessarily promote atherosclerosis, its control may be an important factor decreasing cardiovascular mortality (1). The surgical treatment of endocrine or renal hypertension also reduces this risk factor. In males, successful surgical intervention averts the side effect of impotence caused by antihypertensive drugs (99).

UNCONVENTIONAL THERAPIES

The clinician will encounter queries abut unconventional therapies for atherosclerosis, such as chelation or megavitamin therapy. The former uses an intravenous chelating agent with the intent of causing a resorption of arterial wall calcium to ameliorate atherosclerosis. The reversal of calcification in small arteries with the treatment of secondary hypercalcemia by parathyroidectomy is well known. However, calcification is not often the major plaque component causing obstruction, nor is it a factor in aneurysm formation, though it often exists in aneurysm walls. This therapy depends upon other concurrent risk-factor interventions, mainly the cessation of smoking, which would be beneficial.

Another interesting relationship is the apparent ascorbic acid deficiency in cigarette smokers, so-called smoker's scurvy. In comparison with nonsmokers, smokers have low vitamin C levels in plasma and blood and retain more ascorbic acid during loading tests (100). However, during desaturation periods, the rate of loss of vitamin C in plasma is about the same in both groups. Since most atherosclerotic patients are smokers and as surgical candidates will be subjected to stress and alterations of the diet, I have long used routine vitamin supplements during these periods of dietary alteration. Supplementing the patient's diet with a moderately large dose of ascorbic acid in the immediate preoperative and postoperative period, for example, about 1000 mg/day, does no harm and may replete plasma ascorbic acid levels in smokers and after surgical stress. Whether or not this supplementation favorably affects the arterial wall is unknown.

Medical and Surgical Alternatives

No conflict should exist between medical and surgical alternatives. The ideal management of atherosclerosis varies from patient to patient, depending on the type of involvement of particular arterial beds. Specific therapy should have a demonstrably beneficial effect on the arteries and should prolong survival. The reader should now recognize the dominant role of LDL cholesterol with its apoprotein B complex in lesion initiation and pathogenesis. He or she will also recognize the complex interactions between connective tissue, endothelium, and platelets, which mainly predispose to clinical events such as myocardial infarctions, stroke, and gangrene. The practical problems of compliance with risk-factor interventions and limits of current knowledge have been emphasized in this chapter.

Exercise has not been stressed. It makes patients feel better, improves cardiac function, stimulates collateral growth in the legs, and increases HDL levels but has not been shown to exert a beneficial effect on the atheroma itself. In patients with ischemic heart disease, exercise must be prescribed in a deliberate fashion and monitored by physicians experienced in this field. Walking is the most useful form of exercise to treat occlusive femoropopliteal disease in the absence of critical ischemia. Operative interventions can be avoided in many of these patients with prescriptions for graded walking and the cessation of smoking. On the other hand, it would be foolhardy to prescribe exercise for the patient with a critical left main coronary stenosis or an ulcerated carotid plaque.

Because of their unique knowledge of the pathology and physiology of atherosclerosis, vascular surgeons enjoy an influential role in the control of this disease. They are often required to advise their patients about medical treatment. Medical interventions based on a better understanding of this disease might become as precise as current surgical interventions and thus contribute to better patient survival.

Acknowledgments

The illuminating suggestions about the treatment of hyperlipidemia, about apoprotein B, and about the low-cholesterol–cancer relationship by Dr. John C. LaRosa, associate chairman of medicine and director of the Lipid Research Clinic, the George Washington University School of Medicine, are gratefully acknowledged.

References

1. Levy RI, Moskowitz J: Cardiovascular research: Decades of progress, a decade of promise. Science 1982, 217:121.
2. DeBakey ME, Crawford ES, Cooley DA, Morris GC Jr: Surgical considerations of occlusive disease of the abdominal aorta and iliac and femoral arteries. Ann Surg 1958, 148:306.
3. Dale WA: The beginnings of vascular surgery. Surgery 1974, 76:849.
4. Gordon T, Kannel WB: Predisposition to atherosclerosis in the head, heart and legs: The Framingham study. JAMA, 1977, 221:661.
5. Schettler E, Stange E, Wissler RW: *Atherosclerosis—Is It Reversible?* Berlin, Heidelberg, New York, Springer-Verlag, 1978.
6. DePalma RG: Regression or arrest of atherosclerosis—Does it happen? In Greenhalgh, RM (ed): *Proceedings of International Symposium: Hormones and Vascular Disease,* London, Pitman, 1981, pp 71–92.
7. Armstrong ML, Megan MB: Lipid depletion in atheromatous coronary arteries after regression diets. Circ Res 1972, 30:675.
8. Armstrong ML, Warner ED, Connor WE: Regression of coronary atheromatosis in rhesus monkeys. Circ Res 1970, 27:59.
9. DePalma RG, Bellon EM, Insull W Jr, Roth WT, Robinson AV: Studies on progression and regression of experimental atherosclerosis: Techniques and applications to the rhesus monkey. In Karger S (ed): *Medical Primatology 1972,* Proc 3rd Conf Exp Med Surg Primates, Lyon, part III. Basel, 1972, p. 313.
10. DePalma RG, Hubay CA, Insull W Jr, Robinson AV, Hartman PH: Progression and regression of experimental atherosclerosis. Surg Gynecol Obstet 1970, 131:313.
11. DePalma RG, Insull W, Bellon, EM, Roth WT, Robinson AV: Animal models for the study of progression and regression of atherosclerosis. Surgery 1972, 72:268.
12. Wissler RW, Vessilinovitch D: Studies of regression of advanced atherosclerosis in experimental animals and man. Ann NY Acad Sci 1976, 275:363.
13. Daoud AS, Jarmolych J, Augustyn JM, Fritz KE, Lee KT: Regression of advanced swine atherosclerosis. Arch Pathol Lab Med 1976, 100:372.
14. Malinow MR: Regression of atherosclerosis in humans: Fact or myth? Circulation 1981, 64:1.
15. Ross K, Glomset JA: The pathogenesis of atherosclerosis, N Engl J Med 1976, 295:369.
16. Ross R, Harker L: Hyperlipidemia and atherosclerosis. Science 1976, 192:1094.
17. Insull W Jr, Bartsch GE: Cholesterol triglyceride and phospholipid content of intima, media and atherosclerotic fatty streak in human thoracic aorta. J Clin Invest 1966, 45:513.
18. Hata Y, Hower J, Insull W Jr: Cholesterol ester-rich inclusions from human aortic fatty streak and fibrous plaque lesions of atherosclerosis. Am J Pathol 1974, 75:423.
19. Geer JC, McGill HC: The evolution of the fatty streak. In Brest AN, Moyer JH (eds): *Atherosclerotic Vascular Disease.* New York, Appleton-Century-Crofts, 1967, pp 8–22.
20. Hata Y: Lipids in atherosclerotic lesions. Taishya (Metabolism) 1975, 12:1289.
21. Small DM, Shipley G: Physical-chemical basis of lipid deposition in atherosclerosis. Science 1974, 185:222.
22. Haust MD: The morphogenesis and fate of potential and early atherosclerotic lesions in man. Hum Pathol 1971, 2:1.
23. McGill HC Jr: The geographic pathology of atherosclerosis. Lab Invest 1968, 18:463.
24. Tejada C, Strong JP, Montenegro MR, Restrepo C, Solberg LA: Distribution of coronary and aortic atherosclerosis by geographic location, race and sex. Lab Invest 1968, 18:509.
25. *Report of a Study Group. Classification of Atherosclerotic Lesions.* WHO Technical Report Series 1958, No. 143. Geneva, pp 1620.
26. Lusby RJ, Ferrell LD, Ehrenfeld WK, Stoney RJ, Wylie EJ: Carotid plaque hemorrhage. Arch Surg 1982, 117:1479.
27. Imparato AM. In Discussion. Arch Surg 1982, 117:1488.
28. McMillan GC: Development of arteriosclerosis. Am J Cardiol 1973, 31:542.
29. DeBakey ME: Atherosclerosis: Patterns and rates of progression. In Gotto AM, Smith LC, Allen B (eds): *Atherosclerosis V.* New York, Springer-Verlag, 1980, pp 3–7.
30. Hertzer N: Myocardial ischemia: In symposium on prevention of complications of abdominal aortic reconstruction. Surgery 1983, 93:91.
31. Deweese JA, Rob CG, Satran R, March DO, Joynt RJ, Summers D, Nichols C: Results of carotid endarterectomy for transient ischemic attacks—Five years later. Ann Surg 1973, 178:258.
32. Toole JF, Yuson CP, Janeway R, Johnston F, Davis C, Cordell AR, Howard G: Transient ischemic attacks: A prospective study of 225 patients. Neurology 1978, 28:746.
33. Rosen AJ, DePalma RG, Victor Y: Risk factors in peripheral atherosclerosis. Arch Surg 1973, 107:303.
34. Blankenhorn DH, Brooks SH, Selzer RH, Barndt R Jr: The rate of atherosclerosis change during treatment of hyperlipoproteinemia. Circulation 1978, 57:355.
35. Brooks SH, Blankenhorn DH, Chin HP, Sanmarco ME, Hanashiro PK, Selzer RH, Selvester RH: Design of human atherosclerosis studies by serial angiography. J Chronic Dis 1980, 33:347.

36. Blankenhorn DH, Curry PJ: The accuracy of arteriography and ultrasound imaging for atherosclerosis measurement. Arch Pathol Lab Med 1982, 106:483.
37. DePalma RG, Bellon EM, Klein L, Koletsky S, Insull W Jr: Approaches to evaluating regression of experimental atherosclerosis. In Manning GW, Haust MD (eds): *Atherosclerosis: Metabolic, Morphologic and Clinical Aspects*. New York, Plenum, 1977, pp 459–470.
38. Armstrong ML, Megan MB: Arterial fibrous proteins in cynomolgus monkeys after atherogenic and regression diets. Circ Res 1975, 36:256.
39. DePalma RG, Hubay CA, Insull W Jr, Robinson AV, Hartman PH: Progression and regression of experimental atherosclerosis. Surg Gynecol Obstet 1970, 131:633.
40. DePalma RG, Koletsky S, Bellon EM, Insull W Jr: Failure of regression of atherosclerosis in dogs with moderate cholesterolemia. Atherosclerosis 1977, 27:297.
41. DePalma RG, Bellon EM, Koletsky S, Schneider DL: Atherosclerotic plaque regression in rhesus monkeys induced by bile acid sequestrant. Exp Mol Pathol 1979, 31:423.
42. DePalma RG, Klein L, Bellon EM, Koletsky S: Regression of atherosclerotic plaques in rhesus monkeys. Arch Surg 1980, 115:1268.
43. DePalma RG: Control and regression of atherosclerotic plaques, a commentary. In Dale WA (ed): *Management of Arterial Occlusive Disease*. Chicago, Year Book, 1971, pp 63–64.
44. Brooks SH, Le Croissette DH, Blankenhorn DH: Determinants of atherosclerosis progression and regression. Arch Surg 1978, 113:75.
45. Blankenhorn DH, Sanmarco ME: Angiography for study of lipid–lowering therapy, editorial. Circulation 1979, 59:212.
46. McCullagh KA, Balian G: Collagen characterization and cell transformation in human atherosclerosis. Nature 1975, 258:73.
47. DePalma RG: Angiography in experimental atherosclerosis: Advantages and limitations. In Bond JG, Insull W Jr, Glagove S, Cornhill JF, Chandler AB (eds): *Noninvasive Diagnosis of Atherosclerotic Lesions: Quantitative Evaluation of Morphology, Biochemistry and Pathophysiology*. New York, Springer-Verlag, 1983, pp 99–123.
48. The University Group Diabetes Program: A study of the effects of hypoglycemic agents on vascular complication in patients with adult onset diabetes. Diabetes 1970, 19(suppl 2):747.
49. Bennion LJ, Grundy SM: Effects of diabetes mellitus on cholesterol metabolism in man. N Engl J Med 1977, 296:1365.
50. Goodson WH III, Hunt TK: Studies of wound healing in experimental diabetes mellitus. J Surg Res 1977, 22:221.
51. Jackson RL: Lipid transport and atherogenesis: Role of apolipoproteins. In Crass M (ed): *Vascular Smooth Muscle: Metabolic, Ionic and Contractile Mechanisms*. New York, Academic, 1982, pp 163–196.
52. Levy RI: Cholesterol, lipoproteins, apoproteins and coronary heart disease: Present status and future prospects. Clin Chem 1981, 27:653.
53. Sniderman AD, Wolfson C, Teng B, Franklin FA, Bachorik PS, Kwiterovich PO Jr: Association of hyperapobetalipoproteinemia with endogenous hypertriglyceridemia and atherosclerosis. Ann Intern Med 1982, 97:833.
54. International Collaborative Group: Circulating cholesterol level and risk of death from cancer in men aged 40 to 69 years. JAMA 1982, 248:2853.
55. Levy RI: Cholesterol and disease—What are the facts? Editorial. JAMA 248:2888, 1982.
56. Juergens JL, Barker NW, Hines EA: Arteriosclerosis obliterans: A review of 520 cases with special reference to pathogenic and prognostic factors. Circulation 1960, 21:188.
57. Gordon T, Castelli WP, Hjortand MC, Kannel WB, Dawber TR: Predicting coronary heart disease in middle-aged and older persons: The Framingham study. JAMA 1977, 238:497.
58. Wray R, DePalma RG, Hubay CA: Late occlusion of aorto-femoral bypass grafts: Influence of cigarette smoking. Surgery 1971, 70:969.
59. Robicsek F, Daugherty HK, Mullen DC, et al: The effect of continued cigarette smoking on the patency of synthetic vascular grafts in Leriche syndrome. J Thorac Cardiovasc Surg 1975, 70:107.
60. Schneiderman G, Goldstick TK: Carbon monoxide–induced arterial wall hypoxia and atherosclerosis. In Adams CWM, Kritchevsky D, Seidel D (eds): *Atherosclerosis*. Amsterdam, Elsevier/North-Holland, 1978, pp 1–15.
61. Garrison RJ, Kannel WB, Feinleib M, Castelli WP, McNamara PM, Padgett SJ: Cigarette smoking and HDL cholesterol. Atherosclerosis 1978, 30:17.
62. Koletsky S, Roland C, Rivera-Velezz JM: Rapid acceleration of atherosclerosis in hypertensive rats on a high fat diet. Exp Mol Pathol 1968, 9:322.
63. Veterans Administration Group on Antihypertensive Agents. Effects of treatment on morbidity in hypertension. II. Results in patients with diastolic blood pressure averaging 90 through 114 mmHg. JAMA 1970, 213:1143.
64. DePalma RG, Clowes AW: Interventions in atherosclerosis: A review for surgeons. Surgery 1978, 84:175.
65. Tietze C: New estimates of mortality associated with fertility control. Fam Plann Perspect 1977, 9:74.
66. Butts WC, Kuehneman M, Widdowson GM: Automated method for determining serum thiocyanate to distinguish smokers from nonsmokers. Clin Chem 1974, 20:1344.
67. Greenhalgh RM, Laing SP, Cole PV, Taylor GW: Smoking and arterial reconstruction. Br J Surg 1981, 68:605.
68. Greenhalgh RM: Mechanical and biochemical factors influencing arterial reconstruction. Ann R Coll Surg Engl 1981, 63:400.
69. DePalma RG, Hubay CA, Botti R, Peterka JL: Treatment of surgical patients with atherosclerosis and hyperlipidemia. Surg Gynecol Obstet 1970, 131:313.
70. Barnard RJ, Weber F, Weingarten W, Bennett CM, Pritikin N: Effects of intensive, short-term exercise and nutrition program on patients with coronary heart disease. J Card Rehab 1981, 1:99.
71. Barnard RJ, Lattimore L, Holly RG, Cherny S, Pritikin N: Response of non-insulin-dependent diabetic patients to an intensive program of diet and exercise. Diabetes Care 1982, 5:370.
72. LaRosa JC: The mechanism of action of lipid-lowering drugs. Angiology 1982, 33:562.
73. Buchwald HR, Moore RB, Varco RL: The partial ileal bypass operation in treatment of hyperlipidemias. Adv Exp Med Biol 1974, 63:221.
74. Buchwald H, Moore RB, Matts JP, Long JM, Varco RL, Campbell GS, Pearce MB, Yellin AE, Blankenhorn DH, Holmes WL, Smink RD Jr, Sawin HS Jr: The program on the surgical control of the hyperlipidemias: a status report. Surgery 92:654, 1982.
75. Starzl TE, Chase HP, Porter KA, Putnam CW: Portacaval shunt in hyperlipoproteinemia. Lancet 1973, 2:140.
76. Bilheimer DW, Goldstein JL, Grundy SM, Brown MS: Reduction in cholesterol and low density lipoprotein synthesis after portacaval shunt surgery in a patient with homozygous familial hypercholesterolemia. J Clin Invest 1975, 56:1420.
77. Khachadurian AK, Kawahara FS: Cholesterol synthesis by cultured fibroblasts: Decreased feedback inhibition in familial hypercholesterolemia. J Lab Clin Med 1974, 83:7.
78. Goldstein JL, Brown MS: Familial hypercholesterolemia: Identification of a defect in the regulation of 3 hydroxy-3 methyl glutaryl coenzyme A reductase activity associated with overproduction of cholesterol. Proc Natl Acad Sci USA 1973, 70:2804.

79. Goldstein JL, Brown MS: Lipoprotein receptors, cholesterol metabolism and atherosclerosis. Arch Pathol 1975, 99:181.
80. Hoeg JM, Demosky SJ Jr, Schaefer EJ, Starzl TE, Brewer HB: The effect of portacaval shunt on hepatic lipid and lipoprotein metabolism in familial hypercholesterolemia. Circ Res 1983, 31:192A.
81. Multiple Risk Factor Intervention Trial Research Group: Risk factor changes and mortality results. JAMA 1982, 248:1465.
82. Leren P, Helgeland A, Hjermann I, Holme I: MRFIT and the Oslo study. JAMA 1983, 249:893.
83. Barmeyer J, Buchwalsky R, Blumchen G, Baumeister L, Hansen W, Battke H, Hartung H, Reindell H: Der Verlauf der Arteriosklerose an den Koronarund und Beinarterier. Dtsch Med Wochenschr 1976, 101:443.
84. Kuthan F, Burkhalter A, Baitsch R, Ludin H, Widmer LK: Development of occlusive arterial disease in lower limbs. Arch Surg 1971, 103:545.
85. Blankenhorn DH: Will atheroma regress with diet and exercise? Am J Surg 1981, 141:644.
86. Oblath RW, Buckley FO Jr, Green RM, Schwart SI, Deweese JA: Prevention of platelet aggregation and adherence to prosthetic vascular grafts by aspirin and dipyridamole. Surgery 1978, 84:37.
87. Feins RH, Roedersheimer R, Green RM, Deweese JA: Platelet aggregation inhibition in human umbilical vein grafts and negatively charged bovine heterografts. Surgery 1979, 85:395.
88. McCollum CN, Kester RC, Rajah SM, Learoyd P, Pepper M: Arterial graft maturation: The duration of thrombotic activity in Dacron aortobifemoral grafts measured by platelet and fibrinogen kinetics. Br J Surg 1981, 68:61.
89. Ritchie JL, Stratton JR, Thiele B, Hamilton GW, Warrick LN, Huang TW, Harger LA: Indium-111 platelet imaging for detection of platelet deposition in abdominal aneurysms and prosthetic arterial grafts. Am J Cardiol 1981, 47:882.
90. Hagen P, Wang Z, Mikat EM, Hackel DB: Antiplatelet therapy reduces aortic intimal hyperplasia distal to small diameter vascular prostheses (PTFE) in nonhuman primates. Ann Surg 1982, 195:328.
91. DePalma RG, Bellon EM, Manalo PM: Failure of antiplatelet agents to control dietary atherosclerosis. J Cardiovasc Surg 1981, 22:445.
92. Manalo-Sears P, DePalma RG, Bellon EM: Effect of antiplatelet agents on morphology of dietary induced atherosclerosis in rhesus monkeys. Am J Clin Pathol 1982, 78:280.
93. Bomberger RA, DePalma RG, Ambrose A, Manalo P: Aspirin and dipyridamole inhibit endothelial healing. Arch Surg 1982, 117:1459.
94. Bomberger RA, Wilburn J, DePalma RG: Aspirin and dipyridamole increase intimal thickening after injury. Surg Forum 1983, 34:475.
95. Carson SW, Demling RH, Esquivel CO: Aspirin failure in symptomatic carotid artery disease. Surgery 1981, 90:1084.
96. Lusby RJ, Ferrell LD, Englestad BL, Price DC, Lipton MJ, Stoney RJ: Vessel wall and indium-111-labeled platelet response to carotid endarterectomy. Surgery 1983, 93:424.
97. Chesebro JH, Clements IP, Fuster V, Elveback LR, Smith HC, Bardsley WT, Frye RL, Holmes DR Jr, Vlietstra RE, Pluth JR, Wallace RB, Puga FJ, Orszulak TA, Piehler JM, Schaff HV, Danielson GK: A platelet-inhibitor-drug trial in coronary artery bypass operations. N Engl J Med 1982, 307:73.
98. Nicholls ES, Johansen HL: Implications of changing trends in cerebrovascular and ischemic heart disease mortality, editorial. Stroke 1983, 14:153.
99. DePalma RG: Impotence in vascular disease: Relationship to vascular surgery. Br J Surg 1982, 69:514.
100. Pelletier O: Smoking and vitamin C levels in humans. Am J Clin Nutr 1968, 21:1259.

Chapter 16A

ANTICOAGULANTS (HEPARIN, WARFARIN)

DONALD N. KAPSCH and DONALD SILVER

Anticoagulants are among the most frequently prescribed medications; over a trillion international units of heparin and 974.1 million mg of sodium warfarin (Coumadin*) are utilized annually in the United States (1). Anticoagulants enable the vascular surgeon to alter the coagulation mechanism preoperatively, intraoperatively, and postoperatively according to the needs of the patient. The vitamin K antagonists and the low-dose heparin regimens are the mainstays of deep-vein-thrombosis prophylaxis and have reduced the incidence of deep vein thrombosis and pulmonary embolism in postoperative and other at-risk patients. Despite the increased use of prophylaxis, deep vein thrombosis and its sequelae remain a significant problem: Pulmonary embolism occurs in approximately 630,000 patients in the United States and causes at least 200,000 deaths annually (2). Intravenous or subcutaneous heparin remains the primary therapy of established thromboembolism, with thrombolytic agents or surgical intervention serving as adjuvant measures.

Anticoagulants, when properly administered and monitored, may save life and/or limb but when misused can lead to complications which may threaten survival or significantly prolong recovery from the disease they were used to prevent or treat.

*Data for Coumadin courtesy of IMS America, Ltd., Ambler, Pennsylvania.

Coagulation Mechanism

The coagulation mechanism is composed of a series of interrelated enzymatic reactions, with feedback amplification, that result in the production of the stable hemostatic clot. Of the 12 clotting factors, 7 are proteolytic enzymes; 4 are cofactors responsible for the facilitation, acceleration, and regulation of the reactions catalyzed by the enzymatic factors; and 1 factor, fibrinogen, is converted to fibrin to form the hemostatic clot. All clotting factors with the exception of factor VIII are produced by the liver. Factors II, VII, IX, and X require the presence of vitamin K for their synthesis. The plasma half-life of the coagulation factors varies from 5 to 6 hours for factor VII to 90 hours for fibrinogen and 120 hours for factor XIII. The plasma half-life may be affected by various disease states such as hyperthyroidism or hypothyroidism. All the coagulation factors are found in fresh-frozen plasma. The labile factors, V and VIII, are rapidly depleted in stored plasma.

Activation of the coagulation cascade may occur via the intrinsic and/or extrinsic coagulation pathway(s). Both pathways produce activated clotting factor X_a and share a terminal pathway for the production of fibrin from fibrinogen (Figure 16A-1). The integrity of the extrinsic and intrinsic pathways may be assayed by the measurement of the prothrombin and activated partial thromboplastin times (aPTT), respectively.

Excessive or continued activation of the coagulation mechanism is normally prevented by three mechanisms. Blood flow reduces the local accumulation of activated clotting factors. Activated clotting factors are rapidly removed by the cells of the reticuloendothelial system. And the plasma contains natural anticoagulants, such as antithrombin III, which combine with thrombin and activated factors X, IX, VII, and XI to inhibit their activity. Heparin greatly enhances the rate at which antithrombin III inactivates the activated coagulation factors.

PLATELETS

Platelets play an important role in the initiation and acceleration of the intrinsic and extrinsic coagulation pathways. The platelet membrane adsorbs and transports plasma coagulation factors and provides a reactive surface for their activation. Components of the platelet membrane provide the phospholipid cofactor(s) for several of the reactions of the coagulation cascade. The initial hemostatic plug formed by aggregating platelets is further stabilized by the fibrin network produced by the coagulation system. The contraction of platelet microfilaments in conjunction with activated factor XIII produces clot retraction. Platelet factor IV, with heparin-neutralizing activity, is released during platelet aggregation.

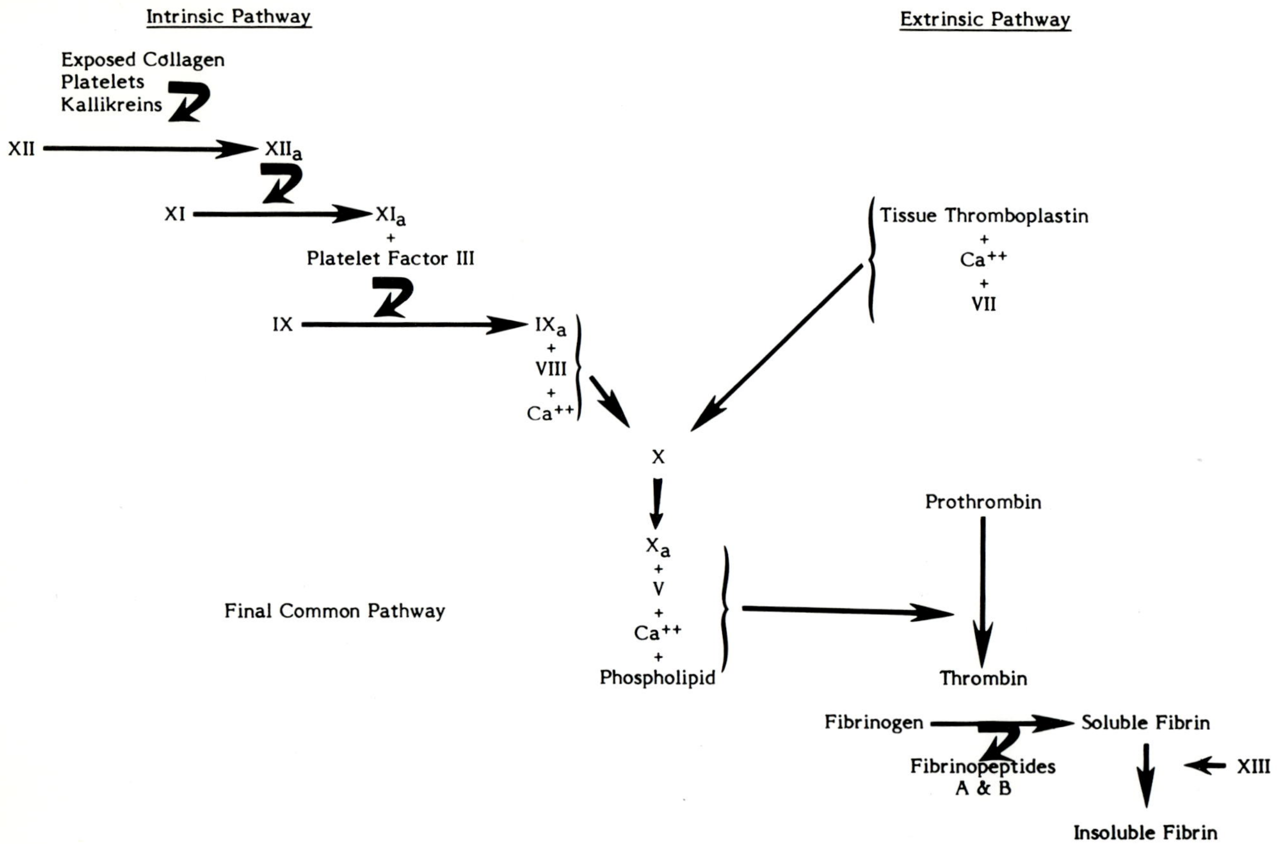

FIGURE 16A-1. The coagulation mechanism.

Anticoagulants

The anticoagulants that are most often utilized clinically include heparin and the vitamin K antagonists. To optimize the benefits of anticoagulant therapy, the clinician must have a thorough knowledge of the pharmacology of each agent, the thromboembolic process in which the agent's usefulness has been demonstrated, and the potential complications associated with each agent.

HEPARIN

Physical Properties

Heparin is a heterogeneous mixture of straight-chain glycosaminoglycuronan sulfate esters with molecular weights ranging from 4000 to 40,000. The glycosaminoglycuronan chains consist primarily of alternating uronic acids and glycosamines with a high degree of sulfation. The sulfation imparts a negative charge to the mucopolysaccharide and is in part responsible for its anticoagulant activity when compared with other glycosaminoglycuronans.

The various molecular weights of heparin have an important effect on its anticoagulant activity. Heparins with molecular weights less than 6000 have minimal anticoagulant activity. Assays of the anticoagulant activity of commercial heparin preparations have demonstrated that up to 70 percent of the preparation by weight, primarily the high-molecular-weight fraction, has less than 15 percent of the anticoagulant activity. The difference in activity appears to be related to the differential binding of the various fractions to the heparin cofactor, antithrombin III (3).

Beef lung and swine intestine mucosa are the primary sources for commercial heparin. The various commercial preparations of heparin have different ratios of high- and low-molecular-weight fractions with differing anticoagulant activities. So that this variation of activity is compensated for, the anticoagulant activity of heparin is expressed as international units rather than by weight.

Mode of Action

Heparin exerts its anticoagulant effect through an interaction with the naturally circulating anticoagulant antithrombin III. Heparin combines with antithrombin III in a 1:1 stoichiometric ratio and produces a conformational change in antithrombin III which makes its active centers more available for binding to thrombin and the other serine proteases of the coagulation cascade. Heparin does not alter the stoichiometric ratio of binding of antithrombin III to thrombin; however, it does increase the rate at which the complex is formed. The high anticoagulant activity fractions of heparin induce conformational changes of the antithrombin III more rapidly than the other fractions. Antithrombin III forms undissociable complexes with the various proteases that it inhibits. After the antithrombin III has neutralized the activated factor, heparin may dissociate from the complex and catalyze other thrombin-antithrombin III interactions (4,5).

The sensitivity of activated factor X to inhibition by the heparin-antithrombin III complex is, in part, responsible for the effectiveness of the low-dose heparin regimens in the prophylaxis of deep vein thrombosis. The inhibition of 1 unit of activated factor X by the heparin-antithrombin III complex prevents the potential generation of more than 50 units of thrombin (2).

The anticoagulant effect of heparin varies from subject to subject and may be a function of circulating antithrombin III concentrations and antiheparin agents such as platelet factor IV. Heparin has limited anticoagulant activity in patients with congenital or acquired antithrombin III deficiencies. Circulating antithrombin III concentrations may fall by up to 12 percent within 4 hours of the initiation of heparin therapy and may be decreased by as much as 33 percent with continued therapy. Patients with preexisting antithrombin III deficiencies may experience an even greater decrease in circulating antithrombin III concentrations with prolonged heparin therapy (5).

Pharmacokinetics

Heparin rapidly binds to plasma proteins, and its early distribution approximates that of plasma. The plasma clearance of heparin is about 0.5 to 0.6 mL/min per kilogram. Heparin is not excreted by the kidney, nor does there appear to be an enzymatic degradation pathway in the liver or plasma. The half-life of circulating heparin is about 90 minutes; the most likely mechanism for its clearance is the transfer of heparin, by active or passive means, to some extravascular space such as the reticuloendothelial system. Heparin attaches to arterial and venous endothelium and may be concentrated there up to 7500 times its concentration in plasma (3,5). The plasma clearance of heparin is dose-dependent in humans and is reduced with increasing doses of the anticoagulant (3).

Higher-molecular-weight fractions of subcutaneously administered heparin are more slowly absorbed than the lower-weight fractions. This may account for the differences in pharmacokinetic properties when the various heparin preparations are given subcutaneously. In addition, the salt to which the heparin is bound may have some effect on its absorption. Although the calcium salts of heparin are said to have slower absorption with lower peak levels compared with the sodium salt (6), some studies have demonstrated the bioequivalence of the two salts of heparin in all routes of administration (3,5).

Since there is minimal renal excretion of heparin, there is no difference in the anticoagulant half-life, or disappearance rate, of heparin in patients with renal failure. Liver disease has no significant effect on the removal of heparin from the plasma, but it may affect the concentrations of antithrombin III and other clotting factors, and, therefore, anticoagulant activity. The disease process for which heparin is being administered may affect its anticoagulant half-life; patients with pulmonary embolism usually have a shorter plasma half-life and require large amounts of heparin for adequate anticoagulation because of the presence of large quantities of activated clotting factors (3,5).

Drug Interactions

Although heparin activates, inhibits, or causes the release of a large number of enzymes, there are no significant drug interactions which directly affect its anticoagulant activity. The high negative charge of heparin makes it incompatible with the concomitant administration of some antibiotics such as erythromycin, aminoglycosides, and tetracyclines, and other drugs such as phenothiazines and nonsteroidal anti-inflammatory agents. Heparin stimulates lipase activity, with a resultant increase in plasma free fatty acid concentrations. The free fatty acids can increase the fraction of unbound propranolol, phenytoin, warfarin, and phenylbutazone in the plasma. Heparin displaces both basic and acidic drugs from their binding sites on plasma proteins (3,5). Heparin has no direct effect on platelets but may interfere with platelet-initiated thrombin generation and with the activity of some of the bioactive amines released by platelets.

Prophylaxis

Minidose heparin regimens have become the preferred prophylaxis against deep vein thrombosis and pulmonary embolism in patients undergoing major surgery, after myocardial infarction, and in patients hospitalized for the treatment of major medical illnesses such as congestive heart failure or stroke. Heparin administered subcutaneously in small amounts has been found to be safe and an effective means of thrombosis prophylaxis and is becoming preferred over the vitamin K antagonists (7–10).

Multiple studies have documented the effectiveness of low-dose heparin regimens (5000 units given subcutaneously 2 hours before the operation and every 8 to 12 hours postoperatively until the patient is ambulatory) in reducing the incidence of postoperative deep vein thrombosis and pulmonary embolism (9,10). The incidence of postoperative deep vein thrombosis in high-risk patients (i.e., patients with a past history of deep vein thrombosis, with malignant disease, or undergoing major abdominal, thoracic, gynecologic, or orthopedic procedures), as determined by the ^{125}I fibrinogen scan technique, has averaged 30 to 50 percent in those not receiving antithromboembolism prophylaxis. In the majority of studies, the incidence of postoperative deep vein thrombosis, similarly determined, was reduced to less than 10 percent in all but orthopedic and open prostatectomy patients when the minidose heparin regimen was instituted preoperatively and continued in the postoperative period until the patient was fully ambulatory or discharged from the hospital (9,10).

The early studies demonstrating no protective effect for patients undergoing total hip replacement have been supplanted by newer trials in which 5000 units of heparin was given subcutaneously every 8 hours rather than every 12 hours, and in which the heparin administration was initiated before surgery. These subsequent trials have demonstrated a decrease in the incidence of postoperative deep vein thrombosis in treated patients from an average of 40 to 50 percent to less than 20 percent (2). More importantly, it was also noted that when deep vein thrombosis occurred in treated patients, there was a lower incidence of bilateral involvement and the thrombotic process usually remained in the calf (2).

A recent study has compared the administration of 5000 units of heparin subcutaneously every 8 hours, on an outpatient basis, with the administration of vitamin K antagonists. The study suggested that the subcutaneous heparin regimen is effective in preventing recurrent deep vein thrombosis when the heparin dose is adjusted to prolong the aPTT to at least $1\frac{1}{2}$ times control values (8). Sharnoff et al. demonstrated that by monitoring the anticoagulant effect of the subcutaneously administered heparin with the whole-blood clotting time, beginning the heparin administration as soon as possible after hip trauma, and giving 2500 to 3500 units of heparin every 6 hours, they could achieve a significant reduction in the incidence of postoperative fatal pulmonary embolism in patients undergoing total hip replacement and repair of hip fractures (11).

Radioiodinated fibrinogen scans and phlebography have demonstrated that the majority of thrombi form in the calf veins and that in only about 20 percent of these patients does the thrombotic process extend proximally into the popliteal, femoral, or iliac veins (9). About half of the group with extension into more proximal veins will suffer an embolic event, but in only 0.5 to 1 percent will it prove fatal (9,10). Multicenter trials have demonstrated a significant reduction in the incidence of fatal and nonfatal postoperative pulmonary embolism in patients receiving heparin prophylaxis compared with untreated controls (9,10). It is estimated that in high-risk patients, 4000 to 8000 postoperative deaths and up to 200,000 deaths from pulmonary embolism could be prevented by heparin prophylaxis (2,9,10,12).

Low-dose heparin prophylaxis is contraindicated in patients suffering from a hemorrhagic diathesis, endocarditis, bleeding of internal organs, or hypertension. Central nervous system and eye surgery are relative contraindications to the use of minidose heparin therapy. Patients receiving perioperative heparin prophylaxis should be given aspirin or other platelet-antiaggregating drugs with caution and should have meticulous hemostasis at the time of operation. Coagulopathies should be corrected before the heparin prophylaxis is begun so that bleeding complications can be avoided.

Our current practice with patients who are at increased risk for deep vein thrombosis is to give 5000 units of sodium heparin subcutaneously 2 hours before operation and to continue with 5000 units given subcutaneously every 8 hours postoperatively until the patient is fully ambulatory. Postmenopausal female patients are given 3000 to 5000 units subcutaneously every 12 hours because of their higher propensity for hemorrhagic complications when given heparin (2). No laboratory monitoring of the anticoagulant effect of heparin is routinely used; however, the platelet count is repeated every 2 to 3 days for 2 weeks, so that the development of heparin-induced thrombocytopenia can be detected before the occurrence of thrombohemorrhagic complications (1).

Therapeutics

Thrombosis involving the major deep veins of the lower extremities and pelvis, and acute pulmonary embolism, are medical emergencies requiring hospitalization and aggressive anticoagulant therapy. These processes are associated with a marked activation of the coagulation mechanism and the generation of large quantities of thrombin and activated clotting factors. Minidose heparin regimens are inadequate. Large initial doses of heparin followed by a continuous intravenous infusion are required to rapidly stop the coagulation process and produce continued inhibition. In patients without contraindications, heparin is frequently administered when the diagnosis of venous thromboembolism is suspected, before confirmation by phlebography, ventilation-perfusion scanning, or both. Patients at increased risk for hemorrhagic complications are given heparin after the diagnosis is established.

Our current management of deep vein thrombosis and acute pulmonary embolism involves the rapid intravenous administration of 300 to 400 units of heparin per kilogram of body weight, followed by continuous intravenous infusion of heparin, usually at 1000 to 1500 units/h. The continuous infusion is subsequently adjusted 8 to 10 hours after the initial bolus, and at regular intervals, to maintain the aPTT at $2\frac{1}{2}$ times the control. Additional heparin may be required to achieve or maintain this prolongation of the aPTT. The continuous-intravenous-infusion method is preferred in the United States because it has been associated with a lower incidence of bleeding complications, it is easier and more accurate to monitor, and it usually requires a smaller amount of heparin to achieve an adequate level of anticoagulation (2,13–15). Continuous-intravenous-infusion therapy also avoids the periods of noncoagulability associated with intermittent intravenous therapy.

In the United Kingdom and Europe, considerable experience has been acquired with the twice-a-day subcutaneous administration of therapeutic doses of calcium heparin. The usual dose of 10,000 to 20,000 units, given as a divided dose twice daily, is adjusted on the basis of the kaolin cephalin clotting time (KCCT) to maintain a clotting time 4 hours following the morning dose in the range of $1\frac{1}{2}$ to 2 times control values. The therapeutic effect of the subcutaneously administered heparin was found to be as beneficial and safe as the continuous-infusion regimen with less patient encumbrance and greater ease of patient care (16). These results have yet to be reproduced in the United States and may be dependent upon the choice of the calcium salt of heparin.

Several laboratory methods have been utilized to monitor the anticoagulant effect of heparin. The Lee-White clotting time (LWCT) has been supplanted by the more reliable aPTT and activated clotting time (ACT). The aPTT is widely available and the most frequently utilized test for regulating the heparin dosage. The maintenance of the aPTT in the range of 2 to $2\frac{1}{2}$ times control values has been shown to stop intravascular coagulation without inducing hemorrhage. The amount of heparin required varies from individual to individual and is dependent upon the thromboembolic process being treated.

The ACT can be determined in a short time in the operating room or at the bedside. Another advantage of the ACT is its linear response to increasing doses of heparin, which allows the construction of a dose-response curve and the calculation of the concentrations of residual plasma heparin. The ACT is useful for the monitoring of the anticoagulant effect of heparin in the treatment of deep vein thrombosis and pulmonary embolism, with values of 150 to 200 s providing adequate anticoagulation (17).

The aPTT or the ACT must be determined several times a day during the initial stages of therapy when large amounts of heparin are required to control the coagulation process, and during the later stages of therapy when the coagulation process becomes controlled and lesser amounts of heparin are required to maintain the level of anticoagulation.

One assumes that the prolongation of the aPTT or the ACT into the therapeutic range is associated with an inhibition of the coagulation process. Factors in the region of the developing thrombus, which include high concentrations of thrombin, other activated clotting factors, and platelet factor IV, may make *local* concentrations of heparin inadequate to prevent thrombosis. Blaisdell and associates have noted that local thrombus propagation, as demonstrated by fibrinogin-consumption studies, may occur in the presence of "adequate" levels of systemic anticoagulation and that additional heparin, up to 4000 units/h, may be required to control the local thrombotic process (18).

It is our current practice to continue the intravenous heparin (with the aPTT maintained at 2 to $2\frac{1}{2}$ times control) for 10 to 14 days, after which most patients' therapy is changed to subcutaneous heparin, 5000 units every 8 hours for the remainder of their hospital stay and for 3 months after discharge. Patients who will not self-administer heparin are treated with oral anticoagulants, which are usually begun on day 7 of the intravenous heparin therapy. The intravenous heparin is continued until a satisfactory hypoprothrombinemia is achieved with the vitamin K antagonists.

A failure to achieve therapeutic levels of anticoagulation with increasing doses of intravenous heparin raises the possibility of an antithrombin III deficiency, excessive concentrations of circulating procoagulants, or the development of heparin-induced thrombocytopenia with the potential for new or recurrent thromboembolic phenomena (2). If the platelet count is greater than 100,000/mm^3, assays of factor VIII and antithrombin III should be done. If factor VIII and antithrombin III assays are not available, the response of the LWCT or ACT to an intravenous heparin infusion should be determined. A normal response with a prolongation of the LWCT or ACT suggests the presence of elevated levels of factor VIII, which can lead to a falsely shortened aPTT. A failure of the LWCT or ACT to respond to the administered heparin often indicates the presence of an acquired or congenital deficiency of antithrombin III. A platelet count less than 100,000/mm^3 raises the possibility of heparin-induced thrombocytopenia (1).

Patients with congenital or acquired deficiencies of antithrombin III are treated with vitamin K antagonists for inhibition of the coagulation process unless immediate anticoagulation is needed for an acute thromboembolic event. When immediate anticoagulation is required, patients may be treated with infusions of fresh-frozen plasma or cryoprecipitate, so that their deficient levels of circulating antithrombin III will be replenished, in addition to heparin (2).

Patients with an active peptic ulcer, ulcerative colitis, diverticulitis, or some other potential or active source of hemorrhage and deep vein thrombosis or pulmonary embolism, or both, may be cautiously anticoagulated with heparin. The initial loading doses are reduced, and the aPTT is maintained at $1\frac{1}{2}$ times the control value. Once the bleeding source is controlled, full therapeutic levels of anticoagulation are utilized. Patients with intracranial bleeding or active gastrointestinal or pulmonary bleeding may require inferior vena cava obstruction to prevent additional thromboembolic events, as anticoagulant therapy is contraindicated in these patients (2).

Intravenous heparin is the drug of choice for the treatment of an acute thromboembolic event during pregnancy, as it does not cross the placenta. Pregnant women who require the continued inhibition of the coagulation mechanism should be managed with subcutaneous heparin until the end of the first trimester, when some may be changed to the vitamin K antagonists to avoid the osteoporosis associated with long-term heparin therapy (19). However, many women in the United States now receive heparin throughout their pregnancies, as the risk of developing osteoporosis during therapy is negligible if they receive less than 10,000 units/day.

The duration of anticoagulation therapy following an acute thromboembolic event remains controversial. Some have recommended the discontinuation of anticoagulant therapy when the acute event resolves, while others have recommended continuing anticoagulation for periods extending to 1 year (2,10). We currently maintain patients with deep vein thrombosis on pulmonary embolism or subcutaneous heparin or oral anticoagulants for 3 months after the acute thromboembolic event. Patients who sustain recurrent thromboembolic events when anticoagulant therapy is discontinued are offered anticoagulation for longer periods of time (Figure 16A-2). Additional measures such as the use of elastic stockings and the avoidance of positions of stasis are utilized to help reduce the incidence of recurrent deep vein thrombosis.

Peripheral Vascular Surgery

Heparin is used by vascular surgeons to prevent clotting in vessel segments during and after clamping. Usually 5000 to 7000 units of heparin is given intravenously immediately before the application of the clamps. Porous vascular prostheses are "clotted" with blood obtained before the heparin is given. Additional heparin, 1000 to 2000 units, is usually administered each additional hour, after the first, that the vascular clamps remain in place. When hemostasis is secure, heparin reversal is rarely needed after clamp removal. Postoperatively our vascular patients, especially those at risk for deep venous thrombosis, e.g., after femoropopliteal or femorotibial bypass, are maintained on subcutaneous heparin, 5000 units every 8 hours, until they are fully ambulatory.

Arterial Thromboembolic Disease

The principal use of heparin in the management of arterial thromboembolic disease is to prevent thrombus propagation and permit collaterals to develop after the acute thromboembolic event. Heparin may also be used to reduce the blood's coagulability after thromboembolectomy while the vascular endothelium is regenerating. So that clot propagation is prevented while appropriate diagnostic and therapeutic measures are being completed, patients with an acute peripheral arterial thromboembolus are usually given 10,000 to 20,000 units of heparin intravenously followed by a continuous intravenous infusion of heparin to prolong the aPTT to 2 or $2\frac{1}{2}$ times baseline values. After thromboembolectomy, the patients are maintained on continuous intravenous heparin for 3 to 4 days to reduce coagulability while endothelial healing occurs. Postoperative hemorrhage is usually not a problem if good hemostasis is obtained intraoperatively and the aPTT is not allowed to exceed 70 to 80 s. Drugs to inhibit platelet adhesion and aggregation are given when the heparin is stopped.

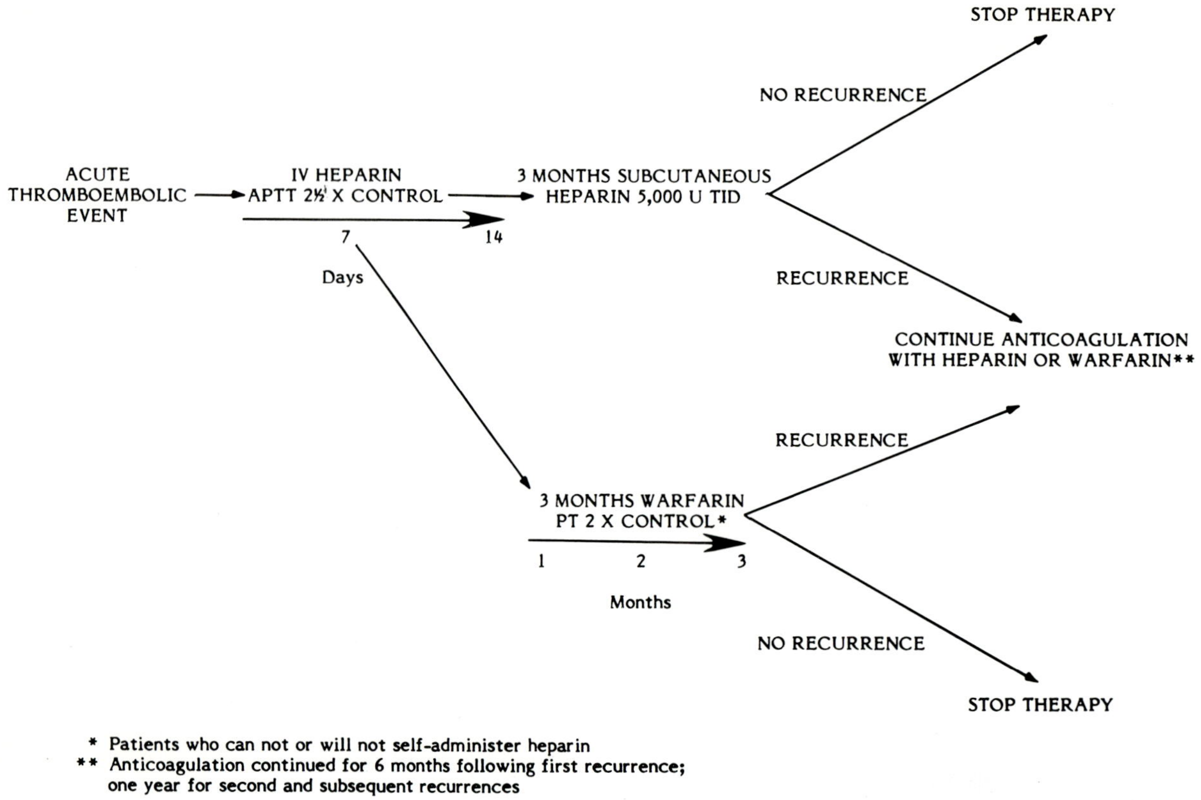

FIGURE 16A-2. Algorithm for the treatment of established deep vein thrombosis and pulmonary embolism.

Provided they do not have a hemorrhagic infarct, patients with an acute cerebral thromboembolic event may benefit from a minidose heparin regimen as prophylaxis against additional thromboembolic sequelae. Such patients should have computed tomography (CT) of the brain before heparin prophylaxis is initiated. If the CT scan does not demonstrate a hemorrhagic infarct, heparin—5000 units subcutaneously every 8 to 12 hours—may be administered with reasonable safety (2,20).

Cardiopulmonary Bypass

Patients placed on cardiopulmonary bypass receive 300 units of heparin per kilogram of body weight before the insertion of the arterial and venous cannulae. For each hour, after the first, that the patient remains on bypass, additional heparin amounting to one-third to one-half the original dose is administered. Alternatively, the heparin dosage may be determined through the use of the ACT. A heparin dosage that produces an ACT of 400 s or greater is considered adequate to inhibit the coagulation cascade during cardiopulmonary bypass (2,17). Patients who are undergoing hypothermic perfusion and who have temperatures less than 32°C may have artificial prolongations of the ACT, due to the low temperature of the blood, and are best managed by the hourly administration of additional heparin (2).

Protamine, 1 mg for every 100 units of heparin administered, is given at the termination of cardiopulmonary bypass to reverse the heparin effect. The return lines to the cardiopulmonary bypass pump must be removed before the administration of the protamine if the surgeon wishes to subsequently transfuse the patient with blood remaining in the reservoir. The ACT, thrombin time, or protamine titration test may be used to determine the adequacy of heparin reversal, with additional small amounts of protamine given when necessary to normalize these tests. Intravenous protamine may produce bradycardia, hypotension, or both and should be administered slowly. One should not give more protamine than is necessary because excess amounts may have an anticoagulant effect.

COMPLICATIONS

The risk of hemorrhage from low-dose subcutaneous heparin therapy is negligible. The risk of bleeding with therapeutic heparinization is 6 percent and is increased in groups such as postmenopausal women and patients with thrombocytopenia, uremia, or preexisting abnormalities of the hemostatic mechanism. The risk of hemorrhage during therapy may approach 50 percent in these patients, in whom heparin administration must be used advisedly and with close monitoring (2,10,13,14). Bleeding rarely occurs with the continuous intravenous infusion of heparin and an aPTT less than 80 to 90 s. The risk of hemorrhage increases markedly when the aPTT remains greater than 100 s (2).

If the hemorrhage is not life-threatening, bleeding secondary to the overadministration of heparin is best managed by discontinuing the heparin. If the bleeding continues or threatens life, the heparin can be neutralized with protamine sulfate. A protamine titration test will help to determine the amount of protamine needed to neutralize the residual heparin. If the protamine titration test is not available, a dose of 1 to 1.5 mg of protamine per 100 units of heparin administered is given slowly until the aPTT or ACT returns toward normal or the bleeding ceases. Usually 30 to 50 percent of the calculated dose is given, slowly and intravenously, to reduce the risk of adverse effects from the protamine. Additional small amounts of protamine are given until the bleeding is controlled or the aPTT or ACT returns toward normal.

An infrequent, but potentially life-and-limb-threatening, complication is the development of thrombocytopenia with thrombosis and hemorrhage. This heparin-induced thrombocytopenia has occurred in 0.6 to 9 percent of patients receiving heparin and is independent of the dose or type of heparin administered (1,21). The thrombocytopenia, which is progressive, usually begins after 6 to 8 days of heparin therapy and is often preceded by increasing heparin requirements to maintain anticoagulation. The thrombocytopenia may begin as early as the second day in patients who have previously received heparin. The appearance of this syndrome is best detected by platelet-count monitoring before the development of thrombohemorrhagic sequelae. If a patient with this syndrome continues to receive heparin, the patient will have a high risk for thromboembolic complications until the heparin is discontinued. The syndrome appears to be caused by the development of a heparin-dependent platelet membrane antibody which is capable of inducing platelet aggregation in the presence of heparin. The thrombocytopenia improves and the thromboembolic complications remit when the heparin is stopped (1).

Sensitivity reactions to heparin have become less frequent with the development of more highly refined heparin preparations. Long-term heparin use may be associated with alopecia and osteoporosis. The concurrent use of vitamin K antagonists is associated with a higher incidence of alopecia. Hair growth usually resumes when the heparin is discontinued. Osteoporosis and pathological fractures have been reported in patients receiving heparin for more than 6 months in dosages exceeding 10,000 units/day.

THE VITAMIN K ANTAGONISTS

Physical Properties

The vitamin K antagonists fall into two groups: the substituted 4-hydroxycoumarins, of which sodium warfarin is the most commonly used member, and the indanediones. The indanediones are rarely used in clinical practice today because of their frequent association with toxic cutaneous and hepatic side effects (19,22).

The 4-hydroxycoumarins are minimally soluble in plasma at pH 7.4; this necessitates protein binding, principally to albumin, of the drugs following absorption. The metabolites of the 4-hydroxycoumarins have better solubilities in plasma and lesser binding to albumin. The high degree of protein binding of sodium warfarin is responsible for its long half-life, volume of distribution, and mode of metabolism and elimination (22).

Mode of Action

The vitamin K antagonists are indirect anticoagulants and bring about a state of hypocoagulability by interfering with the action of vitamin K in the synthesis of clotting factors II, VII, IX, and X by the liver. Reduced vitamin K is a required cofactor in a carboxylase reaction which is responsible for the conversion of glutamyl residues on the clotting-factor percursors to gamma-carboxyglutamyl residues. This conversion is necessary for the binding of calcium, an obligatory cofactor in the reactions catalyzed by the affected factors (19,22).

Patients receiving vitamin K antagonist produce clotting factors that are antigenically similar to the biologically active factors but are without procoagulant activity because of the abnormal calcium-binding characteristics. The effect of the vitamin K antagonists on the vitamin K–dependent carboxylase is reversible and can be blocked by the administration of vitamin K (19,22).

The half-lives of the affected clotting factors range from 6 hours for factor VII to almost 65 hours for prothrombin, and, therefore, a therapeutic reduction of the concentrations of all the affected factors (II, VII, IX, X) may take 3 to 4 days (22). The administration of a large dose of warfarin does not shorten the time span during which therapeutic anticoagulation is achieved but may severely depress concentrations of factor VII; such depression has been associated with a high risk of hemorrhage (2,19,22). The turnover of the clotting factors may be increased in hypermetabolic states such as hyperthyroidism, sepsis, or fever and reduced in hypometabolic states such as hypothyroidism.

During long-term anticoagulant therapy, factor X activity is usually depressed to the greatest degree, and factor IX activity the least. The factor X deficiency is the most common cause of bleeding due to an overdosage of the vitamin K antagonists during long-term therapy (22). When the maintenance dose of warfarin is changed, a new steady-state concentration of each affected factor is achieved. The time required to achieve 90 percent of the total change is 20 hours for factor VII, 65 hours for factor IX, 130 hours for factor X, and 8 days for factor II. The rate of recovery to normal factor concentrations after the discontinuation of anticoagulant therapy follows a similar time course (22).

An additional means by which the vitamin K antagonists may reduce coagulability is by increasing the circulating levels of antithrombin III. The antithrombin III deficiency of patients with low levels of antithrombin III may be corrected after they receive vitamin K antagonists (23). The mechanism for this effect is unknown.

Pharmacokinetics

The absorption of warfarin from the gastrointestinal tract is complete, and peak plasma concentrations occur 2 to 12 hours after a single oral dose. Thus the oral and the intravenous dose are the same. There is considerable variation in the plasma half-life of warfarin, but in most patients it averages 36 to 40 hours. At least 97 percent of warfarin, at therapeutic plasma levels, is bound to albumin. The anticoagulant effect of warfarin antagonists does not correlate with free-drug concentrations or plasma albumin levels, and this suggests that there are other variables involved in the determination of the anticoagulant response (22). There are also differences among individuals in warfarin metabolism, as indicated by the variation in plasma drug concentrations among patients demonstrating similar degrees of anticoagulation (22).

The metabolism of the vitamin K antagonists occurs primarily in the microsomal fraction of the hepatocytes, although soluble enzymes in the hepatic and renal cytosol also contribute. The coumarin metabolites are water-soluble and are excreted in the urine, the principal means for drug clearance. The unchanged parent drugs are not water-soluble and are therefore not significantly excreted by the kidney. There is some evidence for an enterohepatic circulation of coumarin metabolites, but this appears to be of minimal clinical significance (22).

A few patients have a genetically determined resistance to the coumarin anticoagulants. One autosomal dominant trait produces an abnormal vitamin K sensitivity, and another leads to an enhanced metabolism of the drug. Some patients may be hyperresponsive to the coumarin anticoagulants during the first few days following an acute thromboembolic episode and subsequently develop a relative resistance to the anticoagulant effect. For this reason, dosage adjustment is frequently necessary to avoid too much or too little anticoagulation at the beginning of therapy (19,22).

The biological effects of the vitamin K antagonists may be potentiated by certain disease or deficiency states. Patients who are malnourished or who are receiving long-term intravenous alimentation without vitamin K supplementation are often more sensitive to the anticoagulant effects of warfarin because of their vitamin K deficiency. Patients with even mild degrees of liver disease may demonstrate a marked potentiation of the anticoagulant effects of warfarin, as there may be an associated depression of the synthesis of the vitamin K–dependent and non-vitamin K–dependent clotting factors by the diseased liver. Hypermetabolic and hypometabolic states affect the responsiveness to vitamin K antagonists principally by increasing or decreasing the disappearance rates of the vitamin K–dependent clotting factors. Uremia and uncomplicated renal disease do not significantly affect the response to the oral anticoagulants (22).

TABLE 16A-1. Mechanisms of Drug Interactions with Oral Anticoagulants (Partial List)

Drugs	Mechanisms
Potentiators	
Chloramphenicol Ethanol	Enzyme inhibition
Diazoxide Ethacrynic acid Indomethacin Mefenamic acid Nalidixic acid Oxyphenbutazone Phenylbutazone Sulfonamides Tolbutamide	Displacement of bound oral anticoagulant from protein
Clofibrate D-Thyroxine Oral antibiotics*	Reduced availability of vitamin K
Anabolic steroids Quinidine Salicylates	Reduced synthesis of clotting factor
Antagonists	
Barbiturates Meprobamate Griseofulvin	Enzyme induction
Cholestyramine	Reduced absorption
Oral contraceptives Vitamin K (pregnancy)	Increased synthesis of clotting factors

*Especially moxalactam and other second- and third-generation cephalosporins.

Drug Interactions

Several common therapeutic agents, such as aspirin, phenobarbital, and various antibiotics, alter the response of the coagulation system to regularly administered doses of a vitamin K antagonist. This alteration may occur through a decreased absorption from the gastrointestinal tract, a displacement of the drug from its binding site on albumin, an increase in the rate at which it is metabolized by the hepatic microsomes, a decrease in the vitamin K availability, or an increase or decrease in the plasma half-life of the affected clotting factors. Table 16A-1 lists the major drug interactions with the coumarin derivatives. In addition, drugs that affect platelet function, such as aspirin and indomethacin, may increase the risk of hemorrhage by impairing the platelet's ability to participate in the hemostatic process.

Patients who receive additional medications while taking warfarin should have frequent laboratory testing to ensure that the anticoagulant effect is maintained. It may be advantageous to provide patients with a booklet which describes anticoagulant dosage and control, warns about the possible adverse effect of other medications on the activity of warfarin, and provides instructions for actions in the case of hemorrhage.

Prophylaxis

The prophylactic effect of vitamin K antagonists in venous thromboembolism was first demonstrated by Sevitt and Gallagher in 300 patients with hip fractures. The treated group, which received phenindione, had a 3 percent incidence of clinically diagnosed venous thromboembolism, while the control group had a 29 percent incidence of venous thromboembolism. At autopsy, venous thrombosis was found in 83 percent of the control patients, with 10 percent having pulmonary emboli. Only 14 percent of the treated patients who died had evidence of venous thromboembolism; no patient died, while receiving phenindione, as a result of pulmonary embolism (24). Other studies have confirmed this prophylactic effect of warfarin in nonorthopedic surgery, myocardial infarction, and other major medical illnesses which increase the risk of venous thrombosis (25,26). If used for perioperative venous thromboembolism prophylaxis, warfarin must be started 2 to 3 days before surgery to be effective. Prothrombin times $1\frac{1}{2}$ times the control value provide adequate prophylaxis during the immediate perioperative period (2). The prophylaxis is initiated with intravenous or oral doses of 10 to 15 mg of warfarin daily for 3 to 4 days, followed by an adjustment of the dose to maintain the prothrombin time at $1\frac{1}{2}$ to 2 times control values. Full anticoagulation requires 5 to 7 days, when a steady state between drug absorption and effect is achieved. Decreased initial dosages of warfarin, i.e., 2 to 5 mg daily, should be used to begin anticoagulant therapy in elderly patients and in those receiving parenteral nutrition or recovering from surgery. The dosage of warfarin should be subsequently adjusted to maintain the prothrombin time at $1\frac{1}{2}$ to 2 times control values.

The several thromboplastin reagents have differing sensitivities to the clotting-factor changes produced by the vitamin K antagonists. Therapeutic ratios (patient to control) of the prothrombin time may range from 2 to 4 for the British comparative thromboplastin to 2 to 3.5 for the thrombotest reagent and 1.4 to 1.8 for the Ortho reagent (22). It is important, therefore, to be familiar with the reagents that the laboratory responsible for monitoring the anticoagulant effect is using.

Therapeutics

Because of their delayed onset of action, the vitamin K antagonists are infrequently used in the early management of acute venous thromboembolism. They are used when the antithrombin III deficiency is demonstrated or when heparin sensitivity or reaction is present. The vitamin K antagonists are used to maintain outpatient anticoagulation after an acute thromboembolic event in patients who should not receive heparin or who refuse to self-administer it. The vitamin K antagonists are initiated after 5 to 10 days of heparin therapy. Heparin is discontinued when the patient's prothrombin time reaches the therapeutic range of twice the control. Therapeutic anticoagulation is maintained for 3 months following the acute event, after which the risk of bleeding usually exceeds the potential benefits of oral anticoagulation (19). Patients with recurrent thromboembolism may be anticoagulated for 6 to 12 months; these patients are frequently managed with the vitamin K antagonists to avoid the osteoporosis associated with the long-term use of heparin (19,22).

Management of Arterial Thromboembolic Disease

Vitamin K antagonists can reduce the risk of emboli arising from prosthetic heart valves, the enlarged left atria of patients with mitral stenosis, and the atria of patients with chronic atrial fibrillation. Vitamin K antagonists have not affected the incidence of recurrent infarction or the heart-related mortality of patients with recent myocardial infarction; however, the antagonists are useful in reducing the incidence of arterial emboli arising from the mural thromboses in these patients (24). The use of vitamin K antagonists in the management of patients with ischemic cerebrovascular disease has been supplanted by the use of the antiplatelet agents (20). The vitamin K antagonists have no established role in the treatment of chronic peripheral arterial disease.

COMPLICATIONS

The most common complication of the vitamin K antagonists is hemorrhage. Contraindications to therapy are the same as those listed for heparin and include defects in the hemostatic mechanism, active ulcer disease, or other disease processes predisposing the patient to hemorrhage. In addition, patients undergoing therapy with the vitamin K antagonists should have sufficient reliability and intelligence to safely self-administer the drug, return for routine follow-up laboratory testing, and recognize the symptoms of overanticoagulation.

Vitamin K antagonists should not be administered to pregnant women during the first trimester because of the teratogenicity which is related to their interference with the vitamin K–mediated carboxylation reactions necessary for the calcification of bone (19). The coumarins may also cause central nervous system abnormalities. In the United Kingdom, patients who must remain on anticoagulant therapy without pregnancy are given heparin during the first trimester, and the therapy is subsequently changed to warfarin through the thirty-seventh week, when heparin therapy is reinstituted. Heparin is discontinued before delivery and restarted after delivery and continued until the patient is fully ambulatory. Warfarin therapy is substituted for heparin therapy during the midportion of the pregnancy to avoid the maternal osteoporosis associated with long-term heparin use (19). In the United States, however, low-dose subcutaneous heparin is becoming the preferred agent for continued anticoagulation throughout pregnancy and has been associated with a minimal risk of material osteoporosis in dosages up to 10,000 units/day. The vitamin K antagonists should not be given to women who are breast feeding as the drugs are secreted into the milk and could lead to hemorrhagic problems in the breast-fed infant.

The frequency of hemorrhage with the vitamin K antagonists varies widely and is dependent upon the intensity of the anticoagulation and methods for detecting the hemorrhage. The incidence of clinically significant hemorrhage in patients maintained within the therapeutic range was reported by Forfar to be 4.3 percent per treatment year (27). Forfar also noted that severe hemorrhage is more common when the prothrombin time exceeds the therapeutic range and that the risk of hemorrhage is increased in patients in whom control has proved difficult, in men with an aortic valve prosthesis, and in patients anticoagulated for longer than 3 years (11). Other factors which increase the risk of bleeding include advanced age, urologic and gynecologic disorders, the postpartum state, and the initiation of therapy with a large loading dose (19,22,25,27).

The gastrointestinal and urinary tracts, nose, and skin represent the most common sites of bleeding (22). The majority of hemorrhage-related fatalities involve gastrointestinal tract or intracerebral bleeding (22). The site of blood loss is usually clinically obvious but may on occasion be occult, as with bleeding into the retroperitoneal or perinephric spaces. In nearly 20 percent of the hemorrhagic episodes reported by Forfar, bleeding occurred into the retroperitoneal or perinephric space; hemorrhage into the retroperitoneal space was associated with a very high mortality (27). Gastrointestinal and urinary tract bleeding which occur when the prothrombin time ratio is within the therapeutic range should be investigated, since the use of the vitamin K antagonists may have unmasked an unsuspected bleeding source such as a colon or renal carcinoma.

When the patient receiving a vitamin K antagonist bleeds, the anticoagulation may be reversed within 24 hours by the intravenous administration (or, less desirable, the intramuscular administration) of 25 mg of vitamin K_1. Life-threatening hemorrhage is best managed with the replacement of the deficient clotting factors with infusions of fresh-frozen plasma in addition to the intravenous administration of vitamin K_1. Patients who require anticoagulation reversal before the surgery but who will continue to receive the anticoagulant postoperatively are best treated with fresh-frozen plasma before surgery and maintained on subcutaneous heparin until satisfactory anticoagulation with the vitamin K antagonists is achieved postoperatively. The administration of vitamin K to these patients makes them more resistant to the vitamin K antagonists and makes anticoagulation more difficult postoperatively (2).

Less common complications of vitamin K antagonists include alopecia, urticaria, dermatitis, fever, nausea, diarrhea, abdominal cramping, and hypersensitivity reactions. Dermal gangrene of the thigh, breast, and buttocks is a rare complication of oral anticoagulant therapy; the risk of such a complication is increased with high-loading-dose regimens for initiating therapy. Dermal gangrene occurs most frequently in women, and some patients require debridement and grafting, or even amputation (2,19,22).

References

1. Silver D, Kapsch DN, Tsoi EKM: Heparin-induced thrombocytopenia thrombosis and hemorrhage. Ann Surg 1983:301–306.
2. Kapsch DN, Kasulke RJ, Silver D: Anticoagulant therapy: Pharmacology, clinical uses and complications. Vasc Diagn Ther August/September 1981, pp 19–33.
3. Estes JW: Clinical pharmokinetics of heparin. Clin Pharmokinet 1980, 5:204–220.
4. Rosenberg RD: Biologic actions of heparin. Semin Hematol 1977, 14:427–440.
5. Thomas DP: Heparin. Clin Haematol 1981, 10:443–458.
6. Thomas DP, Sagar S, Stomatakis JD, Maffer FHA, Erik A, Kakkar VV: Plasma heparin levels after administration of calcium and sodium salts of heparin. Thromb Res 1976, 9:241–248.
7. Belch JJ, Lowe GDO, Ward AG, Forbes CD, Prenkce CRM: Prevention of deep vein thrombosis in medical patients by low-dose heparin. Scott Med J 1981, 26:115–117.
8. Hull R, Delmore T, Carter C, Hush J, Genton E, Gent M, Turpu G, McLaughlin D: Adjusted subcutaneous heparin versus warfarin sodium in the long-term treatment of venous thrombosis. N Engl J Med 1982, 306:189–194.
9. Kakkar VV: Prevention of venous thromboembolism. Clin Haematol 1981, 10:543–583.
10. Rosenow EC III, Osmundson PJ, Brown M: Pulmonary embolism. Mayo Clin Proc 1981, 56:161–178.
11. Sharnoff JG, Rosen RL, Palazzo PJ, Fethiere AA, Sotudeh S, Alvarez EV, Rosen C: Prevention of fatal pulmonary thromboembolism by small dose heparin prophylaxis in acute hip fracture surgery. Br J Clin Practice 1981, 35:390–392, 427.
12. Council on Thrombosis of the American Heart Association. Prevention of venous thromboembolism in surgical patients by low-dose heparin. Circulation 1977, 55:423A–426A.
13. Coon WW: Management of anticoagulant and thrombolytic agents in deep venous thrombosis. Vas Surg 1982, 16:1–7.
14. Gallus AS: Established venous thrombosis and pulmonary embolism. Clin Haematol 1981, 10:583–611.
15. Kaymeir FJ: Monitoring of heparin therapy. In Lundblad RL, Brown WV, Mann KG, Roberts HR (eds): *Chemistry and Biology of Heparin*. New York, Elsevier/North-Holland, 1981, pp 615–624.
16. Bentley PG, Kakkar VV, Scully MF, MacGregor IR, Webb P, Chan P, Jones N: An objective study of alternative methods of heparin administration. Thromb Res 1980, 18:177–187.
17. Hattersley PG, Mitsuoka JC, King JH: The use of the activated coagulation time (ACT) as a monitor of heparin therapy. In Lundblad RL, Brown WV, Mann KG, Roberts HR (eds): *Chemistry and Biology of Heparin*. New York, Elsevier/North-Holland, 1981, pp 659–664.
18. Blaisdell FW, Graziano CJ, Effeney DJ: In vivo assessment of anticoagulation. Surgery 1977, 82:827–839.
19. Walsh, PN: Oral anticoagulant therapy. Hosp Pract 1983, 18:101–120.
20. Easton JD, Byer JA, Sherman DG: Anticoagulant in cerebrovascular disease. Clin Neurosurg 1981, 28:71–86.
21. Ansell J, Slepchuk N Jr, Raminder K, Lopez A, Southard L, Deykin D: Heparin induced thrombocytopnia: A prospective study. Thromb Haemost 1980, 43:61–65.
22. Winter JH, Douglass AS: Oral anticoagulants. Clin Hematol 1981, 10:459–480.
23. Bern MM, Bothe A Jr, Bistrian B, Batist G, Haywood E, Blackburn G: Effects of low dose warfarin on antithrombin III levels in morbidly obese patients. Surgery 1983, 94:78–83.
24. Sevitt S, Gallagher NG: Prevention of venous thrombosis and pulmonary embolism in injuried patients: A trial of anticoagulant prophylaxis with phenindione in middle-age and elderly patients with fractured neck of femur. Lancet 1959, 2:981–989.
25. Brovic M: Oral anticoagulants: Clinical applications. Semin Hematol 1978, 15:27–34.
26. Salzman EW: Prevention of venous thromboembolism by oral anticoagulants and drugs affecting platelet function. In Bergan JJ, Yao ST, *Venous Problems*. Chicago, Year Book, 1978, pp 545–551.
27. Forfar JC: A seven year analysis of haemorrhage in patients on long-term anticoagulant treatment. Br Heart J 1979, 42:128–132.

Chapter 16B

THROMBOLYSINS IN VASCULAR DISEASE

HENRY D. BERKOWITZ, W. CLARK HARGROVE III, and BROOKE ROBERTS

The management of acute arterial occlusion remains a challenging clinical problem. With the discovery of heparin by J. McLean in 1916, the propagation of thrombi could be prevented, but the removal of thrombus still required mechanical extraction, since the body's intrinsic fibrinolytic system generally does not lyse thrombus rapidly. The use of the Fogarty catheter was a major advance in the mechanical extraction of emboli and thrombus and has enabled surgeons to achieve 90 percent limb salvage rates in patients with acute ischemia. In spite of advances in anesthetic and postoperative care, emergency operation still carries a 15 to 30 percent mortality in these patients. In patients with acute thrombosis secondary to atherosclerotic plaque, the Fogarty catheter is less useful, and bypass grafting is often necessary. In addition, the passage of the Fogarty catheter through occluded vessels produces intimal damage and occasional dissection, even in experienced hands; these problems are intensified when dealing with occluded vein grafts, since intimal viability depends on luminal blood flow, even in established grafts. Although the Fogarty catheter disobliteration of occluded vein grafts is usually successful, long-term graft patency is rarely attained if the occlusion has been present for 24 hours or more. Thrombolytic therapy may provide an alternative approach to emergency operation in some patients with acute and chronic limb ischemia.

In thrombolytic therapy the body's intrinsic fibrinolytic system is activated immediately. It has the potential of lysing clots in the thrombosed vessel or graft as well as clots in distal vascular beds, while preserving the intimal integrity of arterial and vein grafts. It may also reveal, by clearing the lumen of thrombus, the area of an inciting arterial or graft stenosis, making surgery or percutaneous transluminal angioplasty (PTA) a possibility in what may otherwise have been a hopeless or desperate situation.

The fibrinolytic agents currently available are streptokinase and urokinase. Streptokinase was discovered by Tillet and Garner (1) in 1933, when they described the fibrinolytic activity of the hemolytic streptococcus. The first available commercial preparation of streptokinase, Actase, was not a highly purified product, and although it could dissolve thrombi, serious allergic reactions to it were reported. The current product is highly purified, but streptokinase still has the disadvantage of antigenicity in humans. Most adults have some antibody to streptokinase because of previous exposure to β-hemolytic streptococcus.

Urokinase was first isolated from human urine in 1946 (2). It has the chief advantage of being nonantigenic and has proved to be relatively nontoxic and nonpyrogenic. Initially, huge amounts of human urine (about 2500 L) were required in order to supply enough drug to treat a 70-kg man for 12 hours (3), making it very expensive to use. More recently, urokinase has been recovered from tissue cultures of human renal cells. Today urokinase is about six times more expensive than streptokinase (Table 16B-1).

Streptokinase is obtainable as a lyophylized powder under the name of Kabikinase, made by KabiVitrim, Inc., or Streptase, made by Hoechst-Roussel. Urokinase also comes as a lyophylized powder, called Abbokinase, made by Abbott, and Breakinace made by Breon. Both drugs produce clot lysis by the activation of the human fibrinolytic system. Streptokinase combines with the inactive proenzyme plasminogen to form an activator complex (Figure 16B-1). This streptokinase-plasminogen complex then converts available plasminogen to plasmin, the active fibrinolytic enzyme. Urokinase converts plasminogen to plasmin directly. Plasmin has relatively nonspecific activity and degrades fibrin, fibrinogen, prothrombin, and factors V and VIII (4). Both agents convert free and thrombus-bound plasminogen unselectively. Thrombolysis by systemic infusion is dependent on the activation of circulating plasminogen, which nonselec-

TABLE 16B-1. Comparison of the Features of Streptokinase and Urokinase

	Streptokinase	Urokinase
Source	Group C hemolytic streptococcus	Human urine and human renal cells
Size (mol. wt.)	47,000	32,000–54,000
Antigenic	Yes	No
Pyrogenic	Yes, commonly	Rarely
Cost	$9/100,000 units	$50/100,000 units
Allergic reactions	Few	Rare

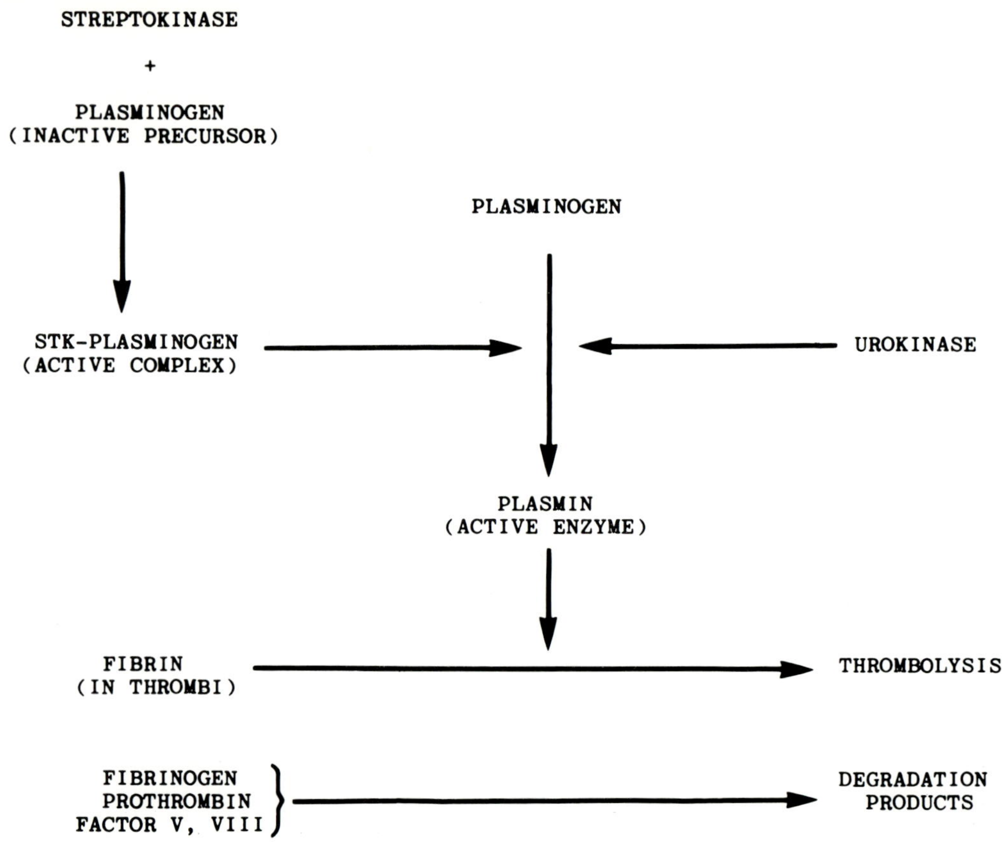

FIGURE 16B-1. Fibrinolysis during thrombolytic therapy. Streptokinase (STK) and urokinase convert plasminogen to the active enzyme plasmin, which then lyses fresh fibrin.

tively lyses thrombi wherever they may occur. High doses of the thrombolytic agent are thus required to overcome systemic inhibitory mechanisms. This is associated with a generalized coagulopathy and a high risk of bleeding complications. Selective infusion has the theoretical advantage of delivering a higher concentration of agent to the clot and activating thrombus-bound plasminogen more effectively (5). This would allow a lower total infusion dose and potentially fewer side effects.

Clinical Use

In the late 1960s, after earlier anecdotal reports had suggested clinical efficacy, controlled studies were undertaken to define the role of thrombolytic therapy in certain clinical conditions. After encouraging reports (6,7) from Europe and the United Kingdom about the use of streptokinase and urokinase in thromboembolic disease, in the United States the National Heart and Lung Institute undertook a multicenter cooperative study comparing thrombolytic agents with heparin in the treatment of pulmonary embolism (8). With both streptokinase and urokinase, the rate and completeness of the dissolution of the embolus and thrombus were enhanced, thus improving the restitution of pulmonary blood flow and lessening any subsequent pulmonary hypertension, when compared with the rate and completeness in controls treated with heparin alone. However, there was no statistical difference in the mortality, as the numbers were small. Likewise, there is evidence that early thrombolytic therapy of phlebitis results in faster resolution and less permanent damage to the venous system than treatment with heparin alone (9,10). Both thrombolytic substances, however, carry the risk of hemorrhagic complications, particularly in patients who have undergone recent major surgery or delivery, a time when phlebitis is common. Because of the risk of hemorrhage, the adverse reactions to streptokinase, and the cost, thrombolytic therapy has generally not been used for phlebitis in the absence of pulmonary embolism.

In the 1960s a number of investigators (11–16) postulated that streptokinase might have a role in the treatment of arterial occlusion. Treatment with systemic therapy in these patients resulted in a high incidence of hemorrhagic complications, and benefit in fewer than 50 percent. Dotter et al. in 1974 (17) reported on the direct intraarterial infusion of streptokinase in the treatment of acute and chronic arterial occlusions. With this technique, he achieved clot lysis with a dosage far lower than that required by systemic infusions. More recently, several groups have reported using local low-dose therapy in acute and subacute arterial occlusions, with good results (18–22). In addition, Hess (23) and coworkers have used a modification of the local low-dose technique in patients whose chronic arterial occlusions were present for up to a year with surprisingly good results.

Other uses of thrombolytic therapy include the treatment of

retinal vein thrombosis, the declotting of intravenous catheters, and the declotting of arteriovenous fistulas used for chronic hemodialysis (1). Intracoronary use in the early postinfarction period is under investigation at a number of centers. Most series report about 80 percent successful lysis of thrombus and salvage of ischemic myocardium if the therapy is started within 3 hours of the onset of symptoms (24).

Contraindications

The risk of hemorrhage, particularly intracranial, from thrombolytic agents has limited their use. Contraindications include a recent cerebrovascular event, particularly within 2 months, severe hypertension, an open wound, active gastrointestinal bleeding, the presence of a coagulopathy, a recent operation (within 10 days), or recent delivery (within 30 days). Relative contraindications include severe liver or renal disease, a history of menorrhagia, and the recent use of anticoagulant drugs, such as warfarin (Coumadin), or even aspirin. Another general precaution to be heeded while thrombolytic agents are being used is the avoidance of intramuscular injections and arterial punctures. Venous punctures may require the application of pressure for prolonged periods. The concomitant use of heparin in conjunction with thrombolytic therapy increases the propensity for hemorrhagic complications. We delay the use of heparin until the thrombin time is not more than twice normal, a delay usually less than 4 hours. Some have reported the use of heparin with streptokinase (21,22,25), and no increase in the incidence of bleeding complications was observed.

Laboratory Studies

Thrombolytic therapy is monitored by standard coagulation tests. The most accurate and easily obtainable is the thrombin time, which is an indirect measurement of the serum fibrinogen level. The partial thromboplastin time (PTT) and prothrombin time (PT) may also be affected. We perform baseline studies before beginning therapy and then repeat the studies on an 8-hour basis. In addition, we obtain daily measurements of the hemoglobin levels, platelet counts, serum fibrinogen levels, and fibrin split product levels. In systemic therapy, a thrombin time between two and seven times the control is desired. If the thrombin time becomes greater than seven times the control, therapy should be terminated at least temporarily. The use of low-dose intraarterial streptokinase has the theoretical advantage of not changing the coagulation profile or fibrinogen level. However, many patients do demonstrate decreased levels of fibrinogen, increased levels of fibrin split products, and decreased levels of plasminogen, despite low-dose therapy (12,22,26,27), but the hemorrhagic complications have not correlated well with these measurements. Nevertheless, we have the studies done and use the results as a guideline for starting cryoprecipitates after thrombolytic therapy has been stopped.

Should spontaneous bleeding occur during thrombolytic therapy, the infusion should be stopped immediately. Fresh-frozen plasma (FFP) may be used to replete fibrinogen levels until the results of the coagulation studies have returned to normal. If volume load is a problem, such as in a patient with severe cardiac disease, cryoprecipitate may be used.

Systemic Treatment

The recommended dosage for systemic therapy with streptokinase is 250,000 units over 20 to 30 minutes as a loading dose, followed by 100,000 units/h. Patients with high levels of antibody against streptokinase may require higher loading doses, but the standard loading dose overcomes antibody resistance in 85 to 90 percent of all patients. Hydrocortisone, 100 mg intravenously, is recommended before streptokinase therapy is begun to lessen the likelihood of allergic or other reactions. After therapy, antibody titers reach their peak in approximately $2\frac{1}{2}$ weeks. A subsequent infusion of streptokinase probably should not be undertaken for at least 6 months. The recommended systemic dosage for urokinase is 4400 units/kg given over 10 minutes, followed by 4400 units/kg per hour. Thus the maintenance urokinase dose is about 3 times the streptokinase dose. Systemic therapy with streptokinase may be continued for up to 24 hours in the treatment of pulmonary embolism and up to 72 hours in phlebitis. Urokinase should be given for from 12 to 24 hours in the treatment of pulmonary embolism. Although equally efficacious, urokinase has not yet been approved by the Federal Drug Administration for the treatment of phlebitis.

Technique of Low-Dose Therapy

The anticipated use of an intraarterial thrombolytic agent entails certain technical considerations. We have found that it is wise to insert the catheter at a site distant from the presumed site of occlusion to avoid having the arterial puncture site near the point of infusion of thrombolytic agents. For example, if the left femoral artery is believed to be occluded, then the right femoral artery is generally used for the introduction of the catheter. If the occasion requires the use of an axillary approach, we recommend the left axilla, as we are hesitant to leave a catheter in the innominate vessel for a prolonged period of time.

Using a standard Seldinger technique, a catheter is inserted, and an arteriogram is obtained to demonstrate the extent of occlusion and the distal vascular bed. The tip of the catheter is then advanced and buried in the clot. Localization is done by the hand injection of contrast material as the catheter is advanced. The administration of streptokinase (5000 units/h) or urokinase (440 units/kg per hour) is begun using an infusion pump. Interval fluoroscopy and x-ray films are used to follow the clinical progress. The infusion may result in a rapid dissolution of fresh clot, in which case the therapy is terminated, but the therapy may be safely continued for as long as 72 hours. We recommend routine arteriography at not more than 12-hour intervals to assess the status of the thrombolysis. In general, the older the clot, the more resistant it is to complete or partial lysis, although the exact response is impossible to predict. Once patency has been reestablished, the arteriogram generally reveals a stenotic lesion, which is the underlying cause of thrombosis. This stenosis may be treated by PTA or by early operation when angioplasty is not deemed feasible. If the stenosis is not relieved, early rethrombosis frequently occurs.

Hess recently reported a variation of this technique (23) in which the thrombus is injected at intervals of 5 to 15 minutes with 1 to 3 mL of a streptokinase solution containing 1000 units/mL and under fluoroscopic guidance the catheter is advanced farther into the clot with repeated small injections. This process is repeated until the catheter reaches the distal reconstituted lumen of the artery and antegrade flow is confirmed by fluoroscopy. With this technique, the duration of the therapy is only 1 to 5 hours, and the total administered dose varies between 4000 and 180,000 units of streptokinase. All the patients in this study had had symptoms for at least 6 days and some for as long as 1 year pretreatment.

Of the 136 patients studied, the reestablishment of patency was demonstrated in two-thirds, with a 2-week patency rate of 50 percent and a 70 percent 1-year patency rate in the vessels which stayed open for at least 2 weeks. An intramural passage of the catheter occurred in 29 of the 136 patients, and in these cases the therapy was immediately terminated (23).

University of Pennsylvania Experience

At the University of Pennsylvania, from August 1981 until August 1983, we treated 31 patients who had peripheral arterial or graft occlusions with low-dose streptokinase infusions. The patient population consisted of 10 patients with arterial occlusions, 17 with vein graft occlusions, and 4 with prosthetic graft occlusions (Table 16B-2). The duration of the therapy was usually 24 hours. The arteriography was repeated, and if complete clot dissolution had not been achieved, the infusions were continued for an additional 24 hours. No patient was treated for more than 72 hours even if complete clot lysis was not achieved.

Complete or partial clot dissolution was achieved in 81 percent of the occlusions, accompanied by significant clinical benefit in 68 percent of the entire group (Table 16B-3). When the results were analyzed by type of occlusion, each showed similar responsiveness to streptokinase. The ultimate clinical benefit was greatest with arterial thrombi (90 percent) and lowest with prosthetic graft thrombi (50 percent) (Table 16B-4).

TABLE 16B-2. Type of Occlusions Treated with Thrombolytic Therapy

	Number of Occurrences	
Arterial occlusions		10
Iliac	2	
Superficial femoral	4	
Popliteal (popliteal aneurysms)	3	
Brachial (embolus)	1	
Vein graft occlusions		17
Femoropopliteal	13	
Femorotibial	4	
Prosthetic graft occlusion		4
Aortic bifurcation graft, Dacron	2	
Femoral-popliteal, PTFE*	1	
Femoral-tibial, PTFE	1	
Total occlusions		31

*PTFE = polytetrafluoroethylene.

TABLE 16B-3. Clot Lysis vs. Clinical Benefit

	Clot Lysis			Clinical Benefit		
	Present			Present		
	Complete	Partial	None	SK*	SK + OP† or SK + PTA‡	None
No. Limbs	21	4	6	2	19	10
Percent	68	13	19	7	61	32
Total percent	81			68		

*SK = streptokinase.

†SK + OP = streptokinase + surgery (6 patients).

‡SK + PTA = streptokinase + percutaneous transluminal angioplasty (13 patients).

TABLE 16B-4. Clot Lysis and Clinical Benefit with Occlusion Type

		Clot Lysis			Clinical Benefit		
		Present			Present		
		Complete	Partial	None	SK*	SK+OP† or SK+PTA‡	None
Arterial thrombi	(10)	8	1	1	2	7	1
Percent		80	10	10	20	70	10
Vein graft thrombi	(17)	12	1	4	0	10	7
Percent		70	6	24	0	59	41
Prosthetic graft thrombi	(4)	1	2	1	0	2	2
Percent		25	50	25	0	50	50

*SK = streptokinase.
†SK + OP = streptokinase + surgery (6 patients).
‡SK + PTA = streptokinase + percutaneous transluminal angioplasty (13 patients).

A total of 90 percent (9 of 10 patients) of the arterial thrombi were successfully lysed with streptokinase therapy, and this resulted in significant clinical benefit. An interesting case of an occluded popliteal aneurysm is illustrated in Figure 16B-2. The patient initially presented with a 5-day history of an ischemic leg. The original arteriogram showed a popliteal artery occlusion with extremely poor distal vessels. Because the distal circulation was so poor, an intraarterial streptokinase infusion was instituted, and after 24 hours the popliteal artery was completely open, revealing a popliteal aneurysm as the cause of the occlusion. The aneurysm was then resected and replaced with a short interposition vein graft. This illustrates two benefits of streptokinase therapy. It allows a more accurate preoperative diagnosis by revealing the cause of the occlusion, and it can often open up the distal occluded vascular bed, allowing a simpler vascular reconstruction than was initially anticipated.

Another example of a successful lysis of an arterial occlusion is shown in Figure 16B-3. A tight stenosis in the right leg was shown on a bilateral femoral arteriogram obtained because of symptoms in the opposite leg. Ten days after a successful femoral–posterior tibial graft, the patient returned to have elective PTA of the stenosis, but the vessel was then occluded. A selective streptokinase infusion was started; this lysed the clot and again revealed the arterial stenosis, which was then dilated successfully.

Although 76 percent of the vein grafts in the University of Pennsylvania study showed significant clot dissolution, only 59 percent (10 of 17 patients) showed clinical benefit (Table 16B-4). Failures to achieve clinical benefit in vein grafts after the successful dissolution of clot were related primarily to catheter complications during the infusion or during subsequent PTA of graft stenoses. Nevertheless, PTA was used in 7 of the 10 successfully treated vein graft occlusions. Figure 16B-4 illustrates a typical vein graft occlusion which was opened with streptokinase infusion. A proximal arterial stenosis was identified as the probable cause of the graft occlusion and was dilated successfully.

A small number of prosthetic grafts were treated in our series, with 75 percent success in clot lysis and 50 percent clinical benefit. Figure 16B-5 is an example of an occluded limb of a Dacron aortic bifurcation graft which was opened with streptokinase infusion, revealing a superficial femoral and deep femoral stenosis which was successfully dilated. Prosthetic grafts present the special problem of transmural bleeding because of the lysis of fibrin in the graft interstices. This is true even with grafts implanted for as long as 6 years (21). We have also seen this with one Dacron graft inserted six years prior to thrombolytic therapy. Extravasation of blood was noted under the fibrous capsule at a subsequent operation, but there was no free bleeding into the surrounding tissue. A more severe complication was noted in a polytetrafluoroethylene graft, used as a femoral-tibial bypass graft, which had been implanted for only 2 weeks (Figure 16B-6). This graft demonstrated a free extravasation of dye through the graft wall, as well as extravasation at the distal suture line during streptokinase infusion. We currently do not recommend thrombolytic therapy for occluded prosthetic grafts which have been in place for less than 3 months.

The majority of occlusions treated in our series were 1 week or less in age (Table 16B-5). In one vein graft, streptokinase therapy was instituted 5 weeks after occlusion, and no significant clot lysis was demonstrated. However, there was no difference in the success of clot lysis related to the age of occlusion up to 2 weeks. Although it is true that acute occlusions will probably show the best response to fibrinolytic therapy (18), some clot lysis will also occur in a smaller percentage of lesions treated more than 2 months after occlusion (13).

TABLE 16B-5. Duration of Vascular Occlusion before Treatment with Thrombolytic Agents

Duration, weeks	Artery	Vein Graft	Prosthetic Graft	Percent
0–1	6	15	3	77%
1–2	4	1	1	19%
>2	0	1	0	4%

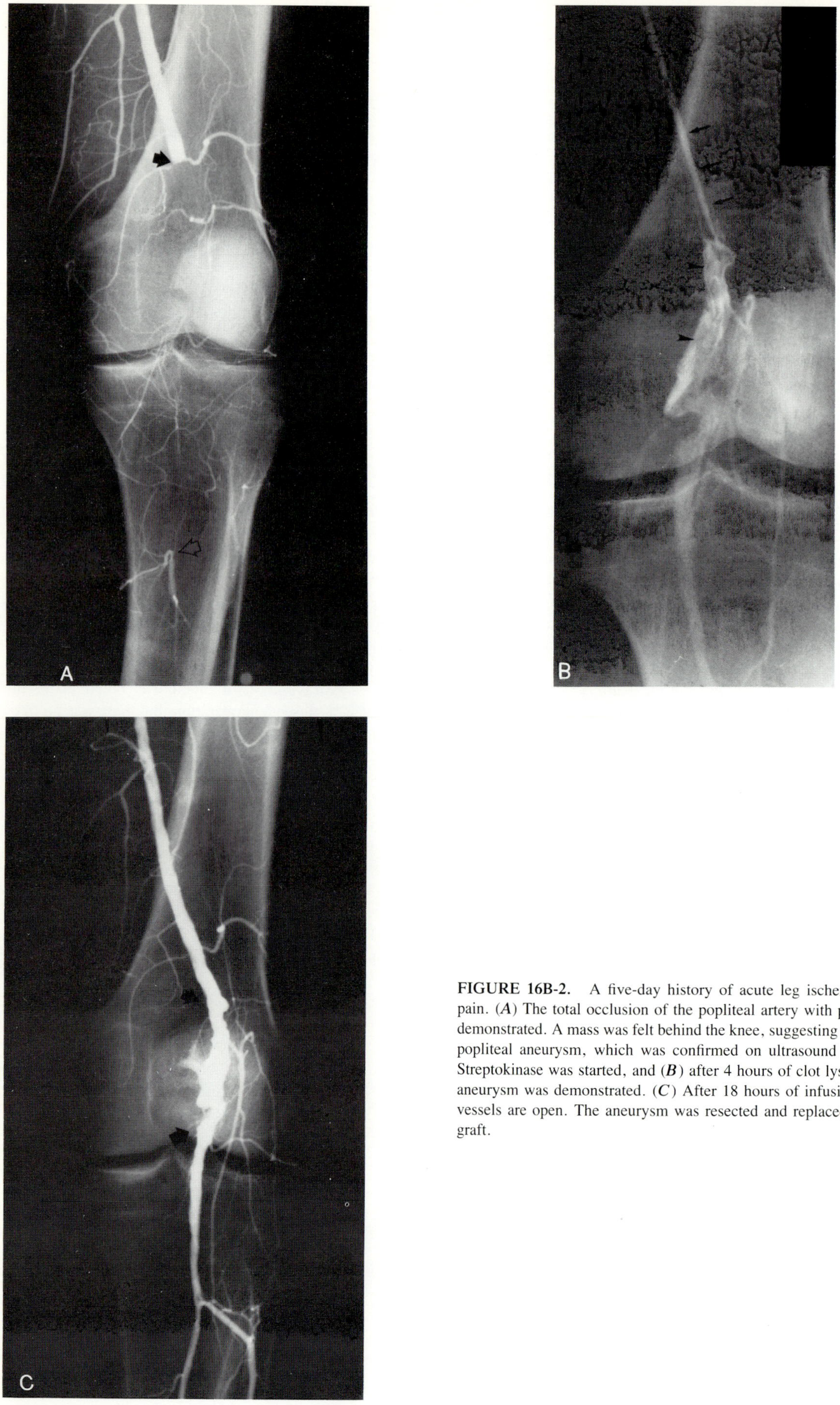

FIGURE 16B-2. A five-day history of acute leg ischemia with rest pain. (*A*) The total occlusion of the popliteal artery with poor runoff is demonstrated. A mass was felt behind the knee, suggesting a thrombosed popliteal aneurysm, which was confirmed on ultrasound examination. Streptokinase was started, and (*B*) after 4 hours of clot lysis a popliteal aneurysm was demonstrated. (*C*) After 18 hours of infusion, the distal vessels are open. The aneurysm was resected and replaced with a vein graft.

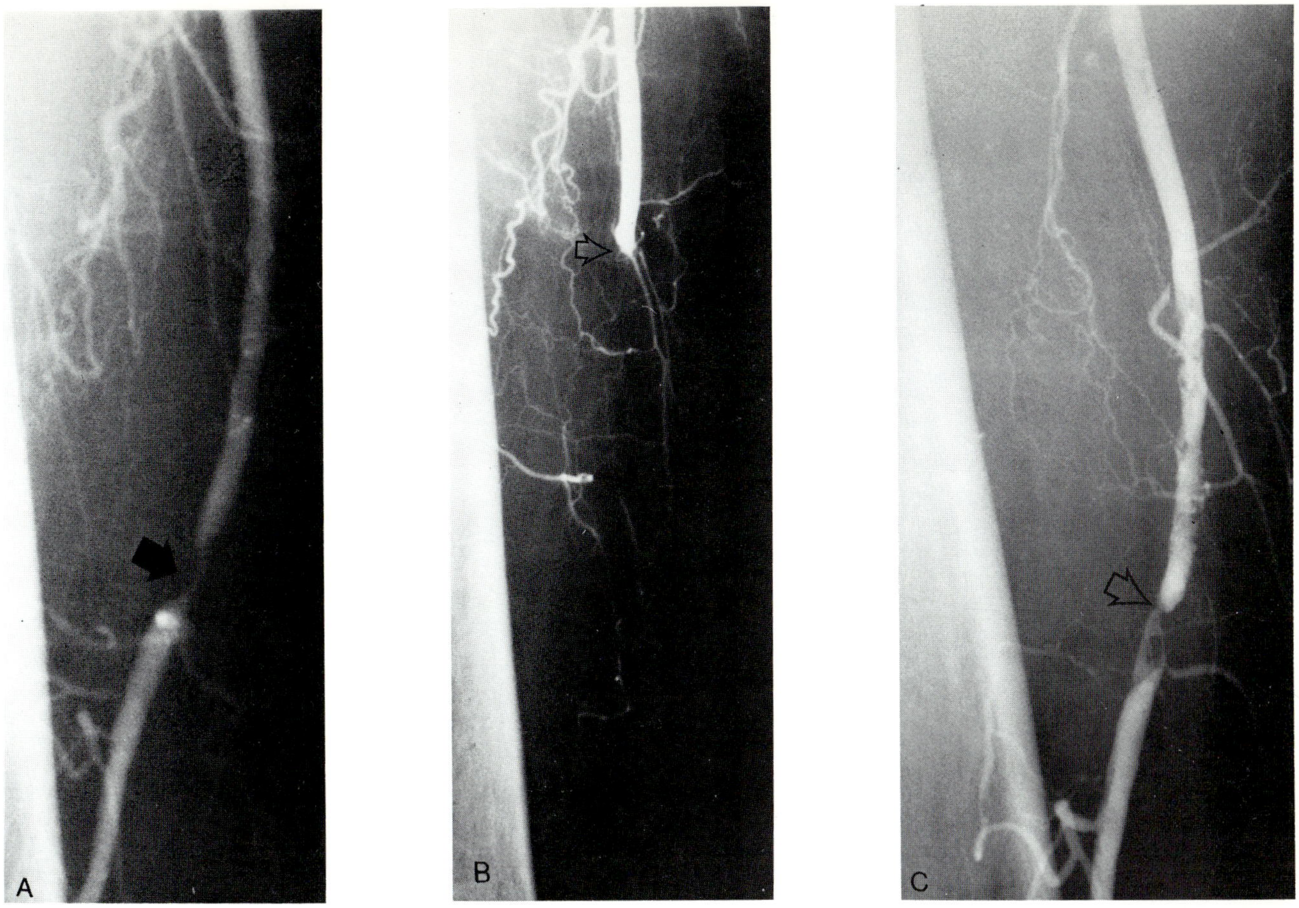

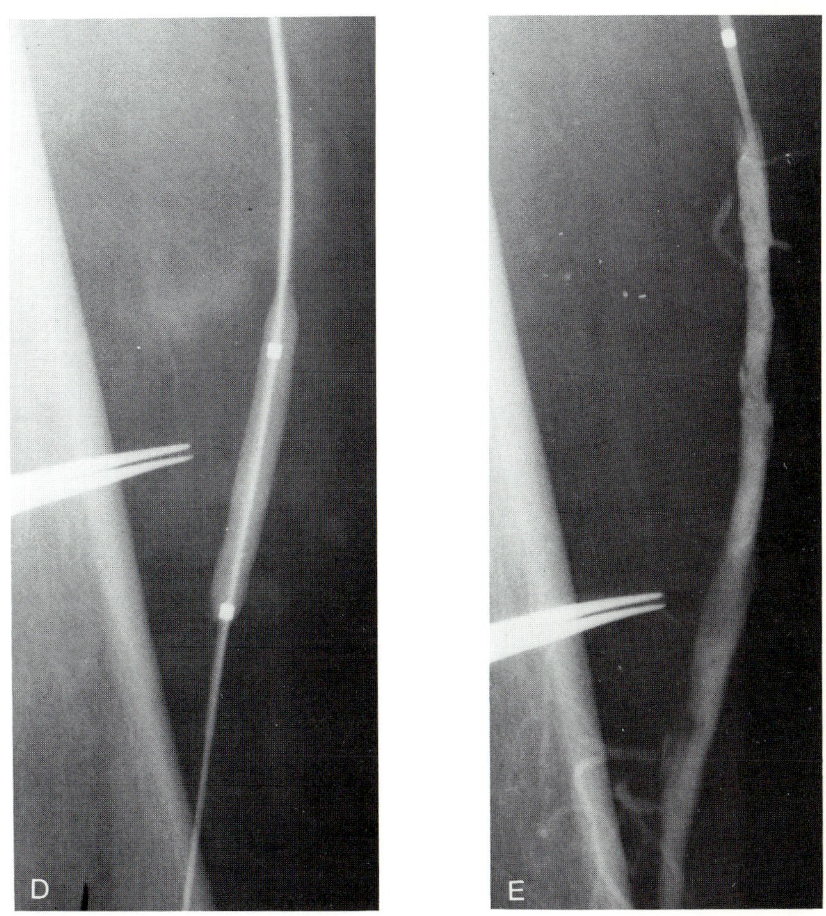

FIGURE 16B-3. (*A*) An arteriogram performed for a symptomatic left leg revealed an unsuspected superficial femoral artery stenosis on the right (*arrow*). (*B*) Ten days postoperatively, the patient had a repeat right femoral angiogram in preparation for PTA and now the SFA was totally occluded (*arrow*). (*C*) After 12 hours of streptokinase infusion at 5000 units per hour, the clot lysed and the tight stenosis was seen again (*arrow*). (*D*) PTA of the stenosis. (*E*) A post-PTA angiogram.

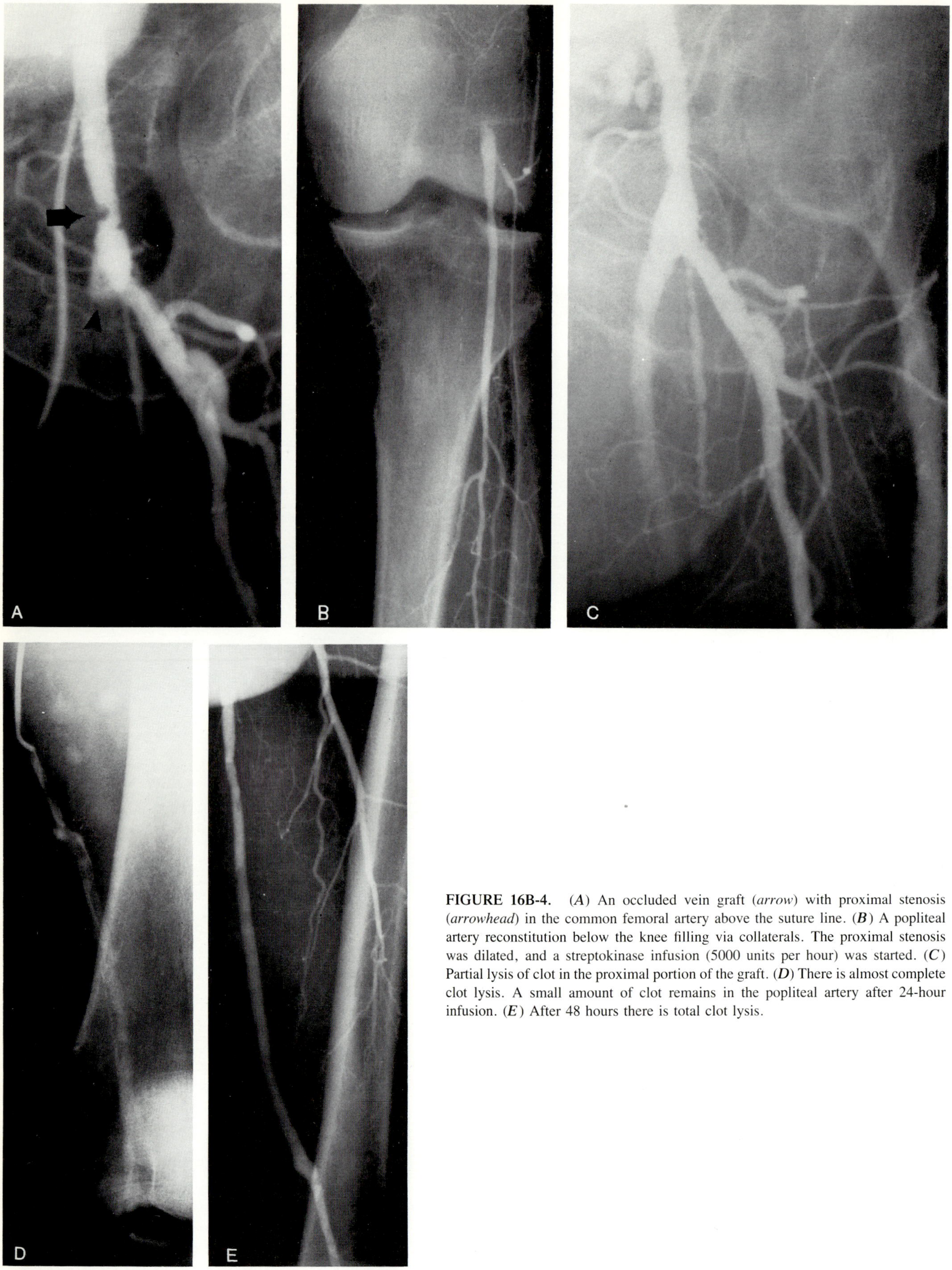

FIGURE 16B-4. (*A*) An occluded vein graft (*arrow*) with proximal stenosis (*arrowhead*) in the common femoral artery above the suture line. (***B***) A popliteal artery reconstitution below the knee filling via collaterals. The proximal stenosis was dilated, and a streptokinase infusion (5000 units per hour) was started. (***C***) Partial lysis of clot in the proximal portion of the graft. (***D***) There is almost complete clot lysis. A small amount of clot remains in the popliteal artery after 24-hour infusion. (***E***) After 48 hours there is total clot lysis.

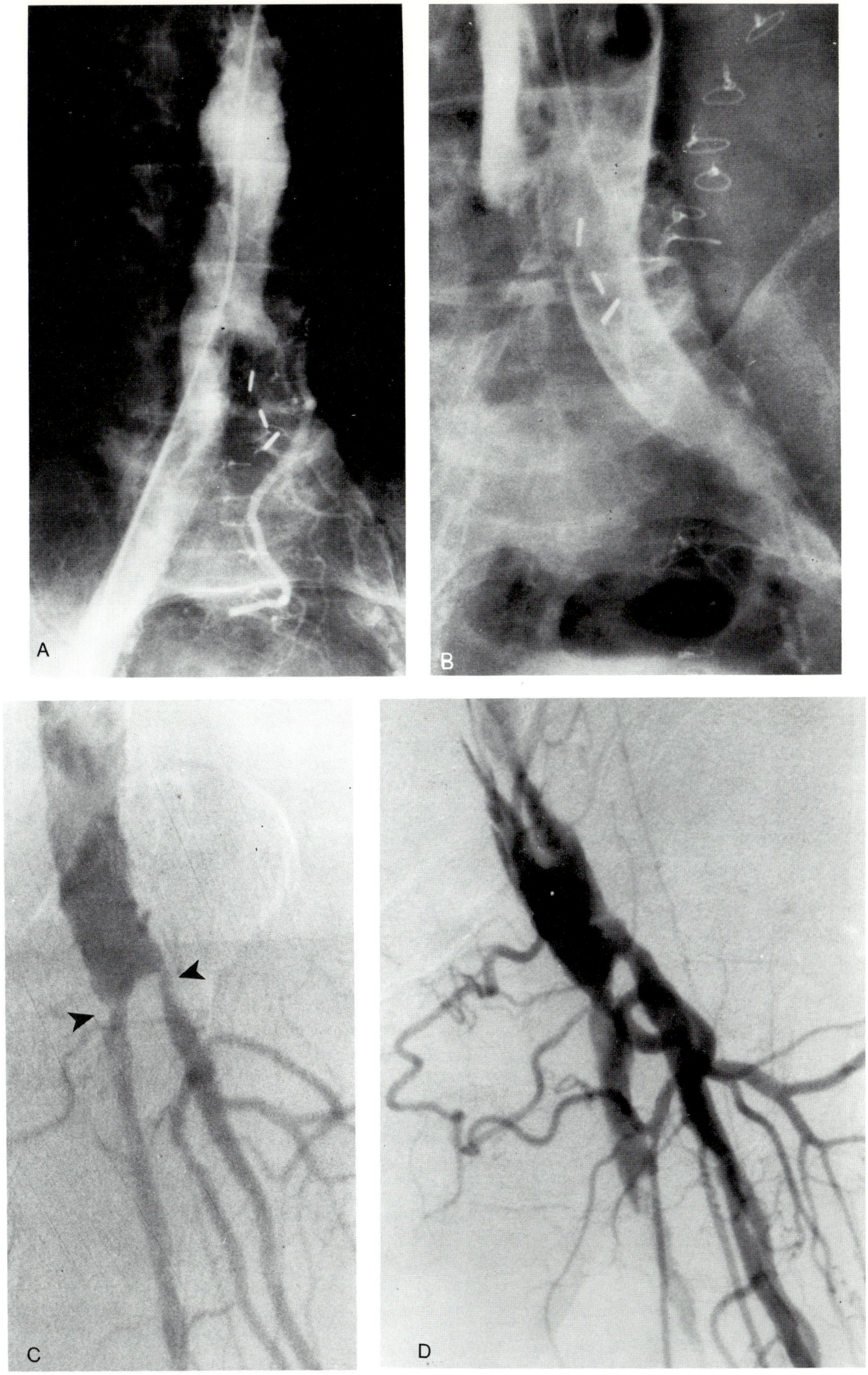

FIGURE 16B-5. A 4-year-old aortic bifurcation graft in a patient with a 4-day history of sudden left leg pain. (*A*) An angiogram showing the occluded left limb of the graft. (*B*) After 55 minutes of streptokinase infusion, at 5000 units per hour. (*C*) Twenty-four hours later, the graft is open and stenosis of the superficial femoral and deep femoral arteries is demonstrated (*arrowheads*). (*D*) A post-PTA of both lesions.

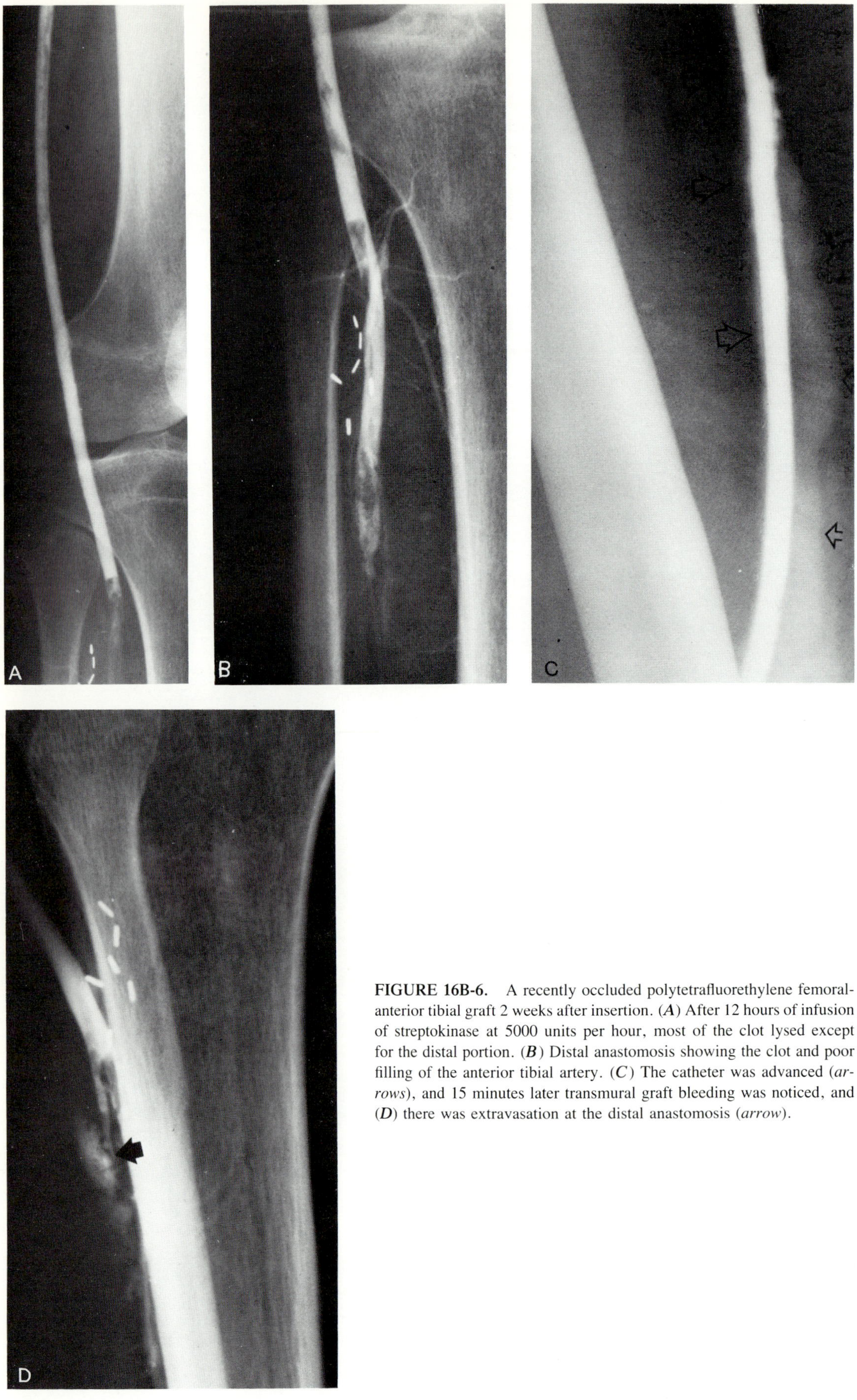

FIGURE 16B-6. A recently occluded polytetrafluorethylene femoral-anterior tibial graft 2 weeks after insertion. (*A*) After 12 hours of infusion of streptokinase at 5000 units per hour, most of the clot lysed except for the distal portion. (*B*) Distal anastomosis showing the clot and poor filling of the anterior tibial artery. (*C*) The catheter was advanced (*arrows*), and 15 minutes later transmural graft bleeding was noticed, and (*D*) there was extravasation at the distal anastomosis (*arrow*).

Complications

The complications of low-dose streptokinase therapy can be divided into those secondary to thrombolytic therapy and those secondary to angiographic procedures. A total of 61 percent of the patients (19 of 31) in our series had some complication (Table 16B-6).

Hemorrhage remains the most serious complication limiting the usefulness of thrombolytic therapy, and it accounted for 71 percent (5 of 7) of our major complications (Table 16B-6). Major hemorrhagic complications have also been reported by others, and their incidence ranges from 12 to 38 percent (17,21,22,27). In our series there were four major groin hematomas that required surgical exploration to evacuate clot and close catheter perforations in the femoral artery. Surprisingly, a definite bleeding site was not always found. The cause of bleeding in two cases was related to the insertion of angiographic catheters on the same side as the occluded vessel, rather than from the opposite side, which is now our preferred practice.

Intracerebral bleeding and stroke has also been a problem which is observed even with selective infusion and has an incidence ranging from 0.7 to 3.5 percent (16,21,22,25). One intracerebral bleed, resulting in complete hemiplegia, was the most serious complication in our series. This patient became very hypertensive, with systolic pressures to 220 mmHg. He gradually became somnolent and developed focal neurologic signs. A massive intracerebral hemorrhage was demonstrated on a CT scan. Careful monitoring in an intensive care setting and the control of blood pressure are mandatory to prevent these complications.

Two vein graft ruptures occurred during the attempted angioplasty of very tight vein graft lesions. Both patients required surgery and are included in our list of major complications.

Minor complications are also listed in Table 16B-6 and bring our total complication rate up to 61 percent which is similar to other reported total complication rates (21). These complications did not require surgical intervention, but in most cases did require the cessation of the thrombolytic therapy.

Catheter complications caused three dissections of the vessel wall and required the cessation of thrombolytic therapy; they were responsible for 3 of the 10 failures. The embolization of lysed clot was not a major complication in our patients. In the one case in which embolus occurred after the lysis of a vein graft occlusion, continued streptokinase infusion lysed the distal clot and embolectomy was not necessary. Following the lysis of a vein graft lesion, one patient had microembolization with lower leg petechiae. These resolved spontaneously with continued streptokinase infusion. Embolization may be a frequent occurrence which has no clinical sequelae because of the lytic powers of the streptokinase infusion.

New thrombus formation on the infusing catheter in the more proximal portions of a previously cleared vessel was seen occasionally in our own series, but has been reported as a common occurrence by others (21). For this reason, the concomitant administration of heparin with streptokinase infusions has been recommended to decrease thrombus deposition on the catheters which sit in a stagnant blood column until the distal occlusion is cleared (21). However, the use of heparin in conjunction with streptokinase remains controversial, and we do not use it routinely; we do start antiplatelet therapy after the streptokinase infusion is stopped.

It remains to be seen whether the benefits of thrombolytic therapy justify the risks of systemic or selective infusions. Although the early results have been dramatic, the long-term benefits are not known, and all the results must be interpreted cautiously in view of the definite dangers of early major hemorrhagic complications. The development of more specific plasminogen activators which only activate thrombus-bound plasminogen may eventually reduce the hemorrhagic complications and give lytic therapy a major place in the treatment of thrombotic occlusive disease (28).

TABLE 16B-6. Complications of Thrombolytic Therapy in 31 Patients

Major			
	Groin hemorrhage	4	
	Intracerebral hemorrhage	1	
	Vein graft rupture	2	
			7 (22%)
Minor			
	Groin hematoma	2	
	Bleeding from suture line	2	
	Bleeding through graft	2	
	Hematuria	1	
	Embolization	2	
	Dissection	3	
			12 (39%)
Total complications			19 (61%)

References

1. Tillet WS, Garner RL: The fibrinolytic activity of hemolytic streptococci. J Exp Med 1933, 58:485–502.
2. MacFarlane RG, Pilling J: Observations on fibrinolysis. Lancet 1946, 2:562.
3. Kwaan HC: *Thrombosis*. Philadelphia: Saunders, 1982.
4. Sharma Gvrk, Cella G, Parisi AF, Sasahara AA: Thrombolytic therapy. N Engl J Med 1982, 306:1268–1276.
5. Chaise LS, Comerota AJ, Soulen RL, Rubin RN: Selective intraarterial streptokinase therapy in the immediate post-operative period. JAMA 1982, 247:2397–2400.
6. Browse NL, James DCO: Streptokinase and pulmonary embolism. Lancet 1964, 2:1039–1043.
7. Hansen PF, Jorgenson M, Kjieldgaard NO, Ploug J: Urokinase—An activator of plasminogen from human urine: Experiences with intravenous application on twenty-two patients. Angiology 1961, 12:367–371.
8. Urokinase-streptokinase embolism trial phase 2 results—A cooperative study. JAMA 1974, 229:1606–1613.
9. Kakkar VV, Howe CT, Laws JW, Flanc C: Late results of treatment of deep vein thrombosis. Br Med J 1969, 1:810–811.
10. Sasahara AA, Sharma GVRK, Tow DE, Armenia RJ, Belko JS: Methodology in diagnosis of pulmonary embolization. In Bergan JJ, Yao JST (eds): *Venous Problems*. Chicago: Year Book, 1978, pp 309–317.

11. Hume M, Gurewich V, Thomas DP, Dealy JB Jr: Streptokinase for chronic arterial occlusive disease. Arch Surg 1970, 101:653–657.
12. Martin M, Schoop W, Zeitler E: Streptokinase in chronic arterial occlusive disease. JAMA 1970, 211:1169–1173.
13. Verstraete M, Vermylen J, Donati MB: The effect of streptokinase infusion on chronic arterial occlusions and stenoses. Ann Intern Med 1971, 74:377–382.
14. Tsapoges MS: The role of fibrinolysis in the treatment of arterial thrombosis: Experimental and clinical aspects. Ann Roy Col Surg, Engl 1964, 34:293:313.
15. Poliwoda H, Alexander K, Buhl V, Holstein D, Wagner HH: Treatment of chronic arterial occlusions with streptokinase. N Engl J Med 1969, 280: 689–692.
16. Amery A, Deloof W, Vermyler J, Verstraete M: Outcome of recent thromboembolic occlusion of limb arteries treated with streptokinase. Br Med J 1970, 4:639–644.
17. Dotter CT, Rosch J, Seaman AJ: Selective clot lysis with low-dose streptokinase. Radiology 1974, 111:31–37.
18. Katzen BT, van Breda A: Low dose streptokinase in the treatment of arterial occlusion. Am J Radiol 1981, 136:1171–1178.
19. Fiessinger JN, Vayssairat M, Juillet Y, Aiach M, Janneau D, Cormier JM, Housset E: Local urokinase in arterial thromboembolism. Angiology 1980, 31:715–720.
20. Hargrove WC, Barker CF, Berkowitz HD, McLean G, Frieman DB, Ring EJ, Roberts B: Treatment of acute peripheral arterial and graft thrombosis with low dose streptokinase. Surgery 1982, 92:981–993.
21. Becker GJ, Rabe FE, Richmond BD, Holden RW, Yune HY, Dilley RS, Bang NU, Glover JL, Klatte EC: Low-dose fibrinolytic therapy. Radiology 1983, 148:663.
22. Mori KW, Bookstein JJ, Heeney DJ, Bardin JA, Donnelly KJ, Rhodes GA, Dilley RB, Warmath MA, Bernstein EF: Selective streptokinase infusion: Clinical and laboratory correlates. Radiology 1983, 148:677–682.
23. Hess H, Ingrisch H, Mietaschk A, Rath H: Local low-dose thrombolytic therapy of peripheral arterial occlusion. N Engl J Med 1982, 307:1627–1630.
24. Rentrop P, Blanke H, Karsch KR, Rutsch W, Schartl M, Merx R, Dorr R, Mathey D, Kuck K: Changes in left ventricular function after intracoronary streptokinase infusion in clinically evolving myocardial infarction. Am Heart J 1981, 102:1188–1193.
25. Martin M: Thrombolytic therapy in arterial thromboembolism. Prog Cardiovasc Dis 1979, 21:351–374.
26. Rush DS, Gewertz BC, Lu CT, Neely SM, Ball DG, Beasley MSN, Zarins CK: Selective infusion of streptokinase for arterial thrombosis. Surgery 1983, 93:828–833.
27. Totty WG, Gilula LA, McClennan BL, Ahmed P, Sherman L: Low dose intravascular fibrinolytic therapy. Radiology 1982, 153:59–69.
28. Weimar W, Stibbe J, Van Seyen J, Billiau A, De Somer P, Collen D: specific lysis of an iliofemoral thrombus by administration of extrinsic (tissue-type) plasminogen activator. Lancet 1981, 2:1018.

Chapter 16C

ANTIPLATELET AGENTS

JAMES A. DeWEESE

There has been increasing awareness of the importance of the platelet in producing vascular problems. It has long been recognized that platelets have a major role in the formation of thrombi, particularly in the arterial system. Their importance in initiating thrombus formation on artificial surfaces such as heart valves or vascular grafts is now well known. It is now appreciated that platelets may indeed be involved in the formation of progressive lesions in the arterial system such as arteriosclerotic plaques, anastomotic thickening in vascular grafts, or recurrent stenosis in endarterectomized arteries (22,31,43,62,82). If the platelet can produce these problems, it would logically follow that agents which interfere with platelet function might prevent these thrombotic and stenotic lesions.

Platelet Function

The formation of acute arterial thrombi apparently occurs in three steps consisting of platelet adherence, platelet aggregation, and then activation of the clotting mechanism (Figure 16C-1). Platelets do not adhere to normal endothelial surfaces. They do adhere to any subendothelial structures exposed by acute or chronic injury, and to artificial surfaces. Adhered platelets undergo a series of morphologic changes resulting in degranulation of the platelet cytoplasm. Products of this *release* reaction include serotonin, adenosine diphosphate (ADP), phospholipase, and the mitogenic factor. Serotonin is of practical importance because of its vasoconstrictive hemostatic activity. ADP plays a primary role in platelet aggregation. The release of phospholipase results in the formation of thromboxane A_2, which is a powerful platelet aggregator as well as a vasoconstrictor. The mitogenic factor, or *platelet growth factor*, is responsible for the secondary migration of smooth-muscle cells and fibroblasts to the site (31). The progressive nature of arteriosclerosis, anastomotic neointimal fibrous hyperplasia, and myointimal hyperplasia in endarterectomized arteries suggests that repeated endothelial injury is producing the continued platelet adherence, platelet aggregation, and smooth-muscle migration to the injured area (14,25,48,51,67,72).

To better understand the way in which antiplatelet agents might affect the formation of these lesions, it is necessary to expand upon the aforementioned simplistic explanation (Figure 16C-2). The pathway between platelet adhesion and degranulation and the formation of thromboxane A_2 apparently begins with the shift of calcium from the platelet membrane into the cytoplasm; this shift is then amplified by the release reaction and liberates phospholipase from the membrane; this in turn results in the liberation of arachidonic acid from accessible phospholipids. Arachidonic acid is then converted to cyclic endoperoxides by cyclooxygenase; this is another calcium-dependent reaction. In the presence of thromboxane synthetase and calcium, thromboxane A_2 is produced. Because of the prime importance of arachidonic acid, this process is frequently termed the arachidonic acid pathway.

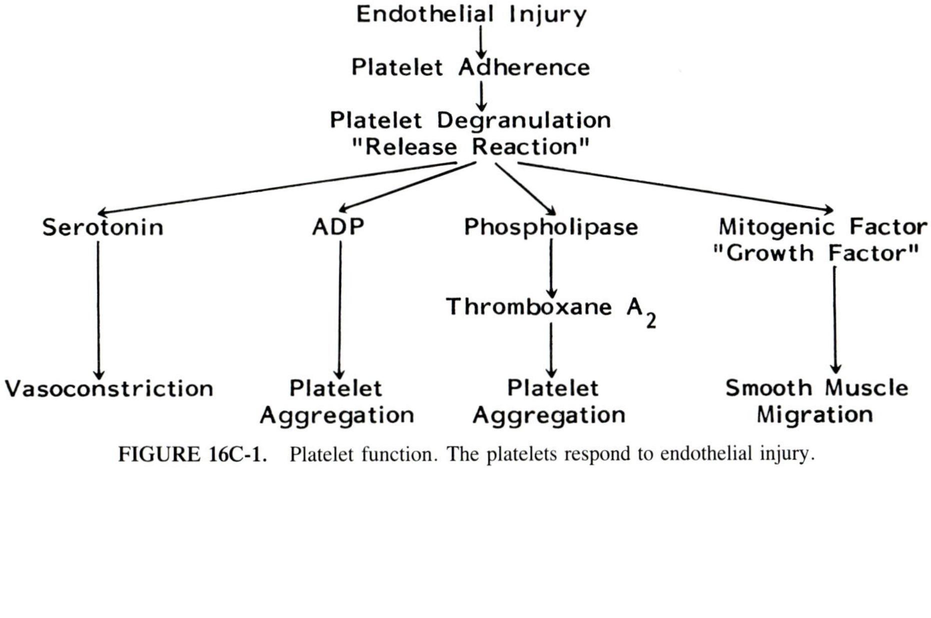

FIGURE 16C-1. Platelet function. The platelets respond to endothelial injury.

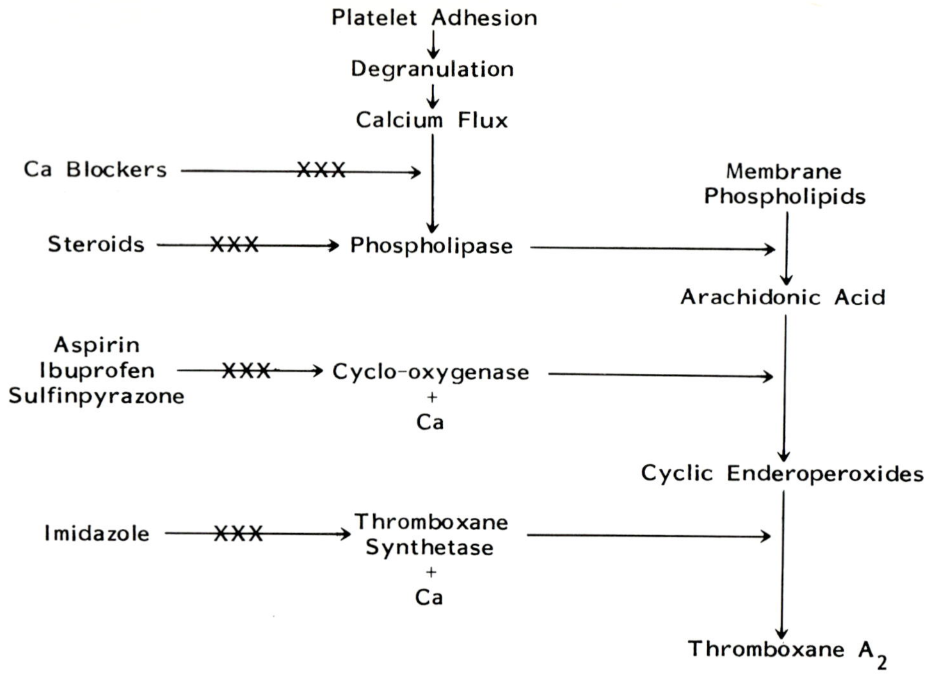

FIGURE 16C-2. Arachidonic acid pathway. The pathway from platelet degranulation to thromboxane A_2 formation, and the sites of action of various antiplatelet agents.

Antiplatelet Agents

There are a number of drugs which may interfere with the arachidonic acid pathway, including aspirin (acetylsalicylic acid; ASA); nonsteroidal anti-inflammatory agents other than ASA; dipyridamole (DPM); steroids; thromboxane synthetase antagonists; and calcium blocking agents (32,33,79,83).

ASA is a most potent blocker of the formation of thromboxane A_2 by irreversibly acetylating the cyclooxygenase that converts arachidonic acid to the cyclic endoperoxides. The antiplatelet effect lasts until new platelets are synthesized, and thus the effect of one dose of ASA lasts for the entire platelet life span of 7 to 10 days. During that time there may be a measurable effect on the bleeding time.

Calcium blockers may interfere with the effect of the calcium flux on the release of phospholipase from the platelet membrane.

Steroids are thought to block phospholipase and inhibit the formation of arachidonic acid from platelet phospholipids.

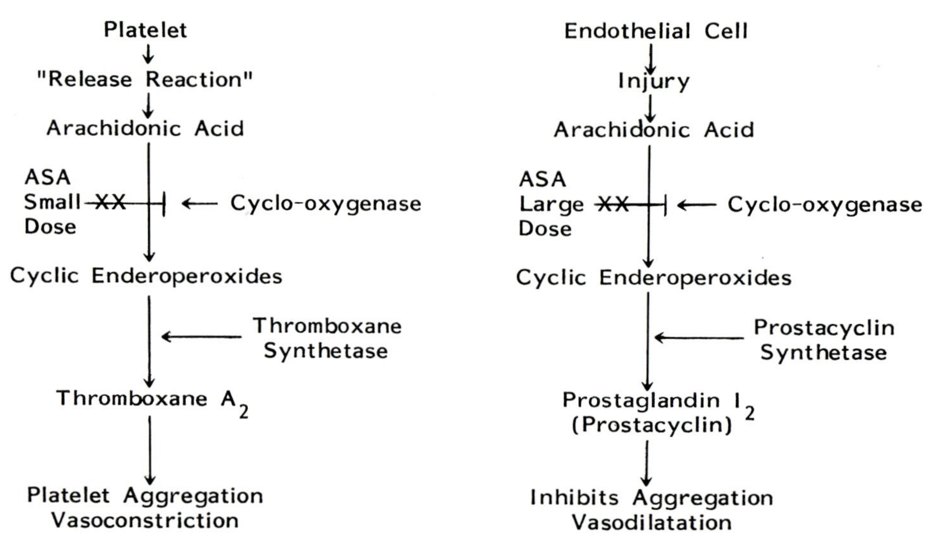

FIGURE 16C-3. Platelet and vessel wall arachidonic acid pathways. The antagonistic results of varying doses of ASA on platelet aggregation and vasoconstriction.

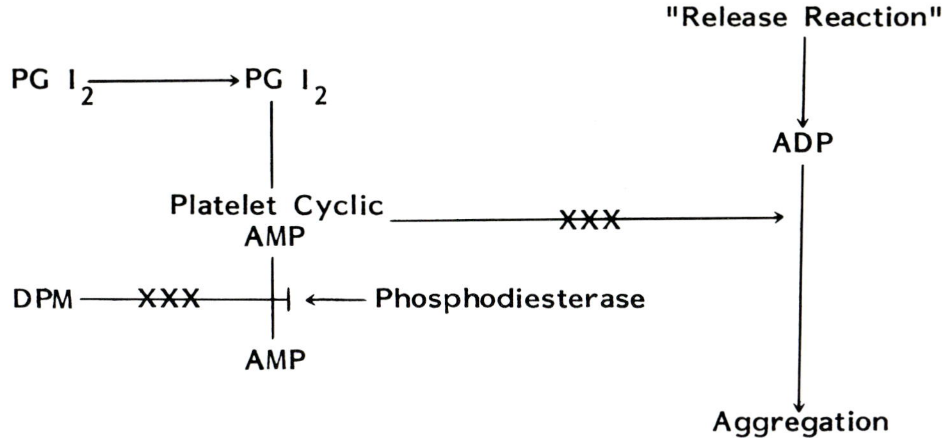

FIGURE 16C-4. Platelet cAMP pathway. This shows the mechanism by which increased levels of circulating PGI_2 or the administration of DPM can increase levels of cAMP and inhibit platelet aggregation.

There are nonsteroidal anti-inflammatory agents other than ASA which inhibit the enzyme cyclooxygenase. These include sulfinpyrazone, ibuprofen, indomethacin (Indocin), and phenylbutazone.

Imidazole can block thromboxane synthetase, which would then exert an antiplatelet activity by inhibiting the formation of thromboxane A_2 from the cyclic endoperoxides.

Arachidonic acid is present in the endothelial cell as well as the platelet, and in response to the same injury that has caused the platelet release reaction and in the presence of cyclooxygenase, cyclic endoperoxides may be produced (Figure 16C-3). Whereas in the platelet, thromboxane synthetase may convert the cyclic endoperoxides to thromboxane A_2, in the endothelial cell, prostacyclin (prostaglandin I_2, PGI_2) synthetase converts the cyclic endoperoxides to prostacyclin. Thromboxane A_2 and prostacyclin have directly opposite hemostatic functions. Whereas thromboxane A_2 causes platelet aggregation and vasoconstriction, prostacyclin inhibits aggregation and causes vasodilatation. ASA blocks the cyclooxygenase from the endothelial cell, as well as the enzyme from the platelet, but the endothelial enzyme is blocked only if larger doses of ASA are administered. It is advisable to administer ASA in small doses to avoid blocking the production of prostacyclin.

There is another pathway which is of some interest (Figure 16C-4). Platelet cyclic adenosine monophosphate (cAMP) inhibits platelet aggregation caused by adenosine diphosphate (ADP) and may also inhibit the adherence of platelets. Prostacyclin is known to increase the level of cAMP in platelets. Of most importance is that phosphodiesterase can convert the cAMP to a nonactive adenosine monophosphate (AMP).

DPM is known to affect platelet aggregation as well as adherence. It is thought that this effect is secondary to an increase in cAMP levels which occurs as a result of DPM's inhibition of platelet phosphodiesterase. There is good experimental evidence that there is a synergistic effect when both ASA and DPM are administered.

Administered prostacyclin may also increase cAMP levels and thereby inhibit platelet aggregation caused by ADP.

Aspirin and Dipyridamole

The antiplatelet agents which have attracted the most attention are ASA and DPM. The theoretical and experimental value of the use of ASA, with or without DPM, as an antiplatelet agent is well-accepted. There is still controversy regarding the optimal dosage, the value of combining the two drugs, the time of administration, and the clinical effectiveness of the treatment.

ASA in large doses may not only inhibit the platelet production of thromboxane A_2 but may also inhibit the synthesis of prostacyclin in the vessel wall. Experimental in vitro studies indicate, however, that dosages of 325 mg/day or less are effective in influencing platelet function without usually decreasing prostacyclin production (68). Intermediate doses of 650 to 1300 mg/day may also not significantly decrease prostacyclin production. DPM alone may also affect platelet function. In dosages of 50 mg of DPM tid, but not 25 mg tid, the collagen-induced platelet aggregation, the platelet adhesion to glass beads, and the availability of platelet factor 4 are inhibited (69). The maximum effect is observed at dosages of 100 mg of DPM tid. There are advantages to using the drugs in combination. They affect platelet function at different sites of metabolism. Smaller dosages are needed when the drugs are used in combination, as demonstrated by increased levels of DPM in the blood when ASA is administered concurrently (33). It is important that as small dosages of ASA as possible are used, since the effect of DPM is thought to be dependent upon prostacyclin's role in increasing cAMP levels (Figure 16C-4). Large doses of ASA may inhibit prostacyclin production (Figure 16C-3). Rajah et al. demonstrated that 180 mg of ASA daily and 50 mg of DPM tid, or 120 mg of ASA daily and 75 mg of DPM tid, give the maximum inhibition of platelet activity without increasing bleeding times (69). Bleeding times are prolonged when ASA is given in dosages of 300 mg daily.

ASA AND DPM AND ARTERIAL GRAFTS

The role of ASA and DPM in preventing thrombosis of grafts used for arterial reconstructions has been extensively evaluated. The early failure of grafts may be secondary to diffuse clot formation on the graft's thrombogenic surface. Occlusion is rare, particularly in high-flow arterial systems (70). Late failure has frequently been related to a progressive anastomotic neointimal fibrous hyperplasia (ANFH) (23,67). The theory that this lesion is platelet-mediated is an attractive one. There is initially adherence and aggregation of white platelet thrombi to anastomoses, presumably because of the presence of artificial graft and suture surfaces as well as traumatized endothelium. This is followed by the maturation of the lesion with hyperplasia of myofibroblasts, which may well be secondary to increased levels of the mitogenic platelet growth factor (72). The localized progressive nature of the lesion is presumably secondary to repeated trauma to the anastomotic surfaces. This trauma may be due to hemodynamic flow factors but is more likely related to mechanical mismatches, with cyclic stress occurring at the junction of noncompliant materials in the pulsating arterial system (1,13, 16,23).

The efficacy of ASA and DPM in decreasing the severity of ANFH and increasing the patency rates of bypass grafts has been demonstrated in several experimental studies. These include studies in which (1) the canine femoral artery was bypassed with polytetrafluoroethylene (PTFE), Dacron, and umbilical vein grafts (28,63); (2) the abdominal aorta of monkeys was replaced with a PTFE graft (38); (3) canine coronary arteries were bypassed with PTFE grafts (39); (4) the iliac artery of monkeys was bypassed with autogenous veins (56); (5) canine iliofemoral arteries were bypassed with knitted Dacron grafts seeded with endothelial cells (73); and (6) canine coronary arteries were bypassed with autogenous veins (60). In a study in which the canine femoral artery was bypassed with autogenous vein and both drugs were not used, DPM alone did not prevent ANFH (9). It is strongly emphasized that in all these studies, treatment was started at least 1 day before the operative procedure. Support for the theory that the antiplatelet activity of ASA and DPM is responsible for decreased graft failure rates includes the following: (1) the adherence of ^{51}Cr-labeled platelets to PTFE and Dacron grafts bypassing the canine femoral artery was decreased in treated animals (63); (2) DPM alone returned the ^{51}Cr-labeled-platelet survival time to near-normal levels in baboons with Silastic femoral arteriovenous shunts (42); and (3) ASA, or ASA and DPM, produced maximal inhibition of platelet consumption and platelet adherence in an artificial circulation in which blood was perfused over a Dacron surface (57).

There have been some clinical studies evaluating the use of ASA and DPM for preventing prosthetic graft occlusions. Combined therapy with ASA and DPM, but neither drug alone, significantly increased the patency rate of arterial reconstructions during the hospital stay (40). The study evaluates only the efficacy of the drugs in preventing early thrombosis. Therapy was started on the first or second postoperative day; this is one of the few studies in which therapy was effective when started postoperatively (40). In a comparative study the patency rate of femoropopliteal PTFE bypass grafts was 72 percent in patients treated with ASA and DPM, as compared with 59 percent in untreated patients. The difference is suggestively but not statistically significant (80). In a controlled double-blind randomized study of patients with femoropopliteal PTFE bypass grafts, with treatment beginning preoperatively, the 1-year patency rates of above-knee grafts were significantly improved in patients receiving ASA alone or ASA and DPM. The patency rates of grafts ending distal to the knee joint were not improved in patients receiving ASA and DPM, but there was a suggestive, but not statistically significant, improvement in patency rates in patients receiving ASA alone (36).

The severity and frequency of ANFH and graft thrombosis has been greater in prosthetic grafts than in vein grafts in comparative studies (23,67). Vein grafts can fail, however, and the widespread use of veins for aortocoronary bypass operations has provided material for several clinical studies. ASA and DPM, or ASA alone, did not improve the patency rates of vein grafts in studies in which the treatment was started on the third postoperative day (58,65). On the other hand, the patency rates were significantly better in treated patients when therapy began on the first postoperative day or preoperatively (15,54).

Support for the theory that the antiplatelet activity of ASA and DPM is responsible for the decreased failure rates of grafts in humans was found in studies in which (1) ^{111}In-labeled-platelet adherence to femoropopliteal Dacron and PTFE grafts for the first 7 postoperative days was significantly decreased in patients receiving ASA and DPM (34), and (2) platelet survival times and graft patencies were significantly increased in patients receiving DPM following saphenous vein aortocoronary bypasses (76).

There are artificial surfaces other than grafts which may be exposed to arterial blood flow, including heart valves and hemodialysis access arteriovenous shunts. Combinations of anticoagulants and ASA or DPM have been found to reduce the incidence of thromboembolic events in patients with prosthetic heart valves (41,77). DPM in dosages of 375 to 400 mg/day plus anticoagulants significantly reduced the incidence of thromboembolism in two separate prospective randomized studies, one of which was blind (49,78). ASA in dosages of 500 to 1000 mg/day plus anticoagulants reduced the incidence of thromboembolism, whereas ASA alone was not effective (2,19). ASA in dosages of 1000 mg/day but not 500 mg/day plus anticoagulants increased the incidence of gastrointestinal bleeding (2,19). Patients with arteriovenous Silastic and Teflon hemodialysis shunts who received 160 mg of ASA daily had a significantly lower thrombosis rate than controls (45).

ASA AND DPM POSTENDARTERECTOMY

An endarterectomy leaves a significant area of exposed subendothelial tissue, and such exposure is known to initiate platelet adherence and platelet aggregation. Smooth-muscle migration then occurs. In endarterectomized canine carotid arteries, ASA and DPM can experimentally significantly decrease the formation of the initial fibrin-platelet coat and subsequent acute thrombosis (20,21). ASA and DPM may also delay endothelial healing in experimental models, but the long-term effect of this phenomenon is not known (6). DPM may actually increase smooth-muscle proliferation and counteract the beneficial effect of ASA (61).

Carotid artery stenosis may recur. Retrospective and some prospective studies suggest that significant lesions appear in approximately 10 percent of the arteries within 5 years (24). Lesions which appear within 2 years are usually white glistening lesions tightly adherent to the vessel wall and histologically appear to be diffuse myointimal hyperplasias. Other lesions have the typical appearance of complicated atherosclerotic plaques, and a suitable plane of dissection within the media permits repeat endarterectomies (24). Although a combination of ASA and DPM has not prevented restenosis in some patients, clinical trials are indicated to fairly evaluate its effectiveness. In a randomized study of patients undergoing endarterectomy or arterial reconstructions with grafts, in-hospital thrombosis was significantly decreased in patients receiving ASA and DPM (40). In one randomized double-blind study of patients treated with ASA following carotid endarterectomy, there was a significant decrease in cerebral infarcts but not transient ischemic attacks (TIAs) or deaths in treated patients (29).

ASA AND DPM AND ARTERIOSCLEROSIS

The role of the platelet in producing the chronic changes of the atherosclerotic plaque as well as acute thromboembolic events is now commonly accepted (43). Atherosclerotic plaques, like ANFH, may well be due to chronic trauma to the vessel wall related to either flow patterns or pulsation against rigid structures (12,43,64). As a result of the trauma and platelet adherence, platelet growth factor is released, and smooth-muscle cells and fibroblasts migrate and produce the simple plaque. The plaque may later become more complicated as a result of lipid deposition or hemorrhage. The deposition of platelet thrombi on the atherosclerotic plaque in secondary ulcerations, or as a result of spasm, may then be the source of embolic phenomena. There are controversial reports on the efficacy of ASA and DPM in preventing experimental atherogenesis (6,61). Despite this, ASA and DPM have been extensively evaluated clinically for their influence on carotid and coronary artery disease.

ASA AND DPM AND CEREBRAL ISCHEMIA

The carotid artery atherosclerotic plaque occurs typically at the bifurcation of the common carotid artery, and the configuration of the plaque suggests that stress secondary to the pattern of blood flow may be responsible for the plaque formation (12). Experimental and clinical demonstrations of platelet thrombi in both carotid arteries and cortical and/or retinal vessels add further support to the theory that the platelet is important in producing acute cerebral ischemia (37,47,55).

There have been at least four reported prospective randomized double-blind clinical trials of ASA in the treatment of patients with TIAs. ASA was administered in dosages of 625 to 1300 mg daily. In the American study, ASA significantly reduced the incidence of TIAs but not the incidence of strokes or deaths (29). In the Canadian study, ASA significantly reduced the incidence of TIAs and of combined strokes and deaths in men (11). In the French study, 16 percent of the patients had TIAs and 84 percent had completed strokes at the time of entrance into the study (7). ASA significantly reduced the incidence of completed strokes. DPM in dosages of 225 mg daily did not improve the results over those with ASA alone. In the Danish study, ASA did not significantly reduce the incidence of strokes, deaths, or TIAs (71). Careful observations of the side effects of the drugs were made in the French study, and 3.5 percent of the patients taking ASA and 5.4 percent of the patients taking ASA and DPM developed either peptic ulcers or bleeding (7).

ASA AND DPM AND CORONARY ARTERY DISEASE

Obstructive atherosclerotic plaques tend to occur at major branches of the coronary arteries, further supporting the concept that hemodynamic trauma to the vessel wall and platelet activity are responsible for the lesions. In addition, the autopsy finding of platelet-fibrin thrombi at the site of previously identified coronary spasm incriminates the platelet as a possible cause of angina, coronary spasm, acute infarction, or sudden death (53). It also raises the possibility that the coronary spasm might be secondary to the release of thromboxane A_2 from aggregated platelets (43). The platelet's role in coronary heart disease is further supported by the finding that about half the patients with symptomatic and arteriographically proven coronary artery disease have shortened platelet survival times (33).

There have been a number of prospective randomized double-blind clinical trials evaluating the use of ASA in dosages of 300 to 1500 mg daily after myocardial infarction (5,8,18,26,27,66). In all but one of six trials there was a favorable trend or statistically significant decrease in the reduction of mortality in the treated patients. For example, in one study by life table analysis, the rates of coronary deaths and nonfatal myocardial infarctions were 21 and 24 percent lower, respectively, in the treated group, which was statistically significant (66). In another study, however, the total mortality was 10.8 percent in the ASA group and 9.7 percent in the placebo group, and the incidence of nonfatal myocardial infarctions was 6.3 percent in the ASA group and 8.1 percent in the placebo group, which was not statistically significant (5). DPM (225 mg) plus ASA (975 mg) daily was equally as favorable as ASA alone in reducing the mortality and nonfatal myocardial infarction rates (66). It should be noted that in two studies, gastric irritation symptoms were noted in 18 to 23.7 percent of the patients receiving ASA, 972 to 1000 mg daily, compared with 13.2 to 14.9 percent of the patients receiving placebos (5,66).

ASA AND DPM AND VENOUS THROMBOEMBOLISM

ASA, 1200 mg daily beginning the day before operation, has been evaluated in the prevention of phlebographically proven deep venous thrombosis following hip replacement. The incidence of thrombosis was significantly less in treated men but not in treated women (44). In a similar study in patients undergoing knee replacement, there was a suggestive but not statistically significant decrease in thrombosis in patients receiving ASA (59). ASA and DPM may be of value in patients with recurrent venous thrombosis, but further trials are indicated (75).

Sulfinpyrazone

Sulfinpyrazone (SPZ), like ASA, inhibits the production of thromboxane A_2 by blocking platelet cyclooxygenase (Figure 16C-2). The SPZ-produced inhibition of platelet consumption and platelet adherence was equivalent to that of DPM in an artificial circulation in which blood was perfused over a Dacron surface (57). ASA was significantly more effective than DPM or SPZ.

The dosage of SPZ is critical. SPZ in dosages of 400 mg daily was ineffective, but in a dosage of 800 mg daily was effective in returning the platelet survival times toward normal in patients with prosthetic heart valves and shortened platelet survival times (81). On the other hand, large doses of SPZ, unlike large doses of ASA, do not significantly decrease the production of prostacyclin by the vessel wall, and thus do not promote clotting (35,50). SPZ also does not prolong bleeding times significantly (81).

Because of its safety, efficacy when taken orally, and sustained effect, SPZ has been evaluated in some clinical studies, although not as extensively as ASA and DPM.

Although there is little reported use of SPZ with prosthetic grafts, its effectiveness in preventing thromboembolism in patients with prosthetic heart valves has been reported. SPZ in daily dosages of 800 mg effectively prevented thromboembolic events in patients who responded to therapy by increasing shortened platelet survival times (77).

SPZ can prolong the platelet survival time in patients with cerebral TIAs (74). However, it was not effective in decreasing the incidence of recurrent TIAs, stroke, or death in patients who had suffered TIAs or reversible ischemic neurologic deficits (11). In the same study, ASA signifcantly decreased the incidence of TIAs as well as stroke and death combined in men but not women.

SPZ increased the platelet survival times and graft patencies in patients receiving SPZ after saphenous vein aortocoronary bypasses (76).

In a prospective randomized double-blind trial, SPZ treatment (800 mg daily) beginning 1 month after myocardial infarction revealed a trend in favor of the treated group. There was also a statistically significant lower incidence of sudden death in the treated group during the first 7 months after myocardial infarction (3,4).

SPZ was effective in returning shortened platelet survival times toward normal in patients with recurrent venous thrombosis (75).

Side effects, particularly gastrointestinal, are rarely reported with SPZ, compared with ASA and SPZ.

Ibuprofen

Ibuprofen, more commonly known as Motrin, like ASA is thought to acetylate platelet cyclooxygenase and block the formation of thromboxane A_2 (Figure 16C-2). Ibuprofen given intravenously for 24 hours significantly increased the thrombus-free surface and patency rate of PTFE graft replacements of short segments of the carotid arteries of sheep (14). The patency rate of PTFE grafts in the abdominal aorta of rats was significantly increased at 30 days by the subcutaneous injection of ibuprofen (17). Mural thrombus formation and pseudointimal thickness were significantly reduced in the canine endarterectomized abdominal aorta by ibuprofen, which was given intravenously preoperatively and orally tid postoperatively (52). Clinical trials are being planned.

Prostacyclin

Prostacyclin (PGI_2) stimulates the production of cAMP, which inhibits platelet aggregation secondary to ADP (Figure 16C-4).

In baboons treated with prostacyclin the uptake of ^{111}In-labeled platelets on Dacron grafts in the carotid artery was markedly decreased (10). When prostacyclin was administered after the platelets adhered, the platelet accumulation on the grafts decreased. In other words, it appears that prostacyclin can not only prevent platelet aggregation but can also cause platelet disaggregation. It is therefore an attractive drug to consider for clinical use.

Miscellaneous Agents

There are a number of other agents which may alter platelet function (79,83). Those of possible practical importance for further investigation include nifedipine and other calcium-channel blockers, imidazole and other thromboxane synthetase antagonists, vitamin E, propanolol, and steroids (79,82). A preliminary experimental evaluation of steroids in canine Dacron femoral bypass grafts indicated that steroids do not significantly alter ANFH and patency rates (46).

References

1. Abbott WM, Bouchier-Hayes DJ: The role of mechanical properties in graft design. In Dardik H (ed): *Graft Materials in Vascular Surgery*. Miami, Symposia Specialists, 1978.
2. Altman R, Boullon F, Rouvier J, Raca R, de la Fuente L, Favaloro R: Aspirin and prophylaxis of thromboembolic complications in patients with substitute heart valves. J Thorac Cardiovasc Surg 1976, 72:127.

3. The Anturane Reinfarction Trial Research Group: Sulfinpyrazone in the prevention of cardiac death after myocardial infarction. N Engl J Med 1978, 298:289.
4. The Anturane Reinfarction Trial Research Group: Sulfinpyrazone in the prevention of sudden death after myocardial infarction. N Engl J Med 1980, 302, 250.
5. Aspirin Myocardial Infarction Study Research Group: A Randomized, controlled trial of aspirin in persons recovered from myocardial infarction. JAMA 1980, 243:661.
6. Bomberger RA, DePalma RG, Ambrose TA, Manalo P: Aspirin and dipyridamole inhibit endothelial healing. Arch Surg 1982, 117:1459.
7. Bousser MG, Eschwege E, Haguenau M, Lefaucconnier JM, Thibult N, Touboul D, Touboul PJ: "AICLA" controlled trial of aspirin and dipyridamole in the secondary prevention of atherothrombotic cerebral ischemia. Stroke 1983, 14:5.
8. Breddin K, Loew D, Lechner K, Uberla K, Walter, E: Secondary prevention of myocardial infarction; comparison of acetylsalicylic acid, phenoprocoumon, and placebo: A multicenter two-year prospective study. Thromb Haemost 1979, 41:225.
9. Brody WR, Brown JW, Reitz BA, Fry DL, Michaelis LL: Effects of dipyridamole and methylprednisolone on intimal thickening in vein grafts. J Thorac Cardiovasc Surg 1977, 73:602.
10. Callow AD, Connolly R, O'Donnell TF Jr, Gembarowicz R, Keough E, Ramberg-Laskaris K, Valeri CR: Platelet-arterial synthetic graft interaction and its modification. Arch Surg 1982, 117:1447.
11. Canadian Cooperative Study Group: Randomized trial of aspirin and sulfinpyrazone in threatened stroke. N Engl J Med 1978, 299:53.
12. Caro CG, Fitzgerald JM, Schroter RC: Atheroma and arterial wall shear: Observation, correlation and proposal of a shear dependent mass transfer mechanism for atherogenesis. Proc R Soc Lond [Biol] 1971, 117:109.
13. Carson S, Demling R, Esquivel C, Talken L, Tillman P: Testing and treatment of arterial graft thrombosis. Am J Surg 1981, 142:137.
14. Carson SN, Esquivel CO, French SW: Experimental carotid stenosis due to fibrous intimal hyperplasia. Surg Gynecol Obstet 1981, 153:883.
15. Chesebro JH, Clements IP, Fuster V, Elverback LR, Smith HC, Bardsley WT, Frye RL, Holmes DR Jr, Vlietstra RE, Pluth JR, Wallace RB, Puga FJ, Orszulak TA, Piehler JM, Schaff HV, Danielson GK: A platelet-inhibitor-drug trial in coronary-artery bypass operations. N Engl J Med 1982, 307:73.
16. Clark RE, Apoltolou S, Kardos JL: Mismatch of mechanical properties as a cause of arterial prostheses thrombosis. Surg Forum 1978, 27:208.
17. Claus PL, Gloviczki P, Hollier LH, Kaye MP: Patency of polytetrafluoroethylene microarterial prostheses improved by ibuprofen. Am J Surg 1982, 144:180.
18. The Coronary Drug Project Research Group: Aspirin in coronary heart disease. J Chronic Dis 1976, 29:625.
19. Dale J, Myhre E, Storstein O, Stormorken H, Efskind L: Prevention of arterial thromboembolism with acetylsalicylic acid: A controlled clinical study in patients with aortic ball valves. Am Heart J 1977, 94:101.
20. Danese CA, Haimov M: Inhibition of experimental arterial thrombosis in dogs with platelet-deaggregating agents. Surgery 1971, 70:927.
21. Deen HG, Sundt TM Jr: The effect of combined aspirin and dipyridamole therapy on thrombus formation in an arterial thrombogenic lesion in the dog. Stroke 1982, 13:179.
22. DeWeese JA: Anastomotic intimal hyperplasia. In Sawyer PN, Kaplitt MJ (eds): *Vascular Grafts,* New York, Appleton Century Crofts, 1978, p 147.
23. DeWeese JA, Green RM: Anastomotic neointimal fibrous hyperplasia. In Bernhard VM, Towne JB (eds): *Complications in Vascular Surgery.* New York, Grune & Stratton, 1981, p 153.
24. DeWeese JA: Long-term results of surgery for carotid artery stenosis. In Bergan JJ, Yao JST (eds): *Cerebro-Vascular Insufficiency.* New York, Grune & Stratton, 1983, p 507.
25. Echave V, Koornick AR, Haimov M, Jacobson JH: Intimal hyperplasia as a complication of the use of the polytetrafluoroethylene graft for femoral-popliteal bypass. Surgery 1979, 86:791.
26. Elwood PC, Cochrane AL, Burr ML, Sweetnam PM, Williams G, Welsby E, Hughes SJ, Renton R: A randomized controlled trial acetylsalicylic acid in the secondary prevention of mortality from myocardial infarction. Br Med J 1974, 1:436.
27. Elwood PC, Sweetnam PM: Aspirin and secondary mortality after myocardial infarction. Lancet 1979, 2:1313.
28. Feins RH, Roedersheimer LR, Green RM, DeWeese JA: Platelet aggregation inhibition in human umbilical vein grafts and negatively charged bovine heterografts. Surgery 1979, 85:395.
29. Fields WS, Lemak NA, Frankowski RF, Hardy RJ: Controlled trial of aspirin in cerebral ischemia. Stroke 1977, 8:301.
30. Fields WS, Lemak NA, Frankowski RF, Hardy RJ: Controlled trial of aspirin in cerebral ischemia. Part II. Surgical group. Stroke 1978, 9:309.
31. Fuster V, Chesebro JH: Antithrombotic therapy: Role of platelet-inhibitor drugs. I. Current concepts of thrombogenesis: Role of platelets (first of three parts). Mayo Clin Proc 1981, 56:102.
32. Fuster V, Chesebro JH: Antithrombotic therapy: Role of platelet-inhibitor drugs. II. Pharmacologic Effects of Platelet-Inhibitor Drugs (second of three parts). Mayo Clin Proc 1981, 56:185.
33. Fuster V, Chesebro JH: Antithrombotic therapy: Role of platelet-inhibitor drugs. III. Management of arterial thromboembolic and atherosclerotic disease (third of three parts). Mayo Clin Proc 1981, 56:265.
34. Goldman MD, Simpson D, Hawker RJ, Norcott HC, McCollum CN: Aspirin and dipyridamole reduce platelet deposition on prosthetic femoro-popliteal grafts in man. Ann Surg 1983, 198:713.
35. Gordon JL, Pearson JD: Effects of sulphinpyrazone and aspirin on prostaglandin (prostacyclin) synthesis by endothelial cells. Br J Pharmacol 1978, 64:481.
36. Green RM, Roedersheimer LR, DeWeese JA: Effects of aspirin and dipyridamole on expanded polytetrafluoroethylene graft patency. Surgery 1982, 92:1016.
37. Gunning AJ, Pickering GW, Robb-Smith AHT, Ross R: Mural thrombosis of the internal carotid artery and subsequent embolism. Q J Med 1964, 33:155.
38. Hagen P, Wang Z, Mikat EM, Hackel DB: Antiplatelet therapy reduces aortic intimal hyperplasia distal to small diameter vascular prostheses (PTFE) in nonhuman primates. Ann Surg 1982, 195:328.
39. Hancock JB, Forshaw PL, Kaye MP: Gore-Tex (Polytetrafluoroethylene) in canine coronary artery bypass. J Thorac Cardiovasc Surg 1980, 80:94.
40. Harjola P, Meurala H, Frick MH: Prevention of early reocclusion by dipyridamole and ASA in arterial reconstructive surgery. J Cardiovasc Surg 1981, 22:141.
41. Harker LA, Slichter SJ: Studies of platelet and fibrinogen kinetics in patients with prosthetic heart valves. N Engl J Med 1970, 283:1302.
42. Harker LA: Platelet mechanisms in the genesis and prevention of graft-related vascular injury reactions and thromboembolism, in Sawyer PN, Kaplitt MJ (eds): *Vascular Grafts,* New York, Appleton Century Crofts, 1978, chap 12, p 153.
43. Harker LA, Ritchie JL: The role of platelets in acute vascular events. Circulation 1980, 62:13.
44. Harris WH, Salzman EW, Athanasoulis CA, Waltman AC, DeSanctis RW: Aspirin prophylaxis of venous thromboembolism after total hip replacement. N Engl J Med 1977, 297:1246.
45. Harter HR, Burch JW, Majerus PW, Stanford N, Delmez JA, Anderson CB, Weerts CA: Prevention of thrombosis in patients on hemodialysis by low-dose aspirin. N Engl J Med 1979, 301:577.

46. Hoepp LM, Elbadawi A, Cohn M, Dachelet R, Peterson C, DeWeese JA: Steroids and immunosuppression: Effect on anastomotic intimal hyperplasia in femoral arterial Dacron bypass grafts. Arch Surg 1979, 114:273.
47. Honour AJ, Russel RW: Experimental platelet embolism. Br J Exp Pathol 1962, 43:350.
48. Imparato AM, Bracco A, Kim GE, Zeff R: Intimal and neointimal fibrous proliferation causing failure of arterial reconstructions. Surgery 1972, 72:1007.
49. Kasahara T: Clinical effect of dipyridamole ingestion after prosthetic heart valve replacement—especially on the blood coagulation system. Nippon Kyobu Geka Gakkai Zasshi (J Jpn Assoc Thorac Surg) 1977, 25:1007.
50. Lewis GP, Westwick J: The effect of sulphinpyrazone, sodium aspirin and oxprenolol on the formation of arterial platelet thrombi. Br J Pharmacol 1975, 55:255P.
51. LoGerfo FW, Quist WC, Nowak MD, Crawshaw HM, Haudenschild CC: Downstream anastomotic hyperplasia: A mechanism of failure in Dacron arterial grafts. Ann Surg 1983, 197:479.
52. Lovaas ME, Gloviczki P, Hollier LH, Kaye MP: Quantitative effects of antiplatelet therapy on healing of the endarterectomized canine aorta. Am J Surg 1983, 146:164.
53. Maseri A, L'Abbate A, Baroldi G, Chierchia S, Marzilli M, Ballestra AM, Severi S, Parodi O, Biagini A, Distante A, Pesola A: Coronary vasospasm as a possible cause of myocardial infarction. A conclusion derived from the study of "preinfarction" angina. N Engl J Med 1978, 299:1271.
54. Mayer JE Jr, Lindsay WG, Castaneda W, Nicoloff DM: Influence of aspirin and dipyridamole on patency of coronary artery bypass grafts. Ann Thorac Surg 1981, 31:204.
55. McBrien DS, Badley RD, Ashton N: The nature of retinal emboli in stenosis of the internal carotid artery. Lancet 1963, 1:697.
56. McCann RL, Hagen PO, Fuchs JCA: Aspirin and dipyridamole decrease intimal hyperplasia in experimental vein grafts. Ann Surg 1980, 191:238.
57. McCollum CN, Crow MJ, Rajah SM, Kester RC: Antithrombotic therapy for vascular prosthesis: An experimental model testing platelet inhibitory drugs. Surgery 1980, 87:668.
58. McEnany MT, Salzman EW, Mundth ED, DeSanctis RW, Harthorne JW, Weintraub RM, Gates S, Austen WG: The effect of antithrombotic therapy on patency rates of saphenous vein coronary artery bypass grafts. J Thorac Cardiovasc Surg 1982, 83:81.
59. McKenna R, Bachmann F, Kaushal SP, Galante JO: Thromboembolic disease in patients undergoing total knee replacement. J Bone Joint Surg [Am] 1976, 58:928.
60. Metke MP, Lee JT, Fuster V, Josa M, Kaye MP: Reduction of intimal thickening in canine coronary bypass vein grafts with dipyridamole and aspirin. Am J Cardiol 1979, 43:1144.
61. Morisaki N, Stitts JM, Bartels-Tomei L, Milo GE, Panganamala RV, Cornwell DG: Dipyridamole: An antioxidant that promotes the proliferation of aorta smooth muscle cells. Artery 1982, 11:88.
62. Niewiarowski S, Rao AK: Contribution of thrombogenic factors to the pathogenesis of atherosclerosis, Cardiovasc Dis 1983, 26:199.
63. Oblath RW, Buckley FO Jr, Green RM, Schwartz SI, DeWeese JA: Prevention of platelet aggregation and adherence to prosthetic vascular grafts by aspirin and dipyridamole. Surgery 1978, 184:37.
64. Palma EC: Hemodynamic arteriosclerosis. J Cardiovasc Surg 1967, 8:198.
65. Pantely GA, Goodnight SH Jr, Shahbudin H, Rahimtoola MB, Harlan BJ, DeMots H, Galvin L, Rosch J: Failure of antiplatelet and anticoagulant therapy to improve patency of grafts after coronary-artery bypass. N Engl J Med 1979, 301:962.
66. The Persantine-Aspirin Reinfarction Study Research Group: Persantine and aspirin in coronary heart disease. Circulation 1980, 62:449.
67. Phillips CE Jr, DeWeese JA, Campeti FL: Comparison of peripheral arterial grafts. Arch Surg 1961, 82:38.
68. Preston FW, Whipps S, Jackson CA, French AJ, Stoddard CJ: Inhibition of prostacyclin and platelet thromboxane A_2 after low-dose aspirin. N Engl J Med 1981, 304:76.
69. Rajah SM, Penny AF, Crow MJ, Pepper MD, Watson DA: The interaction of varying doses of dipyridamole and acetyl salicylic acid on the inhibition of platelet functions and their effect on bleeding time. Br J Clin Pharmacol 1979, 8:483.
70. Sauvage LR, Walker MW, Berger K, Robel SB, Lischko MM, Yates MS, Logan GA: Current arterial prostheses. Arch Surg 1979, 114:687.
71. Sorensen PS, Pedersen H, Marquardsen J, Petersson H, Heltberg A, Simonsen N, Munck O, Andersen LA: Acetylsalicylic acid in the prevention of stroke in patients with reversible cerebral ischemic attacks. A Danish Cooperative Study. Stroke 1983, 14:15.
72. Sottiurai VS, Batson RC: Ultrastructural studies of arterial grafts. In Bergan JJ, Yao JST (eds): *Evaluation and Treatment of Upper and Lower Extremity Circulatory Disorders*. New York, Grune & Stratton, 1984, p 271.
73. Stanley JC, Burkel WE, Ford JW, Vinter DW, Kahn RH, Whitehouse WM Jr, Graham LM: Enhanced patency of small-diameter, externally supported Dacron iliofemoral grafts seeded with endothelial cells. Surgery 1982, 92:994.
74. Steele P, Carroll J, Overfield D, Genton E: Effect of sulfinpyrazone on platelet survival time in patients with transient cerebral ischemic attacks. Stroke 1977, 8:396.
75. Steele P, Ellis J Jr, Genton E: Effects of platelet suppressant, anticoagulant, and fibrinolytic therapy in patients with recurrent venous thrombosis. Am J Med 1978, 64:441.
76. Steele P, Rainwater J, Vogel R, Genton E: Platelet-suppressant therapy in patients with coronary artery disease. JAMA 1978, 240:228.
77. Steele P, Rainwater J, Vogel R: Platelet suppressant therapy in patients with prosthetic cardiac valves: Relationship of clinical effectiveness to alteration of platelet survival time. Circulation 1979, 60:910.
78. Sullivan JM, Harken DE, Gorlin R: Pharmacologic control of thromboembolic complications of cardiac-valve replacement. N Engl J Med 1971, 284:1391.
79. Van Aken WG. In Reitsma WG (ed): *Atherosclerosis, Jonix Lectures*. Excerpta Medica, 1979, p 17.
80. Veith FV, Gupta SK, Samson RH, Scher LA, Fell SC, Weiss P, Janko G, Flores SW, Rifkin H, Bernstein G, Haimovici H, Gliedman ML, Sprayregen S: Progress in limb salvage by reconstructive arterial surgery combined with new or improved adjunctive procedures. Ann Surg 1981, 194:386.
81. Weily HS, Genton E: Altered platelet function in patients with prosthetic mitral valves: Effects of sulfinpyrazone therapy. Circulation 1970, 42:967.
82. Weiss HJ: The pharmacology of platelet inhibition, Prog in Hemostasis and Thromb 1972, 1:199.
83. Weiss HJ. In Koch-Weser J (ed): Antiplatelet therapy (first of two parts), Medical intelligence, drug therapy. N Engl J Med 1978, 298:1344.

Chapter 16D

VASODILATORS

AKSEL G. NORDESTGAARD and RUSSELL A. WILLIAMS

Vasodilator drugs consist of a variety of agents with different modes of action, but which all dilate blood vessels in one or more body region. Based on therapeutic rather than pharmacologic consideration they are subdivided in peripheral, coronary, and antihypertensive vasodilators. This section will be confined to the use of vasodilator drugs in peripheral vascular disease.

Table 16D-1 shows some of the vasodilator drugs that have been used in patients with atherosclerotic obstructive disease or vasospastic disease. Their use in obstructive vascular disease is now generally disapproved; they are ineffective in increasing the muscle blood flow during exercise in patients with intermittent claudication and skin blood flow in patients with skin ischemia (1–3). Indeed blood flow in the affected limb may even be reduced, since most vasodilators tend to lower systemic blood pressure, with a resultant reduction in perfusion pressure and blood redistribution, "stealing" blood from the diseased to perfuse healthy vascular areas that dilate with the drug (1). Removal or bypassing of arterial obstruction is the only treatment at present that effectively restores blood flow in these patients.

TABLE 16D-1. Vasodilator Drugs

Adrenergic neuronal blocking drugs:
Reserpine
Guanethidine
Alpha-adrenergic blocking drugs:
Prazosin
Tolazoline
Phenoxybenzamine
Direct-acting smooth-muscle relaxants:
Papaverine
Nifedipine
Nitroglycerin (topical or sublingual)

Vasospasm implies that the vascular obstruction (constriction) is reversible, and therefore, vasospastic diseases may be more amenable to vasodilator therapy. In Raynaud's syndrome, the most common vasospastic disorder, both sympathetic blocking agents and drugs that directly relax vascular smooth muscle are reported of value. Unfortunately, documentation of objective benefit is incomplete for most of the vasodilators used for treatment for Raynaud's syndrome.

Adrenergic Neuronal Blocking Drugs

RESERPINE

Reserpine depletes stores of the neurotransmitter norepinephrine from the sympathetic nerve endings by interfering with its granular storage mechanisms. Norepinephrine depletion attenuates the vasoconstrictive reflex to cold in both healthy persons and patients with Raynaud's syndrome (4). Reserpine increases total finger blood flow and, most importantly, the nutritional capillary component, which is decreased significantly in patients with Raynaud's syndrome during sympathetic stimulation (5).

Although reserpine has been used for more than 20 years in the treatment of Raynaud's syndrome, no controlled double-blind evaluations of its effect when taken orally have been performed. The dose recommended begins at 0.25 mg per day, increasing to 1 mg or more, depending on the relief of symptoms and the development of side effects.

Single intraarterial injections of reserpine (1.0 to 1.5 mg) have been reported to produce healing of finger ulcers as well as improvement in symptoms which lasts for months (6). Further studies have cast doubts on the occurrence of any long-term benefits, and the use of reserpine by the intraarterial route is suggested only in severe cases of Raynaud's disease in an attempt to postpone amputation or sympathectomy (7,8,9).

Side effects of reserpine therapy include nasal stuffiness, postural hypotension, gastrointestinal symptoms, nightmares, water retention, and depression. Reserpine should never be given to patients with depressive symptoms or a history of depression.

GUANETHIDINE

Guanethidine, like reserpine, diminishes sympathetic activity by interfering with the release of norepinephrine at the sympathetic neuroeffector junction. Unlike reserpine, guanethidine acts only peripherally and is therefore not contraindicated in patients with a history of depression.

Some success has been reported with oral guanethidine in relieving symptoms in Raynaud's syndrome (3), but side effects are frequent with the high doses that are often needed. Starting with 10 mg a day, the daily dose can be increased at 1- or 2-week intervals to 50 mg a day according to response. Using guanethidine (10 mg daily) in combination with prazosin (1 mg twice daily) most side effects of either of these drugs used singly were avoided (10). Intravenous regional sympathetic blockade with guanethidine (12 to 17.5 mg) increases total blood flow in the forearm of healthy humans, indicating this technique may be of value in vasospastic disorders and possibly also as adjuvant therapy in vascular surgery of the extremities (11,12,13).

Side effects include postural or postexercise hypotension, nasal stuffiness, diarrhea, impotence, water retention, and fatigue.

Alpha-adrenergic Blocking Drug

PRAZOSIN

Prazosin (Minipress), a popular antihypertensive agent, has been found effective in reducing the frequency and severity of vasospastic episodes in patients with Raynaud's syndrome, when given in an oral dose of 1 mg tid (14,15). It inhibits vasoconstriction by blocking postsynaptic alpha 2 receptors and is well tolerated by most patients with few of the adverse reactions common to other vasoactive substances.

Side effects include drowsiness, dizziness, headache, nausea, and palpitations. Postural hypotension and syncope may occur but can often be avoided if treatment is instituted slowly with the first dosage of 1 mg given at bedtime.

Direct-Acting Smooth Muscle Relaxants

PAPAVERINE

Papaverine, an opiate with nonspecific smooth-muscle relaxant properties, produces arteriolar dilatation in the systemic, coronary, and cerebral circulations. Oral administration of papaverine or its analogues has not been demonstrated to be of significant therapeutic value in peripheral vascular disease. However, local application, by the intraarterial route, has been used with success in relieving the persistent vasoconstriction present in both nonocclusive and embolic intestinal ischemia (16). A dosage of 30 to 60 mg of papaverine hydrochloride per hour, preceded by a bolus of 60 mg, was used. Animal studies support the favorable clinical reports; using experimentally produced ischemic dog colon, intraarterial papaverine hydrochloride was found to increase the bowel wall blood flow, without producing undesirable systemic effects (17).

Side effects include flushing, cardiac arrhythmias, drowsiness, gastrointestinal symptoms, and headache. Furthermore, it has been reported to have hepatic toxicity (18).

NIFEDIPINE

Among the calcium channel blocking agents, nifedipine has emerged as a potent vasodilator, with effects on both the coronary and peripheral arterial beds. By blocking cellular uptake of calcium, nifedipine decreases vascular tone; skin blood flow increases by 50 to 150 percent in healthy persons, and cold-induced digital vasospasm in patients with moderate to severe Raynaud's syndrome is significantly decreased when nifedipine is given orally (19,20). Several double-blind, controlled clinical trials have documented the usefulness of nifedipine in the treatment of Raynaud's syndrome (20,21,22). However, variability in response to therapy was noticed, with no response at all in some patients. This is in part explained by variation in severity of vasospasm, extent of the anatomic narrowing of the digital arteries, and presence of underlying systemic disease.

Although further studies are needed to determine the efficacy of long-term therapy and the predictors of clinical responsiveness, nifedipine should currently be considered as the first drug in the medical treatment of Raynaud's syndrome.

A dosage of 20 mg tid is recommended and is usually well tolerated. The main side effect is headache. Animal studies have suggested a potential teratogenic effect. Although no similar effect has been reported in humans, contraception should be recommended when nifedipine is prescribed for women of childbearing age (21).

References

1. Hansteen V, Lorentsen E: Vasodilator drugs in the treatment of peripheral arterial insufficiency. Acta Med Scand (suppl) 1974, 556:1–62.
2. Coffman JD, Mannick JA: Failure of vasodilator drugs in arteriosclerosis obliterans. Ann Intern Med 1972, 76:35–39.
3. Coffman JD: Vasodilator drugs in peripheral vascular disease. N Engl J Med 1979, 300:713–717.
4. Kontos HA, Wasserman AJ: Effect of reserpine in Raynaud's phenomenon. Circulation 1969, 39:259–266.
5. Coffman JD, Cohen AS: Total and capillary fingertip blood flow in Raynaud's phenomenon. N Engl J Med 1971, 285:259–263.
6. Romeo SG, Whalen RE, Tindall JP: Intra-arterial administration of reserpine. Arch Intern Med 1970, 125:825–829.
7. Nobin BA, Nielsen SL, Eklov BO, Lassen NA: Reserpine treatment of Raynaud's disease. Ann Surg 1978, 187:12–16.
8. Surwit RS, Gilgor RS, Duvic M, Allen LM, Neal JA: Intraarterial reserpine for Raynaud's syndrome. Arch Dermatol 1983, 119:733–735.
9. Siegel RC, Fries JF: Intra-arterially administered reserpine and saline in scleroderma. Arch Intern Med 1974, 134:515–518.
10. Porter JM, Rivers SP, Anderson CJ, Baur GM: Evaluation and management of patients with Raynaud's syndrome. Am J Surg 1981, 142:183–189.
11. Thomsen MB, Bengtsson M, Lassvik C, Alm A, Elfstrom J: Adjuvant intravenous sympathetic block with guanethidine in construction of arteriovenous fistulas for blood access. Acta Chir Scand 1983, 149:141–145.
12. Thomsen MB, Bengtsson M, Lassvik C, Lewis DH, Elfstrom J: Changes in human forearm blood flow after intravenous regional symapthetic blockade with guanethidine. Acta Chir Scand 1982, 148:657–661.

13. McKain CW, Urban BJ, Goldner JL: The effects of intravenous regional guanethidine and reserpine. J Bone Joint Surg 1983, 65A:808–811.
14. Surwit RS, Gilgor RS, Allen LM, Duvic M: A double-blind study of prazosin in the treatment of Raynaud's phenomenon in scleroderma. Arch Dermatol 1984, 120:329–331.
15. Waldo R: Prazosin relieves Raynaud's vasospasm. JAMA 1979, 241:1037.
16. Boley SJ, Feinstein FR, Sammartano R, Brandt LJ, Sprayregen S: New concepts in the management of emboli of the superior mesenteric artery. Surg Gynecol Obstet 1981, 153:561–569.
17. Williams RA, Wilson SE: Effect of intra-arterial vasodilators on blood flow in ischemic dog colon. Arch Surg 1980, 115:602–605.
18. Gilman AG, Goodman LS, Gilman A (eds): *The Pharmacologic Basis of Therapeutics*, ed 6. New York, Macmillan, 1980.
19. Nilsson H, Jonasson T, Ringqvist I: Treatment of digital vasospastic disease with the calcium-entry blocker nifedipine. Acta Med Scand 1984, 215:135–139.
20. Rodeheffer RJ, Rommer JA, Wigley F, Smith CR: Controlled double-blind trial of nifedipine in the treatment of Raynaud's phenomenon. N Engl J Med 1983, 308:880–883.
21. Smith CD, McKendry RJR: Controlled trial of nifedipine in the treatment of Raynaud's phenomenon. Lancet 1982, 2:1299–1301.
22. Sauza J, Kraus A, Gonzalez-Amaro R, Alarcon-Segovia D: Effect of the calcium channel blocker nifedipine on Raynaud's phenomenon: A controlled double blind trial. J Rheumatol 1984, 11:362–364.

Chapter 16E

PENTOXIFYLLINE

BRUCE E. STABILE

The recent introduction into clinical use of pentoxifylline represents a new and potentially useful chronic medical therapy for peripheral vascular insufficiency. Unlike the various vasodilators which have been prescribed without beneficial effect for intermittent claudication over the past half century, pentoxifylline is characterized as a hemorrheologic agent which improves capillary blood flow by increasing erythrocyte flexibility and thereby reducing blood viscosity. The precise mechanism of pentoxifylline's action remains to be clarified, but the drug's effects on erythrocyte flexibility, blood viscosity, and capillary perfusion purportedly increase oxygen delivery to skeletal muscle. Pentoxifylline is currently being marketed in the United States only for the treatment of intermittent claudication in patients with chronic occlusive arterial disease.

Studies of erythrocytes taken from normal individuals and patients with atherosclerotic peripheral vascular disease have shown decreased flexibility in the atherosclerotic patients (1,2). This impaired flexibility may be due to the presence of a low pH and elevated levels of potassium, calcium, histamine, serotonin, prostaglandins, and various peptides related to the anaerobic metabolism in ischemic muscle beds (3–5).

Muscle contractility has been shown to be impaired when skeletal muscle is perfused by blood with decreased erythrocyte flexibility (6). A good therapeutic rationale therefore appears to exist for reducing the erythrocyte rigidity present in patients with intermittent claudication.

The mechanism of pentoxifylline's effect on the erythrocyte membrane appears to involve increased phosphorylation of membrane proteins by enhanced magnesium-dependent protein kinase activity and by inhibition of calcium-dependent phosphoprotein phosphatase and transglutaminase (7). The increase in phosphoproteins is thought to be responsible for the enhanced membrane flexibility noted after pentoxifylline treatment. Pentoxifylline has also been found to induce vasodilation through inhibition of cyclic adenosine monophosphate (AMP) phosphodiesterase activity and thus increases the cyclic AMP content in vascular smooth muscle (8). The drug indirectly retards platelet aggregation by stimulating prostacyclin formation in blood vessel walls (9).

A number of controlled clinical trials designed to test the efficacy of pentoxifylline for the treatment of intermittent claudication have been conducted abroad and in the United States. These studies generally have shown significant improvements in walking distance with pentoxifylline compared to placebo (10–15) or a vasodilator drug (16). Approximately three-quarters of the pentoxifylline-treated patients demonstrated an improvement in walking distance after 4 to 12 weeks of therapy. The mean increase in walking distance was typically about 100 percent over the pretreatment baseline. Unfortunately, few of these controlled trials included an objective measurement of peripheral perfusion to allow correlation with the symptomatic response.

The largest and best-designed controlled trial comparing pentoxifylline and placebo was the multicenter study reported in 1982 by Porter et al. (10). Eighty-two patients from seven centers in the United States participated in this double-blind, parallel-group, 24-week trial. Initial and absolute claudication distances were measured on a treadmill initially and at 2-week intervals for the initial 8 weeks and then at 4-week intervals throughout the remainder of the study. Forty-two patients were begun on 600 mg daily of pentoxifylline and advanced to 1200 mg daily after the third week. Forty patients received placebo and were followed in an identical manner. Overall the pentoxifylline-treated group showed a mean 45 percent increase over baseline in initial claudication distance and a 32 percent increase in absolute claudication distance, compared to increases of 23 and 20 percent, respectively, for the placebo-treated group. These differences were statistically significant. The pentoxifylline-treated patients showed a greater percentage improvement from baseline than did placebo patients at every follow-up visit throughout the trial period. However, the relief or amelioration of symptoms, including pain, cramping, tiredness, and tightness as well as the patients' own evaluation of their condition, were not significantly different between the two groups. Furthermore, the tibial-brachial systolic blood pressure index after exercise, though not standardized among treatment centers, was not significantly improved at the conclusion of the 24-week trial. Pentoxifylline was found to be as safe as placebo but did cause significantly more nausea.

Pentoxifylline is currently available as a 400-mg controlled-release tablet. The drug is usually administered in a dose of 400 mg three times a day. Side effects such as abdominal discomfort, nausea, and vomiting can be minimized by taking the drug with meals. Rarely do these problems persist and, if troublesome, respond to a diminution in dosage. It is important to continue pentoxifylline for a minimum of 12 weeks in order to obtain the maximum therapeutic effect. No adverse interactions with commonly used cardiovascular, antihypertensive, or antidiabetic drugs have been observed.

Although pentoxifylline has been widely used abroad for over a decade in the treatment of occlusive peripheral vascular disease, it remains to be seen whether further clinical and laboratory evaluation will justify its enthusiastic support in the United States. While solid evidence for pentoxifylline's efficacy in the treatment of claudication remains relatively scant, there is virtually no information on its utility in the management of rest pain or ischemic ulceration. If reduced viscosity of the blood and increased flexibility of erythrocytes in fact improves tissue oxygenation as a result of increased flow through the microcirculation, then hemorrheologic agents like pentoxifylline may become important adjuncts in the medical armamentarium of the physician treating vascular insufficiency. It does not seem likely, however, that hemorrheologic agents will ever replace operative bypass for arterial obstruction. More reasonably, these drugs will probably find applicability in patients with mild symptoms not justifying operation and perhaps also in those with severe nonreconstructible disease.

References

1. Reid HL, Dormandy JA, Barnes AJ, Lock PJ, Dormandy TL: Impaired red cell deformability in peripheral vascular disease. Lancet 1976, 1:666–667.
2. Ehrly AM, Kohler HJ: Altered deformability of erythrocytes from patients with chronic occlusive arterial disease. Vasa 1976, 5:319–322.
3. Weed RI: The importance of erythrocyte deformability. Am J Med 1970, 49:147–150.
4. Braasch D: Red cell deformability and capillary blood flow. Physiol Rev 1971, 51:679–701.
5. Schmid-Schonbein H: Microrheology of erythrocytes, blood viscosity, and the distribution of blood flow in the microcirculation. Int Rev Physiol 1976, 9:1–62.
6. Dormandy J, Ernst E, Bennett D: Erythrocyte deformability in the pathophysiology of the microcirculation. Ric Clin Lab 1981, 11(suppl 1):35–38.
7. Kramer JJ, Swislocki NI: Effects of pentoxifylline on membrane protein phosphorylation in rat erythrocytes. Vas Med 1983, 1:159–174.
8. Stefanovich V: Effect of 3,7-dimethyl-1-(5-oxy-hexyl) xanthine and 1-hexyl-3-7-dimethyl xanthine on cyclic AMP phosphodiesterase of the human unibilical cord vessels. Res Commun Pathol Pharmacol 1973, 5:655–662.
9. Matzky R, Darius H, Schror K: The release of prostacyclin (PGI_2) by pentoxifylline from human vascular tissue. Arzneimittelforsch 1982, 32:1315–1318.
10. Porter JM, Cutler BS, Lee BY, Reich T, Reichle FA, Scogin JT, Strandness DE: Pentoxifylline in the treatment of intermittent claudication: A double-blind trial with objective assessment. Am Heart J 1982, 104:66–72.
11. Volker D: Treatment of arteriopathies with TRENTAL 400. Pharmatherapeutica 1983, 3(suppl 1):135–142.
12. Schubotz R: Double-blind trial of pentoxifylline in diabetics with peripheral vascular disorders. Pharmatherapeutica 1976, 1:172–179.
13. Tonak J, Knecht H, Groitl H: Treatment of circulatory disturbances with pentoxifylline (double-blind trial). Pharmatherapeutica 1983, 3(suppl 1):126–135.
14. Di Perri T, Guerrini M: Placebo controlled double blind study with pentoxifylline of walking performance in patients with intermittent claudication. Angiology 1983, 34:40–45.
15. Feine-Haake G: Assessment of the therapeutic efficacy of TRENTAL 400; double-blind trial in geriatric patients with vascular disorders. Pharmatherapeutica 1983, 3suppl 1:46–51.
16. Accetto B: Beneficial hemorrheologic therapy of chronic peripheral arterial disorders with pentoxifylline: Results of double-blind study versus vasodilator-nylidrin. Am Heart J 1982, 103:864–869.

Chapter 17

THE REVERSIBILITY OF ATHEROSCLEROTIC LESIONS BY MEDICAL TREATMENT

DAVID H. BLANKENHORN and PAMELA J. CURRY

The Definition of Reversibility

This chapter presents evidence for the reversibility of atherosclerotic lesions when risk factors such as smoking, elevated blood pressure, and elevated plasma lipid levels are reduced through medical treatment. Prevention of thrombotic complications with anticoagulant or anti-platelet-aggregation agents is another important aspect of the medical treatment of atherosclerosis and is described in this chapter. The discussion is limited to the effects of therapy on arterial lesions and does not consider whether such risk-factor reduction will ultimately translate into a reduction of morbidity and mortality.

The reversibility of atherosclerosis has been defined in a number of ways. The strictest definition requires the normalization of the anatomy and chemical composition of the vessel wall. At the level of light microscopy, normalization would include (1) restoration of the integrity of the endothelium over plaques, (2) arrest of intimal cell proliferation, (3) decrease in the number of cells within lesions plus decreases in intracellular and extracellular lipid, and (4) decrease in the extent of necrotic foci and calcification (1). A much more liberal definition accepts as proof of reversibility any change which reduces the size on intimal lesions, except those changes which are due to plaque rupture or embolism. In the vast majority of vascular surgery patients, the principal goal of surgery is to remove or bypass obstructive lesions. Given this goal, any reduction in lesion size can be considered to constitute a reversal of the disease. Therefore, this second, more liberal definition of reversibility seems appropriate to a discussion of potential lesion regression in patients who are candidates for vascular surgery. However, in animal models, controlled studies which quantify histologic change over time would argue that reduction in lesion size does not necessarily imply improvement in all cellular elements of the lesion (2).

Four separate lines of investigation provide evidence for a reduction in the size of lesions through risk-factor modification: (1) observations in experimental animal models, including controlled quantitative regression studies (which demonstrate reversibility according to the more rigorous definition as well), (2) observations among patients who are starving or suffering from wasting diseases, (3) anecdotal angiographic human case studies, and (4) controlled clinical angiographic trials in humans. Taken together, these reports provide strong evidence for the reversibility of atherosclerosis—strong enough to indicate that risk reduction should be an integral part of the long-term post-surgical management of the atherosclerotic patient in order to retard or reverse the eventual growth of lesions in operated vessels, bypass grafts, and peripheral vascular beds.

Experimental Animal Models

The first animal to be studied as a model for atherosclerosis was the rabbit. Anitschkow (3) observed that lesions could be induced by feeding rabbits cholesterol and that the continuation of cholesterol ingestion was necessary to sustain the disease. His work demonstrated that regression (or reversibility) was characterized by diminished numbers of foam cells and changes in lesion size and appearance after returning the animals to a normal diet for 18 to 24 months. Recent experience with an inbred strain of spontaneously hyperlipidemic rabbits (Watanabe heritable hyperlipidemic rabbits) corroborates the role of continued elevations of plasma cholesterol in the production of atherosclerosis in this animal (4). With a defective low-density lipoprotein (LDL) receptor system similar to that found in familial type II hyperlipoproteinemia, these rabbits develop persisting severe hypercholesterolemia (14-fold, compared with control animals) on commercial rabbit chow and concomitantly develop progressively severe atherosclerosis. Symptoms of the progressive disease include gross aortic intimal thickening, aortic narrowing, and xanthomas.

A pioneering study of regression in the chicken was published in 1949 by Horlick and Katz (5), who first demonstrated that a semiquantitative relationship exists between the percentage of cholesterol in the diet and both the duration of the induction period and the severity of the resulting disease. Cholesterol feeding was shown to result in a progressive aggravation of the disease over a 6-month period. The cessation of the cholesterol feeding after 10 weeks resulted in the disappearance of foam cells, diminution of stainable lipids, and total remission of lesions in some of the chicks. Birds in whom the disease had progressed to more severe levels were left after the regression diet with some permanent calcification, suggesting that there may be a threshold of damage beyond which total repair of the artery is no longer possible. The authors point out that the ability of each species of animal to remove cholesterol from the arterial walls is a function of the animal's ability to excrete cholesterol. They postulated that the chicken reduces its body stores of cholesterol faster than the rabbit, as evidenced by a more rapid return to normal lipid levels in the chicken after the cessation of an atherogenic diet, and this results in a faster resorption of the early lesions. Previously unsuccessful attempts to demonstrate regression in advanced disease in the rabbit (6,7) were attributed to a relative inability to reduce total body sterol stores and mobilize local deposits.

The White Carneau pigeon, because of spontaneously occurring atherosclerosis (8), has been frequently used in regression studies (9–11). Hrapchak (12) has used this animal to examine disease progression rates. All birds show grossly visible lesions at the celiac bifurcation at 4 years, but lesion development can be accelerated on an atherogenic diet, and Hrapchak has described the time course of the diet-exacerbated atherogenesis with special attention to the effects of hemodynamics on the localization of disease at the carotid bifurcation. Clarkson (9) kept 146 birds on a normal diet supplemented with lard and cholesterol for 1 year and found that the disease can be reversed with dietary manipulation. After returning the animals to a baseline diet, he found an increase in extracellular lipid, a narrowing of the intima, and an increased lumen diameter, compared with age-matched atherosclerotic birds. Reparative changes continued for 8 months, after which no further normalization was observed. Histologic evidence for an improvement in lesion size and severity after lowering cholesterol levels in the pigeon with partial ileal bypass surgery has been reported by several authors (13–15). Peterson and Hirst (16) observed a diet-associated regression of lesions in pigeons and suggested that early lesions might undergo substantial regression after a cholesterol-supplemented diet is stopped; older lesions were shown to be more resistant to repair.

Dogs have served primarily as models for atherosclerosis progression, and reports of disease reversal are limited. The induction of atherosclerotic lesions through diet and thyroid ablation has been described (17–20). DePalma (21) demonstrated consistent lesion production in the dog with sustained serum cholesterol levels of 1500 mg/dL. In one of the few regression studies in dogs, DePalma achieved regression after placing the animals on a combined regimen of dietary cholesterol reduction and internal biliary diversion. The maintenance of serum cholesterol in the range of 100 to 200 mg/dL was necessary to induce regression once plaques had been developed. This suggested a threshold cholesterol level below which arterial lipid deposits may begin to be resorbed, a thesis later supported by DePalma's work with subhuman primates (22).

DePalma developed arteriotomy techniques in the dog to permit repeated visualization of specific lesions over time. This was an attempt to circumvent the necessity of making estimations of lesion growth from a series of single postmortem observations among a group of animals. However, the arterial trauma induced by the surgical procedure proved to be a stimulus for the formation of new atheromas in most vessels, and the authors returned to serial angiographic protocols. The one vascular area which could successfully be inspected at repeated intervals was the mesenteric circulation, as vessels in this area could be observed at laparotomy without physically touching them.

Subhuman primates are the preferred animal for regression studies because of their anatomic, physiologic and metabolic similarities to man. For example, there are minimal differences between humans and macaques in lipoprotein patterns (23). Hyperlipidemia of the rhesus monkey can be compared to human acquired type II hyperlipidemia (22). Whereas other animal models have frequently failed to demonstrate the clinical complications of advanced human disease (24,25), the severely atherosclerotic macaque has been shown to be susceptible to the development of xanthomas (26), myocardial infarction, and severe cerebral ischemia (27,28). Bond (29) observed that the attack rate of symptoms of atherosclerosis in a population of rhesus monkeys undergoing experimentally induced progression was about the same as would be seen in a population of humans with advanced disease.

Species differences in susceptibility to atherosclerosis among primates have been documented. Wissler (30) reported a study in which stump-tailed macaques and rhesus monkeys were treated and caged identically on an atherogenic diet. The percentage of aortic intimal surface area which was raised with atherosclerotic disease in the stump-tailed monkeys was 75 percent; in the rhesus monkeys it was 95 percent. There may, as well, be differences within species in the relative susceptibility to disease of various vascular beds. For example, when challenged with a high-cholesterol diet, *Macaca irus* specimens from the Philippines tend to develop disease in the coronary arteries and little in the aorta. On the other hand, under identical treatment, specimens obtained from Thailand or from Malaysia show a predilection to develop disease equally in these two vessel beds (31).

Portman (32) achieved disease stabilization in squirrel monkeys by returning the animals to regular chow after they had been 3 months on a high-cholesterol diet. Animals returned to the normalizing diet for 3 to 5 months showed significantly fewer coronary lesions than those who remained on the atherogenic diet. In the early 1970s Armstrong (33–35) demonstrated an unequivocal reduction in the size of advancing stenosing coronary lesions in the rhesus monkey. A 17-month induction phase (high-fat, high-cholesterol) was followed by 40 months on a diet which allowed the serum cholesterol to return approximately to baseline levels (140 mg/dL). The lesions produced during dietary induction were found to average 60 percent obstruction in all main epicardial coronary arteries. After the animals had been 40 months on treatment diets, the average coronary lumen obstructions had decreased to approximately 21 percent obstruction. The reduction in the size of the lesion was accompanied by measurable reductions in its lipid and collagen content.

Cellular evidence for strictly defined regression in moderate-sized lesions has been documented in rhesus monkeys. Stary (36) observed the normalization of cell kinetics in arterial lesions during regression attributed to returning the monkeys to a basal diet for 3 to 10 months. Reparative changes included a measurable decrease in intracellular lipid and a return to normal cellular proliferative patterns. Initial signs of disease reversibility were seen as soon as 4 weeks after the serum cholesterol had returned to baseline levels. Foam cell production stopped, and the normalization of smooth-muscle cell morphology was observed. Tucker (37) returned cholesterol-fed monkeys to a basal diet for 4 months and found a resulting decrease in the number of foam cells, a decrease in intracellular lipid levels, and an increase in extracellular lipid levels. A similar lipid depletion was biochemically verified in rhesus monkeys (34) who had undergone experimentally induced atherogenesis. The depletion of total and ester cholesterol, as well as free cholesterol, was essentially completed 20 months into the dietary treatment program.

Wissler's group has shown that experimental lesions in rhesus monkeys can be reversed by treatment with cholestyramine (38–43). Male monkeys were kept on an atherogenic diet for 1 to 2 years. Some were then changed to a low-fat, low-cholesterol diet, with or without the addition of the drug. A final group of animals received the cholestyramine while remaining on the atherogenic diet. The amount of aortic surface area affected with grossly visible lesions was significantly less in all three treatment groups than in the control group (10 to 32 percent versus 66 to 82 percent). The low-cholesterol diet with cholestyramine produced the most favorable results, particularly in the coronary arteries where there was 1 to 5 percent luminal narrowing versus 12 to 36 percent narrowing among animals remaining on an atherogenic diet. The finding of major clinical interest in this study, however, was the substantial regression produced when cholestyramine was added to the high-cholesterol diet. Animals in this group remained on a diet supplemented with cholesterol and peanut oil while being treated with 2.5 percent cholestyramine. After 1 year these monkeys showed luminal narrowing of the same magnitude as those who had been removed to the low-fat, low-cholesterol diet for 1 year (7.5 percent narrowing). Animals remaining on the high-fat diet without the drug demonstrated aortic narrowing of 36.5 ± 4.4 percent. These data suggest that hypocholesterolemic medication may similarly benefit the human patient who does not, or cannot, strictly adhere to a prescribed therapeutic diet.

Whether there may be a threshold serum cholesterol level which determines the presence or the rate of atherogenesis has been considered by several investigators. Bond (44,45) reported that an incomplete return to baseline serum cholesterol levels in rhesus monkeys can be associated with significant lesion regression. Partial reversibility was demonstrated by his team in the moderately elevated cholesterol range of 180 to 220 mg/dL. Armstrong (33) suggested that a serum cholesterol level of 140 mg/dL, if sustained, would permit resorption of advancing lesions in rhesus monkeys. Vesselinovitch observed (46): "It seems likely that advanced atherosclerotic lesions in the primate will regress when serum cholesterol levels are maintained at 175 or below for a number of months." DePalma (47) found that regression of fatty-fibrous plaques occurs in rhesus monkeys when serum cholesterol levels are reduced to the 130 to 160 mg/dL range. It is of interest to note that all these potential threshold levels of serum cholesterol are estimated in ranges which are attainable in humans.

Important advances in quantifying the regressive changes of lesions have been made by Vesselinovitch and Wissler. Morphometric measurements including point counting (48) and computer-assisted digitizing (49) have been used to quantify changes in various lesion components over time, as well as to quantify intimal thickness and the percentage of lumen narrowing. The quantification of such normalization has led to a better description of the pathobiology of atherosclerosis reversibility at different stages of disease severity and has shown that strictly defined regression is characterized by (1) a decrease in cholesterol ester levels, (2) reductions in both intracellular and extracellular lipid levels, (3) the removal of cellular debris from the necrotic core, (4) substantial condensation and remodeling of collagen, and (5) a nearly complete healing of the endothelium. All these changes have been documented and quantified in subhuman primates within 1 year of dietary treatment to lower serum cholesterol levels (50).

Studies of Starved Human Populations

Indirect evidence for the potential reversibility of atherosclerosis in humans comes from retrospective analyses of the consequences of sudden, severe dietary modifications in large groups of people and from studies of starvation due to wasting disease. In 1924, Aschoff (51) inferred that human regression of atherosclerosis might be possible based on European data which showed a lower incidence of atherosclerotic disease in central Europe just after World War I. His suggestion that this was caused by a marked decrease in dietary fats was supported by Beitzke (52), who found a low incidence of atherosclerotic disease at autopsy among populations whose diets had been drastically limited as a consequence of war. After World War II, Malmros (53) and Strom and Jensen (54) related dietary restrictions (fewer calories from eggs and butter) to temporarily reduced mortality figures in the Scandinavian countries. Vartiainen (55) also related a decline in mortality in Finland between 1942 and 1947 to a decreased availability of food, particularly sources of cholesterol. Similar observations were made throughout the Scandinavian countries and in Russia (56). A reported decrease in the number of myocardial infarcts was observed during the siege of Leningrad; the reappearance of a more normal food supply was accompanied by a concomitant increase in the manifestations of coronary disease. Schettler (57) reviewed autopsy findings during three postwar periods and associated progressive decreases in the numbers of atherosclerotic lesions seen at postmortem examination with war-related severe dietary deprivations.

Wilens (58) studied hospitalized patients with marked weight loss secondary to wasting disease. The patients who had suffered more drastic weight losses before death had smaller and less severe lesions. He concluded that lipids were being withdrawn from arterial deposits in relatively short periods of time among those patients, who had lost from 15 to 110 lb within 1 year of autopsy.

Other observations of atherosclerotic improvement associated with wasting disease have been described in studies of anorexia nervosa (59) and carcinoma (60–63).

Angiographic Evidence in Humans: Uncontrolled and Case Studies

Direct evidence of the reversibility of atherosclerotic lesions is apparent in studies which have used serial angiography to detect the stabilization of lesions or the reduction of luminal encroachment. The earliest of these studies was reported by Ost and Stenson (64), who treated 31 hyperlipidemic men for intermittent claudication with large dosages (3 to 6 g/day) of nicotinic acid. Three patients showed a regression in femoral lesions after a treatment period of approximately 3 years. Angiographic improvement was accompanied by increased pulse-volume and improved walking capacities. Although this study is sometimes criticized for not reporting specific lipid levels, it is safe to infer that the dosages of nicotinic acid given probably produced a significant lowering of blood lipid levels.

Serial arteriographic studies have demonstrated the ability to quantify an actual reduction in lesion size in humans. DePalma reported one of the first such cases in a paper appearing in 1970 (21). A 57-year-old diabetic man reduced his serum cholesterol level from 327 to 190 mg/dL, stopped smoking, and began a program of mild exercise. Serial arteriograms taken 9 months apart strongly suggested lessened obstruction in the popliteal artery. Basta (65) reported the case of a 49-year-old hypertensive woman who had smoked a pack of cigarettes per day for 20 years. She was treated for her blood pressure and angina with a regimen of methyldopa and chlorothiazide. Total plasma lipid levels were reduced from 340 to 160 mg/dL, and triglyceride levels were lowered from 157 to 118 mg/dL. During the 2 years of treatment, she also stopped smoking. Pretreatment renal arteriograms showed a 90 percent occlusion on the right and 75 percent on the left. Repeat arteriograms 2 years later showed evidence of marked disease regression on the right and a lesser, but significant, improvement on the left.

Long-term plasma exchange was used by Thompson (66) to treat eight patients with familial hypercholesterolemia. Three of these patients showed a measurable regression of aortic and coronary lesions when angiography was repeated. Functional improvements accompanied the radiographic evidence. Roth and Kostuk (67) reported a case study of a 46-year-old attorney who presented with episodic dyspnea, chest tightness, and a single coronary lesion on arteriography. Through a self-imposed regimen of dietary modifications and increased exercise, the patient reduced his serum cholesterol level from 269 to 201 mg/dL and his triglyceride levels from 205 to 93 mg/dL. Arteriography repeated after 1 year showed decreased stenosis in the left anterior descending artery and a reduction in collateral circulation. Thallium scanning showed an increased myocardial perfusion.

The positive influence of risk-factor reduction was shown by Barndt (68) in an early feasibility study of femoral angiography as an auxiometric tool in a clinical trial. The regression of atheroma was quantified by a study of the superficial femoral artery. In this study 25 hyperlipidemic patients were treated with diet, lipid-lowering medication (primarily clofibrate and neomycin), and antihypertensive medication when necessary. After 13 months, 9 patients showed evidence of atherosclerosis regression. The regression of disease was significantly correlated with reductions in serum cholesterol levels, triglyceride levels, and blood pressure. The average reduction in plasma cholesterol levels observed among the patients who showed a reduction in lesion size was 65 mg/dL, compared with a reduction of 19 mg/dL among those showing a progression of the disease ($p < .001$). The regression patients lowered their triglyceride levels an average of 219 mg/dL; the progression patients showed a lesser lowering of 122 mg/dL. The angiographic changes measured by radiologists were later verified by an automated computer method.

Angiographic Evidence in Humans: Controlled Clinical Trials

One of the earliest of the controlled regression studies in humans, published by Terry and Rouen in 1976 (69), reported that lesions can be stabilized. The nonprogression of disease was shown by these authors in 19 of 22 patients treated with pyridinol carbamate after 2 years and in 16 of 18 patients followed for an additional 2 years. During a continuation period of 27 months, nonprogression was angiographically documented in three patients who had shown progression as control patients before being switched to the treatment group.

Olsson (70) published an early report of a randomized trial in which femoral angiograms were repeated every 6 months. The asymptomatic patients were selected on the basis of elevated blood lipid levels; thus the study was designed to observe early atherosclerotic lesions. The patients were given a therapeutic regimen of moderate dietary intervention followed by major lipid reduction (fenofibrate, 200 mg bid, plus nicotinic acid, 1 g qid). Matched serial femoral angiograms obtained at 6-month intervals were analyzed using a method developed by Crawford (71). The degree of atherosclerotic change seen in the first five patients provided evidence for a regression of disease in all five. Stenosis reduction was correlated with an average decrease of 50 percent in the LDL levels ($r = 0.58$).

In an angiographic study of more advanced disease, Duffield (72) described quantitative evidence of disease stabilization. In this controlled radiologic study, 24 patients with stable intermittent claudication were randomized to a diet-and-drug therapy or to routine care which included weight reduction and smoking cessation when necessary. In the treatment group, mean cholesterol levels were reduced by 25 percent and triglyceride levels by 40 percent. Patients in the usual-care group showed no significant lipid or body-weight changes. Paired, matched femoral angiograms, obtained an average of 19 months apart, were read blindly by two observers, who found significantly fewer arterial segments ($P < 0.01$) exhibiting progression in the treatment group than in the controls. The mean increment in the arterial surface area covered by plaque (square millimeter per segment per year) among treated patients was only 34 percent of that observed among the nontreated patients.

Implications for the Future: Management of the Postsurgery Patient

The patient who has undergone peripheral vascular reconstruction or coronary bypass surgery is at high risk for continued disease progression, which may manifest itself in new clinical symptoms after the initial arterial lesion has been ameliorated with surgery. Accelerated atherosclerotic change, including the formation of nonocclusive concentric fibrous plaques that are morphologically indistinguishable from presurgical atherosclerosis, was demonstrated in all patent saphenous vein coronary artery bypass grafts older than 30 days in a study by Bulkley (73). Bourassa (74) found coronary bypass graft occlusions at 1 year to be the consequence of fibrous intimal proliferation, a phenomenon also responsible for significant stenosis ($P < 0.01$) in 5 to 15 percent of all patent grafts.

The evidence to date indicates that the stabilization and reversal of atherosclerosis can occur in humans. What remains to be learned from controlled clinical trials is: How frequently does reversal happen? How long does it take to become evident? And does the change occur uniformly? Seven controlled randomized clinical trials testing the effect of major plasma lipid reductions on reversibility are now (1986) in progress. Large-scale epidemiologic studies have provided sufficient evidence to indicate that smoking cessation and the control of blood pressure are appropriate in the management of the coronary-prone patient. If these current clinical trials demonstrate the efficacy of lipid lowering, then aggressive lipid reduction should be added to the postoperative regimen for all vascular surgery patients.

In addition to anticipating potential problems which may arise from disease progression in the graft per se, the surgeon should be aware of the high probability of substantial atherosclerosis in other vessel beds (75,76). In a 1962 necropsy study, Mitchell and Schwartz (77) showed that 79 patients with large coronary lesions had more extensive disease, more stenosis, and more plaque ulceration in carotid and iliac arteries than 137 comparably aged unselected patients. These authors concluded that "there is a tendency for the disease to develop in parallel in different arterial systems, and in most of the patients examined, severe disease in one site was accompanied by severe disease elsewhere." The management of the postoperative coronary bypass patient should therefore be augmented with the systematic monitoring of plaque development in other peripheral and coronary vessels.

The improvement of noninvasive and minimally invasive vascular imaging techniques to track the atherosclerotic process in postoperative patients seems certain to have a major impact on the long-term care of the vascular patient. Although the diagnostic value of selective arteriography outweighs its relative risk and discomfort during the preoperative period, its repeated use for continued postoperative monitoring is not appropriate for many patients. Digital subtraction angiography, contrast-enhanced computerized tomography, high-resolution ultrasonography, and nuclear magnetic resonance techniques should soon make it feasible to follow the postoperative course of large peripheral and central vessels in many more patients.

References

1. Malinow MR: Regression in nonhuman primates. Circ Res 1980, 46:311.
2. Armstrong ML: Regression of atherosclerosis. In Paoletti R, Gotto A (eds): *Atherosclerosis Reviews III*. New York, Raven, 1976, pp 137–182.
3. Anitschkow N: A history of experimentation on arterial atherosclerosis in animals. In Cowdry EV (ed): *Arteriosclerosis: A Survey of the Problem*. New York, Macmillan, 1933, pp 271–322.
4. Buja LM, Kita T, Goldstein JL, Watanabe Y, Brown MS: Cellular pathology of progressive atherosclerosis in the WHHL rabbit. An animal model of familial hypercholesterolemia. Arteriosclerosis 1983, 3:87.
5. Horlick K, Katz LN: Retrogression of atherosclerotic lesions on cessation of cholesterol feeding in the chick. J Lab Clin Med 1949, 34:1427.
6. Constantinides P, Gutmann-Auersperg N, Hospes D: Production of advanced cholesterol atherosclerosis in the rabbit. Arch Pathol 1958, 70:712.
7. Friedman M, Byers SO: Observations concerning the evolution of atherosclerosis in the rabbit after cessation of cholesterol feeding. Am J Pathol 1963, 43:349.
8. Prichard RW: Spontaneous atherosclerosis in pigeons. In Roberts JC, Straus R (eds): *Comparative Atherosclerosis*. New York, Harper & Row, 1965, pp 45–49.
9. Clarkson TB, King JS, Lofland HB, Feldner MA, Bullock BC: Pathologic characteristics and composition of diet-aggravated atherosclerotic plaques during "regression." Exp Mol Pathol 1973, 19:267.
10. Wagner WD, Clarkson TB: Effect on regression potential of atherosclerosis produced by intermittent or continuous hypercholesterolemia. Atherosclerosis 1977, 27:369.
11. Wagner WD, Clarkson TB, Foster J: Contrasting effects of ethane-1-hydroxy-1,1-diphosphonate (EHDP) on the regression of 2 types of dietary-induced atherosclerosis. Atherosclerosis 1977, 27:419.
12. Hrapchak BB, Bond MG, Wood LL, Hostetler JR: Time courses of diet-exacerbated carotid artery atherogenesis in the White Carneau pigeon. Atherosclerosis 1980, 35:243.
13. Kottke BA, Unni KK, Carlo IA, Subbiah MTR: Early chemical and structural changes during regression of spontaneous atherosclerotic lesions after intestinal bypass surgery. Circulation 1974, 50:III-93.
14. Gomes MM, Kottke BA, Bernatz P, Titus JL: Effect of ileal bypass on aortic atherosclerosis of White Carneau pigeons. Surgery 1971, 70:353.
15. Subbiah MT, Dicke BA, Kottke BA, Carlo IA, Dinh DM: Regression of naturally occurring atherosclerotic lesions in pigeon aorta by intestinal bypass surgery. Atherosclerosis 1978, 31:117.
16. Peterson JE, Hirst AE: Studies on the relation of diet, cholesterol and atheroma in chickens. Circulation 1951, 3:116.
17. Bevans M, Davidson JD, Kendall FE: Regression of lesions in canine atherosclerosis. Arch Pathol 1951, 51:288.
18. DePalma RG, Bellon EM, Klein L, Koletsky S, Insull W: Ap-

proaches to evaluating regression of experimental atherosclerosis. Adv Exp Med Biol 1977, 82:459.
19. Steiner A, Kendall FE, Bevans M: Production of arteriosclerosis in dogs by cholesterol and thiouracil feeding. Am Heart J 1949, 38:34.
20. Geer JC, Guidry MA: Experimental canine atherosclerosis. In Roberts JC, Straus R (eds): *Comparative Atherosclerosis*. New York, Harper & Row, 1965, pp 170–185.
21. DePalma RG, Hubay CA, Insull W, Robinson AV, Hartman PH: Progression and regression of experimental atherosclerosis. Surg Gynecol Obstet 1970, 131:633.
22. DePalma RG, Bellon EM, Koletsky S, Schneider DL: Atherosclerotic plaque regression in rhesus monkeys induced by bile acid sequestrant. Exp Mol Pathol 1979, 31:423.
23. Wissler RW: Atherosclerosis in nonhuman primates. Vet Sci Comp Med 1977, 21:351.
24. DePalma RG, Koletsky S, Bellon EM, Insull W: Failure of regression of atherosclerosis in dogs with moderate cholesterolemia. Atherosclerosis 1977, 27:297.
25. Adams CWM, Morgan RS, Bayliss OB: No regression of atheroma over one year in rabbits previously fed a cholesterol-enriched diet. Atherosclerosis 1973, 18:429.
26. Mann GV, Andrus SB: Xanthomatosis and atherosclerosis produced by diet in an adult rhesus monkey. J Lab Clin Med 1956, 48:533.
27. Malinow MR, McLaughlin P, Papworth L, Naito HK, Lewis L, McNulty WP: A model for therapeutic interventions on established coronary atherosclerosis in a nonhuman primate. Adv Exp Med Biol 1976, 67:3.
28. Taylor CB, Cox GE, Manalo-Estrella P, Southworth J: Atherosclerosis in rhesus monkeys: I. Arterial lesions associated with hypercholesterolemia induced by dietary fat and cholesterol. Arch Pathol 1962, 74:16.
29. Bond MG, Bullock BC, Bellinger DA, Hamm TE: Myocardial infarction in a large colony of nonhuman primates with coronary artery atherosclerosis. Am J Pathol 1980, 101:675.
30. Wissler RW, Vesselinovitch D, Hughes R: A comparison of the aortic atherosclerotic response in the rhesus and stumptailed monkey using rations rich in vegetable fat, with and without added cholesterol. Am J Pathol 1972, 66:92a.
31. Kramsch DM: Personal communication, 1971.
32. Portman OW, Alexander M, Maruffo CA: Nutritional control of arterial lipid composition in squirrel monkeys. Major ester classes and types of phospholipids. J Nutr 1967, 91:35.
33. Armstrong ML, Warner ED, Connor WE: Regression of coronary atheromatosis in rhesus monkeys. Circ Res 1970, 17:59.
34. Armstrong ML, Megan MB: Lipid depletion in atheromatous coronary arteries in rhesus monkeys after regression diets. Circ Res 1972, 30:675.
35. Armstrong ML, Megan MB: Arterial fibrous proteins in cynomolgus monkeys after atherogenic and regression diets. Circ Res 1975, 36:256.
36. Stary HC: Progression and regression of experimental atherosclerosis in rhesus monkeys. In Goldsmith EF, Morr-Hankowsky J (eds): *Medical Primatology*. Basel, Karger, 1972, pp 356–367.
37. Tucker CF, Catsulis C, Strong JP, Eggen DA: Regression of early cholesterol induced aortic lesions in rhesus monkeys. Am J Pathol 1971, 65:493.
38. Wissler RW, Vesselinovitch D, Borensztajn J, Hughes R: Regression of severe atherosclerosis in cholestyramine treated rhesus monkeys with or without a low-fat, low-cholesterol diet. Circulation 1975, 52:II-16.
39. Wissler RW, Vesselinovitch D: Studies of regression of advanced atherosclerosis in experimental animals and man. Ann NY Acad Sci 1976, 275:363.
40. Vesselinovitch D, Wissler RW: Prevention and regression in animal models by diet and cholestyramine. In Hauss WH, Wissler RW, Lehmann R (eds): *International Symposium on the State of Prevention and Therapy in Human Arteriosclerosis and in Animal Models*. Opladen, Westdeutscher Verlag, 1978, pp 127–137.
41. Vesselinovitch D, Wissler RW, Borensztajn J, Schaffner T: The effect of diets with or without cholestyramine on the lesion components of atherosclerotic plaques. Fed Proc 1978, 37:835.
42. Wissler RW: Current status of regression studies. In Paoletti R, Gotto A (eds): *Atherosclerosis Reviews III*. New York, Raven, 1976, pp 213–229.
43. Wissler W: Evidence for regression of advanced atherosclerotic plaques. Artery 1979, 5:398.
44. Bond MG, Bullock BC, Clarkson TB, Lehner NDM: The effect of plasma cholesterol concentration on "regression" of primate atherosclerosis. Am J Pathol 1966, 82:69a.
45. Bond MG, Bullock BC, Lehner NDM, Clarkson TB: Regression of primate coronary artery atherogenesis at 200 vs 300 mg/dL plasma cholesterol concentration. Stroke 1978, 9:97.
46. Vesselinovitch D, Wissler RW, Hughes R, Borensztajn J: Reversal of advanced atherosclerosis in rhesus monkeys. Part 1: Light-microscopic studies. Atherosclerosis 1976, 23:155.
47. DePalma RG, Klein L, Bellon EM, Koletsky S: Regression of atherosclerotic plaques in rhesus monkeys: Angiographic, morphologic and angiochemical changes. Arch Surg 1980, 115:1268.
48. Vesselinovitch D, Wissler RW: Quantitation of lesions during progression and regression of atherosclerosis in rhesus monkeys. In Naito H (ed): *Nutrition and Heart Disease*. New York, SP Medical & Scientific, 1982, p 121.
49. Wissler RW, Vesselinovitch D, Schaffner JT, Glagov S: Quantitating rhesus monkey atherosclerosis progression and regression with time. In Gotto AM, Smith LC, Allen B (eds): *Atherosclerosis V*. New York, Springer-Verlag, 1980, p 757.
50. Wissler RW: The emerging pathobiology of atherosclerosis. Artery 1979, 5:409.
51. Aschoff L: *Lectures in Pathology*. New York, Hoeber, 1924.
52. Beitzke H: Zur Entstehung der Atherosclerose. Virchows Arch Pathol Anat 1928, 267:625.
53. Malmros H: The relation of nutrition to health. A statistical study of the effect of the war-time on arteriosclerosis, cardiosclerosis, tuberculosis and diabetes. Acta Med Scand 1950, 246(Suppl):137.
54. Strom A, Jensen RA: Mortality from circulatory diseases in Norway 1940–1945. Lancet 1951, 1:126.
55. Vartiainen I, Kanerva K: Arteriosclerosis and war-time. Ann Med Int Fenniae 1947, 36:748.
56. Brozek J, Wells S, Keys A: Medical aspects of semistarvation and Leningrad (siege 1941–42). Am Rev Soviet Med 1946, 4:70.
57. Schettler G: Cardiovascular diseases during and after World War II: A comparison of the Federal Republic of Germany with other European countries. Prev Med 1979, 8:581.
58. Wilens SL: The resorption of arterial atheromatous deposits in wasting disease. Am J Pathol 1947, 23:793.
59. Mordasini R, Klose G, Greten H: Secondary Type II hyperlipoproteinemia in patients with anorexia nervosa. Metabolism 1978, 27:71.
60. London JW, Rosenberg SE, Draper JW, Almy TP: The effect of estrogens on atherosclerosis. Am J Intern Med 1961, 55:63.
61. Rivin AU, Dimitroff SP: The incidence and severity of atherosclerosis in estrogen-treated males and in females with hypoestrogenic or a hyperestrogenic state. Circulation 1954, 9:533.
62. McGill HC: Fatty streaks in the coronary arteries and aorta. Lab Invest 18:560, 1968.
63. Berry JF, Resch JA, Baker AB: Serum lipids and cerebral atherosclerosis in terminal cancer patients. Neurology 1966, 16:673.
64. Ost CR, Stenson S: Regression of peripheral atherosclerosis during

therapy with high doses of nicotinic acid. Scand J Clin Lab Invest [Suppl] 1967, 99:241.

65. Basta LL, Williams C, Kioschos JM, Spector AA: Regression of atherosclerotic stenosing lesions of the renal arteries and spontaneous cure of systemic hypertension through control of hyperlipidemia. Am J Med 1976, 61:420.

66. Thompson GR, Lowenthal R, Myant MD: Plasma exchange in management of homozygous familial hypercholesterolemia. Lancet 1975, 1:1208.

67. Roth D, Kostuk WJ: Noninvasive and invasive demonstration of spontaneous regression of coronary artery disease. Circulation 1980, 62:888.

68. Barndt R, Blankenhorn DH, Crawford DW, Brooks SH: Regression and progression of early femoral atherosclerosis in treated hyperlipoproteinemic patients. Ann Intern Med 1977, 86:139.

69. Terry EN, Rouen LR, Class RH, Katz MC, Redisch W: Attempts to delay progression in occlusive atherosclerosis. Ann NY Acad Sci 1976, 275:379.

70. Olsson AG, Carlson LA, Erikson U, Helmius G, Hemmingsson A, Ruhn G: Regression of computer estimated femoral atherosclerosis after pronounced serum lipid lowering in patients with asymptomatic hyperlipidaemia. Lancet 1982, 2:1311.

71. Crawford DW, Brooks SH, Selzer RH, Barndt R, Beckenbach ES, Blankenhorn DH: Computer densitometry for angiographic assessment of arterial cholesterol content and gross pathology in human atherosclerosis. J Lab Clin Med 1977, 2:378.

72. Duffield RGM, Miller NE, Jamieson CW, Lewis B: A controlled trial of plasma lipid reduction in peripheral atherosclerosis—An interim report. Br J Surg 1982, 69(Suppl):S3.

73. Bulkley BH, Hutchins GM: Accelerated "atherosclerosis." A morphologic study of 97 saphenous vein coronary artery bypass grafts. Circulation 1977, 55:163.

74. Bourassa MG, Campeau L, Lesperance J, Grondin CM: Changes in grafts and coronary arteries after saphenous vein aortocoronary bypass surgery: Results at repeat angiography. Circulation 1982, 65(Suppl II):90.

75. Sternby NH: Atherosclerosis in a defined population. Acta Pathol Microbiol Scand [Suppl] 1968, 194:7.

76. Young W, Gofman JW, Tandy R, Malamud N, Waters E: The quantitation of atherosclerosis III. The extent of correlation of degrees of atherosclerosis within and between the coronary and cerebral vascular beds. Am J Cardiol 1960, 6:300.

77. Mitchell JRA, Schwartz CJ: Relationship between arterial disease in different sites. A study of the aorta and coronary, carotid and iliac arteries. Br Med J 1962, 1:1293.

Chapter 18

PERCUTANEOUS TRANSLUMINAL ANGIOPLASTY

GERALD L. WOLF

Twenty years ago, Charles Dotter and Mel Judkins (1) demonstrated that the hemodynamic effects of atherosclerotic disease in narrowed or even occluded arteries can be modified by the passage of a large angiographic catheter through the lesion. In a series of clinical and experimental studies they speculated that the artheromatous mass is soft and inelastic and can, therefore, be compressed or molded during the passage of this rigid catheter (2–3). Dotter and Judkins called the process percutaneous transluminal angioplasty (PTA) and began the study of a clinical technique that is an alternative to direct surgical intervention for selected patients. Their ideas were seminal but have undergone considerable refinement in recent times, and some investigators believe that further major improvements can be expected. Because their coaxial technique (Figure 18-1) is more frequently utilized for nonvascular interventions today, they have not received just credit for demonstrating that guide wires and catheters can safely be passed through and remain within a vascular conduit narrowed or occluded by plaque. Crossing the lesion with the appropriate wires and catheters remains the biggest technical feat in PTA.

A coaxial catheter produces a large hole at the vascular access site—a technical problem for percutaneous approaches, but not for arteriotomy access sites. Rigid catheters have a potentially large dilating force, but they also produce shearing forces over much of the length of the artery during their passage to and through the treatment site. Except for surgeons in a few European centers, most surgeons feared that the distal embolization of plaques, and other complications, would seriously compromise the result of the treatment. Nonetheless, in the late seventies the Dotter catheter was used to perform several thousand angioplasties in a few enthusiastic centers; there were few significant embolizations, and the results were generally acceptable. While Porstman, Zeitler, and others were steadily increasing their experience with rigid-catheter angioplasty, in 1976 Andreas Gruentzig created the double-lumen balloon catheter that overcame many of the limitations of the Dotter technique and greatly expanded the clinical applications of PTA (4).

Although earlier workers had recognized the potential advantages of a balloon catheter, they were also aware of their limitations. Balloons expand in the direction of least resistance, and very elastic materials, such as latex, tended to track up or down the arterial lumen rather than applying a radial dilating force. Gruentzig's modification (4) utilized polyvinyl chloride—tougher, but still compliant—and could be inflated from a lumen separate from that used for the guide wire and contrast media injections. The method of placing and utilizing the Gruentzig angioplasty catheter is shown in Figure 18-2. Utilizing one lumen, the radiologist can perform the technical maneuvers necessary to position the balloon. Once in place, the balloon can be inflated through the second lumen to accomplish the dilation or recanalization.

The several advantages of the balloon catheter are:

1. It can be introduced through a small percutaneous puncture site.

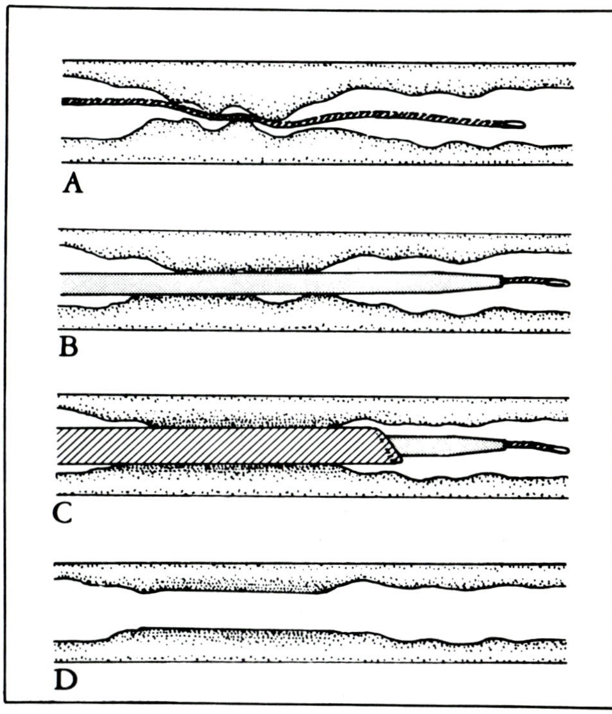

FIGURE 18-1. Coaxial catheter angioplasty. (*A*) A guide wire is manipulated through the stenosis. (*B*) A tapered no. 8-F Teflon catheter is passed over the guide wire, beginning the dilation. (*C*) A no. 12F Teflon catheter is passed coaxially over the no. 8F catheter, completing the dilation. (*D*) The remodeled lumen now permits greater blood flow. (From Ring E, McLean GK: *Interventional Radiology: Principles and Techniques*. Boston, Little, Brown, 1981. By permission of Little, Brown.)

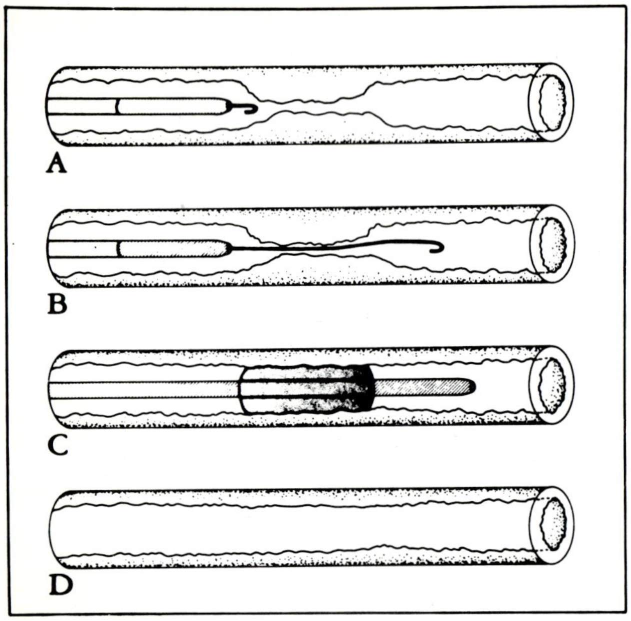

FIGURE 18-2. Balloon catheter angioplasty. (*A*) A catheter and a guide wire are advanced up to a stenotic lesion. (*B*) A guide wire is passed through the lesion. (*C*) A balloon catheter is advanced over the guide wire, and the balloon is inflated in the narrowed area. (*D*) The balloon is deflated, leaving an increased luminal diameter. (From Ring E, McLean GK: *Interventional Radiology: Principles and Techniques*. Boston, Little, Brown, 1981. By permission of Little, Brown.)

2. The dilating force is applied radially.
3. The dilated diameter is large relative to the puncture site.
4. The inflated diameter is variable and under operator control.
5. The surfaces are smooth.
6. The inserting, positioning, and removing of the catheter are all expedited.

In comparison with the rigid catheter, the only apparent disadvantage of the balloon catheter is less dilating force. This disadvantage is being minimized with the use of tougher and less compliant materials for balloon construction. Although better angioplasty catheters will evolve, the clinical applications are not seriously limited by the lack of available dilating force.

Shortly after double-lumen balloon catheters became available, PTA experienced an explosive growth phase, and current balloon catheter sales are in excess of 50,000 per year. It seems unlikely that the majority of these catheters will pass their expiration date unused. Nor is there a dearth of arterial lesions that can be dilated. The medical literature reports, in greater or lesser detail, the results of angioplasty in more than 10,000 cases. Angioplasty has been successful in nearly every named artery in the human body as well as in several other tubular structures, including many surgically created conduits. There are undoubtedly thousands of unreported cases, and an unknown percentage of these have experienced minor or major complications.

Despite this apparent surfeit of information, many important questions remain to be answered. The actual mechanism(s) whereby angioplasty accomplishes its effective enlargement of vessel lumen are still controversial. Potential adjunctive interventions such as drugs, diet, smoking, or exercise could minimize the adverse response to the trauma of either bypass surgery or angioplasty, yet their effects are virtually undocumented. Broad generalizations about the relative merits of surgery, angioplasty, or less invasive treatments have yet to be agreed upon. No randomized controlled trials of bypass surgery or angioplasty in identical populations of patients have yet been reported, and thus direct comparisons of safety and efficacy are not possible.

The individual patient should often consider many factors in selecting from among therapeutic options. Ideally, these options are weighed by a competent team of physicians and presented fairly to the patient for the patient's considered judgment. It is clear that bypass surgery and angioplasty may differ significantly with respect to the risks, indications, durability, costs, and desirability for a particular circumstance. The purpose of this chapter is to present the current state of the angioplastic art to students of vascular surgery. Excellent books on interventional radiology or angioplasty can also be recommended (5,6).

Technical Considerations

There is general agreement that PTA should be restricted to hemodynamically significant lesions that are accessible to the catheter. All the percutaneous approaches commonly used for diagnostic arteriography are also used to insert catheters for angioplasty. Retrograde femoral catheterization is used most for iliac, renal, and supradiaphragmatic arteries. The left axillary approach is usually best for visceral vessels and for the occasional renal artery that arises from the aorta at a very acute angle. The antegrade femoral approach is the most direct route for superficial femoral artery and popliteal dilations. The frequent subcutaneous location of vein bypass grafts for the extremities allows the direct puncture of the graft, if necessary, when treating vein graft stenosis.

In general, the closest and least circuitous path to the lesion is preferred when this avenue does not add risk to the procedure. In special cases, surgical access may be advisable despite the additional costs and risks.

ADVANCING CATHETERS AND GUIDE WIRES THROUGH THE LESION

Most angiographers have already developed the skills of safe selective catheterization under fluoroscopic guidance. Although some blind catheterizations are occasionally possible, and new catheters are being tested that find their own way past an obstruction, the excellent visualization of the catheter, guide wire, and local vascular anatomy is essential for routine angioplasty. Despite interesting research attempts to characterize arterial compliance, our own included, good visualization of the dilated site during and after angioplasty remains important for performing the dilation safely and for deciding when adequate dilation for a particular lesion has been achieved. Angiographic documentation of the immediate results of the procedure is also of great benefit. Thus under most circumstances, angioplasty is best performed where these imaging needs can be met. In most cases, this means in the angiographic suite.

Concentric stenoses in straight vessels are usually not difficult to catheterize, and standard guide wire and catheter techniques are generally successful. When the vessel is tortuous or the plaques are eccentric, the catheterization is more difficult. The lesion is usually approached with a tapered catheter, and then a floppy straight or J-wire is gently pushed across the obstruction. A diagnostic angiogram is used to localize the lesion, often with the aid of skin markers visible by fluoroscopy. The angiographer must be aware of when the wire has passed the lesion, and the tip of the wire must remain within the vessel. Special wires and techniques have been developed to make it easier for the wire to pass the lesion and advance into the distal vessel without inadvertently tracking the subintima or even exiting the vessel completely (7).

Once the guide wire is past the lesion, the catheter is advanced through the obstruction. This begins the dilation process, for the catheter is usually larger than the residual lumen and also affords purchase for the passage of a stiffer wire into the distal site. Before the stiff wire is introduced, drugs such as heparin can be administered since the danger of vessel perforation is by this time considerably diminished.

Then the stiff wire is carefully positioned across the lesion into the distal site, and the tapered catheter is removed with care to minimize abrading motions of the guide wire which would needlessly traumatize the endothelium. The balloon catheter can then be brought down and across the lesion. These catheters do not follow a wire as well as diagnostic catheters and, being a little larger, resist passage both at the puncture site and in crossing the lesion.

Clinical judgment is required when the catheter for dilating the lesion is selected. The tougher polyethylene catheters have been more commonly used than polyvinyl in recent times. The lesion is expected to have some elastic recoil after dilation, so the balloon should be about 10 to 20 percent larger in inflated diameter than the *desired* lumen size. In estimating the size of the normal vessel and the size of the desired lumen after angioplasty, the operator must adjust for the magnification on the diagnostic angiogram. There are usually choices of the length of the balloon as well as the diameter, and one usually selects a length three to four times the length of the stenosis so that the catheter will remain in place during inflation. For long obstructions, such a range of lengths is not available, and one may even have to inflate the longest available balloon of satisfactory diameter several times to treat the entire length of the obstruction.

Mechanisms of Angioplasty

Even though thousands of balloon angioplasties have been performed, it is still a little surprising that the procedure works. To ameliorate clinical symptoms, angioplasty must increase the luminal cross-sectional area, leading to decreased resistance to blood flow. Sometimes the luminal enlargement that relieves symptoms is relatively minimal, yet on occasion, angioplasty can accomplish large increases in lumen size. To be effective, the inflated balloon must induce an irreversible change in the plaque or vessel. In biomechanical terms, maintaining a new shape after the removal of a deforming force is a plastic property of the material. The elastic properties of the artery or plaque oppose effective dilation and complicate experiments to define the mechanism.

The potential mechanisms of enlarging the lumen include (8):

1. Compaction of the plaque
2. Redistributive remodeling of the plaque
3. Embolization of plaque constituents
4. Plastic stretching of the arterial wall
5. Phagocytic removal of volume during healing

COMPACTION OF THE PLAQUE

The explanation first offered for angioplasty was an actual compression of the plaque (2,3). However, the liquids and solids composing the plaque are incompressible. Although the force applied to the plaque is compressive, it is unlikely that "the plaque compresses and nothing is displaced or removed (4)." Histologic sections taken after angioplasty often show concentric rings within the plaque, suggesting compression, but this is undoubtedly due to the molding of the plaque rather than to an actual volume reduction.

REDISTRIBUTIVE REMODELING OF THE PLAQUE

It is not necessary to reduce the volume of the plaque in order to diminish its resistance to blood flow. If the volume is rearranged to occupy less space in the radial direction but more in the linear direction, the resistance will be dramatically lowered. This is because of Poiseuville's law relating resistance to flow directly to length of the tube but inversely to the fourth power of the radius. It is clear that some plaques redistribute (Figure 18-3). We also recognize this process in many clinical cases when careful measurements are possible (Figure 18-4). However, it is common experience that some plaques are soft and some are rock hard. Although some plaques may redistribute, clearly not all of them are capable of this response at pressures less than that necessary to rupture the artery. The process is difficult to study even in actual atherosclerotic vessels obtained at autopsy because the mechanical properties of the plaque and wall are significantly changed by excision or cold storage (9).

EMBOLIZATION OF PLAQUE CONSTITUENTS

The volume of the plaque would be reduced if either liquid or particulate portions of the plaque were released by the abrasion or compression of angioplasty. The endothelium is nearly always desquamated by angioplasty, but this would not enlarge the lumen significantly. The plaque also frequently fragments in situ,

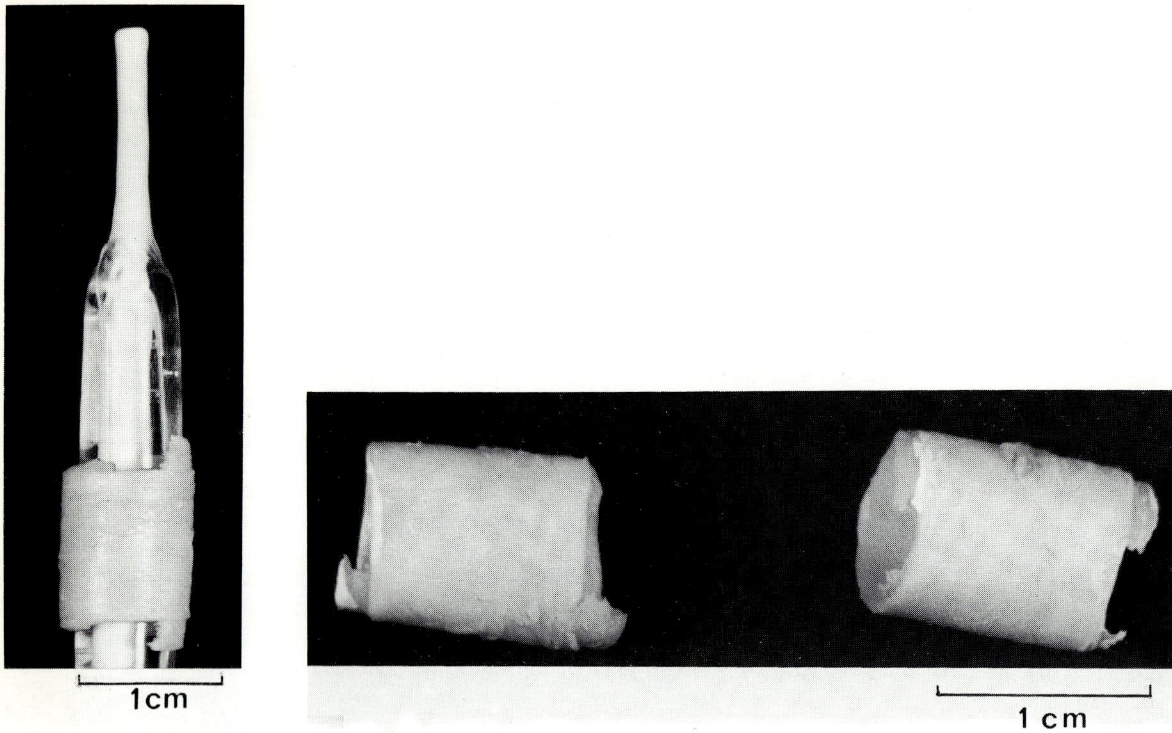

A B

FIGURE 18-3. Distributive plaque remodeling in a postmortem arterial specimen. Atheromatous material is being expressed from inside the artery during balloon inflation (*A*). When the balloon is removed, the plaque retains its new configuration (*B*). (From Wolf GL, LeVeen RF, Ring EJ. Cardiovasc Intervent Radiol 1983, 7:11. By permission of Springer-Verlag.)

but this would do little to the net lumen size unless the plaque were actually stenting the arterial wall. It is perhaps fortunate that these plaque fragments are uncommonly freed for embolization, although this can happen (Figure 18-5).

The very high pressures applied by the balloon could express liquid material from the plaque and/or artery wall. In that event, the arterial lumen would be increased without accompanying evidence of peripheral bed embolization. Squeezing liquid out of the plaque would create the histologic impression of plaque compaction. However, it is unlikely that this occurs commonly in the clinical context of angioplasty.

IRREVERSIBLE STRETCHING OF THE ARTERIAL WALL

If it could be shown that plaque volume and shape were unchanged following dilation, then all the luminal enlargement would have to have occurred by expansion of the arterial tube. Since the plaque is principally in the intima, the media and adventitia may have nearly normal biomechanical properties. If a plastic change can occur in the arterial tube itself, it should be possible to demonstrate it in normal arteries. In fact, the absence of plaque would make the process easier to demonstrate. With appropriate attention to detail, it is easy to dilate normal arteries with balloon catheters, as we show below.

The principal components of the arterial wall are elastin, smooth muscle, and collagen. The properties of elastin suggest that it may be stretched several hundred percent without losing its elasticity. Thus the plastic change we are seeking does not reside in this component, although we must be aware that the lumen will be smaller after the balloon is removed by the amount of residual elasticity. This elasticity of normal arteries complicates quantitative measures in vitro because normal arteries are 80 percent larger in diameter when distended by physiological pressure than they are when removed. Arteries dilated in vivo recoil less, but still an appreciable amount, than arteries dilated in vitro.

The strongest and least elastic structure in the arterial wall is collagen. It is alleged to be virtually inextensible (10). However, our stress-strain experiments on normal arterial strips show that all layers of the artery stretch a considerable amount before they rupture (Figure 18-6). The strength of normal arteries seems ascribable to both the media and the adventitia. Stretching or rupturing collagen seems very dangerous if one views the process as leading to rents in the entire wall or to pseudoaneurysms. Indeed, overzealous angioplasty can do this to normal arteries (see below). However, angioplasty might also stretch or rupture the collagen fibers that connect one smooth muscle cell to the next, leaving an intact adventitial sleeve and some stretched medial bundles.

Finally, the stretch of angioplasty could damage the contractile function of the smooth-muscle cells directly. Smooth muscle does not sustain its contraction when challenged by excessive force, but we are looking for more than a temporary loss of tone. It has been possible to show that stretching the wall of arterial strips in vitro or in vivo blunts or abolishes their contractile

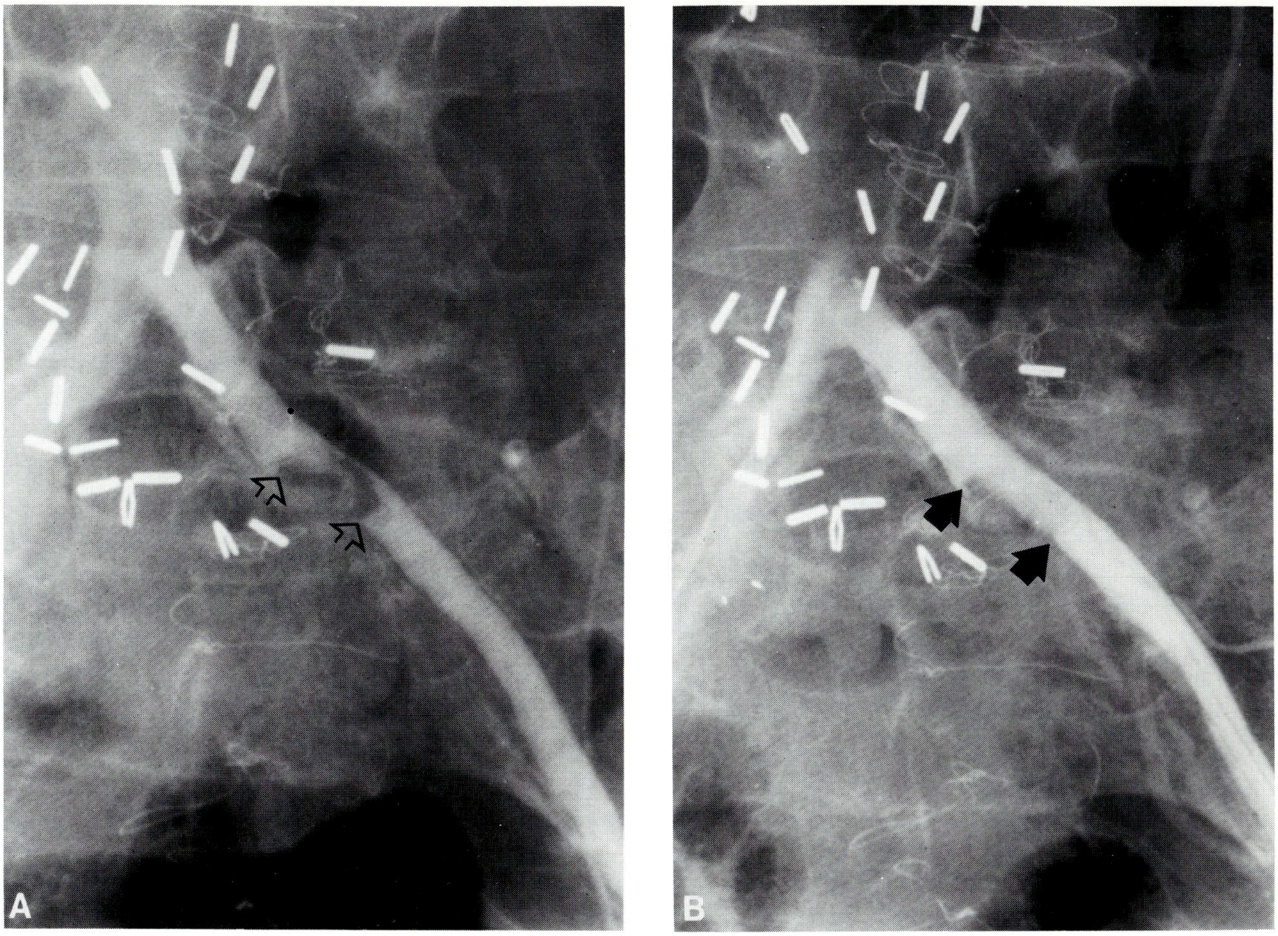

FIGURE 18-4. The length of this iliac lesion increases by 27 percent following angioplasty. (From Wolf CL, LeVeen RF, Ring EJ. Cardiovasc Intervent Radiol 1983, 7:11. By permission of Springer-Verlag.)

response to powerful vasoconstrictors (Figure 18-7) (11–12). Although experiments to date do not define the duration of this functional incompetency nor its mechanism, they do provide important information on how much an artery has to be stretched to enlarge the lumen by this mechanism. Stretching the artery in vivo by 30 percent attenuates the vasoconstrictor response, while stretches over 50 percent abolish the constrictor response to drugs (Figures 18-8, 18-9). Animal studies suggest that effective dilation actually destroys muscle cells at the dilated site. When the debris is removed, the wall is thinner (and the functional lumen more widely patent).

It appears likely that the efficacy of angioplasty does involve the stretching of the arterial tube, and future experiments will define both the benefits and risks that result. These considerations also affect the mechanism and results of angioplasty applied to other biological conduits such as vein grafts, bile ducts, ureters, etc.

REMODELING OF THE "CONTROLLED INJURY"

Although the usual concern about the inevitable trauma that accompanies angioplasty is directed to preventing thrombosis, spasm, and restenosis, it has been observed that films of the site taken some months later are much improved over those obtained immediately after angioplasty. On postangioplasty films there is nearly always some fuzziness reflecting damaged intima and fissures within the plaque or at the plaque-wall interface. This seems not to be a cause for alarm because these surface tears rarely remain patent for long. However, sometimes an extensive remodeling occurs following angioplasty (Figure 18-10). This process is most often seen in fibromuscular dysplasia but is also evident in atherosclerosis. I don't know of a case in which it has turned an incomplete dilation into a clinical success, however.

General Indications for Angioplasty

Physicians agonize over whether and when to perform angioplasty. In our society, this decision belongs to the patient! If angioplasty seems technically feasible, the patient should be offered it as a choice.

Although the physician may recognize that no randomized clinical trial of angioplasty versus surgery has been reported for *any* indication, and may realize that the two therapies are different in important ways affecting the expected outcome for

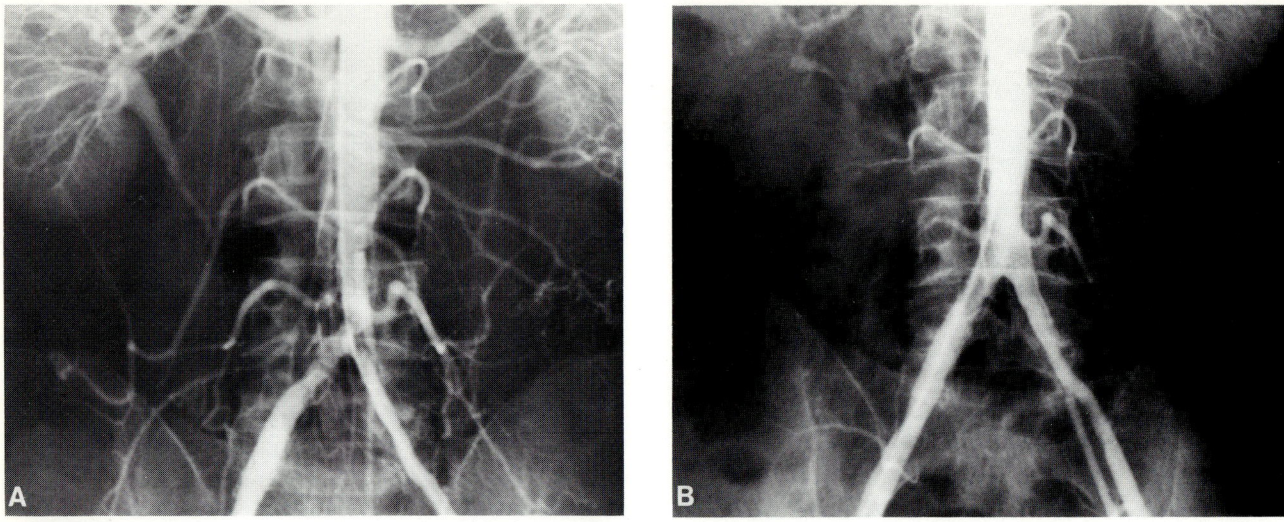

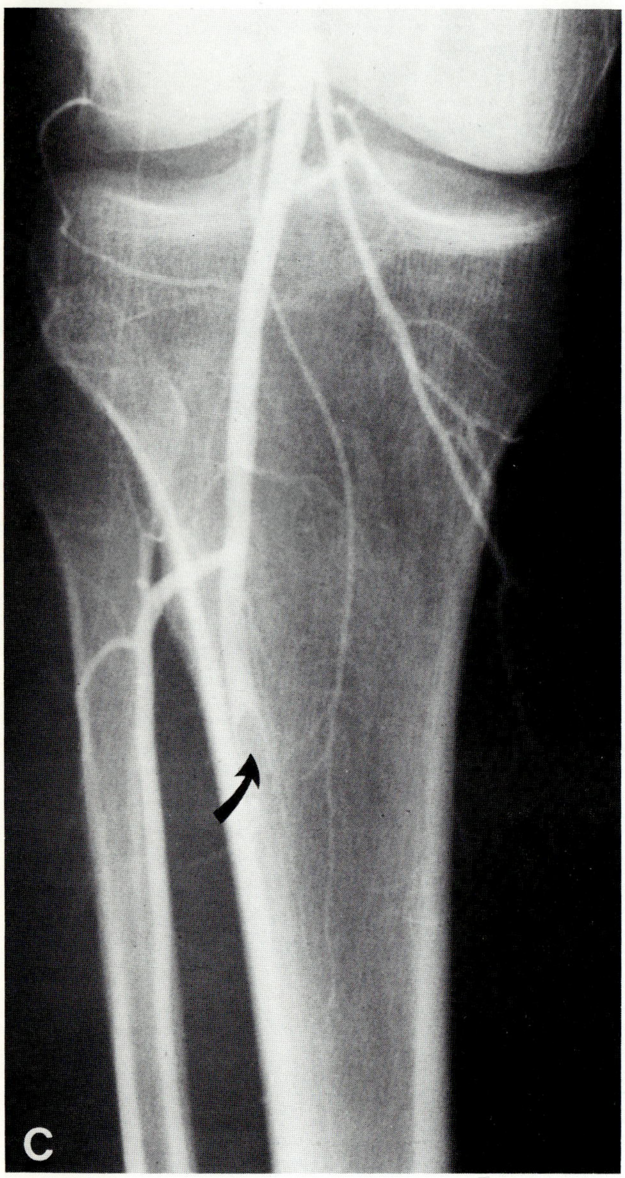

FIGURE 18-5. This patient with proximal iliac disease (*A*) had an excellent local result following angioplasty (***B***), but atheroembolism occurred down the opposite leg (***C***). The embolus was surgically removed, and its atheromatous nature was confirmed histologically. Both the patient and the surgeon were grateful that the final outcome was achieved via iliac PTA and popliteal embolectomy, each accomplished under local anesthesia. (From Wolf GL, LeVeen RF, Ring EJ. Cardiovasc Intervent Radiol 1983, 7:11. By permission of Springer-Verlag.)

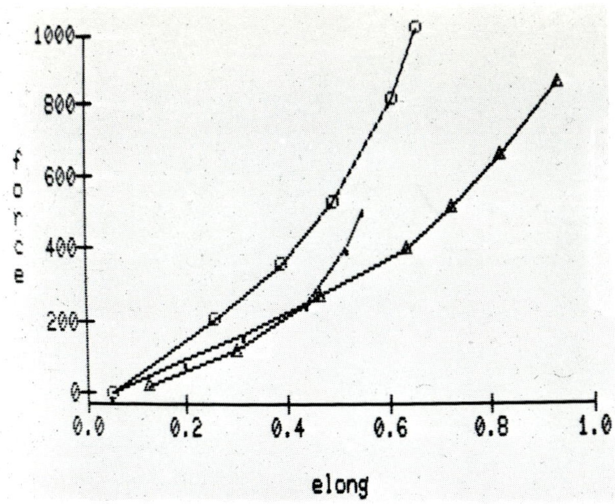

FIGURE 18-6. The stretch response of normal arterial strips. The whole artery (· · · O · · ·) elongates and withstands a large amount of force before rupture. When the intima and media are cut (· · · △ · · ·), the artery elongates more and ruptures with about 20 percent less force. When the adventitia is cut (. . . . . .), the artery still can elongate but ruptures with less force.

individual cases, and may be well aware that patients dread surgery and may select inferior treatment out of the hope that they might ''luck out,'' the physician is still required to present an objective review of the options to the patient for the patient, himself or herself, to select the preferred therapy.

We find that many patients appreciate a discussion of their options from the standpoint of best-case/worst-case considerations. Although one can review the available outcome statistics in terms of durability, complications, costs, hospitalization time, and disability time, the list of imponderables in any given case is usually so formidable that few laypersons could truly judge the odds for their own case. (*N.B.*: This is not a justification to make the decision for them.) Thus our patients want to know what the best that can happen is, what could be done if the worst happened, and what the personal recommendation of the medical team is.

The great attraction of angioplasty is that the treatment can be performed using only local anesthesia and causes less pain than the arteriogram itself. The patient may return to work within 48 hours with minimal postoperative recovery. The procedure carries an extremely low mortality and leads to few major complications. Most important, when a complication occurs after angioplasty, it only rarely makes surgical repair more difficult than it would have been had angioplasty not been attempted. Angioplasty is a focal form of therapy, and very few complications lead to significant deterioration. Distal embolization is the most likely cause of increased ischemia after angioplasty, yet it happened only in 8 of Ring's 1400 patients (13). In each of these cases, the atheromatous embolus was retrieved by an embolectomy, and no limb was lost. Subintimal dissection, with the conversion of a stenosis to an occlusion, occurs in about 2 percent of the cases, but for iliac and lower extremity disease does not usually interfere with preexisting collaterals and therefore does not cause deterioration in the local blood flow. The

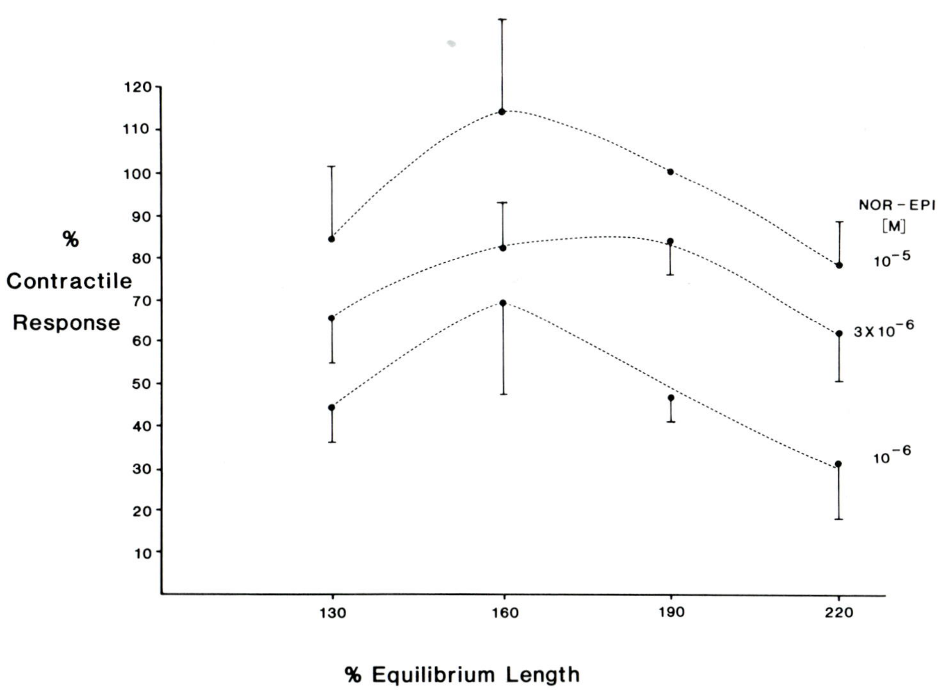

FIGURE 18-7. The influence of in vitro stretch upon the vasoconstrictor response to norepinephrine. Small stretches increase the response, but larger stretches attenuate the response. Arteries in vivo operate at about 160 percent of the in vitro length, so most of the effective dilations probably attenuate the vasoconstrictor response.

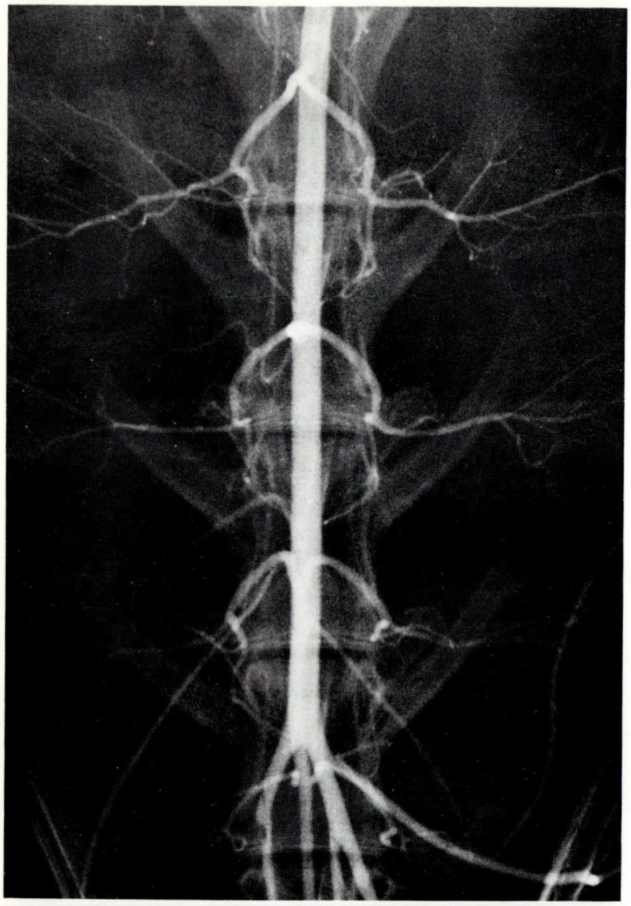

A

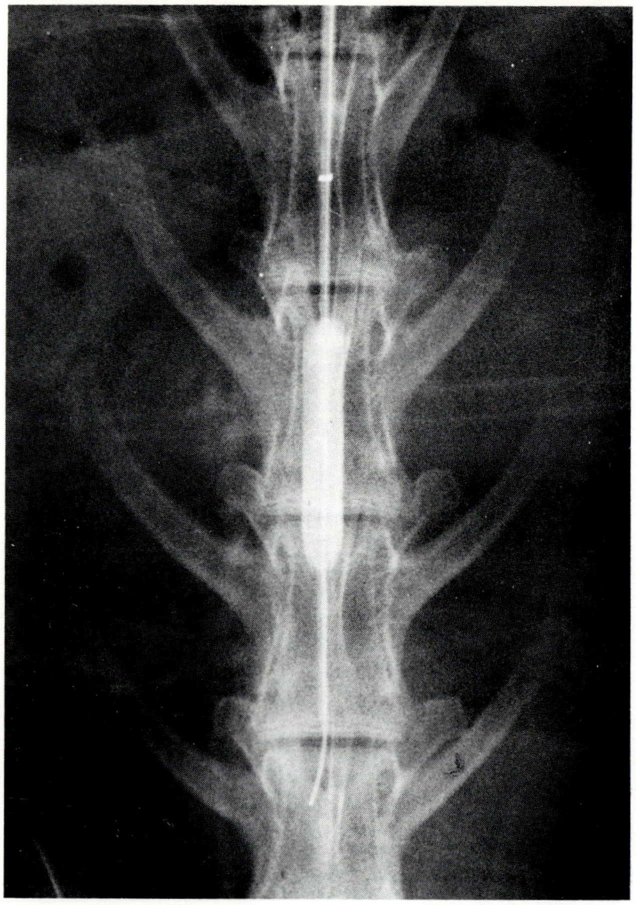

B

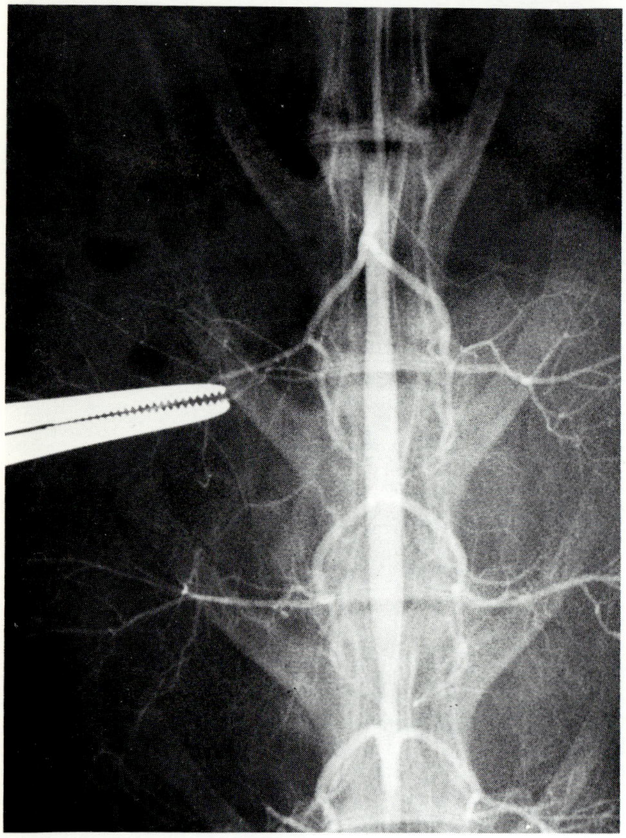

C

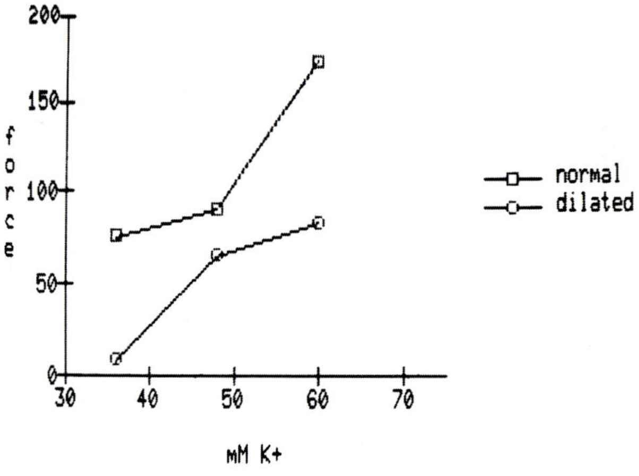

D

FIGURE 18-8. The influence of in vivo stretch upon the vasoconstrictor response in vitro. (*A*) Normal rabbit aorta; (*B*) a 40 percent in vivo stretch resulting in a slight aneurysm after the balloon is deflated (*C*). A vascular strip from the nondilated artery shows the expected dose response to a vasoconstrictor in vitro, while a strip from the dilated site is much less responsive (*D*).

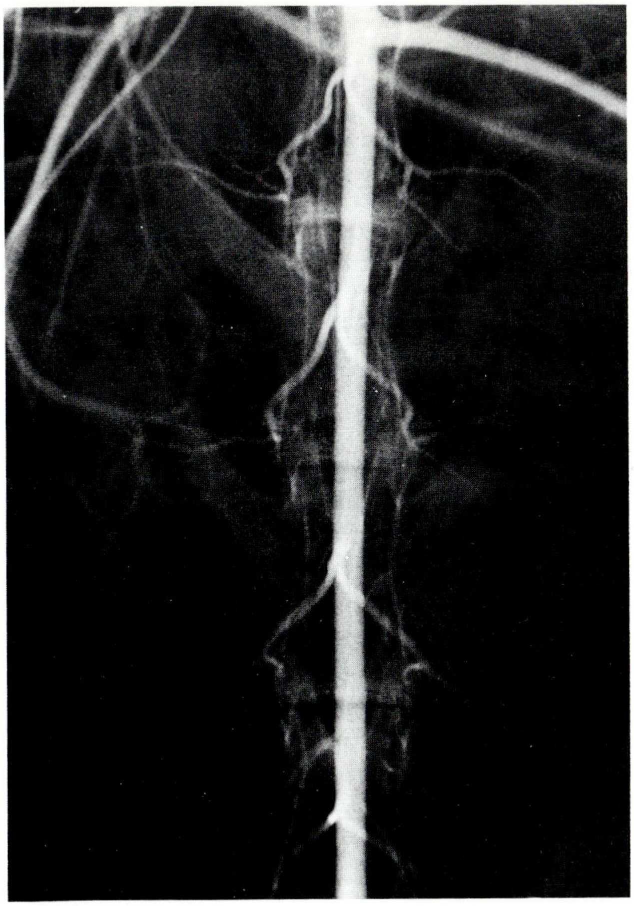

A

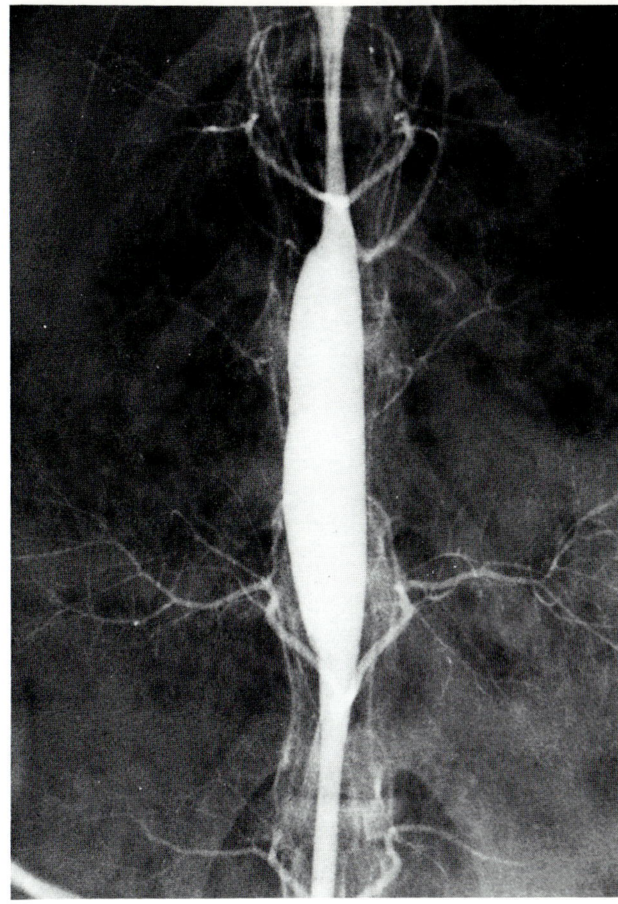

B

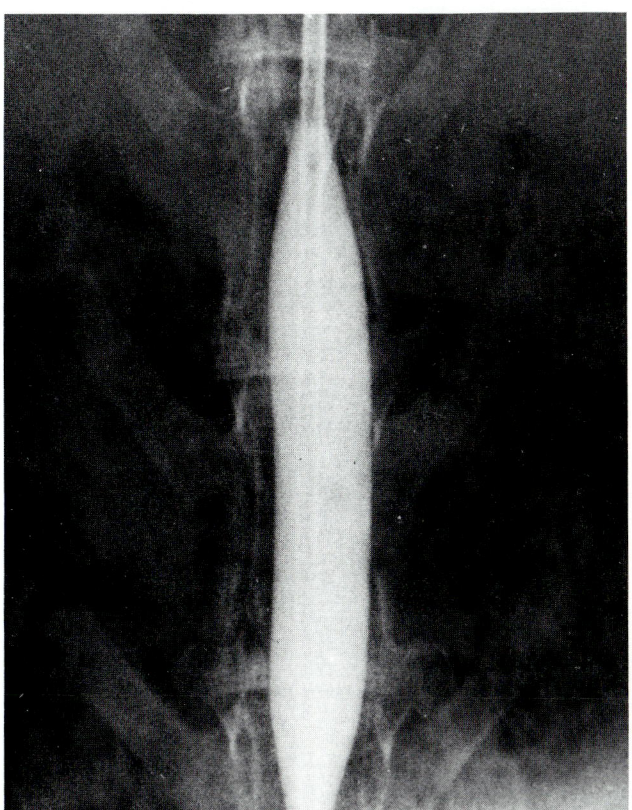

C

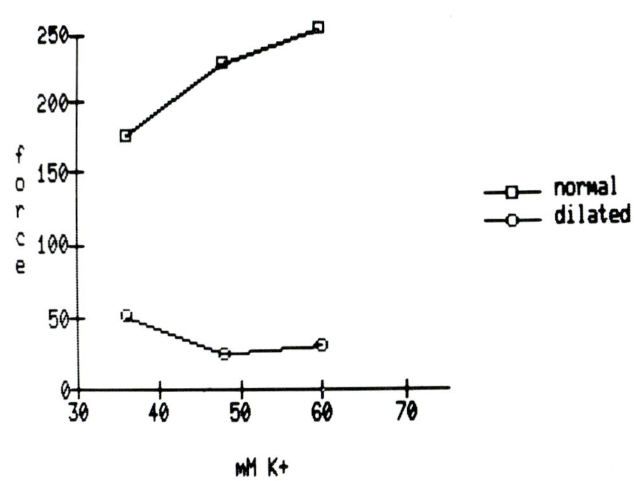

D

FIGURE 18-9. Overzealous angioplasty can create an aneurysm of a normal artery. Same sequence as Figure 18-8.

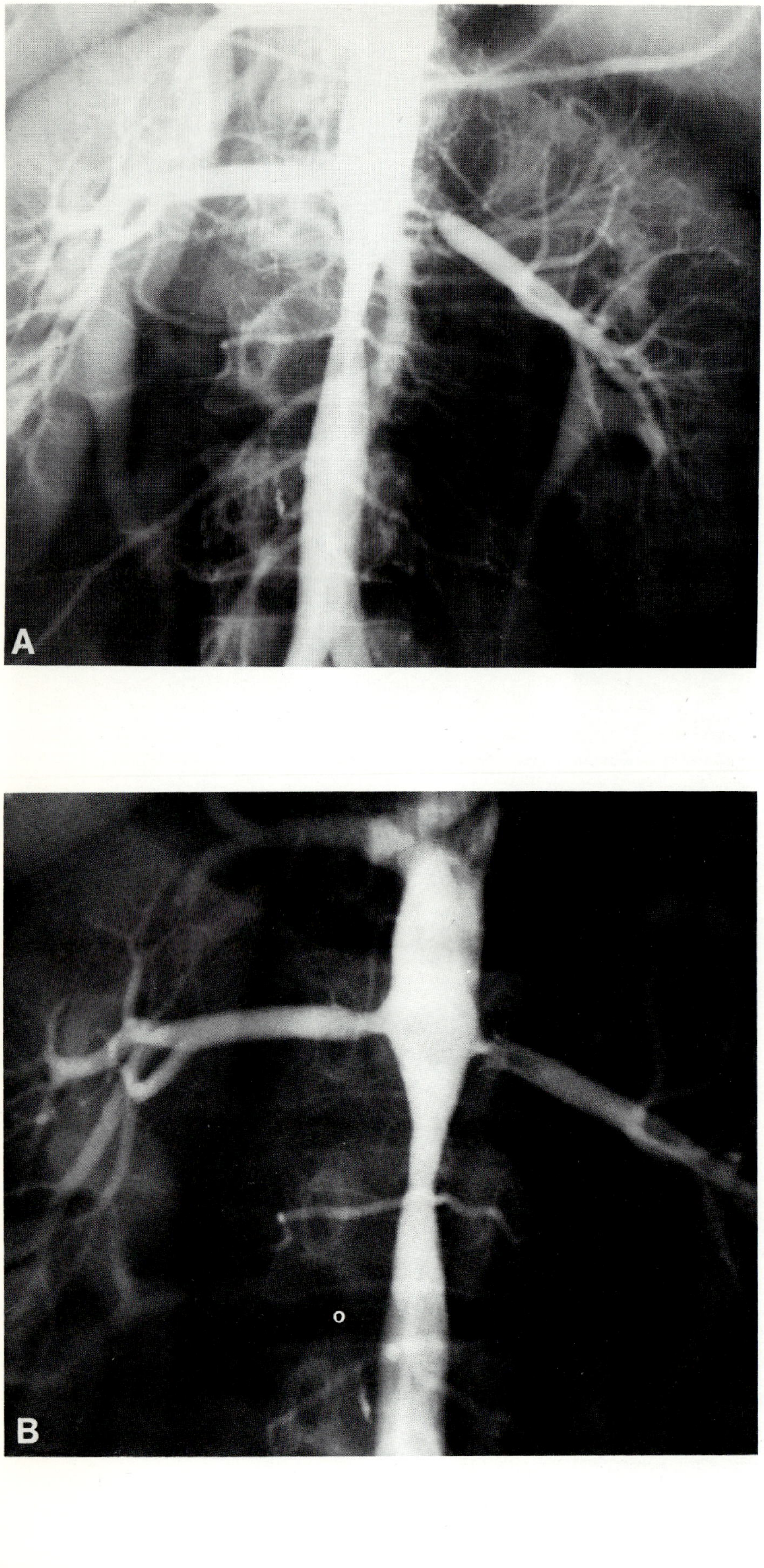

FIGURE 18-10. Patient with Takayasu's arteritis causing hypertension due to left renal artery stenosis (*A*). The patient underwent PTA of the renal lesion and the infrarenal aorta as shown immediately postdilatation. The clinical response was excellent and immediate. Four months later, a follow-up angiogram (*B*) showed striking further improvement in both treated sites.

only cases in which a subsequent operative repair is made more difficult by angioplasty are those in which a subintimal dissection is created which extends beyond the site of preexisting disease. This complication has occurred in 2 of 1400 patients (13).

Iliac Angioplasty

Both bypass surgery and angioplasty have excellent success rates in treating iliac arterial disease. The two interventions are not equivalent. Bypass surgery is often performed bilaterally, while angioplasty is usually unilateral. The surgical approach is a major operation and frequently bypasses disease at many levels in the native circulation, whereas angioplasty is a minor operation and a much more local therapy. In the absence of randomized trials of the two therapies, the reported statistics are informative, but there is no assurance that the populations are comparable.

In the Nuremberg Cooperative Study (14), iliac angioplasty was performed for iliac stenosis in 2,264 cases and for iliac occlusion in 100 cases. In general, short stenoses are considered ideal lesions for angioplasty, and, with experience, angioplasty of occlusions longer than a few centimeters is possible but is being much less frequently attempted. For all cases, the 2-year patency rate is 86.5 percent, and the 5-year patency rate is 84.6 percent. For iliac occlusions, the patency rate is reported to be approximately 33 percent. Angioplasty for long iliac occlusions ($>$ 8 to 10 cm) should be reserved for high-risk or preamputation cases.

Technically, PTA of the iliac artery is usually the easiest angioplasty to perform. When the disease is unilateral and sharply limited, PTA is preferred. PTA is also much more easily repeated than surgery, an important consideration in unilateral disease.

The complication rate for iliac angioplasty is approximately 2 cases per 100 attempts, with a mortality of about 0.1 percent, similar to that of all angioplasty cases. The long-term amputation rate varies with the severity of disease. Using the Fontaine classification, in the Nuremburg trial stage II was followed for 8 years and had a 3.7 percent amputation rate, stage III was followed for 2 years and had a 5 percent rate, and stage IV was followed for 2 years and had a rate approaching 40 percent.

All large studies show considerably less mortality, morbidity, impatency, and cost for angioplasty than for surgery. Diabetics and those who continue to smoke do somewhat worse, but surgery and angioplasty are probably not differentially affected by these risk factors.

Just as all large surgical series show better statistics in later years than at the beginning of the operator's experience, so the learning curve and improvements in adjunctive therapies also affect angioplasty data. The best outcome statistics will undoubtedly result when both surgery and angioplasty are used when appropriate for iliac disease.

There are few absolute contraindications for iliac angioplasty. Occlusions at the aortic bifurcation are worrisome, since it is possible to embolize the less symptomatic leg. If the artery lumen is compromised, but the artery is aneurysmal, then angioplasty is potentially more risky, since the biomechanical strength of the arterial wall is lower and rupture of the artery is more probable.

Femoral Angioplasty

Short of severe rest pain or impending gangrene, it is not as easy to recommend an intervention to claudicant patients. The symptoms may or may not affect the quality of life for a particular patient. However, PTA is clearly less invasive than surgery and could probably be justified earlier in the course of the progressive disease. Femoral angioplasty is a little more technically demanding than iliac angioplasty.

Short segmental stenoses that are responsible for significant hemodynamic impairment and are located anywhere in the superficial femoral artery are ideal angioplasty lesions. As there is less risk of making the patient worse, angioplasty of multilevel stenoses or even 10- to 20-cm occlusions can be attempted (Figure 18-11). These more complicated cases will probably have lower immediate and long-term patency. A surgical approach is preferred for common femoral lesions. Proximal lesions in the profunda femoris artery can be managed a little better with surgery, although there are often unique patient factors that make PTA a better first choice.

Femoral angioplasty in the Nuremberg Cooperative Trial (14) included 1540 stenoses and 1268 occlusions. The overall 1-year patency rate was 79 percent, and at 3 years the rate was 67 percent. There was a 2.5 percent rate of significant complications, about 40 percent of which required surgical intervention. The mortality was 0.17 percent, and no legs were lost acutely. Patients with an advanced Fontaine classification or multilevel disease did worse, but the primary success for the group was 87 percent. The U.S. experience in small series is comparable. Although many authors express their results as the patency rate in successfully dilated lesions, direct comparisons with surgical series are inappropriate unless the trial is randomized to ensure the equivalence of the patient population.

Femoral angioplasty can be very helpful as an adjunct before or after other surgical interventions and as an attempt to avoid amputation, and it will significantly improve patency rates in femoropopliteal vein bypasses by treating an evolving significant stenosis within the graft before occlusion and thrombosis result.

Popliteal Angioplasty

Small balloon catheters (preferred) or even stiff catheters can be used to treat arterial disease in the popliteal or proximal calf arteries. The catheterization is trickier, great gentleness must be employed, and the risks are greater. Spasm or thrombosis is

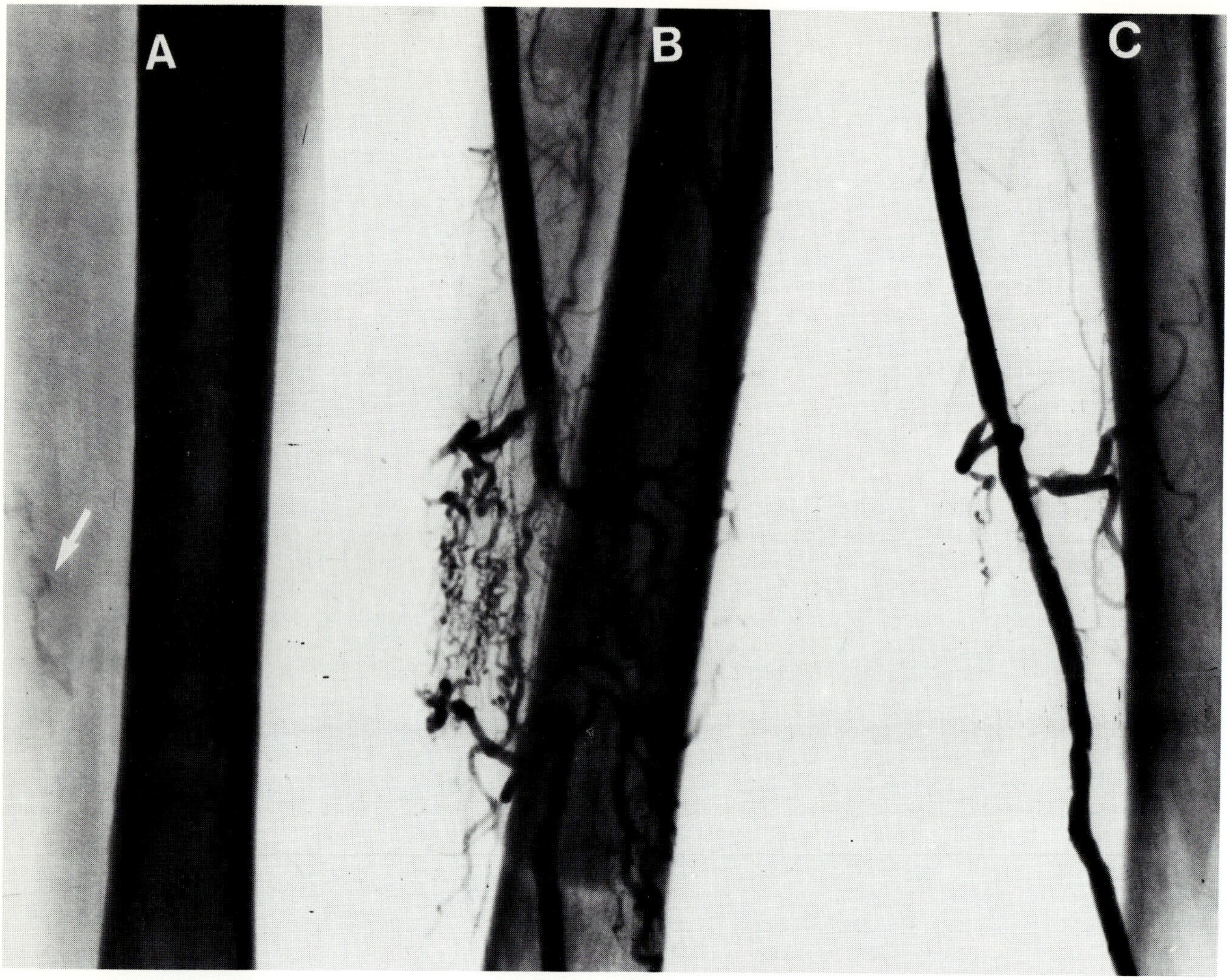

FIGURE 18-11. The response of a calcified, occluded superficial femoral artery to PTA. In the left panel, the calcification is well seen (*arrow*). Extensive collaterals bypass the occlusion but quickly regress after angioplasty. Patency was still present 3 years after the intervention.

more common, and there is less potential collateralization to protect the limb if the angioplasty causes deterioration. The worst-case scenario might also affect available surgical options. Still, in particular clinical circumstances with skilled PTA techniques, popliteal angioplasty can yield excellent immediate results.

Renal Angioplasty

In general, renal revascularization with PTA technique has all the potential benefits of surgery with few of the risks (15,16). It is the treatment of choice for proximal fibromuscular dysplasia. For atherosclerotic lesions of the renal artery it is equally as effective as surgery. The only circumstances in which bypass surgery has a mechanical advantage is in atherosclerosis of the aorta that reduces the orifice size of the renal artery. Although occasionally successful in this circumstance, PTA can rarely alleviate aortic disease by the inflation of a catheter in the renal artery orifice.

In other arterial trees, a bypass intervention can exclude lots of disease in the native circulation, but the renal arteries are sufficiently short that balloon dilation can be just as hemodynamically effective as endarterectomy or bypass surgery. Neither procedure can reverse the systemic effects of sustained hypertension or repair arteriolosclerosis in the downstream renal bed.

Renal angioplasty is technically more difficult than iliac or femoral PTA, and the success rates are higher for fibromuscular stenoses (85 to 90 percent) than for atherosclerosis (60 to 75 percent). Rupture of the artery can occur (probably fewer than 0.3 percent of the cases), and both the radiologist and the surgeon should be prepared to respond to this uncommon disaster. Restenosis rates are variably reported, but occur in about 20 percent of the patients, usually within 6 months. These lesions

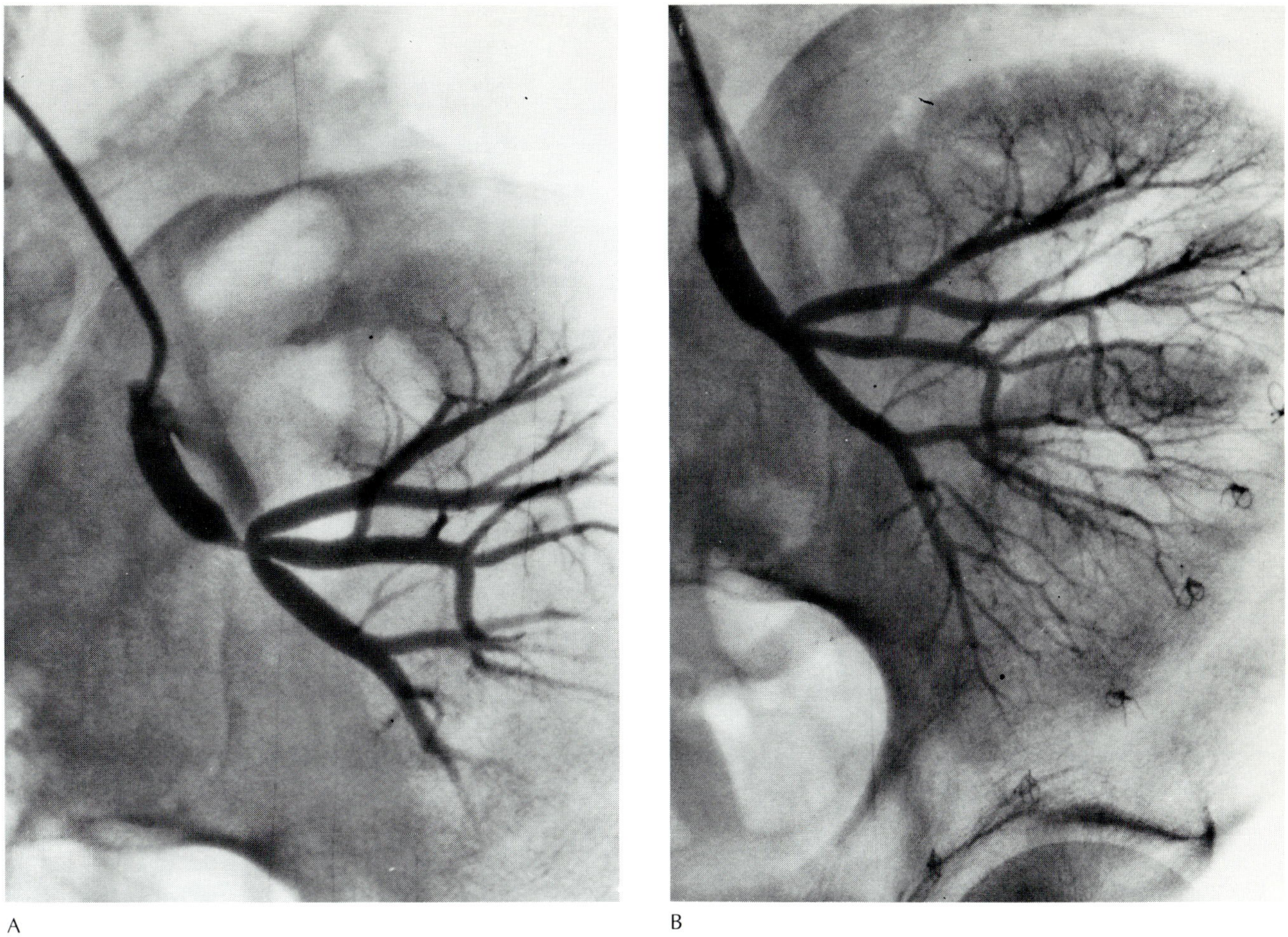

FIGURE 18-12. The successful revascularization of a transplanted kidney is seen on a selective angiogram before (*A*) and after (*B*) angioplasty. The patient's hypertension and diminished urinary function returned to normal within 48 hours.

can be redilated with 80 to 90 percent success. More complete dilation initially, effective antiplatelet medications, and stopping smoking are all potentially important in reducing restenosis.

There are few forms of renovascular hypertension in which the patient should not be offered PTA as a therapeutic choice. On balance, renal PTA seems equally likely to result in cure or improvement as bypass surgery, although no randomized trials have been reported or are in progress. Renal PTA is also useful postoperatively, especially in transplant patients (Figures 18-12, 18-13).

Miscellaneous Angioplasties

Although fibromuscular or atherosclerotic stenosis of the mesenteric circulation is uncommonly dilated, our attempts have been successful to date (Figure 18-14). Often an axillary approach must be used, and this increases the potential for complications somewhat.

The worldwide experience in the supraaortic circulation is fewer than 500 reported cases, and most of these are subclavian artery stenoses. The fear of embolization to the brain and the relatively benign surgical alternatives preclude the routine application of PTA here. Unique clinical circumstances occasionally justify an attempt. The true risk of significant cerebral embolization during or following angioplasty is unknown.

Finally, PTA is often very effective in dilating stenoses that develop in autogenous or artificial grafts. Reoperation is more difficult than the initial intervention, but angioplasty has a privileged access to the lesion. Because PTA is so useful for graft stenosis, the development of new symptoms after successful surgery should indicate repeat angiography to search for a PTA-treatable lesion. Arterial or venous digital subtraction angiography is fully satisfactory for this purpose and is much preferred by patients. Early diagnosis may discover these lesions before the graft thrombosis. With thrombus present, a combination of fibrinolysis (streptokinase or tissue plasminogen activator) followed by PTA to relieve the underlying cause can be effective.

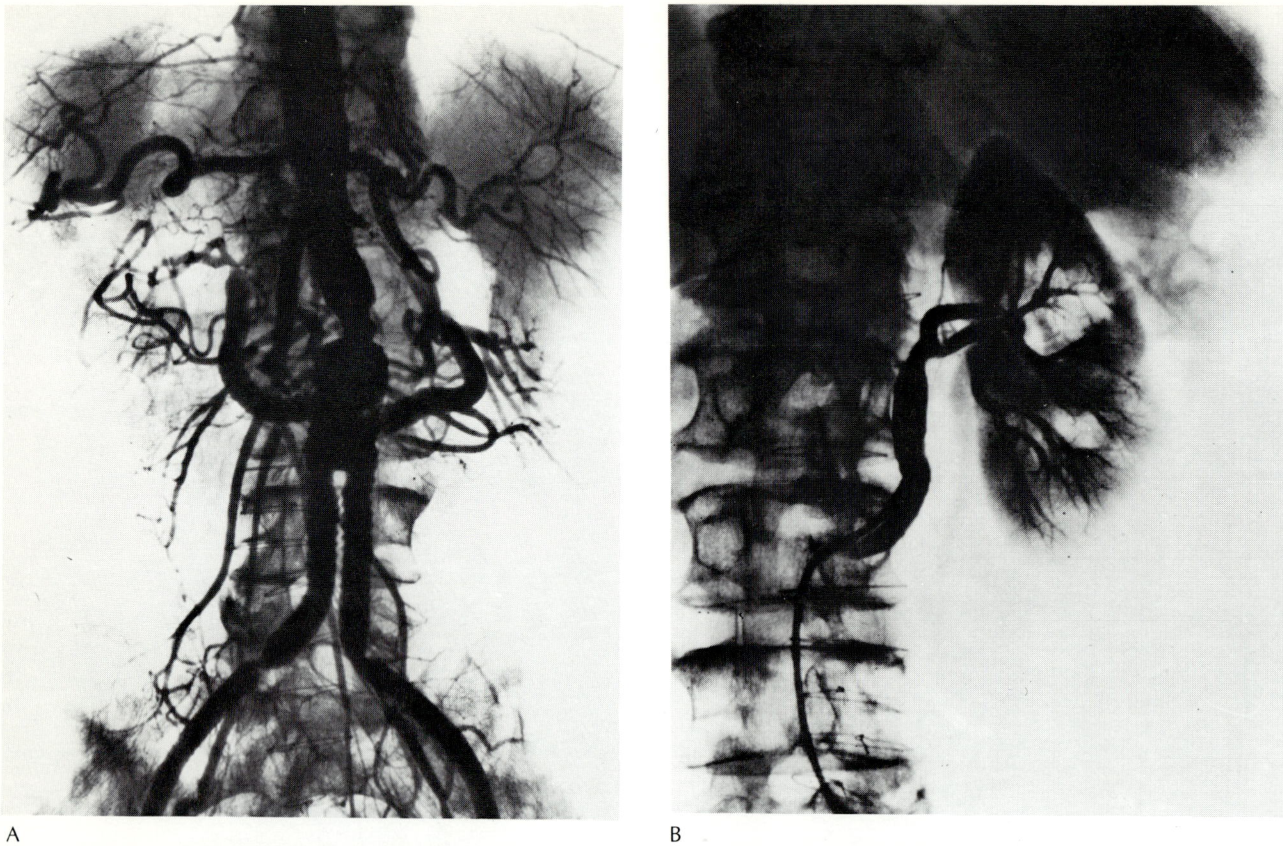

FIGURE 18-13. This patient had a Dacron graft of the abdominal aorta and both renal arteries (*A*) with significant hypertension and claudication. Angioplasty successfully dilated both renal anastomoses (the result of the left renal PTA is shown in *B*) and the right iliac artery.

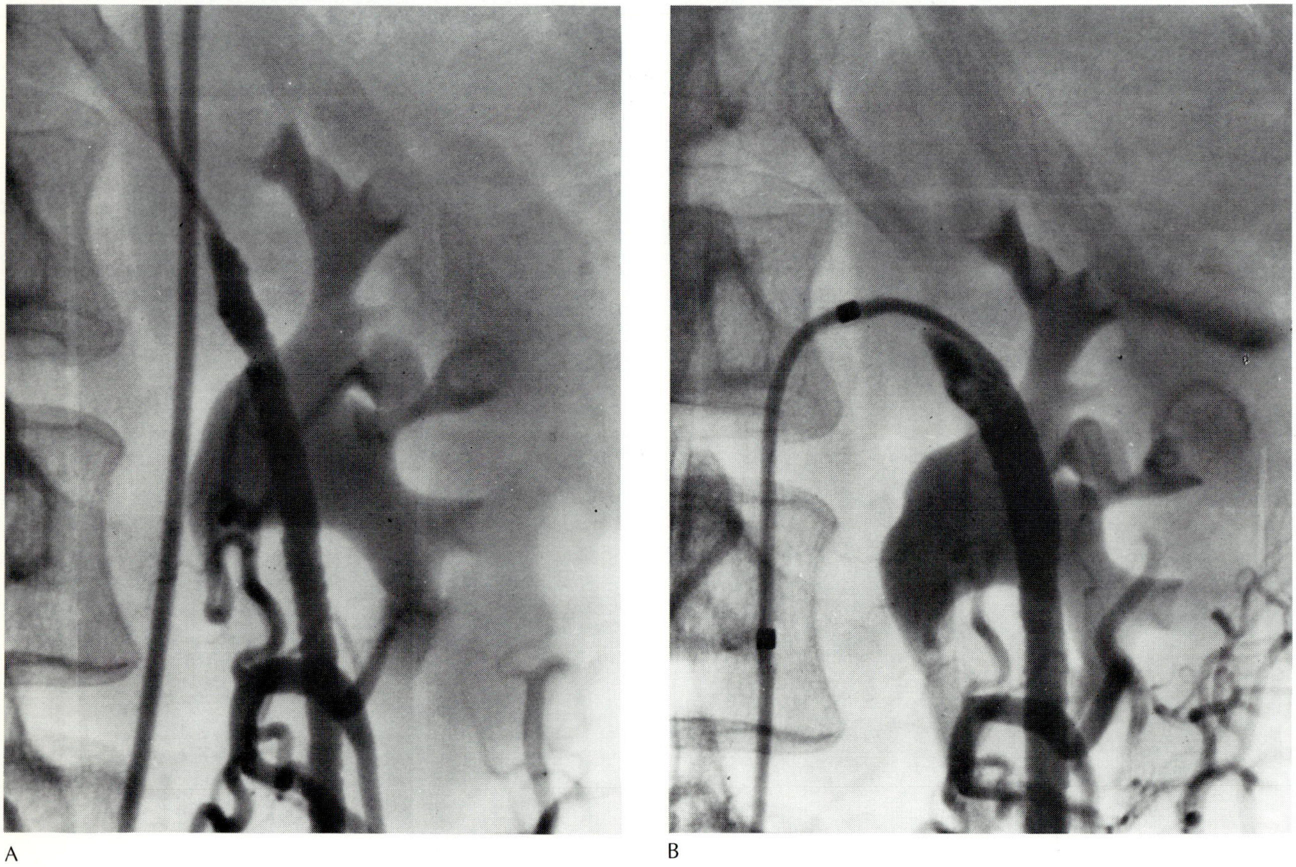

FIGURE 18-14. Fibromuscular dysplasia before (*A*) and after PTA (*B*) of the superior mesenteric artery in a patient with intestinal angina. The symptoms remitted promptly after angioplasty.

Conclusions

Both surgery and angioplasty are continuing to evolve. Further understanding of the mechanism of angioplasty could probably improve the patient outcome but may enhance referral even more. Early explanations of angioplasty were clearly inadequate. PTA is both safe and effective, and should be considered often. When it is technically feasible, it must be presented to the patient for the patient's consideration. Acceptable forms of therapy should not be considered competitive, and, indeed, the best patient outcomes are being achieved when excellent cooperation exists between surgeons and angiographers. Both forms of intervention have much in common, and each discipline can benefit from the further development of drug regimens that reduce thrombosis, platelet aggregation, and restenosis.

References

1. Dotter CT, Judkins M: Transluminal treatment of arteriosclerotic obstructions: Description of a new technique and a preliminary report of its application. Circulation 1964, 30:654.
2. Dotter CT, Rosch J, Judkins MP: Transluminal dilatation of atherosclerotic stenosis. Surg Gynecol Obstet 1968, 127:794.
3. Dotter CT: Catheter techniques in diagnosing and treating femoral artery atherosclerosis. Geriatrics 1974, 29:93.
4. Gruentzig A: Die perkutane Rekanalisation chronischer arterieller Verschlüsse (Dotter-Prinzip) mit einem neuen dopellumigen Dilatationskatheter. Fortsch Roentgenstr 1976, 124:80.
5. Ring E, McLean GK: *Interventional Radiology: Principles and Techniques*. Boston, Little, Brown, 1981.
6. Tegtmeyer C: *Angioplasty*. Chicago, Year Book (in press).
7. Ring EJ, McLean GK, Freiman DB: Selected techniques in percutaneous transluminal angioplasty. Am J Roentgenol 1983, 139:767.
8. Wolf GL, LeVeen RF, Ring EJ: Potential mechanisms of angioplasty. Cardiovasc Intervent Radiol 1983, 7:11.
9. Gow BS, Hadfield CD: The elasticity of canine and human coronary arteries with reference to post mortem changes. Circ Res 1979, 45:588.
10. Strandness DE, Sumner DS: *Hemodynamics for Surgeons*, New York, Grune & Stratton, 1975.
11. Wolf GL, Lentini EA: The influence of short duration stretch on vasoconstrictor response in rabbit aortas. Invest Radiol 1984, 19:269.
12. Wolf GL, Lentini EA, LeVeen RF: Reduced vasoconstrictor response after angioplasty in normal rabbit aortas. Am J. Roentgenol 1984, 142:1023.
13. Ring EJ: Selection of patients for percutaneous transluminal angioplasty. Written communication, June 7, 1984.
14. Zeitler E, Richter EI, Roth FJ, Schoop W: Results of percutaneous angioplasty. Radiology 1983, 146:57.
15. Sos TA, Pickering TG, Sniderman K, Saddakni S, Case DB, Silane MF, Vaughan ED, Laragh JH: Percutaneous transluminal renal angioplasty in renovascular hypertension due to atheroma or fibromuscular dysplasia. N Eng J Med 1983, 309:274.
16. Martin EC, Matlein RF, Baer L, Fankuchen EC, Casarella WJ: Renal angioplasty for hypertension: Predictive factors for long-term success. Am J Roentgenol 1981, 137:921.

Chapter 19

MORPHOLOGIC ALTERATIONS AFTER TRANSLUMINAL ANGIOPLASTY

CHRISTOPHER K. ZARINS and SEYMOUR GLAGOV

Despite the widespread clinical use of percutaneous transluminal angioplasty, the mechanism by which enlargement of the arterial lumen is achieved by this technique has been poorly understood. In their original description of transluminal angioplasty in 1964, Dotter and Judkins attributed the effectiveness of their procedure to compression of the atheromatous plaque against a relatively unyielding artery wall (1). This mechanism was subsequently endorsed by Grüntzig and Kumpe in relation to angioplasty using the balloon catheter (2). The concept of plaque compression or displacement or of herniation of the puttylike atheromatous intima into the artery wall was generally accepted by the early pioneers in transluminal angioplasty. This mechanism did not, however, correspond to clinical and morphologic observations that plaques were generally rigid and calcific rather than plastic and could not readily be compressed or deformed. Angiographic observations before and after dilatation have not always been helpful in defining the mechanism since angiography reveals only the lumen contour and does not provide sufficient information concerning the thickness of the arterial wall or the size, configuration, or precise boundaries of plaques. Although direct observation of lesions and associated artery walls immediately after balloon dilatation could provide the necessary information, such data are difficult to obtain since arteries and plaques are rarely directly inspected after dilatation in the living patient. Knowledge of the morphologic consequences of balloon dilatation in human arteries has therefore been obtained mainly from experimental studies of postmortem arteries and corresponding angiographic images and from specimens obtained from amputated limbs or after death.

Mechanism of Balloon Dilatation: Experimental Observations in Human Peripheral Arteries

The effects of balloon dilatation have been investigated experimentally in both normal and diseased superficial femoral, popliteal, and iliac arteries obtained from amputated limbs or at autopsy. In studies designed to approximate conditions which prevail in the living patient, dilatations have been performed on excised arteries which have been cannulated at both ends, restored to original length, redistended at an intraluminal pressure of 90 to 100 mmHg, and maintained at a temperature of 37°C (3). Angiography was used to locate stenosing plaques and to document the precise position of the balloon as well as the changes in lumen contour associated with dilatation (Figure 19-1). Pressure was maintained throughout the dilatation and visualization procedure, and each artery was subsequently fixed while distended. Transverse histologic sections through the dilated segment were compared with those made at immediately adjacent, nondilated proximal and distal locations and correlated with the angiographic appearances. In such preparations, sites *without* discrete intimal plaques or stenoses showed no significant alteration following balloon dilatation to 4 atm, provided the balloon size is not excessive. When balloons were considerably larger than the normally distended arterial lumen, disruption of the artery wall occurred. The intima and media tended to rupture first, and the adventitia was affected only when balloon diameter was sufficiently great. There was little or no cleavage between intima and media. The absence of such separations, even in

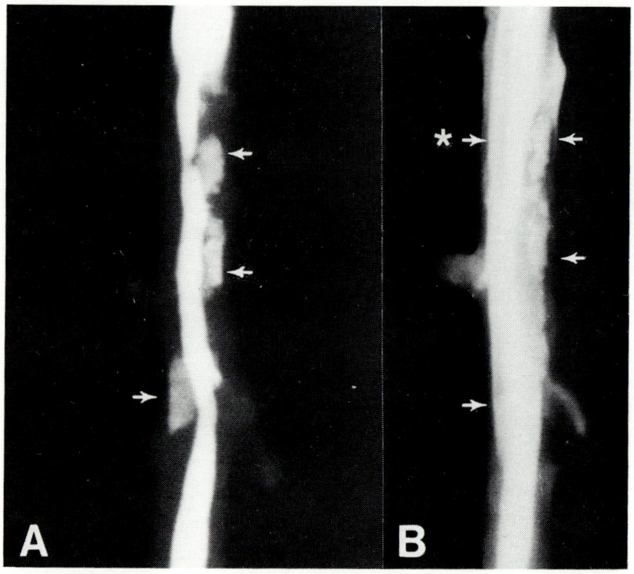

FIGURE 19-1. Postmortem angiogram of excised, redistended superficial femoral artery. (*A*) Before balloon dilatation: Lumen stenosis is evident; note calcification within plaque (*arrows*). (*B*) After balloon dilatation: Note the increase in lumen diameter and the dissection plane (*). The position and length of the calcified plaque are unchanged.

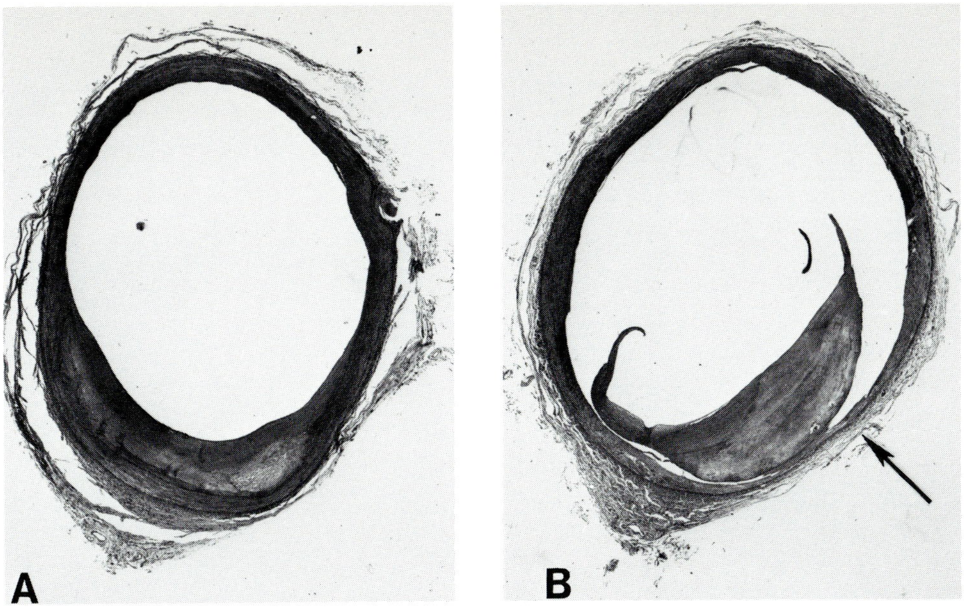

FIGURE 19-2. (*A*) Nondilated segment of superficial femoral artery with relatively small nonstenosing fibrous plaque. (*B*) After balloon dilatation: Note the separation of the plaque from the underlying media, thinning of the media (*arrow*), and protrusion of the plaque into the lumen, leaving an irregular lumen contour but an enlarged lumen cross-sectional area. The plaque remains adherent to the media at its thickest point in most instances, and the plaque shape and contour are not markedly altered.

arteries with moderate uniform fibrocellular intimal thickening, may be due to the similarity in compliance between intima and media in such vessels.

NONSTENOSING PLAQUES

Discrete fibrocalcific but nonstenosing intimal plaques proved to be less compliant than the underlying artery wall, for inflation of the balloon catheter at such locations stretched the uninvolved portion of the artery wall as well as the media beneath the plaque but had little direct effect on the fibrous plaque itself. As a result, a shearing force probably developed at the interface between the plaque and the underlying media, and a plane of separation occurred, beginning usually at the edges of the plaque. The media became thinner as it stretched and sometimes ruptured, leaving only the adventitia at the rupture site to maintain vessel wall continuity. The separated regions of the plaque protruded into the lumen, accentuating the sharp cleavage plane between plaque and media (Figure 19-2). Such cleavages or dissections can be seen on postdilatation angiograms (Figure 19-1) but may be obscured by contrast media within the lumen, depending on the planes of projection.

STENOTIC ARTERIES

Arteries with manifest focal lumen stenoses usually contain eccentric complex fibrocalcific plaques with increased plaque thickness at the stenotic site. The plaque tends to taper in the longitudinal or axial plane of section both proximal and distal to the stenosis, but the lumen contour on transverse section is usually round or oval at all levels (see Chapter 3). Balloon dilatation of such stenoses results in marked detachment of the plaque from the media in both longitudinal and circumferential planes and stretching of the media to enlarge the lumen. The lesion itself does not usually fragment and tends to remain attached at its central thickest portion and for some distance proximal and distal to the dilated area if the lesion is extensive (Figure 19-3). There is little or no evidence of plaque compression, molding, extrusion, or redistribution (3). Persistence of zones of plaque attachment may help to account for the finding that arteries tend to remain patent following balloon dilatation despite extensive plaque dissection away from the media and partial disruption of the artery wall. In instances where an advanced plaque occupies the entire circumference of an artery, the plaque fractures at or near its thinnest point and separation of the remainder of the lesion usually occurs in a plane immediately adjacent to the luminal aspect of the internal elastic lamina. When a plaque is extensive and associated with medial atrophy or degeneration, the dissection plane frequently occurs instead at the outer limit of the media, leaving only the adventitia intact. These are the same planes which are followed to remove lesions when operative endarterectomy is performed. The adventitial layer is nearly always thickened and more compact in arteries with fibrocalcific plaques, and this focal change may contribute to the capacity of the adventitia to contain the arterial pressure and flow adequately.

OCCLUDED ARTERIES

The lumen of a totally occluded artery may be completely replaced by a complex fibrocalcific lesion or it may be partially occluded by a plaque with the remaining lumen obstructed by a thrombus. In the presence of a central thrombotic core, dilatation

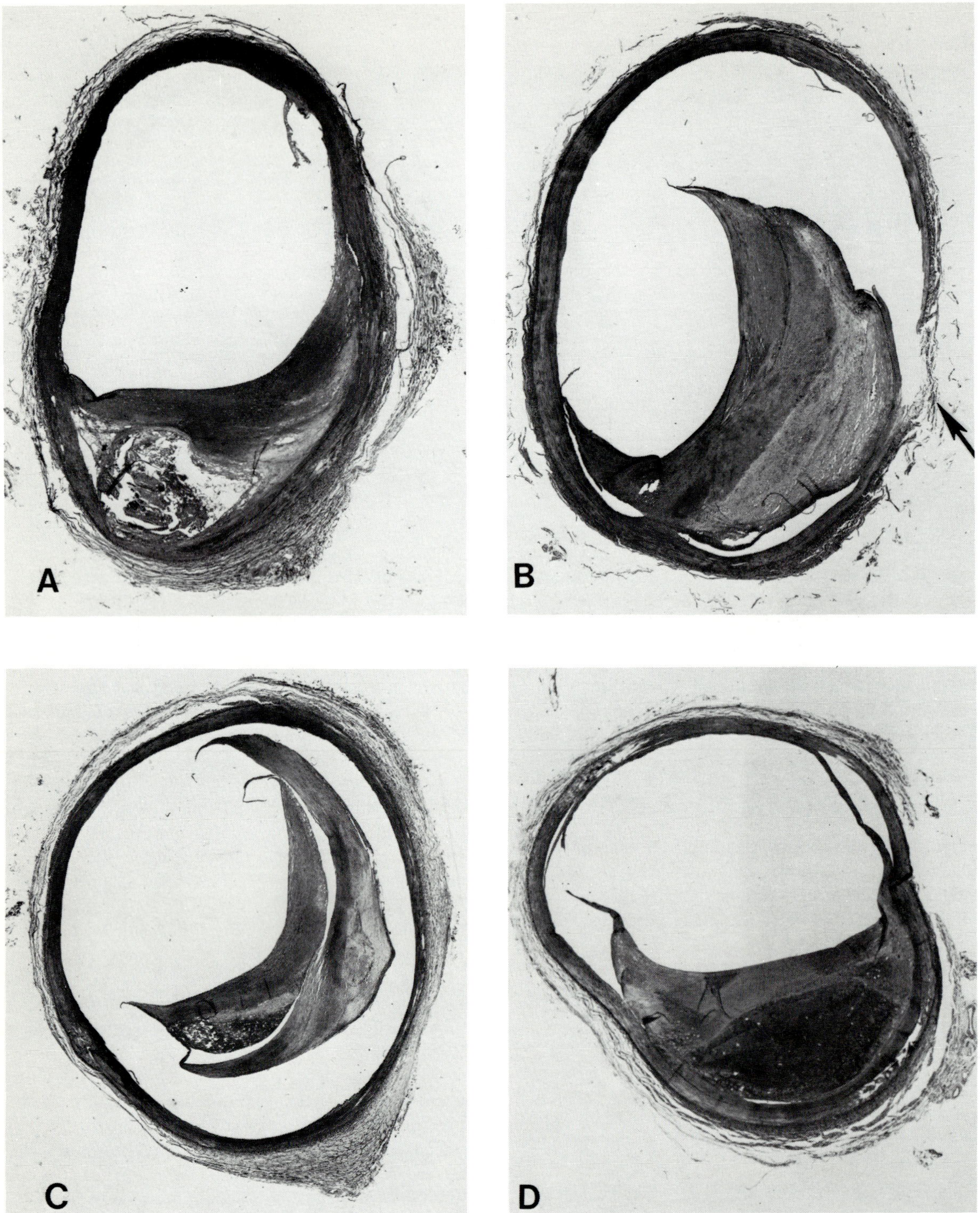

FIGURE 19-3. Balloon dilatation of a stenotic lesion in a superficial femoral artery. (*A*) Proximal nondilated segment of artery with an eccentric fibrocalcific plaque with a prominent fibrous cap and a necrotic core. (*B*) At the site of balloon dilatation the media is stretched and disrupted (*arrow*) and the plaque protrudes into the lumen. [From Zarins CK, Lu CT, Gewertz BL, et al. (5). Reproduced with permission.] (*C*) More distal in the dilated segment, the plaque is entirely separated from the artery wall in an area where the artery wall is maximally stretched. The plaque nevertheless remains intact and attached to the media proximal and distal to the dilated zone. (*D*) Distal to the dilated area the plaque is attached to the vessel wall except for a small flap.

of totally occluded vessels occurs by much the same mechanism as for stenotic vessels. The guide wire travels easily through the thrombotic material, penetrates along the lumen, and the changes in the plaque associated with subsequent dilatation are essentially the same as those which occur in a stenotic vessel. Intimal flaps and lumen irregularities associated with plaque separation and protrusion are seen (Figure 19-4), but additional irregularities may be produced by deformation and fragmentation of the thrombotic core (Figure 19-5). When a plaque occupies the entire lumen, the guide wire frequently travels in a plane between the intima and the atrophic media or between the media and the adventitia, i.e., in the plane of dissection usually employed for endarterectomy. The remaining artery wall is thereby pulled away from the occlusive plaque with the creation of a new or false lumen beneath the plaque. As a result, the usual separation plane may not be discernible on angiography (Figure 19-6). The plaque is therefore effectively "sequestered" away from the new lumen, resulting in a configuration which may resemble that seen in the presence of a usual eccentric plaque which has not been subjected to balloon dilatation (see Figure 19-3*A*). Although many of the morphologic changes noted above have been observed in arteries subjected to dilatation and examined in a nondistended state (4), quantitative evaluations and comparisons with clinical angiograms are likely to require the study of pressure-fixed vessels.

Morphologic Changes following Therapeutic Angioplasty

Examination of arteries which have been subjected to transluminal angioplasty and subsequently obtained at amputation or autopsy also provide information concerning the consequences of balloon dilatation. Although relatively few peripheral vessels have been studied and most are undistended when examined, changes similar to those noted in experimental studies can be identified (5) inasmuch as there is evidence of plaque fracture and extensive plaque separation from the vessel wall (Figure 19-

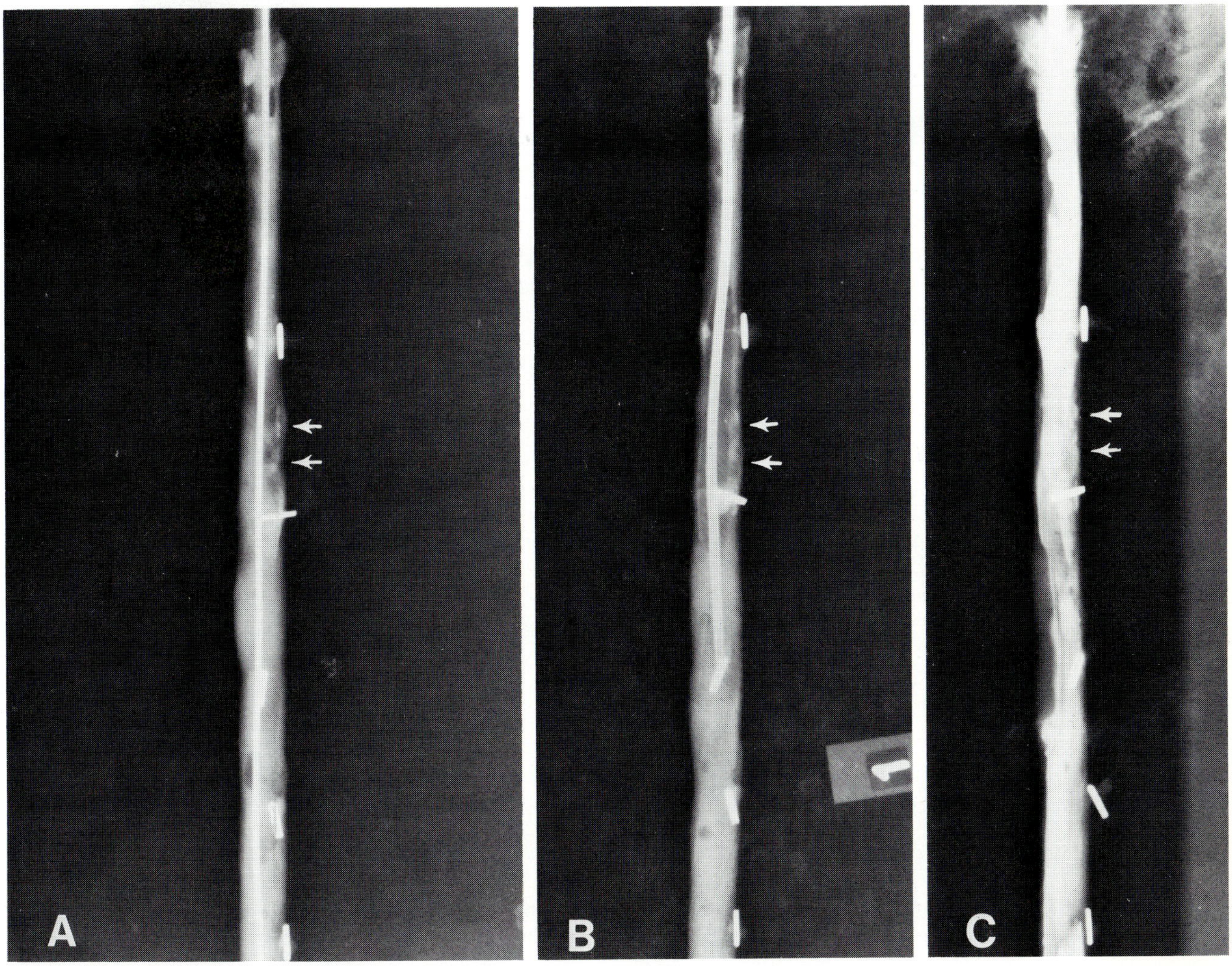

FIGURE 19-4. Experimental dilatation of totally occluded superficial femoral artery. (*A*) The guide wire passed through a thrombotic core: Note calcified plaque (*arrows*). (*B*) The balloon catheter is inflated. (*C*) Angiogram after dilatation shows a patent lumen and dissection planes.

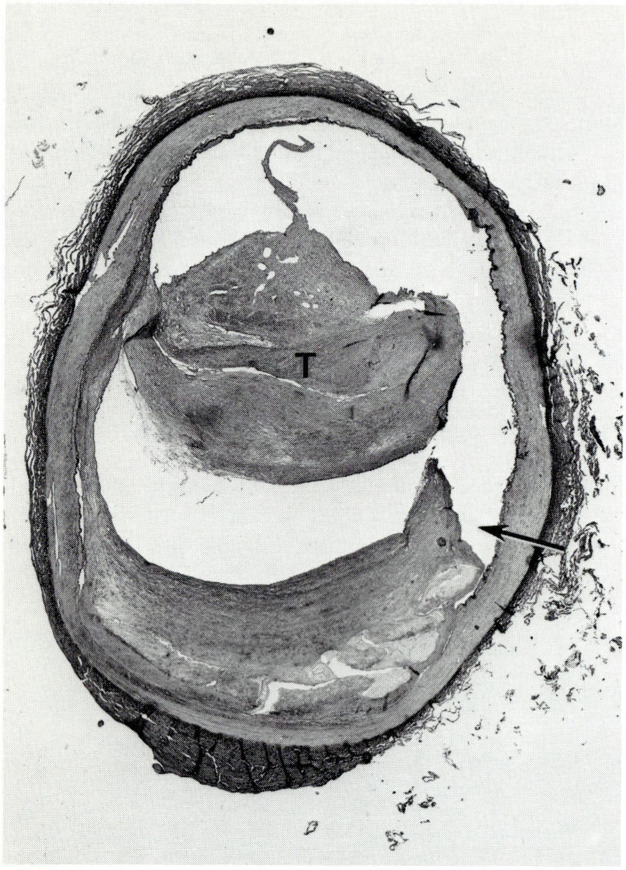

FIGURE 19-5. Totally occluded superficial femoral artery after dilatation. Note plaque separation from media (*arrow*). A thrombotic core (T) has separated from the underlying plaque and creates an additional dissection plane in the vessel.

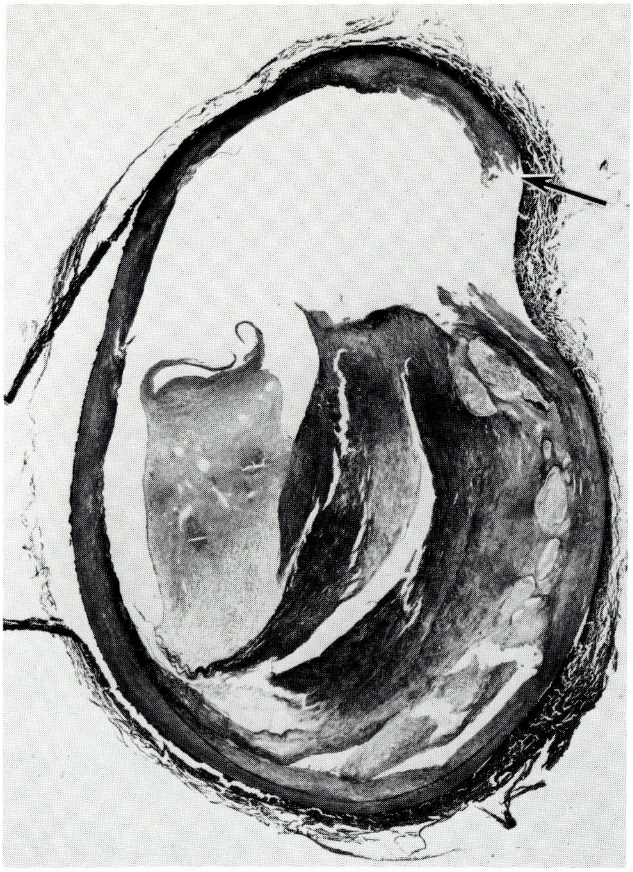

FIGURE 19-6. Totally occluded superficial femoral artery after balloon dilatation. The media is ruptured (*arrow*), and the artery wall is stretched and pulled away from the occlusive plaque. Under these circumstances there may be few or no dissection channels evident. [From Zarins CK, Lu CT, Gewertz BL, et al. (5). Reproduced with permission.]

7*A*). In some specimens, however, very extensive dissection has been noted with little evidence of residual attachment of the plaque to the media (Figure 19-7*B*), providing a basis for complicating obstruction by a loose plaque or a mobile flap. In other specimens, the media is intact, with no evidence of either rupture or stretching, suggesting that vessel dilatation may have been inadequate. Evidence of intimal plaque disruption has been observed on sections as long as 20 months after dilatation (Figure 19-8). In general, specimens which have been in place for extensive periods show little cellular reaction other than increased penetration of vasa vasorum at the site of medial disruption. Nor is there evidence to suggest a marked alteration in plaque configuration other than some curling of the thinnest portion of the separated plaque near its reattachment to the artery wall and blunting of the separated plaque edges. Evidence of ''new plaque'' formation has not been forthcoming in specimens examined thus far.

Angiographic Changes

INTIMAL FLAPS

Lumen contour irregularities, including intimal flaps corresponding to partial plaque separations with protrusion into the lumen and dissection channels beneath plaques, may be seen on 60 to 70 percent of postdilatation angiograms of patients treated by transluminal angioplasty. Intimal flaps may be especially prominent when plaque disruption and dissection have been extensive (Figures 19-9*A*, 19-10). The initial clinical success rate and subsequent restenosis rate do not, however, appear to be related to the presence, absence, or size of the flaps as seen on angiography (6,7). The presence of intimal flaps may instead indicate that sufficient dilatation has been achieved. According to the law of LaPlace ($T = Pr$), the tangential tension (T) tending to keep the

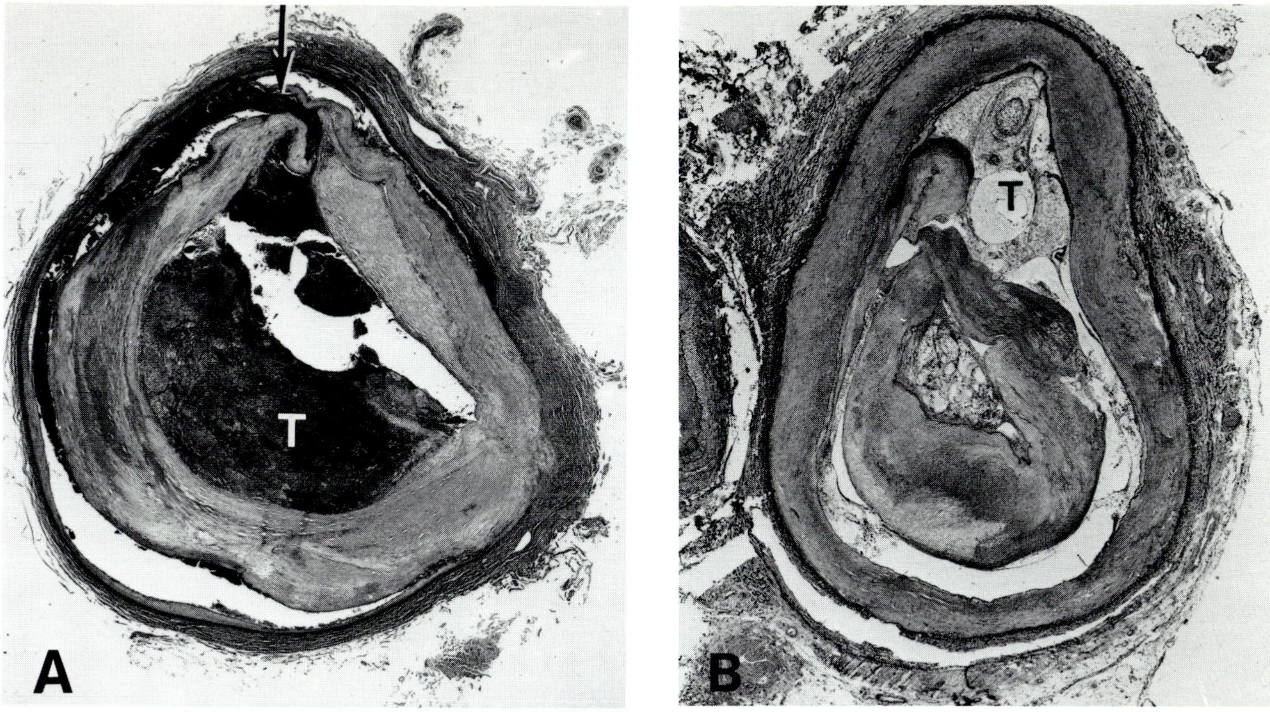

FIGURE 19-7. Totally occluded superficial femoral artery 1 month after balloon dilatation. Patency was restored for 2 weeks, after which the artery was occluded by thrombosis and amputation was performed. (*A*) Proximal zone of dilated segment: Note plaque fracture at its thinnest point with separation of the plaque from the media (*arrow*), rupture of the media, and prominent adventitial fibrosis (compare with Figure 19-3*B*). The lumen is filled with 2-week-old thrombus (T). (*B*) Distal in the dilated segment the entire plaque is separated from the media about its circumference (compare with Figure 19-3*C*), and there is evidence of an older thrombus (T).

vessel lumen open is closely approximated by the product of the intraluminal pressure (P) and the vessel radius (r). Thus, wall tension may be increased both by increasing pressure and by increasing radius (Figure 19-11). The sequence of changes described above suggests that transluminal angioplasty results in an increase in effective lumen diameter due to plaque separation with stretching of the media. Under conditions of marked vessel wall alteration by atherosclerosis, however, the increased level of wall tension resulting from balloon dilatation must be sufficiently high to assure persistence of an adequately patent lumen and increased flow. If such a critical increase in diameter is not achieved, immediate clinical failure or restenosis may result (Figure 19-12). Thus, early restenosis, commonly seen within the first several months after balloon dilatation, may be related to insufficient detachment of plaque corresponding to inadequate stretching of the arterial wall.

The persistence of functionally effective patency for years after angioplasty despite an apparently inadequate angiographic appearance is probably related to the observation that detachment of the most stenotic portion of a plaque may at times occur largely along a longitudinal or axial plane of separation and remain attached proximally and distally. Such a result contrasts with intimal dissections which occur at operation and usually extend in a transverse plane, creating a ''flap-valve'' obstruction.

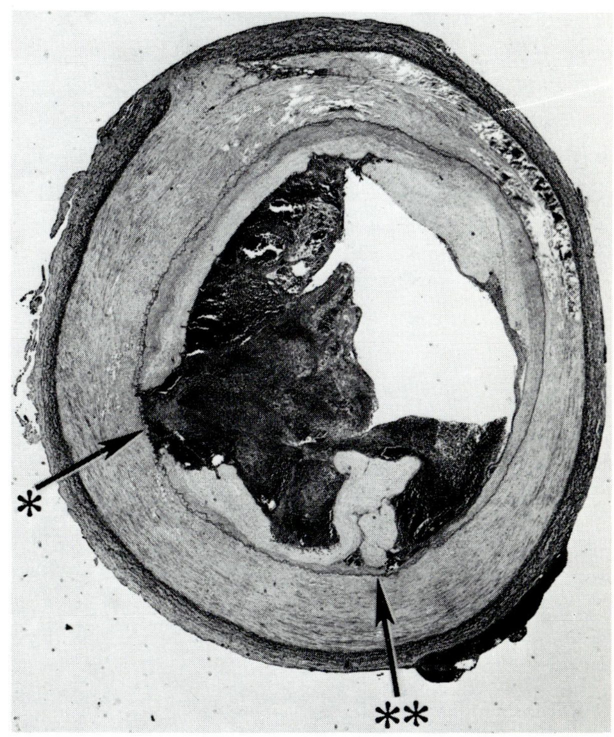

FIGURE 19-8. Superficial femoral artery harvested at autopsy 20 months after balloon dilatation. There is evidence of previous plaque separation (*arrow**) and reattachment of an intimal flap (*arrow***).

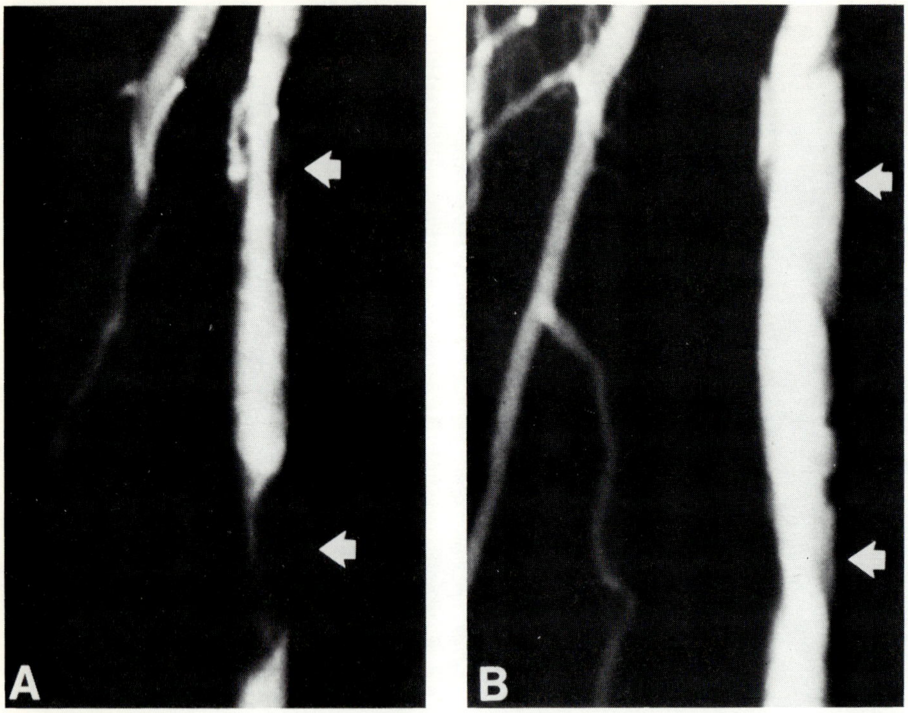

FIGURE 19-9. Postdilatation angiogram demonstrating (*A*) prominent dissection planes (*arrows*) following balloon dilatation, but with poor angiographic appearance. (*B*) One month later there is marked resolution of the intimal flaps and an improved angiographic appearance.

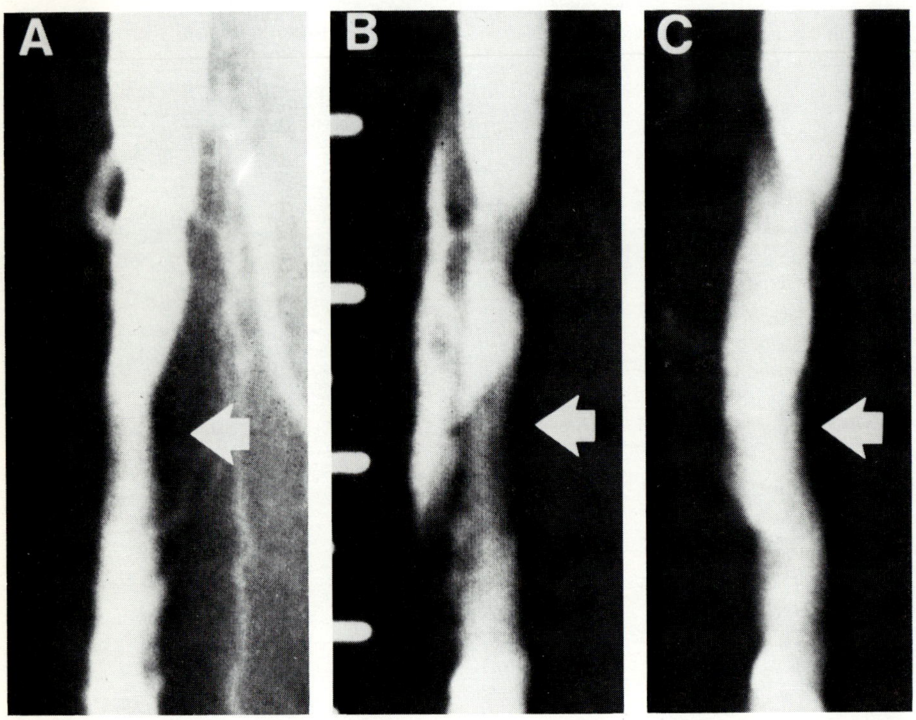

FIGURE 19-10. Superficial femoral artery lesion treated by balloon dilatation. (*A*) Contour of plaque before dilatation. Arrow indicates thickest portion of plaque. (*B*) Postdilatation angiogram reveals plaque disruption with a prominent intimal flap. The contour of the thickest portion of the plaque is unchanged (*arrow*); intimal flaps are located predominantly on the opposite side. (*C*) One year later, the original plaque contour is still unchanged (*arrow*), and continued patency corresponds to ''overdistension'' of the artery wall opposite the thickest portion of the plaque. [From Zarins CK, Lu CT, Gewertz BL, et al. (5). Reproduced with permission.]

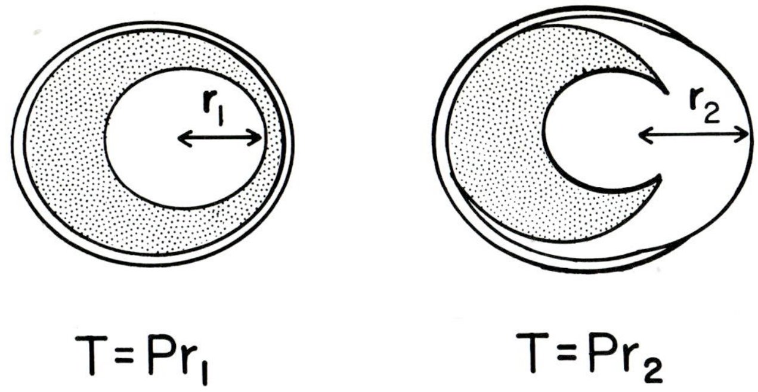

FIGURE 19-11. Diagrammatic representation of the mechanism by which effective lumen radius is increased by balloon dilatation. A critical level of tangential tension (*T*) may be necessary to prevent recollapse.

Since the flaps are freely movable within the lumen immediately after dilatations, fluctuations in ankle systolic blood pressure may occur during the first week following dilatation. When such flaps are prominent, anticoagulation with heparin during the first several days after dilatation may be of benefit.

LUMEN REMODELING

Lumen remodeling occurs rapidly following balloon dilatation. Intimal flaps seen on postdilatation angiograms may be entirely resolved as early as 3 days after the procedure. Subsequent angiography reveals that most dissection planes have resolved by 1 month (Figure 19-9). On occasion, however, residual flaps may persist and protrude into the lumen in association with an unsatisfactory clinical result. Such lesions are usually amenable to repeat dilatation with good long-term results.

Lumen remodeling probably occurs as the intimal flaps readhere at least partially to the vessel wall but may also proceed by thrombus deposition and organization within the dissection dehiscence. There is apparently little change in bulk of the plaque itself, and continued long-term patency appears to depend on persistence of the ''overstretched'' vessel wall (Figure 19-10).

Restenosis

Restenosis is a significant problem following balloon dilatation. The 1-year patency rate for iliac angioplasty has been estimated to be 77 percent, and for femoral angioplasty, 56 percent (8). Failure may occur early due to the presence of untoward dissection planes or inadequate dilatation as noted above. Following successful dilatation, restenosis occurs as an exponentially decreasing function of time, and by 5 years the patency rate is 63 percent for iliac angioplasty and 29 percent for femoral angioplasty (8). Although it has been suggested that balloon dilatation may accelerate atherogenesis and evidence for this has been

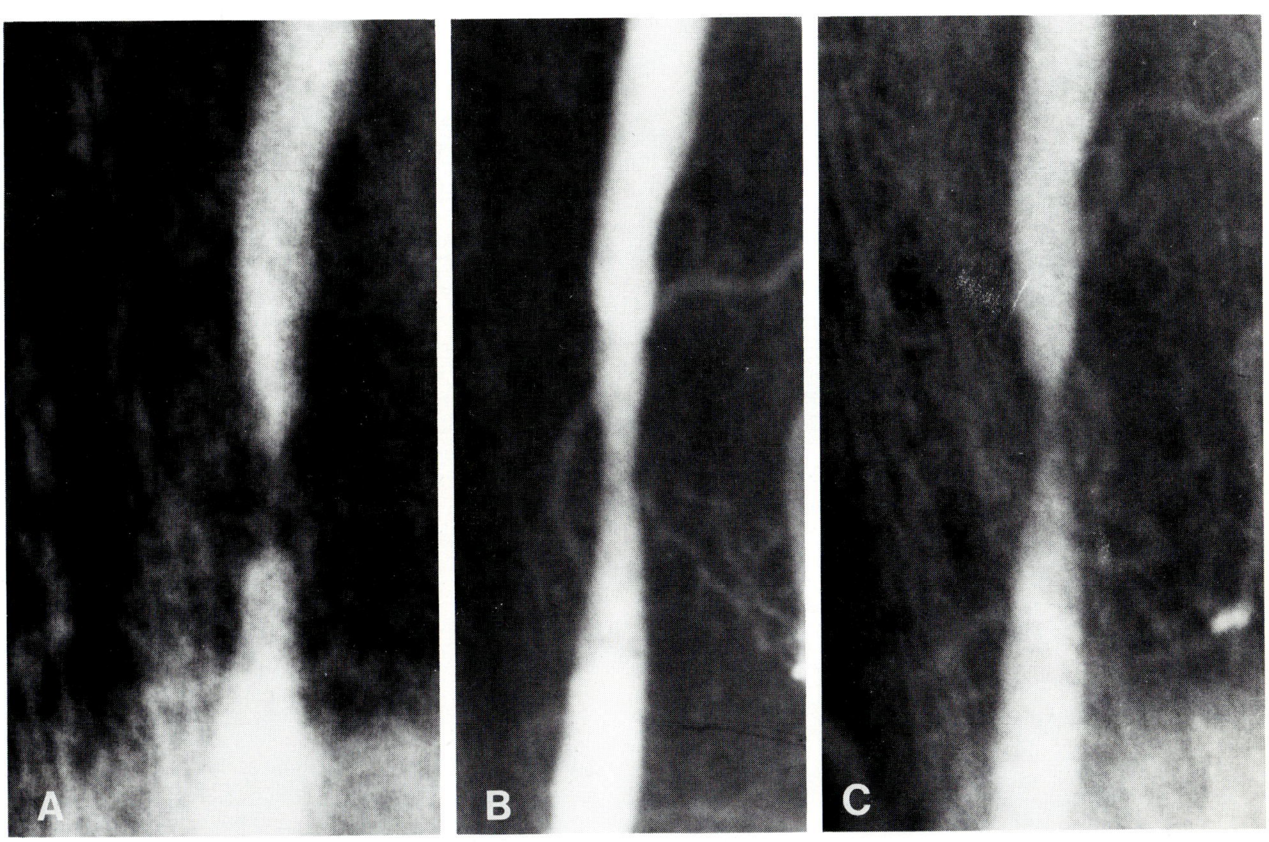

FIGURE 19-12. Superficial femoral artery after attempted transluminal angioplasty with inadequate dilatation. (*A*) Stenosis before dilatation. (*B*) After dilatation, lumen diameter is only slightly increased, and the plaque is not disrupted. (*C*) Restenosis occurred 3 months later.

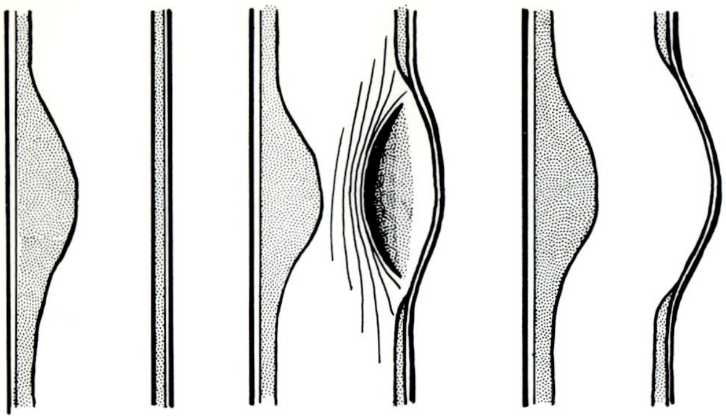

FIGURE 19-13. Mechanism of arterial disruption and remodeling after balloon dilatation. [Zarins CK, Lu CT, Gewertz BL, et al. (5). Reproduced with permission.]

reported in rabbits (9), morphologic studies of human lesions are thus far inconclusive. Configurational alterations of lesions and extension of dissection planes to adjacent undilated segments of the vessel may result in an angiographic appearance of ''progression'' or ''acceleration'' of disease without actual changes in the volume of an intimal plaque. On the basis of current findings, it is likely that restenosis occurs not by new plaque deposition, but by retraction or sclerosis of the disrupted and/or overstretched artery wall, by faulty attachment of the dissected intima, or by thrombus deposition.

Conclusion

Balloon dilatation of human stenotic and occluded arteries occurs by (1) disruption of the plaque and artery wall, (2) separation of the plaque from the wall, and (3) stretching of the artery wall to enlarge the lumen. There is little evidence for plaque compression, molding, herniation or fragmentation, or loss of plaque substance. The acute disruptive changes are followed by remodeling with apparent reattachment of the intimal flaps to the vessel wall. These features are represented in Figure 19-13. Patency is maintained mainly by persistent ''overstretching'' of the vessel wall. Restenosis probably results from contraction, retraction, or sclerosis of the overstretched artery wall or thrombus formation rather than by new plaque deposition.

References

1. Dotter CT, Judkins MP: Transluminal treatment of an arteriosclerotic obstructions: Description of a new technique and a preliminary report of its application. Circulation 1964, 30:654.
2. Grüntzig A, Kumpe D: Technique of percutaneous transluminal angioplasty with the Grüntzig balloon catheter. AJR 1979, 132:547.
3. Lyon RT, Zarins CK, Lu CT, Yang CF, Glagov S: Arterial wall disruption by balloon dilatation: Quantitative comparison of normal, stenotic and occluded vessels. Surg Forum 1981, 32:326.
4. Castaneda-Zunaga WR, Amplatz KA: The mechanism of transluminal angioplasty. In Castaneda-Zunaga WR (ed): *Transluminal Angioplasty*. New York, Thieme-Stratton, 1983, pp 11–19.
5. Zarins CK, Lu CT, Gewertz BL, Lyon RT, Rush DS, Glagov S: Arterial disruption and remodeling following balloon dilatation. Surgery 1982, 92:1086.
6. Turcotte JK, Lu CT, Zarins CK: The role of transluminal angioplasty in limb salvage and claudication. J Surg Res 1981, 30:428.
7. Rush DS, Gewertz BL, Lu CT, Ball DG, Zarins CK: Limb salvage in poor-risk patients using transluminal angioplasty. Arch Surg 1983, 118:1209.
8. Doubilet P, Abrams HL: The cost of underutilization: Percutaneous transluminal angioplasty for peripheral vascular disease. N Engl J Med 1984, 2:95.
9. Faxon DP, Sanborn TA, Weber VJ, Haudenschild C, Gottsman SB, McGovern WA, Ryan TJ: Restenosis following transluminal angioplasty in experimental atherosclerosis. Arteriosclerosis 1984, 4:189.

Chapter 20

ADJUNCTIVE INTRAOPERATIVE DILATATION (ANGIOPLASTY)

JAMES J. ZIMMERMAN and THOMAS J. FOGARTY

The concept of transluminal angioplasty was introduced by Dotter in 1963 (1). In 1964, the first clinical presentation of a patient treated by this technique was reported by Dotter and Judkin (2). Originally, guide wires were passed through an arterial narrowing. Fixed-diameter catheters of increasing size were then passed over these guide wires with a resultant enlargement of the arterial lumen.

Van Andel then used Teflon exchange catheters over guide wires to accomplish dilatation (3). Next, Porstmann used Teflon catheters that could be expanded by latex balloons held within the catheter body (4). In 1974, Gruntzig and Hopff introduced double-lumen coaxial balloon catheters for transluminal arterial dilatation (5). The third generation of catheters now exists for intraoperative and percutaneous usage, the linear extrusion dilatation catheter (6). The development of nonelastomeric balloon dilating catheters has expanded the application and reduced the complications associated with dilatation procedures. Intraoperative dilatation by coaxial systems, i.e., guide wire exchange methods or linear extrusion Fogarty-Chin dilatation catheters, is greatly expanding the forefront of vascular surgery.

Pathophysiological Features of Dilatation

The factors involved in luminal expansion following angioplasty have been defined only recently (Figure 20-1). In our studies, dilatation occurs by separation at the plaque–normal arterial wall junction by cracking within the plaque collinear with the vessel axis and by some arterial wall disruption. This frees the arterial wall to expand under physiological pressures (7). This outward displacement of the wall accounts for 85 to 95 percent of the increased lumen area. Plaque compaction is minimal, contributing less than 2 percent to the increased luminal size. Extrusion of fluid content from the atherosclerotic plaque contributes approximately 10 to 12 percent to luminal size increases.

The concern with any dilatation, whether operative or percutaneous, is that a dissection will develop and cause vessel occlusion. Dissections are the norm in both operative and percutaneous dilatations. In order to understand more fully the reasons for the relatively infrequent vessel occlusion postdilatation, the characteristics of blood flow need be examined.

In nonstenotic vessels, flow is laminar. The flow velocity is essentially zero along the intimal surface at most nonbranch points. Shear stresses (the concentration of frictional force per unit area) are low along these arterial wall–blood interfaces. As the center of the vessel is approached, the velocity of blood flow increases. Blood flow is known to be turbulent, therefore nonlaminar, at bifurcations and other wall irregularities, thus increasing the shear stress and the risk for flap dissection and occlusion. When dilatation occurs, the cracking and separation of the plaque at its junction with the normal artery usually occurs in a longitudinal direction (see Chapter 19). Since the tears are collinear with the flow, there is minimal dissection potential. This also reduces the possibility for distal embolization. Dilatation at a major branch increases the possibility of transverse dissection. Thus angioplasty of stenotic lesions at bifurcations has a significantly increased risk of producing an occlusion.

Because plaques are incompressible, plaque disruption primarily alters the remaining layers of the vessel wall. When the media is stretched beyond a finite limit, it will no longer recover its original shape. When the media distends, it carries the atheromatous plaques along with it (see Chapter 18). The medial

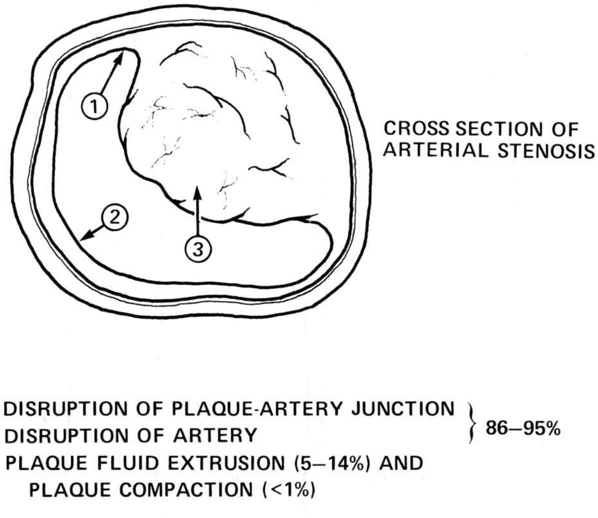

FIGURE 20-1. Mechanisms of vessel enlargement.

muscle fibers become irreversibly stretched, and this is demonstrable histologically by a corkscrew appearance of nuclei which fail to return to their resting state after dilatation (8). After the media is freed from the limiting effect of the atheromata, the vessel lumen remains enlarged under normal physiological pressure. Overzealous dilatation, however, can produce adventitial rupture.

In general, the most severe damage during dilatation occurs to the intima. Following endothelial injury there is deposition of platelets with invasion of the media by platelets and plasma components. This initiates activation of smooth-muscle mitogenicity with proliferation and migration of smooth-muscle cells to the intima. Further deposition of the connective tissue matrix results in eventual development of additional fibromuscular plaque (9). Further maturation of the fibromuscular plaque can proceed with central necrosis, lipid infiltration, hemorrhage, calcification, ulceration, and eventually thrombosis. Such complicated plaques may give rise to stenotic and embolic symptoms. Percutaneous or intraoperative angioplasty and its benefits must be weighed against potential hazards to the segment of vessel less involved in the atherosclerotic process. It is the intent of angioplasty to produce controlled injury with a predictable healing response. Clinical experience indicates this is possible in the majority of cases.

Mechanisms of Balloon Dilatation Catheters

Atherosclerotic vessels are most resistant to deformation in areas of stenosis. Attempts to dilate vessels with an elastomeric balloon, i.e., embolectomy latex balloon catheters, are unsuccessful because the balloon deforms and conforms around a noncompliant stenosis. Unlike embolectomy balloon catheters, nonelastomeric dilatation balloon catheters attain a constant shape independent of the nature of the arterial wall.

Balloon dilatation systems utilize both volumetric and pressure measurements for safe and effective angioplasty. The pressure in a dilating balloon is directly proportional to the force on the syringe piston of the syringe used in the dilatation and is inversely proportional to the cross-sectional area of the syringe barrel. The smaller the syringe diameter, the greater the force applied per unit area.

The balloon catheter dilating forces are related to radial and longitudinal pressures. Dilatation balloons exert greater radial than longitudinal forces. The phenomenon whereby a balloon or any sphere or oval stretches or separates at its circumference when pressure is applied from within is known as "hoop stress" (Figure 20-2).

The dilating force exerted by balloon catheters is also a function of balloon length. The shorter the length of a specific balloon, the more dilating force can be exerted. A balloon 1 cm long may generate 50 percent more force than a balloon 4 cm in length (10).

The characteristics of balloon material composition vary with temperature and multiple inflations. Dilatation elements need to be pliable, nonelastomeric, and of sufficient strength to effectively exert the dilating pressures on a stenosis to effect dilatation.

The force that causes permanent balloon deformation should be very close to its ultimate tensile strength, or the force required to produce bursting. If this is true, overdilatation of the artery during excessive pressure application will be prevented. The diameter of nonelastomeric balloons should change very little during maximum dilating force.

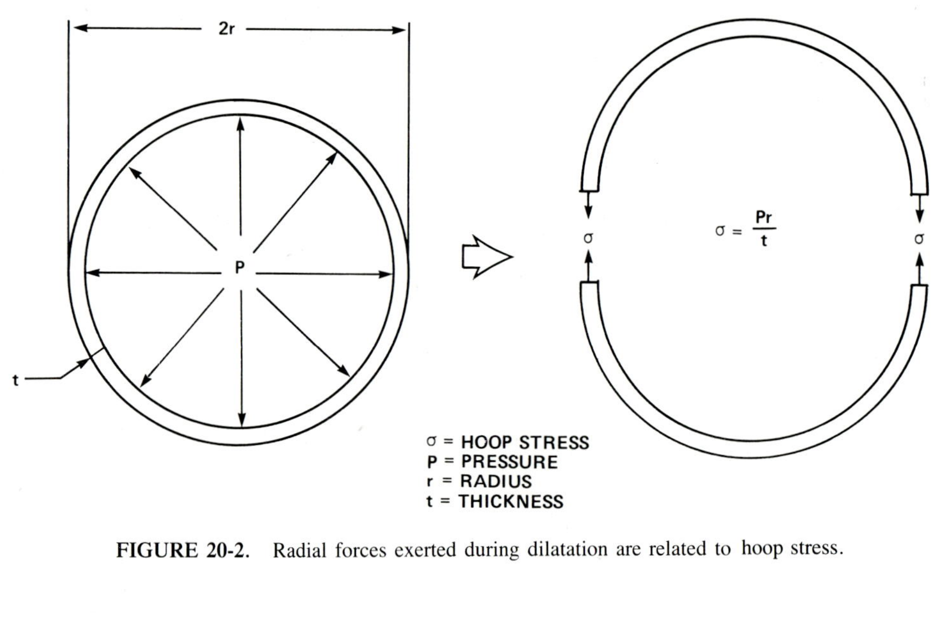

FIGURE 20-2. Radial forces exerted during dilatation are related to hoop stress.

Indications for Operative Dilatation

The primary role of angioplasty is to open an occluded or stenotic vessel and maintain long-term patency. Adjunctive intraoperative angioplasty strives to increase inflow or outflow or to extend reconstruction to the conventionally unreconstructable situation. In significantly compromised and poor-risk patients, the simplified techniques of angioplasty can reduce the risks of extended surgery. The benefit in reducing the number and magnitude of operative procedures in the high-risk elderly patient is obvious.

Preoperative Preparation

The preoperative preparation of the vascular patient for surgical intervention and potential intraoperative dilatation is initiated with a well-performed history and physical. Often, patients are moderately debilitated, long-term smokers with multiple organ involvement. The systemic nature of atheromatous disease makes assessment of the cerebrovascular and cardiac circulation prudent.

The noninvasive laboratory functions as a preoperative indicator and excellent postoperative follow-up tool for the objective assessment of patients undergoing angioplasty. Laboratory evaluations, including complete blood count, prothrombin time, partial thromboplastin time, electrolyte panel, chest x-ray, and cardiograms, are all mandatory prior to elective vascular interventions. Intravenous preoperative hydration and central venous pressure monitoring or Swan-Ganz catheter insertion for adequate cardiac assessment are required for complicated vascular patients.

The role of preoperative antiplatelet therapy is as yet unclear. It has been our policy to pretreat all patients with 5 grains of aspirin a day prior to surgery and postoperatively to continue aspirin 5 grains daily and dipyridamole 75 mg three times daily, for an indefinite period of time after their dilatation.

Operative Management

If intraoperative dilatation is contemplated, the operative management is a team effort involving the surgeon and an anesthesiologist familiar with vascular problems. The operating table should be compatible with radiographic equipment for fluoroscopic or plain-film intraoperative angiograms. Routinely, central venous pressure, urine output, temperature, and arterial pressure are monitored.

Wide operative exposure and adequate vessel dissection facilitate easy, safe access for calibration and dilatation. The site of arteriotomy is dependent upon the operation to be performed and the specific arteriosclerotic pattern within each vessel. Standard techniques for arterial manipulation are used, and performance of planned proximal or distal surgery is carried out prior to the dilatation.

Dilatation is performed through the nearly completed anastomosis prior to the reestablishment of flow. It is our belief that if dilatations are carried out far in advance of the reestablishment of flow, then the advantages of the laminar flow are significantly reduced. The dilated vessel with no flow has a stagnant column of blood which may have a greater predisposition for thrombosis and will not be maximally remodeled by arterial pressure and flow. It is for this reason that we advocate leaving the dilatation catheter in place during the reconstruction.

Catheter Selection

The dilatation catheters presently available for operative use are those of the coaxial and linear extrusion variety. Utilizing coaxial systems, a guide wire must be passed under fluoroscopic guidance for placement beyond a specific lesion. A rigid catheter with an external balloon is then forced through the lesion and the balloon inflated. With the linear extrusion catheter, fluoroscopy is not necessary to transverse tortuous vessels. The rigid portion of the extrusion balloon is placed immediately proximal to the stenotic segment. Dilatation occurs as the balloon evaginates and unrolls concomitant with dilating the lesion.

The shear forces generated are significantly different between coaxial catheters, coaxial balloon catheters, and linear extrusion balloon catheters (11) (Figure 20-3). The results of experiments utilizing model stenoses document that more severe stenoses produce greater shear forces for a given catheter design. In a range of simulated stenoses (69 to 97 percent), the coaxial dilator exerts the highest forces, followed by the coaxial balloon catheter. The linear extrusion catheter exerts the lowest shear forces upon the arterial wall. The reason the linear extrusion system has reduced arterial shear force is that its dilating element is advanced by unrolling, while the coaxial systems all require sliding a rigid catheter over guide wires.

Simultaneous intraoperative dilatation with reconstructive procedures offers operating room sterility, as well as the potential for immediate correction of complications if they are recognized. The choice of the balloon size for dilatation must be appropriate to both the size of the vessel and the amount of plaque present.

It is well known that high-grade stenoses have significant flow reduction. It is not so well appreciated that reestablishment of a normal lumen size in an arteriosclerotic vessel may not be advantageous. Significant increases in flow occur with a minimum reduction in stenosis. A vessel which is 75 to 85 percent stenotic may have a highly significant increase in flow with a return to a 40 to 50 percent stenosis. If attempts are made to return all vessels to a normal diameter, the complication rate significantly

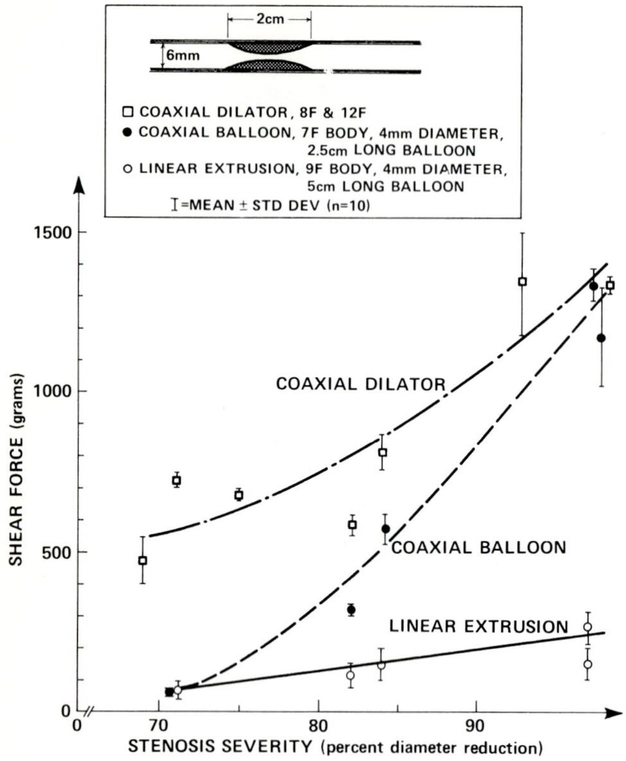

FIGURE 20-3. Sheer stresses generated by dilatation catheters.

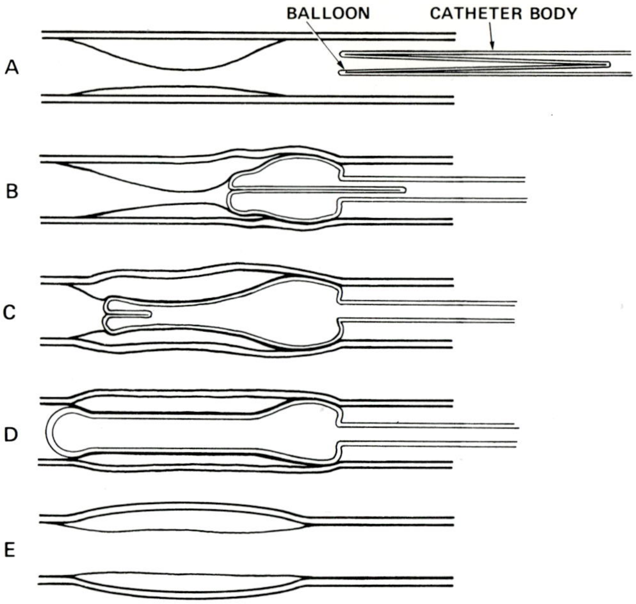

FIGURE 20-4. Mechanisms of action of the linear extrusion dilatation system.

increases. It is not always easy to appreciate the vessel caliber change when dealing with small vessels of the 1- to 3-mm size. Slight increases in small-vessel lumen diameter may produce an important increase in flow.

It is our belief that the linear extrusion catheter system represents the safest and simplest means to reduce complications and improve inflow or improve outflow in patients who need a complicated vascular reconstruction. To understand the dilating element, the catheter may be considered a bag which simply unrolls into a cylinder as it insinuates its way through the stenosis. Overinflation of the balloon by pressure or volume of the balloon will lead to bursting. The actual dilatation of the Fogarty extrusion balloon occurs simultaneously with the unrolling of the dilating element through the lesion and is completed upon full extrusion via inflation (Figure 20-4).

Catheter Placement and the Concepts of Calibration

The basic techniques of dilatation are shown in Figure 20-5. In the figure, the high-grade iliac stenosis would require a more complicated vascular reconstruction to ensure the patency of a femoral distal bypass. The distal anastomosis has been completed and the proximal anastomosis is partially completed. The common femoral, deep femoral, and superficial femoral arteries are isolated and occluded with atraumatic occluding devices. The arteriotomy has been made in the appropriate direction as predetermined by the arteriosclerotic pattern with the vessel.

The calibration procedure is critically important in order to ensure a successful dilatation. Calibration serves to confirm the arteriographic findings, documents the distance the dilatation catheter is to be inserted, and allows one to choose the proper balloon diameter.

The diameter of the dilatation balloon is determined by inflating the balloon calibrator with saline and introducing it to the level of the obstruction. The catheter is withdrawn 1 cm, and additional volume is injected until movement of the catheter is restricted. At this point, the fluid volume injected is noted by making reference to the syringe barrel. The balloon is partially deflated and removed. Reinflation of the balloon outside the artery with the previously documented volume accurately reflects the diameter of the dilatation balloon to be used. Linear extrusion dilatation catheters should not be passed through the lesion. The extrusion should be initiated approximately 1 cm short of the lesion. This distance is determined by passing the partially inflated balloon calibrator until further passage is prevented. This linear length noted on the body of the balloon calibrator minus 1 cm indicates the level to which the dilatation catheter should be passed.

By a combination of this calibration procedure and reference to the preoperative arteriogram, the proper size dilatation catheter is chosen.

The dilatation catheter system is prepared for use by purging it of air with a solution of 50 percent contrast medium and 50 percent saline. A monitoring pressure gauge should be in line during the purging procedure.

The amount of pressure and volume for the different size catheter system is indicated on the individual catheter package. These values should not be exceeded. After calibration, the proper size catheter is selected. The dilatation catheter is introduced to the predetermined level and the system pressurized.

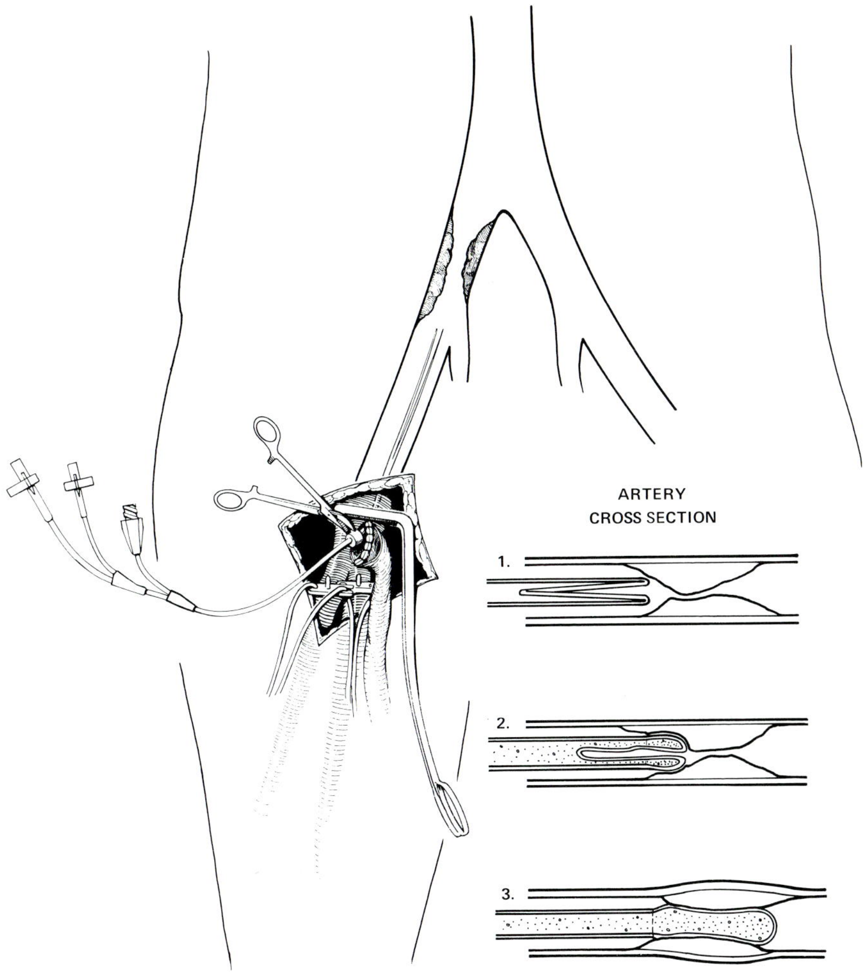

FIGURE 20-5. Technique of intraoperative adjunctive iliac dilatation.

High initial balloon pressures are needed to begin extrusion. A tuberculin syringe may be useful for gaining maximum control in the absence of a gated pressure inflator for the initial 2- to 4-mm extrusion of the balloon. The remainder of the precalibrated volume on the pressure syringe is then injected. As the balloon insinuates through the stenosis, the pressure will be high and will abruptly drop after passing through the stenosis. Additional volume may be required to overcome system compliance and to produce desired plaque deformation. The balloon is then deflated and withdrawn through the arteriotomy. Reinflation of the balloon to maximum inflation pressure and volume confirms complete extrusion. If the predetermined maximum inflation pressure and/or volume is exceeded, bursting or leakage will occur. Adequate antegrade flushing is carried out for removal of any possible debris and to test the adequacy of improved flow. The remainder of the anastomosis is then completed. Operative arteriography either by fluoroscopy or by films may also be used to assess the adequacy of the dilatation. When the success of the surgical procedure depends on adequate inflow, the success of the proximal dilatation should be confirmed. In proximal iliac lesions, improved antegrade inflow may suffice as a guide as to whether a satisfactory dilatation has been accomplished.

Postoperative Management

Immediate postoperative Doppler-determined and pulse volume recordings are important. Although initial spasm or constriction often exists in the distal arterial tree, within several hours a return of pulses or excellent Doppler-determined pressure should be present. In the event that unsatisfactory results are obtained, reoperation with angiography is indicated. Sequential postoperative noninvasive testing is important for the assessment of the long-term results of not only the dilatation but also the reconstructive surgery. These noninvasive tests will serve as valuable guides of the progression or recurrence of the vascular disease. Early ambulation may significantly benefit the results of dilatation by increasing the flow through the lesion and helping to fix it in an optimally dilated position.

Complications

The complications of balloon dilatation, whether operatively or percutaneously, are those of hemorrhage, thrombosis, hematoma formation, vessel rupture, arteriovenous fistula, occlusion of collateral vessels, and extraluminal passage of the catheter system. Unlike percutaneous transluminal angioplasty, operative angioplasty often allows one to deal immediately with complications without the added risks of time delays or indecision.

Results

Although balloon angioplasty in its present form is relatively new, data are accumulating that reasonable patency may be expected, especially in the iliac and upper superficial femoral artery systems. Utilizing extrusion balloons, our early results have demonstrated significant improvement in the iliac system in approximately 90 percent of patients. The ability to simplify operative techniques when intraabdominal procedures would be required may significantly alter the long-term mortality and morbidity rates of complicated vascular patients. The results of extrusion balloons for subclavian stenosis and fibromuscular disease of the carotid and renal artery are still too scanty to evaluate.

Vessels treated with intraoperative extrusion dilatation have been calibrated and demonstrate improvement in vessel diameter ranging from 30 to 166 percent over baseline. The average increase for all vessels in one study was 78 percent (12). Postoperative angiograms were obtained in these patients from 2 months to 3 years after their initial procedure. Significant angiographic improvement was found in 80 percent.

Conclusion

Adjunctive intraoperative dilatation represents a significant advance in the therapeutic modalities available to the vascular surgeon. Intraoperative balloon dilatation, in conjunction with vascular reconstruction, can safely reduce the extent of surgery by improving inflow or outflow.

References

1. Dotter CT: Cardiac catheterization and angiographic techniques of the future. Cesk Radiol 1965, 19:217–236.
2. Dotter CT, Judkins MP: Transluminal treatment of arteriosclerotic obstruction: Description of a new technique and a preliminary report of its applications. Circulation 1964, 30:654–670.
3. Van Andel GJ: *Percutaneous Transluminal Angioplasty*. The Dotter Procedure. *A Manual for the Radiologist*. Amsterdam, Excepta Medica, 1976, pp 114–115.
4. Porstmann W, Wierny L: Intravasale Rekanalisation insperabler arterieller Obliterationen. Zentralbl Chir 1967, 92:1586–1591.
5. Gruntzig A, Hopff H: Perkutane Rekahalisation chronischer arterieller Verschlusse mit einem neuen Dilatationskatheter. Dtsch Med Wochenschr 1974, 99:2502–2505.
6. Fogarty TJ, Chin A, Shoor PM, Blair GL, Zimmerman JJ: Adjunctive intraoperative arterial dilation. Arch Surg 1981, 116:1391–1396.
7. Chin AK, Fogarty TJ, Kinney TB, Hayden WG, Shoor PM, Rurik GW: Pathophysiologic bases for transluminal dilatation. Surg Forum 1981, 32:323–325.
8. Castenada-Zuniga WR, Amplatz K, Laerum F, Formanik K, Sibley R, Edwards J: Mechanics of angioplasty: An experimental approach. Radiographics 1981, 1:1–14.
9. Block PC, Baughman KL, Pasternak RC, Falloon JT: Transluminal angioplasty: Correlation of morphologic and angiographic findings in an experimental model. Circulation 1980, 61:778–785.
10. Abele JE: Balloon catheters and transluminal dilatation: Technical consideration. Am J Radiol 1980, 135:90–96.
11. Kinney TB, Chin AK, Rurik GW, Finn JC, Shoor PM, Hayden WG, Fogarty TJ: Transluminal angioplasty: A mechanical-pathophysiological correlation of its physical mechanism. Radiology 1984, 153:85–89.
12. Zeitler E, Muller R: Erste Ergebnisse mit der Katheter-Rekanalisation nach Dotter bei arterieller Verschlusskrankheit. ROFO 1969, 111:345–352.

Chapter 21

PREOPERATIVE EVALUATION AND PERIOPERATIVE MANAGEMENT OF ASSOCIATED CARDIAC DISEASE IN VASCULAR SURGICAL PATIENTS

ANTHONY D. WHITTEMORE, HERBERT B. HECHTMAN,
and JOHN A. MANNICK

The systemic nature of atherosclerosis imposes a broad challenge to successful perioperative management of patients undergoing vascular reconstruction. That the underlying disease process is systemic has been clearly demonstrated in several studies attesting to the increased prevalence of concurrent manifestations of atherosclerosis in these patients as compared to the general population. Notable among such reports is the Framingham Study, which documented the incidence of coronary artery disease in patients with claudication as two to five times higher than nonclaudicators (1). Claudicants were also characterized by an increased incidence of cerebrovascular and hypertensive disease. Of patients undergoing vascular reconstruction approximately 50 percent have coexistent, clinically evident cardiac impairment, and as many as an additional 18 percent may have highly significant, but clinically silent, coronary artery disease (2–4). In one of the largest series, routine coronary angiography demonstrated surgically correctable disease in 31 percent of patients with aortic aneurysms, 26 percent of those with cerebrovascular disease, and 21 percent of patients with peripheral ischemia (3).

Successful perioperative management of patients undergoing vascular reconstruction is contingent upon minimizing the considerable morbidity and mortality rates associated with an impaired myocardium. It is within this context that the present chapter deals with the perioperative cardiac management of the vascular surgical patient.

Preoperative Evaluation

CARDIAC DISEASE

The incidence of significant antecedent cardiac disease approaches 50 percent among vascular surgical patients, an incidence subsequently reflected in the preponderance of cardiac complications perioperatively. It is therefore incumbent on the surgeon to document the extent of associated heart disease, to properly select both patient and operative procedure, and to provide appropriate preoperative care to reduce existing risk factors.

Coronary Artery Disease

ANTECEDENT MYOCARDIAL INFARCTION. The most significant preoperative risk factor associated with subsequent cardiac morbidity and mortality is a prior history of myocardial infarction. The risk of myocardial infarction associated with general anesthesia and surgery is approximately 0.2 percent for all U.S. adults, in contrast to patients with known ischemic heart disease who have a considerably higher risk rate (5,6). Data generated in the 1970s demonstrated that of individuals with ischemic heart disease, those with preoperative myocardial infarction represented the group at highest risk (6–9). The incidence of postoperative reinfarction correlated with a subsequent mortality rate which ranged from 50 to 83 percent. Patients operated upon within 3 months following a myocardial infarction sustained an approximate 30 percent risk of reinfarction or cardiac death postoperatively. Procedures carried out between 3 and 6 months following infarction were complicated by a 15 percent incidence of postoperative recurrent infarction, and after 6 months the reinfarction rate stabilized at 5 percent. Although early reports indicated a difference in risk between subendocardial as compared with transmural infarctions, more recent data overwhelmingly fail to confirm any significant distinction (9,10). Based on these earlier observations, recent advances in both surgical and anesthetic technique appear to have substantially reduced the postoperative reinfarction rate to 8 percent in patients operated upon within 3 months following infarction and to 3.5 percent in those undergoing procedures between 3 and 6 months (11,12). These more recent reports do not, however, discriminate between vascular patients and other general surgical procedures, yet it is certainly reasonable to assume that with meticulous attention to reducing associated risk factors, such excellent results can indeed be obtained.

It is therefore evident that elective vascular reconstruction should be delayed for 6 months following myocardial infarction to minimize postoperative cardiac morbidity. It is equally evident that truly emergent situations warranting immediate vascular reconstruction will require maximal intensive monitoring and management to reduce the additional risk assumed.

ANGINA. It has been repeatedly shown that patients with angina pectoris are at a higher risk for postoperative cardiac complications than patients with no evidence of ischemic heart disease. Of considerable interest, however, is the fact that stable angina when viewed as an independent predictor of postoperative cardiac complications has not emerged as a significant risk factor after controlling for concomitant manifestations of impaired cardiac function (10). In addition to a myocardial infarction within 6 months, the clinical parameters obtained from history, physical, and routine noninvasive evaluation which carry a significant predictive value for postoperative myocardial infarction consist of advanced age (greater than 70 years), mitral insufficiency, greater than five ventricular ectopic beats per minute, congestive heart failure, and a tortuous or calcified aorta on chest film (9). Patients with chronic stable angina as the only clinical manifestation of ischemic heart disease do not appear to be at a significantly higher risk for postoperative cardiac morbidity and mortality than the normal population.

The perioperative evaluation and management of patients with angina nevertheless remain highly controversial. The controversy stems from differing methods of patient selection in reported series, from differing criteria for establishing the occurrence of a postoperative myocardial infarction given that 50 percent of such infarctions are silent (6,9,13), and from evidence that patients who have undergone coronary artery bypass appear to undergo subsequent noncardiac surgery at a substantially reduced risk (14–16).

Patients with unstable, accelerating, or nocturnal angina are for the most part candidates for coronary artery bypass with or without anticipated noncardiac surgery. It is therefore prudent to proceed with routine cardiac evaluation, including preoperative angiography and preliminary coronary bypass as indicated prior to elective vascular reconstruction. In the event that such patients require emergent vascular surgery, consideration should be given to simultaneous coronary artery bypass. This approach has been used successfully in patients with symptomatic aortic aneurysms (17).

The most controversial patients with ischemic heart disease remain those who are asymptomatic or those with chronic stable angina [New York Heart Association (NYHA) class II]. The routine utilization of preoperative stress testing has been repeatedly proposed, but reservations regarding diagnostic accuracy combined with a small but finite mortality rate impose limitations on their use (18,19). It has also been shown that preoperative resting and pulmonary artery hemodynamic measurements of exercise are not necessarily more accurate in assessing cardiac risk than the judicious utilization of clinically available noninvasive factors (20). Routine preoperative coronary arteriography with prophylactic myocardial revascularization has been recommended, but results following subsequent vascular reconstruction do not necessarily differ from a more selective approach (17,21,22). In addition, it remains difficult to draw firm conclusions from such studies, which have generally been inadequately controlled and utilize a variety of criteria for patient selection. Routine preoperative coronary angiography for patients with stable angina (class II) is, therefore, probably not justified since the risks of infarction or death with catheterization and subsequent bypass surgery may in fact be significantly higher than the risks of the same complications from the anticipated noncardiac surgery (23,24).

Congestive Heart Failure

The second major factor predisposing to postoperative cardiac morbidity is the presence of preoperative congestive heart failure (25). As demonstrated in Table 21-1, only 2 percent of patients with no prior history of congestive failure develop cardiogenic pulmonary edema postoperatively.

In contrast, patients with severe failure manifested by a third

TABLE 21-1. Correlation between Signs and Symptoms of Preoperative Heart Failure and Risk of Perioperative Pulmonary Edema after Major Surgery in Patients over Age 40

Signs and Symptoms	Total Patients, *n*	% Developing Cardiogenic Pulmonary Edema
No history of congestive failure	853	2
History of left heart failure but not evident on preoperative examination or chest film	87	6
Left heart failure by preoperative physical examination or chest film	66	16
Preoperative NYHA functional class for congestive heart failure:		
I	935	3
II	15	7
III	34	6
IV	17	25
History of pulmonary edema	22	23
S_3 gallop	17	25
Jugular venous distension and signs of left heart failure	23	30

SOURCE: Data from Goldman (25).

heart sound or jugular venous distension engender a 30 to 35 percent risk of postoperative pulmonary edema. The incidence of postoperative failure also correlates with the functional classification according to the NYHA. For a NYHA class IV patient, postoperative pulmonary edema developed in 25 percent of Goldman's patients, adversely affecting the operative mortality rate (10). The perioperative mortality rate among these patients is primarily dependent upon the degree of failure present at the time of operation, rather than the maximal severity of decompensation by history. Retrospective analysis suggests that satisfactory control of congestive heart failure preoperatively substantially reduces the risk of cardiac morbidity and mortality (9).

It is therefore mandatory when time allows to provide maximal therapy for congestive heart failure preoperatively. Since this risk reduction involves the use of diuretic therapy with fluid restriction, rapid control of uncompensated congestive heart failure is invariably accompanied by some degree of relative hypovolemia. It is advisable to allow sufficient time preoperatively for reequilibration such that vasodilation attendant to anesthesia does not result in significant hypotension. In urgent situations, diuresis should be restrained to that just sufficient to control congestive failure, and an anesthetic technique designed to minimize vasodilation should be utilized.

Arrhythmias

An increased risk for perioperative cardiac morbidity has been documented in patients with preoperative arrhythmias, most notable among these, frequent premature ventricular contractions (9,10). The cardiac morbidity rate encountered in such individuals relates primarily to the underlying coronary or myocardial disease rather than to the arrhythmia per se. Thus, these patients develop ischemic or congestive complications resulting from the underlying disease process (26,27). Prophylactic pharmacologic control of preoperative arrhythmias is usually not warranted unless the arrhythmia exacerbates coexistent ischemia or left ventricular failure. Therapy with intravenous lidocaine, therefore, would most appropriately be utilized preoperatively for patients with ventricular tachyarrhythmias associated with hypotension by history. In the majority of instances, however, the patient's chronic antiarrhythmic medication should be continued through the morning of surgery, and further therapy instituted as necessary based upon the hemodynamic significance of a particular arrhythmic occurrence.

The patient with established heart block is at considerable risk for perioperative cardiac complications not only because the dysrhythmia reflects underlying myocardial disease, but also because the ability to augment stroke volume in response to stress is impaired (28). This impaired ability to increase cardiac output in response to wide variance in peripheral resistance and left ventricular filling pressure is exacerbated by anesthetic agents which further depress myocardial contractility and/or cause peripheral vasodilatation. The patient with chronic heart block should clearly be provided with at least a temporary pacemaker perioperatively.

A more controversial issue pertains to the patient with chronic bifascicular block. There is no evidence to support a predictable progression from bifascicular to complete block during the perioperative period (9). On the other hand, a significant number of patients during the course of an acute myocardial infarction will indeed progress, often with sudden hemodynamic decompensation. In addition, it is known that approximately 5 percent of patients with established bifascicular block will develop complete heart block annually (29). It would thus seem reasonable to select out a group of patients with established bifascicular block and a history of unexplained syncope for temporary pacing perioperatively. Aside from this select group, patients with chronic bifascicular block are at increased cardiac risk from their underlying myocardial disease rather than from the specific conduction defect.

Valvular Disease

Although there is a slight increase in the incidence of embolization and endocarditis, the cardiac mortality and morbidity of valvular disease are predominantly associated with the degree of underlying myocardial decompensation. Patients who are either asymptomatic, or who have only a mild degree of functional limitation (NYHA class II), appear to be at no added risk and require no additional preoperative therapy with the exception of prophylactic antibiosis for endocarditis. Patients with critical stenosis and significant physical limitations characteristic of NYHA class III or IV are clearly at higher risk for perioperative sudden death or pulmonary edema (30,31). Every effort must be made to identify these high-risk individuals and institute appropriate therapy preoperatively.

Patients with symptomatic aortic stenosis manifested by angina, syncopal episodes, or significant congestive failure should therefore undergo preoperative cardiac catheterization (32). Should critical aortic stenosis be identified (area less than 0.5 cm^2/m^2), preoperative aortic valve replacement should be undertaken, while those with noncritical aortic stenosis in the presence of these symptoms require intensive hemodynamic perioperative monitoring. In similar fashion, patients with severe mitral stenosis, indicated by a mitral valve area less than 1.0 cm^2, should also undergo preliminary mitral valve replacement.

Patients with severe congestive failure resulting from either aortic or mitral regurgitation are also at increased risk for postoperative cardiac complications as in any patient with congestive failure. Such individuals need not necessarily undergo valve replacement prior to vascular reconstruction, provided failure is controlled and adequate hemodynamic monitoring is employed.

Patients with prosthetic valves are often maintained on chronic anticoagulation with sodium warfarin (Coumadin), depending upon the type and position of valve utilized. Several studies, however, have failed to document any significant increase in the number of thromboembolic events when anticoagulants were withheld during the 3 days prior to and following noncardiac surgery (33,34). Chronic anticoagulation should be withheld during the perioperative period to avoid an increased incidence of hemorrhagic complications. Since most bleeding can be controlled, however, whereas the sequela of a single thromboembolic event may well be irreversible, it is not unreasonable to provide some form of anticoagulation throughout the perioperative period, particularly in those patients with valves known to be more highly thrombogenic. Chronic warfarin therapy, therefore, should be discontinued 2 to 3 days preoperatively, and heparin instituted until 4 to 6 h preoperatively and then discontinued. It has been our policy to protect such patients with intravenous dextran during the first few days postoperatively, at which point heparin therapy or oral anticoagulation is resumed.

SURGICAL PROCEDURE

Intuitively one would anticipate that the cardiac morbidity and mortality rates would be directly related to the magnitude of the surgical procedure undertaken. This in fact has proved true, such that intrathoracic and intraperitoneal procedures carry a higher cardiac complication rate than more peripheral procedures (9,10). Numerous surgical series attest to the fact that cardiac complications occur less frequently in extracranial or peripheral vascular reconstruction when compared to transperitoneal aortic procedures. In addition, elective procedures are associated with a reduced cardiac risk when compared to emergent procedures of any nature. Therefore, an emergency transperitoneal aortic procedure will more often place higher demands on the uncompensated myocardium than an elective carotid endarterectomy or distal bypass procedure. In order to reduce the cardiac morbidity and mortality rates associated with emergency aortic procedures, consideration must be given to rapidly correcting the underlying cardiac impairment which may include emergency or simultaneous valve replacement or coronary artery bypass (17,35).

MULTIVARIATE ASSESSMENT

Several parameters of cardiac performance are thus associated with varying degrees of risk, both as single independent factors and when combined with others. It becomes very difficult to quantitate the actual risk of a combination of factors unless some form of multivariate analysis is utilized. Multivariate regression analysis has provided a relative cardiac index to estimate the risk of serious cardiac complications in patients undergoing noncardiac surgery (25).

TABLE 21-2. Computation of Multifactorial Index Score to Estimate Cardiac Risk in Noncardiac Surgery

Factors	Points
S_3 gallop or jugular venous distension on preoperative physical examination	11
Transmural or subendocardial myocardial infarction in the previous 6 months	10
Premature ventricular beats, more than 5/min documented at any time	7
Rhythm other than sinus or presence of premature atrial contractions on last preoperative electrocardiogram	7
Age over 70 years	5
Emergency operation	4
Intrathoracic, intraperitoneal, or aortic site of surgery	3
Evidence for important valvular aortic stenosis	3
Poor general medical condition*	3

*As evidenced by electrolyte abnormalities (potassium, < 3.0 meq/L; HCO_3, < 20 meq/L); renal insufficiency (blood urea nitrogen, > 50 mg/dL; creatinine, > 3.0 mg/dL); abnormal blood gases (P_{O_2}, < 60 mmHg; P_{CO_2}, > 50 mmHg); abnormal liver status (elevated aspartate transaminase or signs on physical examination of chronic liver disease); or any condition that has caused the patient to be chronically bedridden.

SOURCE: Data from Goldman (25).

TABLE 21-3. Incidence of Cardiac Complications following Noncardiac Surgery in 1001 Patients Classified according to Risk Index

Risk Class	Index Points	Fatal, %	Nonfatal, %
I	0–5	0.7	0.2
II	6–12	5	2
III	13–25	11	2
IV	26	2	56

SOURCE: Data from Goldman (25).

In Table 21-2, Goldman lists nine independent variables, each of which is assigned a number of relative risk points. Poorly controlled congestive failure and recent infarction carry the highest number of points, and ''poor medical condition'' the least.

Patients may be grouped into risk classes I to IV based upon their total number of points (Table 21-3). The cardiac risk index may then be used to guide the choice of procedure and to determine the necessity for intensive hemodynamic monitoring. Although the data illustrated were derived retrospectively, the index has proved convincingly accurate when used prospectively and may be more sensitive than other commonly used classifications (36).

HYPERTENSION

Hypertension represents a significant risk factor for noncardiac surgery only when poorly controlled with diastolic pressures greater than 110 mmHg (10,37,38). Approximately 25 percent of patients with a history of hypertension will experience significant perioperative hypertension regardless of the level of preoperative control, and an additional 25 percent of such patients will develop significant hypotension. It has also become increasingly clear, despite prior evidence to the contrary, that chronic antihypertensive medication should be continued to the morning of the anticipated vascular procedure. Considerable evidence suggests that this is not only safe, but may, in fact, provide some protective benefit (39–41). Initial studies suggested that patients treated with beta blockade were less able to respond hemodynamically to volume shifts attendant to major surgery (42). Subsequent studies, however, have disputed this fact and have documented that such individuals have appropriate compensatory responses (43–45). Because of these more recent findings, and the consequences of beta blockade withdrawal, propranolol or similar agents used for the control of either angina or hypertension should be continued to the morning of surgery (46,47).

Patients with poorly controlled (greater than 110 mmHg) of diastolic pressure) or refractory hypertension require more intensive preoperative evaluation. Individuals with recently documented hypertension warrant institution of chronic medical therapy with postponement of elective surgery for a 2-week period of time to allow reasonable equilibration of compartmental volumes as would be true for patients with congestive heart failure. Emergent procedures, however, can be safely undertaken with short-acting intravenous antihypertensives such as sodium nitroprusside. Vascular patients with refractory hypertension warrant careful evaluation since repair of concomitant renal artery stenosis at the time of aortic reconstruction may be undertaken with little added morbidity or mortality (48), and among those individuals with appropriate nonosteal renal artery stenoses, percutaneous transluminal angioplasty prior to anticipated vascular reconstruction may be warranted.

Perioperative Hemodynamic Monitoring

The most frequently encountered serious complications of major vascular reconstruction result directly or indirectly from cardiac dysfunction during the perioperative period. Although the mortality rate from abdominal aortic aneurysm repair, for instance, declined from 10 to 15 percent in the 1960s to 5 percent in the 1970s, this residual mortality remained predominantly cardiac in origin (49–56) (Table 21-4). This is not surprising in view of the 50 percent incidence of clinically evident cardiac disease in these patients, which may be distributed into the various risk categories as outlined in the preceding section. Proper preoperative preparation can reduce the risk in some of these individuals, but life- or limb-saving procedures not infrequently must be undertaken in patients who remain in high-risk categories despite maximal risk reduction or under emergency circumstances where time does not allow optimal preoperative risk reduction. To further reduce this residual cardiac mortality, then, normal perfusion pressure and optimal cardiac output under a variety of circumstances during the perioperative course must be maintained (35,57).

With the advent of invasive monitoring with the thermistor-tipped Swan-Ganz pulmonary artery catheter and routine radial artery cannulation, a group of 10 patients at our institution was

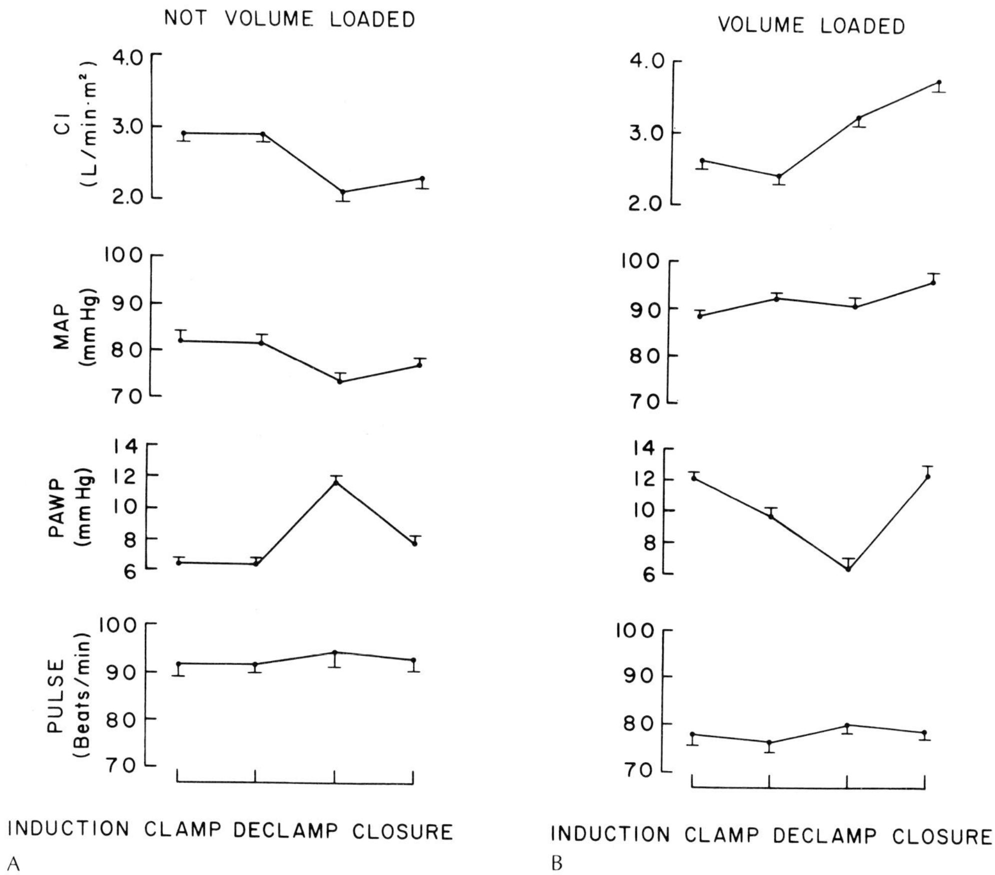

FIGURE 21-1. The intraoperative hemodynamic performance of 10 patients not volume-loaded (*A*) as compared with that of 23 volume-loaded patients (*B*) from the present series. Cardiac index (CI), mean arterial pressure (MAP), pulmonary artery wedge pressure (PAWP), and pulse were measured during induction of anesthesia, 30 minutes following aortic cross clamping, 5 minutes after declamping and during closure of the abdominal incision. Vertical bars indicate the standard error of the mean. In contrast to patients not volume-loaded preoperatively, the volume-loaded group demonstrated improved cardiac performance as evidenced by the increased CI, stable MAP, and diminished PAWP following declamping. This improvement was observed in the absence of pharmacologic manipulation. [From Whittemore, Clowes, Hechtman, et al. (35).]

TABLE 21-4. Operative Mortality Rate for Repair of Intact Abdominal Aortic Aneurysms

Year	Authors	Number of Patients	Operative Mortality Rate, %
1975	Hicks et al. (52)	113	4.2
1975	Thompson et al. (53)	108	5.5
1977	Young et al. (50)	123	5.7
1977	Scobie et al. (55)	137	4.0
1978	Baird et al. (56)	160	5.6
1979	Crawford et al. (51)	329	3.0
1980	Whittemore et al. (35)	110	0
1985	Ruby et al. (17)	227	1.3

studied during elective repair of abdominal aortic aneurysms. Cardiac index, mean arterial pressure, pulmonary artery wedge pressure, and heart rate were observed at the time of induction of anesthesia, 30 minutes after clamping the abdominal aorta, at the time of declamping, and at completion of wound closure. As demonstrated in Figure 21-1*A*, there was a significant decline in cardiac index at the time of aortic declamping associated with a concomitant decline in mean arterial pressure and an increase in pulmonary artery wedge pressure. These observations suggested that aortic declamping resulted in a temporary period of left ventricular failure. This period of relative hypotension attendant to aortic declamping has been termed *declamping shock,* known for many years to correlate with postoperative cardiac and renal complications. It was found retrospectively in this group of 10 patients that the preoperative pulmonary artery wedge pressure remained within the low range of normal. Despite adequate urine output and blood pressure, circulating plasma volume was apparently insufficient. A subsequent series of 23 patients was then investigated with the insertion of pulmonary and radial arterial catheters during the preoperative evening. The pulmonary artery wedge pressure was elevated in incremental fashion with the intravenous bolus administration of either 12.5 g of albumin or 250 mL of Ringer's lactate, and cardiac output was determined at each increment. Individual left ventricular performance curves were then constructed by plotting cardiac index against pulmonary artery wedge pressure. As illustrated by patient A in Figure 21-2, most individuals respond to an increased left ventricular filling pressure with an augmentation of cardiac index. Some were unable to compensate for an increase in wedge pressure as demonstrated by patient B whose performance curve was characterized by an initial rise in cardiac index followed by a decline as the wedge pressure was further increased. It was also found that some patients function optimally at low pulmonary artery wedge pressures such that further increases result in a precipitous decline in cardiac index (patient C). By constructing these individual left ventricular performance curves, it was possible to select a pulmonary artery wedge pressure at which cardiac index would be maximal. Such optimal myocardial function can then be maintained during the various phases of the perioperative course by the appropriate administration of fluid volume and pharmacologic manipulation of afterload and contractility. This group of 23 patients was so managed during subsequent repair of abdominal aortic aneurysms, and similar hemodynamic measurements were made at induction of anesthesia, following aortic cross clamping, 5 minutes following declamping and at the time of wound closure. As demonstrated in Figure 21-1*B*, this second group of patients maintained mean arterial pressure with a concurrent rise in cardiac index and decline in pulmonary artery wedge pressure, indicating a healthier myocardial response to aortic declamping. Monitoring was continued for 48 hours postoperatively and cardiac index maintained at optimal levels during the anticipated postoperative sequestration and subsequent mobilization of third space fluid.

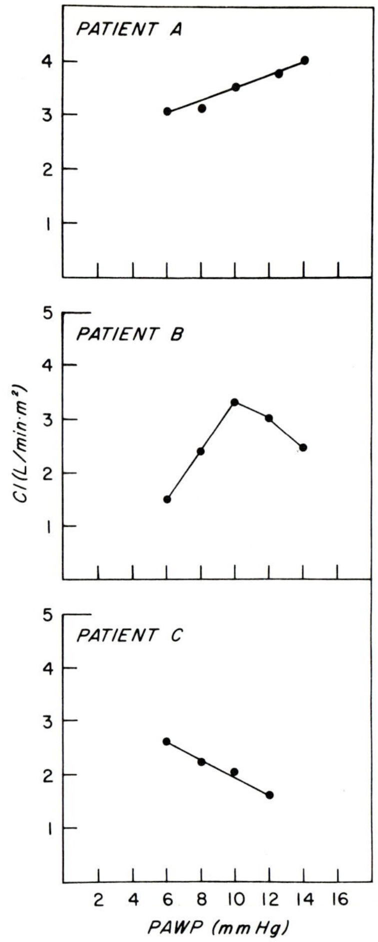

FIGURE 21-2. Three types of preoperative myocardial performance curves are illustrated. During volume infusion, patient A increases cardiac output with each increment in PAWP. In contrast, patient B has a peak in cardiac output such that with further increases in PAWP flow decreases; patient C demonstrates a steady decline in cardiac performance. Volume therapy is designed to raise the PAWP to the point at which cardiac output peaks, or if this does not occur, to a maximum of 12 to 14 mmHg with a cardiac index of more than 2.5. [From Whittemore, Clowes, Hechtman, et al. (35).]

Preoperative volume loading, carefully monitored with pulmonary artery catheterization, then allowed the maintenance of more normal hemodynamics during aortic surgery when compared to individuals who had been managed without preoperative assessment of volume status and cardiac performance. It was then postulated that such monitoring might lead to a substantial reduction in postoperative mortality from cardiac dysfunction in such patients (35). In a subsequent series of 227 consecutive patients undergoing repair of intact abdominal aortic aneurysms, hemodynamic monitoring was routinely employed (17). The

30-day operative mortality rate for this entire group was 1.3 percent, consisting of two patients who sustained fatal pulmonary emboli and one death attributable to a myocardial infarction. This single cardiac death (0.4 percent) represents a substantial reduction in cardiac morbidity and suggests, but clearly does not prove, that this method of perioperative management has merit.

Although a reduction in cardiac index attendant to aortic declamping was minimized in these patients who were adequately volume loaded, a significant fall in cardiac index at the time of aortic cross clamping remained apparent. Although this decline can be minimized with afterload reduction provided by vasodilators, experimental work suggests that circulating levels of prostenoids are elevated in patients undergoing aortic manipulation (58). Such prostaglandins consist of the potent vasodilator prostacycline and thromboxane A_2, a vasoconstrictor which is indirectly associated with a negative inotropic factor in plasma (59). Subsequent studies in patients undergoing abdominal aortic aneurysm repair demonstrated an increase in thromboxane levels following aortic cross clamping (60,61). The observed rise in circulating thromboxane levels could be minimized with the preoperative administration of either aspirin or ibuprofen. Although such studies of prostenoid metabolism may in part explain the decline in cardiac output associated with aortic cross clamping, preoperative blockade of thromboxane synthesis provided no significant difference in clinical outcome when compared to patients who received placebos. In addition, nephrotoxicity associated with a reduction of prostacycline due to cyclooxygenase inhibition may render a relatively ischemic kidney particularly susceptible. The clinical relevance of these observations, therefore, remains unclear, yet suggests that high-risk individuals with compromised cardiac reserve may benefit from modest doses of agents which inhibit thromboxane synthetase during major abdominal aortic surgery.

Anesthesia

The goals for anesthesia during vascular reconstruction include the provision of adequate analgesia and relaxation with the minimum risk of myocardial depression and hypotension. It has become axiomatic that the choice of anesthetic agent is not nearly as important as the proper selection of anesthesiologist. While there are many theoretical advantages and disadvantages to both general and regional anesthesia, and to individual agents utilized, these considerations are far outweighed by the experience of the anesthesiologist directing drug administration.

Most inhalational agents produce depression of myocardial contractility to some extent. Hallogenated agents such as halothane, and to a lesser degree, enflurane (Ethrane), not only produce myocardial depression but also minimal sympathetic stimulation, the summation resulting in relative hypotension (36,62,63). Although these effects may be overcome by appropriate pharmacologic and volume measures, rapid fluctuations of hemodynamic parameters are best minimized by selecting an agent less likely to induce depression. For this reason, nitrous oxide–oxygen technique is more frequently utilized in these patients, along with fentanyl, known to induce minimal myocardial depression (64). Additional relaxation can be obtained with pancuronium which may produce a slight increase in both heart rate and systemic pressure, as opposed to the more likely hypotension resulting from either succinylcholine or D-tubocurarine (64).

Myocardial depression from inhalation agents, however, may be avoided altogether with the use of regional anesthesia in appropriate patients since these agents are not direct myocardial depressants. By virtue of the sympathetic blockade so induced, however, no significant difference in the risk of intraoperative hypotension has been demonstrated when compared with general anesthesia (9,65). The only subgroup of individuals more likely to benefit from regional technique is patients with preoperative congestive heart failure who are less likely to decompensate after spinal anesthesia than general anesthesia. The reason for selecting epidural anesthesia in vascular patients, therefore, concerns the reduction of postoperative pulmonary complications rather than cardiac morbidity. Finally, it has been shown in numerous studies that carotid surgery may be safely undertaken with either general or regional technique (66,67) with comparable results.

Of particular concern is the patient undergoing a transabdominal procedure during which the aorta must be cross-clamped. In the properly volume-loaded patient, optimal cardiac output may be maintained with appropriate fluid administration guided by the pulmonary artery wedge pressure during induction of satisfactory anesthesia (17). When the aorta is clamped, however, afterload reduction may be required. Such reduction should be achieved with a short-acting, easily reversible agent such as sodium nitroprusside or with nitroglycerin, which also augments coronary perfusion. Continuous pulmonary artery wedge pressure monitoring with serial determinations of cardiac output indicate the degree of reduction required, and declamping must be anticipated with appropriate termination of afterload reduction. In the event that cardiac output is not maintained despite adequate volume loading and afterload reduction during clamping, or following declamping, the decompensated left ventricle may require appropriate inotropic agents such as dopamine or dobutamide (68). Finally, intravenous nitroglycerin remains an important adjunct in the maintenance of coronary perfusion should ischemic changes occur in the ECG.

Autotransfusion

While most extracranial and infrainguinal vascular reconstructions do not require blood replacement, homologous transfusion has been necessary during most major aortic procedures. Adjunctive autotransfusion, however, may reduce both the expense and hazards of homologous blood administration, which include infectious complications (69–72); immunologic reactions (71,73,74); increased oxygen affinity with diminished levels of 2,3-diphosphoglycerate (2,3-DPG) (75,76); and coagulopathies (77,78). The many hazards initially associated with autotransfusion such as air embolism, coagulopathy, hemolysis, and microembolism have largely been minimized with the use of a continuous-flow, cell-processing centrifuge system (Haemonetics Cell Saver, Haemonetics Corporation, Natick, Massachusetts). Several series attest to the safety of salvaged autologous blood, and its use routinely in our own experience with aortic reconstruction has led to a dramatic reduction in homologous transfusion. It has been shown that red blood cell survival is satisfactory and that salvaged blood has a significantly increased oxygen-carrying and buffering capacity and a lower microaggregate level (79,80) when compared to bank blood.

Recycled processed blood, however, is essentially devoid of coagulation factors, a disadvantage compounded by the necessity for priming the system with heparin, which results in an unpredictable amount of anticoagulant in each unit. The activated clotting time should therefore be measured after each autologous infusion with appropriate administration of fresh frozen-plasma or heparin neutralization as indicated (81,82).

References

1. Kannel WB, Skinner JJ, Jr, Schwartz MJ, et al: Intermittent claudication: Incidence in the Framingham Study. Circulation 1970, 41:857.
2. Hertzer N: Fatal myocardial infarction following abdominal aortic aneurysm resection. Ann Surg 1980, 192:667.
3. Hertzer NR, Beven EG, Young JR, et al: Coronary artery disease in peripheral vascular patients. A classification of 1000 coronary angiograms and results of surgical management. Ann Surg 1984, 199:223.
4. Hollier LH, Plate G, O'Brien PC, et al: Late survival after abdominal aortic aneurysm repair: Influence of coronary artery disease. J Vasc Surg 1984, 1(2): 290.
5. Plumlee JE, Boettner RB: Myocardial infarction during and following anesthesia and operation. South Med J 1972, 65:886.
6. Tarhan S, Moffitt EA, Taylor WF, et al: Myocardial infarction after general anesthesia. JAMA 1972, 220:1451.
7. Rose SD, Corman LC, Mason DT: Cardiac risk factors in patients undergoing noncardiac surgery. Med Clin North Am 1979, 63:1271.
8. Portal RW: Elective surgery after myocardial infarction. Br Med J 1982, 284:843.
9. Goldman L, Caldara DL, Southwick FS, et al: Cardiac risk factors and complications in non-cardiac surgery. Medicine 1978, 57:357.
10. Goldman L, Caldera DL, Nussbaum SR, et al: Multifactorial index of cardiac risk in noncardiac surgical procedures. N Engl J Med 1977, 297:845.
11. Wells PH, Kaplan JA: Optimal management of patients with ischemic heart disease for noncardiac surgery by complementary anesthesiologist and cardiologist interaction. Am Heart J 1981, 102:1029.
12. Rao TLK, El-Etr AA: Myocardial reinfarction following anesthesia in patients with recent infarction. Anesth Analg 1981, 60:271.
13. Steen PA, Tinker JH, Tarhan S: Myocardial reinfarction after anesthesia and surgery. JAMA 1978, 239:2566.
14. McCollum CH, Garcia-Rinaldi R, Graham JM, et al: Myocardial revascularization prior to subsequent major surgery in patients with coronary artery disease. Surgery 1977, 81:302.
15. Akl BF, Talbot W, Neal JF, et al: Noncardiac operations after coronary revascularization. West J Med 1982, 136:91.
16. Mahar LJ, Steen PA, Tinker JH, et al: Perioperative myocardial infarction in patients with coronary artery disease with and without aorta-coronary bypass grafts. J Thorac Cardiovasc Surg 1978, 76:533.
17. Ruby ST, Whittemore AD, Couch NP, et al: Coronary artery disease in patients requiring abdominal aortic aneurysm repair: Selective use of a combined operation. Ann Surg 1985 (in press).
18. Gage AA, Bhayana JN, Balu V, Hook N: Assessment of cardiac risk in surgical patients. Arch Surg 1977, 112:1488.
19. Fudge TL, McKinnon WMP, Schoettle GP, et al: Improved operative risk after myocardial revascularization. South Med J 1981, 74:799.
20. Bille-Brahe NE, Eickhoff JH: Measurement of central hemodynamic parameters during preoperative exercise testing in patients suspected of arteriosclerotic heart disease: Value in predicting postoperative cardiac complications. Acta Chir Scand 1980, 502:38.
21. Hertzer HR, Young JR, Krawer JR, et al: Routine coronary angiography prior to elective aortic reconstruction: Results of a selective myocardial revascularization in patients with peripheral vascular disease. Arch Surg 1979, 114:1336.
22. Hertzer HR, Beven EG, Young JR, et al: Coronary artery disease in peripheral vascular patients: A classification of 1000 coronary angiograms and results of surgical management. Ann Surg 1984, 199(2):223.
23. Davis K, Kennedy JW, Kemp HG Jr, et al: Complications of coronary arteriography from the collaborative study of coronary artery surgery (CASS). Circulation 1979, 59:1105.
24. Namay DL, Hammermeister KE, Zia MS, et al: Effect of perioperative myocardial infarction on late survival in patients undergoing coronary artery bypass surgery. Circulation 1982, 65:1066.
25. Goldman L: Cardiac risks and complications of noncardiac surgery. Ann Intern Med 1983, 98:504.
26. Schulze RA Jr, Rouleau J, Rigo P, et al: Ventricular arrhythmias in the late hospital phase of acute myocardial infarction: Relation to left ventricular function detected by gated cardiac blood pool scanning. Circulation 1975, 52:1006.
27. Schulze RA Jr, Strauss HW, Pitt B: Sudden death in the year following myocardial infarction: Relation to ventricular premature contractions in the late hospital phase and left ventricular ejection fraction. Am J Med 1977, 62:192.
28. Lyons C: Cardiac arrhythmias as a predictable surgical risk. Surgery 1954, 35:292.
29. Wolf MA, Braunwald E: General anesthesia and noncardiac surgery in patients with heart disease. In Braunwald E (ed): *Heart Disease*. Philadelphia, Saunders, 1980.
30. Skinner JF, Pearce ML: Surgical risk in the cardiac patient. J Chronic Dis 1964, 17:57.
31. Chambers DA: Anesthesia for the patient with acquired valvular heart disease. In Kaplan JA (ed): *Cardiac Anesthesia*. New York, Grune & Stratton, 1979, p 197.
32. Perlroth MG, Hultgren HN: The cardiac patient and general surgery. JAMA 1975, 232:1279.
33. Tinker JH, Tarhan S: Discontinuing anticoagulant therapy in surgical patients with cardiac valve prostheses. JAMA 1978, 239:738.
34. Katholi RE, Nolan SP, McGuire LB: Living with prosthetic heart valves. Subsequent noncardiac operations and the risk of thromboembolism or hemorrhage. Am Heart J 1976, 92:162.
35. Whittemore AD, Clowes AW, Hechtman HB, et al: Aortic aneurysm repair: Reduced operative mortality associated with maintenance of optimal cardiac performance. Ann Surg 1980, 192:414.
36. Zeldin RA: Assessing cardiac risk in patients who undergo noncardiac procedures. Can J Surg 1984, 27:402.
37. Goldman L, Caldera DL: Risks of general anesthesia and elective operation in the hypertensive patient. Anesthesiology 1979, 50:285.
38. Prys-Roberts C: Hypertension and anesthesia—Fifty years on (ed). Anesthesiology 1979, 50:281.
39. Prys-Roberts C, Meloche R, Foex P: Studies of anesthesia in relation to hypertension. I. Cardiovascular responses of treated and untreated patients. Br J Anaesth 1971, 43:122.
40. Prys-Roberts C, Foex P, Greene LT, Waterhouse, TD: Studies of

anaesthesia in relation to hypertension. IV. The effects of artificial ventilation on the circulation and pulmonary gas exchanges. Br J Anaesth 1972, 44:335.

41. Foex P, Prys-Roberts C: Anaesthesia and the hypertensive patient. Br J Anaesth 1974, 46:575.
42. Viljoen JF, Estafanous FG, Kellner GA: Propranolol and cardiac surgery. J Thorac Cardiovasc Surg 1972, 64:826.
43. Moran JM, Mulet J, Caralps JM, Pifarre R: Coronary revascularization in patients receiving propranolol. Circulation 1974, 50(suppl 2):116.
44. Kaplan JA, Dunbar RW, Bland JW Jr, et al: Propranolol and cardiac surgery: A problem for the anesthesiologist? Anesth Analg 1975, 54:571.
45. Kopriva CJ, Brown ACD, Pappas G: Hemodynamics during general anesthesia in patients receiving propranolol. Anesthesiology 1978, 48:28.
46. Nattel S, Rangno RE, Van Loon G: Mechanism of propranolol withdrawal phenomena. Circulation 1979, 59:1158.
47. Goldman L: Noncardiac surgery in patients on propranolol: Case reports and a recommended approach. Arch Intern Med 1981, 141:193.
48. Dean RH, Keyser JE, Dupont WD, et al: Aortic and renal disease: Factors affecting the value of combined procedure. Ann Surg 1984, 200:336.
49. Couch NP, Lane FC, Crane C: Management and mortality in resection of abdominal aortic aneurysms. Am J Surg 1970, 119:408.
50. Young AE, Sandberg GW, Couch NP: The reduction of mortality of abdominal aortic aneurysm resection. Am J Surg 1977, 134:585.
51. Crawford ES, Palamara AE, Saleh SA, Roehm JOF: Aortic aneurysm: current status of surgical treatment. Surg Clin North Am 1979, 59:597.
52. Hicks GL, Eastland MW, DeWeese JA, et al: Survival improvement following aortic aneurysm resection. Ann Surg 1975, 181:863.
53. Thompson JE, Hollier LM, Patman RD, Persson AV: Surgical management of abdominal aortic aneurysms. Ann Surg 1975, 181:654.
54. Kallero KS, Bergqvist D, Cederholm C, et al: Arteriosclerosis in popliteal artery trifurcation as a predictor for myocardial infarction after arterial reconstructive operation. Surg Gynecol Obstet 1984, 159:133.
55. Scobie K, McPhail N, Hubbard C: Early and late results of resection of abdominal aortic aneurysms. Can Med Assoc J 1977, 117:147.
56. Baird RT, Gurry JF, Kellam JF, Wilson DR: Abdominal aortic aneurysms: Recent experience with 210 patients. Can Med Assoc J 1978, 118:1229.
57. Bush HL Jr, LoGerfo FW, Weisel RD, et al: Assessment of myocardial performance and optimal volume loading during elective abdominal aortic aneurysm resection. Arch Surg 1977, 112:1301.
58. Graham LM, Stanley JC, Gewertz BL, et al: Prostaglandin F_{2a} attenuation of aortic declamping hyperemia and hypotension. J Surg Res 1976, 20:413.
59. Karmazyn M, Dhalla NS: Thromboxane B_2: A cardiodepressant of isolated rat hearts and inhibitor of sarcolemma Na^+-K^+ stimulated ATPase activity. Prostaglandins Med 1979, 3:81.
60. Utsunomiya T, Krausa MM, Dunham B, et al: Maintenance of cardiodynamics with aspirin during abdominal aortic aneurysmectomy (AAA). Ann Surg 1981, 194:602.
61. Huval WV, Lelcuk S, Allen PD, et al: Determinants of cardiovascular stability during abdominal aortic aneurysmectomy (AAA). Ann Surg 1984, 199:216.
62. Richards RS: Anesthesia for the patient with cardiac disease. J Am Assoc Nurse Anesthetists 1976, 44:147.
63. Kaplan JA (ed): *Cardiac Anesthesia*. New York, Grune & Stratton, 1979.
64. Bille-Brahe NE, Sorensen MB, Mondorf T, Engell HC: Central haemodynamics during induction of neurolept anesthesia in patients with arteriosclerotic heart disease. Acta Anaesth Scand 1978, 67(suppl):47.
65. Arkins R, Smessaert AA, Hicks RG: Mortality and morbidity in surgical patients with coronary artery disease. JAMA 1964, 190:485.
66. Whittemore AD: Carotid endarterectomy—An alternative approach. Arch Surg 1980, 115:940.
67. Whittemore AD, Kaufman JL, Kohler TR, Mannick JA: Routine electrocephalographic (EEG) monitoring during carotid endarterectomy. Ann Surg 1983, 197:707.
68. Disesa VJ, Browne E, Mudge GH Jr, et al: Comparison of dopamine and dobutamine in the volume-loaded, pressure-loaded and normal ventricle. J Thorac Cardiovasc Surg 1982, 83:256.
69. Alter HJ: The dominant role of non-A, non-B in the pathogenesis of post-transfusion hepatitis: A clinical assessment. Clin Gastroenterol 1980, 9:155.
70. Seeff LB, Zimmerman HJ, Wright EC, et al: VA cooperative study of post-transfusion hepatitis, 1969–1974: Incidence and characteristics of hepatitis and responsible risk factors. Am J Med Sci 1975, 270:355.
71. Myhre BA: Fatalities from blood transfusion. JAMA 1980, 244:1333.
72. Goldsmith MF: Reactions and counter-reactions to transfusion-associated AIDS. JAMA 1984, 251:177.
73. Brezica SM Jr, Pineda AA, Taswell HF: Autologus blood transfusion. Mayo Clin Proc 1976, 51:723.
74. Wilson RF, Mammen E, Walt AJ: Eight years of experience with massive blood transfusions. J Trauma 1971, 11:275.
75. Collins JA: Problems associated with the massive transfusion of stored blood. Surgery 1974, 75:274.
76. Weisel RD, Dennis RC, Manny J, et al: Adverse effects of transfusion therapy during abdominal aortic aneurysmectomy. Surgery 1978, 83:682.
77. Counts RB, Haisch C, Simon TL, et al: Hemostasis in massively transfused trauma patients. Ann Surg 1979, 190:91.
78. Bell WR: Disseminated intravascular coagulation. Johns Hopkins Med J 1980, 146:289.
79. Bennett SH, Geelhoed GW, Terrill RE, Hoye RC: Pulmonary effects of autotransfused blood. Am J Surg 1973, 125:696.
80. O'Hara PJ, Hertzer NR, Santilli PH, Beven EG: Intraoperative autotransfusion during abdominal aortic reconstruction. Am J Surg 1983, 145:215.
81. Kingsely JR, Valeri CR, Peters H, et al: Citrate anticoagulation and cell washing for intraoperative autotransfusion in the baboon. Am J Surg 1976, 131:717.
82. Raines JK, Buth J, Brewtser DC, Darling RC: Intraoperative autotransfusion: Equipment, protocols and guidelines. J Trauma 1976, 16:615.

Chapter 22

INTRAOPERATIVE MANAGEMENT OF THE PATIENT REQUIRING SUPRACELIAC AORTIC OCCLUSION

MICHAEL F. ROIZEN, YUNG J. SOHN, and RONALD J. STONEY

The patient requiring supraceliac aortic occlusion for the repair of visceral arteries often has atherosclerosis of other organs, as evidenced by cardiac, visceral, or cerebral ischemia, or by cardiac, renal, or peripheral artery insufficiency. All these diseases are part of a process that frequently proceeds at different rates in different parts of the arterial tree. Recognizing that atherosclerosis is usually not limited to the celiac trunk but probably exists elsewhere in the arterial tree no doubt aids management. However, even when celiac artery disease is isolated, occluding the aorta can significantly affect renal, spinal cord, hepatic, and myocardial function. Although intraoperative anesthetic or hemodynamic management appears to have little effect on spinal cord or hepatic function after supraceliac occlusion, such management can greatly affect renal and myocardial well-being (1–3).

For example, intraoperative fluid management has almost eliminated postoperative renal failure after supraceliac aortic occlusion (4–6). Nevertheless, even after infrarenal aortic reconstruction, cardiac complications are still common and are the most frequent cause of perioperative mortality and morbidity; cardiac dysfunction accounts for 48 to 100 percent of the perioperative mortality (Table 22-1) (1,7–14). Stress on the heart would be even greater after suprarenal or supraceliac aortic occlusion because of the increase in afterload when a larger portion of the circulation is excluded. We have demonstrated that 92 percent of patients undergoing supraceliac aortic occlusion have signs of myocardial ischemia not revealed by data obtained using an electrocardiogram or pulmonary artery thermodilution catheters (1). Thus methods of avoiding, diagnosing, and treating hemodynamic alterations during temporary supraceliac occlusion are clearly needed. This chapter discusses the physiological challenge presented to the heart by such occlusion, and methods of treating associated abnormal conditions.

Historical Aspects of Thoracoabdominal Aortic Reconstructive Surgery

The literature shows that the outcome of surgery on the aorta at the celiac axis has clearly improved in the past several decades. DeBakey and coworkers reported on resections involving temporary interruption of arterial blood supply to the vital organs supplied by the celiac, superior mesenteric, upper lumbar, lower intercostal, and renal arteries (14–16). Between 1956 and 1966 they reported a perioperative mortality of 26 percent for the first 42 resections and homograft replacements of aneurysms of the thoracoabdominal aorta. This figure is more than three times higher than that for infrarenal reconstructions performed by the Baylor group over the same time period. In 1974 Crawford (17) reported a 4.3 percent operative mortality for 23 patients re-

TABLE 22-1. Percentage of Perioperative Mortality Related to Cardiac Events

Aortic Reconstruction Series	Deaths/ Total No. Patients	Mortality Caused by Cardiac Dysfunction, %
Szilagyi et al. (1966) (7)	59/401	48
Young et al. (1977) (8)	7/144	100
Hicks et al. (1975) (9)	19/225	53
Thompson et al. (1975) (10)	6/108	83
Mulcare et al. (1978) (11)	14/140	79
Whittemore et al. (1980) (2)	1/110	100
Crawford et al. (1981) (12)	41/860	54
Hertzer (1983) (13)	22/523	64

quiring supraceliac interruption. Since 1977 Stoney and coworkers (1,18) have reported a similarly low 7-day mortality.

Outcome has also improved for infrarenal aortic reconstructive surgery. Hicks (9) reported a decrease in mortality from 22 percent between 1955 and 1960 (for 41 patients) to 12.5 percent between 1966 and 1970, and to 4.2 percent between 1970 and 1973. In the series by Scobie and Masters (19), perioperative mortality in elective abdominal aneurysm repair decreased from 12 percent between 1961 and 1969 to 4.1 percent between 1971 and 1975, and to 1.8 percent between 1976 and 1980. Accompanying this decrease in mortality was an increase in the use of certain techniques; the use of venous pressure (fluid) monitoring devices increased from 12 percent between 1961 and 1969 to 100 percent after 1971; after 1975, the use of pulmonary artery thermodilution catheters also increased (19).

Renal morbidity after aortic reconstruction has also decreased. In the report of Porter et al. (20), 47 percent of 183 patients undergoing aortic resections before 1966 had postoperative azotemia and blood urea nitrogen values exceeding 20 mg/dL; 20 percent of their patients who did not survive died of renal failure. In contrast, in a 1983 series of 137 patients that included 38 undergoing suprarenal aortic occlusion, the creatinine levels of only 16 percent increased 0.5 mg/dL (3). No patient died of acute renal failure, and none of the 38 patients required dialysis.

On the other hand, morbidity has not decreased in all areas. The first successful excision and homograft replacement of a thoracic aneurysm in humans was followed by paraplegia (21). Sporadic reports of paraplegia after thoracoabdominal aortic reconstruction continue, and the development of methods to prevent paraplegia is an active area of investigaton (22–24).

Thus mortality and morbidity for aortic reconstructive surgery have greatly decreased over the last three decades. Regarding infrarenal resection, Crawford et al. (12) attributed most of the reduction in morbidity before 1971 to improvements in operative techniques; and after 1971, to improvements in anesthesia, monitoring, and supportive care. However, perioperative mortality from supraceliac aneurysms still exceeds 4 percent, and 92 percent of the patients have signs of myocardial ischemia on the application of a supraceliac cross clamp.

Temporary Aortic Occlusion: Pathophysiological Events

EVENTS ON APPLICATION OF AN AORTIC CROSS CLAMP

Most repairs of suprarenal vessels involve temporarily occluding the aorta at supraceliac levels rather than just occluding the celiac trunk alone. Occlusion of the aorta causes hypertension in the proximal segment and hypotension in the distal segment. During resection of a coarcted aorta, acute occlusion of the thoracic aorta affects cardiovascular variables very little, since extensive collateral vessels have developed around the coarctation. However, without extensive collateral circulation, aortic occlusion increases afterload and peripheral vascular resistance proportional to the level of the occlusion. Thus, myocardial stress varies with the level of occlusion.

Using two-dimensional transesophageal echocardiography, we found that myocardial performance and circulatory variables remained within an acceptable range after the aorta was occluded at infrarenal levels (1). Such data agree with much previous work (25). In 1968 Perry (25) demonstrated that the increase in afterload after temporary infrarenal aortic occlusion had little effect on circulatory variables. The use of newer, more sophisticated techniques has shown that deepening anesthesia or administering vasodilating drugs at the time of infrarenal aortic occlusion keeps indices of myocardial performance within an acceptable range (26–31) even in sick patients (25 percent had severe left ventricular dysfunction prior to aortic surgery). Wall motion abnormalities and changes in the ejection fraction appear to be early signs of myocardial ischemia (31). However, in none of the patients in the infrarenal group did we detect wall motion abnormalities (1). Only one study contradicts the view that myocardial well-being is preserved after infrarenal aortic occlusion. Attia and coworkers (32) report a 30 percent incidence (3 of 10 patients) of myocardial ischemia after infrarenal occlusion. Investigators from the same institution later described a technique that allowed infrarenal aortic occlusion without evidence of myocardial ischemia (33). Therefore, aortic occlusion at the infrarenal level appears to increase afterload only slightly, and current techniques seem to prevent much of the stress on the heart that is associated with such occlusion.

The literature provides little data in humans regarding myocardial and cardiovascular effects of occluding the aorta at the suprarenal-infraceliac or supraceliac level. After occluding the descending thoracic aorta in eight patients, Kouchoukos and coworkers (34) noted increases of 35, 56, 43, and 90 percent in mean arterial, central venous, mean pulmonary arterial, and pulmonary capillary wedge pressures, respectively, and a decrease of 29 percent in the cardiac index. These hemodynamic effects are greater than those we found for supraceliac aortic occlusion, and may be attributable to the more proximal level of thoracic aortic occlusion. Clearly, occlusion at the supraceliac level causes substantially more myocardial stress, as evidenced by wall motion abnormalities, than occlusion at the suprarenal-infraceliac or infrarenal level (Table 22-2). Although systemic pressures and pulmonary capillary wedge pressures were kept normal at all times in 10 of our 12 patients undergoing occlusion at the supraceliac level, 11 patients had left ventricular wall motion abnormalities suggestive of ischemia. These changes may have occurred because of left ventricular dilation secondary to increased afterload, the release of vasoactive substances secondary to intestinal ischemia, or the more than 100 percent increase in peripheral vascular resistance accompanying aortic occlusion at the supraceliac level. Despite low ejection fractions, these patients maintained the cardiac output and the stroke volume by expanding the cavity size of the left ventricle. Because pulmonary capillary wedge pressure frequently does not reflect left ventricular end-diastolic volume accurately, a two-dimensional transesophageal echocardiogram (2-D TEE) allows us to identify and treat myocardial dysfunction that is not detected with conventional monitoring techniques.

TABLE 22-2. Percentage Change in Cardiovascular Variables on the Initiation of Aortic Occlusion

	Level of Aortic Occlusion		
Number of Patients Studied (n)	Supraceliac, % Change (12)	Suprarenal-Infraceliac, % Change (6)	Infrarenal, % Change (6)
Mean arterial blood pressure	54	5*	2*
Pulmonary capillary wedge pressure	38	10*	0*
End-diastolic area	28	2*	9*
End-systolic area	69	10*	11*
Ejection fraction	−38	−10*	−3*
Patients having wall motion abnormalities	92	33	0
New myocardial infarctions	8	0	0

*Statistically different ($p < 0.05$) from group undergoing supraceliac aortic occlusion.

Persistent intraoperative wall motion abnormalities are associated with new myocardial infarctions. Therefore, these changes are important and probably should be treated. Because the anesthetists in our study were aware of the echocardiographic findings, the low incidence of myocardial infarctions (Table 22-2) probably reflects rapid vigorous treatment rather than an overly sensitive testing device.

These pathophysiological changes could result just from the normal flow patterns within the arterial system. For example, 22 percent of the cardiac output usually goes to the renal vessels, and 27 percent goes to the superior mesenteric vessel and celiac trunk (35). Thus the expected decrease in flow and increase in afterload and peripheral vascular resistance after supraceliac aortic occlusion could cause left ventricular dilation. Other factors possibly contributing to myocardial dysfunction during supraceliac occlusion include hypothermia, the release of vasoactive substances from ischemic areas, and the presence of unmetabolized citrate from transfused blood (36).

Studies in animals support the belief that myocardial function is altered after the occlusion of the descending thoracic aorta. Longo and coworkers (37) studied coronary and systemic hemodynamic changes in dogs during suprarenal or infrarenal aortic clamping and unclamping. They found that upon application of the cross clamp to the suprarenal aorta, the peripheral resistance increases two to three times, with immediate proximal hypertension, marked increases in coronary blood flow and pulse pressure, decreases in aortic blood flow and cardiac output, and little change in pulse rate. These results are similar to ours (1). The left ventricles of the dogs in the Longo study dilated upon application of the cross clamp. Mandelbaum and Webb (38) showed that occluding the descending thoracic aorta in dogs decreases left ventricular function. However, occluding the infrarenal aorta is much less stressful, the cardiovascular consequences being (as they are in humans, even those with diseased hearts) only slight (1,38).

In normal dogs, the renal artery can be occluded for an hour before the kidneys are injured even slightly (39). Data from this institution support that observation (3). Preoperative and postoperative renal function in patients undergoing less than 40 minutes of suprarenal cross-clamping did not differ from those functions in patients undergoing infrarenal aortic occlusion (3).

EVENTS ON REMOVAL OF AN AORTIC CROSS CLAMP

Despite the negligible cardiovascular effects of temporarily applying an infrarenal aortic cross clamp, hypotension (declamping shock) occurs upon even the release of an infrarenal cross clamp. These hemodynamic alterations occur even when blood flow is restored to only one leg. Although severe hypotension is rare at large centers (6,33,34), moderate hypotension (i.e., a drop in systolic blood pressure of 40 mmHg) is not uncommon at our institution.

Two hypotheses have been proposed to explain this hypotension. The first suggests that myocardial depression may be caused by the washout of acid, acid metabolites, and vasoactive substances from ischemic extremities when blood flow is restored. This hypothesis has been largely discredited in recent years (26,27,34). Our own work with two-dimensional transesophageal echocardiography supports the second hypothesis, that of relative volume depletion. Reactive hyperemia in the freshly revascularized area decreases vascular resistance, venous return, and blood pressure. Thus hypotension can be ameliorated by volume expansion without decreasing cardiac output, and, in fact, such an expansion may increase it. If hypotension persists for more than 4 minutes after the removal of the clamp, and if blood deficits have been replaced, other causes should be sought. (See the section on the hemodynamic control of the circulation after the removal of the supraceliac cross clamp. A 2-D TEE view of the left ventricle often reveals that venous return is still inadequate, sometimes because of hidden persistent bleeding, and sometimes because of a midjudged replacement of blood deficits.)

Baseline Anesthesia Techniques and Drugs

Virtually all anesthetic techniques and drugs have been used for aortic reconstructive surgery without any demonstrable advantage of one drug or technique to outcome. For this operative procedure, as for other kinds of vascular surgery, maintenance of hemodynamic equilibrium and attention to detail appear more important than the choice of drug (40).

INHALATION ANESTHESIA

Halothane, enflurane, and isoflurane are three halogenated hydrocarbons that have negative inotropic properties when administered to humans not undergoing surgery. However, in humans undergoing surgery, these agents act as vasodilators (41–43), isoflurane being the most potent. This action is both an advantage and a disadvantage: It provides an additional way (besides administration of nitroprusside or nitroglycerin) of controlling afterload and preload, but may lead to increased intravascular volume. This increased volume could be a detriment at the end of the procedure. As anesthetic administration is decreased at the end of surgery, volume could return to the central compartment and cause pulmonary edema. To prevent this problem, we tilt the patient head down for the 30 to 45 minutes of surgical closure, and then slowly return the position to level while gradually turning off the anesthetic agent.

The volatile agents offer several other advantages. They allow careful, deliberate induction, manipulation, and monitoring of hemodynamic variables, and for adjustment of dose. In addition, by providing a degree of muscle relaxation, they decrease the need for muscle relaxants and increase the ease of reversing paralysis. Also, the patient awakens from anesthesia early, allowing the physician to assess limb motor function and sensation if he or she desires to place an epidural catheter to facilitate postoperative analgesia.

In addition, the volatile hydrocarbon anesthetic technique allows intraoperative and postoperative options not available with other techniques. It can be combined with administration of nitroprusside and nitroglycerin to reduce afterload. Also, an epidural catheter can be inserted for postoperative analgesia, or the anesthetic can be continued with alternative drugs such as diazepam and morphine to facilitate prolonged controlled ventilation.

Extubation is usually accomplished by the end of surgery, and the patient is allowed to breathe spontaneously. Thus the stressful stimuli and hypertension associated with continued presence of an endotracheal tube are avoided, and early assessment of neurologic function is facilitated. Also, the patient is able to complain of angina, for which nitroglycerin is administered.

Since the introduction of isoflurane, we have tended to avoid halothane. Halothane can cause hepatitis-like signs and symptoms when the liver is hypoxic (44), and the occlusion of the supraceliac aorta theoretically tends to make the liver hypoxic for a period of time. However, 20 of the first 40 patients we anesthetized for supraceliac aortic revascularization received halothane without any adverse effect being even remotely attributable to the agent.

NARCOTIC ANESTHESIA

All commonly used narcotics produce similar cardiovascular effects (40). The induction of anesthesia with narcotic agents can be accomplished rapidly but decreases the cardiac index by a small but statistically significant amount. In sufficient doses, narcotics can cause anesthesia (produce analgesia and hypnosis) with only slight decreases in cardiac contractility and blood pressure (40). By continuing to infuse narcotics or administering other agents, one can maintain anesthesia throughout the surgical procedure. Surgical stimulation after such anesthetic induction significantly increases heart rate, arterial blood pressure, and systemic vascular resistance. One can add nitroglycerin, nitroprusside, and/or a volatile anesthetic agent to the narcotic to manipulate the circulation during cross-clamping and unclamping.

Nitrous oxide can be used with narcotics as with the inhalation agents. However, it increases afterload and myocardial work while depressing myocardial inotropic performance (43,45). In addition, nitrous oxide may have the potential for a long-lasting toxicity by causing nutritional, neurologic, and immunologic deficits (46).

A disadvantage of using narcotics is that they tend to linger into the postoperative period, thereby necessitating controlled ventilation. However, in over 50 percent of the cases in which we used a narcotic–nitrous oxide anesthetic technique for suprarenal aortic reconstruction, we were able to extubate the trachea in the operating room. An advantage of using high doses of narcotics as the anesthetic is the continued excellent analgesia postoperatively.

EPIDURAL ANESTHESIA

Epidural anesthesia has been used successfully for the resection of infrarenal aortic aneurysms and for aortic reconstruction (47), and it can be combined with general anesthesia for supraceliac aortic reconstruction. A risk with epidural anesthesia is that the administration of heparin might create an epidural hematoma and a subsequent neurologic deficit (48). Such a deficit could be confused with that caused by spinal cord ischemia, thereby delaying correct diagnosis, evacuation of the hematoma, and return of neurologic function. Thus we are reluctant to use epidural anesthesia for supraceliac aortic reconstruction. In addition, the absence of leg sensation and movement postoperatively might create undue worry. This disadvantage can be ameliorated by using, at the end of the operation, concentrations of anesthetic agents that affect only sensory, and not motor, fibers. Epidural anesthesia has another disadvantage: A relative fluid overload can be created, which is a problem as the anesthetic ''wears off'' toward the end of the procedure. As with inhalation agents, we use the head-down tilt toward the end of the procedure so that the fluid status can be normalized as the anesthetic wears off.

The advantages of epidural anesthesia include the provision of excellent muscle relaxation, a smaller bowel (because of the sympatholytic effect) that tends not to obstruct the operative field, and hemodynamic stability once the anesthetic block is fully achieved. However, initiation of epidural anesthetic often decreases blood pressure, cardiac output, and perhaps perfusion to the gut and kidney; the latter may be, in the stenotic state, pressure-dependent. During cross-clamping and unclamping, the circulation can be controlled with volatile anesthetics or intravenous agents that reduce afterload.

MUSCLE RELAXANTS

The choice of muscle relaxants consists of a continuous infusion of succinylcholine or a bolus injection of *d*-tubocurarine, metocurine, or pancuronium. The newer neuromuscular relaxants vecuronium and atracurium have shorter half-lives and grant more hemodynamic stability than the other agents. However, all these agents provide excellent muscle relaxation and have relatively short half-lives. *d*-Tubocurarine is preferable to metocurine or pancuronium when the degree of hypertension is significant, when the vagolytic effect of pancuronium is not desired, or when the renal insufficiency is sufficiently great to prolong the excretion of metocurine or pancuronium.

CONCLUSION

No data indicate that any narcotic, inhalation, or epidural agent is superior in its effect on outcome when used for anesthesia for vascular surgery. Skill and care in the administration of the agent seem to be more critical to cardiovascular outcome than the choice of anesthetic agent.

Preoperative Considerations and Intraoperative Monitoring Techniques

We believe that any drug therapy required before the operation will probably be required during the operative period. Omitting chronic drug therapy can result in a heightened disease condition in the postoperative period, e.g., tachycardia and/or angina if propranolol is omitted, aspiration if L-dopa is omitted, or accelerated hypertension if clonidine is omitted. The patient should be given any antihypertensive medication, including diuretics, before being brought to the operating room (49). Most diabetic patients requiring insulin are given an insulin drip throughout surgery. Preoperative considerations and drug therapy for diabetic patients are described elsewhere (49). Because no particular anesthetic premedication seems indicated or contraindicated for most patients, the patient's anesthetist should determine what is appropriate. We avoid anticholinergic drugs because they produce dry mouth and tachycardia, which increases myocardial oxygen consumption.

Our monitoring practices stress the preservation of myocardial, pulmonary, and renal function. We almost always insert a catheter in the radial artery of the nondominant hand. Also, we monitor the urinary output and some form of ventricular filling pressure, the latter usually via a pulmonary artery catheter. This catheter allows monitoring of systemic vascular resistance, cardiac output, and pulmonary artery wedge pressures. For insertion, we prefer the external jugular route, although many anesthetists use the internal jugular or subclavian route. We use a modified chest lead V_5 (MCL5) to monitor the electrocardiogram (ECG) during the operation, except for patients who have demonstrated myocardial ischemia in areas other than the anterior myocardial wall. In addition, we almost always monitor body temperature and maintain it meticulously by warming all fluids (starting preoperatively), and by placing heating mattresses on the bed. If necessary, we humidify the anesthetic gases. We have found the 2-D TEE to be an invaluable tool for monitoring the myocardial consequences of cross-clamping and unclamping and now use it routinely for supraceliac procedures. We insert this device instead of an esophageal stethoscope. A short-axis cross-sectional view of the left ventricle is obtained at the level of the papillary muscles. Such a view provides an excellent qualitative assessment of left ventricular filling volumes, global ventricular contractility, and regional ventricular function (50). When a discrepancy has existed between the pulmonary artery capillary wedge pressures and the filling pressures obtained by two-dimensional transesophageal echocardiography, we have found the latter to be more reliable and useful (1,51).

Hemodynamic Control of the Circulation before and during Aortic Occlusion

The most important intraoperative goals are to maintain fluid balance, myocardial performance, and perfusion of vital organs.

MANTAINING BLOOD VOLUME

To lessen the incidence of organ ischemia and pulmonary dysfunction, fluid management aims at preventing intraoperative hypotension and minimizing cardiac dilation. Although we have no supporting data, we strongly believe that by ensuring adequate perfusion of vital organs, prehydration of patients undergoing vascular reconstructive surgery minimizes the hemodynamic fluctuations that occur with the induction of anesthesia. During the early dissection, we keep intravascular volume at normal levels by noting cardiac filling on the 2-D TEE or by maintaining normal capillary wedge pressures. To do this, we replace blood losses of less than 10 mL/kg and insensible losses with Ringer's lactate solution. We assume the patient will have insensible losses of 5 to 7 mL/kg per hour during this dissection phase. Blood losses of greater than 10 mL/kg are replaced milliliter for milliliter with whole blood.

The indicators we use for assessing the organ perfusion before cross-clamping are as follows: (1) for the heart, the myocardial contractility, as judged by global and regional wall motion on the 2-D TEE (1,31), by the ST segments of an MCL5 of the

ECG, and by the cardiac output; (2) for the kidney, urinary output (we believe that 2 mL per half hour is adequate, as urinary flow almost always decreases during a dissection around the renal vessels; see the section "Protecting Other Organs") (3); (3) for the central nervous system, eye signs (although the electroencephalogram (EEG) and/or sensory-evoked potentials (52) can be used, we have had little experience with these monitors); and (4) for the lung, gas exchange.

For the half hour immediately before aortic occlusion, we try to keep the patient slightly hypovolemic and are prepared at the time of occlusion to give a vasodilating drug through an intravenous line designated solely for that purpose. This catheter site is often the third lumen of the pulmonary artery catheter. We keep the patient slightly hypovolemic immediately before cross-clamping by examining the ventricular volume using the 2-D TEE or by keeping pulmonary artery pressures from 5 to 12 mmHg.

PROTECTING THE MYOCARDIUM

During early supraceliac dissection, we protect the heart by trying to keep hemodynamic variables within the same range of values as occurred preoperatively. Without evidence to the contrary, we must assume that a little hypertension is as bad as a little hypotension. For example, in an extreme case, we might let the systolic blood pressure of a patient whose preoperative range was 110 to 170 mmHg fall as low as 90 mmHg or rise as high as 190 mmHg. We have a contingency plan should the values approach or exceed that limit: If the blood pressure reaches 150 mmHg, we increase the amount of anesthetic; at approximately 160 mmHg, we start infusing nitroprusside, tilting the table head up if the pressure reaches 165 or 175 mmHg. If the systolic blood pressure drops to 110 mmHg, we decrease the amount of anesthetic and review the possible causes of hypotension. At 105 mmHg, we decrease the amount of anesthetic even more and place the patient in a head-down position. At 100 mmHg, we infuse more fluid, tilt the patient in a more steeply head-down position, review again the possible causes of hypotension, and try to correct the cause. At 90 mmHg, we might add a dilute drip of phenylephrine (10 mg in 500 mL of saline, infused at a rate that brings the systolic blood pressure back to approximately 100 mmHg).

For the heart rate, we again set a range of acceptable values based on the preoperative values. Using a preoperative range of 60 to 90 beats per minute as an example, we might do the following, once these limits were exceeded. At 95 beats per minute, we might increase the amount of anesthetic, give more narcotic, or add an intravenous drip of a beta-adrenergic blocking drug. At 45 beats per minute, we might decrease the amount of anesthetic or give a dilute solution of dopamine (200 mg in 500 mL) to keep the heart rate within the acceptable range. We tend to tolerate bradycardia more than tachycardia during these operations, because we believe that minimizing the myocardial oxygen demand should be of primary importance. By using the 2-D TEE, we have more latitude during the procedure in the range of acceptable values before we intervene. However, we do not allow the pulmonary artery pressures to become abnormal, i.e., below 5 mmHg or above 15 mmHg, during this procedure, assuming these values correlate with our 2-D TEE values. If they do not correlate, we tend to believe the 2-D TEE picture. We aggressively treat increases in the pulmonary artery pressure with nitroglycerin or nitroprusside, depending on whether increases in preload or in afterload are the suspected cause (53,54). For low values, we infuse more fluid, except in the 1 or 2 minutes immediately before the application of the aortic cross clamp.

The application of a cross clamp to the supraceliac aorta is probably the greatest hemodynamic stress ever experienced by a patient. In fact, 92 percent of the patients we studied had ischemia evidenced by wall motion abnormalities (Table 22-2). Normalizing the pulmonary artery pressure and the systemic blood pressure with vasodilating drugs before and during the cross-clamping may not be enough. When myocardial ischemia is indicated by global or regional wall motion abnormalities, we give more vasodilating drugs, taking the systolic blood pressure toward the low end of the normal preoperative range. Once the blood pressure is brought as low as possible (by reducing afterload with nitroprusside), we often attempt to decrease preload with nitroglycerin and, if necessary, to decrease heart rate with intravenous propranolol. If, despite these maneuvers and before the surgeon has actually incised the aorta or its branches, one sees myocardial dysfunction when the cross clamp is placed, one can ask the surgeon to unclamp the aorta partially until myocardial function is more stable. In our study, despite myocardial dysfunction in 11 of the 12 patients undergoing supraceliac cross-clamping, only 1 of those 11 had perioperative myocardial infarction. Therefore, the myocardial pump function seems most affected by ventricular size and protected by keeping vital signs within the normal preoperative range.

PROTECTING OTHER ORGANS

Other investigators have used sensory-evoked potentials and the EEG to gauge spinal cord and cerebral protection (52,55). We have found no benefit in examining the EEG and no evidence that stroke is a predictable consequence of supraceliac aortic reconstruction. However, in rare instances, spinal cord ischemia is a predictable sequence of this procedure. Spinal cord sensory-evoked potentials may prove to be useful for detecting spinal cord ischemia, but we do not have experience in using this technique. Experiments in the research laboratory indicate that isoflurane is probably the best anesthetic to use during temporary occlusion of the blood supply to the spinal cord. Other halogenated and intravenous anesthetics decrease the time the spinal cord can be ischemic before permanent neurologic damage occurs (23).

We do not believe that intraoperative urinary output predicts postoperative renal function (3). In 38 patients undergoing suprarenal aortic reconstruction, we measured the lowest hourly and mean urinary outputs. The pulmonary capillary wedge pressure was kept within normal limits. If the urinary output was less than 0.125 mL/kg per hour, the patients were given crystalloid to raise the pulmonary capillary wedge pressure to a high-normal level, or were given furosemide, mannitol, or nothing. For each patient, the levels of serum creatinine and blood urea nitrogen were assayed on postoperative days 1, 3, and 7. There was no significant correlation between the intraoperative mean urinary output or lowest hourly urinary output and the change from preoperative to postoperative levels of creatinine or blood urea nitrogen.

These patients were part of a larger series of 137 patients. When patients undergoing aortic occlusion at the suprarenal level were compared with those undergoing occlusion at the infrarenal level, postoperative renal function was found not to differ (3). Thus the urinary output, which is believed to be an index of perfusion and therefore is monitored routinely during surgery, does not predict the postoperative renal function in the normovolemic patient.

These results conflict with those obtained in other studies. In patients, and in animal models that impose a period of renal ischemia, pretreatment with mannitol lessened postischemic increases in creatinine levels (56–59). Direct infusion of mannitol into the renal artery sustained renal cortical perfusion (as assayed by the xenon washout technique) in mongrel dogs following infrarenal aortic occlusion (56). In rabbits, pretreatment with mannitol prevented an increase in serum creatinine levels after 60 minutes of renal artery occlusion (59). In dogs subjected to infrarenal aortic clamping and unclamping, an adequate replacement of blood with saline prevents a decrease in the renal blood flow, a result that is consistent with our findings (3). Moreover, furosemide and ethacrynic acid significantly increase both total renal blood flow and the cortical component of renal blood flow, as demonstrated by studies of xenon-133 washout (56). The use of mannitol, furosemide, or ethacrynic acid, however, has not been clearly shown to prevent renal failure. The difference between our results (3) and those of others (56–59) may be due to interspecies variation, to our maintenance of normal intravascular volume, and/or to the insensitivity of urinary output as a measure of the adequacy of renal perfusion. Undoubtedly, preoperative renal function and the maintenance of appropriate intravascular volume and normal myocardial function are the most important determinants of postoperative renal function.

When intraoperative urinary output is less than 0.125 mL/kg per hour, we ensure that no mechanical problems exist in urinary collection, and that left-sided cardiac filling volumes or pressures are adequate. We then continue to monitor the urinary output but do not treat. Urinary output usually returns to acceptable levels within 120 minutes. If it does not, or if we are uneasy about a low urinary output, we administer 2 to 5 mg of furosemide intravenously to stimulate the production of urine.

Thus in aortic occlusion at any level, virtually all studies have concluded that the maintenance of adequate intravascular volume and myocardial function largely prevents renal and other-organ insufficiency from being major clinical problems and are the key to intraoperative perfusion of critical organs.

Hemodynamic Control of the Circulation When Removing the Supraceliac Cross Clamp

MAINTAINING BLOOD VOLUME

When any blood vessel is being dissected, the anesthetist and surgeon must communicate closely: Blood loss can occur with astonishing rapidity, and the attention of the anesthetist may not be directed at the operative field. To ensure adequate volume at the time of cross-clamp removal, we replace blood losses with warmed blood, milliliter for milliliter, during occlusion. We normally have 6 units of whole blood available during this procedure. When greater blood loss is anticipated (e.g., for patients previously operated upon for the same condition), we often have available an autotransfusion setup and a second person to operate that device. After we have given 8 units of blood, or after we have given the sixth unit of blood and are anticipating using more, we have the blood bank type 10 units of platelets for the patient (and occasionally 2 units of fresh-frozen plasma). When no more blood is available and blood is an absolute necessity (that is, when colloid or crystalloid cannot be used), we give the best available type-specific blood. For example, if B-negative blood is needed but not available, we give B-positive blood. We change blood filters every 2 units when the blood we use for transfusion is more than 10 days old, and every 4 units when the blood is less than 10 days old.

Since a large part of the vascular tree is excluded from the circulation during temporary aortic occlusion, blood loss can be considerable during supraceliac cross-clamping without the occurrence of hypotension or tachycardia. Blood loss into the pleural or retroperitoneal cavities may be undetected in the measurements of blood loss that are taken every 5 to 10 minutes. Additionally, the evisceration of bowel, often necessary for optimal exposure of the thoracoabdominal aorta, further depletes intravascular volume. Thus we have to be guided closely by pulmonary artery pressures and/or echocardiographic estimates of left ventricular filling volumes. Just before unclamping the aorta, we allow blood pressure, pulmonary wedge pressure, and filling volumes to go as high as possible without myocardial ischemia's occurring. The surgeon then releases the aortic clamp gradually to ensure that overly severe hypotension does not develop and that too much bleeding does not occur from the suture line.

The pathophysiological events when the aortic cross clamp is removed (see the section "Events on Removal of an Aortic Cross Clamp") are associated with inadequate volume return to the heart, i.e., inadequate preload. Thus immediately before and during the removal of the cross clamp, we stop infusing nitroprusside and start infusing crystalloid or blood; usually 2 units of whole blood is pressured into venous access sites at this time. Guided by filling pressures and/or echocardiographic estimates of volume, we are careful not to dilate the left ventricle to an abnormal size. Another technique for maintaining normal volumes during cross-clamping is controlled volume depletion, i.e., removing a set amount of blood from the patient for a short period of time during the application of the cross clamp. Just before the cross clamp is removed, this amount is replaced. Although we have used this technique, we do not advocate it for routine use until the anesthetist has garnered substantial experience with the technique in less sick patients.

A third technique uses halothane, enflurane, or isoflurane—rather than nitroprusside or nitroglycerin—as the vasodilating agent. Although this is an interesting research technique that usually works (41), it requires very close observation of pulmonary artery pressures and/or the 2-D TEE to ensure that myocardial dysfunction does not occur. Therefore, we do not recommend it for routine use.

It is not uncommon for moderate hypotension (i.e., decreases in systolic pressure of 40 to 60 mmHg) to occur upon removal of the supraceliac aortic cross clamp, regardless of whether the clamp is replaced infrarenally or such that blood flow to only one leg is obstructed. Work with the 2-D TEE supports the belief that such hypotension is caused mainly by relative volume depletion. Reactive hyperemia in the freshly revascularized area decreases vascular resistance, venous return, and systemic blood pressure. If hypotension persists for more than 4 minutes after removal of the clamp and the blood pressure is not returning toward normal after blood deficits have been replaced, other causes should be sought. These include myocardial dysfunction caused by inadequate metabolism of the citrate found in replacement blood; such blood has not yet gone to the liver, where citrate would be metabolized. This problem can be treated by administering calcium, which antagonizes the effect of citrate (36). Other causes include hidden persistent bleeding or a misjudged replacement of blood deficits; in such cases, on an echocardiogram, the left ventricular cavity would be devoid of volume, and on an oscilloscope, the filling pressures reflecting the pulmonary artery pressures would be low. If need be, the surgeon can reclamp or occlude the aorta, preferably below the renal arteries. Thus volume replacement and maintenance are mainstays of therapy just before, during, and immediately after removal of the supraceliac cross clamp. When reinstituting blood flow to the first leg or extremity, volume replacement should also be considered. Removal of the clamp from the artery supplying the second leg usually has few hemodynamic effects, presumably because of the existence of collateral blood vessels across the pelvis.

PROTECTING THE MYOCARDIUM AND OTHER ORGANS

This topic is discussed in the section ''Hemodynamic Control of the Circulation Before and During Occlusion.''

Outcome: Complications and Primary Considerations

An 8 percent incidence of myocardial infarction with no mortality, as we obtained with two-dimensional transesophageal echocardiography, is possible in a group of patients having severe myocardial dysfunction undergoing supraceliac aortic reconstruction (1). However, we think that aiming for the 4 percent mortality that Crawford (17) reports is probably a more realistic goal with current techniques. In patients who have isolated celiac artery disease and little dysfunction in other organs, operation without mortality or morbidity should be possible.

The complications that occur from supraceliac aortic occlusion can usually be linked to the heart, the central nervous system, or the kidneys. We believe that organ dysfunction involving the heart can be minimized by keeping the intraoperative values of the hemodynamic variables within the normal range that occurred preoperatively, by ensuring that cardiac dilation does not occur at any time, and by minimizing episodes of tachycardia. We also believe that vigilance must continue into the postoperative period if the morbidity and mortality are to be reduced.

Renal insufficiency after supraceliac aortic occlusion appears to be greatly reduced. In virtually all studies, the maintenance of adequate intravascular volume and myocardial function prevents renal failure from being a major clinical problem and is a key to the intraoperative perfusion of critical organs.

Perhaps the use of better operative monitoring techniques, i.e., sensory-evoked potentials, may help avoid those instances in which spinal cord dysfunction results after supraceliac aortic occlusion. We do not have enough experience with sensory-evoked potentials to comment on this. The choice of anesthetic agents may make a difference in avoiding spinal cord ischemia.

Thus the primary goals affecting outcome involve keeping intravascular volume and myocardial function at normal levels. We believe that the normal preoperative range of values is the critical guideline to follow. We also believe that the appraisal of the myocardial function with the 2-D TEE prevents myocardial dysfunction that would otherwise go unnoticed intraoperatively and that could lead to major postoperative morbidity.

References

1. Roizen MF, Beaupre PN, Alpert RA, Kremer P, Cahalan MK, Sohn YJ, Shiller N, Cronnelly R, Lurz FW, Ehrenfeld WK, Stoney RJ: Monitoring with two-dimensional transesophageal echocardiography: Comparison of myocardial function in patients undergoing supraceliac, suprarenal-infraceliac, or infrarenal aortic occlusion. J Vasc Surg 1984, 1:300.
2. Whittemore AD, Clowes AW, Hechtman HB, Mannick JA: Aortic aneurysm repair. Reduced operative mortality associated with maintenance of optimal cardiac performance. Ann Surg 1980, 192:414.
3. Alpert RA, Roizen MF, Hamilton WK, Stoney RJ, Ehrenfeld WK, Poler SM, Wylie EJ: Intraoperative urinary output does not predict postoperative renal function in patients undergoing abdominal aortic revascularization. Surgery 1984, 95:707.
4. Barry KG, Mazze RI, Schwartz FD: Prevention of surgical oliguria and renal-hemodynamic suppression by sustained hydration. N Engl J Med 1964, 270:1371.
5. Wheeler CG, Thompson JE, Kartchner MM, Austin DJ, Patman RD: Massive fluid requirement in surgery of the abdominal aorta. N Engl J Med 1968, 275:320.
6. Sabawala PB, Strong MJ, Keats AS: Surgery of the aorta and its branches. Anesthesiology 1970, 33:229.

7. Szilagyi DE, Smith RF, Derusso FJ, Elliott JP, Sherrin FW: Contribution of abdominal aortic aneurysmectomy to prolongation of life. Ann Surg 1966, 164:678.
8. Young AE, Sandberg GW, Couch NP: The reduction of mortality of abdominal aortic aneurysm resection. Am J Surg 1977, 134:585.
9. Hicks GL, Eastland MW, DeWeese JA, May AG, Rob CG: Survival improvement following aortic aneurysm resection. Ann Surg 1975, 181:863.
10. Thompson JE, Hollier LH, Patman RD, Persson AV: Surgical management of abdominal aortic aneurysms: Factors influencing mortality and morbidity—A 20-year experience. Ann Surg 1975, 181:654.
11. Mulcare RJ, Royster TS, Lynn RA, Conners RB: Long-term results of operative therapy for aortoiliac disease. Arch Surg 1978, 113:601.
12. Crawford ES, Saleh SA, Babb JW III, Glaeser DH, Vaccaro PS, Silvers A: Infrarenal abdominal aortic aneurysm. Factors influencing survival after operation performed over a 25-year period. Ann Surg 1981, 193:699.
13. Hertzer NR: Myocardial ischemia. Surgery 1983, 93:97.
14. DeBakey ME, Creech O Jr, Morris GC Jr: Aneurysm of thoracoabdominal aorta involving the celiac, superior mesenteric, and renal arteries. Report of four cases treated by resection and homograft replacement. Ann Surg 1956, 144:549.
15. DeBakey ME, Crawford ES, Garrett HE, Beall AC Jr, Howell JF: Surgical consideration in the treatment of aneurysms of the thoraco-abdominal aorta. Ann Surg 1965, 162:650.
16. Garrett HE, Crawford ES, Beall AC Jr, Howell JF, DeBakey ME: Surgical treatment of aneurysm of the thoracoabdominal aorta. Surg Clin North Am 1966, 46:913.
17. Crawford ES: Thoraco-abdominal and abdominal aortic aneurysms involving renal, superior mesenteric, and celiac arteries. Ann Surg 1974, 179:763.
18. Stoney RJ, Ehrenfeld WK, Wylie EJ: Revascularization methods in chronic visceral ischemia caused by atherosclerosis. Ann Surg 1977, 186:468.
19. Scobie TK, Masters RG: Changing factors influencing abdominal aortic aneurysm repair. J Cardiovasc Surg 1982, 23:309.
20. Porter JM, McGregor F Jr, Acinapura AJ, Silver D: Renal function following abdominal aortic aneurysmectomy. Surg Gynecol Obstet 1966, 123:819.
21. Lam CR, Aram HH: Resection of the descending thoracic aorta for aneurysm. A report of the use of the homograft in a case and an experimental study. Ann Surg 1951, 134:743.
22. Degirolami U, Zivin JA: Neuropathology of experimental spinal cord ischemia in the rabbit. J Neuropathol Exp Neurol 1982, 41:129.
23. Koike M, Roizen MF, Zivin JA, Shnider SM, Krusko N, Joyce JT: Effect of anesthetics on injury to the central nervous system induced by ischemia. Anesthesiology 1982, 57:A312.
24. Zivin JA, Venditto JA: Experimental CNS ischemia: Serotonin antagonists reduce or prevent damage in experimental CNS ischemia. Neurology 1984, 34:469.
25. Perry MO: The hemodynamics of temporary abdominal aortic occlusion. Ann Surg 1968, 168:193.
26. Bush HL Jr, Logerfo FW, Weisel RD, Mannick JA, Hechtman HB: Assessment of myocardial performance and optimal volume loading during elective abdominal aortic aneurysm resection. Arch Surg 1977, 112:1301.
27. Carroll RM, Laravuso RB, Schauble JF: Left ventricular function during aortic surgery. Arch Surg 1976, 111:740.
28. Lunn JK, Dannemiller FJ, Stanley TH: Cardiovascular responses to clamping of the aorta during epidural and general anesthesia. Anesth Analg (Cleveland) 1979, 58:372.
29. Meloche R, Pottecher T, Audet J, Dufresne O, Lepage C: Haemodynamic changes due to clamping of the abdominal aorta. Can Anaesth Soc J 1977, 24:20.
30. Bartowski RR, Aukburg SJ, Greenhow DE, Klineberg PL, Rosenberg H, Andrews R, Roberts B: Comparing anesthetic techniques during aortic cross clamp. Anesthesiology 1979, 51:S136.
31. Pandian NG, Kerber RE: Two-dimensional echocardiography in experimental coronary stenosis. I. Sensitivity and specificity in detecting transient myocardial dyskinesis: Comparison with sonomicrometers. Circulation 1982, 66:597.
32. Attia RR, Murphy JD, Snider M, Lappas DG, Darling RC, Lowenstein E: Myocardial ischemia due to infrarenal aortic cross-clamping during aortic surgery in patients with severe coronary artery disease. Circulation 1976, 53:961.
33. Silverstein PR, Caldera DL, Cullen DJ, Davison JK, Darling RC, Emerson CW: Avoiding the hemodynamic consequences of aortic cross-clamping and unclamping. Anesthesiology 1979, 50:462.
34. Kouchoukos NT, Lell WA, Karp RB, Samuelson PN: Hemodynamic effects of aortic clamping and decompression with a temporary shunt for resection of the descending thoracic aorta. Surgery 1979, 85:25.
35. Guyton AC: Local control of blood flow by the tissues, and nervous and hormonal regulation. In *Textbook of Medical Physiology,* ed 6. Philadelphia, Saunders, 1981, p 252.
36. Olinger GN, Hottenrott C, Mulder DG, Maloney JV Jr, Miller J, Patterson RW, Sullivan SF, Buckberg GD: Acute clinical hypocalcemic myocardial depression during rapid blood transfusion and postoperative hemodialysis. A preventable complication. J Thorac Cardiovasc Surg 1976, 72:503.
37. Longo T, Marchetti G, Vercellio G: Coronary hemodynamic changes induced by aortic cross-clamping. J Cardiovasc Surg 1969, 10:36.
38. Mandelbaum I, Webb MK: Left ventricular function during cross-clamping of the descending thoracic aorta. JAMA 1963, 186:229.
39. Moyer JH, Heider C, Morris GC Jr, Handley C: Renal failure: I. The effect of complete renal artery occlusion for variable periods of time as compared to exposure to sub-filtration arterial pressures below 30 mm Hg for similar periods. Ann Surg 1957, 145:41.
40. Roizen MF: Does choice of anesthetic (narcotic vs. inhalational) significantly affect cardiovascular outcome after cardiovascular surgery? In Estafanous FG (ed): *Opioids in Anesthesia.* Boston, Butterworth, 1985.
41. Roizen MF, Hamilton WK, Sohn YJ: Treatment of stress-induced increases in pulmonary capillary wedge pressure using volatile anesthetics. Anesthesiology 1981, 55:446.
42. Wade JG, Stevens WC: Isoflurane: An anesthetic for the eighties? Anesth Analg (Cleveland) 1981, 60:666.
43. Smith NT, Eger EI II, Stoelting RK, Whayne TF, Cullen DJ, Kadis LB: The cardiovascular and sympathomimetic responses to the addition of nitrous oxide to halothane in man. Anesthesiology 1970, 32:410.
44. Shingu K, Eger EI II, Johnson BH, Van Dyke RA, Lurz FW, Cheng A: Effect of oxygen concentraton, hyperthemia, and choice of vendor on anesthetic-induced hepatic injury in rats. Anesth Analg (Cleveland) 1983, 62:146.
45. Eisele JH, Smith NT: Cardiovascular effects of 40 percent nitrous oxide in man. Anesth Analg (Cleveland) 1972, 51:956.
46. Koblin DD, Watson JE, Deady JE, Stokstad ELR, Eger EI II: Inactivaton of methionine synthetase by nitrous oxide in mice. Anesthesiology 1981, 54:318.
47. Cunningham FO, Egan JM, Inahara T: Continuous epidural anesthesia in abdominal vascular surgery. A review of 100 consecutive cases. Am J Surg 1980, 139:624.
48. Rao TLK, Gorski D, El-Etr AA: Epidural and subarachnoid catheters and anticoagulants. Anesthesiology 1980, 53:S213.
49. Roizen MF: Preoperative evaluation of patients with diseases that require special preoperative evaluation and intraoperative management. In Miller RD (ed): *Anesthesia,* New York, Churchill Livingstone, 1981, vol 1, pp 21–93.
50. Schülter M, Langenstein BA, Polster J, Kremer P, Souquet J,

Engel S, Hanrath P: Transoesophageal cross-sectional echocardiography with a phased array transducer system. Technique and initial clinical results. Br Heart J 1982, 48:67.
51. Beaupre PN, Cahalan MK, Kremer PF, Roizen MF, Cronnelly R, Robinson S, Lurz FW, Alpert R, Hamilton WK, Schiller NB: Does pulmonary artery occlusion pressure adequately reflect left ventricular filling during anesthesia and surgery? Anesthesiology 1983, 59:A3.
52. Laschinger JC, Cunningham JN Jr, Catinella FP, Nathan IM, Knopp EA, Spencer FC: Detection and prevention of intraoperative spinal cord ischemia after cross-clamping of the thoracic aorta: Use of somatosensory evoked potentials. Surgery 1982, 92:1109.
53. Flaherty JT, Magee PA, Gardner TL, Potter A, MacAllister NP: Comparison of intravenous nitroglycerin and sodium nitroprusside for treatment of acute hypertension developing after coronary artery bypass surgery. Circulation 1982, 65:1072.
54. Gerson JI, Allen FB, Seltzer JL, Parker FB Jr, Markowitz AH: Arterial and venous dilation by nitroprusside and nitroglycerin—Is there a difference? Anesth Analg (Cleveland) 1982, 61:256.
55. Rampil IJ, Correll JW, Rosenbaum SH, Quest DO, Holzer JA: Computerized electroencephalogram monitoring and carotid artery shunting. Neurosurgery 1983, 13:276.
56. Abbott WM, Austen WG: The reversal of renal cortical ischemia during aortic occlusion by mannitol. J Surg Res 1974, 16:482.
57. Barry KG, Cohen A, Knochel JP, Whelan TJ Jr, Beisel WR, Vargas CA, Leblanc PC Jr: Mannitol infusion. II. The prevention of acute functional renal failure during resection of an aneurysm of the abdominal aorta. N Engl Med 1961, 264:967.
58. Flores J, Dibona DR, Beck CH, Leaf A: The role of cell swelling in ischemic renal damage and the protective effect of hypertonic solute. J Clin Invest 1972, 51:118.
59. Hanley MJ, Davidson K: Prior mannitol and furosemide infusion in a model of ischemic acute renal failure. Am J Physiol 1981, 241:F556.

PART THREE

Peripheral Vascular Occlusive Disease

Chapter 23

ACUTE ARTERIAL INSUFFICIENCY

G. JEFFREY SMITH, JAMES W. HOLCROFT, and F. WILLIAM BLAISDELL

Whenever the motion of the blood in the arteries is impeded, by compression, by infarction, or by interception, there is less pulsation distally, since the beat of the arteries is nothing else than the impulse of blood in these vessels.

William Harvey

The concept of occlusion or "interception" of arterial flow was introduced by William Harvey in 1628 (1). John Hunter has been credited with proposing embolectomy in 1768 as a procedure for restoring flow (2). One hundred forty years later, Labey performed the first successful embolectomy (3).

The twentieth century has witnessed rapid progress in salvaging limbs that are threatened by acute arterial ischemia, primarily because of two developments. First, heparin anticoagulation has made it possible to limit the propagation of clot distal to the point of occlusion and reduce the incidence of recurrent embolus and thrombosis. Second, the Fogarty balloon catheter, introduced in 1963, has made it possible to extract emboli and thrombi from arteries, the Fogarty catheter being far better suited for this purpose than the devices used in the past, such as corkscrew wires or suction catheters (4).

This chapter describes our current procedures for dealing with acute arterial insufficiency. The chapter describes the etiology, pathophysiology, diagnosis, and treatment of acute arterial insufficiency. The emphasis is on treatment; our bias is toward anticoagulation.

Etiology

Acute arterial ischemia is caused by emboli or by acute thrombosis superimposed on a chronic underlying partial obstruction (Table 23-1). *Emboli* can be of cardiac or noncardiac origin. In the past, 80 percent of all emboli originated from the heart, the majority of these being of left atrial origin in patients with rheumatic heart disease and atrial fibrillation. With the recent decreased incidence of rheumatic heart disease, other embolic sources of acute arterial ischemia are becoming more prevalent. The most common cardiac source of an embolus remains a fibrillating atrium, but the fibrillation is more commonly caused by coronary artery disease. A less common cardiac source of emboli is a left ventricle that is damaged by myocardial infarction: Ventricular aneurysms can harbor a mural thrombus, and an infarcted endocardium can predispose to clot formation. The most common extracardiac sources of arterial emboli include ulcerating atheromatous lesions in the abdominal aorta and common iliac arteries. The lesions may be associated with aneurysmal disease of these vessels as well as more distal vessels. Other sources or causes of emboli are listed in Table 23-1 and include atrial myxoma, endocarditis, prosthetic heart valves, complications of arterial catheterization, and paradoxical embolization.

In approximately 25 percent of cases of acute ischemia caused by embolism, no source for the embolus can be identified. These cases may be due to small ulcerative lesions not demonstrated angiographically or may be caused by paradoxical emboli in which a septal defect cannot be demonstrated.

Thrombosis is the second major cause of acute arterial ischemia and in one recent review, it accounts for 50 percent of all acute ischemic episodes reported (5). Thrombosis usually occurs at a point of narrowing in an atherosclerotic vessel, particularly in association with a flow-related disorder, such as

TABLE 23-1. Etiology of Acute Arterial Occlusion

Embolic
Cardiac
Atrial fibrillation
Valvular heart disease (rheumatic heart disease or endocarditis)
Myocardial infarction (with or without ventricular aneurysm)
Prosthetic heart valves
Left atrial myxoma
Paradoxic embolus
Congestive cardiomyopathy
Hypertrophic cardiomyopathy
Mitral annulus calcification
Mitral valve prolapse
Peripheral
Ulcerating atherosclerotic lesions
Aneurysms (aortic, iliac, femoral, popliteal, subclavian, axillary)
Arterial catheterization complications
Thrombosis
Narrowed atherosclerotic segment (with or without a flow-related disorder)
Intraplaque hemorrhage
Drugs of abuse

congestive heart failure, shock, dehydration, or polycythemia. Additionally, hemorrhage within an atherosclerotic plaque can result in sudden occlusion (6). Traumatically induced ischemia is covered in Chapters 64–67.

Pathophysiology

Emboli of cardiac origin tend to obstruct at bifurcations of large arteries where the luminal diameter suddenly decreases. These arteries are usually more than 5 mm in diameter. Atheroemboli, consisting of debris from atheromatous lesions of the proximal arterial system, are smaller and occlude vessels less than 5 mm in diameter. The size of the obstructed vessel then can help in differentiating between emboli that originate from the heart and emboli that originate from the aorta or common iliac arteries. For example, an embolus that lodges in the common femoral artery is usually of cardiac origin; an embolus that leads to infarction of an isolated toe usually arises from the distal aorta or common iliac arteries.

Once an embolus lodges in an artery, or once a thrombus occludes a previously diseased artery, the vasculature distal to the obstruction goes into spasm. This spasm lasts for approximately 8 hours and then subsides. Clot forms in the arterial system distal to the site of obstruction and propagates distally to the point where collateral blood flow reestablishes patency. Clot also forms proximal to the site of the obstruction, back to the point of adequate collateralization.

Skeletal muscle and peripheral nerves withstand acute ischemia for some 8 hours without permanent damage; skin can withstand severe ischemia for probably as long as 24 hours. The extent of the ischemic necrosis depends on the adequacy of collateral circulation, the patient's underlying cardiovascular function, viscosity of the blood, oxygen-carrying capacity of the blood, propagation of clot into the microvasculature, and effectivensss and promptness of treatment.

If muscle ischemia progresses to necrosis, the muscle becomes paralyzed and acquires a firm, doughy consistency. When peripheral nerves become ischemic, they cease to function, and the affected parts become anesthetic. If the skin undergoes ischemic necrosis, blood suffuses into the interstitium and causes a cyanotic, blotchy appearance. These blotchy, cyanotic areas do not blanch with pressure (7).

The reperfusion of an ischemic extremity poses a threat to the rest of the body. Anaerobic metabolism produces unbuffered acid; dead cells release potassium and myoglobin; microthrombi form in the areas of stasis and acidosis; and platelet aggregates, procoagulants, and kinins accumulate. With reperfusion these toxic factors are washed into the systemic circulation, and remote organ failure can result. The lungs receive the first onslaught of these toxic products (8,9). The patient's mental, cardiac, and renal status can also suffer (10). The degree of insult to the remote organs depends on the degree of necrosis, the suddenness and adequacy of the revascularization, and the underlying condition of the remote organs.

Diagnosis

In most cases a history and physical examination allow identification of the level of obstruction, the probable cause, and the degree of ischemia (Tables 23-2 and 23-3). This information is usually all that is needed to direct the therapy.

The history should review the duration and progression of the symptoms and should document prior cardiac or vascular disease that might complicate the treatment. A history of claudication indicates prior atherosclerotic occlusive disease. A history of not smoking cigarettes makes the diagnosis of aortoiliac occlusive disease unlikely. A history of heart disease, particularly one associated with arrhythmias, makes the possibility of embolization from the heart likely.

TABLE 23-2. Signs of Ischemia

Acute ischemia
Pale extremity at resting position
Temperature change, with sharp line of demarcation
Pain and paresthesias
Decreased sensation
Mottled cyanotic color that blanches with pressure
Mottled cyanotic color that does not blanch
Paresis progressing to paralysis
Firm rigid musculature
Chronic ischemia
Atrophic musculature
Decreased hair
Hypertrophic nails
Pulse deficits
Temperature
Venous troughing*
Slow capillary refill
Prolonged pallor with elevation
Dependent rubor

*Collapse of the superficial veins of the foot.

TABLE 23-3. Patient Evaluation

Cardiac	Vascular
History	
Myocardial infarction	Transient ischemic attack
Arrhythmias—syncope	Amaurosis fugax
Angina	Claudication
Palpitations	Impotence
Medications	Intestinal angina
Congestive heart failure	Prior surgery
Physical Examination	
Rate and rhythm	Pulses:
Murmurs and gallops	Absent
Blood pressure	Aneurysmal
Cardiomegaly	Bruits
Peripheral edema	Signs:
Jugular venous distension	Acute ischemia
	Chronic ischemia
	Dehydration

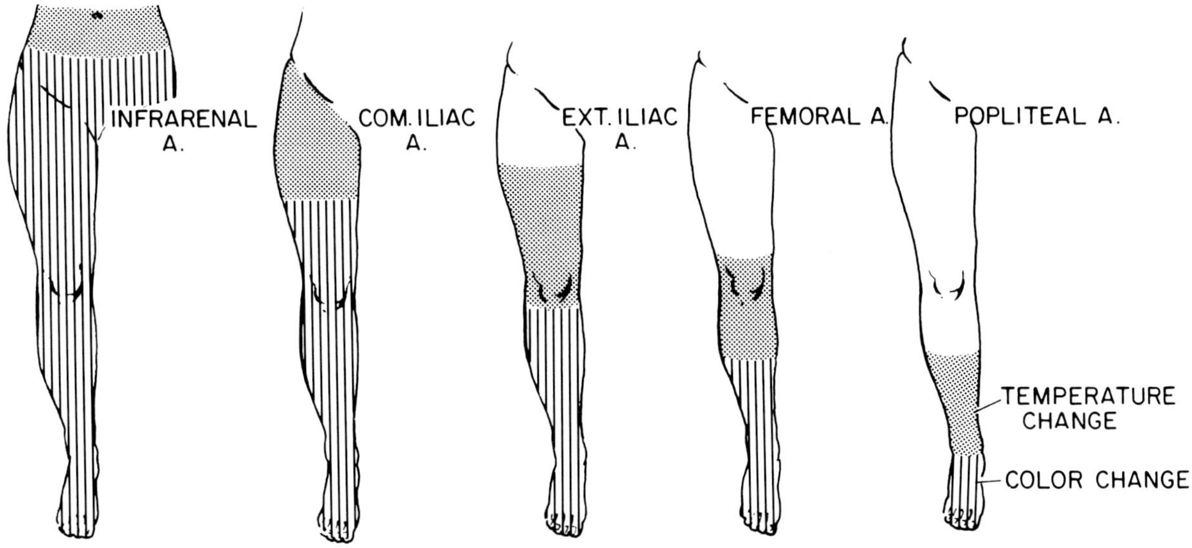

FIGURE 23-1. Level of temperature and color change with occlusion of different arteries.

The physical examination gives information about the heart and the likelihood that the heart is the source of an embolus. Signs of chronic ischemia in the lower extremity—hypertrophic nails, atrophic skin, and hair loss on the feet—indicate previously existing obstructive disease.

The presence of an acute arterial insufficiency is usually manifest by an abrupt temperature change in an extremity, distal to the level of the obstruction (Figure 23-1). The ability to dorsiflex and plantarflex the toes indicates the viability of the musculature in the calves; the inability to move the toes indicates necrosis of at least some of those muscles. Development of doughy, firm musculature, especially if the contralateral side is normal, indicates extensive necrosis of the musculature.

Paresthesias and anesthesia indicate the status of the nerves in the ischemic extremity. Waxy, white skin is characteristic of viable arterioles supplying blood to the skin; blotchy cyanosis that does not blanch with pressure indicates thrombosed capillaries in the subcuticular areas and the establishment of skin necrosis.

Laboratory tests are aimed at evaluating hydration, oxygen-carrying capacity of the blood, renal function, cardiac function, and muscular damage (Table 23-4). A chest x-ray may indicate size of the heart and may identify thoracic aortic disease. A hematocrit can make a diagnosis of polycythemia. A prothrombin time, partial thromboplastin time, and platelet count can aid in initiating anticoagulation therapy. A urinalysis that shows protein and pigment suggests the presence of myoglobin in the urine. The determination of creatinine phosphokinase with isoenzymes can give information about muscle necrosis. An electrocardiogram defines arrhythmias and gives information about the status of the heart. Two-dimensional echocardiography identifies the cardiac chamber size, estimates the ejection fraction, studies the valvular pathology, evaluates the wall motion, and sometimes identifies intracardiac thrombus or tumor (11,12). Echocardiography may also detect a potentially patent atrial septal defect. Echocardiography is not helpful acutely in deciding whether to operate, anticoagulate, or amputate (13). It is of value in discovering underlying cardiac disease that requires attention after successful management of the acute ischemic event. An ultrasound examination of the abdomen may reveal an abdominal aortic aneurysm. Ultrasonography of the popliteal fossa may demonstrate a nonpalpable thrombosed popliteal aneurysm.

We do not obtain arteriograms initially. When an arteriogram is obtained later, however, it can give useful information. An arteriogram sometimes shows a sharp cutoff of a proximally normal artery, indicating an embolus. It may also show preexisting underlying atherosclerotic occlusive disease. Abdominal aortic aneurysms or atheromatous disease involving the distal aorta and common iliac arteries may be demonstrated.

TABLE 23-4. Laboratory Assessment

Hematocrit, PT/PTT, platelets
Electrolytes, BUN, creatinine, glucose
Urinalysis—test for myoglobinuria
CPK with isoenzymes
Chest radiograph
Electrocardiogram
Two-dimensional echocardiogram
Arteriogram

Treatment

All patients with limb-threatening acute arterial insufficiency should be anticoagulated with heparin to prevent distal clot propagation. Heparin is the drug of choice because it is fast-acting, rapidly metabolized, and reversible by protamine sulfate. Many surgeons use conventional dosages of heparin (100 to 200 USP units/kg by bolus, followed by 15 to 30 USP units/kg per hour by constant infusion). We use higher dosages, preferring a bolus of 300 USP units/kg, followed by 60 USP units/kg per hour (14).

An activated clotting time, partial thromboplastin time, or

Lee-White clotting time should be obtained to ascertain that the patient is fully anticoagulated. We do not use these tests, however, to gauge our heparin dose. The degree of anticoagulation distal to an obstruction is not necessarily the same as the anticoagulation of blood taken from an antecubital vein. We use the higher doses of heparin because we want the anticoagulation to proceed in the ischemic areas; we judge the amount of anticoagulation on the patient's clinical response rather than on a laboratory test (15).

Hemorrhage is the major complication of anticoagulation with heparin (16). Patients without surgical wounds and without underlying bleeding dyscrasias seldom bleed on heparin, even high-dose heparin, for the first several days of therapy. Bleeding becomes more common on about the fifth day, when heparin-induced thrombocytopenia can contribute to the anticoagulant effect of the heparin itself. Fortunately, most patients receive most of the benefit from heparin anticoagulation within the first few days of treatment, and if bleeding should develop on the fifth day or later, the heparin can usually be stopped at that time with little danger to the patient's extremity.

Once anticoagulation has been established with heparin, attention should be directed toward cardiovascular function. Many patients have flow-related disorders, are dehydrated, or have arrhythmias compromising flow. Polycythemic patients should be phlebotomized. Patients with congestive heart failure may benefit from the use of cardiotonic medications, and diuresis. Hydration in other patients may help restore perfusion. Patients in shock require aggressive treatment.

We reserve thromboembolectomy for the patients who have a recent onset of ischemia, are a good operative risk, and whose point of occlusion is easily accessible using minimal dissection and Fogarty catheters. We do not operate as an emergency on patients who present with ischemia of longer than 8 hours' duration. If the ischemic insult is severe enough to result in muscle necrosis, the necrosis will be established within 8 hours. Revascularization after this period of time salvages no more muscle beyond that salvaged by anticoagulation, a treatment associated with a lower mortality.

We do not attempt immediate revascularization in patients with serious underlying medical problems. Revascularization of ischemic tissue washes products of ischemia into the central circulation, where those products damage the lungs, heart, kidneys, liver, and perhaps other organs. The patient's medical condition should be considered with respect to the amount of ischemic tissue that would be revascularized. Only a fairly strong patient can tolerate revascularization of an extremely ischemic entire lower extremity; a patient with a modest degree of cardiopulmonary disease will tolerate the establishment of flow into a moderately ischemic foot.

We attempt immediate thromboembolectomy only in the patients whose occlusion is easily accessible as judged by a physical examination. Thromboembolectomy can be performed as a minor procedure and with the patient fully anticoagulated. Meticulous surgical technique keeps the incidence of wound bleeding to an acceptable level, allowing the patient to remain fully anticoagulated postoperatively. In the patient with probable thrombosis superimposed on preexisting vascular disease, full revascularization is delayed until anticoagulation has resulted in as much extremity salvage as possible. An extensive early reconstructive procedure would preclude full heparin therapy postoperatively because of a prohibitively high rate of hemorrhage.

Any patient who presents longer than 8 hours after the onset of acute ischemia, or any patient in poor medical condition with respect to the amount of ischemic tissue, is treated initially with anticoagulation only. No arteriogram is obtained because arterial punctures are likely to bleed with full anticoagulation. The heparin anticoagulation is given to achieve clinical improvement. The improvement can be gauged by the patient's symptoms, by progression of the line of temperature demarcation distally along the leg, by recovery of sensation in the extremity, by maintenance or recovery of skeletal muscle function in the extremity, and by the appearance of the skin. As long as the skin blanches with pressure it is potentially salvageable; when the skin develops blotchy, cyanotic areas that do not blanch with pressure, it will become necrotic.

The heparin should be given for 72 hours at full doses. It should then be decreased and the patient's clinical condition assessed. If the patient's condition remains unchanged with lower doses of heparin, the heparin can be decreased approximately 1000 USP units per hour every 24 hours until the heparin is stopped about 7 days after the initiation of therapy or the patient transferred to oral anticoagulation or low-dose subcutaneous heparin. At that time the extremity is viable or partially necrotic. Amputation, revascularization, or chronic anticoagulation are treatment options in this situation. If revascularization is performed 7 days or more after the acute ischemic insult, it is done to maximize the chance of healing of an amputation or to alleviate symptoms of severe ischemia.

We have found that this treatment, a plan that emphasizes anticoagulation, results in low mortality and salvages extremities as well as those treatment regimens that emphasize immediate revascularization in all patients, both low-risk and high-risk (14). We do perform thromboembolectomy in low-risk patients, and that technique is described in the next section.

Patients presenting with a viable extremity more than 48 hours after the onset of symptoms can be managed like patients with chronic severe obstructive disease. High dose heparin therapy is of limited value, as these extremities have already survived the initial ischemic insult by developing collateral flow. An angiogram to evaluate the vasculature should be obtained. Many of these patients will require revascularization. Some have benefited from embolectomy as a form of revascularization up to 7 weeks after the onset of symptoms (17). Chronic anticoagulant therapy with warfarin (Coumadin) or subcutaneous heparin is indicated in many of these patients.

EMBOLECTOMY

Low-risk patients who present with ischemia of less than 8 hours' duration should have an embolectomy performed if it is likely that the acute ischemia is caused by an embolus. With the patient under local or regional anesthesia, thrombus or embolus can frequently be easily removed via a peripheral incision (18). A Fogarty balloon catheter is passed through the clot or embolus, the balloon inflated gently, and the catheter withdrawn. There are several important aspects to the application of this technique. Proximal and distal control of the vessel should be ensured before arteriotomy. The common femoral, popliteal, and brachial arteries allow access to most vessels with extractable material. Catheter-related complications can be kept to a minimum by continually moving the catheter when the balloon is being manipulated. Because of collateral flow, backbleeding as well as distal pulsation do not guarantee adequate clot extraction. Therefore, an angiogram should be obtained after the removal of the embolus to confirm an adequate clot extraction.

There are four primary complications associated with the use of the balloon catheter: rupture, perforation, intimal injury, and fragmentation of clot resulting in inadequate removal and distal embolization. These complications serve to emphasize another reason for obtaining an angiogram after an embolus extraction. If the angiogram demonstrates an intimal injury compromising circulation, repair is necessary. If there is extravasation of contrast material but good distal perfusion without signs of ongoing hemorrhage, repair may not be necessary. These patients can often be followed clinically and studied later with arteriograms to confirm the resolution of the problem.

POSTOPERATIVE CARE

For at least 24 hours after surgery, the patient should be placed in an intensive care unit so that the distal circulation can be monitored. If evidence of rethrombosis or recurrent embolus is identified, the patient should be returned to the operating room immediately. Pulmonary, cardiac, and renal complications should be treated in standard fashion as they present. Common complications of revascularization are noted in Table 23-5.

TABLE 23-5. Complications of Revascularization

Hemorrhage
Thrombosis
Recurrent emboli
Pulmonary embolus
Microembolic acute respiratory distress syndrome
Extremity edema
Acute renal failure
Cardiac dysfunction—myocardial infarction, arrhythmias
Mesenteric infarction

POSTOPERATIVE ANTICOAGULATION

All patients should be maintained on heparin anticoagulation postoperatively for at least 72 hours, and warfarin (Coumadin) should be started in suitable patients to prevent more emboli. Hemorrhage is a frequent postoperative complication in patients receiving heparin. Postoperative bleeding can be minor, as indicated by melena, hematuria, ecchymosis, or small wound hematomas, in which case the heparin therapy can be continued with monitoring of the hematocrit, platelet count, and partial thromboplastin time. The conversion to oral anticoagulation therapy should be accomplished as soon as possible. If the bleeding is major, the heparin effect should be reversed with protamine. Major bleeding includes that requiring transfusion for stabilization, cerebrovascular accidents, pulmonary infarction, and large wound hematomas. Further anticoagulation therapy should then await the stabilization of the patient and reevaluation.

Acutely, heparin is used in the postoperative period to prevent recurrent embolus or thrombosis. Additionally, one study indicates that mortality is decreased with postoperative anticoagulation (19). The trade-off is a 20 percent incidence of wound complications including an 8 percent incidence of hematomas requiring drainage (20).

FASCIOTOMY

Extremity edema associated with revascularization of an ischemic limb could theoretically threaten distal circulation postoperatively. Fasciotomy has been advocated to release pressure within the compartments and preserve distal circulation (21). The major risk of fasciotomy is infection. Necrotic muscle, which atrophies and resorbs if left alone, is exposed to possible infection, thereby threatening limb salvage and the patient's life. The decision to perform a fasciotomy should therefore be weighed against these risks. When ischemia is associated with significant soft tissue injury in the trauma patient, for example, we occasionally perform a fasciotomy. In the patient with acute ischemia secondary to thromboembolic disease we have never performed a fasciotomy; we believe that the potential complications outweigh the potential benefits.

FIBRINOLYTIC THERAPY

Although we do not use fibrinolytic therapy, others do. Initially, systemic thrombolytic agents, administered intravenously, were evaluated in acute arterial ischemia, and they effectively restored patency in occluded vessels at the expense of hemorrhagic complications. Other forms of systemic anticoagulation, such as heparin, were found to be as effective and safe. More recently, low-dose plasminogen activators have been selectively infused through a percutaneous arterial catheter just proximal to the occlusion (22,23,24). In theory, the hemorrhagic complications of systemic fibrinolytic therapy could be avoided by low-dose local infusion.

Streptokinase is a nonenzymatic protein product of group C β-hemolytic streptococci that combines with plasminogen to form an active enzymatic complex capable of converting plasminogen to plasmin. The low-dose intraarterial regimen provides for 5000 to 10,000 IU per hour to be selectively infused over 12 to 48 hours with the therapeutic effect monitored by physical examination or by serial arteriography. The low-grade fever at times accompanying the treatment is thought to be caused by the antigen-antibody interaction of streptokinase with preformed streptococcal antibodies.

Urokinase is harvested from human renal cells in tissue culture and is not antigenic. It is a trypsinlike protease that directly converts plasminogen to plasmin. Low-dose urokinase at 20,000 IU per hour selectively infused has been effective in restoring vessel patency. It is six times more expensive than streptokinase and therefore has been used rarely.

Ideally, fibrinolytic therapy would be most useful for fresh thrombosis prior to clot organization, propagation, or vessel wall damage. In contrast to heparin, the streptokinase actively lyses clot and therefore might accelerate the return of circulation to normal. Heparin prevents the formation of new clot, allowing fibrinolysis to predominate over clotting. Heparin can be given systemically and, by preventing clot formation, allows collateral circulation to develop while the patient's fibrinolytic system slowly lyses clot. It is unclear at the present time, which form of initial treatment is superior.

Streptokinase therapy has been combined with percutaneous transluminal angioplasty. It has also been successful in restoring patency in vessels occluded for several weeks. The appropriateness of chronic anticoagulation in both these groups of patients should be individualized. In summary, the long-term patency rates for both acute and chronic occlusions treated with streptokinase are under study, and the initial reports are encouraging.

Even with low-dose selective treatment, systemic fibrinolysis can be documented, and complications have been identified. Thrombin time, fibrinogen levels, prothrombin times, partial thromboplastin time, platelet counts, hematocrit, and fibrin split products should be monitored to prevent complications associated with fibrinolytic therapy (Table 23-6). Posttreatment anticoagulation should be monitored because patients have an increased susceptibility to bleeding complications. Although low-molecular-weight dextran has not been evaluated in the clinical setting, it may be preferable to heparin when making the switch from fibrinolytic therapy to oral anticoagulation therapy.

TABLE 23-6. Complications of Fibrinolytic Therapy

Intracranial hemorrhage
Arterial site hematomas
Distal embolization
Extravasation of blood through graft interstices—lysis of pseudointima of Dacron prosthesis
Retroperitoneal hemorrhage
Mild allergic reaction

Upper-Extremity Ischemia

In contrast to lower extremity ischemia, cardiac embolization accounts for the vast majority of cases of upper extremity ischemia (25). Thoracic outlet obstructions at the third portion of the subclavian artery can result in intimal damage, aneurysmal or poststenotic dilation, and subsequent atheroemboli or thrombosis (26). The principles of management of upper-extremity ischemia are similar to those of the lower extremity. Since collateral flow to the upper extremity is extensive, conservative treatment with high-dose heparin is almost always effective. Embolectomy is more dangerous in the upper extremity because of the size of the vessels and because of the danger of dislodging thrombus into the carotid or vertebral arteries. The mortality is lower and the limb salvage rate is higher for upper-extremity compared with lower-extremity ischemia, presumably because the amount of tissue necrosis is less in the upper extremity.

Cerebral Ischemia

Embolism has been estimated to cause 20 to 30 percent of all cerebral infarctions, and the incidence of stroke is five times greater in patients with atrial fibrillation than in the general population (27). Since the risk of recurrent stroke in these patients is approximately 20 percent per year, the treatment is directed at controlling arrhythmias and at preventing further empirical infarctions with oral anticoagulants (28).

Visceral Ischemia

Most visceral ischemia of sudden onset occurs when the superior mesenteric artery is occluded acutely by an embolus or by thrombosis. Abdominal catastrophe associated with cardiac disease is the classic setting. Traditionally, mortality has been 80 percent and treatment has focused on resection of necrotic bowel rather than revascularization. However, revascularization by aortomesenteric bypass, transaortic endarterectomy, or embolectomy may rarely be successful in the acute case. More recently a combination of revascularizaton followed in 20 to 30 minutes by resection of necrotic bowel has been advocated to improve mortality (29). A second-look procedure is always indicated.

References

1. Harvey W: *Exercitatio anatomica de motu cordis et sanguinis in animalibus,* English translation by Leake CD. Springfield, Ill, Charles C Thomas, 1931, p 37.
2. Shor PM, Fogarty TJ: Acute arterial insufficiency. In Miller DC, Avon AJ (eds): *Diagnosis and Management of Peripheral Vascular Disease*. Menlo Park, Calif, Addison-Wesley, 1982.
3. Labey: cited by Mosney M and Dumont NJ: Embolie fémorale au cours d'un rétrécissement mitral pur. Artériotomie. Guerison Bull Acad Med 1911, 66:358.
4. Abbott WM, Maloney RD, McCabe CC, Lee CE, Wirthlin LS: Arterial embolism: A 44 year perspective. Am J Surg 1982, 143:460.
5. Dale WA: Differential management of acute peripheral arterial ischemia. J Vasc Surg 1984, 1:269.
6. Lusby RJ, Wylie EJ: Acute lower limb ischemia: Pathogenesis and management. World J Surg 1983, 7:340.
7. Blaisdell FW in the discussion of Levy JE and Butcher HR: Arterial emboli: An analysis of 125 patients. Surgery 1970, 68:968.
8. Blaisdell FW, Lim, RG, Amberg JR, Choy SH, Hall SD, Thomas AN: Pulmonary microembolism: A cause of morbidity and death after vascular surgery. Arch Surg 1966, 93:776.
9. Stallone RJ, Blaisdell FW, Cafferata HT, Levin SM: Analysis of morbidity and mortality from arterial embolectomy. Surgery 1969, 65:207.
10. Haimovici H: Metabolic complications of acute arterial occlusions. J Cardiovasc Surg 1979, 20:349.
11. Nishide M, Irino T, Gotoh M, Naka M, Tsuji K: Cardiac abnormalities in ischemic cerebrovascular disease studied by two-dimensional echocardiography. Stroke 1983, 14:541.
12. Caplan LR, Hier DB, D'Cruz I: Cerebral embolism in the Michael Reese Stroke Registry. Stroke 1983, 14:530.

13. Robbins JA, Sagar KB, French M, Smith PJ: Influence of echocardiography on management of patients with systemic emboli. Stroke 1983, 14:546.
14. Blaisdell FW, Steele M, Allen RE: Management of acute lower extremity arterial ischemia due to embolism and thrombosis. Surgery 1978, 84:822.
15. Blaisdell FW: Use of anticoagulants in the ischemic lower extremity. In Kempczinski RF (ed): *Management of Lower Extremity Ischemia*. Chicago: Year Book, in press.
16. Gervin AS: Complications of heparin therapy. Surg Gynecol Obstet 1975, 140:789.
17. Jarrett F, Dacumos GC, Crummy AB, Detmer DE, Belzer FO: Late appearance of arterial emboli: Diagnosis and management. Surgery 1979, 86:898.
18. Fogarty TJ, Cranley JJ, Krause RJ, Strasser ES, Hefner CD: A method for extraction of arterial emboli and thrombi. Surg Gynecol Obstet 1963, 116:241.
19. Holm J, Schersten T: Anticoagulant treatment during and after embolectomy. Acta Chir Scand 1972, 138:683.
20. Tawes RL, Beare JP, Scribner RG, Sydorak GR, Brown WH, Harris EJ: Value of postoperative heparin therapy in peripheral arterial thromboembolism. Am J Surg 1983, 146:213.
21. Patman RD, Thompson JE: Fasciotomy in peripheral vascular surgery. Arch Surg 1970, 101:663.
22. Hallett JW, Yrizarry JM, Greenwood LH: Regional low dosage thrombolytic therapy for peripheral arterial occlusions. Surg Gynecol Obstet 1983, 156:148.
23. Hargrove WC, Barker CF, Berkowitz HD, Perloff LJ, McLean G, Freiman D, Ring EJ, Roberts B: Treatment of acute peripheral arterial and graft thrombosis with low-dose streptokinase. Surgery 1982, 92:981.
24. Katzen BT, Van Breda A: Low-dose streptokinase in the treatment of arterial occlusions. Am J Radiol 1981, 136:1171.
25. Haimovici H: Cardiogenic embolism of the upper extremity. J Cardiovasc Surg 1982, 23:209.
26. Haimovici H: Arterial thromboembolism of the upper extremity associated with the thoracic outlet syndrome. J Cardiovasc Surg 1982, 23:214.
27. Sage JI, Van Uitert RL: Risk of recurrent stroke in patients with atrial fibrillation and non-valvular heart disease. Stroke 1983, 14:537.
28. Easton JD, Sherman DG: Management of cerebral embolism of cardiac origin. Stroke 1980, 11:433.
29. Bergan JJ, Dean RH, Conn J, Yao JST: Revascularizaton in treatment of mesenteric infarction. Ann Surg 1975, 182:430.

Chapter 24

ARTERIOARTERIAL ATHEROTHROMBOTIC MICROEMBOLI OF THE LOWER LIMB

ALLASTAIR M. KARMODY, JOHN D. CORSON, DHIRAJ M. SHAH, and ROBERT P. LEATHER

Although recently attention has been paid to atherothrombotic microembolism from atheromatous plaques or from adherent thrombotic material, such pathological occurrences were first mentioned in the German literature over a century ago (1). However, within the last two decades, the pathological implications of this specific entity has come to our attention as a mechanism of serious pathology of the brain, viscera, and both upper and lower limbs. The lodgment of atherothrombotic microemboli (defined as particles of 1 mm size or smaller) into end arteries has now been documented in virtually every part of the human body. The production of stroke or cerebral insufficiency by this mechanism is discussed in Chapter 46, but atherothrombotic emboli are known to cause renal cortical ischemia (2,3), left colonic gangrene (4), and ischemia of the fingers (Chapter 56). This chapter will deal specifically with embolization of this type in the lower limbs.

The sudden appearance of a painful, discolored toe may be very baffling when the rest of the foot appears to be well perfused, particularly when the pedal pulses can be readily felt by digital examination. The confusion has been deepened by the application of a variety of misleading labels to this condition, including vasospasm, "cold injury," localized Raynaud's phenomenon, polymyositis, and idiopathic digital artery thrombosis (5). However, in most of these patients the ischemia has been caused by microembolization to the digital arteries. Crane (6) reported on this entity in three patients in whom distal microemboli were dislodged from atheromatous aortoiliac lesions and were observed in the digital arteries of the toes. Although this possibility has also been mentioned by other authors (2,5,7,8), in general, little attention has been paid to its ultimate pathological implications. Moreover, the natural history of this syndrome was not clearly defined by these observers. The threatened survival of a single toe is not in itself of great clinical consequence, but continuing experience with this pathological entity indicates that when untreated, these episodes are such omens of disaster for the leg that the aim of subsequent diagnostic and therapeutic measures should be promptly concentrated on the location and eradication of the source of microemboli.

Incidence of This Condition

From the literature, it has been difficult to gain any idea of the incidence of this problem. However, examination of our own data tends to offer some perspective on this problem. In the 7-year period (1978–1985), 4820 vascular consultations were made on the Vascular Service of Albany Medical Center, and of these, 120 (2.5 percent) were for suspected microembolism to the lower limbs. Of this entire group, 4043 vascular reconstructions were carried out, and of these 93 (2.3 percent) were done specifically for eradication of emboligenic sources of microemboli to the lower limb. In general, therefore, these data suggest that perhaps 1 in 50 of all vascular reconstructions will be carried out for these purposes in a general vascular service (Table 24-1).

TABLE 24-1. Incidence of Microembolic Sources from Division of Vascular Surgery, Albany, New York

Number of vascular consultations	4820
Number of consultations for atherothrombotic microemboli	120 (2.5%)
Number of vascular procedures	4043
Number of reconstructions for microembolizations	93 (2.3%)

Sources and Nature of Microemboli

A variety of lesions will act as microembolic sources, and these range in location from the infrarenal aorta to the termination of the popliteal artery. Aneurysms of the popliteal artery have long been recognized for this predisposition and are discussed in Chapter 38. Iliac and common femoral aneurysms rarely produce distal embolization and are more prone to acute thrombotic occlusion. In marked contrast, however, atherosclerotic lesions of the iliac, common, and superficial femoral artery are important sources of

TABLE 24-2. Location of Embolic Sources

Author	No. of Cases	Embolic Sources: AAA	Aortoiliac	Femoro-popliteal
Karmody	93	12	18	63
Kwaan (15)	15		15	
Schechter (14)	17	3	9	2
Crane (6)	3		3	
Carvajal (2)	4	4		
Branowitz (7)	4		4	
Kempczinski (13)	10	2	8	
Mehigan (19)	12		5	7

microemboli. While it may be instinctively surmised that pathological degeneration of the larger arteries would be the predominant origin of such arterioarterial emboli, Table 24-2 indicates the somewhat surprising finding that the femoral arteries are the most common emboligenic sources. Apart from popliteal aneurysms, which occupy a special category as previously mentioned, stenotic, irregular, and ulcerated lesions of the iliac and femoropopliteal arteries are frequently microembolic sources, as shown by their relative incidence. However, when there is widespread atheromatous degeneration of the infradiaphragmatic arteries, it can be difficult to precisely identify the specific area which has been responsible for the clinically apparent downstream release of microemboli (9).

Many authors have expressed the view that these microemboli result solely from fragmentation of atheromatous plaques and subsequent dislodgment of the debris (2,3,5,8,10–12). Indeed, atheromatous plaques are known to undergo ulceration and fragmentation, and atheromatous or cholesterol-containing material has been identified in digital vessels and in the smaller arteries of the calf muscles (10). However, many of the microemboli of the lower limb have been identified as being of fibrinoplatelet or thrombotic material. The microemboli which are released from aneurysmal sources (popliteal, aortic, etc.) are part of the flocculent laminated thrombus which lines the arterial flow path. A common surgical finding is that atheromatous plaques are very friable, but the shaggy, frondlike clumps of fibrinoplatelet debris which are invariably present on these lesions are not only impressive but also appear more likely to be dislodged. It has also been confirmed (4,6,7,13) that in addition to cholesterol fragments, fibrinoplatelet aggregates are loosely attached to ulcerated or stenotic atheromatous plaque and are easily swept off. Schechter (14) has recovered a shred of atheromatous plaque (gravel) from a tibial artery and has postulated that after these particles impact, surrounding fibrinoplatelet aggregates and propagated thrombus increase the degree of obstruction.

Branowitz (7) concluded that the clinical and pathological processes involve either distal embolization of atheromatous debris or fibrinoplatelet or thrombotic material. Kempczinski (13) has further clarified this by showing that cholesterol emboli tend

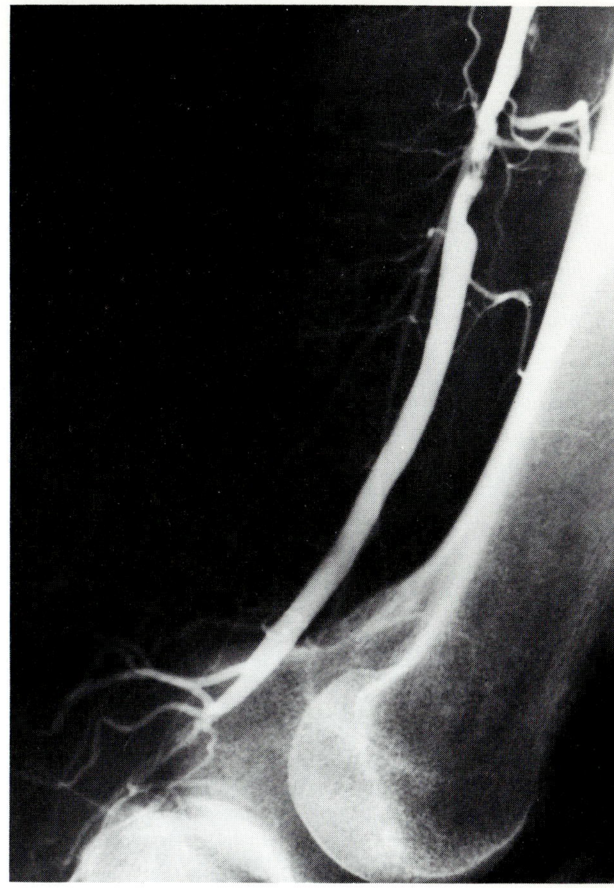

FIGURE 24-1. Good example of emboligenic lesion in mid-superficial femoral from which a distal embolus has occluded the popliteal artery.

to originate in the infrarenal aorta, to be diffuse and to lodge in arteries of 100 to 200 μm in size (e.g., muscular arteries). By contrast, microemboli formed from hemocellular elements tend to be larger and to occlude vessels of up to 1 mm in size. Digital arteries are customarily involved, but emboli have been recovered which were large enough to occlude the tibial, popliteal, and superficial femoral arteries (3,7,15,16) (Figure 24-1). Larger emboli of this type usually arise within the infrarenal aorta in an area of severe atheromatous degeneration which has larger, loosely attached fibrinoplatelet clumps (17). These larger emboli rarely form when compared to the frequency of the smaller microemboli. This clinical entity has been described in various ways in the literature. It has been called the "blue toe syndrome" (18), "atheromatous embolization" (12,14), "acute focal ischemia" (19), and "peripheral atheroembolism" (16). From the foregoing pathological description, the term "arterioarterial atherothrombotic microembolism," although cumbersome, is preferred since it most accurately describes all of the pathological events (17).

Natural History of Atherothrombotic Microembolization

Gore and Collins (20) have shown by autopsy examination that atherothrombotic microembolization is a more frequent clinical problem than has been generally recognized. This option has been confirmed by Maurizi et al. (11), who concluded that the microemboli usually lodged in the lower limbs and that recurrent microembolization which finally led to extensive tissue loss is

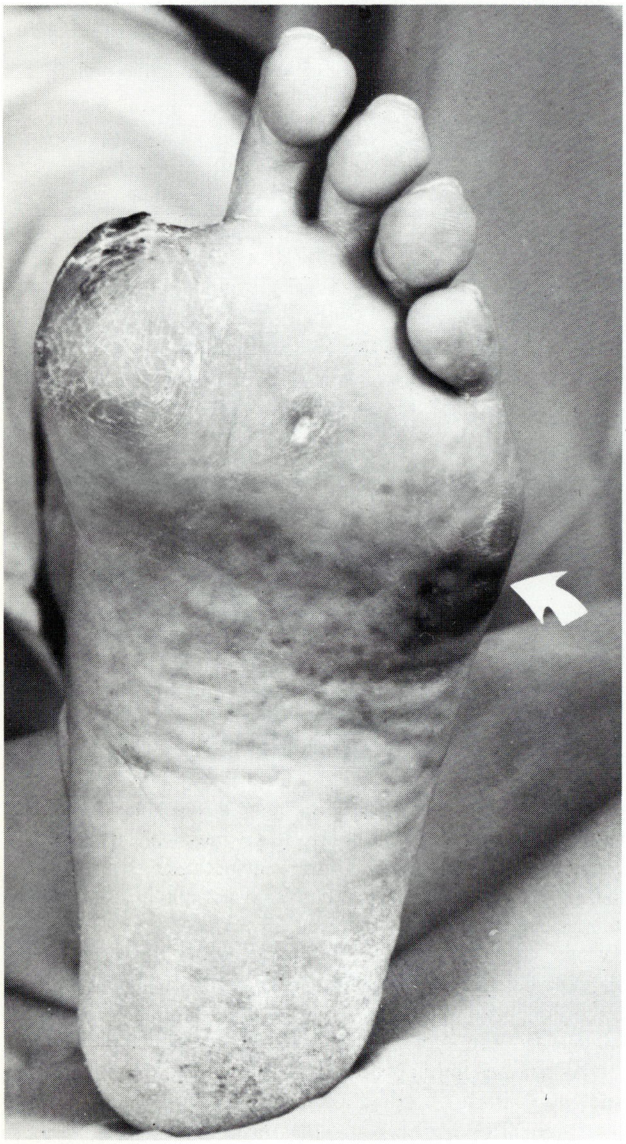

FIGURE 24-2. Natural history of arterial microemboli. The great toe, which was ischemic from the first microembolus, has been hastily amputated, and the wound is healing poorly. In addition, another microembolus has lodged (*arrow*) at the lateral side of the foot. This process will continue until the emboligenic source is corrected.

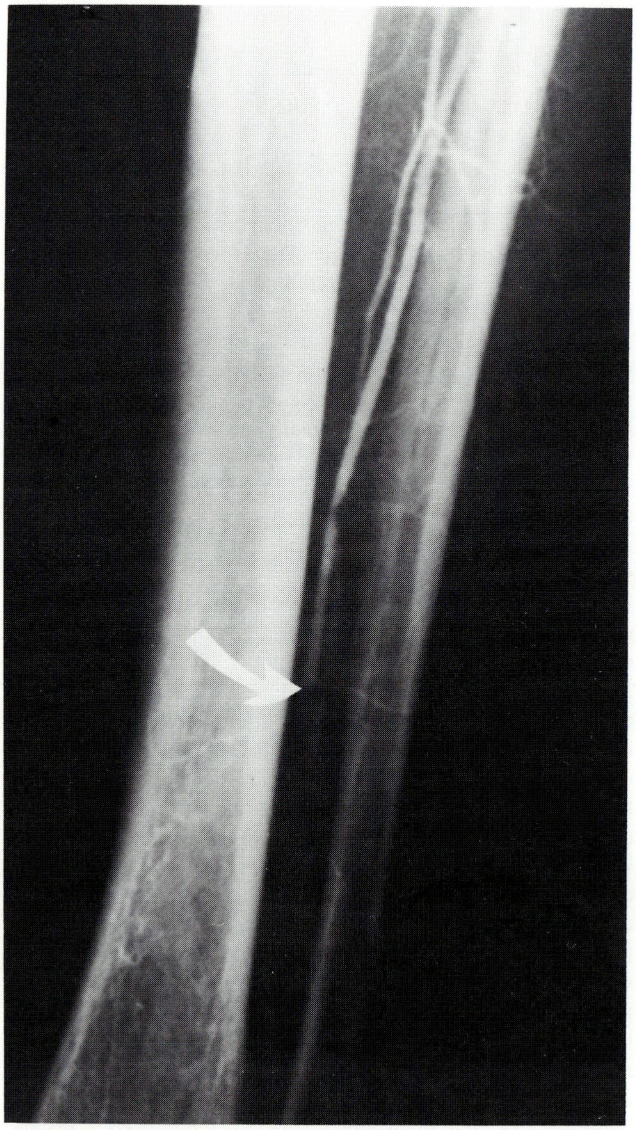

FIGURE 24-3. Occlusion of anterior tibial artery (*arrow*) by microembolus jeopardizing entire foot.

common (Figure 24-2). In 12 of our patients, repeated microemboli to the foot were clinically recognized, and loss of one or more toes occurred in five of these patients. In another patient, the second embolic shower resulted in ischemic death of the forefoot. Schechter (14) reported 11 cases in which there was repeated microembolization, and Mehigan's report (19) contains four patients who also experienced this problem, each with threatened tissue loss, a tendency which has also been confirmed by Branowitz (7) (Table 24-2). Early diagnosis and treatment are, therefore, necessary if recurrence is to be prevented, and it is this aspect of microembolization which enhances its clinical importance and makes recognition and treatment mandatory.

The natural history of atherothrombotic microembolization of the lower limb consists, therefore, of a repetition of embolic episodes. Each successive event causes progressive loss of collateral arteries until tissue necrosis finally occurs. Larger emboli, of course, are likely to occlude the popliteal or tibial arteries and cause acute, profound ischemia of the foot (Figure 24-3). It has been well documented (7,11,13,14,18) that initially both the patient and the physician are frequently lulled into a false sense of security since in most instances the signs are evanescent and recovery is prompt. Further embolization may occur in a few hours, or even after many weeks, but the repetitive tendency remains pronounced in any event.

Although this pattern of events is well recognized in the cerebral circulation, the probable reason that more emphasis has been placed on the carotid lesion relates to the relative ease of identifying serious pathological effects of cerebral microemboli (i.e., stroke potential as compared to less clinical concern about small emboli to the digits or feet). Early and complete eradication of the embolic source has been well established as the definitive treatment in the cerebral arterial system, and these same principles also apply to the peripheral limb arteries because microemboli cause comparable transient ischemic attacks of the foot and also carry a serious threat of tissue loss, which deserves attention similar to that of loss of brain tissue.

Clinical Diagnosis

The typical picture of patients suffering from this condition includes the sudden appearance of a painful digit or small area on the foot (Figure 24-4), which is generally bluish in color (hence the name "blue toe syndrome"), has a sluggish capillary return, and is quite tender to the touch. The discoloration may be either uniform or mottled in character (Figure 24-5). These symptoms may last only a few minutes and cause little noticeable disability, but more commonly, the initial insult will provide symptoms and signs for a few days, although gangrenous changes will rarely occur at this time (Figure 24-6). The eventual outcome is obviously determined by the available collateral pathways, which are themselves determined both by the site of embolic impaction and the effects of previous or unrecognized embolic episodes.

Even if the first or subsequent episodes are short-lived and cause little clinical difficulty, it should be recognized that further emboli are not only probable but also tend to "stream" to the identical area, thus increasing the risk of tissue loss because of progressive reduction of collateral capacity. In many patients, a detailed history will reveal that sudden attacks of pain in the muscles of the lower limbs, particularly in the gastrosoleus muscle complex, have been caused by unrecognized microemboli-

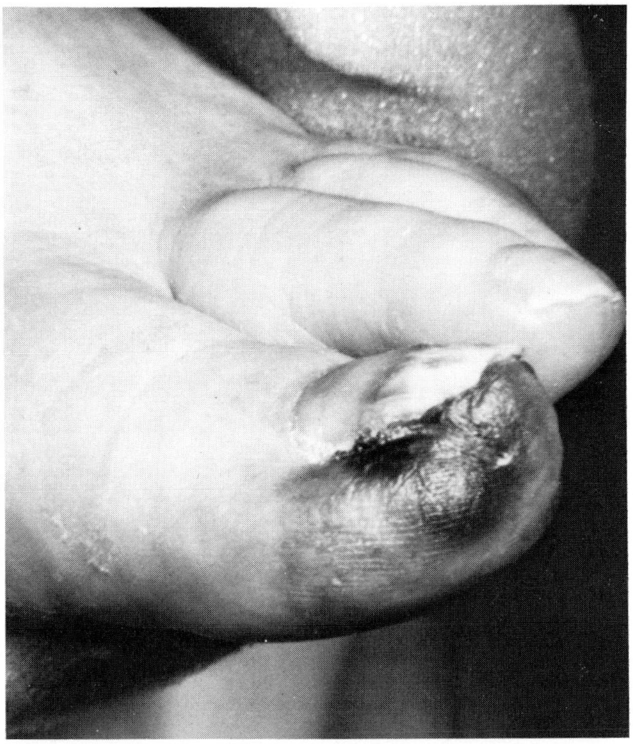

FIGURE 24-4. Most common appearance of microembolic disease consisting of a deep blue painful area of the great toe.

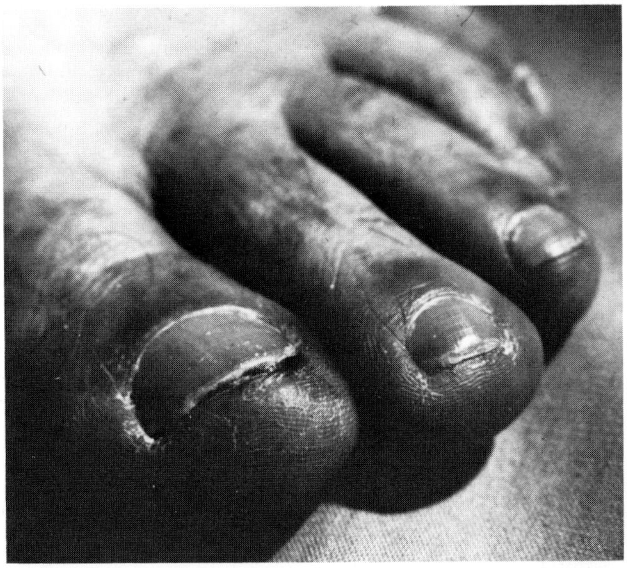

FIGURE 24-5. More diffuse involvement of the foot with uniform discoloration and mottling resulting from embolization of the plantar arch.

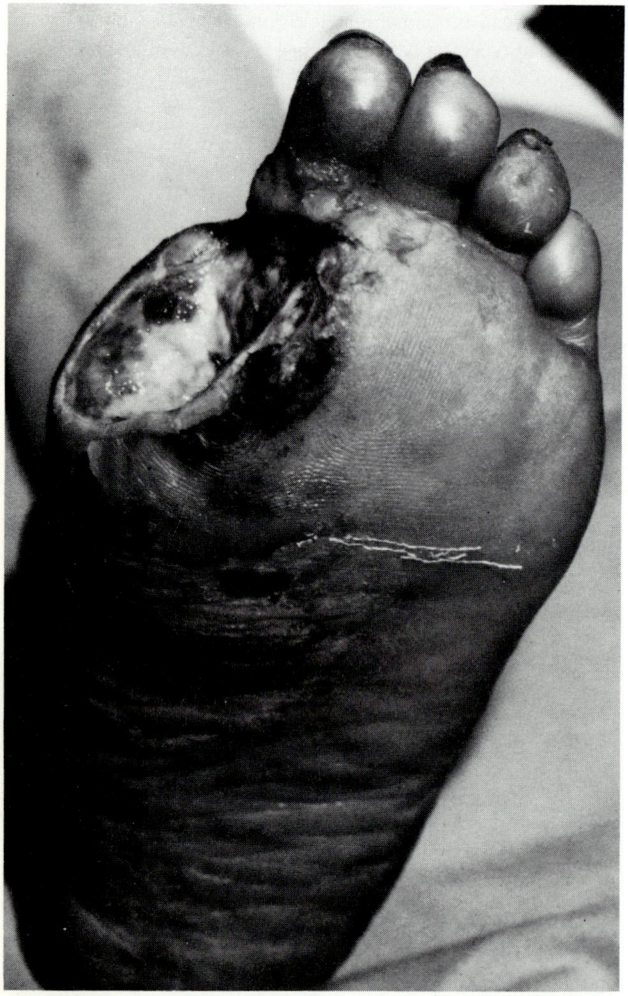

FIGURE 24-6. Nonhealing wound caused by injudicious amputation of great toe without correction of proximal stenotic lesion (cf. Figure 24-2).

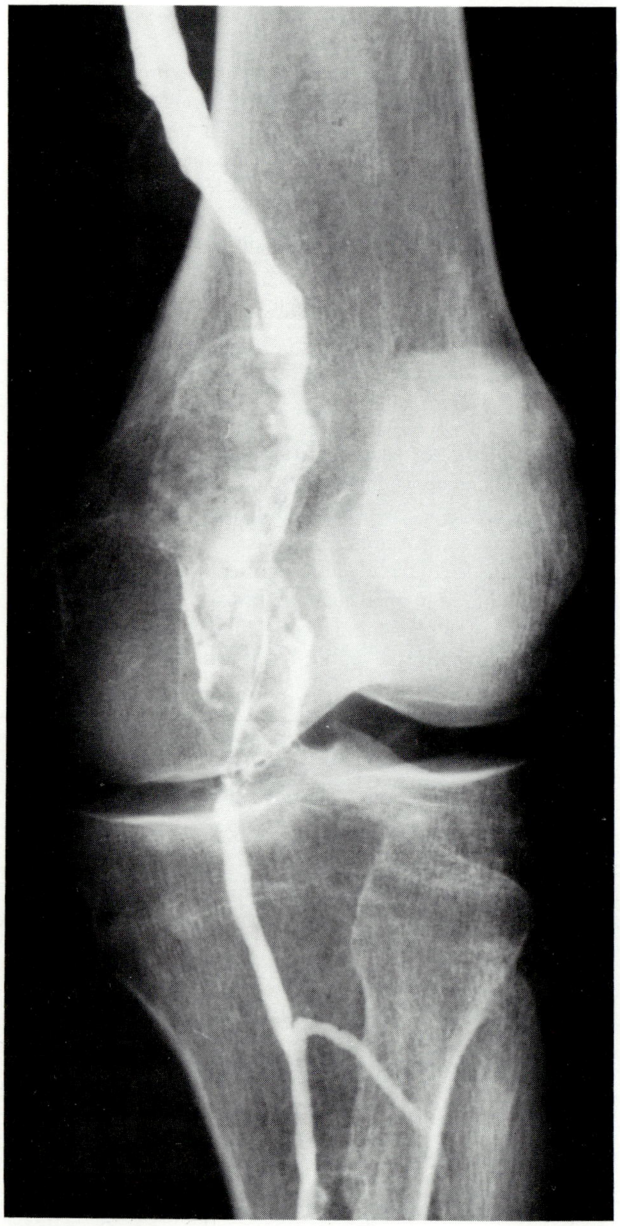

FIGURE 24-7. Typical popliteal aneurysm filled with large quantities of mural thrombus.

zation which preceded the most clinically obvious episodes of digital ischemia (2,10).

Physical examination should include the examination of pulses from the aorta to the foot. As noted previously, the presence of palpable pedal pulses is a rule rather than an exception in these patients, but manual examination of the abdominal aorta and femoral and popliteal arteries may reveal clinically significant aneurysmal enlargement (Figure 24-7). A bruit is frequently present over the affected artery, particularly in the common and superficial femoral vessels. The Doppler ultrasound signal over the distal arteries is usually normally pulsatile, as are the arterial plethysmographic tracings at rest. In many instances in which the toes are affected ultrasound mapping of the course of the digital arteries with a 10-MHz Doppler probe will demonstrate abrupt occlusion of the digital arteries. This may be hard to accomplish in the smaller toes, and for practical purposes, it is useful only in the transmetatarsal arteries and the great toe.

Diagnostic Investigations

When the emboligenic arterial lesion is also hemodynamically significant, the systolic pressures in the pedal arteries with the patient at rest may show such a small gradient that they may not be discernible on digital palpation of pulses. Repeated examination after exercise in most instances will produce a bruit with diminution of the ankle pulses and a measurable decrease in the arterial systolic pressure. Segmental plethysmographic tracings (waveforms) should be obtained at the thigh, calf, ankle, transmetatarsal, and digital levels. As mentioned above, although these may be normal at rest, exercise of the affected limb will commonly produce changes in the waveforms which are clearly diagnostic of a hemodynamic lesion. The use of B-mode duplex ultrasound scanning in the investigation of abdominal aortic aneurysms, particularly in obese patients, and in the common femoral to distal popliteal arteries is especially useful. Computerized tomography body scan may also be helpful, particularly

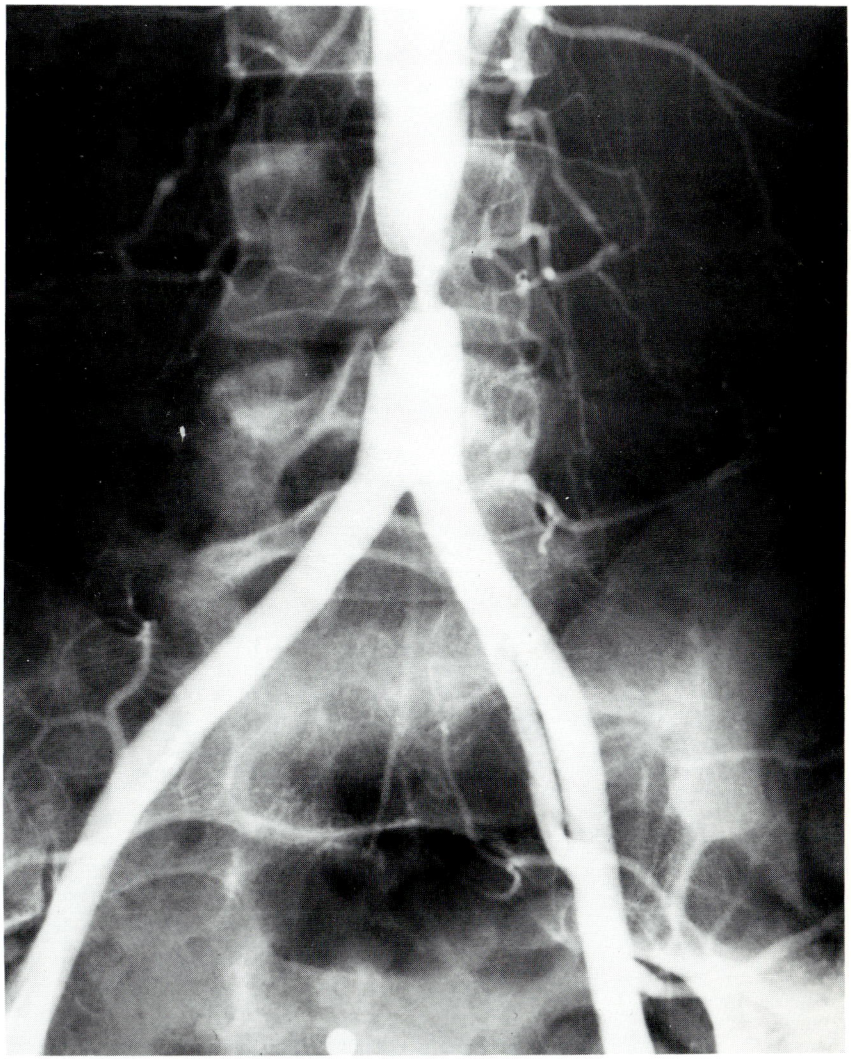

FIGURE 24-8. Well-marked aortic stenosis which was responsible for bilateral microemboli. Treated by endarterectomy.

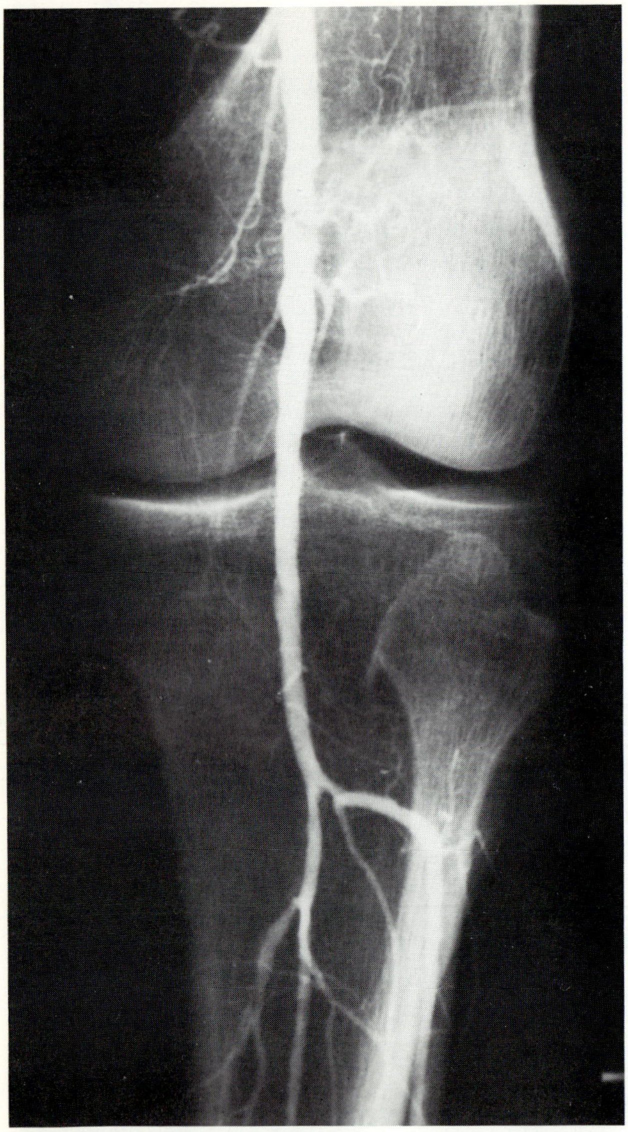

FIGURE 24-9. The other end of the scale (i.e., lesion in distal popliteal). These two figures (Figures 24-8 and 24-9) stress the need for complete angiography.

in the abdominal region. With continued development of these techniques, an increasing ability to obtain more accurate soft-tissue evaluation by newer methods (e.g., nuclear magnetic resonance), it is sometimes possible at present to actually demonstrate intraluminal debris in both the aorta and arteries of the limb.

Muscle biopsies have been used (2,10) as a diagnostic tool in the evaluation of patients with microemboli. The biopsies were taken either surgically or by needle from the gastrocnemius muscle, and a high correlation with the clinical symptomatology has been reported. We have not found this diagnostic method to be so useful, although it may have a place in evaluating patients with atherosclerosis who have obscure symptoms of the calf and foot.

Although in the modern context, angiography should not be considered a diagnostic tool but rather a preoperative measure, in this particular context, biplane angiography is the most accurate of all diagnostic methods. Ideally, this examination should define the arteries from the infrarenal aorta (Figures 24-8 and 24-9) to the toes. Arterial irregularities may be present in many areas, and a complete angiographic examination is necessary if correct clinical decisions are to be made about the most probable source of emboli. The use of high-quality biplane angiograms obtained with a single arterial injection and radiological magnification has greatly improved these studies (Figure 24-10). Although it is generally quite difficult to obtain anteroposterior angiograms of the pedal arches, these can be quite informative (Figure 24-11). However, routine and satisfactory lateral views of the foot can readily be made, and when the obstructions occur within the plantar arch or dorsalis pedis artery, they are easily identified (Figure 24-12).

It should be stressed that one of the prerequisites for the diagnosis of microembolization is the identification of a continuous anatomic arterial channel between the site of the emboligenic source and the point at which the emboli impaction has occurred. While it is also possible that extensive collaterals around an obstructive lesion may be large enough to carry emboli distally, in our experience, such occurrences are rare. The ischemia of the toe or foot which has resulted from microembolic problems should, therefore, be clearly differentiated from the more common form of ischemia which has been caused by extensive proximal obliterative arterial disease.

Management

The foremost principle of treatment of this condition is the removal of the source of emboli. In addition, since many of these emboligenic lesions also cause acute hemodynamic flow reduction, their repair also brings about reversal or improvement of ischemic changes in the foot. The operative procedures for the various aneurysms which are the source of emboli are described in Chapter 36, and the principles of endarterectomy and/or bypass of arterial lesions are also well known. In the highly localized stenotic lesions (1 to 2 cm) of the femoral and popliteal arteries, operative removal of the fibrinoplatelet clumps together with adherent intima (thrombointimectomy) (Figure 24-13) followed by vein patch angioplasty has produced very satisfactory long-term results (Figure 24-14), although all of these arteries inevitably display various degrees of atheromatous degeneration both proximally and distally to their actual stenotic lesions. The great majority of patients treated by this method have maintained patency of these arteries for periods of up to 5 years (9) (Figures 24-15 and 24-16). In patients with longer segments of significant atherosclerotic changes (over 5 cm) vein patch angioplasty is not only tedious but is also less durable, and the standard bypass procedure with the distal interruption of the native artery is the preferable method of treatment (21). When these lesions are identified angiographically, the physician should be alerted to the possibility of microembolic dislodgment, particularly following intraluminal catheter passage during subsequent attempts at intraluminal balloon dilatation.

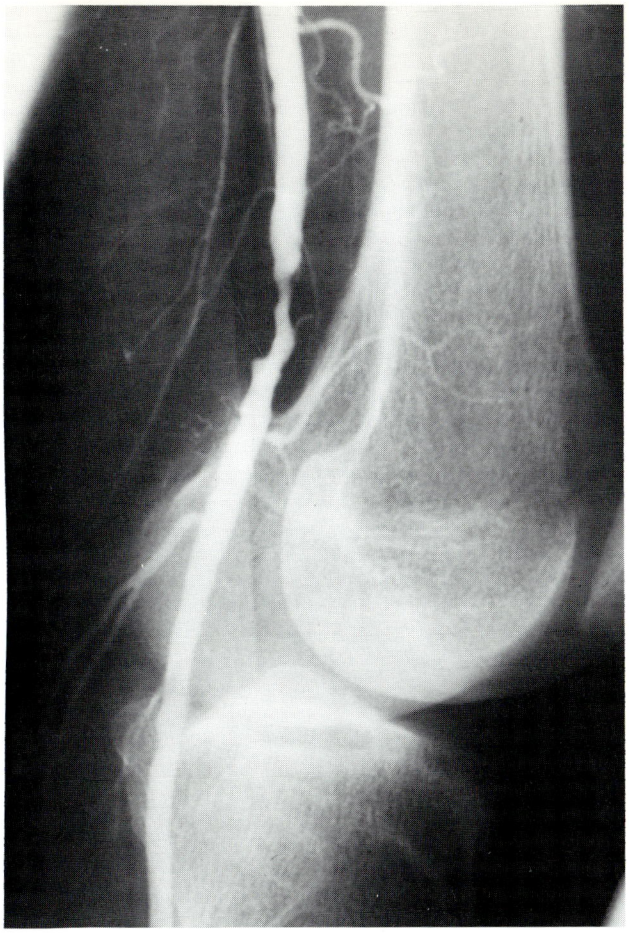

FIGURE 24-10. Lateral view of proximal popliteal showing emboligenic lesion which was poorly identified in the AP projection.

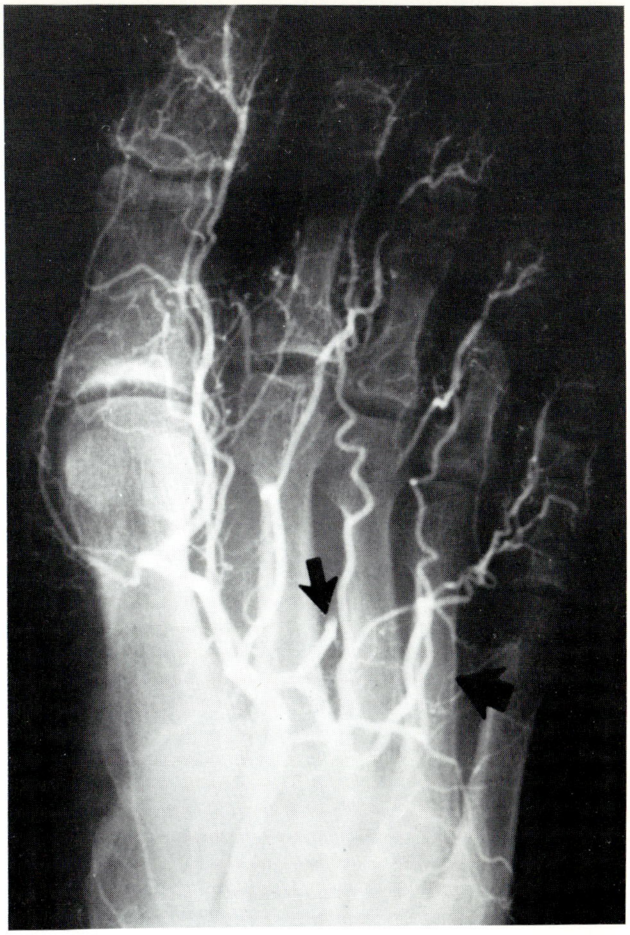

FIGURE 24-11. AP arteriogram of the pedal arch, in which the arrows demonstrate well-defined sites of microembolic impaction.

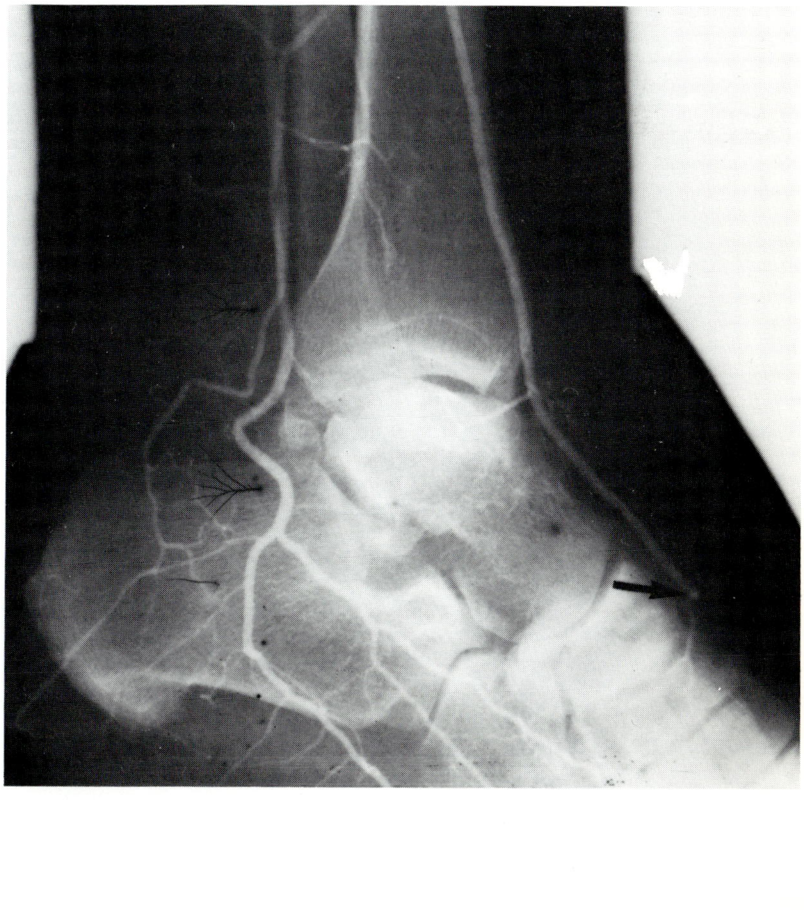

FIGURE 24-12. Lateral view of foot is more easily obtained, and obstruction of the dorsalis pedis (*arrow*) is easily seen.

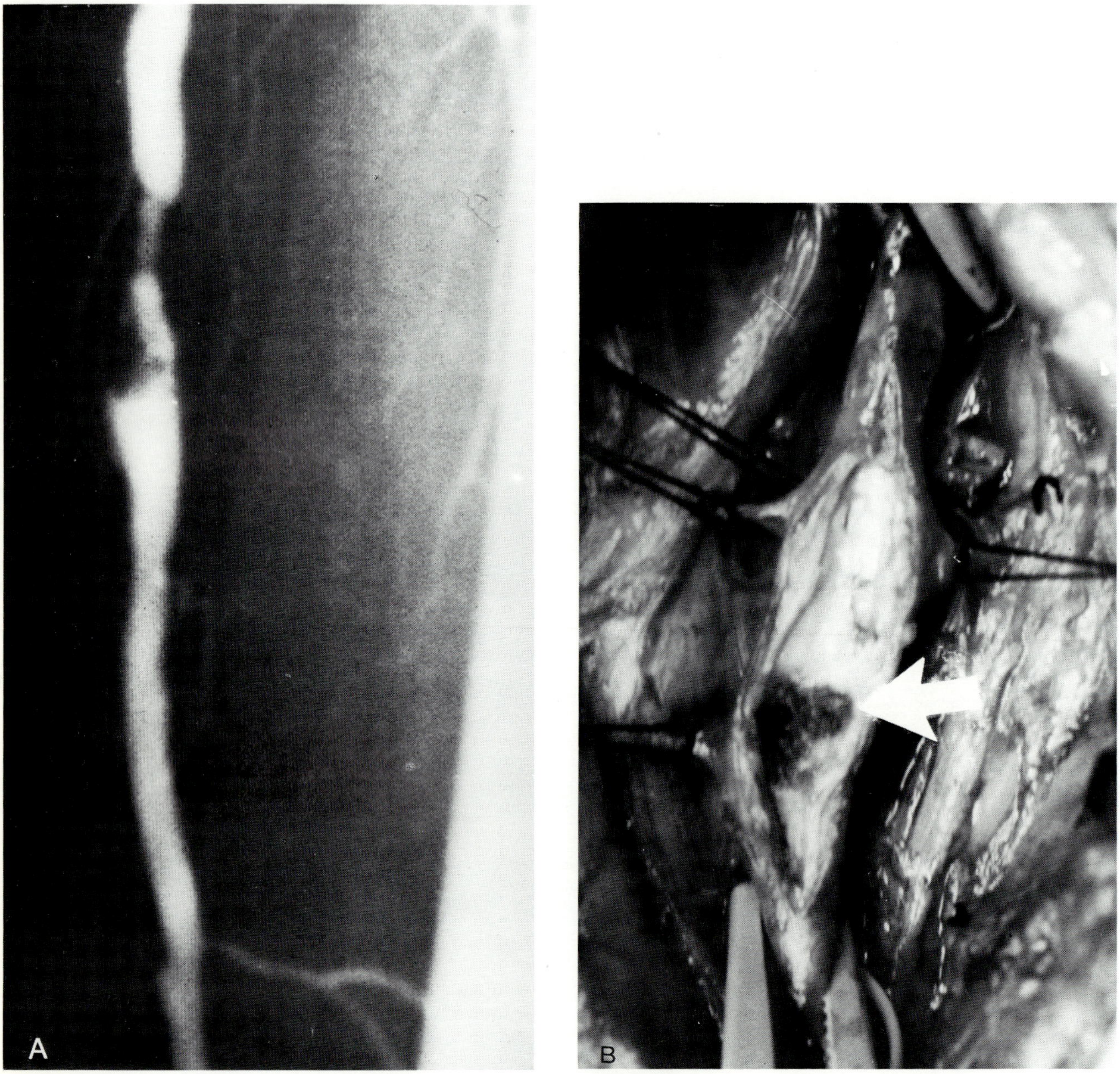

FIGURE 24-13. (*A*) Typical emboligenic lesion in the superficial femoral artery. The stenosis is easily recognized, but immediately distal to it is the characteristic foamy appearance of fibrino-platelet debris, which forms the basis of the emboli. (*B*) Surgical exposure of this lesion. The arrow points to the dark gray fibrino-platelet mass.

In some instances, the exact identification of the emboligenic area can be quite difficult. Flynn et al. (22) have shown that infrainguinal bypasses can be threatened by dislodgment of sizable emboli from the infrarenal aorta and iliac arteries. We have seen this on two occasions, and its onset can be both frustrating and puzzling. Such experiences have led to the suggestion that a total arterial reconstruction may be needed to remove or bypass all the lesions from the infrarenal to the popliteal arterial system. However, this extensive surgical approach is generally not warranted in the management of most of these cases because it is usually not difficult to identify precisely the responsible lesion and treat it by a relatively restricted local procedure.

Special New or Iatrogenic Microembolic Circumstances

DURING FIBRINOLYTIC THERAPY

Fibrinolytic enzymes (e.g., streptokinase, urokinase) are now in reasonably widespread use for the dissolution of thrombi which occur either in native arteries or in grafts. These enzymes are used both as a primary means of treatment of acute occlusion or in an attempt to determine the nature of the precipitating pathological lesion by angiography after thrombolysis. It is now well documented that in some instances, after the majority of thrombus in the conduit has been dissolved, the final residual fragments of thrombus are now exposed to full arterial pressure and may suddenly be dislodged and swept into the distal arterial tree (23). There appears to be no method of prevention of this event, which in some instances may prove to be a fatal blow to the foot.

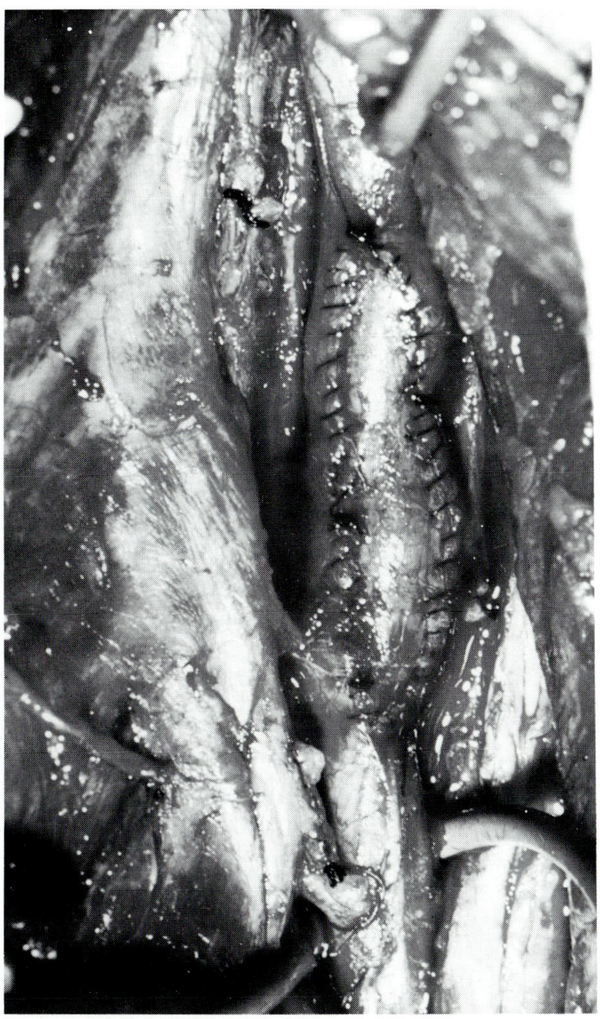

FIGURE 24-14. Treatment of the lesion in Figure 24-13*A* by thrombo-intimectomy and vein patch graft.

PERFORMANCE OF CATHETER ANGIOGRAMS THROUGH DISEASED ARTERIES

The passage of angiographic catheters, particularly of larger size (no. 6 French or greater), and their subsequent manipulation for selective catheterization may in fact cause the dislodgment of fibrinoplatelet clumps or the fragmentation of atheromatous plaques which may embolize distally. This is not a common event but should be recognized by the angiographers and clinicians concerned.

BALLOON ANGIOPLASTY

Balloon widening of stenotic areas in arteries is also widely carried out, but in the lesions which appear to be stenotic, as mentioned previously, fibrinoplatelet clumps may exist as part of the pathology of the lesion, and these when compressed or manipulated by the balloon may, in fact, be suddenly dislodged. Recognition of such lesions on the previous arteriograms should be made wherever possible and is a contraindication to intraluminal instrumentation.

THROMBOTIC OCCLUSION OF SYNTHETIC GRAFTS

We have observed that one of the terminal events following sudden thrombotic occlusion of certain synthetic grafts may in fact be a dislodgment of small thrombi as microemboli distally, thus compromising the collateral circulation and the survival of the foot in addition to the jeopardy already caused by the occlusion of the graft. This unwelcome event usually necessitates even more difficult and more distal arterial reconstructions in order to provide limb salvage.

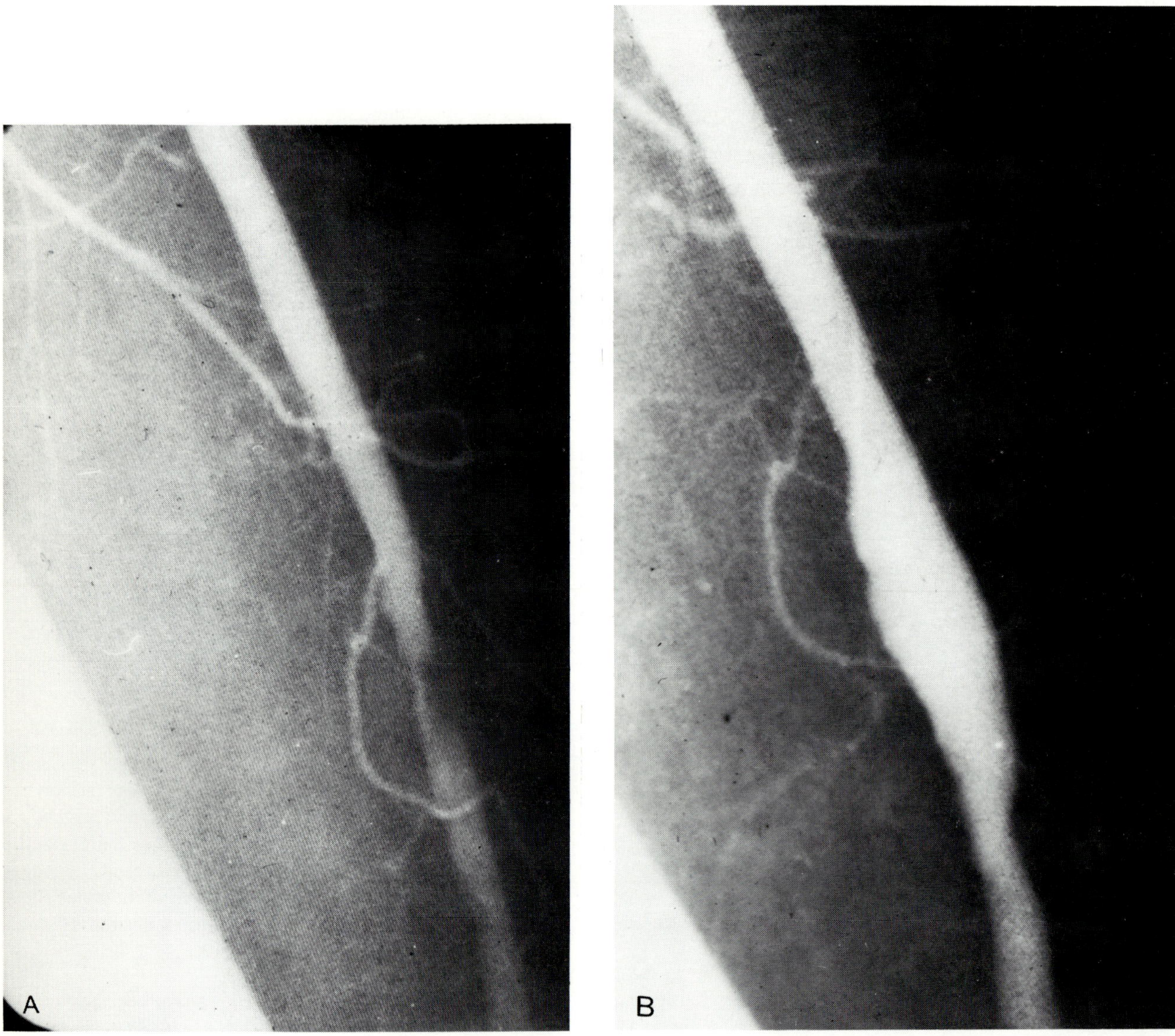

FIGURE 24-15. (*A*) Similar lesion to Figure 24-13*A* treated in the same fashion. (***B***) Five-year follow-up showing durability of reconstruction.

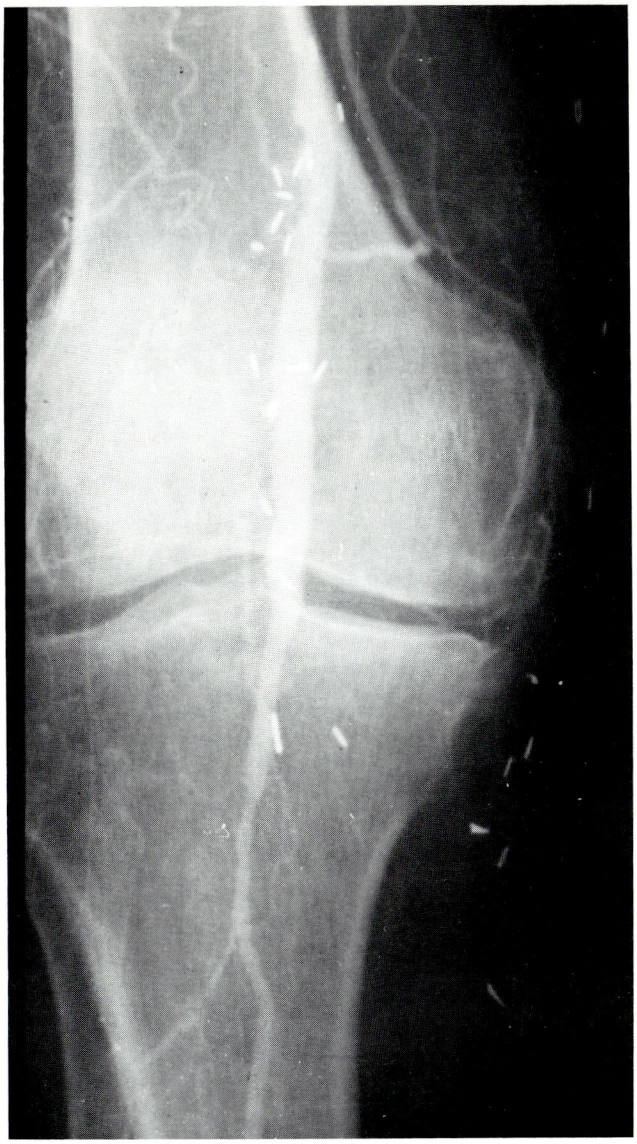

FIGURE 24-16. An example of a longer patch which has lasted for over 7 years.

References

1. Paunam PL: Experimentalle beitrage zur Lehre von deve embolir. Arch Pathol Anat 1962, 25:308.
2. Carvajal JA, Anderson WR, Weiss L, Grismer J, Berman R: Atheroembolism: An etiological factor in renal insufficiency, gastrointestinal hemorrhages and peripheral vascular disease. Arch Intern Med 1977, 119:593.
3. Kaplan K, Millar JD, Canilla PA: "Spontaneus" atheroembolic renal failure. Arch Intern Med 1962, 110:218.
4. Karmody AM, Jordan RF, Zaman SM: Left colon gangrene after acute inferior mesenteric artery occlusion. Arch Surg 1976, 111:972.
5. Haygood TA, Fessel WJ, Strange DA: Atheromatous microembolism simulating polymyositis. JAMA 1968, 203:135.
6. Crane C: Atherothrombotic embolism to lower extremities in arteriosclerosis. Arch Surg 1967, 94:96.
7. Branowitz JB, Edwards WS: The management of atheromatous emboli to the lower extremities. Surg Gynecol Obstet, 1976, 143:941.
8. Kazmie FJ, Sheps SG, Bernatz PE, Sayre GP: Livedo reticularis and digital infarcts: A syndrome due to cholesterol emboli arising from atheromatous abdominal aortic aneurysms. Vasc Dis 1966, 3:12.
9. Karmody AM, Leather RP: Atherothrombotic microemboli of the lower limb. In RB Rutherford (ed): *Vascular Surgery*. Philadelphia, Saunders, 1984, pp 536–546.
10. Anderson WR, Richards AM: Evaluation of lower extremity muscular biopsies in the diagnosis of atheroembolism. Arch Pathol 1968, 86:535.
11. Maurizi CP, Barker AE, Trueheart RE: Atheromatous emboli, a post mortem study special reference to the lower extremities. Arch Pathol, 1968, 86:528.
12. Wagner RB, Martin AS: Peripheral atheroembolism: Confirmation of a clinical concept with a case report and review of the literature. Surgery 1973, 73:353.
13. Kempczinski RF: Lower extremity arterial emboli from ulcerating atherosclerotic plaques. JAMA 1979, 214:807.
14. Schechter DC: Atheromatous embolization to lower limbs. NY State J Med, 79: July 1979, p 1180.
15. Kwaan HJ, Connolly JE: Peripheral atheroembolism. Arch Surg 1977, 112:987.
16. Williams GM, Ricotta JJ, Zimmer M: The extended retroperitoneal approach for treatment of extensive atherosclerosis in the aorta and renal vessels. Surgery 1980, 88:846.
17. Williams GM, Harrington D, Burdick J, White RI: Mural thrombosis of the aorta: An important, frequently neglected cause of large peripheral emboli. Ann Surg 1981, 194:737.
18. Karmody AM, Powers SR, Monaco VJ, Leather RP: "Blue toe syndrome": An indication for limb salvage surgery. Arch Surg 1976, 111:1263.
19. Mehigan JT, Stoney RJ: Lower extremity athromatous. Am J Surg 1976, 132:163.
20. Gore I, Collins DP: Spontaneous atheromatous embolization: Review of the literature and a report of 16 additional cases. Am J Clin Pathol 1960, 33:416.
21. Corson JD, Karmody AM, Shah DM, Naraynsingh V, Young HL, Leather RP: In-situ vein bypasses to distal tibial and limited outflow tracts for limb salvage. Surgery 1984, 96:756.
22. Flynn WR, Harris JP, Rudo MD: Atheroembolism as a cause of graft failure in femoro-distal reconstruction. Surgery 1981, 90:698.
23. Chang BB, Karmody AM, Matulonis UA, Bishop M, Leopold, Corson JD: The effect of streptokinase on endothelial cells in an ex-vivo canine model. To be published, J Vasc Surg.

Chapter 25

AORTOILIOFEMORAL OCCLUSIVE DISEASE

RONALD J. BAIRD, K. WAYNE JOHNSTON, PAUL M. WALKER, RICHARD D. WEISEL, and VERN M. CAMPBELL

Introduction

Atherosclerotic narrowing and occlusion commonly occur at the aortoiliac bifurcation. Coexisting lesions in the coronary, cerebral, and femoral arteries are frequent and affect the indications, risks, and results of surgical intervention.

Two-thirds of the patients are male, and the vast majority have a history of prolonged cigarette smoking. Symptoms usually occur in the mid-fifties, some 5 to 10 years earlier than in patients with more distal disease (1).

The surgical therapy of aortoiliac occlusion has evolved since midcentury. It has been very successful since 1960, and has been relatively standardized since 1970. The purpose of this chapter is to review the development of surgical therapy for aortoiliac occlusion and to discuss the pathophysiology, diagnosis, and complications, and the important decisions to be made before, during, and after such surgery.

Historical Aspects

The possibility of surgical relief from the sequelae of aortoiliac obstruction was suggested by Leriche in 1940 (2), when he described the syndrome of bilateral claudication, sexual impotence, and absent common femoral pulses. Thromboendarterectomy was introduced by dos Santos in 1947 (3) and extended to the aortoiliac area by Wylie in 1952 (4) and by Barker and Cannon in 1953 (5).

Resection of the obstructed segment and its replacement with an arterial allograft was described by Oudot in 1951 (6), Julian et al. in 1952 (7), and DeBakey et al. in 1954 (8). The allografts, however, were cumbersome to obtain and tended to develop late aneurysms. Following Voorhees' introduction of the concept of fabric arterial prostheses in 1952 (9), durable grafts made of Teflon or Dacron were introduced by Edwards (10) and DeBakey (11) and have been in widespread use since 1957. Bypass grafting from the aorta to the external iliac arteries using Dacron prostheses increased in popularity throughout the sixties.

Moore et al. in 1968 (12) and Perdue et al. in 1970 (13) suggested that superior long-term results follow common femoral rather than external iliac anastomoses, and this was confirmed by Baird et al. in 1977 (1). Current operations correct both the aortoiliac problem and the frequently associated deep femoral stenosis to produce excellent long-term relief of symptoms. The current focus is on the durability of the procedure and the prevention of complications.

Pathophysiology

CHRONIC ATHEROSCLEROSIS

Atherosclerosis may produce partial or complete occlusion of the distal aorta and one or both common iliac arteries; the process frequently extends into the proximal portion of the external and/or internal iliac arteries. Usually the plaque is more extensive on the posterior wall, and thus the median sacral and distal lumbar arteries are occluded at an early stage.

Immediately distal to the renal arteries, the aorta is usually free of disease, and the periarterial surgical planes are well-preserved. These features are exploited in the surgical repair: The upper clamp is placed immediately below the renal arteries, and the upper anastomosis is performed about 2 cm distally. In some cases, the disease process extends proximally and involves the orifices of the renal arteries. Involvement in this area must be recognized since exposure at a higher level is more difficult. Clamps must be placed at a higher level, and the arterial supply to the kidneys can be compromised by the embolization of atherosclerotic debris or the inadequate removal of the obstructive material. The origin of the inferior mesenteric artery may or may not be occluded: The status of this vessel influences the design of the operation.

With chronic aortoiliac narrowing, collateral vessels enlarge and compensate to some degree. The potential for collateral flow is higher with aortoiliac obstruction than with femoral, popliteal, or tibial obstruction. Collateral pathways include internal mammary to inferior epigastric; lateral thoracic to lateral circumflex iliac; inferior mesenteric and lumbar to internal iliac; and internal iliac to deep femoral.

As long as the chronic narrowing process is restricted to the aortoiliac region, the distal blood flow is rarely reduced to the point where there are symptoms at rest or where the viability of the extremity is threatened. Thus patients with isolated aortoiliac stenosis generally present with complaints of intermittent claudication and/or sexual impotence. By the time symptoms are noted, half the patients also have obstruction in the femoral popliteal and/or tibial arteries. With tandem disease, symptoms occur at an earlier age, peripheral ischemia is likely to be worse, and the viability of the leg may be threatened (1,14,15).

OCCLUSIVE AND ANEURYSMAL DISEASE

Aneurysmal disease of the aorta or common iliac arteries with coexistent occlusive disease, kinking, or thrombosis of the outflow may produce occlusive symptoms.

HYPOPLASTIC AORTA

The hypoplastic aortoiliac syndrome occurs in women with a history of significant long-standing cigarette addiction. Characteristic features include a high aortic bifurcation, straight iliac arteries without the normal lateral bowing, an aortic diameter less than 14 mm (or less than one-quarter of the diameter of the lumbar vertebrae), and a common iliac diameter less than 7 mm. Collaterals are poorly formed, the femoral and distal vessels are small, and the symptoms of claudication are more severe than expected from the angiographic pattern (16).

ACUTE OBSTRUCTION

Acute aortoiliac obstruction is uncommon. It may result from emboli from the heart, prosthetic cardiac valves, or an aortic aneurysm. Dissecting aneurysms, sharp or blunt trauma, the passage of diagnostic catheters or intraaortic balloons, or failed transluminal dilatation may produce acute obstruction. Since collateral channels are undeveloped, severe ischemia and a risk of tissue loss is usual.

Clinical Diagnosis

Typically, the patients with isolated aortoiliac disease are male cigarette smokers who present with buttock or thigh claudication and some degree of sexual impotence. Complaints of rest pain or cold feet are usually absent unless multilevel disease is present or the occlusion extends up to the renal arteries. On physical examination, one or both femoral pulses are found to be reduced, and iliac or groin bruits are heard. The feet usually appear warm and well-perfused.

An accurate clinical diagnosis of aortoiliac occlusive disease is not usually difficult. However, occasionally it is. One-quarter of the patients with isolated aortoiliac disease complain of calf rather than thigh or buttock claudication; similarly, one-quarter of the patients with normal aortoiliac segments and isolated femoral popliteal disease have thigh as well as calf claudication (17). Groin bruits are present in only two-thirds of the patients with symptomatic isolated aortoiliac obstruction (17).

The differential diagnosis must identify patients complaining of buttock and thigh distress from pathology in the low back or the hip joint. The symptoms of spinal stenosis may be difficult to distinguish from those of aortoiliac occlusive disease. Usually patients with spinal stenosis complain of leg "weakness" on standing or on walking very short distances, and relief is only achieved by sitting or lying down. Numbness and tingling are common and are usually localized in the distribution of one or more nerve roots.

An uncommon clinical presentation of aortoiliac disease is the blue-toe syndrome. These patients present with an ischemic blue and tender toe, and all peripheral pulses are palpable. An ulcerating plaque can usually be demonstrated.

Objective Diagnosis

NONINVASIVE ASSESSMENT

Several noninvasive methods are useful for assessing the severity of aortoiliac disease (17). Measurement of the thigh systolic blood pressure is the most popular. Unfortunately it is not sufficiently accurate, particularly in patients with combined aortoiliac and femoral popliteal disease. It is not possible to place the pressure cuff high enough on the thigh to measure a pressure equivalent to that in the common femoral artery and thus accurately assess the severity of the iliac disease.

Hemodynamically significant aortoiliac disease can be detected through an analysis of Doppler blood flow velocity recordings from the common femoral artery. The Doppler waveform is normally triphasic, with a forward flow, a reverse flow, and a second forward-flow component. If the waveform is dampened (i.e., monophasic), significant iliac disease is likely to be present. The waveforms can be analyzed by subjective evaluation, or a frequency analyzer can be used to provide a *pulsatility index* (defined as a peak-to-peak height of the waveform, divided by the mean height). The pulsatility index has the potential of detecting significant iliac disease with a sensitivity and a specificity of 95 percent (18).

Doppler waveform analysis and the measurement of segmental systolic blood pressures have a role in localizing vascular disease and augmenting the clinical and arteriographic evaluation of its significance. Using the measurement of the ankle-brachial systolic blood pressure ratio, the physician can objectively determine the severity of the vascular insufficiency. Through the use of treadmill-exercise testing, the physician can assess the extent of the patient's disability and distinguish the symptoms of claudication from pain due to orthopedic or neurologic disease.

ARTERIOGRAPHY

If the history indicates that the symptoms are sufficiently disabling to warrant a consideration of transluminal dilation or surgery, an arteriogram is the next diagnostic step. Arteriography is the most important method for evaluating the severity of aortoiliac disease; nonetheless, standard anterior-posterior arteriograms may either underestimate or overestimate the significance of the iliac disease (17,18,19).

The diagnostic accuracy of arteriography is better with the retrograde femoral approach than with the translumbar method, since it is easier to obtain biplane views and to achieve a more rapid injection of a larger bolus of dye. Biplane aortoiliac views are optimum in most patients unless a severe iliac lesion is demonstrated on the single anterior-posterior arteriogram. The aortogram should always be of sufficient quality to allow the surgeon to see adequate detail from the renal arteries to at least the midcalf.

DIRECT PRESSURE MEASUREMENTS

In difficult cases, the best method for assessing the hemodynamic significance of an aortoiliac lesion is to directly measure the aortofemoral pressure gradient. The aortofemoral pressure difference is measured from pressure recordings which are made as the angiographic catheter is withdrawn from the aorta to the level of the external iliac or common femoral artery. A systolic pressure gradient of more than 10 mmHg at rest is considered to be hemodynamically significant. The difference between the femoral systolic pressure at rest and during reactive hyperemia following the intraarterial injection of 30 mg of papaverine can be measured. Normally, the femoral artery systolic pressure does not fall significantly, and a fall of more than 15 percent is indicative of significant iliac disease (19).

Pressure measurements have not become popular because they require additional equipment and skill, prolong the arteriographic procedure, and in some cases are equivocal. However, the radiologist who believes a stenotic lesion is of questionable hemodynamic significance should be prepared to determine this by pressure measurements.

Conservative Treatment

The vascular surgeon must be aware that mild intermittent claudication from aortoiliac disease is not a very disabling symptom: Its natural history is unpredictable but usually favorable. Although major improvement is not likely, stability of the symptoms for many years is common (20). Consequently, no investigation or treatment is necessary in those whose employment and enjoyment of life is not threatened by their claudication.

The discovery of significant atherosclerosis should initiate the control of risk factors such as smoking, hypertension, hyperlipidemia, and diabetes. Vasodilators and megavitamins are not of value. If the patient is obese, weight reduction will reduce the workload. The patient often believes that walking to the point of claudication is harmful to the leg: He or she must be clearly told that exercise therapy is of proven value and frequently improves the claudication distance.

Percutaneous Transluminal Dilatation

The role of percutaneous transluminal dilatation is discussed in detail in Chapters 18 and 19. In our experience with dilatation of the aortoiliac segment, the two-year success rates were 70 percent for the common iliac, 58 percent for the external iliac, and 49 percent for dilatation of both the common and the external iliac arteries (21). Although these results are not as satisfactory as those with surgical repair, the low morbidity of the procedure when performed by an experienced radiologist justifies its use in treating localized iliac stenoses or occlusions, especially if the patient has major associated medical problems.

Surgical Treatment

The surgical repair of atherosclerotic aortoiliac obstruction is achieved by endarterectomy or prosthetic bypass grafting.

ENDARTERECTOMY

Although endarterectomy still has a role in the management of aortoiliac disease, this role has diminished since 1960. Usually the procedure involves an open endarterectomy of the distal aorta and either open or semiclosed endarterectomy of one or both iliac segments.

The long-term results of aortoiliac endarterectomy are comparable to those of bypass grafting; however, since the former procedure is more tedious and time-consuming and is associated with more blood loss and sexual dysfunction, it is usually reserved for specific indications. Although it may be useful in the treatment of localized aortoiliac stenoses, these lesions can often be treated equally satisfactorily by transluminal dilatation (21).

Aortoiliac endarterectomy is useful in treating acute obstruction from catheterization trauma. If the risk of infection is high, endarterectomy is preferable to prosthetic bypass grafting. In selected cases, aortoiliac endarterectomy is useful as a salvage procedure in the treatment of infected aortofemoral bypass grafts, since after the removal of the infected prosthesis the arterial channel to the leg can be reconstituted by endarterectomy of the native vessels combined with patching with pieces of autogenous material (22). Every vascular surgeon should be aware of and competent in the techniques of aortoiliac endarterectomy.

PROSTHETIC ARTERIAL BYPASS

Over the past two decades, bypass grafting has become the standard method for aortoiliac repair. The role of extraanatomic repair is discussed in Chapter 30. Unilateral aortofemoral bypass grafting is rarely indicated but may be useful when the disease is unilateral and not amenable to transluminal dilatation. The standard operation for aortoiliac disease is an aortobifemoral bypass; it is discussed in detail in the following sections.

General Principles of Aortobifemoral Bypass

The aortic anastomosis may be made either end-to-side or end-to-end. End-to-side anastomosis is indicated if (1) a large aberrant renal artery is present; (2) a large inferior mesenteric artery is present, especially if severe bilateral iliac disease is also present; (3) the patient is a male who is concerned about his sexual potency and there is major involvement of the external iliac arteries; or (4) the aorta is hypoplastic. End-to-end anastomosis is indicated in patients with coexisting aneurysmal disease or a complete aortic occlusion extending up to the renal arteries. Although some experienced vascular surgeons routinely use an end-to-side anastomosis to the aorta, most prefer the end-to-end anastomosis. We prefer the end-to-end technique and believe the long-term hemodynamic results to be better, the incidence of intraoperative atheromatous embolization lower, and the risk of subsequent aortoenteric fistulas lessened (14,23–26).

The distal anastomosis is usually made to the common femoral artery. If any narrowing of the deep femoral artery is present, the toe of the graft should be extended into this artery as far as necessary. If the distal anastomosis is made to the external iliac artery, there is an increased chance of requiring a subsequent downstream repair (1,14,23,24).

The Technique of Aortofemoral Bypass

The vascular anesthetist must be fully aware of problems in other organ systems. Important aspects of preoperative preparation and intraoperative management are described in the section Myocardial Infarction, below. The ECG, arterial blood pressure, and central venous pressures are monitored routinely, and a Swan-Ganz catheter is indicated in worrisome cases. A crystalloid infusion is given during induction to increase cardiac preload and urine flow. Prophylactic antibiotics are administered.

The patient is supine and draped so that the groins and legs are exposed with the feet visible in transparent plastic "bowel" bags (1,23,26).

The groins are opened simultaneously by the surgeon and the chief assistant. Each common femoral artery is exposed from the inguinal ligament to the bifurcation. The first 1 to 2 cm of the deep femoral artery is also exposed, and this artery is carefully palpated to confirm the absence of disease at its origin. The posteroinferior 2 to 3 mm of the inguinal ligament is cut, and gentle blunt dissection is used to create a tunnel into the retroperitoneal space in front of the iliac artery and the lateral circumflex iliac vein. The groin wounds are then loosely packed with a moist sponge, and the self-retaining retractors are removed.

The abdomen is opened through a midline incision from the xiphoid to midway between the umbilicus and pubis. Dissection with a blended cautery reduces time spent and blood lost. The abdominal organs are examined, moist sponges are placed to protect the wound edges, and a large abdominal retractor is positioned. The transverse colon is elevated, and the small bowel is gathered to the right (either inside or outside the abdomen) and protected by moist towels.

The surgeon identifies the duodenum and the inferior mesenteric vein and dissects between them directly to the anterior wall of the aorta. The origin of the inferior mesenteric artery is identified but is not dissected, palpated, or manipulated. The anterior and lateral walls of the aorta are exposed up to the level of the renal vein. No attempt is made to divide lumbar arteries or to encircle the aorta.

The type of prosthesis used does not appear to be of great importance. At present, we prefer knitted Dacron grafts of medium porosity either with or without velour surfaces. The grafts are preclotted with blood drawn from the aorta before the anesthetist administers 5000 USP units of heparin intravenously.

The proximal clamp is placed just below the renal arteries, and the distal clamp just above the inferior mesenteric artery. The clamps are placed from an anterior position, and no attempt is made to dissect behind the aorta. The aorta is divided 1 cm above the distal clamp, with care being taken to avoid entering posterior lumbar veins. The distal stump is oversewn with a no. 2-0 or 3-0 monofilament polypropylene suture, starting at the back wall and coming forward with both needles so that only one knot is required. The lower clamp is removed as this suture is pulled tight and tied so that the aortic tissue comes together snugly.

A 1- to 2-cm section of the proximal aorta is removed, leaving 2 to 3 cm of proximal aorta below the upper clamp. Debris in this trunk is carefully removed. The graft is cut so that the aortic trunk is about 2 to 2.5 cm long. It is sewn to the end of the aorta with a double-ended no. 2-0 or 3-0 monofilament polypropylene suture which is started on the left lateral wall and continued across the back wall to the right lateral wall with a "parachute" technique in which the end of the prosthesis is held about 5 cm from the aorta. All tissue bites are taken in a forehand manner, and great care is taken not to exert caudad traction on the aortic stump. The suture is then moistened with saline and tightened. A nerve hook is used to tighten any loose strands, and the final traction is exerted in the plane parallel to the posterior wall of the aorta. The left limb of the suture is then fixed in a taut position over the retractor and held in place by a rubber-shod clamp. The right limb is continued to the midline of the graft, where it is then held tautly while the left limb is continued to meet it. After seven knots have been tied, the suture is held to the left and fixed with a silk suture before being cut. This ensures that the stiff, sharp "rabbit ears" of the monofilament suture point away from the duodenum.

If the thrombotic material extends to the level of the renal arteries, the proximal clamp must be placed on the suprarenal aorta. The exposure of this area is improved if the left renal vein is retracted by vessel loops. The aortic clamp is placed from in front, and the aorta is divided about 2 cm below the renal arteries. When thrombotic material in this area is removed, it is essential that the surgeon clearly see each renal artery orifice and be ensured that it is absolutely clear of loose debris. Thus the aortotomy is frequently extended on the anterior aspect so that this inspection can be done carefully. The trunk of the graft is cut appropriately and sutured as above. Alternatively, the anterior aortic incision can be closed and the clamp placed distal to the renal arteries, thus reestablishing the renal perfusion. With an ischemic time of less than 30 minutes, postoperative renal dysfunction is rarely a problem.

The clamp is temporarily released, and hemostasis is confirmed by inspecting the entire circumference of the anastomosis. Any leaks are repaired with interrupted sutures. A long curved clamp is then passed from each groin to grasp the limbs of the prosthesis and draw them into the femoral areas. Care is taken to make each tunnel behind the ureter and, on the left, behind the inferior mesenteric arterial and venous branches.

The design of each lower anastomosis is determined by the severity of disease in the infrainguinal arteries. If the superficial and deep femoral arteries are normal, the anastomosis is made to the common femoral artery. Narrowing at the origin of the superficial or deep artery is corrected by appropriate arterioplasties. Good-quality preoperative angiograms with oblique views are helpful in predicting stenosis of the origin of the deep femoral artery, but the final decision about a stenosis involving the deep femoral artery is made in the operating room. If there is any doubt about narrowing of the origin of the deep femoral artery, we continue the common femoral arteriotomy into it. The patch angioplasty on this artery is extended as far as necessary. We avoid extensive endarterectomies. The deep femoral artery is often quite fragile and thin-walled; great care must be taken in order to avoid injury to it or its branches.

The groin anastomoses are made with no. 4-0 or 5-0 monofilament polypropylene sutures, starting and finishing on one side of the heel and using a one-knot technique. The groin anastomoses can be made simultaneously if two experienced surgeons are available. Before the anastomoses are completed, adequate flushing of all the vessels is necessary, including the native superficial femoral, deep femoral, and common femoral arteries as well as the graft.

The anesthetist is given 5 to 10 minutes' warning before the graft is opened. The surgeon controls the flow through the new conduit until the blood pressure has stabilized. The heparin is then neutralized with protamine. Hemostasis is checked, the color of the sigmoid colon is noted, and the retroperitoneal space is closed. All blood is removed from the abdomen, a careful sponge and instrument count is completed, and the abdominal incision is closed with a continuous no. 1 monofilament polypropylene suture or a combination of continuous and interrupted Vicryl sutures.

Before the groins are closed, the femoral pulses are checked and the feet inspected to ensure that some misadventure has not occurred. If the surgeon thinks a Fogarty catheter should be passed, this should be done at this time, not several hours later. Groin closure is important and should be done in two or three layers to avoid dead space and lymphatic leaks. Skin closure of all wounds is with skin clips.

In the intensive care unit, the patient is monitored for hemodynamic stability, respiratory function, renal function, and the status of the circulation to both legs. Within 24 hours, the intratracheal tube and the arterial line are removed and the patient is transferred to a step-down unit for another 24 to 48 hours.

Ambulation begins on the second or third day, and most patients are ready for discharge on the eighth or ninth postoperative day. Before discharge, they are checked in the noninvasive laboratory to provide a baseline for followup studies.

Results

The perioperative mortality for aortobifemoral reconstruction is now between 2 and 3 percent (1,23,24). Perioperative myocardial infarction accounts for half the deaths, and stroke, respiratory failure, or renal failure for the remainder (24).

There is general agreement that the expected long-term patency rates of an aortofemoral bypass are excellent. From a consensus of recent reports, we can expect a patency rate of 85 percent at 5 years, 70 percent at 10 years, 60 percent at 15 years, and 55 percent at 20 years (23,24). This represents an attrition rate of 1 to 3 percent per year for aortofemoral bypass grafting compared with about 5 percent per year for femoropopliteal saphenous vein bypass grafting. Ten years after an aortofemoral bypass, the patient has a 70 percent chance of its still working and a 50 percent chance of being alive. In contrast, 10 years after a femoropopliteal bypass with a saphenous vein, the patient has a 50 percent chance of its still working and a 30 percent chance of being alive (23).

Complications and Their Prevention

MYOCARDIAL INFARCTION

Patients with hazardous coronary artery disease can frequently be identified prior to surgery. Cardiac complications of vascular reconstruction can be avoided by careful preoperative preparation, the selection of appropriate operative procedures, and careful intraoperative monitoring.

Recent studies have suggested that preoperative coronary angiography and coronary bypass surgery, in selected patients, may reduce the cardiac risk of peripheral vascular reconstruction (27,28). It seems reasonable to consider coronary angiography in patients with symptomatic coronary artery disease, a strongly positive exercise test, or an abnormality in thallium or radionucleotide angiographic stress tests. Patients who are suitable for coronary revascularization should probably have this revascularization performed before their elective aortofemoral bypass (27,28).

Patients with hazardous coronary disease or severely impaired ventricular function who are not candidates for myocardial revascularization represent the greatest risk. Some patients tolerate aortic surgery if extensive monitoring is used to aid in minimizing the cardiac stress. Others with obviously high risks are better treated by extraanatomic reconstruction. The construction of axillobifemoral or femorofemoral conduits has less risk than an intraabdominal operation and is indicated in such patients.

Preoperative preparation of the high-risk patient can help reduce the myocardial stress involved with aortic surgery. The placement of a Swan-Ganz catheter allows an accurate assessment of myocardial performance and a prediction of the optimum preload to be maintained in the perioperative period (29).

STROKE

Patients with symptomatic internal carotid artery stenosis should have carotid artery repair before their aortoiliac surgery. Those with an asymptomatic bruit should receive their aortoiliac repair; carotid repair is usually delayed until symptoms occur (30).

GRAFT INFECTION

Infection of a prosthetic aortofemoral bypass is a serious complication. Prophylactic antibiotic coverage preoperatively, intraoperatively, and for 48 hours postoperatively has reduced the incidence to about 1 percent (23,24).

As described more fully in Chapter 70, the management of an infected graft usually involves the administration of systemic antibiotics, the removal of all infected prosthetic material, and arterial reconstruction if indicated for limb salvage. If the infection is limited to the graft in the area of the groin and there is no bleeding, a trial of nonoperative treatment is indicated. If this is not successful, a retroperitoneal approach through clean tissue, division of the prosthetic limb near its origin, and extraction of the distal portion via the groin is required. The native groin arteries are closed with a monofilament suture, and the wound is allowed to granulate. If the viability of the limb is threatened, an extraanatomic bypass through clean tissue is indicated—from the axillary artery, the contralateral femoral artery, or the ipsilateral or contralateral limb of the bifurcation graft via the obturator foramen.

When the infection involves the body of the graft and both limbs, complete removal of the prosthesis is necessary. Although aortoiliac endarterectomy and patch grafts may be possible, usually an axillary graft must be taken to the distal profunda, superficial femoral, or popliteal artery (22).

PSEUDOANEURYSM FORMATION

Although pseudoaneurysms may form as a result of groin infection, they usually result from sterile dehiscence of the graft. Predisposing factors include tension on the anastomosis, a poor suture technique, or a thin-walled artery. Since pseudoaneurysms slowly enlarge and will eventually rupture, treatment consists of elective surgery with extension or replacement of the distal portion of the graft. Treatment of pseudoaneurysms of the distal anastomosis consists of control of the arterial inflow and repair of the anastomosis. Once the inflow limb of the prosthesis is clamped, control of the groin arteries is best accomplished by intraluminal occlusion with Fogarty catheters.

A pseudoaneurysm of the proximal anastomosis is rare, irrespective of whether the anastomosis is end-to-side or end-to-end. It is usually asymptomatic and is found during an investigation of a concurrent groin aneurysm. Repair is by resuture or by the replacement of at least the upper end of the graft.

AORTOENTERIC FISTULA

A communication between the aortic prosthesis and a portion of the gastrointestinal (GI) tract is a tragic complication of intraabdominal vascular surgery. It is more common after emergency aneurysm repair than after bypass grafting for occlusive disease (25,26). Of such communications, 75 percent are to the duodenum, 20 percent to the remaining small bowel or to the colon, and 5 percent to the stomach or to a combination of these sites (25). Aortoenteric fistulas result from a sterile or infected perigraft collection which drains into the adjacent bowel, erosion of the mobile viscera by the fixed and immobile prosthetic material of the graft, or erosion by the knot and/or tails of the suture.

The diagnosis must be suspected whenever an episode of GI hemorrhage or septicemia occurs in someone with an intraabdominal prosthetic graft. An upper GI series may show distortion of the terminal portion of the duodenum. Duodenoscopy may visualize the prosthesis or the site of the hemorrhage. An aortogram may demonstrate a pseudoaneurysm or may show the dye passing into the duodenum. Sequential cultures along the graft may reveal one consistently positive site.

The standard method of treatment is the removal of all the prosthetic material, closure of the hole in the bowel, and an axillobifemoral bypass. The overall mortality is 50 to 70 percent (25).

The incidence varies from center to center, and thus attention to prevention is important. We believe that our technique of using a short stump and a high bifurcation with an end-to-end anastomosis serves to keep the graft in the anteroposterior plane of the aorta and avoids contact with the bowel (1,23). We also make sure that the sharp rabbit ears of the monofilament suture point away from the bowel. To cover the upper anastomosis with a cuff of prosthetic material is not likely to be of benefit in preventing this complication. To reattach the terminal portion of the duodenum to the right of the prosthesis and thus avoid contact is rational. The interposition of some free or attached omentum is also reasonable.

LYMPHATIC FISTULAS

The appearance of a draining lymphatic sinus from the groin incision in the first week or two after surgery is worrisome. The complication is avoided by using an incision slightly lateral to the common femoral artery, cauterizing any divided lymph nodes or lymphatics, and careful and complete closing of the groin wound. If a fistula develops, the patient is confined to bed to reduce the lymphatic flow from the leg, appropriate antibiotics are given, and a pressure dressing is applied. Almost all such fistulas close within two to three weeks.

A more aggressive approach may shorten the hospital stay and reduce the chances of wound infection. Operative ligation of the offending lymphatic (facilitated by a preoperative intrapedal injection of Evans blue dye) and primary closure have produced excellent results (31).

UNILATERAL LIMB OCCLUSION

Early limb occlusions result from kinking or twisting the graft, from an error in making the distal anastomosis, or from an inadequate outflow. The problem can usually be corrected by thrombectomy with Fogarty catheters and appropriate refashioning of the distal anastomosis.

The causes of late graft occlusions are fibromuscular dysplasia or a progression of distal disease. If the occlusion is recent, the inflow can usually be reestablished through the use of Fogarty catheters. An endarterectomy curette is useful in removing fibrocollagenous plugs at the prosthetic bifurcation. If an adequate prograde flow cannot be obtained, a cross-femoral bypass is employed or the limb of the prosthesis is replaced. Any outflow stenosis is corrected by graft extension into the deep femoral artery or by femoropopliteal bypass grafting.

DETERIORATION OF THE PROSTHESIS

Sporadic cases of generalized dilatation of the prosthesis or localized pseudoaneurysm formation have been reported, but with current prostheses these risks are minor. The fibers of any arterial prosthesis may be damaged or broken by the application of crushing clamps.

INTERFERENCE WITH SEXUAL FUNCTION

Aortofemoral bypass grafting may affect male sexual function by interference with the preaortic fibers of the sympathetic nervous system or by reducing the pelvic blood flow. The preaortic sympathetic fibers control the closure of the bladder neck during ejaculation, and if they are damaged, ejaculation may be retrograde, resulting in sterility. The surgical techniques described above minimize aortic dissection and reduce the risk of injuring these nerves. In the presence of severe external iliac occlusive disease, a bypass to the common femoral arteries does not increase the flow to the internal iliac arteries and if an end-to-end aortic anastomosis is used, decreases it. In this situation, an end-to-side aortic anastomosis is preferred. It is possible to improve the pelvic blood flow by an internal iliac endarterectomy or an appropriate bypass graft, although there is some risk of autonomic nerve damage during the dissection. This topic has become of increasing interest and concern in the recent surgical literature.

SIGMOID COLON ISCHEMIA

The sigmoid colon is perfused by the inferior mesenteric artery and receives variable but substantial collateral flow from the superior mesenteric artery and the branches of the internal iliac artery. Sigmoid ischemia may result if prograde flow via a large inferior mesenteric artery is diminished. If such an artery is present and will not be perfused with retrograde flow from the groins, the surgeon should consider an end-to-side aortic anastomosis. The sigmoid colon should always be inspected before the abdomen is closed. If it appears ischemic, the origin of the inferior mesenteric artery can be anastomosed to the prosthesis.

In the early postoperative period, left lower quadrant abdominal pain and tenderness, bloody diarrhea, or distension should be investigated, and if ischemia is diagnosed, early decompression or sigmoid resection is indicated. The complications of chronic sigmoid fibrosis or stenosis may appear months to years later and require resection.

URETERIC OBSTRUCTION

Ureteric obstruction and hydronephrosis may result if a taut graft is placed anterior to the ureter or if the periureteric tissue is grasped during the tunneling. Care in tunneling should avoid these complications.

Ureteric obstruction is treated in conjunction with a urologist and involves renal decompression, the lysis of periureteric fibrosis, or the repositioning of the arterial conduit.

TRASH FOOT

Loose intraluminal debris or clot formed in areas of stasis may be washed downstream during the operation. The material may shower in such a way that even with good ankle pulses, distal gangrene may occur. Prevention is important and is achieved by adequately flushing the graft via open arteriotomies.

Summary of Key Points in Surgical Judgment

SELECTION OF PATIENTS FOR ARTERIOGRAPHY

Patients with mild claudication and minimal reduction in the ankle-arm systolic pressure index are usually not candidates for reconstructive surgery and consequently do not require aortography. Instead, they should be reassured, be advised to stop smoking, embark on an exercise program, and lose weight. Patients whose claudication is disabling or who have rest pain or impending gangrene require arteriography and appropriate intervention.

THE HEMODYNAMIC SIGNIFICANCE OF AORTOILIAC STENOSES

The surgeon should carefully weigh the options in patients whose aortogram does not demonstrate severe stenosis. The patient's symptoms and signs will influence the judgment of whether or not a stenosis is significant. Biplane angiography or direct arterial pressure measurements help in deciding the exact significance of an aortoiliac stenosis.

SURGERY OR TRANSLUMINAL DILATATION?

The results of transluminal dilatation of iliac stenoses are quite good, and this procedure must be considered as an alternative to reconstructive surgery in patients with a short isolated lesion. Patients with extensive atherosclerosis, multiple lesions, and severe symptoms, and who also face reasonable operative risks, should have reconstructive surgery rather than dilatation. The experience of the vascular radiologist and his or her rates of success and complications must be considered in this context (21).

SHOULD A PROFUNDAPLASTY BE PERFORMED?

A profundaplasty should be performed whenever there is angiographic or anatomic evidence of proximal stenosis in the deep femoral artery.

SHOULD A FEMOROPOPLITEAL BYPASS BE PERFORMED CONCURRENTLY?

Current practice is to include profundaplasty whenever necessary, but to delay femoropopliteal bypass grafting until the results of the initial procedure are assessed. However, there are some situations in which combined aortobifemoral and femoropopliteal grafting are necessary. Patients with extensive necrosis of the foot or severe claudication, not likely to respond to profunda revascularization in the face of superficial femoral occlusion, may be candidates for combined repair (1).

Conclusion

With proper patient selection and operative technique, gratifying long-term results are achieved by the surgical repair of aortoiliac occlusive disease.

References

1. Baird RJ, Feldman P, Miles JT, Madras PM, Gurry JF: Subsequent downstream repair after aorto-iliac and aorta-femoral bypass operations. Surgery 1977, 82:785–793.
2. Leriche R: De la résection du carrefour aortoiliaque avec double sympathectomie lombaire pour thrombose arterielle de l'aorte: Le syndrome de l'obliteration termino-aortique par arterite. Presse Med 1940, 48:601.
3. Dos Santos JC: Sur la désobstruction des thromboses arterielles anciennes. Mem Acad Chir 1947, 73:409–411.
4. Wylie EJ: Thromboendarterectomy for arteriosclerotic thrombosis of major arteries. Surgery 1952, 4:339–350.
5. Barker WF, Cannon JA: An evaluation of endarterectomy. Arch Surg 1953, 66:488–499.
6. Oudot J: La greffe vasculaire dans les thromboses du carrefour aortique. Presse Med 1951, 59:234–236.
7. Julian OD, Dye WS Jr, Olwin JH, Jordan PH: Direct surgery of arteriosclerosis. Ann Surg 1952, 136:459–474.
8. DeBakey ME, Creech O Jr., Cooley DA: Occlusive disease of the aorta and its treatment by resection and homograft replacement. Ann Surg 1954, 140:290–310.
9. Voorhees AB Jr., Jaretzki A III, Blakemore AH: Use of tubes constructed from Vinyon ''N'' cloth in bridging arterial defects: Preliminary report. Ann Surg 1952, 135:332–336.
10. Edwards WS: Plastic arterial grafts. Charles C Thomas, Springfield, Ill, 1957.
11. DeBakey ME, Crawford SE: Vascular prostheses. Transplant Bull 1957, 4:2–4.
12. Moore WS, Cafferata HT, Hall AD, Blaisdell FW: In defence of grafts across the inguinal ligament: An evaluation of early and late results of aorta-femoral bypass grafts. Ann Surg 1968, 168:207–214.
13. Perdue GS, Long WD, Smith, RB: Perspective concerning aorta-femoral arterial reconstruction. Ann Surg 1970, 173:940–944.
14. Brewster DC, Darling DC: Optimal methods of aortoiliac reconstruction surgery. Surgery 1978, 84:739–748.
15. Imparato AM, Sanoudos G, Epstein JH, Abrams RM, Beranbaum ER: Results in 96 aortoiliac reconstructive procedures: Preoperative angiographic and functional classifications used as prognostic guides. Surgery 1970, 84:610–616.
16. DeLaurentis DA, Friedman P, Wolferth CC Jr, Wilson A., Naide D: Atherosclerosis and the hypoplastic aortoiliac system. Surgery 1978, 83:27–37.
17. Johnston KW, Demorais D, Colapinto RF: Difficulty in assessing the severity of aortoiliac disease by clinical and angiographic methods. Angiology 1981, 32:609–614.
18. Johnston KW, Kassam M, Cobbold RSC: Relationship between Doppler pulsatility index and direct femoral pressure measurement in the diagnosis of aortoiliac occlusive disease. Ultrasound Med Biol 1983, 9:271–281.
19. Brewster DC, Waltman AC, O'Hara PJ: Femoral artery pressure measurement during aortography. Circulation 1979, 11(suppl Cardiovasc Surg):120–124.
20. Bloor K: Natural history of aortosclerosis obliterans in the lower extremities. Ann Roy Coll Surg Engl 1961, 28:36–52.
21. Johnston KW, Colapinto RF, Baird RJ: Transluminal angioplasty. Arch Surg 1982, 117:1604–1610.
22. Ehrenfeld WK, Wieber BC, Olcott CN, Stoney RJ: Autogenous tissue reconstruction in the management of infected prosthetic grafts. Surgery 1979, 85:82–92.
23. Baird RJ: Techniques and results of arterial prosthetic bypass for aortoiliac occlusive disease. Can J Surg 1982, 25:476–478.
24. Crawford ES, Bomberger RA, Glaeser DH, Saleh SA, Russel WL: Aortoiliac occlusive disease: Factors influencing survival and function following reconstructive operation over a 25 year period. Surgery 1981, 90:1055–1066.
25. Perdue GD Jr, Smith RB 3rd, Ansky JD, Costantino MJ: Impending aortoenteric hemorrhage. The effect of early recognition on improved outcome. Surgery 1980, 192:237–243.
26. Baird RJ, Garry JF, Kellam JF, Wilson DR: Abdominal aortic aneurysms: Recent experience with 210 patients. CMA 1978, 118:764–770.
27. Hertzer NR: Myocardial ischemia as a complication of abdominal aortic reconstruction. Surgery 1983, 93:97–107.

28. Crawford ES, Morris GC Jr, Howell JF, Flynn WF, Moorhead DT: Operative risks in patients with previous coronary artery bypass. Ann Thorac Surg 1978, 26:215–221.
29. Whittemore AD, Clowes AW, Hechtman HB, Mannick JA: Aortic aneurysm repair. Reduced mortality with maintenance of optimal cardiac performance. Ann Surg 1980, 192:414–421.
30. Barnes RW, Liebman PR, Marszalek PB, Kirk CL, Goldman MH: The natural history of asymptomatic carotid disease in patients undergoing cardiovascular surgery. Surgery 1981, 90:1075–1083.
31. Kwann J, Bernstein J, Connolly J: Management of lymph fistula in the groin after arterial reconstruction. Arch Surg 1979, 114:1416–1418.

Chapter 26

FEMORAL, POPLITEAL, AND TIBIAL OCCLUSIVE DISEASE

FRANK J. VEITH, SUSHIL K. GUPTA, and ENRICO ASCER

Arteriosclerosis may involve the common femoral artery and its branches, the above-knee and below-knee popliteal artery, any of the infrapopliteal arteries including their terminal branches, or any combination of these arteries. This involvement generally begins early in adult life and progresses slowly to the point where a flow-reducing stenosis or occlusion occurs in one or more of the arteries below the inguinal ligament. As the average age of the population increases, the number of individuals with this hemodynamically significant infrainguinal arteriosclerosis also increases. This chapter deals with the present status of treatment for atherosclerotic occlusive disease of the femoral, popliteal, and tibial arterial systems.

Obviously, this disease is associated, in varying degrees, with arteriosclerotic involvement elsewhere in the body, and this fact must constantly be considered when making therapeutic decisions for afflicted patients. It is this consideration that guides the surgeon correctly to seek palliation rather than cure and to attempt a lesser operation that maintains function rather than one which will restore a normal circulation. The generalized and slowly progressive nature of the disease process and the imperfect results of all interventional treatments should also deter any who might be unwisely tempted to treat asymptomatic or minimally disabling arteriosclerotic occlusive lesions. In the management of the increasingly common entity of infrainguinal arteriosclerosis, diagnostic and therapeutic restraint and the desire to minimize risks and avoid doing harm must be paramount principles if the disease is not producing major functional impairment or tissue necrosis. On the other hand, despite the advanced age and poor generalized condition of the affected population, aggressive intervention for both diagnosis and treatment is justified if limb loss is truly threatened by the disease process.

Clinical Presentation

The human arterial system has an enormous reserve capacity. Hemodynamically significant stenoses or major artery occlusions can exist in the infrainguinal arterial tree with no symptoms or with only minimal symptoms. This is particularly true if collateral pathways are normal or the patient's activity level is limited by coronary arteriosclerosis or other disease processes. Accordingly, the most common manifestation of a short segmental occlusion of the distal superficial femoral artery, the most frequent site of major arteriosclerotic involvement below the inguinal ligament, will be mild intermittent claudication. In many patients, this lesion will be totally asymptomatic, and this is usually the case if only one or two tibial arteries are occluded without other significant lesions. Thus the usual patient who presents with severe disabling intermittent claudication or tissue necrosis has multiple sequential occlusions or so-called combined segment disease with hemodynamically significant lesions at the aortoiliac level and the superficial femoral-popliteal level, or either or both of these combined with severe infrapopliteal disease as well.

STAGING

Patients with hemodynamically significant infrainguinal arteriosclerosis may be classified into one of five stages depending on their clinical presentation as indicated in Table 26-1. Patients in stages III and IV are those whose limbs may be considered imminently threatened, although some patients with mild ischemic rest pain may remain stable for many years and an occasional patient with a tiny patch of ischemic gangrene or a small ischemic ulcer will improve with conservative treatment, i.e., bed rest and antibiotics. With the exception of these few patients, invasive diagnostic angiography is justified for those with stage III and IV disease, which is usually associated with disease at several levels.

Rest pain as an isolated symptom in patients with infrainguinal arteriosclerosis can be difficult to evaluate unless it is accompanied by other findings. Many patients with significant arterial lesions have pain at rest from causes other than arteriosclerosis, such as arthritis or neuritis. Such pain will not be relieved by a successful revascularization. Significant ischemic rest pain must be associated not only with decreased pulses but also with other objective manifestations of ischemia such as atrophy, decreased skin temperature when compared to the other extremity, and rubor and relief of pain with dependency. In some patients with a complex etiology to their rest pain, it may be necessary to perform a noninvasive laboratory and angiographic evaluation before the predominant cause of the symptom can be determined and appropriate treatment instituted. Every patient with pain at

TABLE 26-1. Staging of Infrainguinal Arteriosclerosis with Hemodynamically Significant Stenosis or Occlusion

Stage	Presentation	Invasive Diagnostic and Therapeutic Intervention
0	No signs or symptoms	Never justified
I	Intermittent claudication (> 1 block) No physical changes	Usually unjustified
II	Severe claudication (< $\frac{1}{2}$ block); dependent rubor; decreased temperature	Sometimes justified; not always necessary; condition may remain stable
III	Rest pain; atrophy, cyanosis; dependent rubor	Usually indicated, but patients may do well for long periods without revascularization
IV	Nonhealing ischemic ulcer or gangrene	Indicated

rest and decreased pulses is not a candidate for angiography and an arterial bypass. Some of these patients will be relieved by appropriate treatment for gout or osteoarthritis. Others can be well managed with simple analgesics and reassurance that their limb is not in jeopardy. Such reassurance generally suffices for patients with stage I disease and those with stage II disease who are elderly (> 80 years) or at high risk because of intercurrent disease or atherosclerotic involvement of other organs such as the heart, the kidneys, or the brain.

This conservative approach to patients with stage I involvement from infrainguinal arteriosclerosis is becoming increasingly widespread, although it is not universally so (1). Conservatism appears to be clearly justified by the numerous reports of the benignancy and slow progression of stage I disease to more advanced stages (2–4). Without treatment, 10 to 15 percent of patients in stage I will improve over 5 years, and 60 to 70 percent will not progress over the same period. The 10 to 15 percent who do worsen are, in our opinion, best treated with a primary operation after their disease progresses. We further believe that this conservative approach to stage I disease is justified by the greater surgical difficulty encountered when a bypass for claudication fails in the early or remote postoperative period and the patient then has a threatened limb, a situation that we have observed all too frequently.

The fact that some patients in stage II and stage III and an occasional one with limited stage IV lesions may remain stable and easily managed without operation for protracted periods of one or more years justifies a cautiously conservative nonoperative approach to selected patients in these stages. This often requires hospitalization so that the patient and the progress of the ischemia can be assessed. Moreover, this conservative nonoperative approach is particularly indicated if the patient is elderly and a poor surgical risk from a systemic and a local point of view. An example of this would be an octagenarian with intractable congestive failure in whom a difficult distal small-vessel bypass would be required to alleviate stage III signs and symptoms. Close observation can and often should be the preferred management for such a patient for several months or even years. However, we would not hesitate to revascularize such a patient when rest pain became intolerable or he or she developed a small patch of gangrene which did not improve after 7 to 10 days of hospitalization (5).

DIFFERENTIAL DIAGNOSIS

Intermittent claudication or pain brought on by exertion and relieved by rest is a fairly distinct symptom and usually a manifestation of arteriosclerotic occlusive disease, although mild calf claudication can be produced by a significant stenotic lesion in the superficial femoral artery. An occasional patient will describe the claudication as a sense of heaviness, weakness, or fatigue in the limb without pain, and such patients may be mistakenly diagnosed as having neuromuscular disorders. Sometimes claudication-like symptoms can be produced by lesions compressing the lower spinal cord or cauda equina (6,7). Such *pseudoclaudication* is most often produced by spinal stenosis and can easily be suspected when peripheral pulses are normal. Occasionally, neurologic problems will coexist with arterial occlusive disease, making an exact determination of the cause of the patient's symptoms a difficult challenge for the neurologist and the vascular surgeon. In such circumstances, angiography and myelography may both be necessary.

Some of the difficulties that can be encountered in differentiating pain at rest from *true ischemic rest pain* have already been discussed. Again these difficulties are greatest when arterial occlusive disease coexists with other pathology. Similar difficulties can be encountered in determining the primary cause of ulcerating lesions in the ankle region and on the foot. The typical *venous ulcer* poses no problem in differential diagnosis. It occurs in a setting of chronic venous disease, is associated with stasis changes and normal arterial pulses, is usually relatively painless, and heals with elevation and compressive measures. The typical *arterial* or *ischemic ulcer* is far more painful and is associated with other manifestations of ischemia. It usually has a more necrotic base and is located at an area of chronic pressure or trauma such as over the malleoli or the bunion area. Both conditions may be improved by hospitalization, bed rest, and local care. Differential diagnosis is usually only difficult when chronic venous and arterial disease coexist. Venography and arteriography may be required. In some patients the primary cause of the ulcer can be determined only when arterial reconstruction produces healing after a period of intense conservative management has failed to do so.

When a patient presents with a gangrenous (black) or pregangrenous (blue) toe, several etiologies other than progression of chronic arteriosclerotic occlusive disease must be considered. *Local infection* can be the sole cause or a contributing cause of the toe lesion. This is particularly common in diabetics. If foot pulses or noninvasive tests of arterial function are normal, the gangrenous condition can be presumed to result from local arterial or arteriolar thrombosis secondary to infection. Radical local drainage and excision of all involved tissue will usually result in a healed foot. Diagnosis is more difficult when infection coexists with arterial occlusive disease. Noninvasive studies and arteriography are usually required before it can be determined whether treatment should consist of excision and drainage alone or in combination with an arterial reconstruction. Decision making under these conditions can be among the most difficult in vascular surgery.

Patients with black or blue toes may also have them as the result of embolic processes. Such emboli may originate from the heart, a proximal aneurysm, or any proximal atherosclerotic lesion. In the latter circumstance, small cholesterol, platelet, or fibrin emboli may lodge in interosseous or digital arteries. Peripheral pedal pulses may be normal, and spontaneous improvement of the resulting blue toe often occurs. This sequence of events has been termed "the blue toe syndrome," and its pathogenesis is thought to be analogous to that of transient ischemic attacks from atherosclerotic disease at the carotid bifurcation (8). If a single dominant arterial lesion can be identified by angiography, it should be treated by endarterectomy or more commonly by an appropriate bypass. In our experience, it has been difficult to identify a single lesion in the arterial tree of these patients, and we have usually operated on them only after they have had multiple embolic episodes.

In any patient whose ischemia developed suddenly, the possibility of a *major embolus* from the heart or a proximal aneurysm must be considered. In such circumstances, angiography is indicated even if limb viability is not in question, since major emboli should be removed as soon as they are identified. In the last several decades with progress in cardiac surgery for rheumatic heart disease, most patients with major arterial emboli have had them superimposed on extensive arteriosclerosis. Even with *angiography, which we employ routinely in such cases,* the diagnosis and treatment of embolic disease is difficult and results of surgical treatment are imperfect (9). The only certain diagnostic feature of embolus is multiplicity. Furthermore, the location of the embolus may be atypical, and the vascular surgeon treating a presumed embolus in the presence of extensive arteriosclerosis must be prepared to perform an extensive arterial reconstruction or bypass even if the operation is undertaken soon after the acute event. Because of these facts and because acute thrombosis sometimes cannot be differentiated in any way from embolus, complete preoperative angiography should be mandatory in any suspected embolic occlusion of the lower extremity in a patient who could have arteriosclerosis. Moreover, the care and surgical treatment of such cases should only be undertaken by an experienced vascular surgeon.

Patient Evaluation

LOCAL FACTORS AND EXTREMITY PHYSICAL EXAMINATION

As already indicated, the findings on physical examination of the involved extremity contribute to the staging of the atherosclerotic process and provide a rough guide to whether diagnostic or therapeutic intervention is justified and needed. By revealing discoloration and swelling, physical examination should also provide evidence of the presence and extent of infection in the involved foot. As a general rule, the extent of infection and necrosis deep to the skin is greater than one might expect from an examination of the skin. Reexamination after a short period of soaking to soften the epidermis and dried exudate may also be helpful in revealing purulent collections and subcutaneous necrosis. Exploration of suspicious areas can sometimes be carried out without anesthesia if the patient has diminished sensation from diabetic neuropathy. If not, such exploration and the necessary debridement should be performed under anesthesia in the operating room.

In the initial examination of a patient with suspected infrainguinal arterial disease, careful inspection for previous operative scars is essential since patients may be unaware of a prior sympathectomy or the nature and extent of previous arterial surgery. The site of scars can provide clues as to whether or not the arteries below the knee were violated, whether or not ipsilateral saphenous vein was utilized, and if so, how much is left. Physical examination can also provide evidence of associated chronic venous disease. In evaluating an ischemic limb, particular attention must be given to careful inspection of the heel and between the toes where unsuspected ischemic ulcers or infection may be present. A flashlight is extremely helpful in this regard. The uninvolved extremity must also be examined carefully. Because of the symmetry of atherosclerosis, the opposite extremity may harbor unsuspected ischemic lesions. Moreover, such findings as coolness and bluish discoloration are far more meaningful if they are asymmetrical, since cool, dusky extremities may sometimes be present without major arterial disease.

Pulse Examination

Pulse examination in the lower extremities of a patient with suspected ischemia is extremely important. It requires considerable experience and must be performed with care. The strength of a pulse as assessed by an experienced examiner is a valuable semiquantitative assessment of the arterial circulation at that level. Pulses should be graded from 0 to 4+ and should not be described as "plus or minus" or "questionable." The latter indicates an incomplete exam. A 0 pulse cannot be felt. A 1+ pulse is definitely present but definitely diminished. Both 2+ and 3+ are normal intensities, and 4+ is an abnormally strong pulse such as with an aneurysm or aortic insufficiency. If a pulse is 2+ on one side and 3+ on the opposite side, the 2+ is a decreased pulse, and arterial pressure at that site is probably decreased (unless the 3+ pulse is due to an aneurysm).

In examining a patient with diminished pulses it is extremely helpful to count the pulse to an assistant feeling the radial pulse to be sure the examiner is not feeling her or his own pulse or spurious muscular activity. Before one describes a pulse as being absent, considerable time and effort must be expended and ectopic localization of pulses, such as the lateral tarsal artery pulse, must be examined. In this era of far too frequently performed noninvasive arterial tests, the value of a carefully performed and recorded pulse exam cannot be overemphasized. It provides a basis for comparison if subsequent disease progression occurs, and it is a simple way of accurately assessing the arterial circulation in the lower extremities at a given point in time. It also provides an indicator of what type of approach will be required to save a threatened foot.

Many examples of this value can be cited. If a patient with a gangrenous toe lesion has a pedal pulse, local treatment without reconstructive arterial surgery will almost always be the correct approach to achieve a healed foot. If a patient with a substantial ischemic foot lesion has a normal popliteal pulse but no pedal pulses, some form of infrapopliteal or small-vessel bypass will almost always be required to obtain a healed foot. If a patient with an ischemic foot lesion has a normal ipsilateral femoral pulse without distal pulses, some form of infrainguinal arterial reconstruction, hopefully a femoropopliteal bypass, will probably be required to achieve a healed foot. If such a patient has a diminished femoral pulse, often with an associated bruit, some form of arterial reconstruction or angioplasty above the inguinal ligament will almost certainly be required.

SYSTEMIC FACTORS

Systemic factors which are important in the patient who is a candidate for interventional treatment for infrainguinal arteriosclerosis include all those in the history, physical examination, and routine laboratory tests which might indicate organ failure. Most important are evidence of heart disease, diabetes, kidney disease, hypertension, chronic respiratory disease, and atherosclerotic involvement of arteries to the brain. All of these intercurrent diseases, if present, require appropriate medical management before, during, and after diagnostic and therapeutic interventions so that risks will be minimized. A detailed discussion of this management is beyond the scope of this chapter. However, since all patients with infrainguinal arteriosclerosis also have some degree of coronary involvement and since myocardial infarction is the principal cause of perioperative as well as late mortality in this group of patients, some details of cardiac evaluation and management should be mentioned. Evidence of myocardial ischemia and congestive failure should be sought. If severe angina pectoris is present, some patients should be subjected to coronary arteriography and aortocoronary bypass prior to treating their limb ischemia. Patients with recent myocardial infarctions and those in congestive heart failure should have a Swan-Ganz catheter inserted and have their fluid status and volume replacement optimized before, during, and after operation on the basis of appropriate cardiac output and pressure measurements (10) (see Chapter 21). It is also especially important to monitor renal function repetitively after any angiographic procedure since transient renal failure is common, even though its incidence may be decreased by adequate hydration before and during angiography. If detected and appropriately treated, this is always reversible and rarely a serious problem.

NONINVASIVE VASCULAR LABORATORY TESTS

Although the nature and value of these tests are the subject of another complete chapter (Chapter 8), there are several points that deserve reemphasis because of their particular importance in patients with infrainguinal arteriosclerosis. In the early stages in which interventional measures are not required, segmental arterial pressures and pulse volume recordings provide an objective and semiquantitative assessment of the circulation and help to confirm the diagnosis made by the history and physical examination including a careful pulse exam. These tests also provide a baseline against which future changes can be measured, and a rough index of the localization of occlusive arterial lesions and the degree of ischemia in the foot. However the correlation is not absolute, and flat ankle and forefoot wave tracings with ankle pressures less than 35 mmHg can be unassociated with foot lesions or disabling symptoms. In addition, decreased thigh

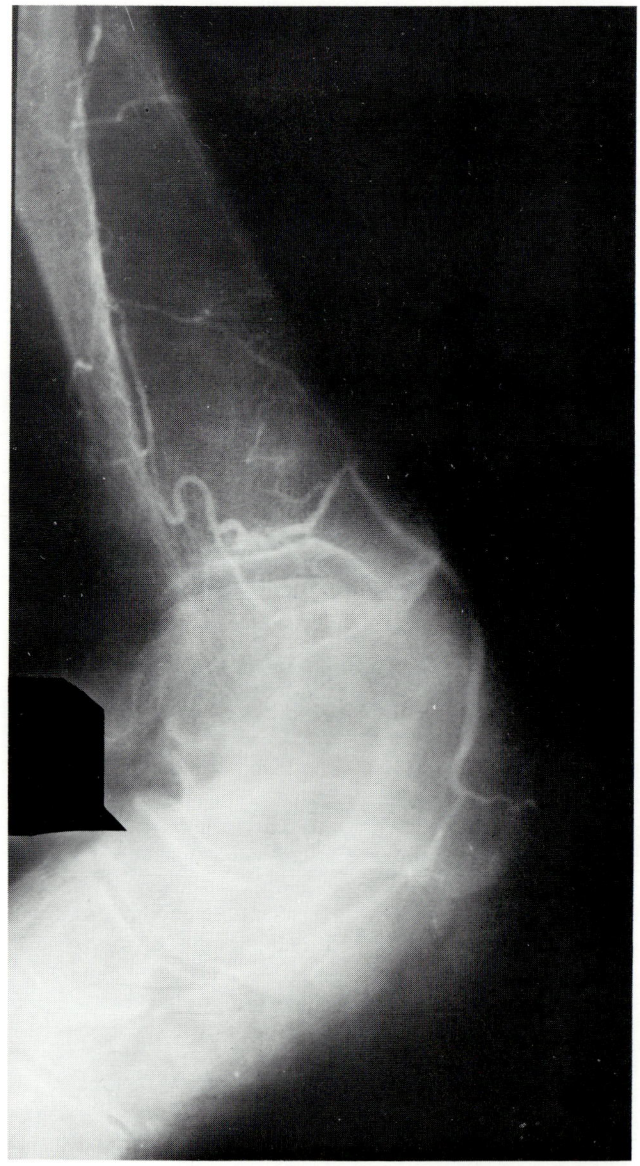

FIGURE 26-1. Arteriogram showing patent segment of posterior tibial artery that was used for a successful bypass in an 89-year-old diabetic who might have been considered unreconstructible with less adequate angiography. A femoral-to-posterior tibial bypass and a concurrent amputation of the gangrenous great toe and first metatarsal head resulted in salvage of a limb which has continued to provide good function for more than 5 years.

waveforms and pressures may be associated entirely with disease below the inguinal ligament as well as with aortoiliac disease. The differentiation between these two types of lesions can only be made by femoral pulse examination and direct intraarterial pressure measurements. Exact localization and definition of lesions can only be made when arteriography, sometimes in two planes, is added to these two determinations.

Noninvasive testing can be extremely helpful in predicting when a toe amputation or local procedure on the foot has virtually no chance of healing. A flatline or almost flatline (1 to 4 mm) forefoot pulse volume tracing with an ankle pressure below 50 mmHg indicates that a toe amputation or other foot operation for an ischemic lesion will not heal without prior revascularization. Because these tests do not evaluate the severity or extent of infection, the opposite is not always true. Good forefoot pulse waves (> 10 mm) and ankle pressures do not guarantee healing of foot operations, although they suggest healing will occur if infection can be eliminated. Furthermore, there is a gray zone of intermediate values in which noninvasive tests are of little value and a therapeutic trial of a local foot procedure is justified and appropriate.

ANGIOGRAPHIC EVALUATION

Arteriography

As in other areas of vascular surgery, proper high-quality arteriography is essential to make the most accurate diagnosis of infrainguinal arteriosclerosis, to determine whether therapeutic intervention is possible and justified by its risks, and to allow planning of the optimal form that this intervention should take (5). Adequate arteriography also defines the localization and extent of arteriosclerotic involvement in the infrarenal aorta and iliac arteries, although for optimal accuracy it may have to be supplemented by direct pressure measurements taken at the time of arteriography or operation.

To provide adequate information, the arterial tree from the groin to the forefoot should be well visualized in continuity, preferably by the transfemoral route. This is generally possible only if a long film changer, multiple exposures, large boluses of contrast medium, and other technical modifications described elsewhere (11) are employed. Oblique views may be required to visualize completely the origin and proximal portion of the deep and superficial femoral arteries. Good preoperative distal artery visualization is, in our opinion, the key to performing optimal bypass surgery to arteries in the foot and lower leg (Figure 26-1). Reactive hyperemia and delayed films may be necessary to achieve the needed visualization. Although others have advocated intraoperative arteriography to achieve this end (12), we have found it less effective and rarely necessary.

Venography

Saphenous venography has been helpful in planning long bypasses (13,14). It may also show a vein defect preoperatively and thereby spare the patient and the surgeon the needless effort of harvesting a saphenous vein that cannot be used. This form of venography is particularly indicated in patients who have undergone prior prosthetic bypasses, since many of these patients have had their vein erroneously injured at their first operation.

Treatment: Principles, Procedures, and Judgmental Issues

Legitimate controversy exists over which patients with symptomatic infrainguinal arteriosclerosis should be treated surgically and how aggressively that treatment should be pursued. The reasons for not operating on most patients whose limbs are not imminently endangered have already been stated. Although disabling claudication is still considered a valid indication for operation or angioplasty in some centers, we and many others consider such interventions usually unnecessary and potentially harmful.

The management of patients with infrainguinal arteriosclerosis that is truly limb threatening is also controversial. Some surgical groups attempt limb salvage in almost all patients with gangrene, a nonhealing ischemic ulcer, or severe ischemic rest pain due to arteriosclerosis below the inguinal ligament; others resort to primary amputation in all or almost all of these patients; and others attempt limb salvage only if distal necrosis is limited and an arterial reconstruction can be performed to a relatively normal popliteal artery with radiographic evidence of good runoff via tibial artery branches.

The history of infrainguinal arterial surgery provides a partial explanation for this controversy. As techniques of arterial surgery evolved in the 1950s and 1960s, endarterectomy and prosthetic bypasses were widely applied for the treatment of superficial femoral artery disease in many centers. Mid- and long-term results following these procedures were poor. Moreover, because the bypass techniques used in these early efforts were less meticulous and refined than those presently available, there was a high incidence of cardiac deaths, early failure and infection resulting in high rates of knee loss, morbidity, and mortality. These negative results from infrainguinal limb salvage surgery prompted a reevaluation of its cost-benefit ratio and recommendations that patients overall would be better served by a primary below-knee amputation (15). The influence of this important reevaluation remains dominant in many areas and centers. However, in the mid and late 1970s, the situation changed once again. Intraoperative and postoperative anesthetic management improved with better monitoring techniques for minimizing anesthetic morbidity and mortality rates in patients with advanced coronary artery disease. More meticulous surgical techniques were developed for performing bypasses to smaller diseased arteries at the popliteal level and below. The superiority of saphenous vein grafts as a conduit for low-flow infrainguinal bypasses became increasingly well recognized. Angioplasty and extraanatomic bypasses became available for treating so-called inflow disease above the inguinal ligament in a low-risk fashion even in sick, old patients. And finally, better angiographic techniques for visualizing distal arteries in the presence of multiple proximal occlusions were perfected (11,12).

All of these developments prompted renewed interest in infrainguinal limb salvage arterial reconstructive techniques, and increasing numbers of centers have found that such aggressive efforts to save limbs have been worthwhile. However, the surgical and nonsurgical management of patients with these problems poses special requirements. Special expertise, training, and commitment is needed to perform the required angiographic and surgical procedures safely and effectively and to achieve good results. Thus controversy remains. It is our belief, however, that aggressive efforts to save limbs, if applied appropriately, are worthwhile. We further believe that this attitude will become increasingly widespread as additional centers demonstrate its applicability and effectiveness by their own evaluations.

In general our approach, which is detailed below, represents the most aggressive effort to salvage limbs that are threatened because of infrainguinal arteriosclerosis. Patients who have ischemic foot lesions or pain but who can be treated successfully by aortofemoral, femorofemoral, or axillofemoral bypass alone should be so treated. These patients are excluded from the following discussion, even though many of them have infrainguinal arteriosclerosis in addition to their more proximal disease.

GENERAL CONSIDERATIONS

According to our aggressive approach to patients whose limbs are threatened because of infrainguinal arteriosclerosis, limb salvage should be considered and attempted if feasible, unless gangrene extends into the deeper tissues of the tarsal region of the foot or unless the patient has severe organic mental syndrome with an inability to ever ambulate, communicate, or provide self-care (5). Patients in the latter categories should undergo primary below- or above-knee amputation.

MEDICAL CONSIDERATIONS

As expected, in these patients there is a high incidence of other arteriosclerotic manifestations, and more than 50 percent in some series have diabetes mellitus. The mean age is over 70 years, and many patients are in their eighties. Many have suffered documented myocardial infarction, some are in uncompensated congestive heart failure or renal failure, some have had myocardial infarctions within 3 weeks of presentation, and some have concurrent carcinomas (5).

The general plan of medical management is to achieve maximal improvement of cardiac, renal, and diabetic status before proceeding with arteriographic examination and operation. In some instances, the urgency of the ischemic situation, coupled with progressive infection in the foot, makes it necessary to perform angiographic examination and operation before ideal medical control can be achieved. In these patients decisions to proceed are made jointly by the surgeon and internist. Almost without exception, age, medical status, incurable malignancy, and/or a contralateral amputation are not considered reasons to withhold arterial reconstruction (5).

SURGICAL CONSIDERATIONS AND CRITERIA FOR RECONSTRUCTIBILITY

Femoropopliteal Bypass

Patients whose limbs are clearly threatened and who have undergone arteriographic examination should undergo femoropopliteal bypass when the superficial femoral or popliteal artery is occluded and the patent popliteal artery segment distal to the occlusion has luminal continuity, on arteriographic examination, with any of its three terminal branches. This is true even if one or more of these branches ends in an occlusion anywhere in the leg. Even if the popliteal artery segment into which the graft is to be inserted is occluded distally, femoropopliteal bypass to this isolated segment (16) is the procedure of choice. If the isolated popliteal segment is less than 7 cm in length or there is extensive gangrene or infection in the foot, a femoral-to-popliteal-to-distal artery bypass or sequential bypass is sometimes performed, in one or two stages (17–21). All femoropopliteal bypasses can be classified on the basis of their relationship to the knee joint and runoff from the popliteal artery, as determined radiographically by previously described criteria (17).

Infrapopliteal Bypass

Bypass to arteries beyond the popliteal (small-vessel bypasses) are performed only when femoropopliteal bypass is not deemed possible, according to the foregoing criteria. These small-vessel bypasses are performed to the posterior tibial, the anterior tibial, or the peroneal arteries, in that order of preference. A tibial artery is generally used only if its lumen runs without obstruction into the foot, although we have recently performed a group of short vein bypasses from the popliteal and tibial arteries to isolated distal tibial segments with patency in some cases persisting over 3 years (Figure 26-2) (22,23). A peroneal artery is used only if it is continuous with one or two of its terminal branches which anastomose with named arteries in the foot. Absence of a plantar arch and vascular calcification *are not* considered contraindications to small-vessel bypasses (Figure 26-3) (5). Very few patients fail to have in their leg or foot an artery which meets these requirements, so that in the past only 6 percent of our patients have been considered unreconstructible on the basis of angiographic findings (5), and this figure has now fallen to less than 3 percent.

With both femoropopliteal and small-vessel bypasses, stenosis of less than 50 percent of the diameter of the vessel is acceptable at or distal to the site chosen for the distal anastomosis. Although an effort is made to find the most disease free segment of artery to use for the distal anastomosis, this may be tempered by the advisability of using the most proximal patent segment possible, to shorten the length of the bypass. For example, a mildly diseased proximal popliteal artery should be used for a distal anastomosis in preference to a nondiseased distal popliteal artery.

The common femoral artery has been generally used as the site of origin for all bypasses to the popliteal and more distal arteries. However, over the last 10 years, we have also used as inflow sites the superficial femoral or popliteal when these arteries were relatively undiseased (Figures 26-4, 26-5) (21,22). These arteries are now used preferentially if possible; and if limited saphenous vein is available, we have also used tibial arteries as origins for distal bypasses (Figure 26-3) (22,23).

Axillopopliteal Bypass

This operation is employed only when amputation is imminent and a more standard arterial reconstruction is not feasible because of groin infection, previous operative scarring, or exten-

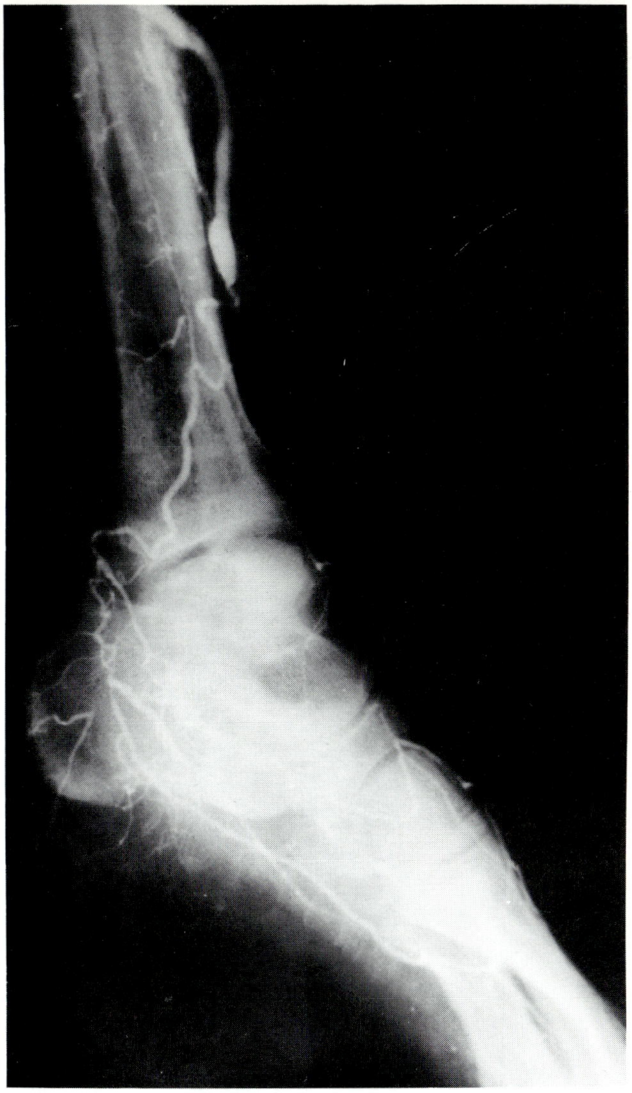

FIGURE 26-2. Arteriogram obtained 6 months after a bypass to an anterior tibial artery segment which is totally obstructed proximally and distally. A large collateral branch supplies the foot. This bypass has remained patent over 3 years. [From Veith, Ascer, Gupta (23) with permission.]

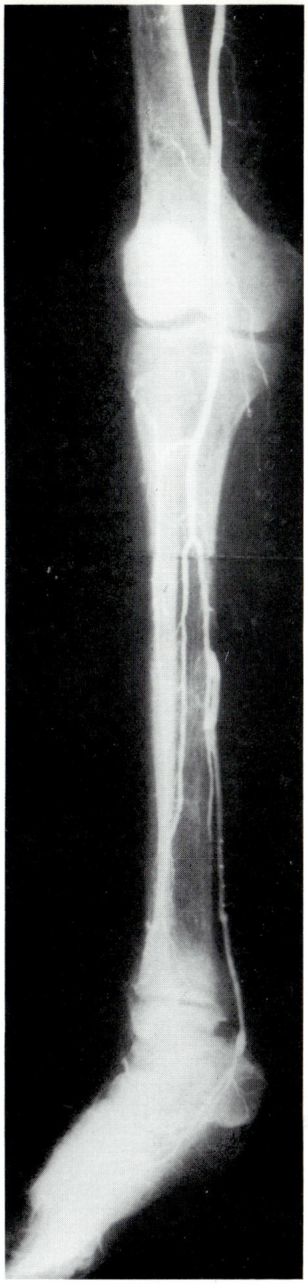

FIGURE 26-3. Arteriogram 3 years after a bypass from the posterior tibial artery in the midleg to a heavily calcified posterior tibial artery distal to the ankle joint. The plantar arch is incomplete, and this patient had only this short segment of saphenous vein available. [From Veith, Ascer, Gupta (23) with permission.]

sive bilateral arteriosclerotic involvement of the iliac and femoral artery systems (24,25).

Profundaplasty

Endarterectomy of the origin and proximal portion of the deep femoral artery is chiefly of value in salvaging threatened limbs when it is combined with some form of inflow operation such as an aortofemoral or axillofemoral bypass (26). As an isolated procedure in patients whose limbs are threatened because of infrainguinal arteriosclerosis, we have found profundaplasty to be of little value. Perhaps it is occasionally justified as the sole procedure if the patient has rest pain without necrosis and a tight stenosis or occlusion of the deep femoral artery *with* a demonstrable pressure gradient across the lesion at operation. In practice we have employed a short bypass to the distal deep femoral artery more frequently than an isolated profundaplasty.

Graft Material

Until 1976, autologous saphenous vein grafts were clearly the graft material of choice, with a variety of Dacron grafts serving as the alternative material if the vein was unavailable. Tubular expanded polytetrafluoroethylene (PTFE) grafts became avail-

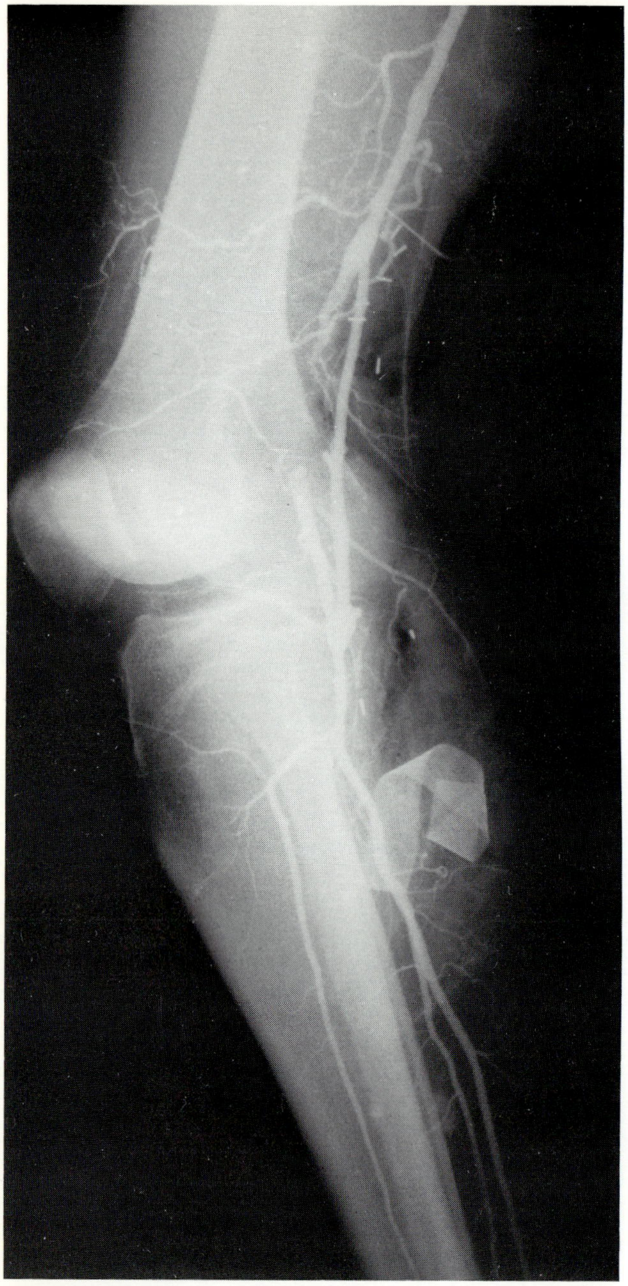

FIGURE 26-4. Intraoperative arteriogram after a proximal popliteal-to-distal-popliteal bypass for a segmental occlusion of the above-knee popliteal artery.

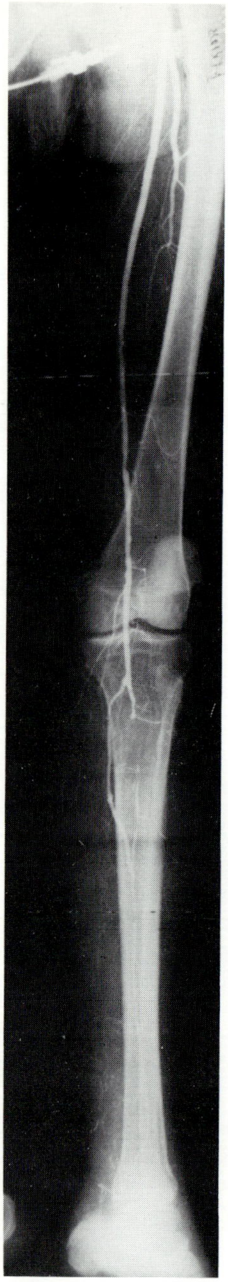

FIGURE 26-5. Arteriogram 1 year after a distal-popliteal-to-peroneal bypass in a patient with no other available saphenous vein.

able in 1976 and were first used only when ipsilateral saphenous vein was unavailable or unusable. Promising early and intermediate results with this material in femoropopliteal bypasses (27–30) prompted liberalization of the indications for its use in this operation to include patients whose probable life expectancy is less than 3 years.

Six years ago we began with Drs. Bergan, Bernhard, and others a cooperative, randomized, prospective study comparing autologous saphenous vein to PTFE grafts in all infrainguinal limb salvage bypass operations. Early results with significant numbers of patients observed up to $2\frac{1}{2}$ years showed that there was no difference in patency between vein and PTFE grafts in the femoropopliteal position, either above or below the knee (31). However, significantly better patency was achieved with vein grafts than with PTFE grafts to infrapopliteal arteries. Substantial numbers of patients at our own institution have now been followed over $3\frac{1}{2}$ years. Although patency differences have emerged between randomized vein and randomized PTFE femoropopliteal grafts (71 vs. 60 percent 4-year primary patency, respectively), these differences are not yet statistically significant ($p < 0.7$). Small-vessel bypass patency is significantly superior with randomized vein than with randomized PTFE grafts (49 vs.

32 percent 4-year primary patency, $p < 0.05$). Because of effective reoperations and other factors, limb salvage rates are approximately 20 percent more than primary patency rates for all groups studied.

Although some vascular surgeons presently regard PTFE grafts as preferable to autologous saphenous vein for femoropopliteal bypass, we do not agree. We believe ipsilateral autologous saphenous vein to be the graft material of choice for femoropopliteal bypass, with PTFE grafts as the best alternative if this vein is unavailable or unsuitable (< 4 mm in smallest diameter), or if the patient's life expectancy is less than 3 years. We also believe that autologous saphenous vein is the best graft material for infrapopliteal bypasses if the vein is more than 3.0 mm in diameter. However, all these opinions are still tentative and may require modification as more data from randomized, prospective, controlled, and refereed studies become available.

Tanned human umbilical vein grafts, if externally supported by a Dacron mesh, have also performed well as femoropopliteal grafts and to a more limited extent as infrapopliteal bypass conduits (32). It is generally agreed that use of these grafts like those of PTFE should be restricted to limb salvage situations in which autologous vein is not available and in which meticulous surgical technique is employed. In addition, late aneurysmal degeneration of these grafts has been observed in some cases.

Operative Technique

All operations are performed with the patient under light general or epidural anesthesia. Care is taken to protect the opposite heel by placing a small pillow under the Achilles tendon. The arterial blood pressure is monitored by a radial artery catheter. Meticulous and careful surgical technique is critically important in determining success. A variety of techniques will work, but it must be remembered that these are special operations and that they require special skills, instruments, and care. Our techniques for performing these operations are described elsewhere (24,28,33), and some important technical details for small-vessel bypass are illustrated in Figures 26-6 to 26-8. Whatever technique is employed, vessels must be occluded with a minimum of force and distortion. Anastomoses must be meticulously constructed with continuous fine polypropylene sutures, with particular care to take small, evenly spaced bites of all layers of the vessel wall, and to exclude all adventitia from the anastomotic lumen. Although others employ it routinely, we use intraoperative angiographic examination only if special problems are encountered since it is difficult to visualize all parts of a complex reconstruction and since angiographic artifacts can be difficult to interpret and can prolong and complicate the operation.

PERIOPERATIVE AND POSTOPERATIVE DRUG TREATMENT

All patients receive prophylactic treatment with 1 g of cefazolin 6 hours preoperatively, during operation, and 12 and 24 hours after operation. All receive heparin, 100 to 150 units per kilogram, during periods of vascular occlusion.

On the basis of the experimental observations of Oblath et al. (34) and the clinical study of Chesebro et al. (35) in aortocoronary vein bypasses, all our patients are given 325 mg of aspirin and 125 mg of dipyridamole three times daily, beginning 48 hours before operation. These drugs are continued throughout the period of hospitalization. When the patient is discharged, the aspirin and dipyridamole dosage is reduced to 325 and 50 mg, respectively, twice daily; these drugs are continued indefinitely if possible.

MANAGEMENT OF FOOT LESIONS

Approximately 75 percent of our patients have gangrenous or necrotic foot or toe lesions (5). Small (< 2 cm^2) uninfected gangrenous lesions on the toe or foot require no local surgical treatment. Larger gangrenous lesions and any area of infection associated with necrosis are extensively debrided at the end of any arterial reconstruction. These debridements often require excision of one or more toes, and frequently consist of a partial (medial or lateral) transmetatarsal amputation. An attempt is made to excise enough bone so there is overhanging skin and soft tissue. These wounds are usually left open, and drying of the soft tissues is prevented by placing the involved portion of the foot in a normal saline wet dressing within a plastic bag. Subsequent debridement of foot lesions is often required on the ward or in the operating room. This is performed to remove all infected or necrotic tissue and exposed cartilage without regard for anatomic landmarks. It is sometimes necessary, particularly in diabetics, to perform multiple secondary operative procedures (up to seven) to achieve a healed foot. Skin grafts are used to cover large cutaneous defects but are placed only when the wound is rendered entirely clean and granulating by debridement and frequent dressing changes. In some patients, particularly those with extensive foot gangrene or infection and a femoropopliteal bypass that is inserted into an isolated popliteal artery segment, it is impossible to achieve healing at the metatarsal or even tarsal level, and below-knee amputation is required. In some similar instances, it has been possible to obtain foot healing by performing a secondary bypass to an artery distal to the popliteal segment (17,18).

REOPERATION

All patients whose limb salvage bypasses thrombose *in the first month after operation* will almost certainly have a threatened foot and should undergo reoperation. The causes of early failure (usually technical or judgmental) and the reoperative techniques employed have been described elsewhere (5,36,37). Intraoperative angiographic examination is used routinely after graft thrombectomy. Vein grafts that fail immediately after operation usually require interposition of a segment of PTFE or total replacement with this material, although we and others (37) have occasionally salvaged all or a portion of a thrombosed vein graft by thrombectomy if the latter procedure is performed within 24 hours of thrombosis and if other lesions are corrected.

Patients whose bypasses thrombose *after the first postoperative month* are considered for aggressive reoperation, and femoral angiography is usually performed. However, the patients are subjected to reoperation only if the bypass failure is associated with a renewed threat to limb viability. If the patient has originally undergone operation elsewhere and details of the first

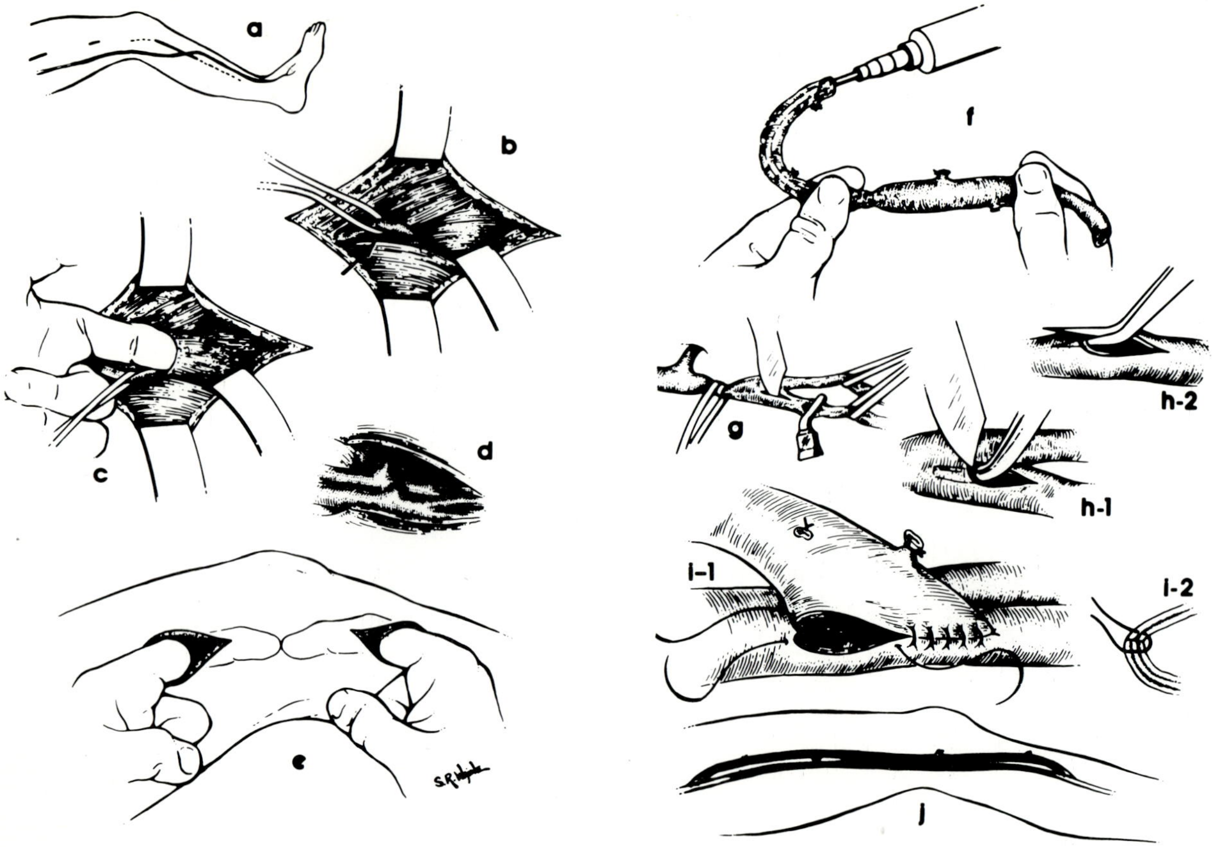

FIGURE 26-6. Small-vessel bypass in the upper and middle third of the leg. This may be performed to the tibioperoneal trunk, the posterior tibial artery, or the peroneal artery, using a medial approach below the knee joint to gain access to these vessels. The anterior tibial artery requires an additional anterior incision shown in Figure 26-7. (*A*) In heavy lines, the position of the incisions required to perform bypasses from the femoral artery to the tibioperoneal trunk or the peroneal or posterior tibial arteries in the upper third of the leg. The upper incision provides access to the common or superficial femoral artery. The above-knee incision allows tunneling under the sartorius muscle and along the course of the popliteal vessels behind the knee. The dashed extension to the lower incision provides access to the posterior tibial and peroneal arteries in the middle third of the leg. If the saphenous vein is to be used, all incisions should be placed over the vein as shown by the double line, and access to deeper structures obtained when needed by raising thick flaps. (*B*) The below-knee incision opened through the skin, subcutaneous fat, and deep fascia of the popliteal space. The gastrocnemius muscle is retracted posteriorly. The more superficial popliteal vein is encircled with a Silastic loop to facilitate dissection of the underlying popliteal artery (*arrow*) which can be seen disappearing deep to the fibers of the soleus muscle. (*C*) A finger or right-angle clamp being placed deep to this muscle prior to cutting it at its origin from the fibrous band that attaches to the back of the tibia. This exposes the origin of the anterior tibial artery and its accompanying vein or veins. (*D*) Division of these veins allows further retraction of overlying veins and exposure of the tibioperoneal trunk and its terminal branches. (*E*) Tunnels are fashioned by finger dissection. (*F*) Details of vein preparation using a long (6-in) cannula to permit the vein to be distended in segments so that leaks can be controlled and recanalized segments detected. (*G*) Elevation of the arteries by Silastic vessel loops and the beginning of the scalpel incision in the artery. In this view only the taut Silastic loops are required to control bleeding, except for the posterior tibial artery which also has a microvascular clip applied to it. (*H*) Placement of a mosquito clamp to facilitate extension of the initial opening in the artery. Alternatively, a microvascular scissors may be used to extend the arteriotomy if the vessel is thin-walled and normal. (*I*) Details of the anastomotic suturing, which is begun at the distal end and continued to the midportion of each side of the anastomosis of the artery and the saphenous vein graft. Equal bites of all layers of each vessel are included in each stitch, which is always placed under direct vision. (*J*) Completed graft in place. If more distal exposure of the posterior tibial or peroneal arteries is required, further separation of the soleus muscle from the posterior surface of the tibia and its overlying muscles provides access to the neurovascular bundles. Careful dissection of the veins with ligation of crossing branches provides access to the more deeply placed arteries. These can be dissected free, taking great care to preserve all branches, so that an appropriate segment of artery can be elevated and controlled to perform the distal anastomosis. [From Veith, Gupta (33) with permission.]

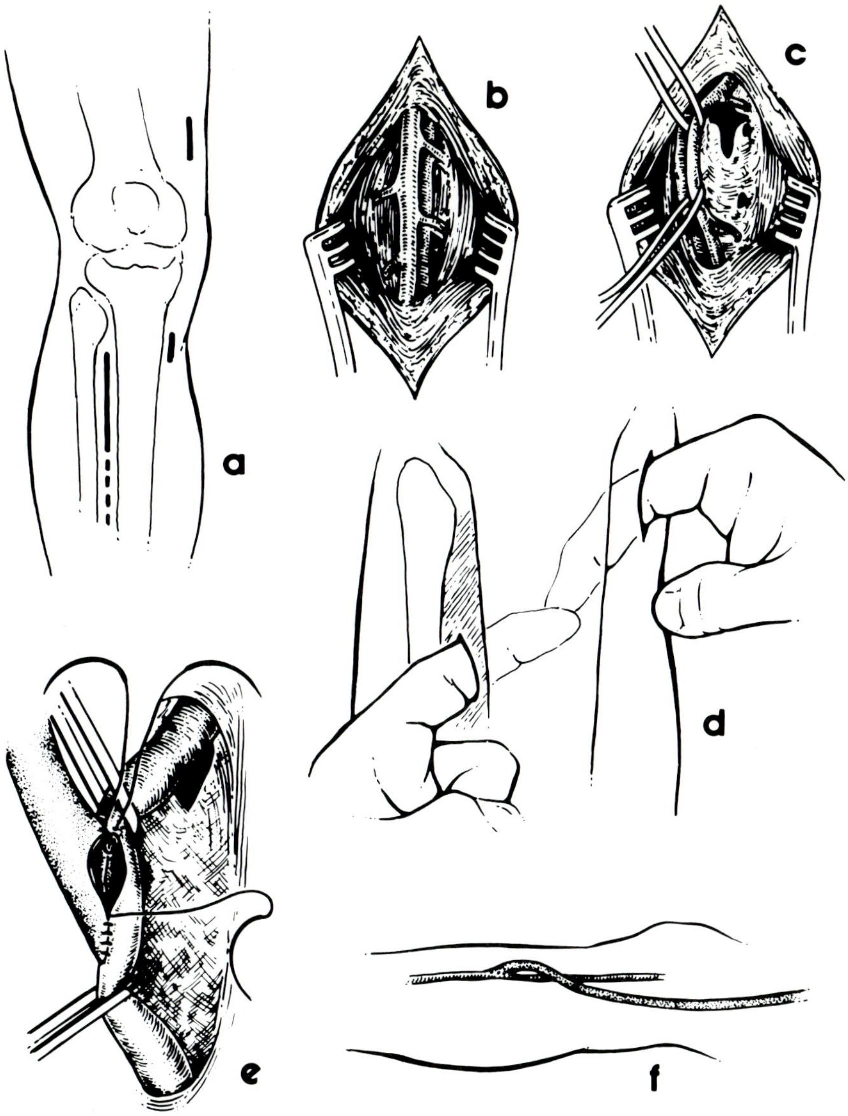

FIGURE 26-7. Bypass to the anterior tibial artery in the upper and middle thirds of the leg. (*A*) This requires an anterolateral incision in the leg midway between the tibia and fibula over the appropriate segment of patent artery. Additional small medial incisions are also required for tunneling. (*B*) The anterior incision is carried through the deep fascia, and the fibers of the anterior tibial muscle and the long extensors of the toes are separated to reveal the neurovascular bundle. Mobilization of accompanying veins with division of branches allows visualization of the anterior tibial artery, which can then be carefully mobilized. (*C*) After the artery is freed, it is elevated and retracted along with the accompanying veins by Silastic loops. This permits further posterior dissection, which allows the interosseous membrane to be visualized and incised in a cruciate fashion. (*D*) Careful blunt finger dissection from this anterior approach and from the popliteal fossa via the medial incision facilitates creation of a tunnel without injuring the numerous veins in the area. Alternatively, the tunnel for the bypass may be placed lateral to the knee in a subcutaneous plane. (*E*) By elevating the anterior tibial artery, a meticulous distal anastomosis can be constructed as already described. (*F*) The resulting graft in place. The anterior tibial artery can also be approached by a lateral incision with fibulectomy, but we believe this approach to be bloodier and more time-consuming than the one we have described. [From Veith, Gupta (33) with permission.]

operation are not known, a totally new bypass is performed. Adequate autologous vein may be available for some of these secondary bypasses. If the first operation has been performed in our institution, operative techniques for late thrombosis of PTFE grafts are as detailed previously (36).

Reoperative Techniques

The prior distal incision is opened, and the distal end of the graft, the distal anastomosis, and the artery proximal and distal to the anastomosis are dissected free. The graft is opened with

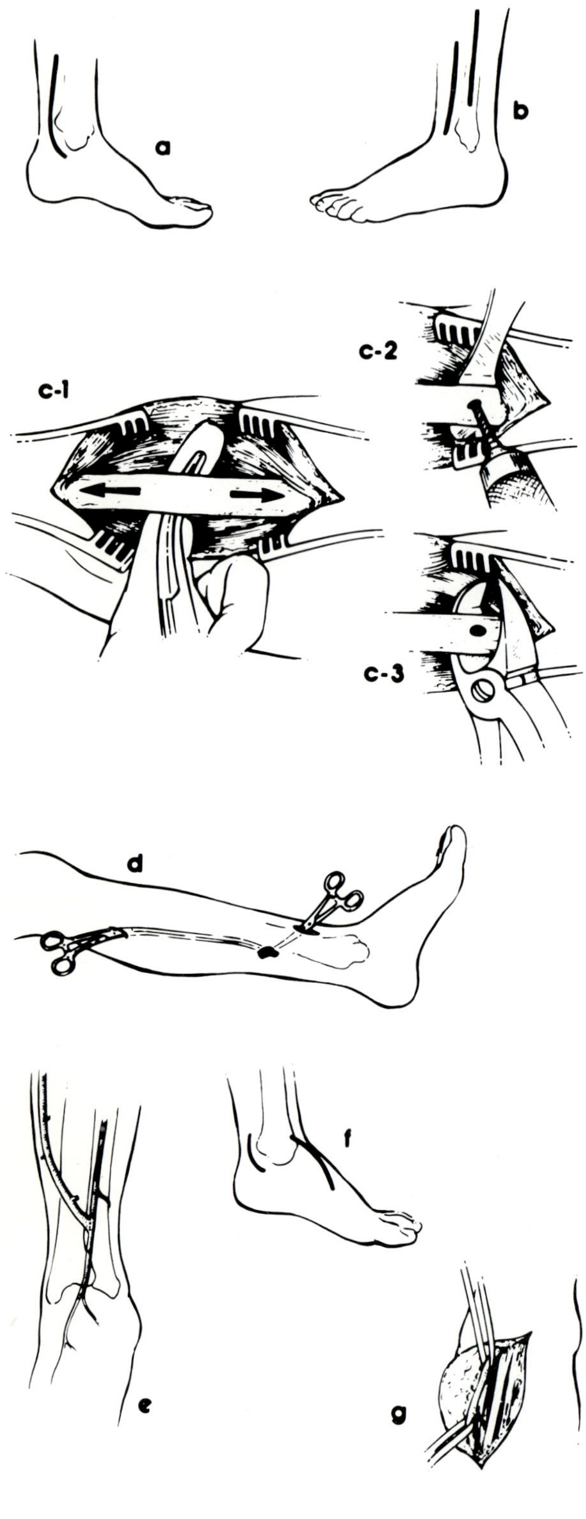

FIGURE 26-8. Bypasses to the distal third of the leg and the foot. Bypasses to the anterior tibial, posterior tibial, or peroneal arteries in the distal leg can be performed by techniques similar to those already described, with the exception of certain features illustrated here. (*A*) The distal posterior tibial artery can be approached by an incision along the posterior edge of the tibia. By deepening this incision along the tibialis posterior muscle and the posterior surface of the tibia, the distal peroneal artery can also be located and isolated just medial to the medial edge of the fibula. By dividing restraining fascia and fibers of the flexor hallucis longus muscle, it is possible to free this artery and elevate it into the wound so that a careful anastomosis can be constructed. However, in its distal third and particularly in patients with a stout calf and ankle, this vessel is approached by a lateral incision with excision of the fibula (*B*). (*C*) This is accomplished by freeing a long segment of fibula from its muscle attachments using a combination of blunt and sharp dissection. Particular care should be taken in the dissection along the medial edge of the bone, since the peroneal vessels are just deep to this edge and are easily injured by instruments. Once a finger has been passed around the fibula, this free edge of bone can be further developed by pushing a right-angled clamp forcefully inferiorly and superiorly. A right-angled retractor can then be passed behind the bone and a hole drilled in it. Then the fibula can be easily and cleanly divided with a rib shears. The peroneal artery can then be dissected free from surrounding veins so that it can be used for construction of a distal anastomosis. Gentle blunt finger dissection is required to develop a tunnel from this lateral wound to the lower popliteal fossa. Great care is taken to avoid injury to the numerous veins in the area. From there, the tunneling to the femoral artery wound is performed in the previously described fashion. Because it is the least accessible of the three leg arteries and normally has the poorest connections with the arteries of the foot, we recommend use of the peroneal artery as a distal implantation site only when the anterior and posterior tibial arteries are not suitable for use. (*D*) The tunnel from the popliteal fossa to the distal posterior tibial artery is made just deep to the deep fascia. This is best accomplished with a long, gently curved clamp. The distal anterior tibial artery is approached by an anterior incision midway between the tibia and fibula (*B*). For bypass to this vessel, a tunnel is made from the distal popliteal fossa, deep to the deep fascia, to a point 5 to 7 cm above the medial malleolus (*D*). From this point, the tunnel is made subcutaneously in a gentle curve across the tibia and adjacent tendons to reach the anterior tibial wound. The underlying tendons are those of the anterior tibial muscle and the long extensors of the toes. The tunnels are marked with umbilical tapes for subsequent identification. (*E*) After completion of the distal anastomosis and drawing the graft through these tunnels, any tendons that distort or compress the graft in its course around the tibia are divided. This is usually required in low anterior tibial bypasses. (*F, G*) When no more proximal procedure is possible, bypasses to the ankle region or foot can be used to salvage limbs. The dorsalis pedis artery can be easily approached via an incision on the dorsum of the foot. We place this incision laterally, curve it, and raise a flap so that the incision will not be directly over the anastomosis. If this artery must be approached at the ankle, it is necessary to divide the extensor retinaculum. Otherwise the operation is performed as already described for distal anterior tibial bypasses. The posterior tibial artery can be approached down to a point several centimeters below the medial malleolus. [From Veith, Gupta (33) with permission.]

a longitudinal incision to within a few millimeters of its distal tip. The graft is then thrombectomized by passage of balloon catheters. Thrombus is gently removed from the distal anastomosis under direct vision, and balloon catheters are passed proximally and distally in the artery using extreme gentleness and care. If no disease or defect is seen within the anastomotic lumen, the opening in the graft is closed and an arteriogram is obtained. If no lesion is found, the operation is terminated. If intimal hyperplasia or other disease is noted at or just distal to the anastomosis, the opening in the graft is extended across its toe and down the artery to a point beyond the disease. A patch graft of vein or PTFE is placed to close this opening, and an intraoperative arteriogram is performed. If graft thrombosis has resulted from progression of arteriosclerosis proximal or distal to an anastomosis, an appropriate graft extension is constructed after removing all clot. Vein grafts that fail more than 1 month after operation require a new bypass with a PTFE graft, or vein graft, although some failed or failing vein grafts may be partly salvaged by operative techniques described by Whittemore et al. (37). These techniques involve use of thrombectomy, intraoperative angiography with vein patching of stenotic lesions, and autologous vein extensions or bypasses for occlusive lesions in the primary vein graft or adjacent arteries. Sources of additional autologous vein in patients with failed or failing bypass grafts include saphenous vein remnants in the ipsilateral leg, the contralateral greater or lesser saphenous veins, and the cephalic or basilic veins in the upper extremities.

Several groups have described the successful use of *intraarterial streptokinase* to reopen occluded grafts with subsequent good results either alone or in concert with subsequent reoperation or angioplasty to correct lesions identified angiographically (38,39). Although we had initial success and enthusiasm for such an approach to occluded grafts, we had several subsequent failures due to distal embolization with resultant limb loss. We therefore believe that this approach is inferior to direct reoperation, which allows immediate revascularization and avoids the risk of embolization.

DETECTION AND MANAGEMENT OF THE FAILING GRAFT

Our group has observed that with careful clinical and noninvasive follow-up of patients with infrainguinal arterial reconstructions, it is often possible to detect failing reconstructions before graft thrombosis has occurred (40). This is possible when the bypass is a PTFE graft as well as a vein graft. The failing state may be produced by the development of lesions within a vein graft (37,41), by intimal hyperplasia at one or both anastomoses, or by progression of atherosclerosis proximal or distal to the bypass graft. Like others, we have found the results of interventions for failing grafts to be superior to those required after graft thrombosis has occurred (37,40,42). In contrast to other studies, we have found that clinical examination alone has been remarkably effective in detecting failing grafts, and we have been able to correct the responsible lesion by percutaneous transluminal angioplasty in more than three-quarters of our 70 cases of failing infrainguinal bypasses (40). The other cases have required a relatively simple proximal or distal extension of the bypass or an interposition graft. The results in terms of augmented bypass patency and limb salvage have been so good that we believe careful close clinical observation of all patients with infrainguinal bypasses is mandatory. Any change in pulse status, symptoms, or noninvasive laboratory parameters mandates urgent arteriography and appropriate intervention to forestall graft thrombosis (40,42).

ROLE OF PERCUTANEOUS TRANSLUMINAL ANGIOPLASTY (PTA)

Opinions regarding the usefulness of this new modality vary considerably, and its exact place in the treatment of infrainguinal arteriosclerosis is still somewhat controversial. Our own and other experience (43–45) suggests that with appropriate patient selection and in skilled hands, the serious complication rate is low. Moreover when complications or failures of PTA do occur, they can generally be well treated by relatively simple surgical procedures with little if any increased patient morbidity or mortality (45).

On this basis we presently will attempt a PTA on any patient with sufficiently severe disease and ischemia (usually stage III or stage IV) to warrant intervention and in whom the procedure is deemed suitable. Patients with stage III or IV ischemia who have a hemodynamically significant segmental iliac stenosis and infrainguinal arteriosclerosis generally have a PTA of the iliac lesion as their first therapeutic intervention. If the PTA is unsuccessful, a bypass to the femoral level is performed. If the PTA is successful, further arterial intervention, usually some form of femorodistal bypass, is performed only if the ischemia is unrelieved and a healed foot cannot be obtained. We do not hesitate to perform a bypass distal to an iliac artery treated by PTA (5,46,47).

PTA is also used as the primary therapeutic intervention in patients without hemodynamically significant iliac artery disease who have a short (< 5 cm) segmental stenosis of the superficial femoral or popliteal artery, if this lesion is judged hemodynamically significant on the basis of pulse examination or noninvasive testing. In more than half of our cases treated by angioplasty, some form of direct arterial surgery has also been required, usually for bypass of a second lesion distal to the one successfully treated by angioplasty (5). As already noted, PTA has also been effective in the treatment of stenotic lesions developing in or proximal or distal to a still functioning vein or PTFE graft (5,40,44).

Results of Treatment

Arteriosclerotic involvement is generally less, both in regard to extent and multiplicity of lesions, in patients with intermittent claudication than in those whose limb is threatened. It is therefore not surprising that the short-term and long-term patency results of infrainguinal arterial bypasses done for intermittent claudication are generally better than those done for limb salvage, and this difference has been documented by virtually every author who evaluated the results on the basis of operative indications (48,49). Since we believe that femoropopliteal bypass should rarely be performed for intermittent claudication and that the other infrainguinal bypasses should never be performed for this indication alone, we will restrict our discussion of results to operations performed because of severe ischemic rest pain, a nonhealing ulcer, or gangrene. However, it must be reiterated that many respected vascular surgeons still believe that femoropopliteal bypasses for disabling claudication are justified by their good results and low risk rate (1).

Results of infrainguinal bypasses clearly vary with the training, technical skill, and commitment of the surgeon. These operations are demanding and should be performed only by surgeons

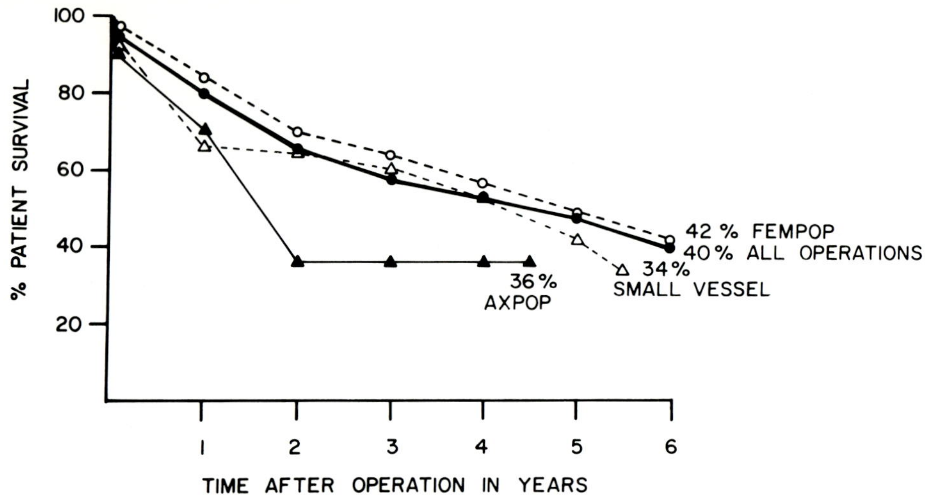

FIGURE 26-9. Cumulative life-table patient survival rates after 318 femoropopliteal, 204 small-vessel (infrapopliteal), and 29 axillopopliteal bypasses. Fifty-two percent of all patients undergoing all reconstructive arterial operations for limb-threatening arteriosclerosis were dead within 5 years. [From Veith, Gupta, Samson, et al. (5) with permission.]

doing them regularly and, more importantly, by surgeons with the skill and commitment to reoperate successfully should a bypass fail in the early or late postoperative period. In deciding whether these operations and an aggressive approach to limb salvage are in fact worthwhile in a given setting, every vascular surgeon should continually examine his or her own results to see if they are good enough to justify continued application of these sometimes difficult operations in these often brittle patients.

OPERATIVE MORTALITY RATE

The 30-day mortality rate for all patients undergoing infrainguinal arterial reconstructions for threatened limbs ranges from 2 to 6 percent (5,50). Operative mortality is slightly greater for infrapopliteal and axillopopliteal bypasses than for femoropopliteal bypasses, probably because the former operations are required in patients with more advanced generalized as well as lower extremity disease. The principal cause of death from these operations is myocardial infarction.

These low operative mortality rates contrast with the high late-death rates reflected in Figure 26-9, which shows that only 48 percent of all patients having arterial reconstructions were alive 5 years later. Almost all late deaths were unrelated to the original operation, most being due to intercurrent arteriosclerotic events, chiefly myocardial infarction. These findings again reflect the advanced stage of generalized arteriosclerosis present in these patients.

LIMB SALVAGE

When the aggressive approach already outlined for the management of patients whose limbs are threatened by infrainguinal arteriosclerosis was used and when only those patients who had organic mental syndrome and extensive local gangrene were excluded, 96 percent of patients underwent arteriographic examination (5). Ninety-four percent of patients who underwent arteriography were suitable candidates for some form of arterial revascularization procedure. With technical innovations and improvements (22,23,51) introduced since 1981, the percentage of unreconstructible patients has fallen below 3 percent, and almost all of these have had prior failed lower extremity arterial reconstructions.

Immediate Limb Salvage

If immediate limb salvage is defined as relief of ischemia and healing of ischemic lesions for 1 month after the first revascularization procedure, immediate limb salvage was achieved in 86 percent of patients in whom revascularization was possible (5).* Multiple (4 to 7) local operations and 2 to 4 months of hospitalization were required to achieve foot healing in 7 percent of our patients. Heel and forefoot gangrene did not preclude ultimate limb salvage, although they could, if extensive, contribute to the need for prolonged hospitalization. Even when the initial procedure attempted to achieve limb salvage failed immediately, the involved extremity could often be saved by promptly performing some secondary procedure (5,36,37,45). This was particularly common if a PTA was technically unsuccessful or failed to improve the arterial supply to the foot (45).

Late Limb Salvage

The cumulative limb salvage rates for all patients having arterial reconstructive operations are shown in Figure 26-10. Sixty-six percent of the patients who survived 5 years after a reconstruc-

*This immediate limb salvage rate was calculated by subtracting from the number of patients who could undergo revascularization procedures those patients who died or whose arterial reconstructive operation and/or angioplasty failed irretrievably within 1 month of the primary procedure, and those patients who required major amputations despite a successful revascularization procedure. The resulting number of patients was divided by the total number undergoing revascularization and multiplied by 100.

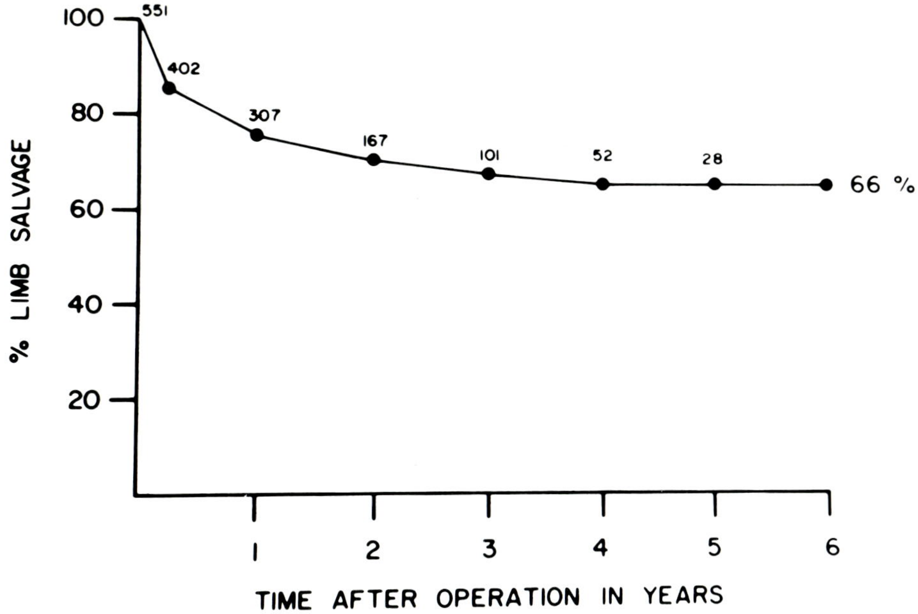

FIGURE 26-10. Cumulative life-table limb salvage rates for all patients undergoing reconstructive arterial operations for limb-threatening infrainguinal arteriosclerosis. The number with each point indicates the number of cases observed with intact limbs for that length of time. [From Veith, Gupta, Samson, et al. (5) with permission.]

tive arterial operation below the inguinal ligament for limb salvage had an intact limb up to that time. The limb salvage rates were significantly better after femoropopliteal bypass than after a small-vessel bypass or an axillopopliteal bypass (Figure 26-11). Even though all operations were performed because the limb was threatened, limb salvage rates (Figure 26-11) could not be equated with bypass patency rates (Figure 26-12). In some patients, gangrene and infection had been healed by the original operation and the limb remained intact when the bypass thrombosed. Moreover, in many instances when the limb was rethreatened, bypass patency could be restored by appropriate reoperation. This was particularly common if the original procedure had been a femoropopliteal bypass (5,36,37,52). On the other hand, limb salvage rates could be rendered lower than bypass patency rates if a major amputation was required despite a patent arterial reconstruction.

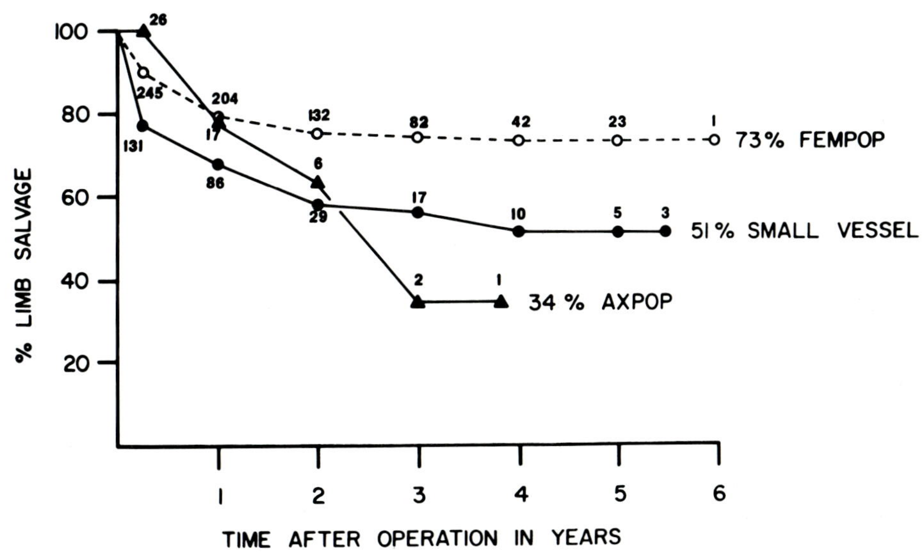

FIGURE 26-11. Cumulative life-table limb salvage rates for 318 femoropopliteal, 204 small-vessel, and 29 axillopopliteal bypasses performed for limb-threatening arteriosclerosis. The number with each point indicates the number of cases observed with intact limbs for that length of time. [From Veith, Gupta, Samson, et al. (5) with permission.]

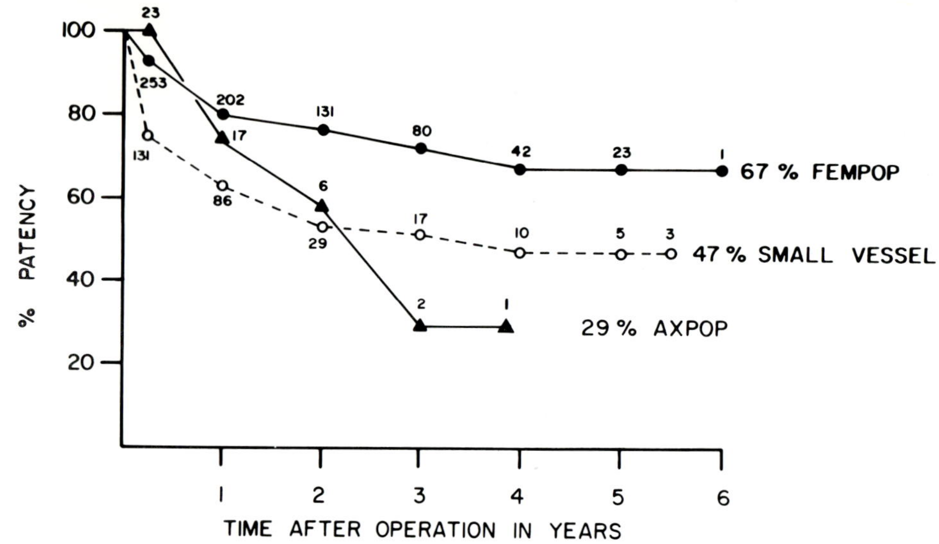

FIGURE 26-12. Cumulative life-table patency rates of 318 femoropopliteal, 204 small-vessel, and 29 axillopopliteal bypasses performed for limb-threatening infrainguinal arteriosclerosis. The number with each point indicates the number of cases observed to be patent for that length of time. [From Veith, Gupta, Samson, et al. (5) with permission.]

PATENCY OF ARTERIAL RECONSTRUCTIVE OPERATIONS

The cumulative life-table patency rates for reconstructive arterial operations are shown in Figure 26-12. Patency rates were significantly better for femoropopliteal bypasses than for small-vessel or axillopopliteal bypasses ($p < 0.01$). Our small-vessel bypass patency rate was not affected by age, sex, hypertensive or diabetic status, or previous ipsilateral bypass. In contrast to reports from other groups, an incomplete plantar arch, a heavily calcified bypass insertion site, an unusable saphenous vein, and a very low ankle pressure did not preclude long-term success, although these factors were associated with a somewhat higher early closure rate (53).

ANGIOPLASTY DURABILITY

Eleven percent of our iliac angioplasties and 8 percent of our femoropopliteal angioplasties were initially unsuccessful (45). If one considers the durability of those angioplasties that were initially successful, cumulative life-table patency at 4 years was 78 percent for the iliac angioplasties and 50 percent for the femoropopliteal angioplasties (45). Repeat angioplasty after late failure had a poor durable success record, and we no longer consider secondary angioplasty with enthusiasm. However, appropriate surgery when an angioplasty failed and a limb was rethreatened resulted in protracted limb salvage in more than 70 percent of cases. Generally, the operative procedure was the same one that would have been performed had the angioplasty not been selected as the initial interventional treatment (45). These facts, coupled with our angioplasty mortality rate of 1 to 2 percent in this elderly, sick group of patients, indicate that the risk of angioplasty failure is not excessive. We therefore continue to regard percutaneous transluminal angioplasty, when performed by a committed radiology-surgery team, as an important part of an aggressive approach to salvaging limbs.

REOPERATIONS

Our past policy of reoperating on all thrombosed *small-vessel* and *axillopopliteal bypasses,* if and when the thrombosis was associated with a threat to the limb, has not resulted in any operative deaths, but has generally been disappointing. The majority of such thromboectomized grafts occluded within a few days, weeks, or months. In occasional instances, comprising approximately 15 to 25 percent of such reoperated cases, patency was restored and persisted over 3 years. Our present policy is to attempt one thrombectomy of a failed small-vessel bypass only if the limb is rethreatened and only if it is not possible to do an entirely new bypass to another unoperated segment of an infrapopliteal artery. Our results with such secondary small-vessel bypasses have not differed greatly from those of primary procedures, although others have not had a similar experience.

The results of aggressive reoperation for failed vein, PTFE, and umbilical vein *femoropopliteal bypasses* have been surprisingly good (5,36,37,54). In our series of 318 femoropopliteal bypasses, 13 failed *during the first month after operation* and all were treated by reoperation. There was one postoperative death and two late deaths among the patients with patent bypasses, 3 and 14 months after operation. Eight of the 10 other bypasses have been patent for 2 to 44 months (mean: 25 months). The ninth patient has a viable limb 26 months after the original operation, although the graft rethrombosed 1 year ago, and the tenth patient also has a viable limb 4 months after the original operation, although her graft reoccluded 2 months after her reoperation.

Thirty-nine of our femoropopliteal bypasses failed *more than 1 month after operation* and were considered for aggressive reoperation. A conservative approach to a failed bypass that did not place the limb in jeopardy has been justified by the continued viability for 2 to 72 months of all 8 limbs in this category. Reoperation was performed on the remaining 31 patients with threatened limbs. In 28 patients, bypass patency was reestab-

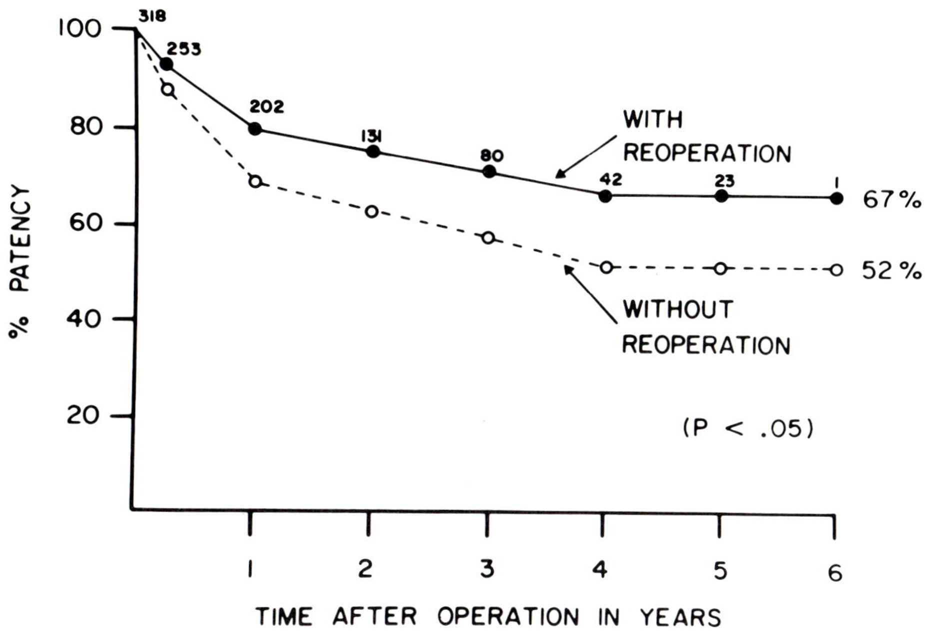

FIGURE 26-13. Cumulative life-table patency rates of 318 femoropopliteal bypasses performed for limb salvage. The upper curve (*secondary patency*) was calculated without regard to whether or not a reoperation was required to maintain patency. The lower curve (*primary patency*) was calculated on the basis of time to first bypass occlusion even if reoperation restored patency. The number with each point indicates the number of cases observed to be patent for that length of time. [From Veith, Gupta, Samson, et al. (5) with permission.]

lished for at least 2 months. In 20 patients, graft patency has persisted until death or the present. The range of patency after reoperation in this group of 20 patients is 2 to 48 months, with a mean of over 17 months, although 7 patients have required a secondary reoperation to maintain bypass patency and limb viability. Sixteen grafts have remained open more than 1 year after reoperation. Only 8 of the 39 patients in whom late graft occlusion occurred ultimately required a major amputation, and in all but two instances this could be successfully performed below the knee. One of the 31 patients died within 1 month of the reoperation.

The sustained effectiveness of appropriate reoperations when limb salvage femoropopliteal bypasses fail in the early or late postoperative period is illustrated by Figure 26-13, which shows that reoperation increased overall patency rates by 15 percent at 5 years. Limb salvage rates were also increased by 15 percent. The efficacy of such reoperations in maintaining durable patency is further shown by the cumulative life-table 4-year patency rate of 56 percent for our 44 femoropopliteal bypasses requiring reoperation for thrombosis. Limb salvage rates were even higher. Similar patency rates and limb salvage rates have also been achieved by Whittemore and his colleagues who employed reoperations in the management of a group of patients with failed vein femoropopliteal bypasses and threatened limbs (37). Both Whittemore's group and we have found that detection of *failing* reconstructions *before* graft thrombosis has occurred permits simpler corrective measures to be used and results in much better long-term graft patency and limb salvage (37,40).

Although Craver and his colleagues showed that reoperation for early postoperative thrombosis of femoropopliteal vein grafts was associated with poor long-term patency rates (55), we have found this not to be the case with PTFE bypasses (36); and Whittemore and his associates have reported similar protracted successes after reoperation for failure of saphenous vein femoropopliteal grafts (37). Appropriate use of intraoperative angiography and other technical details of these reoperations are important in achieving the reported good results (36,37). In both series, clot removal from thrombosed vein and PTFE grafts sometimes allows these conduits to be used effectively for protracted periods if all other lesions encroaching substantially on the lumen are corrected or bypassed (36,37).

ARTERIOGRAPHIC OUTFLOW CHARACTERISTICS OF THE POPLITEAL ARTERY AND PATENCY

With significant numbers of patients now followed 5 years or more, patency rates of femoropopliteal bypasses inserted into popliteal artery segments which appeared on arteriograms to be occluded at both ends were not significantly different from those of bypasses inserted into popliteal arteries that appeared to be continuous with one or more of their main terminal branches. These results support the use of femoropopliteal bypasses to isolated segments of popliteal artery in preference to small-vessel bypasses in most circumstances (17,56). This appears to be true even when the absence of a usable saphenous vein makes it necessary to use a PTFE graft. A major disadvantage of such use of isolated popliteal segments is the high incidence of continued threat to the limb despite a patent bypass. This is particularly common if there is extensive gangrene or infection in the foot (17). In such circumstances, a femoral-to-popliteal-to-small-vessel bypass or sequential bypass is indicated (17–20).

RELATIONSHIP OF POSITION OF ANASTOMOSIS TO PATENCY

In our hands, femoropopliteal bypass patency was not significantly influenced by the position of the distal anastomosis relative to the knee joint (5,17). This was true with both PTFE and vein grafts. However, other authors have observed inferior patency rates with prosthetic grafts extending below the knee.

AMPUTATION LEVEL

When major amputation is required after a revascularization procedure has been performed, every effort should be made to perform it at the below-knee level. This was possible in all our patients who required amputation despite a patent bypass, in 90 percent of patients who required a major amputation when a femoropopliteal bypass occluded, in 69 percent of patients who required a major amputation after a failed small-vessel bypass, and in 30 percent of major amputations required after thrombosis of an axillopopliteal bypass (5). Operative mortality rate for these secondary amputations was 4 percent.

Analysis of Cost-Benefit Ratio of Aggressive Efforts at Limb Salvage

Our results indicate that more than 94 percent of patients whose limbs are threatened because of infrainguinal arteriosclerosis have a distribution of occlusive and stenotic arterial lesions that is suitable for reconstructive arterial surgery which can, in turn, relieve the ischemia at least partially and salvage the limb. The results also show that it is possible to obtain immediate limb salvage in more than 85 percent of the patients in whom revascularization is possible, with an operative mortality rate of less than 4 percent and a low morbidity rate despite the existence in many patients of local and systemic factors which might, in the past, have precluded attempts at revascularization and limb salvage. These factors include advanced age, recent congestive heart failure or myocardial infarction, concurrent malignancy, extensive forefoot or heel gangrene, a contralateral amputation, an isolated popliteal artery segment, absence of a usable saphenous vein, and the presence of a popliteal pulse with three-vessel occlusive disease in the upper, middle, and lower thirds of the leg.

The fact that limbs can now be saved in such circumstances is of interest. Alone it does not mean that limb salvage attempts, which may require multiple operations and prolonged periods of hospitalization to obtain a healed foot, are justified in this group of patients whose life expectancy is known to be poor. Is the cost-to-benefit ratio such that attempts at limb salvage are worthwhile in these patients?

This is a difficult question to answer with certainty since many factors are involved. These include the surgeon's results as well as the surgeon's and patient's philosophy and perspective on subjective factors such as quality of life and the ability of the patient to live and function independently. However, certain objective parameters are relevant. Among these are the durability of limb salvage in surviving patients and the longevity of the patients. Figure 26-9 is an index of patient longevity. Figure 26-10 is a measure of the durability of limb salvage in surviving patients. Of the 48 percent of patients who survived 5 years after operation, two-thirds retained their limb at least that long. It is also relevant to know that of every 100 patients who underwent operation, 68 lived at least 1 year after operation with an intact limb, and 54 lived at least 2 years with a viable, usable extremity (5). Moreover, of the 52 percent of the patients who died within 5 years, 88 percent (range: 81 to 95 percent) retained the salvaged limb until they died (Figure 26-14). Both we and almost all of our patients believe that these benefits outweigh the risks and costs of an aggressive attempt at limb salvage, even if this attempt entails a lengthy period of hospitalization with several operative procedures to achieve a healed foot. Similar conclusions have been reached by Reichle and Tyson, by Maini and Mannick, and by Perdue and his colleagues in their analyses of patients with limb-threatening ischemia (50,57,58).

A case can also be made for performing a primary below-knee amputation in these patients, and relatively rapid rehabilitation may be achieved with such a procedure (15). However, our experience has shown that the older, poor-risk patients do not ambulate easily or quickly with a below-knee prosthesis. Such patients may never walk, and, if they do, they may require 2 or 3 months of institutional training to learn. For some patients, limb salvage offers the only opportunity for them to care for themselves, maintain their independence, and avoid permanent admission to an institution. Furthermore, in many patients the opposite limb soon becomes threatened because of the symmetry of the disease process, and salvage of at least one limb is critical for the patient to maintain independence. Finally, the point has been made that unsuccessful attempts at limb salvage result in a high incidence of loss of the knee (15,49,59). Our data fail to confirm this except after failed axillopopliteal bypass, a procedure performed in patients with the most advanced disease. Thus, we believe that limb salvage should be attempted if suitable vessels for revascularization are present, unless the patient has severe organic mental syndrome or gangrene and infection proximal to the midfoot.

ECONOMIC IMPACT OF LIMB SALVAGE

The dollar cost of our aggressive approach to salvage limbs is high, with a mean cost of $19,000 for femoropopliteal bypass and $29,000 for small-vessel bypass. These figures include all physician, hospital, and rehabilitation costs, including those of reoperations. On the other hand, the mean total cost of below-knee amputation, which in 26 percent of our patients resulted in failed rehabilitation with a need for chronic institutional care or professional assistance at home, was $27,000. Thus, limb salvage surgery is expensive, but no more so than the less attractive alternative of amputation (60).

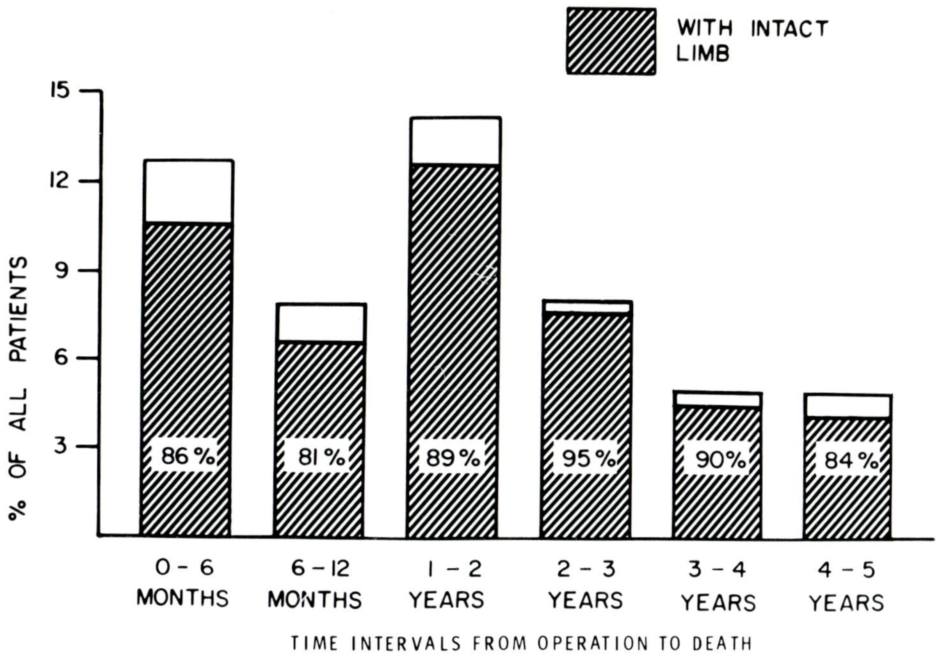

FIGURE 26-14. Percentage of all patients who underwent limb salvage attempts and who died in the various intervals after operation. The cross-hatched areas indicate the proportion of these patients who died without losing their previously threatened limb.

New Developments

Clearly all the principles and practices outlined thus far describe our present attitudes toward the treatment of a complex disease process. As we have tried to point out, many of these attitudes are controversial. More importantly, they are all in a state of constant evolution. As more data and newer methodology become available, our attitudes and those of others interested in the problems caused by femoral-popliteal-tibial arteriosclerosis should and will change. In this section we will describe briefly some of the new developments that have the greatest likelihood of leading to future therapeutic improvements.

DIGITAL (COMPUTER-ASSISTED) VENOUS ANGIOGRAPHY

This method of visualizing the arterial tree using computer-augmented imaging after a central venous injection of contrast medium is gaining increasing popularity since it avoids some of the risks associated with an arterial puncture. It is not yet of great utility as a guide to the treatment of infrainguinal arteriosclerosis because the field of visualization is small and the resolution less than that of the standard arteriography already described. Digital studies have been and may become increasingly useful in assessing graft patency and following patterns of disease progression at and just proximal and distal to anastomotic sites. Moreover, digital image augmentation may improve the visualization of distal small arteries following an intraarterial contrast injection, although we have seldom found it necessary for these purposes. More experience with improved techniques will have to accrue before the role of digital angiography in this field can be assessed with certainty.

IMPROVEMENTS IN ARTERIAL PROSTHETICS

As already mentioned, PTFE grafts currently appear to be the best alternative arterial prosthetic if autologous saphenous vein is unavailable. Many other prosthetics are being evaluated and have shown experimental promise. Among these are the *tanned umbilical vein graft* (32), *externally supported fabric grafts* (61), and the *modified collagen tube graft* (62). Although some promising clinical results have been reported with the umbilical vein graft, more data with careful, prolonged periods of observation are needed before the role and value of all these grafts are known. Clearly, it is unwise to use these or other prosthetics in preference to ipsilateral autologous saphenous vein until appropriate studies comparing the prosthetic to vein have been completed. Many groups, including our own, find it too easy to succumb to the temptation of finding a rationale to use a prosthetic graft preferentially. We believe this temptation must be resisted and encourage randomized study of all promising new prosthetics before they are widely used preferentially. Sixty to 80 percent of patients will have a usable vein if a real effort is made to find it (14,49). On the other hand, many patients do not have an adequate saphenous vein and there are disadvantages to using the vein (41,49) so that continued efforts to develop and study better prosthetics are justified.

Upper extremity veins have been advocated for use as a graft when autologous saphenous vein is unavailable. Although the work of Schulman and Badley show that arm veins are clearly inferior to the saphenous vein in infrainguinal bypasses (63), more recent observations indicate that the cephalic vein can be used with good success in lower extremity arterial reconstructions (64). However, it is thinner walled and more difficult to work with than is the saphenous vein. On the basis of this work and the high degree of symmetry in infrainguinal arteriosclerosis, we believe it is presently justified to use a prosthetic graft in the femoropopliteal position if the ipsilateral saphenous vein is unsuitable or unavailable. For infrapopliteal bypasses, every effort should be made to find usable autogenous vein, although it is still doubtful whether it should ever be obtained from the opposite lower extremity except in young patients.

Endothelial seeding of prosthetic grafts is probably the most important recent development in vascular prosthetics. Methods have been developed to seed fabric prostheses and expanded PTFE grafts with autologous endothelial cells (65). These cells migrate preferentially to, and cover the luminal surface of, the graft and may decrease the tendency to thrombosis and intimal hyperplasia. This technique offers real promise of leading to a substantial improvement in small-diameter vascular prosthetics.

IN SITU SAPHENOUS VEIN GRAFT

The in situ saphenous vein graft was originally described as an infrainguinal arterial graft by Hall (66). It has several theoretical advantages over the more commonly used reversed saphenous vein graft, although the technique is demanding and requires elimination of all venous valves and occlusion of deep communicating branches. Leather, Shah, and Karmody have recently devised new methods for rendering the valves incompetent, and they report excellent results with this graft in infrainguinal arterial reconstructions (67). Although a number of other groups have reported good initial results, the exact role and value of this technique remains to be determined. Moreover, many patients have usable segments of vein which can be used for a reversed vein graft but which could not be used as an in situ graft. Patients with a short good segment of vein in their thigh who are suitable for a popliteal-to-tibial or a tibiotibial bypass are one example. Patients without a usable segment of vein in their threatened leg but with a usable segment of cephalic or contralateral saphenous vein also fall in this category. (In situ vein grafts are discussed more fully in Chapter 27.)

OUTFLOW RESISTANCE MEASUREMENTS

In an effort to predict which infrainguinal bypasses will fail with greater accuracy than has heretofore been possible, Ascer and his associates have begun to measure outflow resistance during femoropopliteal and infrapopliteal bypasses (68,69). This work, which is based on a simple intraoperative method of measurement, has shown that this parameter is a remarkably accurate predictor of early success and failure. Outflow resistance has correlated poorly with angiographic evaluation of so-called runoff characteristics (68). This probably explains why angiographically determined factors have been such a poor predictor of graft patency (5,17,56). Although of little value in femoropopliteal bypasses, outflow resistance measurements have been particularly helpful in small-vessel bypasses in which they can serve as a guide to which patients should have sequential bypasses and which patients should *not* be subjected to reoperation for early graft failure (69).

OTHER NEW DEVELOPMENTS IN TIBIAL BYPASS

Over the last 5 years, because of some of the promising results already discussed, we have been evaluating other procedures to simplify or extend the limits of operability for limb salvage. Some of these new procedures show sufficient promise to deserve mention, although their final evaluation will await larger numbers of cases with longer periods of follow-up observation.

Tibiotibial bypasses are an extension of our concept of using more distal arteries as bypass origins than were previously thought possible (21,23). All these distal origin procedures allow shorter segments of saphenous vein to be used, shorten operative time, avoid dissection in obese or infected groins, and may have superior patency. We have now performed 19 distal vein bypasses to the lower third of the leg or foot using the infrapopliteal (tibial arteries) as inflow sites (23). Many of these grafts remain patent more than 3 years despite their insertion into isolated tibial artery segments and the fact that they were performed with saphenous veins 2.0 to 3.0 mm in smallest diameter (see Figures 26-2 and 26-3).

Use of heavily calcified tibial arteries for distal bypass insertion sites has been possible with a variety of techniques that include crushing of the involved artery to permit occlusion and suture placement. Acceptable early and midterm patency has resulted (51).

INTRAOPERATIVE TRANSLUMINAL ANGIOPLASTY

This has recently been made possible with a new lumen-seeking extrusion balloon catheter devised by Fogarty and his colleagues (70). This procedure should be useful in patients with combined segment disease. The intraoperative dilatation of a stenosis proximal or distal to an occlusive lesion should facilitate shorter bypasses. Although such procedures have considerable theoretical appeal, their value remains to be demonstrated by comparison with standard operative procedures and with percutaneous transluminal angioplasty combined with standard operations.

Reversed versus in Situ Vein Graft

The concept of using the greater saphenous vein as an infrainguinal bypass conduit, by making its valves incompetent and leaving it largely within its bed, has interested vascular surgeons for more than two decades. Technical difficulties in rendering the valves incompetent and in obliterating arteriovenous fistulas have limited application of the procedure. The Albany Medical College group deserves credit for introducing technical innovations that facilitate the performance of in situ vein bypasses in the lower extremity. Because the in situ vein offers potential advantages and because technical details in its preparation are critical, the editors have included a detailed chapter on this operation. Superiority of the in situ vein grafts over the reversed vein graft has not been demonstrated conclusively, although the data are still being collected and weighed. Meticulous attention to technical details is important to the success of all infrainguinal arterial reconstructive operations. Some of the excellent results from both types of autogenous saphenous vein bypass graft may reflect the surgeon's devotion to such operative details rather than intrinsic superiority of the conduit. From a strictly statistical viewpoint, comparison of current results with in situ methods to historical control data for reversed vein grafts may not be justified. Improved techniques for reversed vein grafting have also occurred over the last decade, and equally encouraging results to those reported in this chapter can be achieved with small (2- to 3-mm) reversed vein grafts to disadvantaged outflow tracts. Thus the question of which vein graft is better in a given patient remains unanswered. Both reversed and in situ techniques have potential advantages and disadvantages, the impact of which will be determined only by adequate prospective, comparative studies. The choice of vein graft depends on many considerations, including the surgeon's training and experience. Some patients requiring a bypass in one leg may not have any vein at all remaining in that leg while usable vein is present in the opposite leg, thigh, or arm or the ipsilateral thigh. Thus, optimal vein utilization and optimal results with infrainguinal bypasses can probably be achieved using a combination of surgical methods.

Conclusions

Infrainguinal arteriosclerosis is a common manifestation of this ubiquitous disease. In only a small fraction of afflicted patients does it progress to the point where a lower limb is threatened. Despite this relative rarity, more than 200,000 patients undergo major amputation because of this disease process in the United States every year. Although prevention of atherosclerosis will provide the ultimate solution to this problem, such prevention is not yet at hand. Until it is, committed surgeons and radiologists, using some of the techniques and approaches outlined in this chapter, can make major reductions in the crippling effects of this widespread disease process.

References

1. Donaldson MC, Mannick JA: Femoropopliteal bypass grafting for intermittent claudication. Is pessmism warranted? Arch Surg 1980, 115:724.
2. Boyd AM: The natural course of arteriosclerosis of the lower extremities. Proc R Soc Med 1962, 55:591.
3. Coran G, Warren R: Arteriographic changes in femoropopliteal arteriosclerosis obliterans: A five year follow-up study. N Engl J Med 1966, 274:643.
4. Imparato AM, Kim GE, Davison T, Crowley JG: Intermittent claudication: Its natural course. Surgery 1975, 78:795.
5. Veith FJ, Gupta SK, Samson RH, Scher LA, Fell SC, Weiss P, Janko G, Flores SW, Rifkin H, Bernstein G, Haimovici H, Gliedman ML, Sprayregen S: Progress in limb salvage by reconstructive arterial surgery combined with new or improved adjunctive procedures. Ann Surg 1981, 194:386.
6. Kavanaugh GJ, Svien HJ, Holman CB, Johnson RM: "Pseudo-claudication" syndrome produced by compression of the cauda equina. JAMA 1968, 206:2477.
7. Goodreau JJ, Creasy JK, Flanigan DP, Burnham SJ, Kudrna JC, Schafer MF, Bergan JJ, Yao JST: Rational approach to the differentiation of vascular and neurogenic claudication. Surgery 1978, 84:749.
8. Karmody AM, Powers SR, Monaco VJ, Leather RP: Blue toe syndrome: An indication for limb salvage surgery. Arch Surg 1976, 111:1263.
9. Haimovici HC, Moss CM, Veith FJ: Arterial embolectomy revisited. Surgery 1975, 78:409.
10. Whittemore AD, Clowes AW, Hechtman HB, Mannick JA: Aortic aneurysm repair: Reduced operative mortality associated with maintenance of optimal cardiac performance. Ann Surg 1980, 192:414.
11. Sprayregen S: Principles of angiography. In Haimovici H (ed): *Vascular Surgery. Principles and Techniques*. New York, McGraw-Hill, 1976, pp 39–66.
12. Flanigan DP, Williams LR, Keifer T, Schuler JJ, Behrend AJ: Prebypass operative arteriography. Surgery 1982, 92:627.
13. Sapala JA, Szilagyi DE: A simple aid in greater saphenous phlebography. Surg Gynecol Obstet 1975, 140:265.
14. Veith F, Moss CM, Sprayregen S, Montefusco CM: Preoperative saphenous venography in arterial reconstructive surgery of the lower extremity. Surgery 1979, 85:253.
15. Stoney RJ: Ultimate salvage for the patients with limb-threatening ischemia—Realistic goals. Am J Surg 1978, 136:228.
16. Mannick JA, Jackson BT, Coffman JD: Success of bypass vein grafts in patients with isolated popliteal artery segments. Surgery 1967, 61:17.
17. Veith FJ, Gupta SK, Daly V: Femoropopliteal bypass to the isolated popliteal segment: Is polytetrafluoroethylene graft acceptable? Surgery 1981, 89:296.
18. Flinn WR, Flanigan DP, Verta MJ, Bergan JJ, Yao JST: Sequential femoral-tibial bypass for severe limb ischemia. Surgery 1980, 88:357.
19. DeLaurentis DA, Friedman P: Arterial reconstruction about and below the knee. Another look. Am J Surg 1971, 121:392.
20. Edwards WS, Gerety E, Larkin J, Hoyt TW: Multiple sequential femoral tibial grafting for severe ischemia. Surgery 1976, 80:722.
21. Veith FJ, Gupta SK, Samson RH, Flores SW, Janko G, Scher LA: Superficial femoral and popliteal arteries as inflow site for distal bypasses. Surgery 1981, 90:980.
22. Veith FJ, Gupta SK, Weiser RK, Flores SW, Samson RH, Scher LA, Ascer E: Short vein grafts in limb salvage arterial reconstruction. In Bergan JJ and Yao JST (eds): *Evaluation and Treatment of Upper and Lower Extremity Circulatory Disorders*. New York, Grune and Stratton, 1984, pp 309–317.
23. Veith FJ, Ascer E, Gupta SK, White-Flores S, Sprayregen S, Scher LA, Samson RH: Tibiotibial vein bypass grafts: A new operation for limb salvage. J Vasc Surg 1985, 2:552.
24. Veith FJ, Moss CM, Daly V, Fell SC, Haimovici H: New approaches in limb salvage by extended extra-anatomic bypasses and prosthetic reconstructions to foot arteries. Surgery 1978, 84–764.
25. Gupta SK, Veith FJ, Ascer E, Samson RH, Scher LA, White-Flores S, Sprayregen S, Fell SC: Five year experience with axillopopliteal bypass for limb salvage. J Cardiovasc Surg, In Press.
26. Towne JB, Bernhard VM, Rollins DL, Baum PL: Profundaplasty in perspective: Limitations in the long-term management of limb ischemia. Surgery 1981, 90:1037.

27. Campbell CD, brooks DH, Webster MW, Bahnson HT: The use of expanded microporous polytetrafluoroethylene for limb salvage. A preliminary report. Surgery 1976, 79:485.
28. Veith FJ, Moss CM, Fell SC, Montefusco CM, Rhodes BA, Haimovici H: Comparison of expanded polytetrafluoroethylene and autologous saphenous vein grafts in high risk arterial reconstructions for limb salvage. Surg Gynecol Obstet 1978, 147:749.
29. Gupta SK, Veith FJ: Three year experience with expanded polytetrafluoroethylene arterial grafts for limb salvage. Am J Surg 1980, 140:214.
30. Campbell CD, Brooks DH, Webster MW, Diamond DL, Peel RL, Bahnson HT: Expanded microporous polytetrafluoroethylene as a vascular substitute: A two-year follow-up. Surgery 1979, 85:177.
31. Bergan JJ, Veith FJ, Bernhard VM, Yao JST, Flinn WR, Gupta SK, Scher LA, Samson RH, Towne JB: Randomization of autogenous vein and polytetrafluoroethylene grafts in femoral-distal reconstruction. Surgery 1982, 92:921.
32. Dardik H, Baier RE, Menenaghan M, Natiella J, Weinberg S, Turner R, Sussman B, Kahn M, Ibrahim IM, Dardik II: Morphologic and biophysical assessment of long term human umbilical cord vein implants used as vascular conduits. Surg Gynecol Obstet 1982, 154:17.
33. Veith FJ, Gupta SK: Femoral-distal artery bypasses. In Bergan JJ, Yao JST (eds): *Operative Techniques in Vascular Surgery*. New York, Grune & Stratton, 1980, pp 141–150.
34. Oblath RW, Buckley FO, Green RM, Schwartz SI, Deweese JA: Prevention of platelet aggregation and adherence to prosthetic vascular grafts by aspirin and dipyridamole. Surgery 1978, 84:37.
35. Chesebro JH, Clements IP, Fuster V, Elveback LR, Smith HC, Bardsley WT, Frye RL, Holmes DR Jr, Vlietstra RE, Pluth JR, Wallace RB, Puga FJ, Orszulak TA, Piehler JM, Schaff HV, Danielson GK: A platelet-inhibitor drug trial in coronary-artery bypass operations. Benefit of perioperative dipyridamole and aspirin therapy on early postoperative vein-graft patency. N Engl J Med 1982, 307:73.
36. Veith FJ, Gupta SK, Daly V: Management of early and late thrombosis of expanded polytetrafluoroethylene (PTFE) femoropopliteal bypass grafts: Favorable prognosis with appropriate reoperation. Surgery 1980, 87:581.
37. Whittemore AD, Clowes AW, Couch NP, Mannick JA: Secondary femoropopliteal reconstruction. Ann Surg 1981, 193:35.
38. Hargrove WC, Barker CF, Berkowitz HD, Perloff LJ, McLean G, Freiman D, Ring EJ, Roberts B: Treatment of acute peripheral arterial and graft thromboses with low dose streptokinase. Surgery 1982, 92:981.
39. Van Breda A, Robinson JC, Feldman L, Waltman AC, Brewster DC, Abbott WM, Athanasoulis CA: Local thrombolysis in the treatment of arterial graft occlusions. J Vasc Surg 1984, 1:103.
40. Veith FJ, Weiser RK, Gupta SK, Scher LA, Samson RH, Ascer E, White-Flores S, Sprayregen S: Diagnosis and management of failing lower extremity arterial reconstructions. J Cardiovasc Surg 1984, 25:381.
41. Szilagyi DE, Smith RF, Elliott JP, Hageman JH: The biologic fate of autogenous vein implants as arterial substitutes: Clinical, angiographic and histopathologic observations in femoropopliteal operations for atherosclerosis. Ann Surg 1973, 178:232.
42. O'Mara CS, Flinn WR, Johnson ND, Bergan JJ, Yao JST: Recognition and surgical management of patent but hemodynamically failed arterial grafts. Ann Surg 1981, 193:467.
43. Gruntzig A, Kumpe DE: Technique of percutaneous transluminal angioplasty with Gruntzig balloon catheter. Am J Roentgenol 1979, 132:547.
44. Ring EJ, Alpert JR, Freiman DB, Oleaga JA, Berkowitz H, Roberts B: Early experience with percutaneous transluminal angioplasty using a vinyl balloon catheter. Ann Surg 1980, 191:438.
45. Samson RH, Sprayregen S, Veith FJ, Scher LA, Gupta SK, Ascer E: Management of angioplasty complications, unsuccessful procedures and early and late failures. Ann Surg 1984, 199:234.
46. Alpert JR, Ring EJ, Freiman DP, Oleaga JA, Gordon R, Berkowitz HD, Roberts B: Balloon dilatation of iliac stenosis with distal arterial surgery. Arch Surg 1980, 115:715.
47. Kadir S, Smith GW, White RI Jr, Kaufman SL, Barth KH, Williams GM, O'Mara CS, Burdick JF: Percutaneous transluminal angioplasty as an adjunct to the surgical management of peripheral vascular disease. Ann Surg 1982, 195:786.
48. Deweese JA, Robb CG: Autogenous venous grafts ten years later. Surgery 1977, 82:775.
49. Szilagyi DE, Hageman JH, Smith RF, Elliott JP, Brown F, Dietz P: Autogenous vein grafting in femoropopliteal atherosclerosis. The limits of its effectiveness. Surgery 1979, 86:836.
50. Reichle FA, Tyson R: Comparison of long-term results of 364 femoropopliteal or femorotibial bypasses for revascularization of severely ischemic lower extremities. Ann Surg 1975, 182:449.
51. Ascer E, Veith FJ, Gupta SK: Use of heavily calcified tibial and peroneal arteries for distal bypass: Techniques and results. Unpublished data.
52. O'Donnell TF, Mackey WC, McCullough JL, Jr, Farber SP, Deterling RA, Callow AD: Correlation of operative findings with angiographic and noninvasive hemodynamic factors associated with failure of polytetrafluoroethylene (PTFE) grafts. J Vasc Surg 1984, 1:136.
53. Scher LA, Veith FJ, Samson RH, Flores SW, Sprayregen S, Gupta SK, Ascer E: Prognostic factors influencing patency of femorotibial and femoroperoneal bypasses. Unpublished observations.
54. Boontje AH: Occlusion of femoropopliteal bypasses (Biografts). J Cardiovasc Surg 1984, 25:385.
55. Craver JM, Ottinger LW, Darling RC, Austen WG, Linton RR: Hemorrhage and thrombosis as early complications of femoropopliteal bypass grafts: Causes, treatment and prognostic implications. Surgery 1973, 74:839.
56. Davis RC, Davies WT, Mannick JA: Bypass vein grafts in patients with distal popliteal artery occlusion. Am J Surg 1975, 129:421.
57. Maini BS, Mannick JA: Effect of arterial reconstruction on limb salvage: A ten-year appraisal. Arch Surg 1978, 113:1297.
58. Perdue GD, Smith RB, Veazey CR, Anslery JD: Revascularization for severe limb ischemia. Arch Surg 1980, 115:168.
59. Ramsburgh SR, Lindenauer SM, Weber TR, Kraft RO, Schmidt CM, Fry WJ: Femoropopliteal bypass for limb salvage. Surgery 1977, 81:453.
60. Gupta SK, Veith FJ, Samson RH, Scher LA, Ascer E, Weiser R, White-Flores SA: Cost analysis of operations for infrainguinal arteriosclerosis. Circulation 1982, 66(suppl 2):9.
61. Kennedy DA, Sauvage LR, Wood SJ, Berger K, Davis CC, Smith JC, Rittenhouse EA, Hall DG, Mansfield PB: Comparison of noncrimped, externally supported (EXS) and crimped, nonsupported Dacron prosthesis for axillofemoral and above knee femoropopliteal bypasses. Surgery 1982, 92:931.
62. Sawyer PN, Adamson R, Bhutt K: Long term function of NCGT vascular conduits in a multicenter trial: Evaluation of physical and chemical parameters. Biomater Med Devices Artif Organs 1980, 8:345.
63. Schulman ML, Badley MR: Late results and angiographic evaluation of arm veins as long bypass grafts. Surgery 1982, 92:1032.
64. Harris RW, Andros G, Dulawa LB, Oblath RW, Salles-Cunha SX, Apyan R: Successful long-term limb salvage using cephalic vein bypass grafts. Ann Surg 1984, 200:785.
65. Stanley JC, Burkel WE, Ford JW, Vinter DW, Kahn RH, Whitehouse WM, Graham LM: Enhanced patency of small diameter, externally supported Dacron iliofemoral grafts seeded with endothelial cells. Surgery 1982, 92:994.

66. Hall KV: The great saphenous vein used ''in situ'' as an arterial shunt after extirpation of the vein valves. Surgery 1962, 51:492.
67. Leather RP, Shah DM, Karmody AM: Infrapopliteal bypass for limb salvage: Increased patency and utilization of the saphenous vein used ''in situ.'' Surgery 1981, 90:1000.
68. Ascer E, Veith FJ, Morin L, White-Flores SA, Scher LA, Samson RH, Weiser RK, Gupta SK: Quantitative assessment of outflow resistance in lower extremity arterial reconstructions. J Surg Res 1984, 37:8.
69. Ascer E, Veith FJ, Morin L, Lesser ML, Gupta SK, Samson RH, Scher LA, White-Flores SA: Components of outflow resistance and their correlation with graft patency in lower extremity arterial reconstructions. J Vasc Surg 1984, 1:817.
70. Fogarty TJ, Chin A, Shoor PM, Blair GL, Zimmerman JJ: Adjunctive intraoperative arterial dilatation: Simplified instrumentation technique. Arch Surg 1981, 116:1391.

Chapter 27

IN SITU SAPHENOUS VEIN ARTERIAL BYPASS

ALLASTAIR M. KARMODY, ROBERT P. LEATHER, JOHN D. CORSON, and DHIRAJ M. SHAH

Removal of a vein graft from its bed subjects it to the cumulative injurious effects of surgical manipulation, transmural warm ischemia, contact with nonhemic solutions, and hydrostatic dilatation (1). With the rapid increase in aortocoronary and infrainguinal vein grafting as the stimulus for the evaluation of these injuries (2,3), it has now been shown that there is widespread destruction of the endothelium with alterations in normal prostacyclin and thromboxane production, thus producing a relatively thrombogenic surface. Furthermore, the rate of degeneration in such veins appears to be inversely related to the subsequent rate of flow (4).

All of these factors may contribute to the initial failure rate of these bypass conduits, particularly when the outflow tracts are limited (5). Although the most recent methods of preparation of excised vein grafts have been directed toward the prevention of these injuries (6), none is perfect. At present we believe that the closest approximation of an ideal conduit, i.e., one with normal, viable, physiologically functioning endothelium and a natural taper, is a vein which has been retained in situ and is minimally damaged during its preparation for bypass.

History of in Situ Vein Techniques

In 1962, Hall published the first series of successful in situ bypasses done by the method of valve excision through transverse venotomies (7). This necessarily tedious procedure was practical only because most of the operations were carried out to the above-knee popliteal artery with veins of large size. By 1973, Hall had developed an instrument for serial transluminal retrograde valve disruption (8), as had Cartier (9) and Samuels (10). Valve excision has now been largely abandoned, as has the method of prograde blind blunt valve fracture (11). However, a continuing experience with retrograde valve disruption using the instruments of Hall and Cartier has accumulated in Europe (12–14).

These instruments appear to have two serious disadvantages. The first is that blunt avulsion of the valve leaflets may cause serious damage to the adjacent vein wall. The second is that both instruments must be introduced and withdrawn through the distal divided end of the vein, which invariably has the smallest diameter and is most prone to spasm. Both factors thus combine to produce the greatest potential for injury to the vein wall. These limitations preclude their use in veins less than 4 mm in diameter.

Valve incision achieves the goal of an efficient and minimally traumatic method of valvular incompetence, by division of valve leaflets in their major axes while they are in the functionally closed position.

Preoperative Saphenous Vein Anatomy

An invaluable aid to all saphenous vein operations and in situ techniques in particular has been the use of pre-bypass saphenous venography (13,15,16). This is carried out by injection through a dorsal vein of the foot and not into the saphenous vein itself (Figure 27-1). With soft tissue radiographic technique, the frequently encountered anatomic variations of this vein are accurately portrayed. The most important of these are a variety of double systems, interlacing networks, and large unexpected perforating veins (Figure 27-2). Such anatomical details can be marked on the limb beforehand, thus greatly facilitating the procedure. However, when unrecognized, these details lead to frustrating or even ineffectual surgical explorations. With the patient

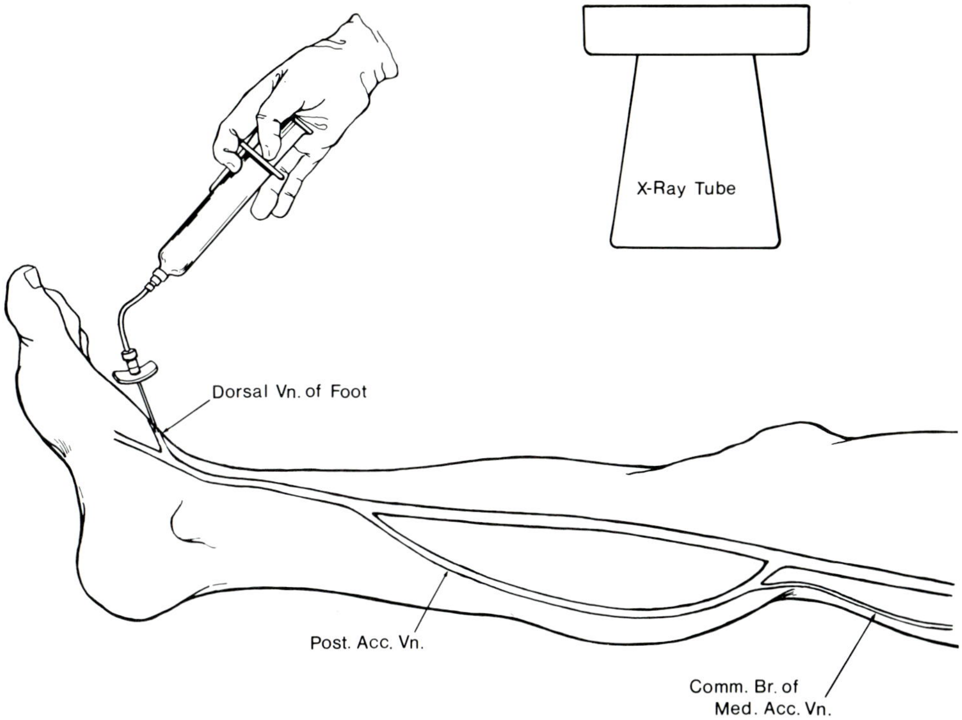

FIGURE 27-1. Technique of venography which is used to determine the details of the anatomy of the greater saphenous vein before operation. Note that the injection is into the dorsal vein of the foot and not into the saphenous vein itself. Note also the common connection of the medial accessory vein to the posterior accessory vein in the calf.

standing, the position of the saphenous vein should also be marked before operation by inducing a pressure wave distally by tapping or brushing the distended vein and detecting its propagation digitally or by Doppler ultrasound methods.

Preparation of the Saphenous Vein for in Situ Bypass

The procedure is readily adaptable to a two-team approach, i.e., simultaneous distal and proximal exposure of both artery and vein (17). The vein is first exposed at the level of the anticipated distal arterial anastomosis by an incision parallel to and 1 cm posterior to the position of the vein. Its size should be determined as soon as it is first identified and before exposure produces spasm, which should be prevented by perivenous infiltration with 1 percent papaverine solution. An acceptable minimal diameter for tibial bypass is 2.5 mm, although terminal segments of 2 mm have also been successfully used (18).

In the groin incision the proximal 5 cm of the saphenous vein is identified and mobilized after careful ligation and division of its tributaries. The saphenofemoral junction is invariably at the level of the common femoral bifurcation (Figure 27-3). Therefore, to enable comfortable anastomosis to the common femoral artery, the entire saphenous bulb is detached from the femoral vein which is repaired by a continuous 6-0 polypropylene suture. Postoperative venography has shown that this does not narrow the femoral vein. The saphenofemoral junction is excised, and the fact that the plane of the valve cusps is invariably parallel to the skin (10) dictates all subsequent attempts at valve incision.

Use of the Valve Scissors

The original instrument used for valve incision was specifically adapted microscissors. Intraluminal access to the vein was gained through its open end and more distally by transverse venotomies at a convenient point proximal to the valve site. Subsequently, the scissors were modified for passage through the larger (>1 mm) branches of the vein. However, both consistent valve defunctioning and instrument maintenance were more difficult, and these have now given way to sturdier scissors designed with a slide action and blunted ball tips (19) (Figure 27-4). The first valve within the vein itself is usually present 2 to 3 cm distal to its bulb and the second at the entry of the prominent medial accessory branch. These valves are identified and closed by gentle distension of the vein through its open end by introduction of a pressurized fluid column. The valves are then incised (19) (Figure 27-5). Freshly drawn heparinized autogenous blood may be best for these purposes, but heparinized dextran 70 has usually been used without apparent adverse effects.

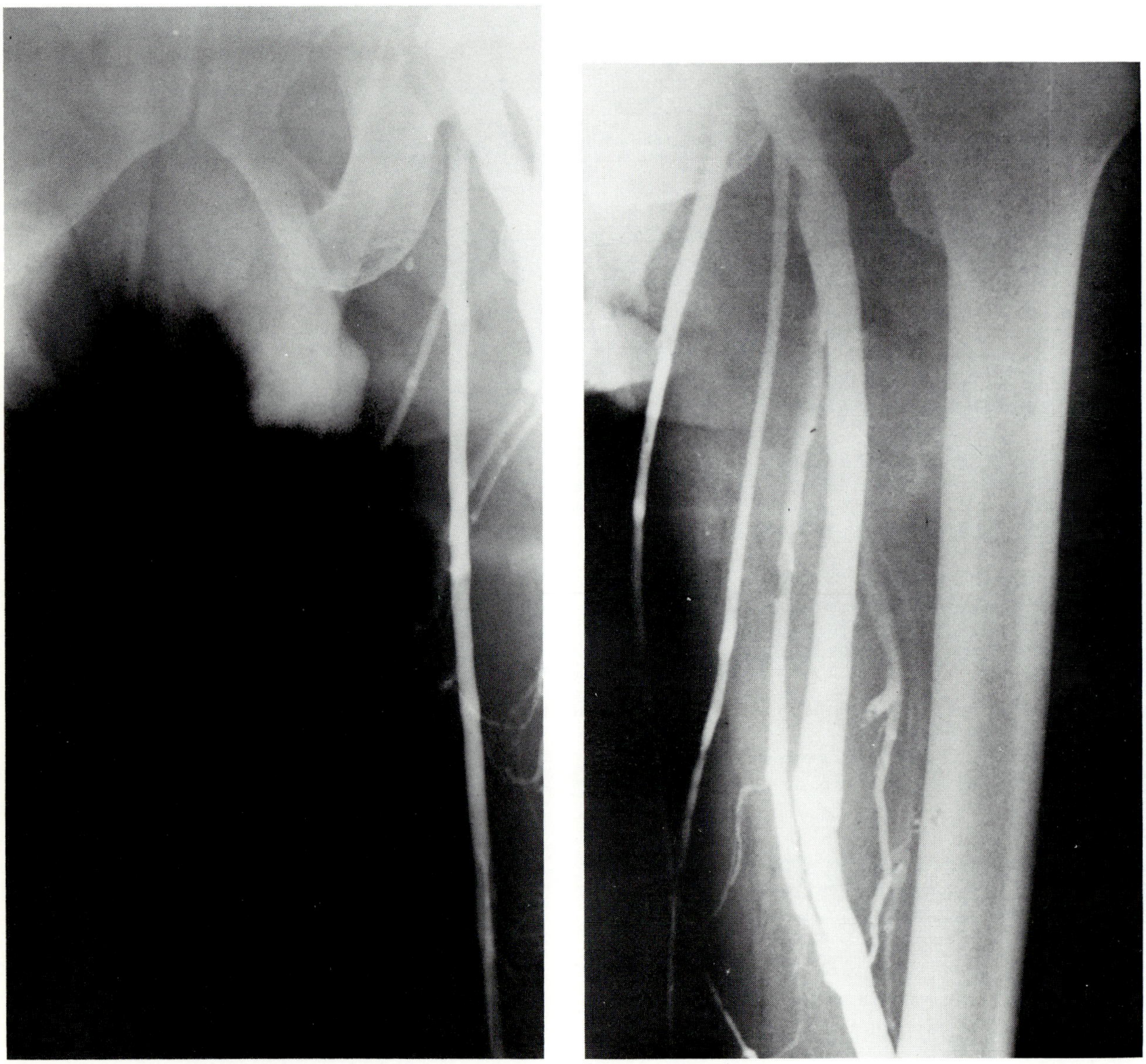

A B

FIGURE 27-2. (*A*) Typical example of a normal single-channel saphenous vein with few branches showing. (*B*) Example of double saphenous system crossing in the midthigh.

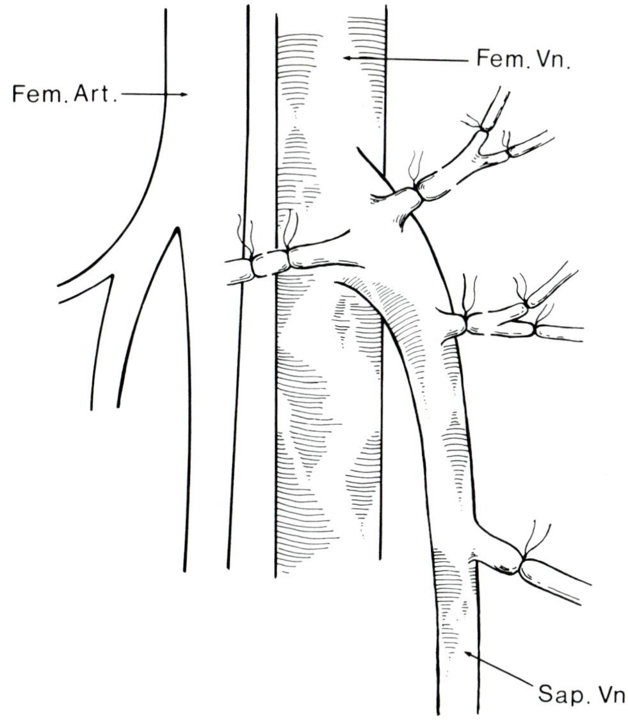

FIGURE 27-3. The saphenofemoral junction has been identified, and all the branches are securely ligated preparatory to its detachment from the femoral vein.

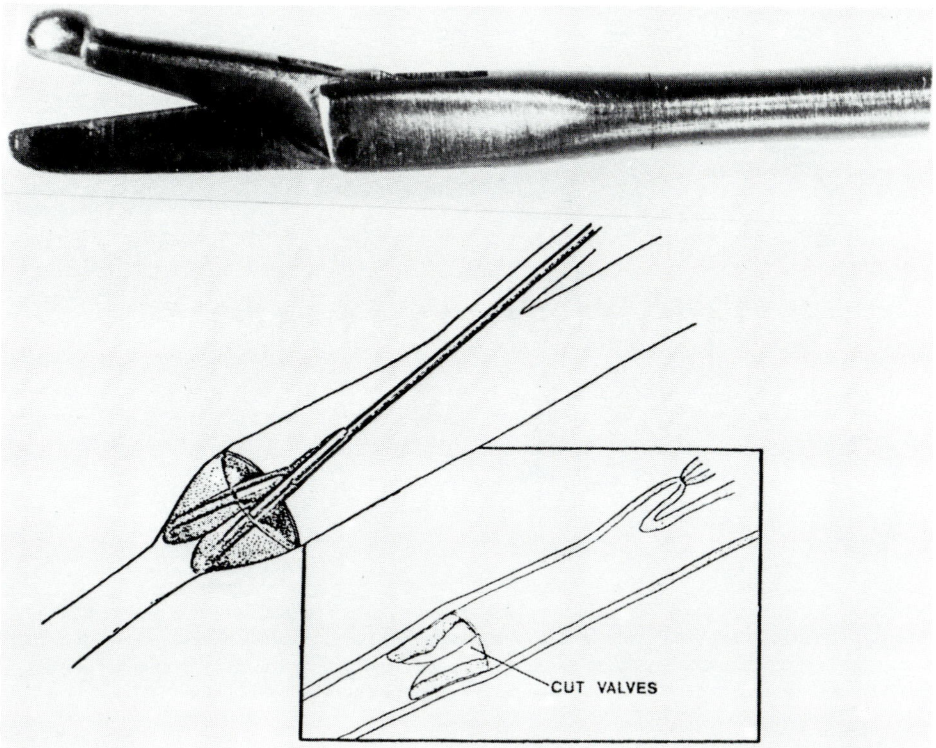

FIGURE 27-4. Current design of scissors used for incision of proximal valves. The ends of both blades are blunt and ball-tipped, while one blade remains stationary and the other moves to effect valve incision.

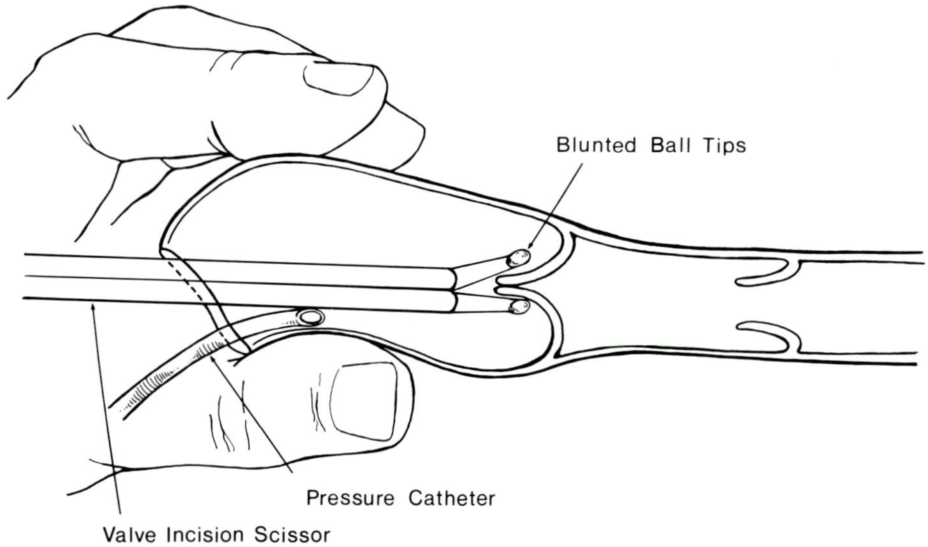

FIGURE 27-5. Diagram of use of scissors. A pressure catheter is used to distend the vein so that it is not abraded by the instrument while the valves are closed. The fingers create a seal around the instrument to maintain the applied pressure while the scissor action on the closed valve takes place. [Copyright © VAMC 1983. Used with permission.]

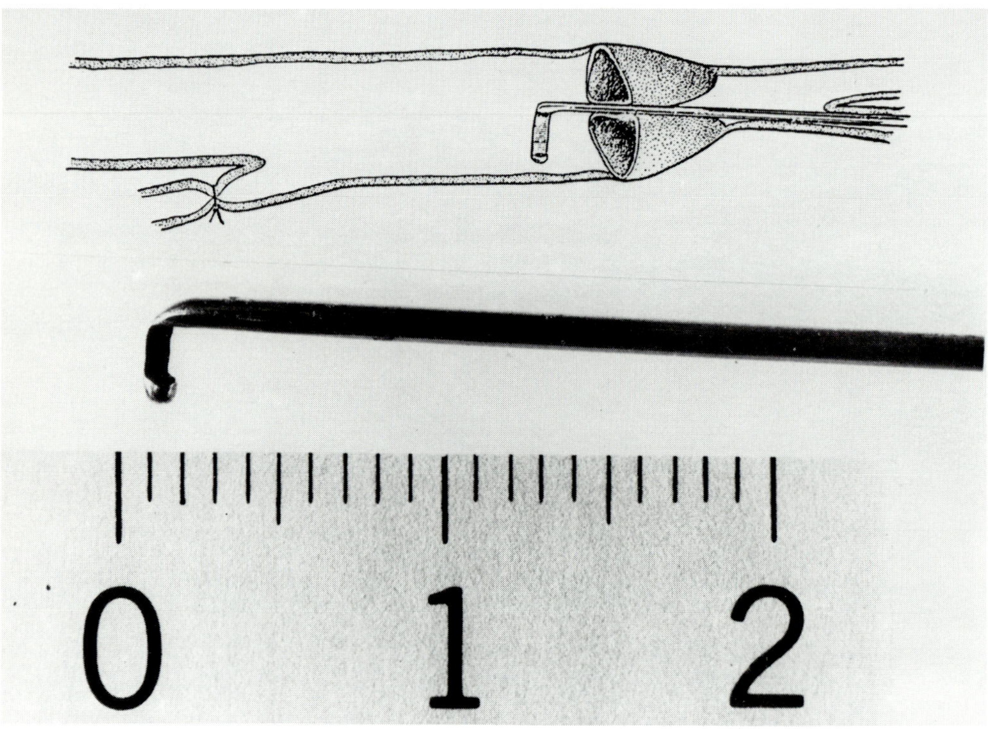

FIGURE 27-6. Photograph of valvulotome and diagram of its use. Note that the valve has been closed by pressure from above and that the vein is distended proximally. The side branch in association with each valve is shown in the diagram. The origin of branches can be accidentally engaged by intraluminal instruments and cause damage to the vein wall. A solution to this problem is shown in Figure 27-7.

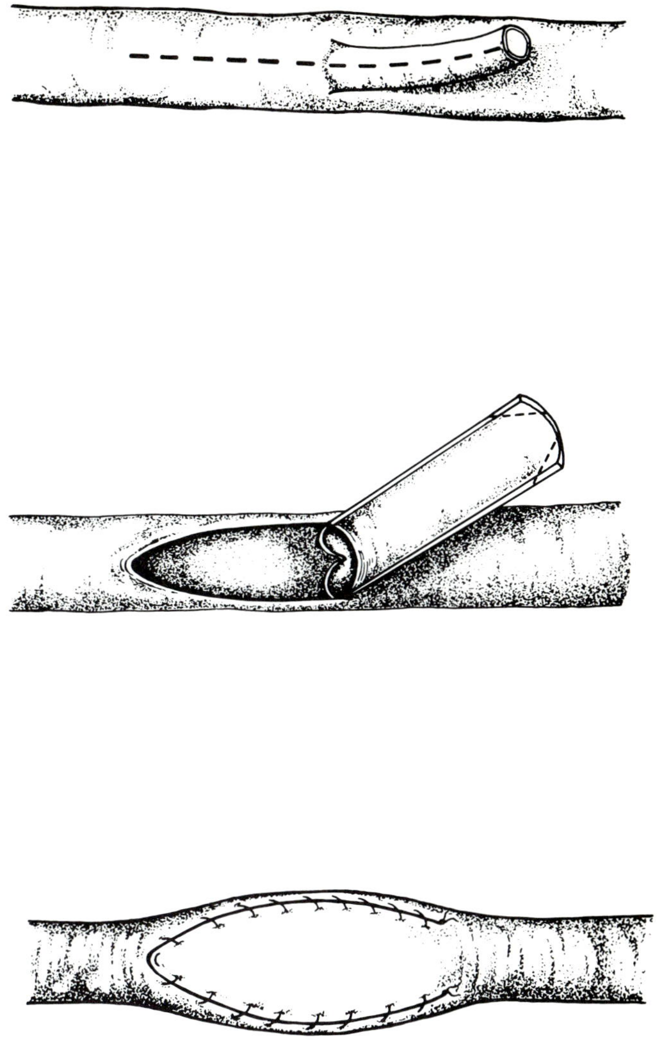

FIGURE 27-7. Use of adjacent vein branch to repair damage to the vein wall or to widen the vein at any desired point.

Use of the Retrograde Valvulotome

The retrograde valvulotome is probably the most efficient instrument designed for valve incision, but it does require surgical visualization of each valve site. It is composed of a narrow (1-mm) springy shaft 20 cm in length with a 3-mm tip, angled at 90° to the shaft and contains a 1.5-mm cutting blade which ends with a ball tip (20) (Figure 27-6). This instrument is introduced distal to the valve through a convenient side branch or through the open end of the vein when it is divided distally. Its size and efficiency make it particularly suitable in veins which are less than 3.5 mm. Surgical exposure of the valve sites is necessary because of the proximity of venous branches to each valve site and the possibility that the origin of a branch can become accidentally engaged by the cutting edge of the valvulotome. If this occurs, downward traction on the shaft will cause laceration of the vein wall. If this occurs, it can be treated by the method of branch angioplasty (21) (Figure 27-7). Each valve should be closed by proximal pressure before it is defunctionalized. Even when the valve cutter is used in the thigh, the retrograde valvulotome is still used to carry out valve incision in the portion of the vein from the knee to the point of its distal transection.

Use of the Valve Cutter

This instrument can save a significant amount of time in the preparation of the thigh segment of the vein from the level of the medial accessory branch to immediately below the knee (i.e., the part of the vein with the largest diameter). The valve cutter safely achieves a more rapid valve incision in this area (Figure 27-8). The concept engineered into its design is that of two blades arranged at 180° to each other in such a way as not to engage the branch orifices (20). It is made of injection-molded polystyrene in two sizes, 3.0 and 2.25 mm, and mounted on a 3 French catheter by means of an internal self-tapping screw thread. The cutter is oriented so that the blades lie at right angles to the plane of valve closure. It is slowly withdrawn distally into

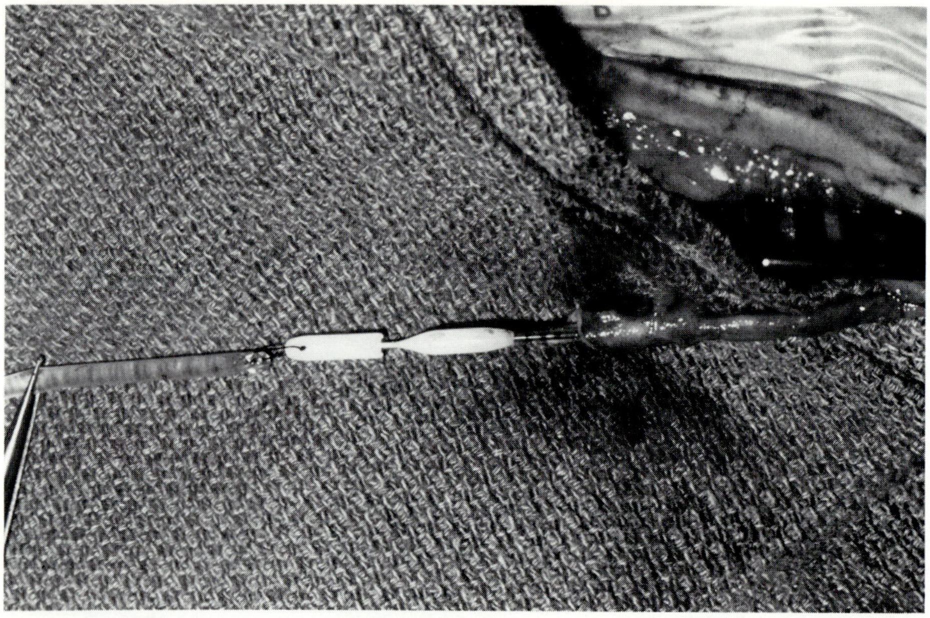

A

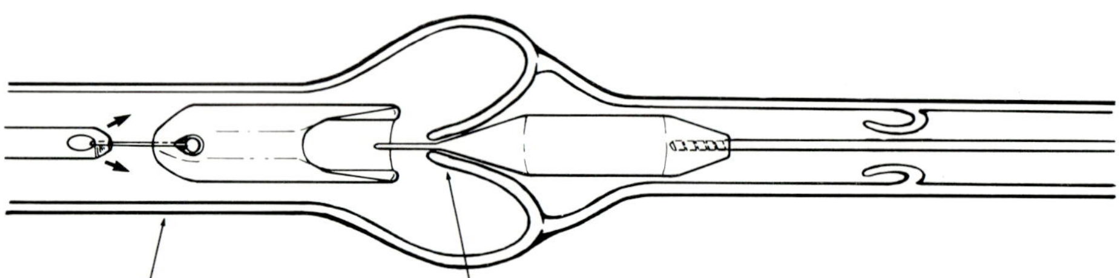

B

FIGURE 27-8. (*A*) Photograph of the extruded polystyrene valve cutter in its present form. From left to right one sees the pressurizing catheter; the attaching suture; the valve cutter itself, which is composed of the follower with two inset blades; a short stem; and the leader, which is attached by means of a self-tapping screw thread to a 3 French balloon catheter stem. The apparatus has been mounted and is about to be drawn into the open end of the vein. (*B*) This diagram shows the action of the valve cutter within the vein. Proximal pressure distension of the vein is important both to allow the cutter to float within the lumen and to not traumatize the walls of the vein while engaging the closed valve cusps cleanly.

the vein; during its passage, each valve is closed by means of the pressure delivered through the proximal catheter and incised by the cutter down to the level of the knee. The cutter should be used only in situations in which the thigh portion of the vein is a single trunk, and its use should be limited to veins which are large enough to allow the instrument to be free-floating within the lumen, thereby minimizing the potential for endothelial shear injury. This is further ensured by the delivery of a sufficient rate of fluid flow, which, in spite of perforator bleedoff, generates sufficient pressure to distend the vein and close the valve cusps for efficient engagement by the cutter blades. At present, these conditions seem to occur in two-thirds of saphenous veins (16).

Early Arterialization of the Saphenous Vein

Our observations suggest that arterialization of the saphenous vein provides both maximum protection of the endothelium and mechanical release of spasm. When only the retrograde valvulotome is used for valve incision, the vein should be arterialized by construction of the proximal anastomosis and release of arterial occlusion as soon as possible to provide these advantages as well as to achieve closure of the distal valves. When the valve cutter is used, arterialization is done immediately after its passage. The proximal anastomosis is made with the common femoral artery whenever possible (Figure 27-9). The already described ''in-continuity'' femoral vein patch is useful in this respect, but if the superficial or profunda femoris artery is to be used as

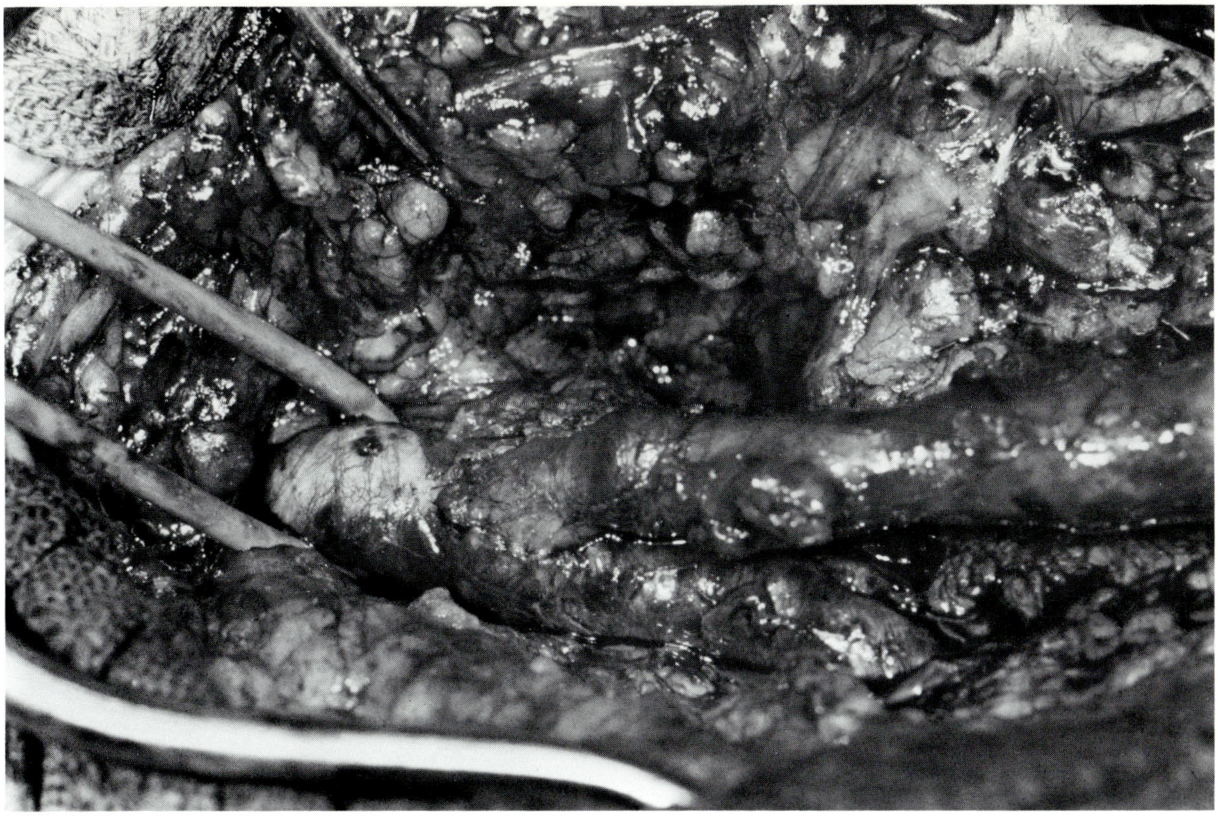

FIGURE 27-9. Photograph of the proximal anastomosis between the common femoral artery and the proximal end of the saphenous vein. Note that the vein reaches comfortably onto the common femoral artery and is easily anastomosed to it because of the close match in size.

an inflow source, then this may not be necessary. Relatively undiseased superficial femoral arteries have been used as inflow sources (30 percent) (22), as has the profunda femoris artery (20 percent), particularly when the common femoral is unsuitable because of calcific disease or previous surgery. Concomitant corrective inflow procedures, e.g., iliofemoroprofunda endarterectomy, are incorporated as needed into the fashioning of the proximal anastomosis. After arterialization of the vein, it should be remembered that its distal pulsations may be considerably diminished by proximal arteriovenous fistulas, particularly those produced by branches which communicate with the deep venous system, i.e., perforating veins. It may even be necessary to occlude these fistulas temporarily to provide a satisfactory pulse. However, the palpation of a distal pulse does not preclude the presence of an incompletely incised valve, the possibility of which should be eliminated by demonstrating unrestricted flow through the open end of the vein for a period of 3 to 5 seconds. However, until completion of the distal anastomosis, arteriovenous fistulas which are present are best left open to allow some degree of arterial flow within the vein. It should also be stressed that after arterialization of the vein, when the last few valves are being defunctionalized, any spasm which occurs during mobilization should be overcome by controlled hydraulic distension so the walls are minimally abraded by passage of the instruments.

Distal Arterial Exposure and Anastomoses

Although lower-extremity arterial exposures and anastomoses have been discussed in Chapter 26, the use of the saphenous vein in situ for arterial bypass imposes certain special considerations. Bypasses to the above-knee *popliteal artery* are not particularly desirable because the placement of an in situ vein graft around the sartorius muscle and its anastomosis to the popliteal artery can be awkward (23) (Figure 27-10). Unless there is no other choice, the anastomosis should therefore be placed in the most distal part of the popliteal artery, i.e., just above the origin of the anterior tibial artery. Exposure of this area is best achieved by division of the soleal tendinous arch (Figure 27-11). This ensures that the angle of approach to the popliteal artery is as small as possible.

The origin of the *anterior tibial artery* can be consistently reached medially through the popliteal fossa, but use of the artery distal to this point necessitates its exposure in the lateral

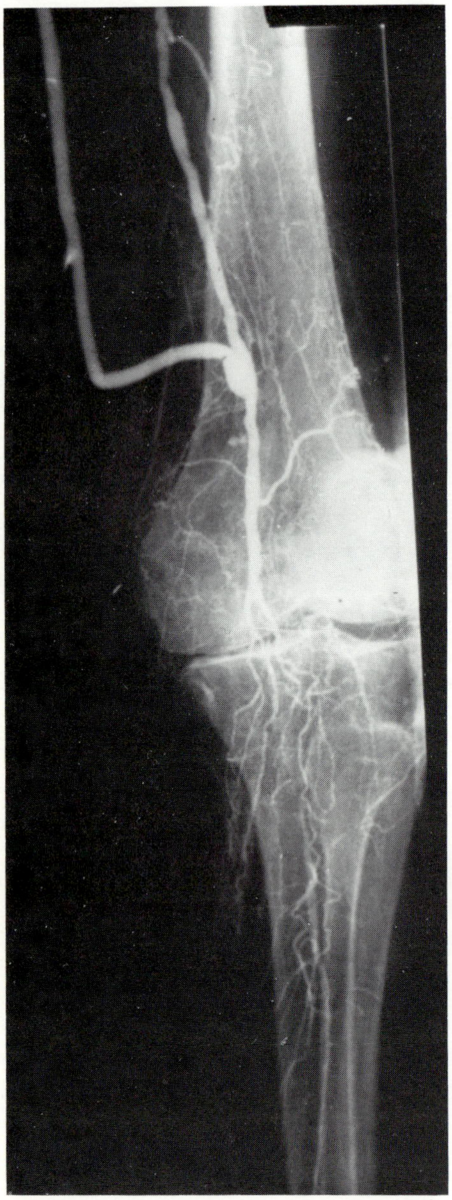

FIGURE 27-10. The difficult geometry of the anastomosis when it is inserted above the knee can be seen from this figure. A considerable length of the vein has to reach the popliteal space around the sartorius muscle.

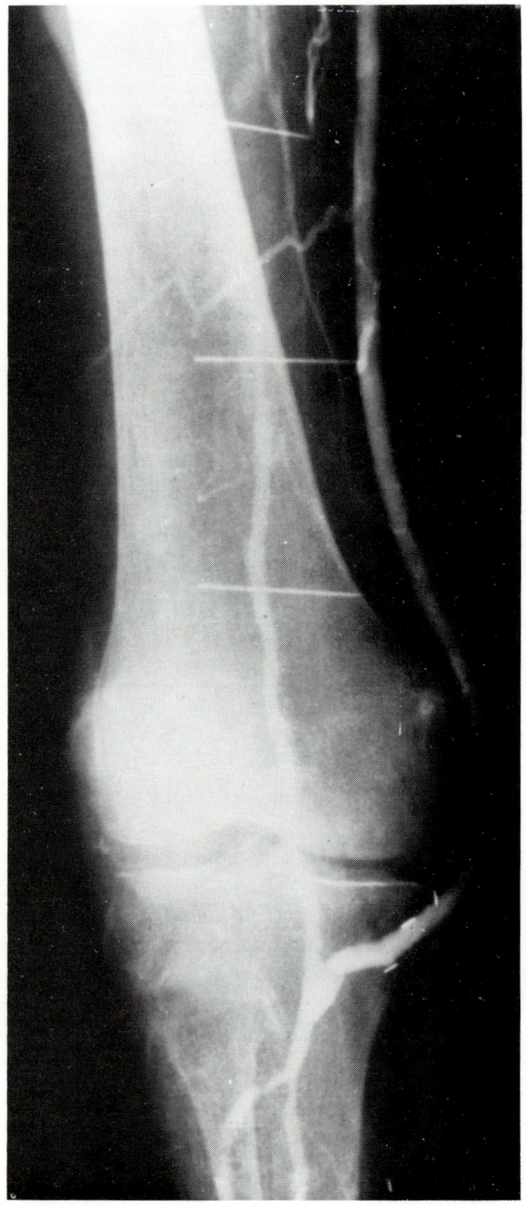

FIGURE 27-11. Preferred placement of the distal anastomosis in the popliteal artery just proximal to the origin of the anterior tibial artery. The smooth curve of the vein is shown here in distinct contrast to that seen in Figure 27-10.

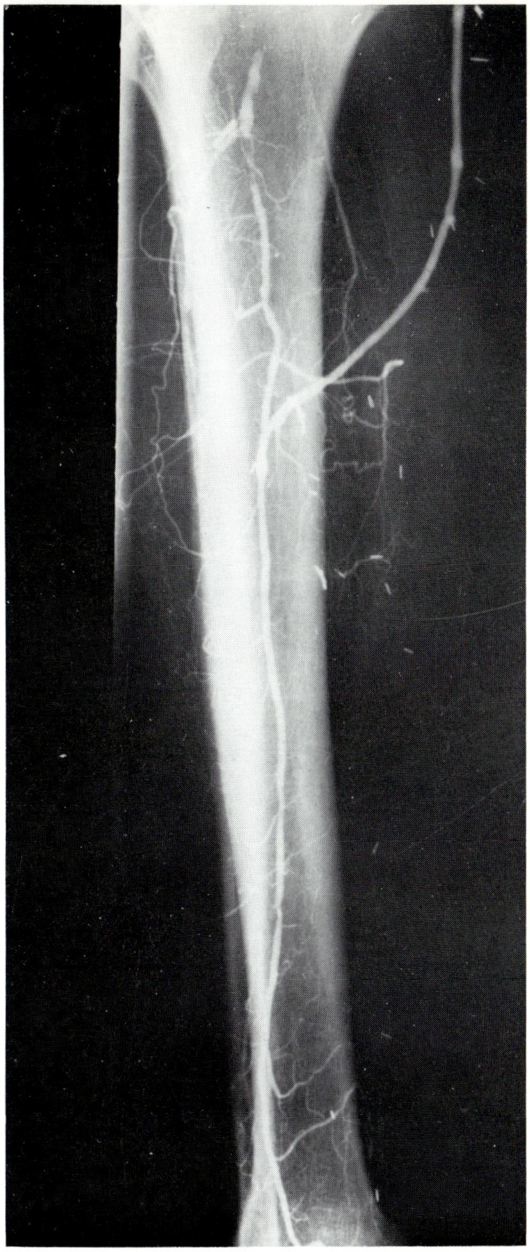

FIGURE 27-12. Insertion of a bypass into the upper third of the peroneal artery. Note that the peroneal artery in this limb is the only patent infrageniculate vessel and that there is a close similarity in size between the peroneal artery (2 mm) and the distal end of the bypass (3 mm).

compartment. For bypasses to the proximal and middle thirds of the anterior tibial artery, we pass the in situ vein through the interosseous membrane, but for its distal third, the vein is best routed over the anterior surface of the tibia (24). Our group has always approached the *posterior tibial and peroneal arteries* medially through the incision which has been used for dissection of the vein. The most convenient bypass is that to the posterior tibial in its middle third. The artery is easily found, and the shortest length of mobilized vein is required. However, we have frequently used the peroneal from the medial approach at all levels with satisfactory results (25) (Figure 27-12).

In our opinion, the distal anastomosis is usually technically easier than with reversed vein or synthetic materials because of the closer matching of sizes of the artery and vein. A loop or parachute technique starts the anastomosis (Figure 27-13) which is completed by continuous suture. As shown in Figure 27-13, small softly sprung clamps (Heifetz, Yasargil) are used for hemostasis both on the artery and on the arterialized vein. Fine polypropylene suture is usually used for tibial anastomoses, which we perform using $\times 6$ optical magnification.

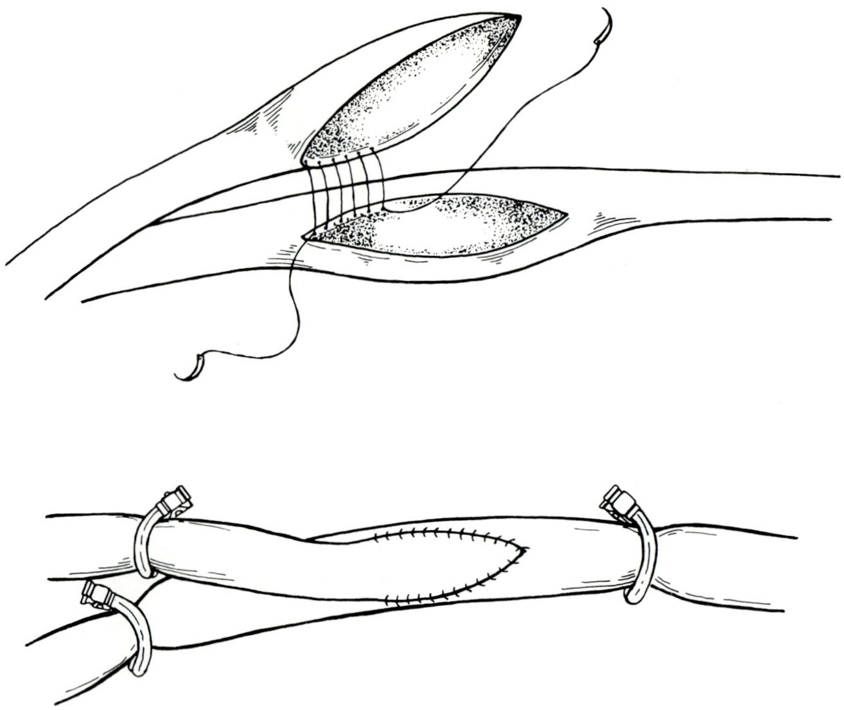

FIGURE 27-13. Use of a parachute technique for performance of the distal anastomosis. This is particularly useful when the space in which the anastomosis is to be performed is limited. [Copyright © VAMC 1983. Used with permission.]

Completion Procedures

The first procedure performed after completing the anastomoses is the location and interruption of hemodynamically significant fistulas; the second is confirmation of a technically accurate anastomosis and detection of platelet adherence within the conduit. These are accomplished by a combination of intraoperative Doppler ultrasound techniques and intraoperative angiography. The method for detection of fistulas by Doppler ultrasound is shown in Figure 27-14. In addition, when the ultrasound probe is accurately placed at the site of a fistula, a continuous or uniphasic sound is heard, particularly when it is a perforating vein. Flow is also checked by ultrasound at the site of the distal anastomosis and proximally and distally in the outflow tract. Unobstructed flow is easily detected by this means, as is flow which is obstructed or nonexistent either at this anastomosis or within the vein.

Technical Requirements or Disadvantages of in Situ Vein Bypass

VALVE DEFUNCTIONALIZATION

Efficient atraumatic functional destruction of the valves which obstruct arterial flow is both the most important and most difficult technical maneuver associated with the procedure. The vein may have a number of valves ranging from 3 to 13, although the usual number for a proximal tibial bypass is between 5 and 7. Valve incision is an efficient technique for rendering the valves incompetent, and the instruments described have increased the ease and speed with which the operation is now performed. Careful follow-up has shown that the incised valve is neither a source of microemboli nor a frequent site of later pathological degeneration.

VENOUS SPASM

Spasm of the saphenous vein is a well-known phenomenon. In excised vein, hydraulic dilatation provides a permanent solution, but the in situ vein retains its neuromuscular activity and thus its propensity for spasm (Figure 27-15). At present, there is no means for determining which patient or vein will exhibit this behavior. All veins are prone to spasm to some degree but in general this is more prevalent and difficult to manage in smaller veins, i.e., below 3 mm. It is better to prevent venous spasm minimizing surgical handling and the topical use of antispasmodic drugs, e.g., papaverine, rather than to correct it after it occurs (26). Apart from its deleterious effect on endothelium

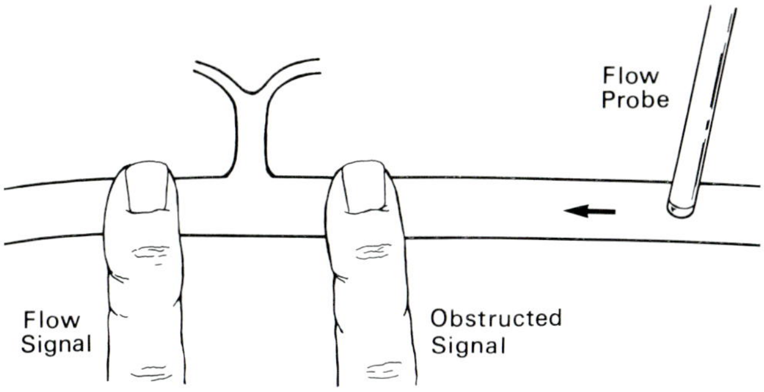

FIGURE 27-14. The use of Doppler ultrasound to detect significant fistulas is shown here. This is the ''null point method'' which is based on cessation of the flow signal in the graft by obstructing it proximal to the fistula while the flow signal persists if the graft is obstructed just distal to the fistula.

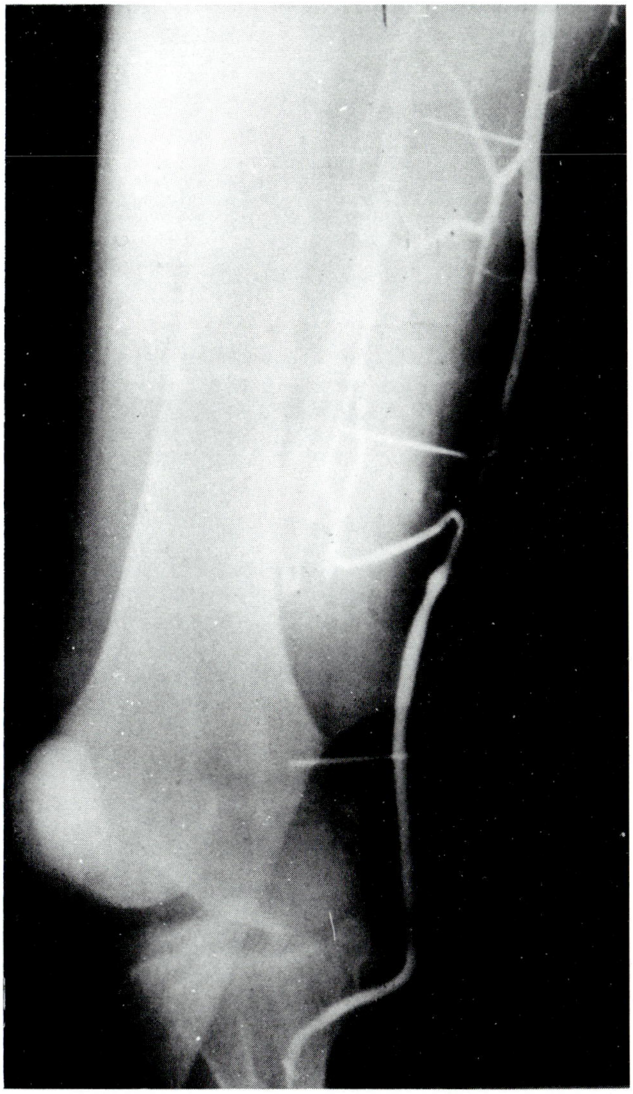

FIGURE 27-15. The intense venous spasm which is occasionally exhibited by veins left in situ after instrumentation is well demonstrated. This can usually be solved by perivenous papaverine infiltration and early arterialization. However, instrumentation through such areas is likely to result in severe endothelial loss with subsequent possible thrombosis.

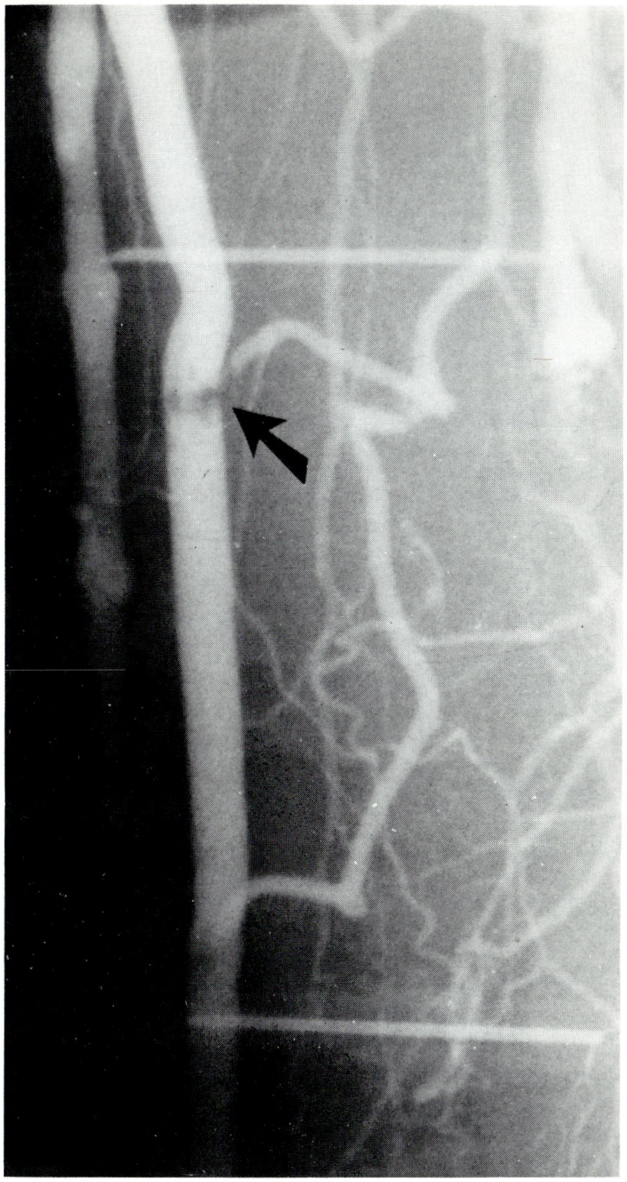

FIGURE 27-16. The arrow shows a small but significant mass of platelets which has been deposited at a probable site of endothelial injury. In addition, several arteriovenous fistulas are shown.

and blood flow, spasm also makes intraluminal instrumentation dangerous because it maximizes endothelial abrasion.

ENDOTHELIAL CONTACT WITH BLOOD

After removal of a vein, blood is usually immediately removed from its endothelial surface. One of the theoretical disadvantages of an in situ bypass is that its endothelial surface necessarily remains more in contact with blood. This, however, is its physiological state and is no cause for concern if this monocellular sheet has not been removed by injudicious instrumentation. Platelet deposition occurs rapidly on these areas of endothelial loss and may subsequently jeopardize arterial flow. Such obstruction can be identified by the diminution of flow by Doppler ultrasound,

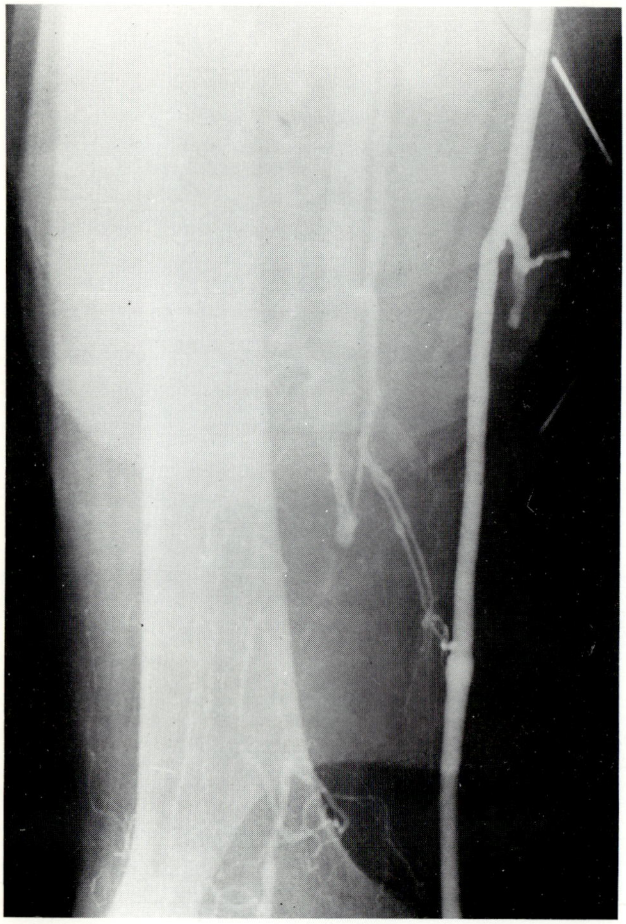

FIGURE 27-17. Example of a completion arteriogram which shows two fistulas via branches. The upper one has only a small outflow tract into the subcutaneous tissue and can generally be left alone since it will undergo spontaneous thrombosis. The lower fistula, although small, communicates directly with the deep venous system and requires interruption because of its propensity to cause swelling of the leg.

the palpation of a solid area within the vein, and/or a characteristic foamy filling defect on the completion angiogram (Figure 27-16). However when the operation is carefully executed, this problem is quite infrequent.

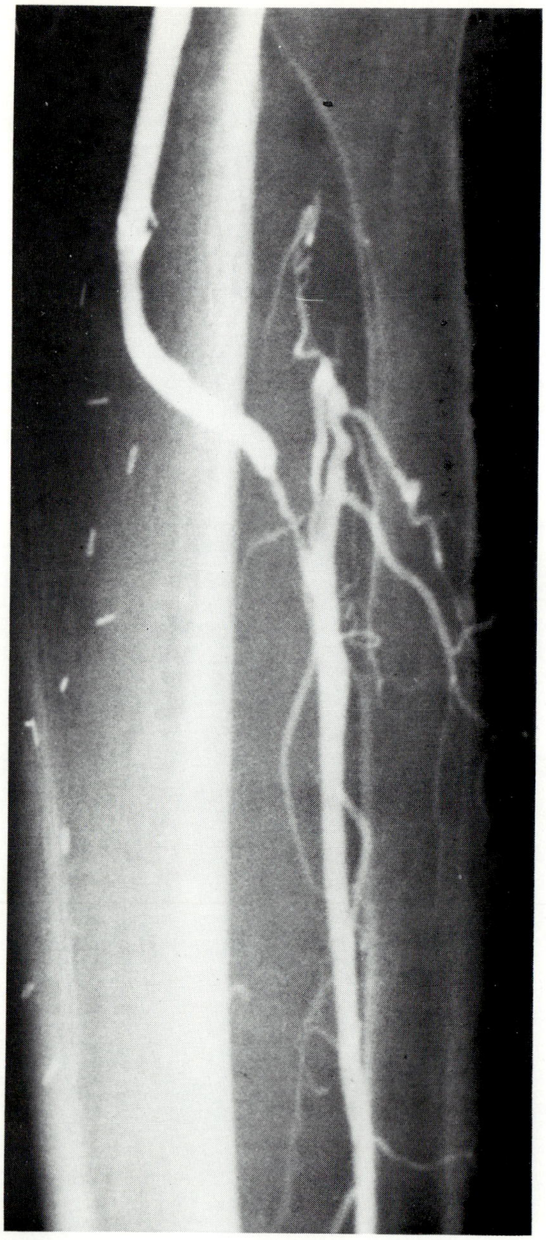

FIGURE 27-18. Typical example of a stenotic lesion just proximal to the distal anastomosis.

ARTERIOVENOUS FISTULAS

Although much stressed in the past, arteriovenous fistula formation is an infrequent clinical problem because most branches of the saphenous vein have competent valves at their entrance into the main channel. The most important arteriovenous fistulas are the perforating veins which, during the operation, may divert so much arterial flow into the deep venous system that the distal pulse becomes markedly diminished. Doppler ultrasound and/or operative angiography will readily identify such fistulas (Figure 27-17). Fistulas into the superficial tissue will in most cases undergo spontaneous thrombosis, and in any event, the degree of flow diversion is generally insignificant. Postoperative fistulas are only of clinical significance when the deep venous system becomes so arterialized that limb swelling or hemodynamic effects (i.e., reduced distal flow) occur (Table 27-1). Their position can easily be determined by either palpation, B-mode ultrasound, or arteriography, and they can be ligated under local anesthesia.

TABLE 27-1. Postoperative Fistulas (29 patients)

No.	Effect	Diagnosis
18	Limb swelling and/or patient anxiety	Stethoscope, Doppler
11	Hemodynamic	Duplex (Angio)

Commentary

As an arterial substitute, the in situ vein graft has many theoretical advantages, particularly when it is to be used for bypasses to extensively diseased infrapopliteal arteries. These advantages include better preservation of endothelial integrity than may be possible with reversed vein grafts. This possibility is supported by experimental observations (26) and by our observation that most stenoses that have been detected in our in situ vein grafts were located in either mobilized end (Table 27-2 and Figure 27-18). Another potential advantage is the distal tapering of vein size which enables the proximal and distal anastomoses to be made between structures that are well matched in size more

TABLE 27-2. Postoperative Stenoses (27 patients)

20/27	Observed within 12 months of operation
15/27	In distal mobilized segment
10/27	In proximal mobilized segment
17/27	In veins 3 mm or less in minimal diameter

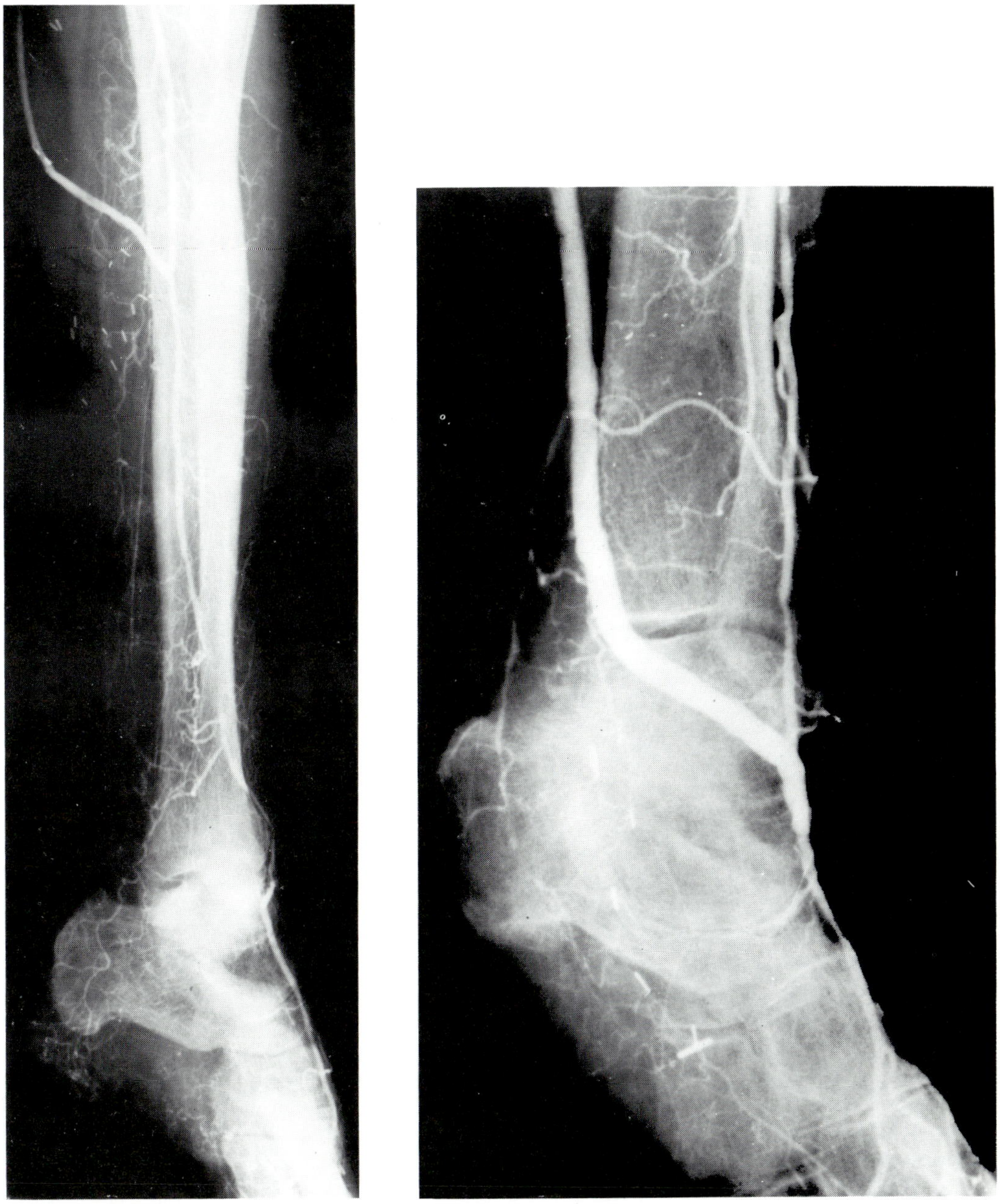

A B

FIGURE 27-19. The use of this method of bypass to disadvantaged outflow tracts. (*A*) An isolated or discontinuous peroneal artery; (*B*) a dorsalis pedis artery with a poor plantar arch.

TABLE 27-3. **Infrapopliteal in Situ Bypasses**

Interval (months)	Grafts at Risk	Occlusions	Interval Patency	Cumulative Patency
0–1	375	15	0.958	0.958
2–12	324	17	0.930	0.891
12–24	146	8	0.928	0.826
25–36	67	3	0.941	0.777
37–48	32	0	1.000	0.777
49–60	22	1	0.938	0.728

frequently than is possible with reversed vein grafts. Possibly as a result of these advantages, we have been able to obtain excellent patency rates up to 5 years when in situ vein bypasses were performed to infrapopliteal arteries in the leg (Table 27-3). Moreover, some of these bypasses were performed using veins that had minimal diameters of less than 3 mm, and others were inserted into outflow tracts which, on the basis of angiographic characteristics, would have to be considered poor or disadvantaged (Figure 27-19) (27).

In view of these results and the potential advantages of using the vein in the in situ position, it is surprising that the procedure has not been employed more widely. Clearly problems with rendering the valves fully incompetent while at the same time not injuring the wall of the vein or its endothelium have discouraged some from using in situ techniques. So also have difficulties in locating and controlling arteriovenous fistulas. Nevertheless, we believe that the possible benefits of in situ vein grafts outweigh the disadvantages of having to master complicated new operative techniques to overcome the difficulties associated with their use.

References

1. McGeachie J, Campbou P, Pendergast F: Vein to artery grafts: A quantitative study of revascularization of vasa vasorum and its relationship to intimal hyperplasia. Ann Surg 1981, 194:100.
2. Abbott W, Wieland S, Anstone WG: Structural changes during preparation of autogeneous venous grafts. Surgery 1974, 76:1031.
3. Brody WR, Kosek JC, Angell WW: Changes in vein grafts following aorto-coronary bypass induced by pressure and ischemia. J Thorac Cardiovasc Surg 1982, 64:847.
4. Baumgartner HR: The role of blood flow in platelet adhesion, fibrin deposition and formation of mural thrombi. Microvasc Res 1973, 5:167.
5. O'Mara CS, Flinn WR, Neiman HL, Bergan JJ, Yao JST: Correlation of foot arterial anatomy with early tibial bypass patency. Surgery 1981, 89:743.
6. LoGerfo FW, Quist WC, Crawshaw HW, Haudenschild C: An improved technique for preservation of endothelial morphology in vein grafts. Surgery 1981, 90:1015.
7. Hall KV: The great saphenous vein used in-situ as an arterial shunt after extirpation of the vein. Surgery 1962, 51:492.
8. Skagseth E, Hall KV: In-situ vein bypass. Scand J Thorac Cardiovasc Surg 1973, 7:53.
9. Cartier P: Personal communication.
10. Samuels PB, Plested WG, Haberfelde GC, Cincotti JJ, Brown CE: In-situ saphenous vein arterial bypass: A study of the anatomy pertinent to its use in situ as a bypass graft with a description of a new venous valvulatome. Am Surg 1968, 34:122.
11. Barner HB, Judd DR, Kaiser GC, Willman VL, Hanlon CR: Late failure of arterialized in-situ saphenous vein. Arch Surg 1969, 99:781.
12. Gruss JD, Bartels D, Vargas H, Karadedos C, Schlechtweg B: Arterial reconstruction for distal disease of the lower extremities by the in-situ vein graft technique. J Cardiovasc Surg 1982, 23:231.
13. Langeron P, Puppinck P, Cordonnier D: La technique de la greffe veineuse in situ dans la chirurgie arterielle restauratrice des membres inferieurs. J Chir 1978, 115:171.
14. Galland RB, Young AE, Jamieson CW: In-situ vein bypass: A modified technique. Ann R Coll Surg Engl 1981, 63:186.
15. Veith FJ, Moss CM, Sprayregen S, Montefusco CM: Pre-operative saphenous venography in arterial reconstructive surgery of the lower extremity. Surgery 1979, 85:253.
16. Shah DM, Chang BB, Leopold PW, Corson JD, Leather RP, Karmody AM: The anatomy of the greater saphenous venous system. J Vasc Surg 1986, 3:273.
17. Leather RP, Powers SR, Karmody AM: A reappraisal of the in-situ saphenous vein arterial bypass. Surgery 1979, 86:453.
18. Leather RP, Shah DM, Karmody AM: Infrapopliteal arterial bypass for limb salvage: Increased patency and utilization of the saphenous vein used in-situ. Surgery 1981, 90:1000.
19. Karmody AM, Corson JD, Shah DM, Young HL, Leather RP: Technique of the in-situ saphenous vein arterial bypass. In Greenhalgh RM (ed): *Atlas of Vascular Surgery*. London, Butterworth, 1984.
20. Leather RP, Shah DM, Corson JD, Karmody AM: Instrumental evolution of the valve incision method of in-situ saphenous vein bypass. J Vasc Surg 1984, 1:113.
21. Corson JD, Leather RP, Shah DM, Karmody AM: In situ vein branch angioplasty. Surg Gynecol Obstet 1984, 159:282.
22. Veith FJ, Gupta SK, Samson RH, Flores SW, Janko, GS, Scher LA: Superficial femoral and popliteal artery as inflow sites for distal bypass. Surgery 1981, 90:980.
23. Karmody AM, Leather RP: The saphenous vein used in-situ for infra-arterial bypass. In Bergan JJ (ed): *Arterial Surgery*. Edinburgh, Churchill Livingstone, 1983.
24. Karmody AM, Powers SR, Leather RP: Surgical guidelines for direct anterior tibial bypass. Am J Surg 1977, 134:301.
25. Karmody AM, Leather RP, Shah DM, Corson JD, Naraynsingh V: Peroneal artery bypass. A reappraisal of its value in limb salvage. J Vasc Surg 1984, 1:809.
26. Buchbinder D, Singh JK, Karmody AM, Leather RP, Shah DM: Comparison of patency rate and structural change of in-situ and reversed vein arterial bypass. J Surg Res 1981, 30:213.
27. Corson JD, Naraynsingh V, Shah DM, Karmody AM, Leather RP: Long bypass to limited tibial outflow tracts for limb salvage. Surgery 1984, 96:756.

Chapter 28

COMBINED AORTOILIAC AND FEMOROPOPLITEAL OCCLUSIVE DISEASE

LARRY A. SCHER, RUSSELL H. SAMSON, and FRANK J. VEITH

Atherosclerosis is a generalized disease often involving multiple segments of the arterial tree. A specific manifestation of the multisegmental nature of this disease is the combined atherosclerotic involvement of the aortoiliac and femoropopliteal arterial segments. The presence of stenoses or occlusions in these two segments is common, and their proper and optimal treatment, although somewhat controversial, remains extremely important in the management of individual patients. Decisions regarding the relative significance of proximal and distal disease may be difficult and tax the surgeon's judgment. Revascularization procedures may have to involve the aortoiliac or femoropopliteal segments alone or in combination. Untreated proximal disease may result in failure of distal vascular operations, whereas treatment of insignificant proximal disease may not benefit the patient and will subject him or her to needless risk. Similarly, untreated distal disease may result in occlusion of a proximal reconstruction or persistence or progression of ischemic symptoms. This chapter will review diagnostic and therapeutic techniques useful in the management of patients with such combined segment arterial occlusive disease involving these two areas.

Incidence

The exact incidence of combined aortoiliac and femoropopliteal disease is unknown, but in most series the majority of patients with arterial occlusive disease of the lower extremities have angiographic evidence of such an association. Femoropopliteal disease is estimated to occur in 20 to 69 percent of patients undergoing aortofemoral reconstruction (1–12). Although this usually occurs in the form of superficial femoral artery (SFA) stenosis or occlusion, atherosclerotic involvement of the deep femoral artery may also occur in up to 15 percent of patients (12).

Patient Characteristics and Prognosis

Many authors have identified a difference in risk factors and general characteristics between patients with isolated aortoiliac disease, localized femoropopliteal disease, and combined segment disease. Although some difference in patient populations between these groups is probable, multisegmental disease may also represent a more advanced phase of a progressive process. On the other hand, some patients may develop advanced femoropopliteal and distal disease without ever developing significant aortoiliac disease.

Normal life expectancy can be anticipated in all three groups in the absence of diabetes and coronary artery disease (13). However, this rarely occurs, and a decrease in life expectancy of 10 or more years has been documented in patients with combined segment disease and coronary artery disease or diabetes (13). Cumulative 5-year life table survival for patients undergoing limb salvage arterial reconstruction for infrainguinal arteriosclerosis with varying degrees of multisegmental involvement has been reported to be as low as 48 percent (14).

Associated risk factors appear to be increased in patients with combined segment disease when compared to those with aortoiliac disease alone. Patients with multisegmental disease were often older (median age 64 vs. 56 years) and had twice the incidence of diabetes (7). It has also been suggested that this group has a greater degree of involvement of the coronary and cerebral vessels than those with localized disease (15). On the other hand, such differences have not been observed between patients with combined segment disease and those with disease restricted to the infrainguinal arteries (14).

Cronenwett et al. (10) reported that women with isolated aortoiliac occlusive disease tended to be younger than those with multisegmental disease (mean age 51 vs. 60 years), were more often normotensive (72 vs. 17 percent), and had a significantly decreased incidence of coronary artery disease (0 vs. 37 percent). However, the incidence of hypoplastic aortoiliac segments or so-called small vessel disease was less when combined segment disease was present.

The prognosis for disease progression also appears to be different in localized aortoiliac and multisegmental disease. Moore et al. (12) and Staple (16) found a definite decrease in the propensity to develop progressive distal occlusive disease in patients with localized aortoiliac disease. Mozersky et al. (17) found a 14 percent incidence of disease progression in patients with aortoiliac occlusive disease alone and a 38 percent incidence of progressive disease in patients with aortoiliac and femoropopliteal disease. Progression of aortoiliac disease proximal to infrainguinal (18) or aortofemoral (19) reconstruction has also been reported. Thus, although some variations in rate of disease progression can be attributed to biologic differences between patient populations, these variations may also represent different stages in a continuum of an ongoing disease process producing increasingly complex lesions.

Evaluation of Segmental Disease

ASSESSMENT OF THE AORTOILIAC SEGMENT

The assessment of the contribution of each segmental lesion to the patient's symptoms is of critical importance in the evaluation of multisegmental disease. The evaluation of the aortoiliac segment is the most difficult and important aspect of this problem (Figure 28-1). Although many patients have some multisegmental arterial occlusive disease, some lesions may be of only radiologic significance, with little or no hemodynamic importance. In patients with combined segment disease, proximal reconstruction alone may be sufficient if inflow disease is hemodynamically significant, but the reconstruction may fail to relieve sympotoms if proximal disease is insignificant (20). In addition, distal reconstructive surgery to relieve femoropopliteal occlusive disease may be doomed to failure if undetected aortoiliac stenosis is present (21). Furthermore, significant distal outflow lesions, particularly in the deep femoral artery, may cause failure of proximal reconstructive operations. And finally, if extensive foot gangrene or infection is present in association with hemodynamically significant disease in both the aortoiliac and femoropopliteal segments, operative correction of both segmental lesions may be required. Although a voluminous literature has attempted to address these issues, the clinical relevance of much of it remains questionable. Several aspects of this problem will be reviewed.

HISTORY

PHYSICAL EXAMINATION
- Pulse examination
- Auscultation for bruits

NONINVASIVE TESTING
- Doppler segmental pressures
- Pulse volume recordings
- Doppler waveform analysis
- Pulsatility index
- Ankle pressure recovery time

INVASIVE TESTING
- Isotope angiography
- Biplane contrast angiography
- Intraarterial pressure
  - Reactive hyperemia
  - Pharmacologic vasodilatation (papaverine)

FIGURE 28-1. Assessment of aortoiliac arterial segment.

A careful *history and physical examination* may help in the assessment of aortoiliac occlusive disease, but several admonitions are in order. Although most patients with significant aortoiliac occlusive disease have thigh claudication, and those with isolated femoropopliteal disease have calf claudication, up to 25 percent of patients may have atypical symptoms (22). Examination of the femoral pulse is important in the assessment of proximal occlusive disease, but it too may be misleading in the presence of obesity, scarring, femoral artery calcification, and even severe distal outflow obstruction (23). Likewise, the presence or absence of an iliac artery bruit may be unreliable. A bruit may be heard in up to 14 percent of patients with hemodynamically normal aortoiliac segments and may be absent in as many as 42 percent of patients with significant aortoiliac disease (22).

Direct *visualization* of the infrarenal arterial tree is critical in planning therapy. Although contrast angiography has been the gold standard for aortoiliac and femoropopliteal evaluation (Figure 28-2), even this may be inaccurate if views in at least two planes are not obtained (20,24). Accordingly, oblique and lateral films may be critical in identifying iliac and femoral arterial stenoses. Isotope angiography received initial enthusiasm (25), but subsequent reports (26) have questioned its value.

In addition to angiographic visualization of luminal defects, hemodynamic information is essential in the evaluation of patients with multisegmental arterial disease. Accordingly, numerous *noninvasive diagnostic tests* have been developed to determine the hemodynamic or functional significance of aortoiliac occlusive disease and to supplement the physical and angiographic examination (see also Chapter 8). Segmental Doppler pressures and pulse-volume recordings are useful in the diagnosis of infrainguinal disease but may be inaccurate in the diagnosis of aortoiliac lesions (2,27). Although it was initially proposed that high and low thigh cuffs would accurately differentiate occlusive disease above and below the inguinal ligament (28), recent studies have questioned the value of even these measurements (29). Determination of calf or ankle pressure following thigh occlusion with resultant reactive hyperemia may also be useful in identifying segmental lesions but is of questionable value in the presence of multisegmental disease (30). Other attempts to evaluate multisegmental disease noninvasively have included the measurement of ankle pressure recovery time after exercise or reactive hyperemia (31,32) or utilization of a femoral cuff technique to assess femoral-brachial pressure indices, wave

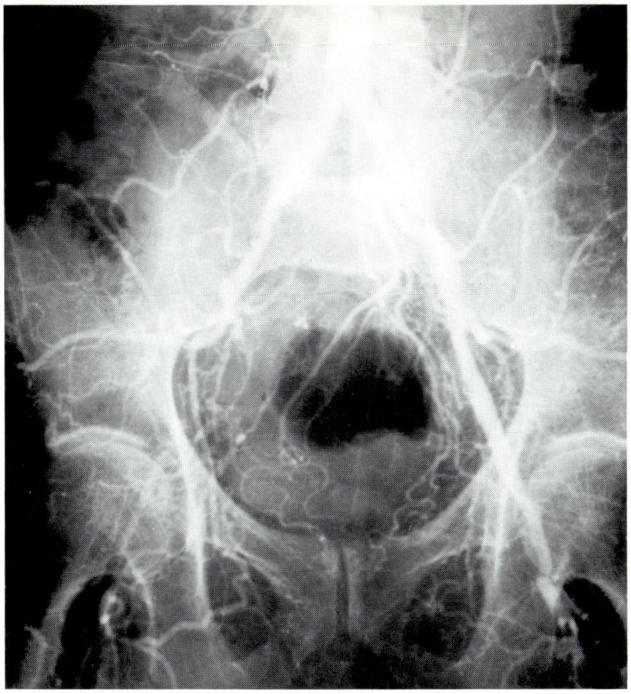

FIGURE 28-2. Translumbar arteriogram demonstrating severe combined aortoiliac and superficial and deep femoral artery disease.

amplitude, and the status of the dicrotic notch (33). Unfortunately, none have proved to be routinely reliable or worthwhile in clinical situations.

Analysis of the femoral Doppler waveform as processed by a zero-crossing detector can also aid in the assessment of the aortoiliac segment (34–36). If the waveform is triphasic and well defined, the proximal arteries probably do not have a hemodynamically significant lesion (Figure 28-3). Based on this, Nicolaides and Angelides (37) have developed a ''waveform index'' and ''resistance factor'' used for the detection of aortoiliac and superficial femoral artery stenosis. The more accurate method of real-time frequency analysis has also been used to assess the spectral broadening and pulsatility index for detection of important proximal stenosis. The pulsatility index (38–41) is calculated as the peak-to-peak height of the wave divided by the mean height. Significant aortoiliac occlusive disease should be present if the pulsatility index is less than 5.5 and absent if it is greater than 6.0. However, the accuracy of this measurement has been questioned in the presence of multisegmental disease (38,40,41). Laplace transformation (38) has also been used to analyze femoral artery Doppler signals to assess proximal stenosis. Although sensitive to even a minimal aortoiliac stenosis of as little as 10 percent (34), Doppler flow velocity analysis has not had the specificity to differentiate mild iliac stenosis from proximal SFA occlusion (35).

Although increasingly sophisticated noninvasive techniques have been developed, none has proved accurate enough to be widely utilized in clinical practice to determine the significance of aortoiliac stenosis in the presence of combined segment disease. We have found that femoral pulse examination supplemented by direct *measurement of femoral artery pressure* is

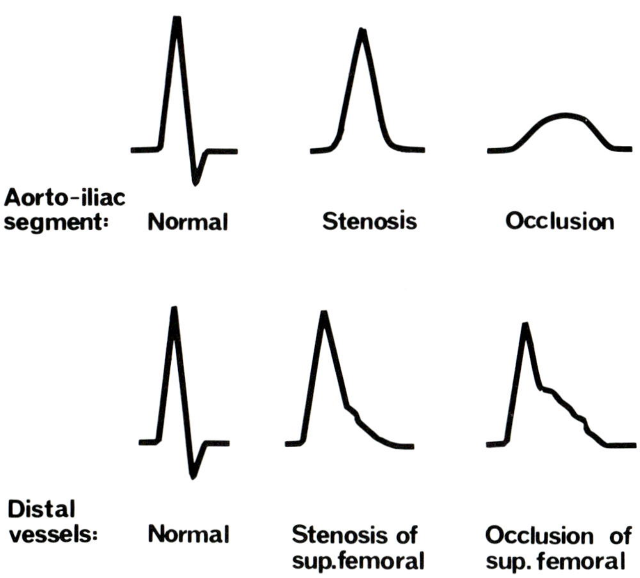

B

FIGURE 28-3. (*A*) Effect of proximal aortoiliac occlusive disease on femoral Doppler waveform. (*B*) Effect of distal femoropopliteal occlusive disease on femoral Doppler waveform. [From Nicolaides (37), by permission.]

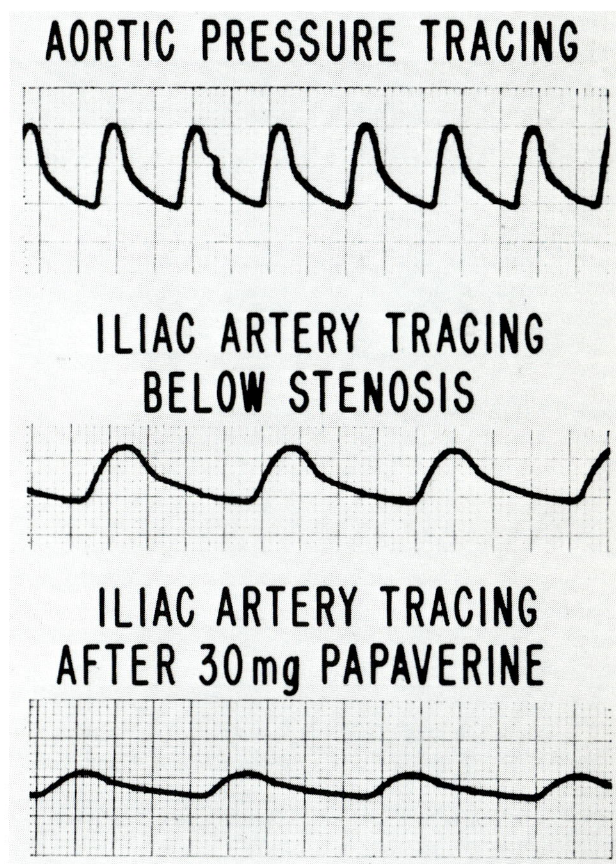

FIGURE 28-4. Direct intraarterial pressure measurement demonstrating a significant iliac artery stenosis and the effect of papaverine-induced peripheral vasodilatation.

unquestionably the most accurate means of assessing the significance of proximal arterial disease (29). This may be accomplished at the time of arteriography (42,43) and may be rendered more accurate by papaverine (44,45) or reactive hyperemia (46,47) induced peripheral vasodilatation (Figure 28-4). A decrease in femoral artery pressure of more than 15 mmHg with or without augmented flow rates suggests hemodynamically significant proximal arterial disease. If therapeutic intervention is justified in patients with this finding, it must first be directed at the aortoiliac segment. However, even in the absence of such a gradient, a distal bypass may increase iliac flow, resulting in a decreased femoral pressure and the need for supplementary correction of the now significant iliac disease.

ASSESSMENT OF THE FEMOROPOPLITEAL SEGMENT

Assessment of the functional significance and relative importance of stenotic or occlusive disease in the femoropopliteal segment is often easier than evaluation of proximal arterial lesions. If insignificant proximal aortoiliac lesions are present with pressure gradients at maximal flow rates of less than 10 to 15 mmHg, then attention should generally be focused at correction of distal disease alone (see Chapters 26 and 27), even if the arteriogram shows extensive stenotic disease in the iliac arteries.

If significant proximal lesions are present, the assessment of distal disease becomes more difficult. The diagnosis of lesions of the superficial and deep femoral arteries is accomplished by combining biplane angiography, segmental limb hemodynamics, and intraarterial pressure measurement when necessary. Doppler-determined segmental arterial pressures and pulse-volume recordings can be used to determine the level and magnitude of gradients resulting from stenotic or occlusive lesions (27). Reidy and his colleagues (2) report a 91 percent accuracy for these hemodynamic tests in the diagnosis of femoropopliteal disease. O'Donnell and his associates (48) utilized the segmental gradient between the thigh, calf, and ankle pulse-volume recording tracings to assess runoff via the femoropopliteal and tibial segments and correlated high gradients with probable failure of a proximal reconstruction. However, we do not believe that current noninvasive hemodynamic tests have significant clinical utility in determining the need for proximal or distal reconstruction in patients with marked combined segment disease. (See Chapter 8 for other views.)

Deep femoral lesions may be of critical importance in the patient with multisegmental disease. Biplane angiography, often supplemented by direct pressure measurement, may be required to accurately define and evaluate stenoses of the deep femoral outflow tract. Archie and Feldtman (45) found that resting profunda femoris gradients of less than 3 mmHg may be associated with angiographic stenosis of 75 percent of the luminal diameter. With increased flow rates, as might be expected after a successful inflow procedure, most lesions with greater than 60 percent stenosis produced gradients of at least 10 mmHg. This reemphasizes the need for careful angiographic and often hemodynamic assessment of this critical vessel. Additional therapeutic considerations are described below.

Treatment

Interventional treatment of patients with combined aortoiliac and femoropopliteal occlusive disease is recommended only for *truly* disabling claudication (i.e., one to two blocks or less or limb-threatening ischemia (i.e., rest pain, nonhealing ulceration, or gangrene). Since some degree of multisegmental involvement is seen angiographically in many patients requiring treatment for limb salvage, therapeutic decisions may be complex and difficult.

If a significant proximal pressure gradient exists, aortoiliac reconstruction is required and may often relieve symptoms without distal revascularization. Techniques available for proximal revascularization include transluminal angioplasty (percutaneous or intraoperative), aortoiliac or aortofemoral endarterectomy or bypass, and extraanatomic (axillofemoral or femorofemoral) bypass. Specific indications, results, and other considerations will be discussed in detail.

Infrainguinal (femoropopliteal or femorotibial) reconstruction alone may be appropriate in the absence of hemodynamically significant proximal disease. Although distal reconstruction will predictably fail if markedly significant aortoiliac disease is present, we have on occasion accepted proximal gradients of up to 30 mmHg after performance of a distal bypass and had the bypass remain patent for several years. On the other hand, if the significance of a proximal lesion is uncertain, a synchronous inflow procedure may be required if a large gradient is produced by an infrainguinal bypass.

The most complex decisions involve selection of patients for combined aortoiliac and femoropopliteal reconstruction. Indications for planned or unplanned synchronous revascularization and the methods utilized will be discussed. Staged proximal and distal revascularization may be required and may offer the advantage of time to fully assess the initial procedure. However, when combined segment revascularization is inevitable, the additional delay and anesthesia required for secondary reoperation is best avoided. These decisions will also be discussed in detail.

TECHNIQUE OF RECONSTRUCTION

Aortoiliac Reconstruction

Percutaneous Transluminal Angioplasty. An important advance in the treatment of patients with combined segment disease has been the adjunctive use of percutaneous transluminal angioplasty (PTA) (see also Chapters 18, 19, and 20). We would agree, to some extent, with suggestions (49) that this modality has been underutilized as an adjunct or an alternative to vascular bypass operations. Results to date have shown that lasting dilatation can be achieved, particularly for iliac PTA (50). We have utilized PTA as the primary treatment modality for most segmental iliac stenoses, even in the presence of distal disease (Figure 28-5). The decision regarding subsequent distal revascularization is then made based on healing of foot lesions and relief of symptoms. Results with up to 3 years follow-up after combined proximal PTA and distal arterial reconstruction have been favorable (51–54). We have also used PTA of femoropopliteal lesions in combination with proximal vascular reconstruction. Furthermore, if surgery is required, the new technology with linear extrusion catheters may eliminate the need for fluoroscopic control and thus allow successful intraoperative dilatation of tandem lesions (55) (see Chapter 20).

Aortofemoral Bypass. This procedure remains the predominant method of aortoiliac revascularization for localized or multisegmental disease (see Chapter 26). Excellent patency rates and clinical improvement can be expected even in the presence of SFA occlusion (56,57). The importance of runoff via the deep femoral artery is further emphasized in the discussion of profundaplasty (vide infra).

Although aortoiliac bypass has been attempted in selected cases, progression of disease in the external iliac arteries in many of these patients with multisegmental disease may affect long-term patency and makes primary bypass to the femoral artery preferable in most instances.

Aortoiliac Endarterectomy. Localized lesions of the aortoiliac segment can be successfully treated by endarterectomy. However, the extensive atherosclerosis present in most patients with combined segment disease makes endarterectomy a complex undertaking (8), and we have advocated its use only in rare instances. Extraperitoneal endarterectomy (58) may be suitable in patients with unilateral iliac occlusive disease but has rarely been utilized since PTA and femorofemoral bypass have been preferred in most patients.

Extraanatomic Bypass for Aortoiliac Revascularization. *Axillofemoral Bypass.* As discussed previously, many patients with combined segment disease are poor surgical risks for anatomic aortoiliac revascularization. Axillofemoral bypass has offered an attractive alternative in the management of these patients (see Chapter 30). Although O'Donnell et al. (59,60) have suggested that axillofemoral grafts do not do as well hemodynamically as aortofemoral grafts in patients with combined segment disease, we have been unable to demonstrate that occlusion of the SFA impairs axillofemoral graft patency (61). We would also disagree with recommendations for routine deep femoral artery reconstruction with axillofemoral bypass (62) and would select patients for both procedures based on previously outlined criteria.

Femorofemoral Bypass. Femorofemoral bypass has become an accepted modality for the treatment of patients with unilateral iliac occlusive disease (63) (see Chapter 30). Donor iliac lesions are clearly associated with poor surgical results in both the donor and the recipient limb (64–66). Although recipient SFA occlusion may again prevent maximal hemodynamic improvement, distal disease in the donor limb should not affect operative results (64,65). McDonald et al. (67) have advocated liberal use of profundaplasty as an adjunct to femorofemoral bypass in limbs threatened by significant synchronous distal disease. Again, we recommend correction of deep femoral lesions only if important origin stenosis is present.

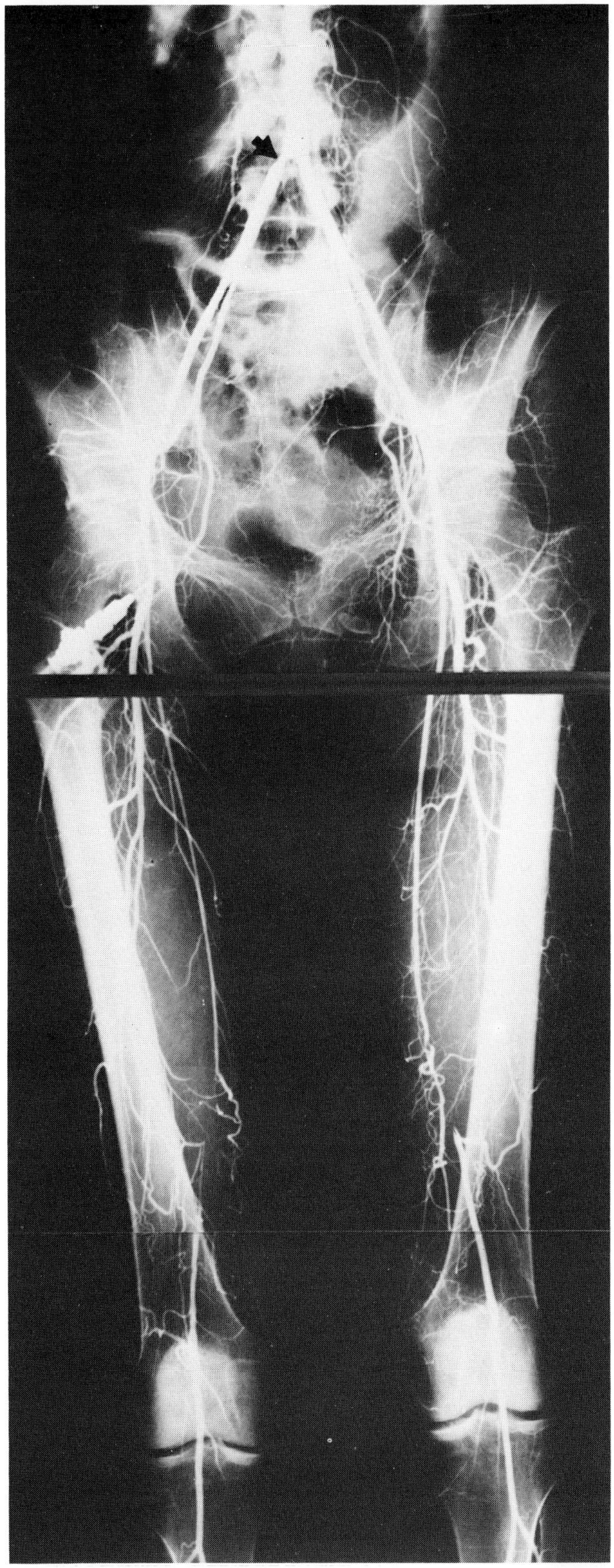

FIGURE 28-5. Arteriogram demonstrating common iliac stenosis (*arrow*) and superficial femoral artery occlusion. Patient improved following percutaneous transluminal angioplasty of iliac artery lesion.

Femoropopliteal Reconstruction

Profundaplasty. The importance of the deep femoral artery as a collateral pathway in patients with multisegmental disease has already been alluded to. Morris et al. (68) demonstrated the value of restoring flow to the deep femoral artery by showing that 40 percent of 102 patients with combined aortoiliac and femoropopliteal disease developed pedal pulses following proximal revascularization despite uncorrected SFA occlusion.

Attempts to predict hemodynamic improvement from profundaplasty (69) have been of limited usefulness in the presence of severe proximal disease. Routine profundaplasty (70) during vascular reconstructions is both unnecessary and meddlesome. We advocate repair of deep femoral stenosis with inflow operations if lesions of greater than 40 percent of luminal diameter are present. Isolated stenosis is repaired only if substantial hemodynamic gradients (i.e., > 15 mmHg) can be documented.

Since extensive lesions of both the deep and the superficial femoral arteries are seen in less than 10 percent of patients with combined segment disease, the deep femoral artery will usually provide acceptable outflow for proximal aortoiliac reconstruction (68,71–74) (Figure 28-6). Fortunately, stenosis of the deep femoral artery is usually limited to the proximal segment (Figure 28-7*A*) and is easily treated by endarterectomy and primary closure (Figure 28-7*B*), patch angioplasty (Figure 28-7*C*), or utilizing the tongue of a proximal graft limb as a vascular patch (Figure 28-7*D*). In fact, profundaplasty is most frequently performed as an adjunct to an inflow procedure such as an aortofemoral, axillofemoral, or femorofemoral bypass (75). Lesions of the mid and distal portions of the deep femoral artery are uncommon and are treated only if significant distal atherosclerosis precludes conventional infrainguinal bypass, which predictably will be more effective if the patient requires revascularization.

Femoropopliteal and Femorotibial Bypass. Revascularization of an occluded femoropopliteal segment may be required if outflow through the deep femoral artery is inadequate for relief of symptoms. This subject is discussed in detail in Chapters 26 and 27. An occasional problem is unrecognized aortoiliac disease which achieves hemodynamic significance only after a distal vascular reconstruction is performed (21). If a large gradient (> 15 mmHg) is confirmed by intraarterial pressure measurements after a femoropopliteal bypass, a synchronous proximal reconstruction or transluminal angioplasty may be required. We have used intraoperative dilatation utilizing specially designed linear extrusion catheters (see Chapter 21) but presently prefer the addition of a femorofemoral or axillofemoral graft to the infrainguinal bypass.

Lumbar Sympathectomy. Lumbar sympathectomy as an adjunct to vascular reconstruction or as a primary modality of treatment in patients with multisegmental disease remains somewhat controversial (see Chapter 32). It has no role in the primary treatment of patients with claudication or extensive gangrene of the foot. It also has been shown to be ineffective in increasing patency rates or decreasing the need for distal reconstruction following aortoiliac reconstruction (76,77).

In patients with severe combined segment disease and lesser degrees of limb-threatening ischemia, numerous predictive tests have been proposed to determine which patients will respond to lumbar sympathectomy (78). None appear to have great value.

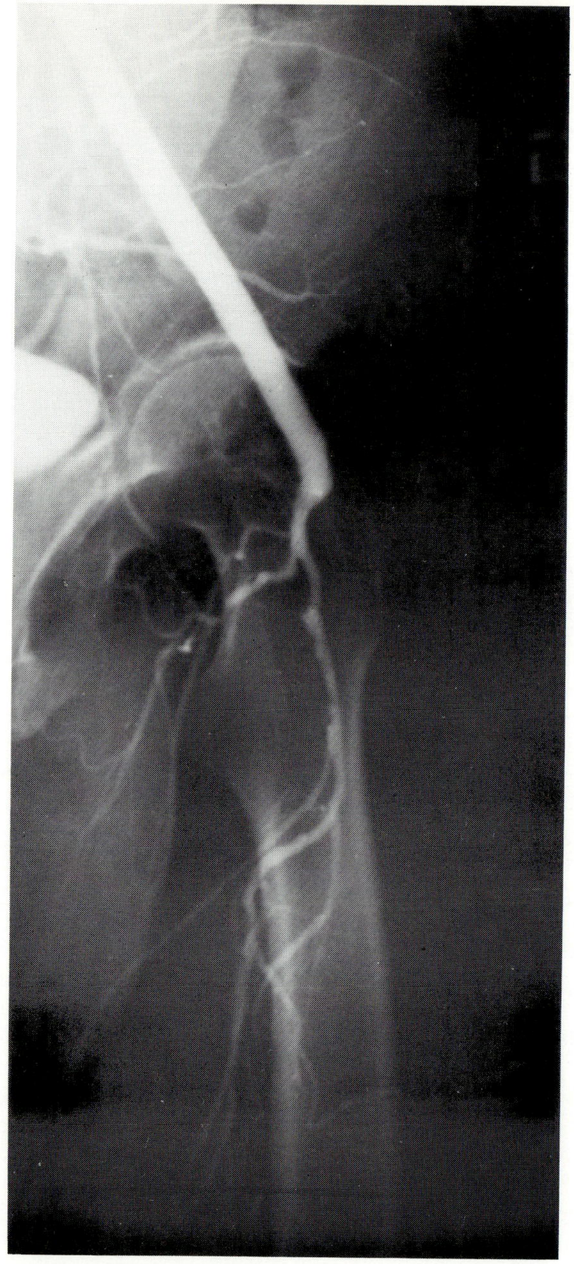

FIGURE 28-6. Arteriogram demonstrating a patent aortofemoral bypass revascularizing the deep femoral artery in the presence of superficial femoral artery occlusion.

Yao and Bergan (79) demonstrated improvement following sympathectomy only in patients with ankle-brachial pressure indices greater than 0.35. However, in our experience, many of these patients have improved following conservative management alone. We currently believe that lumbar sympathectomy either as a primary modality or as an adjunct to vascular reconstruction has little, if any, role in the treatment of combined segment disease.

Combined Segment Bypass

Principles. Ultimately in evaluating patients with multisegmental disease, the need for synchronous or staged combined

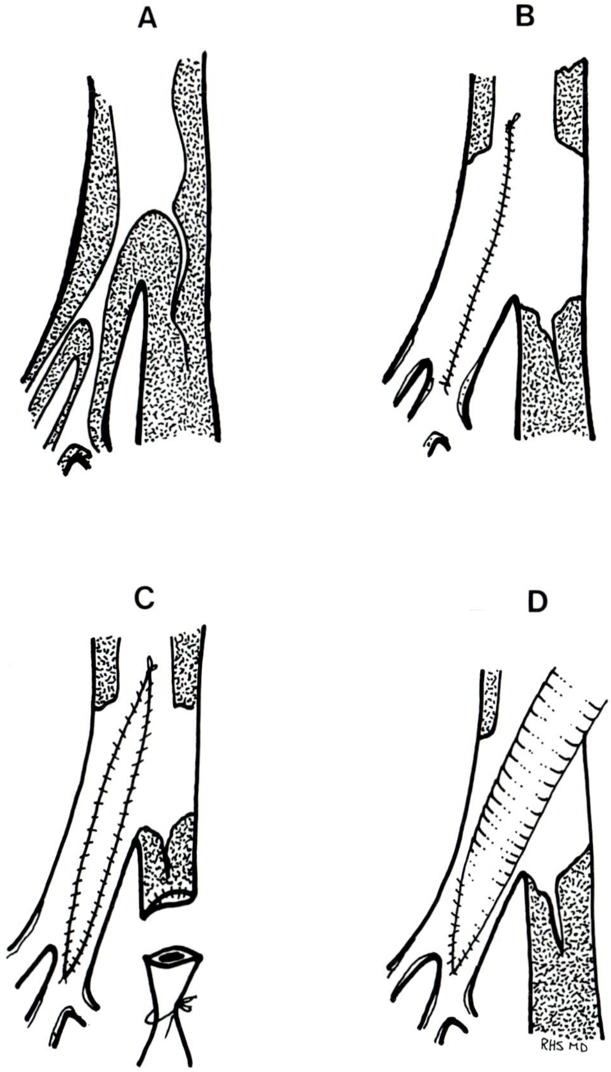

FIGURE 28-7. Profundaplasty. (*A*) Stenosis of proximal deep femoral artery; (*B*) profundaplasty as the sole procedure; (*C*) closure with a patch of endarterectomized superficial femoral artery; (*D*) profundaplasty in combination with a proximal inflow graft such as an aortofemoral bypass.

segment revascularization must be considered. Although numerous clinical and hemodynamic indications for such procedures have been suggested, we have generally reserved synchronous combined segment bypass operations for patients with severe limb-threatening ischemia and occlusions at both the aortoiliac and the femoropopliteal levels. In addition, the selection of patients for planned or unplanned combined procedures is based on the following considerations. The intraoperative assessment of the distal hemodynamic effect of proximal operations may be difficult since coexistent distal occlusive disease may prevent restoration of distal pulses. In addition, since an increase in Doppler ankle pressure (9) and calf blood flow (80) may be delayed for many hours or days after proximal reconstruction, these parameters have also been of limited predictive value. Despite many attempts to identify preoperatively and intraoperatively those patients requiring combined aortoiliac and-femoropopliteal revascularization (5,11,48,59,81–85), we only perform a combined reconstruction when there is severe ischemia and extensive necrosis or infection in the foot. In such circumstances a delay in full revascularization may jeopardize limb salvage, and we perform a planned combined procedure. Otherwise, if significant proximal arterial disease is present as assessed by a diminished femoral pulse or intraarterial pressure measurement, we only perform a revascularization to the femoral level as the primary procedure and reserve any infrainguinal revascularization until it proves to be necessary. Sumner and Strandness (86) also support this approach of isolated proximal reconstruction, and they question the predictive validity of any hemodynamic tests as a guide to combined bypasses.

If minimal proximal disease is present with a pressure gradient of less than 15 mmHg after peripheral vasodilatation, we have advocated femoropopliteal reconstruction alone. On rare occasions an increased, large inflow gradient can be measured *after* femoropopliteal or femorotibial bypass, and this necessitates the addition of a proximal bypass or transluminal angioplasty to treat the now hemodynamically significant inflow disease.

METHODS. Initial attempts to perform synchronous combined segment bypass were unsuccessful, and the procedure was condemned (87). However, improvements, particularly refinements in technique and graft material utilized for femoropopliteal reconstruction (see Chapter 26), have permitted successful aortofemoropopliteal revascularization. We currently prefer to insert the distal end of the proximal bypass into the femoral artery and originate the distal bypass limb from this graft.

Extended extraanatomic reconstruction has produced another possible approach to the performance of combined segment bypass. We have described *crossover femoropopliteal* and *axillopopliteal bypasses* (14,88) which have yielded prolonged periods of limb salvage in selected patients with severe multisegmental disease, and Connolly and his colleagues have reported a similar experience (89). These operations are particularly useful in the presence of heavily scarred or infected groin areas. *Iliopopliteal bypass* has also functioned successfully in appropriate patients (90) and may be performed through a retroperitoneal rather than a transabdominal approach.

Results

Results of treatment of combined segment vascular disease vary widely and are difficult to evaluate. The discrepancies in reported results can perhaps be explained by differences in patient populations, indications for surgery, and definitions of success. Both graft patency and functional improvement (i.e., relief of claudication or limb salvage) must be considered.

AORTOILIAC RECONSTRUCTION IN THE PRESENCE OF FEMOROPOPLITEAL DISEASE

Although Brewster and Darling (8) found that occlusion of the superficial femoral artery (SFA) affected patency rates of aortofemoral reconstruction, Hill et al. (57) could not confirm these results. Mozersky et al. (17) found a slight increase in long-term patency in the absence of distal disease. Deep femoral occlusive disease may significantly and adversely affect aortofemoral graft patency in the presence of SFA disease (91).

Results with extraanatomic bypass are equally controversial. Although Johnson et al. (92) and Ray et al. (93) found axillofemoral patency rates to be worse with SFA occlusion, Ascer et al. (61), reporting our results, were unable to substantiate this finding. Eighty percent of 57 patients who underwent axillofemoral bypass had occlusion of the SFA without any adverse affect on patency. Similarly, Welsh and Repetto (73) found a 90 percent early and 78 percent 5-year patency rate for 236 aortofemoral, axillofemoral, and femorofemoral grafts in limbs with SFA occlusion.

Functional results of proximal reconstruction in the presence of femoropopliteal disease also vary widely. Although extensive gangrene may necessitate synchronous aortofemoral and femoropopliteal revascularization, predictable relief of rest pain and healing of minimal lesions is reported with proximal reconstruction alone in patients with hemodynamically significant aortoiliac disease (7,68,72–74). In addition, femoropopliteal bypass can be performed on a delayed basis with excellent results (94) and is required in only 3 to 21 percent of patients (4,7,10,11,62,95). Relief of claudication following aortofemoral bypass in patients with multisegmental disease is far less predictable, with 26 to 95 percent fully relieved of their claudication (7,11,57,72,73,95,96). Despite these results, subsequent downstream repair is required for persistent disability in only 10 to 20 percent of patients in most series. Brewster and his associates report that 13 percent of 87 claudicants and 29 percent of 90 patients with limb-threatening ischemia required femoropopliteal reconstruction following aortofemoral bypass in the presence of SFA occlusion (11). Similarly, we have found that only 21 percent of 80 axillofemoral and femorofemoral bypasses performed for limb salvage in patients with SFA occlusion required subsequent downstream repair.

FEMOROPOPLITEAL RECONSTRUCTION IN THE PRESENCE OF AORTOILIAC DISEASE

Femoropopliteal reconstruction in the presence of severe, uncorrected aortoiliac occlusive disease is doomed to failure (21). Lesser degrees of inflow disease, even those which produce a small gradient, will presumably influence infrainguinal graft patency less, although proximal disease progression is a recognized cause of late distal graft failure (18). Of recent interest has been the combination of distal arterial reconstruction with PTA of iliac stenoses. Favorable results at least up to 3 years have been reported (51–54), and we have had the same experience.

Summary

Since the majority of patients who present with limb-threatening ischemia or disabling claudication have multisegmental arterial lesions, the management of patients with combined aortoiliac and femoropopliteal occlusive disease is of critical importance. Assessment of the contribution of segmental lesions may be difficult. Angiography and intraarterial femoral artery pressure determinations may provide critical information.

Radiologic lesions without hemodynamic import need not be corrected in most instances. We have preferred segmental reconstruction of hemodynamically significant aortoiliac disease as the initial treatment in most patients. Occasional patients require synchronous combined segment reconstruction for treatment of extensive gangrene. Although many hemodynamic parameters have been proposed to identify patients requiring multisegmental revascularization, we have been disappointed in their utility. We do, however, recognize that requirements for segmental or combined arterial reconstruction are controversial.

Modalities useful in the treatment of patients with combined segment disease have been reviewed. Percutaneous transluminal angioplasty as an adjunct to vascular reconstruction has assumed an increasingly important role. The effect of untreated distal disease on graft patency and functional results has been summarized. Approximately 80 to 85 percent of patients with hemodynamically significant aortoiliac lesions will benefit from proximal revascularization alone. Selected patients require synchronous or delayed femoropopliteal reconstruction for limb salvage and relief of symptoms.

References

1. Haimovici H: Patterns of arteriosclerotic lesions of the lower extremities. Ann NY Acad Sci 1968, 149:997.
2. Reidy NC, Walden R, Abbott WA, Greenfield AJ, L'Italien G, Megerman J: Anatomic localization of atherosclerotic lesions by hemodynamic tests. Arch Surg 1981, 116:1041.
3. Perdue GD, Long WD, Smith RB: Perspective concerning aortofemoral arterial reconstruction. Ann Surg 1971, 173:940.
4. Mulcare RJ, Royster TS, Lynn RA, Connors RB: Long-term results of operative therapy for aortoiliac disease. Arch Surg 1978, 113:601.
5. Imparato AM, Sanoudos G, Epstein HY, Abrams RM, Beranbaum ER: Results in 96 aortoiliac reconstructive procedures: Preoperative angiographic and functional classifications used as prognostic guides. Surgery 1970, 68:610.
6. Edwards WH, Wright RS: A technique for combined aorto-femoral-popliteal arterial reconstruction. Ann Surg 1974, 179:572.
7. Royster TS, Lynn R, Mulcare RJ: Combined aortoiliac and femoropopliteal occlusive disease. Surg Gynecol Obstet 1976, 143:949.
8. Brewster DC, Darling RC: Optimal methods of aortoiliac reconstruction. Surgery 1978, 84:739.
9. Kozloff L, Collins GJ, Rich NM, McDonald PT, Collins JT, Clagett GP: Fallibility of postoperative Doppler ankle pressures in determining the adequacy of proximal arterial revascularization. Am J Surg 1980, 139:326.

10. Cronenwett JL, Dans JT, Gooch, JB, Garrett HE: Aortoiliac occlusive disease in women. Surgery 1980, 88:775.
11. Brewster DC, Perter BA, Robinson JG, Darling RC: Aortofemoral graft for multilevel occlusive disease—Predictors of success and need for distal bypass. Arch Surg 1982, 117:1593.
12. Moore WS, Cafferata HT, Hall AD, Blaisdell FW: In defense of grafts across the inguinal ligament. Ann Surg 1968, 168:207.
13. Malone JM, Moore WS, Goldstone J: Life expectancy following aortofemoral arterial grafting. Surgery 1977, 81:551.
14. Veith FJ, Gupta SK, Samson RH, Scher LA, Fell SC, Weiss P, Janko G, Flores SW, Rifkin H, Bernstein G, Haimovici H, Gliedman ML, Spray-Regen S: Progress in limb salvage by reconstructive arterial surgery combined with new or improved adjunctive procedures. Ann Surg 1981, 194:386.
15. Darling RC, Brewster DC, Hallet JW, Darling RC III: Aortoiliac reconstruction. Surg Clin North Am 1979, 59:565.
16. Staple TW: The solitary aortoiliac lesion. Surgery 1968, 64:569.
17. Mozersky DJ, Sumner DS, Strandness DE: Long-term results of reconstruction aortoiliac surgery. Ann Surg 1972, 123:503.
18. Mozersky DJ, Sumner DS, Strandness DE: Disease progression after femoropopliteal surgical procedures. Surg Gynecol Obstet 1972, 135:700.
19. Robbs JV, Wylie EJ: Factors contributing to recurrent lower limb ischemia following bypass surgery for aortoiliac occlusive disease and their management. Ann Surg 1981, 193:356.
20. Moore WS, Hall AD: Unrecognized aortoiliac stenosis. Arch Surg 1971, 103:633.
21. Charlesworth D, Harris PL, Cave FD, Taylor L: Undetected aortoiliac insufficiency: A reason for early failure of saphenous vein bypass grafts for obstruction of the superficial femoral artery. Br J Surg 1975, 67:567.
22. Johnston KW, Demorais D, Colapinto RF: Difficulty in assessing the severity of aortoiliac disease by clinical and arteriographic methods. Angiology 1981, 32:609.
23. Blaisdell FW, Gauder PJ: Paradoxical variation of the femoral pulse in occlusion of the iliac artery. Surgery 1961, 50:529.
24. Slot HB, Strijbosch L, Greep JM: Interobserver variability in single-plane aortography. Surgery 1981, 90:497.
25. Hurlow RA, Chandler ST, Hardman J: The noninvasive assessment of aortoiliac disease: A comparison of dynamic isotope angiology with thigh/brachial pressure index. Surgery 1978, 84:278.
26. Carson SN, Hunter G, Wong HN, Farrer PA: Dynamic isotope aortoiliac assessment. Arch Surg 1980, 115:859.
27. Rutherford RB, Lowenstein BH, Klein MF: Combined segmental systolic pressures and plethysmography to diagnose arterial occlusive disease of the legs. Am J Surg 1979, 138:211.
28. Heintz SE, Bone GE, Slaymaker EE, Hayes AC, Barnes RW: Value of arterial pressure measurements in the proximal and distal part of the thigh in arterial occlusive disease. Surg Gynecol Obstet 1978, 146:337.
29. Brener BJ, Tiro AC, Alpert J, Brief DK, Parsonnet V, Goldenkranz RJ, Bernstein M, Scher L, Rough WA: Three techniques for assessing iliac artery stenosis. In Diethrich EG (ed): *Noninvasive Cardiovascular Diagnosis,* ed 2. Littleton, Massachusetts, PSG Publishing Company, 1981, pp 261–282.
30. Vandewater JM, Indech CDV, Indech RB, Randall HT: Hyperemic response for accurate diagnosis of arterial insufficiency. Arch Surg 1980, 115:851.
31. Ward AS, Martin TP: Some aspects of ultrasound in the diagnosis and assessment of aortoiliac disease. Am J Surg 1980, 140:260.
32. Yao JST, Hobbs JT, Irvine WT: Ankle systolic pressure measurements in arterial disease affecting the lower extremities. Br J Surg 1969, 56:675.
33. Barringer M, Poole GV, Shircliffe AC, Meredith JW, Hightower F, Plonk GW: The diagnosis of aortoiliac disease: A noninvasive femoral cuff technique. Ann Surg 1983, 197:204.
34. Nicolaides AN, Gordon-Smith IC, Dayandas J, Eastcott HHG: The value of Doppler blood velocity tracings in the detection of aortoiliac disease in patients with intermittent claudication. Surgery 1976, 80:774.
35. Archie JP, Feldtman RW: Determination of the hemodynamic significance of iliac artery stenosis by noninvasive Doppler ultrasonography. Surgery 1982, 91:419.
36. Fronek A, Coel M, Bernstein EF: The importance of combined multisegmental pressure and Doppler flow velocity studies in the diagnosis of peripheral arterial occlusive disease. Surgery 1978, 84:840.
37. Nicolaides AN, Angelides NS: Waveform index and resistance factor using directional Doppler ultrasound and a zero-crossing detector. In Nicolaides AN, Yao JST (eds): *Investigation of Vascular Disorders*. New York, Churchill Livingstone, 1981, pp 291–300.
38. Baird RN, Bird DR, Clifford PC, Lusby RJ, Skidmore R, Woodcock JP: Upstream stenosis—its diagnosis by Doppler signals from the femoral artery. Arch Surg 1980, 115:1316.
39. Bone GE: The relationship between aortoiliac hemodynamics and femoral pulsatility index. J Surg Res 1982, 32:228.
40. Flanigan DP, Collins JT, Goodreau JJ, Burnham SJ, Yao JST: Femoral pulsatility index in the evaluation of aortoiliac occlusive disease. J Surg Res 1981, 31:392.
41. Thiele BL, Bandyk DF, Zierler RE, Strandness DE: A systematic approach to the assessment of aortoiliac disease. Arch Surg 1983, 118:477.
42. Udoff EJ, Barth KH, Harrington DP, Kaufman SL, White RI: Hemodynamic significance of iliac artery stenosis: Pressure measurements during angiography. Radiology 1979, 132:289.
43. Brewster DC, Waltman AC, O'Hara PJ, Darling RC: Femoral artery pressure measurement during aortography. Circulation 1979, 60(suppl 1):120.
44. Flanigan DP, Williams LR, Schwartz JA, Schuler JJ, Gray B: Hemodynamic evaluation of the aortoiliac segment based on pharmacologic vasodilatation. *Surgery* 1983, 93:709.
45. Archie JP, Feldtman RW: Intraoperative assessment of the hemodynamic significance of iliac and profunda femoris artery stenosis. Surgery 1981, 90:876.
46. Brener BJ, Raines JK, Darling RC, Austen WG: Measurement of systolic femoral arterial pressure during reactive hyperemia: An estimate of aortoiliac disease. Circulation 1974, 49(suppl 2):259.
47. Lorentsen E, Hoel BL, Hoel R: Evaluation of the functional importance of atherosclerotic obliterations in the aortoiliac artery by pressure/flow measurements. *Acta Med Scand* 1972, 191:399.
48. O'Donnell TF, Lahey SJ, Kelly JJ, Ransil BJ, Millan VG, Korwin S, Callow AD: Prospective study of Doppler pressures and segmental plethysmography before and following aortofemoral bypass. Surgery 1979, 86:120.
49. Doubilet P, Abrams HL: The cost of underutilization—Percutaneous transluminal angioplasty for peripheral vascular disease. N Engl J Med 1984, 310:95.
50. Samson RH, Sprayregen S, Veith FJ, Scher LA, Gupta SK, Ascer E; Management of angioplasty complications, unsuccessful procedures, and early and late failures. Ann Surg 1984, 184:234.
51. Alpert JR, Ring EJ, Freiman DB, Oleaga JA, Gordon R, Berkowitz HD, Roberts B: Balloon dilation of iliac stenosis with distal arterial surgery. Arch Surg 1980, 115:715.
52. Roberts B, Gertner MH, Ring EJ: Balloon catheter dilation as an adjunct to arterial surgery. Arch Surg 1981, 116:809.
53. Lowman BG, Queral LA, Holbrook WA, Estes JT, Dagher FJ: Transluminal angioplasty during vascular reconstructive procedures. Arch Surg 1981, 116:829.
54. Kadir S, Smith GW, White RI, Kaufman SL, Barth KH, Williams GM, O'Mara CS, Burdick JF: Percutaneous transluminal angio-

plasty as an adjunct to the surgical management of peripheral vascular disease. Ann Surg 1982, 195:786.
55. Fogarty JJ, Chin A, Shoor PM, Blair GL, Zimmerman JJ: Adjunctive intraoperative arterial dilation. Arch Surg 1981, 116:1391.
56. Jones AF, Kempczinski RF: Aortofemoral bypass grafting—A reappraisal. Arch Surg 1981, 116:301.
57. Hill DA, McGrath MA, Lord RSA, Tracy GD: The effect of superficial femoral artery occlusion on the outcome of aortofemoral bypass for intermittent claudication. Surgery 1980, 87:133.
58. Inahara T, Pineda JD: Extraperitoneal endarterectomy for unilateral iliofemoral occlusive disease. Surgery 1974, 75:771.
59. O'Donnell TF, McBride KA, Callow AD, Lahey SJ, Scarpato RA, Kelley JJ, Deterling RA: Management of combined segment disease. Am J Surg 1981, 141:452.
60. O'Donnell TF, Kelly JJ, Callow AD, Lahey SJ, Millan VA: A comparison of the early noninvasive hemodynamic results after aortofemoral or axillofemoral bypass graft. Circulation 1980, 62(suppl 1):7.
61. Ascer E, Gupta SK, Veith FJ, Samson RH, Scher LA, White-Flores SA: Equivalent results with axillo-unifemoral and axillobifemoral bypasses. Surgery 1985, 97:169.
62. DeLaurentis DA, Sala LE, Russell E, McCombs PR: A twelve-year experience with axillofemoral and femorofemoral bypass operations. Surg Gynecol Obstet 1978, 147:881.
63. Dick LA, Brief DK, Alpert J, Brener BJ, Goldenkranz R, Parsonnet V: A 12-year experience with femorofemoral crossover grafts. Arch Surg 1980, 115:1359.
64. Flanigan DP, Pratt DG, Goodreau JJ, Burnham SJ, Yao JST, Bergan JJ: Hemodynamic and angiographic guidelines in selection of patients for femorofemoral bypass. Arch Surg 1978, 113:1257.
65. Harris JP, Flinn WR, Rudo ND, Bergan JJ, Yao JST: Assessment of donor limb hemodynamics in femorofemoral bypass for claudication. Surgery 1981, 90:764.
66. Shin CS, Chaudhry AG: Hemodynamics of extra-anatomical bypass following restriction of inflow and outflow in the donor artery in dogs. World J Surg 1980, 4:717.
67. McDonald PT, Rich NM, Collins GJ, Anderson CA, Kozloff L: Femorofemoral grafts: The role of concomitant extended profundaplasty. Am J Surg 1978, 136:622.
68. Morris GC, Edwards W, Cooley DA, Crawford ES, DeBakey ME: Surgical importance of the profunda femoris artery. Arch Surg 1961, 82:52.
69. Boren CH, Towne JB, Bernhard VM, Salles-Cunha S: Profunda-popliteal collateral index: A guide to successful profundaplasty. Arch Surg 1980, 115:1366.
70. Berguer R, Higgins RF, Cotton LT: Geometry; blood flow and reconstruction of the deep femoral artery. Am J Surg 1975, 130:68.
71. Winegarner FJ, Michl LG, Madura JA, Jesseph JE: Revascularization of the severely ischemic lower extremity by aortoprofunda femoris bypass. Am J Surg 1974, 128:649.
72. Strandness DE: Functional results after revascularization of the profunda femoris artery. Am J Surg 1970, 119:240.
73. Welsh P, Repetto R: Revascularization of the profunda femoris artery in aortoiliac occlusive disease. Surgery 1975, 78:389.
74. Hill DA, Jamieson CW: The results of arterial reconstruction utilizing the profunda femoris artery in the treatment of rest pain and pre-gangrene. Br J Surg 1977, 64:359.
75. Bernhard VM, Ray LI, Militello JP: The role of angioplasty of the profunda femoris artery in revascularization of the ischemic limb. Surg Gynecol Obstet 1976, 142:840.
76. Satiani B, Piapis CD, Hayes JP, Kimmins S, Evans WE: Prospective randomized study of concomitant lumbar sympathectomy with aortoiliac reconstruction. Am J Surg 1982, 143:755.
77. Barnes RW, Baker WH, Shanik G, Maixner W, Hayes AC, Lin R, Clarke W: Value of concomitant sympathectomy in aortoiliac reconstruction. Arch Surg 1977, 112:13251.
78. Imparato AM: Lumbar sympathectomy. Surg Clin North Am 1979, 59:719.
79. Yao JST, Bergan JJ: Predictability of vascular activity relative to sympathetic ablation. Arch Surg 1973, 107:676.
80. Walker PM, Johnston KW: When does limb blood flow increase after aortoiliac bypass grafting? Arch Surg 1980, 115:912.
81. Garrett WV, Slaymaker EE, Heintz SE, Barnes RW: Intraoperative prediction of symptomatic result of aortofemoral bypass from changes in ankle pressure index. Surgery 1977, 82:504.
82. Bone GE, Hayes AC, Slaymaker EE, Barnes RW: Value of segmental limb blood pressures in predicting results of aortofemoral bypass. Am J Surg 1976, 132:733.
83. Baird RN, Davies PW, Bird DP: Segmental air plethysmography during arterial reconstruction. Br J Surg 1979, 66:718.
84. Dardik H, Ibrahim IM, Jarrah M, Sussman B, Dardik I: Synchronous aortofemoral or iliofemoral bypass with revascularization of the lower extremity. Surg Gynecol Obstet 1979, 149:676.
85. Faris I, Tonnesen KH, Agerskov K, Noer I, Sager P: Femoral artery pressure measurement to predict the outcome of arterial surgery in patients with multilevel disease. Surgery 1982, 92:10.
86. Sumner DS, Strandness DE: Aortoiliac reconstruction in patients with combined iliac and superficial femoral arterial occlusion. Surgery 1978, 84:348.
87. Benson JB, Whelen TJ, Cohen A, Spencer FC: Combined aortoiliac and femoropopliteal occlusive disease—Limitations of total aortofemoropopliteal bypass. Ann Surg 1966, 163:123.
88. Veith FJ, Moss CM, Daly V, Fell SC, Haimovici H: New approaches to limb salvage by extended extra-anatomic bypasses and prosthetic reconstructions to foot arteries. Surgery 1978, 84:764.
89. Connolly JE, Kwaan JHM, Brownell D, McCart PM, Levin E: Newer developments in extra-anatomic bypass. Surg Gynecol Obstet 1984, 58:415.
90. Horton RE, Giddings AEB, Parkes AC: Iliopopliteal dacron grafts as an alternative to amputation. Ann Roy Coll Surg 1979, 61:217.
91. Malone JM, Moore WS, Goldstone J: The natural history of bilateral aortofemoral bypass grafts for ischemia of the lower extremities. Arch Surg 1975, 110:1300.
92. Johnson WC, Logerfo FW, Vollman RW, Corson JD, O'Hara ET, Mannick JA, Nabseth DC: Is axillo-bilateral femoral graft an effective substitute for aortic-bilateral iliac/femoral graft? Ann Surg 1977, 186:123.
93. Ray LI, O'Connor JB, Davis CC, Hall DG, Mansfield PB, Rittenhouse EA, Smith JC, Wood SJ, Sauvage LR: Axillofemoral bypass: A critical reappraisal of its role in the management of aortoiliac occlusive disease. Am J Surg 1979, 138:117.
94. Collins GJ, Rich NM, Anderson CA, McDonald PT: Staged aortofemoropopliteal revascularization. Arch Surg 1978, 113:149.
95. Baird RJ, Feldman P, Miles JT, Madras PM, Gurry JF: Subsequent downstream repair after aortoiliac and aortofemoral bypass operations. Surgery 1977, 82:785.
96. Galland RB, Hill DA, Jamieson CW: The functional results of aortoiliac reconstruction. Br J Surg 1980, 67:344.

Chapter 29

ADVENTITIAL CYSTIC DISEASE AND ENTRAPMENT SYNDROMES INVOLVING THE POPLITEAL ARTERY

NORMAN M. RICH, GEORGE J. COLLINS, JR., JERRY R. YOUKEY, JAMES M. SALANDER, HUGH J. DONOHUE, and BRUCE M. ELLIOTT

The popliteal artery in disease and injury remains an enigma and an interesting challenge, in both diagnosis and therapy. It is well documented that despite attempted repair of arteries and associated venous injury when indicated, trauma to the popliteal artery continues to be associated with a relatively high amputation rate when compared to other major extremity arterial injuries in most civilian and military experiences (1,2). During the past 20 years two unusual popliteal arterial lesions have been identified. Initial case reports of adventitial cystic disease of the popliteal artery (3–74) and of popliteal artery entrapment syndrome (75–114) have been recently supplemented with extensive reviews of both entities (115–123).

Although intermittent claudication in patients is usually associated with arteriosclerotic occlusive disease involving lower extremity arteries in elderly males with a long history of smoking, this symptom also occurs in men in their middle forties with adventitial cystic disease of the popliteal artery and in relatively young athletic men with popliteal artery entrapment syndrome.

Noninvasive labortory tests have proliferated during the past 20 years and an extensive literature has evolved. Specifically pertinent to this review is a 1969 contribution by Yao and his associates, who described measurements of ankle systolic pressure in arterial disease affecting the lower extremities (124). In 1972 Barnes and Strandness outlined physiologic observations regarding specific isolated popliteal arterial occlusions (125). Darling and colleagues (85) at Massachusetts General Hospital and McDonald and coworkers (126) at Walter Reed Army Medical Center attempted to correlate noninvasive test results with the angiographic diagnosis of popliteal artery entrapment.

This chapter will review the history and current status of adventitial cystic disease and entrapment syndrome of the popliteal artery. The increasing interest in these two unusual lesions has led to an improved ability to diagnose them. The theraputic implications of this increased identification of these two lesions will be emphasized.

Adventitial Cystic Disease of the Popliteal Artery

HISTORY

Ejrup and Hiertonn in 1954 in Stockholm, Sweden, first described adventitial cystic disease of the popliteal artery (23). In the year preceding their report, Hiertonn, when operating on a patient's popliteal artery, had made a transverse incision in the middle of a thickened area of the popliteal artery and found a mass filled with gelatinous material. Hiertonn regarded this finding tentatively as mucoid degeneration in the media of the popliteal artery. The involved segment of popliteal artery was resected and replaced with a segment of autogenous greater saphenous vein. Hiertonn with coauthors Lindberg and Rob (33) produced a subsequent publication which described cystic degeneration of the popliteal artery. They reviewed four known cases encountered up to 1957. A number of valuable descriptive terms were applied to the lesion including "clear, jelly-like material similar in appearance to that seen in a ganglion;" "the specimen looked like a sausage and was 7 cm in length;" and "the lumen was compressed by an intramural cyst containing jelly under high tension." Hiertonn and his co-authors make reference to a report by Atkins and Key, stating their belief that in 1947 these researchers were the first to report on adventitial cystic degeneration of an artery when they described this lesion in the external iliac artery (5). While the majority of adventitial cystic lesions have been identified in the popliteal artery, other publications have described a similar pathology in a variety of arteries. These include the iliac arteries (127,128), the femoral artery (128), and the radial artery (129). The general subject of cystic adventitial degeneration of blood vessels has also been reviewed (130–132).

An important diagnostic sign was described in 1961 by Ishikawa, Mishima, and Kobayshi (36) when they noted in their report of cystic arterial disease of the popliteal artery that normal distal pulsations were obliterated by complete flexion of their patient's affected knee. These authors noted that the pulses returned to normal immediately after the knee resumed a straight position. They found that this sign was present only in patients whose cystic disease produced a stenosis without total occlusion of the popliteal artery. A year earlier, Jaquet and Meyer-Burgdorff (37) had noted that the cystic lesion might present as a localized stenosis which allowed distal arterial flow through the lesion only at the peak of systolic pressure. In 1963 Eastcott (20) suggested that an arterial murmur over the popliteal fossa was an important sign in establishing the proper diagnosis of adventitial cystic degeneration of the popliteal artery in a young athletic nonsmoker who developed intermittent claudication. In their report of a cyst of the popliteal artery in 1967, Taylor and his colleagues (70) documented that "the sudden onset of symptoms in our case may have been due to the floor of the superficial cyst giving way, resulting in the extrusion of the contents into the dissection plane of the vessel, so forming an internal projection which constricted the lumen" (70). These authors believe that the cysts were similar to ganglia which are degenerative cysts containing collagenous material and which may result from previous trauma.

Despite the increasing recognition of adventitial cystic disease of the popliteal artery during the past 20 years, the true cause remains unknown. The lesion has been treated successfully both by evacuation or aspiration of the cyst when there is associated patency of the popliteal artery and by arterial reconstruction when the popliteal artery is occluded.

INCIDENCE AND DEMOGRAPHICS

The increasing recognition of popliteal artery adventitial cystic disease stimulated Flanigan and his associates (118) to establish a registry for this lesion at Northwestern University and to correspond with authors who had documented previous cases all over the world (118). In 1979 they were able to report a review of the history and findings in 115 cases. Their reference is a classic review of this entity. Approximately 50 percent of their cases came from continental Europe; an additional 12 cases were diagnosed in Scandinavia and 14 in Great Britain. North America and Australia each had identified 13 cases.

Cystic adventitial disease of the popliteal artery is found more frequently in men than in women. The most recent report from Northwestern University in 1984 by Bergan and his colleagues emphasizes that the usual patient is a man who is a high-performance athlete or a heavy manual laborer (116). Although the lesion can occur between 11 and 70 years of age with a mean age of 42 years, it usually presents in patients in their twenties or thirties (116,118).

ETIOLOGY AND PATHOGENESIS

The exact cause of cystic degeneration of the adventitia in the popliteal artery remains uncertain. *Repetitive trauma* is one of three possible causes. However, the lesion's occurrence in childhood makes it unlikely that trauma is the sole cause. A second possible etiology suggests that the lesion is part of a *generalized body disorder* of connective tissue. However, the process has never occurred bilaterally, and generalized connective tissue disorders have not appeared in patients who have been followed after identification of popliteral artery adventitial cystic disease. The third and most likely possibility is that *developmental inclusion of mucin-secreting cells* within the adventitia of the artery could allow a cyst to develop within its adventitia. Several investigators believe that the lesion's pathogenesis is similar to that of the simple ganglion. They have suggested that there can be a developmental mechanism for inclusion of the cells in the arterial wall. There are numerous references that compare ganglia to adventitial cystic disease with representative reports by Clark (133), McEvedy (134), and Parks (135). Recently, there have been suggestions that there can be an enlargement of the knee joint capsular synovial cyst that could develop along a geniculate artery to involve the adventitia of the popliteal artery or that synovial cysts can be sequestered into the arterial wall during development. This could explain why the cysts can be either entirely adventitial or involve other layers of the artery wall and why not all cysts can be enucleated.

PATHOPHYSIOLOGY

Although there is wide variation, the sudden onset of ischemic symptoms in the leg in men in their third decade of life can be associated with cystic adventitial disease of the popliteal artery. The rapid change in the size of the cyst which has been developing over a long period of time causes these sudden symptoms. Some degree of stenosis may be associated with the cyst for a long period of time with preservation of luminal patency in the popliteal artery until the intracystic pressure exceeds that of the artery, causing occlusion with or without thrombosis and the resultant sudden onset of associated symptoms. Intermittent claudication without severe ischemia is a common finding because collateral circulation develops.

The nature of the content of the cyst has been the subject of numerous studies. Endo and his colleagues isolated and identified proteohyaluronic acid in the cyst, and they believe that this represents cystic mucoid degeneration (24). Leaf performed amino acid analysis of the protein present in adventitial cystic disease of the popliteal artery and showed similarities between ganglia and adventitial cysts by both chemical and histologic analyses (41). Both lesions involve mucoproteins and mucopolysacharides.

CLINICAL PRESENTATION

Typically, a patient in his twenties, thirties, or forties presents with the sudden onset of intermittent claudication that is quite limiting. Both the pedal and popliteal pulses may be present if there is only a stenosis of the popliteal artery associated with the cyst. Depending on the degree of stenosis there may be an associated bruit audible over the popliteal fossa. Palpable distal pulses may disappear during acute flexion of the knee. In other patients both pedal and popliteal pulses may be absent, indicating arterial occlusion which is less frequent than stenosis. After the initial sudden onset of cramping pain in the calf, the patient may experience some relief followed by typical intermittent claudication as good collateral circulation develops. This results from the gradual stenosis of the popliteal artery prior to the rapid enlargement of the cyst, which produces either a more significant stenosis or occlusion. Occasionally, ischemic neuropathy may be present.

LABORATORY EVALUATION

Although physical examination as alluded to above is the essential first step of evaluation, the noninvasive blood flow laboratory can be employed to corroborate the initial physical findings by both pressure measurements and waveform analysis (116, 124–126). This evaluation can be performed in a similar manner to that for conventional arteriosclerotic occlusive disease. Comparison with the opposite nonaffected lower extremity will be impressive. In contrast to the normal segmental limb pressures, the affected limb below the cystic lesion will show a decrease in segmental limb pressures. Also, in contrast to the normal pulse waveforms in the unaffected limb, the affected limb will show a flattening of the pulse wave below the cystic lesion. Because of the excellent collateral circulation that usually develops in young men, total absence of pulse waves over the distal tibial arteries is rare.

Angiography, as emphasized by Sutton in 1962 (136), is important. This will outline normal arteries except in the location of the lesion. Frequently, a smooth wall stenosis will be identified, usually at the midportion of the popliteal artery extending from 1 to 8 cm in length. There may be a curvilinear defect, which has been described as a ''scimitar sign'' (Figure 29–1), caused by the displacing the contrast column within the arterial lumen. With expansion of the cyst to encircle the arterial lumen a concentric smooth taper of this lesion has been described as resulting in an ''hour-glass'' appearance. It is important to have both lateral and anteroposterior angiographic views to ensure that the lesion is not missed. In contrast to typical angiographic findings with popliteal artery entrapment, there will be no medial deviation of the popliteal artery with the cystic lesion. The angiographic findings combined with the clinical evaluation of the patient should allow certain diagnosis of the lesion and differentiate if from arteriosclerotic occlusive disease. There may, on occasion, be some confusion with popliteal artery entrapment if total occlusion of the middle portion of the popliteal artery has occurred. Thus, there might be a localized complete occlusion of the midpopliteal artery, with the remainder of the lower extremity arterial anatomy having a normal appearance and with excellent collateral circulation around the limited occlusion. The total occlusion may have a ''beaklike'' appearance of the proximal contrast column (116).

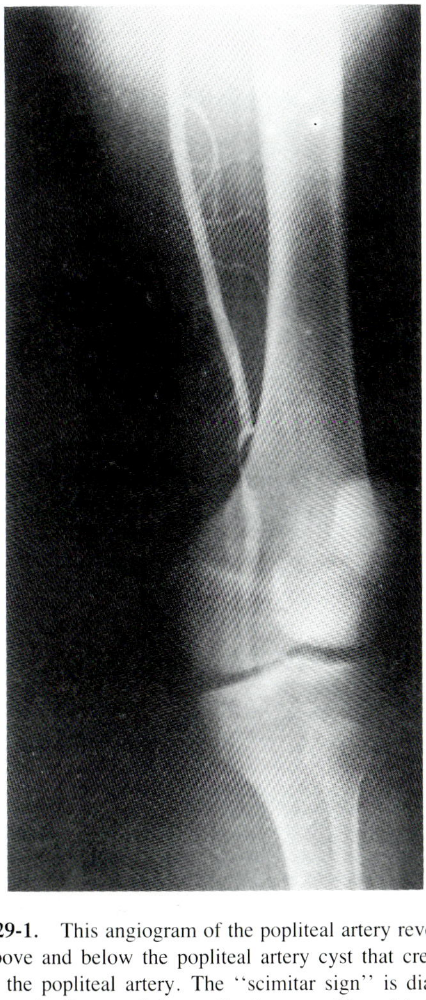

FIGURE 29-1. This angiogram of the popliteal artery reveals smooth tapering above and below the popliteal artery cyst that created severe stenosis of the popliteal artery. The ''scimitar sign'' is diagnostic for adventitial cystic disease of the popliteal artery. (From McAllister HA: Armed Forces Institute of Pathology, Washington D.C. Reproduced with permission.)

TREATMENT

Treatment of adventitial cystic disease of the popliteal artery can be conservative. Adequate experience has documented that *aspiration* of the cyst can be successful in eradicating the cyst and resultant arterial stenosis or occlusion in *some* patients. Bergan and colleagues (116) have emphasized that previous difficulties with aspiration can be avoided by the use of ultrasound needle localization (116). Because the cystic content is quite viscous and gelatinous, aspiration must be done with a relatively large bore needle. However, aspiration can be the treatment of choice if the cyst is diagnosed before the development of total occlusion of the artery (116).

Surgical intervention can also provide effective treatment. Surgical procedures have been divided into nonresectional techniques and resectional techniques. Nonresectional techniques are employed mainly when occlusion of the popliteal artery has not occurred. Evacuation of the cyst or enucleation is the most frequent nonresectional form of therapy (Table 29–1). The popliteal artery can be approached through either a posterior S-shaped incision or a medial incision; however, the posterior approach provides the best exposure of the affected vessel. The normal popliteal artery above and below the lesion can be easily mobilized. The popliteal artery involved by the cystic lesion will be enlarged and sausage-shaped. There may be adhesions binding the cystic adventitial structure to the adjacent vein or to the

TABLE 29–1. **Surgical Treatment of Adventitial Cystic Disease of the Popliteal Artery**

Nonresectional treatment (56 patients)					
	Evacuation	Evacuation with Vein Patch	Evacuation with Synthetic Patch	Aspiration	Total Procedures
Number	41	9	4	2	56
Failures	4/41	2/9	1/4	0/2	7/56
Initial success	90%	78%	75%	100%	89%
Resectional treatment (42 patients)					
	Vein Graft	Synthetic Graft	End–End Anastomosis	Homograft	Total Procedures
Number	30	7	3	2	42
Failures	2/30	1/7	0/3	0/2	3/42
Initial success	93%	86%	100%	100%	93%

Source: Modified from Flanigan DP, Burnham SJ, Goodreau JJ, et al. (118).

posterior aspect of the joint capsule. Although the cyst is usually unilocular, there may be multilocular cysts with septa present (Figure 29–2). An incision into the cyst and evacuation of its contents usually restores arterial patency. The fluid extruding through the incision is usually crystal clear. However, the fluid may be light yellow or even currant jelly in color if there has been recent or old hemorrhage into the cyst.

While evacuation or enucleation of the cyst is preferred if occlusion of the popliteal artery and resultant intimal damage have not occurred, resection and arterial reconstruction may be required if total occlusion of the artery has occurred, with or without thrombosis. Resection and replacement of the involved arterial segment with an autogenous greater saphenous vein graft is the operation of choice for this latter stage of the disease process. Results of such treatment should be excellent.

Recurrent stenosis and/or occlusion of the popliteal artery secondary to cystic adventitial lesions have been treated successfully by needle aspiration, recovering varying amounts of gelatinous material. Many advocate simple evacuation of the cyst by aspiration even for recurrent lesions because of the relatively high degree of success. If this is not successful, a direct surgical approach may be required with evacuation of the cyst or with replacement or bypass of the involved segment of the popliteal artery with an autogenous saphenous vein graft.

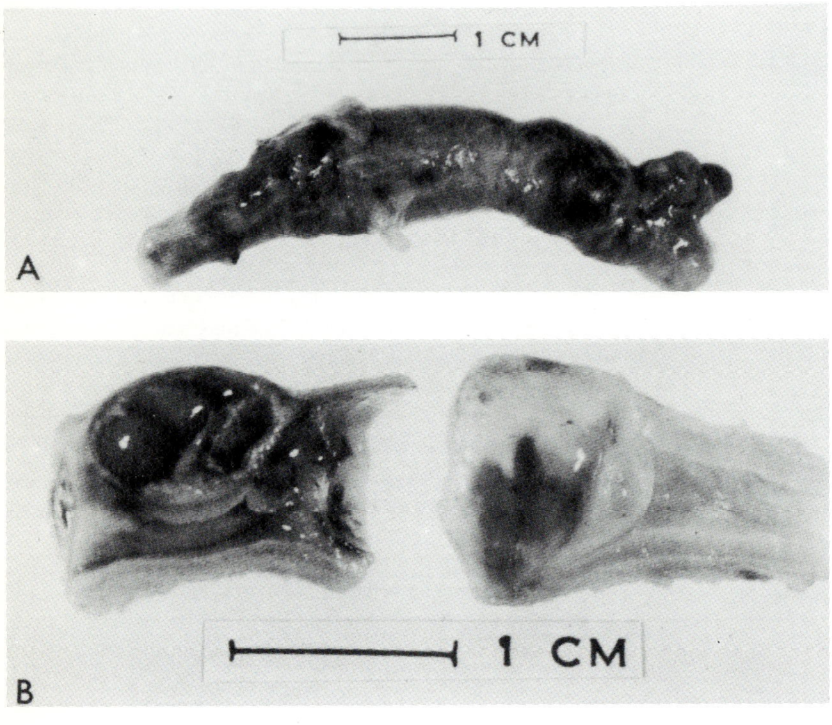

FIGURE 29-2. The gross specimen of the adventitial cyst of the popliteal artery outlined angiographically in Figure 29-1 is demonstrated. Note the sausage-like lesion from the external view (*above*) and the longitudinal transected view which shows the multilocular cystic structure filled with gelatinous material (*below*). These are classic findings of adventitial cystic disease of an artery. (From McAllister HA: Armed Forces Institute of Pathology, Washington, D.C. Reproduced with permission.)

Popliteal Vascular Entrapment Syndromes

Although the usual emphasis in these syndromes is related to entrapment of the popliteal artery, the popliteal vein can also be involved with the artery or, rarely, the popliteal vein can be entrapped alone.

HISTORY

Although there has been considerable interest in and recognition of this anomaly in the past 25 years, it was first described in 1879 by a medical student in Edinburgh, Scotland. T. P. Anderson Stuart was dissecting the amputated leg of a 64-year-old man, and he described the anatomic abnormality associated with the abnormal course of the popliteal artery. The following quotation documents Anderson Stuart's observations (112):

> In May of last year, I was requested by Professor Spence to make for him a preparation of the popliteal space of the limb of a man aged 64, who had had to submit to amputation on account of gangrene of the foot, resulting from a very large popliteal aneurysm. As the dissection proceeded a most striking abnormality in the course of the artery came to light, and so far as I have been able to ascertain, it is now put on record for the first time. The popliteal artery, after passing through the opening in the adductor magnus, instead of, as it usually does, coursing downwards and outwards towards the middle of the popliteal space, so as to lie between the two heads of the gastrocnemius muscle, passes almost vertically downwards internally to the inner head of the gastrocnemius. It reaches the bottom of the space by turning around the inner border of that head, and then passes downwards and outwards beneath it—between it and the lower end of the shaft of the femur. The inner head of the gastrocnemius arises much higher up than usual, namely, from the inner division of the linea aspera about an inch and a half above the condyle, thus leaving a considerable space between it and the condyle, over which space the artery passes. The other structures are normal. The preparation is now in the possession of Mr. Spence (Figure 29-3).

In 1959 Hamming at Leyden University in the Netherlands reported a similar anomaly in a 12-year-old boy (98). However,

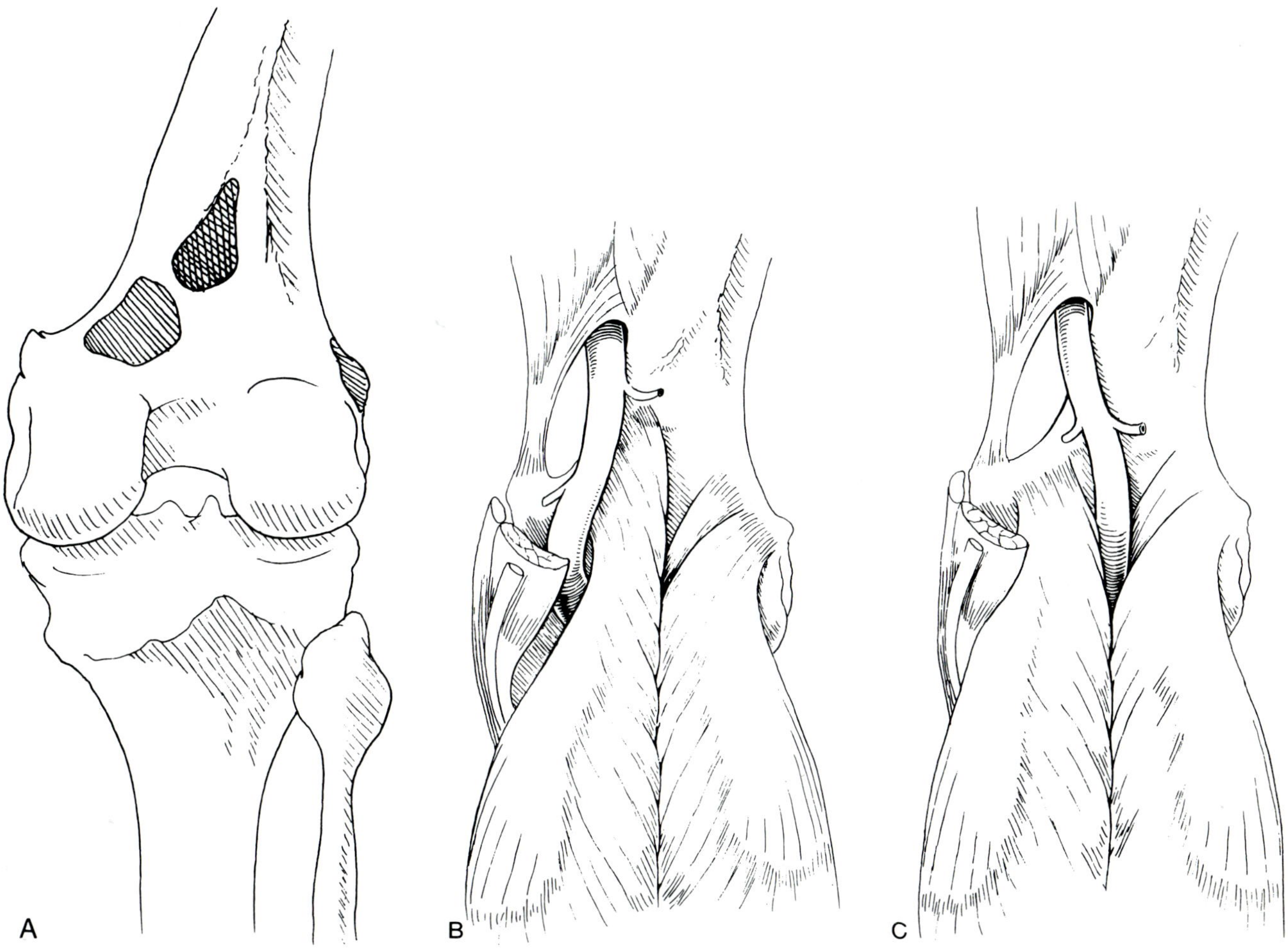

FIGURE 29-3. (*A*), (*B*), and (*C*) represent the artist's interpretation of the written description by T. P. Anderson Stuart in 1879 from the first published observation of a congenital anomaly associated with the resultant abnormal course of the popliteal artery. (*B*) Entrapment. (*C*) Usual course. (With appreciation to the artist, Gary G. Wind, M.D.)

nearly 80 years had passed since the original observation by Stuart. Hamming gave credit to the initial report by Stuart and acknowledged that Chambardel-Dubreuil in 1925 in France had described a case in which the popliteal artery was separated from the popliteal vein by an accessory slip of gastrocnemius muscle. Hamming's case report is a classic reference because it represents the first successful clinical treatment of complications associated with popliteal arterial entrapment. In 1962 Servello at the University of Padua in Italy described a similar patient, a 28-year-old farmer who complained of intermittent claudication (111). Servello had the benefit of reviewing Hamming's article, and he based his diagnosis on this report. In addition, Servello's patient had a small aneurysm of the popliteal artery distal to the entrapped segment in a fashion similar to Stuart's original description in 1879. In the Scandinavian literature, Hall in 1961 described the anomalous insertion of the medial head of the gastrocnemius muscle with circulatory complications in one of his patients (96). In 1964, Hall followed his initial report with an additional report of what he called intravascular gastrocnemius insertion (97). In 1964 Carter and Eban (83) described a case of a bilateral developmental anomaly of the popliteal arteries and the gastrocnemius muscles. In these early reports, most of the patients were young athletic men.

The term *popliteal artery entrapment syndrome* was first used by Love and Whelan in reporting two cases in 1965 from Walter Reed General Hospital (106). Stimulated by this report, Rich and Hughes added an additional case and documented for the first time that the popliteal vein, as well as the popliteal artery, could be involved in a variety of anomalies that frequently include abnormal lateral attachment of the medial head of the gastrocnemius muscle (109). Connell in 1978 first noted that isolated entrapment of the popliteal vein could be one of these anatomic variants (137).

CLASSIFICATION AND ETIOLOGY

There are a variety of *congenital* anatomic variants associated with entrapment of both the popliteal artery and/or the popliteal vein (Figure 29-4). Classification of the anomalies remains confusing; however, this is of little consequence to surgical treatment. An initial attempt at classification was made in 1970 by

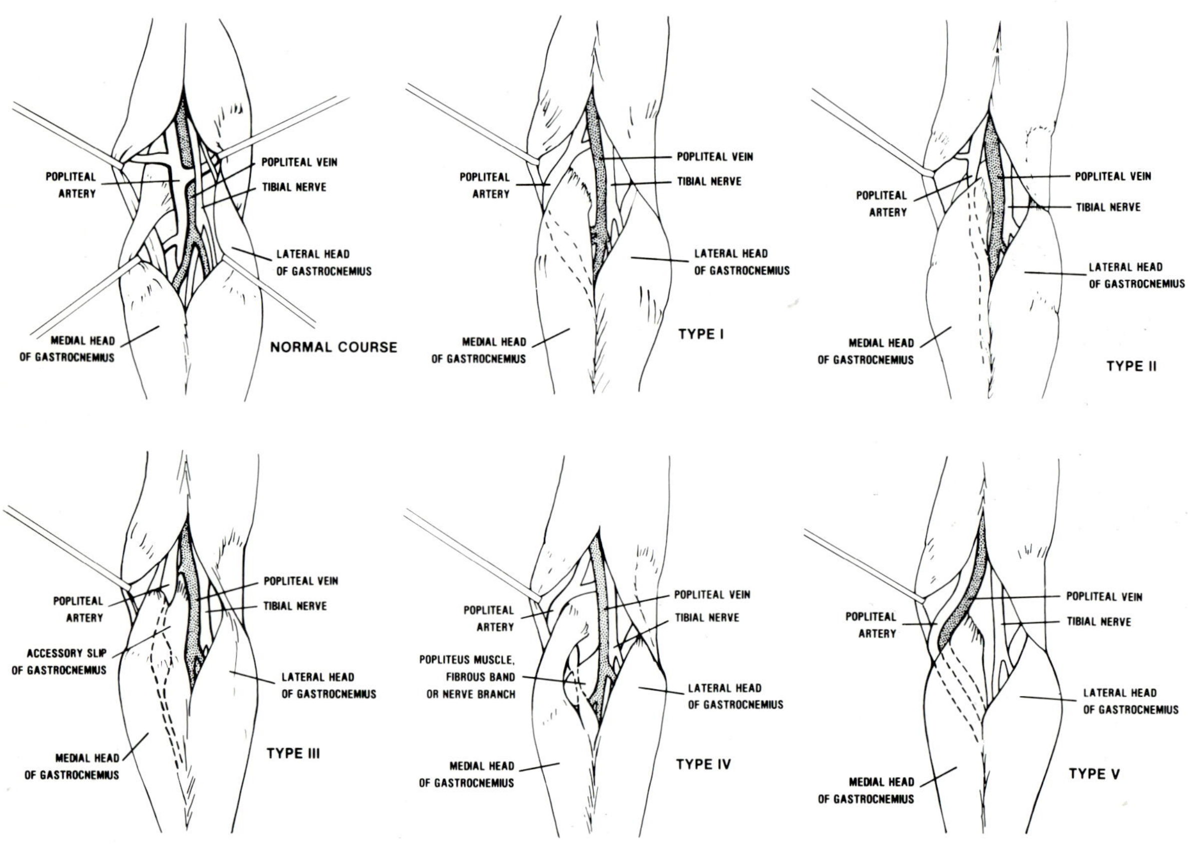

FIGURE 29-4. These drawings outline the normal course of the neurovascular bundle in the popliteal fossa from the posterior approach and show four generally accepted types of anomalies involving entrapment of the popliteal artery. All are usually associated with an abnormal configuration of the medial head of the gastrocnemius muscle. This classification, however, does not satisfy all anatomic variants. Empirically, type IV was expanded to include a branch of the tibial nerve as a structure compressing the popliteal artery, and type V was added to emphasize that the popliteal vein can be entrapped with the artery in all four types. [From Rich NM, Collins GJ Jr, McDonald PT, et al. (122). Reproduced with permission.]

Insua and his associates (103). This was modified subsequently by Delaney and Gonzalez (86). Ferrero and his colleagues extended this classification to a total of 10 lesions (120). In 1979, using the Walter Reed Army Medical Center experiences, Rich and his coworkers identified five major classifications which are outlined graphically in Figure 29-4 (122). In addition, Evans and Bernhard (89) described an unusual variant of vascular entrapment in a patient following injury to the lower extremity (89). These authors could not identify a congenital anomaly or compressive band in their patient who presented with external compression of both the popliteal artery and the popliteal vein. The authors concluded that popliteal vascular entrapment could be caused by massive edema of the heads of the normal gastrocnemius muscle following *trauma*. Baker and Stoney (78) reported another form of acquired popliteal artery entrapment where the popliteal artery entrapment was associated with *arterial bypass surgery*. An interesting question which cannot be answered is the relationship between popliteal artery aneurysms identified in mid- or later life and popliteal vascular entrapment. This relationship will be difficult to clarify since bypass of the aneurysm is now the preferred treatment, and when this is performed via medial incisions, the identification of entrapment is usually not possible. It is also unclear how often muscle abnormalities are present but fail to produce significant signs or symptoms. Gibson and coworkers found three unsuspected cases of popliteal vascular entrapment in 86 cadavers in whom the popliteal artery was dissected (138).

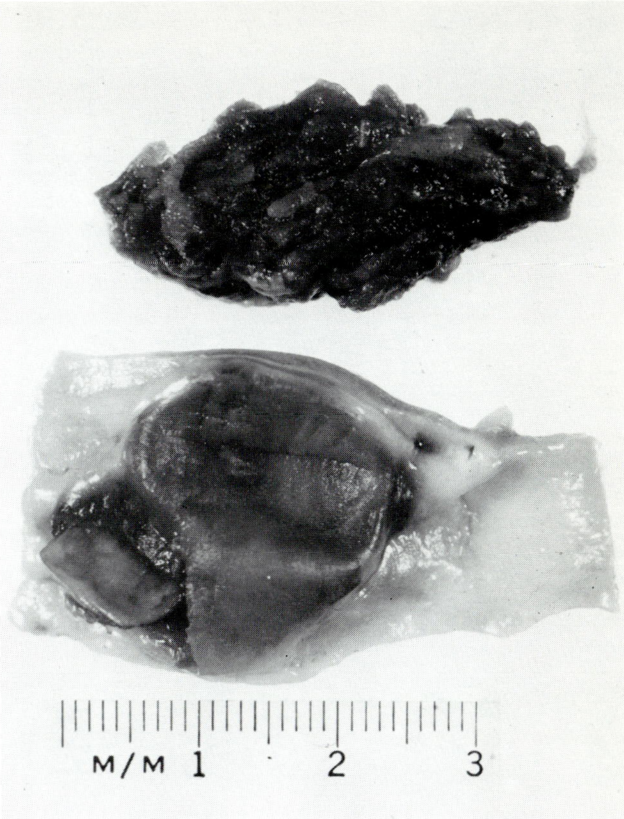

FIGURE 29-5. Longitudinal incision through an aneurysm of the popliteal artery associated with an entrapment syndrome. Laminated clot is present within the lumen. [From Rich NM, Collins GJ Jr, McDonald PT, et al. (122). Reproduced with permission.]

PREVALENCE AND INCIDENCE

There has been international interest in popliteal vascular entrapment syndromes. Although the true incidence of these lesions cannot be established, they are being identified and documented with increasing frequency. Cases have been reported from countries around the world (80,93,94,102,121). This is emphasized by two recent reviews in the surgical literature that provide extensive data regarding this worldwide experience.

PATHOPHYSIOLOGY

The variety of anatomic variants already emphasized can be associated with entrapment of either or both the popliteal artery and the popliteal vein with a variety of effects on normal lower extremity physiology. External compression can vary from minimal in the asymptomatic patient to marked compression that causes a significant stenosis of the popliteal artery or vein. This external compression can advance to total occlusion of the popliteal vessels. This can occur either temporarily with varying positions of the patient's leg and foot, or permanently with intraluminal thrombosis. The arterial pathology associated with external compression of the popliteal artery can range from poststenotic dilatation to the presence of a true aneurysm (Figure 29-5). The potential for embolization of thrombus from the aneurysm to the distal arterial runoff represents an additional threat to the patient's extremity distal to the lesion. Figure 29-6 provides angiographic demonstration of thrombosis of the popliteal artery at the site of entrapment. Midpopliteal arterial occlusion is a classic finding of popliteal artery entrapment with thrombosis. Development of extensive collateral arterial circulation can occur, and the patient may be only mildly symptomatic. Figure 29-7 demonstrates aneurysmal changes that might also develop in the entrapped popliteal vein. Thrombosis of the entrapped vein with resultant venous hypertension and/or chronic venous stasis with associated complications can develop.

An important question remains related to the segment of popliteal artery immediately distal to the area of entrapment. Even after release of the entrapment, will the recurrent trauma from the external compression cause intimal damage and subsequent thrombosis? Certainly the potential exists; however, no study has clarified this relationship. Similarly, it is unclear after release of the entrapment, whether or not the segment of popliteal artery distal to the entrapment, whether it is minimally dilated or not, will progress to a true aneurysm and how long this process will take. Only long-term follow-up of surgically treated cases in which the compression is released and the artery is not replaced will help answer these important questions. There are so few cases of documented entrapment of the popliteal vein that answers to similar questions related to the popliteal vein will probably go unanswered for a long time.

CLINICAL EVALUATION

Diagnosis of popliteal vascular entrapment should be considered and is made most frequently in young, active, athletic men who

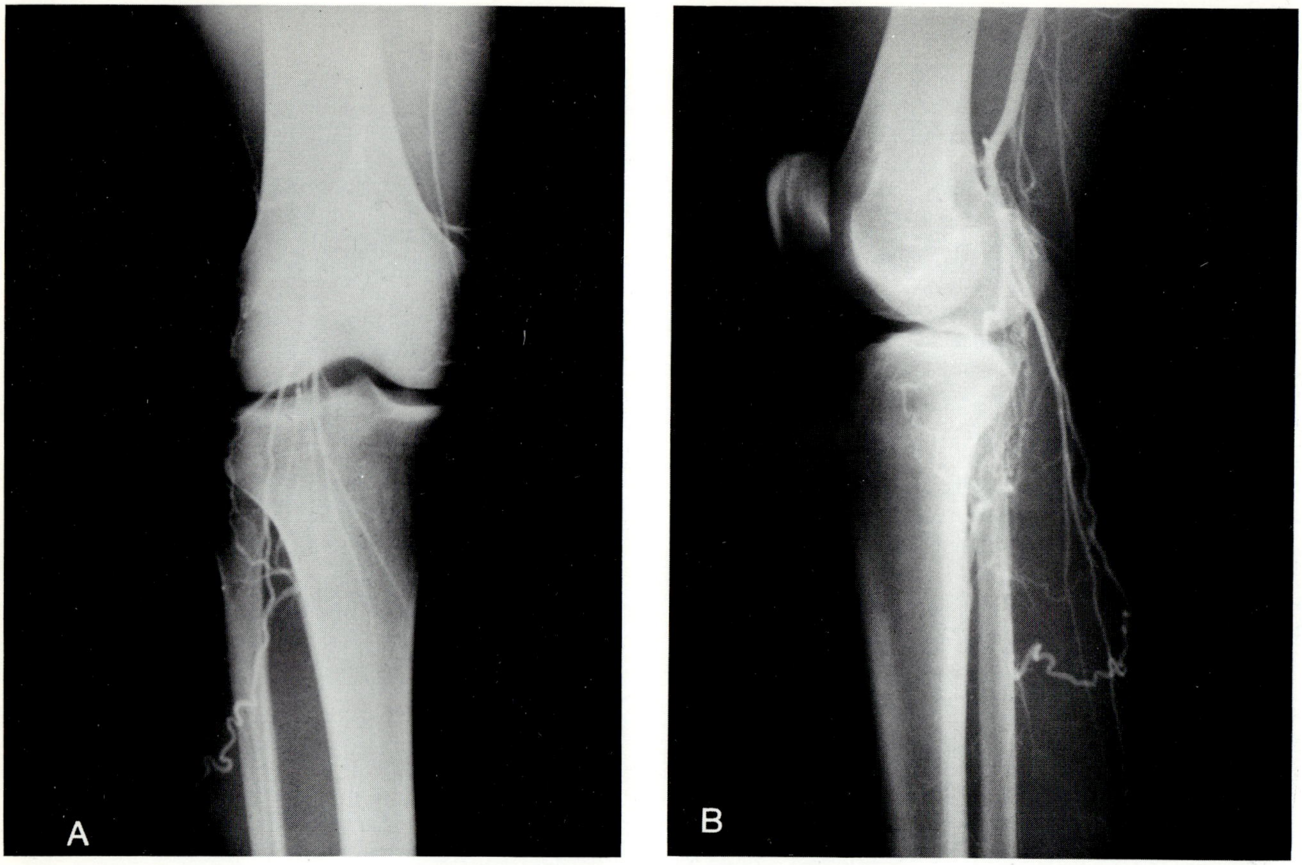

FIGURE 29-6. (*A*) Anteroposterior and (*B*) lateral angiographic views demonstrate medial deviation of the popliteal artery and thrombosis of the midpopliteal artery with development of extensive collateral circulation in a young male that heralded the clinical probability of popliteal vascuar entrapment syndrome. [From Rich NM, Collins GJ Jr, McDonald PT, et al. (122). Reproduced with permission.]

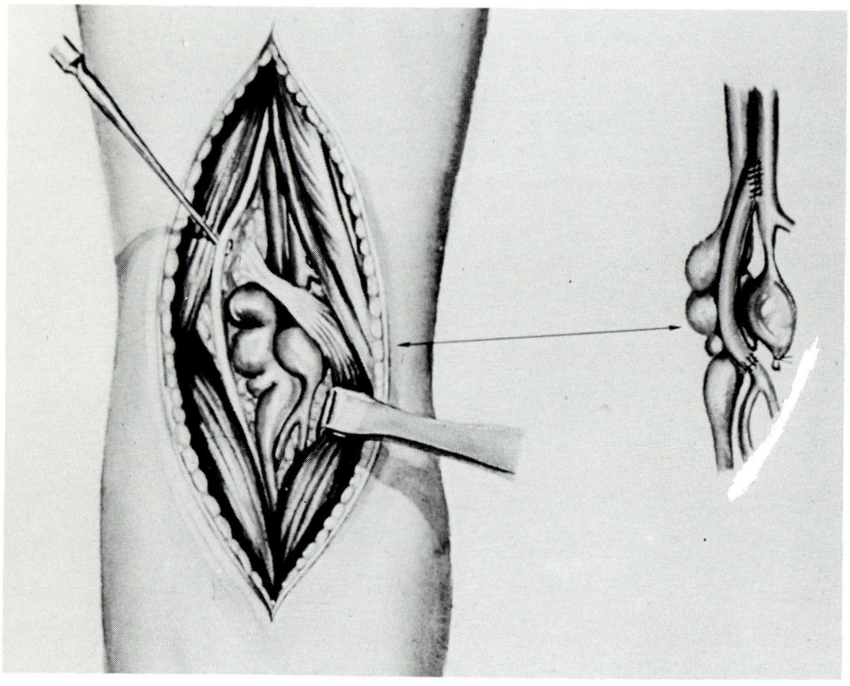

FIGURE 29-7. The drawing shows entrapment with formation of aneurysms in both the popliteal artery and the popliteal vein caused by an accessory slip of the gastrocnemius muscle (*left*). Arterial reconstruction by autogenous greater saphenous vein bypass with ligation of the popliteal arterial aneurysm was performed successfully, (*right*). The accessory slip of muscle was incised near its insertion to release the entrapment of both the artery and vein. [From Rich NM, Hughes CW (109). Reproduced with permission.]

develop intermittent calf claudication with exercise. Despite the male dominance, there are an increasing number of similar lesions being recognized in young athletic women, with the diagnosis of these lesions being made in long-distance runners in an increasing number of cases. With more young men and women jogging and running, it is anticipated that there will be an increasing number of cases identified and reported. In addition, there are also an increasing number of middle-aged patients who are being diagnosed as having popliteal vascular entrapment. In the older population, particularly those who present with a diagnosis of a popliteal artery aneurysm, entrapment of the popliteal artery might also be considered in the differential diagnosis. Although popliteal vascular entrapment was believed initially to be predominately a unilateral lesion, its bilaterality is being recognized with increasing frequency. The syndrome may be present bilaterally in 30 to 40 percent of patients with the anomaly.

DIAGNOSIS

The *history* of intermittent claudication in a young patient during strenuous exercise should raise the suspicion of a tentative diagnosis of popliteal vascular entrapment. Such patients might also have adventitial cystic disease of the popliteal artery. As already emphasized, extensive efforts have been made to establish the diagnosis of popliteal vascular entrapment by *noninvasive techniques* in the vascular laboratory. Results have been accurate in some patients and misleading in others. Table 29-2 illustrates the evaluation of a group of patients at Walter Reed Army Medical Center (126).

Angiographic demonstrations identified classic findings of medial deviations of the popliteal artery as illustrated in Figure 29-6. However, this classic finding may or may not be present. There may also be a midpopliteal artery segmental occlusion as illustrated in Figure 29-6. The angiographic identification of an isolated occlusion of the middle third of the popliteal artery alone should lead one to suspect popliteal arterial entrapment. Although similar occlusions can be associated with adventitial cystic degeneration of the popliteal artery, proximal tapering of the popliteal artery will probably exist with the latter. Phlebograms can also be utilized to outline and identify similar entrapment of the popliteal vein as demonstrated by Connell (137).

TABLE 29-2. Patient Evaluation Representative Findings in Male Soldiers with Leg Symptoms of Possible Arterial Insufficiency

		Ankle/Brachial Pressure Index with Treadmill Exercise Testing								
		Right Leg			Left Leg					
Case No.	Age, yr	Rest	3 min	10 min	Rest	3 min	10 min	Symptoms	Popliteal Arterial Angiographic Findings	Final Diagnosis
1	49	0.8	0.4	—	1.4	1.3	—	Stopped 1 min 45 s due to R foot, calf pain	R occluded 4-cm segment, medial deviation: L normal	R entrapment: L
2	26	0.7	0.5	—	1.1	1.4	—	Stopped 2 min 45 s due to R foot, calf pain	R occluded 3-cm segment; medial deviation: L medial deviation, stenosis with maneuver (Figures 29-2, 29-6, 29-7)	R entrapment: L entrapment
3	21	1.3	1.3	1.2	1.2	1.2	0.6	Completed test complaining of L foot fatigue	R normal: L occlusion with maneuver (Figure 29-3)	R normal: L entrapment
4	27	1.3	1.3	1.4	1.4	1.4	1.4	None	R normal: L normal	Idiopathic leg cramps
5	25	1.1	1.2	—	1.2	1.3	—	Stopped at 3 min due to bilateral leg exhaustion	R normal: L normal	Primary neuromuscular disease
6	23	1.1	1.2	1.1	1.3	1.3	1.1	Minor nonspecific complaints	Not done	Normal
7	38	1.1	1.2	1.1	1.1	1.3	1.1	Minor nonspecific complaints	Not done	Normal
8	31	1.5	1.7	1.3	1.5	1.5	1.2	Minor nonspecific complaints	Not done	Normal
9	32	1.3	1.3	1.1	1.1	1.2	1.3	Minor nonspecific complaints	Not done	Normal
10	30	1.2	1.5	1.4	1.2	1.4	1.4	Minor nonspecific	Not done	Normal

NOTE: The 3-min treadmill exercise was performed at 3 mi/h at a 0 grade. The 10-min treadmill exercise was performed at 4.2 mi/h at a 10 grade. L = left; R = right.

SOURCE: Modified from McDonald PT, Easterbrook JA, Rich NM, et al (126).

TABLE 29-3. Popliteal Vascular Entrapment Treated at Walter Reed Army Medical Center from September 1966 to April 1979

Patient/yr	Age, yr/Sex	Side	Lesion Type	Popliteal Artery	Operation	Result
1/1966	50/M	L	1	Aneurysm	SVG	Excellent
1967	50/M	R	1–3	Aneurysm	SVG	Excellent
2/1967	57/M	L		Aneurysm	SVG	Excellent
3/1968	23/M	L	4	Normal	+	Excellent
4/1970	22/M	L	2	Thrombosis	SVPG-TEA	Excellent
3/1974	29/M	R	4	Normal	+	Excellent
5/1974	59/M	R	1	Normal	+	Excellent
1974	59/M	L	1	Normal	+	Excellent
6/1977	21/M	L	3*	Normal	+	Excellent
7/1978	49/M	R	3	Thrombosis	SVG	Excellent
8/1978	26/M	R	1	Thrombosis	SVPG-TEA	Excellent
1978	26/M	L	1	Normal	+	Excellent
9/1979	35/M	R	4	Normal	+	Good
1979	35/M	L	4	Normal	+	Good

*Although similar to type 3, popliteal vein was also entrapped.

SOURCE: Modified from Rich NM, Collins GJ Jr, McDonald PT, et al. (122).

NOTE: SVG = autogenous saphenous vein bypass graft; + = transection of abnormal gastrocnemius muscle, accessory muscle, fibrous bands, and so forth; SVPG-TEA = autogenous saphenous vein patch graft and thromboendarterectomy.

TREATMENT

Even when these anatomic variants are identified in *asymptomatic* patients, it is now believed that operative intervention should be undertaken to help protect against the later development of complications of the popliteal vascular entrapment. If the vascular involvement extends to thrombosis and/or aneurysm formation, the operative management becomes more difficult and complicated. Operative treatment by release of the entrapping anomalous head of the gastrocnemius muscle, anomalous bands, or associated structures has become widely accepted in both symptomatic and asymptomatic patients.

Although the medial approach to the popliteal artery can be utilized, exact identification of the pathology may not be obvious via medial incisions. We therefore favor a posterior S-shaped incision and have used this approach bilaterally at the same operation in three patients. The S-shaped posterior incision provides adequate exposure for the management of all associated complications such as popliteal artery aneurysm and thrombosis of the midpopliteal artery. The S-shaped incision also provides excellent exposure to identify the variety of anatomic anomaly that is associated with the popliteal vascular entrapment. On the other hand, some surgeons believe that the exact identification of pathology is unimportant and that the midpopliteal artery thrombosis or aneurysm can be adequately managed through the medial approach. Autogenous greater saphenous vein may also be easier to harvest by this approach.

RESULTS

Table 29-3 outlines the most recent Walter Reed Army Medical Center experience. Transection of the anomalous gastrocnemius muscle, accessory slips, fibrous bands, and so forth was utilized successfully in the majority of cases. Either autogenous saphenous vein patch grafts or autogenous greater saphenous vein bypass grafts were used successfully to manage the associated complications of thrombosis and aneurysm. Successful results should be achieved on the management of the majority of patients with popliteal vascular entrapment, whether the entrapment involves the popliteal artery and/or popliteal vein.

PROGNOSIS

Long-term follow-up of patients with popliteal vascular entrapment who have been treated by the operative approach as described remains limited. Initial findings and minimal long-term follow-up of a limited number of patients demonstrate excellent results. Thus successful results should be achieved in the management of the majority of patients with this problem. A long-term follow-up study will be required to answer the question of what happens to the compressed artery and any potentially damaged or weakened artery distal to the compressed segment after the compression is released.

References

1. Rich NM, Spencer FC: *Vascular Trauma*. Philadelphia, Saunders, 1978.
2. Hobson RW II, Rich NM, Wright CB (eds): *Vascular Trauma*. Mount Kisco, New York, Futura, 1983.
3. Alm A: Cystic adventitial degeneration of the popliteal artery. Report of a case. Acta Chir Scand 1975, 141:813.
4. Andersson T, Gothman B, Lindberg K: Mucinous cystic dissecting intramural degeneration of the popliteal artery. Acta Radiol 1959, 52:455.
5. Atkins HJB, Key JA: A case of myxomatous tumour arising in the adventitia of the left external iliac artery. Br J Surg 1947, 34:426.

6. Barnett AJ, Dugdale L, Ferguson I: Disappearing pulse syndrome due to myxomatous degeneration of the popliteal artery. Med J Aust 1966, 2:355.
7. Barnett AJ, Morris KN: Cystic myxomatous degeneration of the popliteal artery. Med J Aust 1964, 2:793.
8. Bartos J, Kalus M, Possner J: Cystische adventitielle degeneration der arteria poplitea. Langenbecks Arch Klin Chir 1966, 314:177.
9. Bliss BP: Cystic myxomatous degeneration of the popliteal artery. Am Heart J 1964, 68:838.
10. Bliss BP, Rhodes J, Harding-Rains AJ: Cystic myxomatous degeneration of the popliteal artery. Br Med J 1963, 2:847.
11. Blum L, Giron F: Adventitial cyst of the popliteal artery with secondary inflammatory entrapment. Mt Sinai J Med 1976, 43:471.
12. Bollinger A, Pouliadis G: Klinik und arteriographie der zystischen adventitia—degeneration peripherer blutgefasse. Vasa 1977, 6:100.
13. Brunner U, Soyka P: Chirurgische gestichtspunkte der arteriellen adventitiazysten. Vasa 1977, 6:105.
14. Chandler JJ: Popliteal artery occlusion by subadventitia pseudocyst. Surgery 1971, 69:474.
15. Chevrier J-L: Un cas de degenerescence colloide de l'adventice de l'artere poplitee. Mem Acad Chir 1962, 88:261.
16. Cousin J, Leleu-Walle M, Cecile J-P, et al: Cystic degeneration of the popliteal artery. Leading article. Br Med J 1970, 4:699.
17. DeLaurentis DA, Wolferth CC Jr, Wolf FM, et al: Mucinous adventitial cysts of the popliteal artery in an 11 year old girl. Surgery 1973, 74:456.
18. Descotes J, Grobert J, Chavent J, et al: Degenerscence colloide de l'adventice de l'artere poplitee. Lyon Chir 1966, 62:898.
19. Dunant JH, Eugenidis N: Cystic degeneration of the popliteal artery. Vasa 1973, 2:156.
20. Eastcott HHG: Cystic myxomatous degeneration of popliteal artery. Br Med J 1963, 2:1270.
21. Eastcott HHG: Cystic degeneration of the popliteal artery. Br Med J 1971, 1:111.
22. Ehringer H, Denck H, Wuketich S, et al: Intermittierender verschluss der arteria poplitea durch zystische adventitiadegeneration. Dtsch Med Wochenschr 1969, 93:2107.
23. Ejrup B, Hiertonn T: Intermittent claudication. Three cases treated by free vein graft. Acta Chir Scand 1954, 108:217.
24. Endo M, Tamura S, Minakuchi S, et al: Isolation and identification of proteohyaluronic acid from a cyst of cystic mucoid degeneration. Clin Chim Acta 1973, 47:417.
25. Faenza A: Cystic adventitial degeneration of the popliteal artery. Arch Chir Thorac Cardiovasc 1976, 33:53.
26. Flanc C: Cystic degeneration of the popliteal artery. Aust NZ J Surg 1967, 36:243.
27. Gedeon A, Puel P, Castany R, et al: Les obliterations non atheromateuses de l'artere poplitee. Chirurgie 1975, 101:355.
28. Gripe K: Intramural cystisk arteriell mukoiddegeneration. Nord Med 1963, 70:1381.
29. Haid SP, Conn J Jr, Bergan JJ: Cystic adventitial disease of the popliteal artery. Arch Surg 1970, 101:765.
30. Hansen JPH: Cystic mucoid degeneration of the popliteal artery. Acta Chir Scand 1966, 131:171.
31. Harris JD, Jepson RP: Cystic degeneration of the popliteal artery. Austr NZ J Surg 1965, 34:265.
32. Hiertonn T, Lindberg K: Cystic adventitial degeneration of the popliteal artery. Acta Chir Scand 1957, 113:72.
33. Hiertonn T, Lindberg K, Rob C: Cystic degeneration of the popliteal artery. Br J Surg 1957, 44:348.
34. Hofmann KT, Consiglio L, Hofmeier G, et al: Die zystische defass-degeneration. Bruns Beitr Klin Chir 1969, 217:284.
35. Holmes JG: Cystic adventitial degeneration of the popliteal artery. JAMA 1960, 173:654.
36. Ishikawa K, Mishima Y, Kobayshi S: Cystic adventitial disease of the popliteal artery. Angiology 1961, 12:357.
37. Jaquet G-H, Meyer-Burgdorff G: Arterielle durchblutungsstorung infolge cystischer degeneration der adventitia. Der Chir 1960, 31:481.
38. Kairaluoma MI, Karkola P, Larmi TKI: Cystic adventitial disease—Cause of intermittent claudication in non-smokers. A case report. Ann Chir Gynaecol 1976, 65:388.
39. Lambley DG: Intermittent claudication due to cystic degeneration of popliteal artery. Br Med J 1963, 2:849.
40. Laurendeau F: La degenerescence adventicielle kystique de l'artere poplitee. Union Med Can 1969, 98:589.
41. Leaf G: Amino-acid analysis of protein present in a popliteal artery cyst. Br Med J 1967, 3:415.
42. Leu HJ: Pathogenese und histologie der zystischen adventitiadegeneration periphereer blutgefasse. Vasa 1977, 6:94.
43. Lewis GJT, Douglas DM, Reid W, et al: Cystic adventitial disease of the popliteal artery. Br Med J 1967, 3:411.
44. Linquette M, Mesmacque R, Beghin B, et al: Degenerescense kystique de l'adventice de l'artere poplitee. Sem Hop Paris 1967, 43:3005.
45. Little JM, Goodman AH: Cystic adventitial disease of the popliteal artery. Br J Surg 1970, 57:708.
46. Marzoli GP, Meyer-Burgdorff G, Jacquet GH: Sulle pseudocisti della parete arteriosa. Chir Ital 1962, 14:291.
47. Mateo AM: Degeneracion quistica de la tunica media de la arteria poplitea. Angiologia 1974, 26:331.
48. Mentha C: Degenerescence kystique adventitelle ou bursite de l'artere poplitee. J Chir 1965, 89:173.
49. Miliken JC: Cystic degeneration of the popliteal artery in a female. Br Med J 1971, 2:769.
50. Morino F, Silverstrini P, Galli T: Un case di cisti dissecante intramurale dell'arteria poplitea. Minerva Chir 1966, 21:786.
51. Muller M, Rodriguez J: Obstruccion da la arteria poplitea por enfermedad quistica mucinosa de la pared arterial. Angiologia 1975, 27:1.
52. Muller-Wiefel H, Papachrysanthou C: Cystic wall degeneration of the popliteal artery. Herz/Kreisl 1974, 6:333.
53. Ohara I, Minaguhi S: Adventitial cystic disease of the popliteal artery. Operation 1973, 27:321.
54. Patel J, Cormier JM: La degenerescence kystique on colloide de l'adventice arteriel. Presse Med 1963, 71:244.
55. Patel J, Facquet J, Piwnica A: Degenerescence kystique on colloide de l'adventice. Presse Med 1958, 66:1164.
56. Pierangeli A, De Rubertis C: Degenerazione cistica avientiziale dell'arteria poplitea. Arch Ital Chir 1966, 92:108.
57. Powis SJA, Morrissey DM, Jones EL: Cystic degeneration of the popliteal artery. Surgery 1970, 67:891.
58. Raithel D, Hacker RW: Die zystische adventitia-degeneration der A. poplitea. Vasa 1975, 4:353.
59. Robb D: Obstruction of popliteal artery by synovial cyst. Br J Surg 1960, 48:221.
60. Savage PEA: Cystic disease of the popliteal artery. Br J Surg 1969, 56:77.
61. Schlesinger A, Gottesman L: Cystic degeneration of the popliteal artery. Am J Roentgenol 1976, 127:1043.
62. Scobie TK, Curry RH: Cystic adventitial disease of the popliteal artery. Can J Surg 1975, 18:46.
63. Shabbo FP: Cystic disease of the popliteal artery. Proc R Soc Med 1976, 69:362.
64. Shannon R: Cystic degeneration of the popliteal artery. Aust NZ J Surg 1971, 40:290.
65. Shute R: Degenerescence colloide de l'adventice de l'artere poplitee traitee par prostese en Dacron. Mem Acad Chir 1963, 89:849.

66. Soots G, L'Hermine C, Lerche E, et al: Degenerescence colloide adventicielle de l'artere poplitee. J Radiol Electrol Med Nucl 1972, 53:85.
67. Sperling M, Schott H, Ruppell V: Die cystische adventitia-degeneration der blutgefasse. Chirurgier 1972, 43:37.
68. Stirling GR, Aarons, BJ: Cystic myxomatous degeneration of the popliteal artery. Alfred Hosp Clin Rep 1967, 14:91.
69. Suy R, Van Osselaer G, Pakdaman A, et al: The pseudocyst of the adventitia of the popliteal artery. J Cardiovasc Surg 1970, 11:103.
70. Taylor H, Taylor RS, Ramsay CA: Cyst of popliteal artery. Br Med J 1967, 4:109.
71. Tracy GD, Ludbrook J, Rundle FF: Cystic adventitial disease of the popliteal artery. Vasc Surg 1969, 3:10.
72. Tytgat H, Derom F, Galinsky A: Degenerescence kystique de l'artere poplitee traitee par greffe en nylon. Acta Chir Belg 1958, 57:188.
73. Vollmar J: Die zystische adventitia—degeneration der schlagadern. Kreis 1963, 52:1028.
74. Zinicola N, Ferrero S, Odero A: Adventitial cyst of the popliteal artery. Case report. Minerva Cardioangiol 1973, 21:474.
75. Albertazzi VI: Popliteal artery entrapment syndrome. JAMA 1969, 209:1087.
76. Albertazzi VI, Elliot TE, Kennedy JA: Popliteal artery entrapment. Angiology 1969, 20:119.
77. Amici F Jr: Un raro caso di decorso anomalo con ostruzione trobotica dell'arteria poplitea. Minerva Ortop 1965, 16:427.
78. Baker WH, Stoney RJ: Acquired popliteal entrapment syndrome. Arch Surg 1972, 105:780.
79. Beebe HG: Popliteal artery entrapment syndrome. Vasc Diag Ther 1981, Feb/Mar 25.
80. Bouhoutsos I, Goulious A: Popliteal artery entrapment: Report of a case. J Cardiovasc Surg 1977, 18:481.
81. Brener BJ, Alpert J, Brief DK, et al: Limb loss in young man due to entrapment of the popliteal artery. J Med Soc NJ 1975, 72:47.
82. Brightmore TGJ, Smellie WAB: Popliteal artery entrapment. Br J Surg 1971, 58:481.
83. Carter AE, Eban R: A case history of bilateral developmental abnormality of popliteal arteries and gastrocnemius muscles. Br J Surg 1964, 51:518.
84. Chavatzas D, Barabas AP, Martin P: Popliteal-artery entrapment. Lancet 1973, 2:181.
85. Darling RC, Buckley CJ, Abbott WM, et al: Intermittent claudication in young athletes: Popliteal artery entrapment syndrome. J Trauma 1974, 14:543.
86. Delaney TA, Gonzalez LL: Occlusion of popliteal artery due to muscular entrapment. Surgery 1971, 69:97.
87. Devin R, Salavert JP, Dor P: Malposition et stenose extrinseque de l'artere poplitee par anomalie d'insertion du jumeau interne. Mem Acad Chir 1969, 95:752.
88. Edmondson HT, Crowe JA Jr: Popliteal arterial and venous entrapment. Am Surg 1972, 38:657.
89. Evans EW, Bernhard V: Acute popliteal artery entrapment. Am J Surg 1971, 121:739.
90. Ezzet F, Yettra M: Bilateral popliteal artery entrapment: Case report and observations. J Cardiovasc Surg 1971, 12:71.
91. Fontanetta AP, Kirshbom E, Fisher MM, et al: Popliteal artery entrapment: Lateral deviation and compression of artery. Vasa 1974, 3:399.
92. Gallagher EG, Hudson TL: Popliteal artery entrapment. Am J Surg 1974, 128:88.
93. Gaylis H, Rosenberg B: Popliteal artery entrapment syndrome. S Afr Med J 1972, 46:1071.
94. Gaylis H, Rosenberg B: The popliteal artery entrapment syndrome: A bilateral case. S Afr J Surg 1973, 11:51.
95. Haimovici H, Sprayregen S, Johnson F: Popliteal artery entrapment by fibrous band. Surgery 1972, 72:789.
96. Hall KV: Anomalous insertion of the medial gastrocnemic head, with circulatory complications. Acta Pathol Microbiol Scand 1961, 148(suppl):53.
97. Hall KV: Intravascular gastrocnemius insertion. Acta Chir Scand 1964, 128:193.
98. Hamming JJ: Intermittent claudication at an early age, due to an anomalous course of the popliteal artery. Angiology 1959, 10:369.
99. Hamming JJ, Vink M: Obstruction of the popliteal artery at an early age. J Cardiovasc Surg 1965, 6:516.
100. Harris JD, Jepson RP: Entrapment of the popliteal artery. Surgery 1971, 69:246.
101. Husni EA, Ryu CK: Entrapment of the popliteal artery and its management. Angiology 1971, 22:380.
102. Inada K, Hirose M, Iwashima Y, et al: Popliteal artery entrapment syndrome: A case report. Br J Surg 1978, 65:613.
103. Insua JA, Young JR, Humphries AWS: Popliteal artery entrapment syndrome. Arch Surg 1970, 101:771.
104. Kessler HJ, McCabe JS, Waller JV: Popliteal artery entrapment syndrome. NY State J Med 1976, 76:80.
105. Laubach K, Trede M, Perera R, et al: Das Kompressionssyndrom der arteria poplitea. Chirurg 1973, 44:74.
106. Love JW, Whelan TJ: Popliteal artery entrapment syndrome. Am J Surg 1965, 109:620.
107. Mark LK, Kiselow MC, Wagner M, et al: Popliteal artery entrapment syndrome. JAMA 1978, 240:465.
108. Mentha C: Malposition et stenose extrinseque de l'artere poplitee par la compression musculotendineuse du jumeau interne. J Chir 1966, 91:489.
109. Rich NM, Hughes CW: Popliteal artery and vein entrapment. Am J Surg 1967, 113:696.
110. Schulze-Bergman G: Zum kompressionssyndrom der arteria poplitea. Vasa 1972, 1:186.
111. Servello M: Clinical syndrome of anomalous position of the popliteal artery: Differentiation from juvenile arteriopathy. Circulation 1962, 26:885.
112. Stuart TPA: A note on a variation in the course of the popliteal artery. J Anat Physiol 1879, 13:162.
113. Turner GR, Gosney WG, Ellingson W, et al: Popliteal entrapment syndrome. JAMA 1969, 208:692.
114. Van Bockel JH, Biemans RGM: Popliteal artery entrapment. Arch Chir Neerl Fac 1976, 28:251.
115. Bergan JJ: Adventitial cystic disease of the popliteal artery. In Rutherford RB (ed): *Vascular Surgery*. Philadelphia, Saunders 1977.
116. Bergan JJ, Yao JST, Flinn WR: Surgical management of young claudicants: Adventitial cyst. In Bergan JJ, Yao JST (eds): *Evaluation and Treatment of Upper and Lower Extremity Circulatory Disorders*. Orlando, Florida, Grune & Stratton, 1984.
117. Cousin J, Leleu-Walle M, Cecile J-P, et al: Degenerescense kystique de l'artere poplitee chez un garcon de 13 ans. J Sci Med Lille 1973, 91:85.
118. Flanigan DP, Burnham SJ, Goodreau JJ, et al: Summary of cases of adventitial cystic disease of the popliteal artery. Ann Surg 1979, 189:165.
119. Biemans RGM, van Bockell JH: Popliteal artery entrapment syndrome. Surg Gynecol Obstet 1977, 144:604.
120. Ferrero R, Barile C, Buzzacchino A, et al: La sindrome da costrizione dell'arteria poplia. Minerva Cardioangiol 1978, 26:389.
121. Ikeda M, Iwase T, Ashida K, Tankawa H: Popliteal artery entrapment syndrome: Report of a case and study of 18 cases in Japan. Am J Surg 1981, 141:726.
122. Rich NM, Collins GJ Jr, McDonald PT, et al: Popliteal vascular entrapment. Arch Surg 1979, 114:1377.

123. Whelan TF Jr: Popliteal artery entrapment syndrome. In Haimovici H (ed): *Vascular Surgery*. New York, McGraw-Hill, 1976.
124. Yao JST, Hobbs JT, Irvine WT: Ankle systolic pressure measurements in arterial disease affecting the lower extremities. Br J Surg 1969, 56:676.
125. Barnes RW, Strandness DE: Isolated popliteal artery occlusion. Physiologic observations. Vasc Surg 1972, 6:103.
126. McDonald PT, Easterbrook JA, Rich NM, et al: Popliteal artery entrapment syndrome. Clinical common noninvasive and angiographic diagnosis. Am J Surg 1980, 139:318.
127. Baumann G, Schmidt FC, Becker HM, et al: Cystische wanddegeneration der arteria ilica external und arteria femoralis communis. Chirurg 1967, 38:520.
128. Campbell RT, McCluskey BC, Andrews MIJ: A case of polycystic adventitial disease of the left external iliac and femoral artery. Br J Surg 1970, 57:865.
129. Backstrom CG, Linell F, Ostberg G: Cystic myxomatous adventitial degeneration of the radial artery with development in the connective tissue. Acta Chir Scand 1965, 129:447.
130. Richards RL: Cystic degeneration. Br Med J 1963, 3:997.
131. Ruppell V, Sperling M, Schott H, et al: Pathological anatomical observations in cystic adventitial degeneration of blood vessels. Beitr Pathol Bd 1971, 144:101.
132. Savage PEA: Arterial cystic degeneration. Postgrad Med J 1972, 48:603.
133. Clark K: Ganglion of the lateral popliteal nerve. J Bone Joint Surg 1961, 43:778.
134. McEvedy BV: Simple ganglia. Br J Surg 1962, 49:585.
135. Parkes A: Intraneural ganglion of the lateral popliteal nerve. J Bone Joint Surg 1961, 43B:784.
136. Sutton D: *Arteriography*. London, Edinburg E. Livingstone, 1962.
137. Connell J: Popliteal vein entrapment. Br J Surg 1978, 65:351.
138. Gibson MHL, Mills MS, Johnson GE, et al: Popliteal entrapment syndrome. Ann Surg 1977, 185:341.

Chapter 30

EXTRAANATOMIC BYPASSES

DONALD K. BRIEF and BRUCE J. BRENER

Revascularization of the brain, ischemic organs, or ischemic upper and lower extremities is traditionally carried out by a direct anatomic approach to the diseased vessels, relieving the occlusive process by endarterectomy, bypass grafting, or a combination of both. Alternative approaches to reconstruction are necessary when a conventional approach would carry too great a risk because of the poor health of the patient, the presence of infection, or other anatomic factors precluding direct exposure of the diseased vessels. The bypass is then carried out at a site remote from the disease.

The donor vessel may generally provide circulation to a different part of the body than that being revascularized, and the graft may lie in an anatomic plane different from the diseased vessel. Despite the objections of some authors, these grafts have been called "extraanatomic," not because they are *outside* the body, but because they are not in the usual location.

Commonly used extraanatomic bypass grafts include carotid-subclavian, axilloaxillary, carotid-carotid, and carotid-vertebral bypasses for brachiocephalic occlusive disease. Because these grafts do not originate from the aorta, they eliminate the need for intrathoracic exposure. Crossover femorofemoral and axillobifemoral grafts, and obturator foramen and lateral femoral bypasses are the commonly used extraanatomic procedures for the lower extremity, which is a more common site for atherosclerosis.

The principles of revascularization of the brachiocephalic system are described in Chapters 42 and 43. The present chapter deals primarily with the indications, hemodynamic principles, techniques, and results of the procedures involved in extraanatomic revascularization of the lower extremities.

General Considerations

INDICATIONS FOR EXTRAANATOMIC BYPASS

The choice of anatomic or extraanatomic reconstruction is based on an evaluation of several factors: severity of the disease; general health of the patient; ease of the reconstructive procedure; anatomical considerations such as severe obesity, scarring from previous surgery, presence of infection; and long-term patency results. The surgeon must weigh each of these factors; some may be more important than others in a given clinical situation. For example, obturator, lateral ileofemoral, ascending aortofemoral, or descending aortofemoral bypass grafting may be more difficult or more taxing to the patient than conventional reconstruction. These extraanatomic procedures are utilized only under specific conditions, such as the presence of infection or in conjunction with open heart bypass procedures. Similarly, axillofemoral bypass may be elected only for limb salvage by some surgeons, whereas femorofemoral bypass may be used more freely for intermittent claudication. The surgeon may believe the patency rate is poorer with axillofemoral procedures than with a conventional approach and will reserve the extraanatomic procedure for limb-threatening ischemia. In contrast, results with femorofemoral bypass may be equal to the anatomic reconstruction, and since this procedure is less taxing, it may be used more widely.

The most common reason for performing axillofemoral or femorofemoral bypass is the presumed lower risk of these subcutaneous procedures. Undoubtedly, some patients in whom this route is used would not survive conventional approaches. This has led Leather et al. (1) to combine axillofemoral grafting and iliac artery ligation to bypass and thrombose abdominal aortic aneurysms. Similarly, we have used the subcutaneous route to revascularize patients with acute lower limb ischemia following recent myocardial infarction, prolonged cardiopulmonary bypass procedures, and intraaortic balloon insertions (2). Evidence of the high-risk nature of the population group undergoing extraanatomic bypass is seen in reports of short- and long-term mortality rates. Livesay et al. (3) have noted a mortality rate of 10 percent at 30 days and 52 percent at 2 years in their patients undergoing axillofemoral bypass.

HEMODYNAMIC CONSIDERATION

An early concern in the performance of extraanatomic bypass grafting was the production of a "steal" phenomenon, that is, a diversion of blood away from the donor artery and the extremity supplied by it (4,5). Initial clinical observations by several workers utilizing axillofemoral and crossover femorofemoral techniques suggested that steal did not occur in the absence of a preexisting stenosis in the donor vessel or one produced at the proximal anastomosis to the donor artery. This has been confirmed by the experiments of Harper et al. (6); Ehrenfeld, Harris, and Wylie (7); Lord and Ehrenfeld (8); Parsonnet, Alpert, and Brief (9); and Trimble et al. (10). In the absence of donor artery proximal disease, no decrease in the donor limb blood flow distal to the crossover was observed despite a 10-fold increase in the flow in the donor artery. This principle has been demonstrated in the human crossover femorofemoral graft on numerous occasions with intraoperative flow measurements.

However, if a proximal stenosis is present in the donor artery, the increased flow created by the new bypass distal to it will increase frictional energy losses across the lesion. The electrical analogue of adding a new low-resistance bed in parallel to the one already in existence is the basis for this increased flow rate. As a result the pressure will be lower in the distal donor and recipient arteries than in the artery proximal to the stenosis. This will be detected as a fall in donor ankle pressure or brachial pressure, depending upon whether the graft is a femorofemoral or an axillofemoral bypass. The greater the stenosis, the greater the fall in donor limb pressure. Furthermore, if the donor limb has a high-resistance "runoff" bed and the recipient limb has a low-resistance outflow bed, the total flow through the donor stenosis may increase more than twofold. This would lead to a greater pressure loss. These physiological changes are not a "steal" of blood from the donor limb through the bypass, but a natural consequence of increased flow through the stenosis.

It is therefore essential that there be no significant disease in the donor segment and that no stenosis be produced by the proximal anastomosis. The presence of ischemia in the donor limb immediately after the performance of an extraanatomic bypass should alert the surgeon to a technical problem at the donor anastomotic site or to the presence in the donor vessel of a stenosis, the importance of which was unappreciated.

An interesting but yet unanswered question is the effect on the donor artery of the markedly increased flow rate proximal to the origin of the extraanatomic bypass. The artery proximal to a large chronic arteriovenous fistula is dilated and often aneurysmal. This has not has been observed in donor arteries supplying extraanatomic bypasses followed up to 15 years. Presumably, this is because the flow rates are lower through the donor artery due to the higher resistance of the arterial system, and therefore dilatation and aneurysmal degenerative processes do not occur. It has been postulated that the increased donor artery flow actually has a protective effect on the donor artery, retarding the atherosclerotic process. There has been a relatively low incidence of late occlusions of crossover femorofemoral grafts because of progressive disease in the donor segment over time. This incidence is less than one might expect on the basis of the fate of the nonbypassed arteries contralateral to unilateral aortofemoral bypass or unilateral aortoiliac endarterectomies, although the relevant evidence on this point is contradictory (11–14).

Graft Materials

There is no conclusive evidence that one graft material is to be preferred over another for anatomic bypass procedures. The majority of reported experience with knitted Dacron grafts in virtually all positions above the inguinal ligament suggests that patency rates are acceptable. Certainly for shorter grafts in the brachiocephalic and crossover femorofemoral positions, long-term patency has been excellent. Recent reports on expanded polytetrafluoroethylene and modified human umbilical vein grafts suggest that these also are satisfactory. The expanded polytetrafluoroethylene graft has the advantages that it is easier to use and to subject to late thrombectomy. Autologous saphenous vein has been used successfully in the crossover femorofemoral position as well as in the brachiocephalic position. The length of graft necessary for axillofemoral operations as well as its relatively small size makes autologous vein impractical, although its use has been reported (15). The optimum diameter of synthetic grafts has not been clearly established. Synthetic grafts become lined with compacted fibrin that often narrows the diameter of the outflow tract. Higher blood flow velocities and thinner fibrin layers are found with 6- and 8-mm grafts than with larger grafts. These diameters are probably adequate for most extraanatomic grafts, and 6-mm grafts may be superior, particularly in settings where bypass flow rates will be relatively low (16).*

Crimped grafts may have a lower patency rate at reduced flows (17). There is some evidence that noncrimped grafts should be used for axillofemoral and femorofemoral bypasses, but this has not been confirmed. Finally, grafts reinforced to prevent compression in the subcutaneous position have been used recently and may give additional longevity to these bypasses, although this is unproved. It would appear that satisfactory long-term patency rates associated with extraanatomic bypass grafts to the ischemic lower extremity relate more to the proper selection of patients, the status of the donor artery, disease progression, and attention to technical details than to the choice of graft material.

*See also Additional References (Sanders et al. and Ascer et al.).

Femorofemoral Crossover Grafts

The earliest reports of femorofemoral crossover grafting for unilateral iliac occlusive disease were by Freeman and Leeds (18), Oudot and Beaconfield (19), McCaughan and Kahn (20), and Vetto (21). Our 12-year experience with femorofemoral grafts in 133 patients is the largest experience with long-term follow-up reported thus far (22). Our current 15-year experience with 154 patients treated for unilateral atherosclerotic iliac occlusive disease continues to support the concept of extraanatomic bypass as a means of dealing with this problem. Crossover femorofemoral grafts have also been useful in revascularizing a limb after unilateral occlusion of an aortobifemoral graft, in continuing support of patients who require intraaortic balloon pumping but whose circulation to the extremity is obstructed by the balloon catheter, and in the management of patients who have an infected kidney transplant and erosion of the iliac artery requiring ligation. The following discussion focuses on the use of crossover femorofemoral grafts for unilateral atherosclerotic occlusive disease since the application of this operation to other clinical settings is obvious and the technical principles are similar to those in occlusive disease.

The indications for crossover femorofemoral grafts are the presence of disabling claudication, rest pain, or gangrene. If the patient's symptoms are primarily unilateral and a strong femoral pulse is present on the unaffected side, the patient is a potential candidate for a crossover femorofemoral graft. Angiography with peak systolic pressure determinations in the aorta and distal donor ileofemoral arterial system is necessary before an accurate final decision to perform this operation can be made. It is often necessary to combine these two studies because conventional arteriography in the anterior-posterior plane may not detect significant obstructive lesions in the iliac system. By performing retrograde transfemoral catheter aortography via the donor femoral artery with oblique views and accurate pressure measurements one can obtain accurate preoperative assessment. Questionable areas of stenosis noted on arteriography may not produce significant pressure gradients at rest. Flow rates in the proposed donor iliac artery can be increased by exercise, vasodilators, or cuff-induced ischemia to elicit or magnify these gradients (23–29). Intraoperative pressure measurements may also be useful (30,31). In our experience if there is no gradient at rest, it is unlikely that a donor lesion would affect the short-term patency of a crossover graft, and the procedure can be used in elderly, poor-risk patients with the expectation of a good result. If a hemodynamically significant stenotic lesion is present in the donor artery, balloon angioplasty can be considered to relieve the stenosis and make the patient suitable for a crossover femorofemoral procedure (32). Most vascular surgeons would reserve this procedure for poor-risk patients and would proceed with an aortobifemoral bypass in good-risk patients.

Should a good-risk patient with hemodynamically significant unilateral iliac disease have a crossover femorofemoral graft as a primary procedure or a unilateral attack on this problem by local endarterectomy, unilateral aortobifemoral bypass, aortobifemoral bypass, or percutaneous balloon angioplasty? In our experience most symptomatic iliac lesions are not isolated, short stenoses in the common iliac artery and therefore are not amenable to balloon angioplasty. Although in skilled hands aortofemoral bypass can be performed with low operative mortality and morbidity rates, even in good-risk patients we still prefer to use the crossover femorofemoral graft as the interventional procedure of choice. This simple operation avoids intraabdominal dissection and potential impotence in the male, produces patency rates comparable to more conventional procedures, does not preclude later aortofemoral procedures if they should prove necessary, and avoids operating on and bypassing a patent artery. The crossover femorofemoral graft will increase flow in the donor iliac system and may exert a protective effect on the development and progression of atherosclerotic changes in this vessel.

TECHNIQUE

The technique for the femorofemoral bypass graft has changed little since its original description and is briefly illustrated in Figure 30-1. The operation can be done under local anesthesia, but we prefer regional or general anesthesia if the clinical situation permits. A two-team approach reduces operating time. After appropriate preparation and draping of the lower extremities and groin areas, vertical incisions are made over the femoral vessels. The dissection is sharply carried down to the femoral arteries, approaching them laterally to avoid severing lymphatic tissue if possible. The vessels are thoroughly dissected, preserving all significant collateral branches, and the deep and superficial femoral arteries are isolated. The subcutaneous suprapubic tunnel is made, and then the patient is given systemic heparin.

The recipient vessel is approached first and carefully palpated. If the superficial femoral artery is occluded and the common femoral artery is patent back to the hypogastric system, the graft is placed in the common femoral artery but carried onto the deep femoral artery to ensure good outflow. If there is significant disease in the orifice of the deep femoral, an appropriate endarterectomy is carried out under direct vision. If both the common femoral and the superficial femoral arteries are occluded and the profunda femoral is the only outflow tract for the graft, an end-to-end or end-to-side anastomosis is carried out. If the deep femoral is a small vessel or is extensively diseased, a concomitant femoropopliteal bypass may be necessary. In our experience this has been necessary in a small percentage of cases, since the deep femoral artery has usually been adequate.

After completion of the recipient anastomosis the graft is tunneled carefully to avoid kinking, and the donor anastomosis is performed in the opposite common femoral artery to allow the graft to lie without kinking or undue tension in a wide inverted U configuration. Care must be taken to avoid creating intimal flaps or clamp trauma in either femoral artery since both may be heavily involved with nonocclusive atherosclerosis. Occasionally some form of endarterectomy or patch angioplasty on the donor vessels is required to ensure adequate inflow. We prefer to use 6-mm or 8-mm Dacron or expanded polytetrafluoroethylene with 6-0 polypropylene sutures for the anastomoses. Optical magnification may be helpful.

When bleeding is controlled and no technical problems are noted, heparin is reversed with protamine sulfate and the wounds are closed without drainage. Occasionally an intraoperative arteriogram is performed. It is important to perform a secure layered closure to avoid dead space and minimize wound sepsis. We employ three layers of running absorbable suture, one to the crural fascia of the femoral sheath, a second to the deep fascia, and the third to the subcutaneous or Scarpa's fascia. The skin is carefully approximated and light dressings applied. In the recovery room baseline plethysmographic tracings and segmental arterial pressures are obtained. Although the graft pulse may not be palpable because of edema, its patency can be confirmed by direct Doppler examination or by hearing a bruit in the suprapubic area. Deterioration in the clinical or noninvasive evaluation in the postoperative period demands immediate reoperation. Graft thrombectomy can be performed and technical defects can be corrected. However, delay may lead to failure of the operation and limb loss.

When the crossover graft is required to provide circulation to a limb rendered ischemic by an intraaortic balloon, the following technique is employed. The occluded common femoral artery is divided distal to the balloon insertion site, and the graft is sutured to it end-to-end. The balloon catheter is isolated from the graft so that it can be removed without further contamination of the graft. No late closures in grafts performed for this indication have occurred in our series. Alternatives to this operation include

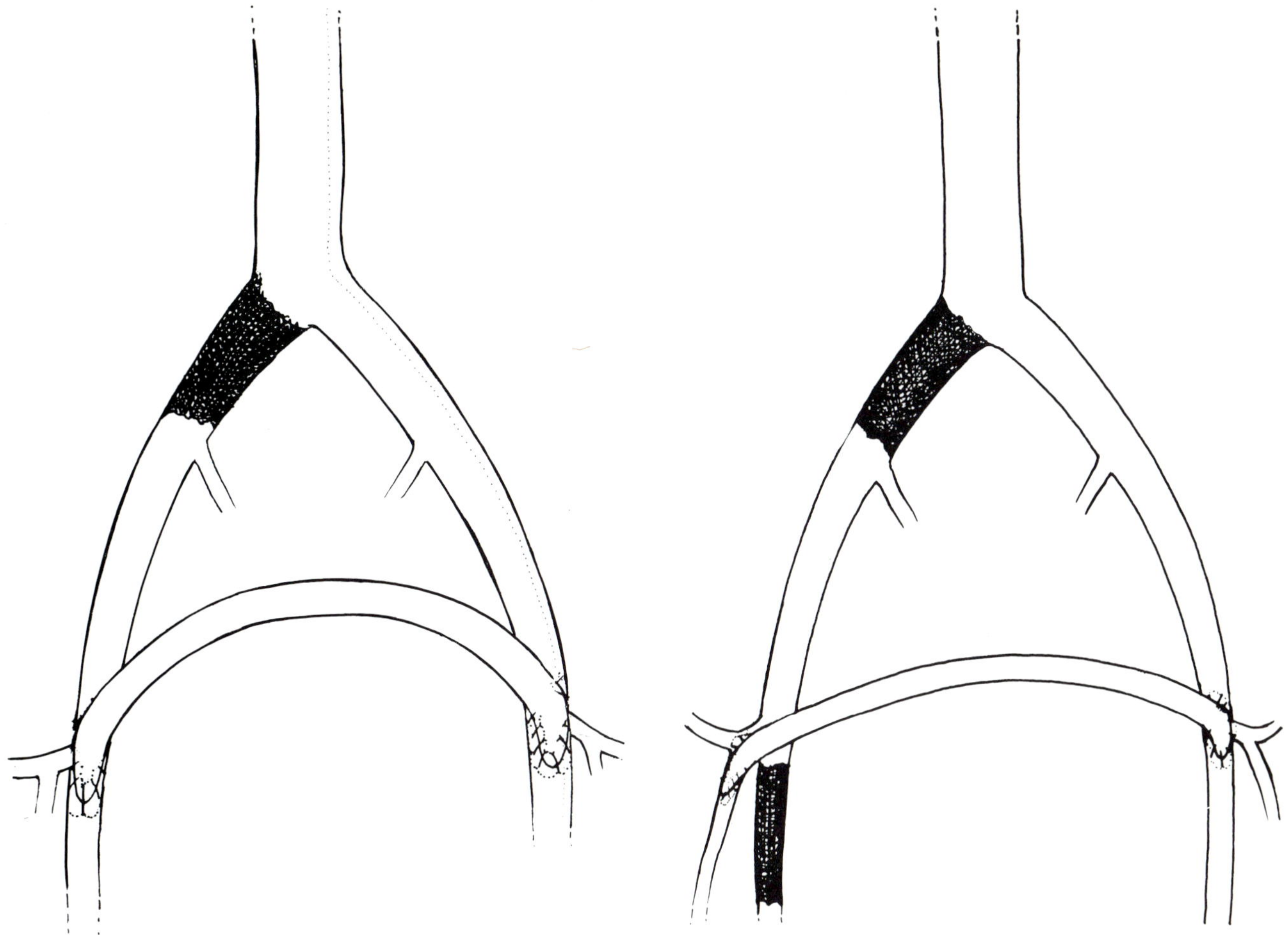

FIGURE 30-1. (*A*) The crossover femorofemoral graft is performed as shown in a wide inverted U configuration. (*B*) Local endarterectomy or patch angioplasty of the profunda femoris artery may be necessary to ensure adequate inflow and outflow when the superficial femoral artery is occluded. The graft is then placed to extend onto this artery.

removal of the intraaortic balloon with thrombectomy and replacement in the ipsilateral or contralateral side.

RESULTS

Patency rates for femorofemoral crossover grafts have been comparable to those for aortofemoral bypass. Results of our 15-year experience and 9 other studies are summarized in Table 30-1. Five-year cumulative patency in over 600 patients averaged about 65 percent, ranging from 45 to 80 percent. In our series of 154 patients, patency was 79 percent at 5, 68 percent at 10, and 60 percent at 15 years, although few patients survived beyond 12 years.

Early in our experience several surgeons expressed doubts that patency would be sustained because of progressive disease in the donor iliac artery. When the principles of patient selection noted above were followed, donor iliac stenosis was unusual. In our 154 cases, graft occlusion due to donor iliac disease occurred only seven times (4.5 percent) in the 15-year experience. Ten cases in our series have had bilateral aortofemoral bypass after late failures of femorofemoral bypass, showing that this more extensive procedure is still feasible after the subcutaneous bypass. To date we have had insufficient experience with balloon dilatation of the donor iliac artery and crossover femorofemoral grafts to know whether these donor arteries will maintain patency. However a number of centers are beginning to report that they will (see Chapters 18, 19, and 20).

In addition to concern about patency, several authors have noted a reduction in donor limb perfusion after crossover grafting (23–25). Harris et al. (25) found a deterioration of either the resting or after-exercise ankle-brachial index in the donor limb in 20 of 44 patients undergoing femorofemoral bypass for claudication. Eighteen of the 20 had patent superficial femoral arteries. Four patients underwent aortofemoral bypass after femorofemoral grafting. Presumably the deterioration in donor limb hemodynamics was not clinically significant in the other patients. This report underlines the importance of careful preoperative evaluation of the donor limb with arteriography in-

TABLE 30-1. Results of Femorofemoral Bypass

Author	Year	Reference	Graft	Number	Operative Mortality Rate, %	Percent Patency at				
						1 Year	3 Years	5 Years	10 Years	15 Years
Plecha	76	34	Dacron	54	15	91				
Brief	76	35	Dacron	99	3	84	76	71		
Eugene	77	33	Dacron	33	15	74	66	45		
Mannick	78	36	Dacron	53	2	91		80		
Livesay	79	3	Dacron	36	6	84		56		
Dick	80	22	Dacron	133	6	90	80	73	64	
Chang	81	37	Dacron	23			62	62		
			PTFE	25			85			
Harris	81	25	Dacron	44			85			
Subram	83	38	Dacron	85	2	91	76	63		
Veith	84	16	PTFE	61		87	84			
Plecha	84	39	Dacron + PTFE + BOV SVG	119	2	98	83	72	55	
Author's current series	84		Dacron + PTFE	154				79	68	60

NOTE: PTFE = polytetrafluoroethylene; BOV = bovine; SVG = saphenous vein graft.

cluding oblique views and intraarterial pressure measurements under conditions of enhanced flow. Preoperative noninvasive tests are usually not adequate to identify iliac lesions in the donor limb, partly because the patient cannot exercise fully due to recipient limb ischemia. Furthermore, standard single-plane angiography can be inaccurate in identifying iliac lesions.

The *operative mortality and long-term survival rates* following femorofemoral grafting depend upon patient selection, since the magnitude of this operation is similar to that of a bilateral hernia repair and can be carried out under regional anesthesia. The high operative mortality rate of 2 to 15 percent (Table 30-1) reflects the operation's use in high-risk patients. Surprisingly, approximately 80 percent of our patients were alive 5 years after the operation and 70 percent after 10 years (22). These figures are similar to survival following aortofemoral bypass (40,41), indicating a similar case mix. This contrasts with a 42 percent 5-year survival rate among patients undergoing crossover grafting reported by Eugene et al. (33).

Axillofemoral Grafts

In 1961, Lewis (42) showed that the axillary artery could supply blood to an ischemic lower half of the body. In 1963 Blaisdell and Hall (43) and Louw (44) reported on the use of axillofemoral grafts to revascularize extremities in poor-risk patients. In 1966 Sauvage and Wood (45) added the femorofemoral extension to the axillofemoral graft for patients with bilateral iliac disease. Subsequent reports by a variety of authors confirm the place of this operation in a variety of clinical settings.

Modern indications for axillofemoral grafts include management of aortoenteric fistula, infected aortic grafts, infected aortic aneurysms, aortic aneurysm in poor-risk patients, and aortoiliac occlusive disease. The selection of this operation rather than aortofemoral bypass for relief of chronic occlusive disease is based on the estimate of the risk status of the patient as well as a variety of anatomic factors already enumerated. The use of this procedure in patients with chronic iliac occlusive disease is usually limited to patients requiring limb salvage. Most patients too ill to undergo aortic surgery do not require bypass for relief of claudication.

Before performing this operation, it is necessary to establish that no occlusive lesion is present in the subclavian or axillary system. If no bruit is heard and cuff blood pressures are equal in both arms, one can usually be certain that either axillary vessel can be used as a donor artery, although some surgeons believe routine arteriography of these vessels should precede this operation.* This left subclavian artery is more frequently the site of disease. If there is any question of adequacy of the inflow vessels, arteriography should be carried out.

TECHNIQUE

The technical principles of axillofemoral bypass for chronic ischemia can be outlined as follows (Figure 30-2). A wide preparation and draping of the patient is necessary. We favor a circumferential prepping of the donor arm so that it can be moved during the procedure to check on tension of the graft and ensure that kinking of the axillary artery does not occur. Although local anesthesia can be used, we favor general anesthesia and a two-team approach to shorten operating time. A subclavicular incision is made over the donor axillary artery by one team and the groin incisions made in the usual manner by a second team. The fibers of the pectoralis major are separated and the pectoralis minor tendon is divided to avoid angulation of the graft. The first and second portions of the axillary artery are dissected and controlled, and an appropriate area is selected for the donor

*See also Additional References (Ascer et al.).

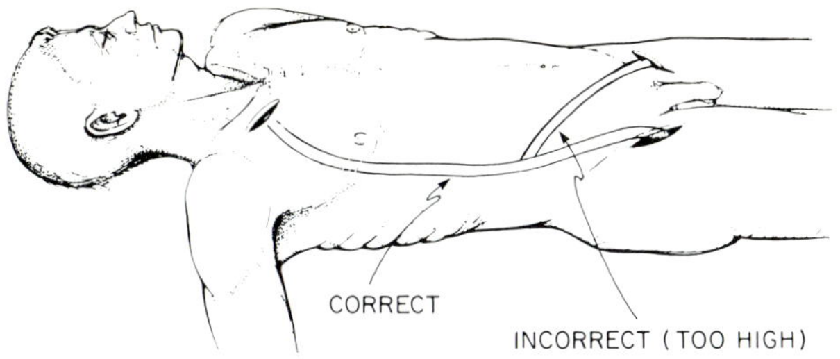

A

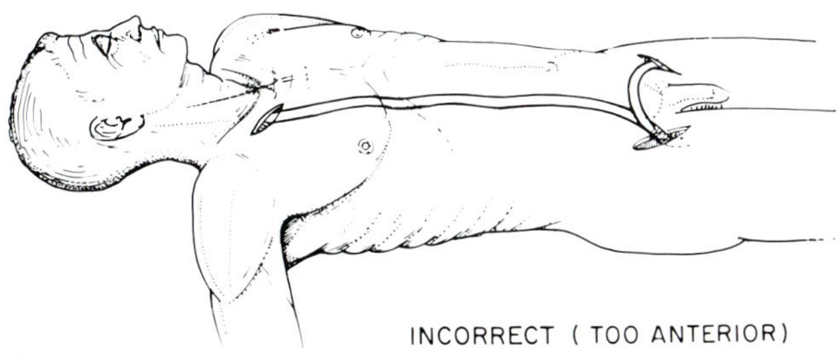

B

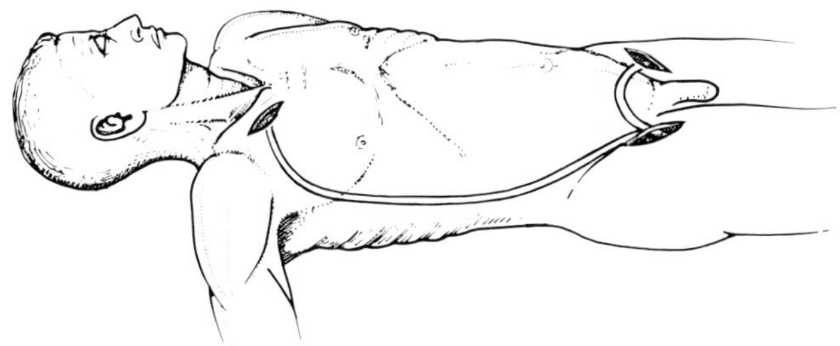

C

FIGURE 30-2. (*A*) The high takeoff of the crossover limb is not optimal because it results in a low flow in too long a portion of the distal axillofemoral limb. (*B*) The axillofemoral graft is in too anterior a position and may kink at the costal margin when the patient is sitting. (*C*) A correctly performed graft with a laterally placed vertical limb and a low takeoff of the crossover limb.

anastomosis. The third portion of the artery is never used since shoulder motion affects this segment. When all dissections are complete, the subcutaneous tunnel is made, curving to the mid-axillary line to avoid angulation over the costal margin in the sitting position. The tunnel is then curved medial to the iliac crest to approach the femoral vessels. Recently Ward and his colleagues (46) described placement of the graft throughout most of its length in the subfascial plane under the pectoralis major muscle and the external oblique fascia. They believe this is a more protected position for the graft, particularly in thin individuals. A subpleural method has been described but has little appeal (47). A counterincision is sometimes necessary to tunnel the graft properly and is generally made inferior to the costal margin. After the vessels are exposed and a suprapubic tunnel is made subcutaneously, the patient is given systemic heparin, and the first anastomosis is carried out to the donor axillary artery. The graft is then tunneled carefully to avoid kinking or tension, and the anastomosis to the femoral artery is performed in a standard fashion. Most authors agree that the crossover component of the graft should originate from the most distal portion of the axillo-femoral graft. Ward et al. (46) have recently suggested sewing the femorofemoral limb either proximal or distal to the axillofemoral anastomosis on the femoral artery. We usually employ an 8-mm graft for the vertical limb and a 6- or 8-mm graft for the horizontal femorofemoral portion. Both Dacron and polytetrafluoroethylene grafts can be used. Externally supported polytetrafluoroethylene grafts are also available.

When an infected groin wound is to be bypassed, the graft is tunneled laterally to the walled off infected wound and is anastomosed to the deep or superficial femoral artery. The axillofemoral wounds are then walled off and the old infected graft removed. When this is done, the femoral artery must be ligated proximally and distally to prevent bleeding.

RESULTS

Patency rates of axillofemoral grafts for occlusive disease have varied considerably (Table 30-2). For example, Eugene et al. (33) reported a 5-year patency of 30 percent, whereas Johnson et al. (48) and Veith (16) have reported 76 to 81 percent 5-year patency rates. These latter figures include as "successful" those grafts whose patency has been restored by thrombectomy. Since both early and late occlusions are not always caused by runoff stenosis and may be related to graft compression, an aggressive attitude toward thrombectomy appears warranted. Johnson et al. (48) reoperated 24 times on 12 out of 56 patients with axillofemoral bypasses. However, each reoperation exposes the patient to further risks and should not be undertaken lightly.

Several authors have postulated that factors which increase flow rates in the graft will increase the likelihood of success. Ray et al. (49) have indicated that a flow rate of over 250 mL/min is necessary for prolonged function. This may explain why the patency in patients with claudication is greater than in those with severe ischemia (49). Similarly, when the iliac flow is severely restricted, there is less competition and therefore a higher flow rate in the graft and increased patency (49). Further, when the superficial femoral artery was patent, Johnson et al. (48) found a success rate of 95 percent as compared with 67 percent when the profunda femoral was the sole runoff vessel. Increased flow in the long vertical limb of the graft would be expected if a crossover femorofemoral graft was added. Several authors have urged this addition (46,48,50,51), but Moore et al. (52), Eugene et al. (33), and Ray et al. (49) have not confirmed the efficacy of this addition.* Ward et al. (46) suggested placing the femorofemoral graft distal to the axillofemoral anastomosis but have used this in only a small number of patients.

Other suggestions to increase patency have included using noncrimped or externally supported grafts. Despite the ease of thrombectomy of polytetrafluoroethylene grafts, three studies have failed to confirm increased patency rates with this material (46,51,53).

Complications associated with these procedures are not unique and include thrombosis of the graft or donor artery, brachial plexus injuries, false aneurysms, and infection. The *operative mortality rate* has remained under 10 percent in most studies. However, as might be expected, the 5-year survival rate in most studies has been limited. Although in the study of Johnson et

*Also see Additional References (Ascer et al.).

TABLE 30-2. **Results of Axillofemoral Bypass**

Author	Year	Reference	Graft	Number	Operative Mortality Rate, %	Percent Patency at 1 Year	Percent Patency at 3 Years	Percent Patency at 5 Years
Mannick	70	55	Uni	37				
			Bi	9				54
Moore	71	52	Uni	24	9		30	
			Bi	22			30	
Cormier	71	56	Uni	29	10	75		
Kruger	71	57	Uni	15	0	67		
Bliss	72	58	Uni	7	0	87		
Pollock	72	57	Uni	17	12	20		
Janish	74	58	Uni	45	7			57
Logerfo	76	50	Uni	64	8			37
			Bi	66				74
Johnson	77	48	Bi	56	2	83*	76*	76*
Eugene	77	33	Uni	35	8	60	40	30
			Bi	24		60	36	36
Ray	79	49	Uni	33	4	75	75	67
			Bi	21		90	85	77
Livesay	79	3	Uni	26	10	77	77	
			Bi	14				
Broome	80	53	Uni	17			75	
			Bi	44				
Burrell	82	51	Uni Dacron	36	8		37/66*	
			Bi Dacron	38			71/97*	
			Bi PTFE			73		
Veith	84	16	Uni PTFE	33				72*
			Bi	29				81*

*With thrombectomy.

NOTE: Uni = unilateral; Bi = bilateral; PTFE = polytetrafluoroethylene.

al. (48) two-thirds of patients were alive 5 years after surgery, survival after 5 years was as low as 26 percent in the report of Eugene et al. (33). Two other groups reported a 50 percent mortality rate at 3 and 4 years (3,51).

The axillofemoral graft has been used with great success in the management of infected aortic aneurysms and grafts and aortic enteric fistulas. It has recently been combined with iliac ligation and induced thrombosis to treat patients with unruptured aortic aneurysms (1) (Figure 30-3). Whether this latter technique will become commonly used remains to be determined, since aneurysm rupture and other complications have been reported.

Functional results after axillofemoral bypass have been studied infrequently. O'Donnell and colleagues (54) reported that in patients with combined aortoiliac and femoropopliteal occlusive disease, axillofemoral bypass resulted in minimal or no improvement in patients with either claudication or severe limb ischemia. In contrast aortofemoral bypass resulted in marked improvement in these patients. Possible reasons for this observation include the degree of collateral circulation, donor subclavian artery stenosis, poor myocardial reserve, or inferiority of the axillofemoral vascular conduit. In the absence of objective criteria such as femoral artery pressure measurements, one might also speculate that the degree of preoperative proximal iliac disease was not equal in the two groups of patients.

Thoracic Aorta to Femoral Artery Bypass

Schumacker first described the ascending aorta to bifemoral artery bypass procedure in 1968 (59) in the treatment of abdominal coarctation of the aorta. Frantz et al. (60) applied this principle and reported ascending aorta to bifemoral artery bypass for the totally occluded infrarenal abdominal aorta in 1974. Others (61–66) have successfully employed this operation in the presence of obesity, horseshoe kidney, abnormal renal arteries, large ventral hernias, thoracoabdominal coarctation, failed aortoiliac repair, and multiple laparotomies. Baird and Oates (67) have reported 16 cases, 17 of whom underwent simultaneous coronary bypass procedures.

In brief the technique involves a sternal splitting incision and the usual groin incisions using a two-team approach (Figure 30-4). A small transverse incision above the arcuate line is necessary to carefully place the graft in the extraperitoneal position deep to the rectus muscle. The ascending aortic anastomosis is performed, using an 8-mm Dacron graft to the more ischemic extremity and a crossover 6- or 8-mm graft to the opposite limb. Although there has been no operative mortality, graft occlusions have occurred. Long-term follow-up has not been reported, but early results suggest that this may be a suitable extraanatomic bypass procedure in selected cases. More data are necessary to determine if this extended graft can be combined with coronary bypass with an acceptable operative risk and mortality rate.

Descending thoracic or upper abdominal aorta to femoral artery bypasses have likewise been used in a number of unusual

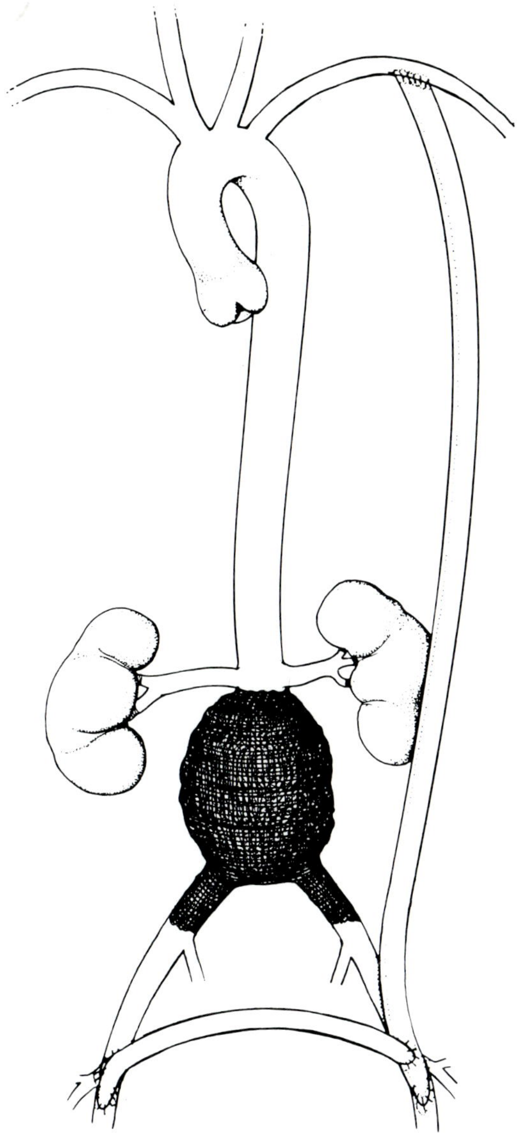

FIGURE 30-3. Axillofemoral grafting has been combined with iliac ligation and induced aortic thrombosis to treat high-risk patients with aortic aneurysms. The place of this technique has not been firmly established.

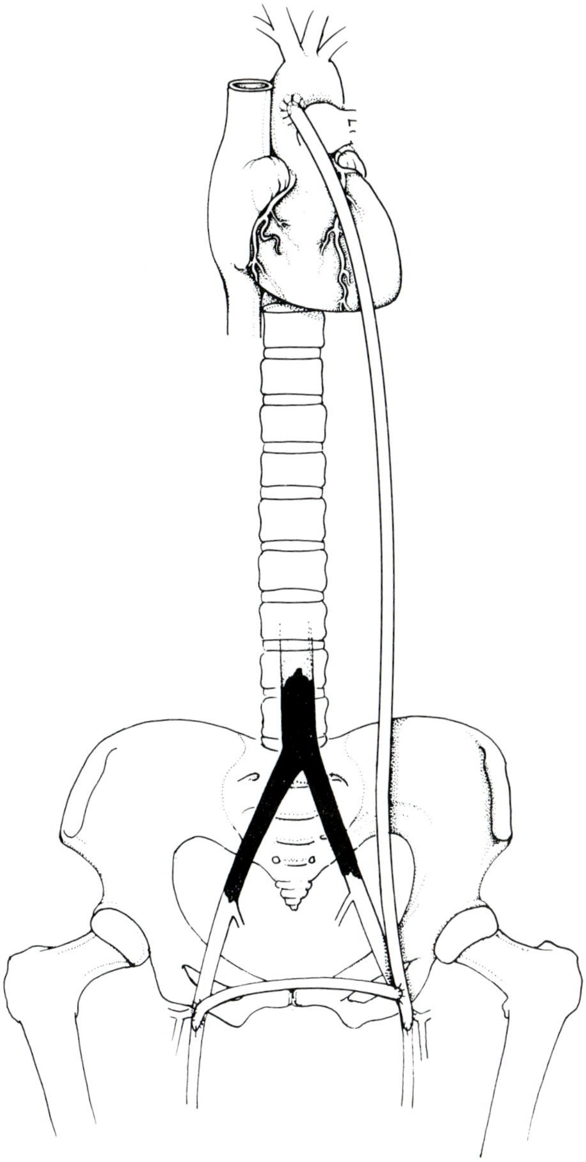

FIGURE 30-4. Ascending aorta to femoral grafting has been carried out to avoid complex abdominal problems and to complement coronary bypass grafting in patients with severe aortoiliac disease.

circumstances including infection, previous graft failures, and adhesions (67–69). These procedures are more complex and pose a greater threat than either the sternal incision or axillofemoral bypass and probably have little role to play except in unusual circumstances.

Obturator Foramen Bypass Grafts

In 1962 Shaw and Baue (70) used the obturator foramen as an extraanatomic route to bypass groin infection in three patients. Since then at least 120 cases have been reported in the literature. VanDet and Brands (71) reviewed results with 66 cases in the literature and added 13 others. Tilson et al. (72), Erath et al. (73), and Feldman and Berguer (74) have recently described 10, 9, and 22 procedures, respectively.

The indications for the procedure have included infections of prosthetic grafts; femoral mycotic aneurysms; septic aneurysms after cannulation, catheterization, or balloon counterpulsation; mycotic embolization into the femoral artery with autolysis of the femoral artery; large aneurysm of the ileofemoral system; scar tissue in the groin following previous vascular surgery; loss of covering tissue as a result of injury, irradiation necrosis, or resection of a malignancy; and a need for revascularization despite suppurative lymphadenopathy.

TECHNIQUE

The technique has been detailed by Guida and Moore (75) and Baue and Tilson (76) (Figure 30-5). The donor artery may be a previously placed aortofemoral limb that is not infected, the aorta, the ipsilateral iliac artery, or the contralateral iliac vessel. The donor vessel is approached either retroperitoneally or transperitoneally through either a vertical incision or preferably a transverse incision. The obturator artery, vein, and nerve penetrate the obturator fascia laterally. The tunnel is created anteromedially to these structures just under the superior ramus of the pubis. The fibers of the obturator internus muscle are separated, and the tough obturator fascia is sharply broken. A tunneling instrument is inserted from above after the superficial femoral or popliteal artery is dissected near the adductor hiatus. The tunneling instrument is placed deep to the adductor longus, but anterior to the adductor magnus and into the enlarged hiatus. The distal anastomosis is placed at the appropriate location. Dacron, polytetrafluoroethylene, and saphenous veins have been used, the latter being preferred in infected cases. Some authors recommend ligation of the external iliac artery below the upper anastomosis and the superficial femoral artery above the lower anastomosis, but we usually prefer to ligate the infected femoral artery directly. This is done after the clean incisions are closed and walled off.

Few reports of the long-term fate of obturator bypass grafts are available. Tilson et al. (72) reported 1 late failure at 10 months in 10 grafts followed 6 months to 9 years. VanDet and Brands (71) found failures at 4 and 7 months in 134 grafts followed up 6 years. Erath et al. (73) noted 3 late failures at 13, 19, and 28 months in 9 grafts observed up to 52 months. All grafts at risk were patent at least 12 months. Late failure may be corrected by insertion of grafts through normal anatomical planes once the infection has been obliterated. In summary the obturator foramen provides a satisfactory route for revascularization where an extraanatomic route to the lower extremity is necessary because of the presence of an infected groin wound.

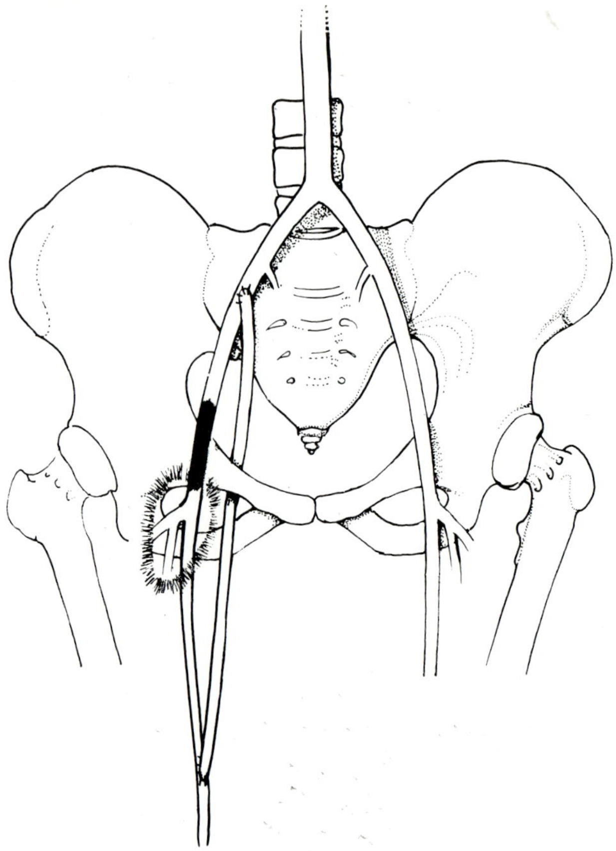

FIGURE 30-5. The obturator foramen bypass is used to revascularize an extremity in which the femoral area is infected or destroyed. The proximal anastomosis may be end-to-end or end-to-side. The infected artery is usually ligated in situ, or the distal external iliac and superficial femoral artery can be ligated separately remote from the groin wound.

Alternatives include femoral artery ligation without reconstruction, immediate or delayed reconstruction through the infected field with autogenous tissue, axillopopliteal bypass (77), or lateral femoral bypass (74,78,79). This technique consists of an extraperitoneal exposure of the iliac artery and a lateral subcutaneous tunnel around the infected groin. We have used all these methods. Individual judgments must be made since each technique has its merits.

Extended Extraanatomic Bypass

The subject of extraanatomic bypass and its role in revascularization of the lower extremities is limited only by the surgeon's ingenuity and resourcefulness. Veith and his colleagues (77,80) summarized his experience with a variety of unusual bypasses necessitated by anatomical and risk factors in 61 patients followed for 12 to 17 months. These consisted of 11 axillopopliteal, 3 crossover axillopopliteal, 5 crossover femoropopliteal or tibial, 8 femoral-popliteal-tibial, and 3 miscellaneous extended extraanatomic grafts. Veith used 6-mm polytetrafluoroethylene grafts in this series of cases with systemic heparinization and 6-0 polypropylene sutures. A similar study was reported by Connolly et al. (81). Recently an axillofemoral left renal bypass was used by McCready et al. (82) to revascularize a left kidney in a patient with an acute aortic occlusion associated with a suprarenal aortic aneurysm. The fact that these operations worked for a significant period of time is indicative of the importance of attention to details of technique and hemodynamic principles as well as the graft materials currently available.

Summary

A variety of extraanatomic bypass grafts are available to the imaginative surgeon when standard bypass procedures cannot be performed safely because the poor operative risk of the patient, the presence of infection, or other anatomic factors obviate standard bypass procedures. In the ischemic lower extremity, axillobifemoral grafts are most commonly used for bilateral lesions and crossover femorofemoral grafts for unilateral disease. Dacron and PTFE grafts, 6 and 8 mm in size, are generally used with nearly equivalent results. The donor artery should be free of a hemodynamically significant lesion, and adequate runoff must be achieved. With meticulous technique satisfactory long-term results can be achieved with results at 5 years only slightly inferior or equal to conventional aortofemoral bypass grafting. Operative morbidity and mortality rates are lower than one would expect if the more extensive intraabdominal operation were carried out in the group of patients. Although infected grafts can be managed by removal without reconstruction or by reconstruction with autogenous material through the infected field, extraanatomic bypass of the infected field will continue to have a major role in the approach to this difficult problem.

References

1. Leather RP, Shah D, Goldman M, Rosenburg J, Karmody AM: Nonresective treatment of abdominal aortic aneurysms. Arch Surg 1979, 114:1402–1408.
2. Alpert J, Goldenkranz R, Brief DK, Brener B, Parsonnet V: Limb ischemia during intra-aortic balloon pumping: Indication for Femorofemoral crossover graft. J Thorac Cardiovasc Surg 1980, 79:5:729–734.
3. Livesay JJ, Atkinson JB, Baker JD, Busuttil RW, Barker WF, Machleder HI: Late results of extra-anatomic bypass. Arch Surg 1979, 114:1260–1265.
4. Foley WJ, Dow RW, Fry WJ: Crossover femorofemoral bypass grafts. Arch Surg 1969, 99:83–87.
5. Warren WD, Foman JJ: Rerouting arterial flow to relieve ischemia: Femorofemoral, axillary-femoral and carotid-carotid artery bypasses. Ann Surg 1966, 163:131–136.
6. Harper JA, Golding AL, Mazzei EA, Cannon JA: An experimental hemodynamic study of the subclavian steal syndrome. Surg Gynecol Obstet 1967, 124:1212–1218.
7. Ehrenfeld WK, Harris JD, Wylie EJ: Vascular "steal" phenomenon. An experimental study. Am J Surg 1968, 116:192–197.
8. Lord RSA, Ehrenfeld WK: Carotid-subclavian bypass: A hemodynamic study. Surgery 1969, 66:521–526.
9. Parsonnet V, Alpert J, Brief DK: Femoro-femoral and axillo-femoral grafts: Compromise or preference. Surgery 1970, 67:26–33.
10. Trimble IR, Stonesifer GL Jr, Wilgis EFS, Montague AC: Criteria for femoro-femoral bypass from clinical and hemodynamic studies. Ann Surg 1972, 175:985–990.
11. Faulkner SL, Fisher RD, Conkle DM, Page DL, Bender HN: Effect of blood flow rate on endothelial proliferation in venous autografts used as arterial substitutes. Circulation 1975, 1(51–52 suppl):163–172.
12. Rittgers SE, Karayannacos PE, Guy JF: Velocity distribution and intimal proliferation in autogenous grafts in dogs. Circ Res 1978, 42:792.
13. Berguer R, Higgins RF, Reddy DJ: Intimal hyperplasia: An experimental study. Arch Surg 1980, 115:332–335.
14. Towne JB, Quinn K, Salles-Cunher S, Bernhard VM, Clowry LJ: Effect of increased arterial blood flow on localization and progression of atherosclerosis. Arch Surg 1982, 117:1469–1474.
15. Stipa S: Axillo-femoral bypass graft with saphenous, cephalic, and basilic veins. Surg Gynecol Obstet 1971, 133:297–300.
16. Veith FJ, Gupta SK: Expanded PTFE vascular grafts. In Rutherford RB (ed): *Vascular Surgery*. Philadelphia, Saunders, 1984, pp. 394–404.
17. Ray LI, O'Connor JB, Davis CC, Hall DG, Mansfield PB, Riffenhouse EA, Smith JC, Wood ST, Sauvage LR: Axillo-femoral bypass: A critical reappraisal of its role in the management of aorto-iliac occlusive disease. Am J Surg 1979, 138:117–126.
18. Freeman NE, Leeds FH: Operations on large arteries. Calif Med 1952, 77:229–233.
19. Oudot J, Beaconfield P: Thrombosis of the aortic bifurcation treated by resection and homograft replacement. Arch Surg 1953, 66:365–374.
20. McCaughan JJ Jr, Kahn SF: Crossover graft for unilateral occlusive disease of the ileo-femoral arteries. Ann Surg 1960, 151:26–29.
21. Vetto RM: The treatment of unilateral iliac artery obstruction. Surgery 1962, 52:342–345.
22. Dick LS, Brief DK, Alpert J, Brener BJ, Goldenkranz R, Parsonnet V: A 12 year experience with femoro-femoral crossover grafts. Arch Surg 1980, 115:1359–1365.
23. Flanigan DP, Pratt DG, Goodreau JJ, Burnham SJ, Yao JST, Bergan JJ: Hemodynamic and arteriographic guidelines in selection of patients for femoral-femoral bypass. Arch Surg 1978, 113:1257–1262.
24. Sumner DS, Strandness DE Jr: The hemodynamics of the femorofemoral shunt. Surg Gynecol Obstet 1972, 134:629–636.
25. Harris JP, Flinn WR, Rudo ND, Bergan JJ, Yao JST: Assessment of donor limb hemodynamics in femoro-femoral bypass for claudication. Surgery 1981, 90:764–770.
26. Weismann RE, Upson JF: Intra-arterial pressure studies in patients with arterial insufficiency of lower extremities. Ann Surg 1963, 157:501–506.
27. Moore WS, Hall AD: Unrecognized aorto-iliac stenosis. Arch Surg 1971, 103:633–638.
28. Brener BJ, Raines JK, Darling RD, Austen WG: Measurement of systolic femoral artery pressure during reactive hyperemia. Circulation 1974, 49(suppl 2):259–267.
29. Brewster DC, Waltman AC, O'Hara PJ, Darling RC: Femoral artery pressure measurement during aortography. Circulation 1979, 60(suppl 1):120–124.
30. Archie JP Jr, Feldtman RW: Intra-operative assessment of the hemodynamic significance of iliac and profunda femoris stenosis. Surgery 1981, 90:876–880.
31. Faris I, Tonnesen KH, Agerkon K, Noer I, Sayer P: Femoral artery pressure measurements to predict the outcome of arterial surgery in patients with multilevel disease. Surgery 1982, 92:10–15.
32. Porter JM, Eidenmiller LR, Pottes CT, Rosch J, Vetto RM: Combined arterial dilatation and femoro-femoral bypass for limb salvage. Surg Gynecol Obstet 1973, 137:409–412.
33. Eugene J, Goldstone J, Moore WS: Fifteen year experience with subcutaneous bypass grafts for lower extremity ischemia. Ann Surg 1977, 186:177–183.
34. Plecha FR, Pories WJ: Extra-anatomic bypasses for aorto-iliac disease in high-risk patients. Surgery 1976, 80:480–487.
35. Brief DK, Alpert J, Brener BJ, Parsonnet V: Crossover femorofemoral grafts. J Med Soc NJ 1976, 73:133–137.
36. Mannick JA, Baini BS: Femoro-femoral grafting: Indications and late results. Am J Surg 1978, 136:190–192.
37. Chang JB: Surgical treatment of aorto-iliac artery disease. Angiology 1981, 32:73–105.
38. Subram AN, Urrutia-S CO, Oh DA, Cooley DA: Femoro-femoral bypass prognostic factors. Tex Heart Instit J 1983, 10:257–261.
39. Plecha FR, Plecha FM: Femorofemoral bypass grafts: Ten-year experience. J Vasc Surg 1984, 1:555–561.
40. Malone JM, Moore WS, Goldstone J: Life expectancy following aorto-femoral arterial grafting. Surgery 1977, 81:551–555.

41. Satiani B, Liapis CD, Evans WE: Aorto-femoral bypass for severe limb ischemia: Long-term survival and limb salvage. Am J Surg 1981, 141:252–256.
42. Lewis CD: Subclavian artery as a means of blood supply to lower half of body. Br J Surg 1961, 48:574.
43. Blaisdell FW, Hall AD: Axillary-femoral artery bypass for lower extremity ischemia. Surgery 1963, 54:563–568.
44. Louw JH: Splenic-to-femoral and axillary-to-femoral bypass grafts in diffuse atherosclerotic occlusive disease. Lancet 1963, 1:1401–1402.
45. Sauvage LR, Wood SJ: Unilateral axillary bilateral femoral bifurcation graft. Surgery 1966, 60:573.
46. Ward RE, Holcroft JW, Conti S, Blaisdell FW: New conception in the use of axillo-femoral bypass grafts. Arch Surg 1983, 118:573–575.
47. Tangpraphephorn V, Spenazzola A, King J: Axillo-femoral bypass: Intra-pleural method. Ann Thorac Surg 1979, 27:80–81.
48. Johnson WC, Logerfo FW, Vollman RW, Coson JD, O'Hara ET, Mannick JA, Nabseter DC: Is axillo-bilateral femoral graft an effective substitute for aortic-bilateral iliac/femoral graft? An analysis of ten years' experience. Ann Surg 1977, 186:123–129.
49. Ray LI, O'Connor JB, Davis CC, Hall DG, Mansfield PB, Rittenhouse EA, Smith JC, Wood SJ, Sauvage LR: Axillo-femoral bypass: A critical reappraisal of its role in the management of aorto-iliac occlusive disease. Am J Surg 1979, 138:117–126.
50. Logerfo FW, Johnson WC, Corson JD, Vollman RW, Weisel RD, Davis RC, O'Hara ET, Nasbeth DC, Mannick JA: A comparison of the late patency rates of axillo-bilateral femoral and axillo-unilateral femoral grafts. Surgery 1977, 81:33–40.
51. Burrell MJ, Wheeler JR, Gregory RT, Snyder SO, Sayle RG, Mason MS: Axillo-femoral bypass: A ten year review. Ann Surg 1982, 195:796–798.
52. Moore WS, Hall AD, Blaisdell FW: Late results of axillary-femoral bypass grafting. Am J Surg 1971, 122:148–154.
53. Broome A, Christenson JT, Eklof B, Norepen L: Axillo-femoral bypass reconstructions in sixty-one patients with leg ischemia. Surgery 1980, 88:673–676.
54. O'Donnell TF, Jr Kelley JJ, Callow AD, Lahey SJ, Millan VA: A comparison of the early noninvasive hemodynamic results after aortofemoral or axillo-femoral bypass graft. Circulation 1980, 62(suppl 1):7–10.
55. Mannick JA, Williams LE, Nabseth DC: The late results of axillofemoral grafts. Surgery 1970, 68:1038–1043.
56. Cormier JM, Bacourt F: Une revascularisation Inhabituelle: Les pontages axillo-femoraux et femoraux-femoraux. Ann Med Interne (Paris) 1971, 122:939.
57. Krieger BJ, Stockman K, Witte C: Der axillofemoral bypass: Ein therapeutisches verfahren bei riskopatienten mit chronischer verschlus krankenheit der arterien im becken abschnitt. Thorax Chir 1971, 19:434.
58. Bliss BP, Barrett BS: Axillo-femoral and axillo-profunda bypass grafts. Ann R Coll Surg Engl 1972, 50:268.
59. Schumaker HB, Nahrwald DL, King H, Waldhausen JA: Coarctation of the aorta. Curr Probl Surg 1968, 1:64.
60. Frantz SL, Kaplitt MJ, Beil AR Jr, Stein HL: Ascending aorto-bilateral femoral artery bypass for the totally occluded infrarenal abdominal aorta. Surgery 1974, 75:471–475.
61. Robinson G, Siegelman S, Attai L: Recurrent dissecting aneurysms of aorta. NY State J Med 1972, 72:2328–2331.
62. Siderys H, Graffis R, Holbrook H, Kasbeckar V: A technique for management of inaccessible coarctation of the aorta. J Thorac Cardiovasc Surg 1974, 67:568–570.
63. Favi P, Massimo D, Diligenti LM: Ascending aorta to femoral arteries bypass without opening the abdominal cavity: Choice treatment in cases of complete occlusion of the infrarenal aorta. J Cardiovasc Surg 1977, 18:475–480.
64. Wukasch DC, Cooley DA, Sandiford FM, Nappi G, Reul J: Ascending aorta-abdominal aorto bypass: Indications, technique and report of 12 patients. Ann Thorac Surg 1977, 23:442–448.
65. Cleveland JC: Ascending aorta to common femoral artery bypass: An unusual but successful method for revascularization of the lower extremity: Report of case. Cardiovasc Dis 1980, 7:74–76.
66. Gelfand ET, Callaghan JC, Sterns LP: Extended aortic bypass. J Thorac Cardiovasc Surg 1980, 79:381–387.
67. Baird RJ, Oates TK: Ascending aorta to bifemoral artery bypass. Can J Surg 1981, 24:415–418.
68. Blaisdell FW: Ligation treatment of an abdominal aortic aneurysm. Am J Surg 1965, 109:560–565.
69. Veith FJ, Hartsuck JM, Crane C: Management of aortoiliac reconstruction complicated by sepsis and hemorrhage. N Engl J Med 1964, 270:1389–1392.
70. Shaw RS, Baue AE: Management of sepsis complicating arterial reconstructive surgery. Surgery 1962, 53:75–86.
71. VanDet RJ, Brands LC: The obturator foramen bypass: An alternative procedure in ileo-femoral artery revascularization. Surgery 1981, 89:543–547.
72. Tilson MD, Sweeney T, Jushey RJ, Stansel HC: Obturator canal bypass grafts for septic lesion of femoral artery. Arch Surg 1979, 114:1031–1036.
73. Erath HG Jr, Gale SS, Smith BM, Deen RH: Obturator foramen grafts: The preferable alternate route? Am Surg 1982, 48:65–69.
74. Feldman AJ, Berguer R: Management of an infected aneurysm of the groin secondary to drug abuse. Surg Gynecol Obstet 1983, 157:519–522.
75. Guida PM, Moore SW: Obturator bypass technique. Surg Gynecol Obstet 1969, 128:1307–1316.
76. Baue A, Tilson MD: Obturator bypasses for lower extremity ischemia. In Rutherford RB (ed): *Vascular Surgery*. Philadelphia, Saunders, 1984.
77. Veith FJ, Moss CM, Daly V, Fell SC, Haimovici H: New approaches to limb salvage by extended extra-anatomic bypasses and prosthetic reconstructions to foot arteries. Surgery 1978, 84:764–772.
78. Smith R, Szilagyi D, Calville J: Surgical treatment of mycotic aneurysms. Arch Surg 1962, 85:674.
79. Leather RP, Karmody AM: A lateral route for extra-anatomical bypass of the femoral artery. Surgery 1977, 81:307–309.
80. Gupta SK, Veith FJ, Ascer E, Samson RH, Scher LA, White-Flores SA, Sarayregen S, Fell SC: Five year experiences with axillopopliteal bypass for limb salvage. J Cardiovasc Surg 1985, 26:321–324.
81. Connolly JE, Kwaan JHM, Brownell D, McCart PM, Levine E: Newer developments of extra-anatomic bypass. Surg Gynecol Obstet 1984, 58:415–418.
82. McCready RA, Hyde GL, Ernst CB: Renal revascularization by extraanatomic bypass. J Vasc Surg 1984, 1:569–572.

ADDITIONAL REFERENCES

Sanders RJ, Kempczinski RF, Hammond W, DiClementi D: The significance of graft diameter. Surgery 1980, 88:856.

Ascer E, Gupta SK, Veith FJ, Samson RH, Scher LA, White-Flores SA: Equivalent results with axillounifemoral and axillobifemoral bypasses. Surgery 1985, 97:169–175.

Chapter 31

SURGERY OF THE PROFUNDA FEMORIS ARTERY

ALLASTAIR M. KARMODY, ROBERT P. LEATHER, JOHN D. CORSON, and DHIRAJ M. SHAH

The majority of blood vessels which are operated upon by vascular surgeons for the relief of ischemia are arteries of conduit, i.e., they are of large caliber, such as the common iliac and common femoral, and have either no or very few branches, such as the external iliac and common and internal carotids. Their function is the rapid passage of blood from an inflow source to arteries of supply (distribution), for example, superficial femoral to popliteal and tibial arteries. All arteries of conduit end by branching into arteries of supply and smaller arteries of conduit, for example, common iliac into internal iliac (artery of supply) and external iliac (artery of conduit). The profunda femoris artery, the subject of this chapter, is an artery of supply, and its primary function is to provide a blood supply to the muscles of the thigh. However, it occupies a special position with respect to arteries of the lower limb because it is actually a separate arterial network which derives its importance because it lies at the crossroads of the entire blood supply of the lower limb. In this crucial position, its importance is such that it has become known as "nature's femoropopliteal graft" (1). To a large extent this is true because of its well-known extensive collateral capacity (Figure 31-1) which comes into play so well when the superficial femoral artery undergoes slow chronic occlusion that the patient may be only dimly aware of any symptoms or signs of this process. However, its function is frequently jeopardized by disease processes which occur (1) proximal to the artery, thus limiting the inflow to an otherwise competent vessel, or (2) by disease processes affecting the profunda femoris artery itself, or (3) worst of all, by a combination of both. This chapter seeks to provide an overview of the current position with respect to improvement or restoration of arterial flow within the profunda femoris artery and the known indications for use of this approach either singularly or in combination with other procedures.

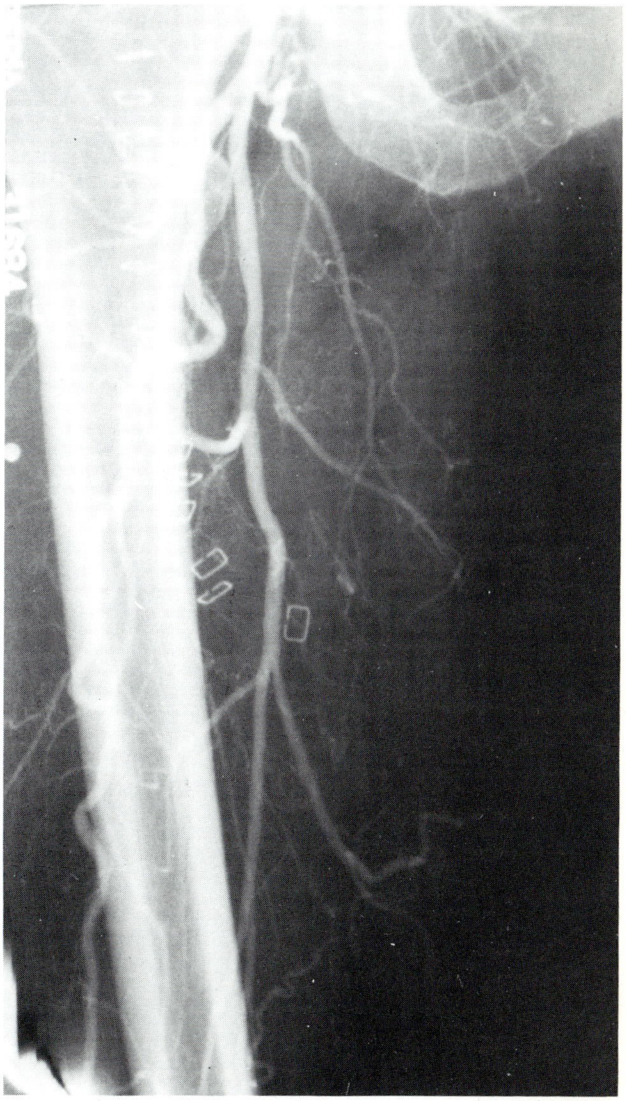

FIGURE 31-1. Patient with superficial femoral occlusion. Note extensive collateral development from profunda femoris artery and especially the parallel system arising from the lateral circumflex branch. Both systems extend beyond the adductor canal.

Anatomy

CLASSIC DESCRIPTION

About 3 to 5 cm below the inguinal ligament the common femoral artery ends in two large divisions, the combined internal diameter of which equals the diameter of the common femoral itself. These arteries are the superficial femoral artery, which continues into the subsartorial space through the adductor canal to the popliteal artery, and the profunda femoris artery, which supplies many branches to the thigh musculature (Figure 31-2). The profunda generally runs posteriorly and very slightly laterally up to its lateral circumflex branch and then curves medially while it passes downward and ends in the region of the adductor hiatus. Its main branches are the lateral circumflex, the medial circumflex, the first, second, and third perforators, and its ter-

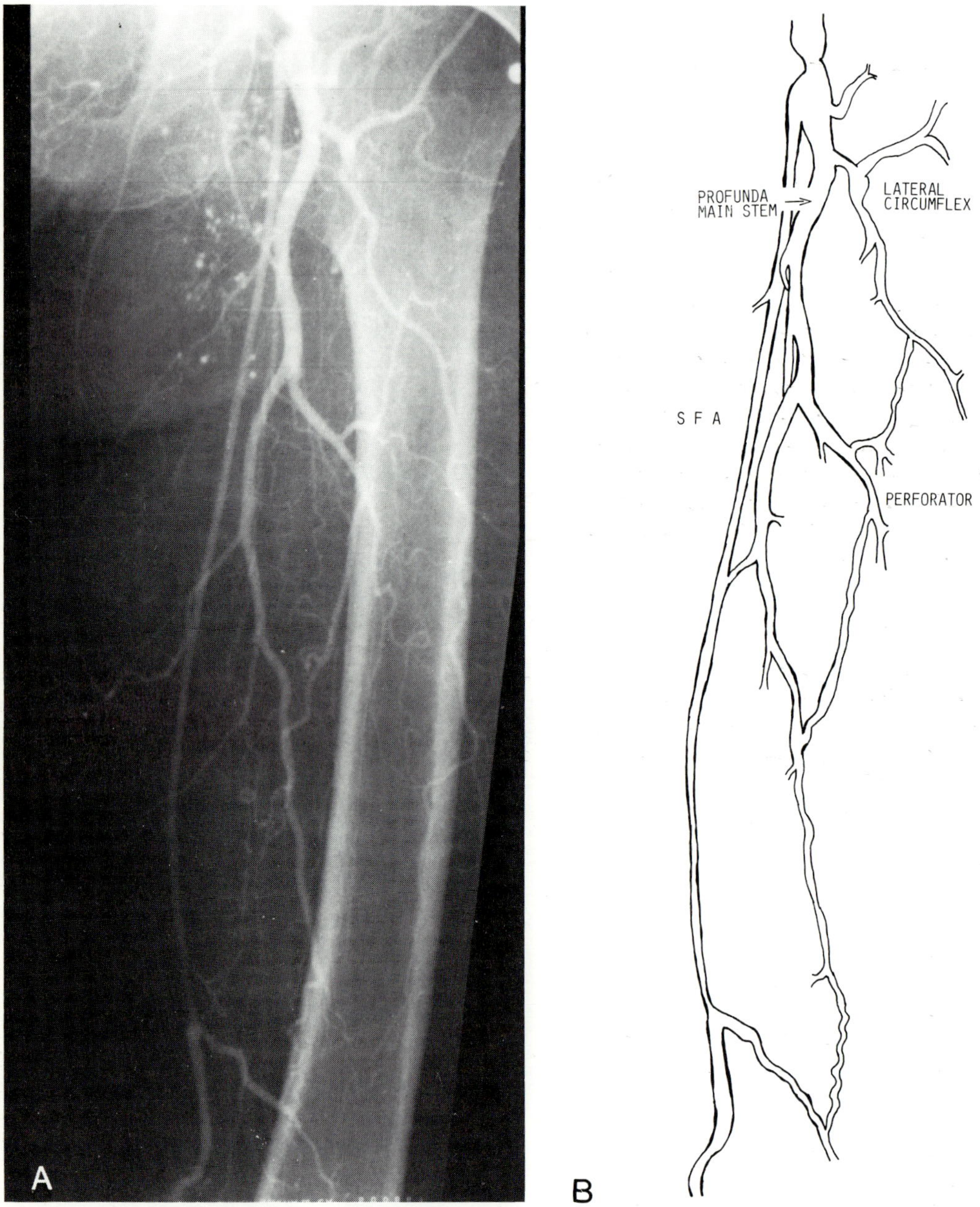

FIGURE 31-2. Angiogram (*A*) and accompanying overprint (*B*) show the 3 parallel systems (SFA, profunda main stem, and descending branch of lateral circumflex). Also shown are the first and second muscular branches and the termination of the profunda in its communication with the superior lateral geniculate branch of the popliteal artery.

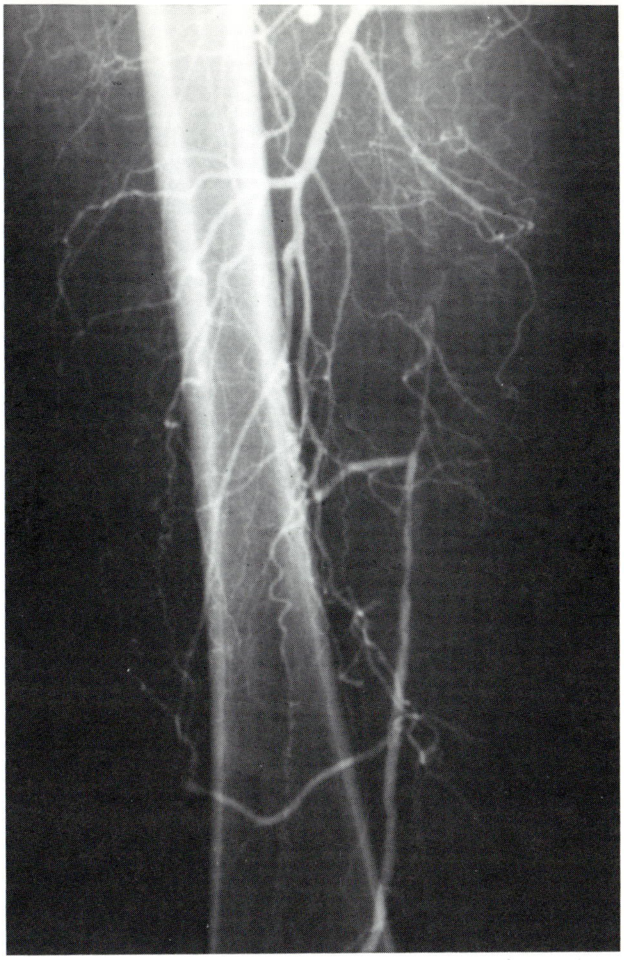

FIGURE 31-3. A further example of extensive communication of profunda femoris with distal superficial femoral and popliteal arteries. In this case the profunda femoris itself communicates with the mid-SFA and popliteal arteries by unnamed collaterals.

minal segment, which ends in two branches that are sometimes referred to as the fourth perforator, and a terminal branch which exits into the back of the thigh. Unnamed intertwining arteries connect these named branches, forming the potentially extensive collateral network which is generally not angiographically visualized in the absence of occlusive disease (Figure 31-3). The lateral circumflex artery is a very important branch of the profunda femoris artery. It is large in size and provides a descending and an ascending branch. This latter forms part of the quadrate collateral anastomosis behind the hip joint, thus providing a very important collateral route to the thigh or beyond even if the profunda femoris artery itself is obstructed (Figure 31-4). Equally important is the role of the descending branch of the lateral circumflex artery as a significant distal pathway which can serve as an alternative even to the profunda femoris artery itself (Figure 31-5). The arterial anatomy in the thigh can, therefore, be considered to consist of three parallel systems which, in descending order of importance, are the superficial femoral artery, the profunda femoris artery, and the descending branch of the lateral circumflex artery.

As it progresses distally the profunda femoris is crossed by a number of large veins, usually in the anterior position. These generally correspond to the branches which have already been described but do not form a profunda femoris vein as such. The more distal veins empty into the superficial femoral vein, and the more proximal veins communicate with the origin of the common femoral vein. In fact, it is the accumulation of these large profunda venous branches which finally constitutes the common femoral vein. Of these venous branches, the most common and anatomically well defined is the vein which corresponds to the lateral circumflex artery and generally is the most proximal of the venous tributaries. This vein is surgically important for the identification of the profunda artery from the lateral approach.

IMPORTANT ANATOMICAL VARIATIONS

The most important anatomical variation is the position of the medial circumflex artery. As will be explained later (see Pathology of the Profunda Femoris Artery, below), this is an important branch of the profunda femoris artery. Although, as Figure 31-1 shows, it classically arises from the profunda femoris artery itself in a position opposite to, and considered to be on the same level as, the lateral circumflex branch, in over 1000 recorded exposures of the femoral arteries in 60 percent of cases, it actually arises from the common femoral artery. In most of these instances, the medial circumflex artery is within 1 cm proximal to the origin of the profunda femoris artery, but it has also been found in the common femoral artery just after its passage under the inguinal ligament. However, its position of origin from the common femoral artery is so common that this should be considered the usual site of origin and not a variant. The second variant is that in 20 percent of instances, the proximal half of the profunda femoris artery does not occupy its usual posterior position with respect to the superficial femoral artery but in fact lies in the lateral position, running in a coronal plane which is almost parallel to the superficial femoral artery (the so-called parallel profunda). In this position, exposure of the proximal profunda femoris artery is technically much easier than in its usual position in which it becomes progressively deeper and more posterior. It is useful to remember that in this ''parallel'' position, the profunda can and has been frequently mistaken for the superficial femoral artery, thus resulting in subsequent operative confusion. Quite rare variations of the profunda are its origin some distance either at or under the inguinal ligament or some distance from it (sometimes as much as 10 cm). Equally rare is the origin of the profunda from the common and superficial femoral arteries as a series of branches rather than a single main stem. As far as we can estimate from our observations, these variations occur in less than 1 percent of profunda femoris arteries.

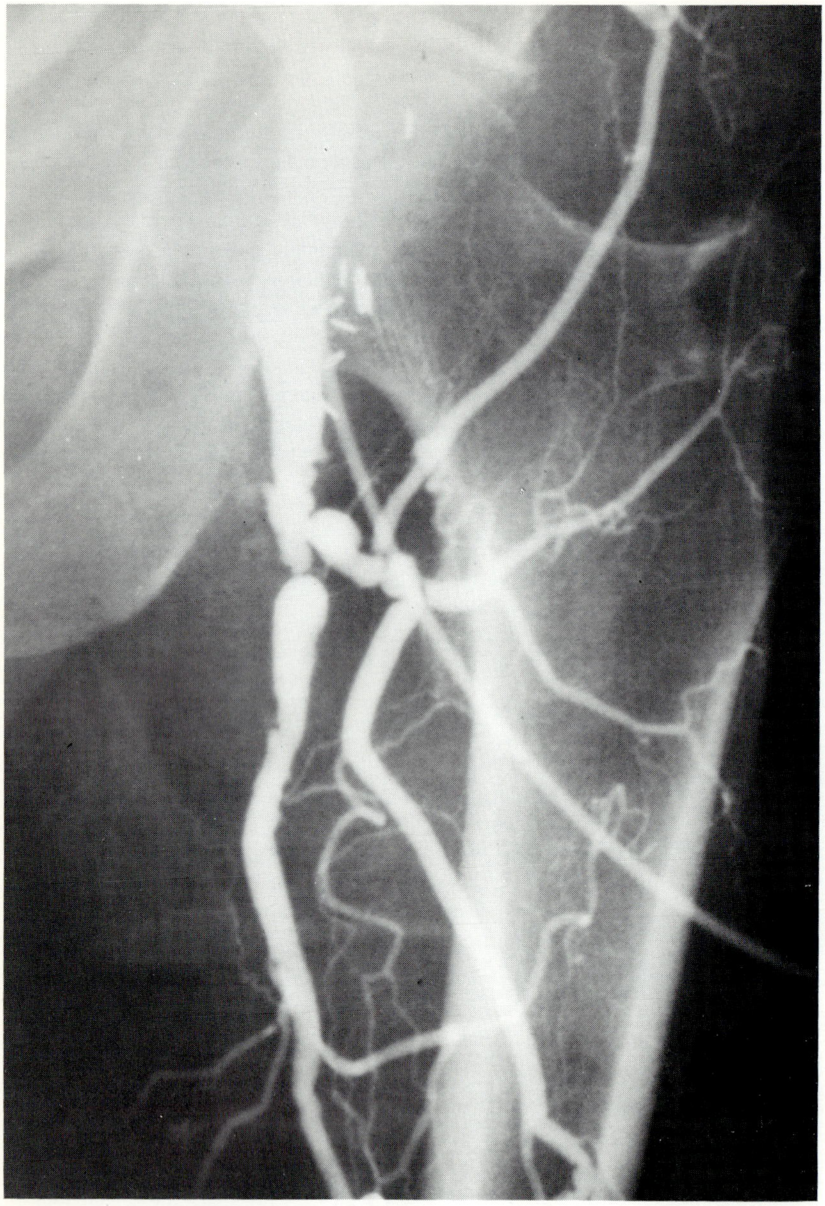

FIGURE 31-4. Angiogram showing profunda orifice stenosis, but most marked is the development of the ascending branch of the lateral circumflex acting as a collateral to the descending branch via the quadrate anastomosis.

Physiological Considerations of the Profunda Femoris Artery

The physiological capacity of the profunda femoris artery as a major collateral to the lower limb has been extensively investigated. Waibel has observed that the pressure in the popliteal artery measured during surgery for the relief of superficial femoral occlusion was further reduced when the profunda femoris artery was cross-clamped (2). Electromagnetic flow studies carried out by Bernhard during operation have confirmed the clinical observations that the collateral function of the profunda femoris artery both is extensive and could effectively compensate for atherosclerotic occlusion of the superficial femoral artery (3). For example, he has observed that the entire flow in the external iliac artery could be handled by the unobstructed profunda femoris artery both when the superficial femoral artery was patent and when it was obstructed either by disease or by vascular clamp. In addition, therapeutic dilatation of the perfusion bed of the profunda femoris with papaverine (effect on more distal perfusion bed at arterial level) has consistently demonstrated the overall normality of its vessel walls and its capacity to respond to increased flow demands. Other authors have shown that restoration of the integrity of the profunda femoris artery has resulted in increases in ankle pressures (4), treadmill tolerance (5), as well as painfree walking distance (6). Nevertheless, it must be pointed out that hemodynamic resistance through the numerous small branches of the profunda femoris artery is additive and is therefore consistently greater than that which is present in the undiseased superficial femoral artery. Using geometric modeling and calculations, Berguer et al. have suggested that since the profunda femoris artery is significantly smaller than the superficial femoral artery and since its orifice is often only 50 percent of this artery, a functional physiological stenosis thus

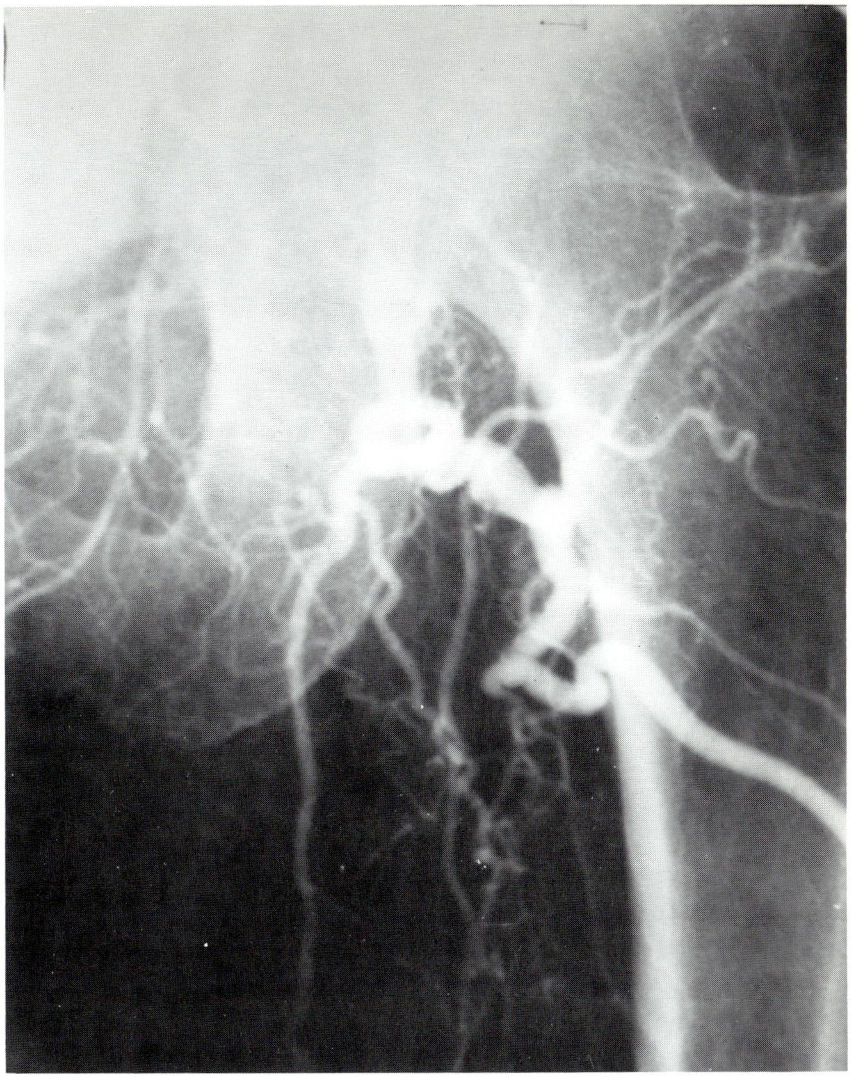

FIGURE 31-5. Excellent example of the entire profunda femoris artery being represented solely by a hugely enlarged descending branch of the lateral circumflex artery and a smaller medial circumflex. Both of these arteries are evidently reconstructable under these circumstances.

exists when the superficial femoral artery is unavailable. These researchers have proposed that under these circumstances a very minor degree of narrowing by the atherosclerotic process produces a disproportionally large reduction in flow into this collateral bed (7). For these reasons they and other authors have suggested that lesser degrees of narrowing of the profunda femoris artery should justifiably be treated more vigorously in order to increase and maintain the flow into the profunda femoris artery, but this concept has never been widely practiced.

Pathology of the Profunda Femoris Artery

In our experience, most instances of failure of the profunda femoris artery to carry out its normal function of arterial inflow to the thigh and subsequently to the lower leg are caused by obstructive lesions at and proximal to its origin. Most proximal lesions are the result of atherosclerotic disease of the iliac vessels, of which the external iliac is most commonly involved along its entire length. Under these circumstances, the common femoral artery is frequently involved in the atherosclerotic process to such an extent that the disease necessarily extends at least into the origin of the profunda femoris artery. More distal lesions usually of the profunda femoris artery itself (i.e., apart from inflow obstructive lesions) are also well recognized. Classically, the most common lesion to be recognized in the profunda system is the orifice lesion, which usually extends no more than 1 cm into the profunda femoris artery itself. Most authors on this subject consider that in over three-quarters of the profunda femoris arteries which are being surgically considered, this is the important lesion that is present. The nature of this lesion will be considered subsequently, but with advances in both the surgery and radiology of the profunda femoris artery and particularly with the use of oblique and lateral projection angiography, lesions involving the entire profunda system are much more frequently seen and in our experience amount to some 40 percent of instances.

Orifice Lesion of the Profunda Femoris Artery

As will be seen from Figure 31-6, the orifice lesion of the profunda femoris artery, which is well known and frequently discussed, is in fact an extension of the atherosclerotic process involving the common femoral artery. Such lesions (e.g., renal artery stenosis, subclavian artery stenosis) are well known in vascular pathology and generally represent extension of the atherosclerotic thickening of the wall of the artery of conduit into the origin of the artery of supply. However in an increasing number of patients, more widespread lesions of the profunda femoris artery are seen on arteriography. Although statistically diabetic patients are more prone to the problem, even nondiabetic patients are frequently seen to suffer from this lesion. The more diffuse lesion of the artery extends throughout its main channel but has its most serious effect in the compromise of the orifice of its individual branches. In this respect, the lateral circumflex artery is so frequently diseased that this artery appears in general to be pathologically unfavorable. Fortunately, the lateral circumflex artery itself is of short length (usually 1 cm) and the disease only infrequently extends into the orifices of the ascending or descending circumflex branches. By contrast, however, the medial circumflex artery is much more favorably disposed. As seen in Figure 31-6, the plaque or atherosclerotic thickening rarely extends beyond its orifice and the artery itself is usually healthy beyond this point. Since this branch is usually quite large, it represents a significant and readily available functional part of the profunda femoris outflow. In severe involvement of the profunda femoris artery, the perforating branches themselves may be so diseased along their length that their occlusion is permanent and irreversible. However, the final bifurcation termination of the profunda femoris artery tends to be less diseased and to remain available as a small but reasonable outflow tract.

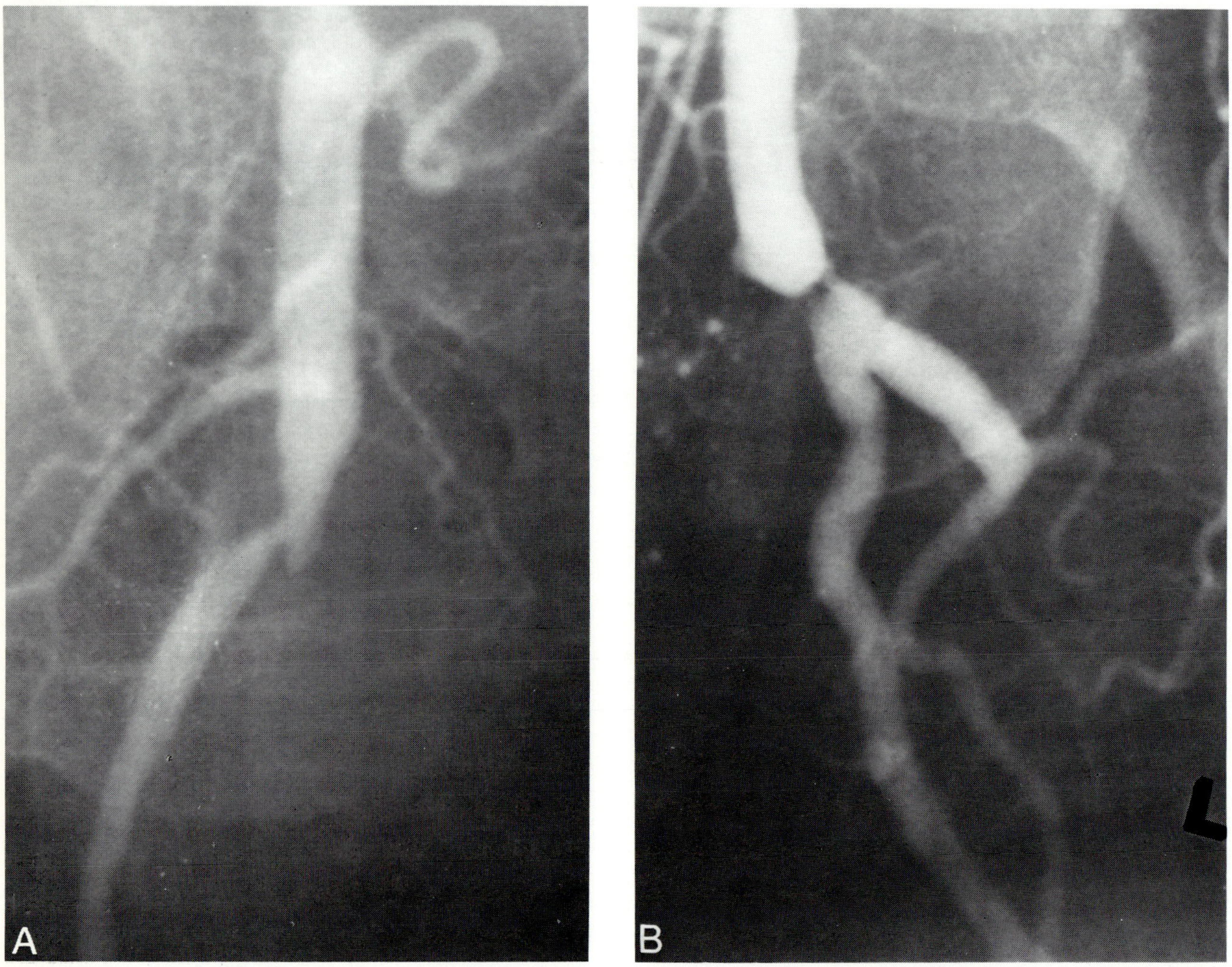

FIGURE 31-6. Two examples of orifice lesions of the profunda. The lesion in (*A*) is smoothly tapered from the plaque in the common femoral artery. The plaque in (*B*) is also extensive but ends in a diaphragmlike obstruction.

Methods of Investigation of the Profunda Femoris Artery

CLINICAL INVESTIGATION

In most circumstances (except for superficially placed parallel profunda arteries), the profunda femoris artery is beyond the reach of the examining finger. When the orifice is narrowed, this may be detected by the presence of a bruit on stethoscopic auscultation. However, such bruits are nonspecific because they may represent lesions of the common femoral artery as well as the proximal part of the branches of the profunda femoris artery itself.

DOPPLER ULTRASOUND

Spectral analysis has been used in an attempt to define these pathological problems but has not been easy to interpret because of the anatomical orientation of the vessels. Doppler ultrasound examination of the profunda femoris arteries has to be carried out carefully in order to prevent confusion with signals arising from the superficial femoral artery. In general, the beam has to be directed away from the superficial femoral artery at a somewhat deeper angle. Since the profunda femoris artery disappears or retreats rapidly in a posterior direction, 5-MHz or longer range ultrasound beams must be employed in order to differentiate profunda from superficial femoral artery flow. Fortunately, since in most instances the superficial femoral artery is occluded, the signal generated by currently available Doppler instruments usually arises from the profunda femoris artery. The descending branch of the circumflex artery is in a strategic position with respect to Doppler examination. Its main physiological function appears to be as a supplier of the sartorius muscle, and as such, it runs under or close to the lateral border of the muscle. It can therefore be consistently sought and found in this position using a 5-MHz instrument, and qualitative information is generally easier to obtain than from the main profunda stem. This examination is of particular importance when this artery represents a significant part of the profunda femoris outflow and the collateral arrangements to the lower limb.

RADIOLOGICAL ASSESSMENT

In the majority of instances, as previously described in the anatomy section, the origin of the profunda femoris artery is posterior to the common and superficial femoral arteries. During the angiographic examination, the dye column in this part of the profunda is therefore frequently obscured by the overlying dye column in both the common and superficial femoral arteries. The classic angiographic paper by Beales (8) pointed out that on routine anteroposterior arteriography, a stenotic lesion of the origin of the profunda femoris artery can therefore be frequently missed. For this reason, biplane views of this bifurcation are necessary either in the 45° oblique position or from true lateral projection. When this anatomical configuration is present, the entire profunda system can be visualized in over 70 percent of instances. In the study referred to above, orificial or proximal stenosis of the profunda was found in 60 percent of patients with lower limb ischemic symptoms. This observation was based on the presence of a 50 percent stenosis, but lesser and presumably clinically unimportant degrees of stenosis were also found. Needless to say, in the smaller percentage of instances in which a true lateral or parallel profunda system is present, anteroposterior arteriogram is all that is required for complete profunda visualization.

INTRAOPERATIVE PARAMETERS

The use of absolute flow measurements in the profunda femoris artery has already been mentioned and will not be discussed further because in practice their interpretation with respect to clinical decisions is difficult. Also, the use of intraoperative pressure measurements in the common femoral and profunda femoris arteries has been reported on by various authors (9,10). However, Archie and Feldtman (11) have pointed out that in spite of all these criteria, the diagnosis of significant profunda femoris artery stenosis may still be difficult. These researchers have measured the pressure gradients across profunda lesions together with intraoperative blood flow before and after pharmacologic vasodilatation. Their results indicate that the low-mean profunda pressure gradients which were measured at resting blood flow show that stenoses of the profunda artery less than 75 percent diameter were significant at rest. After doubling of the blood flow through the artery, even smaller degrees of stenoses appear to be hemodynamically significant, thus providing a more rational basis for surgical treatment of these lesions. In practice, we have found that at rest, pressure gradients of less than 10 mmHg are generally insignificant, pressure gradients of 15 mmHg are moderately significant, and pressure gradients above 25 mmHg have marked physiological significance.

Restoration of Arterial Inflow to Normal Profunda System

The function of the profunda system as the arterial watershed to the lower limb is, in most cases, diminished because of disease in the iliac system, notably the external iliac artery and less commonly in the common iliac and aorta. It is unusual that only the common femoral artery is completely obstructed by atherosclerosis, thus causing a loss of profunda inflow. This situation is usually caused by unrecognized or neglected embolic impaction. The surgical options which are available for iliac occlusion are those of bypass from a suitable proximal inflow source, i.e., aorta or iliac vessel, either directly to the profunda femoris artery or to the common femoral artery, when adequacy of the profunda orifice is ensured either by inspection or by very limited endarterectomy. The choice of bypass material is wide, but synthetic material is usually used. This choice of bypass material also applies to extraanatomic midline crossing grafts from contralateral competent iliac or femoral arteries. At present autogenous

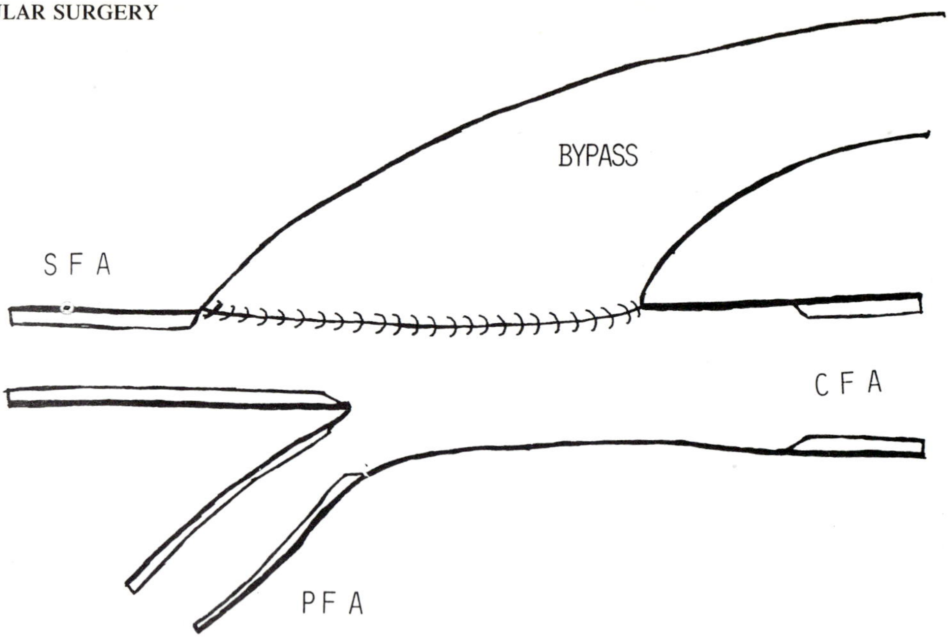

FIGURE 31-7. When arteriotomy is not carried into the profunda femoris artery, diagram shows preferred method of extending it into superficial femoral artery so that profunda orifice can be disobliterated under direct vision before insertion of the bypass.

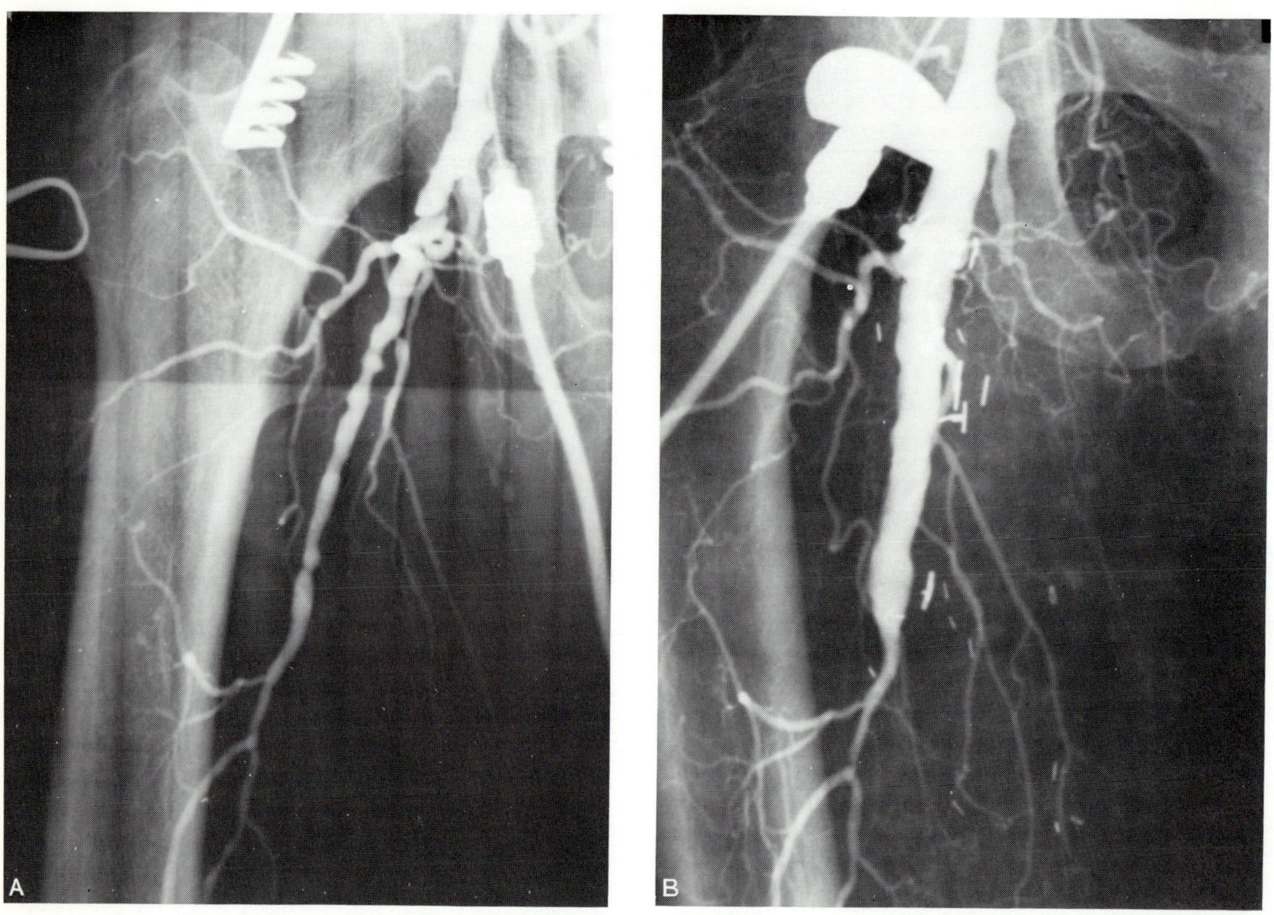

FIGURE 31-8. (*A*) Extensive disease of entire profunda main stem treated in (*B*) by extended endarterectomy of artery with on-lay vein patch. Note that the principles of reconstruction of an artery of supply have been adhered to (i.e., all the branches have been secured as an outflow tract as an essential part of the operation).

reconstitution is only infrequently used, but our extensive experience with endarterectomy from the terminal aorta to the profunda has been almost uniformly good (12).

Endarterectomy of the iliac vessels to provide an inflow source to the common femoral and profunda vessels is one of the traditional uses of this operation. At present, endarterectomy is usually limited to short segment occlusion or stenosis usually occurring in the external iliac system, and most surgeons will not consider this operation beyond the termination of the common iliac artery to the origin of the profunda femoris. However, it is quite feasible to extend this procedure in both directions, i.e., into the aorta as well as distally into the profunda femoris (1) (Figure 31-7). Note that a limited endarterectomy of the common femoral and profunda orifice has been carried out and that the bypass extends into the origin of the superficial femoral, thus allowing the profunda femoris orifice to be clearly examined via the anterior arteriotomy.

Diseased Profunda System with Adequate Common Femoral Inflow

ORIFICE LESION

As mentioned before (see Pathology of the Profunda Femoris Artery, above), one of the most common lesions of the profunda femoris artery is the orifice lesion. This is an extension of the atheromatous degeneration of the wall of the common femoral artery.

The surgical options which are available for an orifice lesion include (1) endarterectomy with primary closure, (2) endarterectomy with application of a patch, and (3) application of a widening patch graft only. These procedures are most commonly used when concomitant lesions exist in the orifices of the superficial femoral arteries and restoration of flow into the superficial femoral is also a reconstructive aim.

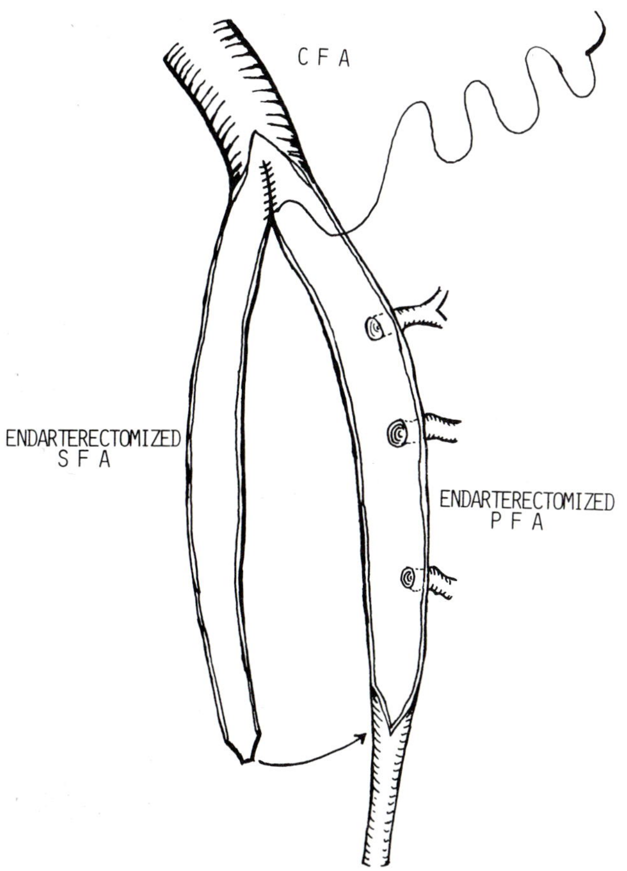

FIGURE 31-9. Diagram to show principle of use of endarterectomized superficial femoral in continuity arterial patch in conjunction with extended profundaplasty.

Most surgeons use some form of patch with or without endarterectomy in order to widen the profunda orifice, but at this level a carefully constructed endarterectomy in a large profunda can frequently be accurately closed without application of a patch graft. The patch materials used are either autogenous vein, endarterectomized artery, or synthetic material.

EXTENSIVE LESIONS WITH COMMON FEMORAL INFLOW

The operation of extended profundaplasty is a relatively new procedure in the field of vascular surgery. Its newness stems from the fact that it is one of the first areas in reconstructive surgery in which a direct planned attack has been made on an artery of supply. In this case, it is defined as a reconstruction which is carried beyond the most distal level of the lateral circumflex origin and usually beyond the first perforating branch (Figure 31-8). In the performance of this operation, certain "rules" have been developed in order to ensure both success of the reconstruction itself and achievement of maximum function of the reconstructed profunda system. These rules are as follows: the reconstruction must preserve as many branches as possible. The integrity of the profunda femoris artery and its function is directly related to the number of outflow branches, and maximum care must be taken to ensure their integrity. The most important branches in order are (1) the lateral circumflex branch, because it serves as an inflow to the descending branch, an important collateral vessel as previously discussed; (2) the medial circumflex branch, because its orifice lesion is easily removed, leaving a large and otherwise normal vessel; note again that this vessel commonly arises in the common femoral artery; (3) the terminal branches of the profunda because of their direct communication to the geniculate arteries (13,14).

The surgical options available are as follows: (1) Endarterectomy without patch. In this procedure, great care must be taken not to jeopardize the orifices of the branches, on which the entire functional integrity of the profunda system depends. (2) Application of an onlay patch. This is usually used after endarterectomy in order to widen the vessel and prevent constriction of its lumen by simple closure, or it is used as a distinct operation on its own without endarterectomy if this procedure is not wise because of the state of the arterial wall or because the surgeon is inexperienced in the creation of a satisfactory end point in the branches. The types of patch are as discussed previously and consist of autogenous excised vein, endarterectomized artery, or synthetic material, at the choice of the surgeon.

A very useful technique for developing patch graft material for extended profundaplasty is to use endarterectomized superficial femoral artery in continuity as an onlay flap shift. This is diagrammed in Figure 31-9. In this procedure, the femoral artery is divided and mobilized at the correctly measured length. It is opened posteriorly along its axis in continuity with the profunda arteriotomy. The superficial femoral is then endarterectomized, all shreds of necrotic muscle being removed until a shiny, external elastic lumen is reached. The lateral edge is trimmed, and as shown in Figure 31-9, the artery is folded over and into the profunda arteriotomy. This procedure provides an excellent patch but has the potential disadvantage that when the superficial femoral artery is used in this way, at a later date there is a loss of its use as an inflow source for a more distal reconstruction after its preparation by thromboendarterectomy.

EXTENSIVE DISEASE OF THE PROFUNDA WITH PROXIMAL (AORTOILIAC) OBSTRUCTION

This condition can be treated by endarterectomy of the profunda, common femoral, and iliac vessels as previously described. However, the most commonly used option is bypass with synthetic material from the most suitably identified inflow source to the profunda together with extended profundaplasty. It has been suggested by Malone et al. (15) that optimally, autogenous material be used as a patch on the profunda femoris itself and up to the point of insertion of the synthetic bypass. However, a synthetic patch in continuity with a synthetic bypass is also frequently used to widen the profunda artery.

Profunda Branch Revascularization

In a small number of instances, the main stem of the profunda femoris artery itself becomes occluded and the usually defined presence of the terminal segment of the profunda femoris artery cannot be identified radiologically. In these instances, the branches of the profunda femoris artery are usually represented angiographically, although the orifices from the main stem of the

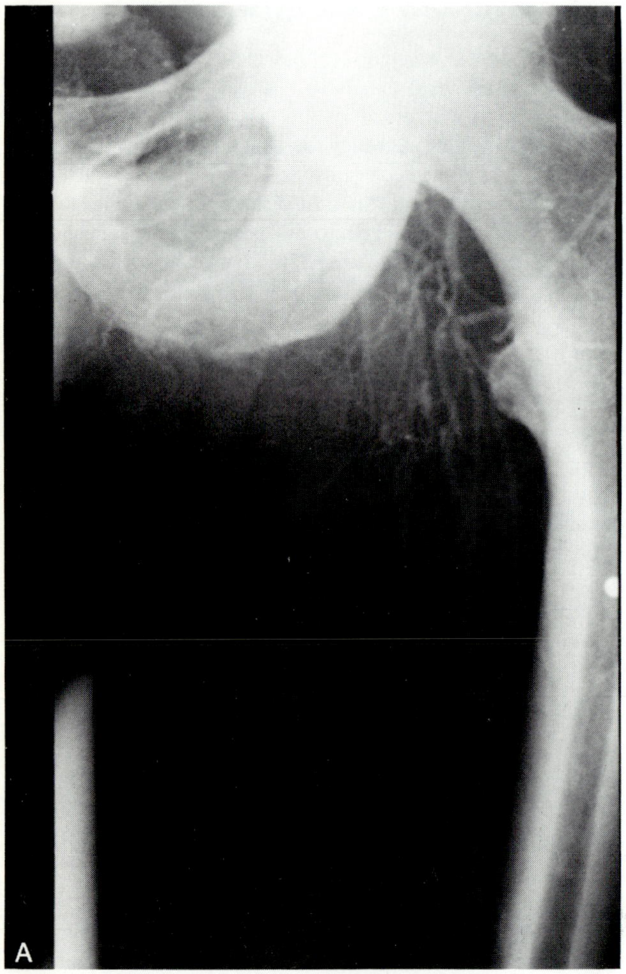

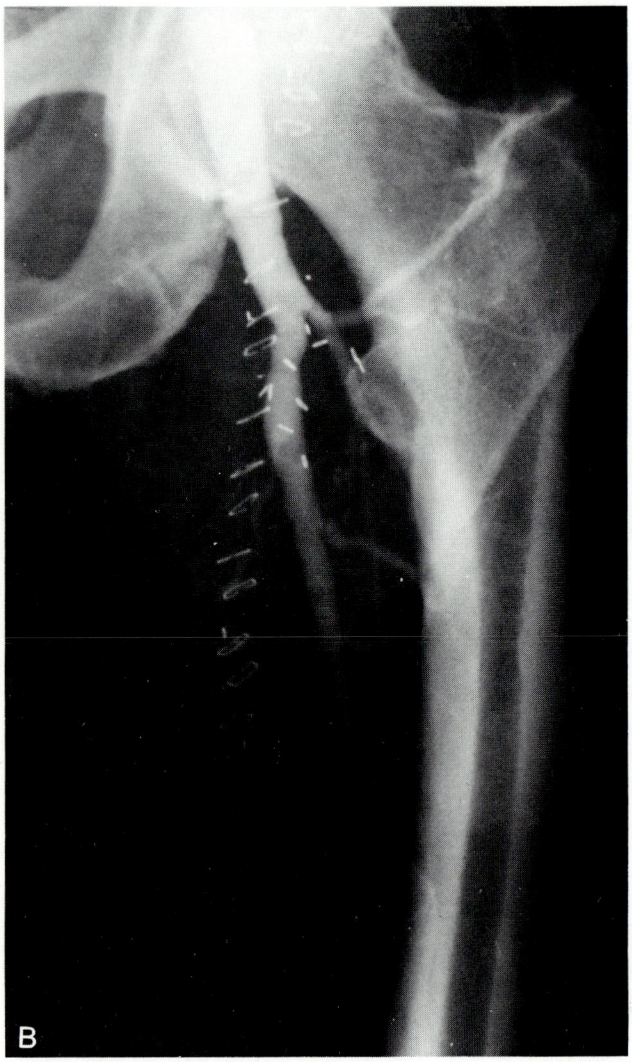

FIGURE 31-10. (*A*) Apparently hopeless and nonreconstructable situation converted into (***B***) (i.e., almost normal profunda system) by exploration and carefully applied extended profundaplasty.

profunda may be diseased (Figure 31-10). In eight such instances, we have attempted to relieve rest pain by revascularization of the anatomically present branches. Unquestionably, the most important of these are the lateral circumflex artery in its entirety, i.e., both the ascending and descending branches of this artery, and the medial circumflex branch (16). Other muscular perforating branches can usually be placed in the circuit but appear to have a much less important role. The favorable pathology of the medial circumflex branch has already been mentioned, and in general, the reconstruction of the lateral circumflex artery has to be carried out across its main trunk into either or both of the ascending or descending branches. In six instances in which autogenous bypass material was used (vein), these attempts were successful, but in the two instances in which Dacron grafts were used, occlusion occurred swiftly and amputation ensued. This experience, therefore, suggests that it is possible using microvascular techniques to achieve very worthwhile distal limb perfusion by rearterialization of the larger profunda femoris branches, which then act as a second parallel collateral network to the distal part of the lower limb. However, our experience also indicates that autogenous bypass material is mandatory for these reconstructions, and if this is not available, the reconstructions should not be attempted because they are doomed to immediate failure.

Commentary

Many of the patients with femoral popliteal occlusion are both elderly and ravaged by the other consequences of cardiovascular degeneration. Restoration of the profunda femoris artery as the flow path to the distal lower limb is an alternative procedure to femoral, popliteal, or infrapopliteal bypass because of its circumscribed nature and the lower operative morbidity rate (17). When significant lesions of the profunda femoris artery can be identified, such reconstructions performed under regional or even local anesthesia may provide very worthwhile palliation in these patients. However, traditional familiarity with femoral distal bypass has diverted attention from the utilization of the full surgical potential of the profunda femoris artery. Our experience has shown that such procedures are excellent for the release of rest pain in both diabetic and nondiabetic patients since all such patients had immediate and relatively lasting clinical improvements (12,14). These results occurred even when there were minimal changes in ankle pressures or waveform amplitude, which is a further indication that rest pain itself requires only a small increment of flow for relief (4). The increase in pain-free walking distance in these patients has also been striking, and in practice this can be used as a simple but practical index of the functional improvement of the postoperative circulation which has not been used in other series (6). We have also found that when tissue necrosis is present in nondiabetic patients, there appears to be a very good chance that this approach will also result in the healing of lesions without recourse to more distal bypass surgery (18,19). In addition, this procedure preserves the important option of more distal bypass surgery if this should later be required. However, we have also found that in diabetic patients with tissue necrosis, particularly when there is concomitant infection, a maximum increment in flow is required to achieve healing (20). In these circumstances, therefore, more direct restitution of pulsatile flow to the popliteal or tibial arteries, in addition to profundaplasty, is the procedure of choice when such vessels are available for reconstruction. In this context, the profundaplasty serves as a backup or "insurance policy" to maintain distal circulation should the bypass itself fail at a later date once healing has taken place.

In the literature, there is some dispute over the value of profundaplasty as a means of achieving the salvage of a profoundly ischemic limb. For example, Bernhard (21), Martin (17), Malone (15), Towne (22), and we have found profundaplasty to be clinically useful, while Rutledge (23) and Jamieson (5) have not been so impressed. After the publication of many papers on the subject of profundaplasty, Jamieson (5) is of the belief that profundaplasty has a limited place in limb salvage when performed alone but is relatively ineffective when combined with a proximal arterial reconstruction. He has also stated that in the presence of superficial femoral occlusion, it does not provide much improvement in pain-free walking distance in many patients. Rutledge (23) has also reported that only a few patients with severe peripheral vascular disease distal to the inguinal ligament (which is unreconstructable by other means) will benefit from primary profundaplasty. However, as they state, they did not consider patients for primary profundaplasty if the distal vasculature allowed reasonable consideration for femoral distal bypass.

From such literature, it is clear that the benefits of profundaplasty appear to be directly related to (1) the technical excellence of the procedure and (2) the presence of some degree of clearly recognizable anatomical outflow vessels distal to superficial femoral occlusion. The sine qua non of successful profundaplasty appears to be the latter factor since in our experience, performance of technically adequate profunda reconstructions in the face of patent superficial femoral arteries in the thigh has never produced any degree of clinical relief concomitant with the surgical effort expended. Therefore, when these conditions apply, profundaplasty can be expected to be worthwhile, but when little or no distal limb runoff vessels can be identified, the results are much less worthwhile. However, the exception to this rule is the revascularization of the profunda femoris artery concomitantly with proximal repair of totally occluded or severely stenotic common femoral or iliac vessels. Under these circumstances, particularly when rest pain is an indication for the reconstruction, the final result is almost always both worthwhile and long-lasting.

The importance of the technical excellence of profundaplasty cannot be overestimated. The vessels involved are usually small, and the final integrity and function of the reconstruction is entirely dependent on preservation of those branches which represent its outflow tract. Reconstruction of vessels of supply (vs. vessels of conduit) is a relatively new concept in vascular surgery. A few reports on reconstruction of the external carotid (24), internal iliac, and secondary and tertiary branches of the renal arteries have appeared, but it is fair to say that general experience with such reconstructions has not yet been developed. With increased surgical care and the use of microvascular techniques, such ventures show a slow but steady expansion. The statement of Towne's (22) that "today's profundaplasty is tomorrow's tibial bypass" is an indication of the value of this limited procedure in preserving limb integrity while allowing for the subsequent performance of a more distal procedure which will extend the useful life of the lower limb.

References

1. Dunlop GR: In discussion of Billig DM, Callow AD, Deterling RA: Surgical considerations in the management of lesions of the profunda femoris artery. Am J Surg 1970, 119:396.
2. Waibel PP, Wolff G: The collateral circulation in occlusions of the femoral artery: An experimental study. Surgery 1966, 60:912.
3. Bernhard VM, Ray LI, Militello JM: The role of angioplasty of the profunda femoris artery in revascularization of the ischemic limb. Surg Gynecol Obstet 1976, 142:840.
4. Strandness DE: Functional results after revascularization of the profunda femoris artery. Am J Surg 1970, 119:240.
5. Jamieson CW, Galland RB: Objective assessment of profunda femoris reconstruction for limb salvage. Cont Surg 1980, 16:39.
6. Fernandes JF, Nicolaides AN, Angelides NA, Gordon-Smith IC: An objective assessment of common femoral endarterectomy and profundaplasty in patients with superficial femoral occlusion. Surgery 1978, 83:313.
7. Berguer R, Cotton LT, Higgins RF: Analysis of deep formal artery hemodynamics and the effect of reconstruction. Cardiovasc Surg 1975, 16:148.
8. Beales JS, Adcock FA, Frawley JS: The radiological assessment of disease of the profunda femoris artery. Br J Radiol 1971, 44:854.
9. Brewster DC, Darling RC: Optimal methods of aortoiliac reconstruction. Surgery 1978, 84:739.
10. Sumner DS, Strandness DE: Aortoiliac reconstruction in patients with combined iliac and superficial femoral arterial occlusion. Surgery 1978, 84:348.
11. Archie JP, Feldtman RW: Intraoperative assessment of the hemodynamic significance of iliac and profunda femoris artery stenosis. Surgery 1981, 90:876.
12. Leather RP, Shah DM, Karmody AM: The use of extended profundaplasty in limb salvage. Am J Surg 1978, 136:359.
13. Martin P, Frawley JE, Barbabas AP, Rosengarten D: On the surgery of atherosclerosis of the profunda femoris artery. Surgery 1972, 71:182.
14. Karmody AM, Shah DM, Leather RP: The distal profunda femoris artery. Its use in limb salvage. Clin Res 1977, 25:651.
15. Malone JM, Goldstone J, Moore WS: Autogenous profundaplasty: The key to long-term patency in secondary repair of aortofemoral graft occlusion. Ann Surg 1978, 188:817.
16. Del Campo C: Profunda-circumflex plasty in the management of severe femoropopliteal occlusion. Tex Heart Instit 1983, 10:152.
17. Martin P, Bouhoutsos J: The medium term results after profundaplasty. Br J Surg 1977, 64:194.
18. Boren CH, Towne JB, Bernhard VM, Salles-Cunha S: Profunda-popliteal collateral index. A guide to successful profundaplasty. Arch Surg 1980, 115:1366.
19. Martin P, Jamieson C: The rationale for measurement after profundaplasty. Surg Clin North Am 1974, 54:95.
20. Karmody AM, Jacobs RL: Salvage of the diabetic foot by vascular reconstruction. Orthop Clin North Am 1976, 7:77.
21. Bernhard VM: The role of profundaplasty in revascularization of the lower extremities. Surg Clin North Am 1979, 59:681.
22. Towne JB, Bernhard VM, Rollins DL, Baum PI: Profundaplasty in perspective: Limitations in long-term management of limb ischemia. Surgery 1981, 90:1037.
23. Rutledge R, Burnham S: Profundaplasty in the ischemic extremity. J Cardiovasc Surg 1983, 24:107.
24. Karmody AM, Shah DM, Monaco VJ, Leather RP: On surgical reconstruction of the external carotid artery. Am J Surg 1978, 136:176.

Chapter 32

LUMBAR SYMPATHECTOMY

DEBORAH A. LANGE, JAMES S. T. YAO, WILLIAM R. FLINN,
and JOHN J. BERGAN

Lumbar sympathectomy has been extensively employed in the treatment of obliterative vascular disease of the lower extremities . . . in spite of the fact, there is still a difference of opinion regarding the value of this operation in the treatment of peripheral vascular disease.
R.H. Smithwick (1)

It is remarkable that lumbar sympathectomy, one of the oldest operations used in the treatment of ischemia of the lower extremities, is still controversial. The opinion above, expressed by Smithwick in 1957 (1), is still true more than 25 years later. The role of lumbar sympathectomy is unsettled, simply because the operation has not been evaluated objectively or with appropriate controls. To do this, it would be necessary to quantitate effects of the procedure performed as a definitive operation, without concomitant arterial reconstruction. This has not been done adequately to date. As a separate consideration, lumbar sympathectomy must also be evaluated when combined with aortofemoral arterial reconstruction, and also when done with reconstruction of the femoral-popliteal-tibial arterial segments. In each instance, the results of the procedure should be evaluated scientifically, without prejudice, using objective measurement, and with control groups of patients not subjected to sympathectomy. There is no reason to repeat past errors of reporting results as "excellent" or "good" without defining these terms. Some studies have been done in recent years which, though nondefinitive, do illuminate the subject. These are the subject of this chapter.

Concomitant Sympathectomy

SYMPATHECTOMY WITH AORTOILIOFEMORAL RECONSTRUCTION

Among the arguments given in favor of performing sympathectomy with aortoiliofemoral reconstruction are the facts that the sympathetic chain is within the operative field, its removal adds very little time to the operation, and it does not increase operative risk or morbidity. Although these facts are true, clear thinking must also include whether the addition of sympathectomy contributes anything to relief of distal ischemia.

Barnes et al. (2), working in the Department of Surgery at the University of Iowa hospitals, studied 51 patients prospectively. These were randomly allocated to sympathectomy or control groups, based on a table of random numbers. In that study, the only significant benefit observed was a decrease in the foot arterial resistance in those patients having sympathectomy. Subjectively, the control subjects failed to demonstrate postoperative reactive hyperemia. The study did not demonstrate a significant difference in early or late postoperative leg hemodynamics, as assessed by the ankle blood pressure or the ankle-brachial index. The study failed to document any significant benefit in patients with intermittent claudication, nor was graft patency improved by lumbar sympathectomy. Although there were postoperative amputations, the numbers did not differ statistically between the nonsympathectomy and the sympathectomy patients. Barnes concluded that, "The results of this study suggest that the only favorable effect of concomitant lumbar sympathectomy is the improvement in pedal circulation that might be sustained for a number of years following operation."

Satiani et al. (3) also performed a prospective, randomized study of concomitant lumbar sympathectomy with aortoiliac reconstruction, entering 93 patients with aortic occlusive disease in the 22-month study. Assignment to the sympathectomy or nonsympathectomy groups was based on hospital number. Eventually, 29 patients received sympathectomy, and 38 did not. Ultimately, distal bypass was required in 11 percent of the patients in the nonsympathectomy group and in 9.4 percent of the patients in the sympathectomy group. Five limbs were amputated 4 to 14 months after aortofemoral bypass. Four of these were in the nonsympathectomy and one in the sympathectomy group. The ankle-brachial index increased significantly after aortofemoral bypass in both groups, but the mean increase after bypass did not differ statistically between the two groups. The conclusion of these authors was that, "In a mean follow-up time of 11 months after aorto-femoral bypass, there was no significant difference in graft patency, need for subsequent distal bypass, or amputation rate between the sympathectomy and nonsympathectomy groups of patients."

SYMPATHECTOMY WITH FEMORODISTAL BYPASS

In an evaluation of sympathectomy in conjunction with infrainguinal bypass, Lee et al. (4) studied 40 patients in whom 50 arterial bypass procedures were done in combination with lumbar sympathectomy. In 32 patients, there were 40 arterial bypass procedures performed without concomitant lumbar sympathectomy. Cumulative patency, as calculated by life table analysis, revealed patency rates of 68 percent in limbs with sympathectomy and 66 percent in limbs without. This study, although not prospective or randomized, and with small numbers of patients and procedures, failed to demonstrate any beneficial effect from concomitant sympathectomy.

LABORATORY STUDIES

In experimental animals and in humans, alterations in blood flow produced by sympathectomy are easily demonstrable. An improvement in the patency of small-vessel anastomoses when sympathectomy was added to the arterial reconstruction has been demonstrated in animals. In humans, Kountz and Cohn (5) showed that bilateral lumbar sympathectomy produced a marked increase in aortic blood flow and that unilateral sympathectomy produced a doubling of blood flow in the superficial femoral artery. However, Weismann and Upson (6) found no beneficial effect when sympathectomy was added to arterial reconstruction, and they concluded that there was "no good evidence that sympathectomy significantly improved the results of arterial reconstructive surgery."

CONCLUSIONS REGARDING SYMPATHECTOMY AND CONCOMITANT ARTERIAL RECONSTRUCTION

Despite excellent experimental evidence that sympathectomy improves limb blood flow, there is no concrete evidence in humans that concomitant lumbar sympathectomy improves graft patency in the aortoiliac segment or in the femoral-popliteal-tibial arterial segments. Although improved foot blood flow can be demonstrated by laboratory techniques and although a decrease in arterial resistance is clearly demonstrable, there is no evident protection of the distal extremity from early or late graft failure, nor is there evidence that a decreased amputation rate or a lower level of amputation is achieved by concomitant sympathectomy.

Lumbar Sympathectomy as Definitive Therapy

Lumbar sympathectomy is generally acknowledged to be effective treatment for causalgia, reflex sympathetic dystrophy, and hyperhidrosis.* One would therefore think that sympathectomy performed alone in the treatment of arterial insufficiency would have been evaluated objectively, and definitive conclusions drawn regarding its efficacy. This, unfortunately, is not true. A number of methods have been used to predict the results of sympathectomy in patients with arterial insufficiency. Reflex vasodilatation was among the earliest tests used, and Cranley (7) and Husni and Simeone (8) confirmed that there was a correlation between the results of sympathectomy and skin temperature response to reflex vasodilatation. Yao and Bergan (9) found that the level of ankle systolic blood pressure and the ankle-brachial index correlated with the ability to prevent amputation by sympathetic ablation. Twenty-six of 27 of their patients with a pressure index <0.20 required amputation following sympathectomy, while all patients with a pressure index >0.35 avoided amputation after lumbar sympathectomy.

Similarly, Lewis and Jamieson, cited by Eastcott (10), found that patients with an ankle-brachial index <0.2 failed to attain good results from sympathectomy, and 70 percent came to amputation. Those with a higher distal pressure experienced relief of rest pain. Moreover, Thulesius and his group (11) found that the ankle-brachial systolic pressure ratio did predict the outcome of sympathetic block in 70 percent of cases and also found that at low ankle pressures, a paradoxical drop in toe temperature was seen in patients undergoing sympathetic block.

However, believing that single tests of sympathetic activity for arterial insufficiency were insufficient to predict the results of sympathectomy, Walker and Johnston (12) measured 7 variables in 72 limbs prior to performing a phenol sympathetic block. The results of discriminant analysis showed that the most important variables in predicting the outcome were the level of ankle systolic pressure, the presence or absence of neuropathy, and the extent of ischemia. In brief, they felt that, if there was no neuropathy, if the ankle systolic pressure was >30 mmHg, and if no extensive tissue damage was present, the phenol block would be successful.

Plecha's group (13) called attention to the fact that patency of the aortoiliac and femoral arterial segments correlated with good results of sympathectomy in patients with severe foot ischemia. In attempting to quantitate this evaluation, they found that limbs with a distal thigh-to-brachial pressure index >0.7 had the best chance for improvement in ankle pressure following sympathectomy. This, in effect, was a confirmation of Smithwick's earlier observations that beneficial effects of sympathectomy would correlate with the presence of a popliteal pulse and absence of distal foot pulses (1).

Our group has had long interest in sympathectomy, reporting on the reasons for increased ischemia following sympathectomy (paradoxical gangrene) in 1962 (14) and the results of hemodynamic prediction of sympathectomy effects in 1972 (9). In the 10 years following the second report, a total of 51 lumbar sympathectomies were performed in 48 patients on our vascular service. In 5 patients, the operation was performed together with direct arterial reconstruction; thus, the results of sympathectomy could not be evaluated. In the remaining 43 patients, there were 24 men and 19 women, of whom 26 were diabetic. Ischemic ulcer was the indication for surgery in 30 patients, rest pain in 10, and superficial gangrene in 4. In all instances, a retroperitoneal sympathectomy, with removal of all ganglia below L2, was performed. All patients were evaluated by arteriography and

*See Additional Reference, by Thompson and Patman.

TABLE 32-1. Listing of Limbs with Significant Ankle-Brachial Index Change following Sympathectomy

	Preoperative			Postoperative		
Patient No.	A-B* Index	Thigh Index	Indication	Change in A-B Index	Change in Thigh Index	Outcome
1	0.52	1.38	Ulcer	+0.45	+0.11	Remained healed 4 years
2†	0.46	1.03	Ulcer	+0.23	−0.01	Required tibial bypass
3†	0.77	0.86	Ulcer	+0.19	+0.22	Healed 7 months
4	0.63	0.82	Gangrene	+0.17	−0.02	Healed
5	0.43	—	Ulcer	+0.15	—	Ulcer healed, patient died after 1 year from myocardial infarction
6	0.67	—	Ulcer	+0.15	—	Healed slowly

*Ankle-brachial.
†Same patient.

Doppler-derived segmental limb pressures, with a calculation of the ankle-brachial index, as well as the thigh-brachial index. In the main, patients were selected for sympathectomy because they matched the hemodynamic criteria previously published by Yao and Bergan (9) and by Plecha et al. (13).

The results of the operation are best evaluated by grouping the patients. Table 32-1 displays the results obtained by sympathectomy in five patients with six limbs undergoing sympathectomy. In each of these, a postoperative increase in the ankle-brachial index >0.15 was obtained. The greatest change in ankle-brachial index was 0.45. In this group, ischemic ulcer was present in five limbs, and superficial gangrene in one. The ultimate outcome was success in five limbs, in which the ischemic ulcers healed in four limbs and the superficial gangrene healed in one. In one of these limbs, the ulcer remained healed for 1 year, at which time the patient died of myocardial infarction.

One other limb might be considered to be a success, since the ischemic ulcers healed and remained healed for 7 months. When they recurred, a tibial bypass procedure was required. In this patient, who had a bilateral sympathectomy, the initial ankle-brachial index changed from 0.46 to 0.69, but later fell as ischemia returned and the tibial bypass was required. In the other limb of the same patient, the ankle-brachial index rose from 0.77 to 0.96, ischemic ulcers healed, and a tibial bypass was not required.

Of tremendous interest to surgeons correlating results of sympathectomy with the presence or absence of diabetes mellitus is the fact that all of the patients in this group were diabetic. Thus, it is clearly shown that an increase in the ankle-brachial index can be obtained by sympathectomy in some diabetic patients.

Table 32-2 displays the results in nine patients undergoing lumbar sympathectomy, all of whom experienced an increase in the ankle-brachial index, but this increase was <0.15. In this group of patients, there were five long-term successes of the procedure. Gangrene healed in one patient, and ischemic ulceration healed in four others. One patient was not followed. Late amputation was performed in the three other limbs, two with rest pain and one with ischemic ulcers as the indication for sympathectomy.

Table 32-3 displays the results of sympathectomy in 16 patients, 3 of whom had no change in the ankle-brachial index postoperatively, and 13 of whom had a decrease in the ankle-brachial index from 0.01 to 0.24. In 5 of the 16 limbs in this group, the operation could be considered a success. However, 8 of the 11 other limbs came to amputation eventually, and in 3 limbs, direct arterial reconstruction was required. One of the patients having sympathectomy followed by limb amputation died following the amputation.

Within the group of patients subjected to sympathectomy during this time interval, there were eight in whom inadequate hemodynamic information was available. The results of the procedure, however, are known. Similar to those in which hemodynamic information followed stratification of patients, the results of sympathectomy were not good in this group. There were

TABLE 32-2. Limbs with Minimal Improvement in Ankle-Brachial Index following Sympathectomy

	Preoperative			Postoperative Change		
Patient No.	A-B* Index	Thigh Index	Indication	A-B Index	Thigh Index	Outcome
7	1.07	1.06	Gangrene	+0.13	+0.14	Healed 10 years
8	0.42	1.11	Rest pain	+0.11	−0.02	Pain relieved, toe amputation later
9	0.32	0.72	Rest pain	+0.11	−0.24	Late amputation
10	0.48	0.94	Ulcer	+0.08	+0.17	Healed
11	0.33	0.7	Rest pain	+0.06	+0.08	Late amputation
12	0.27	—	Ulcer	+0.06	—	One-year success, no late follow-up
13	0.74	0.87	Ulcer	+0.04	+0.27	Healed
14	0.4	0.64	Ulcer	+0.04	−0.08	Long-term healing
15	0.60	1.33	Ulcer	+0.02	+0.12	Late amputation

*Ankle-brachial.

TABLE 32-3. **Limbs with No Change or Worsening of Ankle-Brachial Index following Sympathectomy**

	Preoperative			Postoperative Change		
Patient No.	A-B* Index	Thigh Index	Indication	A-B Index	Thigh Index	Outcome
16	0.83	—	Ulcer	No change	—	Amputation
17	0.21	—	Rest pain	No change	—	Amputation
18	0.00	0.90	Gangrene	No change	−0.18	Amputation
19	0.22	0.56	Rest pain	−0.01	+0.11	Bypass
20	0.24	0.79	Rest pain	−0.02	−0.16	Pain relieved
21	0.24	0.82	Ulcer	−0.02	−0.07	Amputation
22	0.26	0.82	Gangrene	−0.03	+0.01	Local amputation healed
23	0.24	0.67	Ulcer	−0.03	−0.15	Amputation
24	0.46	0.49	Ulcer	−0.03	+0.35	Bypass
25	0.50	1.20	Ulcer	−0.06	−0.32	Amputation
26	0.58	—	Ulcer	−0.08	—	Healed
27	1.07	1.31	Ulcer	−0.11	−0.17	Healed
28	0.39	0.85	Ulcer	−0.12	+0.18	Healed
29	0.47	0.81	Ulcer	−0.15	−0.30	Bypass
30	0.48	0.92	Ulcer	−0.16	−0.06	Reconstruction
31	0.44	0.78	Rest pain	−0.24	+0.09	Bypass

*Ankle-brachial.

two long-term successes. In another patient, an ischemic ulcer healed after profundaplasty. Two patients were dead within a year of sympathectomy, one was not followed, and the remaining two patients had a recurrence of ischemic ulceration and/or amputation.

Within the study group, there were five patients with heavily calcified arteries, in whom the hemodynamic information obtained by noninvasive techniques could not be considered to be accurate. In one of these patients, the ankle pulse velocity waveform appeared to improve after sympathectomy. The patient had an acute myocardial infarction and died within 6 weeks of the procedure. In another patient, ischemic ulceration healed following sympathectomy, but amputation was required 5 months later, when the ischemic ulceration recurred. The other three patients required below-knee amputations.

It can be said that lumbar sympathectomy had a very limited success rate in this group of forty-three patients. When the indication for the procedure was ischemic ulceration, as it was in 30 limbs, the procedure failed in 18. Rest pain should be a good indication for sympathectomy, because a small amount of increased blood flow to the peripheral nerves should relieve ischemic neuropathy. However, of 10 limbs in which the indication for sympathectomy was rest pain without tissue necrosis, amputation or direct arterial reconstruction was avoided in only 4. When the indication for sympathectomy was gangrene, as it was in 4 limbs, the superficial gangrene healed in 3, while in the remaining limb, amputation was required. When all 44 limbs are included, only 19 can be considered to have had a successful outcome after sympathectomy. These 19 had healing of ischemic lesions for 1 year or more.

Of interest is the fact that in the 31 limbs in which adequate hemodynamic data were available, all but 4 fulfilled one or both of the criteria for selection suggested by Yao and Bergan (9) or by Plecha et al. (13). All except 8 had an ankle-brachial index in excess of 0.3, and all but 3 had a thigh index in excess of 0.7, except 6 limbs in which the thigh pressure was not recorded. Studying the tables fails to support the hypothesis that the criteria are helpful in predicting the ultimate results of the procedure.

There are two questions raised by this study. The first is why the patients had such severe ischemia in the presence of relatively elevated preoperative ankle-brachial indices. The second is why the results of sympathectomy in this group of patients are inferior to those reported by other groups in the past. While there is no clear-cut explanation for the presence of the elevated ankle-brachial index in this group of patients, it is true that 26 of the 43 patients were diabetic. It is probable that many of these patients exhibited subtotal calcification of the vessels, and the ankle pressure as obtained was falsely high. Despite this fact, all of the patients who had the greatest positive change in ankle-brachial index following sympathectomy were diabetic, showing that the presence of diabetes alone is not a contraindication to sympathectomy.

The presence of ischemic ulcerations characteristic of 30 of the limbs in this study may be the result of trauma and/or infection in the presence of ischemia, rather than ischemia alone. If so, some of these ulcerations might have healed without sympathectomy. A retrospective view of this group of patients does not clarify this situation.

The reason for the inferior results of sympathectomy in this study is explained by the objective focus on ultimate results, rather than status at postoperative discharge. Also, these patients were a residue left after selection of patients for direct arterial reconstruction. Few were candidates for distal bypass, simply because no distal arterial visualization was obtained on angiography.

In earlier sympathectomy series, the results have been more favorable. Haimovici, Steinman, and Karson (15), for example, stated that cyanosis and coldness was improved in 82 percent of their patients. It is less clear why 71 percent with rest pain were completely relieved of their discomfort. Szilagyi et al. (16), reporting on nearly 300 lumbar sympathectomies, felt that satisfactory rehabilitation occurred in 50 percent, but that the operation could not be recommended for massive gangrene, to alter the level of amputation, or for intermittent claudication. In the 10-year study by Shaw, Austen, and Stipa (17) of patients following sympathectomy, autonomic regeneration was not evident, and 54 percent of the patients who had undergone sympathectomy were dead. Eight patients required amputation after sympathectomy, and progression of the arterial disease, as manifested by the disappearance of peripheral pulses, occurred in one-third of the surviving patients.

It is not surprising that lumbar sympathectomy failed to produce a beneficial effect upon the severe ischemia in the patients at Northwestern University. A number of experimental and clinical observations support this statement. If a sympathectomy is to have a beneficial effect in patients with ischemic ulceration, ischemic neuropathy, or superficial gangrene, it must produce increased nutritive blood flow. Folse, Mack, and Cantrell (18) studied patients in whom epidural blockade produced the effects of sympathectomy. In patients without major arterial occlusion, there was a significant increase in femoral arterial blood flow and a decrease in femoral resistance. On the other hand, the response in patients with occlusive disease varied, but the majority had no significant increase in femoral artery blood flow and only a slight fall in femoral resistance.

Weissenhofer and Schenk (19) studied sympathectomy in an experimental preparation and showed that sympathectomy did produce a significant increase in blood flow through a stenotic blood vessel, but it was accompanied by no increase in regional oxygen consumption. Polacek, Carpenter, and Wagner (20) confirmed this experimental observation clinically in following 30 patients with sympathectomy, all of whom were nondiabetic and were not candidates otherwise for standard arterial grafting procedures. They found that all 30 patients had an elevation in extremity skin temperature immediately following lumbar sympathectomy; that 13 of 30 patients showed an improvement in oscillometric measurements after lumbar sympathectomy as assessed at the foot, ankle, and calf; but that an improvement or increase in arteriovenous (AV) oxygen saturation difference occurred in only 17 patients, with no change occurring in 10, and 3 patients actually showing a decrease in AV oxygen saturation difference. Eventually, within 1 year, 11 of the patients underwent amputation of the compromised limb, and in addition, 2 other patients experienced recurrence of skin ulcerations in the limb, but died before amputation was required. Retrospectively, the femoral AV oxygen saturation differences were a definite prognostic factor. In the 17 patients who had improvement by this parameter, only 1 required a limb amputation within 1 year of follow-up. In contrast, of the 13 patients who showed no change in femoral AV oxygen saturation difference, 10 had amputation, 2 developed recurrent ulcerations, and only 1 had no progression of the ischemic process.

Strandness and Bell (21) evaluated the results of sympathectomy by objective techniques and found that there was evidence of return of sympathetic tone in 12 of the 39 extremities undergoing sympathectomy. Simeone (22) called attention to the medial hypertrophy occurring in arterioles in a sympathectomized limb and emphasized that the resulting reduction in cross-sectional luminal area of the denervated blood vessels might compromise the results of sympathectomy.

It is apparent that the maximum effect of sympathectomy occurs within 24 h of the procedure and that this effectiveness is eroded over the following months and years (Figure 32-1). Some experimental studies are relevant to this discussion. Although experimental studies do not measure the amount of oxygen delivered to the individual cells in the ischemic extremity, Rutherford and Valenta (23) used radioactively labeled microspheres in a canine model. They showed that a total increase in flow to the sympathectomized limb could be obtained, both at rest and following exercise. The increase during exercise was small, and less than that caused by the exercise alone. Increased flow could be demonstrated to the skin, subcutaneous tissues, and bone.

Using a microsphere technique, Delaney and Scarpino (24) studied the extremities of dogs after lumbar sympathectomy and found there was an increase in AV shunting in the lower extremity. Eighteen percent of the blood flow to the leg passed directly through the AV shunts. Their technique did not measure blood flow in skin and subcutaneous tissues.

Cronenwett and Lindenauer (25) used microsphere techniques also and noted an increase in AV shunting in the sympathectomized limb, but they were unable to show an increase in capillary blood flow in the sympathectomized limb. They did emphasize that their model did not examine skin blood flow.

Perry and Horton (26) examined tissue oxygen tension in subcutaneous tissue and muscle in the lower extremities of 10 dogs and 3 patients following bilateral lumbar sympathectomy. They showed that no increase in muscle oxygen tension could be demonstrated and that there were no significant changes in oxygen concentration in the skin and subcutaneous tissue.

These experimental studies support the observation that distal AV shunting is increased in the sympathectomized limb. This would explain an increase in superficial venous blood flow and increases in skin temperature, but it does not indicate that an increase in nutritive blood flow occurs in every limb after sympathectomy.

In a significant experimental observation, Dalessandri et al. (27) tested the hypothesis of Smithwick and the observations of

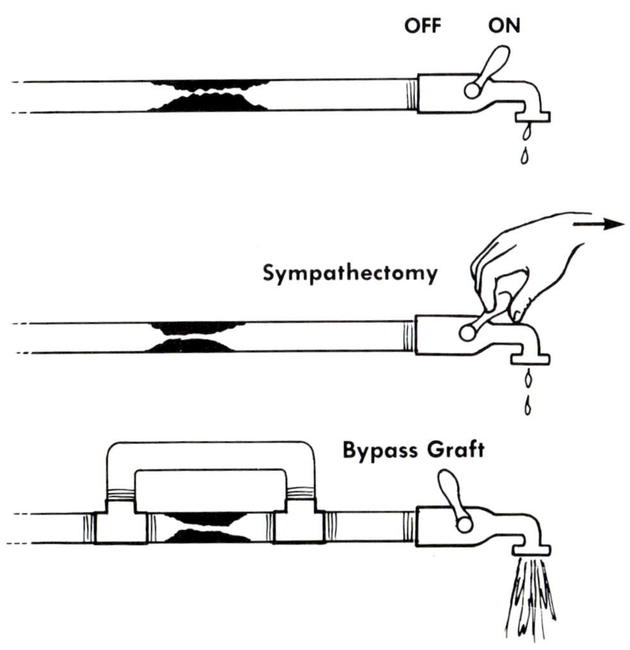

FIGURE 32-1. This illustration, kindly supplied by Dr. David Sumner, vividly portrays the comparative effects of sympathectomy and bypass grafting in the treatment of stenotic and occlusive disease of the lower extremities.

Plecha. In their experimental model, popliteal artery ligation was carried out at the hind limb knee joint, and following ligation, one group of seven animals was kept as a control while another group of seven animals underwent unilateral sypathectomy. Distal pulse-volume recordings and photoplethysmograms were obtained, as well as ankle blood pressure and intraarterial blood pressure. It was found that ligation of the popliteal artery lowered distal hind limb blood pressure to less than half the preoperative value. At 1 week after sympathectomy, the pulse-volume recording amplitudes and pressure showed a transient, but significant rise; however, by 2 weeks after sympathectomy, the arterial pressures and pulse-volume amplitudes had returned to the previous, diminished postligation values. Dalessandri et al. concluded that nutritive capillary skin blood flow increase was questionable following lumbar sympathectomy.

Kreuzer, Keiler, and Salem (28) estimated nutritive blood flow in the experimental animal after sympathectomy and concluded only that lumbar sympathectomy caused opening of AV shunts, which bypassed capillaries, and, therefore, the increased blood flow was of no nutritional significance with regard to regional oxygen consumption.

Nielsen et al. (29), working in Lassen's laboratory in Copenhagen, determined that after sympathectomy, systolic blood pressure in the great toe decreased and also that there was a decrease in subcutaneous blood flow close to gangrenous areas. They concluded that, "Sympathetic denervation might be contraindicated in patients with occlusive arterial disease who have very low distal blood pressure—that is, toe blood pressure below a level of approximately 30 mmHg after a diagnostic blockade."

In a clinical series comparable to our own, Imparato's group (30) reported on 61 patients with lumbar sympathectomy performed for end-stage occlusive disease. They found that the immediate postoperative mortality rate of 6.5 percent was due to cardiac causes and that the early amputation rate was 40 percent in this group of patients. Interestingly, those patients with the best opportunity for good results, those with rest pain, had the poorest prognosis, with an amputation rate of 53 percent.

Conclusion

A review of the available literature on the subject and an analysis of the results obtained by sympathectomy for ischemic ulceration, rest pain, and superficial gangrene at Northwestern University do not support its use as the only procedure done to relieve ischemia. It is apparent that, in the patients who need the procedure most, the results are not long-lasting. In fact, the crtieria most used to predict the success of the procedure fail to do so consistently. Similarly, there is no good evidence to support the use of lumbar sympathectomy as an adjunct to reconstructive arterial procedures.

References

1. Smithwick RH: Lumbar sympathectomy in the treatment of obliterative vascular disease of the lower extremities. Surgery 1957, 42:415–430, 567–578.
2. Barnes RW, Baker WH, Shanik G, Maixner WM, Hayes AC, Lin R, Clarke W: Value of concomitant sympathectomy in aortoiliac reconstruction. Arch Surg 1977, 112:1325–1330.
3. Satiani B, Liapis CD, Hayes JP, Kimmins S, Evans WE: Prospective randomized study of concomitant lumbar sympathectomy with aortoiliac reconstruction. Am J Surg 1982, 143:755–760.
4. Lee BY, Thoden WR, Madden JL, McCann WJ Jr, Trainor FS, Kavner D: Long-term follow-up of bypass procedures with and without lumbar sympathectomy. Contemp Surg 1982, 20:51–55.
5. Kountz SL, Cohn R: Aortic blood flow following lower aortic resection and sympathectomy. Surgery 1963, 53:173–176.
6. Weismann RE, Upson JF: Use of lumbar sympathectomy as an adjunct to reconstructive arterial surgery. Ann Surg 1961, 154:788–790.
7. Cranley JJ: *Vascular Surgery*, vol 1, *Peripheral Arterial Diseases*. New York, Harper and Row, 1972.
8. Husni EA, Simeone FA: Results of lumbar sympathectomy in peripheral vascular disease. Arch Surg 1957, 75:530.
9. Yao JST, Bergan JJ: Predictability of vascular reactivity relative to sympathetic ablation. Arch Surg 1973, 107:675–680.
10. Eastcott HHG: Predicting response to sympathetic ablation. Lancet 1974, 1:634–635.
11. Thulesius O, Gjöres JE, Mandaus L: Distal blood flow and blood pressure in vascular occlusion; influence of sympathetic nerves on collateral blood flow. Scand J Clin Lab Invest 1973, 31(suppl 128):53–57.
12. Walker PM, Johnston KW: Predicting the success of a sympathectomy: A prospective study using discriminant function and multiple regression analysis. Surgery 1980, 87:216–221.
13. Plecha FR, Bomberger RA, Hoffman M, MacPherson K: A new criterion for predicting response to lumbar sympathectomy in patients with severe arteriosclerotic occlusive disease. Surgery 1980, 88:375–381.
14. Bergan JJ, Trippel OH: Arteriograms in ischemic limbs worsened after lumbar sympathectomy. Arch Surg 1962, 85:643–650.
15. Haimovici H, Steinman C, Karson IH: Evaluation of lumbar sympathectomy. Advanced occlusive arterial disease. Arch Surg 1964, 89:1089–1095.
16. Szilagyi DE, Smith RF, Scerpella JR, Hoffman K: Lumbar sympathectomy. Current role in the treatment of arteriosclerotic occlusive disease. Arch Surg 1967, 95:753–761.
17. Shaw RS, Austen WG, Stipa S: A ten year study of the effect of lumbar sympathectomy on the peripheral circulation of patients with arteriosclerotic occlusive disease. Surg Gynecol Obstet 1964, 119:486–494.
18. Folse R, Mack RM, Cantrell JR: Alterations in femoral blood flow and resistance following sympathetic blockade: Hemodynamic evaluation of patients with and without arterial occlusion by dye-dilution technic. Ann Surg 1965, 162:873–880.

19. Weissenhofer W, Schenk WG Jr: Effects of sympathectomy on blood flow through stenotic vessels during exercise: An experimental study in a canine model. Surgery 1973, 74:734–738.
20. Polacek MA, Carpenter B, Wagner M: Limb prognosis in lumbar sympathectomy. Am Surg 1968, 34:303–308.
21. Strandness DE Jr, Bell JW: Critical evaluation of the results of lumbar sympathectomy. Ann Surg 1964, 160:1021–1029.
22. Simeone FA: Intravascular pressure, vascular tone, and sympathectomy. Surgery 1963, 53:1–18.
23. Rutherford RB, Valenta J: Extremity blood flow and distribution: The effects of arterial occlusion, sympathectomy, and exercise. Surgery 1971, 69:332–344.
24. Delaney J, Scarpino J: Limb arteriovenous shunting following sympathetic denervation. Surgery 1973, 73:202–206.
25. Cronenwett JL, Lindenauer SM: Direct measurement of arteriovenous anastomotic blood flow after lumbar sympathectomy. Surgery 1977, 82:82–89.
26. Perry MO, Horton J: Muscle and subcutaneous oxygen tension measurement by mass spectrometry after sympathectomy. Arch Surg 1978, 113:171–178.
27. Dalessandri KM, Carson SM, Tillman P, Talken L, Wong H-N: Effect of lumbar sympathectomy in distal arterial occlusion. Arch Surg 1983, 118:1157–1160.
28. Kreuzer W, Keiler A, Salem G: Nutritional effects following lumbar sympathectomy in peripheral arterial occlusive disease. Bull Soc Int Chir 1975, 6:675–677.
29. Nielsen PE, Bell G, Augustenborg G, Paaske-Hansen O, Lassen NA: Reduction in distal blood pressure by sympathetic nerve block in patients with occlusive arterial disease. Cardiovasc Res 1973, 7:577–584.
30. Grover-Johnson N, Baumann FG, Riles TS, Imparato AM: Effect of surgical lumbar sympathectomy on innervation of arterioles in the lower limb of patients with diabetes. Surg Gynecol Obstet 1981, 153:39–41.

Additional Reference

Thompson JE, Patman RD: Management of posttraumatic pain syndromes: Causalgia and reflex sympathetic dystrophy. In Veith FJ (ed): *Critical Problems in Vascular Surgery*. New York, Appleton-Century-Crofts, 1982.

Chapter 33

PERIPHERAL VASCULAR DISEASE IN THE DIABETIC PATIENT

JOAN WRIGHT, ROBERT SANFORD OZERAN, and STANLEY R. KLEIN

Diabetes mellitus is a disease of worldwide distribution, occurring in 10 million people in the United States alone (1). Multiple therapeutic contributions, especially insulin and oral hypoglycemics, as well as specific remedies for complications, have greatly prolonged the life of the diabetic patient. With this increase in life span, increasingly complex complications of long-standing diabetes involving the eyes, kidneys, nerves, and blood vessels have become common. Overall, vascular disease is responsible for about 75 percent of the deaths in those afflicted with diabetes compared to one-third of deaths in those who are not (2,3,4). In the type II (adult-onset) diabetic patient, up to 15 percent will have some evidence of peripheral vascular disease at the time of diagnosis, increasing to 50 percent after 10 or 15 years of documented disease (6,7). The lower extremities, particularly the feet, represent the site of by far the most frequent clinical manifestation (5). Furthermore, complications of the lower extremities are the most common lesions requiring surgery, accounting for one-fifth of all diabetic hospitalizations (8). Bell's 1952 autopsy study revealed that gangrene of the lower extremity occurred 40 times more frequently in diabetic patients than in nondiabetic ones and was a contributory or principal cause of death in two-thirds of persons with diabetes (3).

PATHOGENESIS

Atherosclerosis in persons with diabetes tends to occur at an earlier age and progresses more rapidly than it does in those not afflicted with the disease (2,4,10). However, clinically significant atherosclerotic lesions are usually unrelated to the duration or severity of overt diabetes and may precede the diagnosis in patients with chemical diabetes (11,12).

Cellular mechanisms relevant to the pathogenesis of atherosclerosis in both diabetics and nondiabetics as well as additional factors unique to the diabetic state have been elucidated by clinical studies and animal models. The current popular theory of Ross, Glomset, and Harker involves injury to the endothelium producing platelet aggregation and subsequent smooth-muscle proliferation. Circulating lipoproteins then deliver lipid to the site of endothelial injury, initiating plaque formation (13,14). Multiple factors in the diabetic are believed to accelerate this basic process (15). Hyperlipidemia with increased levels of triglyceride and cholesterol has been documented in poorly controlled diabetic patients and correlates with accelerated atherogenesis (16,17). Levels of high-density lipoprotein, felt by some to be protective against the deposition of cholesterol and cholesterol esters in peripheral tissues, are often diminished in diabetics, particularly type II non-insulin-dependent diabetics (18,19,20).

Multiple hematologic disturbances leading to a thrombotic tendency in diabetes have been described, including enhanced platelet aggregation and adhesiveness; increased levels of von Willebrand factor; coagulation factors V, VII, X, and fibrinogen; as well as decreased plasma fibrinolytic activity (21,22,23). Increased erythrocyte aggregation and plasma hyperviscosity further contribute to hypercoagulability (23). In addition, hyperglycemia itself may cause tissue hypoxia through increased accumulation of sorbitol in the cell wall, resulting in swelling and subsequent impaired function (24). Glycosylation of hemoglobin A1C is increased to twice normal in diabetes, altering oxygen transport because of the greater hemoglobin-oxygen affinity (25). Finally, glycosylation of collagen alters the function, structure, and turnover of vessel wall collagen by interference with normal cross-linking (26).

In their study of diabetes and associated risk factors, Beach and Strandness found that smoking increased the prevalence of atherosclerosis in diabetic patients by 12 percent and hypertension by 19 percent (27). They found no correlation with obesity, which corresponds to the reports of others suggesting that obesity by itself is not a major risk factor, although it may affect other variables such as hypertension and hyperlipidemia (28,29,30). Hormonal alterations including increased growth hormone level and hyperinsulinism have been implicated in the development of atherosclerosis by several studies (31,32,33). Finally, genetic and racial factors in atherosclerotic disease are interrelated to affect some of the key risk factors, including diabetes per se, but an inherited predisposition to vascular disease has not been proved (34).

PATHOLOGY

Angiopathy in the diabetic involves both large and small vessels. Macrovascular disease is caused by atherosclerosis involving the intima of large arteries and medial calcification of muscular arteries.

Histologically, atherosclerosis in the diabetic is indistinguishable from that in the nondiabetic (35,36). In diabetes, however, the progression of the disease is both centripetal, with steady growth of plaque leading to stenosis and occlusion, and axial, moving distally down the limb to involve collateral arteries and small blood vessels (9). In contrast to the nondiabetic, in whom occlusion tends to involve a single segment of proximal vessels, diabetic patients have diffuse, multisegment involvement. Bilaterality of disease is the rule with 50 percent of patients developing overt lesions in the second leg within 2 years after the first leg is involved (28,37).

The distribution of disease accounts for many of the clinical sequelae occurring in diabetic patients with peripheral atherosclerosis. Aortoiliac involvement is relatively infrequent compared to the nondiabetic patients, while femoropopliteal occlusion occurs commonly in both groups (11,38). Significant disease of the profunda femoris artery, an important collateral in the patient with femoropopliteal disease, occurs in 30 percent of diabetics but in only 10 percent of nondiabetics. Tibioperoneal disease with two of three crural arteries occluded was found in 69 percent of diabetics compared to 35 percent in nondiabetics in one series, with the lowest overall incidence of involvement found in the peroneal artery (39). Significant occlusive disease in the foot has been found, with involvement of 60 percent of plantar arches in diabetics compared to 21 percent of nondiabetics (40). Digital artery disease occurred in 19 percent of diabetics in contrast to only 10 percent of nondiabetics (40). Nonetheless, because of the extensive collateral pathways which exist in the foot, it is uncommon to find enough involvement at this level alone to produce ischemia resulting in tissue necrosis.

Medial calcific stenosis is a morphologically distinct form of arteriosclerosis. It is characterized by calcification of the tunica media of muscular arteries, beginning with the deposition of fine granules of calcium circumferentially distributed about the vessel (35,41). In far advanced cases, the vessel becomes a long, rigid tube of calcium with a classic "pipe stem" or "trolley track" appearance on x-ray (35) (Figure 33-1). This process does not generally involve the intima, so the vascular lumen is uncompromised. However, Christensen and others have demonstrated a reduction in blood flow in the tibialis anterior muscle of diabetic extremities with medial calcification (42). It tends to involve the lower leg and plantar arteries, which become noncompressible and difficult to assess using noninvasive techniques, but occasionally it involves other locations (Figure 33-2).

Microangiopathy in the diabetic is classically characterized by thickening of the basement membrane surrounding capillaries. While not unique to diabetics, it occurs four times more frequently than in nondiabetics (44). Thickened capillary basement membranes can be found throughout the body, but the distribution is patchy, with normal capillaries adjacent to diseased ones (45). The greatest degree of thickening is usually found distally in the leg, suggesting the influence of hydrostatic pressure on the process (43). Because thickness increases with the duration of diabetes mellitus, some feel that the deposition of glycoprotein into the basement membrane is related to carbohydrate intolerance (46). However, several studies show no variation in thickness with severity or degree of control of diabetes (44,47). The exact pathologic significance of thickening of the basement membrane is unknown. These capillaries show increased permeability to fluid and protein, which may interfere with the exchange of nutrients and oxygen across the wall or impede egress of leukocytes into the interstitial fluid (48).

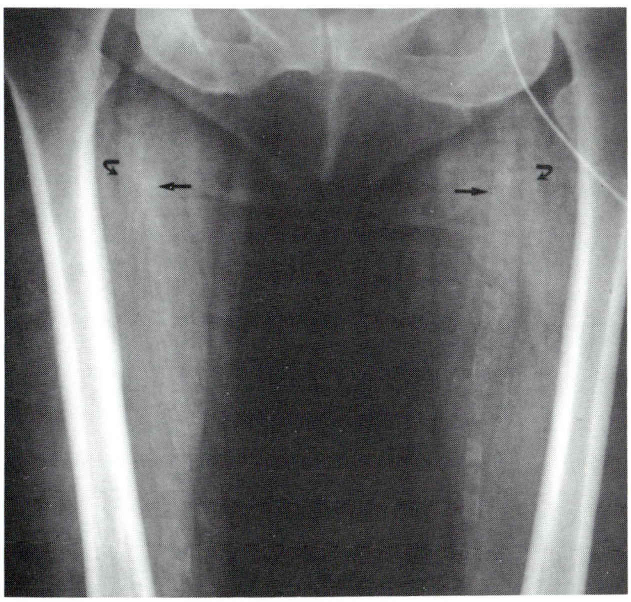

FIGURE 33-1. Type I severe diabetic patient with vascular calcification of the tunica media yielding a classic "trolley track" appearance. This lower extremity x-ray demonstrates the appearance in the superficial (*straight arrows*) and profunda (*curved arrows*) femoral arteries.

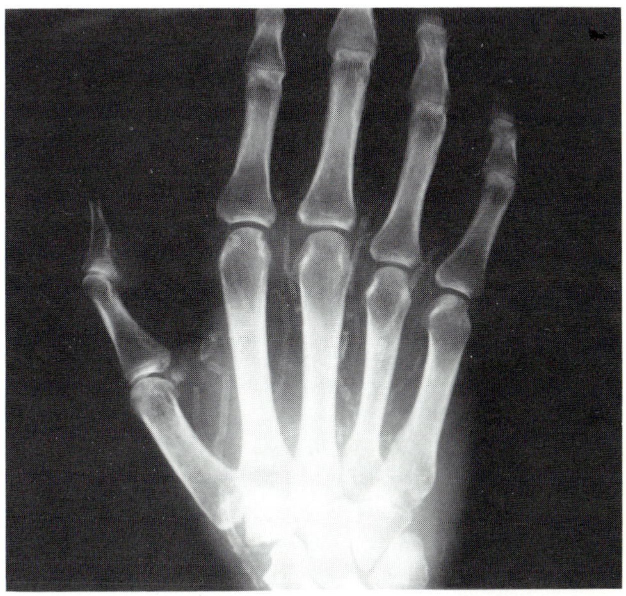

FIGURE 33-2. Type I chronic diabetic patient with vascular calcification observed in the hand vessels. This individual developed a severe infection leading to ultimate amputation of the upper extremity.

Peripheral Neuropathy in Diabetes

Peripheral neuropathy is a ubiquitous complication of diabetes mellitus. Awareness of its manifestations is of importance due to the potential impact regarding differential diagnosis and adverse effect on the outcome of therapy. While clinically significant peripheral neuropathy occurs in up to 30 percent of diabetic patients, abnormalities of nerve conduction have been found in nearly all diabetic patients who are carefully examined (11,25,49,50).

A causal relationship between diabetes mellitus and neuropathy was first described by Marchal de Calvi in 1864 when he identified pain and distal limb sensory loss in patients with diabetes (51). Since that time, many hypotheses concerning the pathophysiology of diabetic neuropathy have been suggested. Direct metabolic damage to the Schwann cell with resultant segmental loss of the myelin sheath has been observed (52). However, it is currently believed that this is secondary to axonal degeneration, which involves both small and large myelinated fibers as well as those that are unmyelinated (53,54). Biochemical abnormalities due to hypoglycemia are implicated in these processes and include depletion of axonal inositol, accumulation of intraneural sorbitol, and impairment of intraaxonal vesicle transport (53,55,56).

The role of vascular disease in the development of diabetic neuropathy has not been established. Thickening of the basement membrane of capillaries and arterioles of the vasa nervorum and supporting cells has been found, but the contribution to nerve dysfunction is speculative (53,57). However, it is widely presumed that the isolated single and multiple mononeuropathies associated with diabetes mellitus result from ischemia, based on the observation of microinfarcts in the vasa nervorum of affected peripheral or cranial nerves (53,58). These neuropathies tend to be acute or subacute in onset, often painful, occur in the older diabetic patient, and have a self-limited course. The most common cranial nerve affected is the oculomotor, and the most frequently involved nerves in the lower extremity are the common peroneal and femoral (59,60).

Diabetic neuropathy encompasses a wide spectrum of neurologic conditions involving sensory, motor, and autonomic functions. Symmetric polyneuropathy occurs most often, with a classic stocking-glove distribution. Initially, it selectively affects either large myelinated fibers subserving proprioception, touch, and vibration, or small myelinated and unmyelinated fibers involving pain and temperature sensation (61). In advanced disease, mixed fiber neuropathy results. Characteristic clinical manifestations include numbness and paresthesias of the feet and lower legs, burning or cold sensation, and deep aching or lancinating pain. Symptoms tend to be more severe at night and are often alleviated by ambulation. The most common objective finding is loss of deep tendon reflexes, with diminished ankle reflexes preceding the loss of the knee jerk (41).

Sensory impairment usually predates motor dysfunction. Motor denervation involves the intrinsic muscles of the foot, with interosseus atrophy causing an imbalance between the long flexors and extensors. This leads to protrusion of the metatarsal heads with clawing of the toes, altering the biomechanics of the feet and changing the normal gait (62). Excessive shearing forces on plantar skin lead to callus formation and subsequent pressure ulceration over the metatarsal heads (63). These neurogenic ulcers, or mal perforans, occur under the first, second, and fifth metatarsophalangeal joints (64) (Figure 33-3). End-stage sensorimotor disease leads to the development of the diabetic Charcot joint (neurogenic arthropathy), most often affecting the tarsal, tarsometatarsal, and ankle joints. Repeated trauma to the foot and ankle results in joint destruction with the production of a "rocker-bottom" foot which is broadened and has lost its longitudinal arch (41).

Abnormalities of the autonomic nervous system can be found in up to 60 percent of patients with sensorimotor dysfunction and may be detectable at the time of initial diagnosis of diabetes (25,49,65). The loss of vasomotor control leads to postural hypotension, an increase in peripheral blood flow, and arteriovenous shunting in the neuropathic foot (66,67). Autonomic fiber injury causes loss of thermal regulation and impairment of sweating, resulting in skin pH changes and dry, scaling, cracked skin with an altered bacterial microflora (11). In the affected extremity, this yields a picture analogous to sympathectomy.

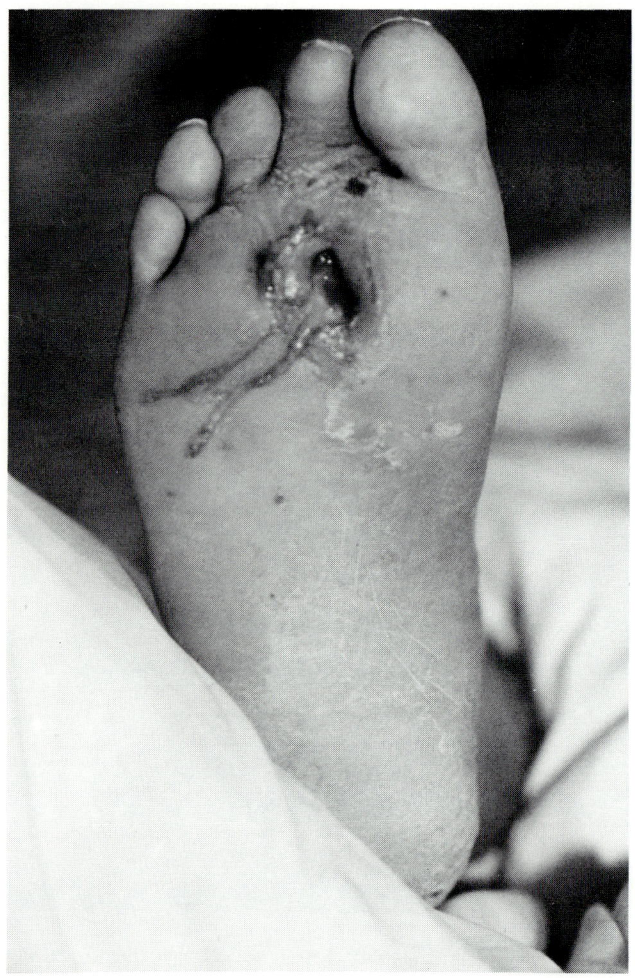

FIGURE 33-3. Type II diabetic patient with a larger "malperforans" ulcer in the characteristic location over the head of the first metatarsal.

Soft Tissue Infection in Diabetes

Several additional factors which complicate the management of peripheral vascular disease in the diabetic are recognizable. Experimental and clinical evidence indicates that patients with diabetes mellitus are more susceptible to infection than nondiabetic controls (68). Defects in host defense mechanisms include impaired chemotaxis (69), phagocytosis (70), intracellular bactericidal activity (71), and serum opsonization (72). Levels of immunoglobulin are normal or high (73), but in the patient with poor glucose control, abnormalities of the cell-mediated response occur (74).

Foot infections are common, accounting for 40 percent of all infections in diabetes mellitus patients (75) (Figure 33-4). Local factors in the wound environment are thought to be responsible for the spectrum of organisms found in the diabetic foot ulcer. Up to 70 percent of diabetics will show superficial dermatophytoses of the interdigital webs of the feet (76). While normal skin flora suppresses most fungi by depletion of glucose, in the presence of hyperglycemia, *Candida* and other species proliferate freely. The resultant breaks in the skin barrier allow portals of entry for pathogenic bacteria (9). Typical aerobes like *Staphylococcus aureus* and streptococci are found along with gram-negative bacilli such as *Escherichia coli* and *Proteus* (77) (Table 33-1). Decreased peripheral blood flow and oxygen tension in

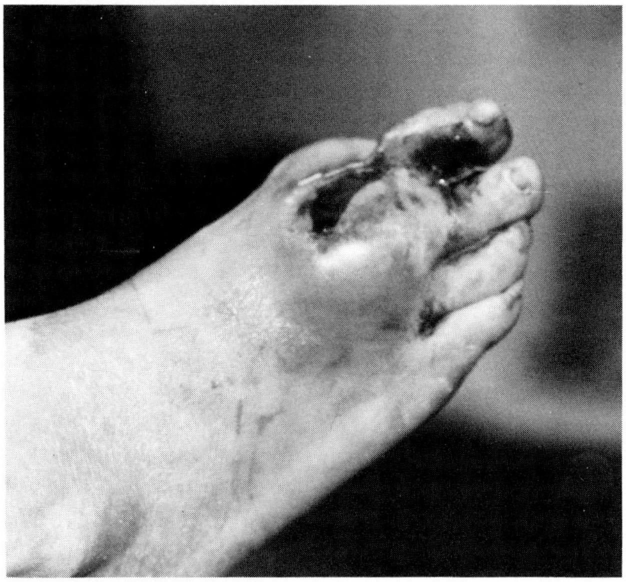

FIGURE 33-4. Type II diabetic patient demonstrating a characteristic foot infection with surrounding edema and erythema.

TABLE 33-1. Frequency of Isolation of Bacterial Species*

	Group I (17 Patients)		Group II (41 Patients)		Group III (42 Patients)	
	No. Patients	Total No. Patients	No. Patients	Total No. Patients	No. Patients	Total No. Patients
Gram-positive aerobes:		15		35		39
S. aureus	9		23		22	
S. epidermidis	6		14		12	
Streptococcus	6		10		13	
Enterococcus	4		12		16	
Diphtheroids	5		7		7	
Total no. isolates	30		66		70	
Gram-negative aerobes:		6		24		21
E. coli	2		3		7	
Proteus	1		10		11	
Klebsiella	1		4		4	
Enterobacter	0		5		3	
Serratia	1		1		0	
Pseudomonas	1		10		3	
Citrobacter	1		1		1	
Acinetobacter					1	
Total no. isolates	7		34		31	
Aerobes:		9		14		29
Clostridium perfringens	0		9		2	
Bacteroides	4		3		6	
Anaerobic cocci	9		13		21	
Total no. isolates	13		16		35	
Total no. isolates	50		116		136	
Average no. isolates per patient	3.0		2.8		3.2	
Necessity of surgery:						
Local	0		20		28	
Amputation (below or above the knee)	0		8		14	

*Microbiology of 100 consecutive diabetic foot ulcers in patients with similar age, duration, and control of diabetes in an attempt to relate the particular pathogens, progression of the ulcer, and necessity of surgical intervention to control either local or systemic sepsis.

SOURCE: From GP Kozak: *Management of Diabetic Foot Problems*. Philadelphia, Saunders, 1984, Table 10-1, p 99.

deep tissues promote the growth of microaerophilic and anaerobic organisms like *Bacteroides*, clostridia, and anaerobic streptococci (78,79,80,81).

Whereas infection in the normal individual leads to vasodilatation, redness, and heat, these changes may be masked in the diabetic with vascular insufficiency. The diabetic response to infection often includes microarterial thrombosis exacerbating ischemia and promoting tissue necrosis. Bacterial fermentation of the high levels of glucose in the soft tissues frequently result in gas formation by coliform organisms (especially *E. coli*), Bacteroides, and enterococci (82). These nonclostridial gas infections occur much more commonly in diabetics than nondiabetics (83). Superficial cellulitis can progress to necrotizing fasciitis with marked systemic toxicity. In the patient with lower extremity edema secondary to congestive heart failure or venous disease, gangrene can rapidly ensue (84). Synergistic gangrene occurs repeatedly in the patient with polymicrobial foot infection, most often when anaerobic streptococci combine with hemolytic *S. aureus* in which both produce potent coagulases (85). Finally, ulceration can extend to the underlying joint and bone, resulting in chronic osteomyelitis, seen most frequently in the toes and small bones of the foot in the diabetic patient (86).

Wound healing in the diabetic is generally impaired, probably as a consequence of defective collagen synthesis and degradation (87). Experimentally, insulin deprivation causes reduced activity of leukocytes and macrophages in the early proliferative stage of wound healing, interfering with fibroblast growth and subsequent collagen formation (88). The effect is improved with insulin administration (89).

Hyperglycemia can also affect the structure and function of skin proteins by the nonenzymatic glycosylation of collagen and keratin (90,91). Increased cross-linkage of protein causes the tissue to become rigid and inflexible, with resistance to enzymatic degradation by collagenase (92). These changes in the skin and subcutaneous tissue lead to limitation of joint mobility and buildup of excessive callus on weight-bearing surfaces (93). Shearing forces from the mechanical trauma of walking on the foot-shoe interface can lead to breakdown in the deep tissues with formation of cavities which eventually ulcerate and become secondarily infected.

Evaluation of Circulation

The symptoms of peripheral vascular disease in the diabetic without concomitant neuropathy vary little from those of other patients with arteriosclerosis obliterans. The picture may be acute or chronic, depending on the status of the collateral circulation (9). Intermittent claudication is quite common, typically occurring in the calves, ranging from mild discomfort to severe pain on walking short distances, and relieved by rest. The level of symptoms can be used to estimate the level of vascular obstruction, with cramping in the buttocks and thighs suggestive of aortoiliac disease. Claudication is not usually seen with isolated distal vessel involvement (94).

With progression of disease, nocturnal ("rest") pain in the area over the metatarsal heads occurs due to diminished tissue perfusion in the elevated extremity (94). This is typically relieved by dangling the involved extremity or walking to augment circulation. Severe vascular insufficiency ultimately produces tissue necrosis which often follows trivial trauma.

Physical examination of the diabetic with vascular insufficiency may reveal cold feet, absence of hair on the legs and feet, atrophy of the skin and subcutaneous tissues, and thickened short nails. However, these findings are nonspecific and may be associated with age alone (94). Diminished or absent pedal pulses are classic signs of occlusive disease but are not conclusive evidence of obstruction, as there is a small incidence of congenital absence of one or both vessels (95). Up to 3 percent of limbs lack an anterior tibial arterial, 2.7 percent are missing a posterior tibial, and 0.3 percent lack both. Conversely, the presence of pulses may occur in the face of significant proximal obstruction due to the development of abundant collateral flow. However, such pulses will diminish or disappear with exercise (96).

Cyanosis and dependent rubor are fairly reliable indicators of arterial insufficiency, especially if unilateral. Pallor on elevation and delayed venous filling time longer than 15 to 20 s also occur with reduced blood supply (8).

Vasculogenic ulcers in the diabetic are often small, superficial, localized to the toes, and with pain out of proportion to the size of the lesion (8). Patchy dry gangrene of the digits may develop with distal occlusion, and extensive gangrene may supervene in the patient with adequate collateral circulation but who incurs an infection.

Laboratory Diagnosis in Peripheral Vascular Disease

The noninvasive laboratory is a valuable adjunct in the evaluation of the peripheral vascular status of the diabetic. The most commonly used examination is the Doppler pulse-volume recording, which measures both blood flow velocity and segmental blood pressure. Systolic pressure in the ankle divided by the brachial systolic pressure yields an index of the degree of arterial disease in the leg. Increased accuracy is achieved with a 1-min postexercise ankle-to-arm ratio measurement (97). Absolute toe pressures have also been reported to be valuable prognostic indicators in occlusive arterial disease (98). However, because of vascular calcification and the resulting noncompressibility in many diabetic extremities, the above measurements frequently may be distorted and are notoriously unreliable (97,99,107).

Direct evaluation of the microcirculation in diabetic vascular disease has been achieved by a variety of perfusion scanning methods (99). Intraarterial injection of technetium-99m–labeled albumin microspheres (100), intravenous injection of technitium-99m–labeled phosphate (101), clearance of radioactive xenon-133 (102), and thallium scanning (103) are available techniques but with limited applicability in most hospitals. Transcutaneous oxygen tension measurements are becoming more widespread in the noninvasive diagnosis of peripheral arterial insufficiency, especially in the diabetic (104,105,106,107).

Arteriography remains the definitive method for delineation of occlusive loci in the peripheral vascular system. Although relatively safe, it entails definite risks and should be reserved to construct a "road map" in the patient for whom surgery is being contemplated. Because peripheral vascular disease in the diabetic is often infrapopliteal, care must be taken by the radiologist to demonstrate the distal runoff and pedal arch, which are frequently the target in reconstructive surgery. Digital subtraction angiography may be useful for this purpose (109).

Complications of angiography include thrombus formation, hematoma or bleeding, and allergic reaction to the iodinated dye. A particular risk in the diabetic is renal failure, occurring most often in the elderly patient with preexisting renal impairment (110). The incidence of involvement varies from 6 percent in the type II nonazotemic diabetic to over 75 percent in the diabetic with a serum creatinine of 2 or above (111,112). While no prophylactic protocol has been found consistently effective, pre-evaluation volume expansion with saline and use of an osmotic diuretic such as mannitol during the contrast exposure appear to offer the best protection (113). In most cases the renal failure is manifested within 48 h as a self-limited oliguria resolving without dialysis (114). The diabetic patient should be monitored closely after angiography with serial creatinine and blood urea nitrogen (BUN) determinations and measurement of urinary output in order to intervene quickly in adjustment of fluid intake should renal deterioration occur.

Peripheral Arterial Surgery in the Diabetic Patient

Following evaluation of the diabetic patient by noninvasive modalities and arteriography, the strategy of revascularization is formulated using the same criteria as in the nondiabetic. Because of the rarity of isolated aortoiliac occlusive disease in the diabetic patient, the primary indication for consideration of surgical bypass is limb salvage including rest pain and gangrene. This therapy might serve to totally ameliorate the patient's problem. Alternatively, reconstruction may permit a lower level of amputation or allow healing of an ischemic lesion with ultimate survival of the limb despite late graft thrombosis (8). In selected patients with femoropopliteal occlusion, severe claudication limiting occupation or lifestyle is a relative indication for revascularization (94).

Appropriate candidates for vascular reconstruction are found less frequently in the diabetic population than among controls for several reasons. Extensive disease involving distal vessels may preclude revascularization, and only about one-third of diabetic reconstructive candidates will have a localized block with enough runoff to accomplish a successful bypass (115). Diabetic patients are frequently poor surgical risks because of generalized vascular disease involving coronary, cerebral, or renal vessels (8). Finally given successful reconstructive vascular surgical procedures with patency rates equal to the nondiabetic, the overall mortality rate in the diabetic is at least 10 percent higher than in controls over a 5-year period (116).

Reconstructive vascular surgery may include endarterectomy, bypass grafting, or both. Endarterectomy is most commonly used for limited areas of disease in the aortoiliac system, although certain lesions in the femoral vessels (particularly the profunda femoris artery) may be amenable (94). With more extensive obstruction in the aortoiliac tree, bypass is usually indicated. Aortoiliac disease is not common in the diabetic, and aortic grafts in this population are required only one-tenth as often as infrainguinal grafts (117).

In the femoropopliteal system, reconstruction in the diabetic has shown comparable results to those in nondiabetics (118–121) (Figure 33-5). Autogenous vein grafts placed for relief of claudication show 70 percent patency at 5 years (122) compared to

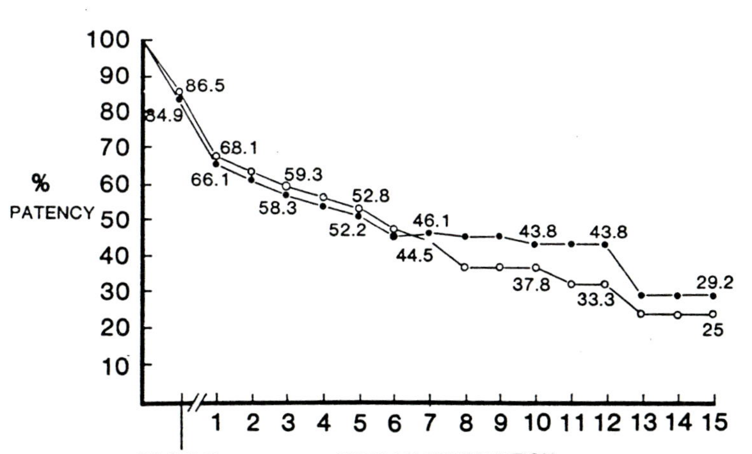

FIGURE 33-5. Cumulative patency rates for nondiabetic and diabetic patients with femoropopliteal and femoroinfrapopliteal arterial occlusive disease following placement of autogenous vein bypass grafts. ○—○, nondiabetic patient (N = 262); ●—●, diabetic patient (N = 335.) (D. Emerick Szilagyi, Surgery 86(6):836–851. With permission of publishers.)

those inserted for limb salvage, yielding patency rates of 47 percent (123). In the latter group the limb salvage rate was 70 percent in spite of many occluded grafts. Autogenous vein grafts, in general, resulted in longer graft patency in contrast to synthetic prostheses (124). The use of Dacron grafts in the elderly diabetic is particularly discouraged, for only 17 percent of such grafts are patent at 3 years (125). Polytetrafluoroethylene (PTFE) grafts frequently show similar early patency to autogenous vein when used above the knee, but markedly worse below the knee (126,127). PTFE grafts inserted into blind popliteal segments in diabetics with extensive gangrene result in a significant limb loss unless an additional graft limb to a more distal artery is placed (128).

Femoroinfrapopliteal bypass in the diabetic patient yields about 10 percent less success in patency rate and limb salvage compared to that in nondiabetics (129,130). Femorotibial bypass results in a slightly higher rate of limb salvage (48 percent at 5 years) than femoroperoneal bypass (38 percent at 5 years) (131). Such small-vessel bypass is efficacious in the diabetic and is indicated in the extremity with tibial or peroneal arteries visualized to the ankle in preference to primary amputation (132).

Adjunctive Therapy

Percutaneous balloon transluminal angioplasty is an attractive therapeutic option in selected cases of diabetic patients with occlusive peripheral vascular disease. The optimal lesions are isolated short stenoses in large arteries which are easily accessible (133). Iliac vessel dilation has the best long-term patency rate, approximately 85 percent at 3 years, dropping to 55 percent in the femoropopliteal tree (134). Diabetic patients show comparable patency rates to nondiabetics (134). Angioplasty may be indicated as the primary procedure in isolated obstructive lesions or in combination with bypass surgery for multilevel disease.

Sympathectomy

The use of sympathectomy in the management of diabetic peripheral vascular disease is controversial. Published indications for its use include severe distal ischemia in the patient with nonreconstructible vascular disease or the uncommon patient with vasomotor instability with periodic sweating and blotchy cyanosis (8). Occasionally sympathectomy in cases of limb threat may improve symptoms, but as a rule it fails to prevent amputation (135). This is attributed to the phenomenon of diabetic autosympathectomy felt to result from sympathetic neuropathy (136). Histologic corroboration is provided by the observation that long-standing diabetics show a decreased number of nerve endings in epineural arterioles of the sural nerve and that this low number is not further reduced after lumbar sympathectomy (137).

Claudication is virtually never improved by sympathectomy, which fails to affect the muscular blood flow (9,138). The role for sympathectomy in conjunction with arterial bypass in the diabetic is likely to have little effect but is still unresolved (139,140).

Amputation

The diabetic patient with progressive lower limb ischemia or infection may require amputation if reconstructive therapy is unsuccessful. The magnitude of this problem is evident from the statistic that 51 percent of amputations performed for occlusive arterial disease occur in diabetics (141). The postoperative mortality rate after major amputation in the diabetic population exceeds 20 percent in most series, primarily attributed to cardiac complications (142,143). A center offering specialized service with a combined medical-surgical team approach to the management of the diabetic patient with peripheral vascular disease has reduced the overall mortality rate to 9 percent in such patients and only 1 percent in those undergoing below-knee procedures (144). The life expectancy for the diabetic amputee is limited, with only 41 percent of patients surviving 5 years (145).

The rate of healing of the diabetic lower extremity amputation is comparable to that of the nondiabetic, so the same indications for surgery and choice of level apply (141). However, because of the diffuse bilateral nature of vascular disease in diabetics, 50 percent will require amputation of the remaining leg within 5 years (145). Therefore, a special attempt at limb salvage surgery is warranted (146). Preservation of the knee joint is critical, for 80 percent of elderly patients will be able to regain independent gait after below-knee amputations compared to only 40 percent of those with above-knee amputations (147). If not successful in salvaging the limb entirely, vascular reconstructive surgery may play a role in lowering the amputation level, but this must be weighed against the risk of failure, necessitating a subsequent above-knee procedure. Several studies demonstrate that most amputations after femoropopliteal bypass will heal below the knee, but those patients with failed distal bypass tend to show an increased rate of above-knee amputation (119,147).

The timing of amputation is influenced by the presence of infection and degree of ischemic symptoms in the limb (148). A period of bed rest, control of blood sugar, and intravenous antibiotics may permit demarcation of gangrene and elective amputation. Unremitting pain requiring narcotic analgesics may force a premature surgical procedure. Active infection with progressive cellulitis, frank purulence, or systemic toxicity requires emergent incision and drainage or guillotine amputation as a first stage (148). Better circulation is needed to heal an open amputation than one that is closed primarily, so in the face of marginal blood supply a distal open amputation may fail and result in ultimate limb loss (149). Therefore, maximal effort must be made to achieve a closed wound at the initial operation.

The goal in amputation is to achieve the lowest level compatible with healing of the stump. Determination of healing potential in the ischemic lower extremity is difficult, and the methodology for prediction is inexact (150). Consideration is given to the general status of the patient, including complicating medical conditions such as blindness or stroke, the presence of flexion contractures, potential for prosthetic use, and condition of the opposite leg (150). The diabetic renal transplant recipient is particularly at risk in the presence of gangrene, for the concurrent immunosuppression compromises the ability to withstand even minor infection. Such patients should be considered candidates for early definitive amputation (148).

Clinical parameters considered in the selection of amputation site include skin condition, color, and temperature, presence of bone or joint involvement, and level of palpable pulses. The absence of palpable peripheral pulses does not imply automatic above-knee amputation, for up to 88 percent of patients with absent popliteal pulses will heal at a below-knee level (151,152).

Noninvasive vascular laboratory criteria predictive of healing include Doppler ankle pressures greater than 70 mmHg and toe pressures above 55 mmHg, values which are higher in diabetics than controls (98,153). An ischemic index of at least 0.45 and positive pulse-volume recordings at the forefoot level also correlate with healing (154,155). Skin blood flow levels of 2.4 mL per 100 g per minute or greater measured by xenon-133 clearance as well as transcutaneous oxygen pressure levels of 50 mmHg are additional indexes of tissue perfusion capable of healing amputations (102,156). However, noninvasive criteria are imprecise in the diabetic, with significant numbers of false-positives and false-negatives, so no patient should be denied an attempt at conservative surgery solely on this basis (152,153,155).

SPECIFIC SITES

Digital amputation may be feasible in the diabetic with localized gangrene or osteomyelitis in a limb with either an intact dorsalis pedis pulse or good collateral circulation (150). In this select group, healing will occur in more than 85 percent of individuals without distal pulses, although 2 percent fail to heal even with a pulse present (149). Amputation at this level retains foot length and preserves nearly normal gait and balance.

Transmetatarsal amputation may be suitable for the patient with gangrene invovling two or more toes and adequate circulation at the forefoot level (150). This amputation yields a comfortable, useful foot which permits ambulation without the need for a prosthesis. Healing will succeed in more than 60 percent of cases (9,115).

Amputation at the ankle level is most commonly performed by the Symes technique, resulting in a shortened stump requiring use of a prosthesis for ambulation (150). Suitable for cases with gangrene extending to the metatarsals or for failed transmetatarsal amputation, it permits improved function with less energy requirement than more proximal amputations (150). While the risk of poor healing and bony nonunion has limited use of Symes amputations in many centers, institutions utilizing a two-stage approach report a success rate of nearly 95 percent (144,150).

If conditions necessitate removal of the foot, a below-knee amputation is suitable for patients capable of using a prosthesis (8). The presence of a popliteal pulse is not required for success, as more than 90 percent will heal at this level (9). This operation is more lengthy than an above-knee procedure, and a certain percentage of patients will experience late stump complications, including ulceration or contracture (150).

Above-knee amputations are the simplest, fastest operations in the poor-risk patient. This level is indicated in the patient with extensive gangrene and infection extending above the ankle or in the nonambulatory patient. There is a high rate of healing even in the absence of a femoral pulse (8), but the rehabilitation period is twice as long as that of the below-knee amputee (147).

The Foot in Diabetes

The diabetic patient is predisposed to the development of foot disorders because of the vascular and neuropathic complications common to this disease (Figure 33-6). These factors enhance the vulnerability of the foot to damage by environmental trauma. Arterial insufficiency resulting in ischemia may produce pathology in the lower extremity by tissue necrosis or may adversely affect the healing of minor injuries or infections. Because of loss of pain and temperature sensation, the diabetic with peripheral neuropathy may fail to perceive minor foot lesions such as blisters, skin cracks, or ingrown toenails. Mechanical trauma caused by localized pressure on the foot from foreign bodies or tight-fitting shoes may be allowed to progress uncorrected. Anatomic foot deformities secondary to motor neuropathy predispose the diabetic to calluses, corns, and pressure ulcers. Decreased resistance to infection may aggravate trivial wounds.

Since the basic problems of diabetic ischemia and neuropathy are not preventable, aversion of serious consequences must aim at avoidance of complications and early recognition of potential problems. Patients and their physicians need to understand and practice preventive foot care. There is a significant relation between the level of patient understanding of the disease and the development of foot lesions (157). Psychological factors play a major role in the determination of outcome of foot lesions, par-

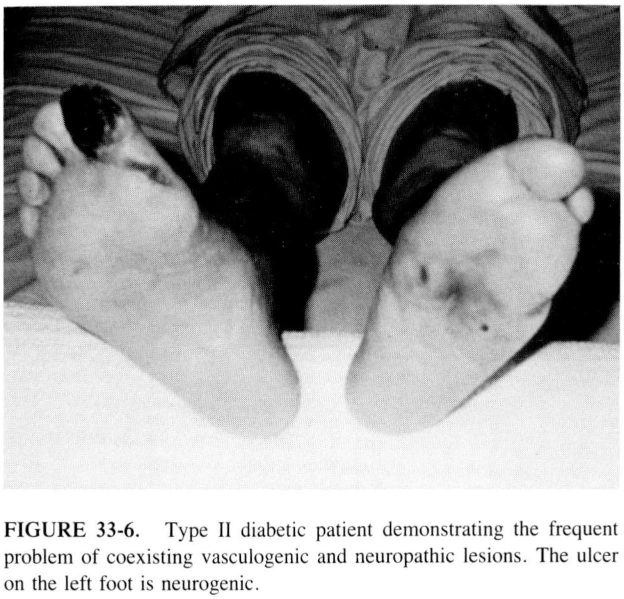

FIGURE 33-6. Type II diabetic patient demonstrating the frequent problem of coexisting vasculogenic and neuropathic lesions. The ulcer on the left foot is neurogenic.

ticularly in the syndrome of "willful self-neglect" which occurs in patients with neuropathy, retinopathy, and ulceration who display indifference to their disease and fail to seek treatment until lesions are far advanced (158). Other patients at risk for developing serious foot lesions include those with poor vision, arthritis, or obesity who are physically unable to adequately care for themselves (159). The physician should incorporate into each office visit a systematic examination of the feet of such patients.

Routine measures for foot care must be taught to the diabetic patient. Daily washing of the feet with warm (not hot) water and mild soap is recommended. Soaking should be avoided as it causes maceration of the skin. After drying with a clean towel, the feet should be carefully lubricated. This ensures that the patient will examine his or her feet and thus recognize calluses, blisters, cuts, and other abnormalities. Lubrication with a lanolin-based preparation helps prevent cracking of skin, but lotion should never be applied between the toes. If tinea pedis is present, antifungal powder should be applied to the digital web spaces. The patient with impaired vision should have such care supervised by a family member or friend. Proper trimming of the toenails is imperative. The traditional directive of cutting the nails straight across results in sharp corners which may injure adjacent toes. The corners should instead be trimmed at a slight angle, never cutting beyond the junction of the lateral nail edge and nail fold. Deformed and thickened nails from fungus infection or arteriosclerosis may require the services of a podiatrist. "Bathroom surgery" of corns and calluses with razor blades, knives, or keratolytic chemicals should be discouraged and the help of a professional sought.

The diabetic patient must be conditioned to avoid trauma to the feet. Bare feet and sandals are not permitted, and proper fitting shoes are essential. New shoes should be worn at only 1- to 2-h intervals, and leather is preferred to vinyl or other plastic material because leather more easily conforms to the shape of the foot (41). Shoes should be inspected before each use for rough lining, nails, or foreign objects. Socks should be carefully checked for wrinkles, and mended stockings should not be worn. Woolen or heavy cotton material offers better protection than nylon, which might result in excessive perspiration. The patient with cold feet should be advised to wear socks at night and never use heating pads or hot water bottles because of the danger of burns to areas with lack of sensation. These patients must be reminded that all injuries to the feet, however minor, may have major consequences and should be reported to the physician immediately.

MANAGEMENT OF FOOT LESIONS

When problems develop in the diabetic foot, they must be evaluated promptly and treated aggressively (161). The examining physician should assess the ulcer depth, presence of infection, and inciting factors such as pressure or trauma (162). Adequacy of arterial supply and degree of neuropathy must be determined. Radiographs of the foot should be obtained to identify bony destruction or soft tissue gas suggestive of advanced infection.

Certain therapeutic maneuvers should be applied to all diabetics with foot lesions regardless of etiology. The extremity must be put at nondependent complete rest with all sources of pressure eliminated. Cigarette smoking should be stopped immediately because it has been associated with an increase in the number of lesions and higher frequency of amputations (157). Control of hyperglycemia and hyperlipidemia is desirable, and favorable results in healing of foot ulcers have been reported with continuous subcutaneous insulin infusion (163). A trial of vasodilating agents is of little or no use in the patient with obstructive vascular disease (164). Peripheral edema should be controlled by treatment of contributing medical conditions such as congestive heart failure and by elevation of the leg, although this may be limited in the presence of ischemia (165).

The need for antimicrobial agents in the treatment of foot ulcers in diabetic patients depends on associated clinical findings. A superficial ulcer without associated warmth or erythema may be managed with local debridement, wet-to-dry saline dressings, and avoidance of pressure (166). If a dry eschar is present, it should be left intact, for it acts as its own biologic dressing and any debridement risks dessication of the underlying tissue and progression of necrosis (8).

In ulcers in diabetic patients complicated by local cellulitis, an oral cephalosporin is usually effective treatment. With deep infection, lymphangitis, or fever, the patient should be hospitalized and placed on parenteral antibiotics. Because of the polymicrobial nature of most diabetic infections, broad-spectrum coverage against aerobic gram-positive and gram-negative bacteria as well as anaerobes is advised after Gram stain and culture are performed. Single-agent therapy with cefoxitin or a combination such as clindamycin plus an aminoglycoside is a useful regimen in treating these infections (166,167,168). However, antibiotics alone will be inadequate, and early surgical drainage of abscesses or debridement of infected bone and tendon is necessary.

The extent of peripheral vascular disease in the diabetic with an advanced foot lesion will determine the available therapeutic options. When a neuropathic ulcer with adequate circulation is present, thorough debridement of necrotic tissue and application of an accommodative Plastazote splint or plaster cast is highly effective in promoting healing (169,170). Once healed, the foot should be protected with regular debridement of callus and specialized shoes containing arch bars for weight redistribution (159). There is a high rate of recurrence of such ulcers despite these measures, and some patients may require metatarsal head resection or even transmetatarsal amputation for relief (171,172).

The diabetic patient with arterial insufficiency and a significant foot lesion should be evaluated for possible revascularization with arteriography. If suitable runoff is present, reconstructive arterial surgery is indicated to optimize limb salvage (36). In the absence of bypassable lesions, early amputation may be necessary to control infection and minimize morbidity.

The select diabetic patient with a foot lesion may be a candidate for reconstruction with local muscle flaps. Island flaps of plantar toe surface have been described for coverage of neurotrophic ulcers of the foot and ankle (173). Lesions of the heel, midfoot, and forefoot in the ischemic extremity have been successfully treated by muscle transposition (174,175). Because the extent of atherosclerosis in the muscular vessels is variable and there are often abundant intramuscular anastomoses, muscles of the foot frequently have satisfactory blood supply for local rotation. However, in the presence of claudication or ischemic lesions extending beyond the metatarsal heads, these procedures are contraindicated (175).

Summary

Peripheral vascular disease is a major cause of morbidity and mortality in the diabetic population. Arterial insufficiency in the diabetic patient occurs early, progresses rapidly, and tends to involve multiple levels in the extremity. Microangiopathy is detectable in many diabetic patients but has an undetermined pathologic significance.

Diabetic neuropathy is ubiquitous and complicates the diagnosis and treatment of vascular disease. Sensory, motor, and autonomic functions are affected. In addition, decreased resistance to infection and impaired wound healing adversely affect the management of peripheral vascular disease in the diabetic patient.

Assessment of vascular disease in the diabetic patient involves clinical parameters and selected noninvasive laboratory studies similar to those used in evaluation of the nondiabetic. Arteriography should be performed selectively only in operative candidates because there is a risk of renal failure. Reconstructive vascular surgery can be performed successfully on appropriate candidates with comparable patency rates to a control population. However, because of the diffuse nature of their vascular disease, fewer diabetics will have adequate runoff to warrant bypass. Amputation is a frequent sequela of ischemic disease in the diabetic patient.

Lesions of the foot occur frequently in the diabetic with vascular disease or neuropathy. The outcome of these ulcers may be tempered by preventive care and early aggressive treatment. Specific therapy is directed at the underlying etiology in each case. Infection of these wounds occurs frequently and tends to be polymicrobial, requiring broad-spectrum antibiotic coverage.

In summary, evaluation and management of peripheral vascular disease in the diabetic patient differs little from that of the nondiabetic one. Specific factors such as neuropathy and susceptibility to infection will temper the physician's management, but accurate and complete clinical evaluation of any patient with peripheral vascular disease and diabetes mellitus is essential to ensure a viable and functioning limb.

References

1. Foster DW: Diabetes mellitus. In Petersdorf RG, Adams RA, Braunwald E (eds): *Harrison's Principles of Internal Medicine*, ed 10. New York, McGraw-Hill Book Company, 1983, p 661.
2. Hirohata T, MacMahon B, Root HF: The natural history of diabetes: I. Mortality. Diabetes 1967, 16:875.
3. Bell ET: A Postmortem study of vascular disease in diabetics, Arch Pathol 1952, 53:445–455.
4. West KM: Epidemiology of diabetes and its vascular lesions, New York, Elsevier, 1978, pp 159–189.
5. Lockwood DH, Prout TE: Diabetes mellitus. In Harvey AM, Johns RJ, Owens AH, Ross RS (eds): *The Principles and Practice of Medicine*, ed 20. New York, Appleton-Century-Crofts, 1980, p 1012.
6. Brandman O, Redisch W: Incidence of peripheral vascular changes in diabetes mellitus. Diabetes 1953, 2:194.
7. University Group Diabetes Program: A study of the effects of hypoglycemic agents on vascular complications in patients with adult-onset diabetes. I. Design, methods and baseline results. II. Mortality results. Diabetes 1970, 19(suppl 2):747, 789.
8. Pratt TC: Gangrene and infection in the diabetic. Med Clin North Am 1965, 49(4):987–1004.
9. Haimovici H: Peripheral arterial disease in diabetes. NY State J Med 1961, 61:2988–2999.
10. Guggenheim W, Koch G, Adam AP, Hoar CS, Wheelock FC: Femoral and popliteal occlusive vascular disease. A report on 143 diabetic patients. Diabetes 1969, 18:428–433.
11. Strandness DE, Bell JW: A comparative evaluation of peripheral arterial disease in the diabetic and nondiabetic. Rev Surg 1965, 22:77–86.
12. Bradley RF: Cardiovascular disease. In Marble A, White P, Bradley RF, Krull LP (eds): *Joslin's Diabetes Mellitus*, Philadelphia, Lea and Febiger, 1971, pp 417–477.
13. Ross R, Harker L: Hyperlipidemia and atherosclerosis. Science 1976, 193:1094–1100.
14. Ross R, Glomset JA: The pathogenesis of atherosclerosis. N Engl J Med 1980, 302:650–654.
15. Colwell JA, Winocour PD, Lopes-Virella M, Halushka PV: New concepts about the pathogenesis of atherosclerosis in diabetes mellitus. Am J Med 1983, 75(5B):67–80.
16. Zimmerman BR, Palumbo PJ, O'Fallon WM, Ellefson RD, Osmundson RJ, Kazmier FJ: A prospective study of peripheral occlusive arterial disease in diabetes. III. Initial lipid and lipoprotein findings. Mayo Clin Proc 1981, 56:233–242.
17. Dunn FL: Hyperlipidemia and diabetes. Med Clin North Am 1982, 1347–1357.
18. Reckless JPD, Betteridge DJ, Wu P, Payne B, Galton DJ: High-density and low-density lipoproteins and prevalence of vascular disease in diabetes mellitus. Br Med J 1978, 1:883–886.
19. Sosenko JM, Breshow TL, Meitten OS, Gabbay KH: Hyperglycemia and plasma lipid levels. A prospective study of young insulin-dependent diabetic patients. N Engl J Med 1980, 302:650–654.
20. Beach KW, Brunzell JD, Conquest LL, Strandness DE: The correlation of arteriosclerosis obliterans and lipoproteins in insulin-dependent and non-insulin-dependent diabetes. Diabetes 1979, 28:836–840.
21. Kazmier FJ, Bowie EJW, O'Fallon WM, Zimmerman BR, Osmundson PJ, Palumbo PJ: A prospective study of peripheral occlusive arterial disease in diabetes. IV. Platelet and plasma functions. Mayo Clin Proc 1981, 56:243–253.
22. Fulleri JH, Keen H, Jarrett RJ, et al: Haemostatic variables associated with diabetes and its complications. Br Med J 1979, 2:964–966.
23. Wautier JL, Paton RC, Wautier MP, Pintigny D, Abadie E, Passa P, Caen JP: Increased adhesion of erythrocytes to endothelial cells in diabetes mellitus and its relation to vascular complications. N Engl J Med 1981, 305:237–242.
24. Morrison AD, Clements RS, Winegard AI: Effects of elevated glucose concentrations on the metabolism of the aortic wall. J Clin Invest 1972, 51:3114–2123.
25. McMillan DE: Deterioration of the microcirculation in diabetes. Diabetes 1975, 24(10):944–957.
26. Rosenberg H, Modrak JB, Hassing JM, Al-Turk WA, Stohs SJ: Glycosylated collagen. Biochem Biophys Res Commun 1979, 91(2)498–501.
27. Beach KW, Strandness DE: Arteriosclerosis obliterans and associated risk factors in insulin-dependent and non-insulin-dependent diabetes. Diabetes 1980, 29:882–888.
28. Beach KW, Brunzell JD, Strandness DE: Prevalence of severe arteriosclerosis obliterans in patients with diabetes mellitus—relation to smoking and form of therapy. Arteriosclerosis 1982, 2(4):275–280.

29. Colwell JA, Halushka PV, Sarji KE, Lopes-Virella MF, Sagel J: Vascular disease in diabetes. Pathophysiological mechanisms and therapy. Arch Intern Med 1979, 139:225–230.
30. Garcia MJ, McNamara PM, Gordon T, Kannell WB: Morbidity and mortality in diabetics in the Framingham population. Diabetes 1974, 23(2):105–111.
31. Merimee TJ: A followup study of vascular disease in growth-hormone deficient dwarfs with diabetes. N Engl J Med 1978, 298:1217–1222.
32. Ledet T: Growth hormone antiserum suppresses the growth effect of diabetic serum. Studies on rabbit aortic medial cell cultures. Diabetes 1977, 26:798–803.
33. Stout RW: Is insulin atherogenic? Mt Sinai J Med (NY) 1982, 49(3):223–226.
34. Ganda OP: Pathogenesis of macrovascular disease in the human diabetic. Diabetes 1980, 29:931–942.
35. Khetty V: Pathology of the diabetic foot. In Kozak GP, Hoar CS, Rowbotham JL, Wheelock FC, Gibbons GW, Campbell D (eds): *Management of Diabetic Foot Problems*. Philadelphia, Saunders, 1984, pp 27–31.
36. Towne JB: Management of foot lesions in the diabetic patient. In Rutherford RB (ed): Vascular Surgery. Philadelphia, Saunders, 1984, pp 661–669.
37. Goldner MG: The fate of the 2nd leg in the diabetic amputee. Diabetes 1960, 9(2):100–103.
38. Strandness DE, Priest RE, Gibbons GE: Combined clinical and pathologic study of diabetic and non-diabetic perhipheral arterial disease. Diabetes 1964, 13(4):366–372.
39. Haimovici H: Patterns of arteriosclerotic lesions of the lower extremity. Arch Surg 1967, 95:918–933.
40. Ferrier TM: Comparative study of arterial disease in amputated lower limbs from diabetics and nondiabetics. Med J Aust 1967, 1:5–11.
41. Faris I: *The Management of the Diabetic Foot*. Edinburgh, Churchill Livingstone, 1982.
42. Christiansen N: Diabetic angiopathy and neuropathy. Acta Med Scand 1972, 541(suppl):13–60.
43. Williamson JR, Kilo C, Crespin SR: Vascular disease. In Levin ME, O'Neal LW (eds): *The Diabetic Foot*. St Louis, CV Mosby Co, 1983.
44. Banson BB, Lacy PE: Diabetic microangiopathy in human toes. Am J Pathol 1964, 45:58.
45. Siperstein MD, Norton W, Unger RH, Madison LL: Muscle capillary basement membrane width in normal, diabetic and prediabetic patients. Trans Assoc Am Physicians 1966, 79:330–347.
46. Williamson, JR, Vogler NJ, Kilo C.: Regional variations in the width of the basement membrane of muscle capillaries in man and giraffe. Am J Pathol 1971, 63:359.
47. Moore JM, Few IDO: Peripheral vascular lesion in diabetes mellitus. Br Med J 1965, 2:19–23.
48. Editorial: Pathogenesis of diabetic microangiopathy. Br Med J 1977, 1:1555.
49. Fraser DM, Campbell IW, Ewing DJ, Murray A, Neilson JMM, Clarke BF: Peripheral and antonomic nerve function in newly diagnosed diabetes mellitus. Diabetes 1977, 26:546–550.
50. Chochinov RH, Vllyot GLE, Moorhouse JA: Sensory perception thresholds in patients with juvenile diabetes and their close relatives. N Engl J Med 1972, 286:1233–1237.
51. Marchal de Calvi CJ: *Recherches sur les Accidents Diabetiques*. Paris, P Asselin, 1964.
52. Thomas PR, Lascalles RG: The pathology of diabetic neuropathy. Q J Med 1966, 35:489–509.
53. Clements RA: Diabetic neuropathy–New concepts of its etiology. Diabetes 1979, 28:604–609.
54. Behse F, Buchtal F, Carlsen F: Nerve biopsy and conduction studies in diabetic neuropathy. J Neurol Neurosurg Psychiatry 1977, 40:1072–1082.
55. Ward JD: The diabetic leg. Diabetologia 1982, 22:141–147.
56. Dyck PJ: The causes, classification and treatment of peripheral neuropathy. N Engl J Med 1982, 307:283–286.
57. Johnson PC, Doll SC: Dermal nerves in human diabetic subjects. Diabetes 1984, 33:244–250.
58. Raff MC, Sangalang V, Asbury AK: Ischemic mononeuropathy and mononeuropathy multiplex in diabetes mellitus. N Engl J Med 1968, 279:17–22.
59. Eliason SGL: Neuropathy and the diabetic foot. In Levin ME, O'Neal LW (eds): *The Diabetic Foot*. St Louis, CV Mosby Co, pp 61–84, 1983.
60. Massey EW, O'Brian JJ: Mononeuropathy in diabetes mellitus. Postgrad Med 1979, 65(5):128–138.
61. Asbury AK, Brown MJ: Clinical and pathological studies of diabetic neuropathies. In Goto Y, Horiuchi A, Kogure K (eds): *Diabetic Neuropathy*. Amsterdam, Exerpta Medica, 1982, pp 50–57.
62. Oakley W, Catterall RCF, Martin MM: Aetiology and management of lesions of the feet in diabetes. Br Med J 1956, 2:953–957.
63. Ctercteko GC, Dhanendran M, Hutton WC, Le Quesne LP: Vertical forces acting on the feet of diabetic patients with neuropathic ulceration. Br J Surg 1981, 68:608–614.
64. O'Neil LW: Surgical pathology of the foot and clinicopathologic correlations. In Levin ME, O'Neil LW (eds): *The Diabetic Foot*. St Louis, CV Mosby Co, 1983, pp 162–200.
65. Dyrberg T, Benn J, Sandahl Christensen J, Hilsted J, Nerip J: Prevalence of diabetic autonomic neuropathy measured by simple bedside tests. Diabetologia 1981, 20:190–194.
66. Watkins PJ, Edmonds ME: Sympathetic nerve failure in diabetes. Diabetologia 1983, 25:73–77.
67. Boulton AJM, Scarpello JHB, Ward JD: Venous oxygenation in the diabetic neuropathic foot: Evidence of arteriovenous shunting. Diabetologia 1982, 22:6–8.
68. Rayfield EJ, Ault MJ, Keusch GT, Brothers MJ, Nechemias C, Smith H: Infection and diabetes: The case for glucose control. Am J Med 1982, 72:439–450.
69. Mowat AJ, Baum J: Chemotaxis of polymorphonuclear leukocytes from patients with diabetes mellitus. N Engl J Med 1971, 284:621–627.
70. Baglader JD, Root RK, Bulger RJ: Impaired leukocyte function in patients with poorly controlled diabates. Diabetes 1974, 23:9–15.
71. Nolan CN, Beaty HN, Bagdade JD: Further characterization of the impaired bactericidal function of granulocytes in patients with poorly controlled diabetes. Diabetes 1978, 27:889–94.
72. Rayfield EJ, Keutsch GT, Gilbert HS, Kovacs I, Smith H: Does diabetic control affect susceptibility to infection? Clin Res 1978, 26:425A.
73. Johnson JE: Infection and diabetes. In Ellenberg M, Rifkin H (eds): *Diabetes Mellitus: Theory and Practice*. New York, McGraw-Hill Book Company, 1970.
74. MacGuish AC, Urbaniak SJ, Campbell CJ: Phytohemagglutinin transformation and circulating lymphocyte subpopulation in insulin-dependent diabetic patients. Diabetes 1974, 23:708–712.
75. Whitehouse FW: Infections that hospitalize the diabetic. Geriatrics 1973, 28:97–99.
76. Greenwood AM, Rickwood EM: The skin in diabetic patients: Further studies. Arch Dermatol Syph 1930, 21:96.
77. Prabhakar P, Rao AB, Hura J: Bacteriological study of diabetic foot ulcers. Trop Geogr Med 1981, 33:249–252.
78. Louie TJ, Bartlett JG, Tally FP, Gorbach SL: Aerobic and anaerobic bacteria in diabetic foot ulcers. Ann Intern Med 1976, 85:461–463.
79. Sharp CS, Bessman AN, Wagner FW, Garland D, Reece E: Microbiology of superficial and deep tissues in infected diabetic gangrene. Surg Gynecol Obstet 1979, 149:217–219.
80. Gibbons GW, Eliopoulos GM: Infection of the diabetic foot. In Kozak GP et al (eds): *Management of Diabetic Foot Problems*. Philadelphia, Saunders, 1984, pp 97–112.

81. Sapico FL, Witte JL, Canawati HN, Montgomerie JZ, Bessman AN: The infected foot of the diabetic patient: Quantitative microbiology and analysis of clinical features. Rev Infect Dis 1984, 6(suppl 1)S171–S176.
82. Spring M, Kahn S: Nonclostridial gas infection in the diabetic; review of the literature and report of three cases. Arch Intern Med 1951, 88:373–377.
83. Rayfield EJ: Can strict glucose control prevent infections in diabetics. Drug Ther Feb 1983, 33–42.
84. Lithner F, Tornblom N: Gangrene localized to the lower limbs in diabetics. Acta Med Scand 1980, 208:315–320.
85. Williams HTG, Hutchinson KJ: Gangrene of the feet in diabetes. Arch Surg 1974, 108:609–611.
86. Little JR, Kobayashi GS, Sonnenwirth AC: Infection of the diabetic foot. In Levin ME, O'Neal LW (eds): *The Diabetic Foot.* St Louis, CV Mosby Co, 1983, pp 133–147.
87. Goodson WH, Hunt TH: Wound healing and the diabetic patient. Surg Gynecol Obstet 1979, 149:700–708.
88. Goodson WH, Hunt TH: Wound healing in experimental diabetes mellitus; importance of early insulin therapy. Surg Forum 1978, 29:95.
89. Goodson WH, Hunt TH: Studies of wound healing in experimental diabetes mellitus. J Surg Res 1977, 22:221–227.
90. Snider SL, Kohn RR: Glycosylation of human collagen in aging and diabetes mellitus. J Clin Invest 1980, 66:1179–1181.
91. Delbridge L, Ellis CE, LeQuesne LP: Nonenzymtic glycosylation of keratin from the diabetic foot. Br J Surg 1985, 70:305.
92. Hamlin CR, Kohn RR, Luschin JH: Apparent accelerated aging of human collagen in diabetes mellitus. Diabetes 1975, 24:902–904.
93. Rosenbloom AL, Silverstein JH, Lezotte DC, Richardson K, McCallum M: Limited joint mobility in childhood diabetes mellitus indicates increased risk for microvascular disease. N Engl J Med 1981, 305(4):191–194.
94. Walker WB: Peripheral arterial surgery in the diabetic. In Levin ME, O'Neal LW (eds): *The Diabetic Foot.* St Louis, CV Mosby Co, 1983, pp 232–257.
95. Lindbom A: Arteriosclerosis and arterial thrombosis in the lower limb. A roentgenological study. Acta Radiol 1950(suppl 80), 7–80.
96. Jacobs R: Neuropathic foot in the diabetic patient. In Bateman JA (ed): *Foot Science.* Philadelphia, Saunders, 1976.
97. Osmundson PJ, Chesebro JH, O'Fallon WM, Zimmerman BR, Kazmier FJ, Palumbo PJ: A prospective study of peripheral occlusive disease in Diabetes II. Laboratory assessment. Mayo Clin Proc 1981, 56:223–232.
98. Holstein P, Lassen NA: Healing of ulcers on the feet correlated with distal blood pressure measurements in occlusive arterial disease. Acta Orthop Scand 1980, 51:995–1006.
99. Rhodes BA, Bader P, Stolz K, White RI, Siegel ME: Assessment of peripheral vascular disease in patients with diabetes. Diabetes 1976, 25(4):307–314.
100. Willard C, Johnson MD, Patten DH: Predictability of healing ischemic leg ulcers by radioisotopic and Doppler ultrasonic examination. Am J Surg 1977, 133:485–489.
101. Lawrence PF, Syverud JB, Disbro MA, Alazraki N: Evaluation of technetium-99m phosphate imaging for predicting skin ulcer healing. Am J Surg 1983, 146:746–750.
102. Moore WS, Henry RE, Malone JM, Daly MJ, Patton D, Childers SJ: Prospective use of Xe-133 clearance for amputation level selection. Arch Surg 1981, 116:86–88.
103. Siegel ME, Stewart CA, Kwong P, Sakimura I: ^{201}Thallium perfusion study of "ischemic" ulcers of the leg: Prognostic ability compared with Doppler ultrasound. Int J Nucl Med Biol 1982, 143:233–235.
104. Cina C, Katsamouris A, Megerman J, Brewster DC, Strayhom EC, Robison JG, Abbott WM: Utility of transcutaneous oxygen tension measurements in peripheral arterial occlusive disease. J Vasc Surg 1984, 1(2):363–371.
105. Byrne P, Provan JL, Ameli FM, Jones DP: The use of transcutaneous oxygen tension measurements in the diagnosis of peripheral vascular insufficiency. Ann Surg 1984, 200(2):159–165.
106. Wyes CR, Matsen FA, Simmons CW, Burgess EM: Transcutaneous oxygen tension measurements on limbs of diabetic and nondiabetic patients with peripheral vascular disease. Surgery 1984, 95(3):339–346.
107. Hauser CJ, Klein SR, Mehringer M, Appel P, Shoemaker WC: Assessment of perfusion in the diabetic foot by regional transcutaneous oximetry. Diabetes 1984, 33:527–531.
108. Levin ME: Medical evaluation and treatment. In Levin ME, O'Neal LW (eds): *The Diabetic Foot.* St Louis, CV Mosby Co, 1983, pp 1–60.
109. Dinerstein C, Mason R, Giron F: Lower extremity complications of diabetes mellitus. Surg Rounds July 1984, 267–42.
110. Kamdar A, Weidman P, Mahoff DL, Massry SG: Acute renal failure following intravenous use of radiographic contrast dye in patients with diabetes mellitus. Diabetes 1977, 26(7):643–649.
111. Der Shieh SE, Hirsch SR, Boshell BR, Pina JA, Alexander LJ, Witten DM, Friedman EA: Low risk of contrast media–induced acute renal failure in nonazotemic type 2 diabetes mellitus. Kidney Int 1982, 21:739–743.
112. Harkonen S, Kjellstrand CM: Intravenous pyelography in nonuremic diabetic patients. Nephron 1979, 24:268–270.
113. Eisenberg RL, Bank WO, Hedgcock MW: Renal failure after major angiography can be avoided with hydration. AJR 1981, 136:859–861.
114. Mission RT, Cutler RE: Radiocontrast-induced renal failure. West J Med 1985, 142(5):657–664.
115. Wheelock FC: Transmetatarsal amputations and arterial surgery in diabetic patients. N Engl J Med 1961, 264(7):316–320.
116. Stipa S, Wheelock FC: A comparison of femoral artery grafts in diabetic and nondiabetic patients. Am J Surg 1971, 121:223–228.
117. Wheelock FC: Management of the diabetic foot. In Najarian JS, Delaney JP (eds): *Vascular Surgery.* Chicago, Year Book Medical Publishers, 1978, pp 73–83.
118. Szilagyi DE, Hageman JH, Smith RF, Elliott JP, Brown F, Dietz P: Autogenous vein grafting in femoropopliteal atherosclerosis: The limits of its effectiveness. Surgery 1979, 86(6):836–851.
119. Raviola CA, Nichter L, Baker JD, Busuttil RW, Barker WF, Machleder HI, Moore WS: Femoropopliteal tibial bypass: What price failure? Am J Surg 1982, 144:115–123.
120. Wheelock FC, Filtzer HS: Femoral grafts in diabetics. Arch Surg 1969, 99:776–780.
121. Ramsburgh SR, Lindenauer SM, Weber TR, Kraft RO, Schmidt CM, Fry WJ: Femoropopliteal bypass for limb salvage. Surgery 1977, 81(4)453–458.
122. Naji A, Barker CF, Berkowitz HD, Chu J, Roberts B: Femoropopliteal vein grafts for claudication: Analysis of 100 consecutive cases. Ann Surg 1978, 188(1):79–82.
123. Naji A, Chu J, McCombs PR, Barker CF, Berkowitz HD, Roberts B: Results of 100 consecutive femoropopliteal vein grafts for limb salvage. Ann Surg 1978, 188(2)162–165.
124. Harmon JW, Hoar CS: Cloth femoral-popliteal bypass grafts in 29 diabetic patients. Arch Surg 1973, 106:282–285.
125. Reinhold RB, Gibbons GW, Wheelock FC, Hoar CS: Femoropopliteal bypass in elderly diabetic patients. Am J Surg 1979, 137:549–555.
126. Simone ST, Dubner B, Safi AR, DelGuercio P, Shah MA, Zagorin L, Reichle FA: Comparative review of early and intermediate patency rates of polytetrafluoroethylene and autogenous saphenous vein grafts for lower extremity ischemia. Surgery 1981, 90(6):991–999k.
127. Bergan JJ, Veith FJ, Bernhard VM, Yao JST, Flinn WR, Gupta SK, Scher LA, Samson RH, Towne JB: Randomization of autogenous vein and polytetrafluoroethylene grafts in femoral-distal reconstruction. Surgery 1982, 92(6):921–930.

128. Veith FJ, Gupta SK, Daly V: Femoropopliteal bypass to the isolated popliteal segment: Is polytetrafluoroethylene graft acceptable? Surgery 1981, 89(3):296–303.
129. Reichle FA, Rankin KP, Tyson RR, Finestone AJ, Shuman CR: Long-term results of femoroinfrapopliteal bypass in diabetic patients with severe ischemia of the lower extremity. Am J Surg 1979, 137:653–656.
130. Kacoyanis GP, Whittmore AD, Couch NP, Mannick JA: Femorotibial and femoroperoneal bypass vein grafts. Arch Surg 1984, 116:1529–1534.
131. Reichle FA, Martinson MW, Rankin KP: Infrapopliteal arterial reconstruction in the severely ischemic lower extremity. Ann Surg 1980, 191(1):59–65.
132. O'Mara CS, Flinn WR, Neiman HL, Bergan JJ, Yao JST: Correlation of foot arterial anatomy with early tibial bypass patency. Surgery 1981, 89(6):743–752.
133. Staple TW: Percutaneous transluminal angioplasty (PTA) of stenosed and occluded lower extremity arteries. In Levin ME, O'Neal LW (eds): *The Diabetic Foot*. St Louis, CV Mosby Co, 1983, pp 258–273.
134. Kumpe DA: Percutaneous transluminal angioplasty for lower extremity ischemia. In Rutherford RB (ed): *Vascular Surgery*. Philadelphia, Saunders, 1984, pp 637–650.
135. DaValle MJ, Baumann FG, Mintzer R, Riles TS, Imparato AM: Limited success of lumbar sympathetctomy in the prevention of ischemic limb loss in diabetic patients. Surg Gynecol Obstet 1981, 152:784–788.
136. Ozeran RS, Wagner GR, Reciner TR, Hill RA: Neuropathy of the sympathetic nervous system associated with diabetes mellitus. Surgery 1970, 68:953.
137 Grover-Johnson N, Baumann FG, Riles TS, Imparato AM: Effect of surgical lumbar sympathectomy on innervation of arterioles in the lower limb of patients with diabetes. Surg Gynecol Obstet 1981, 153:39–41.
138. Krause CA: Thirty-year experience with predictive lumbar sympathectomy. Am J Surg 1985, 150:232–236.
139. Lee BY, Thoden WR, Madden JL, McCann WJ, Trainor FS, Kavner D: Long-term follow-up of bypass procedures with and without lumbar sympathectomy. Contemp Surg 1982, 20:51–55.
140. Satiani B, Leapis C, Hayes JP, Kimmins S, Evans WE: Prospective randomized study of concomitant lumbar sympathectomy with aortoiliac reconstruction. Am J Surg 1982, 143:755–760.
141. Porter JM, Baur GM, Taylor LM: Lower extremity amputations for ischemia. Arch Surg 1981, 116:89–92.
142. Echer ML, Jacobs BS: Lower extremity amputation in diabetic patients. Diabetes 1970, 19:189–195.
143. Cameron HD, Lennard-Jones JE, Robinson MP: Amputations in the diabetic (outcome and survival). Lancet 1964, 2:605–607.
144. Kohn O, Wagner W, Bessman AN: Mortality of diabetic patients treated surgically for lower limb infection and/or gangrene. Diabetes 1974, 23:287–292.
145. Silbert S: Amputation of the lower extremity in diabetes mellitus; a follow-up study of 294 cases. Diabetes 1952, 1:297.
146. Steer HW, Cuckle HS, Franklin PM, Morris PJ: The influence of diabetes mellitus upon peripheral vascular disease. Surg Gynecol Obstet 1983, 157:64–72.
147. Samson RH, Gupta SK, Scher LA, Veith FJ: Level of amputation after failure of limb salvage procedures. Surg Gynecol Obstet 1982, 154:56–58.
148. Pritchard DJ: Amputation in the management of occlusive arterial disease. In Juergens JL, Spittell JA, Fairbairn JF (eds): *Peripheral Vascular Diseases*. Philadelphia, Saunders, 1980, pp 921–929.
149. Sizer JS, Wheelock FC: Digital amputations in diabetic patients. Surgery 1972, 72(6):980–989.
150. O'Neal LW, Wagner FW: Debridement and amputation. In Levin ME, O'Neal LW (eds): *The Diabetic Foot*. St Louis, CV Mosby Co, 1983, pp 274–302.
151. Kohn RB, Warren R, Beebe G: The "geriatric" amputee. Ann Surg 1972, 176(3):305–314.
152. Nicholas GG, Myers JL, DeMuth WE: The role of vascular laboratory criteria in the selection of patients for lower extremity amputation. *Ann Surg* 1982, 195(4):469–473.
153. Carter SA: The relationship of distal systolic pressures to healing of skin lesions in limbs with arterial occlusive disease, with special reference to diabetes mellitus. Scand J Clin Lab Invest 1973, 128(suppl):240–243.
154. Wagner FW: Transcutaneous Doppler ultrasound in the prediction of healing and in the selection of surgical level for dysvascular lesions of the toes and forefoot. Clin Orthop 1979, 142:110.
155. Gibbons GW, Wheelock FC, Hoar CS, Rowbothan JL, Siembieda C: Predicting success of forefoot amputations in diabetics by noninvasive testing. Arch Surg 1979, 114:1034.
156. Katsamouris A, Brewster DC, Megerman J, Cina C, Darling RC, Abbott WM: Transcutaneous oxygen tension in selection of amputation level. Am J Surg 1984, 147:510–517.
157. Delbridge L, Appleberg M, Reeve TS: Factors associated with development of foot lesions in the diabetic. Surgery 1983, 93(1):78–82.
158. Walsh CH, Fitzgerald MG, Soler NG, Malins JM: Association of foot lesions with retinopathy in patients with newly diagnosed diabetes. Lancet 1975, 1:878–880.
159. Frykberg RG: Podiatric problems in diabetes. In Kozak GP, Hoar CS, Rowbotham JL, Wheelock FC, Gibbons GW, Campebell D (eds): *Management of Diabetic Foot Problems*. Philadelphia, Saunders, 1984, pp 45–67.
160. Jacobs RLL, Karmody AM: Office care of the insensitive foot. Foot Ankle 1982, 2:230.
161. Ozeran RS, Reimer TR, Grodon HE: Diabetic foot ulcers: An aggressive approach. Mod Med 1972, 62:65.
162. Kalker AJ, Kolodny HD, Caruoto JW: The evaluation and treatment of diabetic foot ulcers. J Am Podiatry Assoc 1982, 72(10):491–496.
163. Rubinstein A, Pierce CE, Bloomgarden Z: Rapid healing of diabetic foot ulcers with continuous subcutaneous insulin infusion. Am J Med 1983, 75:161–165.
164. Coffman JD: Vasodilator drugs in peripheral vascular disease. N Engl J Med 1979, 300(13):713–717.
165. Dormandy JA: Management of the diabetic foot. Ann R Coll Surg Engl 1979, 61:305–308.
166. Gleckman RA, Roth RM: Diabetic foot infections—Prevention and treatment. West J Med 1985, 142(2):263–265.
167. Fierer J, Daniel D, Davis C: The fetid foot: Lower-extremity infections in patients with diabetes mellitus. Rev Infec Dis 1979, 1(1):210–217.
168. LeFrock JL, Blais F, Schell RF, Carr BB, Jacobs RL, Wirth CR, Kowalsky SF, Tillotson JR: Cefoxitin in the treatment of diabetic patients with lower extremity infections. Infect Surg, May 1983, 361–370.
169. Pollard JP, LeQuesne JP: Method of healing diabetic forefoot ulcers. Br Med J 1983, 286:436–437.
170. Block P: The diabetic foot ulcer: A complex problem with a simple treatment approach. Milit Med 1981, 146:644–646.
171. Singer A: Surgical treatment of mal perforans. Arch Surg 1976, 111:964–968.
172. McKittrick LS, McKittrick JB, Risley TS: Transmetatarsal amputation for infection or gangrene in patients with diabetes mellitus. Ann Surg 1949, 130:826.
173. Morain WD: Island toeflaps in neurotrophic ulcers of the foot and ankle. Ann Plast Surg 1984, 13(1):1–8.
174. Ger R: Muscle transposition in lesions of the ischemic leg. Am J Surg 1983, 145:658–660.
175. Ger R: Newer concepts in the surgical management of lesions of the foot in the patient with diabetes. Surg Gynecol Obstet 1984, 158:213–215.

Chapter 34

BIOLOGIC AND PROSTHETIC MATERIALS FOR VASCULAR CONDUITS: ARTERIAL GRAFTS

W. STERLING EDWARDS

Historical

The field of vascular surgery could not significantly develop until artificial arteries were available to replace or bypass diseased segments containing aneurysms or occlusions.

In 1906 Carrel and Guthrie (1) clearly demonstrated that autogenous veins can adapt as arterial conduits, responding to arterial pressure by a thickening of the walls. Carrel (2) also studied the use of arterial heterografts and methods of arterial preservation by freezing and by chemical preservatives such as formalin. Sporadic reports appeared over the next 40 years, but it was not until 1949, when Kunlin (3) published his classic paper describing the use of autogenous saphenous vein as a femoropopliteal bypass graft, that vein grafts were taken seriously and frequently used.

Gross, Hurwitt, and Bill in 1948 (4) described the use of preserved human homograft arteries in the early surgery of coarctation of the aorta. Human arteries were preserved by freezing and sterilized by cobalt irradiation. Soon other methods of preservation were developed, including freeze-drying and chemical preservation with β-propriolactone. Artery banks were developed in the early 1950s, and vascular replacement or bypass began in earnest. Preserved arterial homografts proved a disappointment—too few young arteries could be obtained to meet the increasing need, and late complications of aneurysmal dilatation, rupture, and thrombosis soon became evident. These problems led to the search for other arterial grafts.

Voorhees, Jaretski, and Blakemore (5) introduced the concept of synthetic (cloth) tubes as arterial substitutes. They proved that tubes tailored from flat pieces of porous Vinyon "N" cloth can be fabricated on a sewing machine into cuffed tubes that remain patent in humans and animals. Edwards and Tapp (6) produced the first off-the-shelf braided nylon tube grafts, including prefabricated bifurcations (7) that were crimped to prevent kinking. Knitted and woven Dacron and Teflon tubes were found to be more durable than nylon and have for 20 years been the principal replacements for larger arteries.

Autogenous Vein

After more than 30 years of searching, vascular surgeons and scientists still have found no better substitute for use in small arteries than the patient's own saphenous vein.

PREPARATION OF SAPHENOUS VEIN

Leg incisions should always be made directly over the vein. Shallow skin flaps undermined to find the vein often result in postoperative sloughs which delay healing and rehabilitation. A single long incision heals just as rapidly and quickly as interrupted incisions if undermining is avoided. Gentle handling of the vein, careful ligation of side branches, and prevention of drying at all times are important features of atraumatic harvesting. The adventitia need not be removed except at the cut edges of the vein to expedite anastomosis, and around side branches to prevent an adventitial stenosis when the side branch is ligated.

Many investigators have studied the effects of mechanical injury to the veins caused by irrigation with crystalloid solutions, distension with high and low pressures, and crushing with clamps. Abbott, Wieland, and Austen (8) found that hydrostatic dilatation causes stiffening of the vein wall which can be minimized by lower pressures. MacGregor, Agarwal, and Silver (9) compared the changes produced in canine saphenous veins distended with saline or blood at high and low pressures. Edema of the vessel wall was seen microscopically in two-thirds of the vein segments distended with saline at either 60 or 300 mmHg, but no edema was seen in veins distended with blood at either pressure. Ramos, Berger, Mansfield, and Sauvage (10) studied 62 canine cephalic vein segments grafted into both femoral arteries of 31 dogs. Half the veins were distended for 2 minutes at 600 mmHg with saline or heparinized blood, while the other half of the veins were not distended before insertion. Specimens examined histologically up to 3 months after grafting showed progressive degenerative changes including endothelial degeneration, desquamation, and reendothelialization plus subendothelial fibrosis. Notably, these changes occurred earlier and were more pronounced in veins distended at 600 mgHg than in veins that were not distended; distension with saline caused more endothelial damage than distension with blood. These authors concluded that distension of veins to overcome spasm should be done gradually with a physiological solution such as blood and only to the degree necessary to overcome spasm. Bonchek (11) has developed a vein distension system which limits the distension pressure to 400 mmHg by incorporating a small balloon.

Another important factor in the satisfactory use of saphenous vein in treating leg ischemia is the physical quality of the vein found at operation. Szilagyi and coworkers (12) performed long-term patency studies on saphenous veins which were graded at implantation as excellent/good or fair/poor based on vein wall structure, vein diameter, presence of varices, fibrotic valves, and diffuse sclerosis. The disastrous effect of poor vein quality on the maintenance of patency was statistically highly significant. It is generally agreed that veins that measure less than 4 mm in outside diameter when distended are more likely to occlude than larger veins (13).

Although the autogenous saphenous vein is the best conduit presently available for femoropopliteal bypass, it is not a perfect graft. The early changes after vein graft implantation into the arterial system are associated with inflammation and repair (14). There is a loss of endothelial cells from the intima and subsequent adherence of fibrin and leukocytes to the denuded area. Edema, focal hemorrhage, and smooth-muscle-cell necrosis appear in the media. Early endothelial regeneration is common and usually covers the intimal surface within 6 weeks. During this period the medial layer undergoes a fibrous transformation with collagen deposition and a decrease in the relative number of smooth-muscle cells. Waddell and associates (15) found that autogenous canine leg veins used as artery grafts lose most of their compliance and elasticity in 1 year and become passive conduits. Szilagyi (12) demonstrated layering of blood clot in human autogenous vein grafts years after implantation, especially if there was distal stenosis causing some stagnation. This finding was present in 21 of 260 veins. Atherosclerosis was evidenced by follow-up arteriograms in approximately 10 percent of vein bypasses (21/260). Valve cusp stenosis in reversed veins was another occasional late complication (15/260). Fibrotic stenosis, probably due to clamping (11/260) and to suturing side branches (8/260), and aneurysmal dilatation (10/260) were also observed in this most careful follow-up study. It is clear from this and many other studies that accelerated atherosclerosis is the most frequent and progressive late complication of saphenous vein grafts used as aortocoronary grafts as well as femoral bypasses. This process usually begins about 3 years after implantation, but occasionally earlier. Szilagyi (16) could find no significant differences in risk factors (smoking, increased serum level of cholesterol, diabetes) in those whose grafts developed arteriosclerosis and those whose grafts did not. It is not yet known whether reduction in risk factors such as dietary cholesterol or smoking can prevent atherosclerotic degeneration of vein grafts.

If an autogenous saphenous vein is not available or is of poor quality, several alternative grafts are available.

Arm Veins

The use of autogenous cephalic veins when no saphenous vein is available was proposed by Kakkar (17). In preliminary studies in cadavers, he found the length of available cephalic veins to vary between 45 and 62 cm, the average length being 54 cm. Measurements in 52 normal persons of different heights showed that the length of the cephalic vein was always sufficient for a femoropopliteal bypass. In every instance the diameter of the great saphenous vein was 2 to 3.5 mm smaller at the lower end than at the upper end. The cephalic vein had a greater diameter at the lower end than the great saphenous vein in the 25 cadavers examined. All veins except varicose veins were capable of withstanding a relatively high intraluminal pressure. None of the cephalic veins ruptured until the intraluminal pressure reached 430 mmHg. The lowest pressure causing rupture of the saphenous veins was 600 mmHg, and some tolerated pressures over 700 mmHg. Varicose veins could not withstand pressures over 115 mmHg.

Several reports (18,19) document that arm veins can be used for grafts, but these thin-walled veins are more difficult to handle and less satisfactory than leg veins. Schulman and Bradley (20) followed a series of arm veins used in the leg for 2 to 10 years and found a 3-year patency rate of 31 percent in femoropopliteal bypasses. There was a higher incidence of elongation, dilatation, and late atheromatous degeneration than has been reported with saphenous vein.

Saphenous Vein Allografts

Saphenous veins from human cadavers have been used as fresh, frozen, or preserved grafts by a number of surgeons with essentially unsatisfactory results, at least by comparison with autogenous veins (21–23). Early thrombosis in the first 6 months and a high incidence of late aneurysmal degeneration have discouraged the use of this type of graft. Allograft failure is apparently due to a rejection reaction, and cryopreservation does not reduce the antigenicity of the graft. Gluteraldehyde tanning appears to reduce the antigenicity of vein allografts but results in a nonviable graft with a thin wall which would appear to be at high risk of aneurysm formation with time, as has happened with other tanned allograft vascular conduits (24).

Bovine Carotid Heterografts

Norman Rosenberg and colleagues (25) in 1956 first reported studies of the treatment of bovine carotid arteries to remove their antigenicity so that they might safely be used in humans. The immune-reactive smooth muscle and other cellular material were removed from the arterial wall by the proteolytic enzyme ficin, which also removed the elastica. The resulting mushy collagen tube was then tanned over a mandril with dialdehyde starch to cross-link the collagen. Follow-up studies of more than 7 years in the dog have shown this graft to withstand pulsatile arterial pressure over the long-term (26). This has been confirmed in humans, with periods of observation over 10 years in clinical sites such as the iliac artery, where progressive obliteration of the distal arterial runoff is not usually a complicating factor (27). In femoropopliteal bypasses, however, other conditions enter the picture. Crossing the knee joint with any graft except autogenous vein leads to an increased incidence of closure due to the stiffening of the graft by the invasion of host fibrous tissue and subsequent kinking of the graft when the knee is flexed. Above-knee femoropopliteal bovine grafts were reported by Rosenberg to have a late patency rate of 41 percent at 3 years. An incidence of aneurysm formation of 3 to 6 percent in bovine grafts in the leg has essentially led to the abandonment of these tubes in this area. The bovine graft is still an effective and useful graft for dialysis access (28). When the bovine graft is used in the upper extremity, the primary infection rate is minimal and late infections in the form of perigraft hematomas are occasional problems. When the graft thromboses, thrombectomy is successful 95 percent of the time. When aneurysms do occur, a segmental excision and replacement can be performed. In this usage, the bovine heterograft is better than autogenous vein because of its durability, better puncture-sealing characteristics, and ease of thombectomy.

Textile Grafts

The outstanding contribution of Voorhees and associates (5) to the development of vascular grafts was their demonstration that porous synthetic cloth tubes could serve as satisfactory arterial conduits. In contrast to cotton and silk cloth, which cause a significant chemical reaction in the body, tubes made of Vinyon "N" cloth were found to be inert. Solid tubes of all kinds had been tried for years and were failures, especially in medium and small arteries. Exactly why porosity is necessary has never been conclusively determined. Autogenous veins or arteries are not porous in the physical sense, yet they function superbly. One prevailing hypothesis is that fibrous-tissue incorporation into the graft is necessary for satisfactory function, and that the larger the pores, the more effective this fibrous-tissue ingrowth is. The claim has been made that the ingrowth of connective tissue is not a mere healing process, but that it serves the purpose of promoting and even initiating the formation of a new, more nonthrombogenic lining of the luminal surface of the prosthesis. There is no convincing proof of this claim, and the best evidence suggests that the new lining of a textile prosthesis is an organized layer of fibrin, whose character is dependent more on hemodynamic factors than on the structure of the blood conduit and the growth of connective tissue through it. The success of the current low-porosity polytetrafluoroethylene (PTFE) grafts and nonporous umbilical vein grafts support this reasoning.

DURABILITY

Durability of the tensile strength of the synthetic graft fiber is another important characteristic. Early grafts of nylon (29) proved unsatisfactory, as chemical reactions of the body fluids resulted in deterioration of the graft fiber and dissolution of the graft wall. Dacron and Teflon tubes proved to be superior to nylon, with Teflon (30) proving to be the most nonreactive and, therefore, most durable graft available. Ultralightweight Dacron tubes did show a tendency to deteriorate and have since been discontinued. Standard-weight Dacron tubes lose about 25 percent of their tensile strength within a year, then stabilize, and seem to maintain strength for a period of at least 20 years in humans (31). Teflon grafts, even after many years, maintain their original strength.

DILATATION

All textile grafts dilate after implantation, sometimes as much as 25 percent of their original diameter (32). This may be due to (1) flattening of the crimps or (2) a rearrangement of the fibers. This dilatation is not dangerous from the standpoint of impending rupture but may predispose to graft thrombosis because of resulting turbulence. Surgeons should anticipate this slight dilatation by using grafts of smaller caliber.

FLEXIBILITY

The flexibility of an artery graft is its ability to bend without kinking. It is especially important in longer grafts that must follow curved or irregular paths. In synthetic grafts, flexibility is obtained primarily by crimping or by use of an elasticized yarn. Unfortunately, this kind of flexibility is temporary—it disappears as the fibrous ingrowth is completed. Flexible crimped grafts across the knee joint, for instance, become rigid tubes in 9 to 12 months, and kink thrombosis can occur.

A new technique to prevent kinking has been introduced by Kenney, Sauvage, and associates (33). Knitted Dacron tubes are encased in an outer spiral polypropylene, which produces a nonkinking tube that maintains its flexibility even after incorporation. A recent report (34) of 100 percent 4-year patency of externally supported Dacron tubes used as axillofemoral grafts is impressive. This graft, however, has not apparently improved the patency rate of femoropopliteal grafts that must cross the knee. The technique of preventing kinking by an outer spiral or by outer plastic rings has recently been introduced in PTFE grafts by their manufacturers. Whether the improved flexibility will result in better long-term graft patency must still be determined.

STANDARD KNIT OR WOVEN GRAFTS VERSUS VELOUR SURFACES

The velour construction creates fibrils that stand up on the graft surface, increase the total surface area, and, therefore, promote a more vigorous connective tissue infiltration. When placed on the outer surface area, the velour provides a thicker outer shell. On the inner surface it is meant to encourage tissue ingrowth into the pores and further extension into the luminal surface, creating a pseudointima that is more resistant to clotting. There is still controversy as to whether the inner velour promotes better development of a nonthrombogenic lining than standard knit grafts (35). The connective tissue shell observed about good standard Dacron or Teflon prostheses appears adequate unless the incorporation has been interfered with by exudate or infection. From a technical surgical standpoint, reoperations which require surgical dissection of velour grafts are more difficult because of the thick, tenacious fibrous sheath that surrounds these grafts.

Dacron and Teflon grafts have been used for over 30 years in larger-diameter applications and have been reasonably successful. Aortoiliac and aortofemoral grafts have success rates above 90 percent for long periods of time, with few complications. Long femoropopliteal grafts have not been as successful, especially when the graft must extend across the knee joint (36). Most vascular surgeons have discontinued the use of textile tubes below the inguinal ligament. Infection in Dacron grafts, though uncommon, is a serious problem. This has been reported in 2 to 5 percent of cases, with infections appearing early or late (from 6 months to 5 years after surgery), indicating that late infection is a continuing risk in Dacron prostheses. In a majority of such cases, removal of the graft is required. False aneurysms at suture lines are occasional problems, which may be related more to the adjacent diseased artery and suture-material failure than to the graft characteristics. There does not appear to be a strong permanent bond between Dacron graft and artery, so a nonabsorbable synthetic suture is required for anastomosis (37).

Graft of Expanded Polytetrafluoroethylene

A relatively new prosthetic graft material is microporous expanded PTFE. This material is Teflon in a nontextile form; it is extruded, not woven or knitted. Originally it was used as an industrial chemical. Since 1972, when Soyer et al. (38) first introduced a type of expanded PTFE as a venous prosthesis, there has been an increasingly active and enthusiastic interest in this material as a vascular prosthesis. However, initial results when tubes of PTFE were used as a small-artery graft were dismal. The lone report of success was by Matsumoto et al. (39), in dogs. Excluding the early thrombotic occlusions due to technical errors, Matsumoto achieved 100 percent patency from 4.5 to 11 months following implantation. However, neither the investigator nor the manufacturers of the material specifically described its structure, especially regarding the internodal distance and the wall thickness.

It was not until Campbell and Goldfarb and associates (40) performed their extensive testing and modifications of various forms of this material and gave detailed descriptions of their work that the properties and functions of PTFE were better understood. After multiple dog implants, these investigators concluded that the optimal internodal distance is 20 to 30 μm, uniform throughout the graft, and the most successful wall thickness is 0.5 mm. When grafts of these characteristics were used, the PTFE lattice frequently showed complete incorporation of fibrous tissue and neocapillaries, accompanied by a smooth neointima extending the entire length of the graft and covering the suture lines. There was also a firm periprosthetic adventitial attachment. In the early clinical evaluation of PTFE, aneurysms occurred. The standards of strength for the prosthesis necessitated the development of a reinforced outer wall. No aneurysms have been reported in reinforced conduits. Manufacturers of PTFE grafts now use a spiral reinforcement that prevents kinking as well as adds strength.

There is now general agreement among surgeons experienced with PTFE grafts that the graft has the following characteristics:

The material is inert and has a low thrombogenic potential.

It needs no preclotting and does not bleed through the pores.

It sutures well and has good pliability.

It does not kink easily, especially with the new spiral wrap. This improves its qualities as an extraanatomic graft.

No aneurysms have been reported since all PTFE grafts have been reinforced.

The incidence of infection in femoropopliteal bypass applications is so low that no published papers cite infection as a problem.

It is easy to perform a thrombectomy even months after the graft is implanted and/or closed (41).

It is available in different diameters and lengths, straight or tapered, which makes it a good extraanatomic graft.

It retains its tensile strength in the body environment and does not lose its structural integrity despite frank infection.

It functions up to 30 months as a femoropopliteal (above-knee) graft almost as well as a saphenous vein (42,43).

Femoropopliteal PTFE grafts to the distal popliteal artery below the knee do not function as well as good veins, but the difference at 30 months is not significant (42,43).

PTFE grafts are much less satisfactory than good saphenous veins if the distal anastomosis is to the tibial or peroneal vessels (42–44).

PTFE grafts make satisfactory dialysis-access grafts with a relatively low incidence of thrombosis or infection. Small-caliber PTFE grafts make excellent aortopulmonary shunts in cyanotic children (45).

A PTFE bifurcation graft has only recently become available, and there is little clinical experience with it yet.

Grafts of Human Umbilical Cord Vein

Another recent addition to the field of vascular grafts is the gluteraldehyde-treated human umbilical vein introduced by Dardik and Dardik (46,47). Because of the thin-walled nature of umbilical cord vein, this graft has been supported by a fine Dacron mesh to prevent dilatation and aneurysms. The gluteraldehyde tanning reduces the antigenicity of these biologic tubes so that rejection is not a problem, and there is reason to believe that these grafts are more resistant to infection than knitted or woven synthetic grafts. Unlike the earlier bovine heterografts, these grafts are not digested with proteolytic enzymes. The muscular component is thus preserved in addition to the collagen layer, adding to the tensile strength of the graft. Umbilical vein grafts are compliant and elastic, but are more difficult to implant than polymer or fabric tubes. When the graft is pulled through tunnels, great care must be taken not to damage the outer cloth sleeve. Careful removal of the alcohol preservative by copious irrigation is necessary immediately before implantation. A final problem is that graft length is often inadequate for the procedure to be performed, and it becomes necessary to combine two grafts with an oblique anastomosis. In femoropopliteal bypass grafting, both umbilical veins and PTFE grafts function equally well, almost as well as a good saphenous vein when the distal anastomosis is above the knee (41). Even below the knee, however, umbilical vein grafts perform almost as well as autogenous vein, and to tibial and peroneal vessels, these grafts reportedly remain patent often enough to be useful when the alternative is amputation. An unanswered question is the long-term biologic fate of umbilical vein grafts—will they undergo aneurysmal dilatation or become rigid tubes as bovine heterografts did? Five- to six-year follow-up studies are encouraging (48).

Autogenous Arterial Grafts

The arterial autograft is an excellent prosthesis in certain situations. It retains viability, it does not degenerate or become aneurysmal with time, it retains flexibility across joints, and it can heal in an infected or contaminated field. When used in children, arterial autografts grow in proportion to the growth rate of the arterial tree. The use of autografts to replace or bypass certain arteries was first proposed by Wylie in 1965 (49). Donor sites for autografts have been (1) the common and/or external iliac artery, which is replaced by a synthetic tube; (2) the hypogastric artery, which does not need replacement; (3) an occluded superficial femoral artery, which is disobliterated by an eversion endarterectomy. Two frequent uses of arterial autografts have been in renal arterial stenosis, especially in children, and in the replacement of infected synthetic grafts in various deep and superficial locations.

An infected aortofemoral bypass graft which has been sutured end-to-side at the proximal end can be completely removed, and leg circulation can be restored by endarterectomy of the aortoiliac system. The anastomotic opening left at the upper anastomosis can be closed with an autogenous arterial patch from a clean donor site such as the superficial femoral artery. This autogenous aortoiliac reconstruction can heal in the face of gross infection. If an infected aortic graft was inserted for aneurysm and the total graft must be removed, direct anatomic continuity may be restored by using endarterectomized superficial femoral arteries even in a purulent field. The advantage of this direct regrafting as opposed to prosthetic extraanatomic bypass is that it prevents aortic stump blowout, which is a frequent cause of death.

Another occasional use of autogenous arterial grafting has been across flexible joints such as the axilla and knee, especially in professional athletes. These grafts maintain flexibility without kinking better than synthetic grafts and may be selected as the graft of choice if an autogenous vein is not available.

The disadvantage of autografts is the time-consuming task of obtaining donor arteries, especially if these arteries must be replaced (50). Nevertheless, arterial autografting is an attractive technique that will quite likely see more usage in the future. The ten-year superior patency of the internal mammary artery for coronary bypass in comparison with autogenous veins is additional testimony in favor of the use of autograft arteries in the other areas (51).

Areas of Current Research

INFECTION-RESISTANT GRAFTS

Significant infections following the implantation of vascular prostheses occur in 2 to 6 percent of patients despite the use of prophylactic systemic antibiotics. The excessive morbidity and mortality associated with established prosthetic infection make the prevention of this complication a compelling goal.

Moore, Malone, and Keown (52) demonstrated in animals that transient bacteremia can result in infected grafts and can explain graft infection occurring late after implantation. They also showed that the susceptibility to infection from bacteremic contamination is a function of the completeness of neointimal healing. Grafts of various designs have been shown to have different rates of healing, to possess various types of histologic lining, and frequently to have large areas of incompletely lined graft surface even 6 months to a year after surgical implantation. These investigators also demonstrated that in dogs a filamentous velour knitted Dacron graft achieved the highest incidence (71 percent) of complete neointimal healing at 3 months, and the lowest infection rate (10 percent) from intravenously injected *Staphylococcus*. By comparison, ultralightweight knitted Dacron, and two types of PTFE grafts, were inferior in both susceptibility to bacteremic infection and completeness of intimal lining. This experimental susceptibility to infection of PTFE may not apply to human implantations, since there are few reports of clinical graft infections of this material in the literature. Certain groups (53) have routinely used PTFE grafts for repairing traumatically injured peripheral arteries, in which contamination is often a complication, and have not reported graft infection.

Despite the demonstration that implanted grafts may become infected by bacteremic challenge, the most common source of infection is contamination at the time of operation. Perioperative antibiotics are helpful but have not completely eliminated the problem (54,55). The graft matrix, a foreign body with no intrinsic blood supply, is the likeliest site for bacterial contamination and proliferation. A new and appealing approach to the problem of graft sepsis has been the development of techniques that would render prosthetic grafts resistant to infection. In 1974 Clark and Margraff (56) reported an experimental study in which prosthetic grafts treated with silver-allantoin-heparin complex significantly resisted infection in dogs and on culture plates. Gott and associates (57) described the direct bonding of heparin to prosthetic surfaces using benzalkonium chloride and graphite as absorbed anchoring molecules. Refinement of this concept has been used in the Gott shunt for nonheparin bypass in removal of thoracic aneurysms. All the heparinized surfaces were based on the noncovalent bonding of the anionic heparin molecule to cationic surfactant. In 1979 Jagpal and Greco (58) demonstrated that a negatively charged antibiotic can be substituted for heparin in the graphite-benzalkonium mode. Later Henry, Harvey, and Greco (59) showed that graphite can be deleted. They produced a benzalkonium-oxacillin-PTFE surface which exhibited superior antibacterial activity in vitro and pointed out that a rather large group of anionic antibiotics are available for this type of bonding. Control PTFE grafts implanted in the dog aorta and then purposely contaminated locally with *S. aureus* were compared with PTFE-benzalkonium-oxacillin grafts similarly treated (60). At 6 weeks the bonded grafts showed statistically significantly fewer bacteria and better graft patency, and the animals with bonded grafts showed better survival. Moore and associates (61) have presented a similar approach in which collagen was used as the vehicle for bonding amikacin to knitted Dacron grafts. These grafts implanted in the canine aorta were much more resistant than controls to the acute challenge of 10^8 organisms of *S. aureus* administered intravenously. This area of graft improvement seems quite promising.

ENDOTHELIAL SEEDING

One area of current experimentation is endothelial seeding of synthetic grafts. Endothelial cells derived either mechanically (62) or enzymatically (63) from dog veins have been mixed with the heparinized blood of recipient animals, and Dacron PTFE grafts have been preclotted with this mixture. Recovered seeded grafts showed much more rapid and complete endothelial coverage than nonseeded grafts. Small-artery Dacron grafts (4 mm ID) (64) showed higher late patency rates if endothelial seeded than if not—in experimental animals. Early patency in these small grafts could only be obtained by using antiplatelet drugs which kept both the control and the seeded grafts open. When the aspirin and dipyridamole were stopped after 2 weeks, significantly more of the seeded small grafts remained open than the controls. Whether grafts in humans will respond in a similar fashion to endothelial seeding is not yet known.

References

1. Carrel A, Guthrie CC: Uniterminal and biterminal venous transplantations. Surg Gynecol Obstet 1906, 2:266–286.
2. Carrel A: Results of the transplantation of blood vessels, organs and limbs. JAMA 1908, 51:1662–1667.
3. Kunlin J: Le traitement de l'artérite oblitérante par la greffe veineuse. Arch Mal Coeur 1949, 42:371.
4. Gross RE, Hurwitt ES, Bill AH Jr: Preliminary observations on the use of human arterial grafts in the treatment of certain cardiovascular defects. N Engl J Med 1948, 239:578–579.
5. Voorhees AB Jr, Jaretski A III, Blakemore AH: The use of tubes constructed from Vinyon "N" cloth in bridging arterial defects—A preliminary report. Ann Surg 1952, 135:332–336.
6. Edwards WS, Tapp JS: Chemically treated nylon tubes as arterial grafts. Surgery 1955, 38:61–70.
7. Edwards WS, Tapp JS: A flexible aortic bifurcation graft of chemically treated nylon. Surgery 1957, 41:723–728.
8. Abbott WM, Wieland S, Austen WG: Structural changes during preparation of autogenous vein grafts. Surgery 1974, 76:1031.
9. MacGregor DE, Agarwal VK, Silver MD: Changes produced in the wall of the saphenous vein of dogs by distending media and pressures. Surg Forum 1972, 23:135.
10. Ramos JR, Berger K, Mansfield PM, Sauvage LR: Histologic fate and endothelial changes of distended and nondistended vein grafts. Ann Surg 1976, 183:205–228.
11. Bonchek LI: Prevention of endothelial damage during preparation of saphenous veins for bypass grafting. J Thorac Cardiovasc Surg 1980, 79:911–915.
12. Szilagyi DE, Hageman JH, Smith RF, Elliott JP, Brown F, Dietz P: Autogenous vein grafting in femoropopliteal atherosclerosis: The limits of its effectiveness. Surgery 1979, 86:836–851.
13. Edwards WS: A technique of femoropopliteal arterial reconstruction. Surgery 1965, 58:496.
14. Fuchs JCA, Mitchener JS III, Hagen PO: Postoperative changes in autologous vein grafts. Ann Surg 1978, 188:1–15.
15. Waddell WE, Vogelfanger IJ, Bose M: Changes in contractility, compliance and elasticity in experimental arterial-vein autografts. Can J Surg 1973, 16:252–260.
16. Szilagyi DE: Atherogenesis in venous bypass grafts. In Sawyer PN, Kaplitt MJ (eds.): *Vascular Grafts*. New York, Appleton-Century-Crofts, 1978, p. 243.
17. Kakkar V: The cephalic vein as a peripheral vascular graft. Surg Gynec Obstet 1969, 128:551–556.
18. Vellar IDA, Doyle JC: The use of the cephalic and basilic veins as peripheral vascular grafts. Aust NZ J Surg 1970, 40:52.
19. Clayson KR, Edwards WH, Allen TR, Dale WA: Arm veins for peripheral arterial reconstruction. Arch Surg 1976, 111:1276.
20. Schulman ML, Bradley MR: Late results and angiographic evaluation of arm veins as long bypass grafts. Surgery 1982, 92:1032.
21. Ochsner JL, DeCamp PT, Leonard GL: Experience with fresh venous allografts as an arterial substitute. Ann Surg 1971, 173:933–939.
22. Haimovici H, Maier N: Autogenous vein grafts in experimental canine atherosclerosis. Arch Surg 1974, 109:95–102.
23. Perloff LJ, Rowlands DT, Baker DF: Studies of the modified venous allograft. Ann Surg 1977, 186:227–232.
24. Axhthelm SC, Porter JM, Strickland S, Baur GM: Antigenicity of venous allografts. Ann Surg 1979, 189:290.
25. Rosenberg N, Gaughran ERL, Henderson J: The use of segmental arterial implants prepared by enzymatic modification of heterologous blood vessels. Surg Forum 1956, 6:242.
26. Rosenberg N, Lord GH, Henderson J: Collagen arterial graft of bovine origin: Seven year observations in the dog. Surgery 1970, 67:951.
27. Rosenberg N: Dialdehyde starch tanned bovine heterografts: Development. In Sawyer PN, Kaplitt MJ (eds): *Vascular Grafts*. New York, Appleton-Century-Crofts, 1978, p 261.
28. Butt KMH: Bovine heterograft for arteriovenous fistula. In Sawyer PN, Kaplitt MJ (eds): *Vascular Grafts*. New York, Appleton-Century-Crofts, 1978, p 278.
29. Edwards WS: Progress in synthetic graft development: An improved crimped graft of Teflon. Surgery 1959, 45:298–309.
30. Edwards WS: Arterial grafts of Teflon. In Sawyer PN, Kaplitt MJ (eds): *Vascular Grafts*. New York, Appleton-Century-Crofts, 1978, p 173.

31. Edwards WS, Snyder R, Botzko K, Larkin J: Dilatation and durability changes in synthetic grafts of Dacron and Teflon. In Bernhard VM, Towne JB (eds): *Complications in Vascular Surgery*. New York, Grune & Stratton, 1980, p 537.
32. Nunn DB, Freeman MH, Hudgins PC: Postoperative alterations in size of Dacron aortic grafts: An ultrasonic evaluation. Ann Surg 1979, 189:749.
33. Kenney DA, Sauvage LR, Wood SJ, Berger K, Davis CC, Smith JC, Rittenhouse EA, Hall DG, Mansfield PB: Comparison of noncrimped externally supported (EXS) and crimped non-supported Dacron prostheses for axillofemoral and above knee femoropopliteal bypass. Surgery 1982, 92:931.
34. Stanley JC, Burkel WE, Ford JW, Vinter DW, Kahn RH, Whitehouse WM Jr, Graham LM: Enhanced patency of small diameter, externally supported Dacron iliofemoral grafts seeded with endothelial cells. Surgery 1982, 92:994.
35. Goldman M, McCollum CN, Hawker RJ, Drolc Z, Slaney G: Dacron arterial grafts: The influence of porosity, velour and maturity on thrombogenicity. Surgery 1982, 92:947.
36. Edwards WS: Late occlusion of femoral and popliteal fabric arterial grafts. Surg Gynec Obstet 1960, 110:714.
37. Edwards WS, Dalton D Jr, Quattlebaum R: Anastomosis between synthetic graft and artery. Arch Surg 1963, 86:477.
38. Soyer T, Lampinen M, Cooper P, Norton L, Eiseman B: A new venous prosthesis. Surgery 1972, 72:864.
39. Matsumoto H, Hasegawa T, Fuse K, Yamamoto M, Saignsa M: A new vascular prosthesis for a small caliber artery. Surgery 1973, 74:581.
40. Campbell CD, Goldfarb D, Detton DD, Roe R. Goldsmith K, Diethrich EB: Expanded polytetrafluoroethylene as a small artery substitute. Trans Am Soc Artif Intern Organs 1974, 20:86.
41. Veith FJ, Gupta S, Daly V: Management of early and late thrombosis of PTFE femoropopliteal bypass grafts: Favorable prognosis with appropriate reoperation. Surg 1980, 87:581–587.
42. Cranley JJ, Hafner CD: Revascularization of the femoropopliteal arteries using saphenous vein, polytetrafluoroethylene, and umbilical vein grafts: 5 and 6 year results. Arch Surg 1982, 117:1543–1550.
43. Bergan JJ, Veith F, Bernhard VM, Yao JST, Flinn WR, Gupta SK, Scher LA, Samson RH, Towne JB: Randomization of autogenous vein and polytetrafluoroethylene grafts in femoral-distal reconstruction. Surgery 1982, 92:921.
44. Hobson RW II, O'Donnell JA, Jamil Z, Mehta K: Below knee bypass for limb salvage. Arch Surg 1980, 115:833.
45. Gazzaniga AB, Lamberti JJ, Siewers RD: Arterial prosthesis of microporous expanded polytetrafluoroethylene for construction of aortopulmonary shunts. J Thorac Cardiovasc Surg 1976, 27:357.
46. Dardik I, Dardik H: The fate of human umbilical cord vessels used as interposition arterial grafts in the baboon. Surg Gynecol Obstet 1975, 140:567.
47. Dardik H, Dardik I: Successful arterial substitution with modified human umbilical vein. Ann Surg 1976, 183:252.
48. Dardik H, Ibrahim MI, Sussman BC, Kahn M, Dardik I: Glutaraldehyde-tanned human umbilical vein grafts. In Stanley JC (ed): *Biological and Synthetic Vascular Prostheses*. New York, Grune & Stratton, 1982, 445.
49. Wylie EJ: Vascular replacement with arterial autografts. Surg 1965, 7:14.
50. Ehrenfeld WK, Stoney RJ, Wylie EJ: Autogenous arterial grafts. In Stanley JC (ed): *Biological and Synthetic Vascular Prostheses*. New York, Grune & Stratton 1982, p 291.
51. Singh RN, Sosa JA, Green GA: Internal mammary artery versus saphenous vein graft: Comparative performance in patients with combined revascularization. J Thorac Cardiovasc Surg, in press.
52. Moore WS, Malone JM, Keown K: Prosthetic arterial graft material: Influence on neointimal healing and bacteremic infectibility. Arch Surg 1980, 115:1379–1386.
53. Vaughan GD, Mattox KL, Feliciano DV, Bell AC Jr, DeBakey ME: Surgical experience with expanded polytetrafluoroethylene (PTFE) as a replacement graft for traumatized vessels. J Trauma 1979, 19:403.
54. Wilson SE, Wang S, Gorden HE: Perioperative antibiotic prophylaxis against vascular graft infections. South Med J 1977, 70:68.
55. Kaiser AB, Clayson KR, Mulherin JL, Roach AC, Allen TR, Edwards WH, Dale WA: Antibiotic prophylaxis in vascular surgery. Ann Surg 1978, 188:283.
56. Clark RE, Margraff HW: Antibacterial vascular grafts with improved thrombo resistance. Arch Surg 1974, 109:159.
57. Gott VL, Whiffen JD, Dutton RC: Heparin bonding on colloidin graphite surfaces. Science 1963, 142:1927.
58. Jagpal R, Greco RS: Studies on a graphite-benzalkonium-oxacillin surface. Ann Surg 1979, 45:774.
59. Henry R, Harvey RA, Greco RS: Antibiotic bonding to vascular prostheses. J Thorac Cardiovasc Surg 1981, 82:272.
60. Greco RS, Harvey RA: The role of antibiotic bonding in the prevention of vascular prosthetic infection. Ann Surg 1982, 195:168.
61. Moore WS, Chvapil M, Sieffert G: Development of an infection resistant vascular prosthesis. Arch Surg 1981, 116:1403.
62. Herring M, Gardner A, Glover J: A single-staged technique for seeding vascular grafts with autogenous endothelium. Surgery 1978, 84:498.
63. Graham LM, Burkel WE, Ford JW, Vinter DW, Kahn RH, Stanley JC: Immediate seeding of enzymatically derived autologous canine endothelium in Dacron velour vascular grafts. Arch Surg 1980, 115:1289.
64. Stanley JC, Burkel WE, Ford JW, Vinter DW, Kahn RH, Whitehouse WM Jr, Graham LM: Enhanced patency of small diameter externally supported Dacron ileofemoral grafts seeded with endothelial cells. Surgery 1982, 92:994.

Chapter 35

VASCULAR PROSTHETIC DESIGN AND THE BLOOD-MATERIALS INTERACTION

RODNEY A. WHITE

Continuing efforts in vascular prosthetic design are focused on understanding the characteristics required for function of small-internal-diameter and low-flow prostheses. The pioneers of vascular surgery developed large-diameter textile prostheses for successful reconstruction of the aortoiliac tree, but fabric grafts function poorly with diameters less than 6 mm. Major advances in small-vessel reconstruction include the use of autogenous vessels for coronary artery lesions, and microvascular repair of digital and cerebral vessels. We believe that future advances in graft design will enable prosthetic repair of 2- to 4-mm-diameter arteries and reconstruction of veins.

Two unsolved problems in the development of cardiovascular biomaterials are definition of the basic mechanisms of blood-material interactions, and development of tests which predict the clinical performance of the materials. Solutions to these problems require a multidisciplinary research effort. An impediment to laboratory progress is that no animal species is accepted as appropriate for predicting the human response to cardiovascular prostheses. Information concerning the function and complications of human implants is best obtained by systematic retrieval and analysis at the time of operative revision or necropsy (1).

This chapter discusses the development of improved synthetic blood-compatible surfaces, with detailed consideration of prosthetic design factors such as pore size, biomaterial, mechanical properties, and thrombogenicity of the blood flow surface.

Porosity and Biomaterial

Porosity is an essential component for the function of small-diameter synthetic vascular prostheses. No material aside from autogenous vessels or collagen tubes remains patent in a solid form. In 1957 Edwards reported that solid polyethylene canine aortic grafts thrombosed and had no luminal healing while perforated tubes had higher patency rates and formed organized neointimal surfaces (2). This observation has been uniformly confirmed. Theoretically, porosity is required for transfer of fluid and ions through the graft matrix, and the porous material provides a scaffold for ingrowth of perivascular tissues.

Porosity is difficult to describe quantitatively. Wesolowski assessed the porosity of fabric vascular prostheses by measuring the volumetric flow of water through the wall of the material at a pressure differential of 120 mmHg (mL/cm^2 per minute) (3). He felt the porosity at implantation should be less than 50 mL/cm^2 per minute to prevent excessive blood loss in the heparinized patient. Calcification of vascular materials diminishes with porosities greater than 5000 mL/cm^2 per minute, and porosities greater than 10,000 mL/cm^2 per minute prevent some of the long-term complications of graft healing. An additional description of porosity is the ratio of open space to solid by volume, area, or weight. Investigators must attempt to describe the porous nature of vascular substitutes as extensively as possible, including the permeability, pore size, dimensions of the interconnections between pores, and the pore-solid ratio so that studies can be compared and interpreted correctly.

Current vascular prostheses are rendered porous by several techniques. Woven or knitted Dacron and Teflon fabrics are the most commonly used materials for large-internal-diameter arterial repairs. Woven fabrics have low porosity (300 to 1000 mL/cm^2 per minute) and are convenient when one wishes to use a prosthesis which does not require preclotting. Knitted prostheses provide a finer, porous lattice (1500 to 4000 mL/cm^2 per minute) which heals more quickly than woven grafts, but they require preclotting to prevent excessive blood loss at implantation. Newer knitted grafts have filamentous velour on the inner and outer surfaces. Microporous expanded polytetrafluorethylene (PTFE) prostheses have a 30- to 40-μm node-and-fibril configuration and are used for 6- to 10-mm diameter vascular reconstructions. Other medical-grade polymers, in particular polyurethanes and silicone rubber, have been evaluated experimentally as vascular prostheses but have not been used clinically. These materials offer improved mechanical and thromboresistant properties compared with Dacron and Teflon. Lyman described precipitated polyurethane grafts (4), and Annis reported electrostatically spun microporous polyurethane fabrications (5). Ashton prepared spun silicone rubber prostheses (6). The different methods of graft preparation produce variations in porosity, and this precludes independent assessment of the effects of pore size and biomaterial on prosthetic function.

The healing of vascular prostheses has been studied primarily in three species—the pig, the dog, and the human. The healing pattern of the luminal surface of vascular prostheses in the human is similar to that in the pig and the dog with the exception that healing of the inner capsule in humans requires approximately 1 year compared with 1 month in the growing pig and 4 months in the adult dog. Keough recently reported that baboons more closely approximate humans with respect to hematologic characteristics and are similar to dogs in healing vascular grafts (7).

Healing of synthetic vascular prostheses in all species increases in speed and extent proportional to the pore size and permeability. Porous grafts are incorporated by the penetration of perivascular fibrous tissue by 1 month in the absence of infection or perigraft hematoma formation. Fibrous-tissue penetration provides vascularity and a tissue substrate for organization of the fibrinous luminal layer. A viable neointima can be maintained by luminal diffusion of nutrients if the neointima is less than 500 μm thick (8). Healing of porous prostheses decreases the susceptibility to infection, anchors the graft to prevent kinking and perigraft seromas, and improves flow surface endothelialization (9).

Wesolowski described the aberrations of long-term healing related to the porous character of the graft (10). In Dacron fabrics with large fibers and large interstices, healing is complicated by cyclic degenerative and regenerative events. Necrosis of tissue ingrowth is caused by strangulation of the vessels by cicatrix or by movement of the graft fibers. Necrotic tissue in the graft matrix has a predisposition to calcification, and this leads to breakdown of the neointimal surface, which either embolizes or progressively thickens by fibrin accumulation. Disruption of healing in the wall of the prosthesis can lead to perigraft hemotoma or seroma formation and sequestration of the graft segment without tissue support. Finer, more porous knitted prostheses improve the healing characteristics and lower the risk of degenerative complications.

In 1971 Sauvage introduced external velour as a filamentous covering for Dacron vascular prostheses (11). The fine porous surface increases the tissue bond between graft and perigraft tissues and improves the rate of tissue incorporation. Sauvage also introduced double-velour Dacron prostheses (12). The internal velour was added to guide ingrowing fibroblasts to the fibrin flow surface. Lindenauer described enhanced healing of double-velour Dacron grafts compared with either internal or external velour surfaces alone (13). Other studies have noted a more adherent outer fibrous layer with double-velour fabrics but no difference in luminal surface healing (14). Clagett reported reduced platelet survival and less pseudointimal development on double-velour grafts compared with knitted surfaces for 42 weeks following surgery (15). At present, improved healing characteristics of velour fabrics, especially in humans, have not been adequately documented.

The relation of tissue response to pore size of vascular grafts is independent of material. Replamineform vascular prostheses are fabricated by reproducing the uniform, microporous configuration of different-pore-size calcium carbonate templates, permitting independent assessment of the effect of pore size and biomaterial on tissue incorporation (16). Using this technology we have shown that silicone rubber and polyurethane vascular prostheses with pore sizes less than 15 μm have minimal tissue ingrowth, prostheses with pore sizes between 15 and 45 μm are incorporated with fibrohistiocytic tissue, and prostheses with pore sizes greater than 45 μm are incorporated with organized fibrous tissue Figure 35-1 (17). The effect of pore size on type of tissue ingrowth is also evident in Dacron and Teflon vascular grafts. The larger void spaces in knitted fabrics become infiltrated with fibrous tissue while the smaller interstices in the filamentous velours have a reactive fibrohistiocytic appearance. The expanded Teflon materials used clinically as vascular grafts have fibril lengths less than 40 μm and become infiltrated with fibrohistiocytic cellular elements (17).

If the pore size of the prosthesis is controlled, the effect of the polymer on graft healing can be independently evaluated. In prostheses with pores of 20 to 30 μm, the biomaterial has a significant influence on the amount and rate of tissue incorporation. Polyurethane fabrications are rapidly incorporated with fibrohistiocytic elements over a 3- to 4-week period, while with silicone rubber prostheses the tissue ingrows more slowly to a maximum of approximately 50 percent (Figure 35-2). During the first 2 weeks of implantation there is a marked inflammatory reaction to the polyurethanes in contrast to less cellular response to silicone rubber. Although the cause of the inflammation has not been identified, it may be surface properties of the polyurethane or by-products from a slow degradation of the polymer.

Hiratzka reported using replamineform silicone rubber and bioelectric polyurethane (polyester polyurethane plus 10 percent carbon black) prostheses with 18- to 25-μm pores as canine aortic interpositions (18). Light and scanning electron micrographs of grafts removed between 1 and 32 weeks demonstrated that organization and endothelialization of the neointima were similar for both polymers and were complete by 4 to 8 weeks. The character of the prosthetic wall ingrowth was strikingly different. The microporous bioelectric polyurethane was rapidly ingrown and fragmented by 32 weeks by continued granulomatous inflammation. Silicone rubber generated minimal inflammatory response and demonstrated slower tissue and capillary ingrowth.

Biochemical analysis of tissues ingrowing vascular prostheses with different porous characteristics demonstrates different patterns of production of total protein, different ratios of collagen to noncollagen proteins, and variation in the synthesis of genetically distinct procollagens (19). Fibrohistiocytic cells from porous implants with 20- to 30-μm pores have high total protein production; approximately 10 percent is type I and type III collagen; type III collagen is associated with organs having elastic properties such as dermis, cardiovascular, and gastrointestinal systems (20). In contrast, in 60- to 120-μm porous prostheses, 50 to 60 percent of the total protein synthesis is type I collagen, the primary constituent of fibrous tissue.

The phenomenon of differential tissue ingrowth patterns (fibrous ingrowth of implants with a pore size greater than 45 μm versus fibrohistiocytic ingrowth of implants with a pore size less than 45 μm) may have important functional significance. Healing of prostheses with fibrous tissue has the potential for long-term contracture, and strangulation of the blood vessels. In contrast, fibrohistiocytic ingrowth appears to have lower mechanical strength and may be more elastic, related to the type III collagen production. By fabricating vascular prostheses with a pore size less than 45 μm, it may be possible to avoid the long-term complications of prosthetic stiffening and tissue cicatrization, in addition to attaining viable tissue incorporation and maintaining compliance.

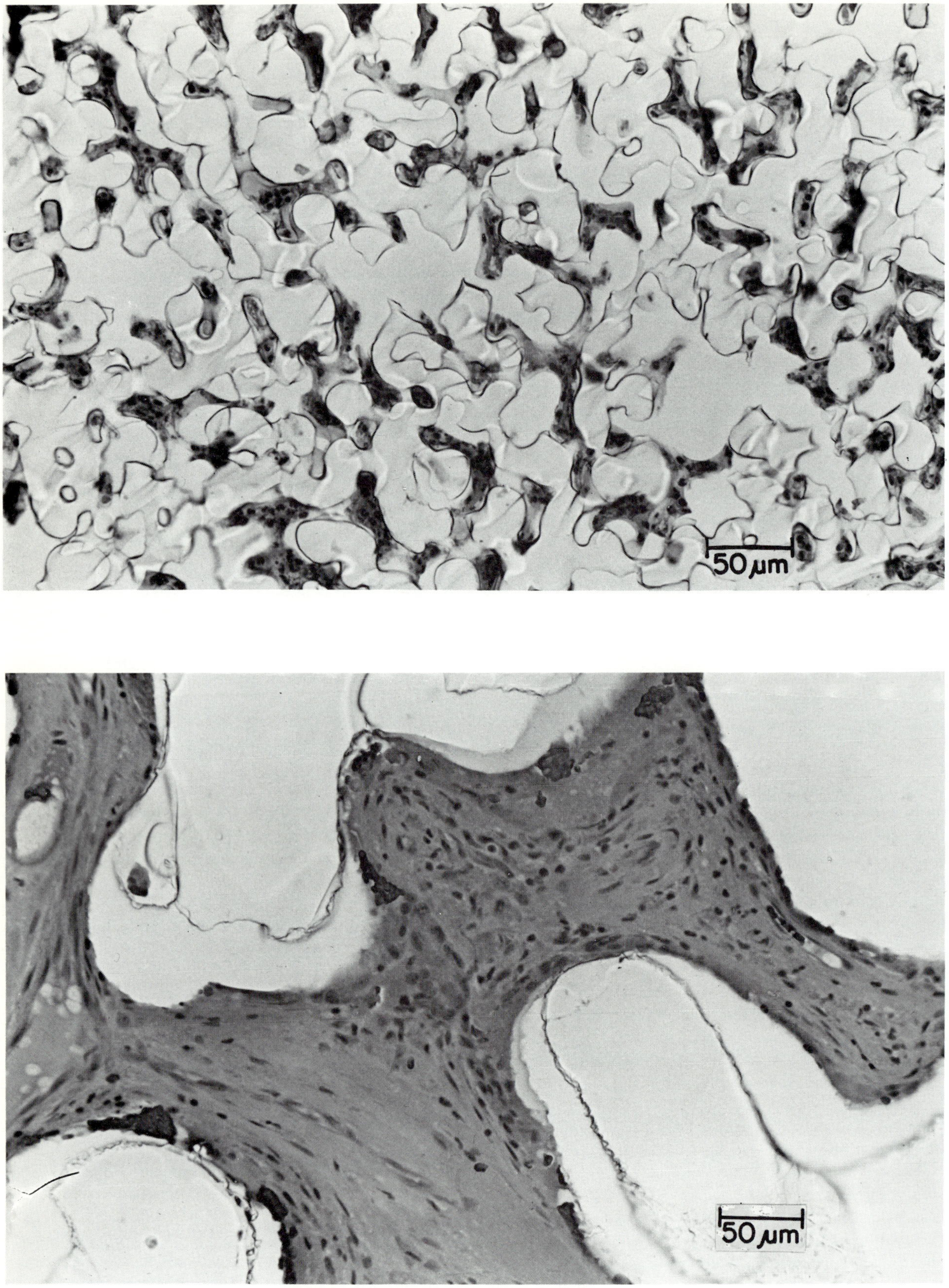

FIGURE 35–1. Fibrohistiocytic cellular incorporation of 20- to 30-μm porous silicone rubber at 12 weeks (*top*) contrasted with fibrous tissue incorporation of 60- to 120-μm porous silicone rubber (*bottom*).

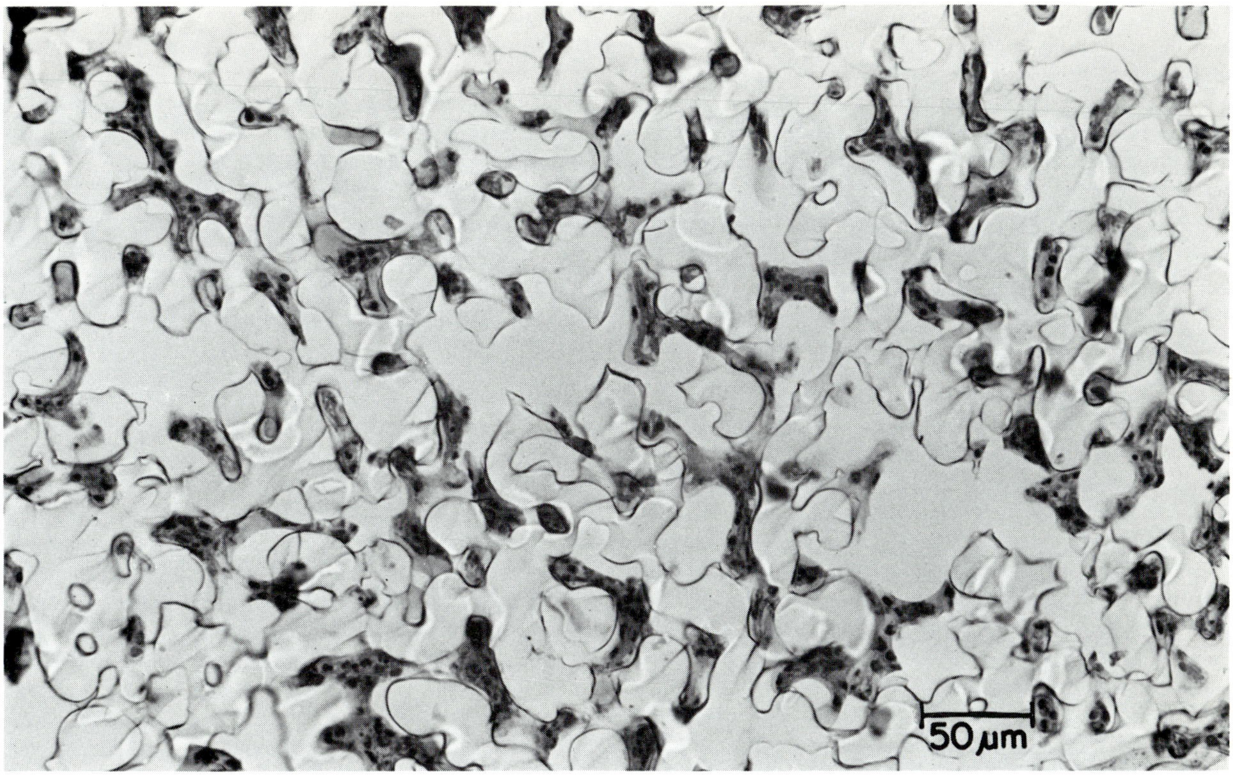

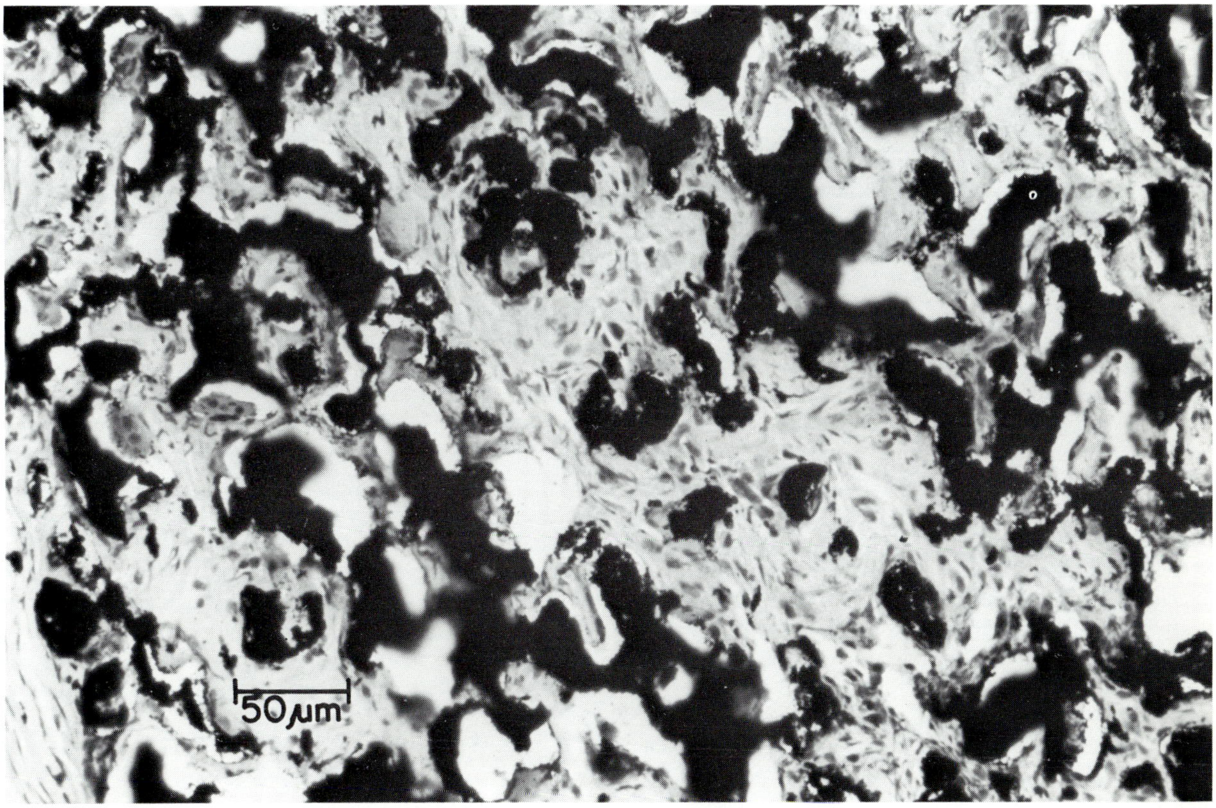

FIGURE 35–2. Effect of biomaterial on tissue incorporation. Minimal fibrohistiocytic cellular ingrowth of 20- to 30-μm porous silicone rubber at 12 weeks (*top*) compared to the completely incorporated, 20- to 30-μm porous bioelectric polyurethane (*bottom*).

It remains undetermined what porous character and subsequent healing pattern is required to obtain long-term patency of small-internal-diameter vascular grafts. The need for ingrowth may be determined by the site of implantation. Large-diameter grafts may require well-incorporated materials to provide stability and resistance to infection. Small-internal-diameter applications may require less well ingrown grafts to maintain compliance and a thin neointimal surface. Szilagyi concluded that connective tissue penetration is not essential for the genesis of a pseudointima, but connective tissue support is critical to its long-term existence (21). He pointed out that although permanent pseudointima is not formed in areas where tissue incorporation is completely absent, it is frequently present in areas where the adjacent connective tissue is minimal. According to these observations, very extensive ingrowth of connective tissue may not be desirable, although some degree of ingrowth is indispensable.

Compliance

The preservation of pulsatile arterial blood flow is important in maintaining optimum function of distal organs (22). Compliance of an artery is the change in the luminal volume (diameter) per unit change in pressure. Arteries are viscoelastic and anisotropic. Elastin provides elasticity, the tendency to return to an original shape following deformation. Viscosity of the arterial wall is supplied by collagen, smooth muscle, and ground substance and confines the limit of distension with pulsations. Arteries are anisotropic because the viscoelasticity is not uniform in all directions.

A mismatch in compliance may contribute to the progression of atherosclerosis. Atherosclerotic lesions occur at bifurcations of arteries and at sites of altered hemodynamics. Plaque formation is thought to depend on the transport of low-density lipoproteins and related macromolecules into the arterial wall which is altered by mechanical factors (23). Recent work has described increased progression of atherosclerosis distal to less compliant PTFE prostheses compared with atherosclerotic progression distal to more compliant autogenous vein in femoropopliteal reconstructions (24).

Decreased compliance is implicated as one of the causes of occlusion of small-internal-diameter arterial replacements (25,26). The importance of this variable is difficult to assess independently because of the overwhelming influence of hemodynamic, thrombogenic, and graft-design factors. The short-term effects of compliance are not well-understood and are apparent only when thrombogenic surfaces are evaluated. With endothelialized surfaces which are less compliant than artery, such as autogenous vein, the thromboresistance of the flow surface provided by the endothelial cell overshadows the effect of compliance on short-term patency. Abbott evaluated the short-term effects of compliance by destroying the endothelium on arterial segments by air-drying (27). He demonstrated a significantly increased thrombosis rate using deendothelialized banded (noncompliant) canine femoral arteries (70 percent), compared with deendothelialized normally compliant segments (10 percent). Seifert confirmed this observation using copolyetherurethane grafts with varying expansile properties (28). Grafts whose elasticity matched the compliance of native artery had the highest patency rates 1 month after implantation.

The long-term effect of an artery-prosthesis compliance mismatch is postulated as one of the causes of anastomotic intimal hyperplasia. Wijesinghe proposed that pseudointimal cellular proliferation in porous prostheses is due, in part, to mechanical stresses at the luminal surface (29). Fluid flux with arterial pulsations at permeable areas of the prosthesis increases the forces at the neointima-substratum interface. He proposed that the mechanical properties of porous prostheses should be matched with those of the attached arteries to reduce or relocate the transmitted forces.

Contemporary graft materials including autogenous vein become less compliant following implantation. Although healing may be a liability to long-term functioning of grafts because of decreased compliance, healing is required for establishment and maintenance of a nonthrombogenic neointimal layer. The following experiments have been performed in our laboratory to study vascular compliance. The compliance of canine native femoral artery has been measured as 10.6 ± 4.5/percent radial change/mmHg $\times 10^{-2}$, $n = 60$ (mean $\pm$ SD). With the overlying skin and perivascular soft tissue removed, repeat compliance values depend on whether manipulation of the artery induces spasm. In general, the compliance of an isolated artery (8.4 ± 3.0, $n = 60$) is less than that of the intact, native artery.

Klein studied the compliance changes related to suture technique at artery-artery anastomoses (30). Running-suture anastomoses as primary repair for transected canine femoral arteries on one side were compared with interrupted-suture anastomoses in the contralateral femoral arteries. Each technique significantly decreases compliance compared to the compliance of native artery ($p < .01$), with running-suture anastomoses being less compliant than interrupted ($p < .05$). In experiments using canine femoral interposition grafts, anastomotic compliance decreases proportional to the compliance of the interposed segment (17). For example, compliance at the proximal interrupted-suture anastomosis of 4-mm internal diameter PTFE vascular grafts was 4.1 1 cm proximal to the anastomosis, 1.0 at the proximal anastomosis, and 0.6 in the graft segment. Compliance measurements distal to the latter point were less than 1.0. When replamineform vascular prostheses with compliance equal to that of native artery were used, the compliance of interrupted-suture anastomoses closely approximated that of the native vessel.

We have studied the effect of vascular graft healing on compliance and patency using 6-cm long and 4-mm internal diameter prostheses with variable healing characteristics in dog femoral arteries (31). The grafts included autogenous vein, PTFE*, replamineform† Biomer‡, and replamineform silicone rubber§ coated with Biolite¶. The replamineform prostheses had porous walls

*W. L. Gore and Associates, Inc., Flagstaff, Ariz.

†Interpore International, Irvine, Calif.

‡Ethicon Corp., Somerville, N. J.

§MDX4-4210, Dow Corning Corp., Midland, Mich.

¶Carbomedics, Inc., Austin, Tex.

with a pore size of 20 to 30 μm. At implantation, compliance of the vein (3.3 ± 7) and PTFE grafts (1.4 ± 0.6) was significantly less than that of the artery, replamineform Biomer (6.2 ± 2.4) was isocompliant to the artery, and replamineform silicone rubber (15.0 ± 4.8) was hypercompliant to the artery.

The compliance of autogenous veins decreased with time, associated with fibrous-tissue encapsulation and progressive luminal thickening. The most significant changes occurred between 2 and 4 weeks, corresponding to the maturation of surrounding fibrous tissue. PTFE prostheses decreased slightly in compliance as healing progressed. Replamineform Biomer grafts remained approximately equal in compliance to the proximal artery for the first 2 to 3 weeks. During this interval the graft matrix was incorporated with fibrohistiocytic cells. After 3 weeks the compliance of the Biomer prostheses decreased and by 8 weeks was approximately half that of the proximal artery. This change in compliance was associated with complete fibrohistiocytic infiltration of the microporous graft and evidence of fragmentation of the Biomer prosthesis by large bands of ingrowing tissue. The silicone rubber prostheses became equal in compliance to the proximal artery over the first 2 weeks as they were encapsulated by a thin fibrous membrane. By 6 to 8 weeks the neointima and outer capsule healed, with dispersed fibrohistiocytic cells ingrowing the graft matrix. Continuing experiments have demonstrated the persistence of isocompliance of the silicone rubber prostheses to 8 months postimplantation, with minimal fibrohistiocytic cellular infiltration of the graft wall persisting for more than 2 years.

Although the expansile quality of arteries decreases with advancing age and as atheromatous changes progress, human femoral arteries from patients 50 years old and older remain compliant (9.1 ± 1.6) (27). Intuitively, matching the compliance of the artery to that of the prosthesis is essential for function of small-internal-diameter arterial grafts. Our data suggest that maintaining compliance of implanted vascular segments is a multifactorial phenomenon. Preserving compliance of the arterial prosthesis appears to be related to the biomaterial, pore size, type of tissue ingrowth, degree of tissue ingrowth of the porous structure, and anastomotic technique.

Thrombogenicity of Blood Flow Surface

The thrombotic process at the vascular (prosthetic) surface is affected by the site of implantation, the rate of blood flow, and the critical surface tension (32). In high-flow applications without turbulence, many materials are acceptable as short-term blood-compatible surfaces. At low flow rates or as shear stresses and exposure times increase, thrombotic and embolic complications limit the clinical applicability of many materials (33). Critical surface tensions of 20 to 30 dyn/cm are the least thrombogenic. Values above and below this range accentuate thrombus formation. Roughness of a material increases the critical surface tension compared with a smooth surface. The attempt is to approximate the critical surface tension of autogenous vessels, which is 25 dyn/cm.

Many investigators have postulated that the thromboresistance of a vascular prosthesis is determined by the chemical composition of the flow surface. Fourier transfer infrared spectroscopy/attenuated total reflectance (FTIR/ATR) and electron spectroscopy for chemical analysis (ESCA) have been used to study the chemical and morphologic structure of the surface before and after implantation (34). Labeling of specific protein fractions, electrophoresis of eluted proteins, and postimplant FTIR/ATR or ESCA evaluations are three techniques that have been used to assess specific protein deposition (35,36). Routine histologic staining methods and scanning electron micrographs have failed to quantitate cellular responses to flow surfaces, although histochemical and immunochemical techniques may demonstrate different cell populations and identify cellular activation (37).

Crystalline polymers are more active with respect to platelet retention and activation than their amorphous or noncrystalline counterparts. Hydrophilic surfaces lacking ionic charge and lacking strongly hydrogen bonding groups are desirable for minimizing platelet activation. These properties have prompted the suggestion that the chemical structure of blood flow surfaces be random, amorphous, perhaps of mobile nature, with nothing in excess on the surface (38).

On exposure to blood the luminal surface of a vascular prosthesis is immediately coated with a layer of serum proteins, the composition of which is dependent on exposed charges at the surface. This reaction is followed by the adhesion of platelets, white cells, fibrin, and red cells. If the process is limited, the prosthesis functions well; however, if the process persists, occlusion eventually occurs from continued deposition of cellular elements and fibrin. Preliminary evidence suggests that surfaces which preferentially absorb albumin are less thrombogenic than surfaces which absorb fibrinogen or gamma globulins (35). The fibronectins, a group of high-molecular-weight glycoproteins, have been implicated in a variety of cell interactions with collagen and fibrin including adhesion of platelets (39). Fibronectin is found in serum and is secreted by a variety of cell types. Fibronectin binds covalently to fibrin through the action of factor XIII and is thought to enhance the reactivity of surfaces with blood. Other serum proteins compete with fibronectin for surface adsorption sites. Fibronectin deposition is enhanced on surfaces which have been exposed to whole blood. Platelet-fibrin meshworks on surfaces are coated with fibronectin, suggesting that fibrin strands formed during clotting are probably a fibrin-fibronectin copolymer. Blood cells other than platelets found in thrombi have no fibronectin on their surface.

Many investigators feel that platelet aggregation initiates the long-term thrombotic complications of prosthetic reconstructions (40). Others have suggested that thrombogenic surfaces bind the enzymatic precursors of coagulation or cause the release of platelet adhesion factors which promote continued thrombosis (41). Platelets and leukocytes are damaged by shear stresses 10-fold less than those encountered physiologically; thus any factors which increase shear stress provoke thrombosis (42,43). Little work has been performed to evaluate the role of white blood cells on graft function. The initial reaction to the prosthetic vascular device is a modified inflammatory reaction to a foreign body. White cell chemotaxis, lysozymes, and immunologic functions may affect thrombosis initiated by a prosthetic surface.

In general, antiplatelet drugs decrease the amount of damage at a given shear rate, but do not prevent cell damage (44). Aspirin and theophylline decrease platelet aggregation (45,46). Aspirin, a cyclooxygenase inhibitor, prevents conversion of arachidonic acid to its physiologically active by-products, either thromboxane A_2 or prostacyclin (45). Theophylline, a phosphodiesterase inhibitor, causes an accumulation of cyclic adenosine monophosphate (AMP) (46). Heparin has little effect on the platelet survival time, but antiplatelet drugs such as dipyridamole and aspirin are effective (47). A number of investigators are dispersing pharmacologic agents or their analogue in polymers in an attempt to control the protein and cellular responses to synthetic vascular prosthetic surfaces.

Porosity or roughness of the luminal surface has an effect on its thrombogenicity. Campbell evaluated the effect of pore size on the patency of 4-mm internal diameter PTFE protheses in dogs and found that grafts with pore sizes less than 22 μm maintain the best patency (48). PTFE prostheses with pore sizes greater than 22 μm have progressively thicker pseudointimal development as the pore size increases, which leads to ultimate occlusion. PTFE prostheses with pore sizes greater than 110 μm are excessively thrombogenic and rapidly occlude on implantation. We have investigated the effects of pore size on patency of small-internal-diameter replamineform vascular prostheses and found that grafts with pore sizes of 60 to 120 μm are more thrombogenic than grafts with pore sizes of 20 to 30 μm (17).

Merrill studied the effect of roughness of a surface on thrombogenicity (49). He showed that surface defects of 0.1 μm stimulate protein adhesion, and defects of 10 to 100 μm also promote adhesion of cells. Rough areas on a surface are sites where entrapped air initiates protein and cellular adhesion (50). Outgassing of implant materials decreases thrombogenicity by removing the entrapped air. Didisheim studied the effect of roughness on the thrombogenicity of Teflon surfaces using smooth expanded PTFE compared with textured Teflon felt (51). The surfaces were otherwise identical except for slightly higher bulk crystallinity in the felt. He demonstrated increased thrombogenicity in the rougher, felt materials by reactivity to von Willibrand factor, total protein absorption, and platelet and leukocyte adhesion.

The controversy over the desirability of smooth surfaces versus textured surfaces for blood compatibility is exemplified by experimental work in total artificial heart design. Some pump bladders are fabricated of cast, smooth polyurethane bags which accumulate a minimal protein layer (52). In this particular high-flow, high-shear application the solid smooth-surface polymers provide an adequate thromboresistant surface. Other prototypes use flocked fabrics or microporous materials which accumulate a limited thromboresistant pseudoneointimal layer (53).

Significant effort has been directed toward development of reliable, cost-effective methods to test and compare the thrombogenicity of biomaterials. Long-term animal-implant studies are inadequate as a screening technique because of prohibitive expense and inability to make rapid evaluations of new materials. Numerous in vitro techniques have been developed which permit controlled evaluation of specific surface variables and blood elements, but they preclude the evaluation of blood-material interactions under normal hemodynamic and hematologic circumstances. In vivo studies using arteriovenous fistulas are being used to simulate natural parameters (54).

Sauvage described a method for evaluating the thrombogenic potential of vascular prostheses by examining the blood-surface interaction following short-term implantation and controlled flow in canine carotid arteries (55). Using a modification of this technique, we have studied the short-term thrombogenicity of preparations of grafts with identical surface microstructure. Various surface treatments alter the thrombogenic response in grafts prepared with the same porous framework (56).

One limitation inherent in laboratory studies is the variability in thrombogenic potential among animals. In an attempt to independently control the variability, we have studied two different graft preparations in the same animal (57). Mongrel dogs had bilateral femoral artery replacements using 6-cm long and 4-mm internal diameter silicone rubber prostheses with 20- to 30-μm pores. In each graft the surface of one-half of the length was coated with a thin membrane of silicone rubber (nonporous surface) and the other half was not coated, leaving a porous configuration with 20- to 30-μm pores. Prostheses were implanted with the nonporous surface proximal in one femoral artery and distal in the contralateral artery. Following 3 hours of implantation, we noted consistent differences in thrombogenic response between nonporous and porous surfaces. Nonporous segments had scattered fibrin strands and adherent platelets, while porous segments had significant white cell and platelet accumulations. The demarcation between surface responses was sharp and independent of location in the blood flow.

This group of experiments addresses several questions regarding small-internal-diameter vascular graft performance. By studying two surfaces in sequence, one can compare the thrombogenicity of surfaces without performing a large number of experiments to rule out the effects of variability among animals. The experiments question the belief that position in the blood flow affects thrombogenicity, as the distinction between responses to each surface was abruptly delineated and equal in intensity regardless of proximal or distal positioning. Most importantly, these results question the reliability of short-term experiments designed to predict the long-term performance of vascular grafts. Solid silicone rubber tubes will not function as vascular prostheses, yet the short-term evaluation of a solid surface in these experiments was favorable. The short-term thromboresistant nature of the solid silicone rubber coating (approximately 100 μm thick) on the inside surface of a microporous prosthesis may be due to exchange of ions across the thin silicone rubber membrane or embolization of accumulated cellular elements.

Further studies have evaluated the thrombogenic events related to independent changes in flow-surface properties. Using the split-graft technique and parallel-blood-flow arteriovenous fistulas, we have independently examined the effect of various flow-surface modifications, including the initial effect of drugs impregnated in the polymer matrix (58). We have demonstrated that smooth porous coatings can be applied to the luminal surfaces of prostheses, improving the thromboresistance by decreasing the surface roughness yet preserving wall porosity.

Investigators studying the thrombogenicity of vascular prosthetic materials know that there is synergism in surface properties such that one cannot vary one property of the luminal surface without simultaneously influencing other surface characteristics. Multiparameter assay of coagulation and thrombotic responses should be combined with multiparameter assay of surface properties. For example, platelet adhesion, which is thought to denote thrombogenicity, correlates inversely with decreasing whole-blood clotting time, illustrating that assessment of any one variable is not indicative of the overall effects.

Future Development

Alternatives for improved cardiovascular surfaces include the development of thromboresistant materials which do not activate blood components, the use of porous, smooth surfaces which accumulate a minimal protein and cellular layer and either endothelialize or become thromboresistant, and endothelial cell seeding.

Recent advances in endothelial cell seeding techniques may offer an interim solution. Initial studies of endothelial seeding demonstrate that Dacron arterial prostheses with water porosities of 1400 to 1600 mL/cm^2 per minute and limited luminal weft-knit are optimum (59). Many medical centers are demonstrating the ability to seed surfaces for clinical trails, and cell-harvesting methods are rapidly improving. Endothelial cell seeding may also extend the use of synthetic prosthetic materials to venous reconstruction. Previous efforts to use synthetic prostheses for venous reconstruction have been uniformly unsuccessful (60). Richardson has demonstrated that the short-term patency of synthetic venous prostheses is dramatically improved by transplanting incorporated prostheses from the aorta to the femoral vein in dogs (61). He showed short-term patencies using this method of 50 percent for Dacron and 82 percent for replamineform silicone rubber grafts.

Despite significant improvement in the reconstruction of large-diameter vascular lesions using natural and synthetic materials, small-diameter grafts (less than 6 mm), including vein, fail at a rate approaching 100,000 per year in the United States alone (62). The need for a prosthesis that will replicate the role of undiseased natural tissue is clear, but the specifications and materials are not yet available. The basic mechanisms of blood- and tissue-material interactions and the consequences of these interactions on long-term function of the graft, and the effects on the distal vascular bed, must be defined. The biology of the human endothelial cell and its role in maintaining blood fluidity remain a major area requiring investigation. Advances in vascular biology, thrombosis research, materials science, and rheology will add to our knowledge of graft design, leading to development of prostheses as well as native vessels.

References

1. Weinstein A, Gibbons D, Brown S, Ruff W (eds), *Implant retrieval: Material and biologic analysis,* Proceedings of conference at National Bureau of Standards, Gaithersburg, MD, May 1–3, 1980. National Bureau of Standards Special Publication 601, Library of Congress Catalog Card Number 80-600194. Washington, DC, US Government Printing Office, January 1981.
2. Edwards WS: The effect of porosity in solid plastic artery grafts. Surg Forum 1957, 8:446–450.
3. Wesolowski SA, Fries CC, Hennigar G, Fox LM, Sawyer PN, Sauvage LR: Factors contributing to long-term failure in human vascular prostheses. J Cardiovasc Surg 1964, 5(6):549–567.
4. Lyman DJ, Albo D, Jackson R: Development of small diameter vascular prostheses. Trans Am Soc Artif Intern Organs 1977, 23:253–260.
5. Annis D, Bornat A, Edwards RO: An elastomeric vascular prosthesis. Trans Am Soc Artif Intern Organs 1978, 24:209–214.
6. Ashton F, Lightwood R, Hardman J: A silicone rubber arterial prosthesis. Br J Surg 1967, 54:709–712.
7. Keough EM, Callow AD, Connolly RJ, O'Donnell TF: Healing pattern of small caliber Dacron grafts in the baboon: An animal model for the study of vascular prostheses. J Biomed Mater Res 1984, 18:281–292.
8. Wesolowski SA: Foundations of modern vascular grafts. In Sawyer PN (ed): *Vascular Grafts,* New York, Appleton-Century-Crofts, 1978, pp 27–49.
9. Moore WS, Malone JM: *Vascular repair,* In Hunt TK, Dumphy JE (eds): *Fundamentals of Wound Management.* New York, Appleton-Century-Crofts, 1979, pp. 476–499.
10. Wesolowski SA, Fries CC, Domingo RT, Liebig WJ, Sawyer PN: The compound prosthetic vascular graft: A pathologic survey. Surgery 1963, 53(1):19–44.
11. Sauvage LR, Berger K, Wood SJ, Nakagawa Y, Mansfield PB: An external velour surface for porous arterial prostheses. Surgery 1971, 70(6):940–950.
12. Sauvage LR, Berger K, Mansfield PB, Wood SJ, Smith JC, Overton JB: Future directions in the development of arterial prostheses for small and medium caliber arteries. Surg Clin North Am 1974, 54(1):213–228.
13. Lindenauer SM, Weber TR, Miller TA, Kahn SP, Wojalik RS: Velour vascular prostheses. Trans Am Soc Artif Intern Organs 1974, 20:314–319.
14. Guidoin R, Gosselin C, Martin L, Marois M, Laroche, F: Polyester prostheses as substitutes in the thoracic aorta of dogs. I. Evaluation of commercial prostheses. J Biomed Mater Res 1983, 17(6):1049–1077.
15. Clagett PC: In vivo evaluation of platelet reactivity with vascular prostheses. In Stanley JC (ed): *Biologic and Synthetic Vascular Prostheses.* New York, Grune & Stratton, 1982, pp 131–152.
16. White RA, White EW, Hanson EL, Rohner RF, Webb WR: Preliminary report: Evaluation of tissue ingrowth into experimental replamineform vascular prostheses. Surgery 1976, 79:229–232.
17. White RA: Evaluation of small diameter graft parameters using replamineform vascular prostheses. In Wright CB (ed): *Vascular Grafting.* Littleton, Mass, John Wright PSG, 1983, pp 315–325.
18. Hiratzka LF, Goeken JA, White RA, Wright CB: In vivo comparison of replamineform silastic and bioelectric polyurethane arterial grafts. Arch Surg 1979, 114:698–702.
19. Long J, Tan E, DeSantis S, Shors E, Klein S, Goldberg L, Nelson R, Uitto J, White R: Implant microstructure and collagen synthesis. Trans Am Soc Artif Intern Organs 1982, 28:195–199.
20. Bornstein P, Sage H: Structurally distinct collagen types. Ann Rev Biochem 1980, 49:957–1003.

21. Szilagyi E, Pfeifer JR, DeRusso FJ: Long-term evaluation of plastic arterial substitutes: An experimental study. Surgery 1964, 55(1):165–183.
22. Milnor WR: Pulsatile blood flow. N Engl J Med 1972, 287:29–34.
23. Chien S: Significance of macrorheology and microrheology in atherogenesis. Ann NY Acad Sci 1976, 275:10–27.
24. O'Donnell TF, Mackey W, McCullough TL, Maxwell SL, Faber SP, Deterling RA, Callow AD: Correlation of operative findings with angiographic and noninvasive hemodynamic factors associated with failure of polytetrafluorethylene grafts. J Vas Surg 1984, 1(1):136–148.
25. Kidson IG, Abbott WM: Low compliance and arterial graft occlusion. Circulation 1978, 58(suppl 1):11–14.
26. Walden R, L'Italien GJ, Megerman J: Matched elastic properties and successful arterial grafting. Arch Surg 1980, 115:1166–1169.
27. Abbott WM, Bouchier-Hayes DJ: The role of mechanical properties in graft design. In Dardik H (ed): *Graft Materials in Vascular Surgery*. Chicago, Year Book, 1978, p 67.
28. Seifert KB, Albo D, Knoulton H: Effect of elasticity of prosthetic wall on patency of small diameter arterial prostheses. Surg Forum 1979, 30:206–208.
29. Wijesinghe AM: Pulsatile pore pressure in vascular prostheses. Trans Am Soc Artif Intern Organs 1979, 25:384–390.
30. Klein SR, Goldberg L, Miranda R, White R: Effect of suture technique on arterial anastomotic compliance. Arch Surg 1982, 117(1):45–47.
31. White RA, Goldberg L, Hirose FM, Klein SR, Bosco P: Effect of healing on small internal diameter arterial graft compliance. Biomat Med Devices Artif Organs 1983, 11(1):21–29.
32. Baier R: The organization of blood components near interfaces. Ann NY Acad Sci 1976, 283:17–36.
33. Anderson GH, Hellums JD, Moare JL, Alfrey CP: Platelet lysis and aggregation in shearfields. Blood Cells 1978, 4:499–507.
34. Barenberg SA, Anderson JM, Mauritz KA: Thrombogenesis: An epitaxial phenomenon. J Biomed Mater Res 1981, 15:231–245.
35. Lyman DJ, Knutson K, McNeil B, Shibatani K: The effect of chemical structure and surface properties of synthetic polymers on the coagulation of blood. IV. The relation between polymer morphology and protein absorption. Trans Am Soc Artif Intern Organs 1975, 21:49–54.
36. Weathersby PK, Horbett TA, Hoffman AS: A new method for analysis of the absorbed plasma protein layer on biomaterial surface. Trans Am Soc Artif Intern Organs 1976, 22:242–247.
37. Sun N: *Hematology: An Atlas and Diagnostic Guide*. Philadelphia, Saunders, 1983, pp 24–49.
38. Andrade J, Coleman DL, Didisheim P, Hanson SR, Mason R, Merrill E: Blood-materials interactions—20 years of frustration. Trans Am Soc Artif Intern Organs 1981, 27:659–662.
39. Grinnell F: *Blood Material Interactions: Adsorption of Fibronectin*. Summary of the Devices and Technology Branch Contractors meeting, December, 1982. NIH Publication No. 84-1651. National Heart, Lung and Blood Institute, 1984, pp 141–142.
40. Fuster V, Chesebro JH: I. Current concepts of thrombogenesis: Role of platelets. Mayo Clin Proc 1981, 56:102–112.
41. Larsson R, Olsson P, Lindahl V: Inhibition of thrombin on surfaces coated with immobilized heparin and heparin-like polysaccharides: A crucial non-thrombogenic principle. Thromb Res 1980, 19:43–54.
42. Joist JH, Stevens DE, Sutera SP: The role of platelet prostaglandin synthesis in shear-induced platelet aggregation, release and lysis. *Blood* 1979, 54:247a.
43. Dewitz TS, McIntire LV, Martin RS, Sybers HD: Enzyme release and morphological changes in leukocytes induced by mechanical trauma. Blood Cells 1979, 5:499–510.
44. Harwick RA, Hellmus JD, Moake JL, Peterson DM: Effects of antiplatelet agents on platelets exposed to shear stress. Trans Am Soc Artif Intern Organs 1980, 26:179–184.
45. Fuster V, Chesebro JH: II. Pharmacologic effects of platelet-inhibitor drugs. Mayo Clin Proc 1981, 56:185–195.
46. Moncada S, Korbut R: Dipyridamole and other phosphodiesterase inhibitors act as antithrombotic agents by potentiating endogenous prostacycline. Lancet 1978, 1:1286–1289.
47. Oblath RW, Buckley FO, Green RM, Schwartz SI, DeWeese JA: Prevention of platelet aggregation and adherence to prosthetic vascular grafts by aspirin and dipyridamole. *Surgery* 1978, 84:37–44.
48. Campbell CD, Goldfarb D, Roe R: A small arterial substitute: Expanded microporous polytetrafluorethylene: Patency versus porosity. Ann Surg 1975, 82(2):138–143.
49. Merrill EW, Properties of materials affecting the behavior of blood at their surfaces. Ann NY Acad Sci 1977, 283:6–16.
50. Ward CA, Koheil A, Johnson WR, Madras PN: Reduction of complement activation from biomaterials by removal of air nuclei from the surface roughness. J Biomed Mater Res 1984, 18:255–269.
51. Didisheim P, Dewanjee MK, Fass DN, Fuster V: *Blood Compatibility of Circulatory Assist Devices*. Second Annual Report, NHLBI Contract HV-92915, April 1, 1980–May 31, 1981. Available from National Technology Information Center, 5285 Port Royal Rd, Springfield, Va 22151.
52. Olsen EK, Shaffer LJ, Pae WE, Pierce WS: Biventricular mechanical assistance in the postcardiotomy patient. Trans Am Soc Artif Intern Organs 1980, 26:29–33.
53. Trono R, Bossart MI, Milan JD, Norman JC: Ultrastructural analysis of blood-interfacing linings formed within partial artificial hearts or abdominal left ventricular assist devices: A qualitative scheme for human pseudoneointimal accretion kinetics. Cardiovasc Dis, Bull Texas Heart Institute 1979, 6(2):153–171.
54. Harker LA, Hanson SR: Graft thrombus formation, detection and resolution. In Stanley JC (ed): *Biologic and Synthetic Vascular Prostheses*. New York, Grune & Stratton, 1982, pp 101–111.
55. Sauvage LR, Fernandez LG, Robel SB: Current status of prostheses for bypass of tibial and coronary arteries. Presented at the 27th Congress of the International Society of Surgery, Kyoto, Japan, September 3–8, 1977. Seattle, Providence Medical Center, 1977.
56. White RA, Klein SR, Miranda RM, Goldberg L, Bosco P, Nelson RJ: Microporous flow surface variation and short term thrombogenicity. *Biomaterials* 1982, 3:145–149.
57. Goldberg L, Bosco P, Shors E, Klein S, Nelson R, White R: Effect of surface porosity on early thrombogenicity using vascular grafts with two surfaces in sequence. Trans Am Soc Artif Intern Organs 1981, 27:517–521.
58. Long, J, DeSantis S, Shors E, Uszler M, Wuest C, Klein S, White R: Thrombogenicity and the interaction of proteins, platelets, and white cells. Biomat Med Devices Artif Organs 1983, 11(1):63–72.
59. Herring M: Endothelial seeding of blood flow surfaces. In Wright CB (ed): *Vascular Grafting*. Littleton, Mass, John Wright PSG, 1983, pp 275–314.
60. Hiratzka LF, Wright CB: Graft materials in the venous system: Recent advances. In Wright CB (ed): *Vascular Grafting*. Littleton, Mass, John Wright PSG, 1983, pp 207–220.
61. Richardson JV, Wright CB, Hiratzka LF: The role of endothelium in the patency of small venous substitutes. J Surg Res 1980, 28:556–562.
62. Megerman J, Abbott WM: Compliance in vascular grafts. In Wright CB (ed): *Vascular Grafting*. Littleton, Mass, John Wright PSG, 1983, pp 334–364.

PART FOUR

Aneurysms

Chapter 36A

AORTIC ANEURYSM: INFRARENAL, AORTOILIAC, AND HYPOGASTRIC

CHARLES G. ROB

In 1957, Barratt-Boyes (1) stated that aneurysms of the abdominal aorta were being diagnosed with increasing frequency. This is still true. One reason may be a real increase in the incidence of this lesion due to the advancing age of our population. In the past, the diagnosis of aortic aneurysms was of less importance, because treatment was largely symptomatic and ineffective. This all changed in 1951, when Dubost, Allary, and Oeconomos (2) were the first to resect an aneurysm of the abdominal aorta and replace the aorta with a homologous arterial graft. The first replacement of the abdominal aorta was reported in 1951, by Oudot (3). He performed the operation for aortic occlusive arterial disease and also used an arterial homograft. The really great advance in the management of abdominal aortic aneurysms was initiated by Voorhees, Jaretski, and Blakemore in 1952 (4). They replaced the aorta with tubes of Vinyon "N" cloth. The results were good; today Dacron is usually used, and many thousands of such prostheses are inserted into patients each year. It is without doubt a most effective operation, and since 1952, countless lives have been prolonged by the resection of an abdominal aortic aneurysm with graft replacement.

Studies by Colt in 1927 (5), Estes in 1950 (6), and many others have been shown that if the patient is age 60 or less at the time of diagnosis, 60 percent of abdominal aortic aneurysm patients rupture the aneurysm within 2 years. If the patient is over 60 years of age, 40 percent of patients rupture their aneurysm within 2 years of diagnosis. This is therefore one of the few lesions where the untreated prognosis in general terms is better in older than in younger patients.

Today, fully 95 percent of abdominal aortic aneurysms are caused by atherosclerosis; less common causes include mycotic aneurysms, syphilis, various forms of arteritis, congenital abnormalities, and trauma. It appears that abdominal aortic aneurysms produce symptoms in a variety of ways, including slow but steady expansion, rapid expansion without rupture, rupture either intraperitoneally or extraperitoneally, dissection into the wall of the aneurysm, thrombosis of the branches of the abdominal aorta arising from the aneurysm, and surprisingly infrequently either embolism or microembolism from the contents of the aneurysm.

Clinical Presentation

Eighty-five percent of patients are men and 15 percent are women. The mean age for both sexes is 67 years. Eighty-three percent are operated upon electively and 17 as an emergency (7). Those who have not ruptured their aneurysm usually present with abdominal pain. The most common presentation is with a boring or throbbing pain in the epigastrium. In some patients, this pain goes through to the back, and in a few, the only pain is in the back. Sometimes this back pain is of considerable severity. In our opinion, pain in the back is often a prelude to rupture, and such patients should be urged to have surgery as soon as possible. Some patients complain of nerve root pain, and this may be severe. Three percent of our patients presented with flank or loin pain and 6 percent with groin pain usually on the left side. This pain may be mistaken for renal colic, but we have never seen the pain of an abdominal aortic aneurysm radiate in the exact manner of renal colic. Twenty-two percent of our patients had noticed an abdominal tumor and complained of it, and 6 of these patients had noted that the tumor pulsated. In a further 17 percent, the referring doctor had found a pulsatile abdominal tumor at this first examination. Therefore, 49 percent were known to have an abdominal tumor after their first medical consultation. In 23 percent, the tumor was known to be pulsatile, and a correct diagnosis was made at this early stage. In many patients this tumor was symptomless or only produced slight discomfort.

About one-quarter of the patients suffer from symptoms of arterial disease elsewhere, the most frequent being those of coronary artery disease. But other problems include cerebrovascular symptoms, ischemia of the lower limb, and renovascular hypertension. In addition, because of the age group involved, other lesions such as chronic cholecystitis with gallstones are common, as well as enlargement of the prostate, and a few patients have an undiagnosed malignant tumor.

Examination of the abdomen reveals a pulsatile abdominal tumor, except for small aneuryms in obese patients and those whose aneurysms have leaked and produced a reduction of blood pressure, coupled often with paralytic ileus. The main source of confusion has been tumors in the upper abdomen which have become attached to the aorta so that they exhibit transmitted pulsation. In this situation, it may be very difficult to distinguish between expansile and transmitted pulsation.

The aneurysm is usually in the center of the abdomen, but it may extend to one side or the other, usually the left. The shape is basically fusiform, but saccular aneurysms are common and in some patients it is possible to palpate separate iliac aneurysms. Abdominal aortic aneurysms vary considerably in size. Some appear to fill almost the whole abdomen, while others are so small that they are hard to detect. As the aneurysm enlarges, the intestines and the mesentry gradually become displaced so that there may be nothing between the sac and the anterior abdominal wall. But it is more usual, particularly in these patients, to see a typical small-bowel pattern lying anterior to the pulsatile tumor. Sometimes there is so much thrombus in the sac that the expansile pulsation is difficult to feel. Auscultation reveals a systolic murmur in one-third of patients; the femoral pulses are absent to palpation in only about 5 percent of patients, although a more distal arterial occlusion in the superficial femoral arteries is common.

A general clinical examination with particular reference to the cardiovascular, pulmonary, urinary, and neurological systems is of great importance. In our practice, 8 percent of patients have been considered unfit for elective resection of an abdominal aortic aneurysm, the vast majority because of myocardial ischemia often combined with severe emphysema.

ULTRASOUND SCAN

Ultrasound scan is a simple and safe way to decide if a patient has an abdominal aortic aneurysm. It is also an accurate means of estimating the size of an aneurysm and therefore is a good way to follow a patient who is being treated conservatively; however, it does not replace aortography as a method of establishing the relationship of an abdominal aortic aneurysm to the branches of the abdominal aorta, and therefore aortography is a better preoperative study. The computerized tomography (CT) scan does show an abdominal aortic aneurysm, but it does not add to the information provided by the much cheaper ultrasound scan. The advantage of the CT scan is that it may show another previously unrecognized intraabdominal problem. Simple anterior, posterior, and lateral x-ray films of the aneurysm show calcification which is frequently present in the wall of the aneurysm.

THE PLACE OF AORTOGRAPHY

At first aortography was performed in a routine manner, but at that time the translumbar route was used and the procedure carried a significant risk of complications or death. It was therefore abandoned unless the aneurysm was thoracoabdominal in position or some other problem was suspected. But with the general use of the Seldinger catheter (8), aortography became safer, and today we use it routinely except in emergency situations, when the aneurysm has ruptured. This means that the surgeon knows before operation not only the diagnosis but also such useful facts as the number and location of the renal arteries, the state of the inferior mesenteric artery, whether it is dominant or not, and the condition of the iliac and other distal arteries.

When aortography was not used routinely, it was possible to diagnose an abdominal aortic aneurysm when in fact their was a retroperitoneal mass such as a lymphoma, or a horseshoe kidney, or a tortuous aorta in a patient with an exaggerated lordosis.

It is possible on clinical grounds alone to decide if an abdominal aortic aneurysm is below the renal arteries. In our experience 96 percent of abdominal aortic aneurysms are below the renal arteries, and if the upper margin of the aneurysm is below the xiphoid process, almost all aneurysms are below the principal renal arteries.

THE PRESENCE OF ASSOCIATED LESIONS WITHIN THE ABDOMEN

Even after a preoperative arteriogram and other studies, it is not uncommon for the surgeon to discover another lesion when she or he opens the abdomen for an abdominal aortic aneurysm. Such lesions include a hiatus hernia, a duodenal ulcer, chronic cholecystitis with gallstones, carcinoma of the colon, diverticulosis or moderate diverticulitis, diverticulitis with a definite abscess, carcinoma of the kidney, carcinoma of the pancreas, and carcinoma with metastatic spread. In the case of hiatus hernia, diverticulosis with or without moderate diverticulitis, or peptic ulcer, it is usually preferable to resect the abdominal aortic aneurysm and treat the other problem medically if possible. Chronic cholecystitis with gallstones presents a different problem because if the gallbladder is not removed, a significant proportion of these patients develop acute cholecystitis during the postoperative period (9). In our opinion the first step should be graft replacement of the abdominal aortic aneurysm with closure of the posterior peritoneum and return of the intestines to the abdomen. Then, if all has gone well and there are no complications, the gallbladder surgery should be performed, before the abdomen is closed. All patients receive prophylactic antibiotics commencing the night before surgery. There is, of course, no place for incidental appendectomy in such patients. Carcinoma of the colon presents a problem which may be managed in one of two ways. First the surgeon resects the aneurysm and closes the retroperitoneal space in the usual manner. He or she may then close the abdomen and 2 weeks later, resect the required segment of the colon. This is the usual procedure, but on many occasions we have carried out a colon resection at the time of aortic aneurysm resection and have not seen a graft become infected. We think that this is an open question justifiably left to the judgment of the operating surgeon. Carcinoma of the kidney is a different matter, because the diagnosis is often known before surgery since the problem will have been discovered during the preoperative arteriogram (Figure 36A-1). In our opinion, it adds little to perform a nephrectomy at the time an abdominal aortic aneurysm is removed. Metastatic carcinoma or carcinoma of the body of the pancreas presents an incurable situation, so an associated abdominal aortic aneurysm should only be removed in the rare situation where the procedure will benefit the patient. The most difficult problem is the discovery of diverticulitis with an abscess and an abdominal aortic aneurysm. The obvious theoretical solution is to drain the abscess and perform a diverting colostomy, deferring the aneurysm surgery. But on three occasions when we have done this, the patient has died from a ruptured aneurysm within 10 days, indicating that the aneurysm was expanding or leaking at the time of the first oper-

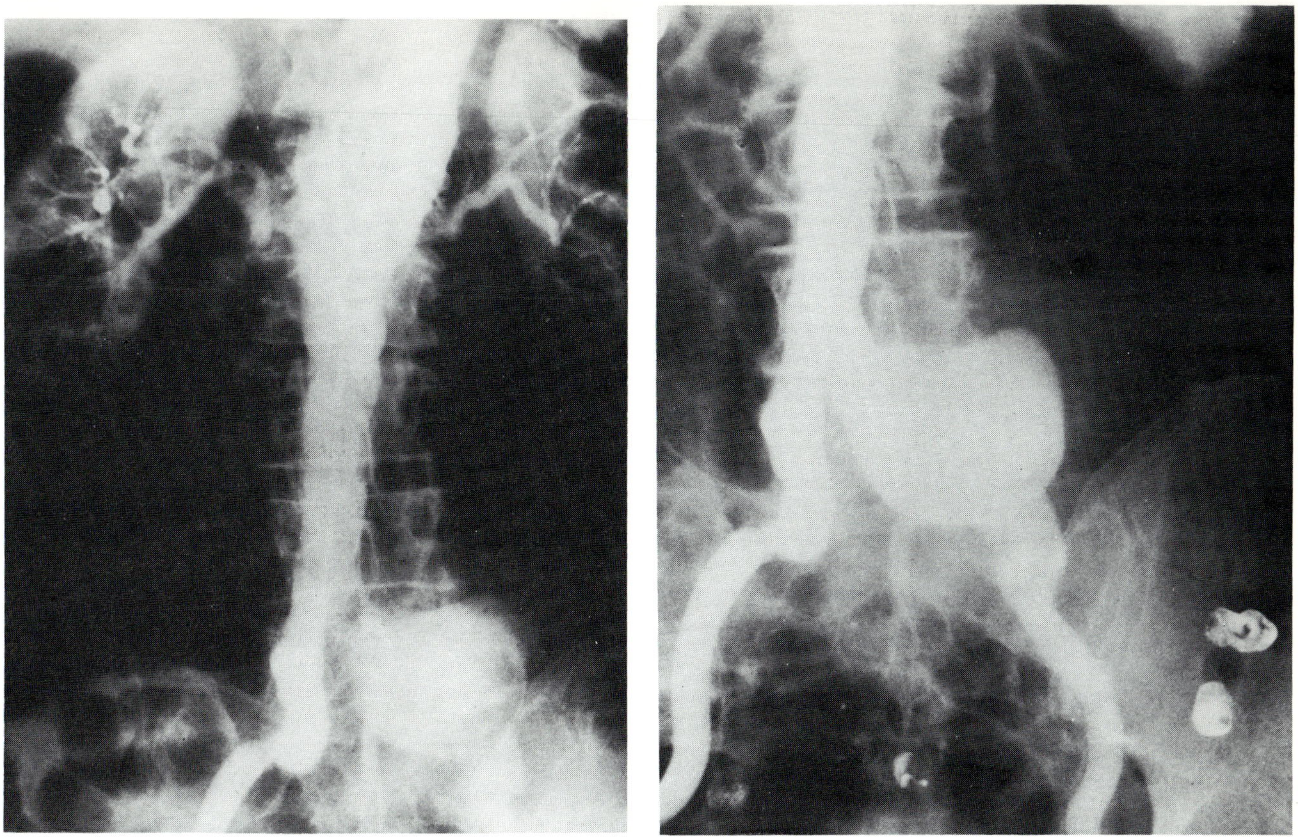

A B

FIGURE 36A–1. Carcinoma of the lower pole of the right kidney in association with a recurrent aneurysm of the left common iliac artery. Twenty years before, the aorta had been replaced with a homologous arterial graft. The kidney carcinoma, the arterial homograft, and the left iliac aneurysm were resected at one operation. Seven years later the patient is alive and now more than 90 years of age. (*A*) Overshot. (*B*) Close-up of aneurysm in homograft.

ation. The solution to this dilemma, we think, is earlier surgery for the aortic aneurysm. While all associated lesions cannot be discussed, many patients also have an inguinal hernia; in this case after completion of the aortic surgery, we invaginate the hernia sac from within the abdomen, excise it, and close the defect from inside the abdomen with interrupted sutures.

RUPTURED ABDOMINAL AORTIC ANEURYSMS

Seventeen percent of our patients have presented with either frank rupture or with an aneurysm leaking into the extraperitoneal space. It is obviously important to diagnose and resect an abdominal aortic aneurysm before it ruptures.

The aneurysm may rupture completely and the patient rapidly exsanguinate into the peritoneal cavity. In other patients the blood loss is slower and remains confined for a period to the retroperitoneal space. This causes severe pain in the back, flank, and abdomen. The abdomen is tender to palpation, often with rigidity, and the patient goes into shock. In such patients, urgent resuscitation followed by surgery is required.

ANEURYSMS OF THE HYPOGASTRIC ARTERY

These are usually seen in conjunction with aortic and iliac aneurysms, but sometimes aneurysms of the hypogastric artery develop as isolated lesions (10). If they remain within the pelvis and are large, they may produce symptoms by pressing upon other pelvic structures including the sacral plexus. They can leave the pelvis by projecting, for example, through the sciatic notch if they involve the gluteal artery. These patients feel a pulsatile sensation when they sit because they sit on the aneurysm. In all patients the aneurysm can be palpated by a rectal examination. Some rupture and major blood loss into the rectum or pelvis can occur.

THE SIZE OF THE ANEURYSM AS AN INDICATION FOR OPERATION

The classic study by Szilagyi et al. (11) in 1966 showed that if an abdominal aortic aneurysm was less than 6 cm in diameter, operation only slightly improved the patient's expectation of life. For larger aneurysms, the benefit of operation was significant.

But the operative mortality rate then was nearly 14 percent. Today the operative mortality rate in many centers is less than 4 percent, and so many surgeons advise operation on small aneurysms, provided that the patient is a good operative risk.

THE PROBLEM OF THE POOR-RISK PATIENT

Old age alone is not a contraindication to operation, but in addition to the aneurysm, many patients have other cardiovascular problems and emphysema is often severe. A particularly difficult situation for the surgeon is to be called to the coronary care unit to see a patient who is recovering from a myocardial infarction and who develops symptoms which suggest that she or he has a leaking abdominal aneurysm. Such a patient is unlikely to survive resection of this aneurysm, and a more conservative approach should be employed. Today, such patients may be treated by inducing thrombosis in the aneurysm and restoring the circulation to the lower limbs and pelvis with an axillary bifemoral graft (12,13).

PREOPERATIVE CARE

We believe that, except in extreme emergencies, every patient should see a cardiologist, or an internist interested in cardiology, before surgery. Some patients require a coronary bypass or carotid thromboendarterectomy before the aortic operation. In addition, associated diabetes often requires control, and patients with severe emphysema benefit from preoperative instruction from a respiratory therapist. It is wise to have 8 units of blood available, 4 of which have been cross-matched. In our hands, the average amount of blood required for transfusion has been less than 3 units when the operation has been elective. Antibiotic coverage should be started the night before operation; our current practice is to give a cephalosporin to cover the perioperative period only.

The anesthesiologist will have seen the patient before the operation. Before surgery, a Foley catheter should be inserted and a nasogastric tube passed into the stomach. In our opinion, it is wise in most patients to insert a Swan-Ganz catheter. The reason is that the measurement of central venous pressure alone is an unreliable index of left ventricular function. The pulmonary capillary wedge pressure in the absence of pulmonary vascular disease is a reliable guide to left ventricular function. The electrocardiogram is monitored throughout the operation, and the blood gases are checked as indicated. It is important to prevent the development of arterial hypotension during the operation and the postoperative period.

The Operation

The aorta may be exposed either transperitoneally or extraperitoneally. The extraperitoneal approach is satisfactory for small and low aneurysms; it provides a smooth postoperative course, and the peritoneaum can be opened and the abdomen explored if the surgeon wishes. The transperitoneal approach through a midline incision is the standard approach. Except in emergency situations a full exploration should be the first step. The surgeon now exposes the aneurysm by opening the posterior peritoneum between the duodenum on the right and the inferior mesenteric vein on the left. This exposure is extended inferiorly along the line of the right common iliac artery.

In the past, it was the standard practice to resect the whole aneurysm including the aortic bifurcation and proximal common iliac arteries in most patients. The reason was that the generation of vascular surgeons who practiced during the decade 1950 to 1960 had been trained as cancer surgeons. They therefore believed that the lesion should be excised. It was soon realized that this was not necessary. Today the aneurysm is not excised. The blood vessel graft is placed within the sac, which is wrapped over it; in our practice at least 55 percent of infrarenal abdominal aortic aneurysms are replaced by a straight tube graft instead of replacing the aortic bifurcation with a bifurcation graft.

The blood vessel graft is usually of Dacron, which either woven or knitted has proved to be an excellent replacement for the abdominal aorta. At one time, we used woven grafts in patients with ruptured aneurysms and knitted grafts when the procedure was elective. A follow-up of our patients has shown that the long-term results are the same. So our opinion today is that the surgeon can use either a woven or a knitted prosthesis with equal confidence, but that the woven graft is best if the aneurysm has ruptured.

The surgeon may use a variety of materials to suture the graft to the aorta or iliac arteries. Prolene is the usual material and gives excellent results, but it is important to place the knot on the left posterolateral side of the anastomosis so that it does not erode into the duodenum. Dacron sutures also give good results, but silk must not be used because it eventually fragments.

THE INFERIOR MESENTERIC ARTERY MAY PRESENT A PROBLEM

If the inferior mesenteric artery is small or normal in size, it can be divided close to the aorta and the blood flow to the intestines will be adequate. If it is large, that is, 5 mm or greater in width, it is probably an important artery, which should be preserved. The first step is to examine the celiac and superior mesenteric arteries; if they are stenosed or thrombosed, this will account for the enlargement of the inferior mesenteric artery because it is an important collateral. This problem is best handled by preserving a circle of aortic wall around the inferior mesenteric arterial orifice and using this to implant the artery into the side of the Dacron graft (Figure 36A-2).

The left renal vein sometimes presents a problem when the aneurysm is high. It is safe to divide this vein to the right of the left adrenal vein and if possible the left gonadal vein. This provides better exposure and apparently does not interfere with the function of the left kidney.

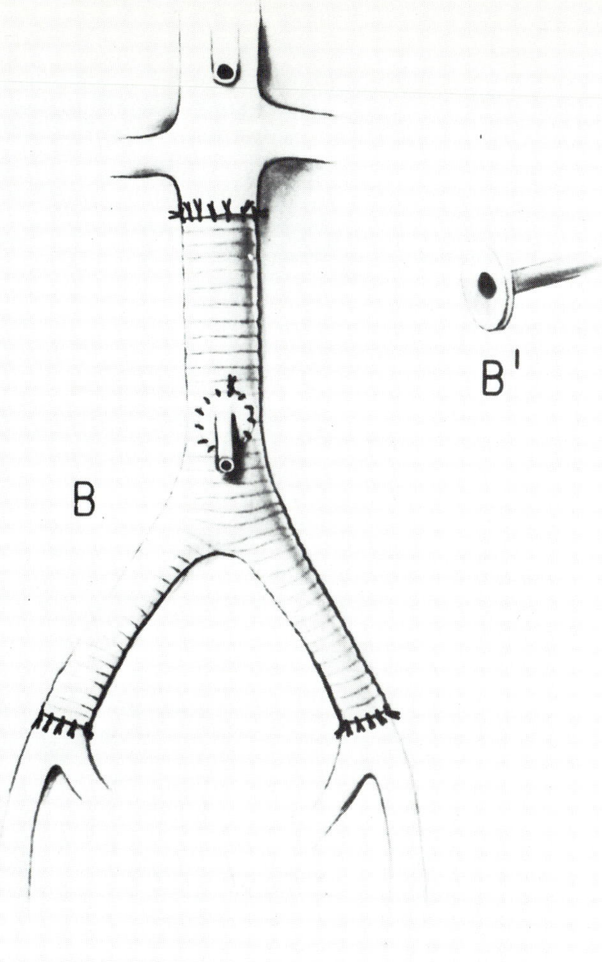

FIGURE 36A–2. If it is decided to reimplant the inferior mesenteric artery into the prosthesis, it is wise to preserve a rim of aortic well around the orifice. This greatly facilitates suturing the artery to the graft.

The lumbar arteries together with the middle sacral artery are controlled from within the sac of the aneurysm. This is best accomplished by oversewing them with a strong suture on a large needle.

If possible it is important to preserve the preaortic plexus of autonomic nerves. Damage to these nerves causes retrograde ejaculation in the male patient (14). Preservation of the sac of the aneurysm aids this objective, but it is particularly important to preserve those nerves which cross in front of the lower aorta and common iliac arteries.

Systemic heparin in a dose of 7000 to 10,000 units is given by the anesthesiologist to every adult patient at the time the aorta is clamped. In the past, local heparin was injected into each iliac artery, but it was soon realized that even after aortic clamping, the collateral circulation was sufficient to equalize the heparin effect in a few minutes on each side of the aortic clamp. Just before the release of the clamps, protamine sulfate is given to counteract the remaining heparin.

HYPOTENSION AT THE TIME OF UNCLAMPING

Sudden removal of the aortic and iliac clamps may cause a major fall in the blood pressure. The following steps are recommended to prevent this: (1) make sure that all lost blood has been replaced before the clamps are removed; (2) give the protamine sulfate slowly; (3) either remove one iliac clamp about 2 minutes before the other, or if both iliac clamps are removed, slowly release the aortic clamp and then manually compress the aorta so that only about 1 pulse beat in 10 is allowed to transmit blood through the graft for 2 minutes or so.

CLOSURE OF THE RETROPERITONEAL TISSUE

This is an important step. The sac is wrapped around the graft. The whole sac can be left in position. This protects the graft, and even partial removal of the sac is rarely practiced today. When this is done, a postoperative x-ray plate will show that the aneurysm is still there. This sometimes requires reassurance of both the radiologist and the referring doctor.

The posterior peritoneum is now closed. At the top, it is important to suture the flap of peritoneum on the side of the duodenum to the peritoneum medial to the inferior mesenteric vein. More distally the peritoneal flaps are larger and the closure is performed more easily. The whole abdomen is now inspected, and the incision in the anterior abdominal wall closed with great care. Paralytic ileus is usual after abdominal aortic surgery, and so a good wound closure is essential.

Postoperative Care

The patient is transferred to an intensive care unit from the recovery room and monitoring continued. Fluid intake must be sufficient to maintain a urine output of at least 30 mL/h. In poor-risk patients, it is wise to keep the patient on a ventilator for the first 24 hours. The nasogastric tube should remain in the stomach until the patient has passed flatus. Most patients can go home on the seventh or eighth postoperative day. As soon as the patient is stable, the Swan-Ganz catheter or central venous pressure line is removed. The Foley catheter can be removed about 48 hours after the operation in most cases. The antibiotics begun the night before surgery are continued for at least 3 days.

Respiratory therapy is important after operation. Pain relief can usually be obtained with meperidine (Demoral).

When the patient goes home, she or he will require an analgesic such as Empracet, and often a hypnotic, such as flurazepam hydrochloride (Dalmane). It is important to stress to patients that it will be at least 3 months before they will fully regain their strength.

Complications

Most complications are due to the patient's primary problem, atherosclerosis, and include myocardial infarction, stroke, mesenteric ischemia, and occlusion of the arteries supplying the lower limbs. Procedures such as preoperative coronary bypass surgery, carotid thromboendarterectomy, and special care to prevent interaoperative embolic or thrombotic occlusion of the lower limb or mesenteric arteries may reduce the incidence of these complications. If after unclamping there is evidence of lower limb ischemia, immediate action is imperative. This usually calls for exposure of the common femoral artery and removal of the arterial obstruction with a Fogarty balloon catheter.

Renal failure used to be more common than it is today. Better hydration before and during surgery has reduced the incidence of this problem, together with better control of the blood pressure during the operation. Should renal failure develop, it is wise to commence dialysis early before more serious problems develop.

Paralytic ileus occurs to some degree in every patient.

Pulmonary atelectosis is common and is best controlled by deep breathing, coughing, and treatment by a respiratory therapist.

References

1. Barratt-Boyes BG: Symptomatology and prognosis of abdominal aortic aneurysm. Lancet 1957, 2:716–717.
2. Dubost C, Allary M, Oeconomos M: Resection of aneurysm of abdominal aorta; re-establishment of continuity by preserved human arterial graft, with result after 5 months. Arch Surg 1952, 64:405–408.
3. Oudot J: La greffe vasculaire dans les thromboses du carrefour aortique. Presse Med 1951, 59:234–236.
4. Voorhees AB, Jaretzki A, Blakemore AH: The use of tubes constructed from Vinyon "N" cloth in bridging arterial defects. Am Surg 1952, 135:332–336.
5. Colt CH: The clinical duration of saccular aortic aneurysms. Q J Med 1927, 20:331–348.
6. Estes JE: Abdominal aortic aneurysm, a study of 102 cases. Circulation 1950, 2:258–264.
7. Rob CG, Williams JP: The diagnosis of aneurysms of the abdominal aorta. J Cardiovasc Surg 1961, 2:55–59.
8. Seldinger SI: Catheter replacement of the needle in percutaneous arteriography: A new technique. Acta Radiol 1953, 39:368–377.
9. Ouriel KO, Ricotta JJ, Adams JT, DeWeese JA: Management of cholelithiasis in patients with abdominal aortic aneurysm. Ann Surg 1983, 198:717–719.
10. Frank IN, Thompson HT, Rob CG, Schwartz SI: Aneurysm of the internal iliac artery. Arch Surg 1961, 83:956–958.
11. Szilagyi DE, Smith RF, DeRusso FF, Elliott JP, Sherrin FW: Contribution of abdominal aortic aneurysmectomy to the prolongation of life. Am Surg 1966, 164:678–686.
12. Berguer R, Schneider J, Wilner HI: Induced thrombosis of inoperable abdominal aortic aneurysm. Surgery 1978, 83:425–429.
13. Leather RP, Shah D, Goldman M, Rosenberg M, Karmody AM: Nonresective treatment of abdominal aortic aneurysms. Arch Surg 1979, 114:1402–1408.
14. May AG, DeWeese JA, Rob CG: Changes in sexual function following operation on the abdominal aorta. Surgery 1969, 65:41–47.

Chapter 36B

AORTIC ANEURYSM: COMPLICATIONS OF ANEURYSMS OF THE ABDOMINAL AORTA AND ILIAC ARTERIES

KENNETH E. McINTYRE, JR., and VICTOR M. BERNHARD

Aneurysms of the abdominal aorta and iliac arteries continue to challenge the vascular surgeon. Because of their insidious onset and growth, these lesions may not become apparent until they produce symptoms. Unfortunately, surgery performed for aneurysms after they have become symptomatic is associated with a higher morbidity and mortality rate than surgery performed electively. For this reason, the goal should be to identify and treat aneurysm disease before symptoms appear.

The natural history of untreated aneurysm has been well documented (1,2,3). Complications may arise from two problems common to all of these lesions. First, with progressive enlargement, tension on the wall becomes greater commensurate with an expanding radius of curvature according to the law of Laplace. Inevitably, the force generated from intraluminal pressure overcomes the tensile strength of the weakened wall, causing disruption. Rupture usually occurs into the retroperitoneum, where surrounding tissue produces temporary tamponade (4). Occasionally, however, perforation may be directed anteriorly into the free peritoneal cavity, or directly into the duodenum or vena cava.

Second, as dilatation occurs, changes in laminar blood flow encourage the formation of laminated clot within the lumen of the aneurysm. In most instances, this laminar clot is stable; however, it may become dislodged and produce distal thromboembolism, causing acute ischemia of one or both lower extremities (5).

Rarely, the laminated clot may expand and encroach upon the lumen, causing total thrombosis of the aneurysm with sudden severe ischemia of the extremities (6,7). This problem is generally related to stasis within the diseased aortic lumen and is commonly associated with poor cardiac output.

It is the goal of this chapter to discuss these complications with the emphasis on earlier diagnosis and treatment to prevent rupture and thromboembolism.

RISK OF ANEURYSM RUPTURE

The most important criterion determining the risk of aneurysm rupture is its size. Rupture occurs when the tangential shear stress on the aortic wall overcomes the tensile strength of the wall itself. According to the law of Laplace, $T = Pr$, where T is the tension on the wall produced by the product of P (dynamic pressure) and r (the radius of curvature). This helps to explain why larger aneurysms are more apt to rupture than smaller aneurysms; also, the risk of rupture is greater in those patients with hypertension.

We know today that an aneurysm with a diameter of 4 cm has less than a 15 percent chance of rupture within 5 years, and an aneurysm with a diameter of greater than 8 cm has more than a 75 percent chance of rupture (8). The risk of rupture seems inordinate to the risk of operation when aneurysms reach 5 cm in diameter; therefore, surgery has been recommended for aortic aneurysms which are greater than this size.

Since there are no reports of aortic aneurysms becoming spontaneously smaller with time, it seems reasonable to operate on smaller aneurysms in otherwise healthy patients. The risk of rupture for aneurysms less than 5 cm is small; however, an average growth rate of 0.4 cm per year has been established (1).

Even though the risk of rupture for small aneurysms is not great, the morbidity and mortality rates from a ruptured aneurysm are excessive when compared with the consistently documented operative mortality rate of less than 5 percent (8–17). Furthermore, small aneurysms may be technically easier to repair. When the aneurysm becomes very large, exposure is more difficult, wider dissection is required, blood loss is increased, and it may be more difficult to interpose a simple tube graft.

Expanding aneurysms produce symptoms due to pressure on adjacent structures such as the lumbar spine and nerve roots which portend frank rupture. Occasionally, the infrarenal aneurysm may have an inflammatory component which causes abdominal pain or obstruction of the ureters. Medial deviation of the ureters seen on an excretory urogram may suggest this diagnosis (18,19,20). Tenderness directly over the aneurysm on palpation may also suggest an inflammatory component.

The most common point of rupture for abdominal aortic aneurysms is into the retroperitoneum. This is fortunate since the surrounding tissue provides a tamponade effect and reduces the rate of blood loss. Occasionally, aneurysms may rupture into the adjacent duodenum or proximal jejunum or even into the adjacent inferior vena cava.

SPONTANEOUS AORTOCAVAL FISTULA

Although an aortocaval fistula may occur in response to penetrating trauma, spontaneous aortocaval fistula is almost always due to erosion of an atherosclerotic abdominal aortic aneurysm into the adjacent vena cava or common iliac vein. The hemodynamic alterations imposed by such a fistula are quite dramatic and demand the utmost in immediate attention to reduce morbidity and mortality. Syme is credited with the first description of an aortocaval fistula in 1831 (21). He reported the classic findings of congestive heart failure associated with a loud abdominal bruit and lower extremity ischemia and edema.

The first surgical attempt at correction was made by Lehman in 1935 (22). Although he was unsuccessful, his attempt set the stage for Beall's successful repair in 1954 (23).

In addition to atherosclerotic degeneration of the aorta, other causes of aneurysm such as syphilis, Ehlers-Danlos syndrome, Marfan's syndrome, and mycotic infection also have been noted to cause erosion into the cava (24). The incidence of aortocaval fistula associated with abdominal aortic aneurysm has been noted to be between 0.3 and 3.0 percent (23,24,25).

The point of erosion of the aneurysm into the vena cava or proximal right iliac vein is usually on its right posterior lateral wall where it produces caval compression (24). Occasionally, fistulization develops between the aneurysm and a left renal vein, which almost invariably is located in an anomalous position behind the aorta (24,26,27).

The clinical findings are always acute and dramatic. Patients may have a known abdominal aortic aneurysm, but more commonly, aortocaval fistula occurs in a patient without this prior diagnosis. A rapidly progressing picture of acute congestive heart failure with a machinery-like bruit and a wide pulse pressure is diagnostic. In association with these findings, the lower extremities may become both ischemic and edematous. The ischemia stems from a "steal" syndrome as blood is short-circuited through the low-resistance fistula rather than flowing distally to supply an arterial bed with a higher resistance. The amount of edema present depends on the degree of vena cava hypertension caused by the compressing aneurysmal bulge and the volume of aortic flow through the fistula which further impedes venous return from the extremities. A fistula developing below a compressing aneurysmal bulge may be associated with more severe evidence of venous obstruction and less prominent cardiac failure.

The rapid onset of severe high-output congestive heart failure is not well tolerated, and standard medical measures for its treatment are not usually helpful. Expeditious surgical intervention is the only hope for patient salvage.

Hemodynamic alterations induced by the fistula affect renal function. Oliguria may occur, again related to renal venous hypertension and impairment of effective renal blood flow. Hematuria has frequently been associated with spontaneous aortocaval fistula and may be a reliable sign, especially when other hemodynamic changes are present (24,27). Hematuria has been ascribed to varices in the renal pelvis or bladder produced by engorgement secondary to venous hypertension. Brewster noted that hematuria was present in 14 of 80 of the reported cases of spontaneous aortocaval fistula (27). The occurrence of hematuria with an aortocaval fistula also suggests the possibility that fistulization of the aneurysm has occurred into an aberrant left renal vein (24,26,28).

Pulmonary embolism has also been reported to occur with spontaneous aortocaval fistula (29,30). The communication between the high-pressure arterial system and the low-pressure venous system provides easy access for thrombotic debris from within the aneurysm to migrate through the arteriovenous orifice into the vena cava and pulmonary tree.

Occasionally, clinical evidence of a fistula is not present prior to surgery and only becomes apparent after the aorta has been opened and laminated thrombus removed during a conventional operation for resection of an abdominal aortic aneurysm. The surgeon should suspect this problem whenever there is the sudden appearance of unexplained venous blood coming from within the aneurysm sac.

Several maneuvers can be employed to facilitate control of hemorrhage during the surgical repair of an aneurysm complicated by aortocaval fistula. It is unwise to try to dissect the aneurysm wall from the vena cava. Fistula closure is more readily accomplished from within the aneurysm sac following arterial occlusion and opening the aorta. If necessary, isolation of the inferior cava just below the renal veins can be easily achieved with a Kocher maneuver to facilitate temporary clamping in order to prevent embolization during aortic manipulation and to reduce retrograde blood loss from the heart. After this degree of major vessel control has been achieved, the aneurysm can be opened. Laminated thrombus and loose debris are quickly removed to better define the fistulous connection. Caval tamponade using sponge sticks from within the aneurysm to compress the cava above and below the aortocaval perforation further controls hemorrhage and facilitates closure of the defect. The use of autotransfusion, as described by Doty et al. (31) and Bernhard (24), is a useful adjunct which may help to reduce the morbidity from multiple blood transfusions. If the defect is very large, Foley catheters with large 30-mL balloons can be inserted through the fistula orifice into the proximal and distal cava and inflated to obstruct the venous lumen. This maneuver controls bleeding until closure can be accomplished.

Considering the acute onset and formidable nature of this problem, the surgical results of treatment are quite good. Mohr reviewed the literature and noted an immediate operative survival rate of 55 percent (32). All patients managed without surgery died within a short time following the onset of symptoms.

PRIMARY AORTOENTERIC FISTULA

Aortoenteric fistula was first described by Sir Astley Cooper in 1829 (33). Little attention was paid to this dramatic problem until Heberer first reported successful surgical correction of a primary aortoenteric fistula in 1957 (34).

Primary aortoenteric fistula in almost all reported cases is related to an aneurysm of the infrarenal abdominal aorta. The intimate juxtaposition of the abdominal aorta and the overlying duodenum appears to contribute to the development of such a fistula due to progressive erosion of an aneurysmal bulge into the overlying bowel. Other rarely reported causes include metastatic carcinoma, duodenal ulcer, and tuberculous mesenteric lymphadenitis, which appear to erode the adjacent walls of these two structures (35,36,37).

Since the development and extensive application of aortic reconstruction, secondary fistula between the prostheses and intestine has become far more common than the primary disease. The appearance of gastrointestinal hemorrhage in a patient with a known aortic prosthesis may bring this diagnosis to mind. However, in a patient without a known abdomminal aortic aneurysm or prior aortic surgery, the more common intrinsic gastrointestinal causes of hematemesis or melena are invariably given primary consideration. Characteristically, the initial presentation is intermittent "herald" bleeding rather than massive continuing blood loss. However, if the true source of bleeding goes undetected, the ultimate outcome is invariably an exsanguinating gastrointestinal hemorrhage.

The diagnosis of primary aortoenteric (usually duodenal) fistula requires demonstration of the underlying aortic pathology. Since this is a rare cause for gastrointestinal bleeding, recognition is usually hampered by a low index of suspicion. Palpation of a pulsatile abdominal mass during preliminary physical examination should immediately suggest the diagnosis. The absence of an actively bleeding site in the esophagus, stomach, or proximal duodenum during upper gastrointestinal endoscopy strengthens this suspicion. If a bleeding erosion is seen in the distal duodenum, especially if an aneurysm is felt, the diagnosis is confirmed. Ultrasound or computed tomographic scanning of the aorta will confirm the nature of the pulsatile mass or rule out an occult nonpalpable aneurysm and should be employed early in the bleeding workup if upper endoscopy is negative. Aortography may also be helpful for demonstrating an aneurysm of the aorta or one of its major branches and should be obtained prior to surgical intervention if the patient's condition is stable. Upper gastrointestinal barium studies usually are not helpful in defining a primary aortoenteric fistula and should be deferred until after endoscopy, scanning, and angiography have failed to identify the cause of the bleeding. This study may demonstrate an extrinsic mass producing a posterior fixed compression of the distal duodenum. On occasion, evidence to support the diagnosis of an aortoenteric fistula or any other cause for intestinal bleeding may be entirely absent, and surgical exploration will be required to find the source and achieve control of hemorrhage.

During surgery, the third and fourth portions of the duodenum should be mobilized completely from the underlying aorta by division of the ligament of Trietz. In addition, any loops of small bowel adhesed to the retroperitoneum should be mobilized if the initial routine exploratory maneuvers do not reveal the cause for bleeding. The pathologic lesion within the aortic wall may be too small to be readily felt by external palpation, thus requiring more direct inspection, as noted by Reckless and in a recent case of our own experience (38). In this instance, a small aneurysmal bleb in the aorta eroding into the duodenum could not be demonstrated by endoscopy, ultrasound, aortography, and prior abdominal exploration and was identified only after dissection of the retroduodenal periaortic area.

Immediate surgical repair of the fistula is the only effective form of treatment. Operative management requires closure of the intestinal defect, resection of the diseased aorta, and reconstruction with a standard retroperitoneal aortic vascular prosthesis. There seems to be a small risk for subsequent graft infection when a prosthesis is placed in the normal anatomic position under these circumstances. Extraanatomic bypass is seldom indicated for this problem. In a collected series, Daugherty et al. reviewed the long-term follow-up on 14 patients who underwent conventional aortic reconstruction and repair of primary aortoenteric fistula (39). A graft-related complication occurred in only one patient. A more recent review by Bunt confirmed these results in 20 of 21 patients (40). However, only slightly more than half of their patients undergoing operation survived.

INFLAMMATORY ANEURYSM

One variant of the common infrarenal abdominal aortic aneurysm has become known as the inflammatory aneurysm because of a dense fibrous reaction around the aortic wall. Very little is known about its pathogenesis. The incidence of this variation has been estimated to be 5 percent of all abdominal aortic aneurysms (19). Medial displacement and/or obstruction of the ureters as well as severe abdominal and back pain in the absence of aneurysm rupture should alert the surgeon to the presence of this problem. In Goldstone's review of this problem, back pain and abdominal pain were the most common symptoms (19). Other symptoms included unilateral leg edema from aneurysmal compression of the iliac vein and constipation. Ureteral deviation with or without obstruction may also be a common presenting problem (18,19,20).

The presence of an inflammatory component can be demonstrated preoperatively by ultrasound, which may reveal a thickened area of relative sonic lucency in the anterior wall of the aneurysmal mass (19,20,35). The characteristic "pearly-white" color of the aneurysm wall and its dense adherence to adjacent structures make the diagnosis obvious at laparotomy.

Although the wall of the inflammatory aneurysm is characteristically thickened, it may be as prone to rupture as the routine aneurysm without an inflammatory component (18,19). The appearance of back or epigastric pain with tenderness over the aneurysm suggests the need for urgent surgical repair; however, most of the time the aneurysm is found to be intact at the time of operation.

The severe perianeurysmal desmoplastic reaction causes significant technical problems during surgery owing to tight adherence to adjacent structures.

Special attention to specific details of operative management is required during repair of an inflammatory abdominal aortic aneurysm. No attempt should be made to separate tightly adherent structures such as the duodenum, the ureters, vena cava, and sigmoid colon from the aneurysm wall, as is done conventionally. Usually, the inflammation ends at or near the renal arteries, and at this point the aorta can be successfully controlled. However, if the inflammatory reaction does not allow the aorta to be safely encircled below the renal arteries, more proximal control may be accomplished at the level of the diaphragmatic hiatus through the lesser omentum. Similarly, the dense inflammatory reaction usually does not involve the iliac arteries or iliac veins. Once vascular control has been established, the aneurysm wall is excised longitudinally, enabling the adherent structures to be retracted laterally with the aneurysm wall. The remainder of the operation progresses in a standard fashion.

INFECTED ANEURYMS

Secondary infection of an established aneurysm or aneurysm formation secondary to a septic process in the aortic wall is far less frequent and dramatic than either thrombosis or rupture.

However, a morbid outcome is inevitable unless the problem is recognized and surgically managed in a timely fashion (41,42,43,44,45).

The first report of an infected arterial aneurysm was described by Koch in 1851 (46). However, Osler, in 1885, was the first to use the term "mycotic" to describe this entity (47). Studies of the pathogenesis of this problem suggest that the most common mechanism involves hematogenous seeding of an abnormal arterial wall from a remote bacteremic focus (43,44). Infection of a relatively normal aortic wall with subsequent degeneration may come from septic arterial emboli. Direct extension from an adjacent infectious process may directly involve a normal or abnormal vessel. Acute bacterial infection of the aortic wall may lead to erosion and rupture even without aneurysmal dilatation or formation of a pseudoaneurysm.

Clinical features which help to make this diagnosis are a history of fever without obvious cause in a patient with a newly diagnosed abdominal aortic aneurysm. In general, these patients have no other evidence of peripheral vascular disease. Both Jarrett and Scher, in their reviews, found a higher percentage of women than the expected male prevalence in atherosclerotic abdominal aortic aneurysms (42,45).

A variety of organisms have been cultured from infected abdominal aortic aneurysms. Jarrett et al. reported a low incidence of aneurysms infected with gram-negative organisms; however, the mortality rate from such infections was quite high (42). *Salmonella* has been found to be the most common arterial pathogen in these infections (44).

Adequate debridement of the infected aortic wall and periaortic tissue is required to control the infectious process and permit reliable suture closure of the proximal aortic stump. Incomplete removal of infected aortic wall will result in early disruption or later aneurysm formation in the proximal aortic stump. Revascularization by extraanatomic techniques such as axillofemoral bypass is required and should be carried out prior to aneurysm excision if the patient is stable and the diagnosis is firmly established. The common-iliac-to-common-iliac anastomosis as described by Ehrenfeld provides an effective and convenient crossover conduit from an axillofemoral bypass graft and eliminates the need for prosthetic material within the abdomen (48). Despite adequate treatment, the mortality rate remains high, Delay in diagnosis as well as the type of organism which has caused the infection affects this mortality rate.

ILIAC ANEURYSMS

Aneurysms of the iliac arteries are most commonly associated with the extension of aneurysmal disease of the abdominal aorta which usually stops at the iliac bifurcation. However, at times, diffuse arteriomegaly may extend to the femoral arteries, causing aneurysmal dilatation of both the external iliac and hypogastric arteries. Aneurysmal dilatation of an iliac artery as an isolated lesion is distinctly uncommon (49,50).

Iliac aneurysms have the same propensity for rupture as other aneurysms; however, the likelihood of this outcome may be proportionately less since there is reduced tangential wall stresses owing to their smaller diameter. Iliac aneurysms may cause localizing symptoms because of their close approximation to adjacent structures such as iliac veins, lumbar nerve roots, or ureters, and the rigid confining walls of the pelvis (49,50,51,52). Compression of the pelvic colon by an iliac aneurysm may cause obstipation or may lead to erosion into the adjacent bowel to produce an iliac-enteric fistula (49,53,54).

The diagnosis of iliac aneurysm by abdominal palpation is much less reliable than for aortic aneurysm owing to the former's deep position in the pelvis. Consequently, these lesions may go undetected until rapid expansion or rupture occur. However, hypogastric aneurysms may be identified by palpation of a pulsatile mass during rectal examination, and plain abdominal radiographs may demonstrate aneurysmal calcification within the pelvis (51,52). The excretory urogram or barium enema may also be helpful by delineating extrinsic compression from an aneurysmal mass. Computerized tomography or ultrasonography provide better estimates of aneurysm size than angiography; however, arteriography is essential to delineate the anatomy of the runoff and to define anatomic variations.

Iliac aneurysms, like those in any other location, are lined with laminated thrombus. Thus, on rare occasions, the first presenting symptom of an iliac aneurysm may be distal thromboembolism, causing obstruction of the major limb vessels and acute leg and foot ischemia. The distal microvasculature may also be affected, producing the "blue toe" or "trash foot" syndrome (55,56). Newly discovered embolic lesions in the distal extremity should suggest the possibility of a proximal aneurysm, especially in patients with no history of prior atherosclerotic occlusive disease and no other obvious sources of emboli. The frequent association of other aneurysms with an abdominal aortic aneurysm supports the need to extend ultrasound examination of the abdomen into the pelvis and popliteal fossae in these cases and to supplement this noninvasive examination with arteriography.

Surgical repair of aneurysms of the common or external iliac arteries does not require any unusual techniques other than the application of standard procedures for excision and graft interposition. On the other hand, hypogastric aneurysms may be very difficult to handle due to their location deep within the pelvis, their adherence to adjacent vital structures, and the entrance of branch vessels into the deep side of the sac. In general, excision of these lesions should be avoided since damage to ureters, pelvic nerve trunks, and deep pelvic veins may occur. A small aneurysm may be effectively treated by ligation of its point of origin from the common iliac to disconnect it from arterial inflow pressure and allow it to thrombose. Larger aneurysms which require debulking to reduce pressure symptoms can be effectively managed by endoaneurysmorrhaphy. After the inflow has been controlled, the dome of the sac is widely incised in an area distant from vital structures. Laminated thrombus is evacuated and the back-bleeding branches are oversewn from within the sac. Autotransfusion is a useful adjunct to salvage blood and improve visualization of the operative field.

THROMBOEMBOLISM

The athermatous and thrombotic debris which line abdominal aortic and iliac aneurysms may embolize into the distal extremity vessels, although this is a much less common occurrence than embolization from popliteal aneurysms. Thrombosis may be less common due to the larger caliber of the proximal arteries and their higher flow rates.

More commonly, embolization of atherosclerotic debris causes multiple localized and limited areas of digital gangrene, often referred to as "trash foot," a descriptive term used to describe this phenomenon. Often, these patients may have no other evidence of peripheral arterial occlusive disease until they present with the acute onset of punctate areas of necrosis in the foot and toes. This phenomenon may occur with or without loss of pedal pulses. Embolization may be tolerated quite well depending on the amount of embolic debris and the adequacy of the collateral circulation. However, trash foot is always accompanied by pain in the distribution of the ischemic areas.

A thorough search for a source of emboli must be undertaken including evaluation of the heart and vascular tree. Although two-dimensional echocardiography has often been recommended for evaluation, we have found it to be distinctly nonproductive in patients with normal sinus rhythm and a normal ejection fraction. Even in patients with an akinetic segment of myocardium, it is extremely difficult to define an intraventricular thrombus by this technique.

Silent aortic, iliac, femoral, or popliteal aneurysm can be discovered with ultrasound examinations of the abdomen and popliteal fossae. Angiography is a valuable technique for demonstrating these occult sources of emboli and is a useful adjunct in preparation for aortic or iliac aneurysm resection. While the diagnostic workup is in progress, systemic heparinization should be employed to prevent further embolization and distal clot propagation. Often, systemic heparin will sufficiently relieve ischemia so that limb viability is not in question and operation can be undertaken electively rather than emergently. Thrombolytic therapy should not be considered under these circumstances since the induction of a systemic thrombolytic state may carry a greater risk of fragmenting the larger, more proximal thrombus and producing a shower of distal emboli.

SUMMARY

Aneurysms of the abdominal aorta and iliac arteries continue to pose a challenge to the surgeon. When repaired surgically under elective conditions, the morbidity and mortality rates of surgical results are quite acceptable. Often, however, aneurysms are not recognized until complications occur. These complications may be related to rupture, thrombosis, embolism, or fistulization into adjacent structures. The mortality rates from these complications are uniformly fatal without surgical attention. However, with prompt diagnosis and timely surgical intervention, such difficult problems as aortocaval or primary aortoenteric fistula can be dealt with satisfactorily.

References

1. Bernstein EF, Dilley RB, Goldberger LE, et al: Growth rates of small abdominal aortic aneurysms. Surgery 1976, 80:765.
2. Darling RC, Messina CR, Brewster DC, et al: Autopsy study of unoperated abdominal aortic aneurysms: The case for early resection. Circulation 1976, 56(suppl II):161.
3. Szilagyi ED, Elliott JP, Smith RF: Clinical fate of the patient with asymptomatic abdominal aortic aneurysm and unfit for surgical treatment. Arch Surg 1972, 104:600.
4. Fitzgerald JF, Stillman RM, Powers JC: A suggested classification and reappraisal of mortality statistics for ruptured atherosclerotic infrarenal aortic aneurysms. Surg Gynecol Obstet 1978, 146:344.
5. Elliott JP, Hageman JH, Szilagyi E, et al: Arterial embolization: Problems of source, multiplicity, recurrence and delayed treatment. Surgery 1980, 88:833.
6. Danto LA, Fry WJ, Kraft RO: Acute aortic thrombosis. Arch Surg 1972, 104:569.
7. Johnson JM, Gaspar MR, Movius HJ, et al: Sudden complete thrombosis of aortic and iliac aneurysms. Arch Surg 1974, 108:792.
8. Rutherford RB: Infrarenal aortic aneurysms. In Rutherford RB (ed): *Vascular Surgery*. Philadelphia, Saunders, 1984.
9. Bickerstaff LK, Hollier LH, Van Peenen HG, et al: Abdominal aortic aneurysms: The changing natural history. J Vasc Surg 1984, 1:6.
10. Crawford ES, Saleh SA, Babb JW III, et al: Infrarenal abdominal aortic aneurysm: Factors influencing survival after operations performed over a 25-year period. Ann Surg 1981, 193:699.
11. Darling RC: Ruptured arteriosclerotic abdominal aortic aneurysms. Am J Surg 1970, 119:397.
12. Estes JE Jr: Abdominal aortic aneurysm: A study of one hundred and two cases. Circulation 1950, 2:258.
13. Foster JH, Bolasny BL, Gobbel WG Jr, et al: Comparative study of elective resection and expectant treatment of abdominal aortic aneurysm. Surg Gynecol Obstet 1969, 129:1.
14. Garrett HE, Anduson J: Management of the Ruptured Abdominal Aortic Aneurysm. In Bergan JJ and Yao JST (eds): *Surgery of the Aorta and Its Branches*. New York, Grune & Stratton, 1979.
15. Hicks GL, Eastland MW, DeWeese JA, et al: Survival improvement following aortic aneurysm resection. Ann Surg 1975, 181:863.
16. Szilagyi DE, Smith RF, DeRusso FJ, et al: Contribution of abdominal aortic aneurysmectomy to prolongation of life. Ann Surg 1966, 164:678.
17. Wright IS, Urdaneta E, Wright B: Re-opening the case of the abdominal aortic aneurysm. Circulation 1956, 13:754.
18. Crawford JL, Stowe CL, Safi HJ, et al: Inflammatory aneurysms of the aorta. J Vasc Surg 1985, 2:113.
19. Goldstone J, Malone JM, Moore WS: Inflammatory aneurysms of the abdominal aorta. Surgery 1978, 83:425.
20. Henry LE, Doust B, Korns ME, et al: Abdominal aortic aneurysm and retroperitoneal fibrosis. Arch Surg 1978, 113:1456.
21. Syme J: Case of spontaneous varicose aneurism. Edinburg Med J 1831, 36:104.
22. Lehman EP: Spontaneous arteriovenous fistula between the abdominal aorta and the inferior vena cava. Ann Surg 1938, 108:694.
23. Beall AC, Cooley DA, Morris GC, et al: Perforation of arteriosclerotic aneurysms into inferior vena cava. Arch Surg 1963, 86:137.
24. Bernhard VM: Aortocaval fistulas. In Haimovici H (ed): *Vascular Emergencies*. New York, Appleton-Century-Crofts, 1982.
25. Dardik H, Dardik I, Strom MG: Intravenous rupture of arteriosclerotic aneurysms of the abdominal aorta. Surgery 1976, 80:647.
26. Yashar JJ, Hallman GL, Cooley DA: Fistula between aneurysm of aorta and left renal vein. Arch Surg 1969, 99:546.
27. Brewster DC, Ottinger LW, Darling RC: Hematuria as a sign of aortocaval fistula. Ann Surg 1977, 186(6):772.
28. Suzuki M, Collins GM, Bassinger GT, et al: Aorto-left renal vein fistula: An unusual complication of abdominal aortic aneurysm. Ann Surg 1976, 184(1):31.

29. Baker WH, Sharzer LA, Ehrenhaft JL: Aortocaval fistula as a complication of abdominal aortic aneurysm. Surgery 1972, 72:933.
30. Hafner CD, Cranley JJ, Krause RJ, et al: Acute abdominal aortal-vena caval fistula. Vasc Surg 1969, 3:149.
31. Doty DB, Wright CB, Lamberth WC, et al: Aortocaval fistula associated with aneurysm of the abdominal aorta: Current management using autotransfusion techniques. Surgery 1978, 84(2):250.
32. Mohr LL, Smith LL: Arteriovenous fistula from rupture of abdominal aortic aneurysm. Arch Surg 1975, 110:806.
33. Cooper A: The Lectures of Sir Astley Cooper on the Principles and Practice of Surgery. London, Westley, 1829.
34. Heberer E: Diagnosis and treatment of aneurysms of the abdominal aorta. Germ Med Monthly 1957, 2:203.
35. Frosch HL, Horowitz W: Rupture of the abdominal aorta into duodenum (through a sinus tract created by a tuberculous lymphadenitis). Ann Intern Med 1944, 21:481.
36. Geary SR, Walunth EZ: Aortoduodenal fistula secondary to metastatic carcinoma, angiographic demonstration. JAMA 1976, 235:2510.
37. Tozer EA: A case of tuberculous aneurysm of the abdominal aorta with rupture into the duodenum. Br Med J 1914, 2:1022.
38. Reckless JPD, McColl I, Taylor GW: Aorto-enteric fistulae: An uncommon complication of abdominal aortic aneurysms. Br J Surg 1972, 59:458.
39. Daugherty M, Shearer GR, Ernst CB: Primary aortoduodenal fistula: Extraanatomic vascular reconstruction not required for successful management. Surgery 1979, 86:399.
40. Bunt TJ: Synthetic vascular graft infections. II. Graft enteric erosions and graft-enteric fistulas. Surgery 1983, 94:1.
41. Brown SL, Busuttil RW, Baker JD, et al: Bacteriologic and surgical determinants of survival in patients with mycotic aneurysms. J Vasc Surg 1984, 1:541.
42. Jarrett F, Darling RC, Mundth ED, et al: Experience with infected aneurysms of the abdominal aorta. Arch Surg 1975, 110:1281.
43. Johansen K, Devin J: Mycotic aortic aneurysms. Arch Surg 1983, 118:583.
44. Perry MO: Infected aortic aneurysms. J Vasc Surg 1985, 2:597.
45. Scher LA, Brender BJ, Goldenkranz RJ, et al: Infected aneurysm of the abdominal aorta. Arch Surg 1980, 115:975.
46. Koch L: Ueber das Aneurysma der Anteria Meseraich, Dissertation. Erlangen, JJ Barfies, 1851.
47. Osler W: Gulstonian Lectures on Malignant Endocarditis. Br Med J 1885, 1:467.
48. Ehrenfeld WK, Wilbur BG, Olcott CN, et al: Autogenous tissue reconstruction in the management of infected prosthetic grafts. Surgery 1979, 85:82.
49. Bernhard VM: Excision of iliac aneurysm. In Nyhus LM, Baker RJ (eds): *Mastery of Surgery*, vol. 2. Boston/Toronto: Little, Brown, 1984, pp 1395–1401.
50. Markowitz AM, Norman JC: Aneurysms of the iliac artery. Ann Surg 1961, 154:777.
51. Short DW: Aneurysms of the internal iliac artery. Br J Surg 1966, 53:17.
52. Silver D, Anderson EE, Porter JM: Isolated hypogastric artery aneurysm: Review and report of three cases. Arch Surg 1967, 95:308.
53. Abramson PD, Jameson JB: Rupture of iliac aneurysm into duodenum. Arch Surg 1955, 71:658.
54. Atin HL: Rupture of an iliac aneurysm into the sigmoid colon. N Eng J Med 1958, 258:366.
55. Kempczinski RF: Lower extremity arterial emboli from ulcerating atherosclerotic plaques. JAMA 1979, 241:807.
56. Kwaan JH, Connolly JE: Peripheral atheroembolism. Arch Surg 1977, 112:987.

Chapter 37

THORACOABDOMINAL AORTIC ANEURYSM

E. STANLEY CRAWFORD and JOHN L. CRAWFORD

Thoracoabdominal aortic aneurysms are those that involve both the thoracic and abdominal aorta in continuity. The latter segment may not but usually does involve the segment from which the visceral vessels arise (Figures 37-1 to 37-4). Graft replacement treatment of thoracoabdominal aortic aneurysm requires thoracoabdominal incisions for exposure and for restoration of flow to the visceral vessels and the lower extremities (1–4). Aneurysms involving the upper abdominal aorta from which the visceral vessels arise pose similar requirements for effective treatment and are considered in the category of thoracoabdominal aortic aneurysms although they may be limited to the abdominal aorta (1) (Figures 37-5 and 37-6). Thus this chapter is concerned with the treatment of aneurysms involving the above specified aortic segment. It is emphasized that involvement at this level may be only a part of a more complex disease consisting of aneurysms involving either extensive segments of the

(*Continued on p. 493.*)

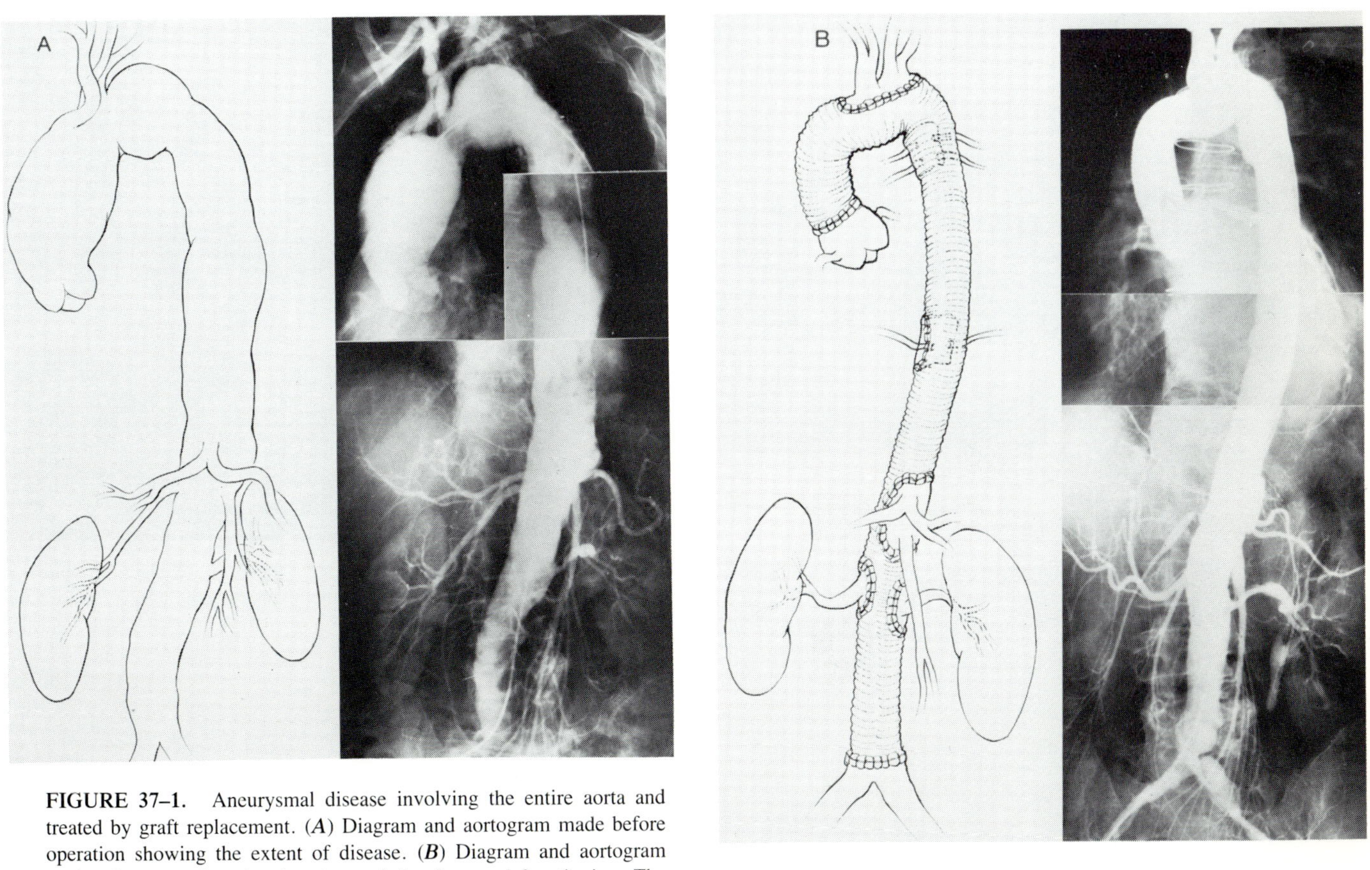

FIGURE 37–1. Aneurysmal disease involving the entire aorta and treated by graft replacement. (***A***) Diagram and aortogram made before operation showing the extent of disease. (***B***) Diagram and aortogram made after operation showing the graft in place and functioning. The ascending and transverse aortic arch was replaced first, and the remainder of the aorta was replaced at a second operation. [Copyright © Baylor College of Medicine 1984. Used with permission.]

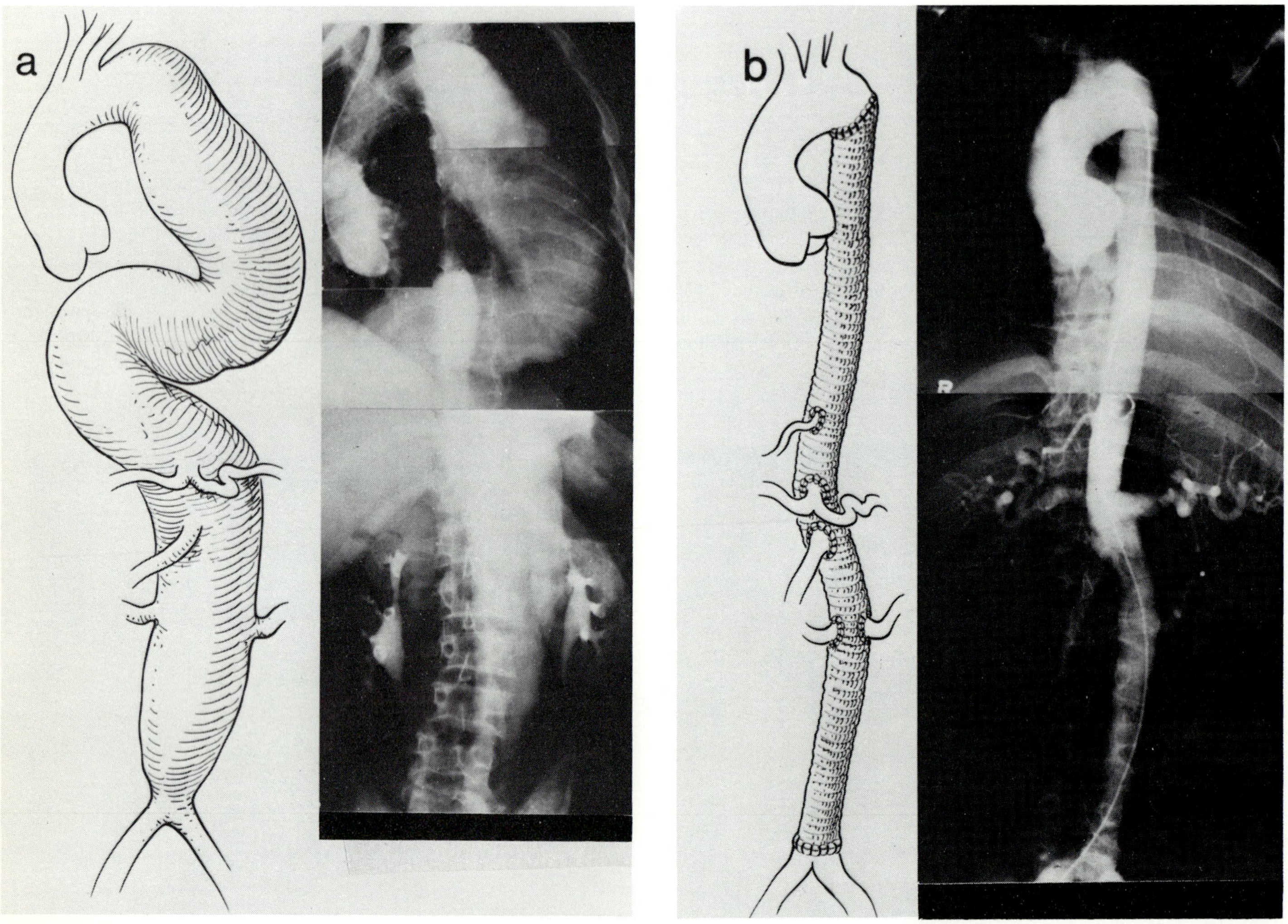

FIGURE 37–2. Aneurysmal disease involving most of the descending thoracic and abdominal aorta and treated by graft replacement. (*A*) Diagram and aortogram made before operation showing the extent of disease. (*B*) Diagram and aortogram made after operation showing the graft in place. [Copyright © Baylor College of Medicine 1982. Used with permission.]

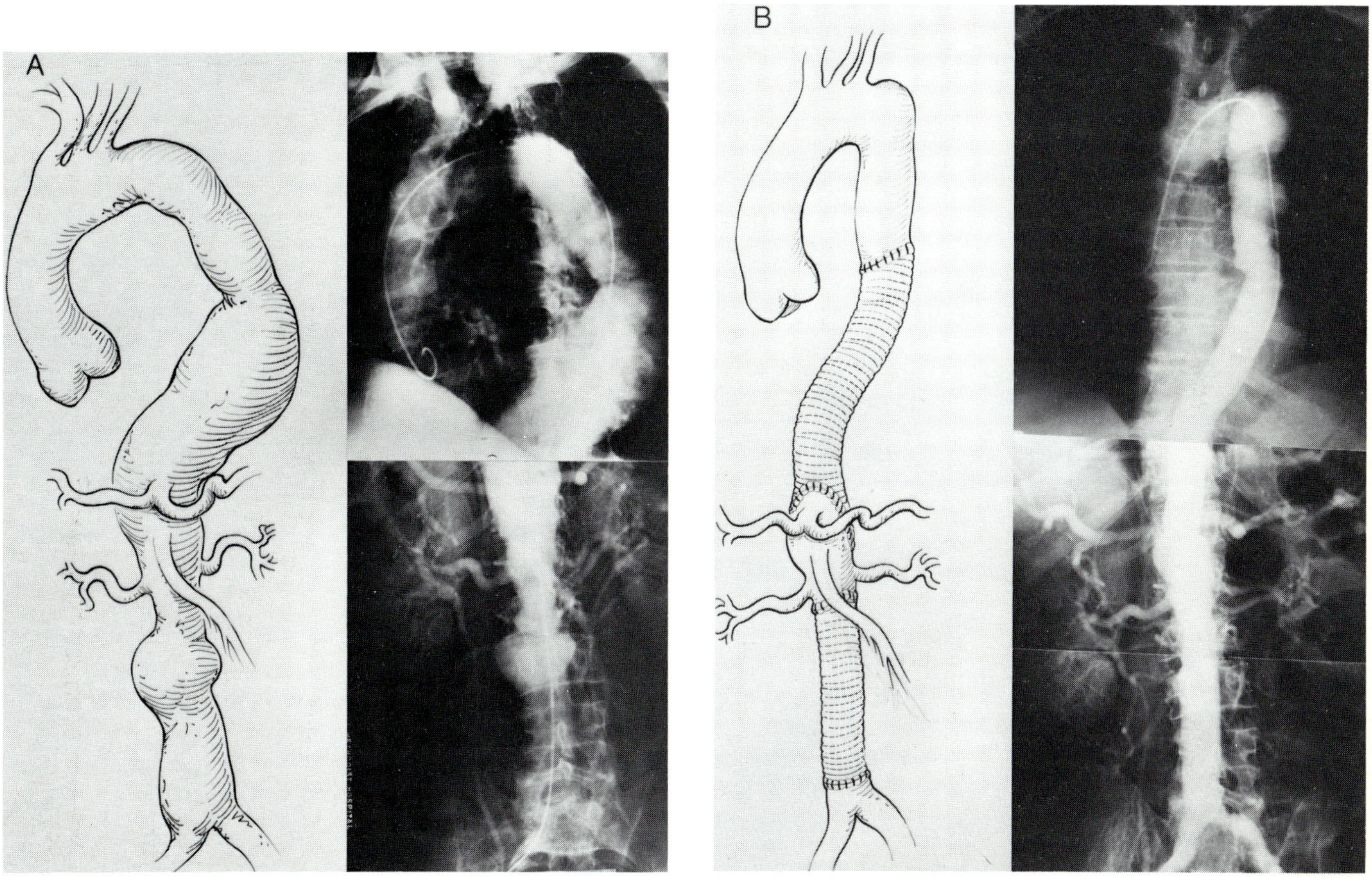

FIGURE 37–3. A thoracoabdominal aortic aneurysm involving the descending thoracic aorta and upper abdominal aorta, and a separate infrarenal abdominal aortic aneurysm; they were treated by separate operations. (*A*) Diagram and aortogram showing the extent of disease. (*B*) Diagram and aortogram made after the second operation showing the grafts in place and functioning. [Copyright © Baylor College of Medicine 1983. Used with permission.]

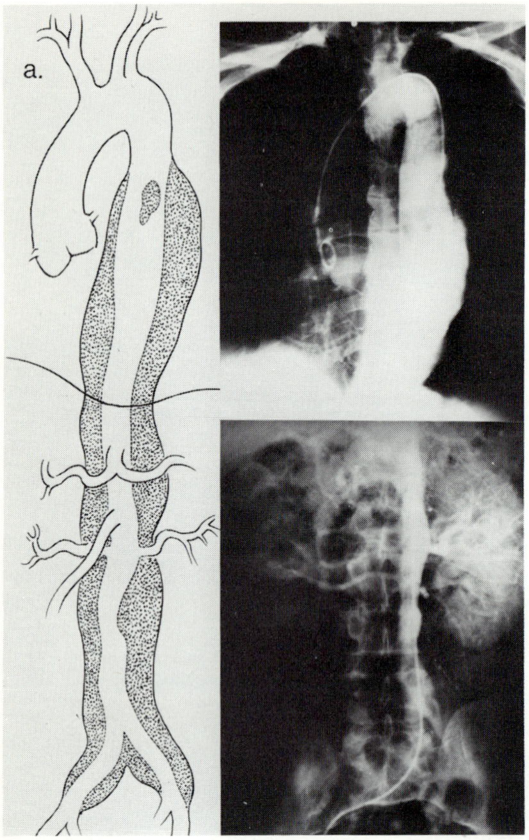

FIGURE 37–4. One method of treating extensive thoracoabdominal aortic aneurysm resulting from chronic aortic dissection. (*A*) Diagram and aortogram showing the extent of aneurysmal disease. (*B*) Drawing showing the method of treatment. (*C*) Diagram and aortogram made after operation. [Copyright © Baylor College of Medicine. Used with permission.]

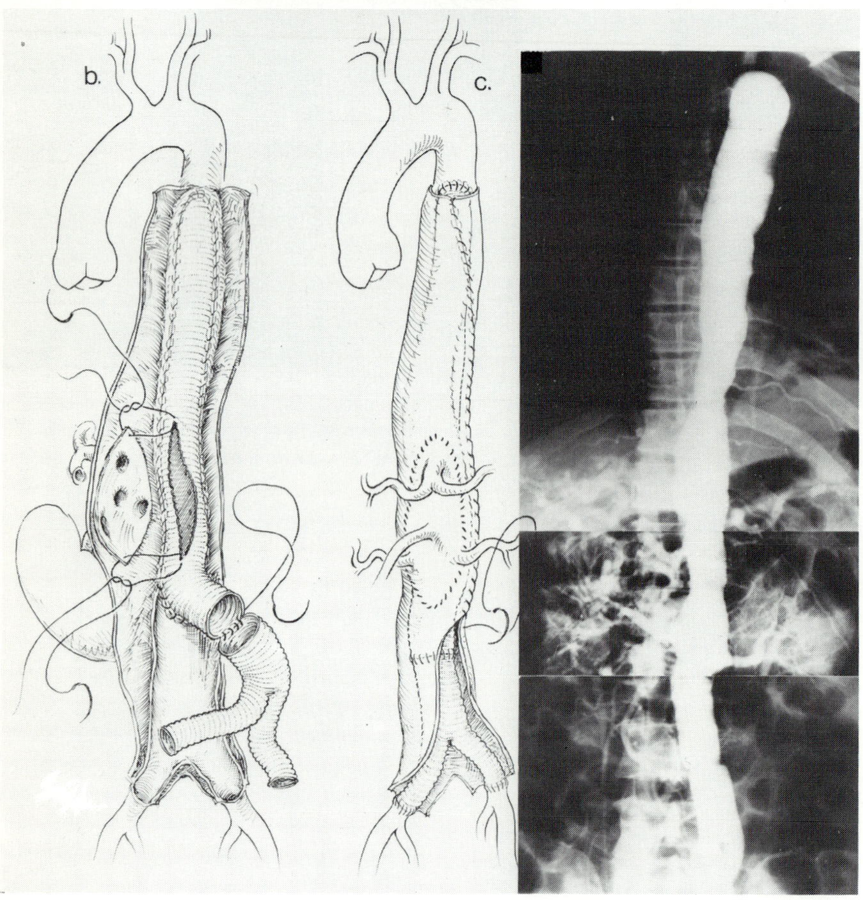

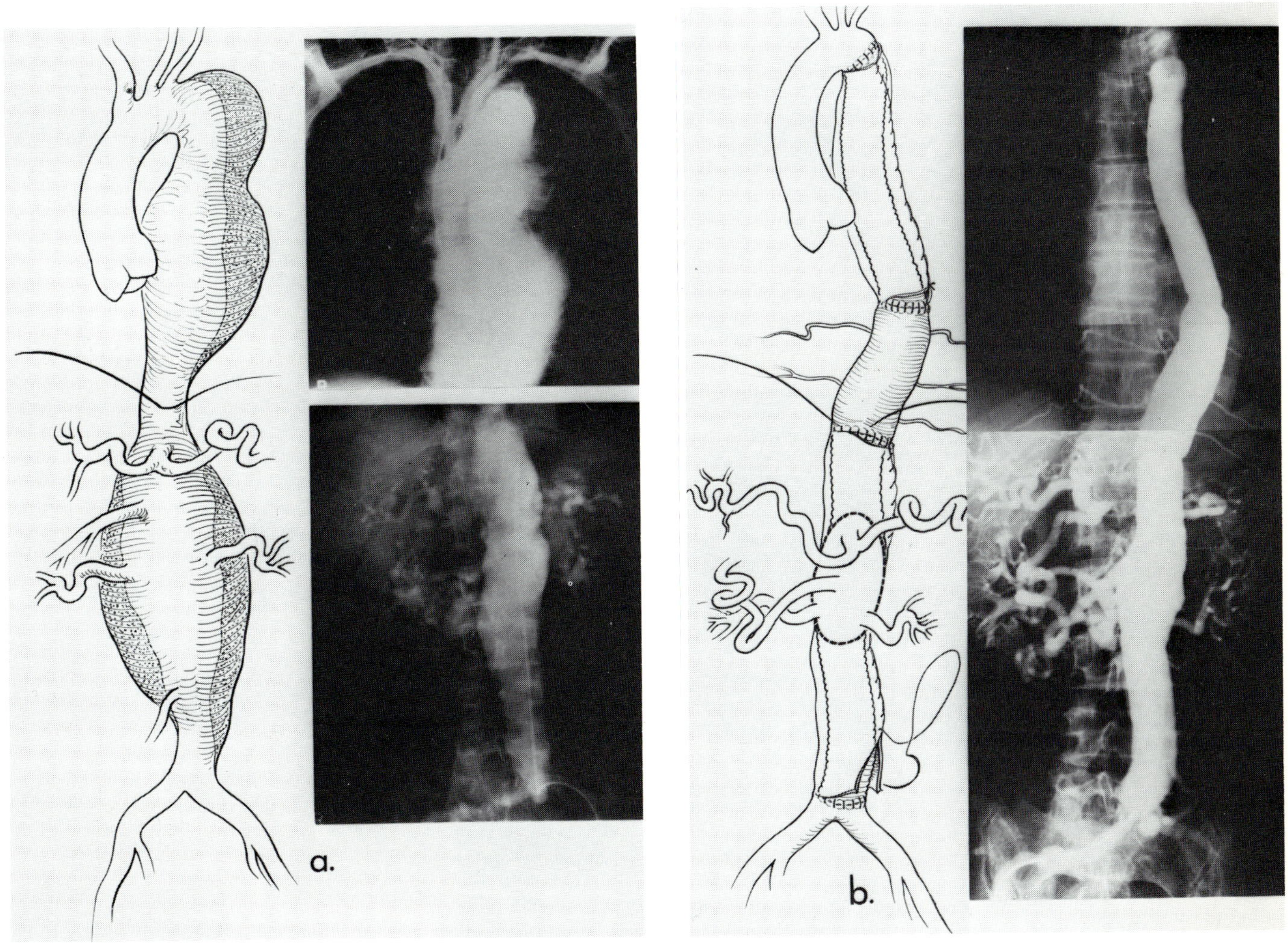

FIGURE 37–5. Treatment of a patient with separate aneurysm of the descending thoracic aorta and the abdominal aorta. (*A*) Diagram and aortogram made before operation. (*B*) Diagram and aortogram made after separate operations, showing the two grafts in place and functioning, with intercostal arteries located between the grafts. [Copyright © Baylor College of Medicine. Used with permission.]

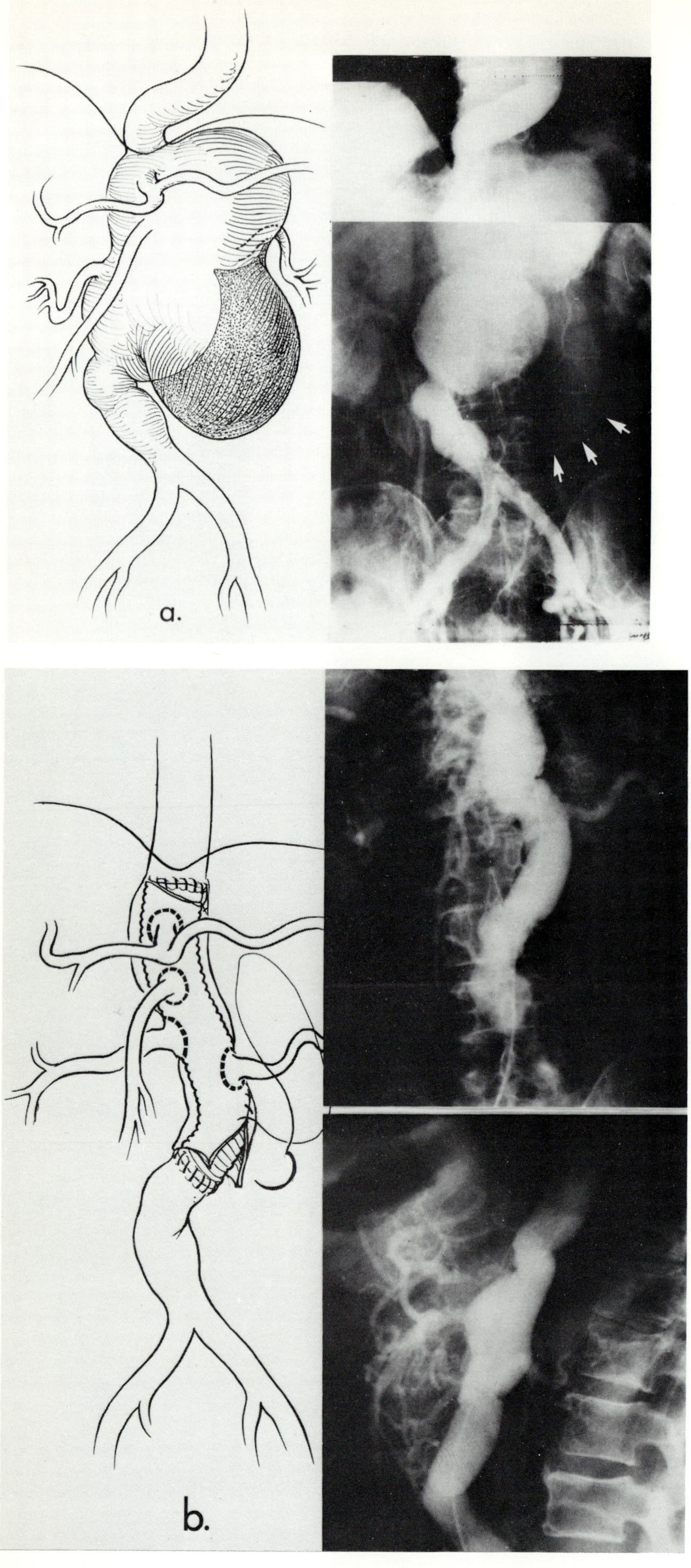

FIGURE 37–6. Treatment of a large aneurysm involving the upper abdominal aorta. (***A***) Diagram and aortogram made before operation showing the location and extent of disease. (***B***) Diagram and aortogram made after operation showing the graft in place. [Copyright © Baylor College of Medicine. Used with permission.]

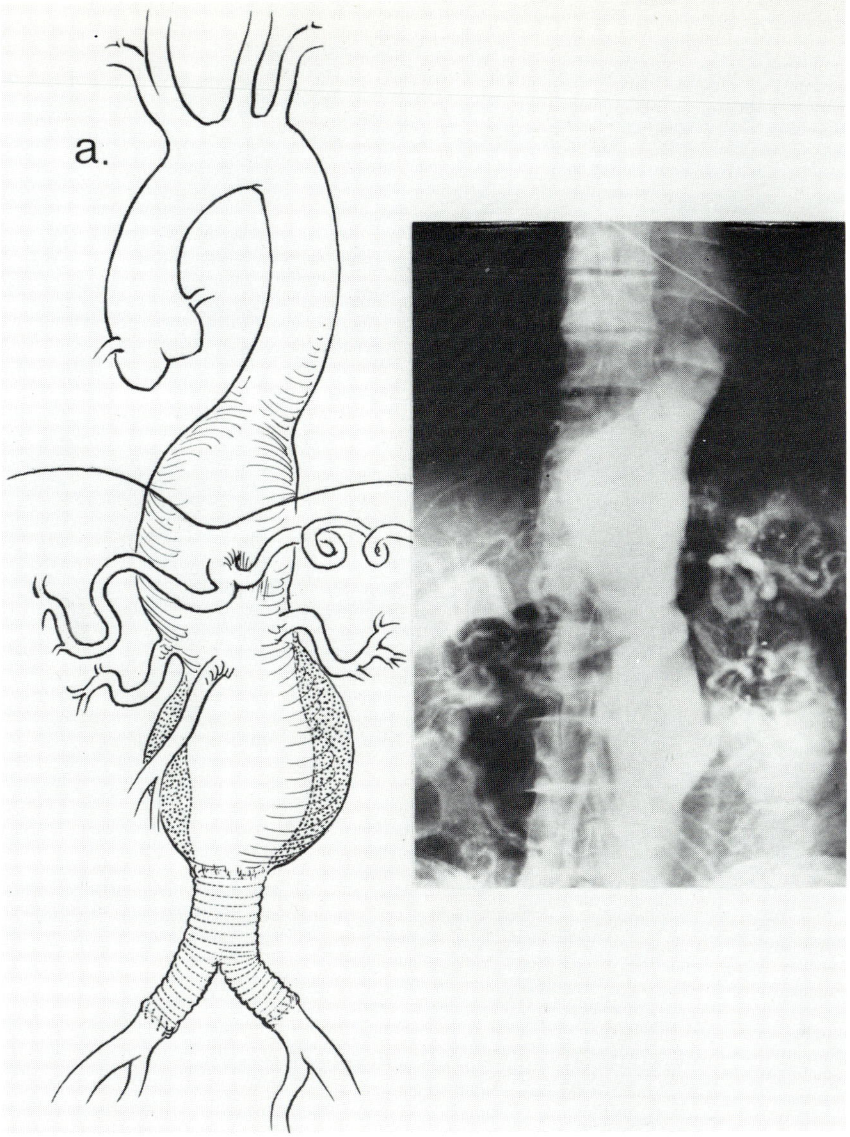

FIGURE 37–7. Aneurysmal disease involving the distal thoracic and abdominal aorta and treated elsewhere by infrarenal abdominal aortic replacement. (*A*) Diagram and aortogram showing the location and extent of disease before the second operation. (*Continued on p. 494.*)

aorta or multiple distant segments that require multiple operations performed at intervals (Figures 37-1, 37-3, and 37-6)(5). In our experience with 544 patients submitted to operation for thoracoabdominal aortic aneurysm, other aortic segments were involved in 284 patients (52 percent). For example, of those having thoracoabdominal operations for abdominal aortic aneurysm involving the visceral branches, 67 had a separate operation at another time for aneurysm of the descending thoracic aorta (Figure 37-5). Similarly, the infrarenal abdominal aorta previously had been or subsequently was removed in 103 patients submitted to operation for aneurysm involving the descending thoracic and upper abdominal aorta (Figure 37-3). In other patients, the infrarenal segment of thoracoabdominal aortic aneurysm had been removed, in the hope that the proximal segment would not enlarge and cause problems (Figure 37-7). The ascending aorta was replaced in 23 patients, the ascending and transverse aortic arch in 26 (Figure 37-1), and other segments in 65. Thus the aneurysmal disease was more diffuse in these patients than implied by the title of this chapter; in fact, the entire aorta was removed in 16 patients (Figure 37-1), and all but the transverse aortic arch in another 13 patients.

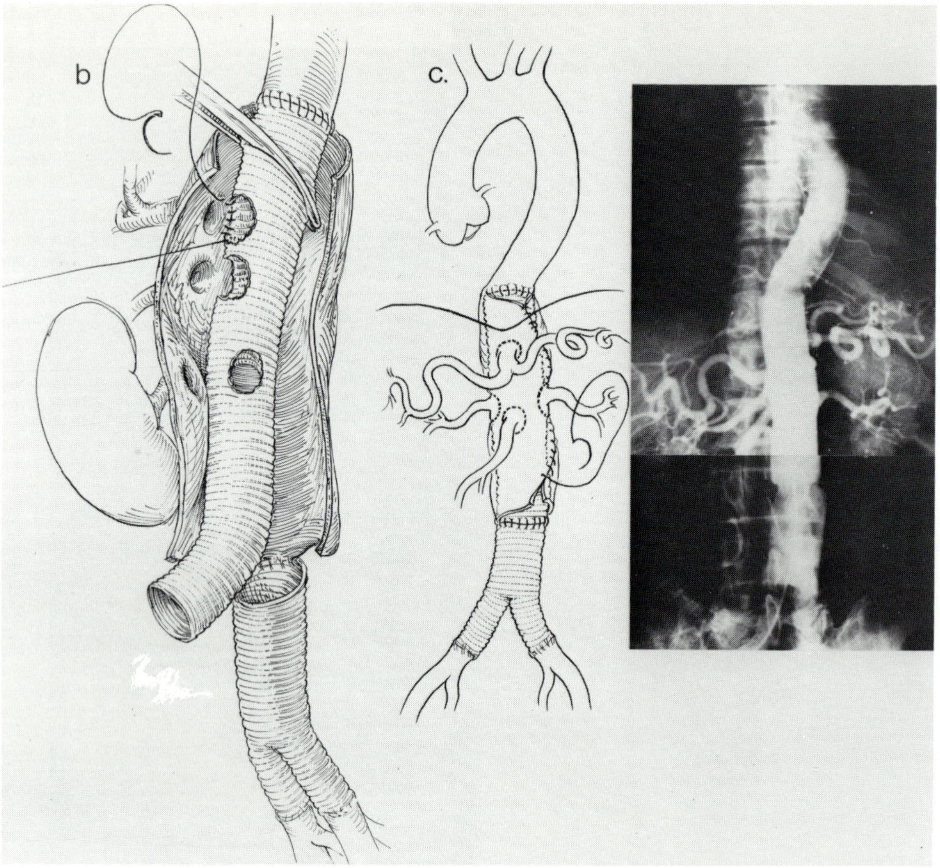

FIGURE 37–7 (*continued*). (*B*) Drawing showing the technique of operation. (*C*) Diagram and aortogram made after the second operation showing grafts in place. [Copyright © Baylor College of Medicine. Used with permission.]

Clinical Features of the Disease

Two-thirds of our patients were men, and one-third were women. Their ages did not differ with the sex of the patient and ranged from 19 to 86, with a median age of 65 years. The most common etiologies were medial degenerative disease (82 percent) and aortic dissection (11 percent). Less common causes were mycotic, false, trauma, and aortitis. Marfan's syndrome was present in 26 of our patients with the first two etiologies, and these were the youngest patients. Associated disease was common; listed in order of frequency such diseases were hypertension, peripheral vascular disease, heart disease, chronic obstructive pulmonary disease, and renal insufficiency.

The disease process produces a pulsating expansile mass that consumes space and presses on adjacent structures. The latter may cause airway or esophageal obstruction, hoarseness from airway obstruction or left recurrent nerve paralysis, hemoptysis, or hematemesis. Back pain may result from erosion of the spine. Chest and abdominal pain may result from simple expansion of the lesion with associated local pressure or stretching. The ultimate fate of these lesions is rupture. Studies of the natural course of aneurysmal disease of both the infrarenal abdominal aorta and descending thoracic aorta indicate that this fatal complication occurs in over half the patients within 2 years (1). Similar results may be expected from thoracoabdominal aortic aneurysms according to our own studies in 105 patients not treated surgically. The rupture is usually into the chest or abdominal cavities; but in our patients, rupture has also occurred into lung, bronchus, esophagus, duodenum, vena cava, and right iliac vein.

Diagnosis

Seventy-five percent of our patients were symptomatic; chest, abdominal, or flank pain was the predominant symptom. Tenderness in the abdominal segment of aneurysm was common, and rupture into either the chest, the abdomen, or other structures had occurred in 4 percent of our patients. The diagnosis was suspected in many cases by palpating an aneurysm in the abdomen in a patient whose chest roentgenogram suggested the presence of an associated thoracic aortic aneurysm. The disease was evident in other patients on plain roentgenograms of the chest, abdomen, or spine made for other reasons, or was found by special examination of the gastrointestinal tract, kidney, ureter, and bladder. Sonographic studies were also helpful in detecting aneurysmal disease of the abdominal aorta, but these studies were less reliable because of air accumulations, inexperience of the operator, and the fact that such studies are less applicable to the chest by present techniques.

Diagnosis is made definitively by CT scanning or aortography. Although we frequently use both to evaluate the actual size of the aneurysm, particularly the suprarenal segment, we always employ aortography because it better displays the lesion for planning and execution of therapy and shows the frequently associated occlusive disease in the visceral and distal vessels. Because of the frequency of either extensive aneurysmal disease or multiple lesions, total aortic examination, preferably by aortography using regular dosage of contrast media delivered by catheter under pressure, is employed. Digital subtraction technique is employed in patients with impaired renal function to reduce the volume of contrast substance needed for examination. This method of examination has the disadvantage of subtracting the calcification frequently seen in the aneurysmal wall. The actual size of the aneurysm thus is not appreciated in this examination in patients whose aneurysms contain clot.

Treatment

The only effective method of treatment is graft replacement, and its application frequently requires either a one-stage replacement of an extensive segment of the aorta or replacement of several segments at different intervals (2,4,6). Thoracoabdominal exposure and multiple vessel reattachments are usually necessary for the thoracoabdominal segment, and equally formidable procedures may be required to replace other segments, such as associated aneurysms of the ascending aorta and transverse aortic arch. Operation is therefore selectively performed based upon operative risks determined by the experience of the team responsible for therapy (1). Elective operation is not generally performed in certain groups of patients. These include most patients over 80 years of age; those with pulmonary disease associated with P_{CO_2} above 50; those with surgically untreatable myocardial diseases and with ejection fractions of less than 30 percent of normal; and those with congestive heart failure. Patients with renal function impairment superimposed on the above conditions are not usually submitted to elective operations. Patients with malignant or other diseases limiting their life expectancy to less than 2 years are not satisfactory candidates for operation. Operation is considered in some members of this group of patients only in the event of intolerable pain or rupture, and then operation is confined to the short segment of dilated aorta in which these complications are located.

Candidates for Operation

Other patients should be considered for operation when the diameter of the aneurysm is twice that of the adjacent uninvolved aorta. Rupture does not correlate well with size; small aneurysms do rupture, and operation should be performed electively to prevent this. The aneurysm was more than twice the size of the uninvolved aortic segment in most of our patients submitted to operation. Most patients had one or more associated diseases, adding to the risk of the procedure. In our series of 544 patients, only 47 (9 percent) were free of associated disease. The survival rate in this small group of patients was 96 percent (45 patients). Survival rates of patients with associated diseases were as follows: hypertension, 90 percent; cerebrovascular disease, 90 percent; heart disease, 88 percent; obstructive pulmonary disease, 86 percent; and renal disease, 83 percent. As indicated previously, 75 percent of those submitted to operation were symptomatic, indicating that rupture was imminent. The total survival rate in our group of 544 patients was 91 percent, which justifies this relatively aggressive approach to the problem.

Preparation of Patients for Operation

Evaluation and preparation of the patient depend upon the nature of the associated disease if any. In hypertensive patients, antihypertensive agents are continued up until the time of operation. Electrolyte disturbances are corrected in these patients; brief-acting agents are given in the immediate operative period, and longer-acting agents that were required before operation are restarted in the period soon after operation when necessary. Aortographic examination is carefully performed to detect renal artery lesions that can be repaired during operation to both relieve hypertension and improve renal function.

A thorough screening of the cardiac status using both invasive and noninvasive studies is performed to detect abnormalities. Patients with mild and stable angina of some duration are considered satisfactory risks for operation provided they have good left ventricular function or ejection fractions over 30 percent. Patients with symptomatic and unstable coronary or valvular heart disease and those with impaired left ventricular function are more extensively evaluated. Suitable candidates are submitted to cardiac operations first, and the aneurysm operation is delayed for several weeks.

Patients with chronic obstructive pulmonary disease are studied by function tests, and those with FEV over 1 and P_{CO_2} less than 45 are considered satisfactory for operation. Patients with bronchoconstrictor components that respond to medical therapy are considered better risk than those who do not. Pulmonary function can frequently be improved in patients with borderline lung function if they stop smoking; are given a short course of antibiotics for bronchitis, the type of antibiotic determined by sputum culture and sensitivity studies; lose weight; and take part in an exercise program. Four to six weeks of this form of treatment may dramatically improve pulmonary funciton.

Patients admitted with elevated blood creatinine levels are evaluated for renal disease. Frequently this abnormality is related to preadmission dehydration and previous contrast studies. Such patients respond well to rehydration and postponement of operation. A history of normal renal function before contrast studies is invaluable, and in such cases operation is delayed until the prestudy or baseline values are regained. Prestudy or persistent elevations of blood creatinine levels do not preclude operation. Operation has been tolerated with values less than 3 mg/100 mL. Operation has been safely performed in four of six patients being treated by chronic hemodialysis. Operation was performed for rupture or severe pain in these patients. Transient hemodialysis has been safely performed in the early postoperative period in others, permitting successful operation in symptomatic patients with impaired renal function (7). In still other patients with renal artery occlusive disease, renal function has been improved or even restored to normal by renal artery operation at the time of aneurysm repair.

Anesthesia, Monitoring, and Blood Replacement

In most cases, patients arrive in the anesthesia area well-hydrated, on digitalis and other long-term drugs except antiplatelet and anticoagulation compounds, and with normal electrolyte and blood gas levels. Bilateral radial intraarterial catheters (one from which to draw blood gases and one with which to continuously measure blood pressure), a central venous line through which to administer drugs, a Swan-Ganz catheter, and four large peripheral venous catheters through which to administer blood, blood products, and electrolyte solution are inserted percutaneously. Intraarterial blood pressure, central venous pressure, pulmonary artery pressure, capillary wedge pressure, cardiac output, electrocardiogram, and EEG are monitored continuously or intermittently. The levels of blood gases and electrolytes are monitored every 30 minutes. Developing abnormalities are corrected by appropriate therapy as they occur.

Anesthesia is obtained with drugs (narcotics) that do not depress the myocardium, and muscle relaxation is achieved by using muscle relaxants. We prefer short-acting agents so that the patient wakes up and resumes muscle activity soon after operation. This permits weaning the patient from the respirator the day of operation or soon thereafter. Unless this is done, the weaker and more frail patients may become "addicted" to the respirator, and days may be spent getting them back on normal unassisted respiration.

A double-lumen bifurcation endotracheal tube is used to deflate the left lung during operation upon the thoracic segment of aneurysm to increase exposure, protect the lung from retraction injury, and avoid cardiac compression during retraction. Electrolyte solutions are started into the various lines mainly to keep the lines open and to administer drugs. Excessive crystalloid administration is to be avoided to prevent overloading and hemodilation of clotting elements in patients who tend to have a disseminated intravascular coagulopathy at the time of admission (one-third have elevated levels of fibrin split products). Ordinarily, Ringer's lactate solution is given except in patients with impaired renal function. Normal saline solution or 5 percent dextrose and water is used in these patients to avoid the potassium present in the Ringer's lactate. Mannitol solution, 25 g, and Mandol, 1 g, are given after induction of anesthesia.

Shunts and bypasses to control proximal blood pressure and distal circulation are not used during operation to avoid their attendant complications. Cardiac hemodynamics are controlled during operation using pharmacologic agents depending primarily upon nitroprusside solution. The aorta is slowly clamped proximally as nitroprusside solution is given intravenously. These two steps of the operation are orchestrated to maintain normal hemodynamics of circulation during and after aortic clamping. As aneurysmal replacement is completed and air is removed from the graft, the administration of nitroprusside solution is discontinued. The aortic clamp is slowly opened as the blood pressure rises. Blood (red cells) accumulated by the cell saver and obtained from the blood bank is given rapidly through all four lines previously inserted for this purpose. Platelets and fresh plasma are also given in the ratio described below. As the blood pressure rises from this expansion of the previously isolated distal arterial bed, the clamp is gradually removed, monitoring normal cardiac and peripheral hemodynamics of circulation. Acidosis and its attendant cardiovascular abnormalities are prevented by continuing the bicarbonate drip started at the time of aortic clamping.

A unit of albumin and 2 units of fresh plasma are given at the onset of operation, and blood replacement is achieved by component transfusion. Autotransfusion using a modified cell-saver unit that permits collection and washing of red cells at a rate of 500 mL per 2 to 3 minutes is employed. Over three-fourths of the red blood cells required for operation are salvaged by this method. Washed red cells are given as blood is lost; after 3 units are given, fresh plasma is given at a rate of 1 unit per 2 units of red cells until 10 units of red cells are given; then unit for unit red cells and plasma are given. Platelets, 10 to 20 units, are given when blood flow is restored through the graft. Coagulation studies are performed at this time, and abnormalities are corrected. The most common needs evident from this examination are fresh plasma, cryoprecipitate, and platelets, in the order listed.

As indicated previously, these patients tend to have abnormalities of bleeding; consequently, heparin is not given at operation. Occasionally, a severe fibrinolysis reaction occurs. Treatment in these cases consists of packing the area of reconstruction to prevent further blood loss and the administration of 40 to 60 units of cryoprecipitate rapidly, i.e., 2 to 3 minutes, in order to "overwhelm" the coagulopathy by replacing more fibrinogen than is being lost through the wound during the period of administration (6). Temporary electrical fibrillation of the heart may be required to prevent severe blood losses from occurring during the period of cryoprecipitate administration. Electrical defibrillation is performed and cardiac function is restored within 2 to 3 minutes to prevent cerebral damage.

Blood loss may be massive in these cases, and from 40 to 120 units of blood elements may be necessary for transfusion.

These and other intravenous solutions are warmed by water bath technique when possible. Other methods to prevent hypothermia of the patient and the development of intraoperative cardiac arrhythmias include a warm room environment (27°C, or 80°F) and frequent vigorous irrigations of the abdominal and chest cavities with warm saline solution. We find that rectal temperature of 34°C prevents hypothermia arrhythmias. Heat blankets and pads have been of little value in our experience and have caused burns in some patients.

Position and Incision

In rare instances we perform operation through an abdominal incision with a counterincision made in the diaphragm to minimize pulmonary dysfunction in a patient with poor lung function and an aneurysm involving the abdominal aorta or one involving the lower thoracic and abdominal aorta. Aneurysms up to the level of the inferior pulmonary vein have been successfully managed in this fashion; however, appropriate exposure is difficult to achieve, and technical intraoperative complications are difficult to manage in the region of the upper part of the reconstruction. Because of these limitations, we prefer routine use of posterolateral thoracoabdominal exposure.

The patient is placed on his or her right side with the chest in maximum vertical position and the abdomen in the maximum supine position and held in place with a beanbag. The chest and abdomen are entered with incision placed according to the extent and level of the aneurysm. A full-length midline abdominal incision curved into the sixth or seventh intercostal space is employed in patients with extensive aneurysms involving both the descending thoracic and the abdominal aorta (Figure 37-8*A*). A similar abdominal incision curved into the eighth intercostal space is employed in patients with aneurysms involving the abdominal aorta or both the abdominal aorta and the lower descending

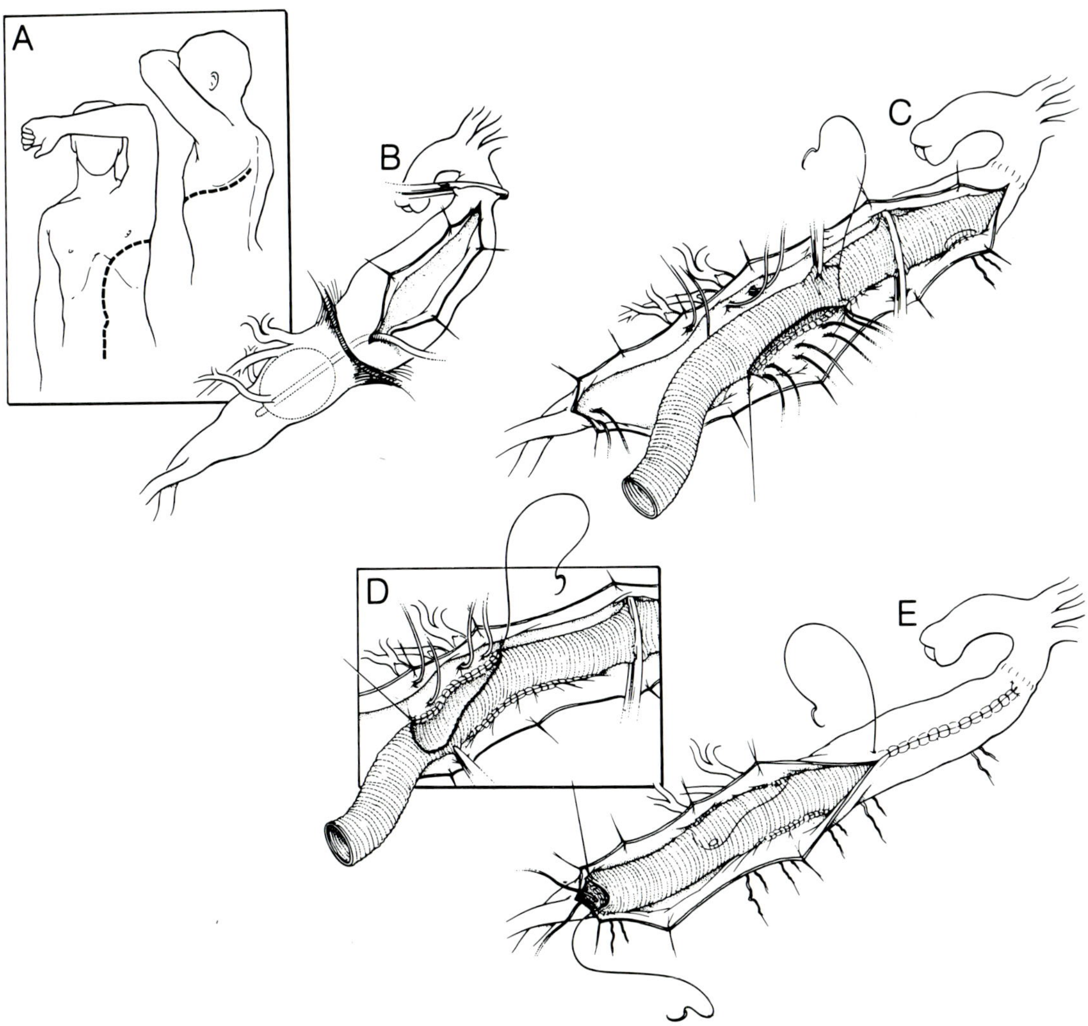

FIGURE 37–8. Drawings showing the technique of treating an extensive aneurysm involving the descending thoracic and abdominal aorta. [Copyright © Baylor College of Medicine 1984. Used with permission.]

thoracic aorta. Aneurysms of the upper abdominal aorta and lower descending thoracic aorta are exposed by a seventh or eighth intercostal space incision extended obliquely across the abdominal wall above or below the umbilicus, depending upon abdominal aortic involvement.

Exposure of the Aneurysm

The uninvolved thoracic aorta above the aneurysm is separated from adjacent structures with minimal dissection to permit clamping. The thoracic component of aneurysm is not separated from adjacent structures. Chest wall adhesions from previous operation or pleuritis may need lysing to permit aortic exposure, but most of the lung adherent to the anterior and lateral aspect of the aneurysm is left intact to prevent troublesome bleeding and to avoid entering the aneurysm.

The abdominal cavity is explored for associated disease, and the abdominal segments of uninvolved and involved aorta are exposed by first incising the peritoneum along the left gutter from the left margin of the esophageal hiatus to the brim of the pelvis. The left iliac artery and the posterolateral wall of the abdominal aorta are exposed retroperitoneally by retracting the left ureter, colon, kidney, body and tail of pancreas, spleen, and fundus of stomach upward and medially. Periaortic dissection is limited, and the aortic arterial branches are not individually exposed.

Reconstruction of Large Degenerative Aneurysm

With the aorta clamped proximally, a longitudinal incision is made in the posterolateral wall of the aneurysm in the thorax and the wall retracted with stay sutures (Figure 37-8*B*). Distal bleeding from the aorta is usually minimal and is controlled with gauze packing. More vigorous bleeding is controlled with an inflated urethral catheter. One end of a woven Dacron tube is attached to the proximal aorta by continuous no. 000 Prolene suture. Intercostal and lumbar arteries T8–L2 are attached to an opening made in the graft, and the visceral vessels are attached to the graft in a similar manner (Figure 37-8*C* and 37-8*D*). The latter are attached according to the distance between their origins. Widely separated vessel origins, as in patients with large aneurysms, are reattached separately (4). Closely located origins, as in patients with dissecting aortic aneurysms or smaller degenerative aneurysms, are attached to one or two openings made in the graft. Most frequently, the celiac axis, superior mesenteric artery, and right renal artery are attached to one opening and the left renal artery to a separate opening (Figure 37-9). The graft

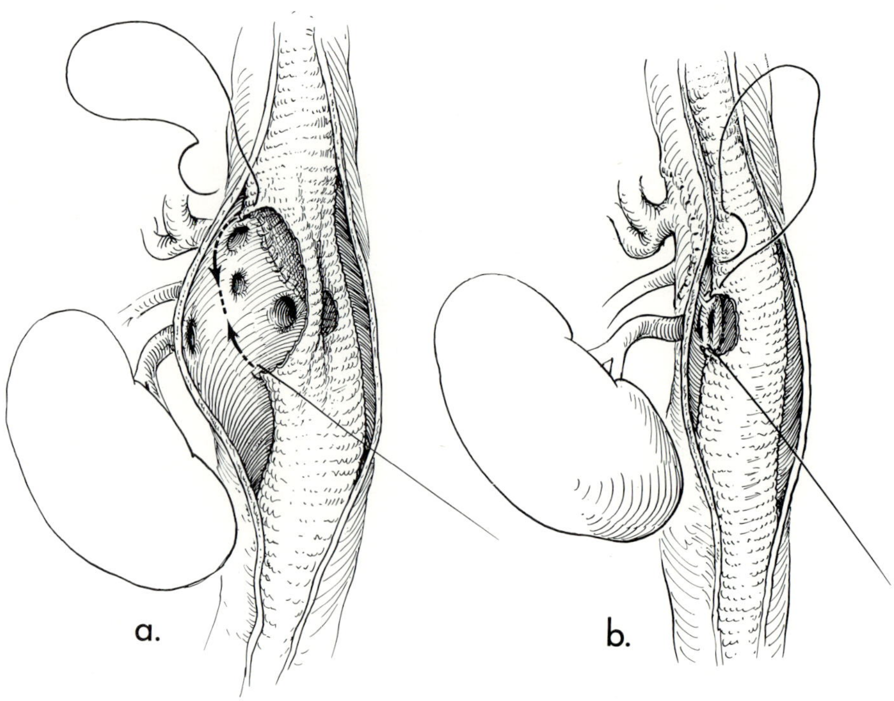

FIGURE 37–9. Drawings showing the most common method of visceral artery attachment to the graft. (*A*) Celiac axis, superior mesenteric artery, and right renal artery are attached to one opening made in the graft. (*B*) The left renal artery is attached to a separate opening made in the graft. [Copyright © Baylor College of Medicine. Used with permission.]

is then flushed by brief loosening of the proximal aortic clamp. With the graft filled with blood and the patient in the head-down position to remove air, the graft is clamped distal to the reattached vessels, and the proximal aortic clamp is removed, restoring visceral arterial circulation. The distal end of the graft is then sutured to either the uninvolved aorta, the iliac arteries, or the common femoral arteries (Figure 37-8*E*).

Reconstruction of Degenerative Aneurysms Involving Shorter Segments of Aorta and Those with Associated Branch Obstruction

Reconstruction of aneurysms involving short segments of the aorta is accomplished as just described. Reconstruction in patients with associated occlusion of the visceral vessels is by endarterectomy in most cases because occlusion is usually due to atherosclerotic lesions arising near the orifices of these vessels. Endarterectomy is performed by entering the cleavage plane between intima and media of the aorta and continuing the dissection in this plane into the involved vessel as gentle traction is applied to the diseased intimal core of involved vessel. When dissection is complete, the specimen suddenly pulls away from the normal distal intima and the distal end of the specimen is typically thinly tapered, indicating a successful operation. The endarterectomized visceral branch is then reattached as previously described.

Reconstruction of Dissecting Aortic Aneurysms

Thoracoabdominal aortic aneurysms resulting from aortic dissection are either chronic type I or type III dissections. These aneurysms involve all the descending thoracic and most of the abdominal aorta and always require extensive reconstructions unless the proximal descending thoracic aorta was replaced in the acute stage (2). Moreover, the intercostal and lumbar arteries remain intact in these cases; the patients are more likely to develop paraplegia after operation and are in greater need of intercostal and lumbar reattachment (8). Anatomically the aorta is "double-barreled," consisting of the normal lumen and the false lumen. The aneurysm is located in the latter and represents dilation of the thinned outer wall of the dissected lumen. The aneurysm is entered as previously described, and the partition between true and false lumen is excised. Reconstruction is performed by either of two methods. In one method the proximal anastomosis is carefully made to the true lumen and distal reconstruction is performed as previously described, reattaching as many intercostal and lumbar arteries as feasible; T8–L2 are probably the most important of these to reattach (9).

In the other method, the dissected aortic circumference is replaced by a long beveled segment of tubular graft down to the midlumbar region to preserve intercostal and lumbar circulation, most of which arises from the nondissected aortic circumference (Figure 37-4). When necessary, the remainder of the aorta and the iliac arteries is replaced with tubular grafts. The visceral vessels are reattached as previously described.

Management Immediately after Operation

The management of these patients immediately after operation is similar to that after any major operation involving the thorax and abdomen, with few exceptions. The patients are monitored about as rigidly during the first 24 hours after operation as during it. The number of intravenous lines is reduced after the patient's condition proves to be stable in the intensive care unit; however, blood volume is determined by pulmonary artery and pulmonary wedge pressures and rigidly maintained at normal limits to prevent renovascular vasoconstriction and acute tubular necrosis. Overloading is treated with dopamine and diuretics. Potassium requirements frequently are high, and serum potassium levels are determined every hour in the patient with large hourly urinary output. Low levels are appropriately treated to prevent onset of cardiac arrhythmias. Normal ventilation and ambulation are begun as soon as possible.

Results

Of the 544 patients in our series submitted to operation for thoracoabdominal aortic aneurysm, as previously defined, 495 (91 percent) survived for 30 days, and complete follow-up indicated that 60 percent were alive at 5 years, the exact results found in our follow-up studies of patients submitted to operation for simple infrarenal abdominal aortic aneurysm. These results are considered encouraging in light of the extent of operation, the mean age of the patients, the frequency of associated disease, and the frequency of other aortic aneurysm operations. Although over half the patients had involvement of substantial segments of the descending thoracic and abdominal aorta, the extent of the lesion and its operation had no influence on survival. Principal factors limiting survival included the associated diseases, described above, the presence of rupture, bleeding after operation, and other complications including infection, respiratory insufficiency, myocardial infarction, and renal failure (10).

The two most dreaded complications in surviving patients were neurologic deficits of the lower extremities and chronic renal failure (7). The former occurred in 10 percent of patients, and the latter in 5 percent. The neurologic deficits occurred most often in patients with extensive replacement of the descending thoracic and abdominal aorta for acute and chronic aortic dissection. The deficit was mild in approximately half the patients and severe in the remainder. The degree of rehabilitation of these cases at 1 year based upon a scoring system numbered 1 to 10 was 10 in 7 patients (21 percent), 9 in 15 patients (45 percent), 8 in 6 patients (18 percent), and less in 5 patients (15 percent).

References

1. Crawford ES, Snyder DM, Cho GC, Roehm JOF Jr: Progress in treatment of thoracoabdominal and abdominal aortic aneurysms involving celiac, superior mesenteric, and renal arteries. Ann Surg 188:404, 1978.
2. DeBakey ME, Creech O Jr, Morris GC Jr: Aneurysm of thoracoabdominal aorta involving the celiac, superior mesenteric, and renal arteries: Report of four cases treated by resection and homograft replacement. Ann Surg 144:549, 1956.
3. DuBost C, Allary M, Oeconomos N: Resection of an aneurysm of the abdominal aorta: Reestablishment of the continuity by a preserved human arterial graft, with results after five months. Arch Surg 64:405, 1952.
4. Etheredge SN, Yee J, Smith JV, Schonberger S, Goldman MJ: Successful resection of a large aneurysm of the upper abdominal aorta and replacement with homograft. Surgery 38:71, 1955.
5. Matas R: An operation for the radical cure of aneurysm based upon arteriorrhaphy. Ann Surg 37:6, 1903.
6. Carrel A, Guthrie C: Resultats du patching des arteres. CR Acad Sci 1009, 1906.
7. Ellis FH Jr, Helden RA, Hines EA Jr: Aneurysm of the abdominal aorta involving the right renal artery: Report of case with preservation of renal function after resection and grafting. Ann Surg 142:992, 1955.
8. Spencer FC, Zimmerman JM: The influence of ligation of intercostal arteries on paraplegia in dogs. Surg Forum 9:430, 1950.
9. DeBakey ME, Crawford ES, Garrett HE, Beall AC, Howell JF: Surgical considerations in the treatment of aneurysms of the thoraco-abdominal aorta. Ann Surg 162:650, 1965.
10. Javid H, Julian OC, Dye WS, Hunter JA: Complications of abdominal aortic grafts. Arch Surg 85:650, 1962.

Chapter 38

POPLITEAL ANEURYSM

WILLIAM E. EVANS AND BLAIR D. VERMILION

The popliteal aneurysm is the most common peripheral arterial aneurysm, accounting for 70 percent of all these lesions. With increased physician awareness of this problem and improvement of diagnostic capabilities, the overall incidence of popliteal aneurysms should increase in the future. Since the first descriptions of the popliteal aneurysm in the second century A.D., their potential for serious complications has been known. This has prompted authors to describe these aneurysms as "vixen . . . sly in apparent benignity"(12) and "sinister harbinger of sudden catastrophe" (9).

Historical Comments

The history of awareness and treatment of popliteal aneurysms dates to the second century A.D., when Antyllus first described the ligation of a popliteal aneurysm proximally and distally, with packing of the aneurysmal sac (1). This method of treatment persisted with slight modifications until 1785 when John Hunter popularized ligation of the superficial femoral artery; thus began the "Hunterian" method of treatment of popliteal aneurysms (1). The next major influence was by Matas, who introduced endoaneurysmorrhaphy. His first report in 1920 described 154 popliteal aneurysms with only a 0.6 percent mortality and a 5.2 percent amputation rate (13). In 1935, Bird advocated preliminary lumbar symphathectomy with subsequent delayed obliteration of the popliteal aneurysm (3). By 1950, methods of bypass grafting were being introduced, and this slowly emerged as the preferred treatment for the popliteal aneurysm (10,11). This technique remains the most popular and successful method of treating this problem. (4,8,15).

Etiology

The most common cause of popliteal aneurysms is atherosclerosis (4,16). However, a small percentage are secondary to trauma, infection, syphilis, and popliteal entrapment (2,4,6,8). In Martin's series of 105 true aneurysms, 102 were atherosclerotic in origin, while in our series of 147 popliteal aneurysms, all were atherosclerotic (4,15).

Since atherosclerosis is the most common cause, it is not unusual to find other associated medical problems. These patients commonly have a history of coronary artery disease, including angina or a previous myocardial infarction (15,16). In addition, there is a relatively high incidence of hypertension, cerebrovascular disease, diabetes mellitus, and ischemic occlusive disease.

Demography

The majority of popliteal aneurysms occur in males. In our series of 87 patients, all but 3 were males (15), while in the series of 152 patients from the Mayo Clinic (16) 148 were male. Ages range from 40 to 98 with the median age of 60 years. However, popliteal aneurysm has been reported in patients as young as 26 years.

Perhaps one of the most interesting aspects of popliteal aneurysms is their frequent bilaterality and their common association with other arterial aneurysms. In a report by Wychulis from the Mayo Clinic (16), 45 percent of 152 patients had aneurysms in extrapopliteal locations. Most commonly seen was an associated abdominal aortic aneurysm (35 percent), but femoral aneurysms were found in 26 percent, while associated iliac aneurysms were present in 18 percent. A similar experience was documented in our series (15) with a 40 percent association with abdominal aortic aneurysms, while 34 percent had a femoral aneurysm and 25 percent had an iliac aneurysm. Over one-half of our 87 patients were noted to have an associated extrapopliteal aneurysm. In addition, bilaterality is quite common in patients with popliteal aneurysms, occurring in 40 to 60 percent of patients (2,6,15,16).

Presenting Symptoms and Complications

The large majority of the popliteal aneurysms will be symptomatic at the time of intitial presentation. In our series (15) 67 percent presented with symptoms attributed to popliteal aneurysm, while Baird noted that 75 percent were symptomatic (2). Most commonly seen was claudication and/or rest pain. In addition, a few patients had distal ulceration due to embolization, while others experienced swelling from venous compression and pain from posterior tibial nerve compression. Table 38-1 shows the presenting symptoms found in our series (15).

Complications of popliteal aneurysms are common and include thrombosis, embolization, rupture, or compression, Wychulis (16) found that 65 of 111 popliteal aneurysms were thrombosed at the time of initial presentation, while 30 had caused venous compression, 28 had ulcerations, 23 embolized, and 6 had ruptured (see Table 38-2). A total of 60 percent of all aneurysms were complicated at the time of initial presentation in this series (16). This compares with an 85 percent incidence of complications reported by Baird (2) and a 69 percent incidence in our series (15) (Table 38-3).

TABLE 38-2. Popliteal Aneurysms: Presenting Complications from Wychulis (16)

Complication	Aneurysms, %
Thrombosis	28
Venous occlusion	13
Ulceration or gangrene	12
Emboli	10
Nerve compression	6
Popliteal thrombosis	5
Rupture	3
Infection	<1

TABLE 38-1. Popliteal Aneurysms: Presenting Symptoms (15)

Symptom	Extremity, %
Asymptomatic	33
Claudication	45
Rest pain	31
Ulceration	7
Venous obstruction	7
Neurologic	8
Total symptomatic	67

TABLE 38-3. Popliteal Aneurysms: Presenting Complications from Evans and Vermilion (15)

Complications	Aneurysms, no.	%	
None	53	36	
Thrombosis*	66	45	69% of total group
Emboli*	34	23	
Rupture	4	3	
Other	1	<1	

*Eleven patients had thrombosis and emboli.

Diagnosis

The diagnosis of a popliteal aneurysm can frequently be made by a careful physical examination, and the diagnosis should be considered if one finds a prominent palpable popliteal artery. Due to the high incidence of associated aneurysms and bilaterality, physical examination must be coupled with further diagnostic procedures when a patient presents with an abdominal aortic aneurysm, a femoral aneurysm, or a contralateral popliteal aneurysm. Ultrasonic evaluation of the popliteal fossa is very helpful in the diagnosis of popliteal aneurysm (14). Ultrasonic scanning of the popliteal fossa has been shown to be more accurate than physical examination or arteriography (5,7). The computerized tomography scan may also be used in this area, but it offers no advantage over ultrasound. We consider a popliteal artery greater than 2 cm in diameter to be aneurysmal. All patients who have popliteal aneurysms documented should have a complete arteriography of the infrarenal aorta and distal vessels to document the existence of other aneurysms and to determine the status of the runoff (8). Many of the aneurysms have embolized extensively prior to the diagnosis of a popliteal aneurysm, and the runoff may be significantly compromised, necessitating distal bypass grafting. As pointed out by Martin (4), the presence or absence of good runoff in these cases is of great prognostic value. His results were much better in patients in whom distal embolization or obstruction had not occurred, as opposed to those who were diagnosed and treated following these complications.

Treatment

The treatment choice is exclusion of the aneurysm with bypass grafting at the time of initial diagnosis. This accomplishes two goals. First, it eliminates the potential for further complication and, second, restores adequate blood flow to the extremity. It is unnecessary and inappropriate to excise the aneurysm unless it is causing compressive symptoms.

Our preference of graft material is to reverse the saphenous vein whenever possible in end-to-side fashion to overcome any size discrepancy. If an adequate vein is not available, either Dacron, polytetrafluoroethylene (PTFE) or umbilical vein may be used. We prefer PTFE. We have found little benefit from sympathectomy alone or in combination with bypass grafting, and no longer employ this. A medial approach to the popliteal artery is utilized. The proximal popliteal artery is isolated through a medial incision in the lower thigh. A lower incision is made parallel to the upper medial tibia and the distal popliteal artery exposed. The aneurysm is ligated proximally and distally and the distal anastomosis completed. The graft is tunneled alongside the aneurysm and anastomosed to the normal popliteal artery above the aneurysm.

Occasionally, complications of an aneurysm will result in nonviability of the leg, necessitating primary amputation. This was necessary in 8 percent of the extremities in our series (15) but may be necessary in as many as 20 percent as reported by Baird (2).

Results

When diagnosis and treatment are accomplished while the aneurysm is asymptomatic, excellent results can be expected. In our series (15) 99 extremities were revascularized. Twenty-nine grafts were placed in asymptomatic limbs with a 96 percent patency rate over the average follow-up period of 26.5 months. Seventy grafts were placed in symptomatic limbs. Over a follow-up period that averaged 37 months, only 70 percent maintained patent grafts. All but 1 of 22 occlusions occurred in an extremity that presented with a symptomatic and complicated aneurysm (15). In addition, primary amputation was necessary in 8 percent of extremities, and secondary amputation was necessary in an additional 15 percent of extremities. All amputations occurred in extremities that were symptomatic and had suffered a complication of the aneurysm. Reports by Wychulis (16), Baird (2), and Crichlow (6) found similar results in their series, and they agree with the concept of early diagnosis and treatment.

Twenty-six aneurysms were followed in our series (15) with no specific treatment. During the follow-up period which averaged 36 months, 31 percent of these extremities developed limb-threatening complications (15). Wychulis (16) reported a 29 percent incidence of complications in asymptomatic aneurysms that were followed.

Summary

1. Popliteal aneurysms are frequently bilateral and commonly associated with other aneurysms.

2. The risk of limb-threatening complications is quite high in symptomatic extremities.

3. Popliteal aneurysms should be ligated and bypassed at the time of initial diagnosis.

References

1. Austin DJ, Thompson JE: Excision and arterial grafting in the surgical management of popliteal aneurysms. South Med J 1958, 51:43.
2. Baird RJ, Swansankar R, Hayward R, and Wilson DR: Popliteal aneurysms: A review and analysis of 61 cases. Surgery 1966, 59:911.
3. Bird CE: Sympathectomy as a preliminary to the obliteration of popliteal aneurysms. Surg Gyn Obstet 1935, 60:926.
4. Bouhoutsos J, and Martin P: Popliteal aneurysms. A review of 116 cases. Br J Surg 1974, 61:469.
5. Collins GJ, Rich NM, Phillips J, Hobson RW, Anderson, CA: Ultrasound diagnosis of popliteal arterial aneurysms. Am Surg 1976, Nov: 853.
6. Crichlow RW, Roberts B: Treatment of popliteal aneurysms by restorations of continuity. Ann Surg 1966, 163:417.
7. Davis RP, Neiman HL, Yao JST, Bergan JJ: Ultrasound scan in diagnosis of peripheral aneurysms. Arch Surg 1977, 112:55.
8. Gaylis H: Popliteal arterial aneurysms: A review and analysis of 55 cases. S Afr Med J 1974, 48:75.
9. Gifford RW, Hines EA, Janes JM: An analysis and follow-up study of one hundred popliteal aneurysms. Surgery 1953, 33:284.
10. Grose RE, Bill AH Jr, Pierce EC II: Methods for preservation and transplantation of arterial grafts. SGO 1949, 88:689.
11. Julian OC, Dye WS, Javid H, Grove WJ: The use of vessel grafts in the treatment of popliteal aneurysms. Surgery 1955, 38:970.
12. Lord JW: Clinical behavior and operative management of popliteal aneurysms. JAMA 1957, 163:1102.
13. Matas R: Endo-aneurysmorrohaphy. SGT 1920, 30:456.
14. Sarti DA, Louis JS, Lindstrom PR, Niles K, London J: Ultrasonic diagnosis of a popliteal artery aneurysm. Radiology 1976, 121:707.
15. Vermilion BD, Kimmins SA, Pace WG, Evans WE: A review of 147 popliteal aneurysms with long-term follow-up. Surgery 1981, 90:1009.
16. Wychulis AR, Spittell JA Jr, Wallace RB: Popliteal aneurysms. Surgery 1970, 68:942.

Chapter 39

SPLANCHNIC ARTERY ANEURYSMS

RUSSELL A. WILLIAMS, JEFFREY C. MILLIKEN, and SAMUEL E. WILSON

Splanchnic artery aneurysms are an uncommon variety of visceral artery aneurysm that mostly involve the foregut vessels. They occur far less frequently than aneurysms of the aorta, iliac vessels, or renal vessels. Nevertheless, every clinician will encounter several or more patients with this problem—most commonly a splenic artery aneurysm.

If specifically sought at necropsy, symptomless, unsuspected splenic artery aneurysms may be found in as many as 10.4 percent of elderly patients (1). Otherwise autopsy findings on more diverse populations show a frequency of splenic artery aneurysms that varies from 0.01 to 0.08 percent (2,3). In 192 patients having celiac angiograms, 8 aneurysms of the splenic artery were demonstrated—an incidence of 4.04 percent (4).

The next common aneurysm develops on the hepatic artery and accounts for about 20 percent of the splanchnic artery aneurysms (splenic artery, 60 percent). Much less common are those of the superior mesenteric artery (8 percent), celiac artery (4 percent), and the gastric, jejunoileal, and colic vessels (2 to 3 percent) (5).

Typically, when these aneurysms present with complications, they are due to compression of surrounding structures or to rupture and abdominal apoplexy. The former is usually associated with a dramatically large aneurysm which may be technically difficult to successfully treat by operation and the latter is a catastrophic and life-threatening, demanding operation. Unfortunately surgical treatment in both situations has a high mortality rate.

At the present time, noninvasive vascular and blood flow studies utilizing magnetic resonance imaging, computed tomography (CT) and ultrasound in addition to computer-assisted venous angiography and selective visceral angiography can detect these aneurysms earlier. Ideally they could then be treated electively by operation or invasive angiographic techniques with a reduced mortality rate, before exigent complications develop.

Splenic Artery Aneurysm

Splenic artery aneurysms have been recognized with certainty since 1770, when Beaussier described one in a woman aged 60, at autopsy (6). Some 50 years ago the first splenic aneurysm diagnosed radiographically was successfully treated by operation (7).

Atherosclerosis is found in the majority, and the fact that these aneurysms develop more commonly in females—a population not especially prone to atherosclerosis, particularly the parturient woman—has led to the suggestion that the atherosclerosis develops secondarily (8). A majority of aneurysms occur within the age group 50 to 70 years, and overall about 87 percent are in females. Some 20 percent are found in patients between the ages of 20 and 50, and in this group the female predominance is 20:1 (9).

Of the women who have a splenic artery aneurysm, only about 20 percent have had a single (12 percent) or no pregnancy (8 percent). The remainder are multiparous. Pregnancy alters connective tissue within the wall of the artery, and it has been suggested that the increase in blood volume and portal congestion of pregnancy, together with the changes in arterial connective tissue, produce irreversible damage in the splenic artery with ultimate aneurysm formation. About one-eighth of women with splenic artery aneurysms were found to have fibromuscular dysplasia of other arteries (8).

Splenic artery aneurysms also develop in patients with portal hypertension and liver cirrhosis or splenic vein thrombosis (2,10). The increased splenic circulation in portal hypertension has been postulated to produce structural changes in the wall of the splenic artery, terminating in dilatation and aneurysm formation. In patients with liver disease the bulk of the celiac artery circulation passes through the splenic artery rather than through the hepatic, and these patients' angiographic diameters may be reversed compared with normal. These aneurysms have thin walls which are mostly fibrous tissue—the muscle and elastic lamina having been largely replaced—and in many the splenic artery shows advanced atherosclerosis, while none is found in the remaining arteries of the body (11).

Some researchers have suggested that congenital defects such as the absence of the internal elastic lamina and media may be associated with spontaneous rupture of the splenic artery where no aneurysm has formed (8). Multiple berry aneurysms have been reported at the branch of the intrasplenic arteries in a small number of patients.

In other cases weakness of the wall, either as a result of trauma or from erosion by an adjacent inflammatory process, such as pancreatitis, has led to a splenic artery false aneurysm (8). Of historical note, President Garfield died secondarily to rupture of a traumatic splenic artery aneurysm produced by a bullet during the attempted assassination of him. Other patients present with hemosuccus pancreaticus—bleeding into the gastrointestinal tract through the ampulla of Vater—and have a pseudoaneurysm of the splenic artery that has formed after an episode of pancreatitis, communicating with the pancreatic duct (12). In fact, this aneurysm may burst into a pancreatic cyst, causing its sudden, massive enlargement and perhaps ultimate rupture. Up to 10 percent of patients with pancreatitis are thought to develop pseudoaneurysms (13).

Mycotic and syphilitic aneurysms have no predilection for development in the splenic artery compared with the superior mesenteric artery or thoracic aorta, respectively.

Splenic artery aneurysms vary in size with an average of about 3 cm in diameter, Mostly they involve the distal main trunk of the splenic arery, much less commonly a branch, and about 70 percent are multiple and 10 percent double (14).

Approximately 70 percent have calcification in their wall, its curvilinear form seen on plain x-ray making the diagnosis of splenic artery aneurysm a simple one (Figure 39-1). However, calcium in the aneurysm wall does not confer protection from rupture.

CLINICAL PRESENTATION

A majority of these aneurysms are asymptomatic. Uncommonly patients complain of left hypochondrial pain not related to meals, which is very rarely associated with a palpable lump in the left hypochondriam. This may not be pulsatile, and any bruit heard is not necessarily related to the aneurysm. On plain film a circular or oval area of the linear calcification outlines the margins of the aneurysm in the majority of cases, and on barium meal there may be a pulsatile deformity of the greater curvature (15). But symptoms and signs are not constant.

At other times patients harboring these aneurysms present with complications, most dramatically and seriously is intraabdominal apoplexy, the aneurysm rupturing spontaneously into the peritoneal cavity. The phenomenon of "double rupture" is recognized in such patients. The aneurysm ruptures initially into the lesser sac and is contained for a period, following which the hematoma breaks free into the general peritoneal cavity or an adjacent hollow viscus, usually the stomach or colon. In one review of 94 collected cases, a little over half had single rupture and the remainder had this two-stage rupture (2,16). With double rupture there may be a sudden, crampy, left upper quadrant pain with nausea and vomiting, and as the lesion expands, so does the area of pain, which can radiate to the left shoulder or to both shoulders. With one-stage uncontained rupture, massive bleeding quickly produces the classic signs of hemorrhagic shock.

Rupture of a splenic aneurysm during pregnancy may be confused with other acute serious complications of pregnancy such as uterine rupture, abruptio placentae, or amniotic fluid embolism. In the pregnant patient about two-thirds of the splenic aneurysm ruptures that occur do so during the last trimester and about 20 percent do so during labor or the puerperium (17,18).

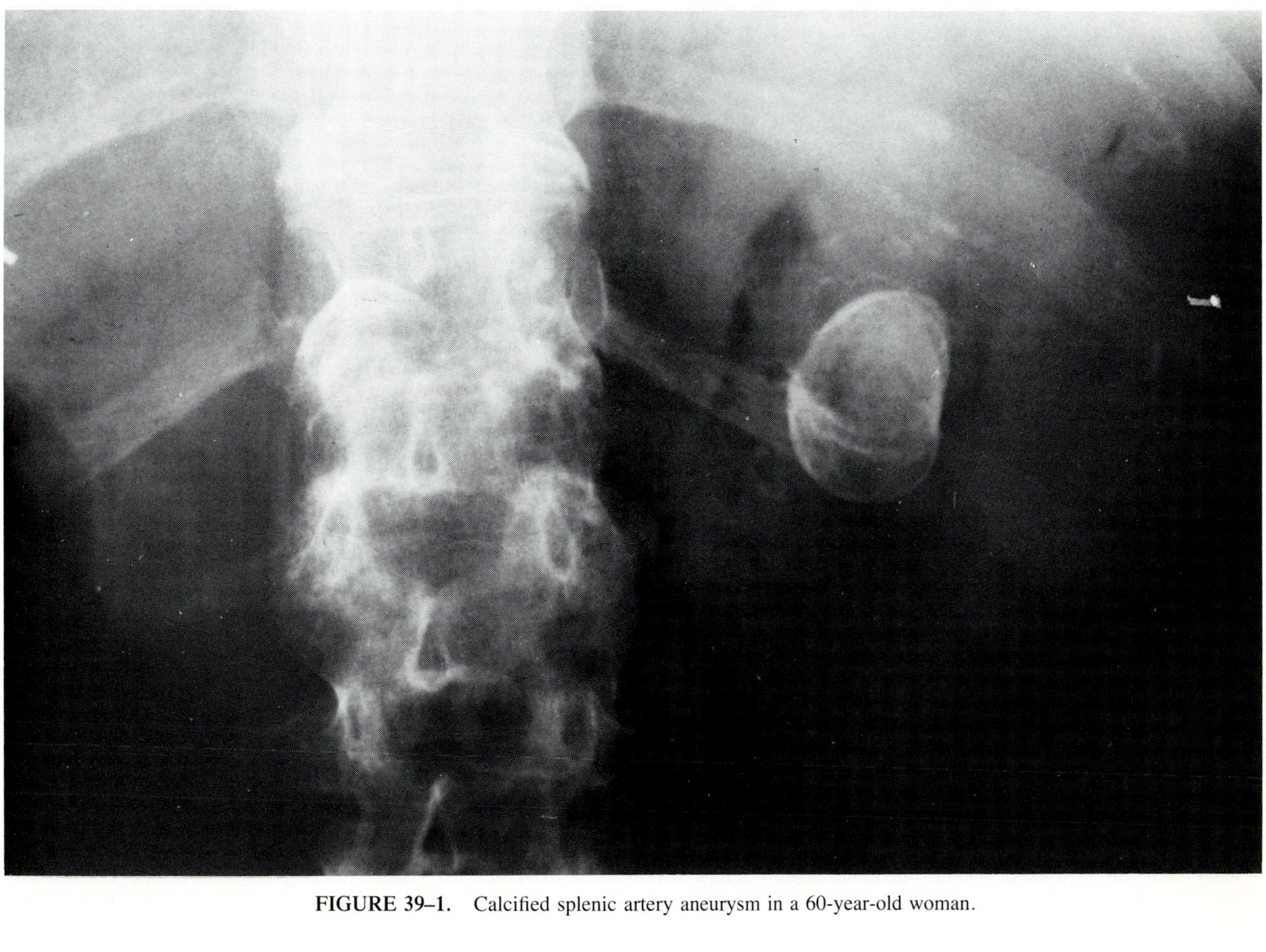

FIGURE 39–1. Calcified splenic artery aneurysm in a 60-year-old woman.

Aneurysms of the splenic artery can also rupture into the gastrointestinal tract, the pancreatic duct, or a pseudocyst. In contrast to the more common true aneurysm of the splenic artery, the pseudoaneurysms formed as the result of pancreatitis develop more often in males.

Hemosuccus pancreaticus was not appreciated as a specific disease until angiography showed it to be from a communication between the pancreatic duct and adjacent vasculature (12). Patients with hemosuccus pancreaticus give a prolonged history of gastrointestinal bleeding, the source eluding routine investigations such as endoscopy but which is finally identified by angiography. A clot in the pancreatic duct may produce pain and a futher episode of pancreatitis that resolves following discharge of the clot through the ampulla of Vater.

Rupture of a splenic artery pseudoaneurysm into a pancreatic pseudocyst can present with abdominal apoplexy, and the blood is found to be contained within the pseudocyst only at laporatomy.

INVESTIGATIONS

The majority of splenic artery aneurysms are found on plain x-ray of the abdomen (Figure 39-1). Their size can be approximated by measurement of the diameter of the semicircular or circular area of calcification. Further information is gained from an ultrasound study of the region or a CT scan. The precise anatomy of the aneurysm, however, is determined with angiography, in particular, selective celiac axis or splenic artery angiography. This shows not only the site but also multiple aneurysms in the splenic artery or in other visceral arteries and the extent of any thrombus replacement of the lumen of the aneurysm.

Angiography is desirable in all patients being considered for operation, In those thought unfit for operation or those who are fit, but as an alternative means for treatment, coils and thrombin may be introduced via an angiogram catheter into the lumen of the aneurysm to induce thrombosis. This form of treatment may be employed particularly if the aneurysm is solitary.

The need for elective treatment of a splenic artery aneurysm depends on its size, the age and fertility of the patient, or occasionally any symptoms and complications. In the older patient or an individual who is unfit for operation, a small asymptomatic aneurysm, less than 2 cm in diameter, may be observed by ultrasound techniques or, if it is calcified, by following the size of the calcific rings on plain x-rays at 6- to 12-month intervals. Catheter embolization may be used to obliterate it, should there be enlargement. In the fit younger patient and in all fertile women, it is recommended that these aneurysms. whatever the size, be treated.

Treatment is strongly recommended for the patient found to have an aneurysm during pregnancy as it is this group in which the aneurysm is prone to rupture. The risk of rupture in patients other than pregnant women has been reported to range between 2 and 10 percent (19). This may be somewhat less among the population at large.

OPERATIONS

Aneurysmectomy for aneurysms of the distal splenic artery usually includes removal of the spleen and perhaps the tail of the pancreas. Those located more proximally on the artery and any aneurysm involved in inflammation or that is very large may be more safely treated by double ligation of its inflow and outflow rather than resection. Interrupting splenic artery blood flow does not jeopardize the viability of the pancreas or spleen, both of which are maintained by an extensive collateral blood supply from the proximal splenic, pancreatoduodenal, and short gastric arteries, provided the spleen has not been removed.

With rupture during pregnancy or the puerperium, the maternal mortality rate may be as high as 70 percent and the fetal mortality rate 95 percent. Other patients with rupture and the hematoma contained in the lesser sac have a mortality rate of about 25 percent. Those patients who have aneurysms operated on electively have a mortality rate that approaches zero (9).

Exposure for the surgical treatment of splenic artery aneurysms is provided by a long upper midline incision, particularly in the thin patient. Alternately a left subcostal incision, which can be extended in a chevron fashion by adding a right subcostal incision, is also useful, especially in the obese or pregnant patient. The latter incision is more time-consuming to perform and inadvisable in an emergency, even if the diagnosis were known. The aneurysm itself is exposed by dividing the gastrocolic ligament to enter the lesser sac. Recent studies in patients with other diseases suggest splenic preservation should be attempted, but this may not be possible if the aneurysm extends into the hilum of the spleen or in an emergency.

Splenic artery aneurysms secondary to pancreatitis may be densely adherent to the pancreas or have ruptured into a pseudocyst or the pancreatic duct. They pose a slightly more difficult problem because the dense inflammatory adhesions usually make operation difficult. Double ligation may even be very difficult, and percutaneous arterial embolism and thrombosis of the aneurysm preferable and safer (20).

Management of the patient with aneurysm rupture into a very large pseudocyst that extends high under the left diaphragm and liver, which may be adherent to the portal vein or even the inferior vena cava, can be extremely difficult. Opening the pseudocyst to control the bleeding point usually leaves the operator with an obscured field that wells full of blood, at times making hemostasis impossible. In this situation the authors have introduced a balloon catheter into the abdominal aorta via the femoral artery to occlude the origins of mesenteric vessels. The gross size and situation of the cyst may preclude the use of a cross clamp of the aorta at the diaphragm hiatus. Once bleeding control is achieved within the pseudocyst, a drain is placed, as many of these cysts communicate with the pancreatic duct and a pancreatic fistula or even pancreatic ascites is a likely sequel.

Splenic artery aneurysms are also induced to thrombose by percutaneous catheter embolization, and an increasing number of successful reports of this technique are emerging. Under local anesthesia the catheter is selectively placed within the lumen of the aneurysm (21). The more commonly used small embolic particles of Teflon, Ivalon, or Silastic are not used in these patients to cause thrombosis as they are not retained in the aneurysm but embolize distally to the spleen. Instead, for this, a Gianturco steel coil which has wooly thrombogenic strands attached is introduced. This expands after extrusion from the catheter, wedging itself within the lumen, making embolization unlikely. Once in place the coil acts as a baffle, and other thrombogenic materials can be injected. This technique may also be useful in patients who have an aneurysm that has formed a fistula with the splenic vein or to avoid operation in patients with portal hypertension due to liver disease.

Clinical experience and laboratory studies on the dog have shown that the spleen has a good collateral blood supply and undergoes no changes when the splenic artery is ligated, analogous to double ligation of a splenic artery aneurysm or thrombosis induced by invasive radiologic techniques (22).

Hepatic Artery Aneurysms

Hepatic artery aneurysms are one-third as common as splenic artery aneurysms and 3 to 10 times more common than aneurysms of the other intestinal vessels (5). They develop two to three times more often in males, the average age of affected patients is 42, and three-quarters of the aneurysms involve the extrahepatic arteries. The hepatic artery proper and the right hepatic artery are about equally likely to be aneurysmal, while the left hepatic, cystic, and gastroduodenal arteries are uncommonly involved (23).

Small aneurysms have a fusiform shape, whereas those of larger size tend to be saccular in configuration. About half the aneurysms are believed to be due to atherosclerotic degeneration of the vessel wall, while another 15 to 20 percent develop following trauma, including operations on the biliary system. About 15 percent are mycotic aneurysms. Penetrating liver trauma is the cause of most intrahepatic aneurysms.

CLINICAL PRESENTATION

How likely hepatic artery aneurysms are to rupture is unknown, but it would seem, from our knowledge of aneurysms, to be a significant risk and certainly potentially lethal. At times they rupture into the peritoneal cavity but more commonly into an adjacent organ such as the liver, bile ducts, portal veins, duodenum, or pancreas. Expansion produces extrinsic compression and obstruction of the bile ducts and can deform the stomach and duodenum seen on barium meal.

An asymptomatic aneurysm may be discovered during operation and may be mistaken for a lymph node in the lesser omentum.

Symptoms usually develop with the onset of a complication and include right upper quadrant pain that may radiate to the right shoulder or have the character of biliary colic if the aneurysm ruptures into the bile ducts. Those patients with aneurysms communicating with the gut lumen via the bile duct, pancreatic duct, or directly (usually the duodenum) present with massive or chronic repeated episodes of bleeding into the gut.

Less commonly, portal hypertension from rupture of a hepatic artery aneurysm into the portal vein results in gastrointestinal bleeding from varices (23).

These aneurysms are rarely felt on physical examination of the abdomen, and if it is heard, a bruit may be unrelated to the aneurysm except where a fistula has formed into the portal vein.

INVESTIGATIONS

On plain film atherosclerotic aneurysms will often appear as a rim of eggshell-like calcification, and ultrasonography and CT scan delineate the aneurysm, showing its relation to the bile ducts or portal vein.

The definitive study that allows for planning treatment is selective celiac or hepatic artery angiography. Angiography delineates the site and extent of the aneurysm, shows an arteriovenous fistula, and demonstrates any arterial collaterals that have formed or enlarged portal venous collaterals if portal hypertension is present. It also outlines the anatomy of the liver blood supply which is via aberrant vessels in up to 40 percent of people. This is important information, as the arterial blood supply to the liver should be maintained following treatment, either through collaterals, normal aberrant arteries, or a prosthetic or autologous vein graft to replace the excised, diseased segment of artery.

OPERATIONS

Aneurysms located on the main hepatic artery proximal to the origin of the gastroduodenal artery may be excised or ligated, the blood supply to the liver being maintained through collaterals from the superior mesenteric artery entering the gastroduodenal branch of the common hepatic artery. Excision, rather than double ligation, is desirable if the aneurysm is infected, very large, and producing obstructive symptoms of the biliary or intestinal system or if it communicates with part of the gastrointestinal tract. In some cases it is safer to only partially remove the aneurysm, reducing its size by "debridement," leaving the sac which may be adherent to adjacent vital tissues. Occasionally patients may have had the gastroduodenal artery sacrificed at a previous operation on the biliary system or more commonly for peptic ulceration of the duodenum. In these patients, where collaterals are likely to be poorly developed, a saphenous vein graft can be used to restore arterial continuity after aneurysm resection.

The 40 percent of patients found on arteriogram to have alternative origins of the hepatic arteries have these from the left gastric or superior mesenteric artery (24–26). Identification of such vessels on preoperative angiography usually precludes the need to restore hepatic artery continuity. At operation, adequacy of arterial collateral blood flow to the liver is demonstrated if there is profuse backbleeding from the distal, divided end of the hepatic artery. Liver blood flow may also be restored by anastomosing the distal divided stump of the hepatic artery to an artery other than the celiac, such as the splenic, utilizing a segment of prosthetic material or a venous autograft.

Invasive angiography has been used to thrombose hepatic artery aneurysms and is the preferred method for treatment of intrahepatic aneurysms that otherwise would be treated by ligation of the right or left hepatic artery or even by hepatic lobectomy (27). Percutaneous embolization and thrombosis is generally not recommended for treatment of an extrahepatic aneurysm because of the importance of maintaining the arterial blood supply to the liver. However, there are reports of extrahepatic aneurysms being successfully treated by arteriographic embolization in patients with additional illnesses such as staphylococcal endocarditis involving several heart valves where multiple mycotic aneurysms had developed (28), patients with liver malignancy (29), or a patient who had previous surgery at which the diagnosis of leaking hepatic artery aneurysm was missed but subsequently found on an angiogram (30). There is one cautionary report of percutaneous hepatic aneurysm embolization being fatal in a 73-year-old man with malignant obstruction of the bile duct treated by introduction of an endoprosthesis for biliary drainage. A hepatic artery aneurysm complicated the initial procedure and was embolized, resulting in extensive hepatic necrosis (31).

Superior Mesenteric Artery Aneurysms

Superior mesenteric artery aneurysms are uncommon, and in contrast to other intestinal artery aneurysms, quite often they have an infective origin—about two-thirds are mycotic aneurysms (32). Most patients have subacute bacterial endocarditis or are intravenous drug addicts, and the streptococcus is commonly grown from the aneurysm, although in drug addicts staphylococcus is also likely (33). In the minority of patients, superior mesenteric artery aneurysms are atherosclerotic in origin and plain x-ray may show ringlike calcification in the upper abdomen near the midline.

CLINICAL PRESENTATION

In patients who have had bacterial endocarditis, the development of a superior mesenteric artery aneurysm should be considered, particularly if they complain of abdominal symptoms, such as epigastric pain, unrelated to meals. In some patients, especially those who are thin, a palpable tender mass which is mobile from side to side may be felt. At times, a pulsation can be appreciated and the patient may have positive blood cultures.

Those with a superior mesenteric artery aneurysm from another cause can present with similar pain but no antecedent history. The aneurysm will then be discovered during investigation (Figure 39-2). With an atherosclerotic aneurysm, a plain radiograph of the abdomen often shows signet-ring-like calcification to the side of the midline with a posterior defect in the circumference, representing the origin of the superior mesenteric artery from the aorta. Otherwise the aneurysm may only be identified at laparotomy.

The natural history of mycotic aneurysms with persistence of infection in the arterial wall is of unrelenting enlargement, and ultimately rupture. That of atherosclerotic or other types of aneu-

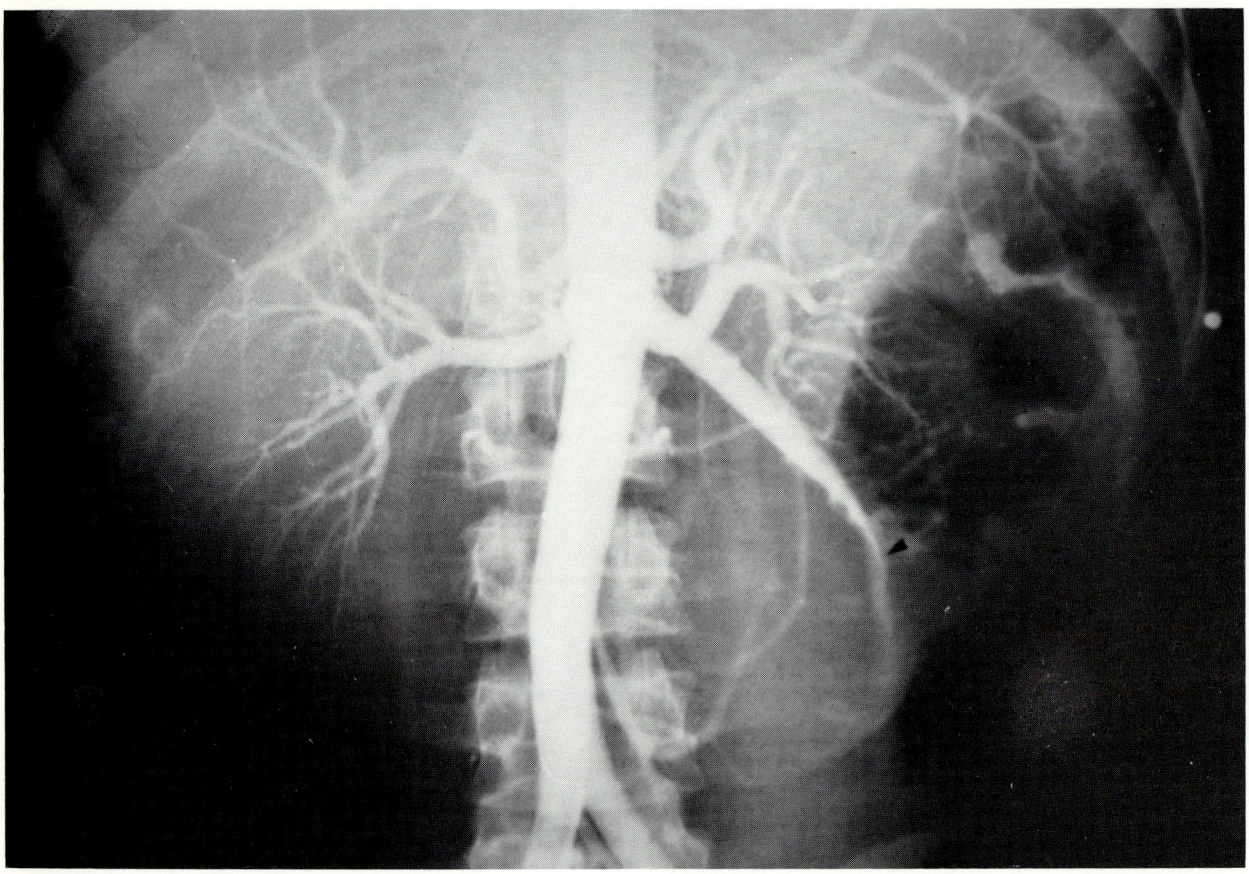

FIGURE 39–2. Mycotic superior mesenteric artery aneurysm in an intravenous drug abuser. (Dr. A. Yellin's case.)

rysms is uncertain, though there is no reason to believe it would be anything other than of progressive enlargement and again ultimately rupture; abdominal apoplexy due to rupture into the peritoneal cavity (34) and rupture of a traumatic superior mesenteric artery false aneurysm into the duodenum some years after an initial penetrating bullet injury to that area have been described (35).

OPERATIONS

The first superior mesenteric artery aneurysm, a mycotic aneurysm, treated successfully was operated on by DeBakey and Cooley in 1949. It was resected, without restoring continuity of the superior mesenteric artery (36).

Following aneurysmectomy, small-bowel viability commonly is not threatened, obviating the need for any additional procedure to restore arterial continuity. Progressive constriction of the aneurysm lumen of the superior mesenteric and other splanchnic arteries is believed to stimulate arterial collateral hypertrophy. However, should aneurysmectomy result in an inadequate blood supply, the jejunal continuation of the artery may be anastomosed to the remaining superior mesenteric artery directly or by interposing a saphenous vein graft.

Following resection of a mycotic aneurysm the use of an inert prosthesis or even a venous homograft especially if it courses through the aneurysm bed is best avoided. If flow needs to be restored, an "extraanatomic" route from an adjacent vessel such as the aorta to the jejunal or ileal segment of the superior mesenteric artery is chosen.

Other techniques for treatment of saccular aneurysms include endoaneurysmorrhaphy: after inflow and outflow control, the aneurysm is opened and its orifice with the main artery, which may be only an ovoid slit, several centimeters long, is oversewn from within the aneurysm, maintaining patency of the native vessel. This technique is particularly recommended for mycotic and traumatic, false aneurysms, which both originate from a limited area of weakness in the arterial wall (37). As part of the management of mycotic aneurysms the infected aneurysm sac and contents are excised or "debrided," but not necessarily excising the native vessel. A prolonged course of the appropriate antimicrobial agent is given, starting before operation and continuing for 6 weeks or more after operation. If this is discontinued too early, residual arterial infection may lead to reformation of an aneurysm.

A variant of aneurysmorrhaphy may be helpful to treat large saccular or fusiform aneurysms: the sac is opened after control of its inflow and outflow, and the orifices of native artery attached to the aneurysmal segment are oversewn from inside the sac. This, in fact, obliterates the involved segment of the artery, and it is ascertained that no distal ischemia results.

Excision of many of these superior mesenteric artery aneurysms may be difficult as they can be adherent to important adjacent structures including the superior mesenteric vein. An injury or deliberate surgical procedure that occludes the superior mesenteric vein is poorly tolerated and may produce small-bowel ischemia. With such an aneurysm, the sac is totally excised except for the section of its wall adherent to the vein.

Operations on the main trunk of the superior mesenteric artery are usually done through a vertical abdominal incision. To expose the artery more proximally and its origin, the duodenojejunal flexure is mobilized and reflected along with elevation of the pancreas. The patient with a ruptured, freely bleeding superior mesenteric artery aneurysm often requires clamp control of the aorta at the diaphragmatic hiatus to stop bleeding and so permit operation on the aneurysm itself. Some very proximally situated aneurysms of the superior mesenteric artery may be operated on by exposing the origin of the artery extraperitoneally, reflecting the left colon and duodenum to the right. In some cases a thoracoabdominal incision facilitates this.

Other Splanchnic Artery Aneurysms

These are very uncommon and include aneurysms of the celiac, gastric, gastroduodenal, and pancreaticoduodenal arteries, the ileal and jejunal branches of the superior mesenteric trunk, and most rarely of all the inferior mesenteric artery. The majority are atherosclerotic degenerative aneurysms. However some arise following trauma to the arterial wall or from local inflammation, particularly in the case of the pancreaticoduodenal and gastroduodenal arteries in patients with pancreatitis.

The rarity of these aneurysms makes them reportable and has led to many sporadic case reports from which recommendations have been extrapolated. Like aneurysms elsewhere it is thought they will all enlarge and, depending on their site, will obstruct adjacent organs, particularly the biliary system, ultimately rupturing (Figure 39-3*A* and *B*).

CELIAC ARTERY ANEURYSMS

Techniques for managing celiac aneurysms usually seek to restore flow to the hepatic branch only (38). At operation the origin of the celiac artery is temporarily occluded, assessing the adequacy of the collaterals, particularly to the liver. Potentially there are a large number of possible collateral pathways, but there is wide variability in the actual collateral blood flow between the mesenteric regions of supply. Many patients with splanchnic aneurysms have generalized atherosclerosis that stimulates hypertrophy of collaterals, and consequently ischemia often does not follow ligation of a principal intestinal artery, including the celiac axis. In fact intentional resection of the celiac axis for radical treatment of cancer of the stomach was not associated with liver ischemia even though the common hepatic artery was not reanastomosed (39).

PANCREATICODUODENAL AND GASTRODUODENAL ARTERY ANEURYSMS

Pancreaticoduodenal and gastroduodenal artery aneurysms in patients with pancreatitis usually present as gastrointestinal bleeding following rupture into the pancreatic duct or the biliary system or adjacent bowel. These should always be considered as a possible origin for intestinal bleeding in patients with pancreatitis (12,13).

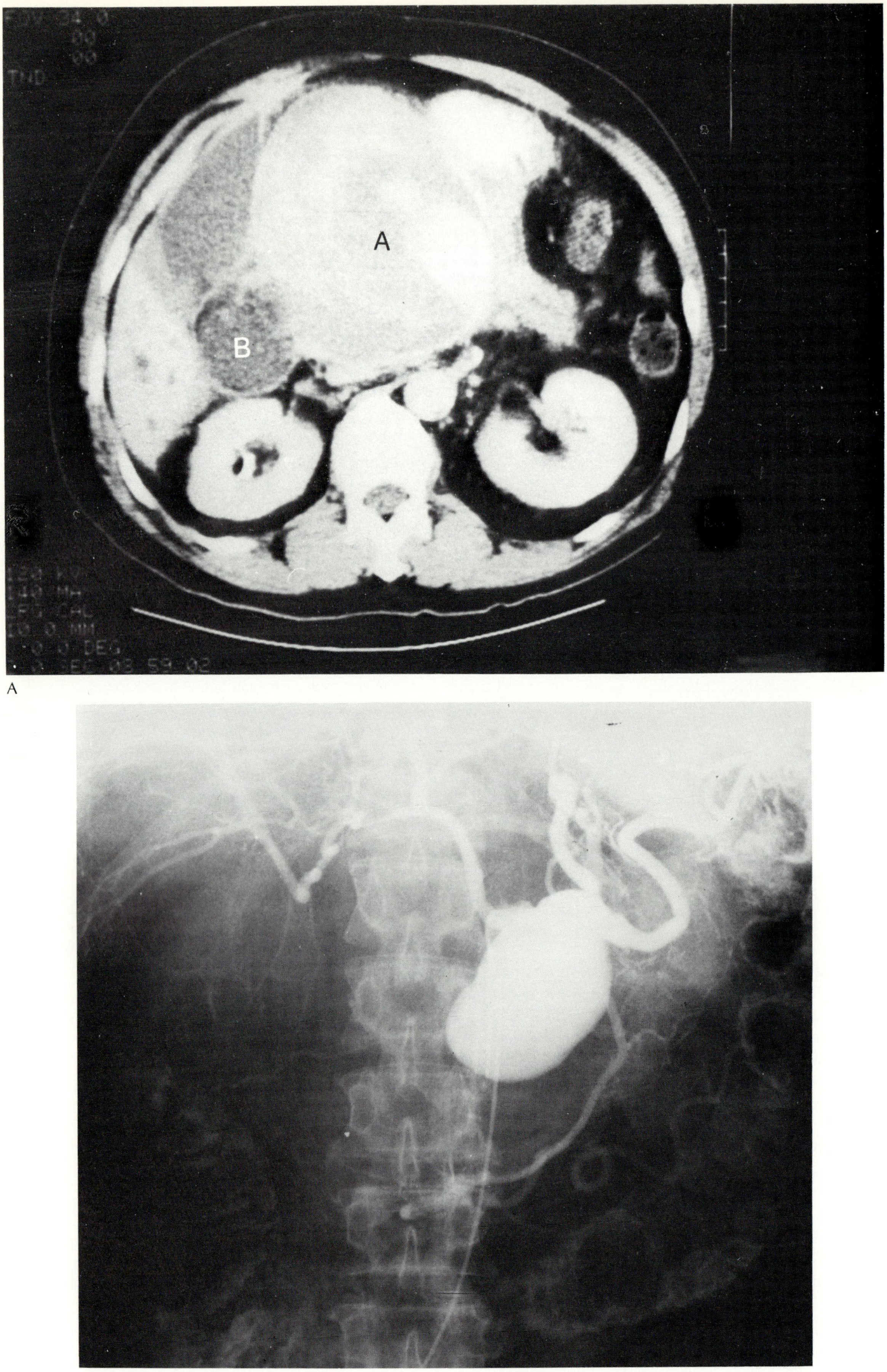

A

B

FIGURE 39–3. (*A*) CT scan with enhancement of celiac artery aneurysm (A) compressing the extrahepatic bile ducts (B) producing biliary obstruction. (*B*) Angiogram of the same celiac artery aneurysm.

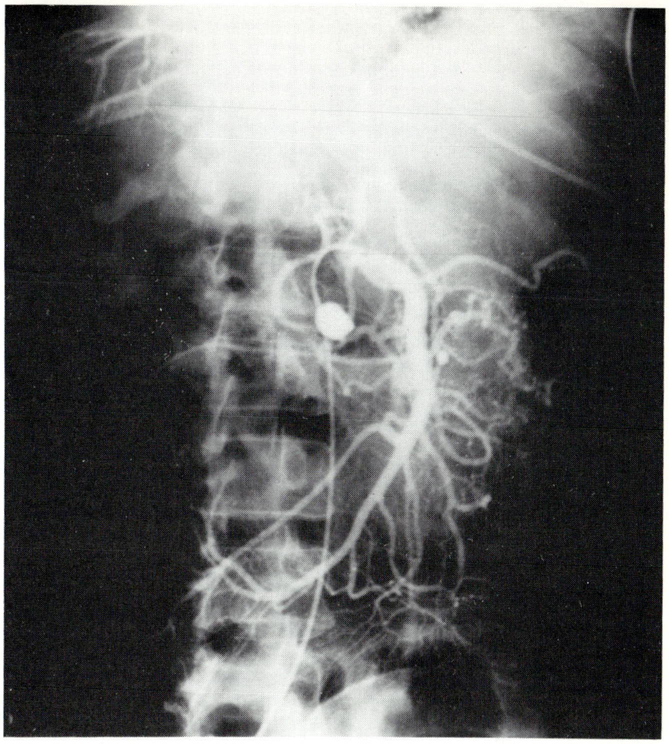

FIGURE 39–4. Pancreaticoduodenal artery aneurysm.

Barium studies have not been useful to detect these aneurysms but will exclude other causes of gastrointestinal bleeding. The same is true of endoscopic studies. Diagnosis is made with mesenteric angiography outlining the aneurysm and in addition possibly showing extravasation of contrast material (Figure 39-4). Transcatheter embolization is an excellent method for treating these aneurysms, avoiding an otherwise difficult operation. Patients who have operative treatment for pancreatitis-related aneurysms and gastrointestinal hemorrhage have approximately a 50 percent mortality rate (20,40).

References

1. Bedford PD, Lodge B: Aneurysm of the splenic artery. Gut 1960, 1:312–320.
2. Owens JC, Coffey RJ: Aneurysms of the splenic artery, including a report of six additional cases. Int Abst Surg 1953, 97:313–335.
3. Foremore SW, Guida PM, Schmacher HW: Splenic artery aneurysm. Bull Soc Int Chir 1970, 29:210–218.
4. Boijsen E, Efsing HO: Aneurysm of the splenic artery. Acta Radiol Scand 1969, 8:29–41.
5. Deterling RA: Aneurysms of the visceral arteries. J Cardiovasc Surg 1971, 12:309–322.
6. Beaussier M: Sur un aneurisme de l'artere splenique dont les parios se sont ossifees. J Med Toulouse 1770, 31:157.
7. Lindboe EF: Aneurysm of the splenic artery diagnosed by x-rays and operated upon with success. Acta Chir Scand 1932, 72:108–114.
8. Stanley JC, Fry WJ: Pathogenesis and clinical significance of splenic artery aneurysms. Surgery 1974, 76:898–909.
9. Trastek VF, Bairolero PC, Joyce JW, Hollier LH, Bernatz PE: Splenic artery aneurysms. Surgery 1982, 91:694–699.
10. Feist JH, Gajaraj A: Extra- and intrasplenic artery aneurysms in portal hypertension. Radiology 1977, 125:331–334.
11. Joske RA: Occurrence of large proximal splenic artery aneurysms in chronic liver disease. Aust NZ J Med 1978, 8:515–517.
12. Clay RP, Farnell MB, Lancaster JR, Weiland LH, Gostout CJ: Hemosuccus pancreaticus. Ann Surg 1985, 1002:75–79.
13. Walter JF, Chuang VP, Bookstein JJ, Reuter SR, Cho KJ, Pulmano M: Angiography of massive hemorrhage secondary to pancreatic disease. Radiology 1977, 124:337–342.
14. Sherlock SPV, Learmonth JR: Aneurysm of splenic artery with account of example complicating Gaucher's disease. Br J Surg 1942, 30:151–160.
15. Sperling L: Aneurysm of the splenic artery: Recovery after removal. Surgery 1940, 8:633–638.
16. Brockman R, Saint L: Aneurysm of the splenic artery. Br J Surg 1930, 17:692–693.
17. McFarlane J, Thorbjarnarson B: Rupture of splenic artery aneurysm during pregnancy. Am J Obstet Gynecol 1966, 95:1024–1037.
18. O'Grady JP, Day EJ, Toole AL, Paust JC: Splenic artery aneurysm rupture in pregnancy. Obstet Gynecol 1977, 50:626–630.
19. Rogers DM, Thompson JE, Garrett WV, Talkington CM, Patman RD: Mesenteric vascular problems. A 26 year experience. Ann Surg 1982, 195:554–565.
20. Stabile BE, Wilson SE, Debas HT: Reduced mortality from bleeding pseudocysts and pseudoaneurysms caused by pancreatitis. Arch Surg 1983, 118:45–51.
21. Probst P, Castaneda-Zuniga WR, Gomes AS, Yonehiro EG, Delaney JP, Amplatz K: Nonsurgical treatment of splenic artery aneurysms. Diagn Radiol 1978, 128:619–623.
22. Tsapogas MJ, Peabody RA, Karmody AM, Chuntrasakuli C, Youssous H, Eckert C: Pathophysiological changes following ischemia of the spleen. Ann Surg 1973, 178:179–185.
23. McKinnon WM, Smith RB, Carter Davis S, Connelly TL, Perdue GD: Ruptured hepatic artery aneurysm with hepatic artery to portal vein fistula. Surgery 1981, 89:626–630.

24. Dwight RW, Ratcliffe JW: Aneurysms of the hepatic artery. Surgery 1952, 31:915–921.
25. Michels NA: Collateral arterial pathways to the liver after ligation of the hepatic artery and removal of the celiac access. Cancer 1953, 6:708–724.
26. Michels NA: Newer anatomy of the liver and its variant blood supply and collateral circulation. Am J Surg 1966, 112:337–347.
27. Kadir S, Athanasoulis CA, Ring EJ, Greenfield A: Transcatheter embolization of intrahepatic arterial aneurysms. Radiology 1980, 134:335–339.
28. Porter LL, Houston MC, Kadir S: Mycotic aneurysms of the hepatic artery: Treatment with arterial embolization. Am J Med 1979, 67:697–701.
29. Wallace S, Gianturco C, Anderson JH, Goldstein HM, Davis JL, Bree RL: Therapeutic vascular occlusion utilizing steel coil. Am J Roentgenol 1976, 127:381–383.
30. Jonsson K, Bjernstad A, Eriksson B: Treatment of a hepatic artery aneurysm by coil occlusion of the hepatic artery. Am J Radiol 1980, 134:1245–1247.
31. Sjovall S, Hoevels J, Sundqvist K: Fatal outcome from emergency embolization of an intrahepatic aneurysm. Surgery 1980, 87:347–350.
32. Wright CB, Schoepfle WJ, Kurtock SB, Corry RJ, Rose EF, Lamberth WC, Cow KC, Khangure MS, Chiu LC: Gastrointestinal bleeding and mycotic superior mesenteric aneurysm. Surgery 1982, 92:40–44.
33. Yellin AE: Ruptured mycotic aneurysm: A complication of parenteral drug use. Arch Surg 1977, 112:981–986.
34. Blumenberg RM, David D, Slovak J: Abdominal apoplexy due to rupture of a superior mesenteric artery aneurysm. Arch Surg 1974, 108:223–226.
35. Maloney RD, Nealon TF, Bonfils Roberts EA: Massive bleeding from a ruptured superior mesenteric artery aneurysm into the duodenum. Arch Surg 1976, 111:286–288.
36. DeBakey ME, Cooley DA: Successful resection of mycotic aneurysm of superior mesenteric artery aneurysm. Ann Surg 1953, 19:202–212.
37. Olcott C, Ehrenfeld WK: Endoaneurysmorrphy for visceral artery aneurysms. Am J Surg 1977, 133:636–639.
38. Haimovici H, Sprayregan S, Eckstein P, Veith FJ: Celiac artery aneurysmectomy: Case report with review of the literature. Surgery 1976, 79:592–596.
39. Appleby LH: The celiac axis in the expansion of the operations for gastric carcinoma. Cancer 1953, 6:704–707.
40. Eckhauser F, Stanley J, Zelenock GB, Borlaza GS, Freier DT, Lindenauer SM: Gastroduodenal and pancreaticoduodenal artery aneurysms. Surgery 1980, 88:335–344.

Chapter 40

INFECTED ANEURYSMS

BRUCE A. PERLER and CALVIN B. ERNST

No problem encountered by the general vascular surgeon is more demanding than management of arterial infection. Despite advances in evaluation and treatment of arterial diseases, an infected aneurysm remains unequaled in terms of risk to life and limb. Although improvements in surgical technique and better antimicrobial prophylaxis have reduced septic complications of vascular reconstruction, spontaneous arterial infection continues to be a challenging problem. Diagnosis is difficult and often delayed, treatment is demanding, and results far from satisfactory. It is the purpose of this chapter to offer a pragmatic definition of infected aneurysms, to highlight the appropriate diagnostic approach, and to outline therapeutic options.

History

Although infection is a far less common cause of arterial aneurysm formation than arteriosclerosis, aneurysms resulting from infection are among the oldest arterial lesions described in the western literature. As early as the sixteenth century, Ambrose Paré recognized that aneurysms could develop secondarily to microbial infection, specifically syphilis.

In 1844, Rokitansky described abscesses in the walls of arteries and proposed that they resulted from the lodgment of infected emboli (1). Koch, in 1851, described a 22-year-old man who died suddenly from a ruptured aneurysm of the superior mesenteric artery while being treated for endocarditis (2). In 1853, Tufnell reported upon a 25-year-old man with endocarditis and a popliteal aneurysm. He believed that the aneurysm resulted from embolization of endocardial vegetations to the popliteal artery (3).

It was upon this background that Sir William Osler, in presenting the first of his Gulstonion Lectures to the Royal College of Physicians in London in March 1885, coined the term "mycotic aneurysm" (4). Osler described several cases in which he believed valvular vegetations characteristic of endocarditis spread directly to the aortic wall and led to aneurysmal degeneration. Osler's work firmly established mycotic aneurysms as a clinical entity and stimulated other workers to make further observations. By 1923 Stengel and Wolferth had identified 217 cases of mycotic aneurysms from a review of the world's literature (5).

TERMINOLOGY

Confusion exists in the literature concerning the classification and categorization of infected aneurysms. Presumably, Osler named these lesions "mycotic" because of the "fresh fungus vegetations" in the multiple beadlike aneurysms he described (4). Although mycotic is synonymous with fungal, the term mycotic aneurysm has been used inappropriately to describe any arterial aneurysm caused by microorganisms, fungal or bacterial. To be accurate and minimize confusion, mycotic aneurysm should be considered a lesion that develops as a complication of bacterial endocarditis, as Osler described.

Eppinger introduced the term "embolomycotic" to describe these aneurysms (6). Although others postulated that embolization of endocardial vegetations led to aneurysm formation through purely traumatic effects, Eppinger identified the same bacterial strains at the site of emboli as found in endocardial vegetations. He postulated that lodgment of bacteria-laden emboli in the arterial wall initiated the development of an exudative periarteritis with subsequent destruction of the elastic and muscular elements of the wall with eventual aneurysm formation. The term embolomycotic recognized both the traumatic and infectious elements in the development of these aneurysms (7).

Although over 90 percent of the mycotic aneurysms reported in the early literature were associated with endocarditis, there were sporadic reports describing patients with infected aneurysms but without endocardial disease (8). In 1937 Crane described a patient with a multilocular aortic aneurysm who had no evidence of endocardial infection (9). He coined the term "primary mycotic aneurysm" to describe this entity. According to Crane, this lesion developed in the wall of an artery without a demonstrable intravascular inflammatory focus, bacterial endocarditis, or any inflammatory or septic process in surrounding tissues. Revell, in a 1943 review of the literature, found only 23 cases of primary mycotic aneurysms and added one of his own (10). Such reports attest to the prevalence of bacterial endocarditis in the preantibiotic era (11). Revell emphasized that a mycotic aneurysm should be classified as primary if it resulted from a bacteremia from an obscure focus. Specifically, he felt there should be no evidence of endocarditis or a septic process adjacent to the arterial lesion, reiterating Crane's definition (9,10).

According to these criteria, Osler's mycotic aneurysms would be classified as "secondary mycotic aneurysms" since they developed as a result of the embolization of infected vegetations or from the direct spread of aortic valve vegetations to the sinus of Valsalva or aortic wall. Likewise, direct spread of sepsis from an infected lymph node or osteomyelitis to an adjacent artery would lead to secondary mycotic aneurysm formation (8).

Compounding the nomenclature confusion was the introduction of the term "cryptogenic mycotic aneurysms" by Blum and Keefer in 1962 (12). They noted infected aneurysms resulted from deposition of organisms upon a diseased intimal surface. In cryptogenic mycotic aneurysms the source of the bacteremia was unknown, as opposed to a known, albeit extravascular, or noncontiguous, source in the primary mycotic aneurysm terminology (13). Since the pathophysiology, bacteriology, clinical presentation, and proper therapy of these lesions are similar to that for primary mycotic aneurysms described in most series (vida infra), this additional terminology seems superfluous.

Rokitansky's observation of abscess formation within the arterial wall remained unnoticed for many years (7). Eventually, however, cases of arterial sepsis without aneurysm formation were reported. Parkhurst and Decker described 12 patients with bacterial infection of the aortic wall, but with aneurysm formation in only 9 (13). In the three without aneurysms, the disease entity was termed "bacterial aortitis." Bardin noted that arterial infection without aneurysm formation represented a midpoint on the continuum from asymptomatic bacterial colonization to invasive infection with aneurysm formation, and he coined the term "nonaneurysmal suppurative aortitis" (14). "Microbial arteritis" has been recently proposed to describe arterial infection without aneurysm development (15).

Classification

Although most of the nomenclature has been well defined by the respective proponents, the multiplicity of terms has led to confusion regarding the appropriate classification of spontaneous arterial infection (Table 40-1). Few authors have attempted to assimilate all forms of spontaneous arterial infection under one comprehensive classification system. Patel and Johnston proposed a comprehensive classification in which an infected aneurysm was categorized according to the preexisting arterial condition: normal, arteriosclerotic, aneurysmal, or arterial prosthesis, and the source of infection intravascular or extravascular (16). Intravascular sources of infection included septic embolism, septicemia, or extension of adjacent endocardial infection. Extravascular sources included spread from adjacent foci or iatrogenic infection. Wilson and his colleagues classified all forms of spontaneous arterial infection into seven categories (Table 40-2) (17).

Review and study of the pathophysiology, bacteriology, and epidemiology of these lesions supports a natural distinction between mycotic aneurysms associated with infective endocarditis as defined by Osler and those arterial infections not associated with infective endocarditis. Therefore, for the purposes of this chapter, these lesions are classified as

Mycotic aneurysms

Infected aneurysms (nonendocarditis):
- Microbial arteritis with aneurysm formation
- Secondarily infected aneurysm
- Microbial arteritis without aneurysm formation

Colonized aneurysms

Traumatic infected pseudoaneurysms, septic arterial emboli, and spontaneous aortoenteric fistula are beyond the scope of this chapter.

TABLE 40-1. Nomenclature for Arterial Infection

Mycotic aneurysm
Primary mycotic aneurysm
Secondary mycotic aneurysm
Cryptogenic mycotic aneurysm
Embolomycotic aneurysm
Bacterial aortitis
Nonaneurysmal suppurative aortitis
Microbial arteritis

TABLE 40-2. Classification of Spontaneous Arterial Infection

I. *Mycotic aneurysm:*
Aneurysm occurring in a normal or atherosclerotic artery resulting from emboli of endocardial origin

II. *Infected aneurysm:*
Established aneurysm infected by bacteremia

III. *Microbial arteritis:*
Infection of normal or atherosclerotic vessel by a bacteremia, often resulting in rupture of the artery and pseudoaneurysm formation

IV. *Traumatic infected pseudoaneurysm:*
Aneurysm caused by trauma (penetrating or blunt); iatrogenic injury; injection sites in narcotic addicts

V. *Contiguous arterial infection:*
Arterial invasion from an adjacent septic focus

VI. *Septic arterial emboli*

VII. *Spontaneous aortoenteric fistula*

SOURCE: After Wilson, Van Wagenen, and Passaro (17).

Mycotic Aneurysms

INCIDENCE

Mycotic aneurysms may occur in a normal or arteriosclerotic artery secondary to embolization or direct extension of septic valvular vegetations in a patient with infective endocarditis (4,17). Prior to the introduction of antimicrobial drugs, this type represented the most common form of arterial infection (5,7). In a 1923 review, Stengel and Wolferth identified 217 patients, of whom 186 (87 percent) developed aneurysms secondary to endocardial infection (5). Pulmonary infection and osteomyelitis were much less frequent causes.

It is difficult to ascertain how frequently mycotic aneurysms develop in patients with infective endocarditis. In one report, 13 percent of patients with endocarditis died of mycotic aneurysm rupture (17). In another, 20 of 442 (4.5 percent) patients treated for subacute bacterial endocarditis died from rupture of a mycotic aneurysm (11).

The introduction of antimicrobial drugs has reduced the mortality and morbidity of bacterial endocarditis. Consequently, a reduction in the incidence of mycotic aneurysms has resulted, although this is difficult to quantitate accurately. In 20,201 autopsies performed at the Mayo Clinic through 1954, 178 abdominal aortic aneurysms were identified and only 6 (3 percent) were infected (18). None were associated with endocarditis. Nevertheless, since endocarditis has not yet been eradicated, the potential for mycotic aneurysm formation remains a concern. This was emphasized by a 1967 report in which 10 of 16 infected aneurysms were secondary to bacterial endocarditis (19). Drug addicts' use of contaminated needles may contribute to an increase in incidence of endocardial disease and subsequent mycotic aneurysms in the future (17).

PATHOGENESIS

Mycotic aneurysms develop from infected heart valves either by direct extension or by embolization. Eppinger was the first investigator to isolate identical bacterial strains from mycotic aneurysms and endocardial vegetations in patients with endocarditis, providing circumstantial evidence in support of the embolic mechanism (6). Direct spread of infection from the aortic valve to the ascending aorta occurs in a substantial number of cases (20,21). Embolization of infected debris also occurs to the vasa vasorum, or to small arterial branches of the main vessel. Finding intact intima in the aorta at sites of mycotic aneurysm development suggests that these intramural abscesses were seeded from vasa vasorum (22–24). Infected emboli may cause thrombosis of the vasa vasorum, and the subsequent vessel wall ischemia, compounded by the local sepsis, initiates degeneration of elastic and muscular elements resulting in aneurysm development (25). This is probably the mechanism responsible for aneurysm formation in large vessels such as the thoracic aorta. Lodgment of septic emboli in small peripheral arterial branches and the subsequent destructive infectious process results in infected aneurysms of peripheral vessels.

In some patients, histological examination of mycotic aneurysms has documented intramural abscesses in the intima and inner portion of the media, areas supplied not by vasa vasorum but by the intraluminal circulating blood (26). Such transmural innoculation leads to intimal and medial damage resulting in aneurysmal dilatation. This mechanism is probably operative in the smaller, more peripheral arteries. The final common pathway is destruction of the arterial wall, with progressive aneurysmal dilatation and eventual rupture.

HISTOLOGY

The grossly normal vessel adjacent to the aneurysm may harbor microscopic signs of inflammation. Although histological findings may be quite variable, the inflammatory reaction is less acute in mycotic than in infected aneurysms. The most characteristic findings in mycotic aneurysms are damage and loss of intima, destruction of elastic lamellae, especially the internal elastic lamina, and periarteritis or mesoarteritis. When the inflammatory reaction is less acute, plasma cells and lymphocytes may predominate. Usually, the inflammatory reaction is most prominent around vasa vasorum, which may be thickened or obliterated in areas of the greatest inflammation. In chronic aneurysms, an infiltration of fibroblasts may be identified as well as calcification (8,18,27).

Infected Aneurysms: Microbial Arteritis with Aneurysm; Infected Aneurysm

INCIDENCE

Coincident with the prompt and effective treatment of endocarditis has been a decline in the incidence of mycotic aneurysms. Paradoxically, infected aneurysms continue to increase. With the aging population and aneurysmal complications of arteriosclerosis on the rise, more patients are being identified with secondary infection of preexisting arterial aneurysms, usually of the abdominal aorta (28,29). In addition, microbial innoculation of a diseased, but nonaneurysmal arterial wall may result in infection, mural weakening, and aneurysm formation. Such lesions are classified as microbial arteritis with aneurysm. Since the pathogenesis and bacteriology of both infected aneurysms and microbial arteritis with aneurysm are similar, and since histological differentiation is often impossible, these lesions should be considered a variant of the same disease process: infected aneurysms.

As with mycotic aneurysms, it is difficult to determine the incidence of infected aneurysms. Most studies have evaluated aortic aneurysms. In an autopsy series from Boston City Hospital covering the years 1902 through 1951, 338 aortic aneurysms were noted and yet only 12 aortic infections (3.5 percent) were recognized. Seven of these were associated with bacterial endocarditis; thus, the incidence of nonendocarditis-associated aneurysms was 1.5 percent (13). A 3.4 percent incidence of infected aortic aneurysms was noted in an autopsy series from the Mayo Clinic (18). Presently, the incidence of infected abdominal aortic aneurysms is estimated to be 3 to 5 percent (30).

PATHOGENESIS

Available data suggest that innoculation of an intimal lesion during transient bacteremia is the mechanism by which both microbial arteritis and infection of a preexisting arterial aneurysm are initiated (27). Since intact intima is known to be highly resistant to bacterial infection, a defect in the intimal surface appears necessary for microbial arteritis to develop (31,32). Arteriosclerosis significantly diminishes resistance of the arterial wall to bacterial infection and is the underlying abnormality in the majority of patients with infected aneurysms (33). Thrombus within arterial aneurysms and the large area of intimal disruption make these lesions particularly susceptible to infection. Whether the infection develops in a nonaneurysmal atherosclerotic plaque or within an aneurysm, results are similar. Localized sepsis results in a disintegration of mural elastic and muscular elements with resultant progressive dilatation of the vessel. Once a nidus of infection is established within a plaque or aneurysm thrombus, it becomes difficult, if not impossible, for systemic antimicrobial agents to eradicate the infection.

Although atherosclerosis is the most common lesion predisposing to development of infected aneurysms, any condition which causes irregularity of the luminal surface such as coarctation may predispose to secondary bacterial infection (34,35). It has been suggested that the thickened intima characteristically located just distal to the coarctation is particularly susceptible to bacterial invasion (36,37).

Infected aneurysms may develop secondary to chronic arteriovenous fistulas (38). Progressive dilatation of the proximal artery and associated degenerative changes of the arterial wall appear to increase susceptibility to bacterial infection (39,40). An infected aneurysm may develop at the reentry site of a chronic aortic dissection (41). Spontaneous arterial infections have also developed in segments of cystic medionecrosis and areas of syphilitic aortitis (17,42).

Some infected aneurysms have been identified with apparently intact intimal surfaces. Under these circumstances it is presumed that hematogenous infection seeded the arterial wall via vasa vasorum (24). An association has been demonstrated between infected aortic aneurysms and both lumbar osteomyelitis and infected paraaortic lymph nodes. In one study, 18 percent of the patients with infected aneurysms of the abdominal aorta also had apparent involvement of adjacent lumbar vertebrae (43). It is possible that infection within the vertebrae or lymph nodes reaches the aorta via the lymphatic channels or the vasa vasorum, although evidence in support of this mechanism is speculative (24).

HISTOLOGY

In addition to differences in pathogenesis, infected aneurysms can usually be distinguished from the classic mycotic aneurysms histologically. In an infected aneurysm, the inflammatory reaction is very localized, in contrast to the diffuse inflammatory involvement in mycotic aneurysms. The inflammatory reaction may be so localized that diagnosis of an infected aortic aneurysm may be missed unless multiple microscopic sections are examined. Whereas the intima may be absent in mycotic aneurysms, identifiable fragments of all layers of the arterial wall are usually found in infected aneurysms. The inflammatory reaction is consistently acute in infected aneurysms, whereas subacute or even more chronic changes may be noted in mycotic aneurysms (28).

Anatomic Distribution

Mycotic and infected aneurysms have involved almost every artery. Although most reports of clinical and autopsy series record solitary aneurysms, occasionally patients have been described with multiple mycotic or infected aneurysms in one or several vessels (4,44). The distribution of these lesions varies among reports (Table 40-3) (5,7,10,31,45,46). Excluding extracranial vessels, the most common sites are the aorta, visceral arteries, and vessels to the arms and legs. As endocarditis with peripheral embolic seeding has declined in etiologic importance, aortic involvement appears to be increasing over that of peripheral lesions (43).

AORTA

All segments of the aorta have been affected, from the ascending thoracic aorta to the bifurcation (Figure 40-1). When bacterial endocarditis was prevalent, mycotic aneurysms frequently developed in the ascending aorta and arch. Either direct extension of infected vegetations from the aortic valve to the aorta or embolization to this site via the vasa vasorum was responsible. As infected arteriosclerotic aneurysms have become more common than true mycotic aneurysms, the abdominal aorta, because of its predilection for arteriosclerotic degeneration, has been more commonly involved (31).

CORONARY ARTERIES

Coronary artery aneurysms are exceedingly uncommon, and sepsis accounts for only a small number. In one review of 89 cases, only 11 percent of coronary aneurysms were mycotic or infected (47). The right and left coronary arteries were equally involved. Most have been true mycotic aneurysms associated with endo-

TABLE 40-3. Anatomic Distribution of Mycotic and Infected Aneurysms

	Stengel (5)	Lewis (7)	Revell (10)	Mundth (31)	Anderson (46)	Total
Aorta	66 (25%)	12 (11%)	21 (75%)	13 (76%)	2 (12%)	114 (27%)
Visceral	69 (26%)	31 (29%)	4 (14%)	1 (6%)	0	105 (24%)
Arm	23 (9%)	13 (12%)	2 (7%)	0	3 (19%)	41 (10%)
Leg	31 (12%)	11 (10%)	1 (4%)	2 (12%)	7 (44%)	52 (12%)
Iliac	10 (4%)	3 (3%)	0	1 (6%)	4 (25%)	18 (4%)
Coronary	9 (3%)	0	0	0	0	9 (2%)
Pulmonary	14 (5%)	0	0	0	0	14 (3%)
Other	42 (16%)	37 (35%)	0	0	0	79 (18%)
Total	264	107	28	17	16	432

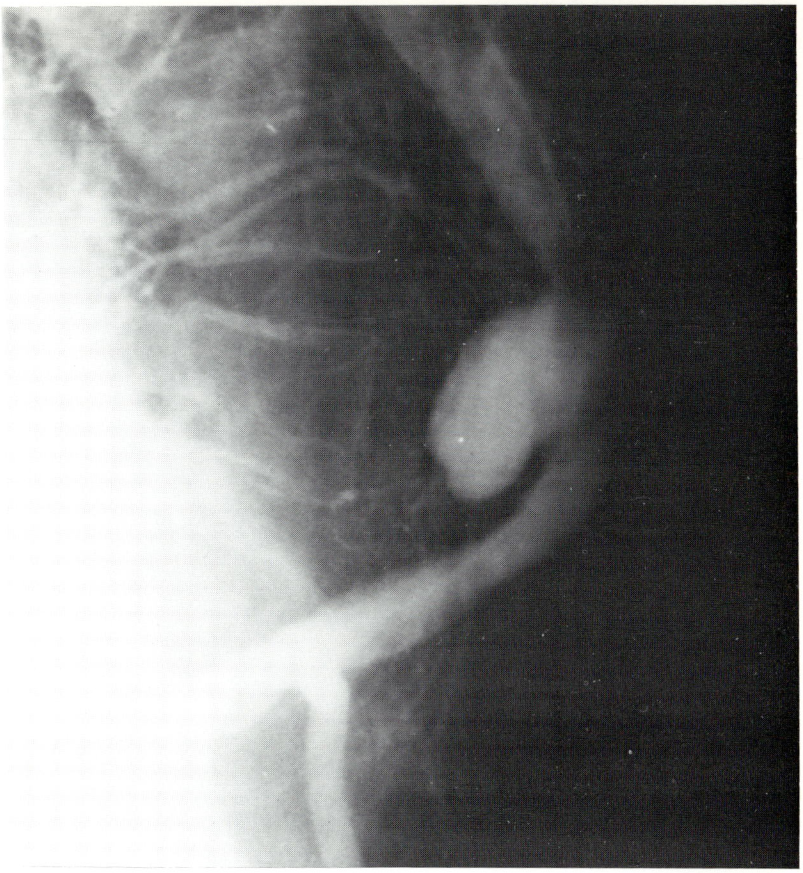

A

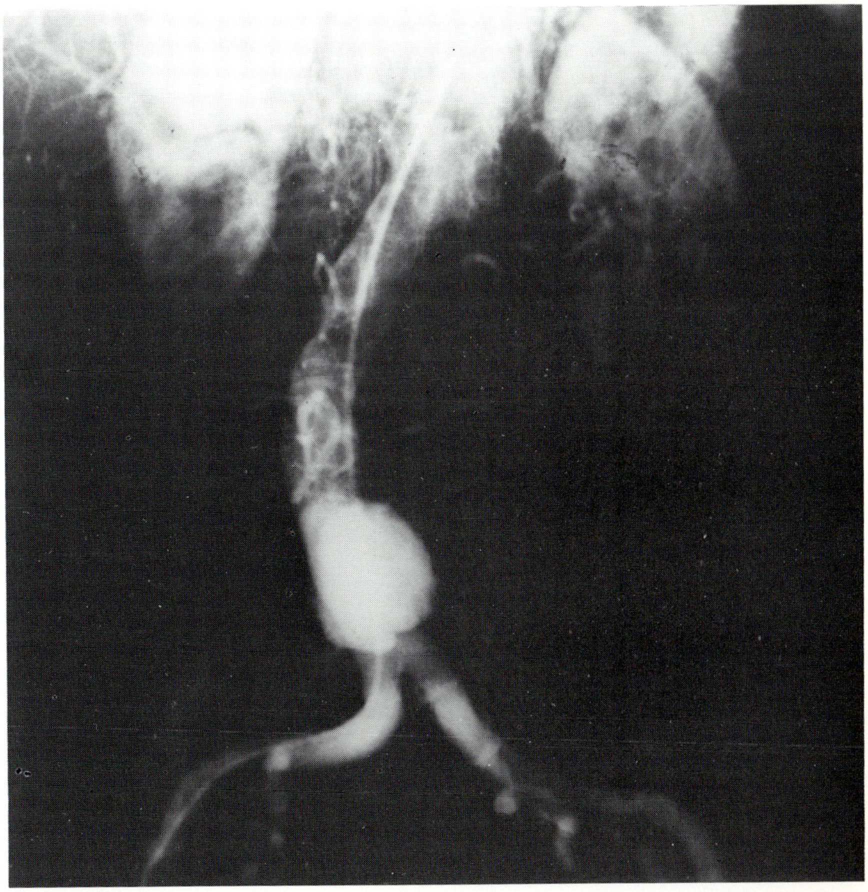

B

Figure 40–1. Lateral (***A***) and frontal (***B***) aortograms showing typical saccular appearance of a mycotic abdominal aortic aneurysm.

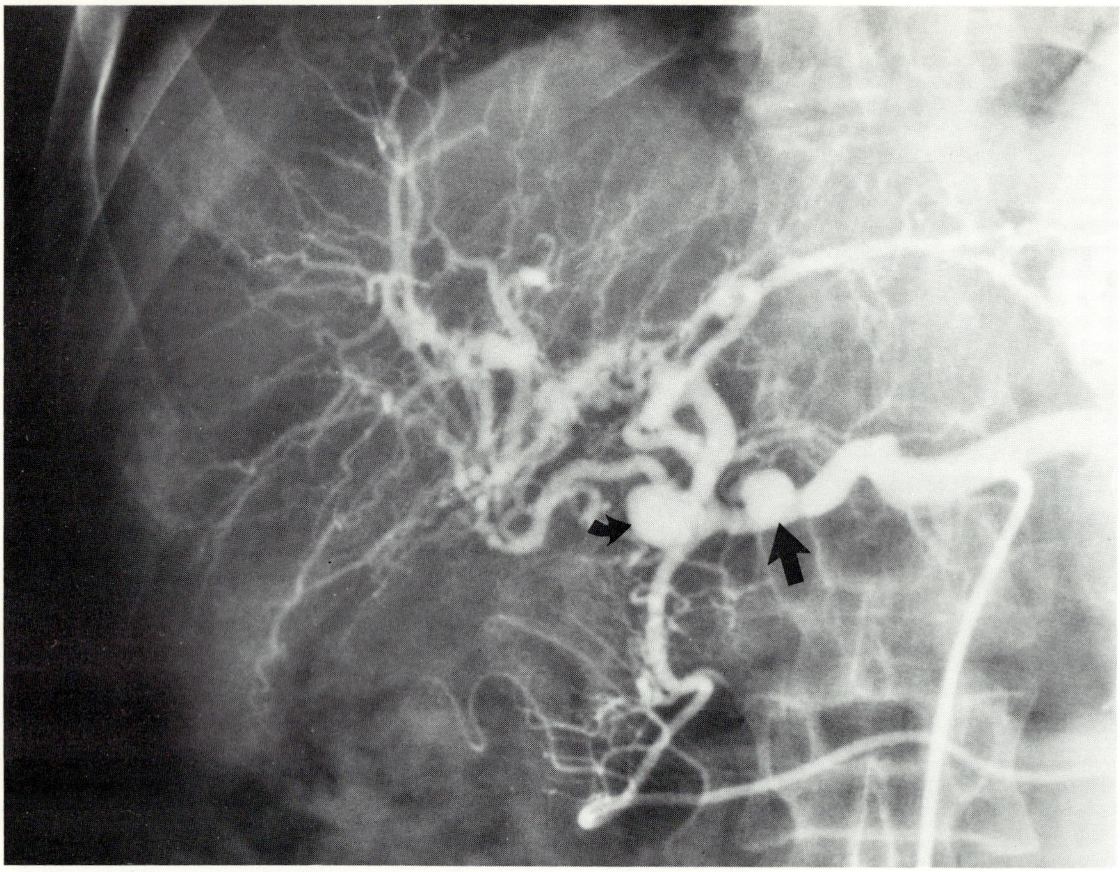

Figure 40–2. Selective celiac arteriogram of mycotic common hepatic (*large arrow*) and proper hepatic (*small arrow*) arterial aneurysms.

carditis, and diagnosis has usually been made at autopsy (48). Infection of arteriosclerotic coronary artery plaques does not appear to be a significant factor in the development of infected aneurysms.

PULMONARY ARTERY

Mycotic and infected aneurysms have been noted in the main pulmonary artery and, more commonly, its peripheral branches. They usually occur with endocarditis or a patent ductus arteriosus (49). Some of these aneurysms develop from direct extension of infection within the lung in addition to bacteremic seeding of the vessel (50). The natural history is of rapid expansion and rupture. Pulmonary angiography remains the definitive diagnostic procedure, enabling differentiation of these aneurysms from other vascular and nonvascular lesions (51).

CAROTID ARTERY

Since they present special problems in management (vida infra), it is fortunate that infected aneurysms involving the extracranial carotid artery are uncommon. Prior to the availability of antimicrobial drugs, many infected carotid aneurysms resulted from pharyngeal or cervical streptococcal infections (51). Spontaneous carotid artery infections have been reported following dental extractions and carotid arteriography and with septic arthritis (52–54). Infected carotid aneurysms may increase in the future secondary to the use of contaminated needles by drug addicts (55).

VISCERAL ARTERIES

Infection remains one of the most common causes of visceral artery aneurysms (56) (Figure 40-2). In the preantibiotic era it was estimated that 20 percent of splenic artery aneurysms were mycotic. Presumably, such aneurysms resulted from emboli from infected cardiac vegetations (57). In a 1969 review of 350 splenic artery aneurysms, 38 mycotic or infected lesions were identified (58). It is not known how often arteriosclerotic aneurysms of the splenic artery become infected.

Although superior mesenteric artery (SMA) aneurysms are not common, infection has been responsible for the greatest number (59). It has been estimated that 63 percent of all SMA aneurysms were mycotic, occurring after an episode of endocarditis (60). Stanley and his colleagues noted that 58 percent of all aneurysms of the SMA reported by 1970 were infected (56). SMA aneurysms may involve the main trunk or branch arteries (61–64).

The hepatic artery is rarely involved (Figure 40-2). As with the SMA, however, infection is the most common cause (65). The majority of hepatic arterial lesions reported have resulted from septic emboli from endocarditis. Since 1960, however, only 16 percent of hepatic artery aneurysms have been infected (56).

EXTREMITIES

Mycotic and infected aneurysms involve arm and leg arteries in about 20 percent of cases (Table 40-3). The brachial and femoral arteries are the most commonly involved vessels. Arteriographic catheterization procedures and drug abuse are responsible for most infected aneurysms at these sites.

Bacteriology

Numerous organisms have been isolated from mycotic and infected aneurysms (Table 40-4). The organism isolated depends upon the etiology of the aneurysm. When bacterial endocarditis was common, nonhemolytic streptococci, pneumococci, and staphylococci were frequently identified (5). In a 1943 study of 24 aneurysms, pneumococci (33 percent), streptococci (33 percent), gonococci (22 percent), and staphylococci (11 percent) were identified (10). In a review of cases recorded prior to 1960, streptococci and staphylococci were found to be the most common offenders (80 percent) followed by pneumococci and enterococci (17).

As endocarditis has become less prevalent, bacteriologic patterns have likewise shifted. The incidence of staphylococcal infection appears to be increasing (Table 40-4). *Salmonella* species have also emerged as frequent pathogens of infected aneurysms, particularly in the aorta. In a 1975 report of infected aortic aneurysms, staphylococci (41 percent) and *Salmonella* (18 percent) predominated (43). Other reports have documented isolation of *Salmonella* from 23 to 66 percent of infected aneurysms (28,31). In addition to the emergence of *Salmonella* and continued prevalence of staphylococcal species as responsible pathogens, other gram-negative organisms and anaerobic bacteria are being identified with increasing frequency (46).

Aneurysm cultures are not always revealing. In one study only 53 percent of aneurysm tissue sampled yielded growth of organisms (28). In another, 71 percent of aneurysm cultures were positive (31). Universal failure to grow organisms from obviously infected aneurysms relates to culture techniques and fragility of the organism being cultured.

TABLE 40-4. Bacteriology of Infected Aneurysms, 1968–1983 (Excluding Colonized Aneurysms)

Organism	No. Positive Cultures
Staphylococcus	23
Salmonella	17
Escherichia coli	10
Streptococcus	7
Pseudomonas	7
Anaerobes	7
Enterobacter	5
Fungal	5
Klebsiella	4
Proteus	4
Pneumococcus	2
Mycobacterium	2
Yersinia	1
Arizona hinshawii	1
Enterococcus	1
Campylobacter fetus	1
Citrobacter	1
Total	98

SOURCE: 14, 15, 29, 31, 32, 33, 38, 41, 43, 46, 49, 52, 55, 57, 67, 73, 81, 88, 91, 96, 98, 124, 127, 131, 149.

In addition to failure to culture organisms consistently, the source of infection has been determined in only 54 to 71 percent of cases (28,31). Osteomyelitis was the most common contributing etiology. Bacteremia secondary to gastroenteritis and endocarditis was also frequently noted. Less commonly encountered were urinary tract sepsis, esophageal fistula, diverticulitis, otitis media, pulmonary infection, and cellulitis. Clearly, transient bacteremias from unknown foci are an important factor in the pathogenesis of infected aneurysms.

In addition to suggesting appropriate antibiotic therapy, culture data may have some prognostic significance. Gram-negative infections of abdominal aortic aneurysms appear more ominous than gram-positive infections. In Jarrett's review, the mortality rate was 84 percent among patients with gram-negative infections, contrasted to only 50 percent when the aneurysm contained gram-positive organisms (43). Rupture of the aneurysm occurred in 5 of 6 patients with gram-negative infections compared to 1 of 10 with gram-positive organisms. The greater tendency for rupture with gram-negative infection and, hence, the increased mortality rate may reflect increased organism virulence.

SALMONELLA INFECTION

One of the more fascinating yet incompletely understood aspects of infected aneurysms, which deserves special comment, is the tendency for *Salmonella* species to cause arterial infection. Three types of vascular lesions may result from *Salmonella* infection. First, a diffuse suppurative arteritis may cause arterial rupture resulting in a saccular or false aneurysm. Second, *Salmonella* may initiate a focal arteritis that leads to weakening of the arterial wall and formation of a true infected aneurysm. Third, *Salmonella* species may infect a preexisting aneurysm. *Salmonella* arterial infections have been reported in the thoracic and abdominal aorta and in the iliac, femoral, popliteal, and coronary arteries (17,66–68). Seventy-five percent of *Salmonella* arterial infections affect the aorta, and 50 percent involve the abdominal aorta (69). Innoculation of the organisms on a diseased intimal surface appears to be the initiating event (70).

Salmonella organisms are gram-negative flagellated bacteria of the family Enterobacteriaceae (71). There are over 2200 serotypes with *Salmonella typhimurium* (33 percent), *S. enteritides* (9 percent), and *S. typhi* (2 percent) predominating (72). The most common isolates from infected aortic aneurysms are *S. choleraesuis* (32 percent), *S. typhimurium* (27 percent), and *S. enteritides* (9 percent) (73). Organism serotype determines the specific clinical syndrome (69). The high incidence of *Salmonella* arteritis caused by *S. choleraesuis* is probably related to its propensity to cause a severe bacteremia (15,74–77). Fifty percent of all *Salmonella* bacteremias are caused by *S. choler-*

aesuis, with localized suppurative infection occurring in 10 percent. In addition to arteritis, meningitis, pleuropulmonary disease, endocarditis, and osteomyelitis, splenic, hepatic, and soft tissue abscesses have been reported (68,77).

The recent increase in *Salmonella* arterial infection has led to rethinking previous dogma concerning antibiotic therapy for *Salmonella* gastroenteritis. Since antibiotics prolong the fecal excretion of *Salmonella* and increase the frequency of resistant stool isolates, most investigators recommend no treatment for this otherwise self-limited gastrointestinal ailment (78). However, in an extensive review of state laboratory records of *Salmonella* bacteremia in Massachusetts, it was noted that 10 of 105 patients with bacteremia developed endothelial foci of infection (79). Four of these 10 patients had preexisting untreated gastroenteritis. Furthermore, all 10 were over 50 years of age. Since only 40 patients older than 50 were noted to have *Salmonella* bacteremia during the study period, the incidence of endothelial infection in this age group was 25 percent. Others have corroborated a predilection of *Salmonella* arteritis for older individuals (80). Therefore, it has been suggested that antibiotic treatment of patients over 50 years old with *Salmonella* gastroenteritis might reduce the incidence of endothelial infection (79).

UNUSUAL BACTERIA

Recently, several unusual organisms have been isolated from infected aneurysms. Plotkin described a 53-year-old man with an infected aneurysm of the internal carotid artery caused by *Yersinia enterocolitica*, an aerobic and facultatively anaerobic, nonencapsulated, rod-shaped gram-negative organism (81). It was presumed that a transient bacteremia in this patient resulted in secondary infection of an arteriosclerotic carotid plaque with eventual aneurysm formation. Although *Yersinia* bacteremia is most commonly noted in patients compromised by malnutrition, carcinoma, hematologic malignancy, diabetes mellitus, and renal or hepatic faiure, it has also been described in healthy individuals.

Two other cases of arterial infection caused by unusual organisms have also been reported. In one, *Arizona hinshawii* was identified and the other *Campylobacter fetus* was isolated (82,83). Bacteria of the genus *Arizona* are among the Enterobacteriaceae that have been noted to cause a variety of diseases in humans, including gastroenteritis, urinary tract infection, cholecystitis, septic arthritis, osteomyelitis, and septicemia. Although taxonomically distinct from other Enterobacteriaceae, these organisms were at one time considered to belong to the genus *Salmonella*, since there are a number of biochemical and serologic similarities between these two groups of organisms (84). *Campylobacter*, like *Salmonella*, lacks the enterotoxin production, cytotoxicity, and invasive properties exhibited by other enteric organisms. Thus, although precise mechanisms of arterial infection are not known, *Campylobacter* and *Arizona* infections may share similar characteristics with *Salmonella*.

FUNGAL INFECTION

Despite the widespread use of "mycotic" (arising from the Oslerian term "fungus vegetations") to describe infected aneurysms, such aneurysms only rarely result from fungal infection. The thoracic and abdominal aorta, as well as the major peripheral and intracranial arteries, may be affected, however. *Histoplasma capsulatum, Aspergillus fumigatus, Candida albicans* and *Actinomyces* and *Penicillium* species are the only reported causative agents (85–88).

Like systemic fungal infections, these arterial infections tend to be associated with chronic immunosuppressive states, diabetes mellitus, and the use of contaminated needles (85,89,90). The precise mechanism of arterial infection varies but is similar to that for bacterial involvement. Innoculation of arteriosclerotic plaques by blood-borne organisms has been documented only for *Histoplasma* (85). Embolization of infected valvular vegetations and contiguous spread from adjacent foci of infection may also be responsible for some cases (85,91). Arterial infection via vasa vasorum, well established for bacterial organisms, has not been conclusively documented for fungi (85).

Fungal infection of arterial aneurysms may occur long after recognition of the original fungal infection. Such aneurysms are usually saccular, and when they involve the abdominal aorta, vertebral body erosion is frequently noted (85). The risk of rupture of these lesions is significant. In a review of aortic aneurysms infected with *Histoplasma capsulatum*, survival was only 33 percent (85). When the diagnosis of fungal infection of an aneurysm is suspected at operation, frozen section specimens should be examined for confirmation. Principles of surgical treatment are similar to those for aneurysms infected with bacteria (vida infra).

COLONIZED ANEURYSM

Three recent reports have documented bacterial growth from aneurysmal contents obtained from arteriosclerotic abdominal aortic aneurysms (92–94). The combined three series totaled 177 patients, and in 26 (15 percent) bacterial growth was identified on such cultures. The predominant organism was *Staphylococcus* (65 percent). In 19 percent of cultures gram-negative organisms were isolated. Principles of management of colonized aneurysms differ from apparently infected aneurysms (vida infra).

Natural History

Complications of infected aneurysms include progressive enlargement and rupture, thrombosis, and embolization. The incidence of rupture is high, averaging 54 percent compared to 20 percent for noninfected aneurysms (95). Furthermore, ruptured infected aneurysms are usually smaller than ruptured noninfected aneurysms, and progression to rupture occurs rapidly. Less commonly, a slow, insidious course precedes rupture of an infected aneurysm. A febrile illness lasting weeks and even months in some cases has been described prior to eventual rupture (28).

Outcome, once an infected aneurysm has ruptured, depends upon the vessel involved. Overall, mortality for a ruptured infected or mycotic aortic aneurysm approaches 95 percent, with only occasional survivors reported (95). Aortocaval and aortoenteric fistulas have also been reported secondary to mycotic and infected aneurysms (82,95). Limited perforation, particularly of a peripheral vessel, results in pseudoaneurysm formation with persistent sepsis.

Prior to rupture, both aortic and peripheral aneurysms may shed emboli, causing septic arthritis and purpura (96). Although less common than rupture, thrombosis of mycotic and infected aneurysms has been noted in both the aorta and the periphery. It has been suggested that thrombosis of these lesions may result in cure, but evidence in support of this contention is limited (8).

Diagnosis

CLINICAL PRESENTATION

The clinical presentation (Table 40-5) of patients with mycotic and infected aneurysms depends upon the pathogenesis, underlying etiology, and vessel involved. Septic arterial lesions have been noted in all age groups from neonates to the elderly (5,21). Early reports documented these lesions most commonly in the second, third, and fourth decades (5). This reflected the causal association with bacterial endocarditis that occurred in young adults. In a 1943 report, 58 percent of infected aneurysms occurred in the third and fourth decades of life (10). Recent studies, however, have documented a shift in incidence to the elderly. In a 1967 study, only 9 percent of infected aortic aneurysms occurred in patients younger than 40 years of age, whereas nearly three-fourths occurred in those over the age of 60 (28). This may reflect the importance of diseased arterial intima, usually by arteriosclerosis, in the pathogenesis of microbial arteritis as well as the rising incidence of infected arteriosclerotic aneurysms. The prevalence of drug abuse and use of contaminated needles may lead to an increased incidence of infectious arterial problems in the future (97).

Most mycotic and infected aneurysms have been reported in males. Stengel and Wolferth noted that approximately two-thirds occurred in men (5). Other studies have documented male predominance ranging from 82 to 91 percent (10,13,28). In contrast, Jarrett and his colleagues noted infected aortic aneurysms in 7 women and 10 men (43).

Fever or a history of a recent febrile illness are the most common complaints in patients with infected arterial lesions. Fever may occur in 70 to 94 percent of patients with proven mycotic or infected aneurysms (31,43,46). The fever may be steady or intermittent and is usually associated with chills and sweats (15). Frequently, a long history of malaise, weight loss, and increasing weakness is present. Pain is almost a universal complaint. In patients with infected aortic aneurysms, the discomfort may be localized to the abdomen or back; in those with peripheral aneurysms, it is usually localized to the site of the lesion where there may be overlying erythema, induration, and tenderness. Nearly 90 percent of infected peripheral aneurysms are palpable, while only 50 to 65 percent of abdominal aortic aneurysms are (31). Fever along with a tender abdominal aortic aneurysm is presumptive evidence of infection since temperature elevation is rarely caused by simple expansion or rupture (43). When pain and tenderness of an infected aortic aneurysm are localized to the flank, differentiation from a perinephric abscess may be impossible (98). Mistaken diagnosis of inflammatory intraabdominal conditions may lead to confusion and catastrophe (99). Hepatic artery involvement may cause right upper quadrant or epigastric pain, suggestive of cholecystitis or pancreatitis. Likewise, SMA lesions may be confused with inflammatory diseases of the small or large bowel. Malabsorption has been reported in association with an infected SMA aneurysm (100).

Infected aneurysms of the peripheral vessels may be confused with localized soft tissue abscesses, cellulitis, or lymphadenitis. A thrombosed infected femoral arterial aneurysm may mimic an incarcerated or strangulated groin hernia. Failure to maintain a high index of suspicion can result in surgical disaster if one approaches these lesions without proper exposure and control (15).

TABLE 40-5. Clinical Characteristics of Infected Aneurysms

Epidemiology:
Males > females (4:1)
All age groups
Bacterial endocarditis; atherosclerosis; illicit drug use
History:
Intermittent febrile episodes
Malaise
Weight loss
Pain
Examination:
Fever with chills (70–94%)
Pain (~100%)
Rapidly expanding mass (50–90%)
Laboratory:
Leukocytosis (65–83%)
Positive blood cultures (50%)
X-ray:
Noncalcified aneurysm
Lumbar osteomyelitis (abdominal aortic aneurysm)
Lobulated, saccular arteriographic appearance
Operative findings:
Thin-walled aneurysm
Surrounding inflammatory reaction
Succulent lymph nodes
Positive Gram stain

LABORATORY DATA

Leukocytosis is the most consistently abnormal laboratory finding in patients with mycotic or infected aneurysms. A leukocytosis above 10,000/mm^3 has been noted in 65 to 83 percent of patients with proven infected aneurysms (28,31,43). Antibiotic therapy, however, may blunt this elevation. Furthermore, leukocytosis may be noted following leakage from a noninfected aneurysm. Elevation of the erythrocyte sedimentation rate is a frequent but nonspecific finding. With infected hepatic arterial aneurysms, liver function tests are usually unremarkable (101).

BACTERIOLOGIC STUDIES

Positive preoperative blood cultures provide strong confirmatory evidence for the presence of an infected aneurysm. Unfortunately, such studies are not consistently found. In one report, only 50 percent of the patients had positive blood cultures (46). In another, positive blood cultures were found in 53 percent of all patients and in only 46 percent of those with infected aortic aneurysms (31). In contrast, Jarrett and his colleagues reported that 70 percent of patients with infected aortic aneurysms had positive blood cultures, and in each patient the organism cultured from the blood was the same as that isolated from the aneurysm (43). Since many patients with infected aneurysms may be receiving antibiotics at the time blood samples are drawn, multiple samples may be required before bacteremia is confirmed. Furthermore, sampling blood from an arterial site downstream from the presumed focus of infection may improve the yield of positive cultures (102,103).

As with preoperative blood cultures, antibiotics may mask bacterial growth from samples obtained at operation. It is critically important, therefore, to perform Gram stain examination in addition to bacterial cultures on material obtained during operation. Positive operative cultures may be obtained in 53 to 94 percent of patients (28,46). In most patients with negative cultures, however, organisms will be identified on histological examination of tissue sections (28). Mundth and his colleagues noted that the responsible organism was isolated in 71 percent of the aneurysm cultures. In the remaining 29 percent, organisms were identified on Gram stain examination of the aneurysm wall or its contents (31).

Radiologic Studies

PLAIN FILMS

Frontal and lateral abdominal x-rays may provide useful information in the patient with a suspected infected aortic aneurysm. An association between osteomyelitis of the lumbar vertebrae and infected aortic aneurysms has been documented (29,43). Since vertebral erosion is rarely noted with an arteriosclerotic aortic aneurysm, such findings should raise a suspicion of aneurysmal infection. In addition, arteriosclerotic abdominal aortic aneurysms are calcified in about 70 percent of cases, and this calcification may be noted on standard lumbosacral spine or frontal and lateral abdominal films (104). Infected aortic aneurysms, however, are less often calcified (43). Therefore, finding a noncalcified aneurysm in a patient with fever and leukocytosis is strongly suggestive of an infected aneurysm. In contrast to prosthetic graft infection, gas bubbles have not been noted on plain films of proven infected aneurysms.

SPECIAL STUDIES

Abdominal ultrasound can confirm the presence of an aneurysm and provide a fairly accurate assessment of its size, even in the absence of calcification (104,105). Ultrasonography is also helpful in documenting intraperitoneal abscesses, a distended gallbladder suggestive of cholecystitis, pancreatic masses, and other intraabdominal inflammatory conditions that must be excluded when evaluating a patient for a possible infected aortic aneurysm. To this end, ultrasonography is a helpful screening procedure. No criteria have been described which confirm aneurysm infection, however.

Computerized axial tomography (CT) may help in the evaluation of intraabdominal masses such as aortic or visceral arterial aneurysms. CT scan documentation of gas adjacent to an aortic graft in a patient with graft sepsis suggests that CT scans may be helpful in evaluation of patients with suspected aortic aneurysm infection (106). However, no CT scan findings have been reported that are specific for an infected aortic or visceral arterial aneurysms (107).

RADIOISOTOPE EXAMINATIONS

Two new methods are currently available for evaluation of septic processes, particularly within the abdomen. Gallium-67 isotopic scans have been used to localize intraabdominal abscesses. Radioactive gallium-67 collects in areas of inflammation and may be detected by external scanning cameras. Successful use of gallium-67 scanning in the diagnosis of a Dacron aortic graft infection and aortoenteric fistulas has been reported (108,109). The inflammatory reaction inherent in a mycotic or infected aneurysm should allow these arterial infections to be detected by gallium scanning, although reports to confirm this suspicion are not available.

Labeling of human leukocytes with indium-111, a gamma emitting agent, is now possible (110). Indium-111 leukocyte scanning is based upon external gamma camera detection of labeled leukocytes that have accumulated at sites of infection or inflammation. This technique has been utilized in recent years to detect intraabdominal abscesses. A recent report has documented the efficacy of leukocyte scanning with indium-111 to identify aortic graft infection (111). Application of this technique to detection of infected aneurysms seems possible but to date has not been confirmed.

ARTERIOGRAPHY

An arteriogram is an essential part of the evaluation of any patient with a presumably infected arterial aneurysm. In addition to providing information for planning reconstruction, arteriography may help confirm the diagnosis of an infected aneurysm. Finding an excessively lobulated, saccular aneurysm arising from an otherwise normal-appearing vessel lacking features of arteriosclerosis is highly suggestive of an infectious etiology (112) (Figure 40-1). The appearance of localized smooth-walled aneurysmal changes, explained by the rapidly progressive transmural inflammatory destructive process, has been emphasized by others (29). A particularly eccentric aneurysm, with a relatively small mouth in comparison to its widest diameter, also suggests infection (113). Despite these characteristic findings in some cases, the aortographic appearance of many infected aneurysms may be indistinguishable from typical arteriosclerotic, traumatic, or congenital aneurysms (114).

Operative Findings

Certain findings at operation suggest infection within the aneurysm, although such features may be quite subtle. Infected aneurysms tend to be saccular, lobulated, and eccentric (113). The wall of the aneurysm is typically quite thin and friable (28). A moderate degree of surrounding inflammation may be noted and large succulent lymph nodes adjacent to the aorta or in proximity to a peripheral aneurysm may be encountered (43). The typical inflammatory aneurysm of the abdominal aorta may also be surrounded by large lymph nodes and may be engulfed in an inflammatory reaction. However, the wall of an inflammatory aneurysm is usually thick and shiny white in contrast to the thin-walled, red mulberrylike infected aortic aneurysm. The general vascular surgeon must maintain a high index of suspicion when encountering unusual-appearing aneurysms in order to make the diagnosis of infected aneurysm.

Treatment

Successful management of the patient with arterial infection presents a great challenge to the general vascular surgeon. The aim of therapy is to eradicate all infection while maintaining adequate circulation. Principles of successful management are independent of the specific lesion (mycotic aneurysm, microbial arteritis with or without aneurysm, and secondarily infected aneurysm), mechanism of infection (transmural bacteremic endothelial innoculation, via vasa vasorum, or direct spread from contiguous sepsis), or organism responsible.

PREOPERATIVE MANAGEMENT

Establishing the correct diagnosis preoperatively is the first step in treatment. Multiple blood cultures should be obtained, including several samples from a source downstream from the presumed site of the aneurysm. Other potential sources of infection such as urine, sputum, and open wounds should be thoroughly cultured. High-dose intravenous organism-specific antibiotic treatment must be started to prevent continued hematogenous spread of infection. Sterilization of the patient's blood is necessary to prevent possible contamination of a vascular prosthesis that might be required for arterial reconstruction. Choice of antibiotic is dictated by the organism(s) isolated. When attempts at identifying the offending organism(s) prove futile, any combination of broad-spectrum bacteriocidal antibiotics for both gram-positive and gram-negative organisms (specifically *Salmonella*) are appropriate. Although sporadic cases of sterilization and spontaneous healing of these lesions with antibiotics alone have been reported, this is the exception, if it occurs at all (31,115). Sudden ruptures of infected aneurysms have been observed while patients were undergoing intensive antibiotic treatment (18,28,112,116). Even aneurysmal sterilization does not preclude progressive enlargement and eventual rupture (11,112,117,118).

OPERATIVE MANAGEMENT

Appropriate intravenous lines should be inserted. If necessary, a Swan-Ganz catheter may be placed to monitor pulmonary artery wedge pressure. A radial artery cannula insertion in the nondominant wrist or the side opposite anticipated axillofemoral reconstruction provides ready access for blood sampling as well as systemic blood pressure measurements.

Once the aneurysm has been exposed, infection must be confirmed. When gross perivascular purulence is encountered, the diagnosis is obvious. In the absence of obvious signs of sepsis, Gram stains should be obtained and frozen sections of the aneurysm wall examined for bacteria or fungi. Identification of microorganisms within the aneurysm wall or contents in the patient with fever, leukocytosis, positive blood cultures, a particularly friable appearing aneurysm, or one surrounded by large lymph nodes is diagnostic of aneurysm infection. Aerobic, anaerobic, and fungal cultures must be obtained and plated immediately in appropriate culture media so the specific offending organism(s) may be identified to assure appropriate antibiotic therapy.

Principles for managing infected aneurysms are similar to those for dealing with infected arterial prostheses. Wide debridement and copious irrigation with antibiotic solution of all involved tissue is required. This includes complete resection of the aneurysm, if technically possible. If rupture has occurred, a wider area will be involved in the septic process and more aggressive debridement may be required. Ligation of arteries should be performed in clean, healthy-appearing tissue with synthetic monofilament or wire sutures. Preoperative vascular laboratory data combined with arteriography help document adequacy of collateral circulation around the infected lesion. If at the initial operation collateral circulation is adequate to support the distal bed without arterial reconstruction, arterial ligation only should be performed. Doppler auscultation of the arteries distal to the site of ligation will be quite helpful in assessing the adequacy of collateral circulation. If vascular reconstruction proves necessary, bypass grafts should be placed through clean tissue planes. This usually requires extraanatomic reconstruction. Autologous tissue is preferred over synthetic grafts (46,119). Specific details of management depend upon the location of the lesion and the extent of arterial involvement.

Abdominal Aorta

Management of an infected abdominal aortic aneurysm is the same as management of a secondary aortoenteric fistula or an infected aortic prosthesis. In general, successful management requires excision of all septic tissue and extraanatomic arterial reconstruction.

Whether dealing with a ruptured or intact infected abdominal aortic aneurysm, secure closure of the proximal aortic stump may prove challenging. Secure closure of the aortic stump distal to the renal arteries is mandatory for successful results. However, this may be the weak link in the operative procedure, since postoperative aortic stump dehiscence may occur in up to 33 percent of patients (120). Healthy tissue that will hold sutures may not be readily available. Under these circumstances, temporary suprarenal aortic occlusion, at the diaphragm through the lesser sac, permits complete mobilization of the infrarenal aorta, unencumbered by an infrarenal aortic clamp. A two-layer aortic closure with monofilament suture has been recommended (15,112). If available, a flap of prevertebral aponeurosis may be included in the closure (121) (Figure 40-3). The suture line may also be covered with omentum (32,122) (Figure 40-3). Although a pedicle of omentum, transposed through the transverse mesocolon, probably provides no buttressing strength, such coverage may facilitate resolution of the periaortic infection. Copious irrigation of the retroperitoneum is performed, and irrigating-drainage catheters may be placed into the aortic bed for drainage and postoperative through-and-through antibiotic irrigation (Figure 40-4). Some authors advocate using povidone-iodine irrigation during the early postoperative period (69).

Although anecdotal reports have described successful management of infected aortic aneurysms by resection without restoring arterial continuity, in the majority of patients arterial reconstruction will be required to prevent distal ischemia (90,123). Several techniques have been utilized, but there is considerable controversy about the optimal method of reconstruction (119).

Efforts to restore arterial continuity through the bed of the infected aortic aneurysm with aortic homografts have proved unsuccessful (74). Bridges and colleagues reviewed 22 patients in whom aortic continuity was restored with either Teflon or Dacron prostheses (124). Fifteen (68 percent) either died or required removal of the prosthesis. Mundth and his colleagues' experience with aneurysm excision and standard aortic reconstruction has been uniquely successful (31). They recorded 4 survivors out of 10 patients operated upon for infected aortic aneurysms. In all four survivors' aortoiliac interposition Dacron grafts were inserted, and the patients were treated for 6 weeks with intravenous antibiotics. They suggested that this method of reconstruction succeeded, despite active sepsis, for two reasons. First, the Dacron graft was isolated from the aortic bed by interposition of the posterior peritoneum between the graft and aortic bed. Second, organisms isolated from these four patients were of low virulence.

Despite this experience and anecdotal reports of successfully employing standard aortic reconstruciton, a growing body of evidence favors performing extraanatomic bypass through clean tissue planes. Axillary-femoral grafting as a means of extraanatomic bypass has gained popularity since first introduced in the United States by Blaisdell and Hall in 1963 (125). Although long-term patency following axillofemoral reconstruction is not as good as aortoiliac or aortofemoral reconstruction, axillobifemoral bypass remains the procedure of choice for lower extremity revascularization when managing infected abdominal aortic aneurysms (33,69,126) (Figure 40-4). When the infected aneurysm is small and limited to the aorta, and following excision and distal closure the aortic bifurcation is preserved, and there is no significant iliac occlusive disease, unilateral axillofemoral reconstruction is appropriate. Under these circumstances, the

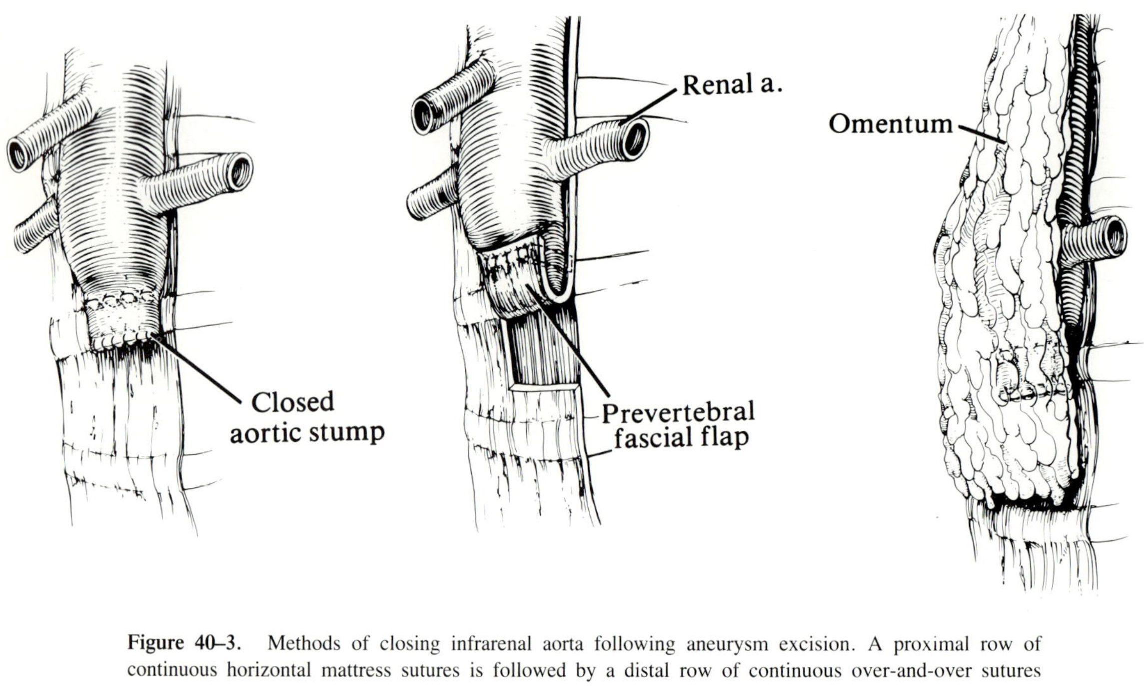

Figure 40–3. Methods of closing infrarenal aorta following aneurysm excision. A proximal row of continuous horizontal mattress sutures is followed by a distal row of continuous over-and-over sutures (*left*). Prevertebral fascial flap buttress sutured over aortic stump (*center*). Omental graft passed through transverse mesocolon provides additional protection (*right*). [By permission of CB Ernst. From H Haimovici (ed): *Vascular Emergencies*. New York, Appleton-Century-Crofts, 1982.]

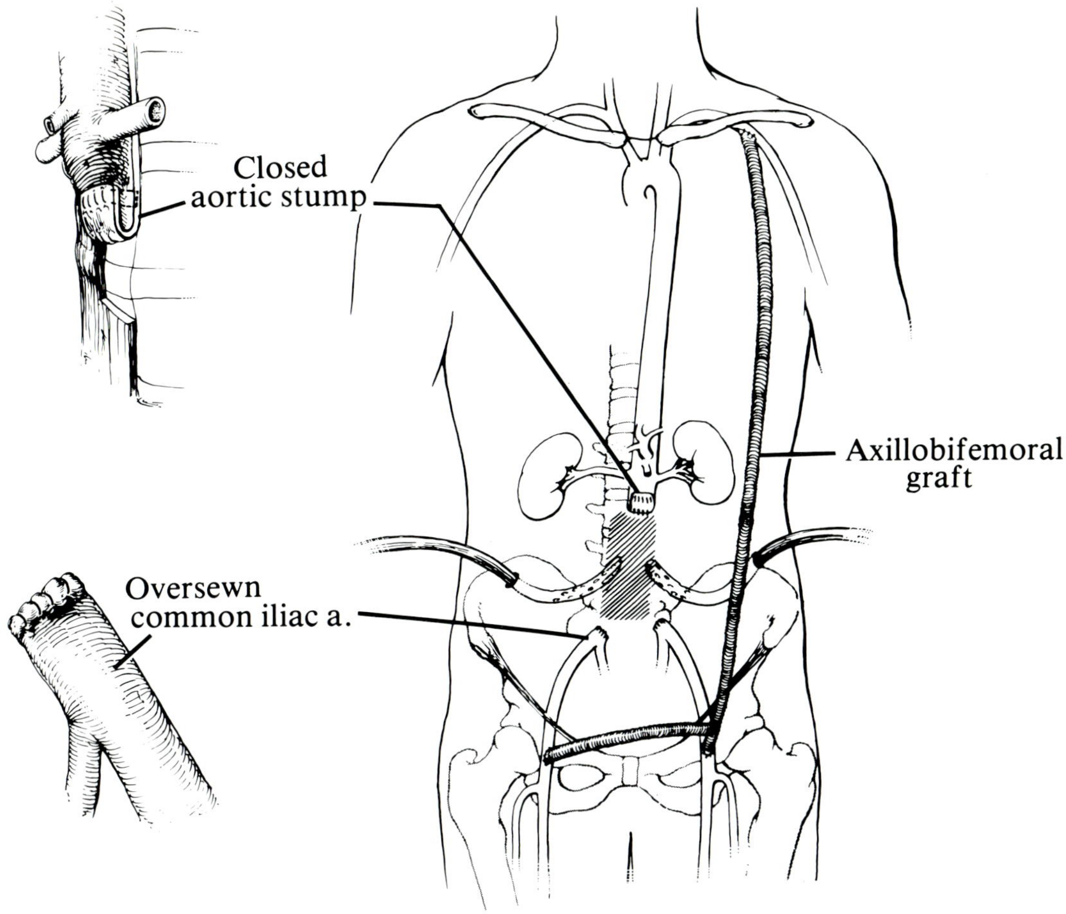

Figure 40–4. Infected aneurysm has been excised. The left axillobifemoral bypass maintains pelvic and leg circulation. Irrigation-drainage catheters are placed in retroperitoneal space (optional). [By permission of CB Ernst. From H Haimovici (ed): *Vascular Emergencies*. New York, Appleton-Century-Crofts, 1982.]

contralateral leg will be perfused retrograde around the bifurcation. If the bifurcation must be excised and the common iliac vessels are free of significant disease, they may be mobilized and anastomosed end-to-end to form a neobifurcation, again allowing use of unilateral axillofemoral reconstructions (29,119).

If late occlusion of the axillofemoral graft becomes a significant problem, anatomic aortic reconstruction may be performed, provided the retroperitoneal infection has completely resolved (112). At least 6 to 12 months should elapse from the original procedure before considering this option.

Controversy exists concerning the proper timing and sequence of excision and reconstruction. When aortic infection is discovered unexpectedly during elective aneurysm repair, and in most cases when it has been suspected preoperatively, the standard has been to perform aneurysm resection and close the abdomen. Then, using different sterile instruments and following repreparation and draping, extraanatomic reconstruction is performed. However, since technical challenges of the intraabdominal procedure may be time-consuming and result in a substantial period of lower extremity ischemia, some surgeons have recommended performing the axillofemoral bypass before aneurysm excision (33,112). Extraanatomic reconstruction may also be accomplished using the thoracic aorta as the donor vessel (127).

When performing preliminary axillobifemoral reconstruction, Cooke and Ehrenfeld have advocated occluding the common femoral artery proximal to the femoral anastomosis to prevent acute graft thrombosis secondary to competitive flow (112). However, based on observations by Blaisdell and his colleagues and Ernst, it appears that axillary-femoral bypass grafts may remain patent for up to 4 months with competitive aortoiliac flow (128,129). Therefore, it does not appear necessary to occlude host vessels proximal to groin anastomoses for fear of failure of extraanatomic reconstruction due to competitive parallel blood flow.

Bacteremic contamination of the newly placed extraanatomic graft has not been a problem. Preliminary axillobifemoral bypass is not an option when dealing with a ruptured aneurysm or one in which the diagnosis of infection is not certain preoperatively.

Visceral Arteries

Infection is the most common cause of visceral arterial aneurysms (Figure 40-2). Their relatively small size and frequency of multiple aneurysms emphasizes the importance of arteriography for diagnosis and preoperative planning (17). The surgical approach required for treatment depends upon the size and location of the lesion as well as the adequacy of collateral development. Goals of operative management are to prevent rupture of the aneurysm while preserving adequate distal perfusion.

Superior Mesenteric Artery. DeBakey and Cooley performed the first successful resection of a mycotic aneurysm of the SMA in 1949 (130). By 1981, 16 patients with infected SMA aneurysms had been successfully treated by ligation with or without aneurysm excision (131). Attempts to excise these aneurysms completely may be hazardous, since they are usually densely adherent to important adjacent structures. With adequate drainage and long-term antibiotic therapy, recurrent infection should not be a problem even with only partial excision and endoaneurysmorrhaphy (132).

Following ligation of the vessel, the bowel should be observed for 30 min to assess viability. Use of the sterile Doppler probe or injection and detection of sodium fluorescein dye may prove useful in assuring bowel viability (133,134). These two techniques are clearly superior to using clinical parameters of mesenteric arterial pulsations, peristalsis, and color to assess viability. Short segments of apparently nonviable intestine must be resected. If long segments of bowel appear compromised, mesenteric revascularization will be required. If such reconstruction is required, autogenous artery or vein conduits are preferred, and the bypass should be performed through noninfected tissue planes, if possible (132). The use of synthetic graft material such as Dacron has been associated with persistent infection and anastomotic disruption (46,135). Therefore, prosthetic grafts are contraindicated.

Endoaneurysmorrhaphy, another method of treating arterial aneurysms, has proved successful in managing infected SMA aneurysms (59,60,132). Restorative endoaneurysmorrhaphy can only be used when managing saccular aneurysms. Restorative endoaneurysmorrhaphy requires obtaining proximal and distal control of the involved artery, opening the aneurysm, and oversewing the aneurysm orifice, performing an arteriorrhaphy which preserves the vessel lumen. An intraluminal shunt facilitates vessel repair by maintaining bowel circulation and provides a stent around which the arteriorrhaphy is performed. The shunt is removed before placing the last few sutures. If the aneurysm is not saccular and involves both afferent and efferent vessels, obliterative endoaneurysmorrhaphy may be performed by oversewing the orifices of these vessels from within the opened aneurysm sac. By limiting dissection and working from within the aneurysm, maximum collateral circulation is preserved. Use of intraluminal balloon occlusion of inflow and outflow vessels facilitates endoaneurysmorrhaphy because extensive dissection required for proximal and distal clamp occlusion is not required.

Hepatic Artery. Most infected hepatic arterial aneurysms can be successfully managed by ligation or ligation with aneurysm excision (136). When the aneurysm involves the proper hepatic artery (the segment distal to the gastroduodenal branch) or when preoperative angiography documents poor collateral development, an attempt at arterial reconstruction should be made to prevent liver ischemia (101,137,138). Saphenous vein or autogenous hypogastric arterial segments are the preferred bypass materials.

Infected aneurysms of intrahepatic arteries have, until recently, been considered curable only by hepatic lobectomy. Porter and colleagues described a 29-year-old man with staphylococcal endocarditis who developed a mycotic aneurysm in a posterior intrahepatic branch of the right hepatic artery (101). This vessel was selectively catheterized, and several methicillin-soaked pieces of Gelfoam were embolized into the aneurysm, resulting in occlusion. Arteriography performed 2 months following embolotherapy confirmed obliteration of the aneurysm. It is suggested that transcatheter arterial embolization may prove useful for treatment of infected visceral arterial aneurysms when surgical intervention is not advisable or technically possible.

Other Visceral Vessels. Mycotic or infected aneurysms involving the celiac, splenic, or inferior mesenteric arteries have been successfully treated by the surgical options described (139). Most splenic arterial lesions may be ligated or excised, with or without splenectomy (57,58). Likewise, rich mesenteric collateral circulation may permit inferior mesenteric artery ligation and aneurysm resection (140). Measurement of inferior mesenteric arterial stump pressure or sterile Doppler auscultation of the colonic mesenteric arterial vessels helps document adequacy of colonic collateral blood flow permitting safe inferior mesenteric artery ligation (141,142).

Carotid Artery

Principles of management of infected aneurysms of the extracranial carotid arteries are the same as for infected arterial lesions elsewhere; namely, excision, wide debridement and drainage, and intensive antibiotic therapy. The necessity for, and optimal methods of, restoring carotid arterial continuity have provoked debate. Risks of neurologic deficit after ligation must be balanced against risks of recurrent infection, arterial disruption, and potentially fatal hemorrhage following arterial reconstruction in a contaminated field.

Sir Astley Cooper performed the first common carotid artery ligation for an extracranial aneurysm in 1805. His patient became hemiplegic and died. However, he performed a second common carotid arterial ligation 3 years later and the patient survived for 13 years (143). Reid reported upon 10 patients treated by ligation. Four died and two of the six survivors developed hemiplegia (144). Moore and Baker recorded mortality and morbidity rates of 17 and 28 percent, respectively, among 104 patients undergoing carotid ligation associated with head and neck tumors (145). In contrast to these disastrous results, Rogers reported transient hemiplegia developing in only 1 of 19 patients undergoing carotid artery ligation (146). Also, James and colleagues recorded only 1 transient deficit among 13 patients after common carotid ligation performed using local anesthesia (147).

Compared to carotid arterial ligation, risks of arterial reconstruction in a contaminated field are also substantial. Anderson and his associates reported a 77 percent failure rate following arterial grafting for the management of infected peripheral aneurysms, the majority of which were femoral (46). Twenty-eight percent of the patients died. Smith and his colleagues reported similar results (135). None of the lesions in these two reports involved the carotid artery, however. Monson and Alexander recently reported successful autogenous saphenous vein interposition after resection of an infected carotid arterial aneurysm (52). Successful primary end-to-end anastomosis following excision of an infected carotid aneurysm has also been reported (148).

The question of arterial reconstruction versus ligation for an infected carotid aneurysm remains unsettled. Most workers favor ligation (149). As an index of adequacy of collateral cerebral blood flow, Ehrenfeld and his colleagues have successfully employed measurement of carotid stump pressure when carotid ligation was required (150). After analysis of data obtained from 24 patients in whom carotid ligations were performed, they concluded that patients whose stump pressures exceed 70 torr systolic tolerate acute carotid ligation, especially if systemic blood pressure was maintained at the same levels as when stump pressure measurements were obtained. Those with intermediate stump pressures of 50 to 68 torr were vulnerable to postligation stroke. It appeared, however, that safety of carotid ligation in these patients was enhanced by systemic anticoagulation with heparin sodium and maintenance of high systemic blood pressure. Furthermore, seven patients also had preoperative stump pressure estimates using ocular pneumoplethysmography (OPG-Gee) with common carotid compression. Close correlation of operative and preoperative measurements were observed in all.

Another alternative to ligation is the application and progressive tightening of a Selverstone clamp around the common or internal carotid arteries. Avellone described a 24-year-old woman in whom the clamp was applied to the internal carotid artery proximal to the aneurysm and progressively tightened over a 72-hour period. This procedure proved successful, but had neurologic symptoms developed, the clamp would have been opened (151). This represents a compromise between ligation and reconstruction.

Should the patient not tolerate carotid occlusion, documented by EEG changes, stump blood pressure measurements, or neurologic instability while awake, a possible alternative for cerebral revascularization is extracranial-intracranial bypass using autogenous saphenous vein (152).

Extremity Vessels

The subclavian or axillary artery between the thyrocervical and subscapular branches can usually be safely ligated because of profuse protective collateral circulation around the shoulder. Resection of lesions involving the distal axillary artery, however, may require reconstruction. When reconstruction is required, autogenous tissue should be used and the grafts should be placed through clean tissue planes (15,153). The brachial artery distal to the profunda branch may be safely ligated. Aneurysms of the radial and ulnar arteries usually can be excised without reconstruction. Documentation of adequacy of collateral circulation through the superficial and deep volar arches by Allen's test or by Doppler auscultation of the nonligated radial or ulnar artery assures safe ligation of these vessels.

When the treatment of infected femoral arterial aneurysms requires sacrifice of the deep femoral artery, reconstruction with autogenous saphenous vein will invariably be necessary to maintain extremity viability (154). Such bypass grafts may be performed through the obturator canal to avoid the contaminated field (154–156). In young patients, common or superficial femoral arterial ligation may be tolerated, although the extremity may be transiently ischemic. If ischemic symptoms persist after the aneurysm infection has resolved, definitive reconstruction may be performed. If, however, the limb appears in severe jeopardy, extraanatomic bypass through clean tissue planes will be required.

Excision of an infected popliteal aneurysm will usually require restoration of arterial continuity. Autogenous saphenous vein is preferred, although the risk of septic complications may be significant (157). Extraanatomic bypass under these circumstances will minimize septic complications.

Postoperative Management

Regardless of the surgical procedure performed, prolonged postoperative antibiotics are mandatory to protect arterial suture lines and vascular grafts from potential reinfection. Although the duration of antibiotic coverage required has not been firmly established, most authors recommend 6 weeks of intravenous organism-specific antibiotic treatment (31,46). Once postoperative antibiotics are discontinued, multiple blood cultures should be obtained over several days to ensure sterility of the blood (31). Some authors have recommended chronic suppressive oral antibiotics in these patients. Although long-term chronic therapy seems reasonable when dealing with fungal infections, its necessity in bacterial infection has not been well established.

Results of Treatment

Prior to the advent of antimicrobial drugs, mycotic or infected aneurysms were invariably fatal. The natural history of these lesions was one of rapid enlargement and early rupture. It has been estimated that the average time from diagnosis to death was approximately 3 months (81). With the introduction of antibiotics, better understanding of the pathophysiology of these lesions, and greater appreciation of the proper therapeutic principles, survival has improved (Table 40-6).

Infected aneurysms of peripheral vessels are more easily diagnosed and, consequently, mortality is less than for lesions in the aorta or visceral circulation. Mundth and his associates recorded a 25 percent operative mortality for patients with infected peripheral aneurysms (31). In Anderson's report of 14 patients with infected peripheral aneurysms, 5 were treated by ligation alone and all survived, although one required amputation (46). Nine patients underwent aneurysm resection and arterial reconstruction. Only two of these patients were cured. The other seven developed bleeding or recurrent sepsis within 1 week. Two of these patients expired, and leg amputation was required in another two after reoperation.

Infected aortic aneurysms present a much greater risk to life than peripheral aneurysms. Among 13 patients undergoing operation for an infected aortic aneurysm 60 percent died (31). A 67 percent operative mortality rate has been noted among patients with *Salmonella*-infected aortic aneurysms (32). In a 1983 review of the English literature only 34 survivors were identified

TABLE 40-6. Results of Surgical Treatment, 1961–1981

Author (Ref.)	Year of Report	No. of Patients	Deaths	Percent
Nabseth (115)	1961	8	2	25
Robb (118)	1962	3	0	
Perdue (19)	1967	10	4	40
Bennett (28)	1967	5	5	100
Mundth (31)	1969	17	10	59
Cliff (45)	1970	3	2	67
Anderson (46)	1974	16	4	25
Jarrett (43)	1975	17	10	59
Scher (29)	1980	2	1	50
Bardin (14)	1981	2	1	50
Total		83	39	47

after operation for infected abdominal aortic aneurysm (69). In 89 percent of the successfully treated patients, the diagnosis was made before operation. Likewise, in 88 percent of these patients operation was performed prior to rupture. In Mundth's study of infected aortic aneurysms, 67 percent of patients with nonruptured aneurysms survived, whereas none with ruptured aneurysms survived (31). It appears that accurate preoperative diagnosis, before rupture has taken place, is mandatory for successful results.

Type of arterial reconstruction has a significant impact on results. The majority of survivors have undergone extraanatomic revascularization (69). In a report of aortic salmonellosis, 70 percent of patients who survived aneurysm resection and standard aortic reconstruction ultimately died of recurrent graft infection (32).

Results of treatment of infected visceral artery lesions are unclear since individual experiences are limited and only anecdotal reports are available for study. In 1981 Howard and Mazer collected 24 patients from the literature who had survived operative treatment for infected SMA aneurysms (131). In 10 patients ligation of the SMA without arterial reconstruction was performed, and 6 of these underwent aneurysm resection. Only 30 percent of this group required bowel resection. Nine patients were successfully treated by aneurysmorrhaphy alone. Five underwent aneurysm resection with some form of revascularization. In two of these patients a Dacron graft was used, and recurrent infection developed in one necessitating replacement with a vein graft. Although the incidence of infected and noninfected lesions was not defined, Stanley reported an operative mortality of 32 percent for hepatic artery aneurysms (56). Eighty-five percent were ruptured at the time of operation.

Colonized Aneurysms

INCIDENCE AND BACTERIOLOGY

A separate, but associated clinical entity from mycotic or infected aneurysms is the bacterially colonized aortic aneurysm. Ernst and his colleagues prospectively studied a group of patients undergoing operation for arteriosclerotic abdominal aortic aneurysms (92). None of the patients had the signs and symptoms of mycotic or infected aortic aneurysms, and none were febrile or had evidence of infection in other organ systems at the time of aneurysm repair. Forty-four patients had asymptomatic aneurysms, 23 had symptomatic but unruptured aneurysms, and 13 patients presented with ruptured aneurysms. All patients but one received parenteral antibiotic therapy and, except for those undergoing emergency operation, antibiotics were started preoperatively. Intraoperative bacterial culture specimens of the aneurysm wall and contents were obtained in 78 patients. In 12 (15 percent) cultures yielded growth of organisms. Aneurysm contents yielded positive cultures in 9 percent of asymptomatic patients, 13 percent of symptomatic patients, and 38 percent of patients with ruptured aneurysms. Gram-positive organisms predominated (81 percent) with *Staphylococcus epidermidis* being most common. *Salmonella* species were not cultured from these aneurysms.

Other works have confirmed these findings. In a similar study, Williams and Fisher defined a 10 percent incidence of positive aortic cultures (93). Gram-positive organisms, most commonly staphylococci, predominated. Scobie and colleagues found bacterial growth in 22.6 percent of aortic aneurysm cultures among 31 patients (94). *Staphylococcus epidermidis* was isolated in 71 percent. The combined three series totaled 177 patients, 26 of whom (15 percent) had bacterial growth on cultures taken from aneurysmal contents.

SIGNIFICANCE

Standard aortic reconstruction with Dacron was performed in all patients with colonized aneurysms (92–94). In Ernst's series, among individuals followed for a minimum of 6 months, late graft sepsis developed in 10 percent of patients with positive aortic cultures, but in only 2 percent of those with negative cultures (92). Neither Scobie nor Williams noted late graft infection in their patients with positive aortic cultures.

It appears that a small group of patients with arteriosclerotic abdominal aortic aneurysms may harbor bacteria within these aneurysms. However, this clinical entity is quite distinct from the classic mycotic or infected aortic aneurysm. If there is an increased risk of late graft sepsis, it is minimal. Adequate treatment consists of standard aortic aneurysmectomy, leaving the posterior aneurysm wall in situ. Wherever practical and possible, after evacuating an intraaneurysmal thrombus, atheromatous material and aortic media should be debrided from the retained posterior aortic wall, leaving viable aortic adventitia as the graft bed. Antibiotic irrigation along with systemic antistaphylococcal antibiotics are recommended. Intraoperative cultures may help direct the appropriate antibiotic choice. In the absence of operative cultures, an antistaphylococcal regimen should be employed. There is no indication for extraanatomic reconstruction in these patients.

References

1. Rokitansky CF: *Handbuch der Paathologischen Anatomie,* 2d ed. 1844, p 55.
2. Koch L: Ueber Aneurysma der Arteriae Mesenterichae Superioris. *Inaug Dis Enlargen,* 1851.
3. Tufnell J: On the influence of vegetation of the values of the heart in the production of secondary arterial disease. *Dublin Q J Med* 15: 371, 1853.
4. Osler W: The Gulstonial Lectures on malignant endocarditis. *Br Med J* 1: 467, 1885.
5. Stengel A, Wolferth CC: Mycotic (bacterial) aneurysms of intravascular origin. *Arch Intern Med* 31: 527, 1923.
6. Eppinger H: Pathogenesis (Histogenesis and Aetiologie) der Aneurysman ein Schliesslich des Aneurysmsa equi Verminosum. *Arch Klin Chir* 35:404, 1887.
7. Lewis D, Schrager J: Embolomycotic aneurysms. *JAMA* 53: 1808, 1909.
8. Barker WF: Mycotic aneurysms. *Ann Surg* 139: 84, 1954.
9. Crane AR: Primary multilocular mycotic aneurysm of the aorta. *Arch Surg* 24: 634, 1937.
10. Revell STR: Primary mycotic aneurysms. *Ann Intern Med* 22: 431, 1943.
11. Cates JE, Christie RV: Subacute bacterial endocarditis. *J Med* 20: 93, 1951.
12. Blum L, Keefer E: Cryptogenic mycotic aneurysm. *Ann Surg* 155: 398, 1962.
13. Parkhurst GF, Decker JP: Bacterial aortitis and mycotic aneurysm of the aorta. *Am J Pathol* 31: 821, 1955.
14. Bardin JA, Collins GM, Devin JB, Hales NA: Nonaneurysmal suppurative aortitis. *Arch Surg* 116: 954, 1981.
15. Wilson SE, Gordon E, Van Wagenen PB: *Salmonella* arteritis. *Arch Surg* 113: 1163, 1978.
16. Patel S, Johnston KW: Classification and management of mycotic aneurysms. *Surg Gynecol Obstet* 144: 691, 1977.
17. Wilson SE, Van Wagenen P, Passaro E, Jr: Arterial infection. *Curr Probl Surg* 15: 5, 1978.
18. Sommerville RI, Allen EV, Edwards JE: Bland and infected arteriosclerotic abdominal aortic aneurysms. A clinicopathologic study. *Medicine* 38: 207, 1959.
19. Perdue GD, Smith RB, III: Surgical treatment of mycotic aneurysms. *South Med J* 60: 848, 1967.
20. Wang Y, Chester E, Korns ME, Edwards JE: Mycotic aneurysms of the left ventricle and ascending aorta. *Minn Med* 51: 395, 1968.
21. Thompson TR, Tilleli J, Johnson DE, Britt W, L'Henreux P, Williams H, Jarvis C, Burke BA: Umbilical artery catheterization complicated by mycotic aortic aneurysm in neonates. *Adv Pediatr* 27: 275, 1980.
22. Bennett DE: Primary mycotic aneurysms of the aorta. *Arch Surg* 94: 758, 1967.
23. Smith G, Hutchinson HE: Lymph borne infection and aneurysm formation. *Surg Gynecol Obstet* 104: 722, 1957.
24. Buxton RW, Holdefer WF, Jr: Primary mycotic aneurysms. *Am Surg* 29: 863, 1963.
25. McCrae J: A case of multiple mycotic aneurysms of the first part of the aorta. *J Pathol Bacteriol* 10: 373, 1905.
26. Saphir O, Cooper GW: Acute suppurative aortitis superimposed on syphilitic aortitis. *Arch Pathol Lab Med* 4: 543, 1927.
27. Hankins JR, Yeager GH: Primary mycotic aneurysm. *Surgery* 40: 747, 1956.
28. Bennett DE, Cherry JK: Bacterial infection of aortic aneurysms: A clinicopathological study. *Am J Surg* 113: 321, 1967.
29. Scher LA, Brener BJ, Goldenkranz RJ, Alpert J, Brief DK, Parsonnet V, Tiro AC: Infected aneurysms of the abdominal aorta. *Arch Surg* 115: 975, 1980.
30. James EC, Gillespie JT: Aortic mycotic abdominal aneurysm involving all visceral branches: Excision and Dacron graft placement. *J Cardiovasc Surg* 18: 353, 1977.
31. Mundth ED, Darling RC, Alvarado RH, Buckley MJ, Linton RR, Austen WG: Surgical management of mycotic aneurysms and the complications of infection in vascular reconstructive surgery. *Am J Surg* 117: 460, 1969.
32. Mendelowitz DS, Ramstedt R, Yao JST, Bergan J: Abdominal aortic salmonellosis. *Surgery* 85: 514, 1979.
33. Davies OG, Thorburn JD, Powell P: Cryptic mycotic abdominal aortic aneurysms. *Am J Surg* 136: 96, 1978.
34. Schneider JA, Rheuban KS, Crosby IK: Rupture of postcoarctation mycotic aneurysms of the aorta. *Ann Thorac Surg* 27: 185, 1979.
35. Oldham HN, Phillips JF, Jewett PH, Chen JT: Surgical treatment of mycotic aneurysm associated with coarctation of the aorta. *Ann Thorac Surg* 15:411, 1975.
36. Clagett OT, Kirkland JW, Edwards JE: Anatomic variations and pathologic changes in coarctation of the aorta. *Surg Gynecol Obstet* 98: 103, 1954.
37. Abbott ME: Coarctation of the aorta of the adult type. *Am Heart J* 3: 574, 1928.
38. Perdue GD, Yancy AG: Mycotic aneurysmla change in the dilated artery proximal to arteriovenous fistula. *South Med J* 65: 1142, 1972.
39. Reid MR: Studies on abnormal arteriovenous communications, acquired and congenital: I. Report of a series of cases. *Arch Surg* 10: 601, 1925.
40. Shumacker HB: Aneurysm development and degenerative changes in dilated artery proximal to arteriovenous fistula. *Surg Gynecol Obstet* 130: 636, 1970.
41. Riester WH, Serrano A: Infrarenal mycotic pseudoaneurysm. *J Thorac Cardiovasc Surg* 71: 633, 1975.
42. Williams MJ: Perforating suppurative aortitis associated with idiopathic cystic medial necrosis: Report of a case. *Am J Clin Pathol* 22: 160, 1967.
43. Jarrett F, Darling RC, Mundth ED, Austen WG: Experience with infected aneurysms of the abdominal aorta. *Arch Surg* 10: 1281, 1975.
44. Liebman E: Cases of mycotic aneurysms. *Trans NY Pathol Soc,* May 1905.
45. Cliff MM, Soulen RL, Finestone AJ: Mycotic aneurysms—A challenge and a clue. *Arch Intern Med* 126: 977, 1970.
46. Anderson CB, Butcher HR Jr, Ballinger WF: Mycotic aneurysms. *Arch Surg* 109: 712, 1974.
47. Daoud AS, Pankin D, Tulgan H, Florentin RA: Aneurysms of the coronary artery. *Am J Cardiol* 11: 228, 1963.
48. Crook BRM, Raftery EB, Oram S: Mycotic aneurysms of coronary arteries. *Br Heart J* 35: 107, 1973.
49. Goh TH: Mycotic aneurysms of the pulmonary artery. *Br Heart J* 36: 387, 1974.
50. Jaffee RB, Condon VR: Mycotic aneurysms of the pulmonary artery and aorta. *Radiology* 116: 291, 1975.
51. Young N: Bleeding from the ear as a sign of leaking aneurysm of the extracranial portion of the internal carotid artery. *J Laryngol* 56: 35, 1941.
52. Monson RL, Alexander RH: Vein reconstruction of a mycotic internal carotid aneurysm. *Ann Surg* 191: 47, 1980.
53. Huebl HC, Read AC: Aneurysmal abscess. *Minn Med* 49: 11, 1966.
54. Wemple JB, Smith GW: Extracranial carotid aneurysm: Report of four cases. *J Neurosurg* 24: 667, 1966.
55. Ledgerwood AM, Lucas CE: Mycotic aneurysm of the carotid artery. *Arch Surg* 109: 496, 1974.

56. Stanley JC, Thompson NW, Fry WJ: Splanchnic artery aneurysms. *Arch Surg* 101: 689, 1970.
57. Dukes HM, Mynors JM: Ruptured mycotic aneurysm of the spleen. *Br J Surg* 59: 572, 1972.
58. Vansant JH: Massive gastric hemorrhage secondary to rupture of mycotic aneurysm of the splenic artery: Resection and survival. *Am Surg* 35: 497, 1969.
59. Alvares JF, Parsonnet V, Brief DC: Mycotic aneurysm of the superior mesenteric artery. *Am J Surg* 111: 237, 1966.
60. McClelland RN, Duke JH: Successful resection of an idiopathic aneurysm of the superior mesenteric artery: Case report and literature review. *Ann Surg* 164: 167, 1966.
61. McNamara MF, Griska LB: Superior mesenteric artery branch aneurysms. *Surgery* 88: 625, 1980.
62. Horton RE: Ruptured mycotic aneurysm of the superior mesenteric artery. *Br J Surg* 46: 541, 1959.
63. Keehan MF, Kistner RL, Banis J: Angiography as an aid in extraenteric gastrointestinal bleeding due to visceral artery aneurysms. *Ann Surg* 187: 357, 1975.
64. Lovezzola MM: Resection of mycotic aneurysm of the small bowel mesentery. *N Engl J Med* 259: 1076, 1958.
65. Guida PM, Moore SW: Aneurysm of the hepatic artery: Report of five cases with a brief review of the previously reported cases. *Surgery* 60: 299, 1966.
66. Sower ND, Whelan TJ: Suppurative arteritis due to *Salmonella*. *Surgery* 52: 851, 1967.
67. Meade RH, Moran JM: *Salmonella* arteritis—Preoperative diagnosis and cure of *Salmonella typhimurium* aortic aneurysm. *N Engl J Med* 281: 310, 1969.
68. Cathcart RS: False aneurysm of the femoral artery following typhoid fever. *South Med J* 2: 593, 1909.
69. Ewart JM, Burke ML, Bunt TJ: Spontaneous abdominal aortic infections: Essentials of diagnosis and management. *Am Surg* 49: 37, 1983.
70. Thompson JE, Garrett WV: Peripheral artery surgery. *N Engl J Med* 302: 491, 1980.
71. Foote SC, Hook EW: *Principles and Practice of Infectious Diseases*. New York, Wiley, 1979, pp 1730–1750.
72. Yoshikawa TT, Herbert P, Oill PA: Salmonellosis. *J Med* 113: 408, 1980.
73. Kanwar JS, Malhotra V, Anderson BR, Pilz CG: Salmonellosis associated with abdominal aortic aneurysm. *Arch Intern Med* 134: 1095, 1974.
74. Zak FG, Strauss L, Saphra I: Rupture of diseased large arteries in the course of enterobacterial (*Salmonella*) infection. *N Engl J Med* 258: 824, 1958.
75. Allison MJ, Dalton HP, Escobar MN: *Salmonella choleraesuis* infections in man: A report of 19 cases and a critical literature review. *South Med J* 62: 593, 1969.
76. DeMuth WE, McConaghie RJ: *Salmonella* infection in ruptured abdominal aortic aneurysm. *Arch Surg* 95: 193, 1967.
77. Reichle FA, Tyson RR, Soloff LA, Lautsch EV, Rosemond GP: Salmonellosis and aneurysm of the distal abdominal aorta: Case report with a review. *Ann Surg* 171: 219, 1970.
78. Aserkoff B, Bennett JD: Effect of antibiotic therapy in acute salmonellosis on the fecal excretion of salmonellae. *N Engl J Med* 281: 636, 1969.
79. Cohen PS, O'Brien TF, Schoenbaum C, Medeiros AA: The risk of endothelial infection in adults with *Salmonella* bacteremia. *Ann Intern Med* 89: 931, 1978.
80. Thorner R, Ellner PE: Thoracic aortitis due to unusual *Salmonella*. *NY State J Med* 76: 1519, 1976.
81. Plotkin GR, O'Rourke JN, Jr: Mycotic aneurysm due to *Yersinia enterocolitica*. *Am J Med Sci* 281: 35, 1981.
82. McIntyre KE, Malone JM, Richards E, Axline SG: Mycotic aortic pseudoaneurysm with aortoenteric fistula caused by *Arizona hinshawii*. *Surgery* 91: 173, 1982.
83. Marty AT, Webb TA, Stabbs G, Penkava RR: Inflammatory aortic aneurysm infected by *Campylobacter fetus*. *JAMA* 249: 1190, 1983.
84. Edwards PR, Fife MA, Ramsey CH: Studies on the *Arizona* group of enterobacteriaceae. *Bact Rev* 23: 155, 1959.
85. Miller BM, Waterhouse G, Alford RH, Dean RH, Hawkins SS, Smith BM: *Histoplasma* infection of abdominal aortic aneurysms. *Ann Surg* 197: 57, 1983.
86. Kakkasseril J, Cabanas V, Saba K: Ruptured actinomycotic aneurysm of the splenic artery: A case report of successful resection. *Surgery* 93: 595, 1983.
87. Myerowitz RL, Friedman R, Grossman WL: Mycotic "mycotic" aneurysm of the aorta due to *Aspergillus fumigatus*. *Am J Clin Pathol* 55:271, 1971.
88. Gladstone JL, Friedman SA, Cerruti MM, Jomain SL: Treatment of *Candida* endocarditis and arteritis. *J Thorac Cardiovasc Surg* 71: 835, 1976.
89. Rose HD, Stuart JL: Mycotic aneurysm of the thoracic aorta due to *Aspergillus fumigatus*. *Chest* 70: 81, 1976.
90. Collins GJ, Rich NM, Hobson RW, Anderson CA, Green D: Multiple mycotic aneurysms due to *Candida* endocarditis. *Ann Surg* 186: 136, 1977.
91. Kriakedes GK, Simmons RL, Najarian JS: Mycotic aneurysms in transplant patients. *Arch Surg* 111: 472, 1976.
92. Ernst CB, Campbell C, Jr, Daugherty ME, Sachatello CR, Griffen WO, Jr: Incidence and significance of intra-operative bacterial cultures during abdominal aortic aneurysmectomy. *Ann Surg* 185: 626, 1977.
93. Williams RD, Fisher FW: Aneurysm contents as a source of graft infection. *Arch Surg* 112: 415, 1977.
94. Scobie K, McPhail N, Barber G, Elder R: Bacteriologic monitoring in abdominal aortic surgery. *Can J Surg* 22: 368, 1979.
95. Hardy JD, Timmis HH: Abdominal aortic aneurysms: Special problems. *Ann Surg* 173: 945, 1971.
96. Merry M, Dunn J, Weismann R, Harris ED, Jr: Popliteal mycotic aneurysm presenting as septic arthritis and purpura. *JAMA* 221: 58, 1972.
97. Geelhoed GW, Joseph WL: Surgical sequelae of drug abuse. *Surg Gynecol Obstet* 139: 749, 1974.
98. Katz ER, Lynne CM, Politano VA: Ruptured mycotic aortic aneurysm. *Urology* 7: 620, 1976.
99. Bass A, Rosenman Y, Adar R: Abdominal aortic aneurysm mimicking acute intraperitoneal inflammation. *Vasc Surg* 14: 334, 1980.
100. Mukerjee A, Nigam M, Awatramann W: Superior mesenteric artery aneurysm. *Br J Surg* 61:233, 1974.
101. Porter LL, Houston MC, Kadir S: Mycotic aneurysms of the hepatic artery. *Am J Med* 67: 697, 1979.
102. Elliott JP, Smith RF, Szilagyi DE: Aortoenteric and paraprosthetic-enteric fistulas. *Arch Surg* 108: 479, 1974.
103. Rosenthal D, Deterling RA, Jr, O'Donnell TF, Callow AD: Positive blood cultures as an aid in the diagnosis of secondary aortoenteric fistula. *Arch Surg* 114: 1041, 1979.
104. Brewster DC, Darling RC, Raines JK, Sarno R, O'Donnell TF, Ezpeleta M, Athanasoulis C: Assessment of abdominal aortic aneurysm size. Circulation 56(suppl 2):164, 1977.
105. Bernstein EF, Harris RV, Leopold GR: Ultrasound and CT scanning in the noninvasive evaluation of abdominal aortic aneurysms, in Bergan JJ, Yao JST (eds): *Surgery of the Aorta and Its Body Branches*. New York, Grune & Stratton, 1979, pp 43–68.
106. Haaga JR, Baldwin GN, Reich NE, Bevin E, Kramer A, Weinstein A, Havrilla TR, Seidelman FE, Namba AH, Parrish CM: CT detection of infected synthetic grafts: Preliminary report of a new sign. *Am J Roentgenol* 131: 317, 1978.
107. Gomes MN, Schellinger D, Hufnagel CA: Abdominal aortic aneurysms: Diagnostic review and new technique. *Ann Thor Surg* 27: 479, 1979.

108. Causey DA, Fajman WA, Perdue GD, Constantino MJ, Sones PJ, Tarcan YA: Ga scintigraphy in postoperative synthetic graft infections. *Am J Roentgenol* 134: 1041, 1980.
109. Perdue GD, Jr, Smith RB, III, Ansley JD, Constantino MJ: Impending aortoenteric hemorrhage: The effect of early recognition on improved outcome. *Ann Surg* 192: 237, 1980.
110. Thakur ML, Coleman RE, Welch MJ: Indium-111 labeled leukocytes for the localization of abscesses: Preparation, analysis, tissue distribution and comparison with gallium-67 citrate in dogs. *J Lab Clin Med* 89: 217, 1977.
111. Stevick CA, Fawcett HD: Aorto-iliac graft infection. *Arch Surg* 116: 939, 1981.
112. Cooke PA, Ehrenfeld WK: Successful management of mycotic aortic aneurysm: Report of a case. *Surgery* 75: 132, 1974.
113. Felson B, Akers DU, Hall GS, Schreiber JT, Greene RE, Pedrosa CS: Mycotic tuberculous aneurysm of the thoracic aorta. *JAMA* 237: 1104, 1977.
114. Weintraub RA, Abrams HL: Mycotic aneurysms. *Am J Roentgenol* 102: 354, 1968.
115. Nabseth DC, Deterling RA: Surgical management of mycotic aneurysms. *Surgery* 50: 347, 1961.
116. Currens JH, Faulkner JM: Gonococcal mycotic aneurysm of the aorta: Report of a case superimposed upon a syphilitic aorta. *Ann Intern Med* 19: 155, 1943.
117. Javett SM, Kahn E: Rupture of a mycotic aneurysm of the thoracic aorta. *Arch Dis Child* 27: 294, 1952.
118. Robb D: Surgical treatment of mycotic aneurysm. *Surgery* 52: 847, 1962.
119. Ehrenfeld WK, Wilbur BG, Olcott CN, IV, Stoney RJ: Autogenous tissue reconstruction in the management of infected prosthetic grafts. *Surgery* 85: 82, 1979.
120. O'Mara CS, Ernst CB, Williams GM: Secondary aortoenteric fistula. *Am J Surg* 142: 203, 1981.
121. Fry WJ, Lindenauer SM: Infection complicating the use of plastic arterial implants. *Arch Surg* 94: 600, 1967.
122. Ernst CB: Aortoenteric fistulas, in Haimovici H (ed): *Vascular Emergencies*. New York, Appleton-Century-Crofts, 1982, pp 365–385.
123. Park I, Pinsky WM, Baker CJ: Ruptured mycotic aneurysm of abdominal aorta: Successful treatment in a child. *Am J Dis Child* 135: 570, 1981.
124. Bridges RA, McTamaney JP, Barnes RW: Recognition and management of ruptured infected aneurysm of the abdominal aorta. *Vasc Surg* 15: 360, 1981.
125. Blaisdell FW, Hall AD: Axillary-femoral artery bypass for lower extremity ischemia. *Surgery* 54: 563, 1963.
126. Moore WS, Hall AD, Blaisdell FW: Late results of axillary-femoral bypass grafting. *Am J Surg* 122: 148, 1971.
127. Finseth F, Abbott WM: One stage operative therapy for *Salmonella* mycotic abdominal aortic aneurysm. *Ann Surg* 179: 8, 1974.
128. Blaisdell FW, Hall AD, Thomas AN: Ligation treatment of an abdominal aortic aneurysm. *Am J Surg* 109: 560, 1965.
129. Ernst CB: Axillary-femoral bypass graft patency without aortofemoral pressure differential. *Ann Surg* 181: 424, 1975.
130. DeBakey ME, Cooley DA: Successful resection of mycotic aneurysm of superior mesenteric artery. Case report and review of literature. *Ann Surg* 19: 202, 1953.
131. Howard TC, Mazer MJ: Mycotic aneurysm of the superior mesenteric artery: Report of a successful repair. *Ann Surg* 47: 89, 1981.
132. Olcott C, Ehrenfeld WK: Endoaneurysmorrhaphy for visceral artery aneurysms. *Am J Surg* 133: 636, 1977.
133. Bulkley GB, Zuidema GD, Hamilton SR, O'Mara CS, Klacsmann PG, Horn SD: Intraoperative determination of small intestinal viability following ischemic injury. *Ann Surg* 193: 628, 1981.
134. O'Donnell JA, Hobson RW, II: Operative confirmation of Doppler ultrasound in evaluation of intestinal ischemia. *Surgery* 87: 109, 1980.
135. Smith RF, Szilagyi DE, Colville JM: Surgical treatment of mycotic aneurysms. *Arch Surg* 85:663, 1967.
136. Kirklin JW, Shocket E, Comfort MW, Huizenga KA: Treatment of hepatic artery aneurysm by excision. *Ann Surg* 142: 110, 1955.
137. McEwen-Alvorado G, Villareal HR, Broders AC, Best EB, Broders CW: Aneurysm of the hepatic artery. *Am J Dig Dis* 12:509, 1967.
138. Rutten APM, Sikkenk PJH: Aneurysm of the hepatic artery: Reconstruction with saphenous vein graft. *Brit J Surg* 58: 262, 1971.
139. Zeppa RH, Petrou P, Womack NA: Collateral circulation to the liver: A case of mycotic aneurysm of the celiac artery. *Ann Surg* 163: 233, 1966.
140. Lau J, Mattox KK, DeBakey ME: Mycotic aneurysm of the inferior mesenteric artery. *Am J Surg* 138: 443, 1979.
141. Ernst CB, Hagihara PF, Daugherty ME, Griffen WO, Jr: Inferior mesenteric artery stump pressure: A reliable index for safe IMA ligation during abdominal aortic aneurysmectomy. *Ann Surg* 187: 641, 1978.
142. Hobson RW, III, Wright CB, O'Donnell JA, Zamil Z, Lamberth WC, Najem Z: Determination of intestinal viability by Doppler ultrasound. *Arch Surg* 114: 165, 1979.
143. Cooper A: Account of the first successful operation, performed on the common carotid artery for aneurysm in the year 1808: With the post-mortem examination in 1921. *Guy's Hosp Rep* 1: 53, 1936.
144. Reid MR: Aneurysms in the Johns Hopkins Hospital: All cases treated in the surgical service from the opening of the hospital to January, 1922. *Arch Surg* 12: 1, 1926.
145. Moore O, Baker AW: Carotid artery ligation in surgery of the head and neck. *Cancer* 8: 712, 1955.
146. Rogers L: Ligation of the common carotid artery: Report of 19 personal cases. *Lancet* 1: 949, 1949.
147. James NJ, Stuteville OH, Tasche C: Elective carotid artery ligation in the treatment of advanced cancer of the head and neck. *Plast Reconstr Surg* 47: 243, 1971.
148. Shea PC, Jr, Glass LF, Reid WA, Harland A: Anastomosis of common and internal carotid arteries following excision of mycotic aneurysm. *Surgery* 37: 829, 1955.
149. Howell HS, Baburao T, Graziano J: Mycotic cervical carotid aneurysm. *Surgery* 81: 357, 1977.
150. Ehrenfeld WR, Stoney RJ, Wylie EJ: Relation of carotid stump pressure to safety of carotid arterial ligation. *Surgery* 93: 299, 1983.
151. Avellone JC, Ahmad MY: Cervical internal carotid aneurysm from syphilis—An alternative to resection. *JAMA* 241: 238, 1979.
152. Samson DS, Gewertz BL, Beyer CW, Jr, Hodosh RM: Saphenous vein interposition grafts in the microsurgical treatment of cerebral ischemia. *Arch Surg* 116: 1578, 1981.
153. Yellin RE: Ruptured mycotic aneurysm. *Arch Surg* 112: 981, 1977.
154. Jarrett F, Darling RC, Mundth ED, Austen WG: The management of infected arterial aneurysms. *J Cardiovasc Surg* 81: 361, 1977.
155. Fromm SH, Lucas CE: Obturator bypass for mycotic aneurysms in the drug addict. *Surg Gynecol Obstet* 130: 82, 1970.
156. Guida PM, Moore SW: Obturator bypass technique. *Surg Gynecol Obstet* 128: 1307, 1969.
157. Dickman FN, Moore IB: Mycotic aneurysms: A case report of a popliteal mycotic aneurysm. *Ann Surg* 167: 590, 1967.

PART FIVE

Cerebrovascular Disease

Chapter 41

NATURAL HISTORY AND MEDICAL MANAGEMENT OF EXTRACRANIAL VASCULAR DISEASE

WILLIAM S. FIELDS

Thromboembolic stroke is a serious health problem in virtually all developed countries. Approximately two out of every five persons who suffer such a stroke will die within the first 30 days, and, of those who survive for a longer period, half will require special care, which places a tremendous economic burden both on the family and on society (1).

In the currently accepted classification of cerebrovascular diseases, ischemic stroke contains a number of categories including transient ischemic attack (TIA), reversible ischemic neurological deficit (RIND), progressing stroke (stroke in evolution), and completed stroke (2). Partial nonprogressing stroke is an additional category that includes small infarcts resulting in minimal residual deficit.

Arteriographic studies of patients entered into the Joint Study of Extracranial Arterial Occlusion (3) demonstrated the frequency with which multiple atherosclerotic lesions were observed and emphasized the importance of extracranial as compared with intracranial vascular lesions and of the frequent embolic origin of intracranial vascular occlusions (see Table 41-1). It is estimated that about 80 percent of ischemic strokes have an embolic basis, and the small number remaining will have some hemodynamic factors underlying the infarction. These factors include orthostatic hypotension; hypotension secondary to myocardial infarction; valvular heart disease, including prolapsing mitral valve; etc.

TABLE 41-1. Sites of Arterial Stenosis and Occlusion

	Incidence of lesions*			
	Stenosis		Occlusion	
Site	Right	Left	Right	Left
Extracranial arteries:				
Internal carotid bifurcation	33.8	34.1	8.5	8.5
Internal carotid (distal to bifurcation)	8.0	9.1	8.6	8.7
Vertebral	18.4	22.3	4.0	5.7
Intracranial arteries:				
Carotid siphon	6.7	6.6	9.0	9.2
Basilar	7.7		0.8	
Middle cerebral	3.5	4.1	2.2	2.1

*Percentages of lesions at designated sites in 4478 patients subjected to angiography (3).

Transient Ischemic Attacks

Episodes of transient strokelike symptoms, which have a rapid onset and which pass in a matter of minutes or hours or occasionally in a day or more, have been recognized at least since the middle of the nineteenth century. A variety of terms have been employed to describe such episodes, including cerebral intermittent claudication, little strokes, and transient cerebral insufficiency. However, in the last two decades the term *transient ischemic attack* (TIA) has displaced all others and has become generally accepted.

The concept of embolism to the eye or brain antedates even the first clear descriptions of TIA. In fact, during the nineteenth century there was considerable interest in both the clinical and pathological features of embolism, but these were for the most part disregarded during the first half of the twentieth century. Excellent descriptions of embolism from the heart can be found in the reports of several authors (4–6) and of embolism from the extracranial arteries in others (7,8).

Traditionally, the source of a "cerebral embolus" has been considered to be the heart. Embolism from this source produces 10 to 15 percent of all cerebral infarcts (9,10). Cardiac emboli vary considerably in size but are commonly large and tend to obstruct major arteries. One variety of large cardiac emboli is seen in association with mitral stenosis, and, when this valvular disorder is accompanied by atrial fibrillation, the incidence of embolism is said to be markedly increased (11). Patients with major cerebral emboli originating from the heart have a poor prognosis, with one in three dying immediately (12). There appears to be a greater risk of recurrence during the first year or two after the initial embolus than is present thereafter.

Mural thrombus associated with myocardial infarction is an

important cause of cerebral embolism, occurring within 6 weeks of the acute event in perhaps as many as 5 percent of patients suffering myocardial infarction. About one-third of the patients die during the immediate postischemic period. However, unless there is recurrent myocardial infarction, the risk of further embolization decreases rather quickly after about 4 to 6 weeks (13).

The link between thrombosis at the common carotid artery bifurcation and embolic occlusion of the distal part of the internal carotid artery was clearly described by Chiari (7), who appears, however, to have been unaware of previous references in the English literature to this connection between extracranial arterial disease and distal thromboembolism. In Allbutt's *A System of Medicine,* embolism from the heart, or from "diseased and roughened" arteries supplying the brain, was described, and it was noted that "in a number of cases recovery from the paralysis which follows embolism is both rapid and complete (14,15).

Unfortunately, after 1914 this knowledge appears to have been largely ignored, only to be revived 40 years later by Fisher (16,17). His theory that embolism could sometimes be a cause of a TIA or stroke was soon supported by evidence coming from other workers (18,19), and the prognostic implications of TIA were emphasized by Marshall (20). It is remarkable that only in the last 30 years have the symptoms of TIA become generally recognized and their prognostic implications with respect to both stroke and coronary heart disease generally understood.

The classification and nomenclature of cerebrovascular disease have never been completely satisfactory, and this is particularly apparent when one attempts to define a TIA. The recognition of a TIA is almost invariably dependent upon the patient's recollection of an event during which apprehension and anxiety may be more prominent features than the focal neurological symptoms. It is rare indeed for a physician to be present when the symptoms occur, and unless the episodes are sufficiently frequent to concern the patient and the doctor has a receptive mind and is familiar with the symptoms of TIA, transient cerebral or ocular symptoms can be completely missed or disregarded. The diagnosis of TIA is almost always based on clinical history, uncommonly on focal signs, and not on any diagnostic tests. It is therefore not too surprising that the definition of TIA is less than satisfactory. Nevertheless, over the past several years there has been a trend toward consensus. The World Health Organization (WHO) (21) proposed in 1978 a definition of TIA as

> Episodes of temporary and focal cerebral dysfunction of vascular origin; rapid in onset (no symptoms to maximum symptoms in less than five minutes and usually less than a minute); and variable in duration, commonly lasting from two to fifteen minutes but occasionally lasting as long as a day (twenty-four hours). The resolution or disappearance of each episode is swift (ordinarily a few minutes at most). A prolonged attack may take longer to clear up. An attack leaves no persistent neurological deficit.

This WHO definition is complex; does not address the issue of transient disturbances of ocular function (amaurosis fugax), which are a specific type of carotid territory TIA; does not specifically exclude focal cerebral dysfunction of other vascular pathology such as hemorrhage; and is rather ambiguous. It is not clear what is implied by dysfunction and deficit, and if both words mean the same thing, it would be more satisfactory to use only one or the other. Furthermore, it is not clear whether it is the neurological symptoms, the neurological signs, or both, that should resolve in 24 hours. Most physicians comprehend the meaning of symptoms and signs rather than dysfunction and deficits, and it is not uncommon to find minimal neurological signs of no functional significance such as reflex asymmetry or a Babinski sign that persists for some hours, days, or even weeks after the symptoms have disappeared. Whether or not such signs are noted will depend upon the thoroughness of the examiner and the length of time that has elapsed after the symptoms have subsided. If these minimal signs are observed, should the episode be called a stroke rather than a TIA? If so, a cohort of patients with focal symptoms lasting less than 24 hours will, if they are adequately examined within a few days, include a large number of individuals who must be classified as having suffered a cerebral infarct. If, on the other hand, they are examined less carefully several weeks after an episode, the same cohort may be considered to contain only TIA patients. The WHO definition would not include a patient with a "persistent neurological deficit" or "minimal residual deficit," leaving uncertainty as to what is really meant by persistent or residual. Does this imply that patients with neurological signs lasting beyond the 24-hour time limit must be excluded from the TIA classification according to the WHO definition?

The 24-hour time limit dividing TIA from stroke is now generally accepted, although it is arbitrary and has no special pathogenetic significance. The limit could have just as easily been 1 or 48 hours. Amaurosis fugax, for example, never lasts for more than a few minutes, and most cerebral hemispheric episodes less than 1 hour. Furthermore, there is no clearly established evidence that even when both symptoms and signs have disappeared by 24 hours, infarction of the brain has not occurred. Evidence obtained from computed tomography now makes it obvious that in some cases infarction and even hemorrhage have occurred. In the final analysis, there is no definitely established knowledge that the pathogenesis, natural history, and clinical management is substantially different in patients whose symptoms have lasted a few minutes, a few hours, or a few days. Whatever difference may be present is probably one of degree. Common practice dictates that however one defines the duration of a TIA, patients whose episodes last somewhat longer than 24 hours tend to be managed in much the same fashion. Whether it is correct to have similar treatment policies for TIA patients and for patients with small cerebral infarcts is not established.

From the foregoing, it might be suspected that it is not necessary or desirable to define a TIA at all. This is certainly not so inasmuch as a consensus definition is required if one is to make comparisons between reports from different centers and for epidemiological surveys. A less ambiguous and simpler definition has been suggested by Warlow and Morris (22): "An acute loss of focal, cerebral or ocular function, with symptoms lasting less than twenty-four hours and which, after adequate investigation, is presumed to be due to embolic or thrombotic vascular disease." If minimal, functionally insignificant physical signs are noted subsequently, the patient can still be deemed to have had a TIA.

There will always be difficulty with the TIA definition until the pathogenesis in each individual case can be determined. Any definition must be kept simple, care must be exercised in excluding other causes for transient neurological episodes, particularly nonfocal episodes, and one must focus attention on the duration of symptoms rather than on the physical signs.

In clinical practice generally, there has been an unfortunate tendency to diagnose TIA in middle-aged or elderly patients suffering transient focal neurological episodes with little concern for the possibility of other etiologies such as migraine and epilepsy. Many general physicians tend to include under the TIA rubric patients who have cardiac arrhythmias with associated transient neurological episodes, as well as those persons with transient nonfocal neurological symptoms. The tendency to utilize the TIA diagnosis for almost any transient neurological dysfunction has resulted in overprescribing so-called vasoactive and antithrombotic medications as well as performing unnecessary examinations for possible surgical intervention. However, the resurgence of medical interest in the whole question of cerebrovascular disease has tended to offset this trend toward overdiagnosis and overtreatment.

It is generally considered that a TIA is an indicator of threatened stroke and must be recognized and appropriately treated in order to reduce the risk for stroke. This indeed is the whole question with respect to the diagnosis and management of TIA patients, namely, the prevention of stroke and of myocardial infarction.

Characteristically there is a return to the preattack status at the termination of the attack. TIAs occur in both the territory of the carotid and the vertebral-basilar arteries. The main distinguishing feature between the two is the presence of lateralized symptoms in the carotid syndrome (e.g., monocular blindness, hemiparesis) compared with nonlateralized symptoms (bilateral or alternating) in patients with the vertebral-basilar syndrome. Care must be taken, however, to differentiate from TIA isolated symptoms such as recurrent vertigo, "drop attacks," transient amnesia, and episodes of unconsciousness. However, such symptoms, when observed together and/or with other brain stem manifestations, suggest a diagnosis of vertebral-basilar TIA.

The pathogenesis of TIA is in one of two major categories: thromboembolic or hemodynamic. Unfortunately, the distinction is not always readily apparent.

THROMBOEMBOLIC PATHOGENESIS

As has already been stated, thrombi can form at the site of an ulcerated atheromatous plaque or in an artery either in or beyond a stenotic segment. Some of these will not be large enough to constitute a major problem. Others will result in the symptoms of a TIA or completed stroke by passing downstream into intracranial branches. Thrombosis in combination with an obstructing atheroma obliterating the arterial lumen will characteristically propagate downstream to the next point of arterial branching. This pathogenetic mechanism is considered to be exceedingly important for TIA because of the potential for instituting corrective medical or surgical management.

Pathologists have known for many years that obstructing atheromas in the cervical portion of the carotid arteries are associated with cerebral infarction. However, it was not until the introduction and widespread use of arteriography as a diagnostic procedure that clinicians began to realize how frequently atherothrombotic lesions in these arteries are associated with cerebral infarction. More recently, there has been increased awareness that stenotic and ulcerated atheromatous lesions, particularly at the cervical carotid bifurcation, may be the site of thrombosis or the source from which emboli may pass into the distal intracranial portions of the cerebral circulation. The term "cerebral embolism" is now used to include emboli from an intraarterial as well as a cardiac course (2). Artery-to-artery emboli are of two main varieties, which may exist either alone or in combination: (1) platelet-fibrin emboli and (2) atheromatous debris.

Platelet-Fibrin Emboli

White bodies have been observed passing through or lodging in the retinal arterioles during an attack of amaurosis fugax (23). Subsequently, this material was studied and shown to contain both platelets and fibrin (24). Identification of platelet-fibrin emboli in the vertebral-basilar arterial territory is more difficult since the distal portion of this circulation is not accessible to direct visual examination as is the case in the territory of the ophthalmic branch of the internal carotid artery. However, it seems reasonable to postulate that a similar mechanism operates in both major arterial circulations to the brain, but in the posterior intracranial circulation the validity of this theory remains to be established.

Atheromatous Material

Fragments of atheromatous debris, when observed in the retinal arterioles, have been referred to as "bright plaques" and are usually associated with the ulceration of a plaque upstream in the carotid artery (25). Irregular atheromas and formation of ulcers may be observed in arteriograms of the cervical arteries of patients with TIAs.

Ulcerated lesions at the cervical carotid bifurcation are located most often on the posterior aspect of the lumen in the distal portion of the common carotid or proximal portion of the internal carotid arteries or both. Such lesions may also be observed, but less frequently, in the carotid siphon or in the vertebral arteries. The importance of extracranial as compared with intracranial vascular lesions has been shown by the above-mentioned results of Hass et al. (Table 41-1) (3).

The clinician, however, even with support provided by arteriography and other examinations, frequently encounters difficulty in deciding whether a specific patient has extracranial arterial disease with embolization into the intracranial arteries, intracranial disease with or without embolization from the aorta or heart, or primary occlusive disease occurring simultaneously in both the extra- and intracranial arteries. It is necessary to examine carefully these diagnostic possibilities in order to select appropriate therapy. In spite of thorough study, the physician is frequently led to the conclusion that although there is ischemia in a certain vascular territory, the exact cause of such ischemia is not readily identifiable.

HEMODYNAMIC PATHOGENESIS

Whenever a clinician is confronted with TIA, she or he should attempt to exclude factors that could be responsible for ischemia on a hemodynamic basis such as orthostatic hypotension, carotid sinus hypersensitivity, low perfusion states, or vascular compression by musculoskeletal structures. Many of these entities are accompanied by diminished cardiac output and are likely to be associated with diffuse disturbances of cerebral function such as impaired awareness or loss of consciousness. Episodes of transient focal ischemia are rare in individuals who are at high risk for stroke, unless there is marked stenosis in one or more of the aortocranial arteries (26,27).

The possibility that vasospasm produces TIA has not proved to be important in the etiology of ischemic stroke. It is clear, however, that on rare occasions a sudden elevation of systemic blood pressure to an excessively high level (diastolic above 130 mmHg) may be associated with transient ocular or cerebral ischemic attacks. Intensive retinal arteriolar narrowing may be observed by ophthalmoscopic examination during such a vascular crisis. Management of the hypertension alone usually brings about cessation of symptoms and disappearance of the ocular changes.

The scientific literature is full of reports of TIA induced by extravascular compression of the vertebral arteries during extreme rotation or hyperextension of the neck by bilaterally situated osteophytes on the cervical vertebrae (28). Tortuous, coiled, or kinked internal carotid arteries have also been suspected. Despite the larger number of reports on the subject, extravascular compression is a very uncommon cause of TIA (29,30).

When it is clear that the pathogenetic mechanism of the cerebral ischemia is hemodynamic, therapy must be directed at the responsible circulatory mechanisms rather than at the thrombotic process. It is absolutely necessary to make this clinical distinction. The impaired circulation resulting from altered hemodynamic phenomena may result secondarily in the initiation of thrombosis, especially in the presence of atherosclerosis. Severe forms of hemodynamic disturbance lead to massive cerebral infarction, and white thrombi made up largely of platelets appear in the pial arteries of the ''waterhsed areas'' in patients who are near death from cardiac failure, cardiac arrhythmia, and severe hypotension.

INCIDENCE, NATURAL HISTORY, AND PROGNOSIS

The natural history of TIA and the prognosis for patients suffering from this disorder have never been clearly delineated because of the inadequacy of available data. The course of the disorder may take one of four possible forms:

1. The attacks may cease spontaneously.
2. The attacks may continue unabated.
3. Cerebral infarction may ensue.
4. The attacks may be associated with some other major vascular catastrophe such as myocardial infarction since the affected population is generally at high risk for vascular disease.

In retrospective studies of patients who have had a completed cerebral infarction, approximately 75 percent reported having had one or more previous TIAs (31). Such information may not always be available, however, since many patients are unable to relate their prior experience after they have suffered a completed stroke.

Prospective studies with follow-up ranging from 1 to 5 years suggest that approximately 35 percent of individuals suffering TIAs will have a completed stroke within 5 years. The first month following the onset of TIAs is the period of most serious risk; approximately 50 percent of the completed strokes will have occurred within the first year (32). However, further data are required on this important subject in order to obtain a more reliable estimate of prognosis.

REVERSIBLE ISCHEMIC NEUROLOGICAL DEFICIT

The differentiation between a reversible ischemic neurological deficit (RIND) and a TIA is merely one of degree or perhaps of definition, since a TIA is said to resolve without neurological deficit within 24 hours, whereas an RIND will last a longer period of time. It serves no useful purpose to discuss the nature, pathogenesis, and treatment of this entity separate from that of TIA since it appears that it is only a temporal extension beyond those limits arbitrarily set for the cessation of transient symptoms (33). Within the past 5 years, there has been an increasing tendency on the part of neurologists to refer to these episodes as prolonged TIA rather than RIND.

PROGRESSING STROKE

The progressing stroke is a clinical state that has never been described with precision. According to the definition suggested by several authors, a progressing stroke is one in which the neurological deficit is still increasing in severity or in distribution after the patient has been admitted to the hospital. Further historical information often reveals that the progression was going on during the period just preceding admission (2). Some authors would restrict the time interval of progression to a few hours, while others would consider it reasonable to include patients who worsened over a period of several days or even several weeks (34,35). A ''stuttering'' or ''stepwise'' stroke progression (to which the term *stroke in evolution* has been ascribed) needs to be included as a clinical variant. Each author has provided a personal definition of progressing stroke, thereby preventing meaningful comparison between reports of frequency, prognosis, and therapeutic measures. In view of the fact that some physicians regard progressing stroke as an indication for the emergency use of heparin, a clearer understanding of the nature of this entity becomes an urgent matter.

COMPLETED STROKE

The term *completed stroke* is ordinarily employed to describe a focal neurological deficit that is abrupt in onset and has become stabilized. The variability in symptoms and the extent of initial disability, as well as the variability in recovery of function, is dependent upon a number of factors, including the adequacy of collateral circulation, the state of cardiorespiratory function, and the presence or absence of major systemic disorders that might critically alter cerebral metabolism (36).

Unilateral and even bilateral carotid occlusion can sometimes be silent events. Arteriographic studies performed on these deficit-free individuals often show remarkable and extensive collateral circulation. Presumably in those who suffer a fixed and severe neurological impairment, the channels for potential collateral flow, although demonstrable, have not functioned with sufficient rapidity to protect the territory of supply of the occluded primary artery.

In the context of the discussion here, it is important to emphasize that some individuals with completed stroke may subsequently suffer a TIA. As a consequence, such individuals may become, once again, candidates for clinical management designed to prevent further cerebral infarction.

Evaluation of Antithrombotic Therapy

Realization that thrombosis or thromboembolism is pathogenetic in many cerebral ichemic events has led to the design of therapeutic approaches for the specific purpose of influencing the thrombotic process. These have included the administration of anticoagulant, platelet-suppressant, or thrombolytic agents depending upon clinical circumstances and therapeutic objectives. The potential for the therapeutic modalities to prevent or alter the outcome of an ischemic stroke will be assessed here from available data collected in controlled clinical trials.

The basic principles that must be considered when designing and executing clinical trials include a clear statement of objectives for the study, a detailed description of the criteria for eligibility and ineligibility, a clear definition of the methods to be used, a description of the outcome variables of interest, and the methods of analysis that will provide information regarding statistical significance. Sample size and randomization are of particular importance in the evaluation of any antithrombotic therapy (37). Unless there is a very strict assignment to the treatment mode in accordance with a predetermined table of randomization, there is a grave risk that bias, on the part of either the observer or the subject, may affect the treatment a particular individual receives.

Because of the large number of subjects required to achieve statistical significance, the evaluation of antithrombotic therapy in ischemic cerebrovascular disease is an especially difficult problem. Since the immediate mortality from cerebral infarction is lower than in other types of stroke, long-term follow-up and large-scale multicentered trials are required. Moreover, the overall frequency of stroke in patients with TIA is approximately 7 percent per year and, if a drug brought about a 50 percent reduction in the incidence of stroke, more than 1000 patient-years would be necessary for a study to be statistically meaningful (38).

ANTICOAGULANT THERAPY

When the pathogenesis of an ischemic episode is presumed to be thrombotic or thromboembolic, the immediate theoretical objective is prevention of further development and propagation of the thrombus in order to minimize the tissue damage. On the other hand, the long-term objective is to prevent a recurrence of local thrombosis of cerebral arteries and further embolization from a remote site (39). Currently available information suggests that anticoagulant therapy should be considered for the patient with ischemic cerebrovascular disease on an individualized basis, depending upon the pathogenesis of the cerebral lesion, the type of disorder, and any concurrent systemic disease (40). The clinician should be familiar with the contraindications to the use of anticoagulants in particular. The clinician who elects to use them should recognize that there is a calculated risk for the patient, namely, the possibility of hemorrhage.

Indications for anticoagulant therapy for TIA remain controversial. In reported clinical trials, this form of treatment has not been demonstrated to increase survival rates or to reduce the incidence of subsequent cerebral infarction. The evidence that anticoagulants are of benefit in reducing the frequency of TIA recurrence is also equivocal (41). In progressing stroke, anticoagulant therapy may have some value in retarding the progress of infarction, but this has never been studied in a controlled fashion. Anticoagulant drugs have not proved to be useful in patients with completed stroke.

It must be remembered that the large-scale trials of anticoagulant drugs for cerebrovascular diseases were conducted between 1958 and 1963. Differential diagnosis between ischemic and hemorrhagic stroke was made on clinical grounds and on the presence or absence of blood in the cerebrospinal fluid. Since the advent of computed tomography scanning, it has become apparent that many small, but strategically located, lesions within the cerebral hemispheres that might have previously been called infarcts are now recognizable as hemorrhages. In such cases, anticoagulants are contraindicated, and so in previously conducted trials they might have been responsible for the catastrophic complications. It would seem reasonable, therefore, to reevaluate the role of anticoagulant therapy while employing more definitive neurological diagnostic tests than were available previously.

Present evidence indicates that patients with emboli from a cardiac source should be placed on anticoagulant therapy unless a serious contraindication exists (42). Both retrospective analysis and prospective randomized and nonrandomized clinical trials suggest that there is an increased chance of survival for these individuals placed on anticoagulant therapy.

THROMBOLYTIC THERAPY

The brain is so sensitive to hypoxia that the catastrophic consequences of thrombotic occlusion are almost entirely the result of reduction in blood flow. Irreversible tissue damage occurs within 10 minutes of total interruption of blood flow and within 1 hour if blood supply is decreased below 20 percent of normal. Therapy directed toward dissolution of the obstructing thrombotic material provides a very attractive approach from the theoretical point of view, since it should restore flow promptly while the tissue is still capable of salvage (43,44). A treatment of this nature should provide a means for dissolution of both single and multiple thrombi in extracranial vessels as well as from surgically inaccessible intracranial vessels. Unfortunately, one seldom sees patients within 60 minutes of the onset of ischemic stroke. By the time they are admitted for observation, there are not only changes in the brain parenchyma but also in the vasculature within the ischemic zone, thereby permitting a breach of the blood-brain barrier. Consequently, the administration of a thrombolytic agent at this point introduces the serious hazard of converting a "white infarct" into a "red or hemorrhagic infarct" when blood flow to the ischemic or infarcted area is reestablished, particularly in patients who are hypertensive. The use of this modality, as attractive as it may appear, is at the present time so hazardous that its clinical value is negated.

PLATELET-SUPPRESSANT THERAPY

The most striking property of platelets is their ability to aggregate (45). When platelets interact with collagen, they first adhere to the collagen fibers; aggregating agents are then released from and synthesized by the platelets, and aggregation ensues. Collagen is present in the subendothelial layer in the walls of blood vessels and is largely responsible for platelet deposition on blood vessels once the endothelial layer has been removed (46). It is widely believed that exposure of subendothelium is a relevant factor in intraarterial thrombosis (47). Once platelets have been induced to aggregate or when they have adhered to collagen or other foreign surfaces, they can undergo the platelet release reaction. This is a secretory process in which the contents of intracellular storage granules are specifically discharged from the platelets into the surrounding plasma (48). The released materials include adenosine diphosphate (ADP), catecholamines, and seratonin. The process is, therefore, one of the mechanisms through which platelets amplify their own aggregation. The same agents that induce aggregation in the release reaction also induce platelets to synthesize prostaglandins and thromboxanes (49–51). This is another mechanism through which platelets can amplify their own aggregation, because some of the intermediate prostaglandins and thromboxanes that are synthesized are potent, though short-lived, aggregating agents (52–55).

Although observations in vitro allow us to speculate on the involvement of platelets in thrombus formation, it is important to appreciate the limitations of such studies. Although valuable biochemical information has been obtained by studying isolated platelets in artificial media, the ways in which platelets behave under such conditions do not fully reflect the ways in which they behave either in anticoagulated plasma or in vivo. Consequently, studies to determine the influence of antiplatelet agents on platelets suspended in artificial media, in the absence of plasma proteins, do not give accurate information on the amount of drug required to affect platelet behavior. Most drugs are highly protein bound, and to effect a given degree of inhibition, higher concentrations are needed in plasma than are needed in a protein-free system.

The walls of blood vessels contain enzymes that convert ADP into materials that do not induce platelet aggregation. Prostaglandin I_2 (PGI_2, prostacyclin) is a potent inhibitor of platelet aggregation (56,57). Vessel walls, therefore, have the capacity to limit any amplification of platelet aggregation that might occur once platelets have been activated. Studies in vitro cannot take account of the modulating effect of the vessel wall.

A considerable number of pharmaceutical agents alter platelet function in vitro, but only a few have potential clinical usefulness when one considers their toxicity, the length of time during which they will affect certain platelet functions, and the dose required to produce a satisfactory clinical response. At the time of writing, three pharmacologic agents have been extensively evaluated in clinical trials—aspirin, dipyridamole, and sulfinpyrazone. Of the three agents, aspirin has the most dramatic effect on platelets in the test tube. Several aspects of platelet behavior are affected, both when the experiments are done wholly in vitro or when the platelets are studied ex vivo after the drug has been ingested. Because of the ease with which the effects of aspirin can be demonstrated, the drug has received a great deal of attention from researchers, and considerable strides have been made toward understanding the mode of action of this agent. The major effects of aspirin on platelets are on the events that follow stimulation of platelets by an aggregating agent. Aspirin completely inhibits the synthesis of prostaglandins and thromboxanes irrespective of the nature of the aggregating agent (54). It also inhibits the release reaction that accompanies the aggregation induced by such agents as adenosine diphosphate, norepinephrine, and low concentrations of collagen (58–61).

The effects of aspirin on prostaglandin and thromboxane synthesis, both in platelets and in the vascular wall, and on the platelet release reaction probably explains most, if not all, of the other effects of aspirin that have been observed in in vitro and ex vivo experiments (58,62).

Aspirin produces gastrointestinal symptoms in approximately 10 to 15 percent of patients on long-term treatment. Although prolonged use is associated with continuing low-grade blood loss from the gut, the evidence that aspirin ingestion produces acute gut blood loss is inconclusive. Furthermore, at the dose levels that have been used in clinical trials to date, neurotoxicity and interaction with other drugs such as anticoagulants have not posed any problems. Although aspirin has been in widespread clinical use for more than 80 years, there are no prospective studies on long-term toxicity that match the requirements for continuous use in patients at risk.

In spite of the fact that aspirin markedly prolongs bleeding time in persons with preexisting hemorrhagic disorders, it prolongs the bleeding time of normal subjects only minimally without producing a clinical hemorrhagic tendency. Furthermore, in the dose recommended thus far for clinical trials (1.0 to 1.3 g daily in a divided dose) there appears to be only slight risk of gastrointestinal hemorrhage unless an active peptic ulcer is present. Consequently, only those persons with a hemorrhagic diathesis, specific aspirin idiosyncrasy, or active peptic ulcer would be considered ineligible for entry into a trial. For these reasons, aspirin has been the most attractive drug to employ in controlled clinical trials in patients with ischemic cerebrovascular disease (63). Unfortunately, it has one serious drawback as an investigational tool because of its widespread use and availability as a nonprescription drug. For these reasons it is difficult to maintain the "double-blind control" unless the taste of both the aspirin and the placebo is disguised.

CLINICAL TRIALS OF ANTIAGGREGANT DRUGS

During the past 6 years, there have been several large-scale multicentered trials conducted to determine the clinical benefits, if any, of platelet-suppressant therapy in both TIA and ischemic stroke. A controlled trial conducted in the United States compared aspirin, 650 mg (two tablets), twice daily with a placebo in subjects who had a definite history of one or more carotid territory TIAs within 12 weeks of entry (64,65). There was a clearly demonstrated marked reduction in transient events, particularly in individuals who had had multiple attacks before entering the trial. An even more striking result was obtained in those subjects in whom there were arteriographically demonstrated lesions in the cervical portion of the carotid artery on the side appropriate to their presenting symptoms. Among those individuals treated medically throughout the duration of the trial, 51 percent had atherosclerotic lesions in the cervical carotid bifurcation that would, in some other clinics, have been considered as surgically accessible lesions requiring operative intervention. In this particular trial, no significant difference was noted in the effect on males versus females with regard to the reduction of TIA, but there was a trend, although not statistically significant, toward less effective protection in females when cerebral infarction was considered.

Coincident with conduct of the trial in the United States, another multicentered controlled trial was carried out under the auspices of the Medical Research Council of Canada, in which aspirin or sulfinpyrazone (Anturane) was tested against placebo and a combination of the two active agents. The published data from this clinical trial clearly indicate a 50 percent reduction in stroke morbidity and mortality in the aspirin-treated group, which appeared, however, to be confined to male subjects (66). The exact reason for this difference in response between the sexes is not clear at this time.

It has been thought by some reviewers that the apparent sex bias resulted from a statistical artifact produced by the small number of females in the study. Two subsequent controlled trials, one positive and one negative for aspirin, have both failed to show any sex difference in clinical response (67,68). Sulfinpyrazone was shown to be about as effective as the placebo, and a combination of aspirin and sulfinpyrazone about as effective as aspirin alone.

When considered together, the results of these two separately conducted trials clearly demonstrate a positive effect by aspirin in a total dosage of 1.3 g daily in male patients with respect to reduced morbidity and mortality from cerebral infarction and in both sexes with respect to a reduction or cessation of carotid TIA. It is suggested, therefore, that TIA and cerebral infarction may have differing pathogenesis, although without question TIA, particularly in the carotid–middle cerebral arterial system, should be considered as a marker for ''threatened stroke.''

Dipyridamole (Persantine), another platelet-suppressant drug, has been used widely as an antithrombotic agent in certain human diseases, but its mode of action is still not clearly understood. Current evidence suggests, however, that its suppressant effect in vitro is mediated by inhibition of phosphodiesterase (69). This inhibition tends to potentiate the effect of PGI_2 on the platelets, a reaction that depends on platelet generation of cyclic AMP. It may therefore be presumed that dipyridamole, as a phosphodiesterase inhibitor, retards the breakdown of cyclic AMP and thereby has an antithrombotic response in vivo. If this can be verified, it will provide a reasonable explanation for why dipyridamole is more active in vivo than in vitro.

As has been previously stated, in humans a single aspirin tablet (325 mg) will reduce the cyclooxygenase activity of platelets by 90 percent, and this effect only begins to disappear 2 days later, presumably with the introduction into the bloodstream of new, unaffected platelets. These observations suggest that smaller daily doses or even large weekly doses of aspirin alone or combined with another antithrombotic agent such as dipyridamole might be of greater therapeutic benefit. Both of these suggested dosage regimens are based on the hypothesis that there is a lesser effect of aspirin against the cyclooxygenase activity in the vessel wall than in the platelet or a more rapid recovery from the effect on the vessel wall.

Role of Prostaglandins in Vascular Disease

When the now-completed North American studies of the use of aspirin in stroke prevention were planned, very little was known about the role of prostaglandins in vascular disease, particularly with respect to platelet–vessel wall interaction. Nearly all of the information now available on this subject was accumulated subsequent to the beginning of recruitment of patients into either trial. The same was true of the German-Austrian trial of aspirin versus phenprocoumon versus placebo (70). For this reason, the daily dose of aspirin selected for administration in all of these trials was between 1.0 and 1.3 g. This dose was selected on the basis of prior experience in clinical practice and because a maximal effect on platelet aggregation observed in vitro could be accomplished with a 0.5 m*M* level of aspirin in the blood (71).

It has been shown subsequently, however, both in experimental models and by in vitro testing, that a much smaller daily dose of aspirin will suffice to produce a significant effect on platelet aggregation. It is claimed that aspirin interferes with the conversion of arachidonic acid into thromboxane A_2 in platelets in a dose approximately one-tenth of that necessary to inhibit the conversion of arachidonic acid into PGI_2, produced in vascular endothelial cells (72). Since thromboxane A_2 is proaggregatory and PGI_2 is antiaggregatory, it would theoretically be advantageous to block the former while sparing the latter. A more recent report (73) demonstrates that this concept is probably unsound and that to recommend low-dose aspirin is unrealistic. The hypothesis is still controversial and has yet to be proved in a clinical trial of patients with symptoms of atherosclerotic vascular disease (74,75).

It has been demonstrated that the amount of thromboxane B_2, the stable end product of thromboxane A_2, can be measured in the blood of persons in whom varying doses of aspirin have been administered (76). From this follows the assumption that a measurable reduction in thromboxane B_2 following the administration of a minimal dose of aspirin, such as 40 mg daily, would indicate that there has been a significant degree of interference with thromboxane A_2 production. Unfortunately, there is only one clinical trial reported to date in which a single daily dose of as little as 160 mg of aspirin was compared with a placebo in patients with renal failure who were receiving dialysis (77). The number of thrombi appearing in the dialysis shunts was sharply reduced in those patients receiving this small amount of aspirin. It cannot, however, be deduced from this observation that a small dose of aspirin would be equally useful in vascular disorders associated with atherosclerosis, since platelet function is altered in uremia and the thrombi occur on artificial surfaces and not within human arteries.

A trial now being conducted in England under the supervision of a neurologist and a biostatistician at Oxford attempts to compare a placebo against two different daily doses of aspirin in patients with transient cerebral ischemic attacks (78). This trial is being conducted in a double-blind fashion with one group receiving two tablets of aspirin (325 mg each) twice daily. The second group receives two placebo tablets in the morning, and one placebo and one aspirin tablet in the evening. The third group receives four placebo tablets, two in the morning and two in the evening. By employing this design, the investigators hope to determine whether or not one 325-mg tablet of aspirin a day is as effective as or more effective than four aspirin tablets, and whether or not either one or both treatment regimens is more effective than a placebo.

The extent to which platelet thromboxane A_2 formation must be inhibited in order to reduce the risk of thrombosis is unknown. It is fair to ssume that the inhibition was close to 100 percent in the clinical trials that employed 1.0 to 1.3 g of aspirin daily. Patrono and associates (79), using control subjects, demonstrated that a ceiling effect is obtained with a single 2-mg/kg dose and that a relatively constant degree of inhibition (greater than 90 percent) can be maintained with such a small dose given every 72 hours. Over a 3-day period, this represents approximately one-thirtieth the dose that is currently employed in clinical trials and that is now recommended by the Food and Drug Administration for clinical use in men. It was also suggested that such an interval between doses would permit the endothelial cyclooxygenase to recover its activity fully, if at all affected, in view of rapid de novo synthesis of the enzyme. It is also possible that platelets of patients at risk of thrombosis may have a different aspirin sensitivity when compared with the platelets of healthy subjects in whom thromboxane B_2 levels have been measured after low-dose aspirin administration (75,80). Furthermore, a sex- or age-related change in aspirin sensitivity may become apparent in older age groups.

It would obviously be advantageous in another trial to utilize low-dose aspirin to achieve an antithrombotic effect in symptomatic patients, since a rational quantitative approach would permit a reappraisal of exclusion criteria, increase medication compliance, and reduce withdrawals by minimizing gastrointestinal complaints. It could be recommended, therefore, that a high priority be given to consideration of another multicenter clinical trial in which the efficacy of 40-mg, 100-mg, and 650-mg daily doses of aspirin could be compared in patients presenting with TIA.

In the United States and Canada during the past several years, many clinicians, largely for empirical reasons, have been employing a combination of aspirin and dipyridamole for the management of both ischemic heart disease and ischemic cerebrovascular disease. Since the validity of this therapeutic regimen still needs to be carefully and thoroughly tested, another multicenter trial was initiated in early 1979 that included institutions in both the United States and Canada. This study compared the efficacy of aspirin, 325 mg, plus dipyridamole, 75 mg, four times daily against aspirin and a placebo. At the conclusion of this controlled trial, 889 subjects had been enrolled (81). Life table data analysis indicated that, for TIA patients taking aspirin, the addition of dipyridamole contributed nothing. The overall end points for both groups were identical (82).

Conclusions

1. Stroke is a very important cause of death and disability in most western nations. Among the various types of stroke, the ischemic variety related to thrombosis or thromboembolism is by far the most common.

2. The clinician should make every endeavor to distinguish between cerebral hemorrhage and cerebral infarction by whatever diagnostic procedures are available. He or she should also attempt to categorize the stroke according to the currently accepted classification [i.e., transient ischemic attack (TIA), reversible ischemic neurological deficit (RIND), progressing stroke (stroke in evolution), and completed stroke.]

3. The clinician should have basic knowledge of the mechanism of blood clotting and the contraindications when one of the various types of antithrombotic therapy is considered in the patient who either has had or is at risk of having a stroke.

4. Currently available information suggests that anticoagulant therapy be considered for the patient with ischemic cerebrovascular disease but that clinical trials of anticoagulant therapy in TIA have failed to demonstrate either an increased survival rate or a reduction in the incidence of subsequent stroke and of TIA recurrence. In progressing ischemic stroke, there may be some value in employing anticoagulant therapy in order to retard the progress of infarction. In patients with completed stroke, present evidence indicates that treatment with anticoagulant drugs is not useful. The use of thrombolytic therapy, although theoretically appealing, has not been shown to provide any significant benefit and is not considered safe.

5. The best available current information suggests that embolism of cardiac origin can be prevented by employing anticoagulants. These agents should not be employed if the patient has long-standing hypertension or a hemorrhagic tendency.

6. The reports of the United States and Canadian cooperative studies on the efficacy of platelet-suppressant therapy indicate that aspirin reduces the frequency of recurrence of TIAs in both male and female patients and provides a 50 percent reduction in stroke morbidity and mortality in males who have suffered a TIA or RIND. The validity of this apparent sex bias in clinical response has been seriously questioned. Subsequent published controlled trials have not demonstrated any difference in response between males and females.

References

1. Joint Committee for Stroke Facilities: I. Epidemiology for stroke facilities planning. Stroke 1972, 3:360–374.
2. Millikan CH, Bauer RB, Goldschmidt J, Goldstein M, Heyman A, Meyer JS, Moosy J, Mount L, Siekert RG, Stallones R, Toole JF: A classification and outline of cerebrovascular diseases II. Stroke 1975, 6:564–616.
3. Hass WK, Fields WS, North RR, Kricheff II, Chase NE, Bauer RB: Joint study of extracranial arterial occlusion: II. Arteriography, techniques, sites and complications. JAMA 1968, 203:961–968.
4. Gowers WR: On a case of simultaneous embolism of central retinal and middle cerebral arteries. Lancet 1875, 2:794–796.
5. Coats G: Obstruction of the central artery of the retina. Royal London Ophthal Hosp Rep 1905, 16:262–305.
6. von Graefe A: Ueber Embolie der Arteria centralis retinae als Ursacht plotzlicher Erblindung. Archiv Ophthalmol 1859, 5:136–157.
7. Chiari H: Uber des Verhalten des Teilungswinkels der carotis communis bei der endarteritis chronica deformans. Verh Dtsch Ges Pathol 1905, 9:326–330.
8. Hunt JR: The role of the carotid arteries in the causation of vascular lesions of the brain, with remarks on certain special features of the symptomatology. Am J Med Sci 1914, 147:704–713.
9. Adams GF, Merrett JD, Hutchinson WM, Pollock AM: Cerebral embolism and mitral stenosis. Survival with and without anticoagulants. J Neurol Neurosurg Psychiatry 1974, 37:378–383.
10. Kurtzke JF: Epidemiology of cerebrovascular disease. Geographic Distr Trans Amer Neurol Assoc 1968, 93:229–231.
11. Hernandez LM: Study of cerebral and peripheral emboli, registered in the National Institute of Cardiology of Mexico. Am Heart J 1947, 33:712.
12. Carter AB: Prognosis of cerebral embolism. Lancet 1965, 2:514.
13. Browne TR III, Poskanzer DC: Treatment of strokes. New Engl J Med 1969, 281:594, 602.
14. Taylor J: Occlusion of cerebral vessels. In TC Albutt (ed): *A System of Medicine*, vol VII. London, Macmillan, 1899, pp 560–576.
15. Welch WH: Embolism. In TC Albutt (ed): *A System of Medicine*, vol VI. London, Macmillan, 1899, pp 228–285.
16. Fisher M: Occlusion of the internal carotid artery. Arch Neurol Psychiat 1951, 65:346–377.
17. Fisher M: Occlusion of the carotid arteries. Further experiences. Arch Neurol 1954, 72:187–204.
18. Millikan CH, Siekert RG, Shick RM: Studies in cerebrovascular disease. V. The use of anticoagulant drugs in the treatment of intermittent insufficiency of the internal carotid arterial system. Mayo Clin Proc 1955, 30:578–586.
19. Gunning AJ, Pickering GW, Robb-Smith AHT, Russell R: Mural thrombosis of the internal carotid artery and subsequent embolism. Q J Med 1964, 33:155–195.
20. Marshall J: The natural history of transient ischaemic cerebrovascular attacks. Q J Med 1964, 33:309–324.
21. World Health Organization: Cerebrovascular disorders: A clinical and research classification. World Health Organization, Offset Publication no 43, Geneva, 1978.
22. Warlow C, Morris PJ (eds): *Transient Ischemic Attacks*. New York, Marcel Dekker, 1982, p 412.
23. Fisher CM: Observations of the fundus oculi in transient monocular blindness. Neurology 1959, 9:333–347.
24. Russell RW: Observations on the retinal blood vessels in monocular blindness. Lancet 1961, 2:1422–1428.
25. Hollenhorst RW: Significance of bright plaques in the retinal arterioles. JAMA 1961, 178:23–29.
26. Brice JG, Dowsett DJ, Lowe RD: Haemodynamic effects of carotid artery stenosis. Brit Med J 1964, 2:1363–1366.
27. Reed RL, Siekert RG, Merideth J: Rarity of transient focal cerebral ischemia in cardiac dysrhythmia. JAMA 1973, 223:893–895.
28. Fields WS, Weibel J: Effects of vascular disorders on the vestibular system. In Fields WS, Alford BR (eds): *Neurological Aspects of Auditory and Vestibular Disorders*. Springfield, Ill, Charles C Thomas, 1964, pp 305–340.
29. Weibel J, Fields WS: Tortuosity, coiling, and kinking of the internal carotid artery. I. Etiology and radiographic anatomy. Neurology 1965, 15:7–18.
30. Weibel J, Fields WS: Tortuosity, coiling, and kinking of the internal carotid artery. II. Relationship of morphological variation to cerebrovascular insufficiency. Neurology 1965, 15:462–468.
31. Drake WE, Drake MAL: Clinical and angiographic correlates of cerebrovascular insufficiency. Am J Med 1968, 45:253–270.
32. Friedman GD, Wilson WS, Mosier JM, Colandrea MA, Nichaman MZ: Transient ischemic attacks in a community. JAMA 1969, 210:1428–1434.
33. Meyer JS, Guiraud B, Bauer R: Clinical and pathophysiological considerations of atherosclerotic and thrombotic disease of the carotid arteries. In Vinken PJ, Bruyn GW (eds): *Vascular Diseases of the Nervous System. Handbook of Neurology*, vol. 11. New York, American Elsevier, 1972, p 327.
34. Jones HR, Millikan CH: Temporal profile (clinical course) of acute carotid system cerebral infarction. Stroke 1976, 7:64–71.
35. Millikan CH: Reassessment of anticoagulant therapy in various types of occflusive cerebrovascular disease. Stroke 1971, 2:201–208.
36. Millikan CH: Treatment of occlusive cerebrovascular disease. In Siekert RG (ed): *Cerebrovascular Survey Report for Joint Council Subcommittee on Cerebrovascular Disease, National Institute of Neurological and Communicative Disorders and Stroke and National Heart and Lung Institute* (revised). Rochester, Minn, Whiting Press, 1976, p 141.
37. Genton E, Gent M, Hirsh H, Harker LA: Platelet-inhibiting drugs in the prevention of clinical thrombotic disease (in three parts). New Engl J Med 1975, 293:1174–1178, 1236–1240, 1296–1300.
38. Marquardsen J: The natural history of acute cerebrovascular disease: A retrospective study of 769 patients. Acta Neurol Scand 1969, 45 (Suppl 38):9–192.
39. Baker RN, Broward JA, Fang HC, Fisher CM, Groch SN, Heyman A, Karp HR, McDevitt E, Scheinberg P, Schwartz W, Toole JF: Anticoagulant therapy in cerebral infarct. Report on cooperative study. Neurology 1962, 12:823–835.
40. Pearce JMS, Gubbay SS, Walton JN: Long-term anticoagulant therapy in transient cerebral ischaemic attacks. Lancet 1965, 1:6–9.
41. Siekert RG, Whisnant JP, Millikan CH: Surgical and anticoagulant therapy of occlusive cerebrovascular disease. Ann Intern Med 1963, 58:637–641.
42. Millikan CH: Therapeutic agents—current status: Anticoagulant therapy in cerebrovascular disease. In Siekert RG, Whisnant JP (eds): *Cerebral Vascular Diseases. Fourth Conference*. New York, Grune and Stratton, 1965, p 181.
43. Atkin N, Nitzberg S, Dorsey J: Lysis of intracerebral thromboembolism with fibrinolysis. Report of a case. Angiology 1964, 15:436–439.
44. Meyer JS, Gilroy J, Barnhard ME, Johnson JF: Therapeutic thromboembolism: Double-blind evaluation of intravenous plasmin therapy in carotid and middle cerebral arterial occlusion. Neurology 1963, 13:927–937.
45. Mustard JF, Packham MA: Factors influencing platelet function: adhesion, release and aggregation. Pharmacol Rev 1970, 22:97–187.
46. Baumgartner HR: Morphometric quantitation of adherence of platelets to an artificial surface and components of connective tissue. Thrombos Diathes Haemorrh Suppl 1974, 60:39–49.

47. Mustard JF, Packham MA: Normal and abnormal haemostasis. Brit Med Bull 1977, 33:187–192.
48. Holmsen H: The platelet: Its membrane, physiology and biochemistry. Clin Haematol 1972, 1:235–266.
49. Hamberg M, Svensson J, Samuelsson B: Prostaglandin endoperoxides. A new concept concerning the mode of action and release of prostaglandins. Proc Nat Acad Sci U.S. 1974, 71:3824–3828.
50. Smith JB, Ingerman C, Kocsis JJ, Silver MJ: Formation of prostaglandins during the aggregation of human blood platelets. J Clin Invest 1973, 52:965–969.
51. Smith JB, Willis AL: Formation and release of prostaglandins in response to thrombin. Brit J Pharmacol 1970, 40:545P–546P.
52. Hamberg M, Svensson J, Wakabayashi T, Samuelsson B: Isolation and structure of two prostaglandin endoperoxides that cause platelet aggregation. Proc Nat Acad Sci U.S. 1974, 72:345–349.
53. Malmsten C, Hamberg M, Svensson J, Samuelsson B: Physiological role of an endoperoxide in human platelets: hemostatic defect due to platelet cyclo-oxygenase deficiency. Proc Nat Acad Sci U.S. 1975, 72:1446–1450.
54. Roth GJ, Stanford N, Majerus PW: Acetylation of prostaglandin synthetase by aspirin. Proc Nat Acad Sci U.S. 1975, 72:3073–3076.
55. Smith JB, Ingerman C, Kocsis JJ, Silver MJ: Formation of an intermediate in prostaglandin biosynthesis and its association with the platelet release reaction. J Clin Invest 1974, 53:1468–1472.
56. Lieberman GE, Lewis GP, Peters TJ: A membrane bound enzyme in rabbit aorta capable of inhibiting adenosine diphosphate induced platelet aggregation. Lancet 1977, 2:330–332.
57. Moncada S, Vane JR: Unstable metabolites of arachidonic acid and their role in haemostasis and thrombosis. Brit Med Bull 1978, 34:129–135.
58. Evans G, Packham MA, Nishizawa EE, Mustard JF, Murphy EA: The effect of acetylsalicylic acid on platelet functions. J Exp Med 1968, 128:877–894.
59. O'Brien JR: Effects of salicylates on human platelets. Lancet 1968, 1:779–783.
60. Weiss HJ, Aledort LM, Kochwa S: The effects of salicylates on the hemostatic properties of platelets in man. J Clin Invest 1968, 47:2169–2180.
61. Zucker MB, Peterson J: Inhibition of adenosine diphosphate-induced secondary aggregation and other platelet functions by acetylsalicyclic acid ingestion. Proc Exp Biol 1968, 127:547–551.
62. MacMillan DC: Effect of salicylates on human platelets. Lancet 1968, 1:1151.
63. Fields WS, Hass WK (eds): *Aspirin, Platelets and Stroke, Background for a Clinical Trial*. St. Louis, Warren H. Green, 1971.
64. Fields WS, Lemak NA, Frankowski RF, Hardy RJ: Coantrolled trial of aspirin in cerebral ischemia. Stroke 1977, 8:301–315.
65. Fields WS, Lemak NA, Frankowski RF, Hardy RJ: Controlled trial of aspirin in cerebral ischemia. Part II: Surgical group. Stroke 1978, 9:309–318.
66. Canadian Cooperative Study Group: A randomized trial of aspirin and sulfinpyrazone in threatened stroke. N Engl J Med 1978, 299:53–59.
67. Moncada S, Korbut R: Dipyridamole and other phosphodiesterase inhibitors act as antithrombotic agents by potentiating endogeneous prostacyclin. Lancet 1978, 1:1286–1289.
68. Breddin K: Multicenter two-year prospective study on the prevention of secondary myocardial infarction by ASS in comparison with phenprocoumon and placebo. In Boissel JP, Klimt CR (eds): *Multicenter Controlled Trials: Principles and Problems*. Paris, INSERM, 1979, pp 79–92.
69. Levy G, Leonards JR: Absorption, metabolism and excretion of salicylates. In Smith MJH, Smith PK (eds): *The Salicylates, a Critical Biographical Review*. New York, Interscience, 1966, pp 5–48.
70. Bousser MG, Eschwege E, Haguenau M, Lefaucconnier JM, Thibult N, Touboul D, Touboul PJ: "AICLA" Controlled trial of aspirin and dipyridamole in the secondary prevention of atherothrombotic ceretral ischemia. Stroke 1983, 14:5–14.
71. Sorensen PS, Pedersen H, Marquardsen J, Petersson H, Heltberg A, Simonsen N, Munk O, Anderson LA: Acetylsalicyclic acid in the prevention of stroke in patients with reversible cerebral ischemic attacks, a Danish Cooperative Study. Stroke 1983, 14:15–22.
72. Masotti G, Poggesi L, Galanti G, Abbate R: Differential inhibition of prostacyclin production and platelet aggregation by aspirin. Lancet 1979, 1:1213–1216.
73. Preston FE, Shipps S, Jackson CA, French AJ, Wyld PJ, Stoddard CJ: Inhibition of prostacyclin and platelet thromboxane A_2 after low-dose aspirin. N Engl J Med 1981, 304:76–79.
74. Pareti FI, D'Angelo A, Manucci PM, Smith JB: Platelets and the vessel wall: How much aspirin? Lancet 1980, 1:371–372.
75. Hogendijk EMG, ten Cate JW: Aspirin and platelets. Lancet 1980, 1:93–94.
76. Anhut H, Bernauer A, Peskar BA: Radioimmunological determination of thromboxane release in cardiac anaphylaxis. Eur J Pharmacol 1977, 44:85–88.
77. Harter HR, Burch JW, Majerus PW, Stanford H, Delmez JA, Anderson CB, Weerts BS: Prevention of thrombosis in patients on hemodialysis by low-dose aspirin. N Engl J Med 1979, 301:577–579.
78. Warlow CB: Personal communication, 1981.
79. Patrono C, Ciabattoni G, Pinca E, Pugliese F, Castrucci G, DeSalvo A, Satta MA, Peskar BA: Low dose aspirin and inhibition of thromboxane B_2 production in healthy subjects. Throm Res 1980, 17:317–327.
80. O'Brien JR, Fincfh W, Clark E: A comparison of the effect of different anti-inflammatory drugs on human platelets. J Clin Pathol 1970, 23:522–525.
81. American-Canadian Co-operative Study Group: Persantine aspirin trial in cerebral ischemia. Stroke 1983, 14:99–103.
82. American-Canadian Co-operative Study Group: Persantine aspirin trial in cerebral ischemia. Part II: Endpoint Results. Stroke 1985, 16:406–415.

Chapter 42

EXTRACRANIAL CAROTID ARTERY OCCLUSIVE DISEASE

SAMUEL E. WILSON, CARLOS E. DONAYRE, and RUSSELL A. WILLIAMS

A stroke is the result of direct or indirect interference with the blood supply of brain tissue. The number of cerebrovascular deaths annually in the United States is about 170,000, ranking stroke as the third leading cause of death after heart disease and cancer. Of the 444,000 patients hospitalized in 1984 for strokes, 330,000 were new stroke victims—an incidence of 141 of every 100,000 North Americans (Table 42-1). If not fatal, the rehabilitation of the majority of patients who have a permanent neurologic deficit is protracted, costly, and requires great physical and emotional support by family members. The prolonged recovery is in sharp contrast to the cataclysmic onset of the stroke. About 40 percent of the patients who do survive require special nursing care and another 10 percent are disabled to such an extent they need to be institutionalized. Approximately 2 million persons in the United States who have survived a stroke are alive (1).

Rationale for Surgery in Stroke

At present there is little a physician can do to influence the recovery of infarcted brain tissue, and accordingly, much emphasis is placed on preventing strokes from developing. Included is treating patients who fit into a statistically developed high-risk profile for development of a stroke. In this category are individuals with diabetes, hypertension, atherosclerosis, or heart disease that may produce emboli, or those who have a history of previous stroke. The treatment of these diseases, particularly hypertension in nonwhite patients, accounts for the modest fall-off in incidence of cerebrovascular disease in recent years. Consideration of these statistically constructed stroke risk profiles has shown that patients within this population have a 40 to 47 percent chance of suffering a stroke within 8 years.

The 14-year Framingham Study of 5000 patients, aged between 30 and 62 at the time they entered the program, indicated that about 5 percent of them developed cerebrovascular disease (2). The majority of this was atherothrombotic, rather than cerebral emboli, subarachnoid hemorrhage, or intracerebral hemorrhage.

The Rochester population study done between 1955 and 1969 showed that the incidence of cerebral ischemia increased with age so that patients over 75 had a rate of 1786 per 100,000 population per year in contrast to patients aged 55 to 64 who had a rate of 277 (3).

One-fifth to one-third of patients die following their first stroke. Over the following 2 years, about 60 percent have a recurrent stroke, and the eventual causes of death after the first stroke are recurrent stroke in 50 percent of patients, other cardiovascular disease in 30 percent, and a miscellaneous group of causes among the remaining patients (4).

Two weeks after the onset of an acute progressing stroke in the carotid region, two-thirds of patients have been found to be still hemiparetic, 14 percent are dead, 15 percent have a residual monoparesis, and only 12 percent are neurologically normal.

After a stroke the treatment of hypertension is the only therapy that has proved useful in preventing recurrent cerebral ischemia, other than the use of anticoagulants to reduce future embolic complications in patients who have cerebral emboli.

These two diagnoses aside, the use of anticoagulants, aspirin, dipyrimadole, or agents to reduce blood lipids have not yet been shown effective in reducing further strokes. In selected patients who have extracranial vascular occlusive lesions that are felt likely to cause further permanent neurologic deficits, surgical correction may be undertaken.

Strokes associated with large-artery thrombosis develop suddenly in about 40 percent of the patients, in a stepwise or stuttering fashion in a third, and in the remainder a smooth, gradual onset or a fluctuating onset occurs with about equal frequency.

The previously described risk profile for the development of cerebral vascular disease is of little use in considering an individual and his or her likely risk for development of stroke or its prevention. Unfortunately, in many patients strokes develop with no preceding cerebral symptoms. However, in some patients, perhaps as many as 50 percent, who have large-artery thrombosis, there is a preceding history of transient ischemic attacks (TIAs). The likelihood of finding a focal TIA with other etiologies for stroke is 23 percent in lacuna strokes, 11 percent in embolism, 8 percent in hematoma, and 7 percent in strokes of aneurysmal origin. There is general agreement that patients who have TIAs should be considered for angiogram and possible surgical correction if correlated pathology is identified in the extracranial carotid system. In the Mayo Clinic, Rochester population study, 31 patients per 100,000 population per year developed TIAs, the incidence increasing with age (3). In the pa-

TABLE 42-1. Acute First Strokes per Year Requiring Hospitalization

Age	Men	Women
Under 35	1650	2660
35 to 44	5215	3355
45 to 54	13,575	10,645
55 to 64	34,670	22,070
65 to 74	44,510	46,235
75 to 84	49,180	53,110
85 and over	17,025	23,415

SOURCE: Data from Barner HB, Rittenhouse EA, Willman VL (1).

tients 65 to 74 years of age, this was 200 patients per 100,000 population per year. About one-third of patients who had TIAs developed a stroke due to cerebral infarction, and 50 percent of these occurred within the first year following the onset of the TIAs. The more recent Canadian cooperative study of patients who had TIAs showed that in the control group of 139 men and women, 20 (14 percent) developed stroke (5). The likelihood of developing cerebral infarction is higher in patients who have multiple hemispheric TIAs rather than a single isolated attack. However in one study of 160 patients the author was unable to differentiate patients who had a benign course following their TIAs from those who ultimately had cerebral infarctions (6).

Carotid endarterectomy will relieve TIAs in 85 to 95 percent of patients, independent of whether or not endarterectomy will prevent strokes. Aspirin has been shown to substantially reduce the risk of stroke in a male experiencing TIAs of all types. No similar advantage was found in women (5). Patients with an extracranial carotid lesion treatable without complication by endarterectomy have a better outlook for not developing stroke than patients treated with aspirin. Angiography and operation should be done with a complication rate (mortality plus stroke) of less than 3 to 5 percent to be acceptable. Over 50 percent of patients with TIAs will be shown on angiogram to have a surgically accessible internal carotid artery lesion.

Patients who have carotid region TIAs but no correctable vascular disease, suggesting another etiology for their problems such as an embolic or a hypercoagulable condition, still have a poor prognosis for stroke. For those who continue to have TIAs on aspirin therapy, treatment may be given in the form of oral warfarin (Coumadin) anticoagulants. With proper anticoagulation the stroke rate and the neurologic complication rate are lower than the stroke rate on no therapy.

Historical Perspective

By the late nineteenth century, astute clinicians had recognized the relationship of stroke to extracranial vascular disease. For example, the *Lancet* of 1875 carried a case report by Gowers of embolism to the middle cerebral artery from an extracranial carotid artery site (7). Hunt's description in 1914 of the role of the carotid artery in the etiology of cerebral infarction and his recognition of episodic cerebral ischemia as "cerebral intermittent claudication" not only established the clinical entity of stroke secondary to extracranial vascular disease but also foreshadowed the current term—transient ischemic attack (8).

The first cerebral arteriogram, performed in Lisbon in 1927 by Moniz (9) was directed at localization of brain tumors, but 10 years later he described four cases of internal carotid occlusion and hemiplegia diagnosed by cerebral arteriography (10). In 1953 Fisher confirmed the importance of extracranial vascular disease in the etiology of stroke by demonstrating on postmortem examination that the carotid artery was completely occluded in 9.5 percent of 432 patients and that more than 40 percent of patients aged 50 or older had at least a 50 percent obstruction of one major cervical artery (11).

As the data linking extracranial vascular disease to stroke syndrome became incontrovertible, surgeons soon adapted vascular reconstruction to its treatment. Credit for the first successful carotid reconstruction is ascribed to the Argentinians Carrera, Molins, and Murphy, who in 1955 reported anastomosis of the external carotid artery to the distal internal carotid artery in a patient with thrombosis of the internal carotid artery (12). The first successful carotid endarterectomy was performed by Michael E. DeBakey on a 53-year-old bus driver who had intermittent episodes of right arm and leg weakness (13). The patient survived 19 years without recurrent cerebral symptoms. Although DeBakey's operation was performed on August 7, 1953, he did not report it until some years later and the first description in the literature of a successful excision of a carotid plaque is that of Eastcott and Robb (14). Eastcott ligated the external carotid artery, transected the common carotid artery and the

TABLE 42-2. Distribution of Atherosclerotic Occlusive Disease

Site		Patients with Atherosclerosis, %	Mean Age	Male, %
I	The coronary arterial bed	32.1	55.4	84
II	In the major branches of the aortic arch	17.	61.7	65
III	The visceral arterial branches of the abdominal aorta	2.6	49.4	60
IV	The terminal abdominal aorta	42.4	59.4	80
V	A combination of two or more of these categories occurring simultaneously	5.7	60.8	73

internal carotid distal to the disease, and anastomosed the internal carotid to the common carotid in an end-to-end technique (15). In the ensuing three decades, carotid endarterectomy has become one of the most common (over 100,000 operations in the United States in 1987) and controversial vascular procedures. The distribution of vascular disease in hospitalized patients is shown in Table 42-2 (16).

Pathogenesis

The pathophysiology of stroke as a result of carotid artery disease continues to defy precise description and is the subject of ongoing research and much spirited debate. What cannot be argued is that a detailed understanding of the pathogenesis of cerebral ischemia is as essential as an accurate knowledge of the natural history of carotid bifurcation stenosis in developing a rational therapeutic program for extracranial vascular occlusive disease.

In the early 1950s Fisher described a variety of pathological changes occurring in the carotid arteries of patients dying of stroke (11). He recognized the two basic mechanisms by which carotid artery lesions produce cerebral ischemia: *embolization* from an irregular luminal surface, usually, but not exclusively, an ulcerated plaque; or *decreased flow* through the narrowed or occluded internal carotid arteries. These observations were verified clinically by the 1968 report of the Joint Study of Extracranial Arterial Occlusions, which showed that approximately 75 percent of over 4000 patients in the study had significant extracranial arterial lesions producing greater than 30 percent stenosis shown by arch and cerebral angiography (17). Stenosis occurred more frequently than occlusion, with the carotid artery bifurcation being the site most frequently involved (34 percent), followed by the vertebral artery origins (20 percent). These findings, together with the then newly recognized significance of Hollenhorst plaques, indicated that cerebral ischemia could occur from either of the two previously mentioned mechanisms.

Atherosclerosis, the most common cause of extracranial cerebral arterial stenosis in humans, is in the simplest terms, the deposition of lipid-laden plaques within blood vessel walls. The initiation and growth of the carotid bifurcation atherosclerotic plaque may be the in vivo lesion which best fits Ross's theory of pathogenesis as described in Chapter 2. Glomset and Ross postulate a "response-to-injury" hypothesis to explain the pathogenesis of atherosclerosis and propose that injury to the endothelium is the initiating event in atherogenesis (18). Endothelium responds to injury in a variety of ways, including endothelial desquamation with loss of nonthrombogenic character and local secretion of growth factors with minimal or no morphologic alteration of the involved endothelium. Platelets adhere to the exposed subendothelial connective tissue and release the contents of their granules. They contain at least two mitogens: epidermal growth factor and platelet-derived growth factor—the latter may be of particular importance in atherogenesis because its chemotactic and mitogenic properties can induce both smooth-muscle migration and proliferation. The monocyte, which develops into the macrophage, a scavenger cell in inflammatory reactions, then becomes involved. In one of the earliest cellular interactions that occurs in hypercholesterolemia, monocytes attach to endothelial cells and there is migration and subendothelial localization of these monocytes which are the first events in fatty-streak formation and thus in atherogenesis. Furthermore, macrophages can release mitogens and have been associated with connective tissue proliferation. Thus, endothelial "injury" at the carotid bifurcation releases chemoattractants and growth factors from endothelial platelets with attachment of platelets and macrophages, all of which lead to migration of smooth-muscle cells from the media into the intima and their subsequent proliferation. These events lead to fibrous plaque formation with further progression of the lesion.

Atherosclerosis shows a predilection for developing in specific vascular sites including the vessels of the circle of Willis and the extracranial carotid artery system. In particular these sites include points of bifurcation and areas of curvature. Hemodynamic injury is thought to cause endothelial injury at these sites. Ideal blood flow is laminar—a column of flowing blood travels in concentric layers along its vascular tube. The core layers travel at the highest velocity with each adjacent layer moving more slowly until a stationary fluid layer is encountered at the vascular wall. This decrease in the velocity of blood flow from core to periphery is known as the velocity gradient. Since each fluid lamina travels at its own speed, it exerts a force on an immediately adjacent lamina traveling at a different speed, referred to as shear stress, which is most pronounced at the vascular wall. The greater the velocity gradient, the greater the shear stress at the wall and the greater the chance of endothelial injury. When the flow velocity increases beyond a critical value, the layered pattern of laminar flow is disrupted and the fluid elements develop irregular motion, tumbling in random local currents called vortices. Blood flow characterized by such irregular patterns of movement is turbulent. Steady flow is most aptly applied to laminar flow through straight vessels and is associated with parabolic flow profiles. The carotid bifurcation, on the contrary, exhibits unsteady flow, a local pressure drop occurs as the carotid divides, and slowing of blood flow follows. Blood velocity near the vessel wall slows and blood in contact with the wall becomes stationary, resulting in a condition of high shear at the wall. Downstream turbulence then arises as a result of decelerating flow.

Endothelial cell injury from shear stress was studied by Fry who showed a strong correlation between sites of endothelial injury and predicted sites of highest shear stress (19). Restructuring of the luminal surface due to endothelial injury occurs and appears to be the result of endothelial cell proliferation. Smooth-muscle-cell migration and proliferation at the intima may then lead to the formation of a stenotic fibrotic plaque. Endothelial desquamation favors platelet attachment and fibrin formation, resulting in red cell thrombi at the site of injury. Blood flowing past this causes a shearing stress and favors detachment of the fibrin-platelet aggregates. In summary, flow alteration at the carotid bifurcation leads to endothelial injury with a resultant stenotic plaque and thrombus formation, causing further hemodynamic changes and an increase in shear stress at the site of injury.

At first, arterial stenosis caused by atherosclerotic plaques was thought to cause cerebral infarction by simply decreasing cerebral blood flow. Arterial stenosis was regarded as ''critical'' if it was flow-limiting and ''subcritical'' if flow volume was maintained. Brice and others measured the pressure gradient and flow in the human carotid artery and concluded that the amount of constriction required to limit flow corresponds to an average reduction of luminal area by about 80 to 85 percent (20). A significant pressure drop does not occur distal to a stenosis of less than 72 percent luminal area reduction. On the other hand, experimental studies have confirmed endothelial cell injury and thrombus formation with arterial stenosis in the 50 to 80 percent area reduction—subcritical stenosis by accepted definition.

Additional factors determine whether a stenosis is critical: pressure and adequacy of collateral circulation to the territory supplied by the affected vessel, increased metabolic demands by the tissue, a drop in systemic blood pressure, or decreased cardiac output. Such factors can modify the demand or supply of the affected tissue for blood and could transform a subcritical stenosis into a functionally critical one.

Imaging techniques such as slow-motion angiography and real-time B-mode imaging have shown vessel wall movement at the level of the carotid bifurcation to be greater than previously appreciated. Lusby demonstrated a greater distensibility of the carotid bulb than the common carotid artery (21). The variations in distensibility indicate differences in compliance, particularly marked at the carotid bulb. Pulsatile flow causes circumferential stress to be greater at the carotid bulb due to this distensibility and may contribute to endothelial injury and the development of atheroma. In addition, a change in elastin and collagen content secondary to atheroma may further contribute to alterations in mechanical properties. These changes in wall structure and the asymmetric nature of atheroma deposition produce imbalances in wall tensions. Sudden alterations in systemic blood pressure may cause abrupt changes in wall tension leading to intraplaque hemorrhage, frank plaque fracture, or luminal thrombosis. Critical stenosis is then really a dynamically changing concept.

The end result is formation of the carotid bifurcation plaque. Imparato analyzed the histologic and gross morphologic characteristics of 69 carotid plaques from 50 symptomatic patients (22). Even though he observed great variability in plaque morphology, some degree of intraplaque hemorrhage was found in 65 percent of the specimens examined. A prospective study of 376 carotid plaques (275 symptomatic, 101 asymptomatic) obtained from endarterectomies in 280 patients was then undertaken to correlate plaque morphology and symptoms (23). Ulceration was the most frequent gross morphologic characteristic of the carotid artery plaques, but hemorrhage was the only gross characteristic that was significantly more frequent in symptomatic patients compared with plaques in asymptomatic patients.

Clinical Presentation

Blood flow through a stenosed lesion is not impaired until over three-quarters of the lumen cross-sectional area has been reduced. This usually takes many years to develop, and during that time collateral blood flow is established beyond the lesion so that asymptomatic occlusion may be the end stage. If the collaterals have developed inadequately, perhaps because of the rapid progression of the carotid lesion, then symptoms of cerebral ischemia will occur.

The clinical presentation may be a *transient ischemic attack* (TIA), lasting typically less than 15 minutes but occasionally up to 24 hours followed by full recovery; a *reversible ischemic neurologic deficit* (RIND), lasting for longer than 24 hours but leaving essentially no residual deficits; or a *permanent fixed deficit* such as hemiplegia in the patient presenting with a cerebral infarction. Pathologically, the difference between a TIA and a fixed neurologic deficit relates to the degree and persistence of ischemia. In the latter there is actual infarction of brain tissue. In the older patient only one carotid artery may be patent, supplying all regions of the brain.

In the region of the carotid artery, TIAs all involve the terminal regions of distribution of the anterior and middle cerebral arteries. Typically, symptoms, including clumsiness, weakness, or paralysis, are experienced on the contralateral side of the body from that of the cerebral ischemia. There may be numbness, anesthesia, or paresthesia, when this occurs in the face, it may be on the opposite side from the body. When the patient's dominant (commonly left) hemisphere is involved, he or she may have motor or perceptive aphasia. Dysarthria may occur if the nondominant hemisphere is involved, and if it is the only symptom, it is more likely to have a vertebrobasilar origin.

Amaurosis fugax, which is a transient loss or blurring of vision in the ipsilateral eye field, is commonly described as being as though a curtain or window shade came down on the visual field or as a quadrant field defect. This is very typically due to a TIA associated with a lesion in the carotid artery. Deviation of the eye to one or the other side is not seen in a TIA. Homonymous hemianopsia associated with any of the forgoing symptoms is usually of carotid origin, but when it occurs alone it may be equally vertebrobasilar in origin.

Headaches and seizures are uncommon as are a loss of consciousness or syncopy. Dizziness, loss of memory, and confusion along with impaired vision are usually not manifestations of a TIA unless they are accompanied by more specific symptoms.

Patients with nonspecific symptoms such as dizzy spells usually have these related to more global cerebral ischemia rather than focal disease. TIAs can readily be differentiated from symptoms due to postural hypotension by taking a careful history. Any of the symptoms described due to TIAs can become permanent as a result of a cerebral infarction.

TIAs due to vertebrobasilar disease are far less specific than those associated with carotid disease. They may include eye field defects, vertigo, ataxia, dysarthria, hoarseness, dysphasia, confusion, hiccups, vomiting, loss of consciousness in conjunction with either postural disturbances or rarely even drop attacks. These symptoms may have a multitude of origins including transient cerebral ischemia.

Noninvasive Testing for Carotid Artery Disease

The role of noninvasive vascular diagnostic techniques in the management of extracranial vascular disease is covered in Chapter 10 and the use of digital subtraction angiography in Chapter 14.

The vascular laboratory is important in evaluating patients with symptoms of cerebral ischemia who may be candidates for surgery. Such complementary studies as oculopneumoplethysmography, Doppler frequency spectral analysis, and B-mode imaging may be used to detect the presence of and determine the morphology and any restriction of a carotid lesion. Patients who have negative tests generally have no lesions notable for surgery and therefore need not undergo angiography. At present duplex scanning, combining B-mode imaging and Doppler frequency spectral analysis, is the most widely used test. The correlation between duplex ultrasonography and digital subtraction angiography (DSA) is absolute in 68 percent of vessels, good in 28 percent, and poor in 4 percent (24). When duplex studies are compared with conventional angiograms, correlations are similar. Duplex scanning tends to overestimate the severity of disease when compared with conventional angiography, whereas DSA tends to underestimate the severity of disease. We use duplex ultrasound (pulse Doppler transducer and real-time ultrasound imaging transducer) for screening patients with suspected carotid artery disease.

There is little use today for older techniques such as carotid phonoangiography and supraorbital Doppler evaluation. In some laboratories the oculoplethysmograph is used as a screening test, but it provides less information than duplex scanning. Duplex ultrasound is also a useful technique for evaluating patients who have recurrent symptoms after carotid endarterectomy. Detection of carotid artery restenosis following endarterectomy is discussed in Chapter 48.

Angiography

It is the exceptional patient who proceeds to operation for extracerebral carotid artery disease without an angiogram. Conversely, because angiography is not an uncomplicated procedure, it is generally not ordered unless operation is under consideration. Noninvasive studies are now accurate enough for diagnosis, and an angiogram is used to confirm the presence of a lesion and determine its suitability for operation.

Intracranial tumors, vascular malformations, or subdural hematomas have all presented with symptoms like TIAs. It is useful to perform computed tomography (CT) of the brain to diagnose the presence of these and to detect actual cerebral infarction if it is present. A hemorrhagic infarct is seen early on CT scan, while that associated with ischemia takes several days to develop. Most patients who are to have angiography should have this preceded by a CT scan.

The full examination of the extracranial vessels includes an arch aortogram in addition to bilateral carotid arteriography. The latter arteries are viewed to their terminal intracranial branches, and biplanar views are routinely included.

Conventional angiography usually includes an aortic arch study to detect lesions at the origins of the cerebral vessels and may indicate the vessels on which the radiologist should focus attention, thus limiting the study to obtaining selective, particularly carotid, angiograms. Well-defined views of the carotid bifurcation may be required at which an ulcerative lesion not producing any hemodynamic abnormality is sought, particularly in a patient with no candidate pathology demonstrated in the extracerebral circulation. This may be seen in only one view of a selective angiogram.

In patients suspected of having subclavian steal syndrome, an aortic arch injection demonstrates the stenotic subclavian lesion and caudad flow direction in the vertebral artery.

DSA may be used if it has been elected to treat a patient who has an asymptomatic carotid stenosis. A symptomatic patient with a carotid stenosing lesion occluding more than 90 percent of the lumen or which appears as a "string" sign on angiography usually requires this to be treated by operation soon after angiogram. Intravenous heparin is administered in the interim to prevent complete thrombosis of this artery which may develop after angiography, possibly due to the dehydrating effect of the intraarterial contrast agents. The operation is done within the next day or so.

If during the study a plaque is shown to have been dissected by the angiogram catheter, even though no neurologic deficit has ensued, there is thought to be a high likelihood of superimposition of carotid artery thrombosis. Prompt carotid endarterectomy is usually recommended. Overall, the risk of stroke following angiography is about 1 percent.

Indications for Carotid Endarterectomy

The indications for surgery of vertebrobasilar insufficiency, management for ulcerative plaques, and operation for asymptomatic stenosis are considered in Chapters 43, 45, and 46. We will discuss the generally accepted indications for endarterectomy for occlusive disease first and then review less-well-defined justifications for surgery.

1. *TIAs*. A focal ischemic episode of neurologic dysfunction typically lasting 2 to 15 minutes, but occasionally as long as 24 hours, resolving without residual disability and producing symptoms involving the carotid system, is considered an accepted indication for carotid endarterectomy. A monocular TIA, amaurosis fugax, is included in the category of the carotid system TIA. On the other hand, certain symptoms such as light-headedness, vertigo, confusion, syncope, dysarthria, or diplopia are generally not indicators of anterior cerebral circulation disease. Patients with these symptoms often do not have clear-cut focal episodes of transient ischemia.

Although most TIAs are due to embolization of platelet-fibrin aggregates or atheromatous debris from the atherosclerotic plaque in the carotid bifurcation, other, less common causes of ischemia are considered in evaluating a patient with TIAs for surgery. Important differential diagnoses include cardiac arrhythmias, embolic phenomena related to the myocardium or subacute bacterial endocarditis, hematologic abnormalities such as polycythemia and sickle cell disease, paroxysmal embolism, and fibromuscular hyperplasia of the internal carotid artery. Because the greatest risk for stroke following TIA occurs in the first year and particularly in the first 2 to 3 months, operation is advisable soon after diagnosis.

2. *RINDs*. Focal cerebral ischemia persisting longer than 24 hours but clearing with little or no residual effect within 7 days fulfills the criteria of a RIND, and when the deficit is anatomically related to an appropriate carotid artery lesion, it is an indication for endarterectomy. Approximately 25 percent of patients with a RIND have a subsequent stroke within 5 years of the initial event.

3. *Completed Stroke*. Cerebral infarction with good recovery and a minimal to modest neurologic deficit is a relative indication for surgery in a patient who is otherwise a good surgical risk. Intracranial small-vessel or large-vessel disorders, emboli arising from distant sources such as the heart, and other systemic disorders must be ruled out. If cerebral angiography identifies pathologic changes in the extracranial vessels related to the symptoms, endarterectomy of the carotid bifurcation may be undertaken to prevent a future additional, possibly further disabling neurologic deficit. Operation is delayed at least 3 weeks after the acute event.

4. *Flow-Restrictive Asymptomatic Carotid Stenosis*. Although the value of carotid endarterectomy has not been proved in patients with asymptomatic stenosis, many surgeons recommend operation for a subcategory of patients with critical or "preocclusive" stenoses. Operation on all patients with narrowing of the carotid artery to more than 50 percent of its diameter has not been shown to be beneficial. A Veterans Administration multicenter cooperative trial is currently investigating the benefit of carotid endarterectomy compared to medical therapy with antiplatelet agents in patients with asymptomatic disease when the stenosis results in a greater than a 50 percent reduction in artery diameter (25).

Certain controversial indications for carotid endarterectomy, not accepted uniformly by neurologists and vascular surgeons, may be appropriately treated by operation in the occasional, carefully selected patient. Although carotid endarterectomy has been advocated for patients with vertebrobasilar disease who have anterior atherosclerotic obstruction, long-term follow-up usually has not demonstrated sustained symptomatic relief. Further investigation of patients with carotid bruits scheduled to undergo a major operative procedure is usually not necessary unless duplex scanning shows a high degree of flow restriction, as correction of non-flow-restrictive asymptomatic stenoses before major procedures does not improve outcome.

Neuropsychological deficits have been observed in patients with extracranial cerebrovascular disease, particularly severe bilateral carotid artery obstruction. Deficits have ranged from emotional instability and personality aberrations to dementia with its associated loss of memory and diminished intellectual and cognitive abilities. Although these intellectual deficits are often associated with a decrease in cerebral blood inflow due to stenosis or occlusion of the extracranial arteries, carotid endarterectomy has not been shown to reliably improve neuropsychological performance. Multiple studies have been conducted on the effect of carotid endarterectomy on pre- and postoperative psychological testing, but the data are still insufficient to support a definite role for endarterectomy in reversing neuropsychological deficits (26).

Carotid endarterectomy is no longer commonly used for treatment of the acute stroke. Surgical management of the acute progressive stroke continues to be a difficult clinical problem. Callow indicates that endarterectomy may be applicable only under extremely limited circumstances, depending on the time of onset of the deficit and the timeliness of surgical intervention (27).

DESCRIPTION OF THE TECHNIQUE

Carotid endarterectomy, arguably the least difficult of the arterial reconstructions, is the most unforgiving of operative error or lapse of judgment in patient selection. Preparation includes an adequate intravenous route for fluid replacement, not necessarily a central venous line, and pharmacologic regulation of the blood pressure. An intraarterial catheter in the radial artery is employed for continuous measuring of blood pressure. The systolic arterial blood pressure is regulated within 20 to 30 mmHg of the patient's baseline pressure to prevent systolic hypertension (over 200 mmHg).

Easy accessibility and predictably situated atherosclerotic disease favor surgical correction of extracranial carotid occlusive disease.

The skin incision may follow the anterior border of the sternocleidomastoid, or alternatively a transverse incision provides improved scar appearance and affords more direct exposure of the carotid bulb. The incision is extended through the platysma and superficial cervical fascia, and the sternocleidomastoid muscle is mobilized along its anterior border.

The transverse facial vein requires division, and the internal jugular vein is displaced laterally and posteriorly by careful placement of a self-retaining retractor, allowing visualization of the carotid sheath. Division of a branch of the ansa hypoglosi supplying the strap muscles of the neck may be unavoidable but does not result in noticeable residual weakness in unilateral operation. The carotid sheath is opened, and the common, external, superior thyroid and internal carotid arteries are isolated by sharp dissection (Figure 42-1). The vessels are manipulated gently to avoid dislodging intraluminal debris. Should bradycardia be reported by the anesthesiologist during dissection of the carotid bulb, 0.5 to 1 mL of 1% lidocaine is injected into the area of the carotid body. Generally dissection is carried superiorly on the internal carotid artery until the hypoglossal nerve is identified. In cases of a low carotid bifurcation, the hypoglossal nerve may cross the internal carotid artery more inferiorly than usual. In high occlusive lesions the hypoglossal nerve may be mobilized gently, displaced anteriorly, and the internal carotid gently mobilized superiorly with gentle downward traction to provide as much exposure as needed.

Difficulty occurs when the bifurcation of the common carotid artery is high and superior exposure of the artery is restricted by

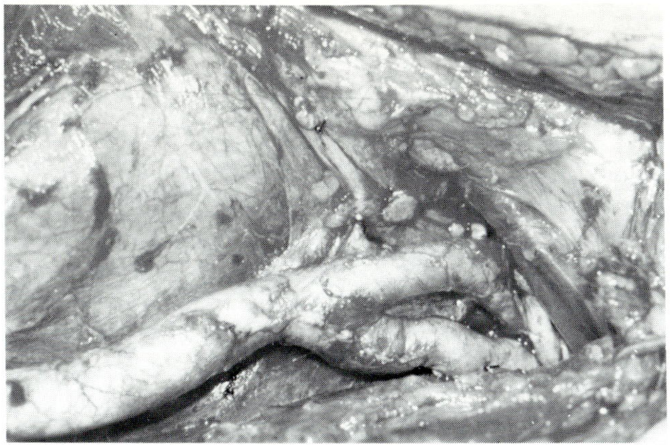

FIGURE 42-1. Exposure of the carotid bifurcation. A small clip has been placed on the superior thyroid artery. The hypoglossal nerve is seen crossing the internal carotid artery.

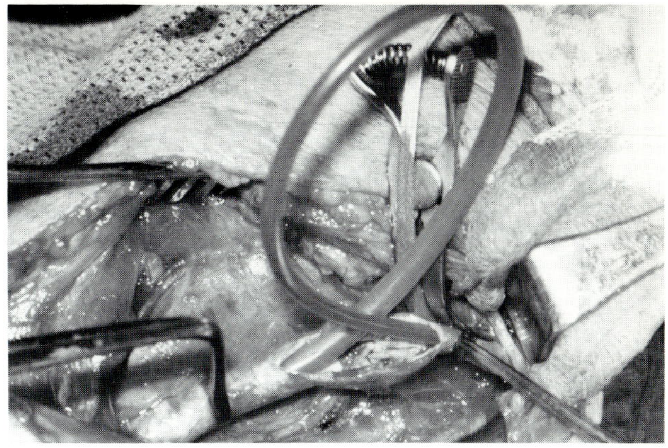

FIGURE 42-3. A Javid shunt has been placed prior to endarterectomy.

the overlying ramus of the mandible; however, careful dissection and mobilization of the twelfth nerve together with gentle downward traction on the internal carotid, usually facilitates exposure. Some have advocated anterior dislocation of the mandible in the rare patient with an exceedingly difficult exposure.

Extension of the atherosclerotic process beyond the usual 2 to 3 cm of the proximal internal carotid renders distal completion of the endarterectomy difficult. In such cases, infrequently the surgeon may trim the tongue of atherosclerotic plaque and secure it to the carotid wall with fine tacking sutures. Laser welding of the distal endarterectomy flap works well in the laboratory, but its clinical usefulness remains to be tested.

After systemic heparinization with 100 units per kilogram, vascular clamps are applied to the distal internal carotid artery, the common carotid artery, and the external carotid artery. The superior thyroid artery is temporarily controlled by the application of a small clip. The arteriotomy is made first in the common carotid artery and continued for approximately 3 to 4 cm, avoiding the carotid body. The arteriotomy is extended beyond the limit of the plaque in the internal carotid (Figure 42-2).

A Javid shunt is inserted, the distal (smaller) end first, to observe collateral backbleeding and expel air from the tubing. It is secured with either a Javid clamp or a Silastic vessel loop; then the other end is inserted into the common carotid (Figure 42-3). The time for arteriotomy and insertion of the shunt (ischemia time) averages 2.5 minutes.

The endarterectomy is begun in the area of the carotid bulb using a plaque elevator and carried distally into the internal carotid. In most cases the arteriosclerotic plaque feathers free in the distal end of the internal carotid artery so that no sutures are needed to reattach the intima. Proximally the plaque is transected sharply with Potts' scissors in the common carotid artery. It may be extracted from the external carotid artery by dissection and traction after release of the vascular clamp securing this vessel. The plaque may be removed in one piece, or if more convenient, it can be divided so that attention is more easily given to its transection at the common carotid end (Figure 42-4).

The ''intimal''(endarterectomized) surface of the carotid is inspected carefully, irrigated with heparinized saline, and shreds of residual tissue removed by gentle teasing in a transverse direction. Arterial closure is begun with the shunt still in place, using a 6-0 polypropylene suture, and continued until approxi-

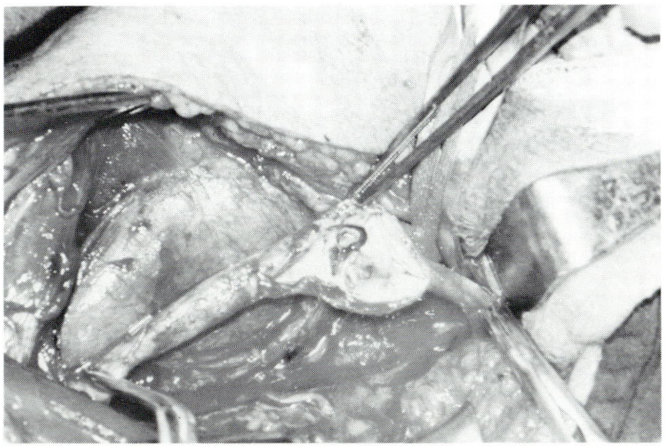

FIGURE 42-2. An arteriotomy has been made exposing the ulcerative plaque.

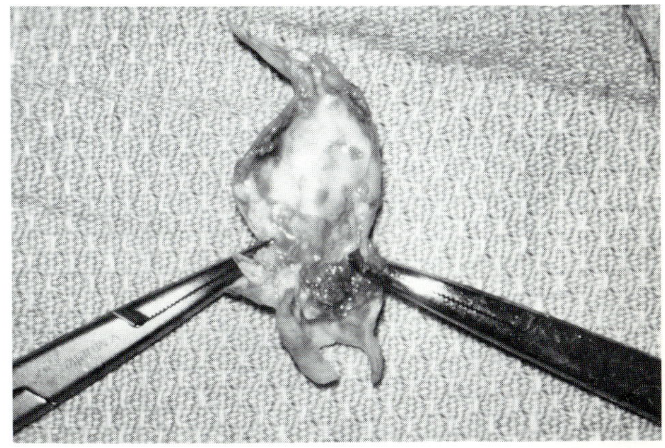

FIGURE 42-4. The operative specimen illustrates the fine tapering of the distal plaque removed from the internal carotid artery.

mately two-thirds of the arteriotomy is closed; the shunt is then removed, the arteries flushed, vascular clamps reapplied, and closure completed within another 2 minutes.

If hemostasis is good, it is unnecessary to reverse the heparin; early adherence of fibrin and platelets to the new endarterectomized surface may be retarded by the heparin's residual effect. A prosthetic patch or vein graft is generally only used for recurrent carotid stenosis. Should there be any doubt about the adequacy of the endarterectomy, an intraoperative arteriogram is obtained. Intraoperative Doppler assessment of the waveform obtained from the internal carotid is a simple method of checking adequacy of flow.

The incision is closed with several interrupted sutures in the subcutaneous tissue and a continuous subcuticular suture for the skin. Drains are not generally employed. On completion of the operation the patient is monitored in the recovery room or intensive care unit for abnormalities in blood pressure or arrhythmias. Hypertension is particularly common.

Most patients are discharged on the third postoperative day. Antiplatelet therapy is often given perioperatively and maintained long-term. Routine use of the shunt provides a margin of safety for some patients during the period of cross-clamping. The advantages and disadvantages of shunting are considered in Chapter 47.

Intraoperative thromboembolic complications can be prevented by gentle dissection of the carotid bifurcation during exposure, careful insertion of the shunt into an area of undiseased artery to prevent dislodgment of a small part of the plaque, and meticulous irrigation and debridement of the endarterectomized surface to prevent residual atheromatous material or thrombus being washed upstream upon resumption of flow.

Thrombosis of the internal carotid artery intraoperatively is unusual, although its true incidence is unknown. This is most likely a consequence of a distal intimal flap and can be detected by the use of Doppler ultrasound probe intraoperatively or by an intraoperative arteriogram. Should an abnormality be discovered with these tests, the artery is reopened and the anatomical abnormality corrected. When a patient awakens in the immediate postoperative period with a neurologic deficit, it is essential to rapidly determine the patency of the operated artery by either noninvasive testing or angiography. One way to accomplish this is to return the patient immediately to the operating room and obtain a direct carotid arteriogram.

COMPLICATIONS

Complications (Table 42-3) can be disastrous, particularly when operations are being performed on patients with TIAs or asymptomatic bruits who have no demonstrable neurologic deficit before operation but suffer a stroke postoperatively which may be permanent or even fatal. A simple method for categorizing the severity of a postoperative stroke is shown in Table 42-4. Cerebral embolization of platelet aggregates or emboli from ulcerated plaques is an important cause of postoperative stroke. Rough or excessive handling of the carotid bifurcation increases the likelihood of such emboli, and the placing of tapes around the arteries is delayed until the final step.

The second cause of operative neurologic deficits is cerebral ischemia. Most patients tolerate temporary carotid clamping without deleterious effects.

TABLE 42-3. Complications of Carotid Endarterectomy

1. Wound
   a. Hematoma
   b. Infection
2. Surgical technique
   a. Carotid artery
      (1) Disruption
      (2) False aneurysm
      (3) Carotid-cavernous arteriovenous fistula
      (4) Graft infection
   b. Cranial nerve injury
   c. Embolism
   d. Cerebral ischemia
3. Postoperative period
   a. Stroke
      (1) Thrombosis of endarterectomized segment
      (2) Hypotension
      (3) Hypertension
   b. Myocardial infarction
   c. Recurrent stenosis

Cerebral ischemia may also result from hypotension during the operative procedure, leading to arterial thrombosis of intracerebral vessels. The most reliable and simplest way to ensure adequate cerebral blood flow during carotid clamping is the use of a temporary bypass shunt. However, it may be used selectively based on neurologic testing with the patient under local anesthesia, when stump pressure is low (less than 50 mmHg), or when EEG changes occur during a period of carotid clamping. Patients with a past history of stroke, multiple large-vessel occlusions, or bilateral carotid disease are shunt candidates. Further, use of a shunt permits unhurried surgery, particularly if the operation is technically difficult, and the shunt prevents narrowing of the arterial lumen when closing the arteriotomy. A detailed review of the efficacy and indications for a temporary shunt are presented in Chapter 47.

TABLE 42-4. Stroke Severity Scale

Severity Grade	Impairment*	Neurologic Symptoms	Neurologic Signs
1	None	Present	Absent
2	None	Absent	Present
3	None	Present	Present
4	Minor, in one or more domains	Present	Present
5	Major, in only one domain		
6	Major, in any two domains		
7	Major, in any three domains		
8	Major, in any four domains		
9	Major, in all five domains		
10	Reduced level of consciousness		
11	Death		

*Impairment in the domains of swallowing, self-care, ambulation, communication, and comprehension. If independence is maintained despite the impairment, it is classified as minor; if independence is lost, it is classified as major (Barnett's method).

Extreme alterations of blood pressure after carotid endarterectomy are a potentially dangerous complication; both transient and permanent neurologic deficits have been ascribed to these. Hypertension was recorded in 19 to 56 percent of patients and hypotension in up to 41 percent of patients after carotid endarterectomy (28). Stimulation of the carotid sinus probably initiates most of these blood pressure changes. Crawford recognized this reflex intraoperative hypotension during carotid endarterectomy and controlled it by injection of local anesthetic around the carotid sinus or phenylephrine (Neo-Synephrine) infusion (29). When a deliberate effort is made to preserve the carotid sinus, postoperative hypotension may be expected and prevented with local instillation of lidocaine (Xylocaine). If surgical destruction of the carotid sinus occurs at the time of endarterectomy, postoperative hypertension may be expected.

Postoperative hypertension has also been found to correlate with preoperative uncontrolled hypertension or a recent antecedent operative procedure. Systolic blood pressure above 200 mmHg should be immediately controlled with intravenous trimethaphan camsylate (Arfonad) or nitroprusside (Nipride) to bring the blood pressure into the range of 140 to 160 mmHg, depending on the patient's baseline value.

Transient postoperative dysfunction of the hypoglossal, recurrent laryngeal, or marginal mandibular branch of the facial nerve has also been reported following carotid endarterectomy. Injury to either the vagus nerve or the recurrent laryngeal nerve produces paralysis of the ipsilateral vocal cord, hoarseness, and loss of an effective cough mechanism. Bilateral recurrent laryngeal nerve injuries may be life-threatening because of airway obstruction. The marginal mandibular nerve lies between the platysma and deep cervical fascia and may be drawn into the operative field when the head is rotated to the opposite side during the operation. Injury is usually due to pressure from a retractor, but a poorly placed incision could damage the nerve. Injury causes drooping of the corner of the mouth. Due to its proximity to the carotid bifurcation, the hypoglossal nerve is most likely to be injured. This paralysis of the ipsilateral tongue musculature results in deviation to the operated side on protrusion and, when severe, clumsiness during speech and mastication. Mobilization of the hypoglossal nerve, by transection of the artery and vein to the sternocleidomastoid that tethers the nerve, provides more protection during the operation. Vagus nerve dysfunction may be due to blunt trauma during dissection and retraction of the carotid artery or its entrapment by a wrongly applied common carotid clamp. Transection injuries should be rare, provided the normal and anomalous courses of the cranial nerves are recognized.

OUTCOME

Unlike peripheral bypass operations that cure symptoms and coronary revascularization operations that prolong life, stroke prophylaxis underlies correction of extracranial carotid artery obstruction. The key issue is whether the risk of stroke or death is less after carotid endarterectomy, with its attendant morbidity and mortality, than if the patient's management is restricted to a reduction of risk factors by medical treatment. With increasingly accurate noninvasive imaging of the carotid bifurcation and correlation of a measured degree of stenosis with flow restriction, we are more able to predict dangerous from quiescent carotid lesions. This has been particularly useful in selective management of the different types of ulcerative plaques as discussed in Chapter 46.

TABLE 42-5. Assessing Risks of Carotid Endarterectomy

Risk Category	Total Morbidity and Mortality, %
Group 1. Neurologically stable patients with no major medical and no angiographically defined risks, with unilateral or bilateral ulcerative-stenotic carotid disease.	1
Group 2. Neurologically stable patients with no major medical risks but with significant angiographically defined risks.	2
Group 3. Neurologically stable patients with major medical risks, with or without significant angiographically defined risks.	7
Group 4. Neurologically unstable patients, with or without associated major medical or angiographically defined risks.	10

SOURCE: From Sundt, Ref. 30.

Consideration of the natural history of carotid bifurcation disease aids correct case selection and ensures surgical treatment. Sundt has developed a risk categorization based on neurologic status, concomitant medical illness and angiographically defined risk factors, which correlates well with operative mortality and postoperative stroke (30) (Table 42-5). The present mortality and complication rate of carotid endarterectomy in the United States is reflected by the statistics of the Cleveland Vascular Registry (31). The operative mortality rate for the 6517 carotid endarterectomies analyzed was 1.5 percent, and the perioperative stroke rate was 1.8 percent. Myocardial infarction was the primary cause of postoperative mortality (53 per 100 deaths).

Thompson's 24-year experience showed that the operative mortality rate is higher for the neurologically compromised patient, 5.1 percent mortality for patients with frank stroke versus 1.1 percent for TIAs and 0 percent for asymptomatic bruits (32). He also followed two groups of patients, one having prophylactic endarterectomy when first seen ($n = 132$) and the other followed medically ($n = 138$) (33). The data on the patients undergoing surgery revealed no operative deaths; a 16-year follow-up showed that 91 percent of the operated patients remained asymptomatic, contrasting with 56 percent in the nonoperated group. The nonfatal stroke rate was 2.3 percent in the operated group, contrasted with a 15 percent incidence in the control group. This differs greatly from the Joint Study of Extracranial Arterial Occlusion, the only published randomized trial of carotid endarterectomy (17). Between 1962 and 1968, 316 patients who had experienced TIAs were randomly allocated to surgery or no surgery. A mean follow-up of 42 months revealed a 12 percent stroke rate in the surgery group and a 27 percent stroke and/or death rate. Comparable figures for the nonsurgical group were 13 and 26 percent, respectively. The trial showed that the risk of carotid endarterectomy was about the same as the risk of conservative management over the follow-up period of 3 to 4 years. This study was criticized as being too small to have reliably detected a modest but clinically worthwhile surgical advantage. Assuming a 4-year mean follow-up and a stroke and/or death risk of 10 percent per year in the nonsurgical group, it would be necessary to randomize about 1000 patients to have an 80 percent chance of detecting a statistically significant reduction of 25 percent in the risk attributable to surgery. The argument is also made that the follow-up was too short to allow any long-term benefit to emerge. However, a strong case to support operation can be made from the very low morbidity and mortality rates associated with carotid endarterectomy in the 20 years since the study.

It is apparent that the presentation and pattern of disease in the individual patient profoundly affects the results of carotid surgery. Postoperative follow-up, extending to 13 years, of patients with frank strokes, has shown that only 30 percent exhibited a normal neurologic status, while 81 percent of TIA patients were normal, as were 91 percent of patients with asymptomatic bruits (34). The incidence of permanent strokes at 5 years was 10.6 percent in the frank stroke group, 5.4 percent in the TIA group, and 4.6 percent in the asymptomatic bruit patients. The principal cause of later death was not stroke but heart disease, followed by cancer; cardiac causes accounted for 41 percent of deaths in the frank stroke group, 61 percent in the TIA group, and 72 percent in the asymptomatic bruit patients.

Cleveland Clinic long-term survival data on patients with carotid disease who had coronary artery disease and carotid endarterectomy showed a 5-year survival of 63 percent in patients who had no prior coronary artery bypass and 85 percent for those with coronary artery bypass (35). Bernstein's study of 456 consecutive carotid endarterectomies confirms that the coexistence of atherosclerosis in other parts of the body, severe enough to warrant surgery, was not associated with either a higher early or late incidence of complications (36). None of the patients undergoing coronary artery bypass pre- or post-carotid endarterectomy developed a stroke, and only 4 percent of them died from a myocardial infarction. Bernstein concluded that the long-term mortality associated with coronary artery disease in certain carotid patients may be modified by appropriate myocardial revascularization.

Over the years, carotid endarterectomy has proved to be a very durable operation with a low incidence of recurrent stenosis. On the basis of angiograms obtained because of new neurologic symptoms or the reappearance of cervical bruits, carotid restenosis sufficiently severe to warrant reoperation was identified in 1 to 4 percent. With the advent of noninvasive studies, routine follow-up has shown recurrence rates of 8 to 15 percent; however, a majority of these patients are asymptomatic and reoperation was required in only 2 to 3 percent, as were those in investigations restricted to clinic assessment. Data at the Cleveland Clinic showed that the incidence of significant recurrent stenosis does not exceed 5 percent even when monitored by noninvasive methods (37). Myointimal hyperplasia accounts for the majority of recurrent lesions encountered within the first two postoperative years, especially among women, whereas late stenosis is caused by recurrent atherosclerosis.

Special Considerations

CONCURRENT CAROTID AND CORONARY ARTERY OCCLUSIVE DISEASE

Recommendations for patients having combined coronary artery and cerebrovascular occlusive disease are controversial. Staged procedures are generally safer for patients with significantly more disease in one system than the other, the more diseased vessels being corrected first. Although several reports indicate that combined coronary artery bypass and carotid endarterectomy can be performed with the same risks as coronary artery bypass alone, the incidence of myocardial infarction, permanent stroke, and mortality tends to be higher in collected series than when either procedure is performed alone. For example, the mortality rate may be as high as 9.5 percent and the perioperative stroke rate 4.5 percent in combined carotid-coronary revascularization (38). Nevertheless, the coexistence of critical symptomatic carotid stenosis with serious coronary artery disease may demand simultaneous repair.

Recommendations have been for conservatism in the patient with an asymptomatic carotid stenosis and angina; coronary artery bypass should be performed first and the carotid lesion evaluated after recovery.

Ordinarily it is safest for patients with abnormal noninvasive tests indicating carotid stenosis which is not severely flow restricting and who have severe angina to have the coronary artery bypass surgery first. Again, in the patient with a totally occluded carotid artery in whom surgical relief is unlikely, it is appropriate to proceed with therapy for the coronary artery disease. A critical or preocclusive, asymptomatic stenosis identified on duplex scan and arteriogram in a patient for whom coronary artery bypass is essential, due to unstable angina, may be the reason for performing both operations at the same time, but some would still delay the carotid procedure.

The patient with recurrent TIAs and stable coronary artery disease should have carotid endarterectomy 1 to 4 weeks before the coronary artery bypass. In the unusual patient who has both symptomatic carotid and coronary artery lesions, combined carotid endarterectomy and coronary bypass can be carried out at the same operation. When this is done, the carotid procedure can be accomplished while the cardiac surgeons harvest the saphenous vein or perform another component of their procedure. When the carotid endarterectomy is completed, the wound should be packed with a gauze dressing and skin closure done after completion of the coronary bypass, to avoid wound hematoma.

CAROTID SIPHON STENOSIS AND ENDARTERECTOMY

The course of the internal carotid artery in the neck extends from its bifurcation to the base of the skull, where it continues intracranially as the petrous segment through the carotid canal in the petrous bone, and the cavernous segment follows the sphenoid bone to emerge intradurally at the circle of Willis. In the cerebral circulation, the carotid siphon is said to be the second site, after the carotid bulb, most likely to develop atherosclerotic changes.

Operation on patients with tandem extracranial and intracranial lesions may carry an increased risk (39). On the other hand, Roederer concluded that patients operated on with a severe carotid bulb lesion and a siphon stenosis were not at greater risk for recurrent symptoms (40). Nevertheless, it is prudent to be conservative in the appoach to carotid endarterectomy when the degree of siphon stenosis exceeds that of the lower carotid lesion.

EXTERNAL CAROTID ENDARTERECTOMY

Cerebral ischemia in the presence of chronic internal carotid artery occlusive disease may be ameliorated by external carotid endarterectomy since the external carotid artery is then an important source of collateral blood flow to the intracerebral circulation. Machleder and Barker demonstrated improvement in intraoperative cerebral perfusion with shunting from the common carotid via the external carotid artery (41). Direct measurement of the pressure in the carotid stump was increased an average of 21 percent with the external carotid artery open rather than clamped. Schuler concluded that external carotid artery revascularization with its low morbidity and low mortality produced a relief of symptoms in 9 of 13 patients (42). Similarly, Hertzer found external carotid endarterectomy useful in the management of selected patients with internal carotid occlusion who had persistent neurologic symptoms or atheromatous ulceration within the carotid bifurcation. There was a low risk for intraoperative stroke and reasonable symptomatic improvement in the four patients reported (43).

References

1. Lavin JH: *Stroke: From Crisis to Victory*. New York, Franklin Watts, 1985.
2. Kannel W: Framingham Heart Study. National Heart Institute, U.S. Department of Health, Education and Welfare, Epidemiology of Stroke. February 1967.
3. Matsumoto N, Whisnaut JP, Kurland LT, Okazaki H: Natural history of stroke in Rochester, Minnesota, 1955 through 1969: An extension of a previous study, 1945 through 1954. Stroke 1973, 4:20.
4. American Heart Association Teaching Collection 1964.
5. A randomized trial of aspirin and sulfinpyrazone in threatened stroke. The Canadian Cooperative Study. N Engl J Med 1978, 299:53–59.
6. Marshall J: The natural history of transient ischaemic cerebrovascular attacks. Q J Med 1964, 131:309.
7. Gowers WR: On a case of simultaneous embolism of central retinal and middle cerebral arteries. Lancet 1875, 2:794–796.
8. Hunt JR: The role of the carotid arteries in the causation of vascular lesions of the brain. Am J Med Sci 1914, 147:704–713.
9. Moniz E: L'encephalographie arterielle son impoortance dans la localisation des tumeurs cerebrals. Rev Neurol (Paris) 1927, 2:72–90.
10. Moniz E, Lima A, deLacerada R: Hemiplegies par thrombose de la carotid interne. Proc Med 1937, 45:977–980.
11. Fisher M: Occlusion of the carotid arteries. Arch Neurol Psychiatry 1954, 72:187–204.
12. Carrera R, Molins M, Murphy G: Surgical treatment of spontaneous thrombosis of the internal carotid artery of the neck. Acta Neurol Latinoam 1955, 1:71–78.
13. DeBakey ME: Successful carotid endarterectomy for cerebrovascular insufficiency. Nineteen year follow-up. JAMA 1975, 223:1083–1085.
14. Eastcott HHG, Pickering GW, Rob C: Reconstruction of internal carotid artery in patient with intermittent attacks of hemiplegia. Lancet 1954, 2:994–996.
15. Connolly JE: Changing concepts in carotid artery surgery: An address to the Society for Clinical Vascular Surgery June 27, 1977. (unpublished)
16. DeBakey ME, Lawrie GM, Glaeser DH: Patterns of atherosclerosis and their surgical significance. Ann Surg February 1985, 201(2):115–131.
17. Fields WS, Maslenikov V, Meyer JS, Hass WK, Remington RD, MacDonald M: Joint study of extracranial arterial occlusion. Progress report of prognosis following surgery or non-surgical treatment for transient cerebral ischaemic attacks and cervical carotid lesions. J Am Med Assoc 1970, 211:1993–2003.
18. Ross R, Glomset JA: The pathogenesis of atherosclerosis. N Engl J Med 1976, 295:369–377.
19. Fry DL: Certain histological and chemical responses of vascular interface to acutely induced mechanical stress in the aorta of the dog. Circ Res 1969, 24:93–108.
20. Brice JA, Dowsett DJ, Lowe RD: The effect of constriction on carotid blood flow and pressure gradient. Lancet 1964,1:84–85.
21. Lusby RJ, Woodcock JP, Machleder HI, Ferrell LD, Jeans WD, Skidmore R, Sheddon EJ, Baird RN: Transient ischaemic attacks: The static and dynamic morphology of the carotid bifurcation. Br J Surg 1982, 69:941–944.
22. Imparato AM, Riles TS, Gorstein F: The carotid bifurcation plaque: Pathologic findings associated with cerebral ischemia. Stroke 1979, 10:238–245.
23. Imparato AM, Riles TS, Mintzer R, Baumann FG: The importance of hemorrhage in the relationship between gross morphologic characteristics and cerebral symptoms in 376 carotid artery plaques. Ann Surg 1983, 197:195–203.
24. Glover JL, Bendick PJ, Jackson VP, Becker GJ, Dilley RS, Holden RW: Duplex ultrasonography, digital subtraction angiography, and conventional angiography in assessing carotid atherosclerosis. Arch Surg 1984, 119:664–669.
25. Veterans Administration Cooperative Study No. 153.
26. Wilson SE, Bennion RS, Owens ML: Effect of carotid endarterectomy on postoperative psychological test performance in 53 patients. J Cardiovasc Surg 1985, 26(1):21–26.
27. Callow AD: Fast or fancy: A twenty year personal perspective on the detection and management of carotid occlusive disease. J Cardiovasc Surg November–December 1980, 21(6):641–658.
28. Bove EL, Fry WJ, Gross WS, Stanley JC: Hypotension and hypertension as consequences of baroreceptor dysfunction following carotid endarterectomy. Surgery 1971, 85:633–637.
29. Crawford ES, DeBakey ME, Blaisdell FW, Morris GC Jr, Fields WS: Hemodynamic alterations in patients with cerebral insufficiency before and after operation. Surgery 1960, 48:76–94.
30. Sundt TM Jr, Sandok BA, Whisnant JP: Carotid endarterectomy: Complications and preoperative assessment of risk. Mayo Clin Proc June 1975, 50:302–306.
31. Plecha FR: Computers for documenting and analyzing results of carotid operations. American College of Surgeons Manual for course on Peripheral Vascular Surgery, page 17, October 1985.
32. Thompson JE: Carotid endarterectomy, 1982—the state of the art. Br J Surg 1983, 70:371–376.
33. Thompson JE, Patman RD, Talkington CM: Asymptomatic carotid

bruit: Long term outcome of patients having endarterectomy compared with unoperated controls. Ann Surg 1978, 188:306–316.
34. Thompson JE, Austin DJ, Patman RD: Carotid endarterectomy for cerebrovascular insufficiency: Long term results in 592 patients followed up to thirteen years. Ann Surg 1970, 172:663–679.
35. Hertzer NR, Loop FD, Taylor PC, Beven EG: Combined myocardial revascularization and carotid endarterectomy: Operative and late results in 331 patients. J Thorac Cardiovasc Surg 1983, 85:577–589.
36. Bernstein EF, Humber PB, Collins GM, Dilley RB, Joseph BD, Stuart SH: Life expectancy and late stroke following carotid endarterectomy. Ann Surg 1983, 198:80–86.
37. Das MB, Hertzer NR, Ratliff NB, O'Hara PJ, Beven EG: Recurrent carotid stenosis: A five year series of 65 operations. Ann Surg 1985, 202:28–35.
38. Babu SC, Shah PM, Singh BM, Semel L, Claus RH, Reed GE: Coexisting carotid stenosis in patients undergoing cardiac surgery: Indications and guidelines for simultaneous operations. Am J Surg 1985, 150:207–211.
39. Schuler JJ, Flanigan DP: The effect of carotid siphon stenosis on stroke rate, death, and relief of symptoms following elective carotid endarterectomy. Surgery 1982, 92:1058–1067.
40. Roederer GO, Langlois YE, Chan ARW, Chikos PM, Thiele BL, Strandness DE: Is siphon disease important in predicting outcome of carotid endarterectomy? Arch Surg 1983, 118:1177–1181.
41. Machleder HI, Barker WF: External carotid artery shunting during carotid endarterectomy: Evidence for feasibility. Arch Surg 1974, 108:785–788.
42. Schuler JJ, Flanigan DP, DeBord JR, Ryan JR, Castronucvo JJ, Lem LT: The treatment of cerebral ischemia by external carotid artery revascularization. Arch Surg 1983, 118:567–572.
43. Hertzer NR: External carotid endarterectomy. Surg Gynecol Obstet 1981, 153:186–190.

Chapter 43

VERTEBROBASILAR INSUFFICIENCY: RECONSTRUCTION OF THE PROXIMAL SUBCLAVIAN AND VERTEBRAL ARTERY

WILLIAM H. EDWARDS AND JOSEPH L. MULHERIN, JR.

Major arteriosclerotic lesions at the origin of the brachiocephalic arteries rarely cause irreversible neurologic changes, but symptoms and disability do occur. Stenotic lesions cause hypoperfusion, while microemboli may arise from ulcerative plaques.

Cerebellar transient ischemic attacks (CTIAs) or basilar artery hypoperfusion are the result of diminished vertebral artery flow. Symptoms include vertigo, ataxia, dizziness, syncope, bilateral paresthesias, visual hallucinations, and "drop attacks." The lesions of the innominate or subclavian arteries may, in addition, produce symptoms in the arm or hand. The excellent collateral to the arm, however, usually minimizes these symptoms. Microemboli, on occasion, do produce ischemic changes in the fingers. Proximal carotid lesions are infrequently encountered and can produce hemispheric TIAs.

Surgical correction of stenotic or ulcerated lesions may relieve symptoms, but the best operative approach will vary depending on the site of the obstruction or the multiplicity of arteries involved. Our plan for the surgical management of these arterial lesions is detailed in this chapter.

Patient Selection

Successful carotid reconstructive surgery was achieved by Eastcott, Pickering, and Rob (9) in England and DeBakey (7) in this country in 1953. Thromboendarterectomy continues to be the best operation to relieve symptoms created by disease at the origin of the internal carotid artery.

Two decades ago, Hutchinson and Yates (12) recognized the role that the extracranial vertebral arteries played in the production of cerebellar and brainstem ischemia. The first successful surgical correction for proximal brachiocephalic occlusive disease was performed by Cate and Scott (3) in 1957.

Several techniques are available for the correction of lesions of the proximal subclavian and vertebral arteries (2,4,16,17). The site and degree of involvement of the extracranial arteries will determine the best surgical procedure and timing of operation. An extrathoracic approach can be used most of the time and offers excellent results with low morbidity and mortality rates.

DIAGNOSTIC STUDIES

In evaluating some 3000 patients with cerebral symptoms, an operation was performed in 498 (16.6 percent) for significant stenosis of the proximal vertebral, subclavian, or innominate arteries, or a combination of these arteries (Figure 43-1). Clinical manifestations ranged from dizziness and ataxia to paresthesias and visual disturbances (Figure 43-2). For the past decade, our operative procedure has been to perform an anastomosis between the end of the subclavian or vertebral artery, distal to the occlusive disease, and the adjacent carotid artery.

Arch aortography is the diagnostic roentgenographic technique used most frequently to visualize subclavian and vertebral lesions. Although we use this method on occasion, we prefer percutaneous retrograde brachial (15) and carotid angiography for high-quality films with detailed visualization of both extracranial and intracranial arterial distribution.

In the early years of evaluating patients with cerebral disease, the origin of the vertebral and subclavian arteries was not routinely visualized. Surgical intervention was more formidable, and most symptoms were thought to be relieved by corrective carotid surgery, when disease was present. The continued occurrence of nonhemispheric symptoms, coupled with better techniques of diagnosis and improved surgical techniques, prompted the complete evaluation of total cerebral flow in all patients evaluated for cerebral symptoms.

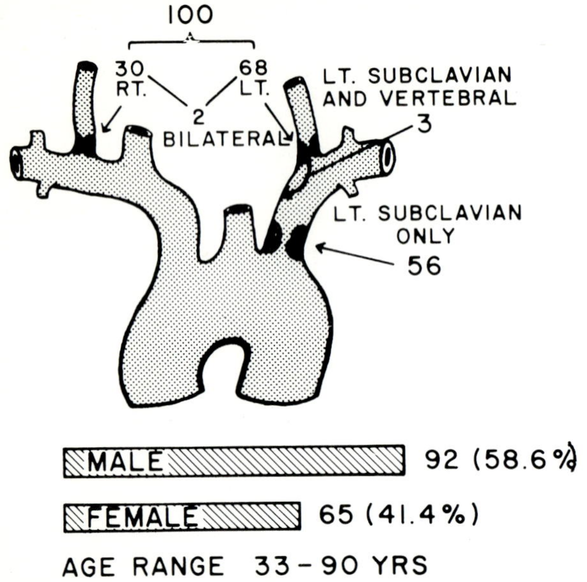

FIGURE 43-1. Sites of involvement in patients who had surgical correction of vertebrobasilar insufficiency.

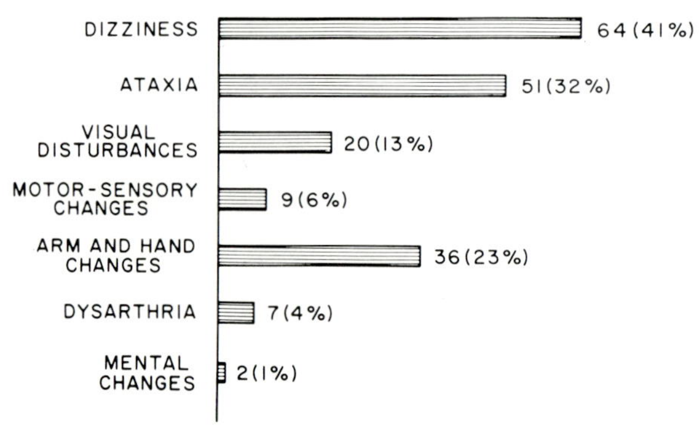

FIGURE 43-2. Clinical manifestations ranged from dizziness and ataxia to paresthesias and visual disturbances.

Operative Approach

The three basic operations of endarterectomy, bypass grafting, or direct arterial anastomosis are all suitable for stenotic lesions of the brachiocephalic or vertebral arteries. The exposure of the origins of the innominate, subclavian, and left carotid are limiting factors in performing an endarterectomy.

An extrathoracic approach is most commonly used in the exposure of the base of the right subclavian and common carotid, but adequate control of the innominate cannot be obtained with this technique. A blind endarterectomy of the proximal innominate is possible, but is fraught with hazards and is not recommended.

A sternal splitting incision gives excellent exposure for the arch of the aorta and the innominate artery. With this approach, the endarterectomy can be performed with partial aortic occlusion. A similar approach and technique can be used for the proximal left carotid artery. The ease and safety of splitting the sternum and the stability achieved on closure makes this an excellent surgical approach.

A somewhat better exposure of the left subclavian is obtained with a left lateral thoracotomy incision. Proximal and distal control of the subclavian can be obtained, but the origin of the vertebral is difficult to deal with in this approach. Also, the depth of the subclavian artery within the thorax makes an endarterectomy a challenging procedure.

Lesions present in the proximal vertebral also may lend themselves to endarterectomy. However, the depth of the vertebral artery in the neck and its right angle origin from the subclavian make an endarterectomy difficult.

OPERATIVE TECHNIQUE FOR ENDARTERECTOMY

Endarterectomy of the vertebral artery requires control of the proximal and distal subclavian artery. Distally, this may require division of the scalenus anticus muscle, as well as the internal mammary artery and thyrocervical trunk. Identification and preservation of the phrenic nerve are necessary. On the left side, any exposure of the vertebral artery needs careful division of the thoracic duct to prevent lymph drainage. Care is taken to avoid injury to the vagus and recurrent laryngeal nerve.

Removal of the diseased intima in the proximal vertebral artery continues to be the operation utilized by many surgeons when operating for vertebral artery stenosis. Either a transsubclavian incision with dissection and extraction of the intima or a combined subclavian and vertebral incision with more direct visualization of the distal intima can be used. Control of the distal intima at the point of termination of the endarterectomy is required. A patch graft is useful in this type of operation to prevent narrowing in what may well be a small vessel. Although possible, shunting is fraught with technical problems and probably is not necessary. Heparinization can be safely achieved with 5000 units intravenously. Reversal at the termination of the endarterectomy is accomplished with 50 mg of protamine sulfate.

With the technical problems involved in an endarterectomy of the vertebral arteries or brachiocephalic vessels, we feel that bypass grafting and direct anastomosis offer safer, better long-term results and can be obtained with an extrathoracic approach.

BYPASS GRAFTING

As advances have been achieved in arterial reconstructive surgery, bypass grafts have, for the most part, supplanted endarterectomy.

The first bypass grafts for proximal innominate and subclavian stenosis were aortic to distal subclavian artery (5). This involved an intrathoracic and extrathoracic incision and the associated difficulties of tunneling a graft through the thoracic outlet. Realization that the distal subclavian and/or the axillary, as well as the ipsilateral carotid, could be used as the donor artery for bypass was a major step in simplification of the treatment of proximal brachiocephalic occlusive disease (1).

For an extrathoracic bypass to be successful, one of the three brachiocephalic arteries should not be involved with significant stenosis. In our experience, this is usually the left carotid followed by the innominate. The proximal subclavian on the left is the most frequently involved (10).

For a left subclavian stenosis, a left carotid to left subclavian bypass will restore flow relieving symptoms. Either synthetic or autogenous tissue may be used, but most surgeons prefer autogenous tissue. Currently, polytetrafluoroethylene (PTFE) is a good second choice. Bypassing in this manner is ineffective if proximal left vertebral stenosis is present along with subclavian disease. For isolated lesions of the vertebral artery, a bypass also may be used. Autogenous saphenous vein functions well.

Similarly for lesions of the right subclavian, the right common carotid can be utilized for bypass.

A patent subclavian artery may be used to originate a bypass graft in the area of the scalenus anticus or, more distally, its axillary segment. There are proponents (11,13) of both subclavian-subclavian or axilloaxillary bypasses. The axilloaxillary is probably the easier and safer to perform and, when completed, leaves a graft with little angulation.

DIRECT ANASTOMOSIS

Some years ago, we discontinued the use of endarterectomy for lesions of the vertebral or proximal brachiocephalic arteries. Since then we have used direct arterial anastomosis alone or in combination with a bypass graft. Our early experience was a side-to-side subclavian to common carotid anastomosis. We subsequently extended the operation to include side-to-side vertebral to common carotid artery. As our operative experience continued, we found that an end of subclavian or vertebral to carotid artery was a better anastomosis with no tension and was also easier to perform. The direct anastomosis, however, cannot be used with innominate stenosis.

The use of the common carotid artery to restore flow to the subclavian or vertebral artery has been criticized because of the potential for siphoning blood from the distal carotid flow (6,8). Experimental studies, as well as our clinical experience, indicate this concern to be unfounded (14). We are careful, however, that there is no internal carotid artery stenosis, as well as being certain that the inflow from the arch is adequate. In our experience, the proximal left common carotid is the least frequently involved of all the extracranial cerebral vessels.

The incision is placed just above the clavicle, extending from the suprasternal notch laterally for 7 to 8 cm (Figure 43-3). The platysma and sternocleidomastoid muscles are divided. This exposes the common carotid artery and the internal jugular vein with the vagus nerve between and deep to the jugular vein. At this point, cephalad and caudad dissection along the course of the jugular vein and carotid artery facilitates the deeper dissection which will follow, as well as preparing a portion of the carotid artery for anastomosis. We generally loop the vagus nerve with a Vesseloop to remind us of its location. Care is taken not to stretch the nerve. The jugular vein and vagus nerve are retracted laterally and the common carotid medially. The exposure from this point on is beneath the deep cervical fascia and does not require exposure of the scalenus anticus muscle or phrenic nerve (Figure 43-4). Visualization of these structures alerts the surgeon that the dissection is too far lateral. On the right side, the recurrent laryngeal nerve looping over the subclavian may at times need identification. The ansa subclavia is usually visualized. On the left side, the thoracic duct is identified, ligated, and divided. If the subclavian is the involved vessel, then a portion of the subclavian proximal to the vertebral must be freed up for the anastomosis. Care is taken not to injure the recurrent laryngeal nerve. It is generally not necessary to disturb the internal mammary or thyrocervical trunk. Preservation of the internal mammary may be important in patients with the potential for coronary artery disease. If the vertebral is the involved vessel, it is unnecessary to expose the subclavian artery. The vertebral artery is the first branch of the subclavian artery, arises from its posterior-superior aspect, and has no branches at this level. This is important in identification. The thyrocervical trunk arises from the anterior aspect of the subclavian, branches almost immediately, and can be mistaken for the vertebral. In an occasional patient, the vertebral may arise from the aortic arch but will follow the same course in the neck to enter the bony canal.

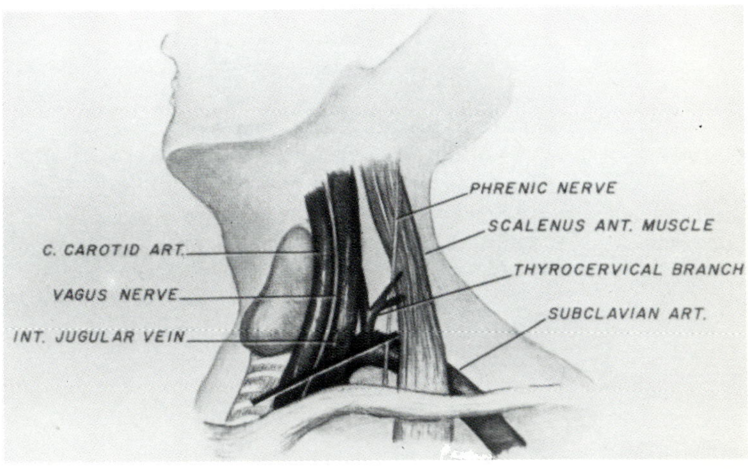

FIGURE 43-3. The incision is placed just above the clavicle to expose the common carotid artery and internal jugular vein. (From Edwards WH, Mulherin JL. Surgery 1980, 87:23. Used with permission.)

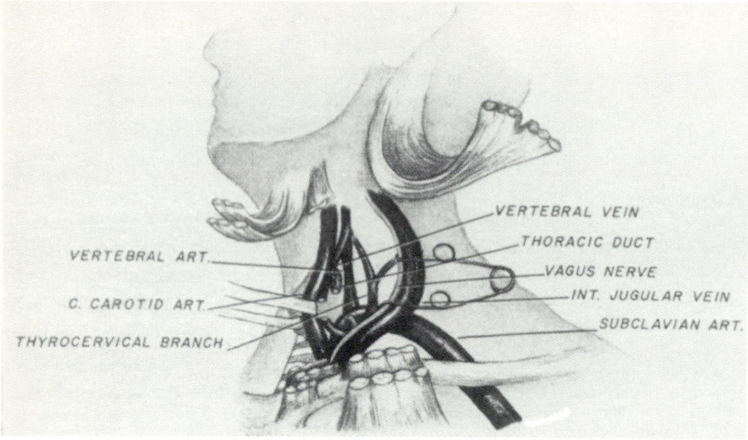

FIGURE 43-4. An incision of the deep cervical fascia exposes the thoracic duct and vertebral vein, both of which are ligated. (From Edwards WH, Mulherin JL. Surgery 1980, 87:23. Used with permission.)

The vertebral is cleared of tissue from its origin to its disappearance behind the longus colli muscle. It is sometimes necessary to divide some of the sympathetic fibers, crossing the vertebral to obtain a sufficient length of the vertebral artery.

The patient is informed of the possibility of a Horner's syndrome occurring. This will depend on the need to divide sympathetic fibers in exposing the vertebral artery. It should not occur in exposure of the subclavian artery. It has not been a long-term problem in any patient.

The common carotid artery, having previously been dissected, is ready for use in the anastomosis. The involved vertebral or subclavian is transected and the stump appropriately occluded. The cut vessel is tailored by incising its medial wall in the case of the vertebral and usually just trimming in the case of the subclavian. The carotid is occluded and opened at the chosen site. We have found that a Goosen punch works well to create an adequate opening in the carotid artery. We use an internal shunt only when a combined internal carotid endarterectomy is performed in conjunction with direct anastomosis. The anastomosis is accomplished with no. 6-0 monofilament nylon on a special small curved needle designed to facilitate the anastomosis in the small vessels. No tension exists on the completed anastomosis (Figure 43-5). Loop magnification is extremely helpful. Following completion of the anastomosis, the wound is closed in layers without drainage.

Total operative time is about 1 hour and 15 minutes, and patients are usually ready to leave the hospital on the third or fourth day after operation.

Both bypass grafting and a direct arterial anastomosis can be employed as long as there is one brachiocephalic artery not involved with stenosis.

SPECIAL SITUATIONS

In patients with multiarterial involvement in the extracranial circulation, innovative combinations of operations may be necessary. This is illustrated by the patient with total occlusion of a carotid artery with stenosis of the contralateral vertebral and internal carotid. In such a situation we feel that combining the direct vertebral to carotid anastomosis with internal carotid endarterectomy is the safest technique to maximize cerebral flow. Use of an internal shunt assures continued flow during occlusion.

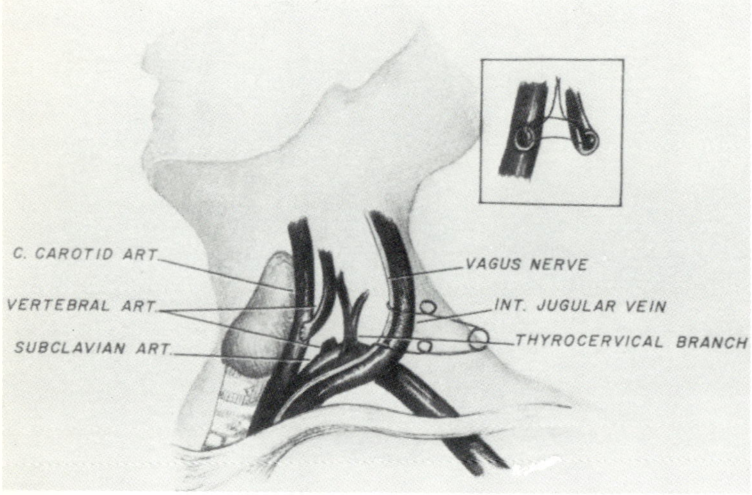

FIGURE 43-5. An adequate length of vertebral (or subclavian) artery must be freed up to prevent tension. (From Edwards WH, Mulherin JL. Surgery 1980, 87:24. Used with permission.)

Comment

We felt there was need for restoration of direct flow into the basilar system, with direct anastomosis of the involved subclavian and/or vertebral artery to its adjacent common carotid artery as described above.

For the past decade, we have performed direct arterial anastomosis when dealing with stenotic lesions of the proximal subclavian or vertebral arteries. The results for both proximal vertebral and subclavian stenotic lesions encourages us to continue to offer this operation to symptomatic patients with significant lesions. There has been no evidence of decreased carotid flow following a subclavian or vertebral anastomosis.

It is our practice to shunt the internal carotid artery when performing an internal carotid artery endarterectomy. We do not, however, shunt in the direct anastomosis and have had no neurologic deficits following operation. We are careful that there is no significant disease in the internal carotid artery prior to cross clamping the common carotid.

The morbidity associated with the operation has been a lymph fistula in one patient and postoperative bleeding in three patients requiring reoperation. One of these was from an improperly secured vertebral stump and the other two were suture line leaks. There has been one cardiac-related death in an elderly woman.

References

1. Barner HB, Rittenhouse EA, Willman VL: Carotid subclavian bypass for "subclavian steal syndrome." J Thorac Cardiovasc Surg 1968, 55:773.
2. Berguer R, Lourdes VA, Bauer RB: Vertebral artery bypass. Arch Surg 1976, 111:976.
3. Cate WR, Scott HW Jr: Cerebral ischemia of central origin: Relief by subclavian-vertebral artery thromboendarterectomy. Surgery 1959, 45:15.
4. Crawford ES, DeBakey ME, Morris GC, Howell JF: Surgical treatment of the occlusion of the innominate, common carotid, and subclavian arteries: A ten year experience. Surgery 1969, 65:17.
5. Crawford ES, DeBakey ME, Morris GC, and Cooley DA: Thrombo-obliterative disease of the greater vessels arising from the aortic arch. J Thorac Cardiovasc Surg 1962, 43:38.
6. Daicoff GR, Lancaster JR, Ranniger K, Moulder PV: Rationale for aorto-subclavian artery bypass. J Thorac Cardiovasc Surg 1965, 49:945.
7. DeBakey ME: Successful carotid endarterectomy for cerebrovascular insufficiency. Nineteen year follow-up. JAMA 1975, 233:1083.
8. Dumanian AV, Frahm CJ, Pascale LR, Teplinsky LL, Santschi DR: The surgical treatment of the subclavian steal syndrome. J Thorac Cardiovasc Surg 1965, 50:22.
9. Eastcott HHG, Pickering GW, Rob C: Reconstruction of internal carotid artery in a patient with intermittent attacks of hemiplegia. Lancet 1954, 2:994.
10. Edwards WH, Mulherin JL Jr: The surgical approach to significant stenosis of vertebral and subclavian arteries. Surgery 1980, 87:20.
11. Forestner JE, Ghosh SK, Bergan JJ, et al: Subclavian-subclavian bypass for correction of the subclavian steal syndrome. Surgery 1972, 71:136.
12. Hutchinson EC, Yates PO: Carotico-vertebral stenosis. Lancet 1957, 1:2.
13. Jacobson JH II, Mozersky DJ, Mitty HA, Brothers MJ: Axillary-axillary bypass for the "subclavian steal" syndrome. Arch Surg 1973, 106:24.
14. Lord RSA, Ehrenfeld WK: Carotid-subclavian bypass: A hemodynamic study. Surgery 1969, 66:521.
15. Marshall TR, Ling JT, Gonzalez R: Additional experiences with direct percutaneous noncatheter brachial angiography-left panarteriography-right cerebral angiography. Radiology 1963, 81:568.
16. Moore WS, Malone JS, Goldstone J: Extrathoracic repair of branch occlusion of the aortic arch. Am J Surg 1976, 132:249.
17. Rob GC: Incipient stroke: Technique of surgical therapy. New York, Grune & Stratton, 1961.

Chapter 44

CEREBRAL REVASCULARIZATION BY EXTRACRANIAL TO INTRACRANIAL ANASTOMOSIS

FERNANDO G. DIAZ and JAMES I. AUSMAN

Although the surgical management of cerebral vascular disease began in the 1950s when carotid endarterectomy was introduced, interest in carotid artery thromboses and cerebral vascular ischemia has existed since the later nineteenth century. In the 1880s, Penzoldt described the pathological changes encountered with thrombosis of the internal carotid artery and W. R. Gowers described the syndrome of carotid artery thrombosis. Then in 1927, Egas Moniz described cerebral angiography, which made it possible to establish the clinical diagnosis of cerebral vascular disease. R. Carrea is credited with performing the first surgical attempt at carotid endarterectomy in 1951. However, the first publicized report of a carotid endarterectomy was by Easton in 1953.

The direct approach to the reconstruction of the intracranial cerebral circulation was initiated by Kredel who described the encephalomyosynangioses, that is, the grafting of muscle directly over the brain surface. The development of microvascular surgery started in 1912 with Carrel, who described the anastomosis of small vessels, without the aid of a microscope. Pioneering work was not implemented in neurosurgery until 1960 when Jacobsen and Suarez introduced microvascular surgery in the management of peripheral blood vessel problems.

In 1951, C. Miller Fisher foresaw the potential for developing an alternative arterial collateral pathway to the brain when he stated

> It is even conceivable that someday vascular surgery will find a way to bypass the occluded portion of the artery during the period of ominous fleeting symptoms. Anastomosis of the external carotid artery or one of its branches, with the internal carotid artery above the area of narrowing should be feasible.

In 1963 Woringer and Kunlin attempted the first extracranial to intracranial bypass with a saphenous vein graft. They anastomosed the vein end to end to the common carotid and then to the internal carotid artery intracranially. Unfortunately, the patient died. Late in 1970, Lougheed finally succeeded with this type of vein graft, and many have reported similar success. Prosthetic grafts have also been tried in the management of intracranial cerebral vascular disease. In 1965, Pool and Potts attempted the use of a prosthetic graft to treat a patient with an aneurysm of the callosomarginal artery. A plastic tube was placed from the superficial temporal artery to the distal portion of the left anterior cerebral artery. Although the graft became occluded as indicated by subsequent angiography, the patient remained asymptomatic.

Finally, in 1967, Donahey and Yasargil were the first to describe the extracranial to intracranial anastomosis as we know it today. Working independently, they performed an anastomosis of the extracranial superficial temporal artery to one of the cortical branches of the middle cerebral artery. Coincidentally, they completed the procedure for a similar problem on the same day, one in Vermont and one in Switzerland.

Clinical Syndromes

Patients with cerebral vascular disease present in different ways, and their symptoms have different causes. The most typical presentation is episodes of transient cerebral ischemia, or transient ischemic attacks (TIA's). These are characterized by repeated episodes of neurological dysfunction which are usually intermittent, completely relieved between events, and repetitive. They are of three predominant types: visual, hemispheric, or brain stem. Episodes of TIA of the eye, called amaurosis fugax, are events of transient visual loss, either complete loss of vision or partial loss. With partial loss, there may be a generalized blurring or dimming of vision, or they may be described as the gradual, progressive descent or ascent of a curtain being drawn over the eye. Sometimes, the loss of vision is permanent. In a few exceptional cases, the visual symptoms are focal quadrantic defects or scotomas. These symptoms usually resolve completely, and the resolution frequently follows a reverse pattern to that of the development.

TIAs in the cerebral hemisphere are characterized by symptoms related to the middle cerebral artery distribution. Patients usually present with contralateral facial palsy and contralateral mono- or hemiparesis. Frequently they have associated contralateral hemihypesthesia which can involve the face, the arm, and the leg. When the ischemic event occurs in the left cerebral hemisphere, there may be associated speech problems, which can be fluent or nonfluent dysphasias. Occasionally, some patients have visual symptoms referable to hypoperfusion of the cerebral visual cortex, characterized by a homonymous or quadrantic visual field defect. In a few cases, the patients present with focal seizures. The identifying characteristic of hemispheric TIAs is that they are always symmetrical, they follow an anatomical distribution, and they are frequently predictable. When amaurosis fugax is associated with episodes of cerebral hemispheric ischemia, the loss of vision is usually on the same side as the cerebral ischemia, and it will therefore be on the side opposite to the hemiparesis.

In brain stem ischemia, the picture is very complicated. These patients usually present with a mixture of symptoms, which can include alternating sensory and motor deficits with ipsilateral facial sensory or motor changes and contralateral body, sensory, or motor changes. These changes are frequently associated with other abnormalities of the cranial nerves, such as diplopia, dysarthria, and dysphagia. Another group of symptoms frequently associated with brain stem ischemia include vertigo, tinnitus, and ataxia. A minimum of two or more of these symptoms occurring in two or more episodes is required for the diagnosis of vertebrobasilar insufficiency.

When ischemic neurological deficits persist for longer than 24 hours, but less than 7 days, they are called reversible ischemic neurological deficits. The symptoms have the same characteristics as those of the TIA, but they last longer. Some authors believe that patients who develop reversible ischemic neurological deficits have small infarcts, but others disagree. No pathological correlation has been made to rule out the possibility of definite, organic neurological destruction.

The clinical presentation of cerebral infarction is of two types. In one type, the patient has a progressive stroke, or stroke in evolution. These patients present with an initial mild deficit, either of the brain stem or a cerebral hemispheric nature. The deficits usually progress gradually but steadily, until the entire ischemic area has become damaged. In some of these patients the neurological deficits are intermittent and recurring; but unlike true TIAs they resolve only partially, and the residual deficit becomes increasingly more severe with each successive event. If untreated, these deficits progress to a permanent, stable neurological deficit once the cerebral ischemia has become established and the area of infarct has developed.

The second type of clinical presentation of cerebral infarction is the completed stroke. This is a sudden, severe neurological dysfunction which occurs abruptly, has severe clinical manifestations, and usually does not show any sign of improvement after it has occurred. These patients experience sudden hemiparesis or hemiplegia or a speech deficit from which they do not recover once the deficit occurs. Any recovery would be very gradual, usually over a matter of weeks or months.

The diagnosis of patients with transient cerebral ischemia must be prompt and aggressive, since once a TIA develops, there is a 35 percent probability that the patient will develop a permanent, stable neurological deficit secondary to cerebral infarction within 4 to 5 years from the onset of symptoms. The diagnosis of patients with TIAs or with a reversible ischemic neurological deficit (RIND) is mostly based on clinical suspicion, since there is usually no residual neurological dysfunction. In patients with progressing stroke, crescendo TIA, or established stroke, the deficit is usually evident to the clinician, and diagnosis can be promptly established. In patients with a crescendo TIA or stroke evolution, the evaluation should be aggressive and very prompt, since a surgically correctable lesion may be encountered, and the progression of the infarct may be arrested or reversed.

Diagnostic Evaluation

Patients suffering from TIAs should have a comprehensive medical and neurological group of tests. Sources other than vascular disease should be excluded as a possible cause of the cerebral vascular ischemic events. These include cardiac and vascular causes, other systemic diseases which may be manifested as transient cerebral ischemia, or other unrelated neurological problems which could mimic transient ischemic events. Diagnostic tools should include a complete electrocardiographic evaluation, including Holter monitoring for 24 to 36 hours, and in some cases echocardiography to rule out embolic sources of cardiac origin. A complete coagulation profile should exclude any hyper- or hypocoagulable states that could lead to a cerebral ischemic event resulting from intravascular sludging or to intracranial bleeding. Other blood tests should determine the serum electrolytes, arterial blood gases, and fasting blood sugar, to exclude the possibility that an intercurrent disease could be manifested as a cerebral vascular ischemic event.

For neurologically related problems, an electroencephalogram will rule out the possibility of a seizure disorder which could mimic transient ischemic events, and a computerized tomographic (CT) scan of the brain will rule out an intracranial, space-occupying lesion that could be responsible for symptoms similar to transient ischemic events. In patients with cerebral infarctions, the CT scan will provide an evaluation of the state of the cerebral parenchyma, although CT scanning is effective only in demonstrating cerebral infarction 2 or 3 days after the event occurred. Isotope brain scanning is also effective in demonstrating the presence of a brain tumor and evaluating a cerebral infarction several days after it has occurred; however, as with CT scanning, isotope brain scanning is not effective in demonstrating cerebral ischemia in the acute stage. Positron emission tomography and nuclear magnetic resonance are two newer diagnostic modalities which could potentially be useful in deciding whether a cerebral infarction has occurred and how extensive it is. However, since these modalities are still not widely available, their application to the everyday management and evaluation of these patients is limited.

If the diagnostic evaluation previously outlined fails to show a source for the episodes of cerebral ischemia, further diagnostic studies including noninvasive and invasive vascular studies are still necessary to establish the diagnosis. Noninvasive tests include auscultation of the neck and supraclavicular areas to rule out the presence of a bruit. Patients with greater than 50 percent but less than 85 percent vessel lumen stenosis will have a local bruit; but if stenosis is greater than 90 percent, the bruit will generally disappear. Bruits in the anterior cervical or supraclavicular area are clues to the possibility of a carotid subclavian or vertebral artery stenosis. A more sophisticated means of evaluating bruits is Doppler sonography, which by ultrasonic techniques can determine the direction of the flow of blood through the vessels. Doppler phonoangiography can provide an image of the carotid artery and can demonstrate abnormalities of carotid vessels with considerable accuracy. These studies are completed by oculoplethysmography, which measures pressures in the central retinal artery and is obtained by the compression of the globe and the detection of the pulse by an electronic inducer applied to the scleral portion of the eye. If greater than a 30 percent difference exists between the two eyes or between the ipsilateral earlobe and the eye, it can be assumed that a hemodynamically significant lesion is present anywhere along the line of flow of the internal carotid artery. Another noninvasive study of the carotid arteries is B-mode or M-mode scanning of the vessels, which demonstrates the diameter of the vessel lumen and the presence of stenotic lesions in the vessel. All of these noninvasive methods have a combined accuracy rate of nearly 90 percent. However, their reported accuracy ranges from as low as 70 percent to as high as 98 percent in different series, and the subjective evaluation of these tests introduces considerable human error.

The definitive diagnostic evaluation of patients with cerebral vascular disease who have had negative medical studies is by means of cerebral angiography. The recent introduction of digital subtraction angiography (DSA) has improved the evaluation of these patients. The procedure is done by intravenous administration of contrast material which uses the computerized summation of images to provide a fairly accurate assessment of the extracranial cerebral circulation. DSA provides a picture similar to that obtained by arch angiography, in which the aortic arch, the greater vessels of the aorta, the carotid arteries, and the carotid bifurcation can be identified and evaluated. However, DSA fails to identify a great number of ulcerative problems, underestimates of the serverity of stenotic lesion, and generally is inadequate to evaluate intracranial vessels.

Precise diagnostic accuracy can be obtained only with selective catheterization of the great vessels as they originate from the arch of the aorta. Selective cerebral angiography with detailed evaluation of the extracranial and intracranial circulation, with the use of different positional radiographs, and with magnification views can provide an accurate, detailed map of the cerebral circulation. Selective cerebral angiography can avoid the possibility of missing an intracranial vascular lesion capable of producing symptoms comparable to those produced by lesions in the extracranial carotid circulation. The risks and potential complications of this procedure are well under 1 percent in competent hands and should not deter the clinician from evaluating these patients completely if other diagnostic tests have failed to demonstrate the source of the problem.

Surgical Indications

At the present time most of the patients who are candidates for extracranial to intracranial (EC-IC) bypass surgery have atherosclerosis involving the carotid, vertebral, or basilar arteries or the major intracranial arteries. The selection criteria for EC-IC bypasses depend on the clinical presentation and angiographic findings. Since no randomized clinical trials have been published to guide patient selection, the criteria have evolved from the experience of many neurosurgeons around the world. In our center a patient presenting with TIAs, prolonged ischemic deficit, or cerebral infarction is thoroughly evaluated. After other nonvascular causes for the symptoms of cerebral ischemia are eliminated, a complete four-vessel angiogram is performed. In patients with hemodynamically significant angiographic lesions, we then obtain a regional cerebral blood flow study to determine the possible effect of the angiographic lesion found.

The angiographic lesions considered suitable for cerebral revascularization include internal carotid artery stenosis in the petrous or cavernous portion of the vessel, internal carotid artery occlusion, middle cerebral artery stenosis or occlusion, bilateral vertebral artery stenosis at the vertebrobasilar junction, bilateral vertebral artery occlusion, basilar artery stenosis or occlusion, and multiple major intracranial vascular occlusions as in Moya Moya disease.

If a stenosis or occlusion in the extracranial or intracranial arteries is found which is consistent with the patient's ischemic events and involves one of the areas described above, the patient is considered a candidate for cerebral revascularization. Patients with bilateral internal carotid artery occlusion generally have a dismal long-term prognosis and are excellent candidates for EC-IC bypass. However, unilateral internal carotid artery occlusion by itself may be compensated by the collateral cerebral circulation and may not be clinically at risk or require a bypass in all cases. The selection of the appropriate patients for cerebral revascularization from this group may be more difficult. In our practice patients with middle cerebral stenosis or occlusion are bypassed regardless of symptoms because we believe that the collateral supply to these areas is usually poor.

Patients with severe neurological deficits are excluded from surgery because they have not been helped by reconstructive vascular surgery in the past.

For posterior circulation ischemia, no treatment is of proven value. Cerebral revascularization of the distal vertebral or basilar circulation has been developed for patients symptomatic for brain stem ischemia.

Cerebral revascularization may be needed in other nonischemic problems, such as in patients with giant intracranial aneurysms with meningiomas of the base of the skull involving the major intracranial arteries or in whom the extracranial internal carotid artery has to be ligated for any major surgical ablative procedure.

Contraindications to the procedure are in general relative; it is discouraged in patients with severe neoplastic disease who have a limited life span. Patients with multiple and advanced medical problems such as severe cardiovascular disease, chronic obstructive pulmonary disease, or severe advanced diabetes mellitus would be generally considered unsuitable candidates for the procedure. The only definite contraindication to cerebral revascularization is the presence of an acute established cerebral infarct because of the potential risk of developing a hemorrhagic infarction.

Surgical Technique

ANTERIOR CIRCULATION REVASCULARIZATION

Different procedures have been designed to revascularize the anterior circulation. The oldest was described by Kredel, who used a portion of the temporalis muscle applied directly on the brain to provide collateral circulation to the ischemic area. The procedure has been used preferentially for patients with Moya Moya disease, especially for young children in Japan. However, this procedure is not widely used.

The most common procedure to revascularize the cerebral circulation is the anastomosis of an extracranial vessel to an intracranial branch of the internal carotid artery, most commonly, the anastomosis of the superficial temporal artery to the middle cerebral artery. The procedure is done in the following manner. After the patient has been anesthetized and placed in a supine position with the ipsilateral shoulder somewhat elevated and the head flat on the table, the superficial temporal artery is traced on the scalp with an ultrasonic Doppler probe (Figure 44-1). The superficial temporal artery has been exposed by different approaches. The earliest was the elevation of a broad scalp flap centered on the superficial temporal artery, extending anterior and posterior to the ear to provide sufficient blood supply through the scalp flap to prevent the development of necrosis (Figure 44-2). Once the flap had been turned down, the superficial temporal artery could be dissected on the undersurface of the flap underneath the galea. This lengthy procedure required rather extensive dissection of scalp and was frequently associated with scalp necrosis, poor healing, and subgaleal hematomas. This approach has, for the most part, been abandoned.

The most common dissection of the superficial temporal artery (STA) is done by an incision made directly over the vessel (Figure 44-3). The STA is exposed immediately below the subcutaneous tissue along its entire length from the most proximal to the most distal area. In general, the posterior or parietal branch of the artery is used, but occasionally when the posterior branch is small or nonexistent, the anterior or frontal branch is used. Once the necessary length has been exposed, an incision is made along the anterior and posterior edges of the vessel to provide a 2- to 3-mm cuff around the STA. All side branches are individually cauterized or ligated with silk sutures and then transected; continuity is thus maintained only at the proximal and distal end of the STA.

The anterior branch of the STA is exposed and dissected with an incision directly over the vessel in a manner similar to that used to expose the posterior branch (Figure 44-4). However, since the anastomosis with the middle cerebral artery is best accomplished with one of the branches emerging in the angular or posterior parietal area, it is necessary to either extend the incision or create a new incision to reach the angular region. A separate incision can be placed directly over the angular region, and the anterior branch of the STA can then be brought to it through a subgaleal tunnel (Figure 44-5). Otherwise, the incision can be extended back diagonally from the preauricular area in

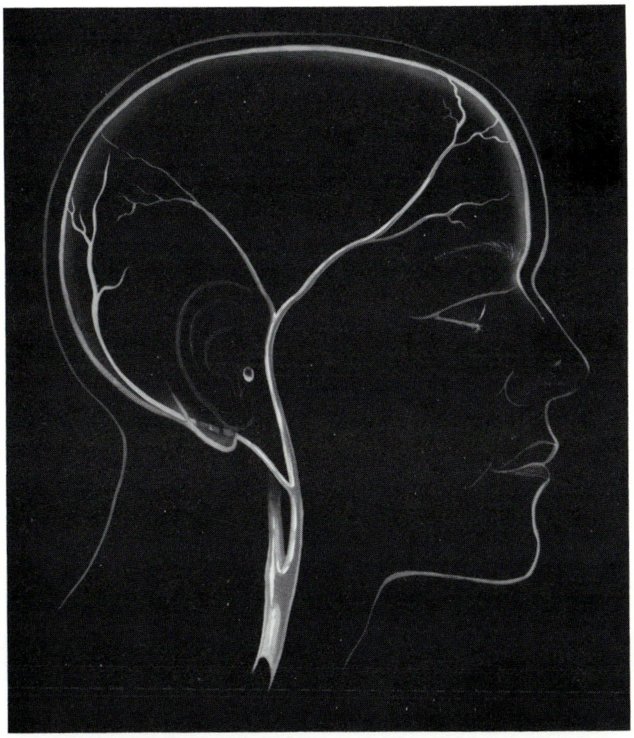

FIGURE 44-1. Superficial temporal and occipital arteries on the scalp.

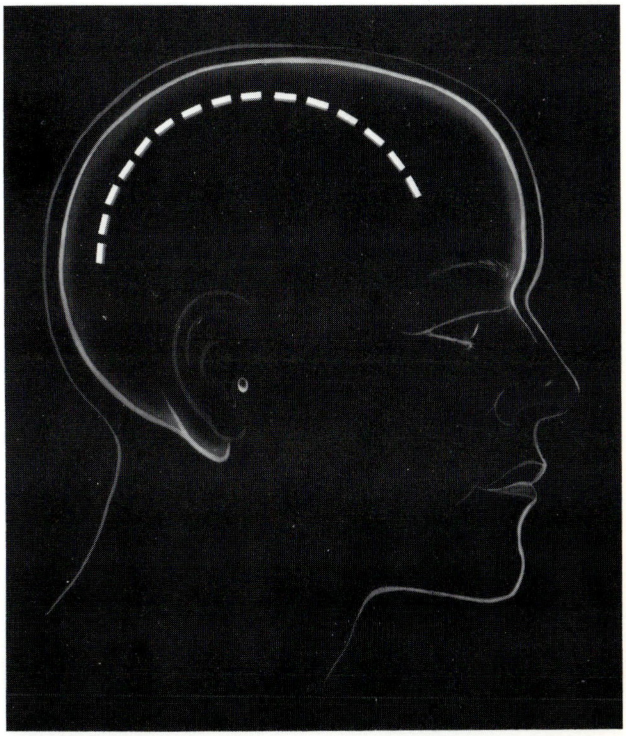

FIGURE 44-2. Scalp flap developed to expose the superficial temporal artery from underneath the galea. The anterior or the posterior branches or both could then be dissected through this approach.

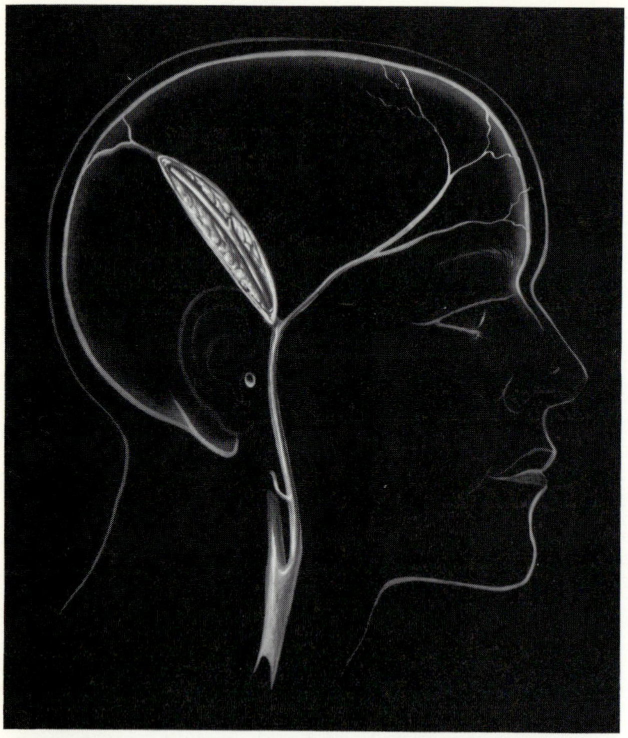

FIGURE 44-3. Incision placed directly over the posterior branch of the STA.

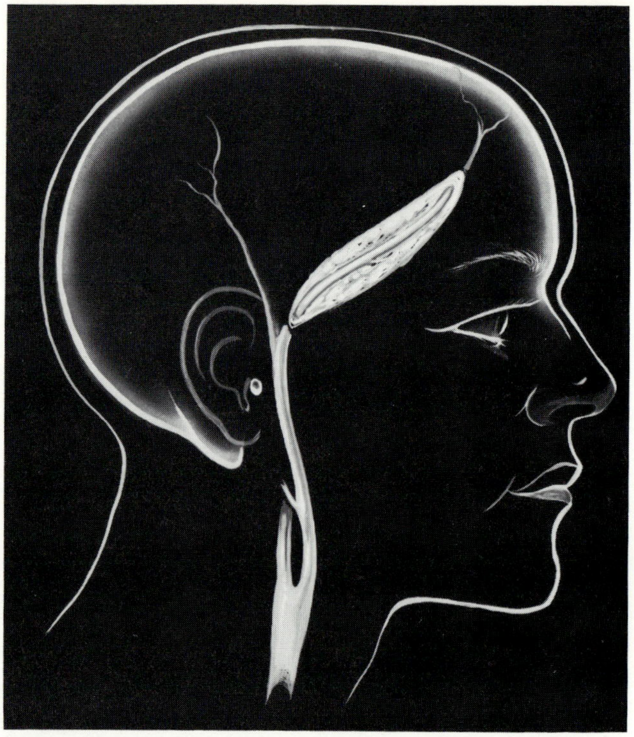

FIGURE 44-4. Incision placed directly over the anterior branch of the STA.

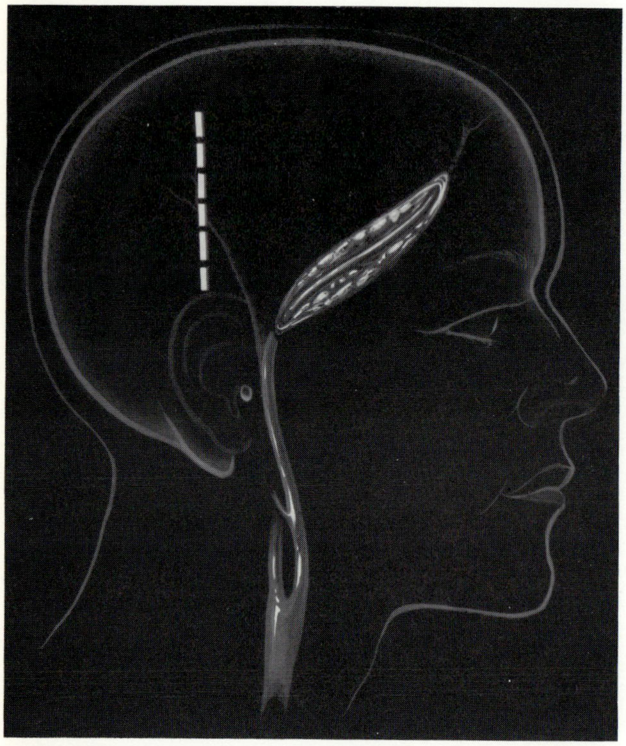

FIGURE 44-5. A separate incision is placed over the area of the angular artery, and the anterior branch of the STA is then tunneled from its original site to the angular area for the anastomosis.

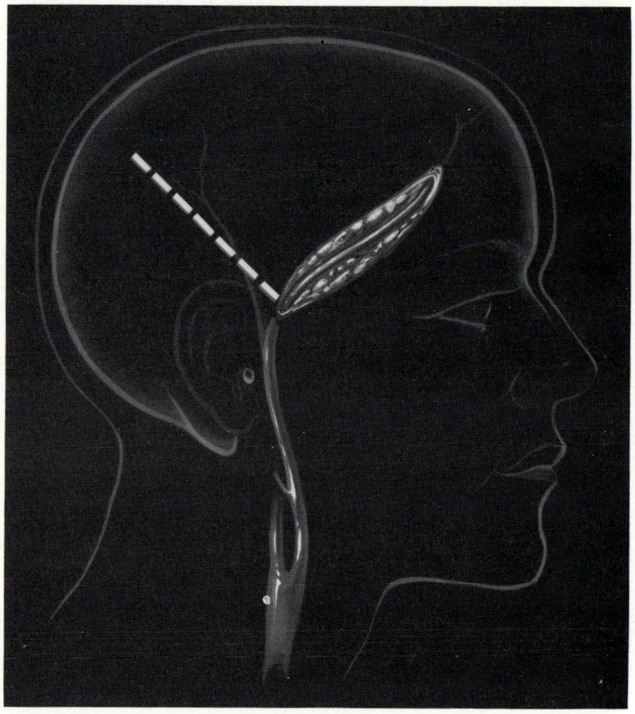

FIGURE 44-6. A connecting incision is placed directly from in front of the tragus to the area of the angular artery developing a V-shaped flap.

front of the tragus to approximately 2 or 3 cm behind the pinna of the ear (Figure 44-6). Either of these two incisions is usually required when the anterior branch of the STA extends very low on the forehead and does not have an ascending branch which curves up into the superior frontal region. In patients in whom the anterior branch has a more superior direction or in whom the main trunk or a large branch of the vessel extends into the superior frontal area, the incision can be extended back in a horseshoe or reverse question mark manner (Figure 44-7). This is preferable to the V-type incision because it provides a broad pedicle for the flap and prevents a sharp corner from developing on the edge at the apex of the V which could potentially become an area of necrosis. The reverse question mark is extended posteriorly approximately 1 or 2 cm behind the posterior margin of the ear.

With any of these incisions, the idea is to expose the posterior and midparietal areas and to center the incision off the temporalis fascia on the line which is directed from the proximal portion of the STA to a point located 6 cm directly above the external auditory meatus. The muscle incision is extended posteriorally in the same direction to the edge of insertion of the temporalis muscle on the superior temporal crest. At this point the muscle is incised along the temporal crest to create two flaps, one anterior and one posterior, which are separated subperiosteally off the bone. When hemostasis is completed and the muscle flaps are retracted, a free bone flap is raised with a craniotome and the dura is tacked to the bone with sutures (Figure 44-8). The dura is opened in a cruciate manner, generally exposing the mid- and posterior portion of the sylvian fissure. When the craniotomy is placed properly, the sylvian fissure bisects the exposed area, the angular branch is located on the central and posterior portion of the flap, and the principal branches of the middle cerebral artery are readily apparent. The largest of the exposed vessels is dissected under the microscope, as few cortical perforators as possible are cauterized and transected to expose an 8-mm segment of dissected vessel, and a small rubber dam is placed under the vessel to facilitate the anastomosis.

At this point, a temporary clip is placed on the proximal section of the STA, and the distal end of the STA is cauterized and transected. A section of approximately $1\frac{1}{2}$ cm is then freed of adventitia, and a fish-mouth stoma is prepared at the required length, allowing for sufficient slack on the vessel, so that both anterior and posterior walls can be anastomosed without tension. A segment of middle cerebral artery (MCA) is then isolated between temporary clips, and longitudinal arteriotomy equal in length to the STA stoma is made on the MCA by removing a small elliptical section of the vessel (Figure 44-9). A small polyethylene stent is placed inside the MCA, and an end-to-side anastomosis is completed between the STA and the MCA, with either interrupted or continuous 10-0 nylon sutures. We have not found any apparent difference between the two techniques (Figure 44-10). When the anastomosis is completed, the temporary clips are removed serially; a small amount of bleeding usually develops after the clips are removed, but it can be controlled by packing gently with cotton. Occasionally, the bleeding will not stop spontaneously, and one or two additional sutures are required to stop it. Whenever possible, we prefer not to add any extra sutures because strictures may develop on the anastomosis.

When the STA is of insufficient caliber or is nonexistent, the

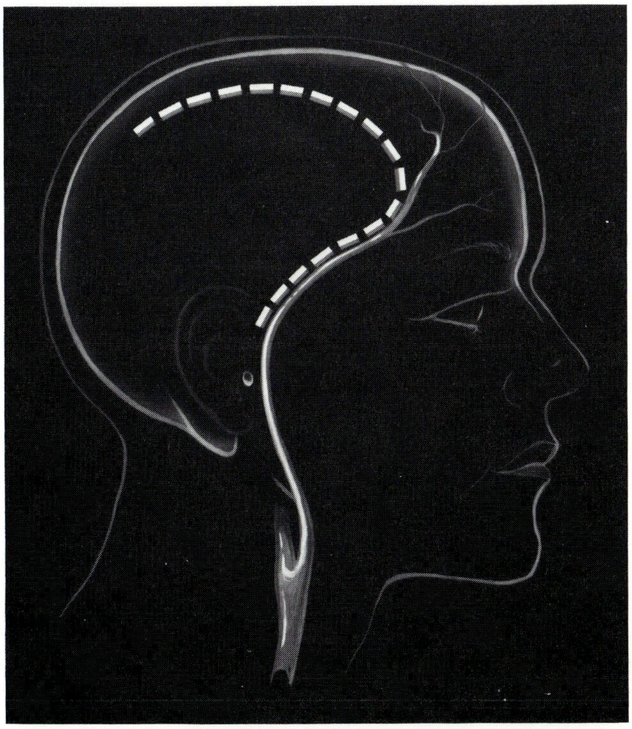

FIGURE 44-7. A question mark incision is developed by extending posteriorly the superior end of the incision which exposed the anterior branch of the STA.

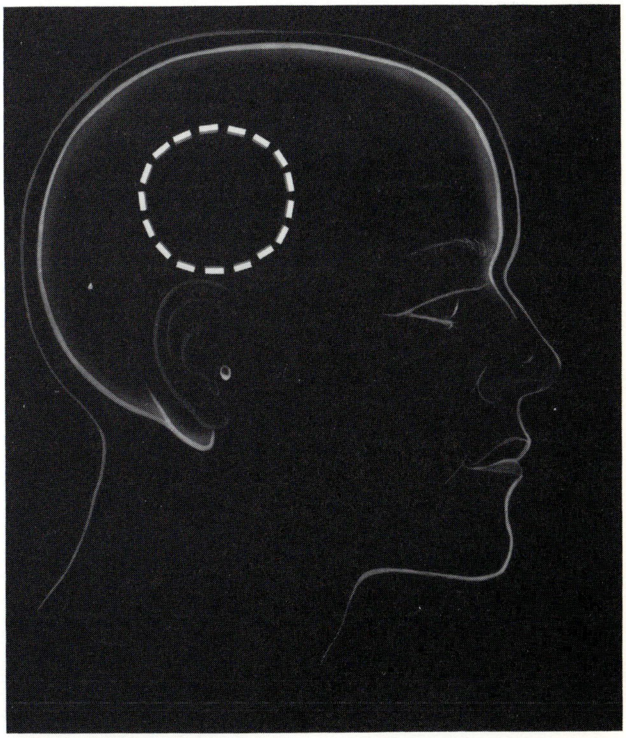

FIGURE 44-8. A circular craniotomy is developed with its center placed 6 cm above the external auditory meatus.

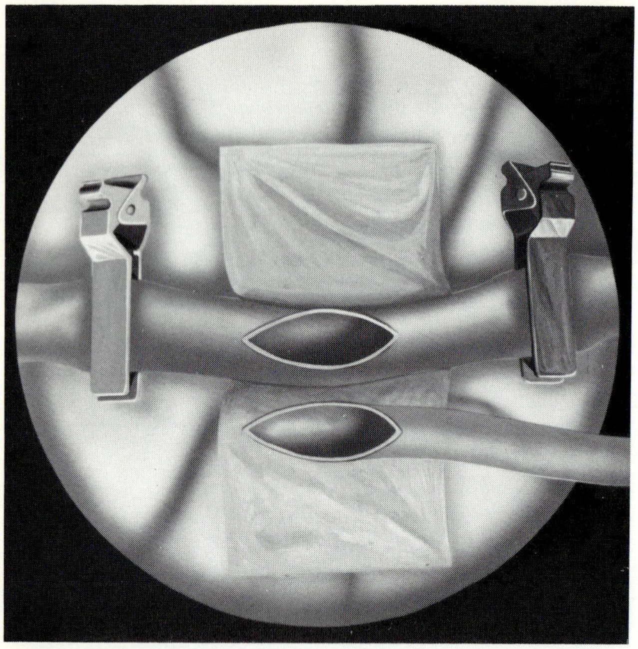

FIGURE 44-9. A section of the largest cortical branch of the MCA has been dissected, a small rubber dam placed under it, and a longitudinal elliptical arteriotomy has been developed. A fish-mouth stoma has been developed on the distal end of the STA to equal in size that of the middle cerebral arteriotomy.

occipital artery must be used to complete the EC-IC anastomosis (see Figure 44-1). The occipital artery orginates from the external carotid artery, underneath the posterior belly of the digastric and under the mastoid process. As it passes the posterior border of the mastoid, it pierces the superficial cervical fascia and becomes associated with the occipital nerve and vein. At this point, it is directed cranially toward the occipital convexity, lying on the galea to its point of termination on the parietal occipital area. The vessel can be dissected from its point of penetration through the occipital muscle to its most distal extent. However, its dissection is generally tedious and difficult because the occipital artery is more tortuous and deeper than the STA. When the dissection is completed, the incision is extended anteriorly to expose the mid- and posterior parietal areas in a manner similar to that used for the STA-MCA anastomosis (Figure 44-11). From this point, the procedure is essentially the same as that used for the STA-MCA anastomosis. It is important to dissect a sufficient length of occipital artery, since the angular artery, which is the most posterior branch of the MCA, is frequently far from the occipital artery.

Another alternative to an extracranial arterial anastomosis is a graft of saphenous vein interposed between an extracranial vessel and the MCA. The graft is obtained from the distal portion of the leg and should be long enough to extend from the subclavian or the common carotid artery to the MCA without tension. The graft is obtained in a conventional manner, and care should be taken to cauterize or ligate side branches without damaging the vein wall. It is also important not to strip the vein clean of all periadventitial tissue, since this could damage the vasa vasorum and result in endothelial necrosis. When dissection is completed, the vein should be gently distended with warm heparinized blood or saline, using a pressure-regulated balloon with no more than 200 to 300 mm of water pressure. The vein is then stored in cold heparinized blood or saline until it is used.

The proximal anastomosis can be completed on the third portion of the subclavian artery, on the common carotid artery, on the external carotid artery, or directly on the most proximal portion of the STA in front of the tragus. An end-to-side anastomosis is generally completed on any of these vessels with 6-0 or 7-0 monofilament nylon. The vein is then tunneled subcutaneously and properly oriented without any kinks. After the MCA has been dissected and temporarily occluded in the manner previously outlined for the STA-MCA anastomosis, the distal anastomosis is completed end to side with continuous or interrupted 10-0 nylon sutures (Figure 44-12). It is extremely important to create a wide stoma on the MCA wall, since the saphenous vein and the MCA differ considerably in size.

On some exceptional occasions, it is necessary to perform an EC-IC anastomosis to a more proximal branch of the MCA. We have found it necessary to anastomose directly to the primary divisions of the MCA in cases where we needed immediate high flow. Direct transpositions of the primary trunks of the MCA have also been completed in cases of giant aneurysms of the MCA trifurcation. These deep anastomoses are more complicated because they require more extensive dissection of the MCA trunks and primary divisions and can be associated with significant cerebral edema because of the direct manipulation of the brain.

POSTERIOR CIRCULATION

Different procedures have been designed to revascularize the vertebral basilar circulation. Vertebral endarterectomies have been performed in patients with highly stenotic areas in the third and

FIGURE 44-10. (*A*) A series of interrupted sutures is placed on the perimeter of the anastomosis and tied down individually. (*B*) A continuous running suture is placed on the perimeter of the anastomosis using two separate sutures for the anterior and for the posterior walls. (*C*) (*left*) Preoperative angiogram shows a right MCA occlusion. (*right*) Postoperative carotid angiogram demonstrating a patent STA-MCA anastomosis completed with interrupted sutures. (*D*) (*left*) Preoperative left carotid angiogram showing a severe MCA stenosis. (*right*) Postoperative carotid angiogram demonstrating a patent STA-MCA anastomosis completed with running sutures.

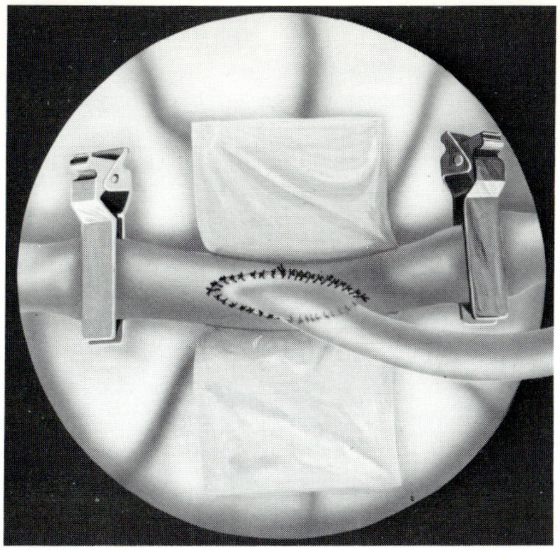

A

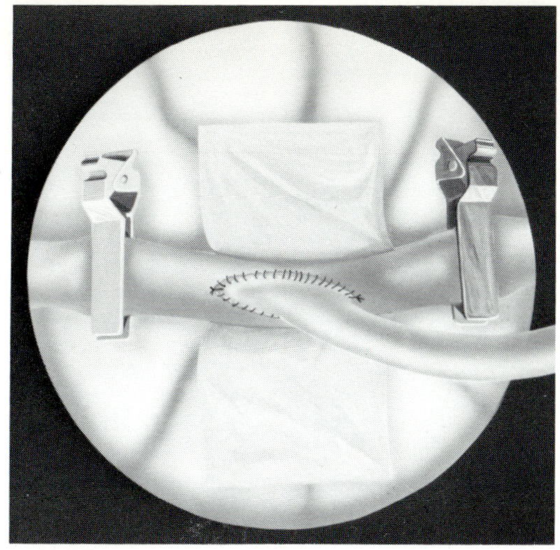

B

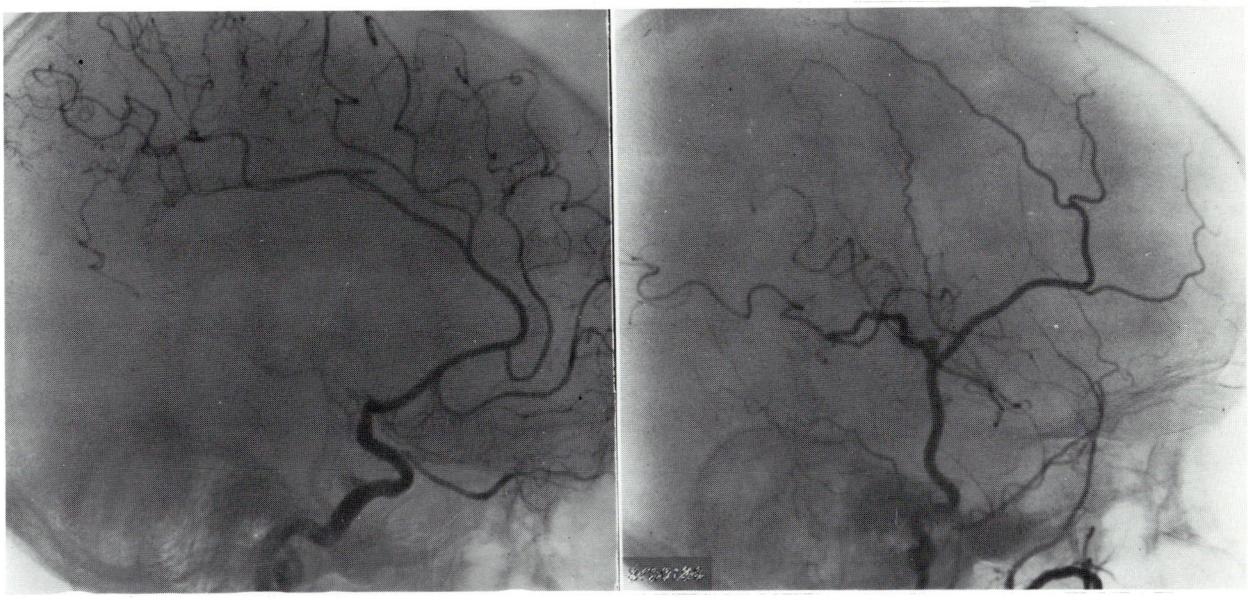

C

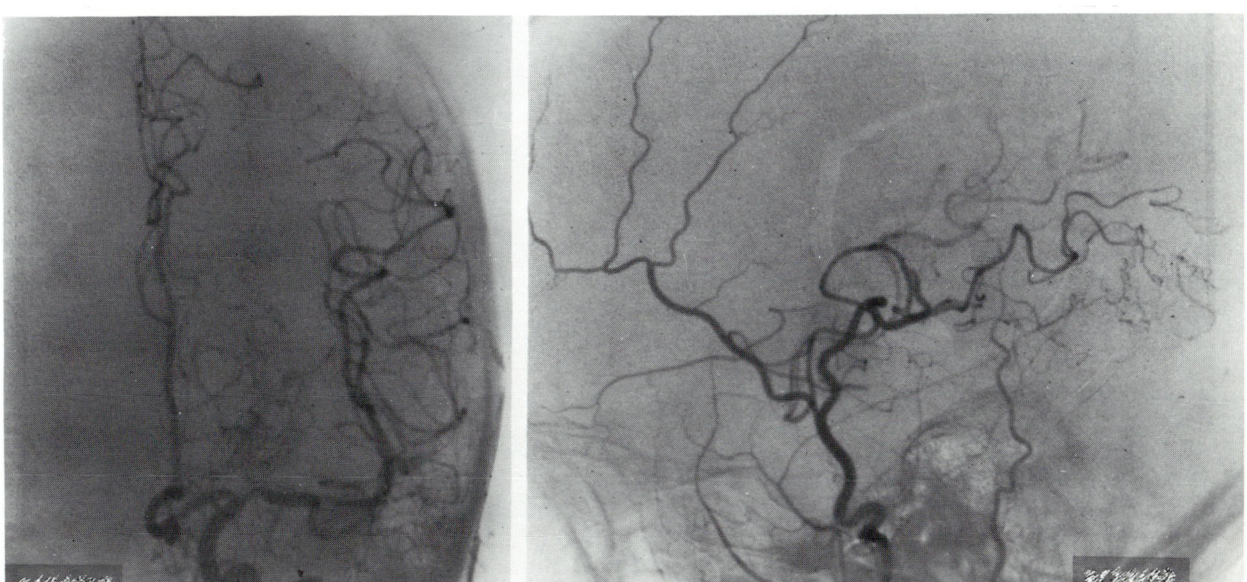

D

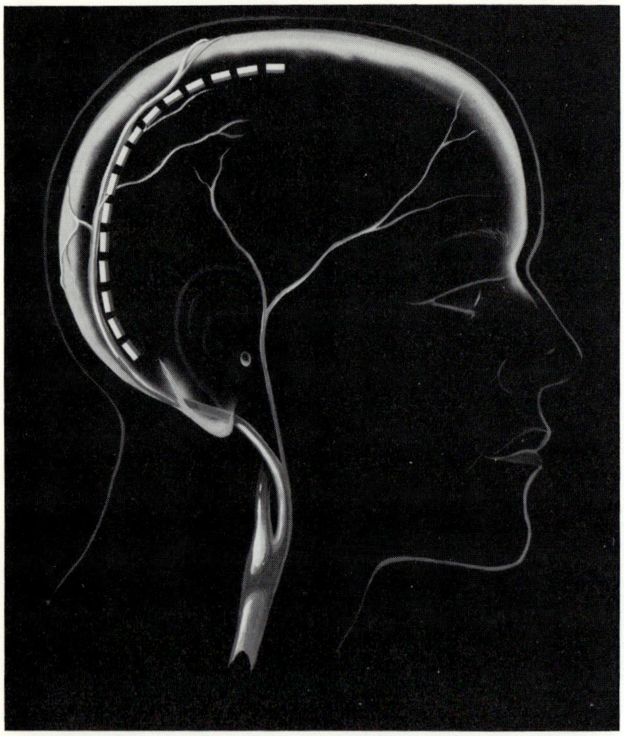

FIGURE 44-11. An incision is placed directly over the occipital artery, extending the superior end toward the area of the angular artery.

fourth portions of the vertebral artery, usually associated with contralateral or high-grade stenosis or vertebral artery occlusion. The vertebral artery is approached through a suboccipital craniotomy performed with the patient lying in a three-quarter prone position. A midline approach is carried down and extended laterally until the vertebral artery is exposed, and the artery is dissected from its exit from the first transverse process to its entry into the dura through the atlantooccipital membrane. The vertebral artery is surrounded by a venous plexus which must be carefully dissected, cauterized, and transected. When dissection is completed, the dura is opened from the midline in the direction of the vertebral artery entry. The perimedullary portion of the vertebral artery is dissected to expose the origin of the posterior inferior cerebellar artery (PICA). If a vertebral endarterectomy is required, the artery can be clipped proximally at C1 and distally prior to the PICA. A longitudinal arteriotomy is made (Figure 44-13), and the plaque is dissected under the microscope. After the plaque is removed, the arteriortomy is closed with running 6-0 or 7-0 polypropylene sutures. During the occlusion period, patients receive an intravenous bolus of 250 mg

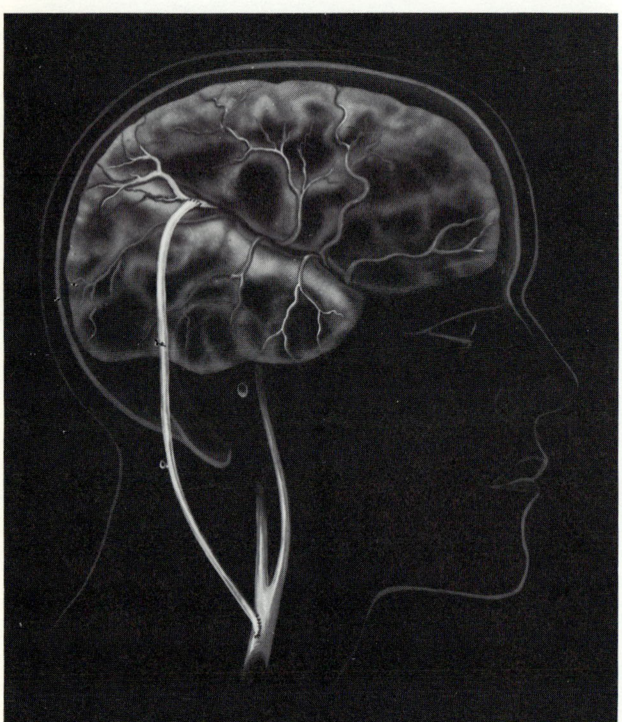

A

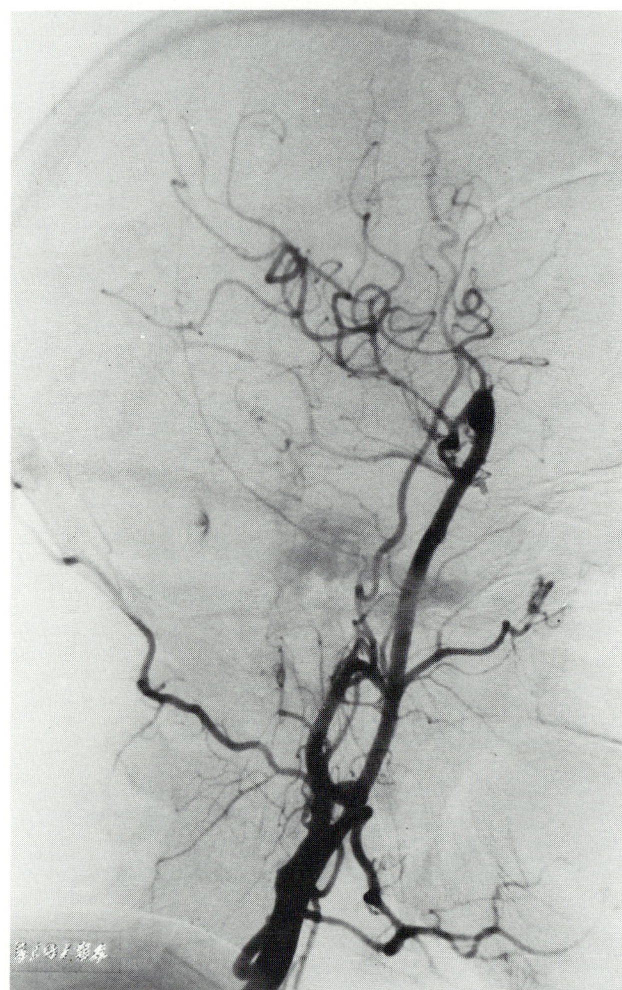

B

FIGURE 44-12. (*A*) A saphenous vein graft is anastomosed proximally to the common carotid artery in the neck and distally to the angular branch of the MCA. (*B*) Postoperative carotid angiogram showing a patent saphenous vein graft filling the MCA.

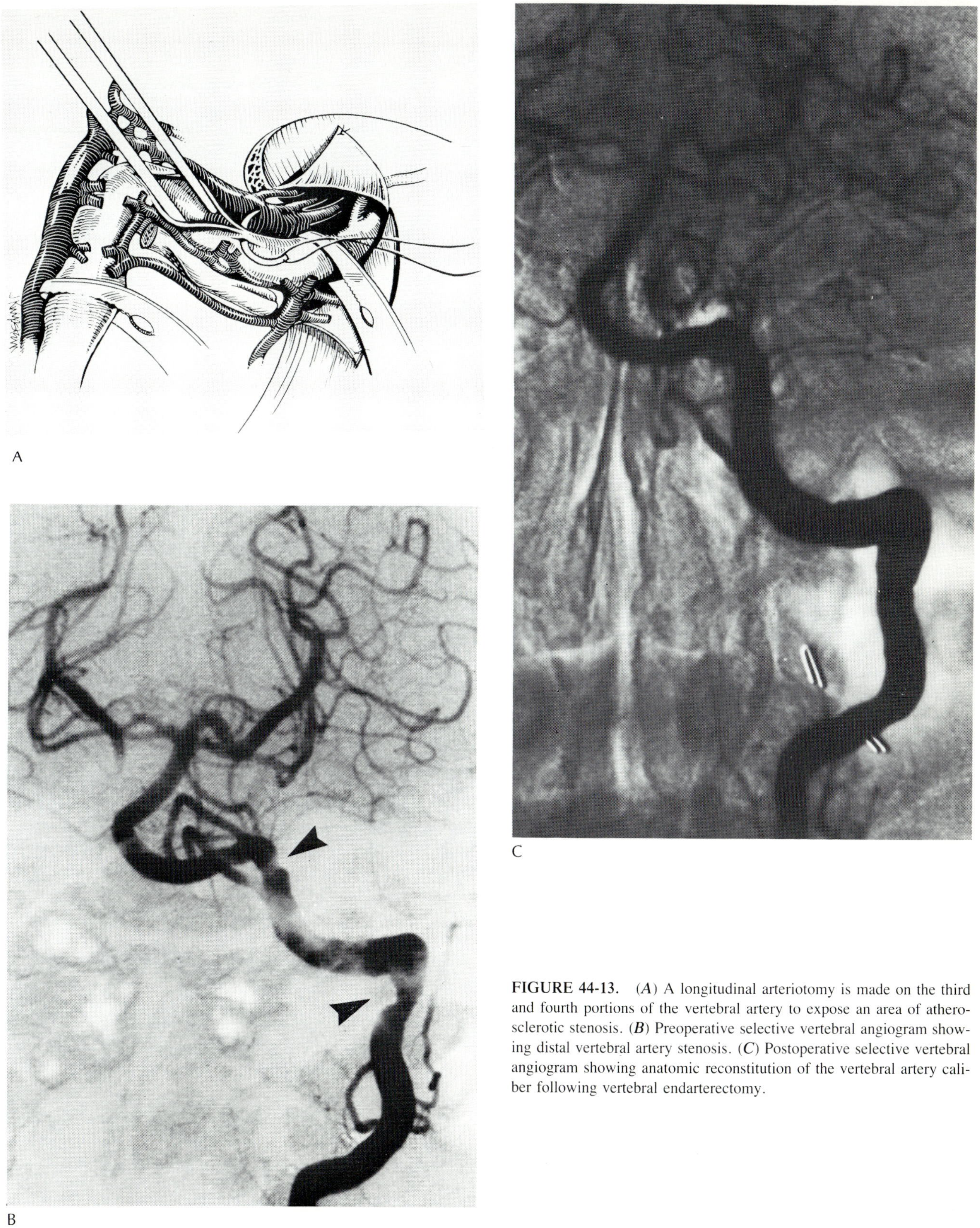

A

B

C

FIGURE 44-13. (*A*) A longitudinal arteriotomy is made on the third and fourth portions of the vertebral artery to expose an area of atherosclerotic stenosis. (*B*) Preoperative selective vertebral angiogram showing distal vertebral artery stenosis. (*C*) Postoperative selective vertebral angiogram showing anatomic reconstitution of the vertebral artery caliber following vertebral endarterectomy.

of thiopental, 100 mg of lidocaine (Xylocaine), and 5000 units of heparin.

For occlusive lesions of the vertebral artery proximal to the PICA, the vertebral basilar circulation can be reconstructed by an anastomosis of the occipital artery to the PICA itself. The patient is placed in a park bench or lateral position, and the occipital artery is dissected in the same way as previously outlined for the anterior circulation. However, the dissection is extended to the level of the mastoid to obtain sufficient vessel length. After the incision has been carried down through the suboccipital musculature, a unilateral suboccipital craniectomy is completed from the foramen magnum to the transverse sinus and from the edge of the mastoid to the midline. Generally it is not necessary to remove the arch of C1. After the dura is opened and tacked to the bone, the cerebellum usually falls away by its own weight after the cisterna magna has been drained of spinal fluid. When the perimedullary portion of the PICA has been identified on the lateral medullary area and either the rostral or the caudal branches of the PICA have been dissected, a section of the vessel devoid of any branches is isolated, and a temporary clipping is done in a similar manner to that described above. An end-to-side anastomosis of the occipital artery to the perimedullary portion of the PICA is then completed (Figure 44-14).

When the vertebral arteries are occluded distal to the PICA or when a high-grade stenosis of the vertebral artery is distal to the level of the PICA, the EC-IC anastomosis must be completed to the anterior inferior cerebellar artery (AICA). The exposure is essentially the same as that for the anastomosis to the PICA, and the dissection of the occipital artery is completed in a similar manner. The cerebellum must be gently retracted laterally to expose the area of the seventh and eight cranial nerves. The prepontine portion of the AICA is identified as it extends from in front of the foramen of Luschka and is directed toward the anterior surface of the cerebellum. At this point the vessel has already divided on its rostral and caudal branches. Choosing the anastomotic site, we prefer to use the branch without collateral branches to the brain stem. After the chosen branch is dissected carefully and isolated, an anastomosis is completed from the occipital to the AICA in a manner similar to that described for other EC-IC microanastomoses (Figure 44-15).

In patients who have a stenosis or an occlusion of the proximal or midportion of the basilar artery without collaterals from the anterior circulation, any of the previously described procedures will not bypass the problem. These patients require an anastomosis to the superior cerebellar artery or to the posterior cerebral artery. In either case, the patient is positioned supine with the ipsilateral shoulder elevated and the head flat on the table. The STA is traced on the scalp with a Doppler. Since a minimum of 15 cm is required to reach the perimesencephalic area from the scalp surface, the largest of the artery's two branches is dissected to gain as much length as possible. Centered on the ear, a subtemporal craniotomy is completed, flush with the middle cranial fossa. It is necessary to extend this craniotomy a minimum of 3 cm in front and 3 cm behind the external auditory meatus to have enough room to manipulate the instruments for the anastomosis (Figure 44-16). After the dura has been opened, the temporal lobe is elevated. Care must be taken to preserve the temporal veins since if the temporal veins are injured, postoperative swelling and cerebral contusions are common. We prefer to preserve these veins at all costs by gently retracting on the brain and applying moistened Gelfoam strips over them. To expose the superior cerebellar artery, we incise the tentorium by exposing first the fourth cranial nerve under the tentorial incisura and extending the incision toward the petrous apex from approximately 2 cm from the insertion of the tent on the posterior clinoid process. The two flaps of the tentorium are then retracted laterally and sutured back to the dura. This permits us to expose the perimesencephalic portion of the superior cerebellar artery, which at this point usually has no branches and divides on its rostral and caudal branches. The most available and largest of the two branches is carefully dissected and isolated. At this point, the distal end of the STA is transected, and a temporary clip is placed at the base. The fish-mouth stoma is prepared in a similar manner to that outlined above to ensure that all of the length available for the STA is used, since otherwise the anastomosis cannot be completed. An end-to-side anastomosis is then completed from the STA to the superior cerebellar artery in a similar manner to that previously described.

In patients in whom the superior cerebellar artery is of insufficient caliber, the posterior cerebral artery is used. We prefer not to use the posterior cerebral artery because its collateral circulation is not as extensive as that of the superior cerebellar artery. Also, the risk of a cortical injury with secondary cortical blindness is greater than that of a cerebral deficit when the superior cerebellar artery is used. The posterior cerebral artery is found in the perimesencephalic area just beneath the edge of the uncus of the hippocampus. The vessel is usually large and easy to isolate, although much more retraction is needed to identify and separate the posterior cerebral artery. The vessel has less mobility than the superior cerebellar artery, and the cortical perforators cannot be cauterized since they are usually large. Once the vessel has been isolated and temporarily clipped, an anastomosis is then completed with the STA or a saphenous vein graft to the posterior cerebral artery in a manner similar to that described previously (Figure 44-17).

Performing any of the anastomotic procedures for the posterior fossa requires complete cerebral relaxation. This is obtained by the placement of a lumbar subarachnoid drain, the intravenous administration of mannitol and furosemide, and the gentle retraction of the brain. The anastomoses are very difficult to perform because of the depth at which they are done. In general, not only do they require the use of very long instruments, but they are also taxing on the surgeon and require considerable skill to complete.

Postoperative Results

Many surgical series have been published since the procedure of EC-IC anastomosis was first introduced. However, with the exception of the EC-IC bypass study group, most surgical series reported to date have not been compared with patients treated medically, and therefore conclusions regarding the therapeutic value of the EC-IC procedure are controversial. Nevertheless, the results available suggest the possible value of the procedure in carefully selected patients.

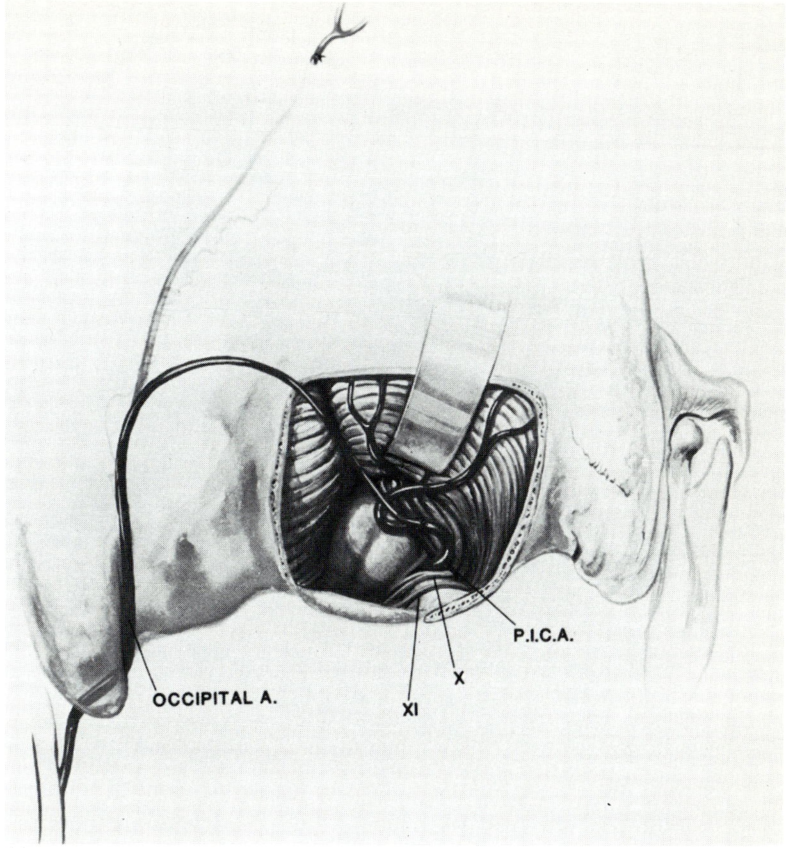

A

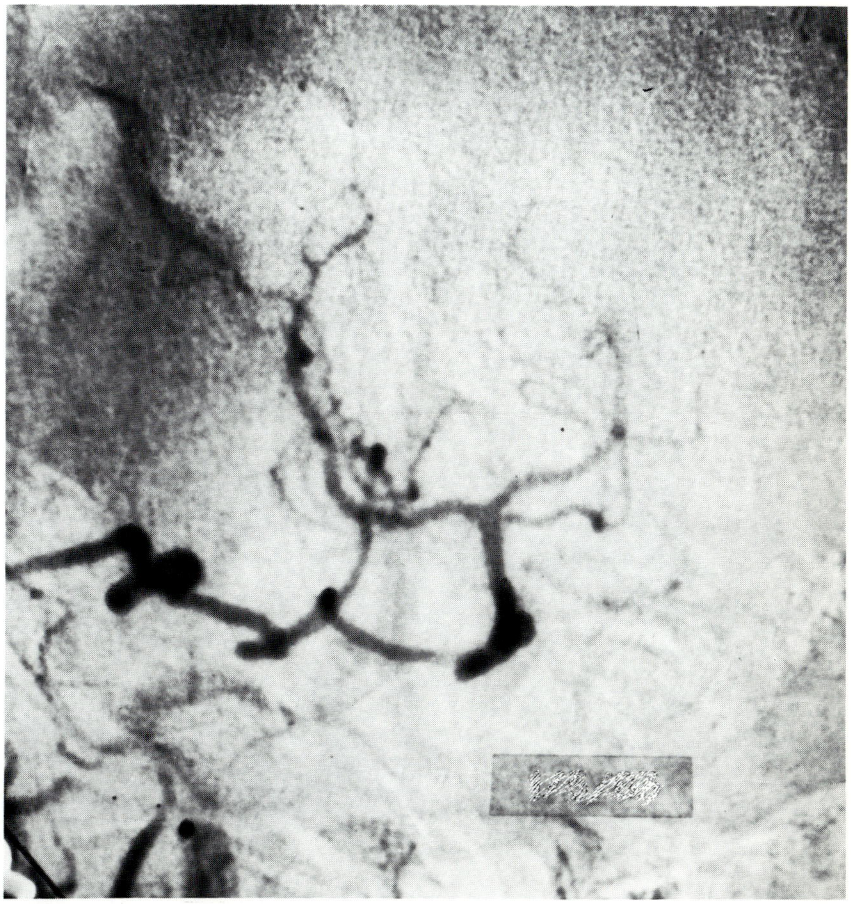

B

FIGURE 44-14. (*A*) The occipital artery is dissected and anastomosed to the posterior inferior cerebellar artery through a suboccipital craniectomy. (*B*) Postoperative angiogram showing filling of the vertebrobasilar tree through a patent OA-PICA anastomosis.

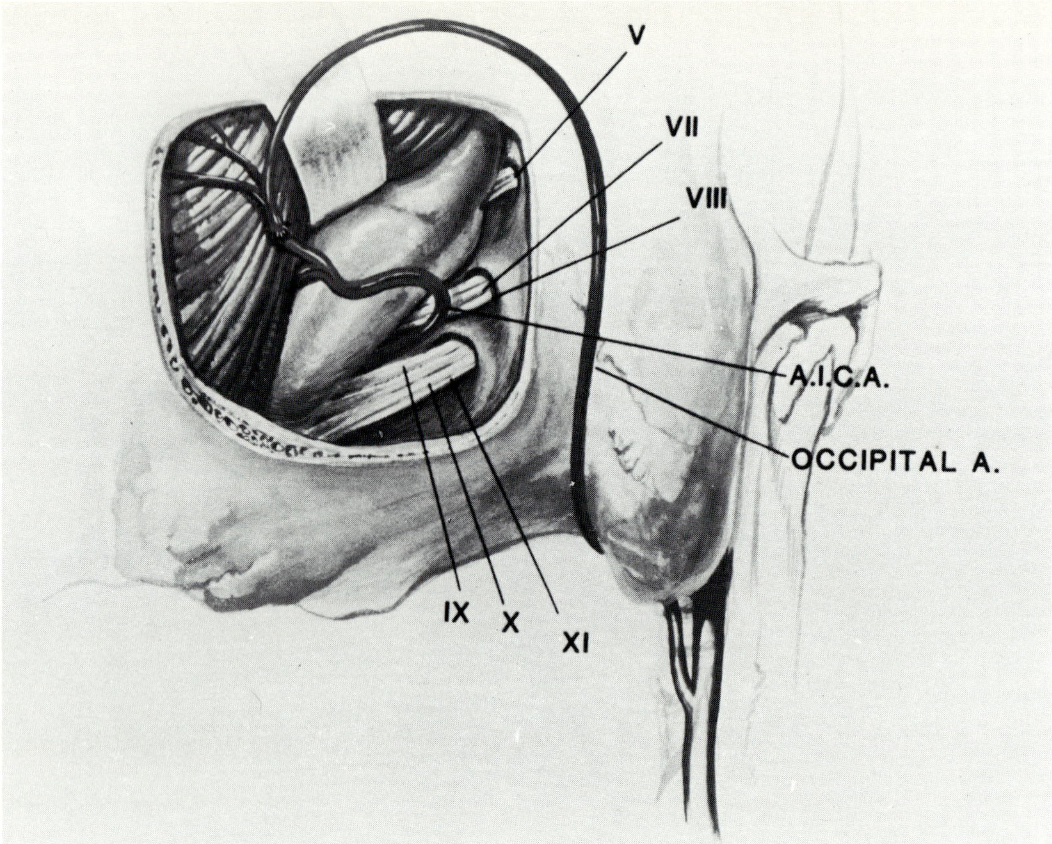

A

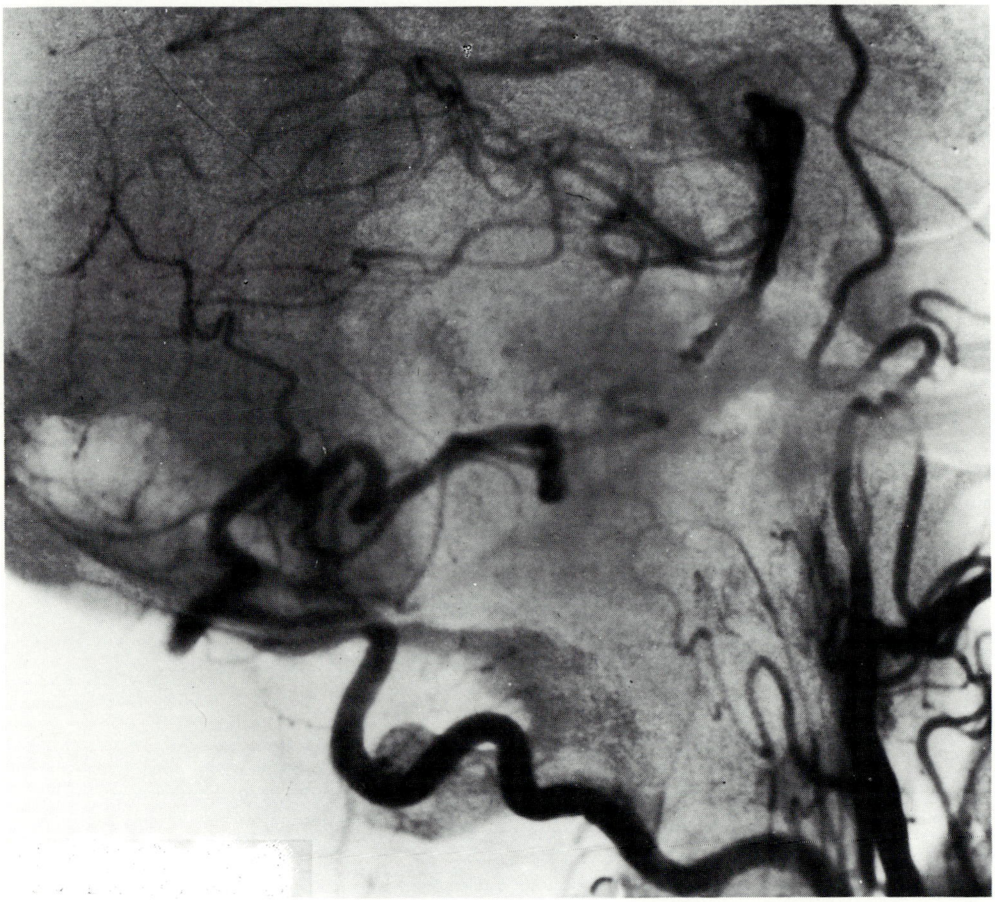

B

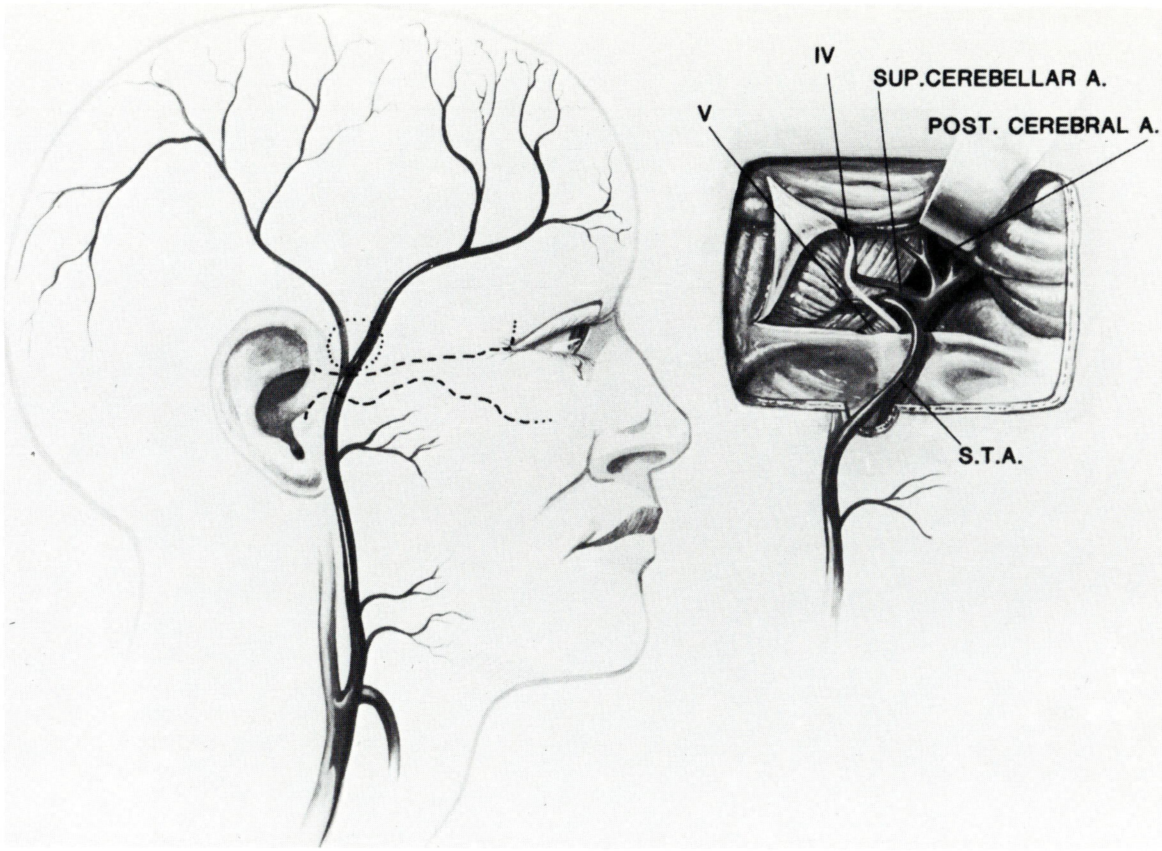

A

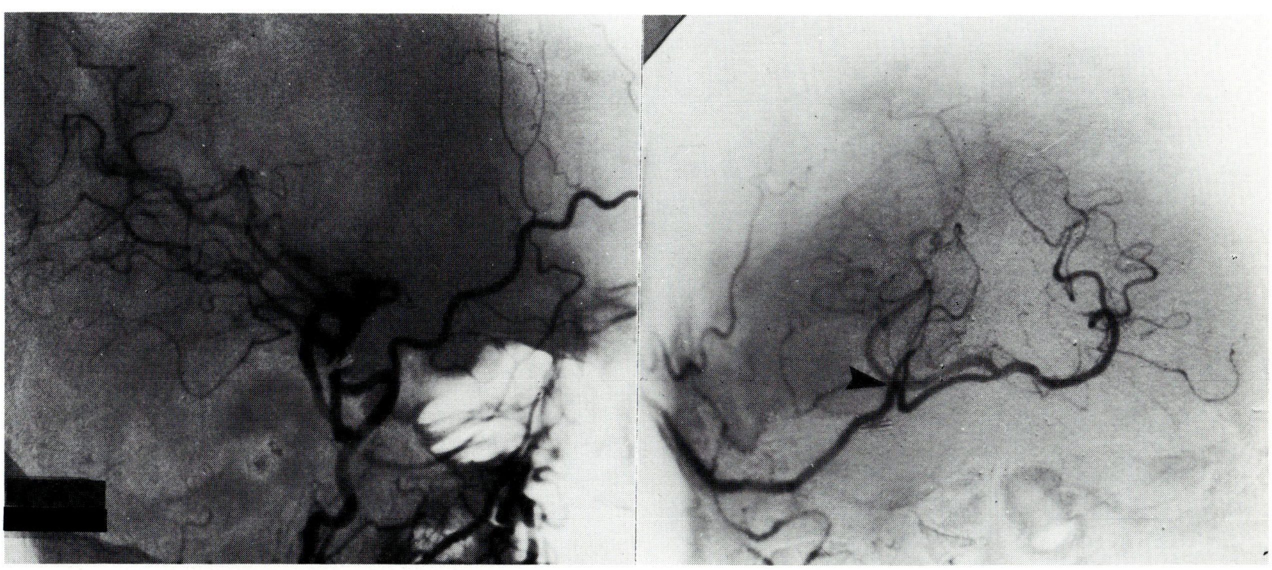

B

FIGURE 44-16. (*A*) The STA is dissected and anastomosed to the superior cerebellar artery through a subtemporal craniotomy. (*B*) Postoperative angiogram (2 views) showing filling of the distal basilar artery through a patent STA-SCA anastomosis (*arrowhead*).

FIGURE 44-15. (*A*) The occipital artery has been dissected and anastomosed to the anterior inferior cerebellar artery through a suboccipital craniectomy. (*B*) Postoperative angiogram shows filling of the vertebrobasilar tree through a patent OA-AICA anastomosis.

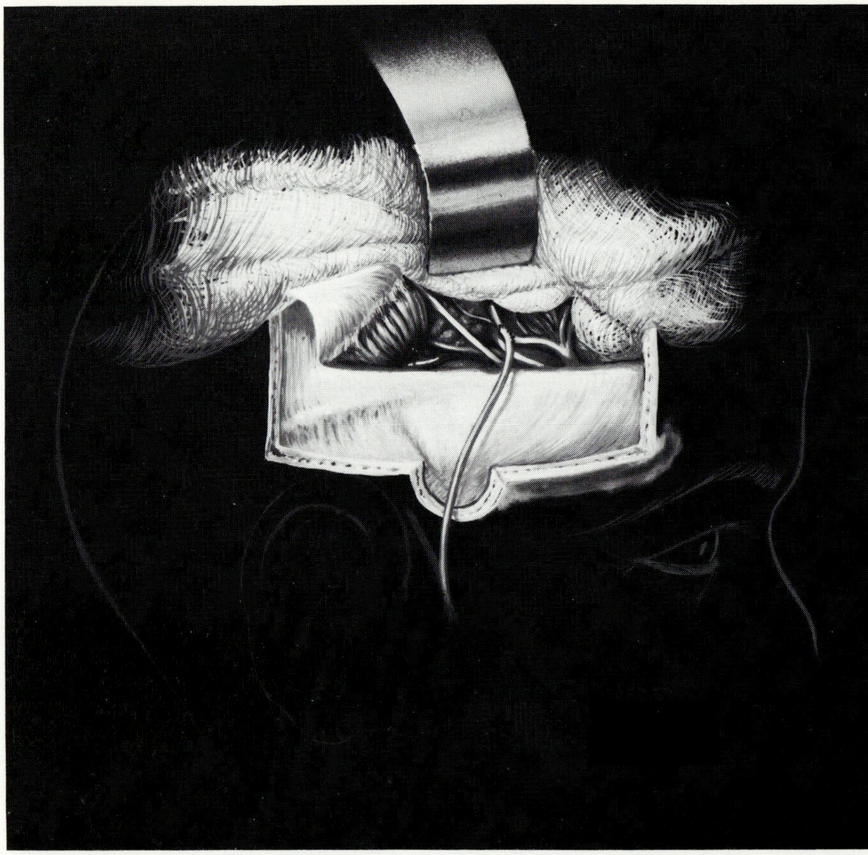

A

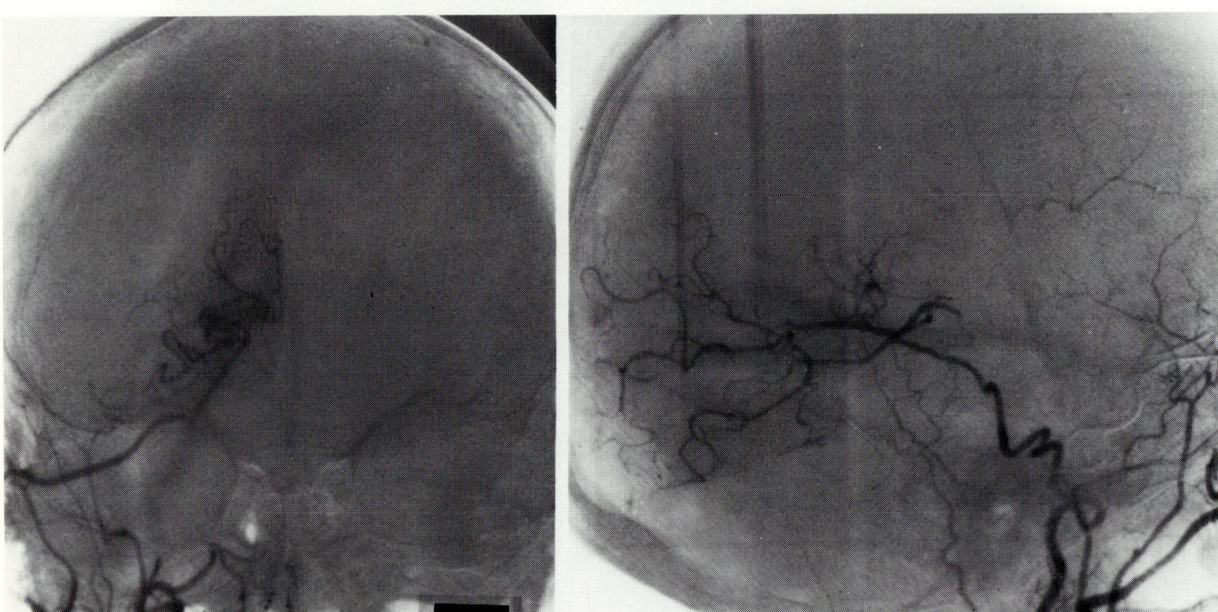

B

FIGURE 44-17. (*A*) The STA is dissected and anastomosed to the posterior cerebral artery (PCA) through a subtemporal craniotomy. (*B*) Postoperative angiogram (2 views) shows filling of the posterior cerebral artery through a patent STA-PCA anastomosis.

The surgical results compiled from 17 fully documented series and our own (a total of 1559 operations) are encouraging. The neurological complications which developed following surgery included transient neurological deficits which were not present before surgery and did not resolve after 24 hours in 66 patients (4 percent). The reported operative mortality occurring during the first 30 days after surgery included 40 patients (3 percent) of which 20 were cardiac, 10 were pulmonary, and 10 were stroke-related.

Other surgical morbidity of nonneurological type has been reported (Table 44-1). Scalp necrosis leads the list, probably because in most early series a scalp flap was developed to harvest the STA. Since most surgeons have now switched to a direct incision over the STA, this is no longer a significant problem. Subdural hematomas are found because it is necessary to maintain an opening on the dura mater to allow free passage of the arterial pedicle and this may allow the leakage of blood from the extradural space into the subdural space. This opening in the dura also permits free flow of spinal fluid outside the dura, which can result in the leakage of spinal fluid through the wound and the development of an intracranial infection or even meningitis when the patient has a concurrent wound infection.

Postoperative seizures cannot always be explained by a demonstrable structural lesion on patients who had an anastomosis to the cerebral cortex. In these patients, it is possible that the seizure focus may be caused by the local hyperemia produced by the EC-IC anastomosis when this is completed on an area which does not have fully reestablished autoregulation. When we have found postoperative seizures in patients who underwent an anastomosis to the superior cerebellar artery for basilar ischemia, these patients have always had associated temporal lobe contusions.

TABLE 44-1. Nonneurological Postoperative Complications Among 1559 EC-IC Anastomoses

Complications	No. of Patients
Scalp necrosis	37
Subdural collection	28
Seizures	27
Wound infection	10
Pulmonary embolism	5
Cerebral spinal fluid	8
Deep venous thrombosis	2
Others*	30
Total	147(9%)

*Subgaleal fluid collection, transient atrial fibrillation, intracerebral hematoma, hemorrhagic softening, subendocardial infarction, fever (one case).

The cumulative morbidity rate including neurological and nonneurological complications is 16 percent; however, only 2 percent of the total group of complications had any residual neurological deficit once the problem had been resolved.

Once the patients have passed beyond the immediate acute surgical morbidity and mortality, their outlook is similar to that of other patients of similar age. Chater (1983) reported a late stroke incidence of 2 percent per year on follow-up in a large group of patients followed for up to 10 years after surgery, and only 0.9 percent of these were ipsilateral to the bypass. The causes for delayed mortality among the reported series are predominantly cardiac, 52 (49 percent); but some of these deaths were due to recurrent fatal strokes, 25 (25 percent). The remaining 30 (27 percent) patients died of other causes, including pulmonary insufficiency, renal failure, cancer, and others.

In conclusion, cerebral revascularization appears to have a limited role in the management of patients with cerebral vascular disease. A variety of procedures have been developed for patients suffering from anterior or posterior circulation ischemia and who have vascular lesions that have been considered surgically inaccessible. Any level of the cerebral circulation can now be revascularized with different and innovative procedures designed specifically for individual areas of the brain. These procedures can be completed with low morbidity and minimal mortality rates, but they do require a competent surgical team with experience in the procedures and equipped with all possible ancillary services necessary to evaluate the patients pre- and postoperatively and to provide intensive care management to these critically ill patients. In carefully selected patients EC-IC bypass can provide symptomatic relief and has the potential to provide additional circulation to the brain. The procedure may not decrease the incidence of stroke in symptomatic patients with specific vascular lesions. The international randomized trial conducted by the EC-IC Bypass Study Group compared the best medical treatment with EC-IC bypass, joining the superficial temporal artery and the middle cerebral artery, in 1377 patients. Their results failed to show any reduction in the rate of subsequent strokes and stroke-related death.

Bibliography

CLINICAL PRESENTATION

1. Bannister CM: The influence of carotid artery pathology on the planning of procedures for cerebral revascularization. Acta Neurochir 1982, 64:292.
2. Kim SH, Nishikawa M, Tsukahara T: Cerebral vertigo caused by ischemia in the carotid artery distribution. Report of three cases. Acta Neurochir 1982, 66:55–59.
3. Penzoldt F. Ueber thrombose (autoch-thone oder embolische) der carotis. Deutsches Arch Klin Med Leipz 1881, 28:80–93.
4. Gowers WR: *A Manual of Diseases of the Nervous System*, vol 2. London, Churchill, 1888.
5. Moniz E: Rev Neurol 1927, 2:72.
6. Carrea R: Acta Neurol Latinoamericana 1955, 1:71.

NATURAL HISTORY AND EPIDEMIOLOGY

1. Acheson J. Hutchinson EL: Observations on the natural history of transient cerebral ischemia. Lancet 1964, 2:871–874.
2. Auer L: Surgical treatment of cerebrovascular insufficiency—A follow-up study. Acta Neurochir 1979, 46:85–92.
3. Barnett HJM: In answer to the question: "As compared to what?" A progress report on the EC/IC Bypass Study. Stroke 1980, 11(2):137–140.
4. Barnett HJM: Is there a place for cerebral revascularization? Clin Neurosurg 1979, 26:314–329.
5. Fields WS, Lemak NA: Joint study of extracranial arterial occlusion: X Internal carotid artery occlusion. JAMA 1976, 235:2734–2738.

6. Fisher CM: The natural history of middle cerebral artery trunk occlusion. In Austin GM (ed): *Microneurosurgical Anastomoses for Cerebral Ischemia*. Springfield, Illinois, Charles C Thomas, 1976, pp 146–154.
7. Furlan AJ, Little JR, Dohn DF: Arterial occlusion following anastomosis of the superficial temporal artery to middle cerebral artery. Stroke 1980, 11:91–95.
8. Grillo P, Patterson RH: Occlusion of the carotid artery: Prognosis (natural history) and the possibilities of surgical revascularization. Stroke 1975, 6:17–20.
9. Hinton RC, Mohn JP, Ackerman RH, Adair LB, Fisher CM: Symptomatic middle cerebral artery stenosis. Ann Neurol 1979, 5:152–157.
10. Mehdorn HM, Hoffman WF, Chater NL: Microneurosurgical arterial bypass for cerebral ischemia: The San Francisco experience. In Peerless SJ, McCormick CW (eds): *Microsurgery for Cerebral Ischemia*. New York-Heidelburg-Berlin, Springer-Verlag, 1980, pp 350–356.
11. Olteanu Berbe V, Schmiedek P, Gratzl O, Marguth F: Extra-intracranial arterial bypass surgery in patients with bilateral internal carotid artery occlusion. In Peerless SJ, McCormick CW (eds): *Microsurgery for Cerebral Ischemia*. New York-Heidelberg-Berlin, Springer-Verlag, 1980, pp 292–296.
12. Pasztor E. Nyary I, Vajda J, Horvath M: Dependency on bypass circulation: A case study. Acta Neurochir 1982, 62:277–283.
13. Peerless SJ, Chater NL, Ferguson GF: Multiple vessel occlusions in cerebrovascular disease. A further follow-up of the effects of microvascular bypass on the quality of life and the incidence of stroke. In Schmiedek P (ed): *Microsurgery for Stroke*. New York-Heidelberg-Berlin, Springer-Verlag, 1977, pp 251–259.
14. Wassmann H, Friedrich J, Fischdick G: Cerebrovascular disease in patients over 60 years of age—Is vascular surgery helpful? Acta Neurochir 1983, 68:146 (abstract).
15. Whisnant JP, Matsumoto N, Elveback LR: Transient cerebral ischemic attacks in a community, Rochester, Minnesota, 1955 through 1969. Mayo Clin Proc 1973, 48:194–198.
16. Winkler D: The results of vascular surgery under the special aspect of higher age. Acta Neurochir 1983, 68:145 (abstract).
17. Ziegler DK: Prognosis in patients with transient ischemic attacks. Stroke 1973, 4:666–673.

MORBIDITY AND MORTALITY

1. Conley FK: Embolization of a superficial temporal artery to middle cerebral artery bypass: Case report. Neurosurgery 1983, 12(3):342–345.
2. Donaghy P: Pitfalls in extracranial-intracranial blood flow diversion. In Austin GM (ed): *Microneurosurgical Anastomoses for Cerebral Ischemia*. Springfield, Illinois, Charles C Thomas, 1976, pp 304–307.
3. Fleischer AS, Faria MA, Hoffman JC: Pseudoaneurysm complicating superficial temporal artery–middle cerebral artery bypass. Surg Neurol 1979, 12:305–306.
4. Heros RC, Nelson PN: Hemorrhagic infarction after microsurgical cerebral revascularization. In Peerless SJ, McCormick CW (eds): *Microsurgery for Cerebral Ischemia*. New York-Heidelberg-Berlin, Springer-Verlag, 1980, pp 333–340.
5. Reichman OH: Complications of cerebral revascularization. Clin Neurosurg 1976, 23:318–335.

DIAGNOSTIC STUDIES

1. Hartmann A, Menzel J, Rommel T, Winter R: Regional cerebral blood flow in patients with extra-intracranial bypass operation. Acta Neurochir 1983, 68:151 (abstract).
2. Heilbrun MP, Anderson RE: Preoperative evaluation of STA-MCA anastomosis candidates with r CBF studies. In Schmiedek P (ed): *Microsurgery for Stroke*. New York-Heidelberg-Berlin, Springer-Verlag, 1977, pp 202–213.
3. Williams RW: Experience in the diagnosis and surgical management of cerebral stroke. A 12-year self-performance assessment. Vasc Surg pp 148–171, 1982.

ANTERIOR CIRCULATION REVASCULARIZATION

1. Agnoli A, Maira G, Pola P, Rossi GF, Ruggieri S, Savi L, Vignati A: Extra-intracranial arterial anastomosis in ischemic completed stroke. Acta Neurochir 1981, 57:131 (abstract).
2. Boone SC: The surgical management of bilateral carotid artery occlusive disease. In Peerless SJ, McCormick CW (eds): *Microsurgery for Cerebral Ischemia*. New York-Heidelberg-Berlin, Springer-Verlag, 1980, pp 297–304.
3. Chater N: Neurosurgical extracranial-intracranial bypass for stroke: With 400 cases. Neurol Res 1983, 5(2):1–9.
4. Chater N, Popp J: Microsurgical vascular bypass for occlusive cerebrovascular disease: A review of 100 cases. Surg Neurol 1976, 6:115–118.
5. Deruty R, Bret P, Lecuire J. Lapras C, Capdeville J: L'anastomose arterielle extra-intracranienne. Bilan d'une experience clinique de 40 cas. Neurochirurgie 1978, 24:355–359.
6. Donaghy RMP: What's new in surgery. Neurological surgery. Surg Gynecol Obstet 1972, 134:269–271.
7. Donaghy RMP: Evaluation of extracranial-intracranial blood flow diversion. In Austin GM (ed): *Microneurosurgical Anastomoses for Cerebral Ischemia*. Springfield, Illinois, Charles C Thomas, 1976, pp 256–274.
8. Donaghy RMP, Yasargil MG: Extra-intracranial blood flow diversion. Presented at the American Association of Neurological Surgeons. Chicago, Illinois, April, 1968.
9. Galibert P, Grunewald P: Extra-intracranial anastomosis in patients with completed stroke. Acta Neurochir 1979, 28 (suppl):306–307.
10. Grunewald P, Lepage M, Mizon JP, Froissart M, Galibert P: Reflexions sur les anastomoses extra-intracraniennes. A propos d'une serie de 65 cas. Rev Neurol 1979, 135:467–471.
11. Guegan R, Deruty R, Rey A, Lagarrigue J: EICA in transient ischemic attacks and neurological deficits. Acta Neurochir 1979, 28 (suppl):304–305.
12. Jerva MJ, Pintozzi N: Cerebral microvascular surgery in completed stroke. In Peerless SJ, McCormick CW (eds): *Microsurgery for Cerebral Ischemia*. New York-Heidelberg-Berlin, Springer-Verlag, 1980, pp 283–285.
13. Kikuchi H, Karasawa J: Extra-intracranial arterial anastomosis in ten patients with Moya-Moya syndrome (occlusion of the circle of Willis). In Schmiedek P (ed): *Microsurgery for Stroke*. New York-Heidelberg-Berlin, Springer-Verlag, 1977, pp 260–263.
14. Khodadad G: Extracranial-intracranial bypass procedures for occlusive cerebrovascular disease. Acta Neurochir 1979, 51:135–136 (abstract).
15. Lazar ML, Clark K: Microsurgical cerebral revascularization: Concepts and practice. Surg Neurol 1973, 1:355–359.
16. Merei TF, Bodosi M: Microsurgical anastomosis for cerebral ischemia in 90 patients. In Schmiedek P (ed): *Microsurgery for Stroke*. New York-Heidelberg-Berlin, Springer-Verlag, 1977, pp 264–270.
17. Ojemann RG, Crowell RM: *Surgical Management of Cerebrovascular Disease*. Baltimore/London, Williams & Wilkins, 1983.
18. Salazar JL, Amine ARC, Sugar O: Intracranial neurosurgical treatment of occlusive cerebrovascular disease. Stroke 1976, 7:348–353.

19. Samson DS, Boone S: Extracranial-intracranial arterial bypass: Past performance and current concepts. Neurosurgery 1978, 3:79–86.
20. Shaw D: Extracranial-intracranial anastomosis in cerebrovascular disease. In Peerless SJ, McCormick CW (eds): *Microsurgery for Cerebral Ischemia*. New York-Heidelberg-Berlin, Springer-Verlag, 1980, pp 341–343.
21. Spetzler RF: Extracranial-intracranial arterial anastomosis for cerebrovascular disease. Surg Neurol 1979, 11:157–161.
22. Spetzler RF, Chater N: Occipital artery–middle cerebral artery anastomosis for cerebral artery occlusive disease. Surg Neurol 1974, 2:235–238.
23. Spetzler RF, Zabramski J: Revascularization of anterior and posterior circulation ischemia. Clin Neurosurg 1982, 29:575–593.
24. Sundt TM, Siekert RG, Piepgras DG, Sharbrough FW, Houser OW: Bypass surgery for vascular disease of the carotid system. Mayo Clin Proc 1976, 51:677–692.
25. Kredel FE: Collateral cerebral circulation by muscle graft technique of operation with report of three cases. South Surg 1942, 11:235–244.
26. Yasargil GM, Yonekowa Y: Results of microsurgical extracranial-intracranial arterial bypass in the treatment of cerebral ischemia. Neurosurgery 1977, 1:22–24.

INDICATIONS AND PATIENT SELECTION

1. Auer LM, Heppner F: Indications for surgery in patients with several cerebrovascular lesions. In Peerless SJ, McCormick CW (eds): *Microsurgery for Cerebral Ischemia*. New York-Heidelberg-Berlin, Springer-Verlag, 1980, pp 305–316.
2. Chater N: Patient selection and results of extra-intracranial anastomosis in selected cases of cerebrovascular disease. Clin Neurosurg 1976, 23:287–309.
3. Engel S, Ferraz H: Indications and results of extra-intracranial arterial bypasses. Int Surg 1983, 68:197–200.
4. Reichman OH: Selection of patients and clinical results following STA-cortical MCA anastomosis. In Austin GM (ed): *Microneurosurgical Anastomoses for Cerebral Ischemia*. Springfield, Illinois, Charles C Thomas, 1976, pp 275–280.
5. Rodreiguez Y, Baena R, Brambilla GL, Rainoldi F, Sangiovanni G, Locatelli D: Re-evaluation of the indications for cerebral revascularization surgery after three years' experience. Acta Neurochir 1981, 57:319 (abstract).

RESULTS AND FOLLOW-UP

1. Austin G, Hayward W, Laffin D: Modification of cerebral ischemia by microsurgical intracranial anastomosis. In Austin GM (ed): *Microneurosurgical Anastomoses for Cerebral Ischemia*. Springfield, Illnois, Charles C Thomas, 1976, pp 281–294.
2. Chao Ya-tu: A cooperative study of surgical treatment of ischemic cerebral disease. Acta Neurochir 1982, 64:276 (abstract).
3. Chater N: Surgical results and measurements of interoperative flow in microneurosurgical anastomoses. In Austin GM (ed): *Microneurosurgical Anastomoses for Cerebral Ischemia*. Springfield, Illnois, Charles C Thomas, 1976, pp 295–304.
4. Deruty R, Lecuire J, Bret P, Capdeville J: Results in 51 patients with EC-IC bypass. Technical and clinical considerations. In Peerless SJ, McCormick CW (eds): *Microsurgery for Cerebral Ischemia*. New York-Heidelberg-Berlin, Springer-Verlag, 1980, pp 344–349.
5. Gratzl O, Schmiedek P: STA-MCA bypass: Results 10 years postoperatively. Neurol Res 1983, 5:11–18.
6. Gratzl O, Schmiedek P, Olteanu-Nerbe V: Long-term clinical results following extra-intracranial arterial bypass surgery. In Schmiedek P (ed): *Microsurgery for Stroke*. New York-Heidelberg-Berlin, Springer-Verlag, 1977, pp 271–275.
7. Gratzl O, Schmiedek P, Steinhoff H, Enzenback R: Microneurosurgical anastomoses for cerebral ischemia in 39 patients—Clinical results, angiography and regional cerebral blood flow. In Austin GM (ed): *Microneurosurgical Anastomoses for Cerebral Ischemia*. Springfield, Illnois, Charles C Thomas, 1976, pp 308–319.
8. Lee MC, Ausman JI, Diaz FG, Klassen AC, Latchaw RE: STA-MCA anastomosis: Further analysis of long-term results—A neurologist's view. In Peerless SJ, McCormick CW (eds): *Microsurgery for Cerebral Ischemia*. New York-Heidelberg-Berlin, Springer-Verlag, 1980, pp 257–261.
9. Levinthal R: Extracranial-intracranial bypass in the elderly. Neurosurgery 1981, 8:517–519.
10. Mizukami M, Kin H, Sakuta Y, Nishijima M, Araki G: Cortical arterial pressure in occlusive cerebrovascular disease and results of bypass surgery. In Schmiedek P (ed): *Microsurgery for Stroke*. New York-Heidelberg-Berlin, Springer-Verlag, 1977, pp 233–239.
11. Schmiedek P, Gratzl O, Olteanu Nerbe V, Steude U, Marguth F: Nine years' experience with extra-intracranial bypass surgery for cerebral ischemia. Acta Neurochir 1979, 46:310 (abstract).
12. Schmiedek P, Olteanu Nerbe V, Gratzl O, Leaschem D, Marguth F: Extra-intracranial arterial bypass surgery for cerebral ischemia in patients with normal cerebral angiograms. In Peerless SJ, McCormick CW (eds): *Microsurgery for Cerebral Ischemia*. New York-Heidelberg-Berlin, Springer-Verlag, 1980, pp 268–274.
13. Yasargil GM, Yonekawa Y: Results of microsurgical extra-intracranial arterial bypass in the treatment of cerebral ischemia. Neurosurgery 1977, 1:22–24.
14. Yonekawa Y, Yasargil MG: Extra-intracranial arterial anastomosis: Clinical and technical aspects. Results. Adv Tech Stand Neurosurg 1976, 3:47–78.
15. The EC/IC bypass study group: Failure of extracranial-intracranial arterial bypass to reduce the risk of ischemic stroke. N Engl J Med 1985, 313:1191–1200.

POSTERIOR CIRCULATION REVASCULARIZATION

1. Allen GS, Cohen RJ, Preziosi TJ: Microsurgical endarterectomy of the intracranial vertebral artery for vertebrovasilar transient ischemic attacks. Neurosurgery 1981, 8:56–59.
2. Ausman JI, Diaz FG, de los Reyes RA, Pak H, Patel S, Boulos R: Superficial temporal to proximal superior cerebellar artery anastomosis for basilar artery stenosis. Neurosurgery 1981, 9:56–60.
3. Ausman JI, Diaz FG, de los Reyes RA, Pak H, Patel S, Boulos R: Anastomosis of occipital artery to anterior inferior cerebellar artery for vertebral basilar junction stenosis. Surg Neurol 1981, 16:99–102.
4. Ausman JI, Diaz FG, de los Reyes RA, Pak H, Patel S, Mehta B, Boulos R: Posterior circulation revascularization. Superficial to superior cerebellar artery anastomosis. J Neurosurg 1982, 56:766–776.
5. Ausman JI, Diaz FG, Pearce JE, de los Reyes RA, Leuchter W, Mehta B, Patel S: Endarterectomy of the vertebral artery from C2 to posterior inferior cerebellar artery intracranially. Surg Neurol 1982, 18:400–404.
6. Ausman JI, Lee MC, Chater N, Latchaw RE: Superficial temporal artery to superior cerebellar artery anastomosis for distal basilar artery stenosis. Surg Neurol 1979, 12:227–282.
7. Ausman JI, Lee MC, Klassen AL, Seljeskog EL, Chou SN: Stroke: WHat's new? Cerebral revascularization. Minn Med 1976, 59:223–227.
8. Ausman JI, Nicoloff DM, Chou SN: Posterior fossa revasculari-

zation anastomosis of vertebral artery to PICA with interpost radial artery graft. Surg Neurol 1978, 9:281–286.

9. Khodadad G: Occipital artery–posterior inferior cerebellar artery anastomosis. Surg Neurol 1976, 5:225–227.
10. Khodadad G: Short- and long-term results of microvascular anastomosis in the vertebrobasilar sysem, critical analysis. Neurol Res 1981, 3:33–65.
11. Sundt TM, Piepgras DG: Occipital to posterior inferior cerebellar artery bypass surgery. J Neurosurg 1978, 48:916–928.
12. Sundt TM, Piepgras DG, Houser OW, Campbell JK: Interposition saphenous vein grafts for advanced occlusive disease and large aneurysms in the posterior circulation. J Neurosurg 1982, 56:205–215.

Chapter 45

ASYMPTOMATIC CAROTID STENOSIS

JOHN B. LONG, THOMAS G. LYNCH, and ROBERT W. HOBSON II

Cerebrovascular disease is the third leading cause of death in this country and accounts for 9 percent of the total deaths in the United States. The associated morbidity results in approximately $8 billion in related health care costs each year. It is estimated that 10 to 46 percent of these patients will have a transient ischemic attack (TIA) as the first sign of impending cerebral ischemia; the remainder, however, will have a cerebrovascular accident (CVA) as the first manifestation of otherwise asymptomatic vascular disease (1,2). The Joint Study of Extracranial Arterial Occlusion (3) documented that 75 percent of patients with cerebrovascular ischemia had a surgically accessible lesion and that stenosis of the common carotid artery, its bifurcation, or the internal carotid artery was present in approximately 50 percent of the patients in whom these segments were visualized arteriographically. Theoretically, if these patients could be identified prior to a CVA, prophylactic carotid endarterectomy might potentially reduce the incidence of stroke.

Carotid endarterectomy is widely accepted as the treatment of choice for patients with symptomatic extracranial stenosis. A patient experiencing TIAs has a 30 percent risk of subsequent stroke (4); patients who have had a stroke have a 30 percent recurrence rate (5). The morbidity and mortality associated with a carotid endarterectomy are significantly less than those associated with the progression of cerebrovascular disease in these patients (6–15).

Fundamental to the current management of patients with an asymptomatic carotid stenosis is the assumption that this lesion predisposes these patients to an increased risk of stroke. In a retrospective analysis published in 1978, Thompson et al. (16) concluded that the asymptomatic carotid bruit was associated with an increased risk of stroke, which could be significantly reduced by prophylactic endarterectomy. In their series, the nonoperated group had a 27 percent incidence of TIAs and a 17 percent incidence of stroke, compared with 4 and 5 percent, respectively, in the operated group (Figure 45-1). This landmark paper has served as a stimulus for the further study of patients with asymptomatic carotid disease. Currently there is controversy regarding the association between asymptomatic carotid stenosis and the incidence of subsequent cerebrovascular events, the percentage of patients that will develop CVAs as the first manifestation of their lesion, and the ability of prophylactic carotid endarterectomy to reduce the incidence of stroke.

Definition

The hemodynamic significance of a stenosis is a function of flow, the geometry of the stenosis, the distal resistance, and the extent of collateral circulation. Experimentally a hemodynamically significant stenosis is characterized by a 10 percent decrease in distal mean flow (17) and a 5 percent fall in distal mean pressure (18). May et al. (19) determined that a stenosis of the carotid artery does not result in a significant decrease in pressure until it exceeds 75 percent of the cross-sectional area or 50 percent of the diameter. Crawford (20) also concluded that a hemodynamically significant flow reduction is associated with a 50 percent diameter-reducing stenosis. Young (21) observed that flow across an arterial stenosis is variable and may be related to the distal arterial resistance. Moore (22) has shown that a significant stenosis is not a fixed percentage, but varies directly with the cross-sectional area of the artery and inversely with the flow rate. Thus no absolute stenosis can be defined as hemodynamically significant, but in most cases at least a 50 percent reduction in the diameter of the carotid artery is required.

	Asymptomatic	TIAs	Stroke Nonfatal	Stroke Fatal	Length of Follow-up
Operated: 132 patients	120 90.9%	6 4.5%	3 2.3%	3 2.3%	6 to 184 months mean—55.1 months
Nonoperated: 138 patients	77 55.8%	37 26.8%	21 15.2%	3 2.2%	To 180 months mean—45.5 months
Significance	$p < 0.01$	$p < 0.01$	$p < 0.01$		

FIGURE 45-1. Long term follow-up data, reported by Thompson et al. (16), comparing the cerebrovascular morbidity and mortality in groups of operated and nonoperated patients presenting with an asymptomatic bruit.

A carotid bruit is not necessarily synonymous with a hemodynamically significant stenosis, although it may be indicative of a flow disturbance and can be associated with a carotid stenosis varying from 30 to 95 percent. Kartchner and McRae (23) reported that only 36 percent of 668 patients with cervical bruits had a hemodynamically significant carotid stenosis. This was also confirmed by Roederer et al. (24). Using duplex scanning techniques to screen patients with cervical bruits, they observed that more than half of the arteries with an associated bruit did not have hemodynamically significant lesions. Similarly, Hennerici et al. (25), Ziegler et al. (26), and Riles et al. (27) have concluded that the clinical evaluation of cervical bruits does not provide reliable information regarding the presence or hemodynamic significance of an associated carotid stenosis. In addition, hemodynamically significant disease may not be associated with a carotid bruit. Jain et al. (28) have reported that 50 percent of their patients with hemodynamically significant disease had no associated bruits, while Barnes et al. (29) observed this association in only 27 percent of arteries found, by noninvasive evaluation, to be significantly obstructed.

The clinical significance of a carotid bruit has been evaluated in several epidemiological studies. The Framingham Study (30) concluded that the incidence of bruits increased with age, the presence of hypertension, and diabetes mellitus. The stroke rate was more than twice the expected incidence, but half were contralateral to the side of the bruit. Myocardial events and a decreased survival were also closely linked to the detection of a bruit. In the Evans County, Georgia, study (31), the presence of a carotid bruit was associated with a higher risk of stroke in men but not in women. There was, however, poor correlation between the location of the bruit and the subsequent stroke. A cervical bruit was most predictive of an increased risk of death from coronary artery disease. These studies again confirm that bruits may be from noncarotid sources and do not reflect the degree of stenosis, the presence of ulceration, or the status of collateral circulation.

Diagnosis

Noninvasive diagnostic studies have become an appropriate means with which to screen asymptomatic individuals for the presence of hemodynamically significant carotid stenoses. Such noninvasive studies may include an indirect assessment of hemodynamic significance, as well as spectral analysis and direct arterial imaging. O'Leary et al. (32) assessed the impact of noninvasive testing upon patient management and found that their use resulted in a significantly higher percentage of positive arteriographic studies. Arteriographic studies demonstrating less than 49 percent stenosis decreased from 49 to 19 percent ($p < 0.001$), and those studies identifying 75 to 99 percent stenosis increased from 20 to 62 percent ($p < 0.001$).

As outlined in Chapter 10, indirect techniques reflect the hemodynamic consequences resulting from a significant carotid flow obstruction. These include the periorbital Doppler evaluation of carotid collateral circulation (cerebrovascular Doppler examination, CDE) and the plethysmographic determination of ocular pulse delay (OPG-K) or ophthalmic artery pressure (OPG-G). The CDE and both of the oculoplethysmographic techniques are sensitive to the presence of hemodynamically significant carotid disease, but they cannot quantitate the degree of stenosis or differentiate between significant stenosis and occlusion. Spectral analysis provides a means with which to analyze the Doppler flow-velocity profiles from the common and internal carotid arteries, permitting the quantitation of carotid stenoses. Barnes et al. (33) showed that spectral analysis was sensitive to 98 percent of hemodynamically significant disease and correctly discriminated 77 percent of carotid occlusions, 96 percent of stenoses greater than 50 percent diameter reduction, and 70 percent of stenoses less than 50 percent diameter reduction. Ultrasonic imaging yields additional information regarding the morphology of the carotid lesion, as well as the patency of the carotid artery (34).

Currently, there is also interest in the role of venous digital subtraction angiography (VDSA) in the evaluation of asymptomatic carotid disease. In over 5000 studies, Little et al. (35) demonstrated its usefulness in a wide range of cerebrovascular disease entities. Russel et al. (36) compared arteriography and VDSA, concluding that VDSA studies were uninterpretable in 10 to 15 percent of cases and obviated arteriography in only 34 percent. Tans et al. (37) evaluated the role of VDSA in 168 patients with carotid disease confirmed by Doppler studies and angiography. They concluded that VDSA reliably detected therapeutically relevant obstructive disease, but angiography was still required prior to anticipated surgery. Zwiebel et al. (38) concluded that the accuracy of ultrasound (continuous-wave Doppler and B-mode imaging) and VDSA were comparable. The sensitivity to those stenoses exceeding 50 percent was 79 percent using ultrasonic techniques and 85 percent using VDSA. When the stenosis exceeded 70 percent, the sensitivity was 95 percent for both of the techniques. Since VDSA is costly, does not provide selective carotid views, and requires the same contrast load as standard arteriographic techniques, its value as a screening test for asymptomatic patients would seem to be limited.

Arteriography remains a standard for the diagnosis of carotid arterial disease, although it provides only a biplanar characterization of a three-dimensional process. While the morbidity associated with arteriography has been reduced significantly by the use of percutaneous femoral techniques and appropriate patient preparation, there does remain the necessity of arterial puncture and the need for hospitalization; therefore its use in screening and follow-up is limited. The sensitivity and specificity associated with noninvasive diagnostic techniques, however, as well as the ease with which these studies may be repeated, make them ideal for screening and following the asymptomatic patient. VDSA and arteriography are reserved for symptomatic patients or those with noninvasive evidence of hemodynamically significant stenosis.

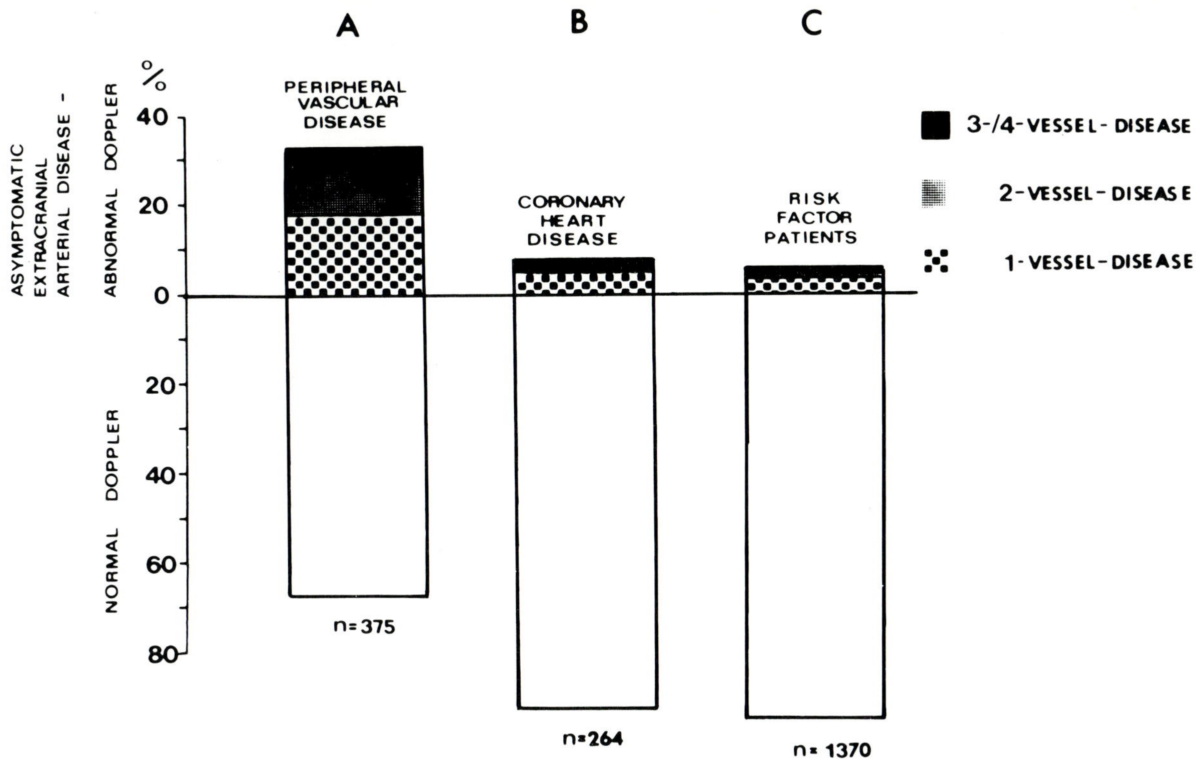

FIGURE 45-2. The incidence of asymptomatic extracranial arterial disease, determined by noninvasive examination, in patients admitted with peripheral vascular disease (32.8 percent), in patients with severe coronary artery disease (6.8 percent), and in patients with risk factors for atherosclerosis (5.9 percent). Approximately one-half (48.8 percent) of the patients with peripheral vascular disease and one-third of those with coronary artery disease or significant risk factors had abnormalities in two or more cerebral vessels on Doppler examination. (From Hennerici et al., Ref. 25.) (By permission of the American Heart Association, Inc.)

Asymptomatic Stenosis

The incidence of asymptomatic carotid stenosis is difficult to define for the population at large but is probably very low. Certain subgroups are at increased risk, including smokers, diabetics, hypertensive patients, and patients with other forms of vascular disease. Hennerici et al. (25) screened over 2000 neurologically asymptomatic patients using a direct continuous-wave Doppler technique. Significant extracranial arterial disease was identified in 32.8 percent of patients with peripheral vascular disease, in 6.8 percent of patients with coronary artery disease, and in 5.9 percent of patients with significant risk factors (Figure 45-2).

The natural history of hemodynamically significant carotid stenosis has not been defined clearly. Javid (39) in 1970 attempted to characterize the natural history of carotid bifurcation disease. He obtained serial arteriograms in 86 patients with previously documented carotid occlusive disease. Two-thirds had progression of the disease, one-third increasing by more than 25 percent each year and one-quarter increasing by less than 25 percent. Roederer et al. (24) evaluated, noninvasively, disease progression in 167 patients presenting with asymptomatic cervical bruits. Using B-mode imaging and spectral analysis they observed an 8 percent mean annual rate of disease progression from a less than 50 percent to a more than 50 percent diameter lesion. After 3 years some evidence of disease progression was apparent in 60 percent (cumulative rate) of the population (Figure 45-3). Risk factors associated with progression included cigarette smoking, diabetes, and an age of less than 65 years. In a related study, Roederer et al. (40) observed similar findings in a group of 134 patients, followed after carotid endarterectomy for evidence of disease progression on the side contralateral to the operation.

A few studies have attempted to noninvasively screen asymptomatic patients and follow those with hemodynamically significant stenoses; unfortunately not all have documented the degree of stenosis, its progression, or the relationship of subsequent ischemic events to the stenotic lesion. Kartchner and McRae (41) reported a 12 percent stroke rate, after 2 years, in a group of asymptomatic patients with hemodynamically significant stenoses identified by OPG-K and carotid phonoangiography (CPA). A significant percentage (53 percent) of the patients were nonrandomly selected for prophylactic endarterectomy, however, and thus strokes occurred in 22 percent of those patients without intervening surgery. Forty-one percent of the strokes were unrelated to the stenotic lesion. Cullen et al. (42) used the

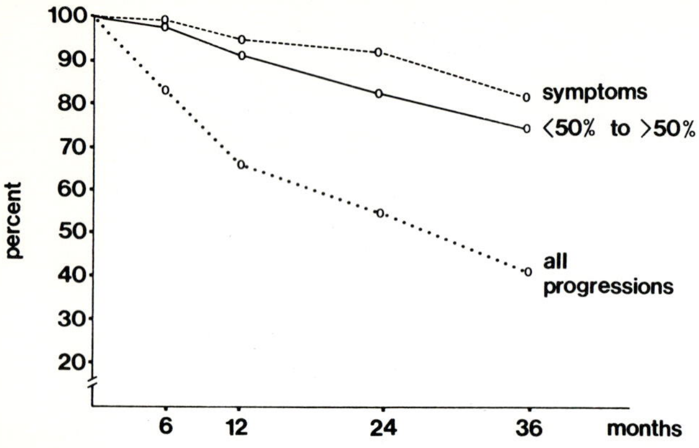

FIGURE 45-3. In 167 patients presenting with asymptomatic cervical bruits, the mean annual rate of progression from a less than 50 percent to a greater than 50 percent lesion was 8 percent. When disease progression in all categories was considered, about 60 percent of the sides progressed after 3 years of follow-up. Symptoms occurred at an annual rate of 4 percent. (From Roederer et al., Ref. 24.) (By permission of the American Heart Association, Inc.)

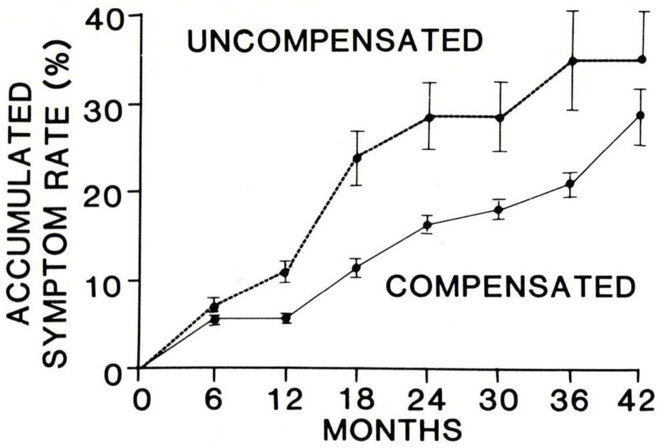

FIGURE 45-4. Patients with an uncompensated, hemodynamically significant stenosis developed symptoms at a higher rate than did those with compensated stenoses. A difference was observed after 6 months and was apparent for 36 months. At the end of 42 months, however, there was no difference between the groups. (From Cullen et al., Ref. 42.) (By permission of the American Heart Association, Inc.)

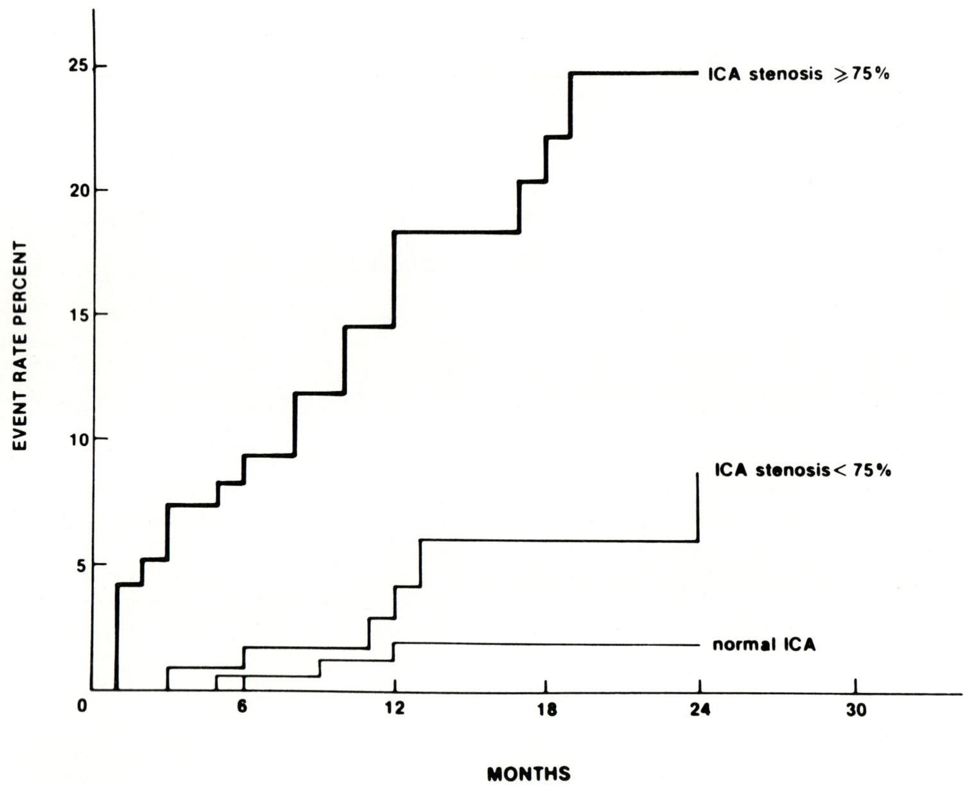

FIGURE 45-5. Neurological events and carotid stenosis. Neurological ischemic events, in patients with an internal carotid artery stenosis greater than 75 percent, occurred at a rate of 15 percent per year. In patients with stenoses of less than 75 percent, however, the rate was 3 percent per year, and in patients without evidence of disease the rate was 2 percent per year. (From Chambers, Norris, Ref. 44.) (By permission of the American Heart Association, Inc.)

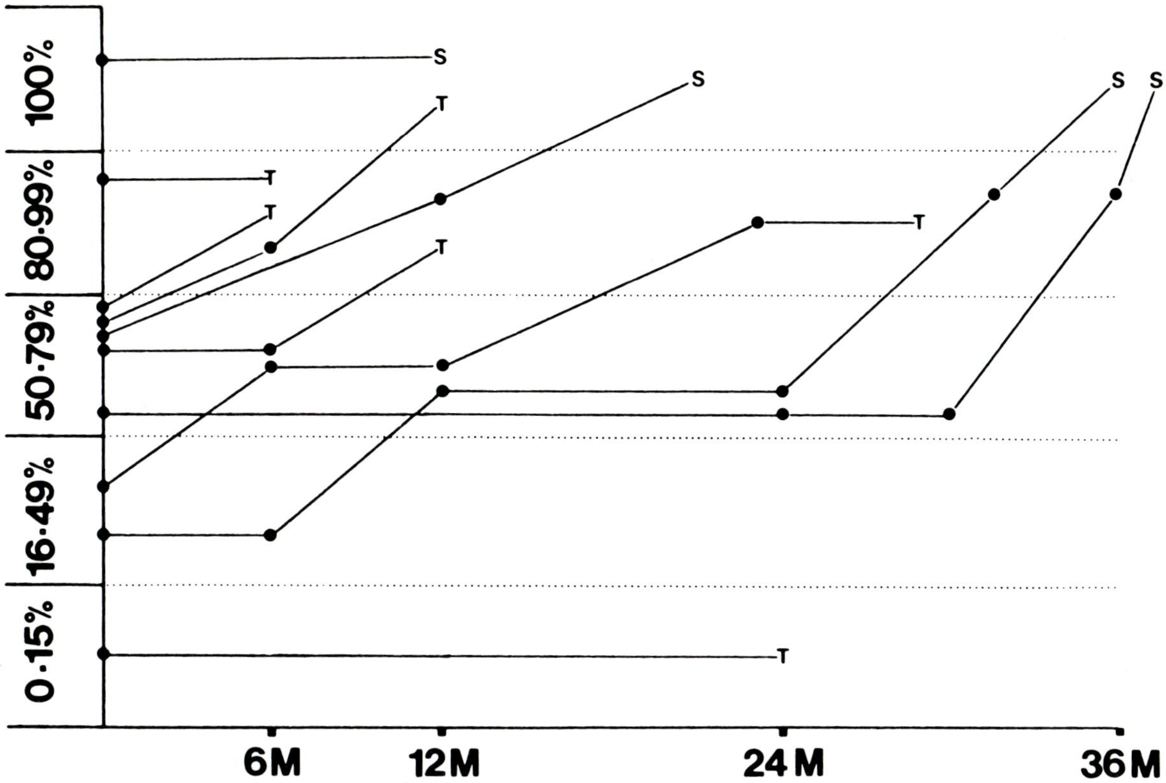

FIGURE 45-6. In 167 patients presenting with asymptomatic cervical bruits, there was a strong association between disease progression and the occurrence of TIAs (T) and stroke (S). (From Roederer et al., Ref. 24.) (By permission of the American Heart Association, Inc.)

OPG-G to identify 77 patients with hemodynamically insignificant carotid stenoses and 29 with hemodynamically significant stenoses. Follow-up at 18 months demonstrated that 11 percent of those without significant stenoses had become symptomatic compared to 24 percent of the group with significant stenoses. While the relative proportion of strokes was not reported, this series does demonstrate a higher percentage of cerebral ischemic events occurring in patients with hemodynamically significant carotid stenoses (Figure 45-4). Busuttil et al. (43) also reported an increase in the incidence of strokes (7 percent) and a significant ($p < 0.05$) increase in the incidence of TIAs (29 percent) in 45 patients with asymptomatic and hemodynamically significant carotid stenoses followed for an average of 19 months. In 28 patients with asymptomatic and hemodynamically insignificant bruits, there were no strokes and a 7 percent incidence of TIAs.

Barnes et al. (29), using Doppler ultrasound, identified a group of patients, awaiting cardiac or peripheral vascular surgery, with evidence of a hemodynamically significant carotid stenosis and/or a cervical bruit. Within 2 years, 10 of 72 patients (14 percent) with an asymptomatic stenosis or bruit had had a TIA, and one patient had had a stroke. Eight of the events were ipsilateral to the previously identified disease. In comparison, only 1 percent of the 254 patients without stenosis or bruit had had a TIA. Of 500 patients followed in the Toronto Asymptomatic Cervical Bruit Study (44), the ischemic cerebrovascular event rate in patients with stenoses greater than 75 percent was 15 percent per year compared with 3 percent per year in those patients with stenoses of less than 75 percent (Figure 45-5). Of those patients who subsequently developed symptoms, 93 percent (26 of 28) presented following a TIA, and only two patients had a stroke without a prior history of TIA. In their prospective evaluation of disease progression, Roederer et al. (24) also identified a significant correlation between the development of symptoms and an initial stenosis exceeding 80 percent or the subsequent progression to a stenosis exceeding 80 percent (Figure 45-6). Seventy percent of the patients in their series presented with a TIA, while 30 percent had an unheralded stroke.

Contralateral Asymptomatic Lesions

In the patient with symptomatic carotid artery disease, the contralateral side provides a unique opportunity to evaluate the natural history of asymptomatic carotid stenosis. Unlike the previous noninvasively evaluated series (24,29,41–44), patients with contralateral disease will have had arteriography. Many will have stenoses which exceed 50 percent, and in some the stenosis on the asymptomatic side will be greater than that on the symptomatic side.

TABLE 45-1. Incidence of Late Cerebral Events Associated with Asymptomatic Contralateral Stenosis of 50 to 75 Percent

Author (Ref.)	Follow-up, yrs	Arteries	TIAs	CVAs
Podore (45)	5	22	3(14%)	2(9%)
Humphries (46)	0–13	182*	29(16%)	1(0.5%)
Durward (47)	4	31	4(13%)	0
Levin (48)	0–20	147†	9(6%)	0
Johnson (49)	1–4	22‡	2(9%)	0
Total		404	47(12%)	3(0.7%)

*Of the arteries, 111 were contralateral to a symptomatic stenosis; 66% of the arteries had a stenosis measuring between 50 and 70%, 19% had a stenosis between 71 and 90%, and 15% had a stenosis exceeding 90%.

†Of the arteries, 85% had a stenosis measuring between 50 and 90%, 15% between 91 and 99%, and 8% had nonstenotic ulcerative disease. Five patients had prophylactic repair of the asymptomatic artery prior to repair of the symptomatic side, and five had prophylactic endarterectomy prior to coronary bypass.

‡This series includes arteries with stenoses of 51 to 99%. Both of the TIAs were associated with 60% stenoses.

In the literature, five series specifically address the problem of asymptomatic contralateral stenosis. Podore et al. (45) retrospectively evaluated 67 patients whose arteriograms had demonstrated a contralateral stenosis. Forty-two percent (28 of 67) of the stenoses exceeded 50 percent. While the authors observed an increased incidence of ischemic cerebrovascular events (21 percent), the majority of these patients presented with a TIA. There was, in addition, no correlation between the initial degree of stenosis and the subsequent incidence of symptoms. Humphries et al. (46) followed 168 patients with 182 asymptomatic stenoses of greater than 50 percent. One hundred eleven (61 percent) of these stenoses were contralateral to symptomatic carotid disease. Eighty-one percent of the patients remained asymptomatic, 17 percent had a subsequent TIA, and 1 percent an unheralded CVA. Durward et al. (47) identified 50 patients with contralateral asymptomatic stenoses which exceeded 50 percent. Sixteen percent developed symptoms of cerebral ischemia on the previously asymptomatic side; however, 75 percent of the initial events were TIAs. Of 147 patients reported by Levin et al. (48), 9 developed lateralizing symptoms related to the asymptomatic hemisphere. While there were no CVAs, 10 patients (7 percent) underwent prophylactic endarterectomy because of "very tight stenoses" or anticipated coronary artery bypass surgery. Similarly, Johnson et al. (49) reviewed 103 patients who had undergone carotid endarterectomy. Of 22 patients with asymptomatic contralateral stenoses, 9 percent subsequently had a TIA and none had a CVA.

Table 45-1 summarizes the data for stenoses in the range of 50 to 75 percent. There is an average stroke rate of 0.7 percent and a 12 percent incidence of TIAs. These averages are only an estimate, because the groups may not be comparable and may vary in the length of follow-up (range, 0 to 13 years). Nonetheless, the data do suggest that patients with stenoses of less than 75 percent can be managed nonoperatively. A significant percentage (12 percent) will eventually become symptomatic, but the overwhelming majority will present with TIAs. Thus prophylactic endarterectomy would not seem to provide a significant benefit in this group.

The incidence of cerebral events associated with carotid stenoses exceeding 75 percent may be significantly higher than that associated with 50 to 75 percent stenoses, but no available series or composite data allow a valid comparison. Each of the previous studies has included only a few patients with stenoses exceeding 75 percent, and some have nonrandomly selected those patients with the most stenotic lesions for prophylactic endarterectomy. This is true for 4 percent of the patients reported by Johnson et al. (49), 7 percent of those reported by Levin et al. (48), and 12 percent of those reported by Podore et al. (45). Each study is, in addition, retrospective, and, while Durward et al. (47) did observe significant disease progression in six patients who were restudied following the onset of new symptoms, the other authors failed to document disease progression or the degree of stenosis at the time the patient became symptomatic. Roederer et al. (24) have approached these latter questions noninvasively. In a prospective study of 167 patients with asymptomatic cervical bruits, 3 of 4 patients had evidence of disease progression prior to a CVA and 6 of 7 TIAs followed progression to a stenosis exceeding 80 percent. Therefore, it can be recommended that stenotic lesions of less than 75 percent diameter reduction should be followed until symptoms develop. Lesions of greater than 75 percent diameter reduction can be considered for prophylactic endarterectomy, until larger series are available.

Asymptomatic Carotid Stenosis in the Preoperative Patient

The risk of perioperative stroke is about 0.3 percent in general surgical patients, 1 percent in patients undergoing peripheral vascular reconstruction, and 1 to 5 percent following coronary artery bypass grafting (50). Intraoperative hypertension, combined with carotid occlusive disease, is the mechanism most commonly postulated for cerebral hypoperfusion and stroke. Hart and Hindman (51), however, reviewed their experience, as well as the available literature, on the mechanism of perioperative cerebral infarction. They concluded that 83 percent of strokes occurred in the postoperative period and were unrelated to hypotension; that carotid occlusive disease was not predictive of perioperative stroke; and that cardiogenic emboli and/or an altered coagulability in the postoperative period were of potential importance.

It has been well documented that there is no relationship between the presence of a carotid bruit and the subsequent incidence of perioperative stroke (52–54). The perioperative risk of stroke in the asymptomatic patient with a hemodynamically significant carotid stenosis, however, has not been well established.

Barnes et al. (29) used spectral analysis and the cerebrovascular Doppler examination to evaluate 449 patients undergoing cardiac or peripheral vascular surgery. Fourteen percent of the patients had a carotid stenosis which exceeded 50 percent of the arterial diameter; however, the range and distribution of these stenoses are not detailed. There was no correlation between the presence of stenosis and the incidence of perioperative stroke. The incidence of postoperative death from myocardial infarction, however, was significantly increased in this group of patients. Turnipseed et al. (55) evaluated 330 patients prior to cardiac or vascular reconstruction and identified 103 patients with significant stenosis or occlusion. Perioperatively, however, this latter group did not have a significant increase in the incidence of stroke or TIA. Kartchner and McRae (56), using oculoplethysmography, studied 234 patients prior to planned cardiovascular surgical procedures and reported a 1 percent stroke rate in patients with a normal OPG-K and a 17 percent incidence in those with an abnormal study. Only 47 percent of the patients were asymptomatic, however, while 27 percent had nonlateralizing symptoms, 18 percent TIAs, and 8 percent a previous stroke. In addition, a number of patients had been nonrandomly selected for prophylactic endarterectomy. Brener et al. (57) studied 2026 patients prior to coronary artery bypass surgery using a combination of carotid phonoangiography, OPG-G, OPG-K, and the CDE. During the latter part of the study, spectral analysis and duplex scanning were also employed. Fifty patients (2.5 percent) were identified who had hemodynamically significant disease. This incidence is significantly ($p < 0.001$) less than the 12.3 percent identified by Barnes et al. (29) and the 11.8 percent by Turnipseed et al. (55). There was a 15 percent incidence of perioperative neurologic deficit associated with significant carotid occlusive disease, compared to a 2 percent incidence in the patients with no carotid disease. Of the seven patients with perioperative deficits and associated carotid occlusive disease, however, three had had a previous CVA, one deficit was contralateral to the identified stenosis, and one was associated with combined bypass and endarterectomy.

While these studies reached differing conclusions, the two studies (29,55) confined to the evaluation of asymptomatic patients concluded that a noninvasively defined carotid stenosis is not associated with a significant increase in the incidence of perioperative stroke. A significant percentage of patients in Kartchner and McRae's (56) study had had previous cerebrovascular events or had been selected for a prophylactic endarterectomy. Additional reports exist, but differences in diagnostic evaluation, operative procedures, and the range and distribution of stenoses make conclusions difficult. Larger series will be required, with a wide range of stenoses, particularly those exceeding 75 percent. In addition, the work of Hart and Hindman (51) strongly suggests that mechanisms other than hypotension may be involved in perioperative stroke and concludes that a causal relationship between carotid stenosis and perioperative stroke has not been established.

Surgical Therapy

The justification for any prophylactic procedure is based upon the supposition that its associated complications are less than the expected morbidity and mortality of the nonoperated population. For carotid endarterectomy this must take into account perioperative complications, restenosis, and the cumulative stroke rate. Thompson's series (16) clearly demonstrates that the procedure can be accomplished with a low perioperative morbidity. In that series, there was a 2 percent incidence of perioperative morbidity, and no operative deaths. This experience is similar to that reported by White et al. (58) in a retrospective comparison of the operative morbidity and mortality for symptomatic and asymptomatic patients undergoing carotid endarterectomy. In their series of 44 endarterectomies for asymptomatic lesions, there were no operative deaths or postoperative neurologic complications. Immediate and long-term results following carotid endarterectomy in the asymptomatic patient also have been evaluated by Moore et al. (59). There were no operative deaths or perioperative strokes in this series, and there was a 95 percent stroke-free status in surviving patients. Table 45-2 presents a composite of the data for carotid endarterectomy in asymptomatic patients (60–63).

The incidence of symptomatic carotid restenosis, following endarterectomy, is approximately 1 percent. Lynch et al. (64) using B-mode ultrasonography and the OPG-G found a 13 percent incidence of recurrent disease following operation. Only two of the seven patients were symptomatic, and three of the seven had hemodynamically insignificant lesions. Kremen et al. (65), using the OPG-G, observed a 9.8 percent incidence (170–173) of recurrent stenosis following 173 endarterectomies. Only 2 percent (3 of 173) were symptomatic. Cantelmo et al. (66) combined ultrasonic arteriography with oculoplethysmography, reporting a 12 percent incidence of restenosis. Sixty-two percent of the stenoses were asymptomatic, and 25 percent were hemodynamically insignificant (<50 percent). Nicholls et al. (67) used a duplex scanning technique and identified recurrent high-grade stenosis in 22 percent of 145 operated arteries. Subsequent follow-up suggested regression of the restenosis in seven, for a persistent rate of 17 percent. There was no consistent association between the development of symptoms and the occurrence of restenosis.

Cardiac complications are the principal cause of perioperative and late mortality in the patient undergoing carotid endarterectomy. The epidemiological studies of asymptomatic carotid bruits document a high frequency of cardiac complications in this group (30,31). Burke et al. (68) assessed perioperative risk factors in patients undergoing prophylactic endarterectomies. Eighty-three

TABLE 45-2. Morbidity and Mortality of Carotid Endarterectomy for Asymptomatic Carotid Disease

			Morbidity	
Author (Ref.)	Operations	Mortality	Transient	Permanent
Sargent (12)	43	1(2.3%)	1(2.3%)	
Thompson (16)	167	0	2(1.2%)	2(1.2%)
White (58)	44	0	0	0
Moore (59)	78	0	2(2.6%)	0
Hertzer (60)	94	2(2.1%)	0	0
Whitney (61)	279*	3(1.1%)	5(1.8%)	6(2.2%)
Kremer (62)	53	0	0	0
Javid (63)	65	1(1.5%)	1(1.5%)	1(1.5%)

*Procedures included standard endarterectomy (62%), shortening procedure with eversion endarterectomy (23%), shortening procedure (7%), dilatation (3%), subclavian to carotid transposition (2%) and vein graft replacement (1%).

percent had at least one cardiac risk factor, and more than 50 percent of the late deaths were due to cardiac causes. These authors concluded that patients with a total of three cardiac risk factors, including hypertension, a history of myocardial infarction, and diabetes mellitus, have a much higher incidence of late cardiac events and should not be candidates for prophylactic endarterectomy because of their decreased survival rate.

Prophylactic carotid endarterectomy can be accomplished with an acceptably low perioperative and long-term morbidity. In attempting to identify those patients who will benefit from a prophylactic endarterectomy, it is necessary to consider not only the estimated stroke rate without surgery, but also the individual's cardiac risk factors. The data of Kartchner and McRae (41), Cullen et al. (42), Roederer et al. (24), and Chambers et al. (44) indicate that those patients with a hemodynamically significant carotid stenosis are at highest risk for cerebral ischemic events. This subset of patients may represent a group which would benefit from prophylactic endarterectomy if cardiac risk factors are not prohibitive.

Medical Therapy

The medical treatment of asymptomatic carotid stenosis presupposes that the surface of the carotid lesion induces secondary platelet aggregation, resulting in arterioarterial embolism and/or occlusive thrombosis. Aspirin is an active inhibitor of collagen-induced platelet aggregation. It appears to interfere with the conversion of arachidonic acid into thromboxane A_2 at a dosage approximately one-tenth of that necessary to inhibit the synthesis of prostacyclin by vascular endothelial cells (69,70). Since the balance between thromboxane A_2 and prostacyclin regulates platelet aggregation, thrombus formation, and, perhaps, subsequent smooth-muscle proliferation, it is theorized that low-dose aspirin may be of clinical benefit in many atherosclerotic conditions.

Data currently available on the use of aspirin in the treatment of patients with cerebrovascular disease are drawn in large part from two controlled trials in patients presenting with TIAs. The Canadian study (71) demonstrated that aspirin reduced the combined incidence of stroke and death in patients who had experienced at least one cerebral or retinal ischemic attack. The incidence of stroke in both the treated (15.3 percent) and untreated (14.4 percent) groups was not evaluated as an independent end point, however, and the efficacy attributed to aspirin was sex-dependent, being observed only in male patients without a prior history of myocardial infarction. The American study (72,73), conversely, could demonstrate no differences between the aspirin and placebo groups when the end points included death from any cause, cerebral infarction, and/or retinal infarction. The study did demonstrate a significant reduction in the subsequent incidence of TIAs in the group treated with aspirin, however. Aspirin appears to be of greatest efficacy in male patients without a previous myocardial infarction who have had multiple anterior circulation TIAs. This group will also respond to carotid endarterectomy with results which are significantly better than those reported for aspirin alone (73).

Although no current studies comparing the medical and surgical treatment of asymptomatic carotid stenosis are available, a prospective randomized trial (74) is now underway and may clarify these controversial issues in the future. However, no modalities exist to prevent or reverse the atherosclerotic progression of carotid lesions. The use of aspirin in patients with asymptomatic carotid stenosis is empiric, and there is no evidence to suggest that it is any more efficacious than placebo. On the contrary, the work of Carson et al. (75) suggests that the use of aspirin potentially may mask the progression of carotid disease and accelerate the process of atherosclerosis by inhibiting the synthesis of prostacyclin by the arterial wall. Future studies will have to determine the role of antiplatelet agents in patients with asymptomatic carotid disease and whether there is any impact on the natural history of asymptomatic carotid stenosis.

Summary

The use of noninvasive screening techniques has permitted the identification of an increasing number of patients with asymptomatic carotid stenoses. The management of these patients must be individualized, as the preferred method of therapy has not been established. Such a solution ultimately requires a prospective randomized trial to define the natural history of these lesions and to establish the role of prophylactic carotid endarterectomy. Currently, a prospective randomized trial comparing endarterectomy and aspirin versus aspirin therapy alone in patients with hemodynamically significant asymptomatic carotid stenoses is under way in United States Veterans Administration Hospitals (74). Specifically, the relationship between subsequent ischemic cerebrovascular events and the degree of stenosis, progression of stenosis, contralateral disease, and the influence of operative intervention are being studied. This study will not be completed for 5 years, however, so that other current guidelines must be sought.

It is essential that any surgeon considering prophylactic carotid surgery demonstrate combined morbidity and mortality figures approximating 3 percent (44). The patients being considered must also be an acceptable cardiac risk, as myocardial infarction represents the most common fatal postoperative complication. Until prospective data are available with detailed analysis of the degree of stenosis, presence of ulceration, and ultimate clinical course, the surgeon undertaking prophylactic endarterectomy must carefully screen patients and concentrate on high-risk groups. This is especially important as more data become available on the significant incidence of carotid restenosis.

The work of Kartchner and McRae (41), Cullen et al. (42), and Busuttil et al. (43) suggests that those patients with hemodynamically significant stenosis, identified noninvasively by OPG techniques, are at a greater risk for cerebral ischemic events than those patients without significant stenosis. In addition, Kartchner and McRae (76) have concluded that disease progression, demonstrated by OPG-K/CPA, is associated with a 17.5 percent incidence of stroke and a 33 percent incidence of TIAs. Roederer et al. (24,40) also suggest that disease progression or the presence of a stenosis which exceeds 80 percent is associated with a greater risk of ischemic cerebral events.

Currently, specific groups that appear to be at greatest risk include patients with a stenosis exceeding 80 percent, patients who demonstrate progression of atherosclerotic disease on serial noninvasive evaluation, and those with poorly compensated lesions by OPG. These groups are chosen because inadequate collateral circulation is potentially a major risk factor in the development of a stroke. These groups should encompass those patients most at risk for developing a stroke as the first clinical manifestation of carotid stenosis, with the full realization that the majority of these patients will present first with TIAs.

References

1. Kuller LH, Sutton KC: Carotid artery bruit: Is it safe and effective to auscultate the neck? Stroke 1984, 15:944–947.
2. Whisnant JP: The role of the neurologist in the decline of stroke. Ann Neurol 1983, 14:1–7.
3. Fields WS, North RR, Hass WK, Galbraith JG, Wylie EJ, Ratinov G, Burns MH, MacDonald MC, Meyer JS: Joint study of extracranial arterial occlusion as a cause of stroke. I. Organization of study and survey of patient population. JAMA 1968, 203:955–960.
4. Whisnant JP, Matsumoto N, Elveback LR: Transient cerebral ischemic attacks in a community. Rochester, Minnesota, 1955 through 1969. Mayo Clin Proc 1973, 48:194–198.
5. Matsumoto N, Whisnant JP, Kurland LT, Okazaki H: Natural history of stroke in Rochester, Minnesota, 1955 through 1969: An extension of a previous study, 1945 through 1954. Stroke 1973, 4:20–29.
6. Baker WH, Littooy FN, Hayes AC, Dorner DB, Stubbs D: Carotid endarterectomy without a shunt: The control series. J Vasc Surg 1984, 1:50–56.
7. Bernstein EF: Influence of preoperative factors on late neurological events after carotid endarterectomy. In *International Vascular Symposium Program and Abstracts*. New York, Macmillan, 1981.
8. Chung WB: Long-term results of carotid surgery for cerebrovascular insufficiency. Am J Surg 1974, 128:262–268.
9. DeWeese JA, Rob CG, Satran R, Marsh DO, Joynt RJ, Summers D, Nichols C: Results of carotid endarterectomy for transient ischemic attacks—five years later. Ann Surg 1973, 178:258–264.
10. Fields PL: Effective stroke prevention with carotid endarterectomy: A series of 400 cases with two year follow-up. In *International Vascular Symposium Program and Abstracts*. New York, Macmillan, 1981.
11. Lees CC, Hertzer NR: Postoperative stroke and late neurologic complications after carotid endarterectomy. Arch Surg 1981, 116:1561–1568.
12. Sergeant PT, Derom F, Berzsenyi G, DeRoose J, Hamerlynck O: Carotid endarterectomy for cerebrovascular insufficiency: Long-term follow-up of 141 patients followed up to 16 years. Acta Chir Belg 1980, 79:309–316.
13. Thompson JE, Austen DJ, Patman RD: Carotid endarterectomy for cerebrovascular insufficiency: Long-term results in 592 patients followed up to 13 years. Ann Surg 1970, 172:663–679.
14. Duke LT, Slaymaker EE, Lamberth WC, Wright CB: Carotid arterial reconstruction: Ten year experience. Am Surg 1979, 45:281–289.
15. Nunn DB: Carotid endarterectomy: An analysis of 234 operative cases. Ann Surg 1975, 182:733–738.
16. Thompson JE, Patman RD, Talkington CM: Asymptomatic carotid bruit: Long-term outcome in patients having endarterectomy compared with unoperated controls. Ann Surg 1978, 188:308–316.
17. Archie JP, Feldtman RW: Critical stenosis of the internal carotid artery. Surgery 1981, 89:67–72.
18. Berguer R, Hwang NHC: Critical arterial stenosis: A theoretical and experimental solution. Ann Surg 1974, 180:39–50.
19. May AG, Vandeberg L, DeWeese JA, Rob CG: Critical arterial stenosis. Surgery 1963, 54:250–257.
20. Crawford ES, Wukasch DW, DeBakey ME: Hemodynamic changes associated with carotid artery occlusion: An experimental and clinical study. Cardiovasc Res Cent Bull 1962, 1:3–10.
21. Young DF, Cholvin NR, Roth AL: Pressure drop across artificially induced stenoses in the femoral arteries of dogs. Circ Res 1975, 36:735–743.

22. Moore WE, Malone JM: Effect of flow rate and vessel calibre on critical arterial stenosis. J Surg Res 1979, 26:1–9.
23. Kartchner MM, McRae LP: Noninvasive evaluation and management of the "asymptomatic" carotid bruit. Surgery 1977, 82:840–847.
24. Roederer GO, Langlois YE, Jager KA, Primozich JF, Beach KW, Phillips DJ, Strandness DE: The natural history of carotid arterial disease in asymptomatic patients with cervical bruits. Stroke 1984, 15:605–613.
25. Hennerici M, Aulich A, Sandman W, Freund H: Incidence of asymptomatic extracranial disease. Stroke 1981, 12:750–758.
26. Ziegler DK, Zieleli T, Dick A, Sebaugh JL: Correlation of bruits over the carotid artery with angiographically demonstrated lesions. Neurology 1971, 21:860–865.
27. Riles TS, Lieberman A, Kopelman I, Imparato AM: Symptoms, stenosis, and bruit. Arch Surg 1981, 116:218–220.
28. Jain KM, Hobson RW, Jamil Z, Marsters C, Berry SM: Clinical screening of preoperative patients for carotid occlusive disease by oculoplethysmography. Am Surg 1980, 192:679–685.
29. Barnes RW, Liebman PR, Marszalek PB, Kirk CL, Goldman MH: The natural history of asymptomatic carotid disease in patients undergoing cardiovascular surgery. Surgery 1981, 90:1075–1083.
30. Wolf PA, Kannel WB, Sorlie P, McNamara P: Asymptomatic carotid bruit and the risk of stroke. JAMA 1981, 245:1442–1445.
31. Heyman W, Wilkinson WE, Heyden S, Helms MJ, Bartel AG, Karp HR, Tyroler HA, Hames CG: Risk of stroke in asymptomatic persons with cervical arterial bruits. A population study in Evans County, Georgia. N Engl J Med 1980, 302:838–841.
32. O'Leary DH, Clouse ME, Potter JE, Wheeler HG: The influence of noninvasive tests on the selection of patients for carotid angiography. Stroke 16:264–267, 1985.
33. Barnes RW, Rittgers SE, Putney WW: Real-time Doppler spectrum analysis: Predictive value in defining operable carotid artery disease. Arch Surg 1982:52–57.
34. Hobson RW, Berry SM, Lynch TG: Applications of B-mode ultrasonography in the diagnosis of carotid occlusive disease. In Bergan JJ, Yao JST (eds): *Cerebrovascular Insufficiency*. New York, Grune & Stratton, 1983.
35. Little JR, Furlan AJ, Modic MT, Weinstein MA: Digital subtraction angiography in cerebrovascular disease. Stroke 1982, 13:557–566.
36. Russel JB, Watson TM, Modi JR, Lambeth A, Sumner DS: Digital subtraction angiography for evaluation of extracranial carotid occlusive disease: comparison with conventional angiography. Surgery 1983, 94:604–611.
37. Tans JT, Hoogland PH, Jonkman EJ: The role of venous digital subtraction angiography of the carotid bifurcation in the evaluation of patients with reversible ischemic attacks or stroke. Stroke 1985, 16:435–440.
38. Zwiebel WJ, Strother CM, Austin CW, Sackett JF: Comparison of ultrasound and IV-DSA for carotid evaluation. Stroke 16:633–643, 1985.
39. Javid H, Ostermiller WE, Hengesh JW, Dye ES, Hunter JA, Najafi H, Julian OC: Natural history of carotid bifurcation atheroma. Surgery 1970, 67:80–86.
40. Roederer GO, Langlois YE, Lusiani L, Jager KA, Primozich JF, Lawrence RJ, Phillips DJ, Strandness DE: Natural history of carotid artery disease on the side contralateral to endarterectomy. J Vasc Surg 1984, 1:62–72.
41. Kartchner MM, McRae LP: The clinical use of oculoplethysmography and carotid phonoangiography. In Baker WH (ed): *Diagnosis and Treatment of Carotid Artery Disease*. Mt. Kisco, Futura Publishing Company, 1979.
42. Cullen SJ, Correa MC, Calderon-Ortiz M, Walburn FJ, Raines J: Clinical sequelae in patients with asymptomatic carotid bruits. Circulation 1983, 68(suppl II):83–87.
43. Busuttil RW, Baker JD, Davidson RK, Machleder HI: Carotid artery stenosis-hemodynamic significance and clinical course. JAMA 1981, 245:1438–1441.
44. Chambers BR, Norris JW: The case against surgery for asymptomatic carotid stenosis. Stroke 1984, 15:964–967.
45. Podore PC, DeWeese JA, May AG, Rob CG: Asymptomatic contralateral carotid endarterectomy. Surgery 1980, 88:748–752.
46. Humphries AW, Young JR, Santilli PA, Beven EG, DeWolfe VG: Unoperated asymptomatic significant internal carotid artery stenosis: A review of 182 instances. Surgery 1976, 80:695–698.
47. Durward QJ, Ferguson GG, Barr HWK: The natural history of asymptomatic carotid bifurcation plaques. Stroke 1982, 13:459–464.
48. Levin SM, Sondheimer FK, Levin JM: The contralateral diseased but asymptomatic carotid artery: To operate or not? An update. Am J Surg 1980, 140:203–205.
49. Johnson N, Burnham SJ, Flanigan DP, Goodreau JJ, Yao JST, Bergan JJ: Carotid endarterectomy: A follow-up study of the contralateral nonoperated carotid artery. Ann Surg 1978, 188:748–752.
50. Corman LC: The preoperative patient with an asymptomatic cervical bruit. Med Clin North Am 1979, 63:1335–1340.
51. Hart RG, Hindman B: Mechanisms of perioperative cerebral infarction. Stroke 1982, 13:766–773.
52. Evans WE, Cooperman M: The significance of asymptomatic unilateral bruits in preoperative patients. Surgery 1978, 83:521–522.
53. Ropper AH, Wechsler LR, Wilson LS: Carotid bruit and the risk of stroke in elective surgery. N Engl J Med 1982, 307:1388–1390.
54. Hart RG, Easton JD: Management of cervical bruits and carotid stenosis in preoperative patients. Stroke 1983, 14:290–297.
55. Turnipseed WD, Berkoff HA, Belzer FO: Postoperative stroke in cardiac and peripheral vascular disease. Ann Surg 1980, 192:365–368.
56. Kartchner MM, McRae LP: Carotid occlusive disease as a risk factor in major cardiovascular surgery. Arch Surg 1982, 117:1086–1088.
57. Brener BJ, Brief DK, Alpert J, Goldenkranz RJ, Parsonnet V, Feldman S, Gielchinsky I, Abel RM, Hochberg M, Hussain M: A four-year experience with preoperative noninvasive carotid evaluation of two thousand twenty-six patients undergoing cardiac surgery. J Vasc Surg 1984, 1:326–338.
58. White JS, Sirinek KR, Root D, Rogers W: Morbidity and mortality of carotid endarterectomy in asymptomatic and symptomatic patients. Arch Surg 1981, 116:409–412.
59. Moore WS, Boren C, Malone JM, Goldstone J: Asymptomatic carotid stenosis: Immediate and long-term results after prophylactic endarterectomy. Am J Surg 1979, 138:228–233.
60. Hertzer NR, Beven EG, Greenstreet RL, Humphries AW: Internal carotid back pressure, intraoperative shunting, ulcerated atheromata, and the incidence of stroke during carotid endarterectomy. Surgery 1978, 83:306–312.
61. Whitney DG, Kahn EM, Estes JW, Jones CE: Carotid artery surgery without a temporary indwelling shunt. Arch Surg 1980, 115:1393–1399.
62. Kremer RM, Ahlquist RE: The prophylactic carotid thromboendarterectomy. Am Surg 1979, 45:703–708.
63. Javid H, Ostermiller WE, Hengesh JW, Dye WS, Hunter JA, Najafi H, Julian OC: Carotid endarterectomy for asymptomatic patients. Arch Surg 1971, 102:389–391.
64. Lynch TG, Hobson RW, Berry SM: The role of real-time B-mode ultrasonography and ocular pneumoplethysmography following carotid endarterectomy. Am Surg 1983, 49:31–36.
65. Kremen JE, Gee W, Kaupp HA, McDonald KM: Restenosis or occlusion after carotid endarterectomy: A survey with ocular pneumoplethysmography. Arch Surg 1979, 114:608–610.

66. Cantelmo NL, Cutler BS, Wheeler HB, Hermann JB, Cardullo PA: Noninvasive detection of carotid stenosis following endarterectomy. Arch Surg 1981, 116:1005–1008.
67. Nicholls SC, Phillips DJ, Bergelin RO, Beach KW, Primozich JF, Strandness DE: Carotid endarterectomy: Relationship of outcome to early restenosis. J Vasc Surg 1985, 2:375–381.
68. Burke PA, Callow AD, O'Donnell TF, Kelly JJ, Welch H: Prophylactic carotid endarterectomy for asymptomatic bruit: A look at the cardiac risk. Arch Surg 1982, 117:1222–1227.
69. Moncada S, Vane JR: Arachidonic acid metabolites and the interactions between platelets and blood vessel walls. N Engl J Med 1979, 330:1142–1147.
70. Masotti G, Pogesi L, Galanti G, Abbate R, Neri Serneri GG: Differential inhibition of prostacyclin production and platelet aggravation by aspirin. Lancet 1979, 2:1213–1216.
71. Canadian Cooperative Study Group: A randomized trial of aspirin and sulfinpyrazone in threatened stroke. N Engl J Med 1978, 299:53–59.
72. Fields WS, Lemak NA, Frankowski RF, Hardy RJ, Bigelow RH: Controlled trial of aspirin in cerebral ischemia. Circulation 1980, 62(suppl V):90–96.
73. Thompson JE: Correspondence to the editor. N Engl J Med 1978, 299:954.
74. Hobson, RW: Veterans Administration Cooperative Study Group: Role of carotid endarterectomy in asymptomatic carotid stenosis.
75. Carson SN, Demling RH, Esquivel CO: Aspirin failure in symptomatic atherosclerotic carotid artery disease. Surgery 1981, 90:1084–1092.
76. Kartchner MM, McRae LP: Carotid phonoangiography and oculoplethysmography. In Nicolaides AN, Yao JST (eds): *Investigation of Vascular Disorders*. New York, Churchill Livingstone, 1981.

Chapter 46

MANAGEMENT OF ULCERATIVE LESIONS OF THE CAROTID ARTERY: SYMPTOMATIC AND ASYMPTOMATIC

WESLEY S. MOORE

Significance of the Problem

The majority of territorial transient ischemic attacks and hemispheric infarctions secondary to extracranial atheromatous lesions are caused by embolic material emanating from a strategically placed atheromatous plaque (1–4). Embolization happens primarily during the fragmentation process that occurs with plaque degeneration or secondarily from the ulcer crater created by plaque degeneration. The presence of an ulcer, as seen on angiography, usually represents the condition of the plaque after the fact; that is, degeneration and primary embolization have already occurred. This process may have produced a temporary or permanent neurologic deficit, or the emboli may have gone to silent areas of the brain and therefore occurred in an asymptomatic fashion.

Angiographic work-up after the embolic event often identifies an irregular or ulcerated plaque on the symptomatic side or reveals the presence of an unsuspected ulcer on the contralateral or asymptomatic side. The current problem revolves about the likelihood of further plaque degeneration from these ulcerated lesions or the possibility of secondary embolization of platelet aggregate or thrombotic debris accumulating in the ulcer crypt which may later be dislodged by pulsatile blood flow.

This chapter focuses on the potential of secondary embolization from ulcerated plaques that were either symptomatic from the primary embolic event or have demonstrated plaque instability by the presence of large areas of ulceration that are discovered on the contralateral side and are "asymptomatic" when first identified. Data are presented to support the embolic theory as well as the potential for recurrent emboli leading to stroke. The therapeutic alternatives are reviewed, and finally the results are compared so that a rational program of evaluation and management can be developed.

Historical Aspects

The history of the relationship between degeneration of atheromatous plaques leading to embolization and specifically cerebral embolization makes a fascinating review and emphasizes the fact that new concepts are often simply newly rediscovered bits of obscure historical data.

The relationship between atherosclerotic plaques and emboli is first credited to Panum who, in 1862, described plaque degeneration and suggested that fragments of the degenerating atherosclerotic plaque had the capability of downstream embolization (5). The actual proof of Panum's hypothesis awaited a report by Flory who, in 1945, reported on a series of autopsies in which atheromatous emboli were actually recovered in the vascular beds of kidneys, spleen, and thyroid; these occurred downstream from degenerating atheromatous plaques. These atheroma emboli had produced infarction of tissues distal to the site of vascular obstruction (6).

The possibility that atheromatous plaques in the carotid bifurcation might produce emboli was first suggested by Chiari in 1905 (7). However, the proof of this hypothesis awaited a report by Handler who, in 1947, noted the concomitant occurrence of encephalomalacea in patients with demonstrable atheroma emboli to other organs (8).

The in vivo observation of atheroma embolism was described by Hollenhorst in 1961 who described "bright plaques" in retinal vessels and suggested that these were actually cholesterol emboli emanating from eroded atheromatous plaques (9). This hypothesis was further strengthened in the same year by a report of Ross Russell who described two patients with transient monocular blindness and suggested that these events were caused by retinal emboli (10). The first surgical correlation between plaque morphology and cerebral embolization was made by Julian and colleagues in 1963 who noted the presence of ulceration from plaques removed from a group of patients undergoing carotid endarterectomy. These authors suggested that there may be a relationship between the patient's symptoms and embolization from these ulcerative lesions (11).

Further support for the embolic theory was provided in a report from Gunning and colleagues who observed a high incidence of mural thrombus adhering to carotid bifurcation plaques in patients suffering from monocular or hemispheric ischemic events. They concluded that many instances of transient or permanent neurologic deficits come from embolization emanating from carotid bifurcation plaques (12).

Ehrenfeld and coworkers reported on a series of patients who were relieved of transient monocular blindness by surgical removal of stenotic, ulcerative lesions from the carotid bifurcation (13).

While the concept of arterial embolization appeared quite reasonable, it was a difficult theory to prove on the basis of available surgical evidence because the criteria for selecting patients for carotid endarterectomy inevitably included the presence of a high-grade, hemodynamically significant stenosis. Thus the relief of symptoms could equally be credited to improvement in blood flow as well as the removal of an embolic source.

The first surgical series that isolated the embolic from the hemodynamic contributions to transient ischemic attacks was reported by Moore and Hall in 1968 (1). We reported on a group of 12 patients suffering from monocular or hemispheric transient ischemic attacks in whom the only identifiable lesions seen on angiography were nonstenotic, ulcerative plaques in the carotid bifurcation. Removal of these ulcerative lesions by carotid endarterectomy produced abrupt cessation of the ischemic attacks. We updated this series in 1970 with a large number of patients and longer follow-up. Our patients remained asymptomatic, which led us to the conclusion that the removal of an embolic source was the responsible act since these low-profile plaques had no effect on blood flow (2).

Pathophysiology

Atherosclerotic plaques can undergo softening and degeneration. This leads to fragmentation of the plaque, disgorgement of plaque contents into the bloodstream, and embolization. Following fragmentation, the plaque surface is irregular or ulcerated. This raw surface is thrombogenic and leads to platelet aggregation or mural thrombus formation. These aggregates are unstable and can be dislodged by pulsatile blood flow producing further embolization.

Because of the dynamic changes in plaque morphology, cerebral embolization of atheromatous plaque origin can be divided into primary and secondary embolic events. Primary embolic events come about from the initial plaque degeneration process. Why some plaques undergo degeneration and embolization while others remain smooth and stable is not fully understood. There is probably a relationship between the actual composition of the atherosclerotic plaque, the balance between cholesterol, calcium salts, and fibrous tissue, that makes some plaques firm and stable and others subject to degeneration and embolization.

There is a growing body of evidence to suggest that one of the contributing features to plaque degeneration is hemorrhage into the plaque substance (14). Hemorrhage into an atherosclerotic plaque produces a sudden expansion leading either to acute arterial stenosis or to intimal rupture with discharge of the plaque contents into the bloodstream. The material that is discharged is made up of a mixture of old thrombus, calcium salts, and cholesterol crystals. The consequences of plaque discharge depend upon particle size and the destination or terminal vascular bed that will be the recipient of this primary embolic discharge.

Once a plaque is evacuated, a central crypt or ulcer is left behind. The presence of an ulcer is visible evidence of two important facts: (1) there has already been a primary embolic event, and (2) the plaque containing an ulcer has the proper composition that makes it susceptible to further degeneration and embolization. These ulcerated plaques can undergo further degeneration and embolization of the core content, or the ulcer itself can be the nidus for platelet aggregation or clot formation with the risk of secondary embolization. Because of these dynamic events, the composition of emboli emanating from carotid bifurcation plaques may be either platelet aggregate material, thrombus, or atheromatous debris.

Clinical Presentation

The clinical presentation of ulcerating lesions of the carotid bifurcation can be divided into two groups, symptomatic and asymptomatic lesions. The symptoms associated with lesions that are actively shedding emboli are territorial transient ischemic attacks or cerebral infarction, which may include monocular events, hemiplegia, hemidysesthesia, or single limb involvement. It is conceivable that multiple emboli to silent or intellectual centers of the brain may result in progressive intellectual impairment, but this has never been proved.

Asymptomatic ulcerative lesions, particularly in the absence of hemodynamically significant stenosis, had been of little clinical concern until 1978 when Moore and colleagues reviewed the natural history of these lesions in a retrospective study. Patients who were found to have asymptomatic ulcerative lesions, discovered serendipitously while undergoing angiographic study for a contralateral symptomatic lesion or because of asymptomatic bruit, constituted our study group. Because it had not been our practice to operate on asymptomatic ulceration in the absence of a hemodynamically significant stenosis, we were able to review retrospectively the natural history of patients with these lesions. We classified the ulcers into group A (small ulcers), group B (large ulcers), and group C (large, multiple or compound ulcers) (15). We updated this study with a larger and more meaningful series in 1982. Our most recent results demonstrate that the asymptomatic A ulcers carried a benign prognosis with an insignificant stroke incidence on long-term follow-up. However, patients with B ulcers had a stroke rate of 4.5 percent per year, and those with C ulcers had a stroke rate of 7.5 percent per year. Of particular concern was the fact that all patients who went on to develop a stroke failed to have warning transient ischemic attacks prior to the event (16).

At this point, we do not know whether the established, angiographically visible ulcer itself is the responsible feature for this stroke incidence or if it simply serves as a marker for those plaques that have the potential for further degeneration and embolization.

Noninvasive Studies

At the present time, there are no noninvasive methods available to identify ulceration per se. It is hoped that as the quality of resolution of B-mode or duplex scanning improves, it may be possible to identify ulcerated areas on the arterial wall by noninvasive means.

Some investigators have also attempted to tag platelets with radioactive indium oxine in the hope that tagged platelet aggregates would accumulate in areas of ulceration. This does occur, but not with significant frequency to be an accurate diagnostic test.

It is important to recognize the fact that hemispheric or monocular symptoms can be caused by embolization in the absence of a hemodynamically significant stenosis (1–4,17). Since noninvasive studies are of no help in this instance, the only accurate method available to identify nonstenotic ulceration is conventional angiography. Thus, patients with hemispheric or monocular events require angiography for adequate evaluation, regardless of the results of noninvasive studies.

Angiography

The angiographic documentation of ulceration is dependent upon placing the maximum ulcer depth in profile. An ulcer may only be seen in a single angiographic projection. Therefore, several angiographic views may be required before an ulcer is visualized. This is best accomplished by selective carotid angiography.

Occasionally, embolization may take place from shallow ulceration that is not visible by angiographic criteria (17). In addition, an ulcer crypt may be filled with thrombolic or platelet aggregate material and therefore remains hidden from angiographic survey. In these two instances, the presence of an atherosclerotic plaque in patients with a well-documented history of territorial transient ischemic attacks may be the only evidence of the source for these embolic events.

In order to better quantitate the three categories of ulcer, we developed a numerical method of identification. The length of the ulcer, in millimeters, is multiplied by the ulcer depth. An A ulcer measures 10 mm^2 or less. A B ulcer can range in size from 11 to 40 mm^2, and a C ulcer is identified by its compound nature or is an ulcer that measures greater than 40 mm^2 (16).

Medical Management

The only effective medical management is the use of antiplatelet or anticoagulant drugs. The only effective antiplatelet drug that has been studied in a randomized trial is aspirin. The best therapeutic dose of aspirin is controversial, with recommendations ranging from 3 grains daily to 10 grains twice daily. The efficacy of antiplatelet drugs has only been established in comparison to drug placebo. There have been no trials comparing antiplatelet drugs with carotid endarterectomy.

Warfarin (Coumadin) anticoagulation has been advocated by some investigators. In two randomized studies, warfarin reduced the frequency of transient ischemic attacks but had no effect on the overall stroke rate and actually increased the mortality rate.

Both antiplatelet and anticoagulant drugs can only be effective against emboli of platelet aggregate or thrombotic origin. It is inconceivable that drug therapy will have any beneficial effect in reducing plaque degeneration or preventing atheroma embolization. In fact, there is one report which suggests that aspirin has an accelerating effect on plaque degeneration by increasing the incidence of intraplaque hemorrhage.

Operations

The usual technique of carotid endarterectomy is applicable to ulcerated lesions with and without stenosis. However, endarterectomy for nonstenotic ulceration is a more exacting procedure because the development of an intimectomy plane is more difficult with a less bulky lesion.

Results

The results with well-performed carotid endarterectomy in properly selected patients are excellent. When the indications for operation are transient ischemic attacks or an asymptomatic ulcer, the combined neurologic morbidity and mortality should be less than 3 percent. The late stroke rate in patients having undergone successful operation is reduced to 1 percent per year, in contrast to the natural history of the disease which carries a stroke risk ranging from 6 to 10 percent per year.

Key Points in Management

1. Good risk patients with territorial transient ischemic attacks or stroke with significant recovery should be studied with selective carotid angiography.

2. Patients with symptomatic ulcerative lesions, with or without stenosis of hemodynamic significance, are best treated by carotid endarterectomy, provided the surgeon's personal results carry a risk of morbidity and mortality of less than 3 percent.

3. Asymptomatic ulcerative lesions, in the B or C category, carry a significant stroke risk and should be treated by prophylactic carotid endarterectomy, provided that the risk of morbidity and mortality is less than 3 percent.

References

1. Moore WS, Hall AD: Ulcerated atheroma of the carotid artery. A cause of transient cerebral ischemia. Am J Surg 116:237, 1968.
2. Moore WS, Hall AD: Importance of emboli from carotid bifurcation in pathogenesis of cerebral ischemic attacks. Arch Surg 101:708, 1970.
3. Hertzer NR, Beven EG, Benjamin SP: Ultramicroscopic ulcerations and thrombi of the carotid bifurcation. Arch Surg 112:1394, 1977.
4. Thiele BL, Young JV, Chikos PM, Hirsch JH, Strandness DE: Correlation of arteriographic findings and symptoms in cerebrovascular disease. Neurology 30:1041–1046, 1980.
5. Panum PL: Experimentelle beitrage zur lehre von der embolie. Virchows Arch [Pathol Anat] 25:308, 1862.
6. Flory CM: Arterial occlusions produced by emboli from eroded aortic atheromatous plaques. Am J Pathol 21:549, 1945.
7. Chiari H: Ueber das verhalten des tielungswinkels der carotis communis bei der endarteriitis chronica deformans. Verh Dtsch Ges Pathol 9:326, 1905.
8. Handler FP: Clinical and pathological significance of atheromatous embolization, with emphasis on an etiology of renal hypertension. Am J Med 20:366, 1956.
9. Hollenhorst RW: Vascular status of patients who have cholesterol emboli in the retina. Am J Ophthalmol 61:1159, 1966.
10. Russell RWR: Observations on the retinal blood-vessels in monocular blindness. Lancet 2:1422, 1961.
11. Julian OC, Dye WS, Javid H, Hunter JA: Ulcerative lesions of the carotid artery bifurcation. Arch Surg 86:803, 1963.
12. Gunning AJ, Pickering GW, Robb-Smith AHT, Russell RR: Mural thrombosis of the internal carotid artery and subsequent embolism. Q J Med 33:155, 1964.
13. Ehrenfeld WK, Hoyt WF, Wylie EJ: Embolization and transient blindness from carotid atheroma. Surgical considerations. Arch Surg 93:787, 1966.
14. Imparato AM, Riles TS, Gorstein F: The carotid bifurcation plaque: Pathologic findings associated with cerebral ischemia. Stroke 10(3):238–245, 1979.
15. Moore WS, Boren CB, Malone JM, Roon AJ, Eisenberg R, Goldstone J, Mani R: Natural history of nonstenotic asymptomatic ulcerative lesions of the carotid artery. Arch Surg 113:1352–1359, 1978.
16. Dixon S, Pais SO, Raviola C, Gomes A, Machleder HI, Baker JD, Busattil RW, Barker WF, Moore WS: Natural history of nonstenotic asymptomatic ulcerative lesions of the carotid artery: A further analysis. Arch Surg 117:1493–1498, 1982.
17. Edwards J, Kricheff II, Riles T, Imparato A: Angiographically undetected ulceration of the carotid bifurcation as a cause of embolic stroke. Radiology 132:369–373, 1979.

Chapter 47

CEREBRAL PROTECTION DURING CAROTID ARTERY SURGERY

ALLAN D. CALLOW

Carotid appears to be derived from the Greek *karos* meaning heavy sleep and from *karoun* meaning to stupefy. Pressure on the artery was believed to result in unconsciousness and possibly death. The ancient Greek physicians labeled this vessel the artery of sleep (1). The human brain claims only 2 percent of the body weight but requires 15 percent of the cardiac output and 20 percent of the inspired oxygen in the resting state (2). Of the 900 mL of oxygenated blood that flows through the normal adult brain every minute, each internal carotid supplies approximately 300 to 400 mL to the ipsilateral orbit and cerebral hemisphere. Less than 200 mL flows through the two vertebral arteries. The transit time from common carotid to jugular vein is approximately 7 s, and it is estimated that each unit of blood spends only about 2 s in its capillary bed (3).

Anatomy

The anterior and middle cerebral arteries constitute the anterior circulation and supply the eyes, the basal ganglia, most of the hypothalamus, the frontal lobe, the parietal lobe, and most of the temporal lobe. The middle cerebral artery provides approximately 80 percent of the total brain blood supply. It has been labeled the artery of aphasia and is the one most frequently associated with infarction.

The posterior circulation derives from the paired vertebral arteries coming together to form the basilar artery from which arises the posterior cerebral arteries. The circle of Willis, composed of the paired posterior communicating arteries which link the anterior and posterior systems, together with the single transversely situated anterior communicating artery, which links the two hemispheres, is classically configured in fewer than 50 percent of individuals. Congenital anomalies include lack of connection of the two hemispheres, isolation of the anterior and posterior systems, and many anomalies of lesser flow significance (4).

Additional collateral pathways consist of the leptomeningeal anastomoses, a network of arteries in the watershed areas of the anterior, middle, and posterior cerebral arteries; anastomoses from the anterior and middle meningeal arteries; and various cervical branches of the external carotid and vertebral vessels. The existence and the functional capacity of these collaterals in the patient with carotid occlusive disease are not discernible by clinical examination or conventional diagnostic means.

The cerebral circulation comprises two types of vessels: the superficial or conducting arteries which course and interlace with one another on the surface of the brain, and nutrient or penetrating arteries arising from them to enter the brain parenchyma. Only the long circumferential arteries, or approximately 10 percent of intracranial vessels, are demonstrable on the standard arteriogram (3).

Physiology

A remarkable feature of the cerebral circulation is, first, its autoregulatory ability to keep brain blood flow constant. Neither an increase in cardiac output during exercise nor moderate changes in arterial blood pressure are accompanied by a great change in brain blood flow. Simultaneous adjustment of the resistance of small cerebral arteries and arterioles keeps perfusion pressure constant. Arterioles must be supplied with an adequate perfusion pressure in order to function normally. Severe, prolonged hypotension, hypoxia, and excessive concentrations of drugs impair autoregulation, and cerebral blood flow becomes dependent upon perfusion pressure. Thus, during carotid cross clamping, systemic arterial blood pressure should not be permitted to fall below the patient's normal level. Second, this ability of the brain to closely regulate its own blood flow severely limits the effect of induced hypertension during carotid endarterectomy. The caveat that the brain can tolerate not more than 4 minutes of anoxia before irreparable damage occurs assumes zero flow and zero pressure. Such may be the case during cardiac arrest but is unlikely during periods of reduced flow coincident with carotid cross clamping. Infarction that may develop within minutes of zero flow may actally take hours to occur in regions of marginal flow. Areas of borderline flow may benefit from and infarction may be avoided or contained if appropriate therapy such as maintenance of an adequate PaO_2, $PaCO_2$, and systemic pressure is given.

The localized vasodilatation which occurs in the early stages of regional hypoxia may not be a compensatory response but rather may be more accurately described by the term "cerebral vasoparalysis." Autoregulation of vascular resistance is lost, and blood flow changes passively with pressure. There is "uncoupling" of the relationship between function and flow. The metabolic demands of the hypoxia region are low, and restoration of normal perfusion pressure results in a local hyperemic state. Flow exceeds need resulting in a state of "luxury perfusion" (5).

Carbon dioxide is a potent vasodilator, and moderate degrees of hypoxia are associated with increased flow. Prolonged hypoxia, however, is associated with a decrease in flow velocity and an increase in viscosity, sludging, and cortical pallor. Arteriolar spasm, unresponsive to carbon dioxide, vasodilating drugs, and stellate ganglion block, supervenes. The failure of these measures to relieve arteriolar spasm is probably because the mechanisms responsible for vasorelaxation are energy-dependent. Until the substrates which provide for normal vasomotor metabolism are restored, vasoconstriction cannot be reversed (2).

Pathology

Inspection of the brain 4 to 6 hours after an ischemic episode reveals no gross changes. Between 6 and 48 hours, however, the gray matter and white matter become swollen, the cortex becomes browner as a consequence of vasodilatation, and within the next 7 days, the swollen infarcted tissue becomes friable and soft. There may be liquefaction of the necrotic white matter. On microscopic examination at 24 to 48 hours, the capillary endothelium becomes swollen and hemorrhagic transformation develops. By 48 hours, activated microglia from monocytes enter the infarcted tissue. Astroglial fibers are laid down on the borders of the infarct, the necrotic material is removed, macrophages decrease, and the interstices become filled with fluid.

Carotid endarterectomy performed too soon after stroke may transform what might become a dry or ischemic infarct into a hemorrhagic infarct accompanied by extension of the neurologic deficit (6). There may be uncertainty as to whether the patient has suffered a transient ischemic attack (TIA), a reversible ischemic neurologic deficit, or a frank stroke. Cerebral protection would indicate that restoration of flow not be attempted until some degree of stability has been introduced into the infarcted area by the fibroglial fibers. This may not occur for a minimum of 4 to 6 weeks. In patients with carotid stenosis so severe as to be "preocclusive," such a delay may permit thrombotic occlusion with loss of opportunity to restore flow. Should the event, however, not be a completed stroke, but a severe TIA, a distinction not always possible without contrast computer-assisted tomography, delay may be hazardous because of the increased frequency of stroke reported to follow upon a recent TIA (7).

Cerebral Protection

The most ominous perioperative complication is hemiplegia or any lesser neurologic deficit of more than a few hours' duration. The risk varies with the neurologic status of the patient, being highest in the patient with a stroke in evolution; less frequent but still in substantial numbers in the patient with a fixed preoperative deficit; and least in the patient with a normal neurologic status at the time of operation (8). A high incidence has also been reported when the contralateral carotid is occluded (9). Many methods have been devised in attempts to prevent cerebral hypoxia during endarterectomy. The most popular is the routine use of a temporary indwelling shunt (10). It permits the use of general anesthesia, maintains normal blood flow, eliminates the need for any type of monitoring system, and avoids a sense of haste (11). Shunts may predispose to embolization, limit exposure, and are unnecessary in most patients, hence their use by some surgeons on a selective basis (12). The efficacy of the collateral circulation is easily and effectively assessed by using a regional cervical block to monitor the level of consciousness in the awake patient (11,13,14). Indirect assessment consists of measurement of the pressure of the internal carotid artery distal to the occluding clamp, the so-called back or stump pressure (15,16), a safe level usually specified as 50 mmHg, but more recently as 25 mmHg (17), by oculoplethysmographic monitoring (18), and by continuous electroencephalographic surveillance (19–21). Measures to alter the metabolism of the brain in the vain attempt to render it less susceptible to ischemia, to improve collateral flow by induced hypertension (22,23), or to reduce intracerebral vascular resistance by induced hypercarbia (24) have been abandoned as ineffective and even dangerous. Induced hypertension places an additional burden upon the myocardium of the patient with coexisting coronary artery disease. Hypercarbia may cause postoperative intracerebral hemorrhage (9).

General endotracheal anesthesia is considered the optimal method for managing patients undergoing carotid endarterectomy. It provides good airway control, permits higher PaO_2 levels, better regulation of the $PaCO_2$ level, and far better control of cardiac rate and blood pressure than is possible in the patient under regional or local anesthesia. In addition, there is freedom from pain and anxiety for the patient and avoidance of undesirable added tension for the operating team. Several studies have suggested the unreliabilty of the stump pressure (11,25–27). In a series of 125 patients operated on under local anesthesia, Connolly (28) found that 24 lost consciousness within 1 minute of cross clamping. Eight patients (33 percent) had stump pressures above 55 mmHg. In our series of 289 consecutive carotid endarterectomies during which the stump pressure was measured during continuous electroencephalographic monitoring, 17, or 6

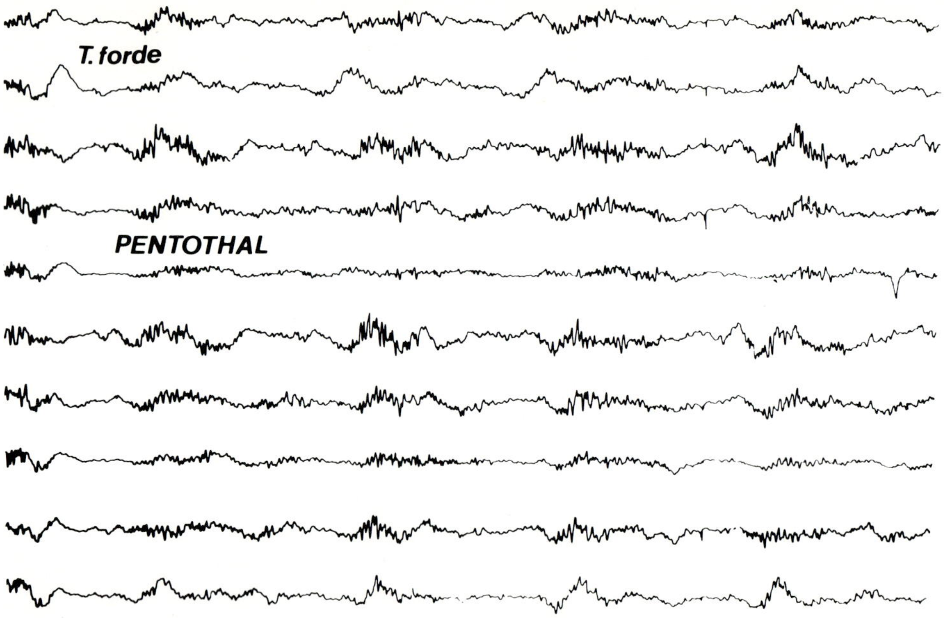

FIGURE 47-1. Ten lead electrodes (upper 5 left, lower 5 right cerebral hemispheres) showing bursts of suppression effect of intravenous bolus of thiopental (Pentothal). (Courtesy of Dr. Allan Callow.)

percent, of the patients were found to have ischemic changes on the electroencephalogram (EEG) despite stump pressures greater than 50 mmHg. Conversely, 7 percent, or 21, of the patients had a normal EEG despite stump pressure of less than 50 mmHg. In this group there was zero incidence of neurologic deficit. Clearly, cerebral blood flow does not always correlate with stump pressure. In each of two categories of patients, those with a history of completed and recovered stroke, and those with vertebral basilar insufficiency symptoms plus carotid artery stenosis, 24 percent developed ischemic EEG changes and required a shunt. In all instances where a temporary shunt was utilized, it was done solely on the basis of EEG criteria and irrespective of the back pressure. Eleven percent of individuals operated on because of an asymptomatic bruit displayed EEG ischemic changes on the EEG and required a shunt (29).

In a series of 335 consecutive patients undergoing 390 carotid endarterectomies from 1969 through 1973, Lees and Hertzer (30), who were using hypercarbia with no intraluminal shunting, noted that postoperative neurologic complications were most common among patients with previous neurologic symptoms and those with subtotal stenosis or occlusion of the contralateral artery. Conversely, the introduction of routine carotid shunting and normal carbia anesthesia during a subsequent series of 626 procedures was associated with significantly fewer operative strokes within comparable groups of patients.

Rampil and associates (31) state that ischemic EEG events occur within 15 to 30 s of onset of cerebral hypoperfusion. EEG changes associated with inhalation anesthetics, however, are more gradual and usually occur over several minutes because of the relatively slow change in anesthetic partial pressure in the brain. Changes in ventilation and body temperature also cause changes in the EEG, but these, too, are gradual. Conversely, changes in EEG following a bolus injection of fentanyl or thiopental are swift and profound and may simulate the rapid onset of an ischemic EEG event (Figure 47-1). Such pharmacologic interventions must be announced and recorded. Only gross changes in postoperative neurologic status are detected by the customary clinical examination. This holds true in Rampil's study (31). With more refined testing, such as provided by psychometrics, a higher incidence of new postoperative deficits may be detected. These more subtle deficits may be heralded by a less prolonged or less pronounced EEG change. In order to increase EEG sensitivity, their detection may require a change in the event-recognition protocol, including additional EEG channels for analysis.

Method

A 16-channel Grass EEG console utilizing 20 gold electrodes glued to the scalp and to each earlobe is standard equipment. The EEG is recorded continuously in 10 leads from prior to induction to ending with extubation. In rare instances it may be continued in the recovery room and for the first few postoperative days. A careful log is kept of all medications and anesthetic agents administered preoperatively and throughout the operation together with blood pressure variations. A variety of anesthetic agents may be used, depending upon the experience and preference of the anesthesiologist. These include halothane, ethrane, and furane. In patients who are at high risk because of coexisting coronary artery disease, a so-called narcotic technique utilizing fentanyl, morphine, oxygen, and nitrous oxide is preferred together with a Swan-Ganz catheter. An intraarterial monitoring line is placed to permit continuous monitoring of arterial pressure and blood gases.

Although the EEG may vary widely from one person to another and brain activity in the same subject changes from moment to moment, an individual's EEG as a whole remains remarkably constant during adult life. With adequate cerebral perfusion, the basic symmetric pattern consists of sustained rhythmic activity of 10 to 14 Hz and ranges between 25 and 100 μV (32).

Four major frequencies, alpha, beta, theta, and delta, named in order of their discovery, are customarily identified in the EEG. [Figure 47-2 (33)]. On the normal EEG, the 8- to 13-Hz rhythm, alpha, is the most prevalent finding [Figure 47-3 (34)]. The beta band is in excess of 13 Hz and in the presence of hypoxia may be depressed or even absent. The delta band, sometimes referred to as slow wave activity, is under 4 Hz and becomes prominent with hypoxia and increasing depth of anesthesia (33,35). During early stages of anoxia, the delta band becomes the prevailing rhythm coinciding with a decrease of approximately 65 to 70 percent of cerebral metabolic rate for oxygen. Slowing of the EEG occurs when the cerebral metabolic rate is decreased by about 30 percent and rapidly deteriorates with further decrease (36). With progressive anoxia, equally as striking as the appearance of the delta wave is the gradual suppression and eventual loss of the beta band. If anoxia is severe and prolonged, electrical silence appears. These two changes—diminution and eventual disappearance of fast wave activity, that is, the beta band, and the simultaneous appearance of the slow wave, or delta, activity—are taken as urgent and absolute indications for a temporary shunt. Depth of anesthesia must be carefully observed lest the EEG become dominated by slow waves (Figure 47-4). Patients with preexisting EEG abnormalities are more vulnerable to reductions in cerebral blood flow than patients with a normal EEG. The severity of blood flow reduction during surgical carotid occlusion is mirrored in the EEG (37,38). The more severe the changes in the EEG, reflecting a greater degree of ischemia, the longer period of time is required for the EEG to return to its preocclusion pattern.

No new postoperative deficit was seen in the EEG that was not predicted by the EEG during operation or immediately following it. Although patients with TIAs may have normal tracings, no prolonged or fixed deficit occurred in our experience without an associated EEG abnormality. The converse, however, apparently is not true; namely, that focal EEG changes in silent areas, the temporal and frontal lobes, have been seen with no recorded fixed deficit detectable in the patient postoperatively. Significant transient or permanent ipsilateral EEG changes occurring suddenly during or immediately after surgery usually indicate thromboembolism from or thrombosis at the endarterectomy site.

Our experience from 1968 to 1983 with continuous EEG monitoring is summarized in Table 47-1 (34). Of 1262 operations for a variety of indications, transient deficits occurred in 36 instances for an incidence of 2.8 percent. Permanent or prolonged but not always severe deficits, but lasting beyond the time of hospital discharge, usually the fourth or fifth postoperative day, occurred in 17 patients for an incidence of 1.3 percent. There were 6 deaths for an incidence of 0.48 percent. Each of these was due to myocardial infarction. None was a primary stroke death.

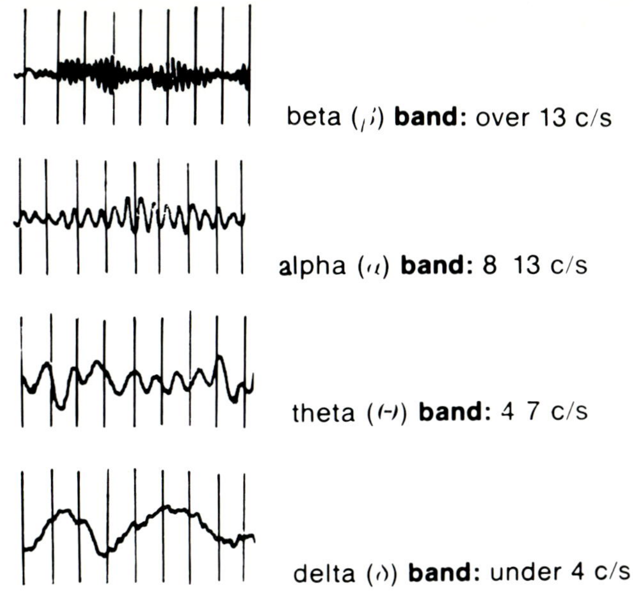

FIGURE 47-2. The four major EEG frequencies. [From Hess (33), by permission of Sandoz Limited.]

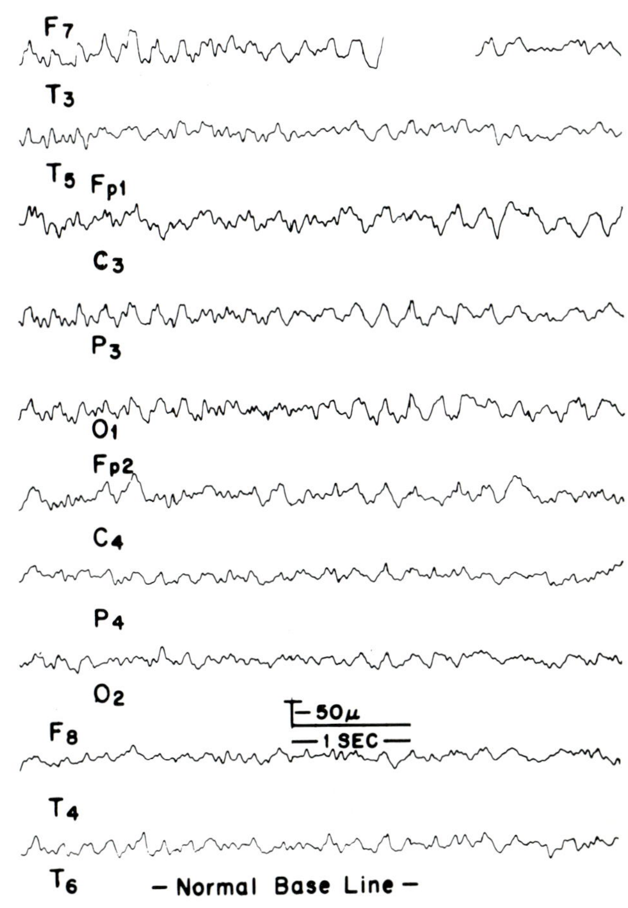

FIGURE 47-3. Normal baseline EEG. [From Callow and O'Donnell (34), by permission of Pitman Books Limited.]

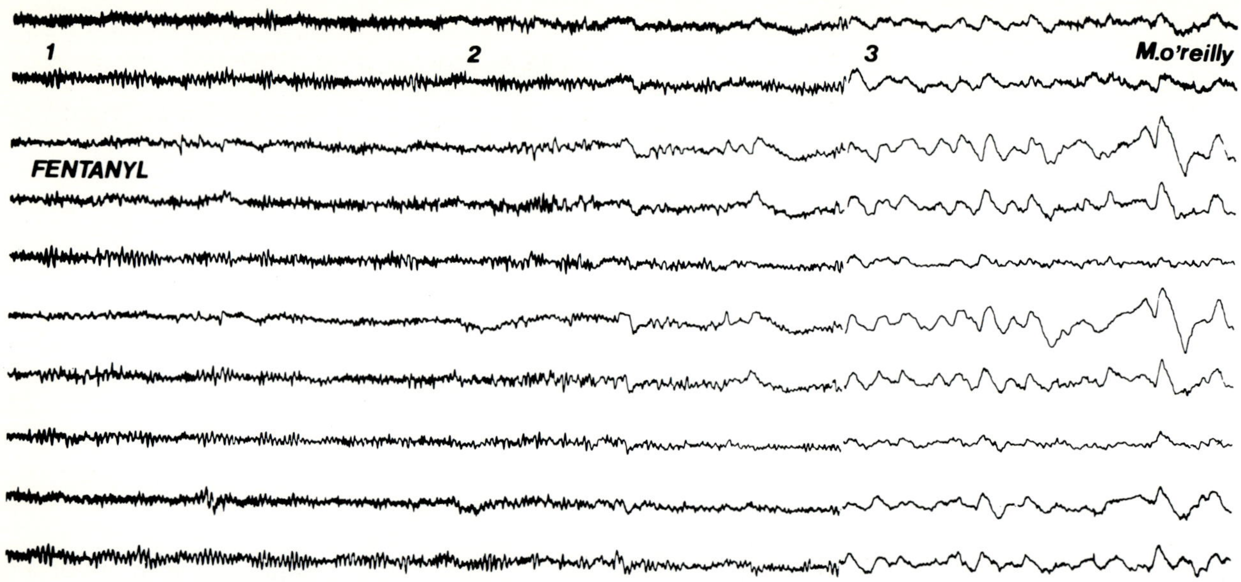

FIGURE 47-4. Suppression of electrical activity, particularly fast wave (point 3), after intravenous injection of fentanyl. (Courtesy of Dr. Allan Callow.)

The EEG provides close correlation between cerebral perfusion and electrical activity (22,26,27,39); provides continuous surveillance of cerebral flow; avoids reliance on a single stump or back pressure measurement; avoids a sense of haste; and provides adequate protection for all patients irrespective of undetected variations in collateral flow, depth of anesthesia, and transient or permanent cardiac malfunction under anesthesia. It is an accurate indicator of cortical ischemia during general anesthesia, provided the depth of anesthesia is closely monitored. Close cooperation between surgeon, anesthesiologist, and electroencephalographer is essential. Its disadvantages, which appear trivial, are added expense and time.

TABLE 47-1. **Carotid Endarterectomies, 1968 to January 1, 1983**

	Deaths		Transient Deficits		Permanent Deficits	
Operations, No.	No.	%	No.	%	No.	%
1262	6*	0.48	36	2.8	17	1.3

SOURCE: Data from Callow and O'Donnell (34).
*All myocardial infarction deaths.

Discussion

In an earlier series from 1958 through 1967 [Table 47-2 (21)] in 266 carotid endarterectomies performed under a variety of techniques including induced hypertension, induced hypercarbia, hypothermia, regional block and local anesthesia, and general anesthesia with selective use of an indwelling shunt based upon stump pressure, note was made of a handful of patients who, despite no detectable postoperative motor or sensory neurologic deficit, had apparently suffered some diminution of higher cortical function. Subtle, usually minimal, changes were noted such as, for example, occasional confusion as to orientation in place and time, mild memory loss, change of mood, and mild personality change. Often these changes were more apparent to

TABLE 47.2. **1958 to 1967 Series of 266 Cartoid Endarterectomies**

		Improved		Unchanged		Worse		Expired	
Type	Operations, No.	No.	%	No.	%	No.	%	No.	%
TIA	216	188	87	21	10	5	2	2	1
Completed	20	2	10	14	70	3	15	1	5
Acute	30	8	26	8	26	8	26	6	20

SOURCE: Data from Callow (21).

family members than to the patient. In an attempt to study the problem, a battery of psychometric tests was adminstered both preoperatively and postoperatively. The incidence of preoperative and postoperative change in performance was so small as to cause discouragement on the part of the investigators. More recently, Archie and Feldtman (40) have assumed that somewhere between 20 and 35 percent of patients operated on without the use of an internal shunt have some degree of cerebral ischemia during the clamp period. The insensitivity of the gross neurologic deficit as an end point plus the short cross-clamp times and prompt reperfusion are offered to explain the infrequency with which a temporary or permanent neurologic deficit is found (21,31). Archie and Feldtman's study indicates that patients undergoing carotid endarterectomy under general anesthesia have a mean ipsilateral collateral cerebral perfusion pressure of 29 mmHg but with a wide and skewed standard deviation. Twenty-five percent had a cerebral perfusion pressure less than 18 mmHg and theoretically are in a high-risk group. The carotid back pressure alone identified only two-thirds of this group. According to Archie and Feldtman, "Clearly, patients with carotid back pressures as high as 40–45 mmHg but with high jugular venous pressures as well may have a perfusion pressure less than 18 mmHg and thereby be at risk for cerebral ischemic injury."

Utilizing xenon-133, Boysen has demonstrated that a regional cerebral blood flow of less than 18 mL/110 g per minute occurs in approximately 20 to 25 percent of patients who undergo carotid endarterectomy. Such low flow is associated with ischemic EEG changes and neurologic deficits (41). Normal regional cerebral blood flow (22,42) is 50 to 55 mL/100 g per minute. Because the autoregulatory lower limit of cerebral perfusion pressure in humans is 50 to 55 mmHg (43), perfusion pressures below 18 mmHg should correlate with flows below 18mL/100 g per minute. Thus, a pressure of 18 mmHg may be the cutoff point for safe perfusion pressure in humans with a normal cerebral vascular bed and a normal hemoglobin and hematocrit. The lower limit of the safe perfusion pressure, however, may be higher than 18 mmHg in a region of the brain with a high vascular resistance and in a region that has lost its autoregulatory ability, as for example, in both instances, in and around a zone of previous infarction. Collateral circulation may be compromised because of a previous stroke, coexisting vertebral basilar insufficiency, severe stenosis or occlusion of the contralateral carotid, intracranial occlusive disease, and congenital anomalies of the circle of Willis. These individuals will require higher perfusion pressures.

A contrary opinion, that neither intraoperative monitoring nor the use of internal shunts is necessary to avoid intraoperative stroke, is expressed by several reviewers (44–47). Ferguson states that the usual cause for stroke is embolization, "Although monitoring provides interesting data, the parameters cited in the literature for ischemic tolerance do not, in fact, correlate with clinically detectable postoperative deficits. This should not be totally unexpected as the situation in carotid endarterectomy is not one of arrest of cerebral circulation but rather a relative reduction in flow" (47). Tolerance will be a function of the extent and duration of the flow reduction (48). "Skillful general anesthesia together with a relatively short occlusion time are sufficient to prevent failure of energy metabolism and irreversible damage" (47).

Consideration of cerebral protection must include not only the technical features of the operation but also the selection of patients. In order to advance understanding of the cerebral protection problem, achieve further reduction of operative morbidity and mortality, and provide for wider acceptance of the operation for patients who may benefit from it, it is urged that standardization of categories of patients be established (8). It is possible to classify patients into risk groups based upon their neurologic status; the coexistence of coronary or other disease, including hypertension and diabetes mellitus; the status of the contralateral carotid artery; the delineation on arteriogram of collateral channels such as anterior and posterior communicating arteries; and the results of contrast computer-assisted tomography to determine the presence of infarcts, whether lacunar or larger, despite what appears clinically to be a classic TIA. Additional risk factors include the history of a previous stroke, the coexistence of vertebral basilar insufficiency symptoms, and the presence as determined by four-vessel arteriography of coexisting vertebral basilar stenotic lesions. Because of this need for large amounts of data—clinical, angiographic, and intraoperative—concerning the several categories of patients, and because of the possible additional risk which is assumed to be present and may be associated with the concept, we do not support nor find justification for recent reports advocating the conduct of carotid endarterectomy without a shunt and with no monitoring support whatsoever. For the same reasons, recommending and performing carotid endarterectomy solely on the basis of noninvasive evaluation, specifically the withholding of angiographic assessment, as has been recently reported, seems unwarranted and unnecessarily hazardous (49). Better to improve one's angiography capability than to accept a less reliable, although safer, substitute.

References

1. Callow AD, O'Donnell TF: EEG monitoring in cerebrovascular surgery. In Bergan JJ, Yao JST (eds): *Cerebrovascular Insufficiency*. New York, Grune & Stratton, 1983, pp 327–341.
2. Sundt TM: Blood flow regulation in normal and ischemic brain. *Curr Concepts* Upjohn Co, 1979.
3. Toole JF, Patel AN: *Cerebrovascular Disorders*. New York, McGraw-Hill, 1967.
4. Abrams HL: *Angiography*, vol 1. Boston, Little, Brown, 1961, p 62.
5. Lassen NA: The luxury-perfusion syndrome and its possible relation to acute metabolic acidosis localized within the brain. Lancet 1966, 2:1113.
6. Wylie EJ, Hein MF, Adams JE: Intracranial hemorrhage following surgical revascularization for treatment of acute strokes. J Neurosurg 1974, 21:212–215.
7. Pressin MS, Hinton RC, Davis KR, Duncan GW, Robertson, GH, Ackerman RH: Mechanisms of acute carotid stroke. Ann Neurol 1979, 6:245–252.

8. Thompson JE: Operative mortality following carotid endarterectomy. Letter to the editor. Stroke 1983, 14:115.
9. Imparato AM, Ramirez A, Riles T, Mintzer R: Cerebral protection in carotid surgery. Arch Surg 1982, 117:1073–1078.
10. Thompson JE, Patman RD, Talkington CM: Carotid surgery for cerebrovascular insufficiency. Curr Probl Surg 1978, 15(12):1–68.
11. Kwann JHM, Peterson GJ, Connolly JE: Stump pressure. An unreliable guide for shunting during carotid endarterectomy. Arch Surg 1980, 115:1083.
12. Hunter GC, Sieffert G, Malone JM, Moore WS: The accuracy of carotid back pressure as an index for shunt requirements. A reappraisal. Stroke 1982, 13:319–326.
13. Rich NM, Hobson RW: Carotid endarterectomy under regional anesthesia. Am Surg 1975, April:253–259.
14. Hobson RW, Wright CB, Sublett JW: Carotid artery back pressure and endarterectomy under regional anesthesia. Arch Surg 1974, 109:682.
15. Hays RJ, Levinson SA, Wylie EJ: Intraoperative measurement of carotid back pressure as a guide to operative management for carotid endarterectomy. Surgery 1972, 953–960.
16. Moore WS, Hall AD: Carotid artery back pressure. Arch Surg 1969, 99:702.
17. Moore WS: Controversy in neurovascular surgery. Letter to the editor. Stroke 1983, 14:115.
18. Gee W: Physiologic principles of ocular pneumoplethysmography. In Bernstein EF (ed): *Noninvasive Diagnostic Techniques in Vascular Disease*. St Louis, CV Mosby, 1978, pp 57–67.
19. Baker JD, Gluecklich B, Watson W, Marcus E, Kamat V, Callow AD: An evaluation of electroencephalographic monitoring for carotid surgery. Surgery 1976, 78:787–794.
20. Matsumoto GH, Baker JD, Watson CW, Gluecklich B, Callow AD: EEG surveillance as a means of extending operability in high risk carotid endarterectomy. Stroke 1976, 7:554–558.
21. Callow AD: An overview of the stroke problem in the carotid territory. Am J Surg 1980, 140:181.
22. Boysen G, Engell HC, Henriksen H: The effect of induced hypertension on internal carotid artery pressure and regional blood flow during temporary carotid clamping for endarterectomy. Neurology 1972, 22:1133.
23. McHenry LC, West JW, Cooper ES, Goldberg HI, Jaffe ME: Cerebral autoregulation in man. Stroke 1974, 5:695–706.
24. Ehrenfeld WK, Hamilton FN, Larson CP: Effect of CO_2 and systemic hypertension on downstream cerebral arterial pressure during carotid endarterectomy. Surgery 1970, 67:87–96.
25. Rowed DW, Vilaghy MI: Intraoperative regional cerebral blood flow during carotid endarterectomy. Can J Neurol Sci 1981, 8:235–241
26. Boysen G: Cerebral hemodynamics in carotid surgery. Acta Neurol Scand 1973, 49 (suppl 52):46.
27. Kelly JJ, Callow AD, O'Donnell TF: Failure of carotid stump pressures. Its incidence as a predictor for a temporary shunt during carotid endarterectomy. Arch Surg 1979, 114:1361–1366.
28. Kwann JHM, Peterson GJ, Connolly JE: Stump pressure. An unreliable guide for shunting during carotid endarterectomy. Arch Surg 1980, 115:1083–1085.
29. Callow AD: The Leriche Memorial Lecture. Fact or fancy: A twenty year personal perspective on the detection and management of carotid occlusive disease. J Cardiovasc Surg 1980, 21:641–658.
30. Lees CD, Hertzer NR: Postoperative stroke and late neurologic complications after carotid endarterectomy. Arch Surg 1981, 116:1561–1568.
31. Rampil IJ, Holzer JA, Quest DO, Rosenbaum SH, Correll JW: Prognostic value of computerized EEG analysis during carotid endarterectomy. Anesth Analg 1983, 62:186–192.
32. Westmoreland BF: Normal and benign EEG patterns. Am J EEG Tech 1982, 22:3.
33. Hess R: *EEG Handbook* (Sandoz Monographs). EEG Laboratory of University Hospital. Zurich, Sandoz Limited, 1966.
34. Callow AD, O'Donnell TF: The detection of cerebral ischemia during carotid endarterectomy by continuous electroencephalographic monitoring. In Greenhalgh RM (ed): *Progress in Stroke Research, 2*. London, Pitman Books Limited, 1983.
35. Spehlman R: *EEG Primer*. Amsterdam, Elsevier/North-Holland Biomedical Press, 1981.
36. Constant S: Understanding hypoxia and its effects on the EEG recordings. Am J EEG Tech 1982, 22:33.
37. Sundt TM, Sharbrough FW, Piepgras DG: The significance of cerebral blood flow measurements during carotid endarterectomy. In Bergan JJ, Yao JST (eds): *Cerebrovascular Insufficiency*. New York, Grune & Stratton, 1983, pp 287–307.
38. Sundt TM, Sharbrough FW, Piepgras DG: Correlation of cerebral blood flow and electroencephalographic changes during carotid endarterectomy with results of surgery and hemodynamics of cerebral ischemia. Mayo Clin Proc 1981, 56:533–543.
39. Sharbrough FW, Messick JM, Sundt TM: Correlation of continuous electroencephalograms with cerebral blood flow measurements during carotid endarterectomy. Stroke 1983, 4:674.
40. Archie JP, Feldtman RW: Determinants of cerebral perfusion pressure during carotid endarterectomy. Arch Surg 1982, 117:319–322.
41. Boysen G, Engell HC, Pistolese GR: On the critical lower level of cerebral blood flow in man with particular reference to carotid surgery. Circulation 1974, 49:1023.
42. Boysen G, Ladegaard-Pedersen HJ, Engell HC: Cerebral blood flow studies during carotid surgery. In Brock M, Fieschi C, Ingvar DH (eds): *Cerebral Blood Flow*. New York, Springer-Verlag, 1969, p 155.
43. Fieschi C, Angoli A, Battistina N: Derangement of regional cerebral blood flow and its regulatory mechanisms in acute cerebrovascular lesions. Neurology 1968, 18:1166.
44. Rosenthal D, Stanton PE, Lamis PA: Carotid endarterectomy. The unreliability of intraoperative monitoring in patients having had stroke or reversible ischemic neurologic deficit. Arch Surg 1981, 166:1569–1575.
45. Whitney DG, Kahn EM, Estes JW: Carotid artery surgery without a temporary indwelling shunt. Arch Surg 1980, 115:1393–1399.
46. Baker WH, Dorner DB, Barnes RW: Carotid endarterectomy: Is an indwelling shunt necessary? Surgery 1977, 82:321–326.
47. Ferguson GG: Intra-operative monitoring and internal shunts: Are they necessary in carotid endarterectomy? Editorial. Stroke 1982, 13:287–289.
48. Astrup J, Siesjo BK, Symon L: Thresholds in cerebral ischemia—the ischemic penumbra. Stroke 1981, 12:723–725.
49. Sandmann W: Carotid artery surgery without angiography: Risk or progress? In Greenhalgh RM (ed): *Progress in Stroke Research, 2*. London, Pitman Books Limited, 1983.

Chapter 48

INTRAOPERATIVE ASSESSMENT OF CAROTID ENDARTERECTOMY AND RECURRENT CAROTID STENOSIS

R. EUGENE ZIERLER

Intraoperative Assessment of Carotid Endarterectomy

The major determinants of morbidity and mortality in carotid endarterectomy are patient selection, timing of operative treatment, and technical aspects of the procedure. In general, neurologic complications result from either inadequate cerebral blood flow or embolization. The factors that contribute to neurologic complications are listed in Table 48-1. These factors are all related, at least in part, to surgical technique. The presence of a large intimal flap, residual atherosclerotic plaque, or suture stenosis is an unacceptable technical result which can be safely corrected only if it is recognized immediately. Since a postoperative neurologic deficit may be permanent even when technical errors are later identified and corrected, it is not sufficient to wait until the patient is awake to assess the result of surgery. The detection of technical problems before neurologic sequelae develop requires the use of intraoperative methods to assess the technical adequacy of the arterial reconstruction.

TABLE 48-1. Factors Contributing to Neurologic Complications after Carotid Endarterectomy

Inadequate cerebral blood flow:
Failure to use a shunt
Shunt thrombosis
Intimal flap
Residual atherosclerotic plaque
Clamp injury
Suture stenosis
Internal carotid artery spasm
Embolization:
Excessive manipulation of the diseased artery
Shunt emboli

Visual inspection and palpation of the carotid bifurcation are highly subjective and are not sufficient for the detection of technical errors. More reliable methods for intraoperative assessment are based on either some type of anatomic imaging or flow detection.

IMAGING TECHNIQUES

Operative Arteriography

Operative arteriography is the standard method for identifying technical errors during both peripheral arterial reconstruction (1,2) and carotid endarterectomy (3–5). Although completion arteriography is commonly performed after vascular operations in the lower extremities, the similar practice of operative arteriography after carotid endarterectomy has not been widely adopted. The reluctance to perform routine operative arteriography is related to inexperience with the technique, lack of suitable equipment and personnel, concern over prolonging the operation, and the potential complications.

TECHNIQUE. The patient should be positioned on an operating table that will accept an x-ray cassette placed directly below the head and neck. A scout film is taken to assure proper placement and exposure of the film. After completion of the endarterectomy and restoration of arterial flow, all retractors and vessels loops are removed to allow the artery to assume its natural configuration. A 19-gauge "butterfly"-type needle is attached to one end of a length of intravenous infusion tubing, and the other end is connected to a syringe filled with heparinized Ringer's lactate or saline solution. The needle is inserted into the common carotid artery proximal to the arteriotomy. Although the needle can be inserted with the point directed either proximally or distally, the proximal orientation helps to assure adequate mixing of the injected contrast material. Retention of the needle within the artery is facilitated by the wings on the needle, clamping the tubing to a surrounding drape, and bending the needle slightly approximately 1.5 cm from its tip. Throughout the procedure extreme care must be taken to remove all air bubbles from the system and avoid air embolism.

The position of the needle is confirmed by aspirating arterial blood, and a syringe filled with 60% methylglucamine iothalamate (Conray 60) is attached to the infusion tubing. Methylglucamine solutions have been advocated as the contrast media of choice for cerebral angiography since they are less toxic than the sodium compounds (6). The operative field is covered with a sterile plastic sheet, and the x-ray machine is moved into position. Standing behind a sterile-draped x-ray shield, the sur-

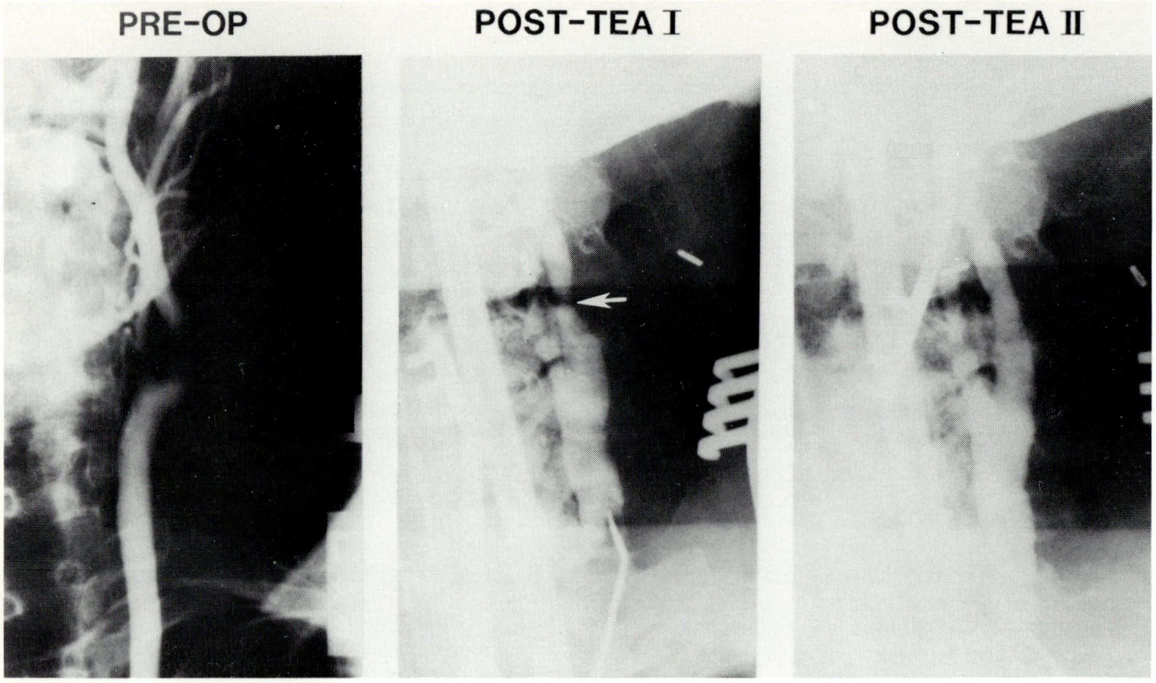

FIGURE 48-1. Sequence of arteriograms illustrating the management of a technical error. The preoperative internal carotid stenosis is shown on the left. The initial operative arteriogram (Post-TEA I) shows a stenosis at the distal end of the arteriotomy closure (*white arrow*). A repeat operative arteriogram after patch angioplasty (Post-TEA II) shows a widely patent internal carotid artery.

geon injects the contrast material as rapidly as possible, and the film is exposed as the injection proceeds after a volume of 12 to 15 mL has been infused. A 6-0 polypropylene suture is placed in the adventitia around the needle and is tied down as the needle is removed. The film is developed immediately and can be available for review within 3 to 5 minutes.

Results. The surgeon's interpretation of the operative arteriogram is always somewhat subjective, and immediate repair is not considered necessary for every arteriographic defect. For example, in the study by Zierler and associates (7), abnormalities were noted in 23 of 150 operative arteriograms (15 percent); however, only 10 (7 percent) of the arteriographic abnormalities were surgically repaired. In general, the technical result should be considered unacceptable if the operative arteriogram shows complete occlusion or greater than 30 percent stenosis of any carotid bifurcation vessel, intraluminal thrombus, residual atherosclerotic plaque, or intimal flap. These problems are most likely to occur at the distal extent of the endarterectomy in the internal and external carotid arteries. Correction of defects in the internal carotid usually requires opening the arteriotomy and reinserting the shunt if one was originally used; most external carotid defects can be repaired without occluding the internal carotid by clamping the origin of the external and making a small, separate arteriotomy. The arteriographic appearance of a luminal defect facilitates the surgical repair by indicating whether tacking of an intimal flap, additional endarterectomy, patch angioplasty, or removal of thrombus will be necessary. An arteriographic finding which has rarely been mentioned is spasm of the internal carotid artery. Spasm was identified by Lye and coworkers in approximately 10 percent of operative arteriograms (8). The severity of spasm varied considerably, and it usually involved the internal carotid distal to the area of operative exposure. Although this is probably a transient event in most cases, extremely severe spasm may be associated with postoperative internal carotid occlusion.

In the case illustrated in Figure 48-1, the initial operative arteriogram (Post-TEA I) shows a stenotic lesion at the distal end of the arteriotomy closure. A patch angioplasty was performed, and a repeat operative arteriogram (Post-TEA II) shows a widely patent internal carotid artery. Figure 48-2 is an example of a normal operative arteriogram; there is some irregularity of the luminal surface in the endarterectomized segment, but there is no evidence of intimal flap, stenosis, thrombus, or plaque.

In 1967, Blaisdell and associates reported a 25 percent incidence of unacceptable technical results in a series of operative arteriograms obtained during 100 carotid endarterectomies (5). As shown in Table 48-2, subsequent studies based on operative arteriography have indicated an incidence of unacceptable defects between 5 and 10 percent (3,4,7,9,10). This probably represents the minimum incidence of technical errors that can be expected by experienced surgeons performing carotid endarterectomy. The arteriographic defects occur with approximately equal frequency in the internal and external carotid arteries; the common carotid is rarely involved.

The risk of operative arteriography is associated mainly with the injection of contrast material and includes subintimal injec-

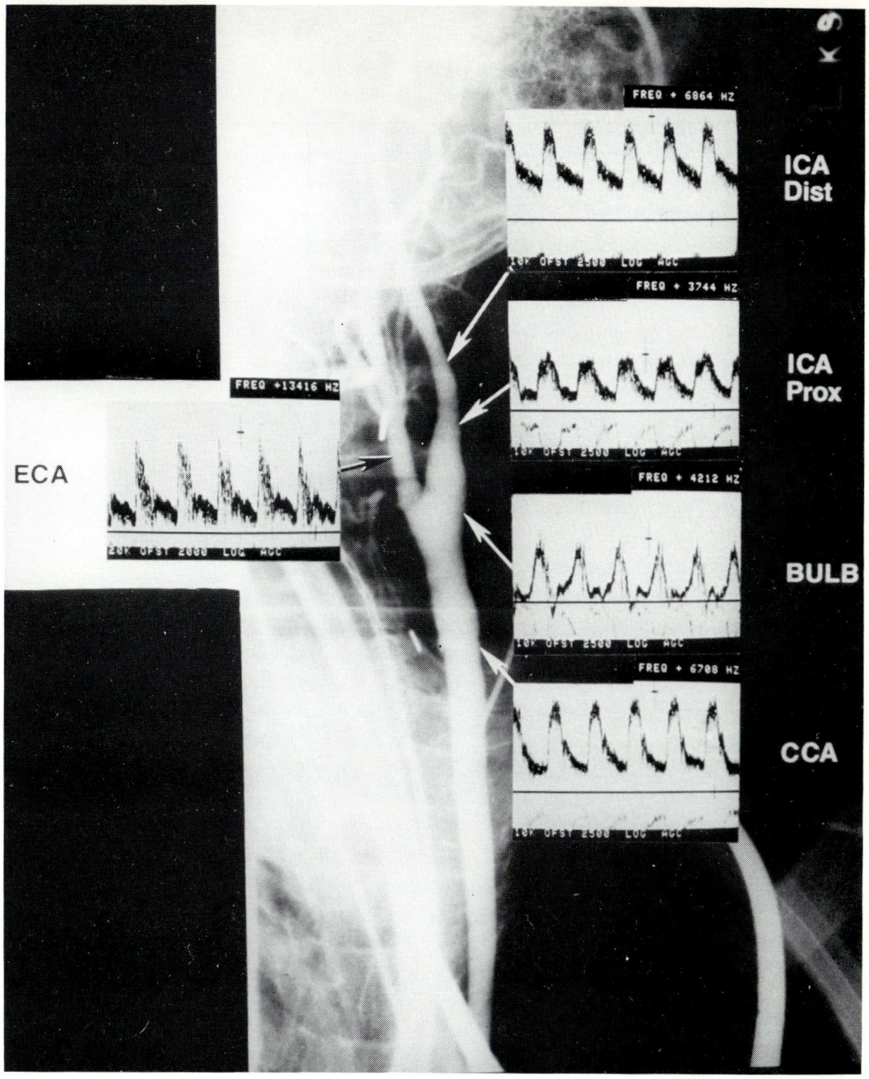

FIGURE 48-2. This normal operative arteriogram shows some irregularity of the endarterectomized segment but no evidence of intimal flap, stenosis, or plaque. The corresponding spectra obtained with a 20-MHz pulsed Doppler show a narrow band of frequencies with a "clear area" under the systolic peak. [From Zierler, Roederer, and Strandness (31), by permission of Grune and Stratton, Inc.]

tion, embolization, and allergic reaction. Although these complications are extremely uncommon, their occurrence has discouraged some surgeons from performing routine operative arteriography (4,11). A selective approach to operative arteriography has been advocated in which arteriograms are obtained only when the endarterectomy has been difficult and a technical error is suspected (4). Whenever operative arteriography is performed, it is absolutely essential to have an experienced radiology technologist and to make sure that the entire surgical team understands the procedure. If the proper equipment and personnel are readily available, operative arteriography can be performed rapidly and with a very low risk of complications (7,10).

TABLE 48-2. Incidence of Unacceptable Technical Results during Carotid Endarterectomy Based on Operative Arteriography

		Site of Defect			
Author (Ref.)	Number of Operations, *n*	Internal Carotid, %	External Carotid, %	Common Carotid, %	Total, %
Andersen (4)	131	1.5	2.3	1.5	5.3
Blaisdell (5)	100	—	—	—	25
Hobson (9)	50	4	6	—	10
Larson (10)	457	3.9	3.1	1.1	8.1
Rosental (3)	260	3	4	1	8
Zierler (7)	150	5	2	—	7

B-Mode Scanning

The technique of anatomic imaging with B-mode ultrasound has been successfully applied to the diagnosis of a variety of vascular and nonvascular diseases (12). B-mode scanning has also been used intraoperatively during biliary, pancreatic, and vascular surgical procedures (13–15). When used for the intraoperative assessment of carotid endarterectomy, B-mode scanning avoids many of the risks associated with operative arteriography.

TECHNIQUE. The B-mode instrument is a compact small-parts scanner with a hand-held probe that is gas-sterilized and connected to the main ultrasound unit by a flexible cable (16). Either a 7.5- or a 10-MHz imaging frequency may be used. Acoustic coupling is achieved by filling the operative incision with warm saline solution. The available scan angles are limited by the size of the incision; however, both transverse and longitudinal images can usually be obtained. The real-time B-mode images are viewed on a television monitor, and they can be recorded for later review on videotape or Polaroid film.

RESULTS. The criteria for determining the significance of a defect seen on the B-mode image are subjective and depend on the experience of the examiner. An experimental study by Coelho and associates showed that B-mode ultrasound was highly accurate in the detection of intimal flaps, strictures, and thrombi (17). The challenge is to decide which intravascular defects require immediate surgical correction. This decision must be based on the size, type, and location of the defect. Flanigan and coworkers (16) used high-resolution B-mode scanning to examine 48 carotid arteries after endarterectomy and noted defects in 13 (27 percent). However, only 2 of these 13 defects (4 percent) were considered severe enough to require repair, and all 13 patients had uneventful postoperative courses. In a similar study by Lane and Appleberg (18), B-mode scanning showed defects in 9 of 60 carotid arteries (15 percent), but only 3 (5 percent) of the defects were corrected. It should be noted that the incidence of defects requiring immediate repair in these studies is similar to the incidence of unacceptable technical results found on operative arteriography.

The main disadvantages of intraoperative B-mode scanning are the relatively high equipment costs, the need for the surgeon to learn a new technique, and the inability to evaluate arterial segments beyond the edges of the operative incision. Another limitation of B-mode scanning is that it does not differentiate between fresh thrombus and flowing blood (19), so a completely thrombosed artery may appear patent on B-mode scan. This error is easily avoided by using some method for flow detection (7,14). The advantages of intraoperative B-mode scanning are its high accuracy when used by an experienced examiner and the opportunity to avoid exposing the patient to the risk of operative arteriography.

Vascular Endoscopy

Endoscopic techniques have been used during biliary surgery (20), urologic procedures (21), and vascular reconstructions (22–24). Towne and Bernhard used a rigid choledochoscope and arthroscope to evaluate the technical results of 42 carotid endarterectomies prior to completion of the arteriotomy closure (22). Atheromatous shreds capable of embolizing were found in 2 internal carotid arteries (5 percent), and 17 external carotids (40 percent) had elevated distal intimal flaps. The endoscopic examination required only a few minutes and was not associated with any significant morbidity.

For surgeons who are experienced with the technique and have access to the proper equipment, vascular endoscopy is an alternative to operative arteriography for the assessment of carotid endarterectomy. The only disadvantage of the endoscopic technique is that the examination cannot be performed after the arteriotomy is closed and the flow restored. While this may be a minor drawback, an optimal method for intraoperative assessment is one that can be used on the completed arterial reconstruciton under physiologic conditions of pressure and flow.

FLOW DETECTION

A major limitation of operative arteriography and the other imaging techniques is that they provide no direct information on the rate or pattern of flow in the endarterectomized vessel. Since the success of carotid endarterectomy ultimately depends on the adequacy of blood flow in the carotid system, techniques that detect flow are potentially useful methods for intraoperative assessment.

Electromagnetic Flowmeter

Although the electromagnetic flowmeter has been used to assess both peripheral artery reconstruction (25) and carotid endarterectomy (9,26), the technique has not gained wide acceptance. Hobson and coworkers measured internal carotid blood flow before and after 25 endarterectomies performed under regional anesthesia (9). The mean flow was 126 $\pm$ 17 mL/min before endarterectomy and 159 $\pm$ 15 mL/min after endarterectomy; however, this increase in flow was not statistically significant ($p > 0.1$). While improvement in flow rates did occur in some patients, particulary those with severe preoperative carotid stenoses, this technique was not discriminating enough to establish a minimally acceptable increase in flow for carotid endarterectomy. The explanation for this observation is that a stenosis of approximately 75 percent area reduction (50 percent diameter reduction) or greater is necessary before a measurable drop in flow rate will occur in the internal carotid artery (27). Since many surgically correctable lesions produce less than this critical degree of stenosis, measurement of flow rates is not suitable for the routine intraoperative assessment of carotid endarterectomy.

Continuous-Wave Doppler Ultrasound

The intraoperative assessment methods which utilize a continuous-wave Doppler instrument are the supraorbital Doppler examination and audible interpretation of signals from the reconstructed arterial segment (28–30). The supraorbital Doppler examination is only capable of detecting lesions which reduce pressure and flow in the carotid system, and false-positive results may occur in patients with ophthalmic artery occlusion (28). Consequently, this technique is of limited value in the intraoperative assessment of carotid endarterectomy.

A gas-sterilized Doppler probe can be brought into the operative field and acoustically coupled to the outer surface of a vessel with a small amount of blood or saline solution. By listening to the quality of the Doppler signal, the experienced examiner can learn to recognize the normal arterial flow pattern and the harsh, high-frequency flow pattern associated with stenotic lesions. Keitzer and associates used this technique to assess 93 peripheral vascular reconstructions and compared the results to 49 operations performed without using the intraoperative Doppler (30). Reoperation was necessary in 31 percent of the patients in the latter group, but only 9 percent of the patients in the former group. Both the reoperation and death rates were significantly lower for those patients who had the benefit of intraoperative Doppler assessment. Barnes and Garrett used audible interpretation of continuous-wave Dopper signals to assess the results of 42 carotid endarterectomies (28). All the internal carotid signals were considered normal; however, obstructive signals were noted in three external carotid arteries. In these three cases, the external carotid lesion was repaired and a satisfactory result confirmed by repeat Doppler examination. The audible interpretation of continuous-wave Doppler signals is extremely subjective and depends primarily on major frequency shifts to indicate the presence of a stenotic lesion. The main advantages of the technique are that it is simple to perform, does not prolong the operation, and requires relatively inexpensive equipment.

Pulsed Doppler Ultrasound and Spectral Analysis

The use of a pulsed Doppler instrument and signal processing by spectral analysis can provide more objective, quantitative data than is possible with the continuous-wave technique already described (31). Unlike the continuous-wave Doppler which examines an entire vessel, a pulsed Doppler detects blood flow at a discrete site referred to as the ''sample volume.'' Positioning the sample volume in the center of the arterial stream avoids the velocity gradients adjacent to the vessel wall and provides a signal which is better suited for spectral analysis than that from a continuous-wave device. A spectrum analyzer displays the entire frequency and amplitude content of the Doppler signal. Various characteristics of the center stream Doppler spectrum have been correlated with the severity of carotid artery disease (31,32). A widening of the frequency band, or ''spectral broadening,'' occurs when arterial lesions disrupt the normal laminar flow pattern and produce a state of disturbed flow. An increase in peak systolic frequency with spectral broadening reflects the increased flow velocity and turbulence associated with a high-grade stenosis.

A direction-sensitive 20-MHz pulsed Doppler has been designed specifically for intraoperative use (7,31,33). The probe for this instrument consists of a small ultrasonic transducer mounted on the end of a 16-gauge needle, and the sample volume is approximately 0.2 mm^3. During the examination, the transducer is placed directly on the outer surface of the artery, and the sample volume is positioned in the center of the flow stream. The Doppler spectra are visually monitored with a real-time spectrum analyzer. Zierler and associates used this technique and routine operative arteriography to assess the results of 50 carotid endarterectomies (7). Comparison of internal carotid spectra before and after endarterectomy showed improvement of the flow pattern in the majority of cases. Flow disturbances consistent with technical errors were noted in seven internal carotids, and in two of these cases operative arteriography showed defects which required immediate repair. No other technical errors were encountered, and there was no neurologic morbidity or mortality in any patient studied. Figure 48-2 is an example of normal postendarterectomy spectra and the corresponding operative arteriogram. At each site in the common and internal carotid arteries, the spectrum shows a narrow band of frequencies with a ''clear area'' under the systolic peak. The intraoperative spectra for the arteriograms shown in Figure 48-1 are given in Figure 48-3. The spectrum prior to endarterectomy (Pre-TEA) shows spectral broadening and increased frequencies in the distal internal carotid artery. The initial examination after endarterectomy (Post-TEA I) is essentially unchanged, and the operative arteriogram confirms the presence of a stenotic lesion. After a patch angioplasty, the internal carotid spectrum is improved (Post-TEA II), although a minor degree of spectral broadening persists.

Intraoperative assessment with pulsed Doppler and spectral analysis is a sensitive method for detecting technical errors. Since the examination can be performed rapidly with no inherent risk, it may be valuable in selecting those patients who are most likely to benefit from operative arteriography. The technique has the characteristics of an ideal screening test—no false-negative results and a high negative predictive value—and the occurrence of some false-positive assessments is not a serious disadvantage. Although pulsed Doppler with spectral analysis permits a more detailed assessment than is possible with continuous-wave Doppler and audible interpretation, the method is still somewhat subjective. As with many of the other intraoperative assessment techniques, there is a ''learning curve,'' and the proper acquisition and interpretation of pulsed Doppler data require considerable experience.

CONCLUSIONS

Anatomic imaging and physiologic flow detection techniques for intraoperative assessment are actually complementary, since they examine different aspects of the completed carotid endarterectomy. For example, combining one of the Doppler techniques with B-mode scanning or operative arteriography provides information on both blood flow and the configuration of the arterial wall. Because the incidence of technical errors requiring immediate correction is low and neurologic complications are relatively uncommon after carotid endarterectomy, the practical value of intraoperative assessment is difficult to prove. Even the absence of a postoperative neurologic deficit does not necessarily mean that a satisfactory technical result has been obtained (3). Still, technical errors which could potentially cause thrombosis or embolism are clearly undesirable, and every reasonable effort should be made to achieve the best possible result during the initial procedure. Therefore, the routine use of intraoperative assessment techniques is justified if they are safe and result in the correction of technical errors which could lead to neurologic complications.

The performance of carotid endarterectomy can be recommended only if the perioperative mortality and morbidity rates are extremely low; operative mortality should be less than 1 percent, and the incidence of neurologic complications should not exceed 4 percent (34). Since the difference between acceptable and unacceptable complication rates is small, the identification of technical errors in only a few percent of operations should be considered beneficial. Operative arteriography is clearly

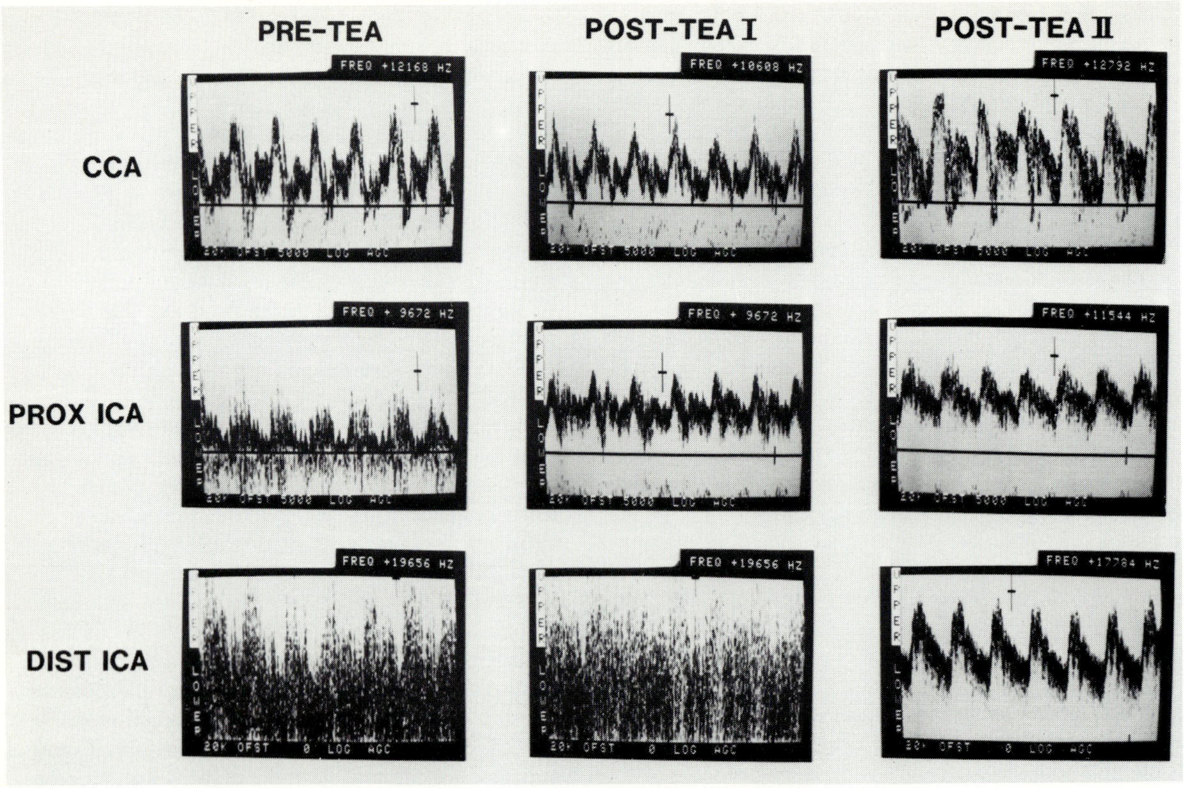

FIGURE 48-3. 20-MHz pulsed Doppler specta corresponding to the arteriograms in Figure 48-1. Before endarterectomy (Pre-TEA) there is marked spectral broadening and increased frequencies in the distal internal carotid (Dist-ICA). The initial examination after endarterectomy (Post-TEA I) is unchanged, but after a patch angioplasty the internal carotid spectrum is improved (Post-TEA II).

the standard method for intraoperative assessment, and it can be safely used for the routine evaluation of carotid endarterectomy (3,5,7,8,10). If operative arteriography is to be applied selectively, one of the less invasive methods such as continuous-wave or pulsed Doppler could be used as a screening tool. Continuous-wave Doppler has the advantages of simplicity and availability. It must be emphasized, however, that all the assessment techniques described are somewhat subjective and need to be interpreted by the operating surgeon. The safety and accuracy of a particular method should increase with experience. Intraoperative assessment is particularly important for documenting the technical result of operations performed on a teaching service. The routine use of intraoperative assessment techniques is a constant reminder of the need for meticulous surgical technique in carotid endarterectomy.

Recurrent Carotid Stenosis

Stenosis of the carotid artery after endarterectomy can theoretically result from a variety of technical and biologic factors. The technical factors that may contribute to recurrent stenosis include vascular clamp injury, incomplete removal of plaques, intimal flaps, and suturing faults. Proliferation of cells in the arterial wall and reaccumulation of atherosclerotic plaque are biologic processes that could contribute to the formation of stenotic lesions. As discussed in the preceding section, the incidence of significant technical errors is low in carotid endarterectomy, particularly when intraoperative methods are used to assess the surgical result. Consequently, technical errors are probably not a major cause of recurrent carotid stenosis (35,36). The problem with much of the available data on stenosis following carotid endarterectomy is that it is based predominantly on those patients having arteriography for recurrent neurologic symptoms. Since arteriography is an invasive procedure which is generally indicated only for the evaluation of symptomatic patients, the majority of patients who remain asymptomatic are excluded from study. Thus, it is possible that the incidence of recurrent carotid stenosis has been underestimated. More representative data would be obtained by serial follow-up of an unselected series of patients after carotid endarterectomy. Some of the recently developed noninvasive testing methods are capable of detecting carotid artery stenosis with a high degree of accuracy and are ideally suited for this type of study. Therefore, whenever recurrent carotid stenosis is considered, a clear distinction must be made between those lesions that are asymptomatic and those lesions that are only evident on invasive or noninvasive tests.

TABLE 48-3. Incidence of Recurrent Carotid Stenosis in Studies Based Primarily on Patients with Recurrent Neurologic Symptoms

Author (Ref.)	Number of Operations, *n*	Incidence of Stenosis, %	Time Interval to Stenosis: 2–24 mo, %	Time Interval to Stenosis: > 2 yr, %
Cossman (36)	361	3.6	100	—
Hertzer (37)	1250	1.3	56	44
Stoney (38)	1654	1.5	35	65

INCIDENCE OF RECURRENT CAROTID STENOSIS

The incidence of recurrent carotid stenosis in studies based primarily on patients presenting with recurrent neurologic symptoms is between 1 and 4 percent (Table 48-3) (36–38). Stenosis at the site of a previous carotid endarterectomy may also be discovered when a patient is being evaluated for disease of the contralateral carotid artery. Although a midcervical bruit is often associated with carotid artery stenosis prior to endarterectomy, it is generally not considered to be a reliable sign of recurrent stenosis (39). Bruits over the carotid bifurcation are relatively common postoperatively and are probably related to scarring and other changes in the wall of the endarterectomized segment that produce turbulent flow. A bruit is more likely to be significant if its quality changes suddenly, it disappears completely, or it is associated with recurrent symptoms. Noninvasive tests should be used to determine the hemodynamic significance of postoperative cervical bruits; arteriography can then be considered when the noninvasive tests are positive.

When noninvasive tests are used to examine patients after carotid endarterectomy, the incidence of recurrent stenosis is considerably higher than estimates based on symptomatic patients (Table 48-4). While the incidence of symptomatic recurrent stenosis is less than 5 percent, the total incidence by noninvasive testing is between 9 and 19 percent (35,40–44). One reason for this wide variation in results is the different methods and criteria used for the noninvasive evaluation of carotid stenosis. Some studies rely on direct tests such as Duplex scanning (35) or ultrasonic arteriography (43), and other studies use indirect tests like the supraorbital Doppler examination or oculoplethysmography (42,44). A few reports are based on combinations of direct and indirect noninvasive tests (40,41). The diagnostic accuracy of noninvasive testing depends not only on the method chosen, but also on the skill of the examiner and the specific criteria used to interpret the results. Some of the studies listed in Table 48-4 only reported stenoses severe enough to reduce pressure and flow (35,42,44), while others included lesser degrees of stenosis (40,41). The accuracy of noninvasive testing for recurrent carotid stenosis was evaluated by Roederer and associates (45). In their study, Duplex scanning with spectral analysis was compared to carotid arteriography and found to be 94 percent accurate in detecting stenoses of 50 percent or greater diameter reduction and total internal carotid occlusions.

It should be pointed out that the majority of studies listed in Table 48-4 did not include serial follow-up of individual patients after carotid endarterectomy. In the group of patients examined by Duplex scanning (35), serial tests indicated that some high-grade stenoses initially noted in the early postoperative period became less severe during follow-up. This observation is consistent with the formation and regression or remodeling of proliferative myointimal lesions. Thus, the postoperative carotid artery is a dynamic structure, and a single examination may not provide complete follow-up data.

TABLE 48-4. Incidence of Recurrent Carotid Stenosis in Studies Using Noninvasive Tests

Author (Ref.)	Number of Operations, *n*	Testing Method(s)	Total Incidence of Stenosis, %	Incidence of Symptomatic Stenosis, %
Baker (40)	133	SOD, OPG-K, CPA, Direct Doppler	10*	3.0†
Cantelmo (41)	199	OPG-K, CPA, UA	12	4.5
Kremen (42)	173	OPG-G	10	1.7
Salvian (44)	105	OPG-G	11	4.8
Turnipseed (43)	80	UA	9	2.5
Zierler (35)	89	Duplex scan	19	4.5

*Excludes patients with an abnormal result on the initial examination.

†Includes patients operated on for symptomatic recurrent stenosis.

SOD: Supraorbital Doppler examination; OPG-K: Kartchner oculoplethysmography; CPA: carotid phonoangiography; UA: ultrasonic arteriography (Doppler imaging); OPG-G: Gee oculoplethysmography.

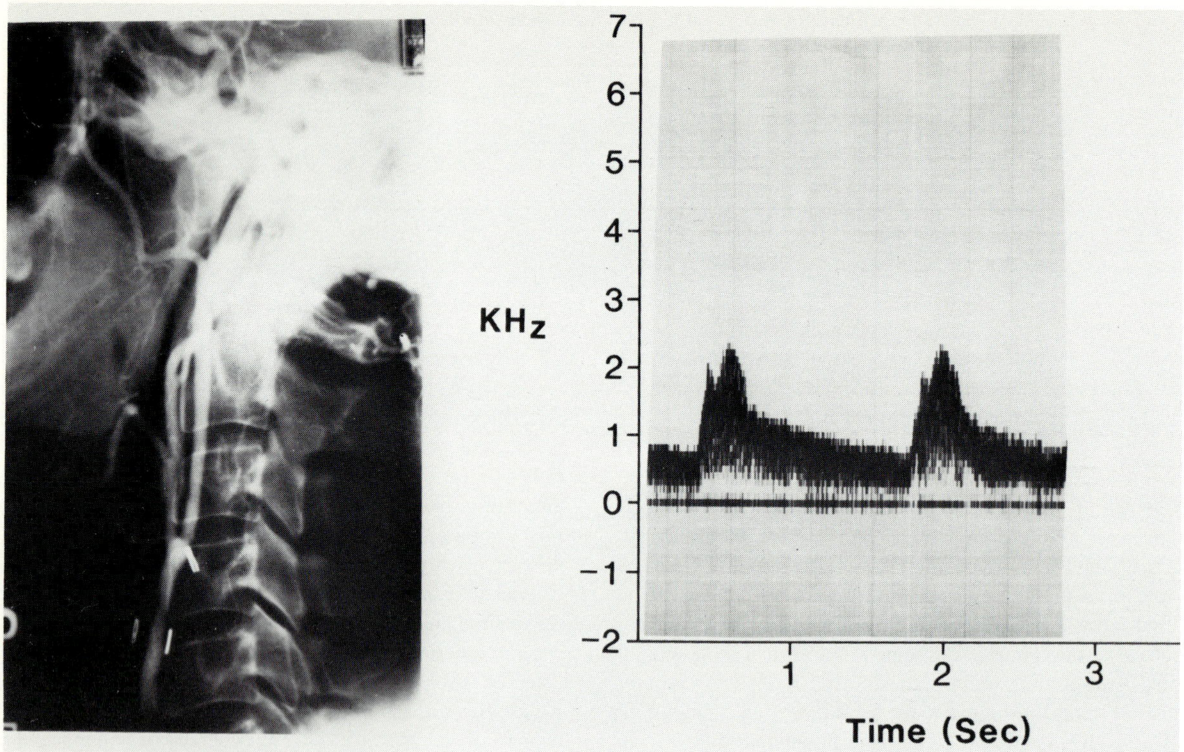

FIGURE 48-4. Arteriogram of left carotid artery 7 months after endarterectomy shows some irregularity of the common carotid and filling in of the carotid bulb without significant stenosis. The internal carotid spectrum shows normal peak frequency, but spectral broadening is present. [From Zierler, Bandyk, Thiele, and Strandness (35), by permission of Archives of Surgery.]

ARTERIOGRAPHIC STUDIES

The changes documented by serial Duplex scanning are consistent with two arteriographic studies that showed improvement in early postoperative carotid lesions (46,47). Arteriographic features of the early postoperative carotid bifurcation include a filling in of the carotid bulb, minor irregularities of the endarterectomized segment, and smooth stenoses involving the distal common and proximal internal carotid arteries (35). The irregular plaques and focal stenoses characteristic of atherosclerotic lesions are usually absent. These observations support the conclusion that the lesion of early recurrent stenosis is a distinct entity. Figures 48-4 and 48-5 are examples of postoperative arteriograms and corresponding internal carotid spectra obtained with the Duplex scanner. In Figure 48-4, there is some irregularity of the common carotid and filling in of the carotid bulb without significant stenosis. A recurrent internal carotid stenosis 7 months after endarterectomy is shown in Figure 48-5.

The recently developed technique of digital subtraction arteriography (DSA) has also been applied to the postoperative carotid artery. Acher and coworkers compared the results of DSA and noninvasive testing (Doppler imaging) after 49 carotid endarterectomies (48). DSA of the carotid bifurcation was normal in 45 cases (92 percent); however, significant lesions were identified in two internal carotids (4 percent) and two external carotids (4 percent). Although serial follow-up was not given for the surgically treated arteries, this study also showed that noninvasive testing was comparable to DSA for the detection of significant recurrent stenoses. Hertzer and associates performed DSA after 255 carotid endarterectomies prior to discharge from hospital (49). Approximately 94 percent of the internal carotids and 93 percent of the external carotids were considered normal. Minor defects were noted in 3.6 percent of the internal carotids, while significant internal carotid stenosis or occlusion were observed in 0.8 and 1.9 percent, respectively. The results of postoperative DSA are similar to the previously discussed incidence of unacceptable defects on operative arteriography. This is further evidence that technical errors are relatively uncommon after carotid endarterectomy and that they are not responsible for the majority of recurrent carotid stenoses.

PATHOLOGY

The healing process in the arterial wall after carotid endarterectomy was studied in a canine model by Dirrenberger and Sundt (50). Immediately after restoration of flow, a fibrin-platelet layer formed on the endarterectomized surface. This layer was initially covered by a typical thrombus, however by 48 hours after operation active thrombus formation had ceased and reendothelialization was noted. At 1 week most of the mural thrombus had disappeared, and reendothelialization was complete by 3 months after surgery. The formation of mural thrombus was significantly reduced by intraoperative heparinization. French and Rewcastle

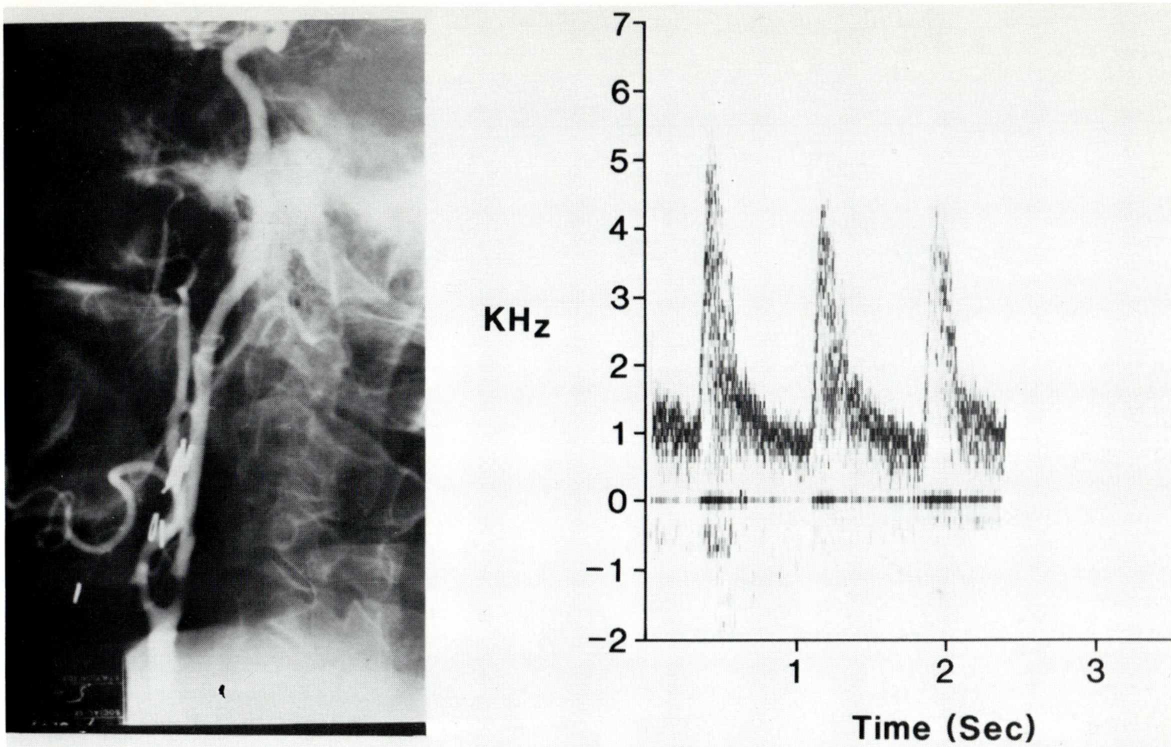

FIGURE 48-5. Arteriogram of left carotid artery 7 months after endarterectomy shows internal carotid stenosis of approximately 60 percent diameter reduction. The internal carotid peak frequency is abnormally increased (above 4 kHz), and spectral broadening is also present. [From Zierler, Bandyk, Thiele, and Strandness (35), by permission of Archives of Surgery.]

examined carotid arteries at postmortem after endarterectomy had been performed from 1 hour to 11 years previously (51). The changes observed between 1 hour and 6 days after operation included adventitial inflammation, medial necrosis, and mural thrombus deposition. This acute phase was followed by organization of the mural thrombus, reendothelialization, and formation of new elastic tissue. By 30 days after operation the endarterectomized segment was completely covered by new intima; however, this layer tended to increase in thickness with the passage of time.

There are two histologic types of stenotic lesions that occur after carotid endarterectomy. The early lesion, which appears during the first 24 months, consists of an exuberant proliferation of myointimal cells (36,38,39). These lesions do not contain hemosiderin or fibrin, and there is little or no lipid present. This distinct appearance excludes atherosclerotic plaque and organized mural thrombus as the cause of early recurrent stenosis. Stenotic lesions developing later than 24 months after surgery tend to resemble typical atherosclerotic plaque. It is likely that the early proliferative lesion is a manifestation of the arterial repair process that follows carotid endarterectomy (52). The operation exposes a large area of smooth muscle and collagen that may interact with platelets and coagulation factors to induce a proliferative response in the arterial wall (51). This mechanism could be responsible for the relatively high incidence of early postoperative stenosis documented by noninvasive testing. The early lesion found at reoperation for recurrent carotid stenosis has been described as firm, smooth, nonulcerated, and without definite cleavage planes. This is similar to the neointimal fibrous lesion associated with abnormal hemodynamic patterns after arterial reconstructions (53). Since the regression of injury-induced intimal lesions has been described in an experimental model (54), it is possible that the early lesion of recurrent stenosis may also decrease in severity over a period of time. The dynamic nature of early recurrent stenosis has been suggested by noninvasive testing (35).

SURGICAL TREATMENT

Since operations for recurrent carotid stenosis are rarely necessary, no firm guidelines have been established for the evaluation and treatment of this problem. This issue is further complicated by the fact that recurrent symptoms are not always associated with stenotic lesions and recurrent stenoses may be asymptomatic (35). Arteriography is justified in patients who develop neurologic symptoms appropriate to a carotid artery that has undergone endarterectomy. In those patients who are asymptomatic but have recurrent stenosis demonstrated by arteriography or noninvasive testing, the proper approach is not clear. Since some early postoperative stenoses appear to regress over a period of time, these lesions should be followed by serial noninvasive testing. When noninvasive tests show persistence or progression of recurrent stenosis, the need for further evaluation may depend on the status of the other cerebral arteries, the necessity for a major surgical procedure, or individual risk factors. So, at present, the decision to reoperate on a carotid lesion must be based primarily on clinical criteria.

Reoperative carotid surgery is more tedious and difficult than the initial procedure because of scar formation and loss of the normal anatomic planes of dissection. Particular care must be taken to identify and protect the cranial nerves in the vicinity of the carotid bifurcation. In spite of these technical problems, there is no clear evidence that neurologic complications are more common after reoperation than after initial carotid endarterectomy (39). Repeat endarterectomy is generally not possible in early recurrent stenoses of the fibrous, proliferative type. These lesions will require patch angioplasty using either autogenous vein or prosthetic material (55). When operating for late recurrent stenosis, a typical atherosclerotic plaque may be found which is amenable to endarterectomy. However, even in these cases, a patch angioplasty is recommended to further enlarge the stenotic segment. When difficulty is encountered with either of these surgical approaches, resection of the diseased segment and replacement with a vein bypass graft should be considered (38,56). Intraoperative assessment is a vital component of reoperation, just as it is for initial carotid endarterectomy. Since reoperation presents a greater technical challenge, it is especially important to document the result of surgery. Operative arteriography is the most objective and reliable of the methods described and is the method of choice for the immediate assessment of reoperative carotid surgery.

CONCLUSIONS

The data presented indicate that recurrent carotid stenosis is a more frequent event than the incidence of recurrent neurologic symptoms suggests. Although the hemodynamic and anatomic consequences of carotid endarterectomy are poorly understood, a number of factors can contribute to recurrent stenosis. Technical errors obviously play a role in some cases; however, the routine use of intraoperative assessment should minimize this problem. The early lesion of myointimal cell proliferation is apparently related to the repair process in the arterial wall following endarterectomy. This cellular response could also be influenced by hemodynamic factors and elements in the circulating blood. While abnormal flow patterns have been observed in the carotid bifurcation after a technically adequate endarterectomy, their significance is not known (33). There is experimental evidence that antiplatelet therapy decreases intimal hyperplasia related to intimal injury and vascular grafts (57,58). However, the effect of these agents after carotid endarterectomy has not been determined, and recurrent stenoses have occurred in patients receiving anticoagulants or antiplatelet drugs (55,59). The influence of patch angioplasty during the initial carotid endarterectomy on the incidence of recurrent stenosis also merits further study.

Late recurrent stenosis can usually be attributed to the underlying atherosclerotic disease process. The systemic risk factors found in association with recurrent carotid stenosis are those common to any group of patients with atherosclerosis. These include hypertension, hyperlipidemia, and diabetes mellitus. While it is always prudent to control these factors, there is no general agreement on their specific contribution to recurrent stenosis (39).

It is evident that all carotid stenoses do not have the same potential for causing neurologic symptoms, and a smooth myointimal lesion is not as dangerous as an ulcerated atherosclerotic plaque. Unfortunately, there is no completely reliable means for predicting which lesions will follow a benign course and which will produce neurologic sequelae. The clinical significance of asymptomatic lesions is especially relevant to the use of endarterectomy for asymptomatic carotid stenosis. If recurrent stenosis is more common than previously recognized, then the indications for endarterectomy in asymptomatic patients must be analyzed carefully. It must be shown that the natural history of asymptomatic carotid disease is improved by operation and is not adversely affected by recurrent stenosis.

The information available on recurrent carotid stenosis is clearly incomplete. Continued clinical and noninvasive follow-up is needed to document the anatomic changes in the endarterectomized vessel, the incidence of neurologic symptoms, and the role of systemic risk factors. Serial testing is particularly important during the early postoperative period when many recurrent stenoses develop. If possible, noninvasive evaluation should be performed at 3- to 6-month intervals through the first and second postoperative years. When these data are analyzed, a more rational approach to the problem of recurrent carotid stenosis will be possible.

References

1. Courbier R, Jausseran JM, Reggi M: Detecting complications of direct arterial surgery—The role of intraoperative arteriography. Arch Surg 112:1115, 1977.
2. Plecha FR, Pories WJ: Intraoperative angiography in the immediate assessment of arterial reconstruction. Arch Surg 105:902, 1972.
3. Rosental JJ, Gaspar MR, Movius HJ: Intraoperative arteriography in carotid thromboendarterectomy. Arch Surg 106:806, 1973.
4. Andersen CA, Collins GJ, Rich NM: Routine operative arteriography during carotid endarterectomy: A reassessment. Surgery 83:67, 1978.
5. Blaisdell FW, Lim R, Hall AD: Technical result of carotid endarterectomy—Arteriographic assessment. Am J Surg 114:239, 1967.
6. Fischer HW, Cornell SH: The toxicity of the sodium and methylglucamine salts of diatrizoate, iothalamate, and metrizoate—An experimental study of their circulatory effects following intracarotid injection. Radiology 85:1013, 1965.
7. Zierler RE, Bandyk DF, Thiele BL: Intraoperative assessment of carotid endarterectomy. J Vasc Surg 1:73, 1984.
8. Lye CR, Marrow IM, Downs AR: Carotid artery spasm—A cause of postendarterectomy thrombosis? Arch Surg 117:1531, 1982.
9. Hobson RW, Rich NM, Wright CB, Fedde CW: Operative assessment of carotid endarterectomy—Internal carotid arterial back pressure, carotid arterial blood flow, and carotid arteriography. Am Surg 41:603, 1975.

10. Larson SR, Movius HJ, Bell OD, Gaspar MR, Rosental JJ, Lemire GG: Intraoperative arteriography in cerebrovascular surgery. In Bergan JJ, Yao JST (eds): *Cerebrovascular Insufficiency*. New York, Grune and Stratton, Inc, 1983, pp 353–365.
11. Collins GJ, Rich NM, Andersen CA, McDonald PT: Stroke associated with carotid endarterectomy. Am J Surg 135:221, 1978.
12. Bernstein EF, Dilley RB, Goldberger LE, Gosink BB, Leopold GR: Growth rates of small abdominal aortic aneurysms. Surgery 80:765, 1976.
13. Sigel B, Coelho JCU, Machi J, Flanigan DP, Donahue PE, Schuler JJ, Beitler JC: The application of real-time ultrasound imaging during surgical procedures. Surg Gynecol Obstet 157:33, 1983.
14. Lane RJ: Intraoperative B-mode scanning. J Clin Ult 8:427, 1980.
15. Sigel B, Coelho JCU, Flanigan DP, Schuler JJ, Spigos DG: Ultrasonic imaging during vascular surgery. Arch Surg 117:764, 1982.
16. Flanigan DP, Sigel B, Schuler JJ: Intraoperative ultrasonic carotid artery imaging. In Bergan JJ, Yao JST (eds): *Cerebrovascular Insufficiency*. New York, Grune and Stratton, Inc, 1983, pp 343–352.
17. Coelho JCU, Sigel B, Flanigan DP, Schuler JJ, Spigos DG, Tan WS, Justin J: An experimental evaluation of arteriography and imaging ultrasonography in detecting arterial defects at operation. J Surg Res 32:130, 1982.
18. Lane RJ, Appleberg M: Real-time intraoperative angiosonography after carotid endarterectomy. Surgery 92:5, 1982.
19. Anderson JC, Baltaxe HA, Wolf GL: Inability to show clot—One limitation of ultrasonography of the abdominal aorta. Radiology 132:693, 1979.
20. Shore JM, Berci G, Morgenstern L: The value of biliary endoscopy. Surg Gynecol Obstet 140:601, 1975.
21. Vatz A, Berci G, Shore JM: Operative nephroscopy. J Urol 107:355, 1972.
22. Towne JB, Bernhard VM: Vascular endoscopy—Useful tool or interesting toy? Surgery 82:415, 1977.
23. Vollmar JF, Storz LW: Vascular endoscopy—Possibilities and limits of its clinical application. Surg Clin North Am 54:111, 1974.
24. Towne JB, Bernhard VM: Vascular endoscopy—An adjunct to carotid surgery. Stroke 8:569, 1977.
25. Dean RH, Yao JST, Stanton PE, Bergan JJ: Prognostic indicators in femoropopliteal reconstruction. Arch Surg 110:1287, 1975.
26. Owens ML, Wilson SE: Prevention of neurologic complications of carotid endarterectomy. Arch Surg 117:551, 1982.
27. May AG, Van de Berg L, DeWeese JA, Rob CG: Critical arterial stenosis. Surgery 54:250, 1963.
28. Barnes RW, Garrett WV: Intraoperative assessment of arterial reconstruction by Doppler ultrasound. Surg Gynecol Obstet 146:896, 1978.
29. Mozersky DJ, Sumner DS, Barnes RW, Strandness DE Jr: Intraoperative use of a sterile ultrasonic flow probe. Surg Gynecol Obstet 136:279, 1973.
30. Keitzer WF, Lichti EL, Brossart FA, DeWeese MS: Use of the Doppler ultrasonic flowmeter during arterial vascular surgery. Arch Surg 105:308, 1972.
31. Zierler RE, Roederer GO, Strandness DE Jr: The use of frequency spectral analysis in carotid artery surgery. In Bergan JJ, Yao JST (eds): *Cerebrovascular Insufficiency*. New York, Grune and Stratton, Inc, 1983, pp 137–161.
32. Fell G, Phillips DJ, Chikos PM, Harley JD, Thiele BL, Strandness DE Jr: Ultrasonic Duplex scanning for disease of the carotid artery. Circulation 64:896, 1978.
33. Zierler RE, Bandyk DF, Berni GA, Thiele BL: Intraoperative pulsed Doppler assessment of carotid endarterectomy. Ult Med Bio 9:65, 1983.
34. Thompson JE, Talkington CM: Carotid endarterectomy. Ann Surg 184:1, 1976.
35. Zierler RE, Bandyk DF, Thiele BL, Strandness DE Jr: Carotid artery stenosis following endarterectomy. Arch Surg 117:1408, 1982.
36. Cossman D, Callow AD, Stein A, Matsumoto G: Early restenosis after carotid endarterectomy. Arch Surg 113:275, 1978.
37. Hertzer NR, Martinez BD, Beven EG: Recurrent stenosis after carotid endarterectomy. Surg Gynecol Obstet 149:360, 1979.
38. Stoney RJ, String ST: Recurrent carotid stenosis. Surgery 80:705, 1976.
39. McBride K, Callow AD: Recurrent stenosis after carotid endarterectomy—A limited survey. In Bernhand VM, Towne JB (eds): *Complications in Vascular Surgery*. New York, Grune and Stratton, Inc, 1980, pp 259–273.
40. Baker WH, Hayes AC, Mahler DM, Littooy FN: Durability of carotid endarterectomy. Surgery 94:112, 1983.
41. Cantelmo NL, Cutler BS, Wheeler HB, Herrmann JB, Cardullo PA: Noninvasive detection of carotid stenosis following endarterectomy. Arch Surg 116:1005, 1981.
42. Kremen JE, Gee W, Kaupp HA, McDonald KM: Restenosis or occlusion after carotid endarterectomy—A survey with ocular pneumoplethysmography. Arch Surg 114:608, 1979.
43. Turnipseed WD, Berkoff HA, Crummy A: Postoperative occlusion after carotid endarterectomy. Arch Surg 115:573, 1980.
44. Salvian A, Baker JD, Machleder HI, Busuttil RW, Barker WF, Moore WS: Cause and noninvasive detection of restenosis after carotid endarterectomy. Am J Surg 146:29, 1983.
45. Roederer GO, Langlois Y, Chan ATW, Breslau P, Phillips DJ, Beach KW, Chikos PM, Strandness DE Jr: Post-endarterectomy carotid ultrasonic Duplex scanning—Concordance with contrast angiography. Ult Med Bio 9:73, 1983.
46. Schutz H, Fleming JFR, Awerbuck B: Arteriographic assessment of carotid endarterectomy. Ann Surg 171:509, 1970.
47. Diaz FG, Patel S, Boulos R, Ausman JI: Early angiographic changes following carotid endarterectomy. Stroke 11:135, 1980.
48. Acher CW, Turnipseed WD, Sackett JF, Strather CM, Crummy A, Mistretta C: Digital subtraction angiography and continuous-wave Doppler studies. Arch Surg 118:462, 1983.
49. Hertzer NR, Beven EG, Modic MT, O'Hara PJ, Vogt DP, Weinstein MA: Early patency of the carotid artery after endarterectomy—Digital subtraction angiography after two hundred sixty two operations. Surgery 92:1049, 1982.
50. Dirrenberger RA, Sundt TM: Carotid endarterectomy—Temporal profile of the healing process and effects of anticoagulation therapy. J Neurosurg 48:201, 1978.
51. French BN, Rewcastle NB: Sequential morphological changes at the site of carotid endarterectomy. J Neurosurg 41:745, 1974.
52. Callow AD: An overview of the stroke problem in the carotid territory. Am J Surg 140:181, 1980.
53. Imparato AM, Bracco A, Kim GE, Zeff R: Intimal and neointimal fibrous proliferation causing failure of arterial reconstructions. Surgery 72:1007, 1972.
54. Moore S, Friedman RJ, Gent M: Resolution of lipid-containing atherosclerotic lesions induced by injury. Blood Vessels 14:193, 1977.
55. Cossman DV, Treiman RL, Foran RF, Levin PM, Cohen JL: Surgical approach to recurrent carotid stenosis. Am J Surg 140:209, 1980.
56. Sproul G: Recurrent carotid stenosis or false aneurysm—A simple approach. Am J Surg 144:573, 1982.
57. McCann RL, Fuchs JCA: Aspirin and dipyridamole decrease intimal hyperplasia in experimental and vein grafts. Ann Surg 191:238, 1980.
58. Oblath RW, Buckley FO, Gran RM, Schwartz SF, DeWeese JA: Prevention of platelet aggregation and adherence to prosthetic vacular grafts by aspirin and dipyridamole. Surgery 84:37, 1978.
59. French BN, Rewcastle NB: Recurrent stenosis at site of carotid endarterectomy. Stroke 8:597, 1977.

Chapter 49

FIBROMUSCULAR DYSPLASIA OF THE CAROTID ARTERY

DAVID J. EFFENEY, WILLIAM C. KRUPSKI, RONALD J. STONEY, and WILLIAM K. EHRENFELD

Fibromuscular dysplasia was described, but not named, by Leadbetter and Burkland in the renal arteries of a young boy in 1938 (1). In 1958 McCormack et al. described four types of obstructive lesions of the renal arteries associated with hypertension and called one of these fibromuscular hyperplasia (2). For many years the disease was thought to be confined to the renal vessels, but in 1964 Palubinskas and Ripley (3) described fibromuscular dysplasia in the internal carotid artery. It is now known that many medium-sized arteries can be affected by fibromuscular disease (4). An increasing number of reports (5–12) document fibromuscular disease as a cause of the symptoms of cerebrovascular insufficiency. The carotid and vertebral arteries may be involved with fibromuscular disease, although it appears that the vertebral artery is infrequently, if ever, a cause of symptoms. The lesions of fibromuscular disease have been described in the intracranial vessels as well as the cervical carotid, and the disorder is associated with an increased incidence of intracranial aneurysms. (12,13).

Clinical Features of Fibromuscular Disease

The clinical findings presented here were compiled after the review of 101 patients, aged 27 to 86 years, who were operated upon at the University of California, San Francisco, for symptomatic fibromuscular disease. Tables 49-1 and 49-2 show the major symptoms and the physical findings in this group of patients.

It is clear that fibromuscular disease is associated with a wide variety of symptoms. However, we do not know what proportion of patients who have the disorder develop symptoms. It was disturbing that a completed stroke had occurred in 22 percent of the patients prior to presentation, and almost 9 percent of the group had a residual neurologic deficit at the time operation was undertaken. This is a very significant incidence of neurologic events in a relatively young group of people. A recent report from Kelly and Morris (8) described 4 of 25 patients they had operated on who presented with a stroke, a figure almost identical to that noted in our group of patients. Likewise, they confirmed that localizing symptoms such as transient ischemic attacks and amaurosis fugax occurred more commonly in that patient population than did nonlocalizing neurologic events. There was a marked preponderance of females in the patient group we treated, and the mean age of the group was 58 years, almost 10 years younger than patients with atherosclerotic disease operated on during the period of review.

A loud bruit, which was heard by the patient, was a principal complaint in almost 25 percent of the group, and a loud, high-pitched bruit heard by the examiner over the internal carotid was the most common physical sign. A third of the patients were hypertensive with diastolic blood pressures greater than 110 mmHg on admission or were receiving continuing treatment with antihypertensive medications.

TABLE 49-1. Fibromuscular Disease of the Internal Cartoid Artery

Symptoms	Percent
Transient ischemic attacks	41
Nonlocalizing neurologic events	31
Bruits heard by patient	23
Amaurosis fugax	23
Completed strokes	22
Asymptomatic bruits	8
Prolonged ischemic attack	2
Other	6

TABLE 49-2. Fibromuscular Disease of the Internal Carotid Artery

Physical Findings	Percent
Carotid bruit	77
Hypertension	37
Neurologic deficits	9
ECG abnormalities	17

Arteriographic Findings

We reviewed the arteriograms of 86 of our patients, and the main features are illustrated in Figures 49-1 through 49-3. We have previously noted (14,15) that the internal carotid arteries affected by fibromuscular disease were longer than normal. The carotid bifurcation is usually lower than in patients with atherosclerotic disease, being at the C-4 to C-5 disk level or below in the majority of the films. When the bifurcation was high in the neck, the internal carotid was frequently coiled or kinked. The most striking feature, however, was that fibromuscular disease affected the middle and distal third of the cervical portion of the artery, and the lesions were most commonly seen and were worst opposite the C1 or C2 vertebral bodies. The proximal and distal portions of the internal carotid artery was spared the manifestations of fibromuscular disease. The angiographic appearance of fibromuscular disease is usually present bilaterally, although one side is frequently more severely involved than the other. Three types of appearances of this disorder are recognized: the classic string of beads, a tubular form of the dysplasia, or a very localized lesion with only one or two bands (13,16,17). The finding of a carotid dissection (Figures 49-4 and 49-5) at the time of arteriography after an acute neurologic event should lead the examiner to visualize the other vessels known to be at risk for fibromuscular disease (14,15). Table 49-3 documents the distribution of the other arteries affected by fibromuscular disease in this patient population. Approximately 20 percent of the patients with fibromuscular disease will have concurrent atherosclerosis of the carotid bifurcation.

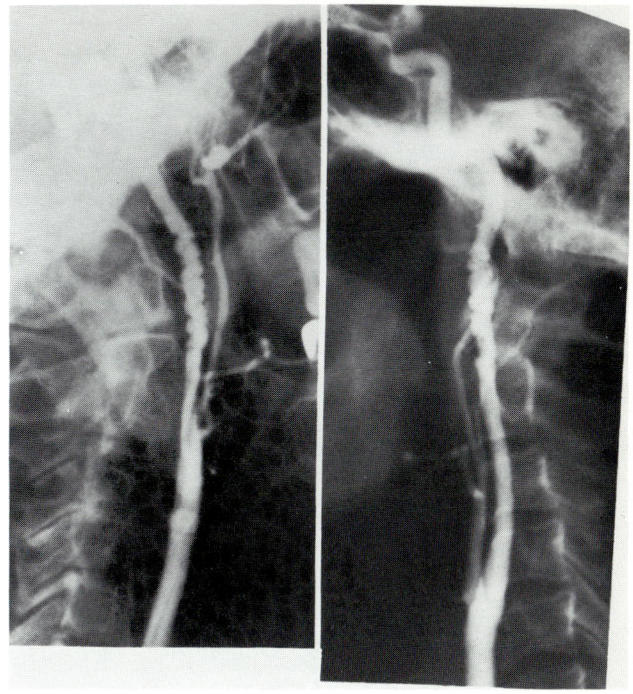

FIGURE 49-2. Left and right carotid angiograms showing more advanced cervical carotid fibromuscular dysplasia. This appearance corresponds to the classic "string of beads" pattern.

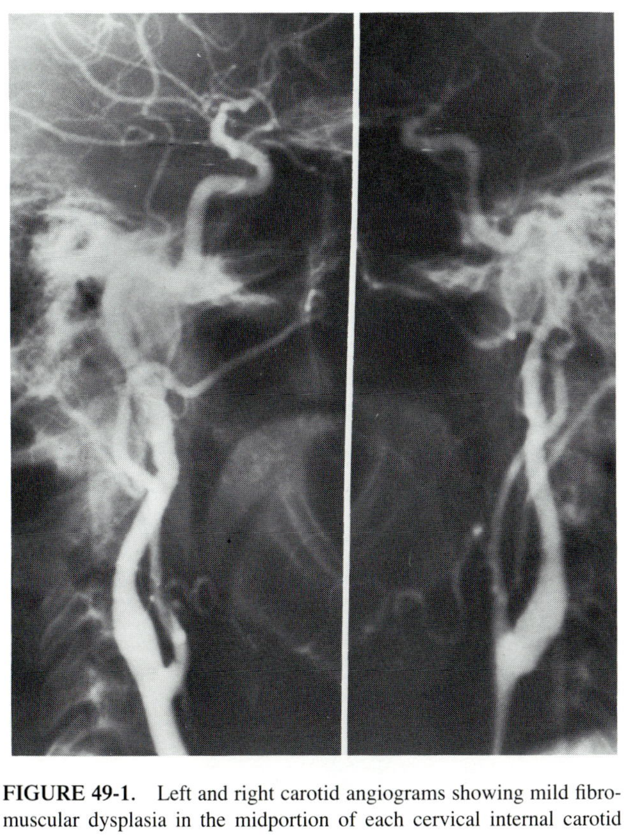

FIGURE 49-1. Left and right carotid angiograms showing mild fibromuscular dysplasia in the midportion of each cervical internal carotid artery.

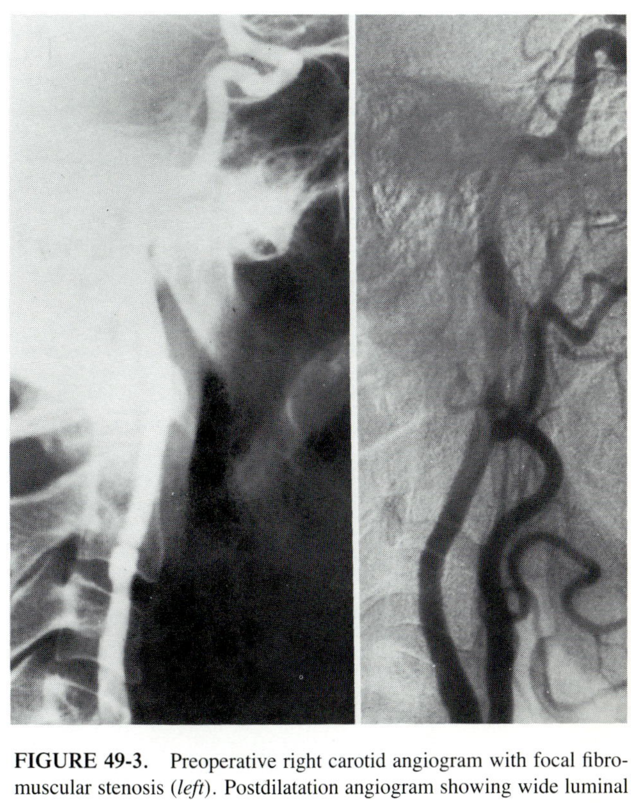

FIGURE 49-3. Preoperative right carotid angiogram with focal fibromuscular stenosis (*left*). Postdilatation angiogram showing wide luminal patency without evidence of stenosis (*right*).

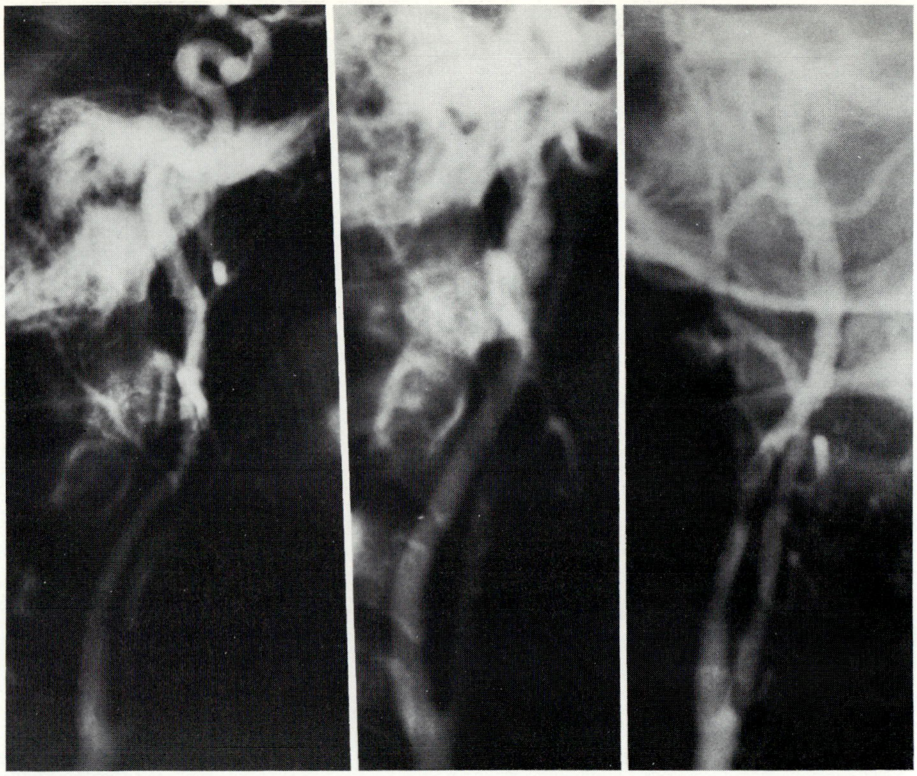

FIGURE 49-4. Carotid angiogram showing a dissection within an area of fibromuscular dysplasia (*left*). Angiogram of same patient, 2 months later, showing some resolution of the dissection (*middle*). Angiogram at 6 months showing virtually complete resolution of the dissection (*right*).

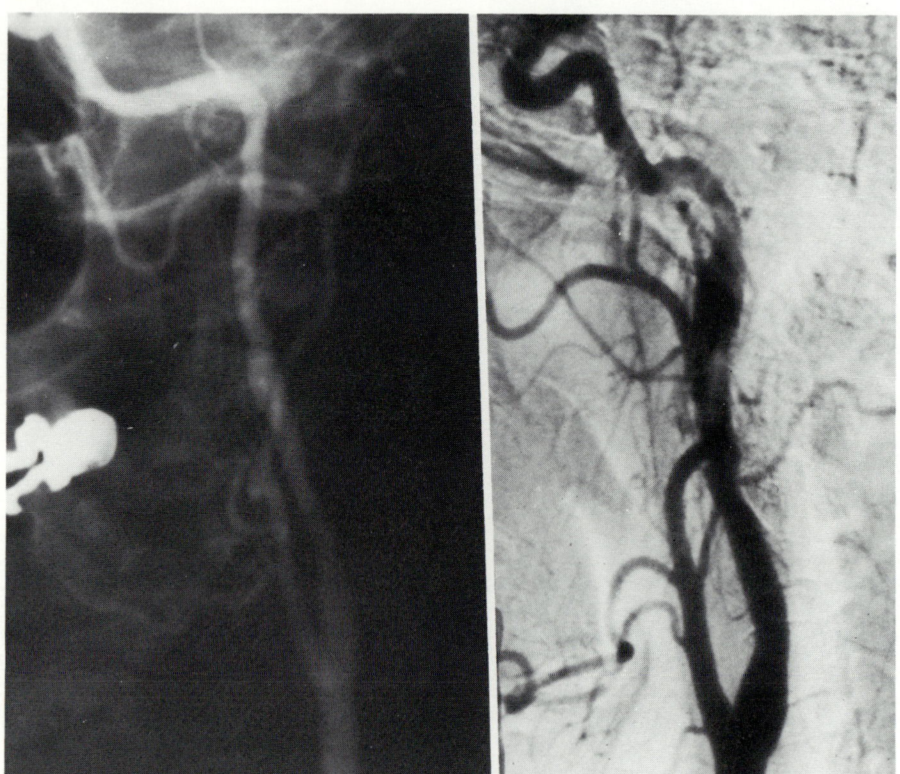

FIGURE 49-5. Carotid angiogram showing localized dissection in area of fibromuscular dysplasia (*left*). Same patient 6 months later showing persistent postdissection aneurysm (*right*).

TABLE 49-3. **Other Arteries Affected by Fibromuscular Disease in a Series of 101 Patients with Carotid Involvement**

Renal artery	27
External iliac	8
Vertebral arteries	6
Intracranial aneurysms	5*

*Of 35 patients having intracranial views.

Pathology and Pathogenesis

Although four distinct histologic types of fibromuscular disease have been described, the most common of these is medial fibroplasia (18). In Stanley's classification the other types are intimal fibroplasia, medial hyperplasia, and perimedial dysplasia. The disease is a nonatherosclerotic angiopathy of unknown etiology. It is not, however, a generalized dysplasia in the arteries. Fibromuscular disease affects segments of long arteries that have few primary branches. The predominance of the disease in the female has caused considerable speculation about the role of estrogens and other hormones in the pathogenesis of fibromuscular disease. There is no evidence at present to incriminate oral contraceptives or postmenopausal estrogen therapy as causative agents, but female sex hormones may have a facilitative role in the development and progression of this disorder. The observations of pathology specimens as well as some experimental work (18) have led to a concept of pathogenesis. In this hypothesis, it is suggested that normal intraarterial stresses act on a segment of artery that is somewhat longer than normal and that has a relatively poorer supply derived from vasa vasorum because of a lack of primary arterial branches. The damaged media progresses to one or other of the histologic types of dysplasia, depending on which artery is involved, the depth of medial injury, and the mechanisms of attempted repair. All of these factors may be modified by the hormonal environment (14,18).

Surgical Methods

The technique of graduated intraluminal dilatation first described by Morris (9) has been used as the treatment modality for symptomatic fibromuscular disease almost exclusively since 1970 (Figure 49-6 and 49-7). The internal carotid artery is mobilized in the neck to the level of the styloid process, and, if required, the carotid sinus nerve is divided to allow for retraction caudally. The internal carotid is straightened during the dilatation. A short vertical arteriotomy is made in the carotid bulb, and the blood vessel is dilated with a 1.5- or 2-mm Bakes dilator. This instrument is advanced until resistance is felt. Gentle pressure is applied, and the advance of the instrument is accompanied by loss of the resistance. The artery is progressively dilated with 3-, 3.5-, and 4-mm dilators, usually, with less resistance being encountered. If the internal carotid is a small vessel, the maximum size dilator we use is 3.5 mm, and normally we do not dilate any artery beyond 4 mm. The artery is allowed to "bleed back" through the arteriotomy to flush out any accumulated debris or thrombus. A clamp is applied to the internal carotid above the arteriotomy, and the vessel is closed using continuous suture technique. Standard techniques of arterial resection and end-to-end anastomosis or vein grafting have been used to treat patients with accessible carotid fibromuscular disease (19). Two patients underwent resection of a redundant carotid artery combined with distal intraluminal dilatation. Ipsilateral carotid endarterectomy for atherosclerosis was performed on 18 percent of our patients during their dilatation. Four percent of the patients required an endarterectomy of the contralateral carotid which was minimally affected by the dysplasia.

Results of Therapy

The 101 patients in our series have undergone 150 operations without death. There have been three strokes in the early postoperative period, nine patients had transient neurologic deficits or episodes of amaurosis fugax. Thus the results would support the conclusion that treatment of symptomatic fibromuscular disease by surgery is safe. We have followed the patients from 1 to 18 years. Two patients have had strokes in this time, one of which was known to be due to an embolus 6 months after operation. This embolus lodged in the right middle cerebral artery and arose from an intimal disruption high in the internal carotid artery. The cause of the other stroke is not known. There have been two subarachnoid hemorrhages from associated intracranial aneurysms. Three patients have continuing generalized neurologic symptoms and probably represent inappropriate patient selection for operation. We have performed arteriography routinely after dilatation to confirm early patency. Some patients have been studied for up to 5 years after their original dilatation. The durability of the procedure has been confirmed in these studies for in only one patient was a previously dilated artery found to be occluded. There was one patient who presented with three episodes of transient ischemia 1 year after the first dilatation and who required re-dilatation of that carotid artery for a persistent band of fibromuscular disease.

The nonneurologic complications of the surgical management of fibromuscular disease are those associated with carotid endarterectomy and occur with about the same frequency as is reported in major series reviewing endarterectomy. There is, however, one intraoperative complication peculiar to dilatation. This is the risk of perforation. This complication occurred once, and its occurrence reinforces the need to straighten the artery and pass the dilator gently. In the one instance, the perforation occurred in an inaccessible portion of the carotid, immediately below the base of the skull where the artery had not been completely mobilized and straightened. The bleeding was controlled by local packing, and the patient did not develop false aneurysm at the site of the perforation.

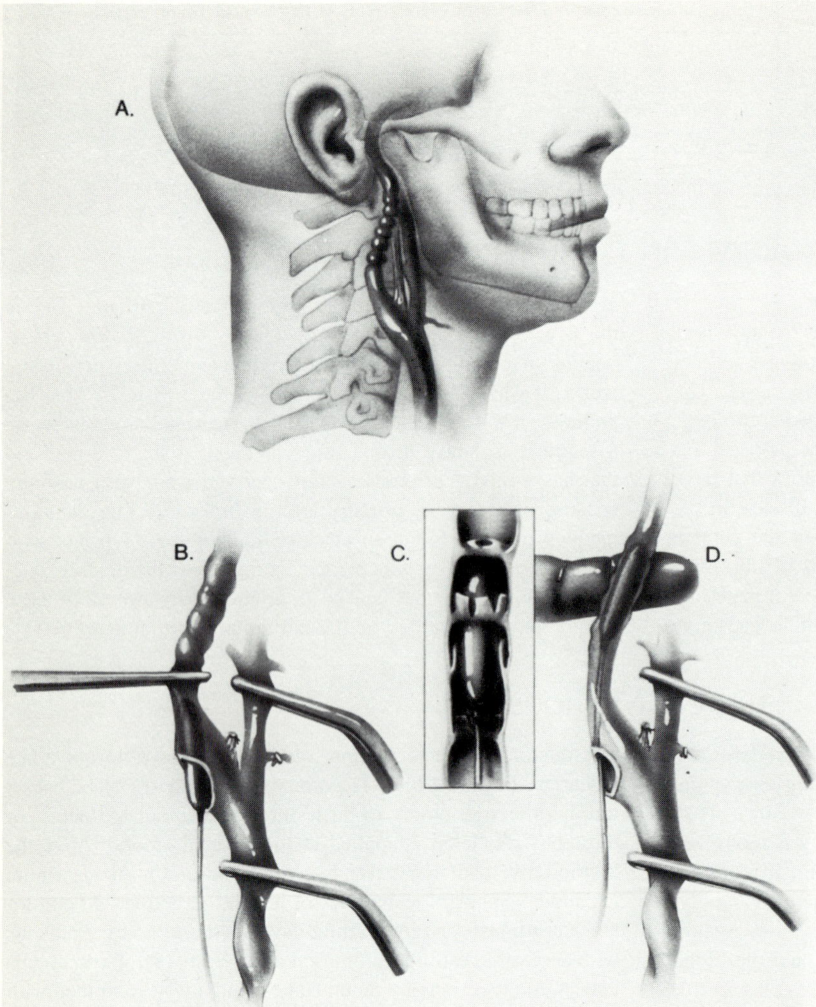

FIGURE 49-6. Summary of operative technique of intraluminal dilatation. (*A*) The classic appearance of fibromuscular disease opposite the C1 to C2 vertebral bodies. (*B*) The artery is mobilized, the carotid sinus nerve divided, and a short vertical arteriotomy is made in the carotid bulb. (*C*) The insert depicts the initial rupture of the membranes with a small dilator. (*D*) The passage of a larger dilator. Note that the index finger of the left hand supports the internal carotid during dilatation.

Discussion

Although there are reports of a frequency of 0.25 to 0.68 percent (13,16) of fibromuscular disease in patients undergoing carotid arteriography, the incidence of fibromuscular disease is not precisely known. It is a disease of women primarily, with females accounting for more than 90 percent of the reported cases. The disorder affects women earlier in life than atherosclerosis.

The clinical dilemma of fibromuscular disease is that the natural history is not known. It is certain that many patients remain asymptomatic even with advanced morphologic changes of fibromuscular disease, while in others the first symptom of extracranial fibromuscular disease may be a stroke with residual neurologic deficit. In our patients once fibromuscular dysplasia became symptomatic, it was no longer a benign disease, since almost 25 percent of them had suffered a stroke prior to their surgical correction.

The clinical presentation of these patients lends support to a thromboembolic cause for symptoms. However, other possibilities include hypoperfusion, phenomena related to hypertension, intracranial fibromuscular disease, or the associated aneurysms. The true cause of symptom production in the disorder remains unknown. The variety and severity of the antecedent neurologic events in symptomatic patients underscores a need for careful and critical evaluation of each patient.

The initial clinical and radiological assessment should be complete. A detailed physical examination after a careful history is, of course, mandatory. The initial radiological assessment of patients with suspected extracranial fibromuscular disease should include intracranial views to look for aneurysms and an arch injection to document possible vertebral disease as well as the standard views of the extracranial carotid vessels themselves. We also recommend a midstream aortogram to visualize the renal and external iliac arteries—common sites for fibromuscular disease in this subset of patients. The only major vessel in which fibromuscular dysplasia occurs and is not visualized using this approach is the superior mesenteric artery. The extra runs required and the low yield from investigation of this vessel have led us to conclude that it is not worthwhile in all patients.

Most of our patients have been treated with aspirin and many with dipyridamole. There are however no data to confirm or deny that medical therapy is efficacious in the management of

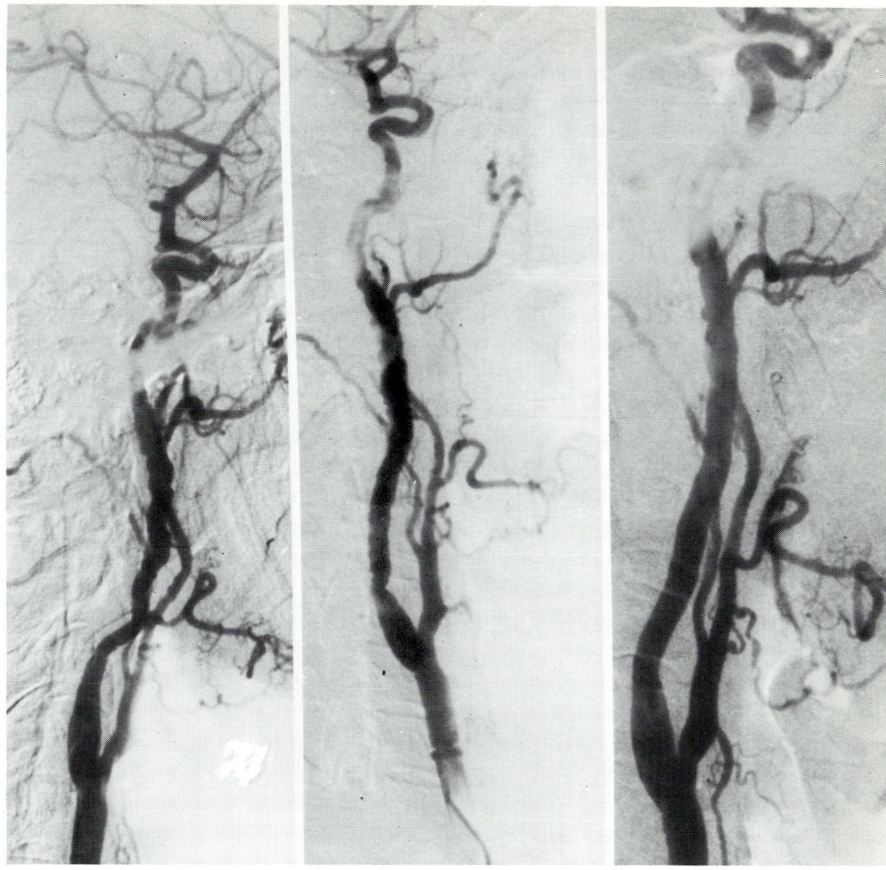

FIGURE 49-7. *Left* and *middle* panels show right carotid fibromuscular dysplasia in two projections. The right panel was obtained 6 months after graduated transluminal dilatation. Wide patency without significant defect is apparent.

fibromuscular disease. We continue to use aspirin in asymptomatic patients and recommend surgery for patients with symptoms.

The spectrum of symptoms seen in fibromuscular disease is a valid indication for operation in patients with atherosclerotic disease. We have extended the same indications to patients with fibromuscular disease, and it seems valid to assess the results of therapy using accepted criteria for operations performed for atherosclerosis of the carotid bifurcation. Intraluminal dilatation fulfills the need for surgical accessibility and removes the need to replace a segment of the carotid artery that is difficult to expose and control. The dilatation operation can be performed with acceptably low morbidity and mortality rates. In our large series, we have had no deaths and the morbidity from the procedure is about that of carotid endarterectomy. Postoperative arteriography has proved the early patency, and follow-up studies 5 years after dilatation have confirmed that the repair is durable. It is interesting that years after dilatation, the appearance of the vessel is improved with the ragged appearance of the arteries in the studies performed shortly after dilatation has been undertaken.

The clinical response has paralleled the apparent maintenance of satisfactory anatomical repair. The majority of patients have had no further neurological events. Two patients have had subarachnoid hemorrhages. Neither of these had intracranial views at the time of original study, which is an important reminder of the requirement for the complete initial radiological assessment. The long-term stroke rate has been satisfactorily low, and patient selection has been appropriate with only three patients complaining of persistent nonlocalizing neurologic symptoms in the presence of satisfactory anatomic repair.

It has been suggested (10) that operation is unwarranted in all patients with fibromuscular disease until the natural history of the disease is ''more clearly defined.'' This statement is difficult to dispute while the patient remains asymptomatic, and we do not recommend prophylactic surgery in asymptomatic patients. However, the results of surgical treatment have been gratifying in terms of symptom relief, stroke prevention, the durability of the anatomic repair, and the sustained clinical response after operation. We therefore, continue to recommend surgical treatment to patients with symptomatic fibromuscular disease.

References

1. Leadbetter WF, Burkland CE: Hypetension in unilateral renal disease. J Urol 1938, 39:611–626.
2. McCormack LJ, Hazard JB, Poutasse EF: Obstructive lesions of the renal artery associated with remedial hypertension (abstract). Am J Pathol 1958, 34:582.
3. Palubinskas AJ, Ripley HR: Fibromuscular hyperplasia in extra renal arteries. Radiology 1964, 82:451–455.
4. Nunn DB: Fibromuscular hyperplasia of the internal carotid artery. Am Surg 1974, 40:309–314.

5. Connett MC, Lansche JM: Fibromuscular hyperplasia of internal carotid artery. Report of a case. Ann Surg 1965, 162:59–62.
6. Ehrenfeld WK, Wylie EJ: Fibromuscular dysplasia of the internal carotid artery. Surgical management. Arch Surg 1974, 109:676–681.
7. Harrington OB, Crosby VG, Nicholas L: Fibromuscular hyperplasia of the internal carotid artery. Ann Thorac Surg 1971, 9:516–524.
8. Kelly TF, Morris GC: Arterial fibromuscular disease. Am J Surg 1982, 143:232–236.
9. Morris GC, Jr, Lechter A, DeBakey ME: Surgical treatment of fibromuscular disease of the carotid arteries. Arch Surg 1968, 96:636–643.
10. Patman RD, Thompson JE, Talkington CM, Garrett WV: Natural history of fibromuscular dysplasia of the carotid artery (abstract). Stroke 1980, 2:135.
11. Perry MO: Fibromuscular dysplasia. Surg Gynecol Obstet 1974,139:97–104.
12. Stanley JC, Fry WJ, Seeger JF, Hoffman GL, Gabrielsen TO: Extracranial internal carotid and vertebral artery fibrodysplasia. Arch Surg 1974, 109:215–222.
13. Osborn AG, Andersen RE: Angiographic spectrum of cervical and intracranial fibromuscular dysplasia. Stroke 1977, 8:617–626.
14. Effeney DJ, Ehrenfeld WK, Stoney RJ, Wylie EJ: Fibromuscular dysplasia of the internal carotid artery. World J Surg 1979, 3:179–186.
15. Effeney DJ, Ehrenfeld WK, Stoney RJ, Wylie EJ: Why operate on carotid fibromuscular dysplasia? Arch Surg 1980, 115:1261–1265.
16. Houser OW, Baker HL: Fibrovascular dysplasia and other common diseases of the cervical carotid artery: Angiographic aspects. Am J Roentgenol 1968, 104:201–211.
17. Palubinskas AJ, Perloff D, Newton TH: Fibromuscular hyperplasia: An arterial dysplasia of increasing clinical importance. Am J Roentgenol 1966, 98:907–913.
18. Stanley JC, Gewertz BL, Bove EL, Sottiurai V, Fry WJ: Arterial fibrodysplasia: Histopathologic character and current etiologic concepts. Arch Surg 1975, 110:561–566.
19. Ehrenfeld WK, Stoney RJ, Wylie EJ: Fibromuscular hyperplasia of the internal carotid artery. Arch Surg 1967, 95:284–287.

Chapter 50

CAROTID ARTERIAL TORTUOSITY, KINKS, AND SPONTANEOUS DISSECTION

J. TIMOTHY FULENWIDER and ROBERT B. SMITH III

If the carotid of one side should be obstructed, then the vessels of the other side might provide for either Province . . . further, if both the carotids should be stopt, the offices of each might be supplied through the vertebrals (1).

The above quotation by Thomas Willis illustrates his precocious knowledge of the brain's collateral arterial flow. Cerebral vascular anatomy was described in detail by Willis in *Cerebri Anatome,* in which his friend, Sir Christopher Wren, provided drawings demonstrating the intracranial communications of the anterior and posterior cerebral circulation. Willis also recognized that complete carotid arterial occlusion could occur without symptoms. The earliest human application of this knowledge occurred in 1808 when Sir Astley Cooper performed the first successful carotid operation: ligation of the common carotid artery of a 50-year-old man who presented with a painful pulsatile swelling at the left mandibular angle (2). Postmortem examination 13 years later corroborated Willis' views of the importance of the intracranial collateral circulation because the patient's left posterior communicating artery had markedly enlarged allowing persistent perfusion of the left cerebral hemisphere from the vertebral artery.

In 1913, Dr. Ramsay Hunt of Columbia University, addressing the American Neurological Association, first emphasized the significance of obstructive lesions of the cervical carotid arteries in the causation of cerebral infarction (3). Twenty-four years later, the development of the technique of cerebral angiography by Dr. Egaz Moniz of Portugal allowed visualization of the carotid arterial pathways. Using direct thorotrast injection into the carotid artery, Moniz identified a thrombosis of the carotid artery, leading to the speculation that total occlusions occurred more frequently than clinically suspected (4). Following neuropathological investigations at the Massachusetts General Hospital, Drs. Miller Fisher and Raymond Adams suggested that many of the deaths from cerebral infarction were secondary to cerebral embolism and that emboli were responsible for some of the transient neurological phenomena prior to death (5). Subsequently, observations of retinal cholesterol emboli by Hollenhorst and further recognition of the association of ulcerative carotid atheromas and transient neurological deficits supported the conclusions of Drs. Fisher and Adams (6). Based on these observations, the modern era of carotid arterial reconstruction began in the mid 1950s. Since that time carotid endarterectomy has proved clinically efficacious in the relief of transient neurologic dysfunction and the prevention of ischemic brain infarction.

The overwhelming majority of extracranial carotid stenoses are secondary to atherosclerosis, typically involving the carotid bulb and proximal 1 to 2 cm of the internal and external carotid artery. Initiated by hemorrhage into the carotid atheroma or accretion of platelets and fibrin in an ulcer niche, embolization is the probable cause of most carotid-related cerebral ischemic events; however, stenoses reducing the carotid lumen area to 25 percent of normal may also produce cerebral ischemia—especially during periods of systemic hypotension or reduced cardiac output.

Although most carotid stenoses are due to atheromatous plaques, certain congenital and acquired deformities and arteriopathies of the carotid system may also be responsible for cerebral ischemia and infarction. The carotid loop or coil, the carotid kink, and spontaneous dissection of the internal carotid are among these infrequent causes of cerebral ischemia. Each of these entities shares the common pathologic potential of impairing cerebral blood flow by either hemodynamic or thromboembolic mechanisms. This chapter examines the carotid loop or coil, the carotid kink, and spontaneous carotid dissection individually.

The Carotid Loop

Extracranial internal carotid tortuosity is a relatively common angiographic finding (7–9). The carotid loop, defined as a 360° coil or spiral configuration, or as an elongation and redundancy resulting in a sigmoid curvature, is felt to be congenital in origin (Figure 50-1) (10–14). Development of this anomaly is best explained by defective embryogenesis of the carotid artery (15). Normally, extensions of the endocardial heart tubes form the embryonic dorsal aortas, which assume an arched configuration in the fetal pharyngeal region due to rotation of the cardiogenic plate and fusion of the endocardial heart tubes. Central to an

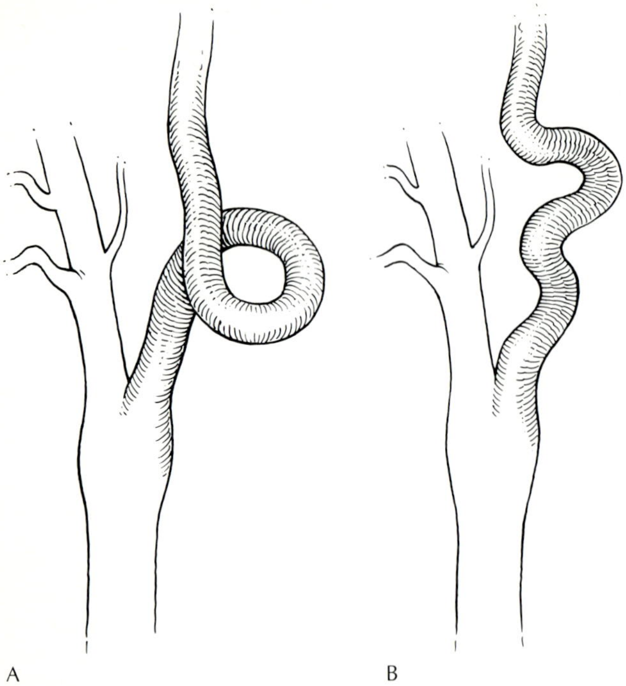

FIGURE 50-1. Artist's rendition of a 360° loop of the internal carotid artery and of marked tortuosity without coiling. *A,* elongation (loop); *B,* tortuosity.

understanding of development of the arterial tree is an appreciation of the development and retrogression of the dorsal aortas, appearing initially as symmetrical and parallel conduits destined to transform into the adult vascular form by as early as the 14-mm embryo stage. The dorsal aortas run parallel to the primitive foregut and fuse with the truncus arteriosus, forming the aortic sac which contributes branch arteries to each developing pharyngeal arch. The third aortic arch ultimately forms the common carotid artery and the proximal internal carotid artery; the distal internal carotid system is formed by the cranial portion of the dorsal aorta. The external carotid artery sprouts from the third aortic arch, which joins with remaining portions of the first and second arches.

Early in development, the communication between the third and fourth aortic arches, the carotid duct, becomes obliterated, and the extracranial carotid system assumes its adult configuration. These primordial vascular changes and cardiogenesis occur in the cephalad region of the embryonic pharynx. Developmental elongation of the fetal neck subsequently leads to descent of the heart into the mediastinum with elongation of the innominate and carotid arteries. Maldescent of the heart or persistence of embryonic anatomy is felt responsible for subsequent looping and redundancy of the internal carotid artery (9). Evidence for the congenital origin of the carotid loop is based upon its identification in fetal postmortem examinations. The anomaly is found in approximately 15 percent of children studied, with the prevalence rising to 25 percent of adults (16). Degenerative changes of the arterial wall with secondary elongation are probably responsible for the higher prevalence in aging populations. Others have identified elastic tissue dysplasia of the tunica media of the carotid artery, a finding supportive of the congenital origin of carotid loops and tortuosities (17,18). The etiologic significance of degenerative changes secondary to arteriosclerosis with accentuation by chronic arterial hypertension and other hyperdynamic circulatory states remains speculative.

Although anatomists of the mid-eighteenth century accurately described elongation of the carotid arteries in autopsy examinations, Dr. Brown Kelly in the *Glasgow Medical Journal,* in 1898, was among the first to observe the condition and to forewarn unwary surgeons of the significance of the bulging pharyngeal wall behind the posterior tonsillar pillar (19). Edington, also, in an autopsy of a 34-year-old man who had died from chronic Bright's disease, identified bilateral, tortuous internal carotid arteries abutting each ipsilateral posterior pharyngeal wall and speculated that the condition was secondary to the arteritis of chronic nephritis; however, he noted that abnormal persistence of portions of the embryonic arches could not be excluded etiologically (19). In 1925, Kelly reported 150 consecutive cases of tortuous or redundant internal carotid arteries and ascribed the condition in young individuals to developmental abnormalities (11). He stressed the infrequency of progressive enlargement and alleviated fears of spontaneous rupture. On a number of occasions, tortuous internal carotid arteries have been misdiagnosed as peritonsillar abscesses with fatal exsanguination following surgical drainage.

Since the first successful surgical correction of a tortuous extracranial carotid artery by Riser in 1951, controversy has persisted concerning the potential association of tortuous or coiled internal carotid arteries and the risk of cerebral ischemia and infarction (20,21). While precise figures are unavailable, the relatively high prevalence of tortuosity, looping, and coiling of the cervical internal carotid artery is noteworthy. In patients with cerebral symptoms undergoing carotid arteriography, 4 to 31 percent of adults and 15 to 43 percent of children have demonstrated extracranial internal carotid tortuosity, coiling, or looping (7,16,22,23). The tortuosity frequently occurs in association with atheromatous plaques in adults. It is probable that tortuosity or carotid looping alone is rarely a primary cause of neurologic symptoms in adults; however, Sarkari has described several children with seizures, transient hemiparesis, hemianopia, and dysphasia in association with an ipsilateral internal carotid loop (14). Unfortunately, Sarkari, who theorized that the carotid anomaly was responsible for the severe neurologic deficits, provided no pathological studies of the vessels involved. Additionally, most other series affirming the association of carotid tortuosity and coiling with cerebral ischemia have not provided convincing evidence of such a cause and effect relationship. The available data suggest that carotid coiling, whether unilateral or bilateral, rarely accounts for cerebral ischemic symptoms in the absence of atherosclerotic occlusive disease in the carotid, vertebral, or basilar arteries (7,24). Thus far, proof is lacking that the risk of stroke in unselected patients with carotid tortuosity and coiling exceeds the risk of neurologic injury or death associated with operative intervention (7).

Most patients presenting with cerebral ischemic symptoms who are found to have redundancy or looping of the extracranial carotid artery are middle-aged with peak incidence of approximately 60 years. Approximately one-fourth of adults have bilateral lesions, whereas up to 50 percent of children with tortuous vessels have bilateral coiling or elongation which may be associated with other arterial anomalies such as aortic coarctation.

For unknown reasons, women with elongation of the common carotid are four times more likely than age-matched men to have this vascular anomaly (25).

Presenting symptoms mimic those from extracranial carotid atherosclerotic lesions and include both focal and global transient ischemic events, fluctuating deficits, and fixed neurologic damage of variable severity (26,27). Not infrequently symptoms are most intense while the patient is supine in bed or immediately upon awakening. Symptoms are usually considered to be secondary to hemodynamic consequences, and most frequently are provoked by ipsilateral cervical rotation. However, contralateral cervical rotation, flexion, and extension may also lead to impairment of carotid flow. As demonstrated arteriographically, cervical rotation manuevers may reduce or cease carotid flow by causing critical angulation or compression of the vessel by parapharyngeal soft tissue or osseous structures (28). While extrinsic compression by the atlas, mandible, vertebral bodies, or fibrous bands is thought to limit carotid flow with cervical motion, the possibility of distal embolization has not been excluded in these cases. Albanese recently reported finding elastic tissue dysplasia of a coiled internal carotid artery in a 48-year-old man who suffered two episodes of transient left cerebral hemispheric ischemia prior to the development of a left hemispheric infarction. The extracranial carotid coil demonstrated a paucity of elastic fibers in the tunica media; however, in addition to focal areas of intimal hyperplasia, a small area of endothelium was covered by recent thrombus—a possible source for cerebral embolus (17). Theoretically, flow disturbances in looped, high-flow arteries may occur, creating areas of high luminal surface shear stress potentially sufficient to denude the endothelium and allow disposition of platelet-fibrin aggregates with cerebral embolic potential.

Although there are no pathognomonic neurologic changes attributable to carotid tortuosity and coiling, symptoms of either hemispheric or global neurologic symptoms and vertebrobasilar insufficiency provoked by cervical rotation, extension, or flexion are important clues. Moreover, transient or permanent cerebral hemispheric signs in children should *always* arouse suspicion of the presence of internal carotid coiling. There are also no pathognomonic signs of internal carotid tortuosity. A prominent cervical pulsation below the mandibular angle that becomes pronounced with head turning may rarely be found and is best appreciated using bidigital, peritonsillar palpation. Rarely, a bruit or thrill may be appreciated during cervical rotation maneuvers. Carotid compression tests, as recommended by Derrick, add little diagnostically and are potentially hazardous, since four of his patients developed acute neurologic deficits with these compression maneuvers (29). The diagnostic potential of the noninvasive vascular laboratory in identifying flow-reducing carotid loops and coils remains controversial. Specifically, the sensitivity of oculoplethysmographic (OPG) determinants (ophthalmic systolic pressures and eye-ear pulse arrival discrepancies) during cervical positional testing is unknown; however, reproduction of symptoms by positional-OPG testing lends further credence that the carotid anomaly may be responsible for cerebral ischemic symptoms. Although real-time, B-mode ultrasound arteriography may visualize the carotid loop and associated atheroma, noninvasive tests dependent upon Doppler frequency shifts and spectral analysis predictably would be difficult to interpret because of flow disturbances related to the geometry of the coil. Most authorities agree that complete, four-vessel cerebral angiography is essential and should include multiple views taken in flexion, extension, and bidirectional rotation (7,24,29,30). Examples of typical internal carotid tortuosity and looping are presented in Figures 50-2 and 50-3.

Prior to assignment of the carotid loop as causal in producing cerebral symptoms, other possibilities must be excluded. The most common of these include cerebral neoplasm, intracranial vascular disease, cardiogenic emboli and arrhythmias, subdural hematoma, orthostatic hypotension, and other possible causes of cerebral ischemia. The natural history of the tortuous, or coiled, extracranial internal carotid artery is unknown, yet it is generally agreed that these anomalies, if symptomatic and discovered coincidentally, may be safely observed without significant threat of cerebral ischemia.

Once the decision is made that the tortuous carotid is responsible for cerebral symptoms, operative correction should be considered, since the roles of systemic anticoagulation and antiplatelet compounds have not been determined. The goal of operative therapy should be to eliminate the tortuosity or loop of the carotid artery and also to remove any intrinsic obstruction from atherosclerotic plaque. Restoration of unimpeded carotid arterial flow is essential. Originally described by Riser, carotid arteriopexy to the sternocleidomastoid muscle to straighten the elongated artery has been abandoned (21). Presently, resection

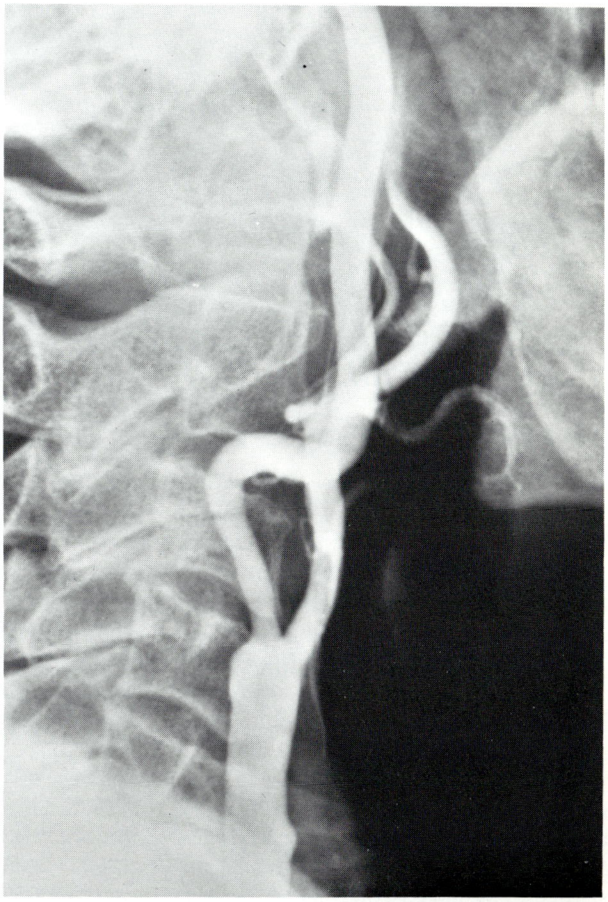

FIGURE 50-2. Lateral view angiogram of the extracranial carotid system, demonstrating a smooth atheromatous plaque of the proximal internal carotid artery and a sigmoid curve in the vessel at the level of the angle of the mandible.

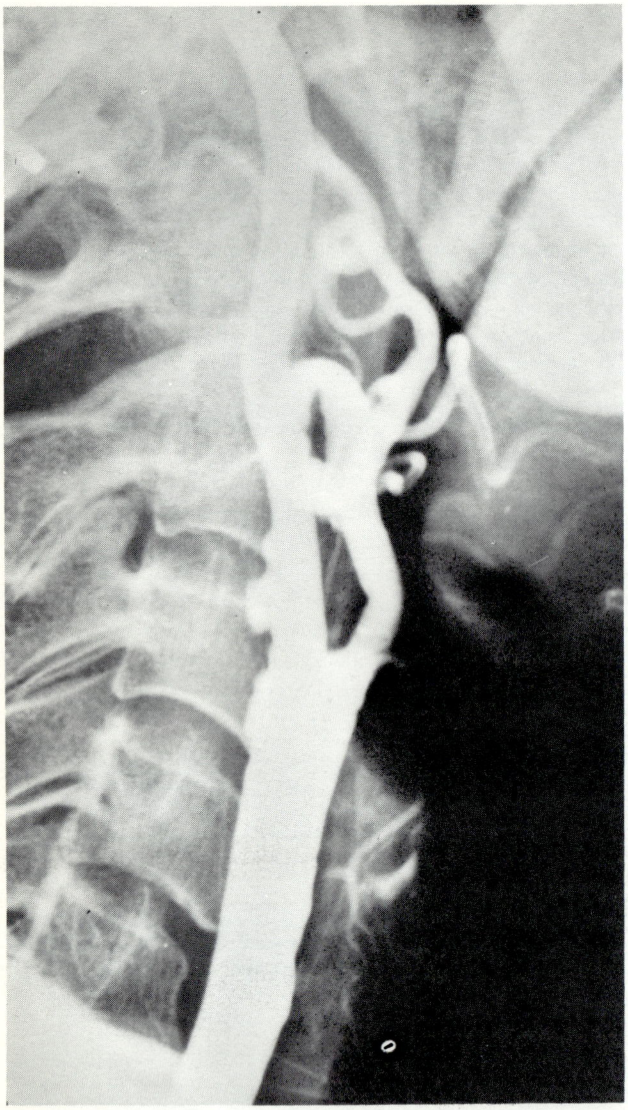

FIGURE 50-3. Lateral angiogram showing an ulcerated atheroma in the proximal internal carotid artery and a 360° loop just cephalad to the plaque.

of the elongated carotid artery is the operation of choice and demands proper assessment of the redundant arterial length. This determination is facilitated by complete mobilization of the distal internal carotid artery with lysis of all fibrous bands which tether the artery near the base of the skull. Gentle manipulation of the thin-walled, friable, internal carotid artery is mandatory to prevent possible dislodgement of atherothrombotic material and to minimize endothelial injury. Endarterectomy of coexistent atheromas is as essential as complete mobilization and precise geometric planning to eliminate possible kinking.

In order to minimize the dangers of suture line disruption of the friable internal carotid artery, some authors have advocated resection of the common carotid artery, placing the anastomosis in this vessel of larger caliber and greater structural integrity. However, this technique frequently necessitates sacrifice of the external carotid artery—an important route of cerebral collateral blood flow and possible donor vessel for subsequent extracranial-intracranial bypass. To preserve the external carotid artery, others have recommended ligation at the origin of the internal carotid artery with translocation of the orifice of the internal carotid artery more proximally onto the anterolateral common carotid surface (31). The authors prefer instead to excise a segment of proximal internal carotid artery, to apply caudad traction and detorsion in order to eliminate the redundancy, and then to construct a new anastomosis over an indwelling shunt as previously recommended by Najafi et al. (32). Caution is essential during insertion of the internal carotid shunt; the redundant length of internal carotid artery must be straightened prior to shunt insertion to minimize the risk of creating an endothelial flap. The internal carotid artery and common carotid artery are spatulated to create an elliptical anastomosis that is two times the length of the diameter of the internal carotid artery. The anastomosis is constructed with continuous monofilament suture, and the shunt is removed immediately prior to completion of the anastomosis.

Because of the extensive dissection necessary, general anesthesia is routinely employed, but local or regional block anesthesia is also suitable for some patients. In properly selected patients, the results of carotid arterioplasty for congenital loops and coils are quite acceptable with approximately 80 percent completely relieved of symptoms; perioperative neurologic morbidity and mortality rates should be under 5 percent (27).

The Carotid Kink

Kinking of the extracranial internal carotid artery is defined as an acute bending or angulation of the artery, often described as "buckling." Acute angulation of the internal carotid artery is almost invariably associated with atherosclerosis, with the distal tip of the atheroma corresponding to the vertex of the carotid angle (23). Kinking of the carotid is most frequently an acquired condition which appears later in life and occassionally coexists with tortuous changes of the internal carotid (16). The relative fixation of the proximal common carotid artery by the aortic arch and the distal internal carotid artery at the base of the skull predisposes the more flexible internal carotid to angulation, particularly when elongation of the artery occurs as a result of congenital lengthening or acquired degeneration secondary to chronic hypertension. The exact incidence of acute angulation of the carotid artery is unknown; however, in selected patients with cerebral symptoms, the incidence varies from 4 to 20 percent (7,8,22,23). Even more confusing is the matter of stroke risk from the carotid kink alone, since the overwhelming majority of patients with carotid kinks also demonstrate significant extracranial carotid atherosclerotic disease. Nonetheless, most authorities agree that a demonstrated carotid kink represents a greater threat of ischemic stroke than does elongation or coiling of the internal carotid artery.

The first direct operation for correction of an internal carotid artery kink was performed by Hsu and Kistin in 1956, but was unsuccessful (33). In 1959, Quattlebaum, Upson, and Neville successfully resected the common carotid artery in three symptomatic patients with kinked internal carotid arteries (34). In

1962, Derrick and Smith postulated that carotid kinking was more frequently causal of cerebral infarction than previously recognized and endorsed a more aggressive attitude toward investigation and operative correction of carotid kinks (35). More recently, Vannix reemphasized the potential lethality of cerebral complications associated with the internal carotid artery kink and urged operative correction of this potentially disabling condition (9). Contrariwise, others have deemphasized the importance of carotid kink alone in the production of neurologic symptoms and have correctly pointed out the high prevalence of concomitant atherosclerosis and other coexisting nonvascular pathology as potentially responsible for the apparent cerebral ischemia (7). The role of the noninvasive vascular laboratory in screening for significant carotid kinks remains controversial (36). Stanton et al. were among the first to popularize oculoplethysmography (OPG) during cervical rotation, flexion, and extension as potentially useful in screening (37). These authors, utilizing the electromagnetic flowmeter intraoperatively with recordings obtained during bidirectional rotation, hypertension, and flexion, confirmed the hemodynamic significance of the carotid kink with reductions of arterial flow from 30 to 80 percent during testing. According to their report, correction of the kink by segmental resection restored normal OPG scores with positional testing. Interestingly, each of the 16 patients undergoing operation had atherosclerotic stenoses and presumably underwent concomitant endarterectomy of an associated carotid atheroma (37). While positional OPG testing for screening of carotid kinks has not been universally accepted, these data indicate that internal carotid kinks may account for symptomatic flow impairment. Nonetheless, as elaborated by Metz, it is difficult to be certain of the relevance of any factor in the production of cerebrovascular symptoms (22). He stated that the cessation of symptoms after the removal of a suspected factor does not necessarily establish a causal relationship between the two. Many, in fact, believe that removal of carotid plaque by endarterectomy alone is sufficient to relieve cerebral symptoms and that correction of redundant length is rarely necessary (7).

Symptoms produced by the kinked internal carotid artery are virtually indistinguishable from those transient and permanent neurologic deficits of atherosclerotic origin. It is generally accepted that the hemodynamic theory of cerebral hypoperfusion is operative in the majority of symptomatic cases; however, microembolic events cannot be excluded with certainty. Kinking of the vertebral or innominate arteries also may coexist. Historical clues suggestive of the presence of a carotid kink typically include the precipitation of cerebral symptoms with extremes of cervical motion. Development of an audible bruit with cervical rotation may be observed, but physical examination of the cervical region is most often entirely normal.

The definitive diagnostic test is the four-vessel carotid and vertebral angiographic examination with complete intracranial views (Figure 50-4). Positional angiography may confirm the anatomic significance of carotid kinks, whereas physiological information may be obtained by using positional OPG. Parenthetically, it must be stated that while positional OPG, if positive, supports the hemodynamic significance of the carotid kink, operative correction may not be curative; also, negative positional OPG testing does not necessarily preclude successful operative correction. While most would agree that correction of an incidental, asymptomatic carotid kink is not indicated, some

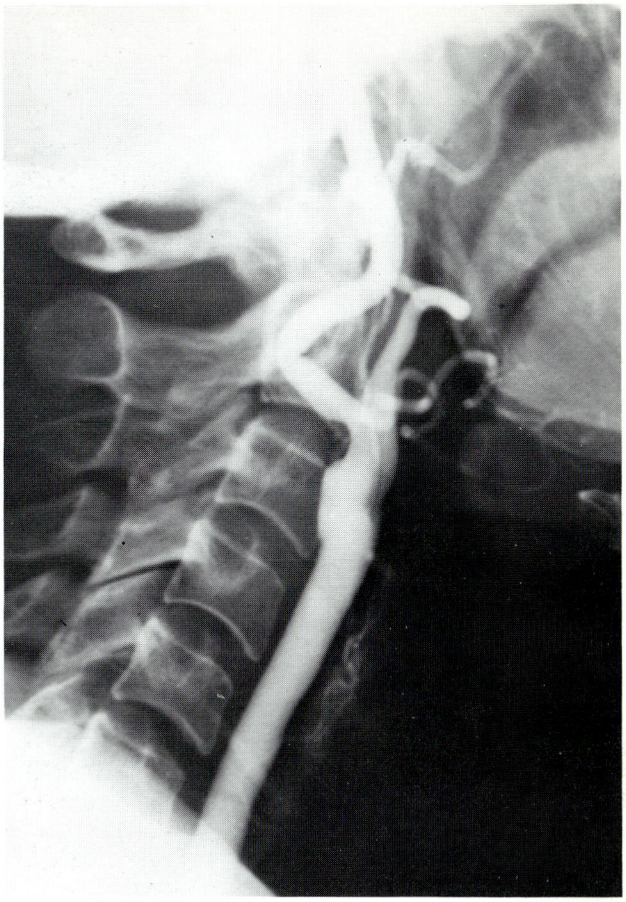

FIGURE 50-4. Angiogram with coexisting atheromatous stenosis of the proximal internal carotid artery and a 90° forward angulation of the vessel just distal to the rigid segment.

have recommended corrective arterioplasty if positional OPG testing suggests a significant reduction in carotid flow. The authors endorse the more conservative approach to the asymptomatic kink, for it appears that the natural history of this lesion, even in the presence of atherosclerosis, is less morbid than operative correction.

Generally accepted indications for the correction of internal carotid artery kinks are the following: (1) Evidence that the kink may be responsible for cerebral ischemia by reproduction of symptoms on head rotation, flexion, or extension. (2) Exclusion of other craniocerebral vascular, neoplastic, or developmental abnormalities which might account for similar symptoms. In actual practice, most patients with extracranial carotid kinks undergo operation primarily for correction of ulcerostenosing atheromas of the carotid with coincidental angulation of the artery noted at the apex of the rigid atheroma. Following endarterectomy and primary or patch closure of the arteriotomy, the acute angulation is frequently relieved. On rare occasions, acute angulation of 90° or less is observed after performance of the endarterectomy. If such a kinked vessel creates a harsh thrill or produces significant intraoperative pressure reduction in the distal internal carotid artery, the angulation should be corrected. A variety of shortening techniques have been advocated, but direct arteriopexy is rarely indicated. The authors' preferred technique

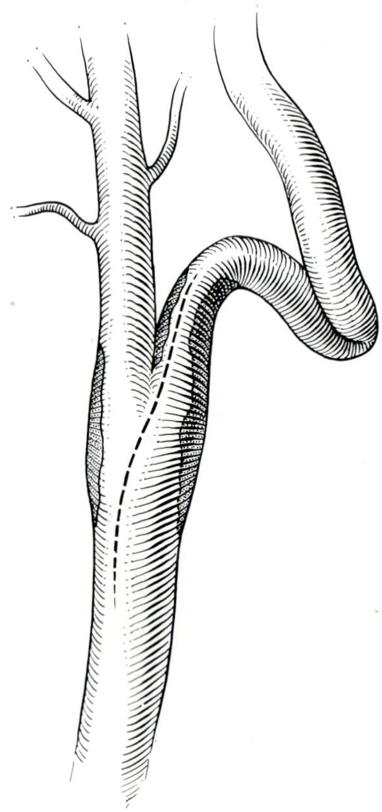

FIGURE 50-5. Operative repair of a carotid bifurcation atheroma with associated redundancy and kinking: location of the arteriotomy.

of arterioplasty for correction of acute angulation is similar to that described earlier for the correction of the internal carotid artery loop (Figures 50-5 to 50-10). Following endarterectomy, if required, resection of a cuff of proximal carotid is performed over an indwelling shunt. An elliptical end-to-end anastomosis (length to diameter ratio of 2:1) is then constructed with running monofilament vascular sutures. Despite the infrequent need for correction of a carotid kink, operative morbidity and mortality rates are acceptably low and should parallel that of simple carotid endarterectomy in experienced hands.

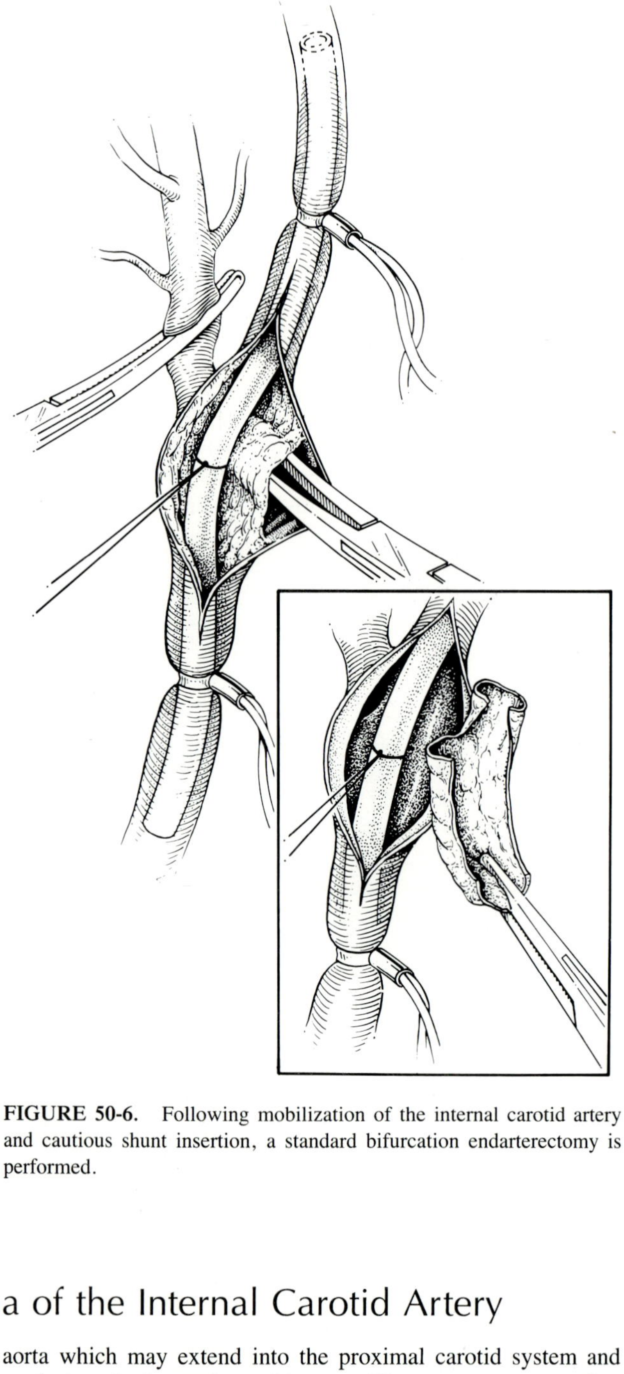

FIGURE 50-6. Following mobilization of the internal carotid artery and cautious shunt insertion, a standard bifurcation endarterectomy is performed.

Spontaneous Dissecting Hematoma of the Internal Carotid Artery

Dissecting hematomas of the extracranial internal carotid artery are rare yet potentially devastating causes of cerebral ischemia. The term ''spontaneous'' implies the occurrence of internal carotid dissection without recognizable traumatic antecedent, although, not infrequently, spontaneous dissections are observed in association with fibromuscular dysplasia, cystic medial necrosis, and arteriosclerosis (38–40). Since the original description by Anderson and Schechter in 1959 (41), approximately 72 cases have been reported, and over half of the reported cases are from the series of Ehrenfeld et al. and Fisher et al. (42,43). Blunt and penetrating cervical trauma, and acceleration-deceleration cervical injuries are well-recognized causes of arterial dissection, but are excluded from this consideration. Likewise excluded are dissecting aneurysms of the ascending and transverse aorta which may extend into the proximal carotid system and rarely into the internal carotid artery. The term spontaneous has been applied to carotid dissections thought to be initiated by cervical hypertension or flexion occurring during vigorous exercise or following ''head banging''—the rhythmic flexion and extension of the neck in cadence with rock music as reported by Jackson who described the fatal case of a 15-year-old boy indulging in head banging while enjoying a rock concert 1 day before death (44). In this patient, massive left cerebral infarction found at autopsy was ascribed to ischemia secondary to spontaneous left internal carotid artery dissection. Rare examples have also been reported following violent coughing paroxysms, presumably as a result of cervical hyperextension causing disruption of the intima of the internal carotid artery (43). In the

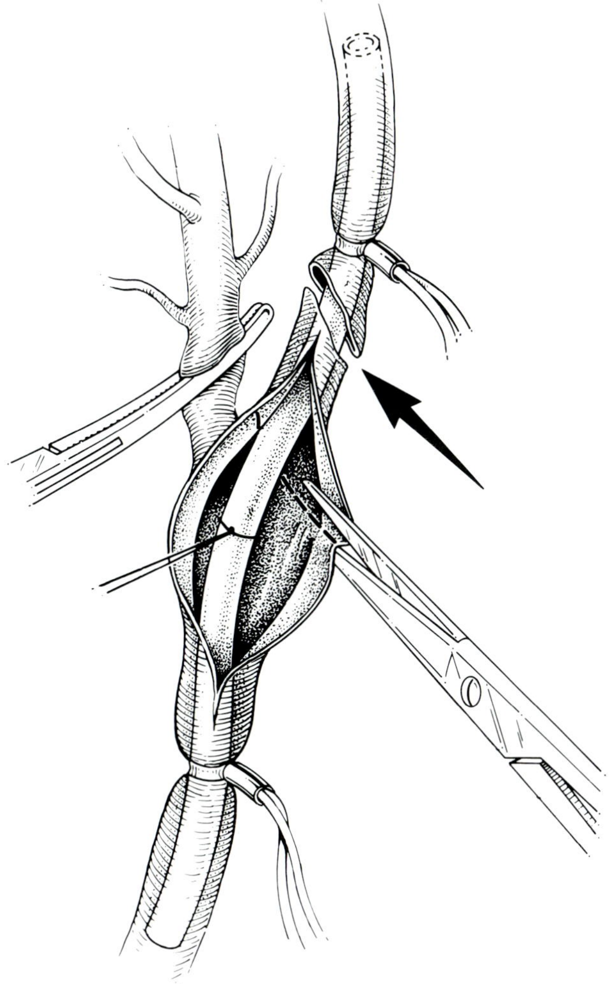

FIGURE 50-7. An appropriate length of redundant internal carotid is excised, taking care to prepare the ends for an oblique reanastomosis.

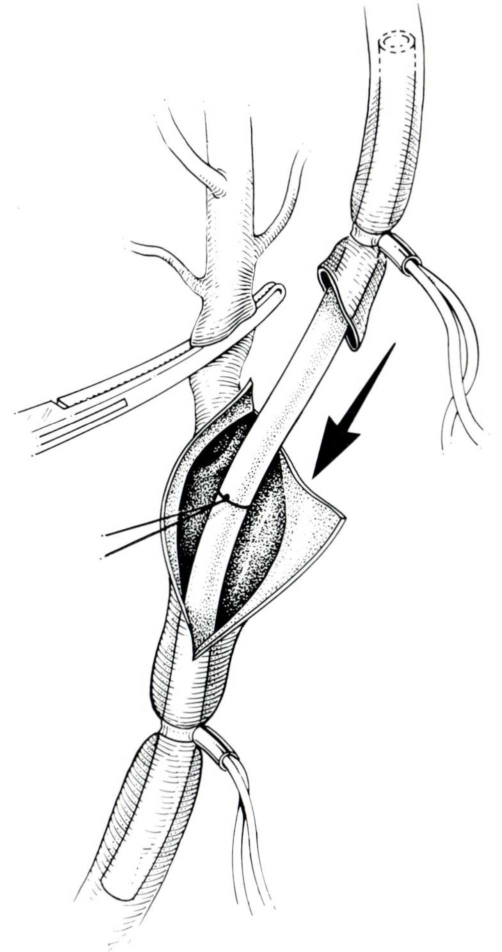

FIGURE 50-8. Using gentle traction while advancing the indwelling shunt, the internal carotid stump is positioned at the cut edge of the common carotid artery.

majority of patients, however, the etiology is unknown (45). Males and females appear to be afflicted at similar rates with the mean age at diagnosis of 46 years (range, 11 to 74 years) (42,43).

Presenting clinical manifestations of internal carotid dissection include focal cerebral neurologic deficits—either transient or permanent—in over 80 percent of cases, but it appears that the regional extent of neurologic complaints in this condition is greater than that attributable to atherosclerotic embolization (43). Thus, many patients present with signs of both retinal ischemia and contralateral hemiparesis or hemihypesthesia, in addition to multiple cranial nerve palsies. Noteworthy physical symptoms and signs of carotid dissection may include the rapid onset of severe hemicrania; Horner's syndrome; Raeder's trigeminal syndrome; scalp hyperalgesia; dysgeusia; central VI, VII, and XII cranial nerve palsy; as well as contralateral focal sensory and motor deficits. These neurologic features may occur singly or in variable combinations. Dysgeusia is felt to result from involvement of the chorda tympani branch of the VIIth cranial nerve. Importantly, the evolution of a complete Horner's oculosympathetic palsy may occur asynchronously or may be incomplete. The acute onset of ipsilateral head and facial pain in the frontal, parietal, or periorbital area may be followed in 24 to 72 hours by the development of one or more features of Horner's syndrome with anhydrosis most frequently absent. The headaches are typically nonthrobbing, fluctuating in intensity, and frequently require 2 to 6 months to resolve completely. During this interval, rarely is there complete relief of the cephalalgia. Other complaints include pulsatile or machinery vascular tinnitus (42,43,46).

Physical findings of carotid dissection vary enormously. The multiplicity of neurologic findings mentioned above, in addition to tenderness over the carotid bulb and an evolving cervical bruit, are strongly suggestive of the diagnosis. The origin of the internal carotid dissecting hematoma usually occurs 2 to 3 cm distal to the carotid bulb. Through the usually vertically oriented intimal rent, the hematoma pulsates deep into the media, creating a subadventitial cleavage plane (42,43). The entire arterial circumference is rarely involved; however, thrombosis of the false channel severely compromises the true lumen, leading either to markedly reduced flow or to secondary complete thrombosis. The dissection seldom extends beyond the base of the skull, but

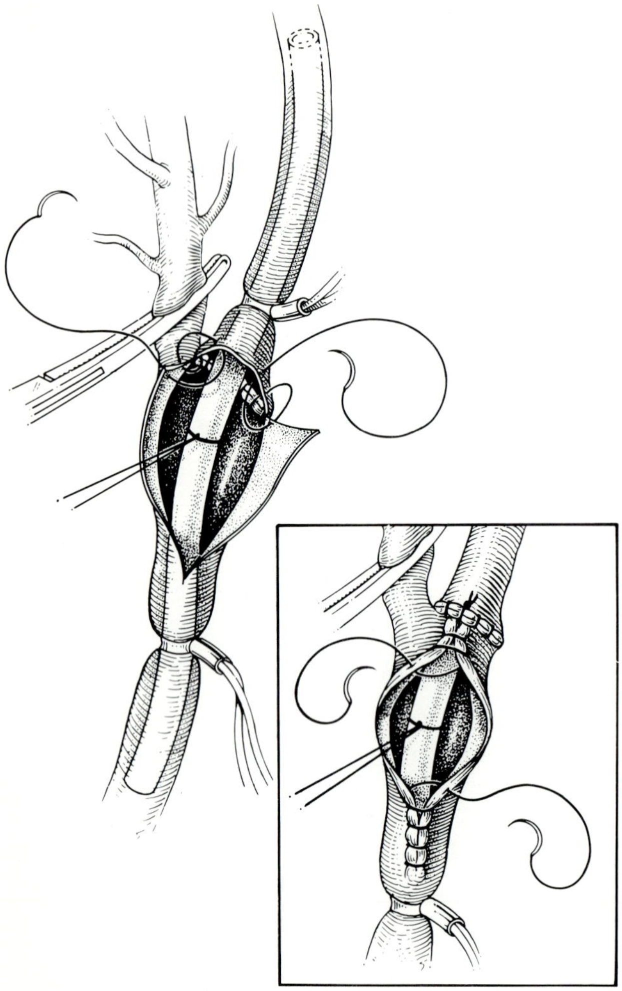

FIGURE 50-9. Reanastomosis is performed by use of a continuous monofilament vascular suture producing a "T-shaped" closure.

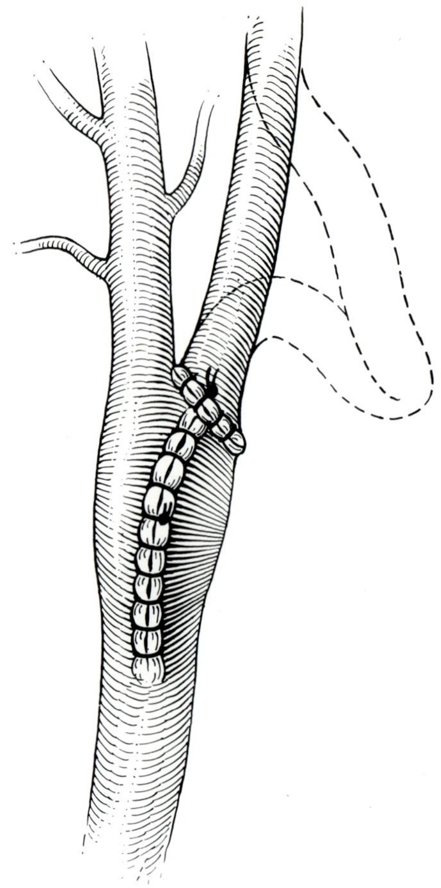

FIGURE 50-10. Completed endarterectomy and internal carotid shortening procedure. Note that the continuity of the external carotid is preserved by this technique.

cavernous sinus extension has been reported. On rare occassions, reentry of the hematoma into the true lumen may occur acutely, restoring arterial flow.

The experience of Ehrenfeld and Wylie in 10 patients with dissecting aneurysms has provided the best description of the typical gross pathology (42). A consistent finding in their experience was a sharp transition between the normal color and size of the internal carotid artery and the dark blue discoloration and moderate cylindrical dilatation produced by the dissection. Only four patients of their series experienced termination of the dissection at a level easily visualized from the cervical incision, whereas the other six experienced dissections beyond the limits of surgical accessibility. Three patients had an arteriotomy performed, and each demonstrated the short, vertical, intimal rent marking the origin of the dissection. Microscopically the typical features included organizing hematoma in the deeper layers of the tunica media with reduction of elastic tissue and fragmentation of internal elastic membranes. Smooth-muscle cells were widely separated and diminished in number. Mucopolysaccharide stains demonstrated the deposition of mucoid material indicative of degenerative changes. Atherosclerosis was consistently absent (42).

In 1972, Ojemann suggested that the long, stenotic segment of extracranial internal carotid artery visualized angiographically ("string sign") might be a reliable indicator of carotid dissection (47) (Figures 50-11 and 50-12). Adopting this radiographic feature, radiologists became convinced that spontaneous carotid dissection was clearly not as rare as previously suspected. Typically, the angiogram of the carotid dissection reveals an irregular, extremely narrow column of contrast beginning slightly above the carotid bulb with a gradual taper ending at the base of the skull. Usually there is little, or no, evidence of atherosclerotic plaque. These radiographic features are highly suggestive of carotid dissection, but the "string sign"' may also occur with other types of vascular disease such as atherosclerosis, fibromuscular dysplasia, arteritis, moya moya, and vasospasm (43). Although the degree of stenosis is usually high-grade, the length of the angiographic stenotic segment can be variable. Occasionally a small cul-de-sac projecting cephalad and posterior is identified angiographically and is thought to represent the residual lumen at the origin of the intimal tear. If spontaneous organization of the false channel hematoma develops, retraction of the intima occurs at variable rates, producing scalloped or undulating angiographic margins of the recanalizing carotid artery walls. Bilateral carotid dissections are extremely rare (43).

Early experience with this condition included a variety of urgent attempts to restore cerebral arterial flow. These included resection of the involved segment with saphenous vein inter-

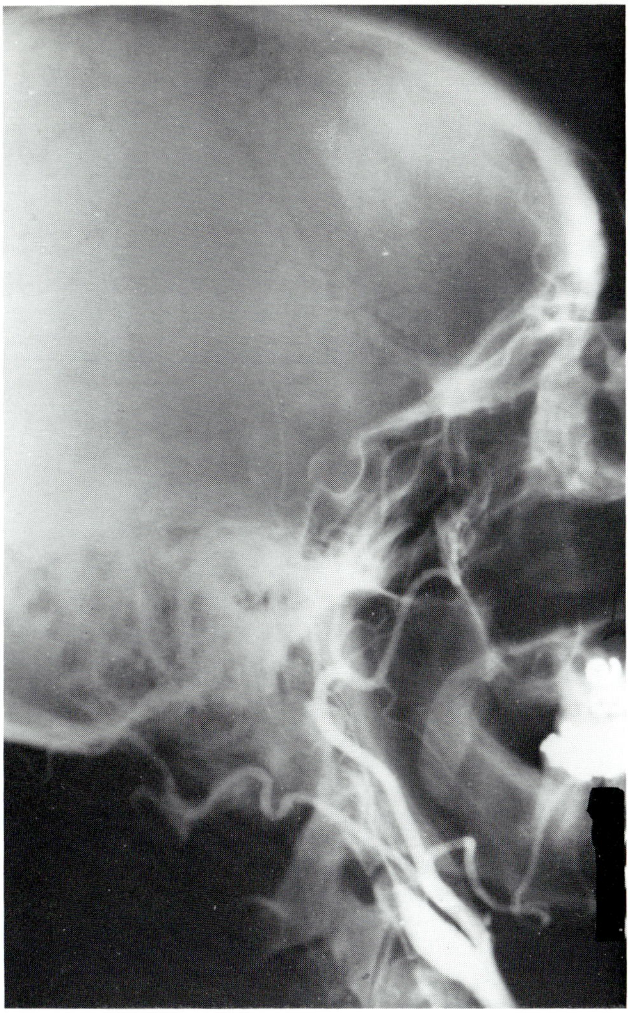

FIGURE 50-11. Lateral carotid arteriogram of a young patient with carotid dissection showing severe tapering of the internal carotid lumen and a "string sign" extending cephalad. Note the absence of atherosclerotic changes.

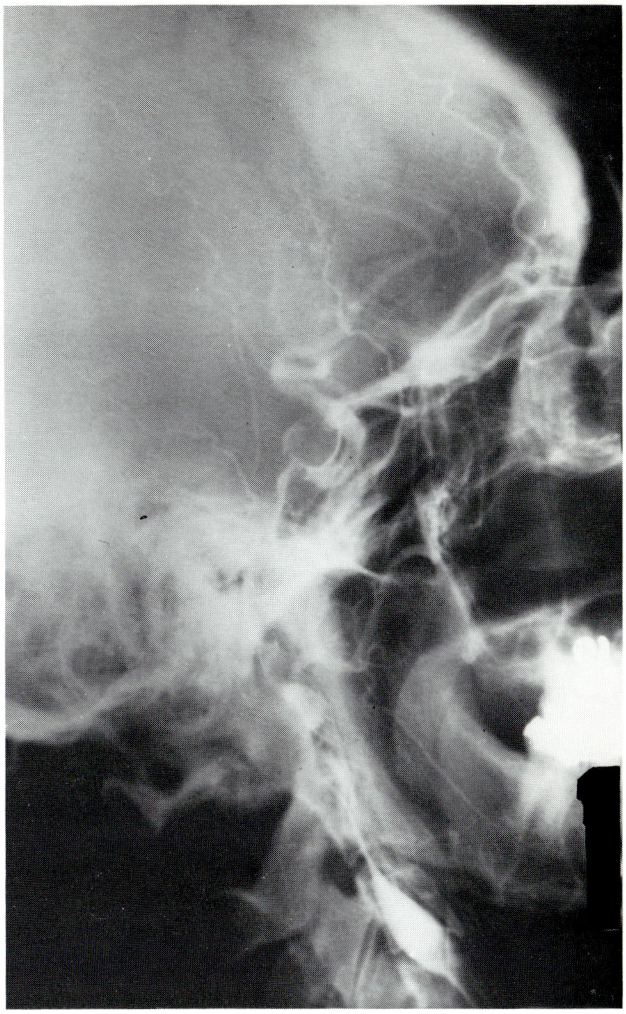

FIGURE 50-12. Later film from the same angiographic sequence demonstrating eventual filling of the carotid siphon and suggesting patency of the severely narrowed lumen.

position grafting, dilatation, balloon catheter thrombectomy, or ligation of the internal carotid artery, provided a stump pressure of greater than 65 torr was identified (42). The majority of these operations were unsuccessful due to technical difficulties with exposure of the distal point of dissection, the presence of residual thrombus with cerebral embolic potential, or progression of frank stroke as a result of acute revascularization of a bland cerebral infarct. Taking a new approach, in 1976, Ehrenfeld and Wylie described experience with seven patients in whom the carotid artery was not disturbed surgically. Three of these patients underwent cervical exploration only, and four were managed nonoperatively. Surprisingly, none of the patients had further progression of neurologic symptoms with up to 3 years follow-up. Repeat arteriography was obtained in six of these patients from 2 to 16 months following the original arteriogram. One carotid progressed to total occlusion, whereas the remaining five had increased to essentially normal caliber (42). Others have since reported favorable results with nonoperative therapy (45); however, the optimum therapeutic protocol is presently unknown. Although the exact role of heparin, warfarin, and antiplatelet drugs is uncertain, a consensus of the recent literature suggests that the initial approach should be nonsurgical. In the absence of massive cerebral infarction, systemic heparinization should be initiated and theoretically may facilitate resolution of the hematoma and minimize the threat of distal cerebral embolization. It has been suggested that a minimum of 3 weeks of heparin therapy is necessary (48); however, continuing heparinization until there is normalization of the ophthalmic systolic pressure by OPG testing is a logical approach (45). Operative intervention is reserved for medical failures: Persistence of transient ischemic neurologic events with failure of recanalization may necessitate graft replacement of the diseased carotid artery or ligation, preferably preceded by extracranial-intracranial bypass. Bilateral extracranial carotid dissections may require extracranial-intracranial bypass grafting for symptoms of the low-flow endangered brain.

The initial dismal results with this rare disorder have been supplanted recently by more optimism, since the condition appears to be self-limited and amenable to medical therapy in the majority of cases.

References

1. Symonds C: The circle of Willis. Br Med J 1955, 1:119.
2. Cooper A: Account of the first successful operation, performed on the common carotid artery, for aneurysm, in the year 1808: with the post mortem examination, in 1821. Guys Hosp Rep 1836, 1:53.
3. Hunt JR: The role of the carotid arteries, in the causation of vascular lesions of the brain, with remarks on certain features of the symptomatology. Am J Med Sci 1913, 147:704.
4. Moniz E, Lima A, de Lacerda R: Hémiplégies par thrombose de la carotide interne. Presse Med 1937, 45:977.
5. Fisher M, Adams RD: Observations on brain embolism with special reference to the mechanism of hemorrhagic infarction. J Neuropathol Exp Neurol 1951, 10:92.
6. Hollenhorst RW: Significance of bright plaques in the retinal arterioles. JAMA 1961, 178:23.
7. Perdue GD, Barreca JP, Smith RB: The significance of elongation and angulation of the carotid artery: A negative view. Surgery 1975, 77:45.
8. Brosig H-J, Vollmar J: Chirurgische korrektur der knickstenosen der A. carotis interna. Munch Med Wochenschr 1974, 116:969.
9. Vannix RS, Joergenson FJ, Carter R: Kinking of the internal carotid artery. Clinical significance and surgical management. Am J Surg 1977, 134:82.
10. Desai B, Toole JF: Kinks, coils and carotids: A review. Stroke 1975, 6:649.
11. Kelly AB: Tortuosity of the internal carotid in relation to the pharynx. J Laryngol Otol 1925, 40:15.
12. Gass HH: Kinks and coils of the cervical carotid artery. Surg Forum 1958, 9:721.
13. Ohara I, Iwabrehi T, Yaegashi S: Abnormally twisted cervical internal carotid artery, probably congenital. Vasc Surg 1969, 3:1.
14. Sarkari NBS, Holmes JM, Bickerstaff ER: Neurological manifestations associated with internal carotid loops and kinks in children. J Neurol Neurosurg Psychiatry 1970, 33:194.
15. Gray SW, Skandalakis JE: The thoracic aorta (chapter 26). In *Embryology for Surgeons, the Embryological Basis for the Treatment of Congenital Defects*. Philadelphia, Saunders, 1972, pp 809–857.
16. Weibel J, Fields WS: Tortuosity, coiling, and kinking of the internal carotid artery. I. Etiology and radiographic anatomy. Neurology 1965, 15:7.
17. Albanese V, Spadaro A, Iannotti F: Elastic tissue dysplasia of coiled internal carotid artery in an adult. J Neurosurg 1983, 58:781.
18. Ochsner JL, Hughes JP, Leonard GL: Elastic tissue dysplasia of the internal carotid artery. Ann Surg 1977, 185:684.
19. Edington GH: Tortuosity of both internal carotid arteries. Br Med J 1901, 2:1526.
20. Robicsek F, Daugherty HK: Redundancy of the carotid artery combined with intrinsic occlusion. Vasc Surg 1970, 4:101.
21. Riser MM, Geraud J, Ducoudray J: Dolicho-carotide interne avec syndrome vertigineux. Rev Neurol (Paris) 1951, 85:145.
22. Metz H, Murray-Leslie RM, Bannister RG: Kinking of the internal carotid artery in relation to cerebrovascular disease. Lancet 1961, 1:424.
23. Bauer R, Sheehan S, Meyer JS: Arteriographic study of cerebrovascular disease. II. Cerebral symptoms due to kinking, tortuosity and compression of carotid and vertebral arteries in the neck. Arch Neurol 1961, 4:119.
24. Weibel J, Fields WS: Tortuosity, coiling, and kinking of the internal carotid artery. II. Relationship of morphological variation to cerebrovascular insufficiency. Neurology 1965, 15:462.
25. Schecter DC: Dolichocarotid syndrome. Cerebral ischemia related to cervical carotid artery redundancy with kinking: Parts I and II. NY State J Med 1979, 79:1391, 1542.
26. Harrison JH, Davalos PA: Cerebral ischemia: Surgical procedures in cases due to tortuosity and buckling of the cervical vessels. Arch Surg 1962, 84:85.
27. Quattlebaum JK Jr, Wade JS, Whiddon CM: Stroke associated with elongation, and kinking of the carotid artery: Long-term follow-up. Ann Surg 1973, 177:572.
28. Freeman TR, Lippitt WH: Carotid artery syndrome due to kinking: Surgical treatment in forty-four cases. Am Surg 1962, 28:745.
29. Derrick JR: Carotid kinking and cerebral insufficiency. Geriatrics 1963, 18:272.
30. Robicsek F, Daugherty HK, Sanger PW: Intermittent cerebrovascular insufficiency. A frequent and curable cause of stroke. Geriatrics 1967, 22:96.
31. Rundles WR, Kimbrell FD. The kinked carotid syndrome. Angiology 1969, 20:177.
32. Najafi H, Javid H, Dye WS: Kinked internal carotid artery. Arch Surg 1964, 89:134.
33. Hsu I, Kistin AD: Buckling of the great vessels. Arch Intern Med 1956, 98:712.
34. Quattlebaum JK Jr, Upson ET, Neville RL: Stroke associated with elongation and kinking of the internal carotid artery. Ann Surg 1959, 150:824.
35. Derrick JR, Smith T: Carotid kinking as a cause of cerebral insufficiency. Circulation 1962, 25:849.
36. Henrikson J: The carotid kink. Bruit 1983, 8:33.
37. Stanton PE, McClusky DA, Lamis PA: Hemodynamic assessment and surgical correction of kinking of the internal carotid artery. Surgery 1978, 84:793.
38. Mettinger KL, Ericson K: Fibromuscular dysplasia and the brain. Observation on angiographic, clinical and genetic characteristics. Stroke 1982, 13:46.
39. Boström K, Liliequist B: Primary dissecting aneurysm of the extracranial part of the interal carotid and vertebral arteries. Report of three cases. Neurology 1967, 17:179.
40. Luken MG, Ascherl GF, Carrell JW: Spontaneous dissecting aneurysms of extracranial internal carotid artery. Clin Neurosurg 1979, 26:353.
41. Anderson R, Schechter M: A case of spontaneous dissecting aneurysms of the internal carotid artery. J Neurol Neurosurg Psychiatry 1959, 22:195.
42. Ehrenfeld WK, Wylie EJ: Spontaneous dissection of the internal carotid artery. Arch Surg 1976, 111:1294.
43. Fisher CM, Ojemann RG, Roberson GH: Spontaneous dissection of cervicocerebral arteries. Can J Neurol Sci 1978, 5:9.
44. Jackson MA: "Headbanging" and carotid dissection. Br Med J 1983, 287:1262.
45. Gee W, Kaupp HA, McDonald KM: Spontaneous dissection of internal carotid arteries. Spontaneous resolution documented by serial ocular pneumoplethysmography and angiography. Arch Surg 1980, 115:944.
46. Maitland CG, Black JL, Smith WA: Abducens nerve palsy due to spontaneous dissection of the internal carotid artery. Arch Neurol 1983, 40:448.
47. Ojemann RG, Fisher CM, Rich JC: Spontaneous dissecting aneurysm of the internal carotid artery. Stroke 1972, 3:434.
48. McNeill DH, Dreisbach J, Marsden RJ: Spontaneous dissection of the internal carotid artery. Its conservative management with heparin sodium. Arch Neurol 1980, 37:54.

Chapter 51

EXTRACRANIAL CAROTID ARTERY ANEURYSMS

JAMES A. GILLESPIE

Carotid artery aneurysms are uncommon, but their clinical significance has long been recognized. Indeed, surgical treatment was first employed successfully in 1808 by Sir Astley Cooper (1), a London surgeon, using the technique of proximal ligation, even then widely practiced in dealing with peripheral aneurysms. His patient lived for another 13 years. Since that time, reports of carotid aneurysms have appeared regularly in the literature, Winslow (2) collecting some 106 cases up to 1925. However, it was not until 1952 that a reconstructive surgical technique was used to deal with a carotid aneurysm (3), and since that time the number of cases reported has increased considerably. Reconstructions, by maintaining carotid blood flow, reduce the risk of a cerebrovascular accident, so often the sequel of simple ligation, and the various surgical techniques are now fairly well standardized.

The Incidence of Carotid Artery Aneurysms

The actual total incidence of extracranial carotid artery aneurysms is relatively small, and this is perhaps best indicated by Schechter's recent detailed survey (4). He found reports of a total of only 853 carotid aneurysms in the literature up to 1977. The low incidence of carotid artery aneurysms compared to that of other extracranial aneurysms is also well demonstrated, for example, in figures from DeBakey's unit in Houston (5), where there were only 37 carotid aneurysms out of a total of 8500 aneurysms which they treated surgically in the 20 years up to 1977. Another group in Ohio reported 41 carotid aneurysms from a total of 1118 peripheral aneurysms which they evaluated over a 30-year period (6). Yet another report states that while 500 patients with occlusive carotid disease had been dealt with over a 24-year period, only 19 carotid aneurysms were treated in the same period (7). Most reports of carotid aneurysms in the literature have been concerned with only one or two new examples, however, and it is therefore a relatively rare condition which has a special importance because of the threat of hemorrhage, stroke, or death that it poses.

Pathology of Carotid Artery Aneurysms

Many causes of carotid aneurysms have been described, but the two most important are undoubtedly atherosclerosis and trauma. Before considering these in more detail, some of the other less common etiologies may be noted. Syphilis was an important cause in the last century and first part of this one, but rarely is today. Loss of elastic tissue in the arterial wall in Marfan's syndrome has been the cause of some reported carotid aneurysms, as has cystic medial necrosis, where carotid aneurysms are frequently associated with other peripheral aneurysms. Similarly, carotid aneurysms may occur with renal artery aneurysms in fibromuscular hyperplasia. Congenital carotid aneurysms, perhaps bilateral, have been reported, and so also have primary or spontaneous dissecting aneurysms, as opposed to traumatic dissecting ones, though their etiology is somewhat obscure (9). Carotid aneurysm has also been associated with polyarteritis nodosa. Mycotic carotid aneurysms are occasionally caused by infected emboli in bacterial endocarditis, but more usually result from spread of infection from a nearby area of cellulitis, or from a peritonsillar or mastoid abscess. Mycotic aneurysms also may follow a septic penetrating injury, perhaps from a heroin injection in an addict (8). Diabetes seems to have been only rarely mentioned in patients with carotid aneurysms. Finally, carotid aneurysms have been described after irradiation for cervical malignancy (10).

ATHEROSCLEROTIC CAROTID ANEURYSMS

These aneurysms usually occur in elderly patients and are frequently associated with atherosclerotic aneurysmal or occlusive arterial disease elsewhere. Many of these patients are hypertensive, and the aneurysm wall is frequently calcified. These aneurysms may be bilateral, are usually fusiform rather than saccular, and tend to occur in the region of the carotid bifurcation (10).

TRAUMATIC CAROTID ARTERY ANEURYSMS

These aneurysms are the second most common type, after atherosclerotic aneurysms. They may result from blunt trauma, penetrating injuries, sudden neck hyperextension and rotation, or they may follow previous carotid artery surgery for stenotic or occlusive disease. Penetrating injuries may lead occasionally to arteriovenous aneurysms, and, if infection enters, mycotic aneurysms. Traumatic aneurysms are often of saccular type, but dissecting ones occasionally may result. Blunt trauma may cause intimal tears and medial disruption with consequent weakening of the arterial wall. Traumatic carotid aneurysms can also result from damage to the arterial wall from bone splinters, and examples in association with mandibular fractures are reported. While traumatic aneurysms involve mostly the common carotid artery, some occur in the high internal carotid artery, often extending up to the base of the skull. It is likely that fixation of the internal carotid artery as it passes into the bony carotid canal in the base of the skull base is an important factor when the more distal part of the artery is deformed and twisted by blunt trauma. Many posttraumatic aneurysms are actually false aneurysms, especially those occurring as a result of penetrating injuries and after surgery for carotid stenosis. The latter most commonly occurs when the original arteriotomy was closed with a patch graft, and seldom when it was closed directly. False aneurysms have also, very rarely, been reported after needling the carotid vessels in arteriography. Aneurysms of any type involving the external carotid artery are rare, just over 2 percent of all (11).

Effects of Carotid Artery Aneurysms

Like other peripheral aneurysms carotid aneurysms may occlude spontaneously, may liberate emboli distally, or, less commonly, may rupture. Their special danger lies in the effect of emboli or sudden ischemia on the brain, while rupture and hemorrhage may occur into the oropharynx with desperate airway consequences. Carotid aneurysms pose a very real threat to life, and Winslow (2) in his extensive early survey of these lesions made the point that four out of every five patients treated conservatively eventually died from a complication of their aneurysm, though few authorities would put the figure so high today.

Clinical Presentation

The most common presentation of a carotid aneurysm is a swelling in the neck, which is usually felt to be pulsatile. Pain in the area is also a frequent complaint, especially when the aneurysm is expanding or dissecting, and here the mass is likely to be tender to palpation. Reports on brain damage vary greatly, some suggesting that perhaps up to half of all patients present with some neurological feature, such as a stroke, transient cerebral ischemic attacks (Figure 51-1), or a visual defect due to embolization (12). The patient sometimes complains of a buzzing in the ear, and auscultation over the neck may reveal a loud systolic bruit. Hoarseness can result from vagal or recurrent laryngeal nerve compression, or from Horner's syndrome from similar compression of the cervical sympathetic nerves.

Some internal carotid aneurysms project into the oropharynx (Figure 51-2), occasionally giving dysphagia or dyspnea. It has long been recognized that here a carotid aneurysm may resemble a peritonsillar abscess and disaster attends attempted lancing. Occasionally, fatal spontaneous rupture into the oropharynx has occurred. Small, high internal carotid aneurysms may not be palpable in the neck and can be a rare cause of unexplained facial pain. Occasionally they may rupture to give rise to profuse epistaxis or to bleeding from the ear. For these reasons otolaryngologists especially recognize the importance of carotid aneurysms (13).

Differential Diagnosis

In most cases the diagnosis can be made clinically without much difficulty. However, enlarged cervical lymph nodes, branchial cysts, and carotid body tumors may occasionally be confused, and if the aneurysm bulges into the oropharynx, it may be misdiagnosed as a peritonsillar abscess. Perhaps the greatest difficulty in differential diagnosis arises where the carotid artery in an elderly and often hypertensive patient is elongated and kinked outward, pulsation and swelling being both visible and easily palpable. Here it may only be possible to prove or refute the diagnosis of aneurysm with arteriography or ultrasound scanning.

Investigation of Carotid Aneurysms

While diagnosis often is certain on clinical examination, it can sometimes be difficult, for example, with high, small internal carotid aneurysms. Investigations include plain x-rays of the neck to show a soft tissue mass and perhaps calcification in the aneurysm wall. Ultrasound scanning demonstrates aneurysms well and is the best noninvasive investigative method. Examination of the fundi may reveal retinal artery emboli in patients with aneurysms complicated by transient visual field defects or transient cerebral ischemia. Flow-through aneurysms can be measured by the Doppler flowmeter.

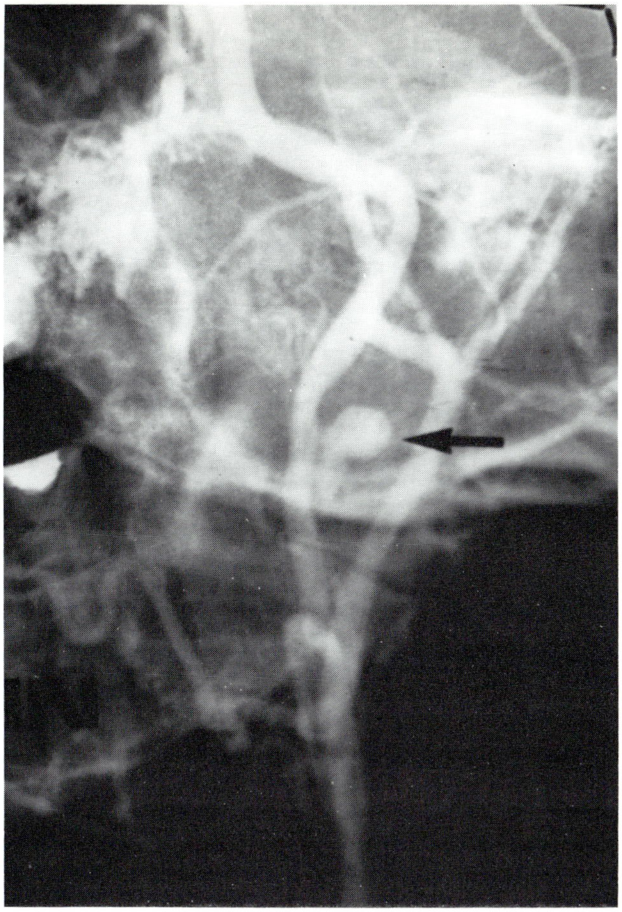

FIGURE 51-1. Traumatic high internal carotid aneurysm (arrow) in a 28-year-old male patient. He was briefly unconscious following an auto accident, but made an apparently complete recovery. Two months later he presented with transient strokes. A CT scan showed small brain infarcts.

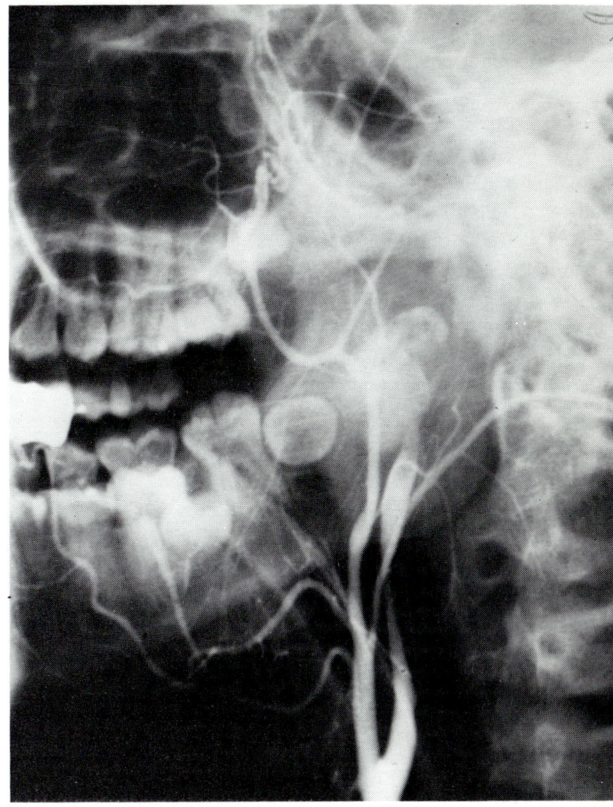

FIGURE 51-2. Three weeks after an apparently trivial injury to the left side of his neck this 15-year-old male patient presented in the ear, nose, and throat unit with a mass in the left tonsillar region. On needle aspiration blood was obtained. Arteriography showed a large, false internal carotid artery aneurysm. This ruptured into the esophagus immediately before surgery was to be undertaken, but he was resuscitated and the common carotid artery ligated. He made a complete recovery.

Arteriography, however, is the essential investigative method when surgical intervention is planned. The proximal and distal carotid artery, as well as the aneurysm, must be visualized. Arteriography can be performed either by selective carotid catheterization via an arm artery, or contrast can be injected by direct needle puncture into the lower common carotid artery in the neck. The aneurysm itself should not be needled. Arteriography shows dissecting aneurysms well (Figure 51-3), a common appearance being a tapering narrowing with a fine string of contrast extending distally.

Treatment of Carotid Aneurysms

Treatment is essentially surgical, there being little to offer of a nonsurgical nature that is likely to be helpful. Patients who are for other reasons unfit for operation, those who have small and symptomless aneurysms discovered by chance, and those whose aneurysms extend right to the base of the skull, may merely be observed. However, a conservative approach to carotid aneurysms in general is likely to result in a considerable morbidity, mainly because of neurological complications, but occasionally from rupture. For example, Winslow (2) found that of 106 patients treated conservatively, 71 percent died as a result of a complication of their aneurysm. Even though the only active treatment then was proximal ligation, he concluded that carotid aneurysm was "strictly a surgical problem." Perhaps an occasional exception to this rule of active treatment arises in dealing with the rather rare dissecting aneurysms without cerebral embolic complications. Here reports suggest that the caliber of the arterial lumen may return spontaneously to normal in time, as has been shown arteriographically (9). Long-term anticoagulation or aspirin therapy with the aim of preventing cerebral embolic symptoms in conservatively treated patients does not appear to have been employed, and it seems unlikely that it would be effective. Mycotic aneurysms require intensive antibiotic therapy but also need urgent surgical treatment because of the high risk of rupture, and the same applies to false aneurysms, which in general are liable to continue to expand and possibly to rupture.

Techniques of Surgical Treatment

The techniques for surgical treatment fall into two main types, namely simple ligation and reconstructive surgery.

SIMPLE LIGATION

As has been noted, treatment of a carotid aneurysm by ligation was carried out successfully over 175 years ago, and ligation remained virtually the only surgical option available until the advent of reconstructive arterial techniques. Ligation may be done just proximal to the aneurysm or both proximal and distal to it, or the common carotid may be ligated. Wherever the ligature is placed, however, it has long been recognized that there is a high risk of cerebral infarction postoperatively. In the early literature, for example, death rates of over 50 percent were reported as a sequel to common carotid ligation. However, more recent reports put the incidence of serious neurological damage at a lower figure, and ligation is still the only feasible surgical treatment in certain patients. The best example of this situation is that in which there is a symptom-producing high internal carotid aneurysm with no possibility of making a distal anastomosis.

Two methods have been employed to try to reduce the risk of neurological sequellae following ligation in those patients in whom it has to be employed. One is to occlude the artery slowly over several days using a Selverstone clamp in the hope of allowing an adequate collateral circulation to develop before occlusion is complete. The patient is anticoagulated throughout this period to reduce the risk of embolization. When the clamp is finally removed, a ligature is applied in its place (14). If ischemic signs appear at any time, the clamp is slackened. The other method is to try to estimate the likely risk of brain damage by preligation investigations and only to subject the patient to ligation if it seems likely to be safe. These investigations will be described later. Simple proximal ligation is of course a good technique for dealing with the uncommon external carotid aneurysms, where there is no risk of producing cerebral ischemia.

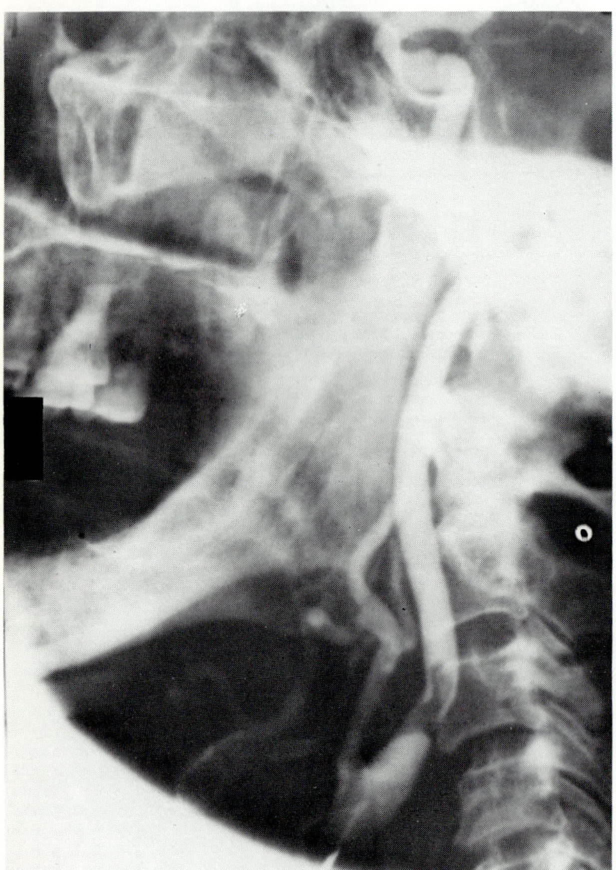

FIGURE 51-3. Right carotid angiogram showing a partial occlusion due to dissection of the proximal part of the right internal carotid artery in a patient who developed hemiplegia following a traffic accident. He sustained multiple facial fractures including a fracture of the right mandibular ramus.

RECONSTRUCTIVE APPROACH TO CAROTID ANEURYSM SURGERY

However carefully simple ligation is performed, the risk of cerebral damage remains sufficiently high to make those techniques by which carotid blood flow can be maintained the first choice, and reconstruction was first employed successfully in 1952. Several procedures have now been described, the most preferable being excision of the aneurysm with primary end-to-end reconstruction of the artery. This is quite often feasible, but it does require the availability of a sufficient redundant length of artery. If there is not a sufficient length, interposition of a vein or prosthetic tube graft is necessary. An occasionally applicable technique for avoiding the use of an interposition graft in dealing with low internal carotid aneurysms is to divide the external carotid artery at such a level that its proximal end can be anastomosed to the distal end of the internal carotid after excision of the aneurysm.

Saccular aneurysms often have a relatively narrow neck, especially those saccular false aneurysms arising after previous carotid endarterectomy. Here the small defect in the arterial wall left after excision of the aneurysm may be closed with a vein or prosthetic patch graft. Mycotic aneurysms require special additional measures including antibiotic cover, vein rather than prosthetic graft material, and complete excision of all the infected aneurysm wall. A vein bypass rather than an interposition graft may occasionally be feasible when removing mycotic aneurysms to avoid having suture lines in the infected area (15).

In conclusion, two other surgical techniques may be mentioned. One is wrapping carotid aneurysms with cellophane or plastic sheets. This is now obsolete because reconstructive methods are technically no more difficult, the results are superior, and wrapping cannot prevent embolization. The other is Matas's endoaneurysmorrhaphy. Perhaps the only situation in which this may still usefully be employed is in dealing with high internal carotid aneurysms where a distal anastomosis at the base of the skull is not technically possible. In these patients a Matas repair is done over a temporary internal shunt. This shunt may be a tapered one to allow better wedging of it into the distal internal carotid artery as it passes through the bony carotid canal in the base of the skull (16). Much ingenuity has also been displayed in planning the distal anastomosis of grafts even in this very difficult situation (17).

MEASURES TO MINIMIZE THE RISK OF CEREBRAL EMBOLIZATION AND ISCHEMIC DAMAGE DURING SURGERY

Cerebral embolization may occur during surgery as a result of handling an aneurysm which contains laminated and loose thrombus. It is therefore essential to disturb aneurysms as little as possible during their dissection. When an internal shunt is to be used, a clamp is first applied distal to the aneurysm, which is then incised so that the thrombotic material inside can be removed quickly before the shunt is inserted. Intravascular clotting during surgery can be minimized by the use of heparin, and heparin therapy is essential for the whole period of gradual occlusion during which a Selverstone clamp is applied postoperatively. This clamp should, of course, be tightened only when the patient is fully conscious.

Many techniques for avoiding cerebral ischemic injury, or predicting its likely occurrence, have been described, and it is also generally agreed that cerebral protection during the operation is essential routinely.

The degree of risk of cerebral ischemic damage after simple ligation or during reconstructive procedures may be predicted preoperatively by such procedures as oculoophthalmodynamometry with carotid compression; or intraoperatively by continuous EEG monitoring, xenon cerebral blood flow measurements (18), and carotid stump pressure measurements. In the latter a pressure of 50 to 70 mmHg probably indicates an adequate cerebral collateral circulation. Anesthetic measures to try to protect the brain from ischemia during operation include using hypercarbia and a hypertension-producing technique. Hypothermia has also been used.

However, by far the best way of avoiding brain ischemia is to insert an internal shunt during any reconstructive procedure, and, indeed, this is now standard practice. Where an interposition vein or prosthetic graft is to be used, this is passed over the shunt before the shunt is inserted. The distal anastomosis is then completed first and the shunt is removed just before the last sutures are placed in the proximal anastomosis. Occasionally an external shunt is more applicable. However used, a shunt means that internal carotid blood flow is only arrested for 1 or 2 minutes.

SURGICAL ANATOMY OF THE CAROTID ARTERIES

The left common carotid artery is intrathoracic in its lower part on the left side, and in the neck each common carotid artery is covered by the sternomastoid muscle. Surgical exposure is achieved by an incision through the skin and platysma in line with the anterior border of the sternomastoid. The vagus nerve and cervical sympathetic chain lie behind the common carotid, as does the jugular vein. The internal carotid artery is closely related to the ninth to twelfth cranial nerves, as well as to the internal jugular vein and the carotid body. The uppermost third of this artery is deeply placed below the base of the skull, the temperomandibular joint, and the parotid gland. It is crossed superficially by the stylohyoid ligament, the posterior belly of the digastric muscle, and the styloglossus and stylopharyngeus muscles. The mastoid and styloid processes lie behind it, as do the longus capitus muscle and the prevertebral fascia. The external carotid artery lies behind the stylohyoid muscle and the posterior belly of the digastric muscle, and passes up toward the parotid gland. It is closely related to the superior laryngeal, facial, hypoglossal, and glossopharyngeal nerves, and to the pharyngeal branch of the vagus.

Care must be taken to avoid injury to all these nerves during exposure of aneurysms. To lessen the risk of nerve damage when dealing with large nonmycotic aneurysms, portions of the aneurysm wall with adherent nerves can safely be left in situ when the bulk of the aneurysm is removed.

RESULTS OF SURGERY FOR CAROTID ANEURYSMS

Apart from damage to adjacent nerves and the risk of local infection, the only serious complication of surgery is cerebral damage from ischemia or embolization. If this does not occur, the operation can be judged successful. However, the risk of neurological damage in association with surgery remains significant, though just exactly how significant it is difficult to say because widely varying figures appear in the literature. Simple ligation appears to be followed by cerebral damage in about 30 percent of patients in collected series (19), while its reported incidence after reconstructive operations varies widely, for example, from 10 to 25 percent.

The severity of this neurological damage ranges from the massive fatal stroke to lesser defects with later partial or complete recovery. Occasionally, evidence of neurological damage does not appear immediately after operation but becomes manifest after several days, presumably because of late distal thrombosis of the internal carotid or its intracranial branches, occlusion of the reconstruction, or late embolization.

Conclusions

Aneurysms of the extracranial carotid arteries are uncommon, but they have a special significance because of the threat they pose of cerebral embolic phenomena and, less commonly, of rupture. They appear to have been increasingly recognized, and to have generated much interest, over the last 10 or 15 years, judging by the number of case reports and reviews which have appeared in the surgical literature. The present tendency is to treat them actively, preferably by reconstructive vascular techniques.

References

1. Cooper A: Account of the first successful operation performed on the common carotid artery for aneurysm in the year of 1808 with post mortem examination in the year 1821. Guy's Hosp Rep 1:53, 1836.
2. Winslow N: Extracranial aneurysm of the internal carotid artery. Arch Surg 13:689, 1926.
3. Dimtza A: Aneurysms of the carotid arteries. Report of two cases. Angiology 7:218, 1956.
4. Schechter DC: Cervical carotid aneurysms. NY State J Med 79:892, 1979.
5. McCollum CH, Wheeler WG, Noon GP, DeBakey ME: Aneurysms of the extracranial carotid artery. Am J Surg 137:196, 1979.
6. Welling RE, Taha A, Goel T, Cranley J, Krause R, Hafner C, Tew J: Extracranial carotid artery aneurysms. Surgery 93:319, 1983.
7. Busuttil RW, Davidson RK, Foley KT, Livesay JT, Barker WF: Selective management of extracranial carotid arterial aneurysms. Am J Surg 140:85, 1980.
8. Ledgerwood AM, Lucas CE: Mycotic aneurysm of the carotid artery. Arch Surg 109:496, 1971.
9. Campbell FC, Robbs JV: Spontaneous dissecting aneurysm of the internal carotid artery. J R Coll Surg Edin 26:286, 1981.
10. McCready RA, Hyde GI, Bivins BA, Mattingly SS, Griffen WO: Radiation-induced arterial injuries. Surgery 93:306, 1983.
11. Kaupp HA, Haid SP, Jurayj MN, Bergan JJ, Trippel OH: Aneurysms of the extracranial carotid artery. Surgery 72:946, 1972.
12. Boddie HG: Transient ischaemic attacks and stroke due to extracranial aneurysm of internal carotid artery. Br Med J 3:802, 1972.
13. Lane JR, Weisman RA: Carotid artery aneurysms: An otolaryngologic perspective. Laryngoscope 90:897, 1980.
14. Webb RC, Barker WF: Aneurysms of the extracranial internal carotid artery. Arch Surg 99:501, 1969.
15. Monson RC, Alexander RH: Vein reconstruction of a mycotic internal carotid aneurysm. Ann Surg 191:47, 1980.
16. Rhodes EL, Stanley JC, Hoffman GL, Cronenwett JL, Fry WJ: Aneurysms of extracranial carotid arteries. Arch Surg 111:339, 1976.
17. Pellegrini RV, Manzetti GW, DiMarco RF, Bekoe S, Arena SA, Marrangoni AG: The direct surgical management of lesions of the high internal carotid artery. J Cardiovasc Surg 25:29, 1984.
18. Mokri B, Piepgras DG, Sundt TM, Pearson BW: Extracranial internal carotid artery aneurysms. Mayo Clin Proc 57:310, 1982.
19. Rittenhouse EA, Radke HM, Sumner DS: Carotid artery aneurysm. Arch Surg 105:786, 1972.

Chapter 52

CAROTID BODY TUMORS

FRANK T. PADBERG, JR., and ALFRED V. PERSSON

Few vascular surgeons will encounter this treacherous neoplasm in large numbers, but all should be familiar with its management. Although the carotid body tumor is relatively uncommon, its treatment has generated considerable clinical controversy. Technical advances and an improved understanding of the tumor's natural history now provide the basis for a rational surgical approach.

Advocates of nonsurgical management once emphasized the high incidence of devastating neurologic sequelae incurred by carotid ligation. Development of carotid arterial reconstruction, now safely performed on a routine basis, has significantly reduced the need for such drastic measures. Precise description of the natural history of the untreated carotid body tumor has been hindered by the difficulty in establishing an accurate initial diagnosis. Arteriography, if obtained, will now correctly identify these lesions prior to operative exploration. The high incidence of histologic malignancy described in some reports correlated poorly with the low incidence of clinically malignant behavior described in others. Prolonged observation and development of strict clinicopathological criteria for malignancy now permit more accurate description of the growth patterns and potential for mortality from tumors of the carotid body.

Historical Aspects

In 1743, Von Haller published an anatomic description of the carotid body. The first surgical resection of a tumor of the carotid body was attributed to Reigner in 1880; his patient succumbed to hemiplegia 3 days following resection with carotid ligation. Tumor excision with survival was described in 1886, as was resection without significant neurologic sequelae (1). The carotid body tumor excised in 1887 by Gay was probably both the first to be excised in the United States and the first to be removed without sacrificing the carotid artery. Lund recorded the first uncomplicated bilateral resection on the same patient in 1917 (2).

Evolution of an appropriate approach to this lesion developed slowly because tumors of the carotid body were seen only infrequently. Since the diagnosis was rarely made prior to operative exploration, no surgeon or clinic could develop a large experience. At the beginning of the twentieth century, surgical resection, usually including the carotid bifurcation, was recommended (1–3). Enthusiasm for this procedure was soon tempered, however, by the high complication rate (4). A 1929 review by Bevan and McCarthy (5) concluded that nonresective treatment was preferable if ligation of the carotid arteries was required. In support of this approach, they cited a single case of tumor regression following radiation. Unfortunately neither histological confirmation of the lesion nor subsequent long-term follow-up were included in this influential report.

In 1940 Harrington, Clagett, and Dockerty (6) described microscopic malignancy in 50 percent of their patients. On the basis of these pathological findings, they again recommended routine surgical resection. The surgical options had been expanded and now included subadventitial dissection of the tumor with carotid preservation. This report described an overall reduction in the incidence of complications from tumor resection, but the mortality rate for those patients who required carotid ligation remained unacceptably high. Although a significantly greater number of these tumors could be removed without sacrificing the carotid arteries, predicting which lesions would require carotid ligation was not possible until virtually the entire dissection had been completed.

In 1947, Lahey and Warren (7) reported a 33 percent mortality rate and a 50 percent incidence of neurologic sequelae in their patients who required carotid ligation. LeCompte thoroughly reviewed these tumors for the Armed Forces Institute of Pathology and reported that he could find no conclusive evidence of malignancy (8). Since the available information suggested that the natural history of this tumor was generally benign and since the risks of ligation were unacceptable, these authors again recommended that resection be abandoned if carotid ligation was required. Hayes Martin, succinctly reiterating this philosophy, stated that "since the carotid body tumor is rarely malignant, little benefit is conferred on the patient by removing it except to establish the diagnosis" (9).

Subsequently, advances in vascular surgical practice have significantly reduced the risks of excision. Successful resection and reanastomosis of the carotid bifurcation for carotid body tumor was first reported in 1938 (10). However, it was only after a similar procedure was reported in 1954 by Eastcott, Pickering, and Rob for an atherosclerotic lesion, that carotid reconstruction became commonplace (11). Preservation of cerebral blood flow during carotid occlusion was achieved by development of the intraluminal shunt.

Accurate diagnosis prior to operation is provided by arteriography, which is now a relatively low risk procedure. In addition to facilitating appropriate perioperative planning, precise identification of the lesion permits more accurate description of the natural course of the carotid body tumor. Reports of fatal outcomes directly related to continued growth of carotid body tumors demonstrate that this lesion is not invariably benign in terms of either local extension (12–14) or metastasis (15–18). Accordingly, an aggressive surgical approach is now the recommended therapy (12,19,20).

Pathophysiology

The surgical literature most commonly refers to this lesion as a *carotid body tumor*. Confusion with respect to nomenclature arose because many similar terms have been applied and because pathologic classification has related it to other paraganglionic tumors. In the current *Atlas of Tumor Pathology*, Glenner and Grimley (21) refer to this lesion as a carotid body paraganglioma; as such, it is the most common of the extraadrenal paraganglionic tumors. LeCompte, in the previous edition of the atlas, classified the tumor of the carotid body as a separate entity because of its chemoreceptor function (8). Glenner's return to the unified paraganglionic system of tumor classification was supported by electron microscopic data confirming that these structures were derived from neuroectoderm. Less commonly used terms (perithelioma, glomus caroticum, endothelioma, chemodectoma, chromaffinoma, and nonchromaffin paraganglioma) have been deleted from general usage.

The normal carotid body is a small (3 by 6 mm) organ of neuroectodermal origin located between the bifurcating vessels of the carotid artery. Embryologically, the carotid body develops between the adventitia and media of the arterial wall, deriving its blood supply predominantly from the external carotid artery (22). It is highly vascular, with a blood flow proportionately greater than that of the brain (23). The cells are responsive to changes in P_{O_2}, P_{CO_2}, and pH and probably function primarily in the control of respiration.

The described pathology of this organ encompasses hypertrophy and tumor development. Physiologic hypertrophy of the carotid body may occur with chronic hypoxia and has been associated with habitation at high altitude, cyanotic heart disease, and chronic obstructive lung disease (24,25). Carotid body tumors have been reported in patients with cyanotic congenital heart disease (26). These tumors also occur with greater frequency in populations residing at altitudes greater than 6000 ft (27). Thus, although a correlation is established between chronic hypoxic stimulation and tumor development, the vast majority of these lesions have no such predisposing factors. On gross examination the carotid body tumor has a firm consistency with a poorly defined capsule. Histologically, the characteristic appearance is that of clumps of cells (Zellballen) contained in a stroma richly interspersed with capillary endothelium. There is no histologic criterion which reliably defines malignancy. This determination is made only by clearly documented nodal or distant metastatic foci.

There is no longer any reasonable doubt that this tumor is capable of metastatic behavior (21). The reported incidence of malignancy ranges from 2 percent (16) to 30 percent (13,28). In part, this variation in incidence has been attributed to differences in policies of patient follow-up (12,13,21). Since metastases may not become apparent for 10 to 20 years, prolonged patient observation may be an important factor in explaining the observed variation. It has been suggested that curative resection of the early lesion may effectively prevent subsequent clinical manifestations. In addition, the differentiation of true metastatic lesions from multicentric primary paragangliomas represents a significant problem when attempting to accurately define the incidence of malignancy.

Although local extension does not fulfill the above criteria for malignancy, the net effect on the patient can be of equally significant importance. Death has been described from asphyxia (12) and intracranial extension (13,14) of these tumors. Several authors have estimated that a 25 to 30 percent overall mortality rate results from the combined effects of metastatic and local tumor growth (12,14,28).

Clinical Presentation

Almost all cases present as an asymptomatic cervical mass. Complaints of pain or discomfort vary greatly but if present are generally mild and nonspecific. A history of slow enlargement is frequently elicited. The average lesion has been present for approximately 6 years at the time of surgical intervention (15,16,29). Although tumors have been described in infants (14) and in patients over 70 years of age (12), the average patient will be in the late forties at the time of presentation. There is no predisposition to either sex. Bilaterality occurs most frequently when the tumor is familial (30).

Specific physical findings with this lesion are limited. The diagnosis should be considered with any lateral cervical mass. Due to its attachment to the underlying artery, the carotid body tumor tends to be more mobile in the horizontal than in the vertical plane. It is usually firm and rubbery on palpation. Due to its intimate arterial attachment, it is often pulsatile. Although absent in the majority of cases, a bruit may be audible but is not pathognomonic and may indicate more common conditions, such as atherosclerotic occlusive disease. Cranial nerve dysfunction from a previously unoperated carotid body tumor is uncommon, but vagal, hypoglossal, and sympathetic involvements have been described (19,31).

Differential diagnosis is critical in the assessment of a solitary lateral cervical mass. Branchial cleft cysts may be distinguished by fluctuation on palpation or a dimple produced by tension on the sinus tract. Most inflammatory adenopathies will initially be tender; usually size and tenderness will decrease slowly when the lesion is observed. Tubercular adenopathy, which can be mistaken for a lesion of the carotid body, is fortunately rare. Lymphoma rarely presents as a solitary cervical node but when present is indistinguishable from the carotid body tumor on physical examination. Epithelioid carcinomas may metastasize to a single cervical node; however, they possess a distinctive hardness, and a diligent search will often identify a primary in the oral cavity. Thyroid carcinoma may also present as a solitary lateral cervical mass. A true carotid artery aneurysm is very rare and is characterized by its expansile quality. Solid tumors which may present as solitary masses in this location include neurofibromas, schwannomas, and other cervical paraganglia (jugular, vagal, sympathetic).

Bilateral carotid body tumors and multicentric paragangliomas (12,16) are most commonly encountered with tumors which have occurred in a familial pattern. Bilaterality is noted in 25 percent of familial carotid body lesions and 4 percent of randomly occurring tumors (30). However, the multicentric potential of a paraganglioma is present in any of these patients with such a tumor. The vast majority of carotid body tumors do not secrete circulating hormones. The presence of hypertension or an increased secretion of catecholamine metabolites should stimulate the search for additional paragangliomas, particularly pheochromocytomas.

Diagnostic Considerations

Solitary, midlateral neck masses of several months' duration should be considered carotid body tumors until proven otherwise. Patients with such masses should have contrast arteriography early in their evaluation; this exam is virtually 100 percent accurate in establishing the diagnosis of carotid body tumor (12,15,17,19,31). An early tumor blush, located at the bifurcation of the common carotid artery, will characteristically splay apart the origins of the internal and external carotid arteries. The importance of clearly establishing the diagnosis of carotid body tumor preoperatively cannot be overemphasized. Excision of this tumor requires extensive preoperative and intraoperative preparation, which is usually not necessary for most other midlateral neck masses.

Percutaneous needle biopsy or incisional biopsy under local anesthesia is ill advised and inaccurate (31,32). Arterial injuries reported from these procedures have produced significant hemorrhage (12), pseudoaneurysms (19), and carotid thrombosis (32).

B-mode ultrasonic imaging has been helpful in identifying branchial cleft cysts, thyroid cysts, or the widened lumen of the rare carotid aneurysm but is of little value in definitive diagnosis of this tumor. Although noninvasive vascular studies are not helpful in establishing the diagnosis, they are uniquely suited to preoperative assessment of the physiologic consequences of carotid ligation. Gee has accurately predicted successful, uncomplicated carotid ligation by oculoplethysmography (OPG) during common carotid compression (33). Thus, these noninvasive studies provide an objective assessment of the patient's ability to withstand acute carotid occlusion.

Therapeutic Considerations

Primary surgical excision is the preferred treatment for the carotid body tumor. Most of the considerations which earlier led clinicians to advocate a conservative, nonoperative approach have been effectively countered by subsequent developments. These tumors were once thought to be largely benign, relatively innocuous lumps in the neck (5,7,8,13). More recent reports have now described the delayed appearance of distant metastases and significant local growth in 20 to 30 percent of carotid body tumors (12,13,14,21). Inability to predict which patients would require carotid ligation and the prohibitive mortality rate accompanying this surgical procedure once provided the most cogent argument against routine resection. Significant reductions in the operative mortality rate have been attributed to advances in surgical technique (17,19,31). A greater frequency of successful subadventitial resection has been achieved. The development of a reliable technique for carotid reconstruction has provided a superior alternative to ligation. It is unwarranted to assume that all of these lesions are malignant, but since differentiation of malignancy is not possible histologically, complete resection is indicated when a carotid body tumor is diagnosed.

Conservative treatments are not curative and have not generally been efficacious. Radiation therapy has been applied to these lesions sporadically, but with little substantive benefit. Chemotherapy has not been proved to be of value. Selective intravascular embolization of the external carotid has been advocated for reduction of tumor bulk prior to surgery, or as definitive treatment (34). Although potentially offering an attractive alternative in the difficult situation, the procedure is not without risk of mortality (35). Partial resection of tumors deemed unresectable has been followed by persistent enlargement, intracranial extension, and metastases (31, 36). However, there will still be lesions with bulk and extension that prevent reconstruction, but with inadequate collateral to permit ligation. In this situation, these therapeutic options may require reconsideration.

Preoperative preparations for resection of the carotid body tumor differ significantly from those of other cervical lesions. The diagnosis can be established by angiography, which is not usually required for other masses in this vicinity. Physiologic evaluation of the collateral cerebral circulation is recommended when it is anticipated that carotid ligation may be required. Rational therapeutic decisions can then be based on knowledge of the tumor's natural history and the relative risks of surgery. Arrangements for adequate supplies of bank blood and the autotransfusion system are made. Preoperative preparation should include both the neck and the lower extremity, so that the saphenous vein can be harvested if required.

Surgical Technique

Small carotid body tumors can generally be excised with modest blood loss and without interruption of cerebral blood flow. Accordingly, the risk of excision in these patients is relatively low. However, larger tumors more commonly come to surgery. Extensive blood loss, averaging 2000 mL (12), can be anticipated. To prevent coagulation in the surgical field and to facilitate retrieval by the autotransfusion system, the patient is given 3000 to 5000 units of heparin. Although most of these tumors can be excised through a subadventitial plane, the surgeon must be prepared to replace the internal carotid artery if it cannot be spared. Therefore, it is important to have an adequate conduit available and the saphenous vein is thus exposed.

The neck is explored through an S-shaped incision made along the anterior border of the sternomastoid muscle. First the common and then the internal carotid arteries are exposed, and Dacron umbilical tape is placed around each for control. Control of the external carotid artery is not sought since the tumor generally involves the entire artery. An intraluminal arterial shunt is prepared prophylactically. As the dissection progresses, the hypoglossal and the vagus nerves (Figure 52-1) are identified and preserved. Once the tumor has been exposed and arterial control established, resection is begun. A subadventitial plane is developed on the common carotid artery, and the dissection proceeds upward. The external carotid artery is ligated at its origin, and the tumor is freed from the internal carotid artery in the same subadventitial plane (Figure 52-2). The various branches of the external carotid artery are identified and ligated. At the end of the dissection, the common and internal carotid arteries should be left intact, and the hypoglossal and vagal nerves undamaged.

Resection of the carotid bifurcation is often necessary when

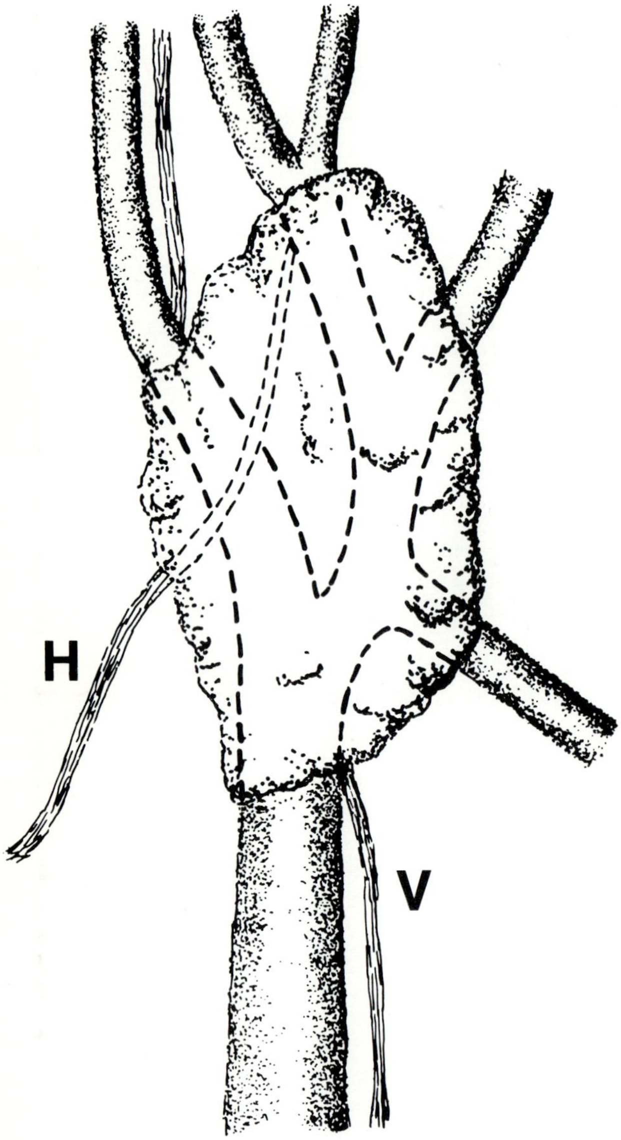

FIGURE 52-1. The carotid body tumor is shown in relationship to the carotid artery, the vagus nerve (V), and the hypoglossal nerve (H).

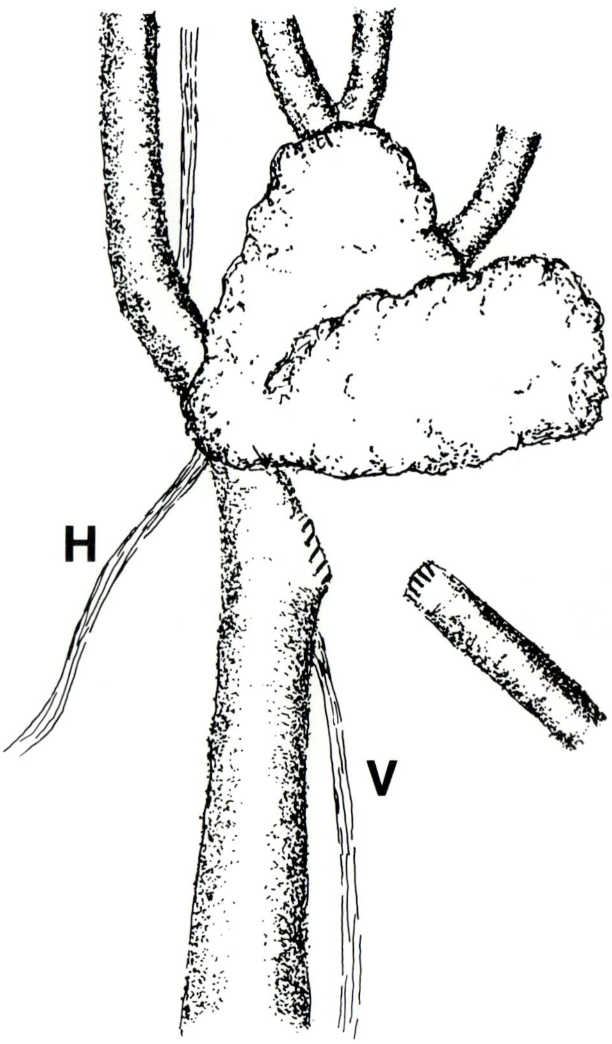

FIGURE 52-2. The carotid body tumor being removed from below. The external carotid artery has been sacrificed. Care has been taken to spare the vagus (V) and hypoglossal (H) nerves.

large tumors are encountered. In such patients, as much as possible of the tumor is exposed. The upper end of the internal carotid artery is carefully dissected. A segment of saphenous vein is harvested and an internal shunt is placed in its lumen. Supplemental heparin may be required to maintain patency of the shunt. The internal carotid artery is transected above the tumor, an arteriotomy is made in the common carotid artery, and the shunt is inserted expeditiously. The internal carotid artery is anastomosed to the saphenous vein end-to-end with a running 5-0 or 6-0 vascular suture. The next step varies with the logistics of the tumor and its relationship to the arteries. Since the tumor usually blocks the surgical field, the vein must be draped over the tumor to connect it to the common carotid artery. Therefore an attempt is made to complete the resection prior to constructing the proximal anastomosis. If the tumor can be excised first, the length of saphenous vein can be adjusted properly. Proximal anastomosis between the saphenous vein and common carotid artery is also fashioned end-to-end. The saphenous vein is cut tangentially because of the discrepancy in the size of the two vessels.

In very large tumors which have grown up to the base of the skull, vascular reconstruction may be impossible because the distal internal carotid artery is rendered inaccessible (Figure 52-3). In such cases, the internal carotid artery must be sacrificed if the tumor is resected. Preoperative assessment of the collateral capabilities of the cerebral circulation are important, because it is better to leave the patient with a large tumor than to leave her or him hemiplegic.

After the tumor has been excised, meticulous care should be taken with hemostasis. The heparin is reversed to avoid postoperative hematomas, and the wound is generally not drained. If the patient has a concomitant carotid stenosis, an endarterectomy is not performed unless the patient is symptomatic. We use the same procedure for the endarterectomy as we would in a patient without a carotid body tumor.

Outcome and Prognosis

Primary surgical excision of the carotid body tumor is generally curative. Following successful resection the vast majority of patients will have no further complaints related to the tumor. However, there is a small but definite incidence of contralateral tumors. Likewise, diligent examination of the patient's relatives may also detect carotid body tumors.

Periodic clinical observation is warranted for detection of multicentric lesions as well as further definition of the natural history of this tumor. Since histologic criteria are inaccurate for diagnosis of malignancy, regular clinical evaluation assumes a significant role in defining this threat. Descriptions of malignant carotid body tumors are characterized by low-grade malignancy with delayed appearance of metastatic foci often occurring after the standard 5-year interval. Although tumor expansion has been responsible for a number of deaths, such extensive growth has also required many years. Similarly, patients may also live for more than 5 years following identification of metastatic deposits (28). The true incidence of malignancy with these lesions is difficult to define accurately but is probably between 20 and 30 percent.

Complications

Complications arising from treatment of the carotid body tumor may be minimized by reasonable application of diagnostic and technical expertise. Although the diagnosis may be established by other methods, contrast arteriography is clearly the method of choice. Both safe and accurate, arteriography requires only that the clinician maintain a high level of suspicion for these uncommon tumors. Thus, percutaneous needle biopsy or local excisional biopsy can be avoided, along with their attendant potential for significant hemorrhage and pseudoaneurysm formation (Figure 52-4). When these problems occur, treatment of the tumor becomes significantly more complex. The unprepared surgeon is faced with a difficult therapeutic decision when a carotid body tumor is diagnosed at the time of cervical exploration. However, when the lesion is recognized preoperatively, the surgeon can make necessary preparations for resection. Blood loss can be anticipated as well as carotid arterial reconstruction.

Cranial nerve injury is more commonly associated with excision of the carotid body tumor than with other cervical procedures such as carotid endarterectomy. The precise incidence is difficult to determine since most reports describe multiple procedures at multiple institutions. However, the incidence of cranial nerve involvement approaches 35 percent, when abnormalities noted both at presentation and following treatment are considered together (17,19,29). The probability of injury increases in proportion to the size of the tumor, and with prior attempts at resection. Although injuries of the vagal and hypoglossal nerves are the most frequently encountered, accessory, facial, and cervical sympathetic nerve damage has also been reported. Earlier series reporting tumor resection without arterial reconstruction were characterized by a prohibitive incidence of major cerebral deficits. In more recent reports emphasizing arterial reconstruction, this problem has virtually been eliminated.

Summary of Key Points in Judgment

The innocuous presentation of the carotid body tumor subtly disguises the potential for significant complications arising from treatment of these uncommon, highly vascular tumors. Preoperative diagnosis is essential for counseling the patient and planning appropriate management. Early identification requires a high level of suspicion and a low threshold for angiography which

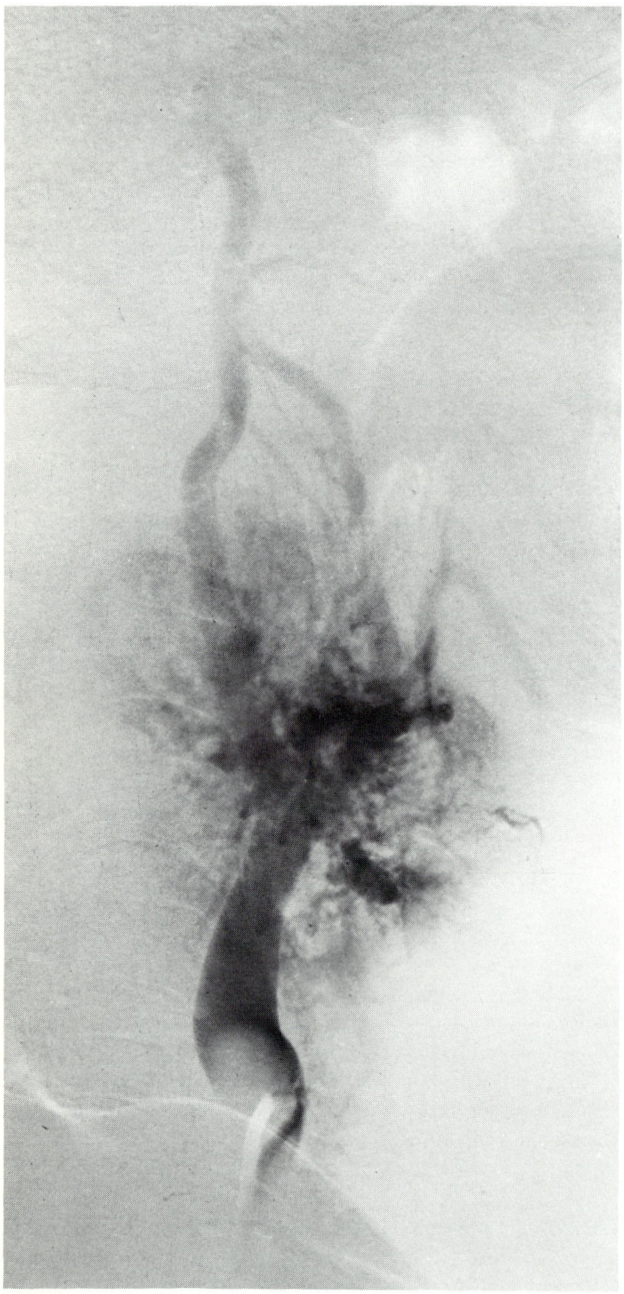

A

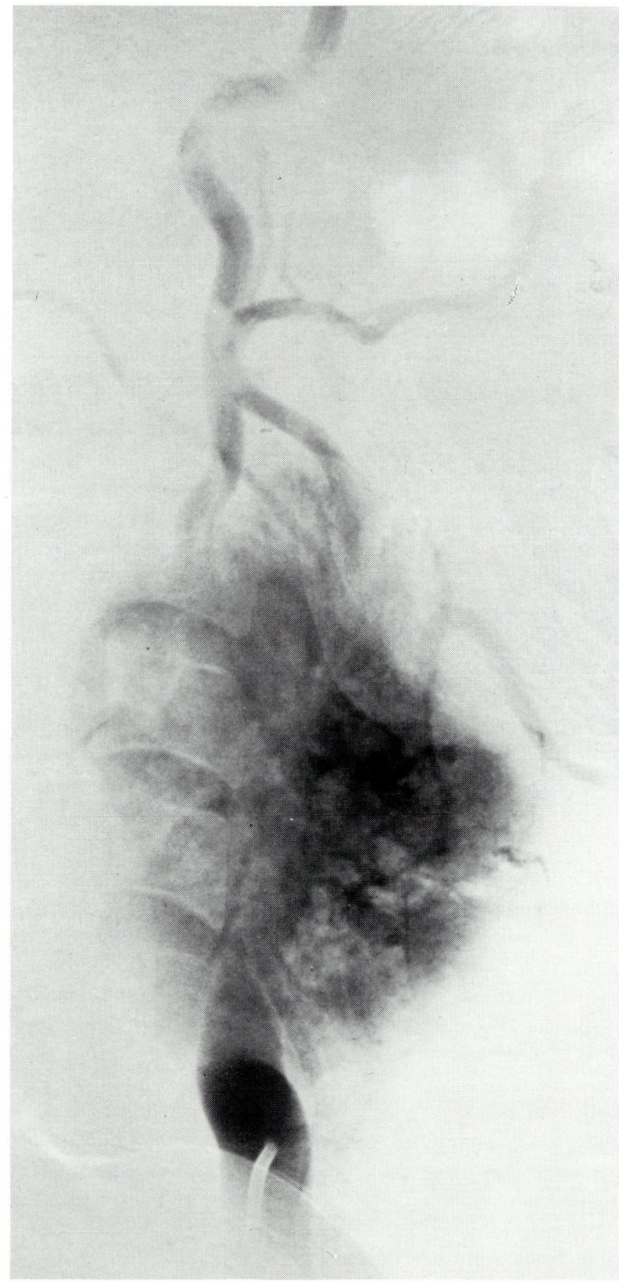

B

FIGURE 52-3. Arteriogram of patient with large carotid body tumor. Note its relationship to the carotid vessels.

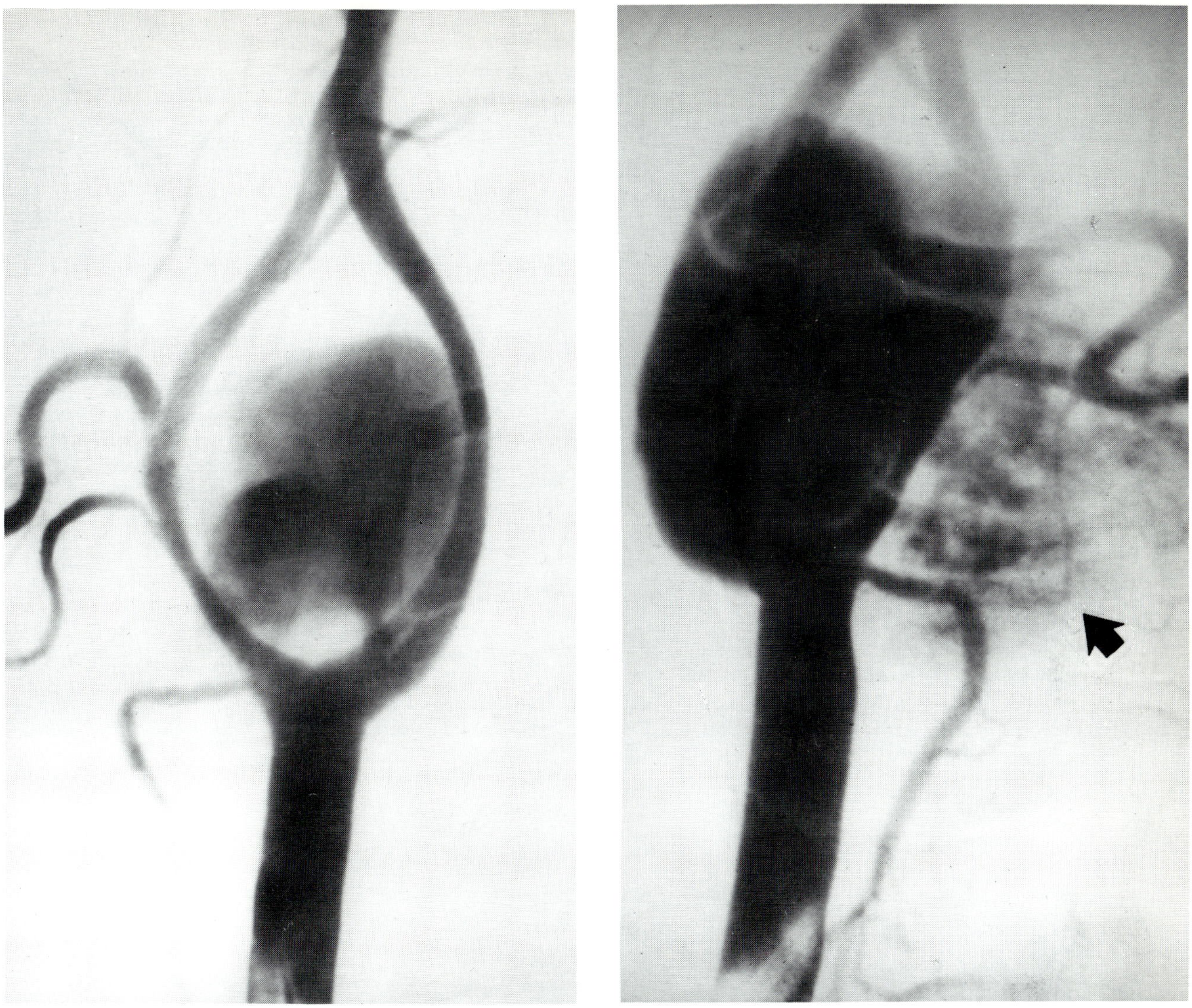

A B

FIGURE 52-4. This carotid body tumor demonstrates splaying of the carotid bifurcation. The typical tumor blush (*arrow*) appears behind a pseudoaneurysm, which resulted from direct biopsy.

confirms the diagnosis. Although the incidence of malignancy is low, insidious local growth has also proved life-threatening. Surgical complications are less likely when the tumor is relatively small and preoperative preparation has been complete. Refinement of vascular surgical techniques has facilitated safe excision of larger tumors and those which require arterial reconstruction. Surgical resection is the recommended treatment for the carotid body tumor and is preferably undertaken before the lesion has attained excessive bulk.

References

1. Gratiot JM: Carotid body tumors: Collective review. Surg Gynecol Obstet (Intern Abs Surg) 1943, 77:177–186.
2. Lund FB: Tumors of the carotid body. JAMA 1917, 69:348–352.
3. Scudder CL: Tumor of the intercarotid body. Am J Med Sci 1903, 126:384–389.
4. Chase WH: Familial and bilateral tumors of the carotid body. J Pathol Bacteriol 1933, 36:1–12.
5. Bevan AD, McCarthy ER: Tumors of the carotid body. Surg Gynecol Obstet 1929, 49:764–779.
6. Harrington SW, Clagett OT, Dockerty MB: Tumors of the carotid body. Ann Surg 1941, 114:820–833.
7. Lahey FH, Warren KW: Tumors of the carotid body. Surg Gynecol Obstet 1947, 85:281–288.
8. LeCompte PM: Tumors of the carotid body and related structures (chemoreceptor system). In *Atlas of Tumor Pathology,* section 4, fascicle 16. Armed Forces Institute of Pathology, 1951.
9. Martin H: *Surgery of Head and Neck Tumors*. New York, Hoeber-Harper, 1957, p 20.

10. Enderlen E: Originalmitteilungen, operation der carotisdrusengeschwulste. Zentrallbl Chir 1938, 46:2530–2531.
11. Eastcott HHG, Pickering GW, Rob CG: Reconstruction of internal carotid artery. Lancet 1954, 2:994–996.
12. Dent TL, Thompson NW, Fry WJ: Carotid body tumors. Surgery 1976, 80:365–372.
13. Martin CE, Rosenfeld L, McSwain B: Carotid body tumors: A 16 year follow-up of seven malignant cases. South Med J 1973, 66:1236–1243.
14. Monro RS: Natural history of carotid body tumors and their diagnosis and treatment. Br J Surg 1950, 37:445–453.
15. Lahey FH, Warren KW: A long-term appraisal of carotid body tumors with remarks on their removal. Surg Gynecol Obstet 1951, 92:481–491.
16. Shamblin WR, ReMine WH, Sheps SG, Harrison EG: Carotid body tumor (chemodectoma). Am J Surg 1971, 122:732–739.
17. Lees CD, Levine HL, Beven EG, Tucker HM: Tumors of the carotid body. Am J Surg 1981, 142:362–365.
18. Gould VE, Memoli VA, Warren WH: Diagnosis of human tumors. Case 5 metastatic paraganglioma in lung. Ultrastruct Pathol 1983, 5:299–306.
19. Padberg FT Jr, Cady B, Persson AV: Carotid body tumor. Am J Surg 1983, 145:526–528.
20. Javid H, Chawla SK, Dye WS, Hunter JA, Najafi H, Goldin MD, Serry C: Carotid body tumor—Resection or reflection. Arch Surg 1976, 111:344–347.
21. Glenner GG, Grimley PM: Tumors of the extraadrenal paraganglion system (including chemoreceptors). In *Atlas of Tumor Pathology*, second series, fascicle 9. Armed Forces Institute of Pathology, 1973.
22. Boyd JH: The development of the human carotid body. Contrib Embryo 1937, 26:1–31.
23. Daly M de Burgh, Lambertsen CJ, Schweitzer A: Observations on the volume of blood flow and oxygen utilization of the carotid body in the cat. J Physiol 1954, 125:67–89.
24. Heath D, Edwards C, Harris P: Postmortem size and structure of the human carotid body. Thorax 1970, 25:129–140.
25. Edwards C, Heath D, Harris P: The carotid body in emphysema and left ventricular hypertrophy. J Pathol 1971, 104:1–13.
26. Hirsh JM, Killien FC, Troupin RH: Bilateral carotid body tumors and cyanotic heart disease. Am J Radiol 1980, 134:1073–1075.
27. Saldana MJ, Salem LE, Travezan R: High altitude hypoxia and chemodectomas. Hum Pathol 1973, 4:251–263.
28. Gaylis H, Mieny CJ: Incidence of malignancy in carotid body tumors. Br J Surg 1977, 64:885–889.
29. Krupski WC, Effeney DJ, Ehrenfeld WK, Stoney RJ: Cervical chemodectoma, technical considerations and management options. Am J Surg 1982, 144:215–220.
30. Rush BF Jr: Familial bilateral carotid body tumors. Ann Surg 1963, 157:633–636.
31. Farr HW: Carotid body tumors—A 40 year study. CA 1980, 30:260–265.
32. Engzell U, Franzen S, Zajicek J: Aspiration biopsy of tumors of the neck. II cytologic findings in 13 cases of carotid body tumor. Acta Cytol 1971, 15:25–30.
33. Gee W, Mehigan JT, Wylie EJ: Measurement of collateral cerebral hemispheric blood pressure by ocular pneumoplethysmography. Am J Surg 1975, 130:121–127.
34. Schick PM, Hieshima GB, White RA, Fiaschetti FL, Mehringer CM, Grinnell VS, Everhart FR: Arterial catheter embolization followed by surgery for large chemodectoma. Surgery 1980, 87:459–464.
35. Pandya SK, Nagpal RD, Desai AP, Purohit AV: Death following external carotid artery embolization for a functioning glomus jugular chemodectoma. J. Neurosurg 1978, 48:1030–1034.
36. Warren KW: Some observations on carotid body tumors. Surg Clin North Am 1959, 39:621–635.

PART SIX

Visceral Arterial Disease

Chapter 53

RENOVASCULAR HYPERTENSION

RICHARD H. DEAN

Although hypertension has been recognized for centuries, the importance of its identification and treatment has been appreciated only during the past 150 years. Most commonly, hypertension is a silent process and is manifested only by sequellae of acceleration in the rate of atherogenesis and the frequency of cardiovascular morbid and mortal rates. Uncommonly, the hypertension may be so severe that the elevated pressure itself produces vessel wall injury and the clinical picture of malignant hypertension. Although most physicians appreciate the potentially lethal nature of this malignant variety and the importance of its control, physician apathy toward the merits of aggressive diagnostic evaluation and management of asymptomatic patients with less severe hypertension continues to limit the impact of current knowledge on the populationwide success of treatment of this disorder.

The incidence of renovascular hypertension (RVH), the necessity for its identification, and the value of operative management remain poorly defined. Some centers are routinely evaluating hypertensive patients for a renovascular origin and are submitting suitable candidates to operative treatment. Other centers seldom study patients for RVH and even more uncommonly select operative management for this form of hypertension. Several factors have led to this disparity in approaches. Among these reasons are reports emphasizing a low frequency of a renovascular cause of hypertension, the low cost effectiveness of diagnostic investigation, the infrequent cure of hypertension by operation, and improvements in management by drug therapy. Unfortunately, the inappropriately biased collection of data and conflicting results of studies in these areas have perpetrated the lack of uniformity in concepts regarding the value of diagnostic study and merits of operative treatment. In this chapter, diagnostic studies and methods of management of the respective causes of renovascular disease and RVH will be reviewed with emphasis on the current status of their value and results of their use.

Incidence of Renovascular Hypertension

Renovascular hypertension (RVH) is generally thought to account for 5 to 10 percent of the hypertensive population. Recently, Tucker and his associates (1) have suggested an even lower prevalence. Likewise, Shapiro et al. (2) have suggested that the identification and successful operative treatment of RVH in patients over the age of 50 years is so unlikely that diagnostic investigation for a correctable cause in that group should be undertaken only when hypertension is severe and uncontrollable. Estimates of the prevalence of hypertension in the United States from all causes vary from 15 to 30 million people, and it may be present in 10 to 15 percent of the adult population. Indeed, the incidence of RVH is undoubtedly low in this general hypertensive population if all patients with even mild hypertension are included. Since RVH tends to produce relatively severe hypertension, its prevalence in the large subpopulation of mildly hypertensive patients (diastolic blood pressure <105 mmHg) is probably negligible. In contrast, however, it is a frequent cause of hypertension in the smaller group of severely hypertensive people. Hollifield (3) recently investigated 137 patients with previously unrecognized hypertension who were uncovered in a shopping center screening program (Table 53-1). Diagnostic study in these patients included arteriography and, when appropriate, renal vein renin assays and split renal function studies. None of the 102 patients with a diastolic blood pressure between 90 and 115 mmHg had RVH. In contrast, 9 of the 35 patients (26 percent) with a diastolic blood pressure of 118 mmHg or higher had RVH. Further, if one breaks down these numbers according to race, the results were even more striking. In the more severely hypertensive group, none of the 13 black patients had RVH, whereas RVH occurred in 9 of the 22 (41 percent) white patients in this group. Similarly, Davis et al. have shown a 31 percent incidence of RVH in 85 patients initially evaluated in our center for malignant hypertension (4).

In our experience, the presence of severe hypertension at the two extremes of life carries the highest probability of being RVH. Our review of the causes of hypertension in 74 children admitted for diagnostic evaluation over a 5-year period showed that the hypertension in 78 percent of those who were less than

TABLE 53-1. Results of Screening 137 New Hypertensive Patients

Diastolic Blood Pressure	No. of Patients	No. with RVH	Percent
90–115 mmHg	102	0	0
>117 mmHg:	35	9	26
Blacks	13	0	0
Whites	22	9	41

Supported in part by NIH Grant 14192-12, SCOR in Hypertension.

5 years old had a correctable renovascular origin (5). Interestingly, after childhood, the age group which has the next highest probability of having RVH is the elderly. In our center, 33 percent of patients over 60 years old admitted for evalution have had RVH. Certainly, the elderly age group admitted for evaluation is skewed toward the more severe spectrum of hypertension, for less severe levels likely would not have led to referral of such patients to our center.

Based on this data it is inappropriate to view hypertensive patients as a homogeneous group with respect to the prevalence of RVH. Rather, the probability of finding RVH correlates with the severity of hypertension. Accordingly, the search for RVH should be directed to the subset of patients who have the more severe degree of hypertension. It must be remembered, however, that severity of hypertension is based on its level without medication interference and does not refer to the difficulty of control by drug therapy.

Pathophysiology of Renovascular Hypertension

The kidney is a dominant site of blood pressure regulation because of its influence on circulating plasma volume as well as its activity in modulation of vasomotor tone. To examine the pathophysiology of renovascular hypertension, it is appropriate to first review the normal homeostatic activities of the kidney in the regulation of blood pressure.

The renin-angiotensin-aldosterone system is a complex feedback mechanism which, in its normal state of activity, maintains a stable blood pressure and blood volume under varying conditions. Richly innervated, modified smooth-muscle cells located along the afferent arterioles in juxtaposition to the renal glomerulus (juxtaglomerular apparatus) are sensitive monitors of perfusion pressure. Diminished perfusion pressure stimulates these cells to release renin, a proteolytic enzyme. Renin, in turn, interacts with an alpha 2 globulin (angiotensinogen) manufactured in the liver to produce angiotensin I. Angiotensin I, an inactive and labile decapeptide, is converted to the potent vasoconstrictor, angiotensin II, by a converting enzyme found primarily in the lungs. In addition to its potent vasoconstrictor properties, angiotensin II also increases blood pressure through its stimulation of aldosterone release from the zona glomerulosa of the adrenal cortex. This, in turn, increases plasma volume by increasing sodium and water resorption in the renal tubules. Through these actions of angiotensin II, blood pressure, plasma volume, and plasma sodium content are increased. In addition, the adjacent cells of the distal convoluted tubule (macula densa) may play a role by acting as a sensor of sodium concentration in the distal tubules and thereby exerting a positive feedback mechanism on renin release. As these mechanisms increase perfusion pressure to the juxtaglomerular cells, further renin production and release is suppressed and blood pressure is modulated within a narrow range.

Potentially, two forms of hypertension may be produced by the development of renovascular disease. These are (1) renin-dependent hypertension and (2) volume-dependent hypertension. Through the mechanisms just described, decreased perfusion activates the renin-angiotensin-aldosterone axis of vasoconstriction and volume expansion. Current information regarding the nature of renovascular hypertension suggests that a functionally significant unilateral renal artery stenosis activates both the angiotensin II–mediated increase in peripheral resistance and blood pressure as well as aldosterone-mediated volume expansion. When the contralateral renal artery and kidney are normal, the normal feedback mechanisms in the normal kidney produce an effective naturesis and compensatory reduction in circulating plasma volume. In this scheme, an angiotensin II–vasoconstrictive source of hypertension is created.

In contrast, when the contralateral renal artery or kidney is also diseased, this compensatory diuresis is lost and volume expansion occurs, producing an angiotensin-aldosterone–mediated volume-dependent hypertension. Modification of renal perfusion by renal revascularization can effectively diminish or abolish the underlying mechanism producing either of these two varieties of renovascular hypertension.

Characteristics of Renovascular Hypertension

Due to the relative infrequency of renovascular hypertension (RVH) in the entire hypertensive population, many reports have focused on the value of demographic factors, physical findings, and screening tests as discriminants between essential hypertension (EH) and RVH on which to base the decision for further diagnostic study. The most frequently quoted discriminating factors which suggest the presence of RVH and a need for further study are the recent onset of hypertension, a young age, a lack of a family history of hypertension, and the presence of an abdominal bruit.

In the review of the first 122 patients with RVH treated in our center, 52 percent had a family history of hypertension, 46 percent had no audible abdominal bruit, and ages ranged from 4 months to 69 years (mean, 46 years) (6). Since RVH can be secondary to any of several processes affecting the renal artery and since each of these diseases has its own clinical characteristics, it is not surprising that the use of demographic or physical findings such as age, abdominal bruit, and duration of hypertension as discriminants to exclude patients from study has a high risk of inappropriately excluding patients with RVH from further study. Therefore, one should base the decision for diagnostic study primarily on the severity of hypertension. Mild hypertension has a minimal chance of being renovascular in origin. In contrast, the more severe the hypertension, the higher the probability that it is from a correctable cause. With this in mind, we submit all patients with diastolic blood pressures greater than 105 mmHg who would be acceptable operative candidates to evaluation for a correctable origin of hypertension.

Diagnostic Evaluation

The general evaluation of all hypertensive patients is shown in Table 53-2. Electrocardiography is important to gauge the extent of secondary myocardial hypertrophy or associated ischemic heart disease. Serum electrolytes and serial serum potassium determinations can effectively exclude patients with primary aldosteronism if potassium levels are greater than 3.0 mg/dL. One must remember, however, that hypokalemia is most often due to salt-depleting diets and previous diuretic therapy. Estimation of renal function is mandatory. Preexisting renal disease may reduce renal function and cause hypertension. Further, hypertension from any cause may produce intrarenal arteriolar nephrosclerosis and subsequent depression of renal function. Finally, assessment of the urinary 17-hydroxy- and ketosteroid and vanillylmandelic acid (VMA) levels will effectively identify the rare patient with a pheochromocytoma or a functioning adrenocortical tumor.

SCREENING STUDIES

A number of screening diagnostic studies have been advocated for the recognition of the patient with RVH. They include peripheral plasma renin assays, the rapid sequence intravenous pyelogram, isotope renography, and renal arteriography. Each of these studies is useful in the evaluation of hypertensive patients. With the exception of renal arteriography, however, none of these screening tests has the necessary sensitivity to serve as the single study on which the necessity for more definitive diagnostic evaluation can be determined. Previous review of the results of these other proposed screening studies has shown that over 30 percent of patients with RVH would have been missed if further evaluation had been undertaken solely on the basis of these results (7).

RENAL ARTERIOGRAPHY

There continues to be controversy over the use of aortography and renal arteriography in the routine screening of hypertensive individuals. Some feel it should be reserved for select groups of patients. We do not share this conservative view and proceed with arteriography in any patient who would be a candidate for renal artery revascularization if a lesion were found, irrespective of other screening tests. As a general rule, we have required that the patient have documented diastolic blood pressures in excess of 105 mmHg, and the majority have had pressures in excess of 120 mmHg.

Both aortography and selective renal arteriography using multiple projections are necessary to adequately examine the entire renal artery. The proximal third of the left renal artery usually courses anteriorly, the mid third transversely, and the distal third posteriorly, whereas the right renal artery pursues a more consistent posterior course. Previous review of these factors has underscored the necessity of oblique aortography and oblique selective renal arteriography to project these portions of the vessels in the profile and identify the stenosis (8).

Through the introduction of computer-assisted subtraction angiography (digital venous angiography), one can now obtain anatomic definition of the renal vasculature as an outpatient screening procedure. Unfortunately, further technologic refinements are required before this study can replace conventional arteriography. Currently, it does not identify fibromuscular dysplastic lesions with accuracy and frequently provides a picture which underestimates the severity of atherosclerotic lesions. Nevertheless, further instrumental development is awaited with enthusiasm.

TABLE 53-2. General Evaluation of Patients with Hypertension

History and physical examination
Hemogram; SMA-12; urinalysis, urine culture; serum K, 3 times
Electrocardiogram and chest x-ray
Analysis of 24-h urine collection for creatinine clearance, electrolytes, catecholamines, VMA, and 17-OH-steroids and ketosteroids
Rapid sequence intravenous pyelogram
Renal arteriography

FUNCTIONAL STUDIES

Renal Vein Renin Assays

When an obstructive lesion is found by renal arteriography, its functional significance should be evaluated. Most centers now rely solely on renal vein renin assays (RVRA) to establish the diagnosis of RVH. The unfortunate consequence of this trend is that one must presume that all patients with RVH will have lateralizing RVRA. The results of evaluation of this study in our center underscore the fallacy of this presumption. There are many factors that affect the results of RVRA which, if not properly managed, will lead to erroneous results.

The effect of antihypertensive medications and unrestricted sodium intake on renin release and, thereby, RVRA is widely recognized. Many antihypertensive medications, especially those which function through beta-adrenergic blockade, suppress renin output and can lead to false nonlateralization of RVRA. Before one can consider that there is no drug interference in the release of renin, all such medications must have been withheld for at least 5 days prior to the measurement of RVRA. Similar effects on renin levels are seen when sodium intake is not restricted. For this reason, the patient must be on no more than a 2-g sodium diet for at least 2 weeks prior to the study. The preparation of patients for RVRA in our center is summarized in Table 53-3.

Vaughn has stressed the importance of expressing RVRA in relation to the systemic renin activity rather than simply evaluating the ratio of renin activity between the two renal veins (9).

TABLE 53-3. Patient Preparation for Renal Vein Renin Assays

1. Chronic salt restriction (2-g sodium diet)
2. Discontinue all antihypertensive drugs except diuretics for at least 5 days prior to study
3. Oral furosemide (40 mg) diuresis night before the study
4. Nothing by mouth for 8 hours prior to study
5. Strictly flat bed rest for 4 hours before and during study
6. Prestudy sedation with intramuscular diazepam (Valium) (5 mg)

In patients with RVH secondary to unilateral renal artery stenosis one should find hypersecretion of renin from the ischemic kidney and suppression of renin secretion from the normal kidney. Through application of this hypothesis, Stanley and Fry have shown a statistically significant difference in the renal–systemic renin indices in patients who were cured of RVH by operation when compared to those who were only improved (10). Although this method has appeal as a predictor of the extent of benefit, its value in patients with bilateral renal artery lesions is limited. Since both lesions may be producing RVH, both this method and RVR ratios have reduced validity as predictors of response to operation. Further, the risk of hypertension is more directly related to its severity rather than to its absolute presence or absence. If one bases the decision for operative management solely on whether or not absolute cure is to be expected, then many patients who would receive the benefit of reduction in severity of hypertension to a mild, easily controlled level would be dropped from consideration as operative candidates. Therefore, this method of RVRA interpretation should be considered only as an additional predictive tool and not an alternative to the evaluation of RVR ratios. We consider a 1.5:1 ratio between the involved and uninvolved sides to be a positive test and, when positive, to have functional proof that the renovascular lesion is causing RVH.

Split Renal Function Studies

With the advent of RVRA, most centers have stopped using split renal function studies (SRFS) because of the associated discomfort, possible complications, and confusing results. Valuable information can be obtained from SRFS that is not obtained from RVRA. Information regarding the likelihood of viability of a severely ischemic kidney and data suggesting the most severely affected side in bilaterally stenotic kidneys are among the benefits of SRFS. Classically, a positive test shows a 40 percent reduction in urine volume, a 50 percent increase in creatinine concentration, and a 100 percent increase in *para*-aminohippuric acid concentration on the involved side. Further experience with this test, however, shows that these criteria are much too rigid (11). We now feel that this test is positive if there is consistent lateralization in each of three samples with a decrease in urine volume and an increase in *para*-aminohippuric acid and creatinine concentration. When either the RVRA or the SRFS is positive, the diagnosis of renovascular hypertension is established.

Treatment of Renovascular Hypertension

THERAPEUTIC OPTIONS

Identification of the optimal method of treating patients with RVH remains an elusive goal. Advocates of drug therapy, operative management, and, more recently, percutaneous transluminal angioplasty (PTA) separately defend their viewpoint with selective data from the literature to strengthen the validity of their argument. A majority of the medical community still only evaluate patients for RVH when medications are not tolerated and hypertension remains severe and uncontrolled. Although we are currently conducting a randomized, prospective study comparing drug therapy to surgery, it is not completed; and no similar randomized comparative trial is available in the literature. The study by Hunt and Strong (12) is the most informative one currently available to assess the comparative value of drug therapy and operation. In their study, they compared the results of operative treatment in 100 RVH patients with the results of drug therapy in 114 similar patients. After 7 to 14 years of follow-up, 84 percent of the operated group were alive as compared to 66 percent in the drug therapy group. Furthermore, of the 84 patients alive in the operated on group, 93 were cured or significantly improved, while 16 (21 percent) of the patients alive in the drug therapy group had required operation for uncontrollable hypertension. Another seven patients remained uncontrolled without operation. Death during follow-up was twice as common in the medically treated group. These differences were statistically significant ($p < 0.01$) in both patients with atherosclerotic lesions and those with fibromuscular lesions of the renal artery.

Additional information influencing the decision for operative management of RVH in the atherosclerotic patient is the anatomic and renal function changes that occur during drug therapy. We recently reported the results of serial renal function studies which were performed on 41 patients with RVH secondary to atherosclerotic renal artery disease who had been randomly selected for nonoperative management (Table 53-4) (13). In 19 patients, serum creatinine levels increased between 25 and 120 percent. The glomerular filtration rates dropped between 25 and 50 percent in 12 patients. Fourteen patients (37 percent) lost more than 10 percent of renal length. In four patients (12 percent), a significant stenosis progressed to total occlusion. Seventeen patients (41 percent) had deterioration of renal function or loss of renal size that led to operation. One patient required

TABLE 53-4. Frequency of Severe Deterioration in Parameters of Renal Function during Drug Therapy, 40 Patients

Parameter	Patients Followed	Mean Follow-up, mo	Failure Event	Number Affected	Percent Affected
Renal length	38	33	≥10% decrease	14	37
Serum creatinine	41	25	≥100% increase	2	5
Glomerular filtration rate or creatinine clearance	30	19	≥50% decrease	1	3
Total	41			17	41

removal of a previously reconstructible kidney. Of the 17 patients with deterioration, 15 had acceptable blood pressure control during the period of nonoperative observation. Therefore, we feel that progressive deterioration of renal function in nonoperatively treated patients with atherosclerotic renal artery stenosis and RVH is common and occurs even in the presence of blood pressure control with drugs.

The detrimental changes that occur during drug therapy and the current excellent results of operative management (14) argue for an aggressive attitude toward renal revascularization in the treatment of RVH. Our indications for operative management of RVH have been outlined in detail elsewhere (15). Nevertheless, in brief, all patients with severe, difficult to control hypertension should be considered for operation. This includes patients with complicating factors such as branch lesions and extrarenal vascular disease, and patients with associated cardiovascular disease which would be improved by blood pressure reduction.

Young patients with moderate hypertension and no complicating diseases who have an easily correctable atherosclerotic or fibromuscular main renal artery stenosis also are candidates for operation. The chance for cure of moderate hypertension is quite good in such patients who have no complicating factors. It remains to be proved that drug control is ever as good as the complete cure of hypertension. In fact, one might argue that reduction in the driving pressure of blood flow across the stenosis by successful drug therapy might accelerate deterioration in renal function by further reducing renal perfusion.

Finally, there is no clear evidence that age (at least under 60 years), type of lesion (whether atherosclerotic or fibromuscular), duration of hypertension, or the presence of bilateral lesions by themselves have proven value as determinants of operative risk or likelihood of successful operative management. Therefore, they should not be used as deterrents to such management.

Certainly the atherosclerotic patient with a 20-year history of easily controlled, mild hypertension who experiences acceleration in severity secondary to the development of renovascular hypertension is unlikely to be cured by operation. We believe, however, that removal of severe, difficult to control hypertension by operation with reversion back to a mild, easily controlled variety is equally valuable in reducing the risk of cardiovascular morbid events secondary to hypertension.

In addition, risk of operation must be considered when determining the most appropriate therapeutic option. This consideration is of greatest pertinence when both renal and aortic disease must be managed simultaneously. In our center, renal revascularization, when done alone, is associated with a risk of less than 1 percent. Similarly, elective repair of infrarenal abdominal aortic aneurysms or aortoiliac occlusive disease alone also has an associated operative mortality rate of less than 3 percent. These risks are in contrast to a 12 percent risk when performing combined aortic and renal procedures. To assess preoperative factors possibly predictive of operative risk for combined procedures, we recently reviewed the 50 patients who underwent such procedures over a 10-year period.

There were six operative mortalities (12 percent). Factors associated with increased mortal risk were azotemia (43 vs. 7 percent), associated complex renal or visceral procedures (31 vs. 5 percent), treatment of aortic aneurysm vs. occlusive disease (17 vs. 5 percent), positive electrocardiogram (ECG) (19 vs. 4 percent), age over 60 years (20 vs. 4 percent), and a history of diffuse peripheral vascular disease (18 vs. 7 percent). None of these differences by themselves, however, had statistical significance. Through discriminate analysis with assignment of weighted scores to the five most powerful predictors of operative death (complex procedure, 4; azotemia, 4; aortic aneurysm repair, 3; positive ECG, 2; history of diffuse vascular disease, 2), a weighted score of ≥ 10 predicted operative death with an 83 percent sensitivity and 93 percent specificity ($p = 0.003$). Although advanced age, diabetes, severity of hypertension, and history of heart disease were associated with increased operative risk, they contributed minimal discriminate value to that provided by the preceding five variables. This was because these weaker risk factors were usually found in association with the predictors in the discriminate score. There were no deaths in the group with a weighted score of five or less. Nevertheless, this study suggested that in patients with high weighted discriminate scores (≥ 10), consideration of operative risk is particularly important in the evaluation of the proposed value of combined procedures. In contrast, however, many patients can undergo such combined procedures with a negligible operative risk.

Finally, management of patients with bilateral disease warrants special comment. When patients have severe bilateral atherosclerotic orificial stenoses, we currently proceed with simultaneous bilateral revascularization even when functional data lateralize to one side. If functional data do not lateralize, we only proceed to operation for bilateral disease when hypertension is severe and difficult to control. Similarly, in these circumstances we will correct both sides. In contrast, if severe fibromuscular dysplasia (FMD) is present bilaterally, we will only revascularize the side to which the functional data lateralize. In the absence of lateralization we will only correct the side which appears angiographically to be most severe. This apparent paradox in bias toward unilateral repair of FMD relates to the increased operative time and small branch repair frequently necessary when managing FMD and the theoretical increase in risk of technical error when managing such branch disease. In any event, if hypertension persists after unilateral repair, functional studies are repeated and contralateral repair is undertaken if the data then lateralize to the uncorrected side.

PREOPERATIVE PREPARATION

Antihypertensive medications are reduced during the preoperative period to the minimum necessary for blood pressure control. Frequently, patients requiring large doses of multiple medications for control outside the hospital setting will have significantly reduced drug requirements while hospitalized. If continued therapy is required, then alpha methyldopa is the drug of choice. There is little effect on hemodynamics when this agent is combined with anesthesia. We have also commonly continued low-dose propranolol therapy as well without any adverse effects. If the patient's diastolic blood pressure is 120 to 140 mmHg, it is essential that the pressure be brought under control and that operative treatment be postponed until this is accomplished. Recently, if blood pressure has been difficult to control, we have transferred the patient to the intensive care unit where intravenous nitroprusside therapy with continuous intraarterial monitoring of blood pressure is instituted for the 24 h prior to operation. Similarly, if the patient has a significant history of heart disease, pulmonary artery wedge and cardiac output are monitored to maintain optimal cardiac hemodynamics and recognize and correct adverse changes before they become critically significant.

OPERATIVE TECHNIQUES

A variety of operative techniques have been used to correct renal artery stenoses. From a practical standpoint, two basic operations have been most frequently utilized: aortorenal bypass and thromboendarterectomy. We favor aortorenal bypass, preferably with saphenous vein, and limit endarterectomy to orificial lesions of accesory renal arteries or in an occasional case with severe bilateral orificial stenoses. Uncommonly, the renal artery will be redundant after it has been circumferentially mobilized. In such patients with orificial lesions, renal artery reimplantation also has been used with gratifying results (Figure 53-1).

Certain measures and maneuvers are applicable in almost all renal arterial operations. Mannitol, 12.5 g, is administered intravenously early in the operation. Just prior to renal artery cross clamping, heparin, 75 mg or 7500 units, is given intravenously. Protamine is occasionally required for reversal of the heparin at the end of the reconstruction.

Exposure of the renal arteries is the most difficult yet important aspect of renal artery surgery. A midline xiphoid to pubis incision provides excellent access to either renal artery. To expose the left renal artery, the posterior peritoneum overlying the aorta is incised longitudinally, the duodenum is mobilized to the patient's right, and the left renal vein dissected out and mobilized (Figure 53-2). By extending the posterior peritoneal incision to the left along the inferior border of the pancreas, an avascular plane behind the pancreas can be entered. The inferior mesenteric vein courses obliquely through the left peritoneal area. This vein is often ligated and divided to facilitate this exposure. (When this is done, one must be certain that an ascending branch of the inferior mesenteric artery is not accompanying the vein. Ligation of such an ascending arterial branch may compromise colonic perfusion if visceral artery atherosclerotic occlusions are present.) This allows excellent exposure of the entire renal hilum on the left and is of special significance when distal lesions are to be managed. The artery lies behind the left renal vein. In some cases, it is easier to retract the vein cephalad in order to expose the artery. In others, caudal retraction of the vein provides better access. Usually, the gonadal vein and adrenal vein which enter the renal vein have to be ligated and divided to facilitate exposure of the artery. Another frequent tributary is a lumbar vein which enters the posterior wall of the left renal vein and is easily avulsed unless special care is taken in mobilizing the renal vein.

The proximal right renal artery can be exposed through the same retroperitoneal exposure at the base of the mesentery by

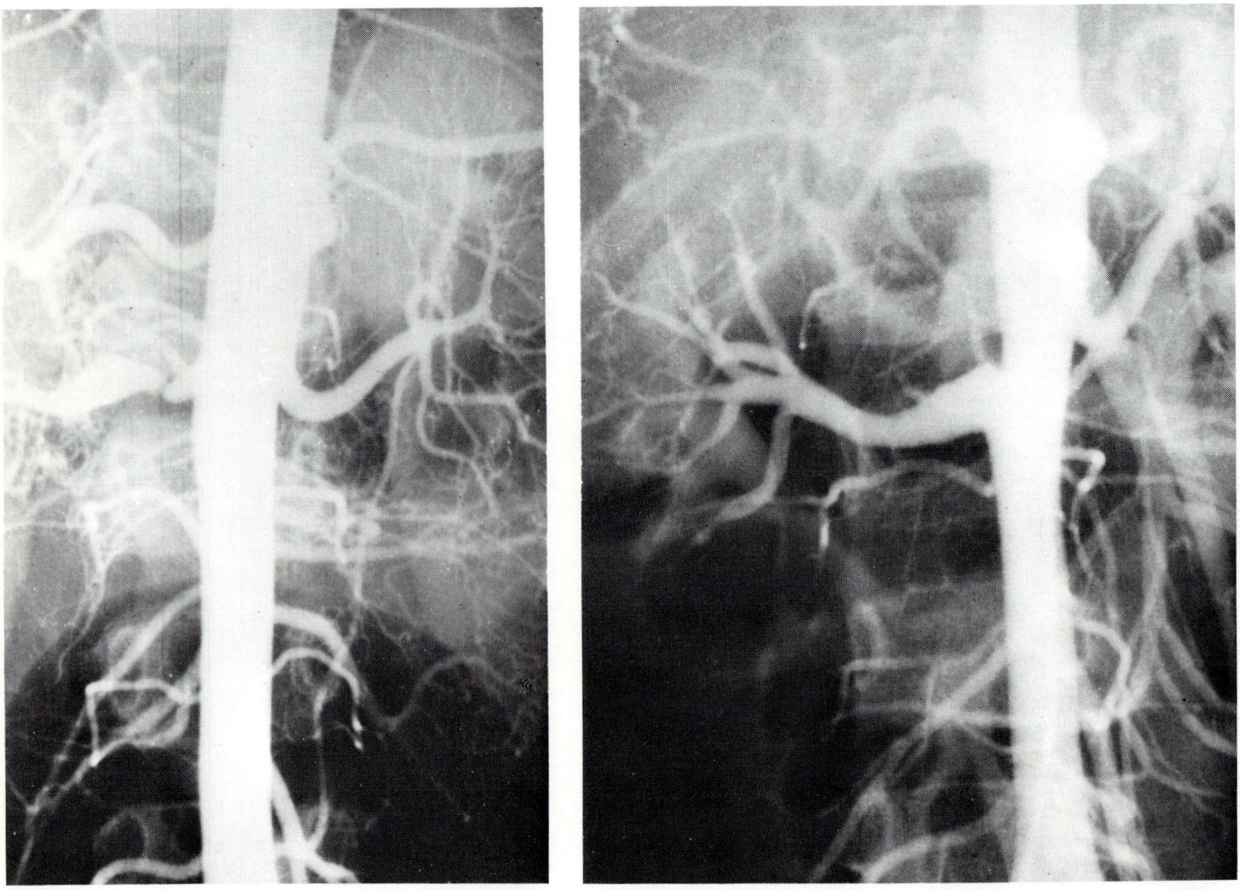

FIGURE 53-1. Preoperative and postoperative arteriograms in a 5-year-old child who underwent right renal artery reimplantation.

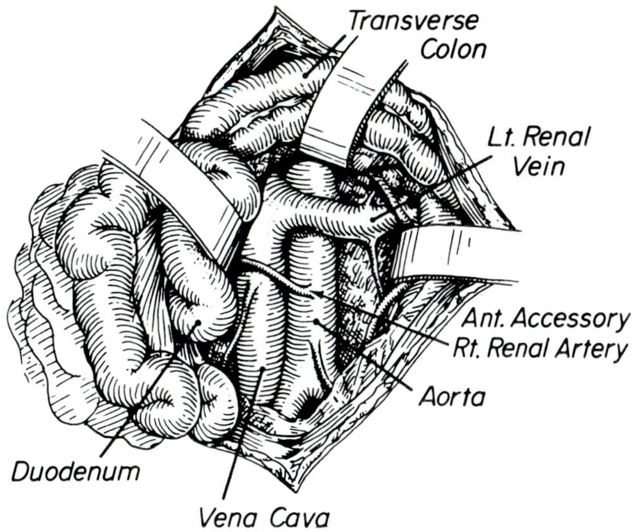

FIGURE 53-2. Exposure of the retroperitoneum through the base of the mesentery.

ligating two or more pairs of lumbar veins and retracting the vena cava to the patient's right and the left renal vein cephalad. Usually, however, the right renal artery is best exposed by mobilizing the duodenum and right colon medially. The right renal vein is mobilized and usually retracted cephalad in order to expose the artery. In some patients, there is an accessory right renal artery which arises from the anterior wall of the aorta about 1 in above the origin of the inferior mesenteric artery. This artery is unusual in that its course is anterior to the vena cava and then over to the lower pole of the right kidney instead of the retrocaval course of the normal right renal artery. The accessory artery can easily be injured if one is unaware of its presence.

Aortorenal Bypass

Three types of graft are usually available for aortorenal bypass: (1) autologous saphenous vein, (2) autologous hypogastric artery, and (3) synthetic prosthesis. The decision as to which graft should be used depends on a number of factors. We use the saphenous vein preferentially. However, if it is small—less than 4 mm in diameter—the hypogastric artery or a synthetic prosthesis may be preferable. A 6-mm polytetrafluoroethylene graft is quite satisfactory when the distal renal artery is of large caliber.

When an end-to-side renal artery bypass is used, the anastomosis between the renal artery and the graft is done first. Silastic slings can be used to occlude the renal artery distally. This method of vessel occlusion is especially applicable to this procedure. In contrast to vascular clamps, these slings are essentially atraumatic to the delicate renal artery. The absence of clamps in the operative field is also advantageous. Further, when tension is applied to the slings, they lift the vessel out of the retroperitoneal soft tissue for more accurate visualization.

The length of the arteriotomy should be at least three times the diameter of the renal artery to guard against late suture line stenosis. A 6-0 or 7-0 monofilament polypropylene (Prolene) suture material is employed with loop magnification.

After the renal artery anastomosis is completed, the occluding clamps and slings are removed from the artery and a small bulldog clamp is placed across the vein graft adjacent to the anastomosis. The aortic anastomosis is then done. First, an ellipse of the anterolateral aortic wall is removed, and then the anastomosis is performed. If the length of the graft is too long, it may result in kinking of the vein and subsequent thrombosis. If there is any element of kinking or twisting of the graft after both anastomoses are completed, the aortic anastomosis should be taken down and redone after appropriate shortening or reorientation of the graft. In certain instances, an end-to-end anastomosis between the graft and the renal artery provides a better reconstruction. Fry et al. (16) prefer the end-to-end anastomosis. We routinely employ end-to-end renal artery anastomosis when combining aortic replacement with renal revascularization. In this circumstance, the saphenous vein is attached to the Dacron aortic graft prior to its insertion. After the aortic graft is attached and flow is restored to the distal extremities, the renal artery can be resected and attached to the end of the saphenous vein graft without interrupting aortic flow.

Thromboendarterectomy

This procedure is employed only for atherosclerotic renal artery stenosis. It is not applicable in fibromuscular disease. Transaortic endarterectomy of bilateral main renal artery lesions has been strongly advocated by Wylie and Stoney (17). In this procedure, the proximal aortic clamp must usually be placed above the superior mesenteric artery. If it is placed below this artery, it will seriously compromise the exposure of the orifices of the renal arteries. Visualization of the distal end of the renal artery endarterectomy, however, is often difficult or impossible with this procedure. Because of this, we currently prefer a transverse aortotomy carrying the incision across the stenoses and into each renal artery. By this method, the entire endarterectomy can be performed under direct vision (Figure 53-3).

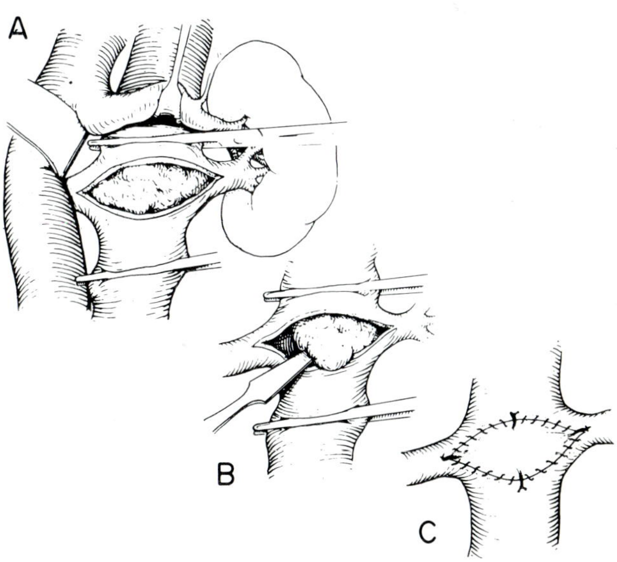

FIGURE 53-3. Drawing of arteriotomy for bilateral renal artery thromboendarterectomies.

Nephrectomy

Nephrectomy is a procedure that should be limited to a subgroup of patients with RVH in whom the kidney responsible for the hypertension has nonreconstructible vessels and has negligible or no residual excretory function. In these circumstances of unretrievable renal function, nephrectomy can provide benefit in control of hypertension while not diminishing overall excretory function. In all other circumstances in which there is significant residual excretory renal function, the price of nephrectomy (loss of functioning renal mass) is greater than the potential benefit. Exception to this rule occurs only when hypertension in uncontrollable on maximal drug therapy and residual pressures consistently are severely elevated (>120 mmHg). This extreme conservatism for the role of nephrectomy is based on the knowledge that greater than 35 percent of patients with atherosclerotic lesions will develop contralateral severe lesions during follow-up. Such lesions will place such a patient at risk for clinically severe renal failure and recurrent hypertension. This is of even greater importance in children: 50 percent of those who initially present with a unilateral lesion subsequently will develop contralateral disease.

POSTOPERATIVE CARE

The patient is usually kept in the surgical intensive care unit for 2 or 3 days. Body weight is measured daily. Central venous pressure is monitored, as is hourly output. These measurements are used to gauge fluid balance. Long-standing hypertension usually results in some degree of cardiac compromise. Congestive failure or pulmonary edema as the result of fluid overload is a frequent occurrence in the poorly monitored patient. Elastic stockings, leg exercise, subcutaneous miniheparin, and early ambulation are used to avoid thromboembolic complications. Postoperative hypotension is usually the result of inadequate blood replacement. Severe hypertension is commonly encountered and is treated with antihypertensive medications. Fifty percent of the patients who are eventually classified as cured, require antihypertensive drugs for several weeks or months postoperatively. If there is rapid acceleration of the hypertension in the postoperative period, thrombosis of the renal artery reconstruction should be suspected and an arteriogram obtained. Even though a bypass graft may have thrombosed, the distal renal artery may remain patent and a second reconstruction may be feasible.

Effect of Operation on Hypertension

Most of the controversy surrounding the role of the operative treatment of RVH relates to the risk of operation, an unacceptable frequency of technical failures, and a low rate of favorable blood pressure response to operation. Certainly the literature adequately documents the fact that poorly performed operations in poorly selected patients will result in an infrequent favorable blood pressure response. Current results of operative intervention in centers experienced with management of RVH, however, underscore the predictability of success. Although our experience stems over 20 years and includes the operative management of over 600 patients, a recent 5-year period (Table 53-5) exemplifies current expectations.

During the period 1977 to 1982, we undertook operative management in 182 patients. Operative risk has been low with only one patient (0.5 percent) dying as a result of renal revascularization. Technical success also has been highly predictable. Based on the results of routine postoperative angiography, 97 percent of patients have had a patent reconstruction without technical errors.

TABLE 53-5. Early (6-Mo) Results of Operation, 1977–1982, 182 Patients

Result	Percent
Technical success	97
Operative mortality rate (1)	0.5
Graft stenosis (2)	1.6
Graft occlusion (2)	1.1
Beneficial blood pressure response (cure or improved)	94
Cure:	
Atherosclerosis	31
FMD	77

Blood pressure response to operation is dependent on three factors: the preoperative documentation of the causal relationship between renal artery stenosis and the hypertension, the technical success of renal revascularization, and the underlying disease. We insist that the results of RVRA or SRFS confirm the presence of RVH before operation is undertaken. Having identified the functional significance of the renovascular lesion preoperatively, a beneficial blood pressure response has been achieved in 94 percent of patients undergoing successful operation in our center. Although significant improvement in the severity of hypertension is predictably high, regardless of the underlying pathology, patients with FMD have a much higher chance of a total cure of hypertension than do patients with atherosclerosis as the source of renovascular disease (77 vs. 31 percent). Many patients with atherosclerotic lesions have a background of previous mild essential hypertension, and most such patients have microscopic evidence of arteriolar nephrosclerosis. These factors frequently limit the likelihood of cure by renal revascularization but do not prevent improvement by reduction of severe, difficult to control hypertension to a mild variety easily controlled with minimal medications. Since the risk of morbid cardiovascular events secondary to hypertension is severity-related, we feel that such a reduction in the severity of hypertension in the majority of atherosclerotic patients (63 percent) is almost as beneficial as cure.

Effect of Renal Revascularization on Renal Function

Absent from most discussions of the management of RVH is the long-term adverse effect of uncorrected renal artery occlusions on renal perfusion and excretory function. Since renal artery occlusions can produce both secondary hypertension and alterations in renal function, proper treatment of patients with RVH also requires understanding of the natural history of changes in

TABLE 53-6. Effect of Revascularization on Excretory Function

	Preoperative Creatinine Clearance Groups		
	0–10 mL/min 7 patients	11–20 mL/min 9 patients	21–30 mL/min 9 patients
Preoperative creatinine clearance	3 ± 2.4 mL/min	16 ± 2.9 mL/min	25 ± 1.9 mL/min
Postoperative creatinine clearance	37 ± 27 mL/min	32 ± 8.3 mL/min	30 ± 1.9 mL/min
Significance of difference	$p < 0.02$	$p < 0.01$	$p > 0.05$

renal function during nonoperative treatment and the effect of revascularization on renal function. If one considers that changes in renal function during follow-up may be independent of, or even adversely affected by, drug-induced blood pressure reduction, knowledge of the probability of stability or deterioration in excretory function during nonoperative treatment is of even greater importance.

In contrast to the detrimental changes in renal function which may occur during drug therapy in many patients with renovascular hypertension is the response in renal function to revascularization of the poorly functioning kidney. Through the routine use of preoperative SRFS we have been able to compare individual kidney excretory function before and after revascularization. No change in excretory function after revascularization has been seen in kidneys with creatinine clearances greater than 30 mL/min (18). Conversely, however, we have demonstrated a statistically significant improvement in excretory function after revascularization of kidneys with less than 20 mL/min creatinine clearances. Table 53-6 summarizes our 1979 report (19) of the preoperative and postoperative SRFS in 25 patients who underwent successful revascularization of kidneys with less than 30 mL/min creatinine clearance. The type of renal artery lesion was atherosclerotic in 21 patients and fibromuscular dysplastic in 4 patients. Eight individuals had total renal artery occlusion. Preoperative creatinine clearances in the affected kidneys ranged from 0.27 to 30 mL/min (mean: 16 ± 16 mL/min). Fifteen of the 16 kidneys with preoperative creatinine clearances less than 20 mL/min had improvement in renal function following revascularization ($p < 0.01$). Improvement (60 percent) or cure (36 percent) in hypertension followed revascularization in 24 of the 25 patients. The most dependable predictor of successful management of both hypertension and retrieval of renal function in these patients was the arteriographic demonstration of a patent distal vessel without evidence of severe intrarenal stenoses.

This experience has led us to employ renal revascularization rather than nephrectomy whenever the distal artery is visualized and reasonably free of severe branch artery disease, regardless of the degree of excretory renal function impairment or the status of the contralateral renal artery. Obviously, this approach would have greatest application when contralateral renal function is reduced or contralateral renal artery disease is present. Nevertheless, since progression of apparently insignificant contralateral lesions or the development of new lesions during follow-up occurs in over 40 percent of patients undergoing operative management of renovascular hypertension, concern over protection of renal function should not be limited to patients with severe contralateral disease at the time of the initial evaluation. Indeed, if renal function in the poorly functioning kidney is retrievable by revascularization, then nephrectomy would be an inferior choice of operative management, regardless of the status of the contralateral kidney.

Such an aggressive attitude toward the role of revascularization in managing these patients with renovascular hypertension requires that both the operative risk and the frequency of graft thrombosis be low. Nevertheless, enthusiasm for revascularization of poorly functioning kidneys in older patients must be weighed against the operative risk when severe associated cardiovascular disease is present. Currently, however, nephrectomy is employed primarily only when intrarenal disease is severe, hypertension is otherwise difficult to control, and residual excretory function in the affected kidney is negligible.

Finally, the role of renal revascularization in severely azotemic patients requires special comment. Obviously, retrieval of renal function by revascularization is of greatest practical importance in this group. Although none of the patients in this study were severely azotemic, all had renovascular hypertension. This was predicted in each instance by the results of RVRA and SRFS and was proved by the response to operation. In this setting, severe reductions in the excretory function of one kidney were also improved by revascularization. Therefore, if a patient with a renal artery stenosis and severe azotemia has positive RVRA or SFRS, a benefit in overall excretory function should be expected from renal revascularization. Clearly, this beneficial effect would have the greatest practical significance if bilateral renal artery stenoses existed and could be corrected.

Late Follow-up of Reconstructions

From our 20-year experience with the operative management of RVH, 1- to 14-year follow-up sequential angiography of 176 reconstructions is available for evalution (Table 53-7). Four saphenous vein grafts and two hypogastric autografts have undergone aneurysmal dilatation. Only one of these, a hypogastric autograft, has required replacement (Figure 53-4). The remaining five have stabilized, and the patients have remained cured of hypertension. Aneurysmal dilatation of autogenous grafts (vein or artery) has occurred only in children in our experience. Al-

TABLE 53-7. Sequential 1- to 14-Year Follow-up Arteriography, 176 Reconstructions

Status	No. of Grafts	Percent
No adverse change	139	90
Aneurysmal dilatation	6	3
Stenosis	8	5
Occlusion	2	1
False aneurysm	1	<1

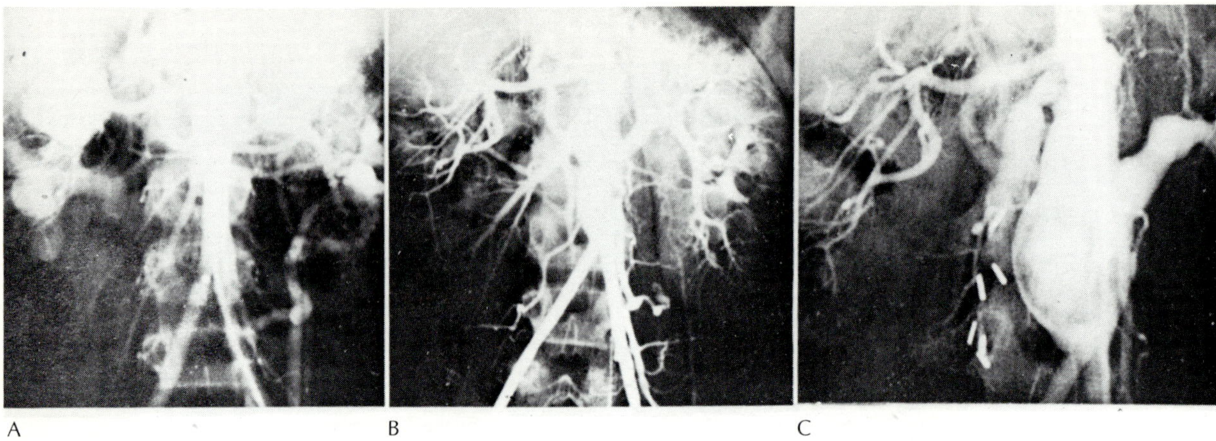

FIGURE 53-4. Sequential follow-up arteriogram of a 10-year-old child who underwent a hypogastric autograft to the left renal artery and an iliac vein autograft to the superior mesenteric artery. Ultimately, both grafts required replacements. (*A*) preoperative, 1970. (*B*) postoperative, 1970. (*C*) postoperative, 1973.

though the incidence of aneurysmal degeneration is low in our overall experience, all occurred in children, which suggests that the saphenous vein is particularly susceptible to this phenomenon in this age group. For this reason, we prefer the normal hypogastric artery as the conduit of choice in this group. Interestingly, in the two instances of autogenous arterial graft aneurysmal degeneration, FMD of the donor hypogastric artery was identified in retrospective microscopic evaluation.

Eight grafts have developed suture line or midgraft stenoses (Figure 53-5) requiring revision from 1 to 8 years after the initial

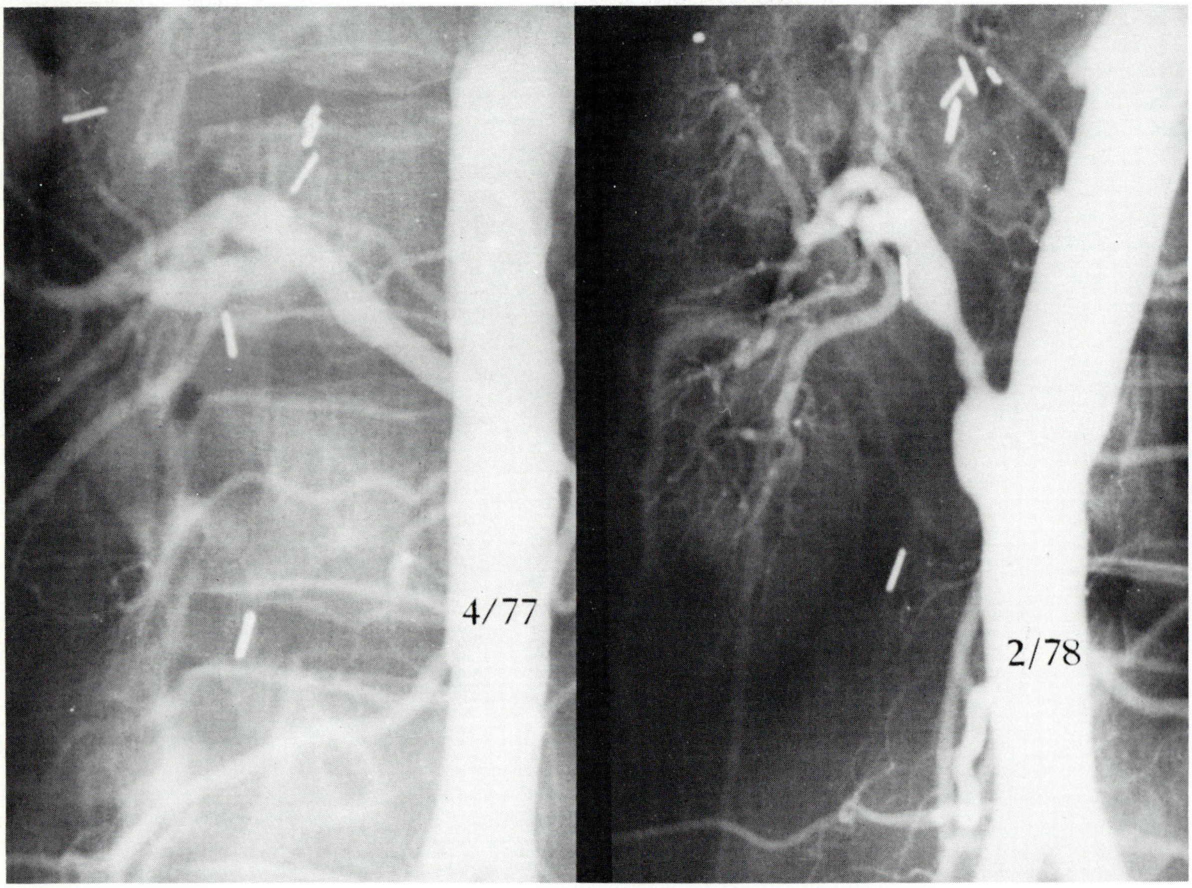

FIGURE 53-5. Postoperative arteriograms showing fibrous narrowing of the saphenous vein graft secondary to subendothelial fibroblastic proliferation.

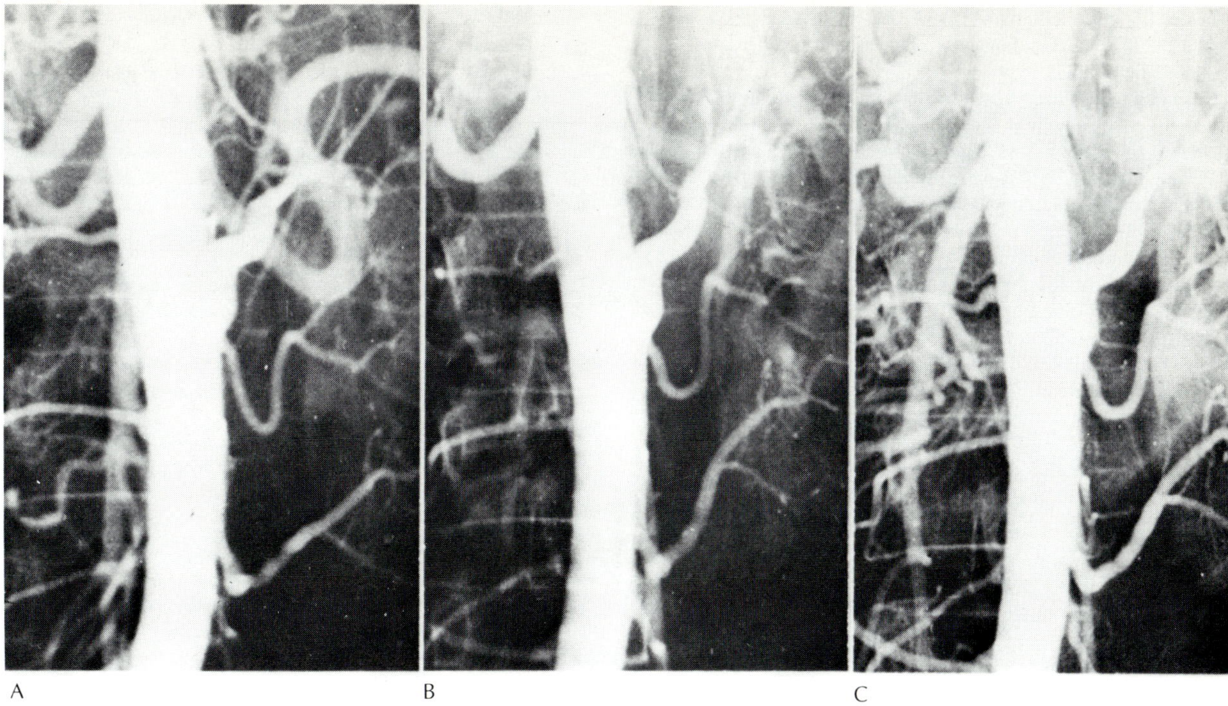

FIGURE 53-6. Sequential follow-up arteriograms after autogenous vein aortorenal bypass showing its long-term durability. (*A*) 1 year. (*B*) 4 years. (*C*) 9 years.

operation. Three patients have had graft occlusions during follow-up and probably represent missed graft stenoses which progressed to occlusion. One patient required correction of an aortic anastomotic false aneurysm in a Dacron graft 8 years postoperatively. The remaining 159 grafts (90 percent) have had no untoward changes with continued patency of the reconstruction during follow-up (Figure 53-6).

Follow-up angiography also has shown progression of mild to moderate contralateral renovascular disease in 38 percent of the patients. This is most important in children, where 7 of 15 with FMD had bilateral involvement (5). Only three of these seven children had the contralateral disease demonstrated at the time of the initial evaluation and operation. The remaining four children had documentation of the development and progression of contralateral disease subsequently. This occurrence of subsequent contralateral stenosis had led us to perform nephrectomy in children only if blood pressure is uncontrollable and revascularization is impossible. Since the longest follow-up in this group is only 10 years, the true incidence of subsequent contralateral disease requires additional longitudinal follow-up.

In summary, current experience with operation and percutaneous transluminal angioplasty (PTA) in respective centers devoted to their use suggests that both modalities can be performed safely and that both are initially successful methods of treating RVH. The occasional use of either modality, however, cannot be expected to produce the results reviewed in this discussion. Since control of hypertension by renal revascularization is most commonly employed for its long-term benefit in reducing associated risk factors, interventional therapy (operation or PTA) should provide a durable, long-term result. Although available data strongly support the role of operative management as a permanent method of renal revascularization and resolution of renal ischemia, PTA appears to be a method that achieves only temporary benefit in many patients with atherosclerotic lesions. Certainly, such a technique may play an important role in a subgroup of high-risk patients in whom short-term improvement is an acceptable goal of management. Its position among available therapeutic options, however, remains incompletely defined at this time. With this background, the euthusiasm for PTA as a standard mode of treatment and its current widespread use appear to be premature.

References

1. Tucker RM, Labarthe DR: Frequency of surgical treatment for hypertension in adults at the Mayo Clinic from 1973 through 1975. Mayo Clin Proc 1977, 52:549.
2. Shapiro AP, Perez-Stable E, Scheib ET, Bron K, et al: Renal artery stenosis and hypertension. Am J Med 1969, 47:175.
3. Hollifield JW: Unpublished data.
4. Davis BA, Crook JE, Vestal RE, Oates JA: Prevalence of renovascular hypertension in patients with grade III or IV hypertensive retinopathy. N Engl J Med 1979, 301(23):1273.
5. Lawson JD, Boerth RK, Foster JH, et al: Diagnosis and management of renovascular hypertension in children. Arch Surg 1977, 112:1307.

6. Foster JH, Dean RH, Pinkerton JA, et al: Ten years' experience with the surgical management of renovascular hypertension. Ann Surg 1973, 177:755.
7. Dean RH: Renal artery repair—Errors in patient selection and evaluation. In Bernhard VM, Towne JB (eds): *Complications in Vascular Surgery*. New York, Grune & Stratton, 1980, pp 167–210.
8. Dean RH, Burko H, Wilson JP, Mulherin JH, Foster JH: Deceptived patterns of renal artery stenosis. Surgery 1974, 76(6):872–881.
9. Vaughn ED, Buhler FR, Larach JH, et al: Renovascular hypertension: Renin measurements to indicate hypersecretion and contralateral suppression, estimate renal plasma flow, and score for surgical curability. Am J Med 1973, 55:402.
10. Stanley JC, Fry WJ: Surgical treatment of renovascular hypertension. Arch Surg 1977, 112:1291.
11. Davidson J, Lowe B, Dean RH, Rhamy RK: Variability of split renal function studies in essential and renovascular hypertension. Surg Forum 1979, 30:574.
12. Hunt JC, Strong CG: Renovascular hypertension. Mechanisms, natural history and treatment. Am J Cardiol 1973, 32:562.
13. Dean RH, Kieffer RW, Smith BM, Oates JA, Nadeau JHJ, Hollifeld JW, DuPont WD: Renovascular hypertension. Arch Surg 1981, 116:1408.
14. Dean RH: Operative management of renovascular hypertension. In Bergan JJ, Yao JST (eds): *Surgery of the Aorta and Its Body Branches*. Philadelphia, Grune & Stratton, 1979.
15. Dean RH: Indications for operative management of renovascular hypertension. J South Carolina Med Assoc December 1977, p 523.
16. Fry WJ, Brink BE, Thompson NW: New techniques in the treatment of extensive fibromuscular disease involving the renal arteries. Surgery 1970, 68:959.
17. Wylie EJ, Perloff DL, Stoney RJ: Autogenous tissue revascularization techniques in surgery for renovascular hypertension. Ann Surg 1969, 170:416.
18. Dean RH, Shack RB, Rhamy RK, Wilson JP, Foster JH: The effect of renal revascularization on kidney function. J Surg Res 1977, 22:443.
19. Dean RH, Lawson JD, Hollifield JW, Shack RB, Polterauer P, Rhamy RK: Revascularization of the poorly functioning kidney. Surgery 1979, 85(1):44–52.

Chapter 54

ACUTE MESENTERIC VASCULAR DISEASE

SCOTT J. BOLEY and EDWARD B. BORDEN

Acute Mesenteric Ischemia

During the past 25 years there has been increasing recognition of the importance and frequency of intestinal ischemia. In part this is because of a real increase in its incidence; more importantly, it is the result of the belated realization that many clinical manifestations have as their common etiology interference with intestinal blood flow. Acute ischemia of the intestines is far more common than chronic ischemia and occurs in approximately 1 per 1000 admissions to major medical centers.

Reduction in blood flow to the intestine may be a reflection of generalized poor perfusion, as in shock or with a failing heart, or it may result from either local morphologic or functional changes. Narrowings of the major mesenteric vessels, emboli of atheromatous material or blood clot, thromboses, vasculitis as part of a systemic disease, or mesenteric vasoconstriction can all lead to inadequate circulation at the cellular level. However, whatever the cause, intestinal ischemia has the same end results—a spectrum ranging from completely reversible functional alterations to total hemorrhagic necrosis of portions or all of the bowel.

In spite of the great interest focused on acute mesenteric ischemia and the tremendous advances in roentgenologic and surgical techniques, the lethality of this intraabdominal catastrophe has with few exceptions remained as high (1,2) as in 1933 when Hibbard reportedly a mortality rate of 70 percent (3). This lack of improvement can be attributed to three main factors: (1) failure to diagnose ischemia before intestinal gangrene occurs, (2) the progression of bowel infarction after the primary vascular or systemic problem has been corrected, and (3) the number of patients with nonocclusive mesenteric ischemia with its reported mortality rate of over 90 percent (1).

Acute intestinal ischemia is especially important to vascular surgeons not only as a primary clinical problem but also because it frequently complicates other vascular conditions and operations. Examples are the occurrence of colonic ischemia after aortic aneurysmectomy or aortoiliac reconstruction, and the common association of superior mesenteric and peripheral arterial emboli.

HISTORICAL BACKGROUND

The first description of mesenteric thrombosis is attributed to Antonio Beniviene of Florence in the fifteenth century, but Tiedenman's clinical case report in 1843 first stimulated interest in this problem. The first successful bowel resection for intestinal infarction was reported by Elliott in 1895. In 1906 Delbet suggested the possibility of revascularization for superior mesenteric artery (SMA) obstruction. Although Ryvlyn in 1943 and Blinov in 1950 described patents in whom SMA embolectomy was unsuccessfully attempted (4), Klass is generally credited with establishing the feasibility of this operation. In 1951 he described two patients who underwent successful embolectomy but died of cardiac causes postoperatively (5). One year later Stewart performed the first SMA embolectomy with survival (6). Successful operative approaches to acute SMA thrombosis as well as chronic mesenteric ischemia were reported in the 1950s. Ende in 1958 first described nonocclusive mesenteric ischemia (NOMI) (7), and during the 1960s various attempts to treat this condition using local and regional anesthetic blocks as well as systemic and intraarterial vasodilators were reported.

PATHOPHYSIOLOGY

The intestines are protected from ischemic injury to a great extent by their abundant collateral circulation. Collateral pathways around occlusions of smaller mesenteric arterial branches are provided by the primary, secondary, and tertiary arcades in the mesentery of the small bowel, and the marginal arterial complex of Drummond in the mesocolon. Within the bowel wall itself, there is a network of communicating submucosal vessels which can maintain the viability of short segments of the intestine whose extramural arterial supply has been lost. There is good clinical evidence that in gradual occlusions of the major mesenteric arteries, and in acute occlusions when mesenteric vasoconstriction does not supervene, the collateral blood supply is adequate to maintain intestinal viability.

When a major vessel is occluded, collateral pathways open immediately in response to the fall in arterial pressure distal to the obstruction. Increased blood flow through this collateral circulation continues as long as the pressure in the vascular bed distal to an obstruction remains below the systemic arterial pressure. If vasoconstriction develops in the distal bed, the arterial pressure there rises, the pressure differential narrows, and flow diminishes. Similarly, if normal blood flow is reconstituted, flow through collateral channels ceases.

Vasoconstriction of the mesenteric vascular bed has been postulated as the mechanism for NOMI and also has been demonstrated experimentally, angiographically, and intraoperatively in association with acute occlusions of the SMA. The occurrence of persistent or sustained vasoconstriction after the initiating cause is corrected, however, has only recently been identified. We have demonstrated such persistent vasoconstriction following a controlled decrease in mesenteric blood flow in a series of experiments performed on more than 200 anesthetized dogs (8–10).

The flow in the SMA was decreased 50 percent with a hydraulic occluder and maintained at this level while alterations in cardiac output, intestinal perfusion, oxygen consumption, systemic and mesenteric arterial pressures, and blood flow through other arteries of the splanchnic circulation were measured. Following acute diminution in SMA to 50 percent of control values, the mesenteric arterial pressure (MAP) in the peripheral bed immediately fell a mean of 49 percent (range, 36 to 71 percent), and in several instances the decrease in MAP exceeded the decrease in blood flow. When SMA flow was maintained at 50 percent, the MAP returned to control levels within 1 to 6 hours while celiac artery flow, which initially had increased, returned to normal. If the occluder was released when MAP first returned to its control value, the SMA flow immediately rose to control levels. However, if the SMA occlusion was continued for 30 minutes to 4 hours after MAP had returned to control, SMA flows remained at 30 to 35 percent of control, even after removal of the occluder. These low SMA flows persisted for up to 5 hours of observation. However, in several of the experimental animals with persistent vasoconstriction, injection of papaverine into the SMA relieved the vasoconstriction and produced an immediate return of SMA flow to control levels. In other animals, when papaverine was infused continuously (30 to 60 mg/h) into the SMA while 50 percent flow was maintained in this vessel, the MAP remained low during the entire 4 hours of the experiment, and SMA flow returned to normal promptly upon releasing the occluder.

Thus mesenteric vasoconstriction probably plays a significant role both during an acute occlusive or nonocclusive episode and for varying periods after correction of its cause. The effectiveness of locally administered vasodilators in preventing and reversing the persistent vasoconstriction following low SMA flow suggested that local intraarterial papaverine could be used clinically to treat the vasoconstriction of the "low-flow" syndrome. Although other methods and drugs have been used, direct intraarterial papaverine has been most consistent and effective in relieving this vasoconstriction. Currently a host of new vasodilators including prostacyclin, vasoactive intestinal polypeptide, and angiotensin converting enzyme inhibitor are being investigated as alternatives to papaverine.

Thus, low SMA flow initially produces mesenteric vascular responses that tend to maintain adequate intestinal flow, but if the diminished flow is prolonged, active vasoconstriction develops and may persist even after the primary cause of mesenteric ischemia is corrected. Such persistent vasoconstriction appears to violate the concept of autoregulatory escape but is not unique to the gastrointestinal circulation. A similar potential for persistent vasoconstriction has been described in the kidney in humans (11).

One of the puzzling characteristics of intestinal necrosis caused by low flow states is the frequent lag between correction of the primary systemic problem and the onset of abdominal symptoms and signs. It has been postulated that the bowel is injured during an episode of diminished cardiac output or hypotension, and with correction of the primary problem, mesenteric blood flow returns to normal. This would not explain the operative finding of persistent bowel ischemia without venous or arterial occlusion in patients whose cardiovascular problems have been corrected. The paradox can be explained, however, by our experimental observation that an episode of low mesenteric blood flow of as short as 2 hours' duration can produce mesenteric ischemia which may persist for many hours after correction of the primary problem.

CLINICAL PRESENTATIONS

Early identification of acute mesenteric ischemia (AMI) depends upon recognition of those patients who are at risk of developing this catastrophe. AMI is most likely to develop in patients over 50 years of age with heart disease and long-standing congestive heart failure (especially with unsatisfactory control of digitalis therapy or prolonged use of diuretics), cardiac arrhythmias, recent myocardial infarctions, or patients with hypovolemia or hypotension, e.g., brought on by burns, pancreatitis, or hemorrhage. The development of abdominal pain in a patient with one of these conditions should raise the suspicion of AMI. Previous or simultaneous arterial emboli increases the possibility of the ischemia being caused by an SMA embolus.

Abdominal pain is present in 75 to 98 percent of patients with intestinal ischemia, but varies in severity, nature, and location. Patients with SMA thrombosis commonly have postprandial abdominal pain for several weeks or months preceding the acute episode. A characteristic early clinical feature of AMI is a disparity between the severity of the pain and the paucity of significant abdominal findings. Sudden severe pain accompanied by forceful intestinal emptying is strongly suggestive of an acute arterial occlusion, especially when there are minimal or no abdominal findings. Mesenteric venous thrombosis is associated with abdominal pain, nausea, and vomiting which may be present for 2 to 3 weeks before abdominal signs develop.

Unexplained abdominal distension or gastrointestinal bleeding may be the only indication of acute intestinal ischemia, since pain may be absent in up to 25 percent of patients, especially those with NOMI. Distension, while usually absent early in the course of mesenteric ischemia, may be the first sign of impending intestinal infarction. Gastrointestinal bleeding may precede any other symptom of mesenteric ischemia, and stools are positive for occult blood in up to 75 percent of patients.

Early in the course of an ischemic episode there are no abdominal findings, but, as infarction develops, increasing tenderness, rebound tenderness, and muscle guarding reflect the progressing intestinal changes. Significant abdominal findings are strong evidence for the presence of nonviable bowel. Nausea, vomiting, fever, rectal bleeding, hematemesis, intestinal obstruction, back pain, shock, and increasing abdominal distension are other late signs.

LABORATORY FINDINGS

Leukocytosis above 15,000 cells per cubic millimeter occurs in approximately 75 percent of patients with AMI, and a metabolic acidosis is present in about 50 percent. Elevations of serum amylase and of peritoneal fluid intestinal alkaline phosphatase and inorganic phosphates have all been reported, but the sensitivity and specificity of these findings have not been established. Leukocytosis (especially out of proportion to the physical findings), elevated hematocrit, and blood-tinged peritoneal fluid, often with a high amylase content, are all signs of advanced intestinal necrosis.

DIAGNOSTIC STUDIES

Several potentially diagnostic radioisotopic techniques utilizing ^{99m}Tc pyrophosphate (12) or diphosphonate (13) and ^{99m}Tc colloid sulfur labeled leukocytes (14) have been developed in animal studies. These are being evaluated clinically but have not yet been proved reliable. Laparoscopy is another diagnostic modality, especially useful for patients too ill to undergo angiography. This technique is potentially hazardous, however, since profound decreases in SMA flow occur with intraperitoneal pressures over 20 mmHg. Lower pressures for brief periods produce only minimal alterations in flow (15). Unfortunately, laparoscopy enables visualization of only the serosal aspect of the bowel. Thus, while this modality is useful for identifying transmural infarction, it is not reliable for diagnosing earlier stages of mucosal ischemia when the serosa appears normal.

Angiography has been successfully employed to diagnose AMI, but until recently its role has been limited to identifying an embolus or acute thrombosis, both of which might be successfully treated by prompt operation. In 1974, we reported on a series of studies aimed at establishing criteria for the angiographic diagnosis of mesenteric vasoconstriction, the presence of which suggests NOMI (16). Mesenteric vasoconstriction was produced in dogs and the resulting angiographic abnormalities identified. Subsequently, selective superior mesenteric angiograms of a control group of 65 patients were examined to determine if the observed angiographic abnormalities occured in the absence of vasoconstriction. The reliability of these angiographic signs of vasoconstriction was then evaluated in patients with AMI.

Based upon these studies, four reliable angiographic criteria for the diagnosis of mesenteric vasoconstriction were identified:

1. Narrowing at the origins of multiple branches of the SMA
2. Irregularities in intestinal branches
3. Spasm of arcades
4. Impaired filling of intramural vessels

While mesenteric vasoconstriction occurs with hemorrhage, pancreatitis, and other conditions, its presence in patients with suspected intestinal ischemia who are not in shock or receiving vasopressors is strong evidence for the presence of NOMI. Thus, if angiography is performed sufficiently early in their course, patients with both occlusive and nonocclusive AMI can be identified before bowel infarction occurs.

PLAN FOR DIAGNOSIS AND THERAPY

Selection of Patients

Patients over 50 years of age with any of the previously enumerated conditions predisposing to AMI, who develop sudden onset of abdominal pain lasting more than 2 or 3 hours, are started on the management protocol. Less absolute indications for an aggressive investigation are unexplained abdominal distension, gastrointestinal bleeding, or metabolic acidosis. These broad selection criteria are essential if early diagnosis and treatment are to be achieved, because the presence of more extensive and specific signs and symptoms usually signifies irreversible intestinal damage.

Initial Preparation

Initial treatment is directed toward correction of predisposing or precipitating causes of the mesenteric ischemia. Relief of acute congestive heart failure, correction of cardiac arrhythmias, and replacement of blood volume must precede any diagnostic studies. In general, efforts at increasing intestinal blood flow will be futile if low cardiac output, hypotension, or hypovolemia persist. Plain roentgenographic studies of the abdomen are then obtained, and subsequent abdominal angiography is routinely performed unless some other intraabdominal condition is diagnosed on the plain film examination. Based on the angiographic findings and the presence or absence of signs of peritoneal irritation on physical examination, the individual patient is then treated according to the proposed plan outlined in Figure 54-1.

Even when a decision to operate has been made based on clinical grounds, an angiogram must be obtained to manage the patient properly at operation. Moreover, the relief of mesenteric vasoconstriction is an integral part of the therapy for emboli and thromboses, as well as the low flow states and can best be achieved by intraarterial infusion of papaverine through the angiography catheter in the SMA.

Treatment Plan

General Principles. When papaverine is used, it is infused at a constant rate of 30 to 60 mg/h using an infusion pump. Systemic arterial pressure and cardiac rate and rhythm are monitored because these amounts of papaverine may have systemic effects. The duration of the infusion varies with both the purpose for its use and the clinical and angiographic response of the patient.

Laparotomy is indicated during the course of AMI either to restore intestinal arterial flow, after an embolus or thrombosis, or to resect irreparably damaged bowel. Revascularization should precede any evaluation of intestinal viability since bowel that initially appears infarcted may show surprising recovery after restoration of blood flow.

After revascularization, any nonviable or questionably viable short segments of bowel are resected. If extensive segments of bowel are involved, only the frankly necrotic bowel is resected and a planned reexploration ("second look") is performed within 12 to 24 hours.

A decision to perform a second look is made at the initial laparotomy if there is questionable viability of either a major portion or multiple segments of intestine. The purpose of the second look, as proposed by Shaw is "not just to allow a clear definition between dead and live bowel to take place, but also to allow time for the institution of supportive measures which may render more of the bowel viable" (17).

The use of anticoagulants in the management of AMI is controversial. We do not employ heparin anticoagulation in the perioperative period, except for venous thrombosis, because of the

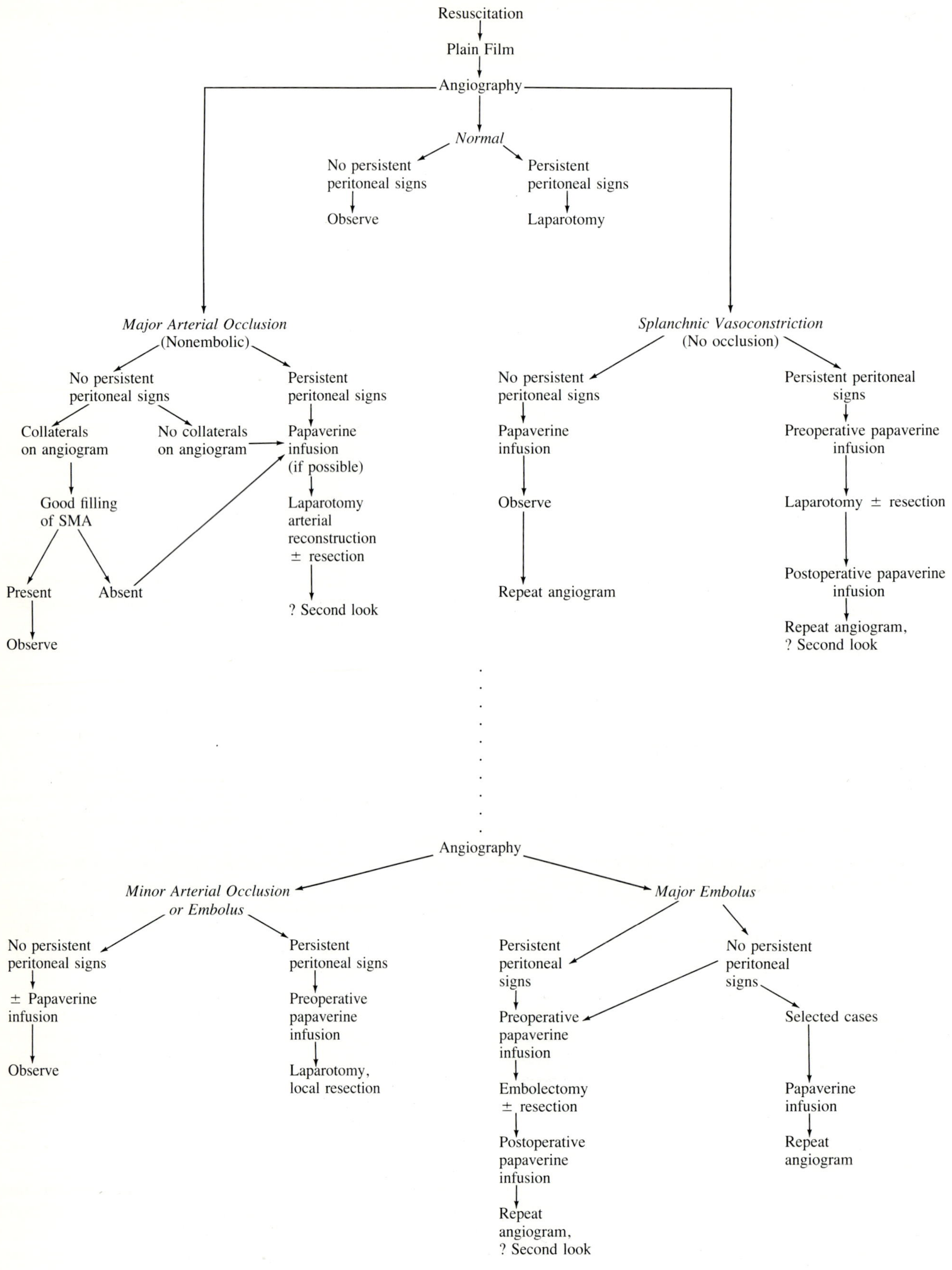

FIGURE 54-1. Proposed plan for diagnosis and treatment of acute mesenteric ischemia.

danger of intestinal hemorrhage. Thromboses late in the postoperative period, however, have prompted us to start anticoagulation 48 hours postoperatively following embolectomy or arterial reconstruction.

The value of both systemic and locally administered antibiotics to improve the viability of compromised bowel is well accepted. For this reason, and because of the high incidence of positive blood cultures with AMI, systemic antibiotics are started as soon as the diagnosis is established.

Superior Mesenteric Artery Embolus (SMAE). Emboli to the SMA are responsible for 40 to 50 percent of episodes of AMI and usually originate from a mural or atrial thrombus. In the past, such thrombi were most commonly associated with rheumatic valvular disease, but today arteriosclerotic heart disease is the most frequent cause. Many patients have a previous history of peripheral arterial embolism, and approximately 20 percent have synchronous emboli in other arteries.

SMAE tend to lodge at points of normal anatomic narrowings usually just distal to the origin of a major branch (Figure 54-2).

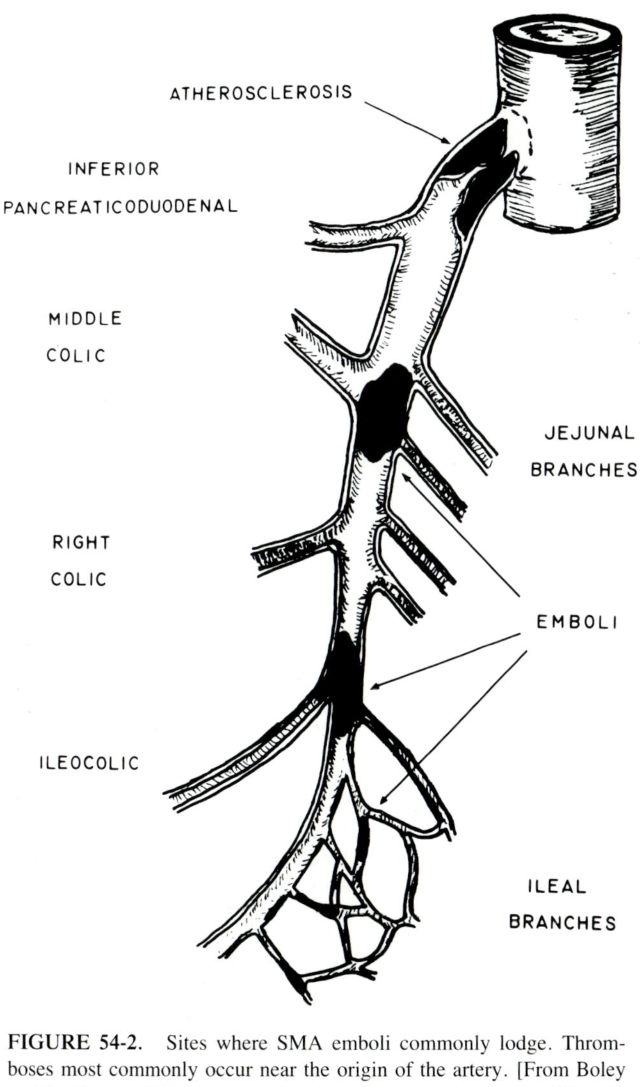

FIGURE 54-2. Sites where SMA emboli commonly lodge. Thromboses most commonly occur near the origin of the artery. [From Boley and Veith, in JD Hardy (ed): *Hardy's Textbook of Surgery*, 1983, by permission of J.B. Lippincott Company.]

In 10 to 15 percent of patients the emboli are more peripheral in the SMA or in branch arteries.

An embolus may completely occlude the artery, but more often it only partially obstructs blood flow. Mild to marked vasoconstriction is frequently present in arteries both proximal and distal to the embolus (Figure 54-3) and affects the retrograde filling of the SMA and its branches distal to the embolus.

If an embolus is identified on the angiogram, a papaverine infusion is begun through the angiographic SMA catheter which is secured in place. The patient is then managed according to the plan in Figure 54-1 based upon the site of the embolus, the presence or absence of peritoneal signs, and the state of perfusion of the vascular bed distal to the embolus as determined from a repeat angiogram after an intraarterial bolus of 25 mg of tolazoline.

Minor emboli are those limited to branches of the SMA or to the SMA distal to the origin of the ileocolic artery. Patients with major emboli who are selected for management only by papaverine infusions are those with compelling medical reasons for avoiding operation, no peritoneal signs, and angiographically demonstrated good perfusion of the vascular bed distal to the embolus after the bolus dose of tolazoline. Thrombolytic agents infused through the angiographic catheters have been employed successfully in a few patients with SMAE, but this approach is still experimental.

Embolectomy is performed before assessing intestinal viability. We prefer to approach the embolus directly, or less optimally through a proximal arteriotomy. The proximal SMA is exposed by drawing the transverse colon superiorly and anteriorly, and packing off the small intestine inferiorly. The inferior leaf of the transverse mesocolon is incised, and the proximal SMA is identified by dissection between the pancreas and duodenum. The origin of the middle colic artery is identified and isolated, and the main SMA freed for a distance of 2 to 3 cm proximal and distal to the origin of this branch. After identifying the site of the embolus, the vessel is occluded proximally and distally with double-looped tapes, gentle vascular clamps, or bulldog clamps (Figure 54-4). A longitudinal arteriotomy is made over the embolus or just proximal to it. The embolus is removed and the proximal and distal occlusions released to flush out retained fragments of clots. A Fogarty balloon catheter is then passed proximally and distally to remove all residual clots. The arteriotomy is closed carefully with or without a vein patch.

Following embolectomy, if no second look is planned, the papaverine infusion is continued for 12 to 24 hours, and an angiogram obtained immediately prior to removing the catheter. When a second look is scheduled, the infusion is maintained until that procedure is completed.

Nonocclusive Mesenteric Ischemia. After 1958, when Ende first described NOMI (7), the proportion of mesenteric vascular accidents resulting from this entity rose from 12 to over 50 percent in the 1970s. More recently the incidence of NOMI has been declining. The pathogenesis of NOMI is believed to be splanchnic vasoconstriction occurring in response to a decrease in cardiac output, hypovolemia, dehydration, vasopressor agents, or hypotension. This vasoconstriction may persist even after the initiating cause has been corrected. Predisposing conditions include myocardial infarction, congestive heart failure, aortic insufficiency, renal and hepatic disease, or major abdominal or cardiac operations. In addition, a more immediate pre-

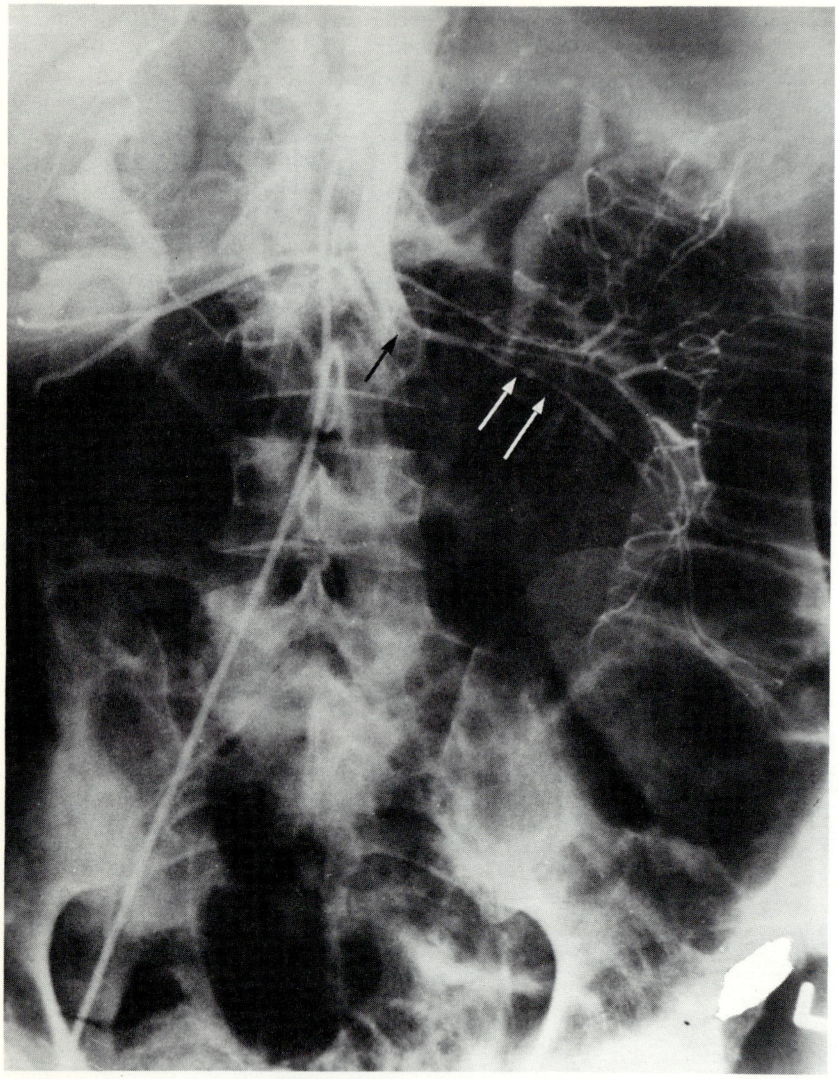

FIGURE 54-3. Superior mesenteric artery angiogram of a patient with an embolus at the origin of the middle colic artery (*black arrow*) with vasopasm of the unobstructed arterial branches (*white arrows*). [From Brandt and Boley, in LD MacLean (ed): *Advances in Surgery*, 1981, by permission of Yearbook Medical Publishers.]

cipitating cause such as pulmonary edema, cardiac arrhythmias, or shock is usually present, although the intestinal ischemic episode may not be manifested until hours or days later.

Angiographically, NOMI is diagnosed when the signs of mesenteric vasoconstriction are seen in a patient who has a clinical picture suggestive of intestinal ischemia, but who is neither in shock nor receiving vasopressors. The angiographic findings may vary from localized spasm to a ''pruned'' appearance of the entire mesenteric tree.

A papaverine infusion is begun on all patients with NOMI as soon as the diagnosis is made (Figure 54-1), and in patients with persistent peritoneal signs the infusion is continued during and after laparotomy.

At operation, manipulation of the SMA is kept to a minimum. Obviously necrotic bowel is resected and a primary anastomosis is performed. If bowel of questionable viability is left behind, a second look is scheduled. It is better to leave bowel of doubtful viability than to perform a massive small bowel resection, for in many instances the circulation will have improved by the time of the second exploration.

When papaverine infusion is used as the primary treatment for NOMI, it is continued for approximately 24 hours. A repeat angiogram is then performed 30 minutes after changing the infusion to isotonic saline without papaverine (Figure 54-5). Based on the clinical course of the patient and the response of the vasoconstriction to therapy as noted on the angiogram, the infusion is discontinued or maintained for another 24 hours; the patient is then reevaluated. Infusions have been continued for up to 5 days but usually can be stopped after 24 hours. When papaverine is used in conjunction with laparotomy for nonocclusive disease, a second look is frequently necessary. In such cases the infusion is continued as described previously for second look operations following embolectomy. The papaverine infusion is discontinued when no signs of vasoconstriction remain on an angiogram obtained 30 minutes after the vasodilator infusate is replaced by saline alone. The SMA catheter is removed promptly when the intraarterial infusion is stopped.

Acute Superior Mesenteric Artery Thrombosis (SMAT). The incidence of SMAT varies in different reports. While Ottinger (18) and Jackson (19) found thromboses to be almost as common as emboli, in most recent reports emboli were three to four times more frequent. SMAT almost always is superimposed upon severe atherosclerotic narrowing, most often in the region of the origin of the SMA. Since the acute episode represents the

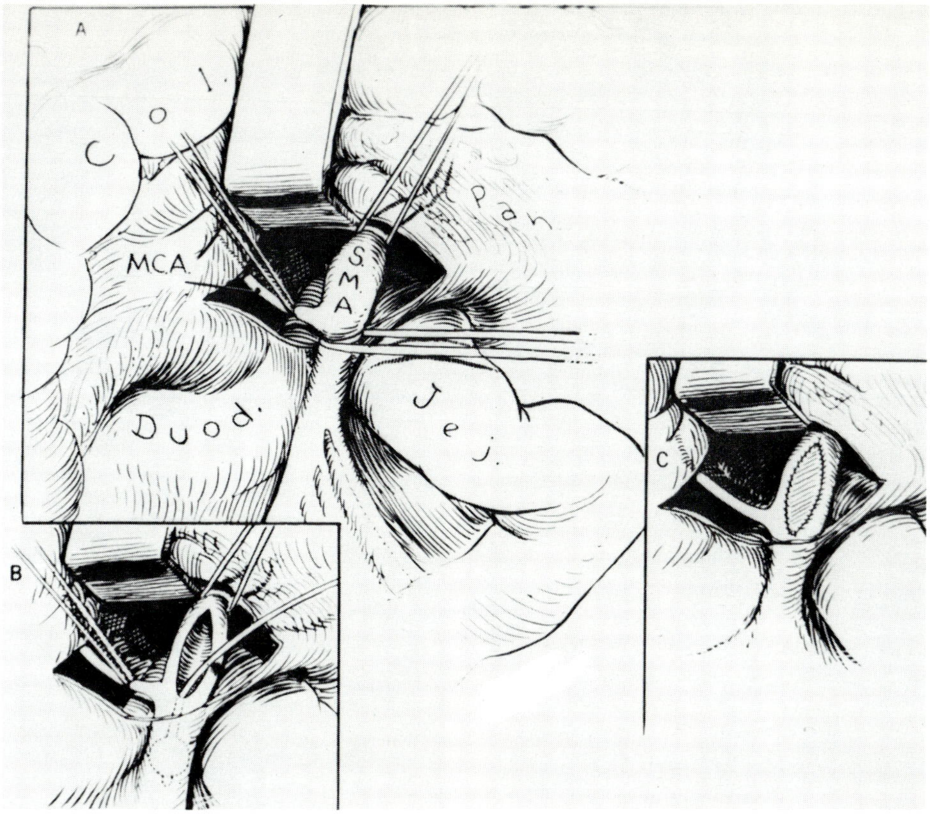

FIGURE 54-4. Technique of superior mesenteric artery embolectomy. *(A)* The artery has been isolated at the base of the transverse mesocolon and controlled with tapes. *(B)* Longitudinal arteriotomy placed proximal to the origin of the middle colic artery. A Fogarty catheter has been passed distally. *(C)* The arteriotomy closure using a vein patch. The patch is usually not required. [From Boley et al., in LM Nyhus (ed): *Surgery Annual,* 1973, by permission of Appleton-Century-Crofts.]

end stage of a chronic problem, it is not surprising that 30 to 50 percent of patients have had abdominal pain during the preceding weeks to months. Most patients have severe diffuse atherosclerosis and a prior history of coronary, cerebral, or peripheral arterial ischemia.

Identification of SMAT is usually made from the flush aortogram which most often shows total occlusion of the SMA within 1 to 2 cm of its origin. Some filling of the artery distal to the obstruction is almost always present because of collateral circulation. Branches both proximal and distal to the occlusion may show local spasm or diffuse vasoconstriction. Angiographic differentiation between a thrombosis and an old embolus may be difficult; in such instances the patients are treated initially as if they have emboli. A more difficult problem arises when total occlusion of the SMA is demonstrated by angiography in a patient with abdominal pain but no abdominal findings. In such an instance, it is important to be able to differentiate an acute occlusion from a long-standing one, because the latter may be coincidental to an unrelated present illness. The presence or absence of prominent collaterals between the superior mesenteric and celiac and/or inferior mesenteric circulation is the most helpful finding. If large collaterals are demonstrated on the angiogram (Figure 54-6), chronic occlusion is most likely and is confirmed by good filling of the SMA in late films. In the absence of any peritoneal signs, such patients are treated expectantly. The absence of collaterals indicates acute occlusion, and prompt intervention is indicated whether or not peritoneal signs are present.

If the position of the angiographic catheter permits, papaverine infusion is started preoperatively and maintained during and after the arterial reconstruction.

Revascularization procedures for SMAT are similar to those used for chronic mesenteric ischemia and are discussed in detail in Chapter 55. Thrombectomy and endarterectomy or some form of bypass graft to the SMA distal to the obstruction is employed. While a short graft from the aorta to the SMA is the easiest and most satisfactory operation in our opinion, extensive aortic disease may make this impossible. Often a common or external iliac artery may be the best source of inflow, and we have had success with prosthetic grafts from either to the SMA.

Acute Mesenteric Venous Thrombosis (AMVT). Mesenteric venous thrombosis was considered the most frequent cause of intestinal infarction 57 years ago (20), when infarction in the absence of arterial occlusion was interpreted as being the result of venous thrombosis. Today NOMI is recognized as the cause of most of these cases.

Mesenteric venous thrombosis may be primary (''agnogenic'') or secondary to a variety of conditions incuding hematologic disorders, hypercoagulable states, intraabdominal sepsis, local venous stasis, and abdominal trauma. Recently there has been a spate of reports of minor and major mesenteric venous throm-

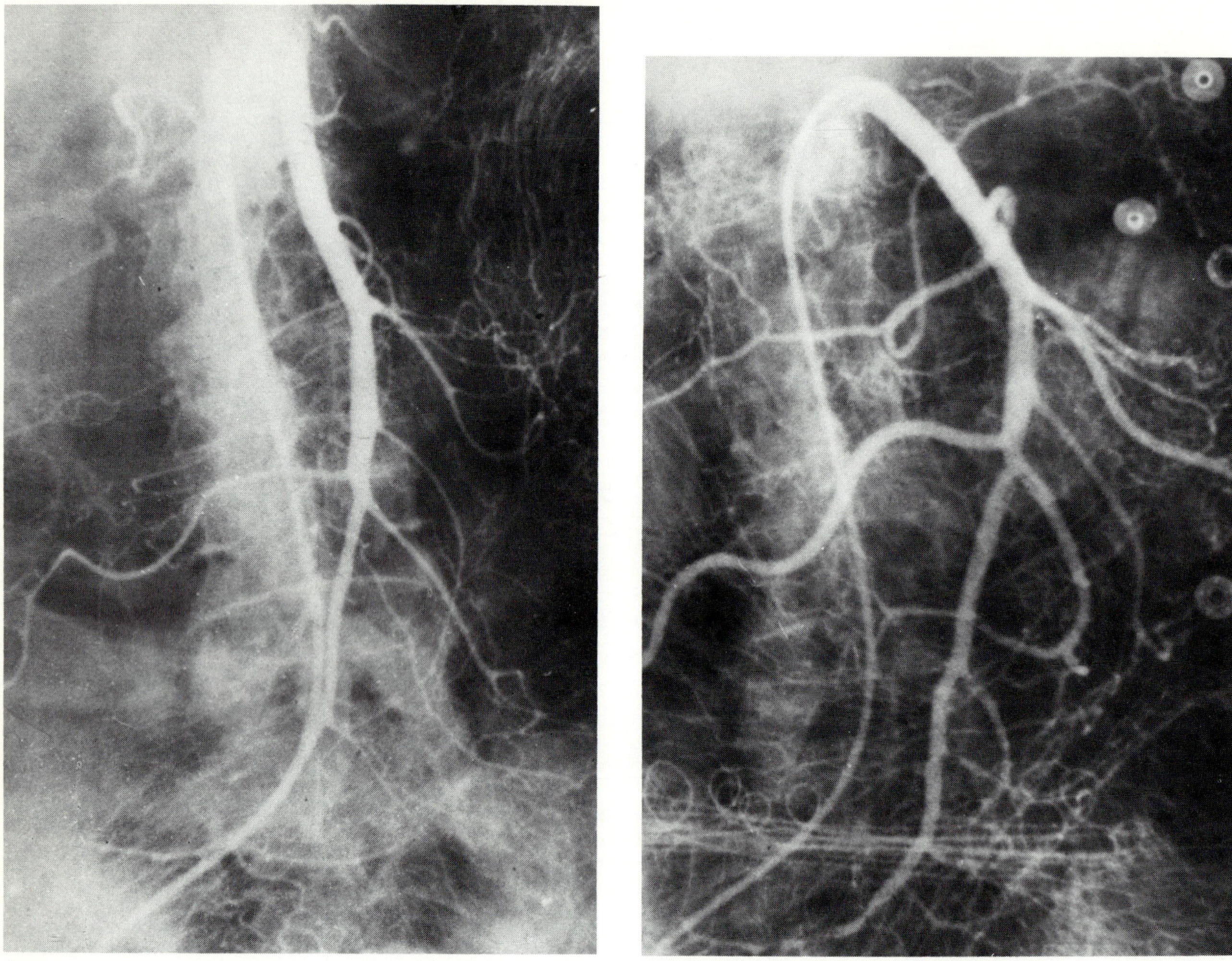

A B

FIGURE 54-5. Patient with nonocclusive mesenteric ischemia managed with papaverine infusion for 3 days. *(A)* Initial angiogram showing spasm of main superior mesenteric artery, origins of branches, and intestinal arcades. *(B)* Angiogram after 36 hours of papaverine infusion. This study was obtained 30 minutes after papaverine was replaced with saline. At this time the patient's abdominal symptoms and signs were gone. [From Boley, Brandt, and Veith in MM Ravitch (ed): *Current Problems in Surgery,* 1978, by permission of Yearbook Medical Publishers.]

boses in patients taking oral contraceptives. The angiographic diagnosis of AMVT has only rarely been made in the clinical setting.

Mesenteric venous thrombosis is most often diagnosed at laparotomy. Angiography is usually nondiagnostic, and laparotomy is performed because of the presence of peritoneal signs. The thrombosis may involve the superior mesenteric vein (SMV) and portal vein, but more frequently involves a segmental jejunal or ileal vein. At operation the diagnosis can be confirmed by mesenteric venous angiography and pressure measurements performed through a peripheral venous branch.

Localized segments of infarcted intestine are resected and primary anastomoses performed. When most of the small bowel is involved but not frankly infarcted, a thrombectomy should be attempted. If thrombosis of the SMV and/or portal vein is identified, the SMV is dissected out just below the pancreas and proximal and distal control obtained. Through a transverse venotomy in the SMV, a Fogarty catheter is passed up to the liver and clot from the portal vein removed. Clot from the intestinal side of the venotomy is removed by massaging the intestines and mesentery and by passage of a small Fogarty catheter. Good blood flow must be obtained from both the portal and peripheral ends of the venotomy. The venotomy is closed with simple interrupted sutures without a patch graft (21). AMVT is the one condition for which anticoagulants are used routinely postoperatively to prevent the recurrent venous thromboses which are frequent.

PROGNOSIS AND COMPLICATIONS

Although mortalities from AMI of 70 to 90 percent have been reported through 1980 using traditional methods of diagnosis and therapy, the aggressive approach described above can reduce these catastrophic figures (22). Of the first 50 patients managed

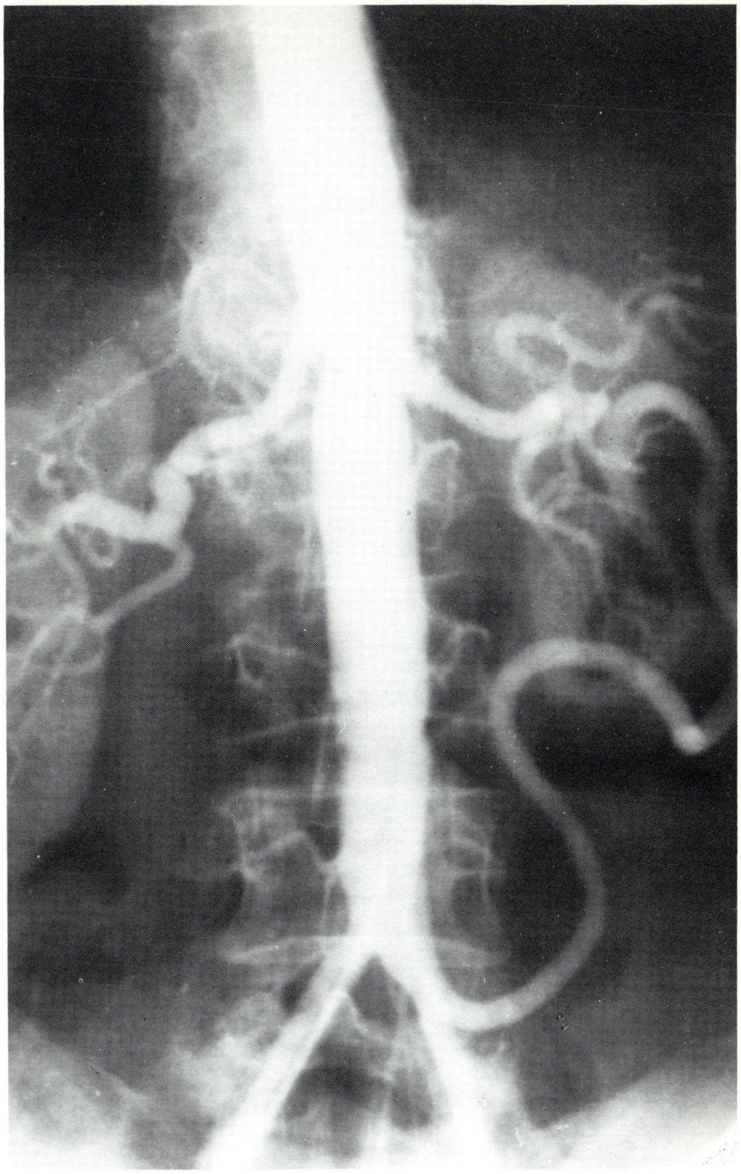

FIGURE 54-6. Angiogram from patient with superior mesenteric artery occlusion. The prominent "meandering artery" shows that collateral channels have been present for some time and the occlusion is not acute. [From Boley, Brandt, and Veith in MM Ravitch (ed): *Current Problems in Surgery,* 1978, by permission of Yearbook Medical Publishers.]

by this approach, 35 (70 percent) proved to have AMI. Of these, 33 had angiographic signs of ischemia. The remaining two patients had normal angiograms. Nineteen (54 percent) of the patients with AMI survived, including 9 of 15 patients with NOMI, 7 of 16 patients with SMAE, 2 of 3 patients with SMAT, and 1 patient with AMVT. Seventeen of the 19 survivors lost no bowel or less than 3 feet of small intestine.

In a more recent review of 47 patients with intestinal ischemia resulting from SMA emboli (23), a survival rate of 55 percent was achieved in patients managed according to our aggressive protocol, whereas only 20 percent of those treated by traditional methods survived. Intraarterial papaverine as the primary treatment was successful in four patients; two were not operated upon, and the other two had normal intestine at the time of delayed laparotomy.

The complications from angiographic studies and prolonged infusions of vasodilator drugs have not been excessive. Three of our first 50 patients developed transient acute tubular necrosis following angiography and treatment of their mesenteric ischemia. One patient developed arterial occlusions in both lower extremities during a papaverine infusion for an SMAE. These probably represented other emboli from his primary source of embolization, but the SMA catheter could not be excluded as a factor. There were several local hematomas at arterial puncture sites, but no major problems were encountered with blood flow to the lower extremities.

Problems with prolonged papaverine infusions have been minimal. Infusions for more than 5 days have been used without significant systemic effects. Fibrin clots on the arterial catheter have been observed commonly but have not caused any difficulty. Three catheters clotted and had to be removed, but this complication can be avoided if a continuous infusion pump is used. Catheter dislodgment occurred several times requiring replacement.

Ninety percent of patients with AMI who had angiography but no physical signs of peritonitis have survived, demonstrating the potential value of early diagnosis. Ideally all patients with AMI should be studied before physical signs develop, and when the plain films of the abdomen are normal.

KEY POINTS IN TREATMENT

1. Always obtain an angiogram, even when laparotomy is already scheduled, and leave the catheter in place. This establishes the diagnosis of AMI and its cause and provides a "road map" for revascularization. The catheter provides access for intraarterial infusion of vasodilators.

2. Always revascularize when there is occlusion of the SMA above the origin of the ileocolic artery unless all of the small bowel is necrotic. This rule applies even if all the bowel appears viable at laparotomy.

3. Postoperative infusions of papaverine should be employed following revascularization procedures and for NOMI when laparotomy is performed for resection of infarcted intestine.

4. When short segments of bowel are of questionable viability after revascularization or with NOMI, resection is advisable; but when a major portion of the small bowel is involved, a second look is preferable. Every attempt to prevent a "short bowel" syndrome is worthwhile.

Colonic Ischemia

Colonic ischemia (CI) is rarely an indication for a vascular surgical procedure, but not infrequently it is a problem during and after aortic operations. However, while ischemia of the colon is probably the most common vascular disorder of the intestines, only a small fraction of cases result from vascular operations.

CI results from many causes: iatrogenic or noniatrogenic, occlusive or nonocclusive, and systemic or local. Although a cause of the CI, or a site of occlusion, is sometimes recognized, in the majority of cases no specific etiology or occlusion is identified. The great frequency of colonic ischemic lesions in older age groups suggest a relationship to degenerative changes in the vascular tree, but angiography in these disorders only rarely demonstrates a significant occlusion or abnormality.

Prior to the late 1950s most reports of intestinal vascular disease were related to catastrophic mesenteric vascular accidents involving the small and, only rarely, the large intestine. In the 1950s the increasing number of operations for aortic aneurysms and the introduction of ligation of the inferior mesenteric artery (IMA) during resections of colonic carcinomas resulted in numerous instances of large bowel ischemia, resulting in gangrene, stricture, and colitis (24,25). Experimental and clinical studies during the last 20 years have led to the recognition of both the full gamut of pathologic changes produced by intestinal ischemia and the protean clinical manifestations with which it may present. In 1963, based upon a series of laboratory and clinical investigations, Boley, Schwartz, and coworkers first identified the spontaneous and reversible nature of some episodes of CI and described the radiological criteria for their early diagnosis (26,27). The ability to diagnose CI in its early stages enabled those investigators to observe the natural history and late results of acute ischemic insults and led to their emphasis of the vascular origin of segmental colitis in the aged, of nonspecific colonic ulcers, and of colonic strictures (26–28).

Many names have been applied to the various clinical forms of CI, but an appropriate overall designation is *colonic ischemia*, which can be applied to both reversible and irreversible lesions. Terms such as "ischemic colitis" (29) and "colonic infarction" are not entirely suitable, for the milder reversible ischemic episodes are not inflammatory but hemorrhagic, and coagulation necrosis (infarction by definition) is often absent.

PATHOPHYSIOLOGY

Regardless of its cause, bowel ischemia produces a single spectrum of pathologic, clinical, and radiologic manifestations. The pathologic changes evoked by ischemia range from simple submucosal edema to infarction and necrosis. Between these extremes are gradations of tissue damage which form the basis for the diverse clinical courses that individual episodes of CI may take (Figure 54-7). Varying with the severity of the episode, mild ischemia produces morphologic changes which regress and ultimately disappear or heal, a sequence of events reflected clinically and radiologically by transient or reversible colonic findings. More severe ischemia may result in irreparable damage, with gangrene, perforation, or persistent colitis; if healing occurs, it does so with scarring, fibrosis, and resultant stricture.

The ultimate outcome of an episode of CI depends on many factors. Among these are

1. The cause, i.e., occlusion or low flow
2. The level of the occlusion
3. The duration and degree of the ischemia
4. The rapidity of onset of the ischemic process
5. The adequacy of the collateral circulation
6. The state of the general circulation
7. The metabolic requirements of the affected bowel
8. The presence of bacteria within the lumen
9. The presence of associated conditions, such as colonic distension

While the end results of the interaction of all these factors are obviously multifold, the initial response to ischemia may be the same regardless of its severity. *It is, therefore, impossible to predict the progression of the ischemic process from the initial physical, radiologic, or sigmoidoscopic evaluation.*

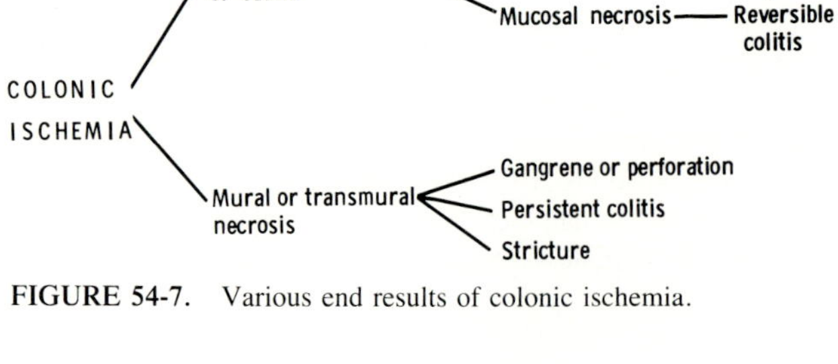

FIGURE 54-7. Various end results of colonic ischemia.

CLINICAL PRESENTATION

Most episodes of CI produce clinical, radiologic, and pathologic changes which are completely reversible. Recognition of the nature and reversibility of these lesions will prevent unnecessary operations and the use of improper medical therapy which may aggravate an otherwise self-limited condition. Irreversible damage resulting in gangrene, perforation, stricture, or chronic colitis may have the same clinical onset as reversible episodes, but the greater severity of the lesion soon becomes apparent.

Typically, CI presents with sudden onset of mild lower abdominal pain, usually crampy in nature and localized to the left side. The pain is frequently accompanied by tenesmus and is followed within 24 hours by passage of dark or bright red blood per rectum or by bloody diarrhea. Less commonly, the pain can be severe, especially with irreversible lesions, while in other patients it may be minimal or absent. Characteristically, the blood loss is minimal. Although massive bleeding has resulted from CI, its presence militates against this diagnosis.

Initially, the only physical finding is abdominal tenderness over the area of the involved colon, most commonly on the left side. Signs of peritoneal irritation have been noted with ultimately reversible lesions, but if these persist for more than a few hours, they should be considered evidence of irreparable tissue damage. Fever and leukocytosis are usually present and, together with the physical findings, are parameters to be followed in assessing the progress of ischemic lesions. Early and serial barium enema studies are the keys to diagnosing CI, but colonoscopy is being employed with increasing frequency. When colonoscopy is used, extreme care is necessary because high intraluminal pressures may lead to further ischemia or perforation of the already damaged colon.

COLONIC ISCHEMIA COMPLICATING ABDOMINAL AORTIC RECONSTRUCTION

The occurrence of postoperative CI was recognized early in the history of abdominal aortic surgery. This sometimes fatal complication has been reported to occur in 1 to 10 percent of patients undergoing aortoiliac reconstruction. One to 2 percent of patients have had clinically evident CI, while a greater incidence has been noted when routine colonoscopy was performed. Although the incidence of postoperative CI appears low, it is responsible for up to 10 percent of the deaths following aortic surgery. Factors found to contribute to the occurrence of postoperative ischemia include (30)

1. Ruptured aneurysm
2. Episodes of hypotension
3. Operative trauma to the colon
4. Hypoxemia
5. Arrhythmias (supraventricular and ventricular)
6. Prolonged cross-clamp time
7. Improper management of the IMA

The most important aspect of management of CI following aortic surgery is its prevention. Collateral blood flow to the left colon after occlusion of the IMA comes from the SMA via the arc of Riolan (''meandering artery'') (Figure 54-6) or the marginal artery of Drummond, and from the internal iliac (hypogastric) arteries via the middle and inferior hemorrhoidal arteries (31). If the surgeon assures that these collateral pathways are intact, postoperative colonic ischemia can be minimized.

Aortography and full mechanical and antibiotic bowel prep are preoperative measures to prevent CI. While antibiotic therapy will not prevent colonic infarction, multiple studies have shown that it can ameliorate the effects of CI and reduce the length of bowel damage. Aortography is essential to determine patency of the celiac axis, SMA, IMA, and internal iliac artery, and to idenfity collateral circulation when it exists. Visualization of a meandering artery has been stated by some authors to be an indication that reimplantation of the IMA is not necessary. However, this collateral vessel can be enlarged because of obstruction of either the IMA or the SMA, and in our experience more often results from collateral blood flow *from the IMA to the SMA*. Hence, the presence of a meandering artery suggests that ligation of the IMA is safe only when the direction of flow is from the SMA to the IMA. Its presence is an absolute indication for both reimplantation of the IMA and revascularization of the SMA when the IMA is the source of inflow, that is, when the SMA is either tightly stenosed or occluded.

If preoperative angiograms show occlusion of both hypogastric arteries, the rectum is usually dependent on collateral blood flow from the IMA or from the SMA via a meandering artery. In such patients, reconstitution of flow to one or both hypogastric arteries is desirable.

At operation cross-clamp time should be kept to a minimum, and episodes of hypotension should be avoided. If a meandering artery is present, it is carefully preserved. The appearance of the colon after occlusion of the IMA is not a reliable indicator of collateral blood flow, and various methods have been suggested to determine the need for reimplantation of the IMA. Ernst et al. measured the IMA stump pressure after transection (32). They found that a pressure greater than 40 mmHg or an IMA/systemic pressure ratio greater than 0.40 was an accurate indication of adequate collateral circulation and obviated the need for reimplantation. Hobson et al. found that Doppler ultrasound flow signals present at the base of the mesentery and at the serosal surface of the colon during temporary IMA occlusion were reliable in assessing the need for IMA reimplantation (33).

When IMA reimplantation is deemed necessary, the IMA should be excised with a patch of aortic wall and sutured into the side of the graft. Revascularization of the SMA, in addition to reimplantation of the IMA, should be performed whenever the SMA is occluded. This can best be accomplished by a jump graft from the aortic graft to the side of the SMA.

Prediction of the development of ischemic changes in the colon following aortic reconstruction can be difficult because of diverse factors which may influence their occurrence. The difficulty in accurately assessing this danger and the significant mortality associated with it have prompted the recommendation of postoperative colonoscopy in those patients considered at high risk. Such patients include those with

1. Ruptured abdominal aortic aneurysms
2. Prolonged cross-clamp time or hypotension
3. A preoperative angiogram demonstrating a patent IMA
4. Failure to reestablish hypogastric artery pulses at operation
5. Diarrhea after operation

Colonoscopy carefully performed 2 or 3 days after operation should identify CI early enough to permit treatment before major complications develop (34).

TREATMENT

Proper treatment of ischemic lesions of the colon is based upon early diagnosis of ischemic damage, continued monitoring of the patient, and the radiologic or endoscopic appearance of the colon. If a presumptive diagnosis of CI is made, and the physical findings do not suggest intestinal gangrene or perforation, the patient is observed for fever, a rising white blood cell count, or changes in abdominal signs. Systemic antibiotics are administered and blood and fluids replaced when indicated. In the early stages of the disease it is best to place the bowel at rest and provide fluids intravenously. If the colon appears distended, it is decompressed with a rectal tube and careful saline irrigations, since increased intraluminal pressure may further compromise the intestinal blood supply. Contrary to their efficacy in ulcerative colitis, systemic corticosteroids are not only of no value but also are contraindicated since they increase the possibility of intestinal perforation and secondary infection.

Serial barium studies or endoscopy of the colon are an essential part of the therapy since they definitely establish the diagnosis of ischemia and will either verify the reversibility of the colonic damage or demonstrate progression to an ischemic colitis or stricture.

If deterioration in the clinical course is suggested by increasing abdominal signs, fever, and leukocytosis, or if the diarrhea, bleeding, or both persist for more than 2 weeks, irreversible damage almost certainly has occurred and surgical intervention is indicated. Reversible lesions should improve within 7 to 10 days, and continued symptoms beyond this period warrant a change from a very conservative therapeutic approach to a very aggressive one. In our experience, such patients with persistence of diarrhea and bleeding have often gone on to perforation and peritonitis.

An asymptomatic patient with a stricture should be observed, because strictures may improve spontaneously after several months. When symptoms of obstruction are present, however, surgical intervention is necessary.

The operative treatment of irreversible ischemic lesions of the colon is local resection of only the involved area with restitution of intestinal continuity by primary anastomosis. The specimen should be opened immediately by the surgeon or by the pathologist to be certain that all of the involved colon has been removed. Bowel with mucosal damage should be excised even though it may have a normal external appearance, since anastomoses through it may leak. Moreover, if such ischemic colon is retained, it may go on to stricture.

Thus, the treatment of CI consists of early identification and continued surveillance, an ultraconservative approach were reversibility is probable, and a very aggressive surgical approach where permanent ischemic damage has probably occurred.

References

1. Ottinger LW, Austen WG: A study of 136 patients with mesenteric infarction. Surg Gynecol Obstet 124:251, 1967.
2. Vellar ID, Doyle JC: Acute mesenteric ischemia. Aust NZ J Surg 47:54, 1977.
3. Hibbard JS, Swenson JC, Levin AG: Roentgenology of experimental mesenteric vascular occlusion. Arch Surg 26:20, 1933.
4. Blinov NI, Shaak TV: Ob embolii aorte na meste ee bifurkastii i embolektomii verhnei brejiichnoi arterii. Vestn Khir Grekov 70:59, 1950.
5. Klass AA: Embolectomy in acute mesenteric occlusion. Ann Surg 134:913, 1951.
6. Stewart GD, Sweetman WR, Westphal K, Wise RA: Superior mesenteric artery embolectomy. Ann Surg 151:274, 1960.
7. Ende N: Infarction of the bowel in cardiac failure. N Engl J Med 258:879, 1958.
8. Boley SJ, Treiber W, Winslow PR, Gliedman ML, Veith FJ: Circulatory response to acute reduction of superior mesenteric arterial blood flow. Physiologist 12:180, 1969.
9. Everhard ME, Regan JA, Veith FJ, Boley SJ: Mesenteric vasomotor response to reduced mesenteric blood flow. Physiologist 13:191, 1970.
10. Boley SJ, Regan JA, Tunick PA, Everhard ME, Winslow PR, Veith FJ: Persistent vasoconstriction—A major factor in non-occlusive mesenteric ischemia. Curr Top Surg Res 3:425, 1971.
11. Hollenberg NK, Epstein M, Rosen SM, Basch RI, Oken DE: Acute oliguric renal failure in man: Evidence of preferential renal cortical ischemia. Medicine 47:455, 1968.
12. Schimmel DH, Moss AA, Hoffer PB: Radionuclide imaging of intestinal infarction in dogs. Invest Radiol 11:277, 1976.
13. Ortiz VN, Sfakianakis G, Haase GM, Boles ET: The value of radionuclide scanning in early diagnosis of intestinal infarction. J Pediatr Surg 13:616, 1978.
14. Bardfeld PA, Boley SJ, Sammartano RJ, Bontemps R: Scintigraphic diagnosis of ischemic intestine with technetium 99m sulfur colloid labelled leukocytes. Radiology 124:2, 1977.
15. Kleinhaus S, Sammartano RJ, Boley SJ: Variations in blood flow during laparoscopy. Physiologist 19:255, 1976.
16. Siegelman SS, Sprayregen S, Boley SJ: Angiographic diagnosis of mesenteric arterial vasoconstriction. Radiology 122:533, 1974.
17. Shaw RS: The "second look" after superior mesenteric arterial embolectomy or reconstruction for mesenteric infraction. In Ellison EH, Friesen SR, Mulholland JH (eds): *Current Surgical Management*. Philadelphia, W.B. Saunders Co, 1965, p 509.
18. Ottinger LW: The surgical management of acute occlusion of the superior mesenteric artery. Ann Surg 188:721, 1978.
19. Jackson BB: Occlusion of the superior mesenteric artery. Monograph in *American Lectures in Surgery*. Springfield, Illinois, Charles C Thomas, Publisher, 1963.
20. Cokkinis AJ: *Mesenteric Vascular Occlusion*. London, Bailliere, Tindall & Cox, 1926.
21. Inhara T: Acute superior mesenteric venous thrombosis: Treatment by thrombectomy. Ann Surg 174:956, 1971.
22. Boley SJ, Sprayregen S, Siegelman SS, Veith FJ: Initial results from an aggressive roentgenological and surgical approach to acute mesenteric ischemia. Surgery 82:848, 1977.
23. Boley SJ, Feinstein FR, Sammartano RJ, Brandt L: New concepts of management of superior mesenteric artery emboli. Surg Gynecol Obstet 153:4, 1981.
24. Moore SW: Resection of the abdominal aorta with defect replaced by homologous graft. Surg Gynecol Obstet 99:745, 1954.
25. Young JR, Humphries AW, DeWolfe VG, LeFevre FA: Complications of abdominal aortic surgery. Arch Surg 86:51, 1963.
26. Boley SJ, Schwartz S, Lash J, Sternhill V: Reversible vascular occlusion of the colon. Surg Gynecol Obstet 116:53, 1963.

27. Schwartz S, Boley SJ, Lash J, Sternhill V: Roentgenologic aspects of reversible vascular occlusion of the colon and its relationship to ulcerative colitis. Radiology 80:625, 1963.
28. Boley SJ, Schwartz S, Krieger H, Schultz L, Siew FP, Allen AC: Further observations on reversible vascular occlusion of the colon. Am J Gastroenterol 44:260, 1965.
29. Marston A, Pheils M, Thomas MC, Morson BC: Ischaemic colitis. Gut 7:1, 1966.
30. Kim MW, Hundahl SA, Dang CR, McNamara JJ, Straehley CJ: Ischemic colitis after aortic aneurysmectomy. Am J Surg 145:392, 1983.
31. Michels NA, Siddharth P, Kornblith PL, Parke WW: The variant blood supply to the descending colon, rectosigmoid and rectum based on 400 dissections. Its importance in regional resections: A review of medical literature. Dis Colon Rectum 8:251, 1965.
32. Ernst CB, Hagihara DF, Daugherty ME, Griffen WO: Inferior mesenteric artery stump pressure: A reliable index for safe IMA ligation during abdominal aortic aneurysmectomy. Ann Surg 187:641, 1978.
33. Hobson RW, Wright CB, Rich NM, Collins GJ: Assessment of colonic ischemia during aortic surgery by Doppler ultrasound. J Surg Res 20:231, 1976.
34. Ernst CB, Hagihara PF, Daugherty ME, Sachatello CR, Griffen WO: Ischemic colitis incidence following abdominal aortic reconstruction: A prospective study. Surgery 80:417, 1976.

Chapter 55

CHRONIC MESENTERIC ISCHEMIA AND SURGERY FOR CHRONIC VISCERAL ISCHEMIA

RONALD J. STONEY, LINDA M. REILLY, and WILLIAM K. EHRENFELD

The reduction of visceral blood flow by one of several pathologic processes may produce the clinical syndrome of chronic intestinal ischemia. Although the pathologic lesion was described over a century ago (1), a clinical correlation was first established by Dunphy in 1936 (2). Twenty years later Mikkelsen coined the term *intestinal angina* and suggested that a surgical approach to the chronically occluded vessels was feasible (3). Within a year the first successful operation for visceral occlusive disease was performed (4). The causative lesions may be atherosclerotic, extrinsic, inflammatory, dysplastic, or congenital in nature. Of these the most common cause is atherosclerosis.

Anatomic Considerations

Normally the blood supply to the gastrointestinal tract is provided by three aortic branches—the celiac axis, the superior mesenteric artery (SMA), and the inferior mesenteric artery (IMA). In the physiologic state, 90 percent of the splanchnic blood flow is provided by the celiac axis and the SMA. There is potential for extensive collateralization of these vessels, involving any or all of the three systems (Figure 55-1). Terminal branches of the gastroduodenal and superior pancreaticoduodenal arteries anastomose with similar branches of the inferior pancreaticoduodenal artery to provide the collateral pathway between the celiac axis and SMA. Similarly the superior mesenteric–inferior mesenteric collateral flow is carried by terminal branch connections of the middle colic artery and left colic artery, respectively. Finally, the IMA collateral flow from the iliac system (via the hypogastric arteries) is provided by the sigmoidohemorrhoidal anastomoses.

The celiac axis and SMA arise from the ventral surface of the midabdominal aorta and may be compromised by atherosclerotic disease of the aortic wall or of the vessel origin. Typically these orifice lesions do not extend more than about 2 cm into the visceral vessel. This sparing of major branches allows the development of extensive collateral blood flow, using the previously described normal anastomotic pathways. Infrarenal aortic atherosclerotic disease is very common, frequently occludes the IMA origin, and also compromises iliac flow. The multiple vessels supplying the gastrointestinal tract and the many collateral pathways imply that visceral vessel occlusive disease should be extensive before symptoms will result.

Clinical Presentation

The diagnosis of abdominal pain caused by mesenteric ischemia is difficult because the clinical presentation and physical findings are nonspecific. Classically, the affected patient presents with a history of postprandial, crampy, midabdominal or epigastric pain. There is a 3:1 female predominance, and the patient is usually between 50 and 60 years old. Although abdominal pain is universally present in visceral ischemia, 10 percent or more of patients will not demonstrate the described classic pattern (5,6). As the pain episodes increase in frequency and severity, the patient develops a food aversion resulting in weight loss, the most common physical finding. Although a substantial number of patients will complain of gastrointestinal motility disturbances (nausea, vomiting, episodic diarrhea, or constipation), documented malabsorption is rare.

Physical findings are rarely diagnostic. Seventy-five percent of patients have a midabdominal or epigastric bruit, and approximately one-third of patients have findings suggesting atherosclerotic peripheral vascular disease. Abdominal examination is usually quite unremarkable, even during episodes of pain. Laboratory studies are nonspecific, though occasionally there is occult blood in the stool.

This vague presentation and insidious progression of symptoms often mimic visceral malignancy or are mistaken for functional bowel disease. If a thorough evaluation of weight loss and

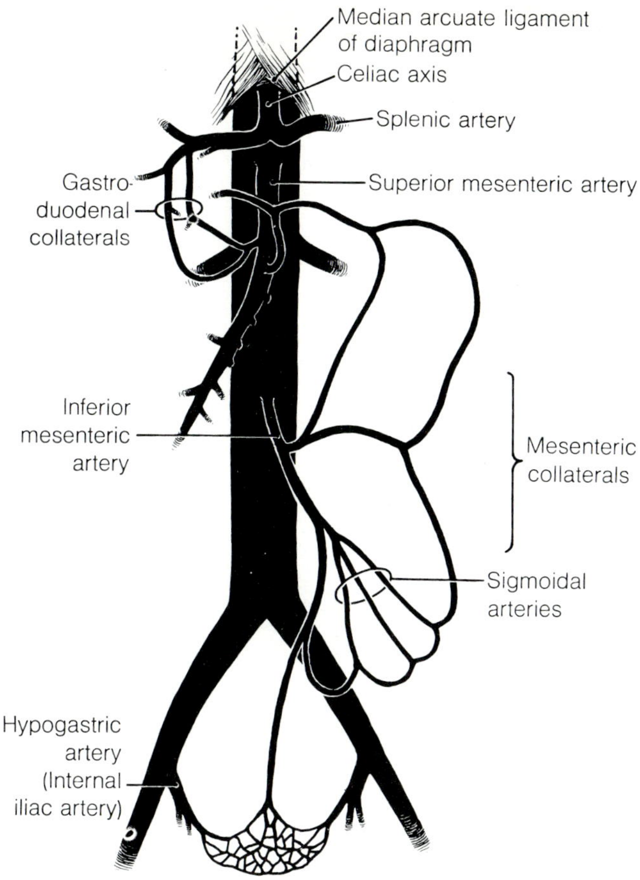

FIGURE 55-1. Intestinal vascular supply with collateral pathways.

abdominal pain has failed to provide an etiology, intestinal ischemia should be strongly considered. Abdominal aortography is required to confirm the diagnosis. Other procedures such as contrast gastrointestinal studies, endoscopy, and computerized tomography (CT) scanning serve to exclude other intraabdominal pathology. Since the origins of the celiac axis and SMA overlie the aorta in the anteroposterior (AP) plane, lateral projections are necessary to visualize these orifices in profile (Figure 55-2). The AP projection may demonstrate large collaterals developing between anastomotic beds or occasionally may be remarkable for the absence of any significant aortic visceral branches (Figure 55-3). The IMA orifice is usually best seen on an oblique projection (Figure 55-4).

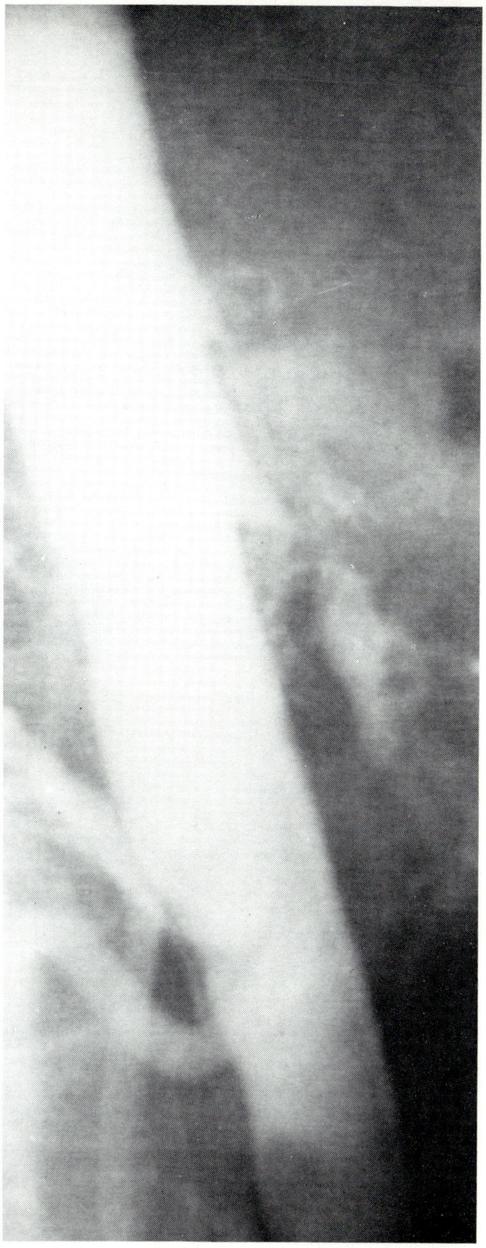

FIGURE 55-2. Lateral aortogram showing occlusion of the celiac artery and stenosis of the superior mesenteric arteries.

Pathophysiology

The pathophysiology of the postprandial pain of mesenteric vascular origin is poorly understood. Experimental evidence does suggest that mesenteric blood flow increases following food ingestion. However, intestinal motor activity probably has a greater influence on mesenteric blood flow. During peristalsis resistance changes in the intramural vessel segments lead to decreased arterial inflow and increased venous outflow. In a patient with impaired splanchnic circulation, this balance of increased flow and increased resistance after a meal may be disturbed, leading to tissue hypoxia and true visceral pain.

Because the development and capacity of the intestinal collateral circulation are difficult to predict, the exact percentage of patients with atherosclerosis involving the visceral arteries, who will utlimately become symptomatic, is unknown. In general at least two of the three visceral vessels must be significantly diseased for symptoms to develop. Eighty-five percent of symp-

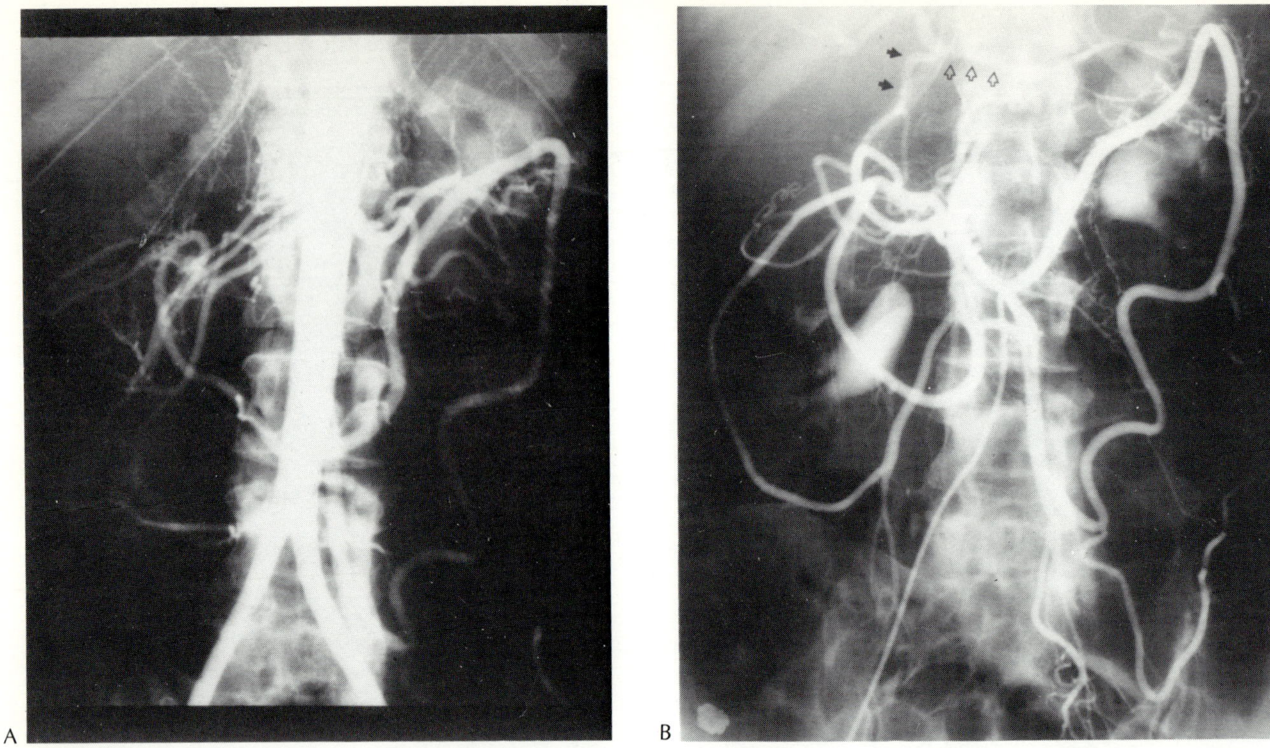

FIGURE 55-3. *(A)* Anterioposterior aortogram showing absence of significant abdominal aortic branches (''pruned'' aorta) and large wandering collateral. *(B)* Selective IMA injection demonstrates extensive collateralization with reconstitution of the celiac branches (*open arrows*) via the gastroduodenal (*solid arrows*).

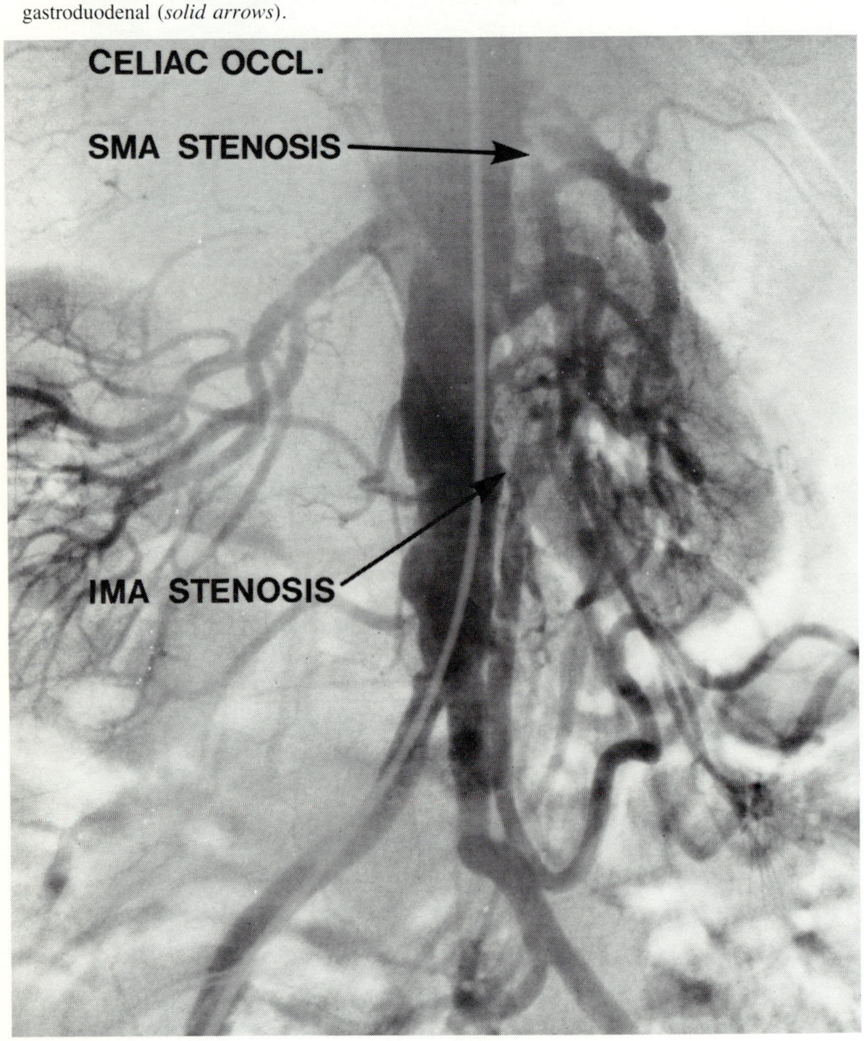

FIGURE 55-4. Oblique projection demonstrating celiac occlusion and stenosis of the superior and inferior mesenteric arteries.

tomatic patients undergoing operation at our hospital (63 of 75) had angiographically demonstrated critical stenosis or occlusion of both the celiac axis and SMA. Although it is rare for single-vessel disease to produce symptoms (5–8), eight patients were symptomatic with only celiac axis disease and two patients had only critical SMA disease.

Surgical Revascularization

Although many techniques for visceral revascularization have been described, there are three basic procedures: reimplantation, bypass, and endarterectomy. To alleviate ischemic symptoms and prevent bowel infarction, revascularization of both the celiac axis and the SMA is preferred, since these two branches supply most of the splanchnic flow under normal conditions. In addition long-term symptom palliation has been correlated with the completeness of the revascularization (5). If the operative repair must be limited, celiac reconstruction is performed. The justification for this choice is provided by two observations. First, isolated celiac disease is a more common cause of symptoms than isolated SMA disease. Second, when a major visceral branch reconstruction (celiac or SMA) failed postoperatively, only those patients with celiac reocclusion experienced recurrent symptoms.

REIMPLANTATION

Revascularization of the major visceral branches can be performed by transecting the artery distal to the orifice lesion and reimplanting the normal vessel into an adjacent segment of aorta or graft. There are two inherent difficulties with this approach. First, the location and short length of the celiac trunk, and its proximity to the SMA, make its reimplantation technically difficult. Second, the presence of atheroma on the ventral surface of the aorta makes anastomosis of either the celiac or SMA difficult and allows for later restenosis or occlusion secondary to disease progression in the aortic wall. Therefore reimplantation as the definitive procedure for visceral occlusive disease is rarely performed. Occasionally, following aortic replacement with prosthetic graft, visceral reimplantation will be performed to an adjacent graft segment.

BYPASS

Occlusive visceral lesions may be bypassed using autogenous tissue or a prosthetic graft, and the bypass may be constructed for antegrade flow or retrograde flow.

Retrograde Bypass

The standard aortomesenteric bypass, as originally designed, runs cephalad from the ventral surface of the infrarenal aorta to the side of the SMA distal to the diseased area. Because the SMA is mobile, it is difficult to ensure that a graft in this position will not be redundant or kink as a result of movement of the mesentery. Additionally the site of origin on the infrarenal aorta may be involved with atherosclerosis or become so at a later date, contributing to late graft failure. Finally, retrograde flow seems to be associated with a greater degree of turbulence, an additional factor which may play a role in late graft occlusion. Several large series have reported a significant incidence of symptom recurrence and late graft occlusion (6,8–11) which may have resulted in part from these technical disadvantages of the retrograde bypass. For these reasons we now place all grafts to allow antegrade flow.

Autogenous Antegrade Bypass

VENOUS Six antegrade autogenous vein grafts have been used to revascularize the celiac axis or SMA, and five have failed within 2 years (Table 55-1). Three were successfully converted to prosthetic grafts with resultant relief of symptoms. Fibrosis and stricture, not progressive or recurrent atherosclerosis, was the cause of occlusion and recurrent symptoms in these patients. Because of this experience and other reports of aneurysmal degeneration and late occlusion of aortorenal vein bypass grafts, we have abandoned the use of vein conduits for visceral reconstruction. However, occasionally a vein patch is used to close an SMA arteriotomy in order to prevent narrowing.

ARTERIAL Arterial autografts are reliable conduits in many other settings, but their use for visceral reconstruction poses two problems. First, the hypogastric artery, the most frequently harvested donor vessel, is an important collateral pathway for intestinal perfusion. Therefore, it may not be possible to sacrifice it. Second, since bypass to more than one vessel is frequently required and since antegrade flow is preferred, obtaining an ade-

TABLE 55-1. Operations for Visceral Atherosclerosis, 1959–1982

Procedure	Patients	Arteries Repaired	Late Occlusions*
Transaortic endarterectomy	41	72	3
Antegrade prosthetic bypass	18	28	1
Transarterial endarterectomy	7	9	2
Vein bypass	5	6	5
Arterial autograft bypass	2	2	1
Reimplantation	2	3	0
Total	75	120	12

*All occurred more than 1 year postoperatively.

quate length of arterial autograft for reconstruction poses a difficult problem. These relative contraindications make arterial autografts an undesirable choice for visceral vessel disease.

Prosthetic Antegrade Bypass

Antegrade prosthetic visceral bypass involves grafting from the undiseased, supraceliac aorta to the divided visceral branch, distal to the area of disease. Knitted Dacron prostheses, 5 or 6 mm, are preferred for single-vessel bypass. Bifurcated grafts (10 × 5 or 12 × 6) are used when both the celiac axis and SMA are revascularized. Initial concern about possible visceral erosion by these grafts has resolved since no such complication has occurred in the 18 patients (28 vessels) treated with this procedure and followed from 1 to 4 years.

The operative approach to the supraceliac aorta and celiac axis is through the gastrohepatic ligament. The left lobe of the liver is retracted to the right and the esophagus mobilized to the left to expose the crura of the diaphragm. Separation of these fibers provides exposure of the distal thoracic aorta (Figure 55-5). Dissection continues caudally with division of the median arcuate ligament and the celiac ganglia to expose the celiac axis out to and including the trifurcation. Further dissection of the anterior surface of the aorta below the celiac axis, with elevation and caudad reflection of the body of the pancreas, allows access to the proximal SMA (Figure 55-6).

The supraceliac aorta is temporarily occluded below the diaphram and above the celiac origin. If a single bypass to the celiac or SMA is planned, an elliptical segment is excised from the midventral aortic wall (Figure 55-7). If a bypass to both vessels is planned, the aortotomy is placed at an oblique angle on the right anterolateral aspect of the aorta to allow proper alignment of the graft limbs (Figure 55-8). A preclotted, knitted, flanged tubular graft (single bypass) or bifurcation graft (double bypass) is anastomosed to the aorta using a 4-0 Dacron suture. The graft is then clamped and aortic flow is restored. The mean aortic occlusion time is 24 minutes (range, 16 to 45 minutes). The vessel to be bypassed is then clamped and transected, and the proximal end is oversewn. An end-to-end anastomosis is fashioned between the graft limb and the distal, nondiseased

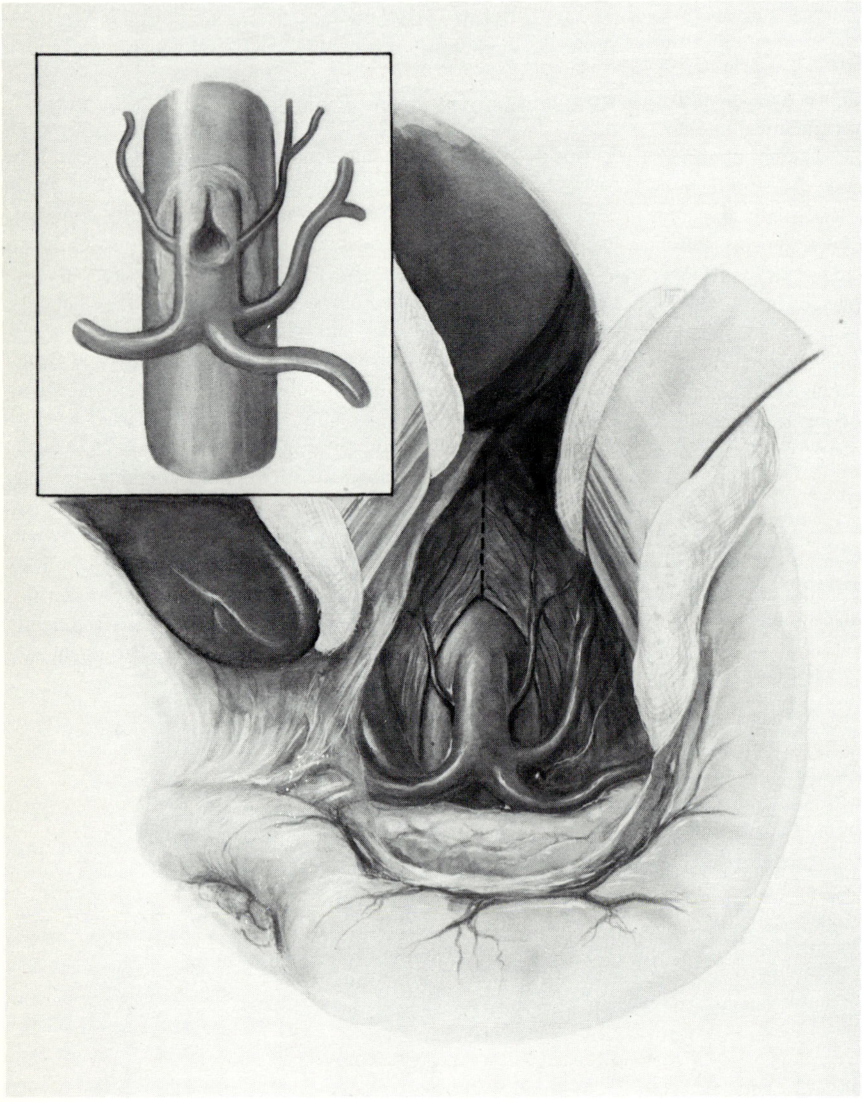

FIGURE 55-5. Transabdominal anterior approach to the supraceliac aorta showing line of division of crural fibers. *Inset:* typical celiac orifice lesion. [Reproduced with permission from Wylie EJ, Stoney RJ, Ehrenfeld WK: Manual of Vascular Surgery Vol. I, New York, Springer-Verlag, 1980, p. 210.]

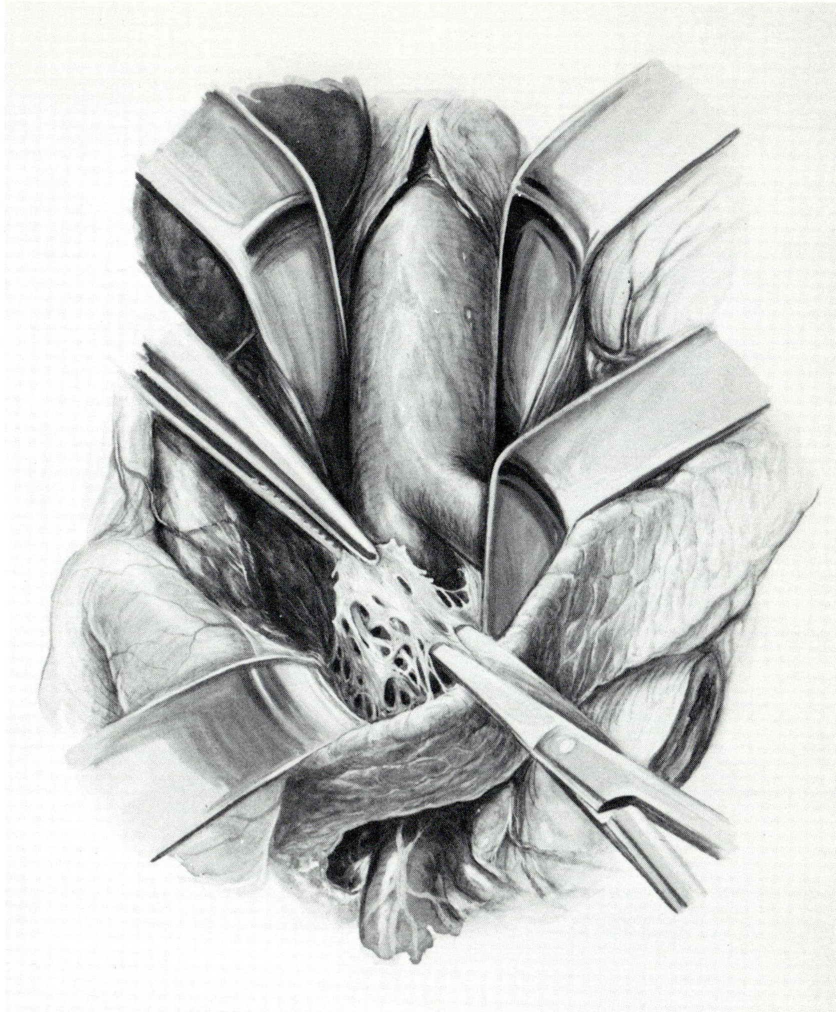

FIGURE 55-6. Mobilization and caudad retraction of body of the pancreas. [Reproduced with permission from Wylie EJ, Stoney RJ, Ehrenfeld WK: Manual of Vascular Surgery Vol. I, New York, Springer-Verlag, 1980, p. 213.]

visceral vessel using 5-0 suture. The right (SMA) limb of the bifurcated graft travels along the right anterolateral aspect of the aorta, behind the pancreas to parallel the course of the SMA and allow proper orientation (Figure 55-9).

Intraoperative assessment of the reconstruction is accomplished using electromagnetic flow probe measurement and recently ultrasound B-mode imaging with Doppler flow velocity measurement. This latter procedure offers promise of accurate assessment of vessel patency and flow while avoiding the complications and difficulties of lateral aortography in a supine patient. Postoperative assessment is routinely obtained prior to discharge using conventional or arterial digital aortography (Figure 55-10).

Antegrade prosthetic visceral bypass is advantageous because of the absence of disease in the parent aorta, the short graft segments involved, the antegrade flow, and the avoidance of mobilization of the diseased infrarenal aorta. The entire procedure is accomplished transabdominally and is well tolerated by patients with significant operative risk, even though temporary supraceliac aortic occlusion is required. Among 18 patients who underwent this procedure, there was one death and one patient with transient renal failure (Table 55-2). Careful intraoperative monitoring of cardiac function, recently using a transesophageal two-dimensional ultrasound probe, and manipulation of preload and afterload (see Chapter 21) have contributed greatly to this improved outcome. Symptom relief was obtained in all 17 pa-

TABLE 55-2. Results of Visceral Reconstruction (Current Procedures)

Procedure	Operations	Morbidity	Mortality	Symptom Relief
Transaortic endarterectomy	41	3	4	37
Antegrade bypass	18	1	1	17
Total	59	4	5	54

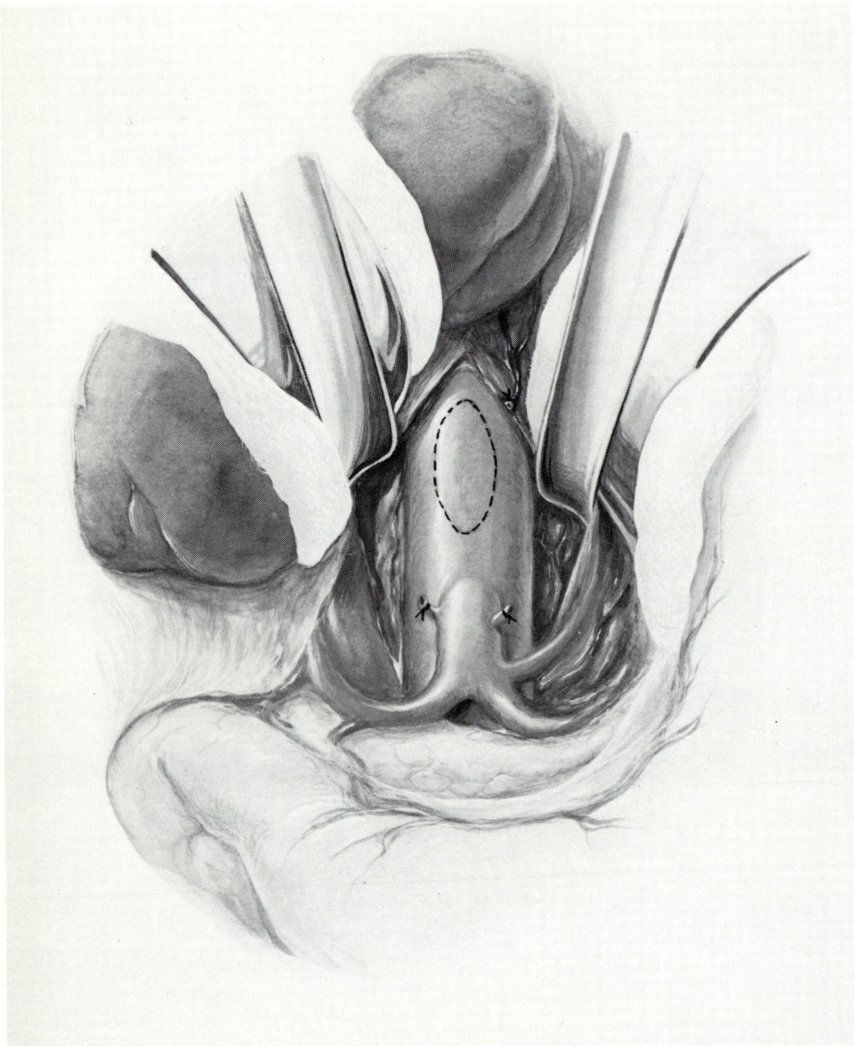

FIGURE 55-7. Position of elliptical aortotomy for antegrade aortoceliac bypass. [Reproduced with permission from Wylie EJ, Stoney RJ, Ehrenfeld WK: Manual of Vascular Surgery Vol. I, New York, Springer-Verlag, 1980, p. 211.]

tients who survived. However, 1 of 28 vessels bypassed demonstrated late occlusion which was clinically silent (Table 55-1).

ENDARTERECTOMY

Shaw and Maynard first used endarterectomy in 1958 to disobliterate the SMA and thus effect the first operative cure of intestinal angina (4). Although this approach is theoretically attractive, there are certain limitations. The difficulties of surgical access initially prompted endarterectomy via the diseased vessel itself (transarterial). However, attempts to remove the diseased aortic intima surrounding the visceral vessel orifice by this route are generally unsuccessful. The frequency of failure of these reconstructions suggests that aortic wall disease progression may be responsible. Additionally, distal embolization from loose, incompletely removed, atheromatous fragments is possible. Transaortic endarterectomy, originally introduced for the treatment of renal disease, has therefore been adopted. However, transabdominal aortic endarterectomy is difficult owing to the vertical orientation of the visceral branches and the position of overlying organs which makes safe exposure a formidable problem. These considerations have led to the development of the thoracoretroperitoneal exposure. This approach affords unrestricted access to the lower thoracic and entire abdominal aorta and all of its branches.

The patient is supine on the operating table, but the left chest is elevated 45°. A posterolateral thoracic incision is made in the eighth interspace and carried across the costal margin to the abdominal midline. The retroperitoneum is bluntly entered and the peritoneum and its contents displaced medially. The diaphragm is divided circumferentially leaving a 2- to 3-cm cuff along the chest wall. The crural fibers overlying the aorta are divided parallel to the aorta, exposing the supraceliac aorta. Further exposure of the aorta is obtained by dividing the celiac ganglia and dissecting away the retroperitoneal tissue to provide access to the midabdominal aorta and the renal and visceral branches. Extension of the abdominal incision in the midline to the pubis allows exposure of the entire abdominal aorta and iliac vessels.

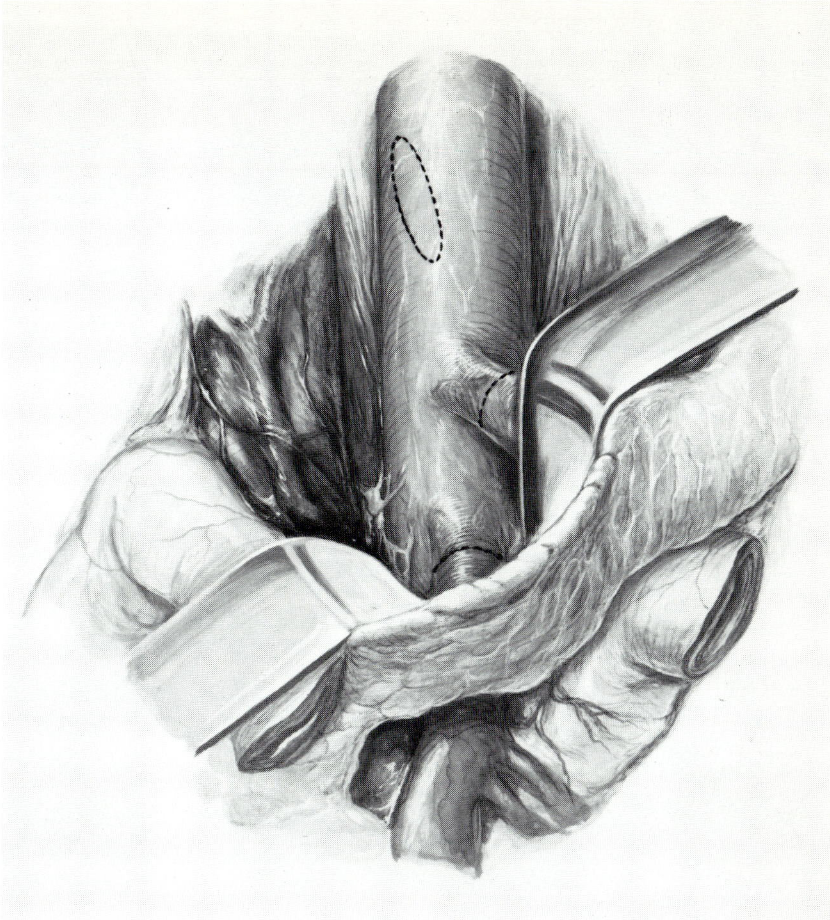

FIGURE 55-8. Position of aortotomy for antegrade bifurcated graft to celiac and SMA. [Reproduced with permission from Wylie EJ, Stoney RJ, Ehrenfeld WK: Manual of Vascular Surgery Vol. I, New York, Springer-Verlag, 1980, p. 213.]

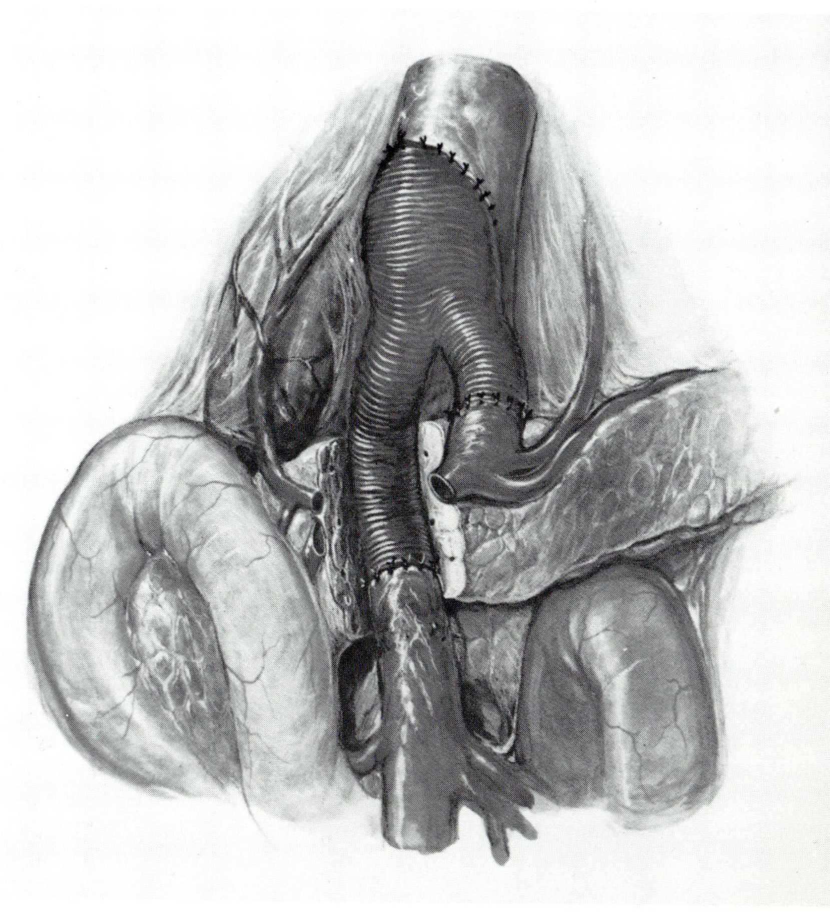

FIGURE 55-9. Final alignment of bifurcated graft (pancreas cutaway to show course of graft limbs). [Reproduced with permission from Wylie EJ, Stoney RJ, Ehrenfeld WK: Manual of Vascular Surgery Vol. I, New York, Springer-Verlag, 1980, p. 214.]

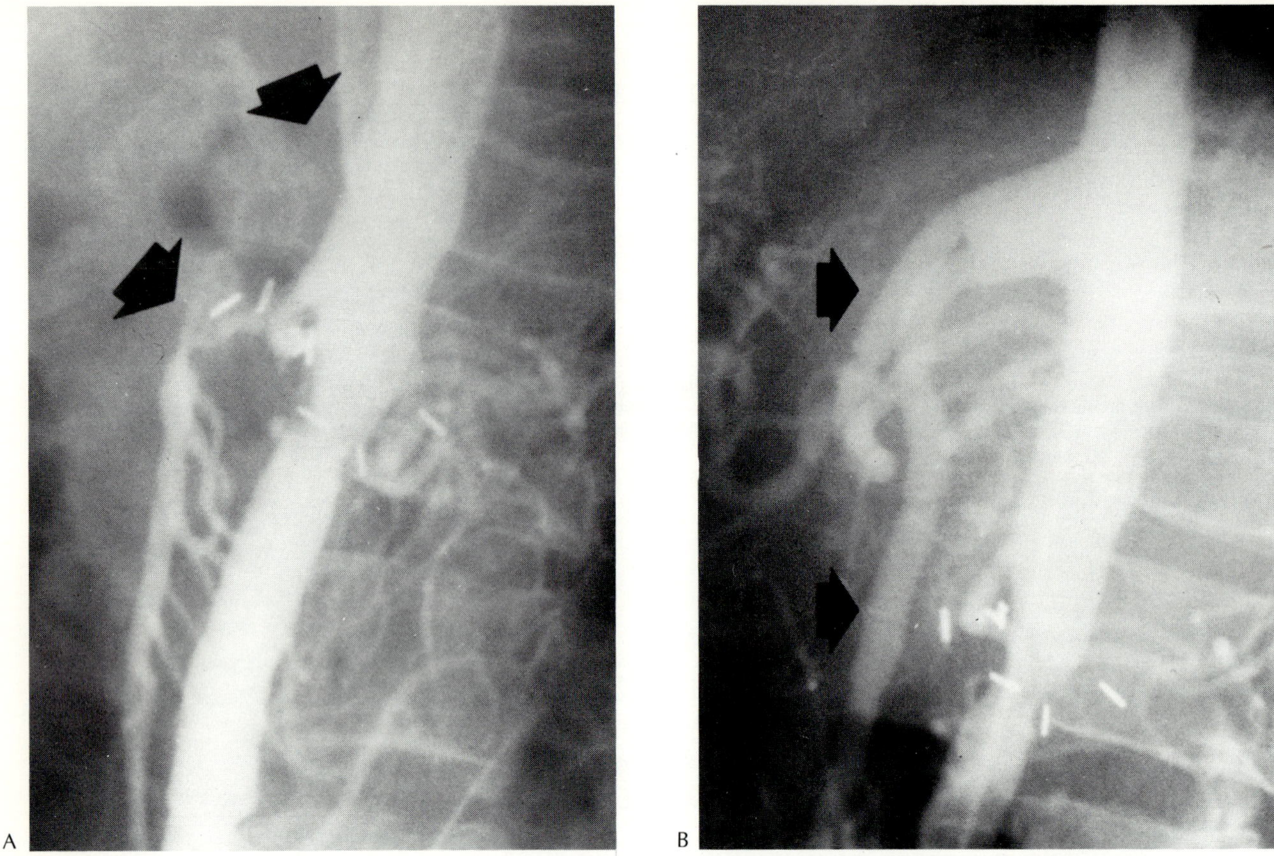

FIGURE 55-10. *(A)* Preoperative study showing celiac occlusion and SMA stenosis. ***(B)*** Postoperative angiogram of antegrade aortoceliac-SMA bypass. [Reproduced with permission from Wylie EJ, Stoney RJ, Ehrenfeld WK: Manual of Vascular Surgery Vol. I, New York, Springer-Verlag, 1980, p. 216.]

Direct transaortic exposure of the celiac and SMA orifices is obtained using a trap-door aortotomy in the anterolateral aortic wall, following control of the aorta and its branch vessels (Figure 55-11). If the atheroma is localized to the ventral aortic wall, a trap-door endarterectomy is performed. If the disease is circumferential, often seen with coexistent renal disease, a sleeve aortic endarterectomy is performed (Figure 55-12). The distal aortic end point is obtained by sharp-beveled dissection. The endarterectomy is extended into the visceral trunks and the atheromatous core extracted. All of the visceral branches, as well as the renal vessels, can be disobliterated in this manner. Following this, the aortotomy is closed using 4-0 suture, and flow is restored to the viscera, kidneys, and lower extremities. If distal aortic disease is present, aortoiliac or aortofemoral reconstruction by endarterectomy or bypass may be performed at this point without further renal or intestinal ischemia. The mean supraceliac aortic occlusion time is 26 minutes (range, 14 to 47).

When SMA occlusion rather than stenosis is present, thrombus usually propagates to the first branch orifice. To remove this completely and provide a clean end point, a separate longitudinal SMA arteriotomy is required. Following completion of the thromboendarterectomy this incision is closed with a saphenous vein patch to prevent narrowing of the SMA trunk (Figure 55-13).

As with antegrade bypass, intraoperative assessment is performed using the electromagnetic flow probe and ultrasound imaging, and a postoperative aortogram is obtained prior to discharge (Figure 55-14).

Transaortic endarterectomy has provided consistent symptom relief and long-term patency. There have been 4 deaths among 41 patients, secondary to myocardial infarction, hemorrhage, and cerebral hypoxia (Table 55-2). All patients surviving the perioperative period have been cured of their symptoms. There were three late visceral artery occlusions and two were symptomatic (Table 55-1). Reoperation and antegrade aortovisceral bypass were successful in relieving symptoms again in both cases. Morbidity consisted of myocardial infarction (two patients) and transient renal failure (one patient). No patient experienced spinal cord ischemia, either with this approach or with antegrade bypass. The technique is advantageous because it is entirely autogenous and anatomic, but the extensive nature of this dissection restricts its use to good risk patients. Additionally it allows simultaneous correction of coexistent multiple vascular lesions (Table 55-3).

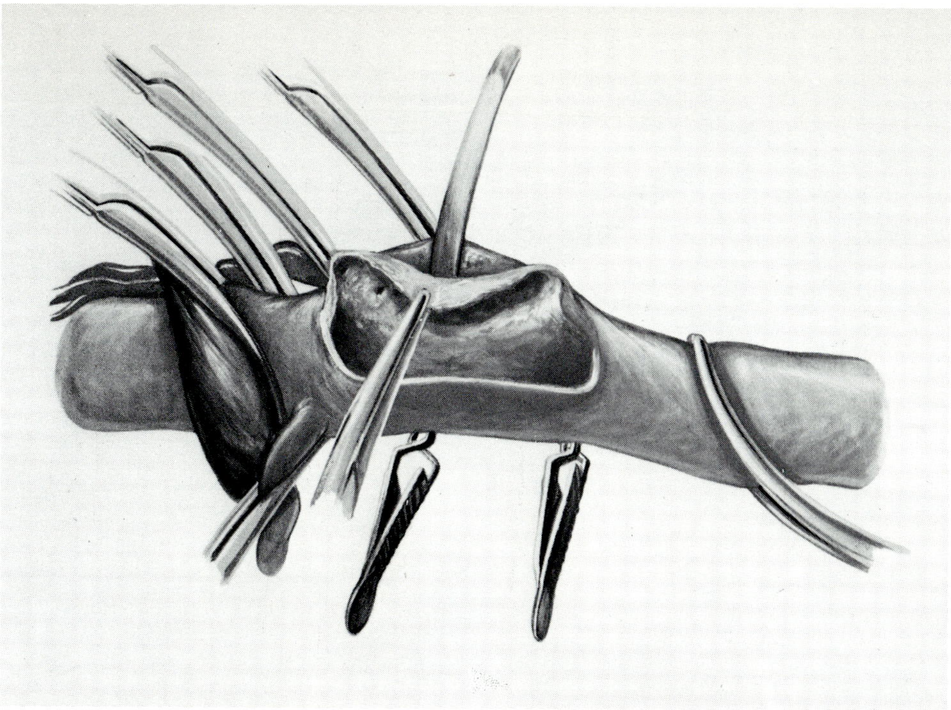

FIGURE 55-11. Development of endarterectomy plane through anterolateral trapdoor aortotomy. [Reproduced with permission from Wylie EJ, Stoney RJ, Ehrenfeld WK: Manual of Vascular Surgery Vol. I, New York, Springer-Verlag, 1980, p. 217.]

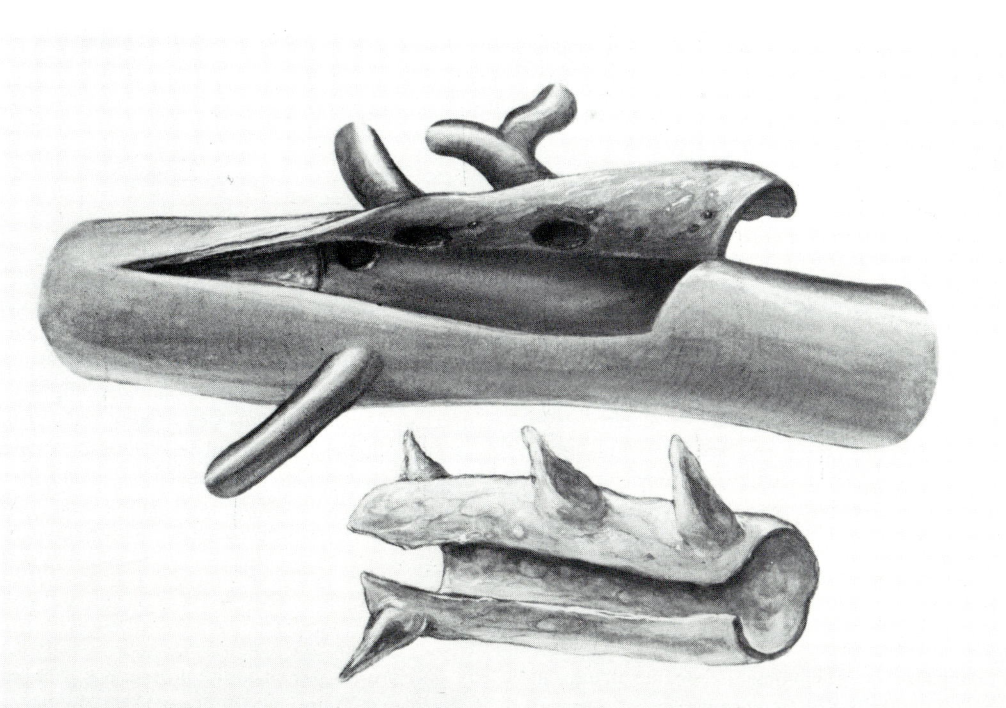

FIGURE 55-12. Combined visceral and renal endarterectomy with sleeve aortic endarterectomy. [Reproduced with permission from Wylie EJ, Stoney RJ, Ehrenfeld WK: Manual of Vascular Surgery Vol. I, New York, Springer-Verlag, 1980, p. 217.]

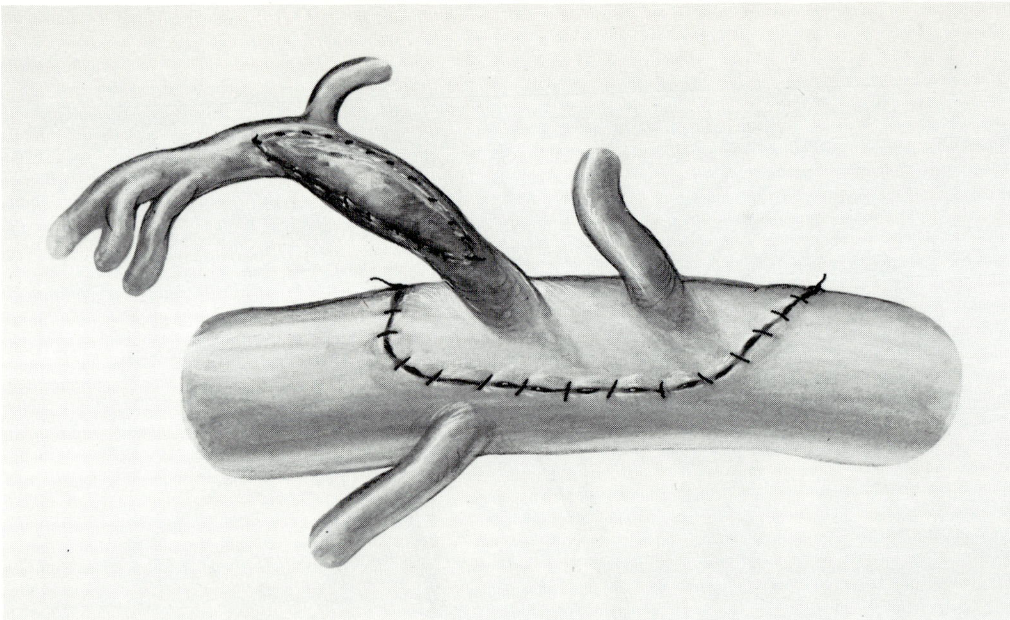

FIGURE 55-13. SMA endarterectomy completed through a separate arteriotomy and closed with a vein patch.

TABLE 55-3. Visceral Revascularization and Associated Reconstructions

Approach	Patients	Arteries Repaired		
		Celiac-SMA	Celiac-SMA-Renal	Celiac-SMA-Renal-Aortic
Thoracoretroperitoneal	41	23	8	10
Transabdominal	34	32	0	2

Nonoperative Therapy

Medical treatment of visceral ischemic symptoms is quite limited. Some patients have experienced symptomatic improvement using long-acting nitrates with meals. The mechanism of action is unclear but may be related to alterations in mesenteric vascular resistance. It is unknown whether patients so treated have an improved long-term outcome, since obviously, this treatment does not alter the underlying disease process. Similarly, dietary manipulation may reduce symptoms but should be regarded as a method of maintaining nutrition while evaluation and preparation for definitive treatment continue.

Percutaneous transluminal balloon dilatation of visceral lesions has been successful in reducing obstruction, but at present the durability of this approach remains unproved (12). The orifice location of atheromatous disease reduces the likelihood of successful dilatation. Also distal embolization remains a concern. The technique can be beneficial in temporizing for the poor risk patient and allowing some nutritional recovery in the cachectic patient prior to definitive treatment.

Discussion

Since the natural history of asymptomatic visceral atherosclerosis is unknown, revascularization in these patients is a consideration only when an indicated aortic operation would further jeopardize intestinal blood flow. In such patients, preservation of collateral flow or reconstruction of the involved visceral branch may be indicated. Incidentally discovered visceral disease may be safely followed since the presence of disease does not imply clinical significance and does not invariably progress to intestinal infarction.

For the symptomatic patient the decision for surgical revascularization is influenced by the extent of disease, the severity of the symptoms, and the general patient condition.

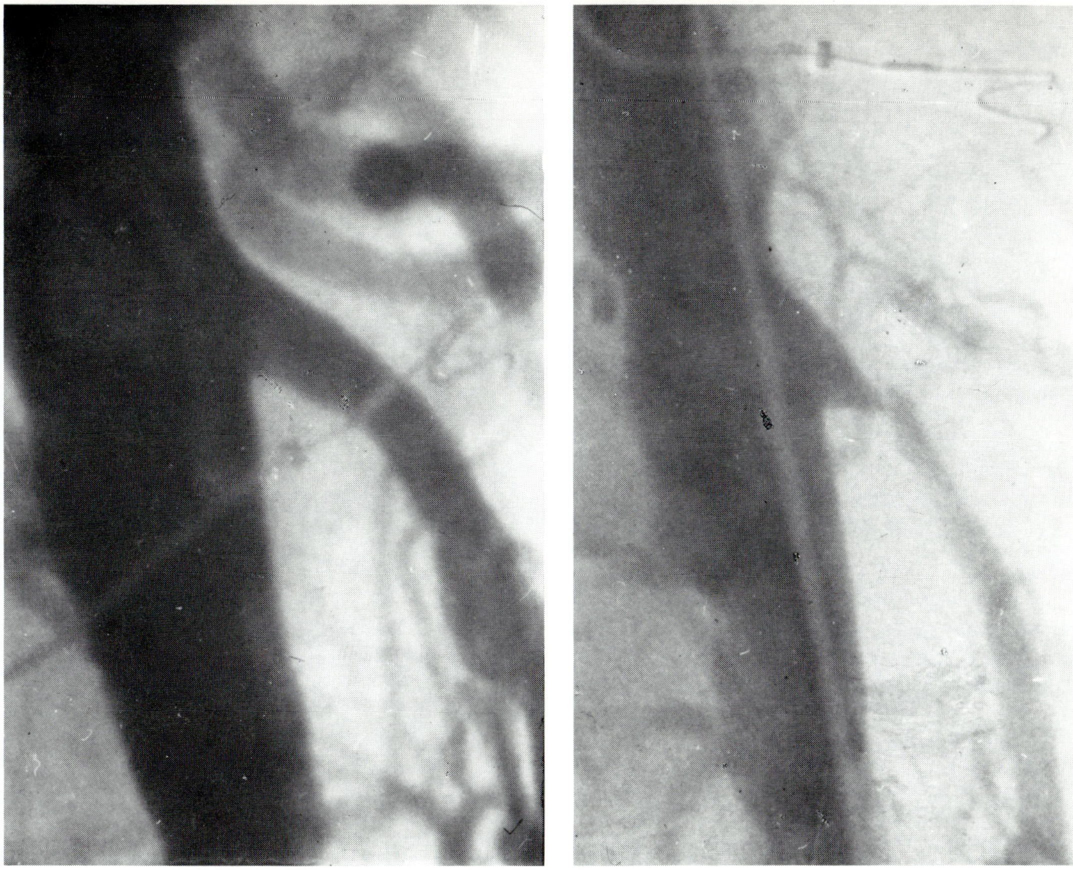

A B

FIGURE 55-14. Postoperative arteriogram showing patent SMA and celiac after endarterectomy. *(A)* Postoperative. *(B)* Preoperative.

Classic, severe symptomatology in the presence of significant and appropriate lesions on angiography demands aggressive operative treatment to avoid intestinal infarction with fatal consequences (13). Considerable judgment is required in deciding for or against surgery in a patient who has atypical symptoms and mild atherosclerotic visceral disease on aortography. Single-vessel disease (or mild two-vessel disease) takes on a different significance if one suspects that collateralization may be impaired secondary to previous gastrointestinal surgery or associated severe aortoiliac disease (14,15). Unfortunately no simple method exists for determining if the demonstrated lesions are sufficient to produce the symptoms experienced.

The nutritionally impaired patient requires preoperative preparation with either intravenous hyperalimentation or dietary manipulation until an anabolic state is restored. The technique and operative approach selected are dictated by the patient's operative risk and the distribution of the disease to be corrected (16).

In good risk symptomatic patients, we prefer thoracoretroperitoneal transaortic endarterectomy. The wide exposure provides safe access to and control of the entire abdominal aorta and its branches. Definitive treatment of complex renal, visceral, and aortoiliac atherosclerotic or aneurysmal disease may be performed with a single operation. Properly selected patients will have no increased mortality or morbidity, and the reconstructions are durable and long-term (17).

The transabdominal approach for an antegrade prosthetic bypass is an appropriate second choice for higher risk patients. The limited dissection, single-cavity procedure is better tolerated in this patient group. Although this technique has been used in a smaller number of patients, the early results suggest it may provide equally good symptomatic relief and protection against visceral infarction as does the transaortic endarterectomy (18).

Conclusion

In summary, chronic intestinal ischemia is most often caused by atherosclerotic involvement of the visceral arteries, with multiple vessel involvement in at least 85 percent of cases. Aortography is required to make the diagnosis, which is frequently delayed because of the nonspecific symptoms and minimal physical findings. Since the preponderance of splanchnic flow is carried by the celiac axis and SMA, revascularization of both of these vessels is performed whenever possible. However, sustained symptom relief and intestinal protection can be obtained with celiac revascularization alone.

The technique and operative approach chosen for a given case is determined by the extent of disease involvement and the patient's operative risk. The best results in terms of low operative mortality and morbidity, sustained symptom relief, and long-term patency have been obtained with thoracoretroperitoneal transaortic endarterectomy and with antegrade aortovisceral prosthetic bypass. Both procedures require temporary supraceliac aortic occlusion. This requires careful intraoperative management but was well tolerated by our patients without significant renal ischemia and with no spinal or intestinal ischemic complications.

The thoracoretroperitoneal approach requires a good risk patient but provides the opportunity for one-step correction of complex, multivessel, atherosclerotic disease. It is also an autogenous repair. The transabdominal antegrade prosthetic bypass is appropriate for a poorer risk patient, and early results suggest excellent long-term results, comparable to the transaortic endarterectomy.

References

1. Chiene J: Complete obliteration of celiac and mesenteric arteries: Viscera receiving their blood supply through extraperitoneal system vessels. J Anat Physiol 3:65, 1869.
2. Dunphy JE: Abdominal pain of vascular origin. Am J Med Sci 192:102, 1936.
3. Mikkelson WP: Intestinal angina. Its surgical significance. Am J Surg 94:262, 1957.
4. Shaw RS, Maynard EP III: Acute and chronic thrombosis of mesenteric arteries associated with malabsorption. Report of two cases successfully treated by thromboendarterectomy. N Engl J Med 258:874, 1958.
5. Hollier LH, Bernatz PE, Pairolero PC, Payne WS, Osmundson PJ: Surgical management of chronic intestinal ischemia: A reappraisal. Surgery 90:940, 1981.
6. Reul GJ Jr, Wukasch DC, Sandiford EM, Chiarillo L, Hallman GL, Cooley DA: Surgical treatment of abdominal angina: Review of 25 patients. Surgery 75:682, 1974.
7. Hertzer NR, Beven EG, Humphries AW: Chronic intestinal ischemia. Surg Gynecol Obstet 145:321, 1977.
8. Zelenock GB, Graham LM, Whitehouse WM Jr, Erlandson EE, Kraft RO, Lindenauer SM, Stanley JC: Splanchnic arteriosclerotic disease and intestinal angina. Arch Surg 115:497, 1980.
9. McCollum CH, Graham JM, DeBakey ME: Chronic mesenteric arterial insufficiency: Results of revascularization in 33 cases. South Med J 69:1266, 1976.
10. Stoney RJ, Ehrenfeld WK, Wylie EJ: Revascularization methods in chronic visceral ischemia caused by atherosclerosis. Ann Surg 186:468, 1977.
11. Stoney RJ, Wylie EJ: Recognition and surgical management of visceral ischemia syndromes. Ann Surg 164:174, 1966.
12. Golden DA, Ring EJ, McLean GK, Freiman DB: Percutaneous transluminal angioplasty in the treatment of abdominal angina. AJR 139:247, 1982.
13. Bergan JJ, Dry L, Conn JJ, Trippel OH: Intestinal ischemic syndrome. Ann Surg 169:120, 1969.
14. Stoney RJ, Wylie EJ: Surgery of celiac and mesenteric arteries. In Haimovici H (ed): *Vascular Surgery Principles and Techniques*, ed 2. New York, McGraw-Hill, 1976, pp 668–679.
15. Fry WJ, Kraft RD: Visceral angina. Surg Gynecol Obstet 117:417, 1963.
16. Perdue GD, Smith RB: Intestinal ischemia due to mesenteric arterial disease. Am Surg 36:152, 1970.
17. Stoney RJ, Olcott C IV: Visceral artery syndromes and reconstruction. Surg Clin North Am 59:637, 1979.
18. Connolly JE, Kwaan JHM: Management of chronic visceral ischemia. Surg Clin North Am 62:345, 1982.

PART SEVEN

Vascular Disorders of the Upper Extremity

Chapter 56

THORACIC OUTLET DISORDERS: THORACIC OUTLET COMPRESSION SYNDROME AND AXILLARY VEIN THROMBOSIS

HERBERT I. MACHLEDER

The term *thoracic outlet compression syndrome* first appeared in the medical literature as used by Rob and Standeven in 1958 (1). The significance of this change in nomenclature was the impetus it gave at a critical point to categorization of a group of painful disorders involving the shoulder and upper extremity. The idea of unifying a group of diverse neurovascular compression syndromes arising at the shoulder girdle was ready for acceptance, and in subsequent literature there was an attempt to define the underlying anatomical variations which resulted in the symptom complex in the majority of these patients.

Although there was now a clear tendency to focus attention on some common basic structural relationship, long-standing biases which crossed interdisciplinary lines continued to confuse the diagnosis and therapy of thoracic outlet compression syndrome. For about a century prior to this pivotal period, neurovascular compression phenomena around the shoulder girdle were classified relative to either the suspected specific compressive component or the suspected etiologic abnormality. A diffuse literature, therefore, exists describing the costoclavicular syndrome, cervical rib syndrome, scalenus anticus syndrome, subclavius tendon syndrome, pectoralis minor muscle syndrome, and effort thrombosis or Paget-Shroetter syndrome.

The syndrome is characterized by symptoms of neurovascular compression at the thoracic outlet and occurs widely within the population in a spectrum ranging from mild numbness and tingling of the fingers when the arms are placed in certain stress positions to severe functional disability and incapacitation, venous hypertension, and arterial insufficiency to a degree where digital gangrene and ischemic tissue loss become manifest. In a recent epidemiologic study, thoracic outlet compression was considered ''an important often neglected cause of cervical brachial pain, weakness and sensory disturbance'' (2).

Historically, the evolution in recognition of thoracic outlet compression has moved synchronously with changing concepts of etiology and therapy. The earliest well-recognized description in the English literature was the neurovascular compressive effects of a cervical rib. The opportunity to identify a distinct anatomic characteristic in this particular group of individuals focused attention on the cervical rib as the dominant structural abnormality for many years. In 1861, Holmes Coote resected a cervical rib in a patient hospitalized at St. Bartholemew's in London and demonstrated its clear-cut relationship with a large subclavian aneurysm (3,4). With the perfection of radiographic techniques the identification of the cervical rib became more common, and reports in the medical literature subsequent to this initial description were authored by John B. Murphy and William S. Halsted. By the early 1920s, thoracic outlet neurovascular compression by cervical rib was a well-accepted concept (5,6).

With increasing interest and attention focused on the problem, it became evident that a large group of patients presented with fairly typical symptoms of neurovascular compression at the thoracic outlet without evidence of an accompanying cervical rib or any other demonstrable musculoskeletal structural abnormality. It was also clear that although some patients presented with signs and symptoms predominantly of arterial insufficiency, a small group of patients presented with evidence of intermittent venous obstruction, and still the largest group of patients presented predominantly with symptoms of nerve compression of the brachial plexus. Despite these vagaries it was evident that the compressive phenomenon was located at the thoracic outlet where the neurovascular bundle passes between the clavicle and first rib.

In 1938 Naffziger introduced the concept of the scalenus anticus syndrome as one of the group of anomalies encompassed by the broader category of thoracic outlet compression. It was thought that the scalenus anticus muscle compressed the brachial plexus and vascular structures by tension and eventual fibrosis and adhesions (7). Acceptance of this concept by the medical and surgical community was widespread, and division of the scalenus anticus muscle in the neck gained favor as a therapeutic maneuver for a large group of patients suffering from thoracic outlet compression with or without an accompanying cervical rib (8). Treatment, however, continued to be plagued by a high rate of symptomatic recidivism, and the quest continued for more effective means of decompression or enlargement of the thoracic outlet.

Telford and Stopford reported that the compression syndrome

could be relieved by resection of the normal first rib, postulating that this structure formed the underlying unyielding base of the thoracic outlet tunnel (9). Concomitant with this new concept there were reattempts to identify specific manifestations of compression with more specific abnormalities of thoracic outlet configuration. Notable in this regard were the studies of McCleery, who felt that intermittent compression and obstruction of the subclavian vein was most likely caused by impingement on the vein by the subclavius muscle and tendon at the most medial aspect of the thoracic outlet channel. He recommended resection of the subclavius tendon as an effective method of decompression of the proximal thoracic outlet (10).

The surgical approach to the thoracic outlet was brought around full circle, anatomically, when Rosati and Lord recommended claviculectomy as a method of removing the roof of the thoracic tunnel, thereby providing adequate and effective long-term decompression. The operation, however, was rather disfiguring from a cosmetic standpoint and was not popular, particularly in the young individuals who seemed to have a much higher incidence of thoracic outlet compression requiring surgical correction (11).

As follow-up of patients improved and long-term results were analyzed, the pivotal role of the first thoracic rib began to take on much greater significance as a common structure to all of the manifestations of thoracic outlet compression. Whether the compressive phenomena were medially, centrally, or laterally located, resulting in either venous arterial or brachial plexus compression, the first rib seems to be a common underlying structure with the accessory component being the subclavius tendon, scalenus anticus muscle, a rudimentary or well-developed cervical rib, or an exostosis of the first rib. Resection of the first rib gained increasing acceptance then as the procedure which would most likely provide long-term and adequate decompression along the whole lower dimension of the thoracic outlet.

Resection of the first rib by the posterior approach was reintroduced and described by Clagett in 1962 (12). Based on this work and the excellent results afforded by first thoracic rib resection, Roos popularized the transaxillary approach which is retained today as the most common surgical method of first thoracic rib resection. The relative ease of operation coupled with low morbidity and excellent cosmetic result has served to establish this procedure as the standard for first rib resection (13).

Pathologic Anatomy

The historical evolution of therapeutic and diagnostic concepts in thoracic outlet compression is best understood by reviewing the anatomical structures which form the boundaries of the thoracic outlet (Figure 56-1). The thoracic outlet can be visualized in a triangular configuration with the apex directed toward the manubrium of the sternum. The base of the triangle is made up of the first thoracic rib, and the hypotenuse or superior limb is made up of the clavicle and underlying subclavius muscle and tendon. The medially disposed apex of the triangle can also be thought of as the fulcrum of a pair of scissor blades such that

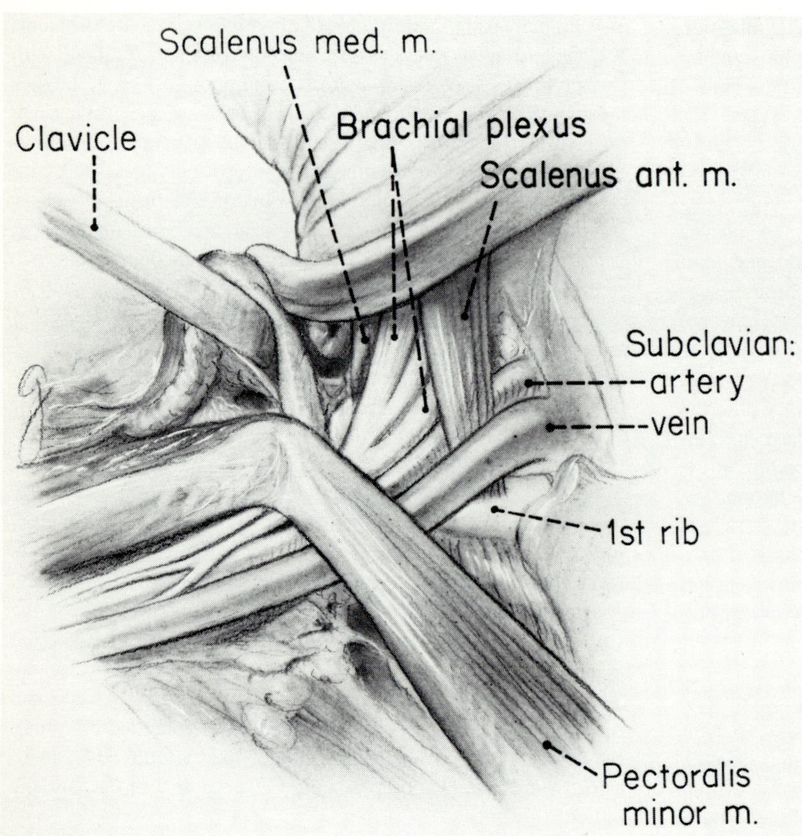

FIGURE 56-1. Anatomic configuration of thoracic outlet as seen from an anterior perspective. The clavicle has been reflected laterally from the manubrium, hinged on its acromial attachment. The first rib can be seen underlying the thoracic outlet structures and attaching to the manubrium of the sternum, and the pectoralis minor tendon inserting on the coracoid process. (From HI Machleder: *Vascular Disorders of the Upper Extremity*. Mt. Kisco, New York, Futura Press, 1983.)

they form a more or less acute apical angle depending on arm position. It is this scissor movement that accounts for the symptoms and signs which occur in the various stress position maneuvers (Figure 56-2). At the most medial aspect of the thoracic outlet, the subclavian vein exits the thorax and demarcates the entrance to the thoracic outlet tunnel. At this point the first rib and clavicular head join the manubrium of the sternum in a fibrocartilaginous joint. The subclavius tendon, which lies just beneath the clavicle, inserts at the junction of the first rib and clavicle, and with enlargement and hypertrophy can serve to indent the subclavian vein at that acute apical angle.

The structure of the thoracic outlet continues laterally, as the clavicle and subclavius muscle form the roof, and the generally flat, smooth superior surface of the first rib forms the floor. A more or less prominent tubercle occurs at the superior posterior surface of the first rib at the site of insertion of the scalenus anticus muscle, which is the second structure to enter the thoracic outlet just lateral to the subclavian vein. The scalenus anticus muscle has a fairly consistent insertion on the posterior margin of the thoracic rib. This insertion may vary in its extent along the rib margin and probably accounts for some elements of neurovascular compression when the muscle is particularly hypertrophic or is accompanied by posttraumatic or congenital fibrotic bands. The section of first rib which lies laterally and adjacent to the scalenus anticus insertion is a common site of fusion for either a well-developed cervical rib or the rudimentary fibrocartilaginous bands which have been implicated in many instances of thoracic outlet compression. The subclavian artery is the third structure entering the normal thoracic outlet, just lateral to the insertion of the scalenus anticus muscle. The artery enters the thoracic outlet from a somewhat more cephalad location, as the innominate artery branches to form the arch of the subclavian and right common carotid arteries. An apparently high arching subclavian artery is a fairly distinctive characteristic of thoracic outlet compression. This relatively high arch may be related to descent of the clavicle toward the first rib position and may well be significant to the development of thoracic compression in those patients with this propensity. Insertions of cervical ribs and fibrocartilaginous bands are also observed just lateral to the subclavian artery, and occasionally a synostosis or exostosis will be found in this portion of the first thoracic rib. Lateral to the subclavian artery, the brachial plexus enters the thoracic outlet with the C7 and T1 roots disposed inferiorly and the C4, C5, and C6 roots oriented superiorly. Lateral to the brachial plexus, the scalenus medius muscle has a rather broad and variable attachment to the first rib and may be traversed by the long thoracic nerve innervating the serratus anterior muscle.

Although multiple abnormalities can account for reduction of the available space in the thoracic outlet, the rigid boundaries are formed by the clavicle superiorly and the first rib inferiorly. It has remained evident that the most effective decompression, irrespective of the specific site of impingement, will be a surgical procedure directed at one of the rigid structures.

Clinical Presentation

Despite advances in the therapy of thoracic outlet compression syndrome and careful attention to anatomic details, the basic underlying pathophysiology remains enigmatic. Even the readily demonstrable cervical rib has an unclear relationship to the basic disease process. Cervical ribs occur with considerable frequency in the asymptomatic population and make up only as many as 25 percent of patients who have well-established thoracic outlet compression symptoms. The symptoms which begin in the second, third, and fourth decades of life may arise spontaneously. More commonly, relatively minor shoulder or cervical trauma can precipitate the entire symptom complex in a previously asymptomatic individual. It has been noted at the time of surgery that congenital fibrocartilaginous bands traverse the brachial plexus and enter various portions of the thoracic outlet. Clavicular fracture and hyperextension neck injuries also seem to result in rather typical symptoms of thoracic outlet compression.

There are developmental changes in the clavicular sternal angle over the passage of time, particularly after adolescence, that bear some relationship to changes in anatomic configuration of the thoracic outlet and probably account for the peculiar age distribution of this syndrome. It would seem likely that in some individuals the close tolerance of clearance space existing in the thoracic outlet is easily upset by cervical-brachial trauma, with the resultant muscle spasm generating a cycle of pain, spasm, and increasing disability which often cannot be interrupted without surgical intervention.

The spectrum of thoracic outlet compression symptoms ranges from mild to disabling, as previously described. The specific symptom complex of the compressive phenomena can be attributed to the region of the neurovascular bundle affected. Arterial compression is perhaps the least common, comprising only 1 percent of all cases seen. These patients may present with typical Raynaud's type symptoms or indeed may have intermittent ischemia and rubor of their hands and digits. Occasionally peripheral embolization and frank gangrene of the fingertips will arise from arterial compression at the thoracic outlet.

Venous compression occurs slightly more commonly and often may present rather suddenly. Although deep venous thrombosis in the upper extremity is uncommon (approximately 2 percent of all cases of deep venous thrombosis) and occasionally is associated with congestive heart failure and metastatic or mediastinal tumors, it is most commonly associated with effort thrombosis.

Spontaneous thrombosis of the subclavian vein was described by Sir James Paget in 1875 and again by Von Schroetter in 1884. This event has often been referred to as the Paget-Schroetter syndrome (14,15). The syndrome, however, is most likely secondary to thoracic outlet compression and occurs generally after extreme effort involving the upper extremity, such as in weight lifting, tugging, and stressful activities with the arms in the abducted, externally rotated position. Clinically the patient may have a painful injury in the shoulder region followed in several days by swelling of the fingers, forearm, or entire upper extremity, with great difficulty using the arms in abduction or external rotation. The clinical course is rather protracted with continued disability being the rule rather than the exception. Collateral

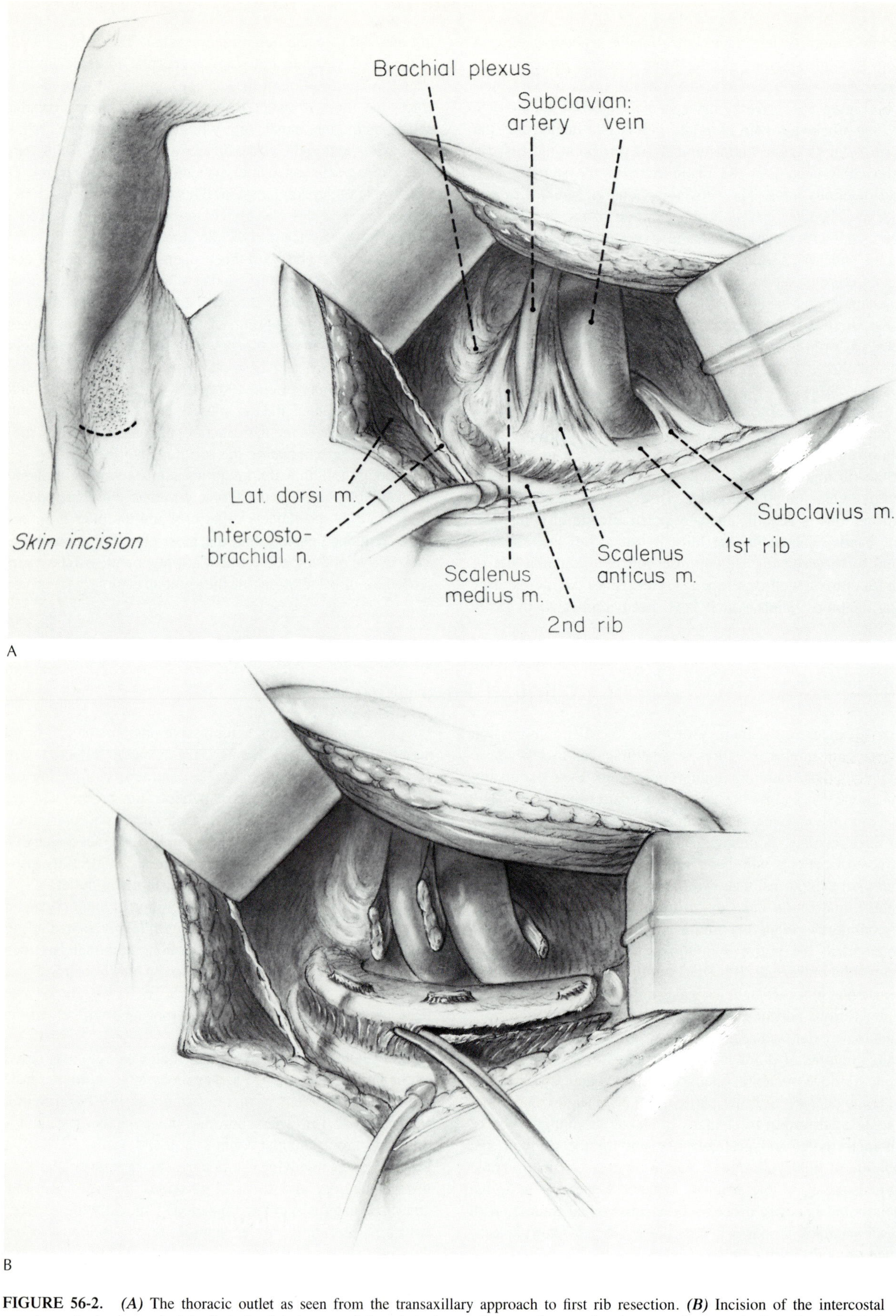

FIGURE 56-2. *(A)* The thoracic outlet as seen from the transaxillary approach to first rib resection. ***(B)*** Incision of the intercostal muscles, prior to removal of the first rib. Attachments of the subclavius, scalenus anticus, and scalenus medius muscles have been divided. (From HI Machleder: *Vascular Disorders of the Upper Extremity*. Mt. Kisco, New York, Futura Press, 1983.)

venous channels do develop over time, but normal activity is rarely feasible in the presence of chronic subclavian vein occlusion.

Patients who develop acute thrombosis of the subclavian vein should be hospitalized immediately for an attempt at thrombolytic therapy. Two approaches have been utilized: first, the use of systemic fibrinolytic drugs such as streptokinase; or second, heparinization as a temporizing measure which will rarely result in lysis of the thrombus or significant improvement in the patient's symptoms. The objectives of heparinization are to prevent propagation of thrombus during the early period of stabilization and to avoid the loss of important collateral veins in the supraclavicular and thoracic outlet area. More recently, direct intravenous local fibrinolytic therapy has been utilized with varying success. The catheter is placed via the antecubital veins directly into the axillosubclavian vein thrombus, and streptokinase therapy is begun with lower doses than are required for general systemic therapy. The streptokinase activates plasminogen to plasmin, and clot lysis should take place over a period of 12 to 24 hours. This should be followed by heparin, and then dicumarol anticoagulation for maintenance of patency and prevention of rethrombosis. Arm elevation should be avoided in these instances because it generally exacerbates the symptoms and may also complicate the compressive phenomena at the thoracic outlet. These patients whose thrombosis is based on thoracic outlet compression should then be considered for early decompression by first rib resection or scalenectomy. Venography is very helpful in demonstrating compression after the vein has regained patency.

Perhaps the most frequent manifestation of thoracic outlet compression involves the brachial plexus. Two patterns of brachial plexus compression have emerged: first is that affecting the upper cords, and generally presenting with pain in the side of the neck, head, and suprascapular area of the trapezius muscle, as well as the lateral shoulder and radial nerve distribution of the arm. The second type of brachial plexus compression involves predominantly lower plexus involvement and is likewise characterized by pain in the suprascapular area of the trapezius muscle, the neck and shoulder, and the ulnar aspect of the arm from axilla down to the ulnar nerve distribution in the fingers (16).

In all of the various manifestations of thoracic outlet compression, patients typically complain of specific physical or occupational disability. The syndrome is particularly stressful in waitresses, who are unable to maintain their arms in abduction and external rotation in carrying trays of food and dishes; plumbers, carpenters, and mechanics, who work with their arms above their heads, also find particular disability relative to their occupational requirements. Driving poses considerable difficulty related to numbness and tingling of the fingers. Women will often complain of pain and weakness when reaching for objects above their heads, fixing or washing their hair, and other activities of a similar nature. The syndrome is seen with particular severity in certain athletes, especially baseball pitchers and swimmers. Even sedentary activities can be significantly affected by thoracic outlet compression and can lead to occupational disability in typists and keyboard operators who develop rapid tiring, and reduction of speed and accuracy in addition to pain and weakness. In these sedentary workers particularly, thoracic outlet compression symptoms must be differentiated from other peripheral nerve entrapment such as carpal tunnel syndrome, which entraps the median nerve at the wrist and may give rise to very similar hand, wrist, and forearm symptoms. Ulnar nerve entrapment at the olecranon groove may also present in a similar manner. Generally these conditions are easily differentiated by clinical evaluation and physical examination.

Epidemiologically there appears to be a bimodal distribution of individuals with thoracic outlet compression. One group is composed of individuals with extensive muscle development around the shoulder and upper arm whose compression is very likely related to muscle hypertrophy and the stress of their activities. Another group are individuals of very asthenic habitus, this latter group being more responsive to physical therapy and attempts to restore the normal postural relationships of the upper thorax.

Noninvasive Vascular Laboratory Evaluation

Although the majority of patients present with neurologic rather than vascular impairment, various stages of vascular compressive phenomena can be demonstrated in most patients with documented thoracic outlet compression syndrome. This hemodynamically significant compressive phenomenon can be documented using appropriate thoracic outlet maneuvers, and the pulse volume and pressure changes can be verified by simple tests available in the peripheral vascular laboratory with the simplest test being measurement of bilateral brachial artery pressure using the Doppler flowmeter. The Doppler flow signal can be assessed at either the brachial, radial, or ulnar arteries. A reduction of 20 mmHg or more from the neutral to the stress position, or when comparing one side to the other, is considered indicative of a positive test.

Digital plethysmography can be utilized as an alternative to direct pressure measurement, and the damping factor of the systolic waveform shape can be noted with various thoracic outlet maneuvers.

As a consequence of extensive potential collateralization around the subclavian artery, there will often be a palpable or Doppler-detectable radial or ulnar pulse despite complete obstruction of the subclavian artery at the level of the thoracic outlet. A pressure discrepancy or abnormality detected in the neutral position should indicate to the clinician the desirability of angiographic investigation to better evaluate the presence of a significant stenosis, poststenotic dilatation, or atherosclerotic degeneration of the vessel at the point of trauma.

Significant venous obstruction in the upper extremity can be detected using the Doppler flowmeter, although clinically this approach is not applied very frequently. Changes in venous flow pattern with the arm placed in various thoracic outlet maneuvers has enabled some investigators to diagnose venous obstructive phenomena accurately and consistently (17).

A number of electrophysiologic tests have been used in an attempt to further delineate the thoracic outlet syndrome, but results have been quite variable. It is generally conceded that nerve conduction times and electromyography have relatively little value in establishing a definitive diagnosis of thoracic outlet compression. Nerve conduction across Erb's point, the olecranon groove, and the carpal tunnel is useful in establishing other causes for apparent neurologic dysfunction of the upper extremity. These studies are of particular usefulness in separating thoracic outlet compression symptoms from carpal tunnel median nerve compression, which occasionally presents with a similar pattern and overlapping disability. Carpal tunnel compression syndrome of the median nerve occurs in about 10 percent of patients with well-documented thoracic outlet obstruction. Early experience using somatosensory evoked potentials suggests that this method of evaluating peripheral nerve function may prove more helpful in documenting the neurologic abnormalities seen with thoracic outlet compression syndrome.

Physical Examination

Physical examination of the patient with complaints suggestive of thoracic outlet compression should include a complete examination of the head and neck to detect signs of cervical spine disease and discogenic disease with radiculopathy, as well as cervical osteoarthritis with neuroforaminal compression. Although neck pain is quite common with thoracic outlet compression syndrome, restriction of normal neck movement and flexibility or tenderness over the cervical spine is not usually seen. Compression of the disk spaces by downward pressure on the head rarely elicits symptoms in patients with thoracic outlet compression syndrome but may be quite useful in demonstrating cervical discogenic disease. Muscle spasm and tenderness can often be encountered in patients with thoracic outlet compression, particularly at the lateral border of the trapezius muscle and along the lateral border of the sternocleidomastoid muscle, over the course of the scalenus anticus muscle and brachial plexus. Tenderness to pressure over the brachial plexus is also characteristically found in patients with thoracic outlet neurovascular compression. Clavicular percussion on the symptomatic side will often provoke symptoms, whereas it is generally easily tolerated on the noninvolved side. Palpation of the radial pulse, with the arm in the neutral position, then using the various thoracic outlet maneuvers—Adson's maneuver, costoclavicular maneuver, and scalenus anticus maneuver—and the abduction external rotation (AER) position, is useful to detect changes in pulse volume. Very often the positional change will evoke the symptom complex, particularly with abduction and external rotation.

With the arm in the abducted and externally rotated position (as with a hand raised in a greeting) rapid clenching and unclenching of the hand will lead to fatigue, tiring, and inability to maintain the position for more than 60 to 90 s. Normally this type of activity is well tolerated for 3 to 5 minutes. A bruit is very commonly heard at the lateral third of the infraclavicular area as the arm is brought from neutral into the abducted, externally rotated position. Occasionally the bruit is better heard at the lateral portion of the supraclavicular fossa. The bruit typically extends through only a short range of movement, and unless auscultation takes place continually, as the arm is moved from neutral to abduction and external rotation, the bruit may well be missed as the pulse is obliterated and the volume flow reduced.

Although one or another of these signs may be elicited in normally asymptomatic individuals, which has prompted some investigators to denigrate the value of positional evaluation, it is the constellation of signs, the presence of concomitant symptoms, together with a fairly typical history, that establishes the diagnosis of thoracic outlet compression. The isolated finding of one abnormality on physical examination is generally insufficient to diagnose thoracic outlet compression reliably. It has been demonstrated in the past that a number of asymptomatic individuals obliterate their pulse with extreme abduction or hyperabduction. Additionally the finding of a cervical rib, on routine chest x-ray, does not establish the diagnosis of thoracic outlet compression.

Adson's test, for example, long the hallmark of thoracic outlet compression, has been reported to be positive in less than 3 percent of patients diagnosed, treated, and cured of the syndrome (18). The hyperabduction maneuver, for years an important diagnostic feature of this syndrome, was demonstrated by Wright to be positive in more than 80 percent of normal individuals (19). Supernumerary ribs occur in 0.5 to 1 percent of the asymptomatic population (20). The clinical significance of this lack of specificity of the diagnostic tests is diminished when placed in the context of the complete clinical evaluation.

Angiography

Although the vast majority of patients suffering from thoracic outlet compression present with symptoms of brachial plexus nerve compression, vascular presentations, such as acute axillosubclavian vein thrombosis, or acute ischemic events associated with intermittent subclavian artery obstruction or distal embolization are indications for angiography.

Patients who have unequivocal signs of arterial insufficiency, such as evidence of peripheral embolization, Raynaud's syndrome, asymmetry of resting brachial artery pressures in the neutral position, or evidence of a subclavian bruit in the neutral position, should undergo arteriography to delineate significant arterial damage, particularly atherosclerotic stenosis at the point of compression, or poststenotic dilatation and aneurysm formation. Typically, angiography is performed via the transfemoral arterial route with the patient in the supine position, although it is occasionally difficult to demonstrate any areas of compression using this technique even when the patient has unequivocal clinical signs of arterial compression. This problem has been clarified with the advent of digital intravenous angiography, and we have found that patients having normal arteriographic findings in the abducted, externally rotated position while supine will demonstrate unequivocal compression in the sitting position. The difficulty of doing standard angiography in the sitting position has limited its usefulness in this regard, and the greater mobility of the patient during digital angiography has helped us recognize this limitation. The patient should be studied arteriographically with arms in the neutral position and also in positions of thoracic outlet stress such as abduction and external rotation.

Although evidence of axillosubclavian artery compression can be demonstrated in asymptomatic individuals, this generally requires that the arm be placed in a relatively extreme degree of hyperabduction. Nevertheless, the angiogram must be interpreted cautiously where there is no clear-cut evidence of arterial damage or evidence of poststenotic dilatation. It is important to reiterate that the angiogram is best interpreted in light of the clinical evaluation, history, and physical assessment. As an isolated finding, it has unfortunately relatively little specificity. This underscores the lack of a single objective test which will help diagnose thoracic outlet compression syndrome.

Venography should be undertaken in patients with thoracic outlet compression whose symptoms suggest intermittent compression of the subclavian vein or actual axillosubclavian vein thrombosis. As with arteriography, the study should be performed with the arm in the neutral and then in the abducted, externally rotated position. Injection can be done in one of the hand veins using 30 to 40 mL of meglumine diatrizoate or by direct injection into the brachial vein. Evidence of collateralization is very important in interpreting these venographic studies.

Medical Therapy

In general, once the diagnosis of thoracic outlet compression is established, a course of conservative therapy should be instituted prior to consideration of surgical intervention. It has been our experience that patients who develop the syndrome in the setting of occupational strain or muscular hypertrophy derive little benefit from a program of exercise and physical therapy. Patients in certain occupational categories such as plumbers, carpenters, mechanics, and athletes with extensive shoulder girdle development are generally relieved of their symptoms during a period of suspension of occupation or muscular stress. This is particularly true when the syndrome has been precipitated by some acute soft tissue trauma in the head and neck region. If the period of rest is followed by progressive rehabilitation using multimodal therapy such as diathermy, massage, and muscle relaxants, the program can often be quite beneficial. Those individuals who have posture deformities and an asthenic habitus will generally respond to a series of thoracic outlet exercises designed for postural rebalance and strengthening of the shoulder girdle (21). In general, the response is quite prompt, and the symptoms are either severely exacerbated or the patient notes rather early beneficial signs. In those who have severe exacerbation of their symptoms, we have found it unproductive to persist with physical therapy. A number of exercises are designed for reestablishment of muscular balance of the thoracic outlet, particularly overcoming scalenus or sternocleidomastoid muscle spasm. There are certain therapeutic modalities which have a particular propensity for exacerbating symptoms and in general these should be avoided. Cervical collars and cervical traction will very often cause considerable discomfort. One subgroup of patients becomes quite symptomatic at night. Generally, these patients sleep on their abdomens with their arms placed above the head or beneath the face. They often awaken with dysesthesias during the night, and occasionally severe vascular symptoms lead to digital ischemia. Retraining these patients to sleep with their arms at their sides and even passing a loose band around the waist, through which the arms are inserted at night, has been found to alleviate symptoms successfully. Episodes severe enough to cause digital gangrene have, in fact, been controlled using these conservative measures alone (19).

Significant changes in occupation or sports activities are an obvious means to avoid symptomatic exacerbation. We have often found that patients do make these modifications and adjustments after unsuccessfully seeking medical relief for their symptoms. Many patients, in fact, develop protective maneuvers and activities which significantly modify symptoms and may obviate the requirement for any additional therapy. At the more modest end of the symptom spectrum, patients can be reassured and quite tolerant of their mild symptoms when educated as to the nonsystemic nature of this process. Often patients are concerned that a progressive degenerative neurologic disease is developing, and that anxiety coupled with the lack of objective confirmatory evidence of disease becomes very unsettling. As a consequence, the physician is often faced with a neurotic and distraught individual. Surprisingly, a significant improvement in these individuals can be expected with patient and careful explanation on the part of the physician. As is so often the case, patients with even modest chronic pain suffer an indolent but progressive psychological disability which acts as an impediment to their medical care and very often exacerbates interfamily and professional stresses. The fact that many of these patients have been quite successful and well adjusted prior to the onset of their symptoms should suggest considerable caution on the part of the physician in labeling any of these symptoms psychosomatic. In our experience, neurotic patterns are more commonly a result of the chronic debilitating nature of unremitting pain rather than the achievement of significant secondary gain from development of the painful disabling syndrome.

Despite the effectiveness of conservative therapy in most patients, it has been reported in the literature that between 10 and 30 percent of patients presenting to the physician with thoracic outlet compression syndrome eventually require surgical therapy for control of their symptoms (22). The presence of progressive arterial symptoms should particularly indicate the necessity for surgical therapy. Evidence of intermittent venous obstruction which continues despite conservative measures should also lead to the consideration of surgical therapy. Spontaneous obstruction of the subclavian vein is quite difficult to reverse, and the progression of symptoms after subclavian vein thrombosis is particularly disabling and unresponsive to therapy. In this group of patients early intervention is probably well indicated.

Surgical Therapy

Current surgical practice in the treatment of thoracic outlet syndrome remains controversial. Specifically there are three major approaches. The first is resection of the first rib; the second is scalenectomy alone; and the third is a combination of first rib resection and scalenectomy done during the same operative procedure.

The most effective single surgical procedure is probably resection of the first thoracic rib. Two anatomic approaches have been utilized in recent years: the posterior approach as popularized by Clagett and the transaxillary approach described by Roos. In the transaxillary approach the patient is positioned in the lateral decubitus position and an incision made between the lateral border of the pectoralis major and the medial border of the latissimus dorsi muscle at the lower portion of the axilla. The rib and accompanying superior periosteum are removed after dividing the insertions of the scalenus anticus muscle and subclavius muscle tendon. The adequacy of the operation depends on removing the rib far posteriorly so that residual compression of the brachial plexus is obviated. Recuperation is generally fairly prompt, and patients usually leave the hospital by the third postoperative day (Figure 56-2). Occasionally entrance into the pleural cavity during the operative procedure does result in pneumothorax, which is resolved by tube drainage through the incision. The tube is removed at the completion of the procedure. Residual pneumothorax may require aspiration at the time of the upright chest film in the recovery room. Two major complications have been reported with this procedure, although the exact incidence is not known. The long thoracic nerve can be injured in its position traversing the scalenus medius muscle, resulting in winging of the scapula. The other major neurologic deficit has been reported as partial, partial-temporary, or occasionally protracted paresis of the extremity from injury to the brachial plexus.

Several other approaches to the first rib have been utilized, specifically the posterior and the anterior supraclavicular approaches. Insufficient numbers of these cases have been reported to assess the effectiveness when compared with the transaxillary approach.

It is generally reported that between 85 and 95 percent of patients have good or excellent results, and approximately 5 to 10 percent of patients represent failures in therapy. Major complications have rarely been reported, but in a survey done by Dale there is the implication that after first rib resection, a significant number of major or minor neurologic deficits, which are not reflected in the medical literature, may occur (22).

The second major surgical approach to thoracic outlet compression syndrome is division of the scalenus anticus muscle or in fact resection of the lower portion of the muscle. This approach has been described by Sanders (23). The procedure of scalenectomy involves division of the scalenus anticus muscle in the supraclavicular area and removal of the entire lower portion to the attachment of the first rib. The scalene muscle overlies the brachial plexus, and very often fibrotic cords or tense bands can be seen compressing the brachial plexus from above. There seem to be numerous small attachments of the scalenus anticus muscle to the perineurium of the brachial plexus, and these generally must be divided with great care as the muscle is dissected back toward the insertions on the transverse processes of the cervical vertebrae. Reported complications of this procedure have been uncommon, although phrenic nerve injury has been observed. Early reports of success with this procedure are in the neighborhood of 85 percent excellent results with 15 percent of the patients either unrelieved of their symptoms or experiencing only modest relief of pain.

It seems clear that if the precise site of compression could be identified preoperatively or by objective testing, one or more of the various operative procedures might be more suitably tailored to the patient's particular pathologic anatomy and symptom complex. Nevertheless, identification of the exact site of compression has remained elusive, and it seems evident that scalenectomy and first rib resection benefit two different groups of patients: those whose primary symptoms are upper plexus compression benefited by scalenectomy, and those whose primary symptoms are lower plexus compression benefited primarily by first rib resection. This observation has encouraged a number of surgeons to apply a combined approach, with first rib resection followed by scalenectomy at the same operative sitting. Long-term results of these combined procedures are not yet available for analysis (24).

Most recent reports indicate that although excellent results can be anticipated initially, by the end of 2 years the recurrence rate exceeds 15 percent for either scalenectomy or first rib resection. Further recurrences after that period of time are not well documented, and it is unclear whether patients are lost to follow-up or whether there is no further attrition of those who have achieved excellent or satisfactory results.

The foundation of successful treatment of patients with thoracic outlet compression syndrome rests on careful diagnostic evaluation, the basis of which is a meticulous history and physical examination, particularly in the absence of reliable specific objective tests. Other nerve entrapment processes must be carefully ruled out in the evaluation of these patients, particularly cervical radiculitis, discogenic disease, and nerve compression at the neuroforamina. Ulnar nerve entrapment and median nerve entrapment at the carpal tunnel are occasionally confusing diagnostic entities with similar presentations. It should be obvious that careful and meticulous operative technique is necessary, particularly when working around the delicate neurovascular structures and brachial plexus, to minimize postoperative fibrosis and scarring.

After diagnosis, a careful program of physical therapy is generally advisable prior to the recommendation for operative intervention. This will enable the surgeon to observe the patient over a somewhat longer period of time than that afforded by an initial consultation. In general, at the time these patients reach the surgeon for therapy, they have undergone numerous consultations, diagnostic tests, and a wide spectrum of therapies of varying effectiveness and legitimacy. Very often, the patients are psychologically disabled by this course of events, and the surgeon should be prepared to deal with this difficult and challenging aspect of management.

References

1. Rob CG, Standeven A: Arterial occlusion complicating thoracic outlet compression syndrome. Br Med J 1958, 2:709–712.
2. Waris T: Epidemiologic screening of occupational neck and upper limb disorders; methods and criteria. Scand J Work Environ Health 1979, 5:25–28.
3. Coote H: Exostosis of the 7th cervical vertebrae surrounded by blood vessels and nerves. Lancet 1861, 1:360–361.
4. Hutchinson J, Jackson JH, Coote H: Pressure on the axillary vessels and nerve by an exostosis from the cervical rib; interference with the circulation of the arm, removal of the rib and exostosis; recovery. Med Times Gaz 1861, 2:108.
5. Murphy JB: Case of cervical rib with symptoms resembling subclavian aneurysm. Ann Surg 1905, 41:399–403.
6. Halsted WS: An experimental study of circumscribed dilation of an artery immediately distal to a partially occluding band, and its bearing on a dilation of the subclavian artery observed in certain cases of cervical rib. J Exp Med 1916, 24:271–286.
7. Naffziger HC, Grant WT: Neuritis of the brachial plexus, mechanical in origin: The scalenus anticus syndrome. Surg Gynecol Obstet 1938, 67:722–730.
8. Ochsner A, Gage M, DeBakey N: Scalenus anticus [Naffziger] syndrome. Am J Surg 1935, 28:669–695.
9. Telford ED, Stopford JSP: The vascular complications of the cervical rib. Br J Surg 1937, 18:559–564.
10. McCleery RS, Kesterson JE, Kirtley JA, Love RB: Subclavius and anterior scalenus muscle compression as the cause of intermittent obstruction of the subclavian vein. Ann Surg 1951, 133:588–602.
11. Rosati LM, Lord JW: Neurovascular compression syndromes of the shoulder girdle. In *Modern Surg Monographs*. New York, Grune and Stratton, 1968.
12. Clagett OT: Presidential Address; research and prosearch. J Thorac Cardiovasc Surg 1962, 44:153–166.
13. Roos DB: Transaxillary approach for 1st rib resection to relieve thoracic outlet syndrome. Ann Surg 1966, 163:354–358.
14. Hughes ES: Venous obstruction in the upper extremity. Int Abst Surg 1949, 88:89–127.
15. Adams JT, Deweese JA: "Effort" thrombosis of the axillary and subclavian veins. J Trauma 1971, 11:923–301.
16. Roos DB: The place for scalenectomy and 1st-rib resection in thoracic outlet syndrome. Surgery 1982, 92:1077–1085.
17. Sumner DS: Vascular laboratory diagnosis and assessment of upper extremity vascular disorders. In Machleder HI (ed): *Vascular Disorders of the Upper Extremity*. Mt. Kisco, New York, Future Press, 1983.
18. Roos DB: Pathophysiology of congenital anomalies and thoracic outlet syndrome. Acta Clin Belg 1980, 79:353–361.
19. Wright IS: The neurovascular syndrome produced by hyperabduction of the arms. Am Heart J 1945, 29:1–19.
20. Pollak EW: Surgical anatomy of the thoracic outlet syndrome. Surg Gynecol Obstet 1980, 150:97–103.
21. Rosati LM, Lord JW: *Neurovascular Compression Syndrome of the Shoulder Girdle*. New York, Grune and Stratton, 1961.
22. Dale WA: Thoracic outlet compression syndrome, critique in 1982. Arch Surg 1982, 117:1437–1445.
23. Sanders RJ, Monsur JW, Gerber WF, Adams WR, Thompson N: Scalenotomy vs. 1st rib resection for treatment of thoracic outlet syndrome. Surgery 1979, 85:109–121.
24. Wylie EJ: Discussion in Roos: The place for scalenectomy and 1st rib resection of thoracic outlet syndrome. Surgery 1982, 92:1084.

Chapter 57

RAYNAUD'S SYNDROME, UPPER EXTREMITY VASOSPASTIC DISORDERS, AND SMALL ARTERY OCCLUSIVE DISEASE

STEVEN P. RIVERS and JOHN M. PORTER

Raynaud's syndrome defines a clinical condition characterized by episodic digital ischemia occurring in response to cold or emotional stimuli. The hands and fingers are most affected in a large majority of patients, although the toes, cheeks, and ears are occasionally involved. Episodic digital ischemia has occupied the interest of generations of vascular physicians, following the initial description of the syndrome by Maurice Raynaud in 1862. This interest has been prompted by several factors, including the recent recognition of the high frequency of Raynaud's syndrome in the population and the realization that Raynaud's syndrome constitutes the classic clinical model for the study of vasospasm, a condition of increasingly recognized clinical importance and one about which so little is known.

Raynaud's syndrome, regardless of severity, is often found in association with a variety of seemingly unrelated disorders, as shown in Table 57-1. Until recently the understanding of Raynaud's syndrome has been confused by a failure to recognize both of the two discrete pathophysiologic mechanisms producing episodic digital ischemia and the relationships between the myriad of conditions listed in Table 57-1 and these pathophysiologic mechanisms. In this chapter we will review the pathophysiology, clinical presentation, diagnosis, and treatment of both Raynaud's syndrome and the related topic of digital ischemic ulceration.

TABLE 57-1. Disorders Which Have Been Reported in Association with Raynaud's Syndrome

I. Immunologic and connective tissue disorders	IV. Drug-induced Raynaud's syndrome without arteritis
A. Scleroderma	A. Ergot
B. Mixed connective tissue disease	B. Beta-blocking drugs
C. Systemic lupus erythematosus	C. Cytotoxic drugs
D. Rheumatoid arthritis	D. (?) Birth control pills
E. Dermatomyositis	V. Miscellaneous
F. Polymyositis	A. Vinyl chloride disease
G. Hepatitis B antigen-induced vasculitis	B. Chronic renal failure
H. Drug-induced vasculitis (hypersensitivity angiitis)	C. Cold agglutinins
I. Sjögren's syndrome	D. Cryoglobulinemia
II. Obstructive arterial diseases	E. Monoclonal gammopathy
A. Arteriosclerosis	F. Neoplasia
B. Thromboangiitis obliterans	G. Neurologic disorders
C. Thoracic outlet syndrome	1. Central
III. Environmental conditions	2. Peripheral
A. Vibration injury	*a.* Polyneuropathy
B. Direct arterial trauma	*b.* Neurofibromatosis
C. Cold injury	H. Endocrinologic disorder
1. Frostbite	I. Thrombocytosis/hypercoagulability
2. Chronic cold exposure	

Historical Aspects

In 1862, the French physician Maurice Raynaud described a series of patients with finger ischemia which he attributed to vasospasm (1). He was unaware of the existence of palmar and digital arterial occlusive disease and postulated that vasospasm was the principal pathogenetic mechanism based on the finding of a normal radial pulse in most of his patients. Detailed reevaluation of the patients described by Raynaud indicates that most if not all had advanced arterial occlusive disease with associated ischemic digital ulceration. It is likely that none of the patients actually suffered from idiopathic, or spastic, Raynaud's syndrome, as currently defined. Hutchinson was the first to question the theory that digital vasospasm represented a single disease process, and, in 1901, he observed accurately that fixed arterial occlusive disease may be associated with episodic digital vasospasm (2). Thus, by the turn of the century, the two major pathogenetic factors in Raynaud's syndrome, obstruction and spasm, had been identified.

A very important study by Allen and Brown in 1932 addressed the issue of the clinical significance of Raynaud's syndrome (3). They noted that in some patients episodic digital ischemia appeared as an isolated event, while in others the digital vasospasm was associated with a systemic disease process. These investigators categorized the former patients as having Raynaud's disease and the latter as having Raynaud's phenomenon. In the following year, Lewis and Pickering utilized this classification to report that approximately 70 percent of their patients with episodic digital vasospasm (4) had primary Raynaud's disease.

This stratification of episodic digital vasospasm into Raynaud's disease or Raynaud's phenomenon dominated the thinking of the medical community for the next three decades. The recognition of associated diseases appearing long after the onset of supposedly uncomplicated Raynaud's disease was first reported by Gifford and Hines in 1957 (5) and by deTakats and Fowler in 1962 (6), who also noted that earlier methods of diagnosis of associated connective tissue disease were relatively unsophisticated. The development of sensitive laboratory tests in recent years for the detection of immunologic disorders has revealed a surprising variety of subtle abnormalities in many of these patients.

Although the ultimate clinical significance of these immunologic abnormalities is still under investigation, the findings do suggest that any arbitrary classification of patients based on early follow-up data and the clinically evident expression of associated systemic disease is unsatisfactory. Thus, we have abandoned the older arbitrary classification of Raynaud's disease and Raynaud's phenomenon, terms which frequently implied far more than was actually known. We now use the term *Raynaud's syndrome* to describe patients with temperature- or stress-related episodic digital vasospasm. Our present inability to recognize associated abnormalities in certain of these patients may reflect only the inadequacy of our current diagnostic techniques.

Epidemiology

Surprisingly little is known about the prevalence of Raynaud's syndrome in the general population, although preliminary information suggests that it is a common disorder. Undoubtedly, numerous people are troubled by cold sensitivity and do not seek medical attention. Whether or not these mildly affected individuals will exhibit immunologic abnormalities with the same frequency as the more severely affected patients studied in referral centers is unknown. In one study, 22 percent of healthy women aged 21 to 50 years in Copenhagen described symptoms of Raynaud's syndrome (7), while a survey in Oregon revealed that nearly 30 percent of persons interviewed described some cold-induced digital color changes (8). These areas both have cool, damp climates, an observation which may be of considerable importance in the clinical expression of symptoms.

There is a clear predilection for Raynaud's syndrome to affect women. In most series 60 to 90 percent of the patients are female (9). Female patients typically present at a young age and are likely to have either an associated connective tissue disease or the primary form of Raynaud's syndrome without any associated disease process. Men usually develop symptoms of Raynaud's syndrome later in life. Many of these older men have associated arteriosclerosis, with digital symptoms on the basis of palmar and digital atherosclerotic occlusive disease. Raynaud's syndrome appears more prevalent in cooler climates (10). The important issue remains unsettled whether persons in different climates have episodic digital vasospasm with equal frequency but differing climate-related expressivity or whether a cold climate actually causes episodic digital vasospasm with greater frequency.

The only well-studied subsets of the general population are those groups whose occupation is associated with a high incidence of Raynaud's syndrome. Between 40 and 90 percent of workers using certain types of vibratory equipment, such as miners or loggers, develop Raynaud's symptoms (11,12). In one intriguing report correlating cold exposure with the development of Raynaud's syndrome, 50 percent of workers in a fish packing plant exposed to alternating hot and cold temperatures had symptoms of cold sensitivity, while persons exposed to a continuous cold environment had the same low rate of symptoms as the office workers in the same plant (13). Additional clarification of the relationship of environment and occupation to the causation of Raynaud's syndrome has great potential medicolegal significance.

Pathophysiology

Two distinct pathophysiologic mechanisms, arterial obstruction and vasospasm, are capable of producing episodic digital ischemia. Fixed organic obstruction of the palmar or digital arteries, with a resultant decrease in the intraluminal distending pressure, produces vessel closure and complete cessation of blood flow in the face of a normal vasoconstrictive response to cold or emotional stimulation (Figure 57-1). A systolic brachial-to-finger pressure drop of approximately 10 mmHg (with 15 mmHg being the upper limit) is observed in normal individuals (14). A brachial-to-finger gradient of more than 15 mmHg, an absolute finger pressure of less than 70 mmHg, or a difference of more than 15 mmHg between any two fingers implies the presence of significant arterial obstruction (15). In most patients such distal arterial obstructions result either from arteriosclerosis or from

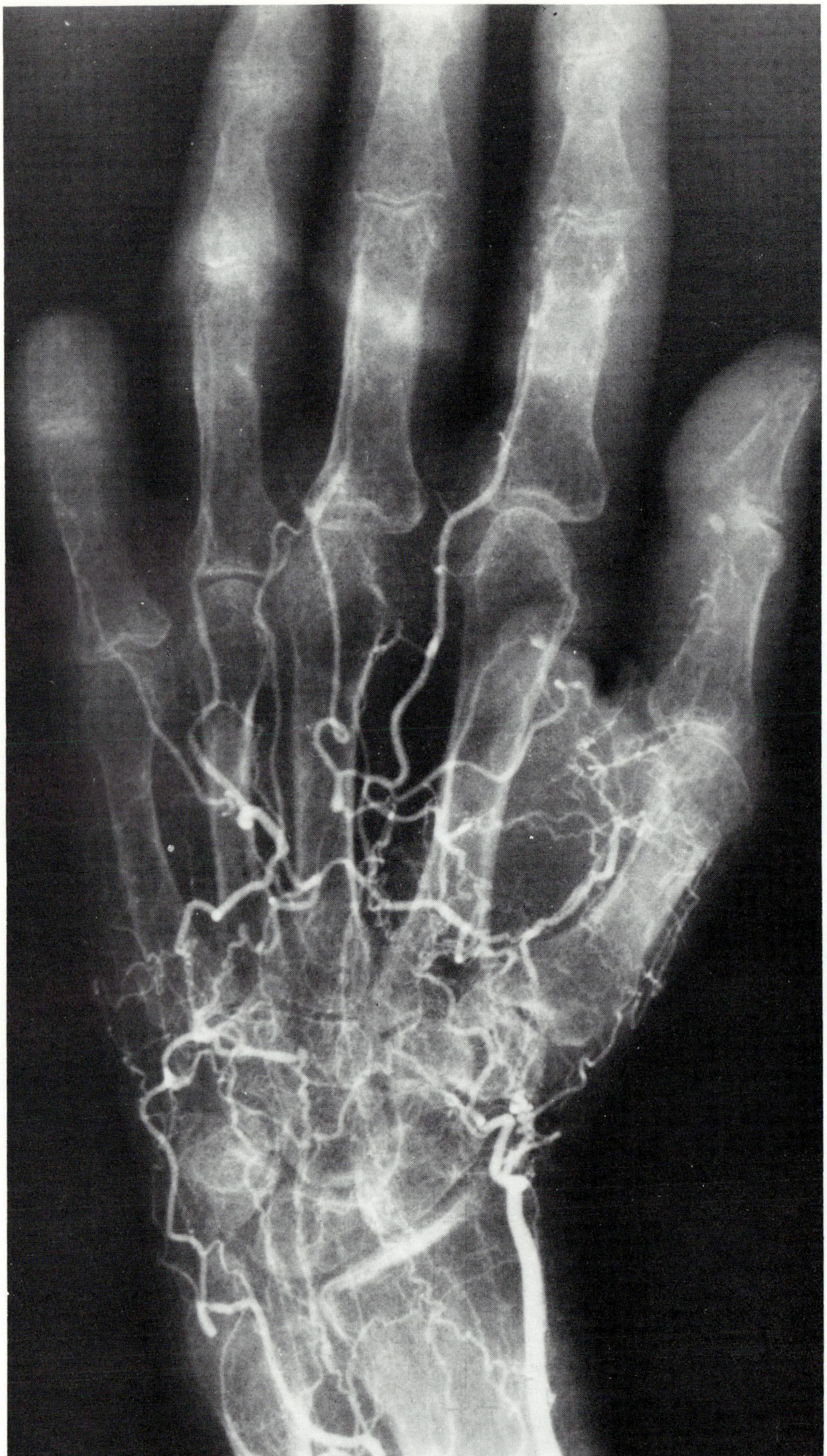

FIGURE 57-1. Resting hand arteriogram of patient with obstructive Raynaud's syndrome showing advanced arterial obstructive disease and associated digital vasospasm.

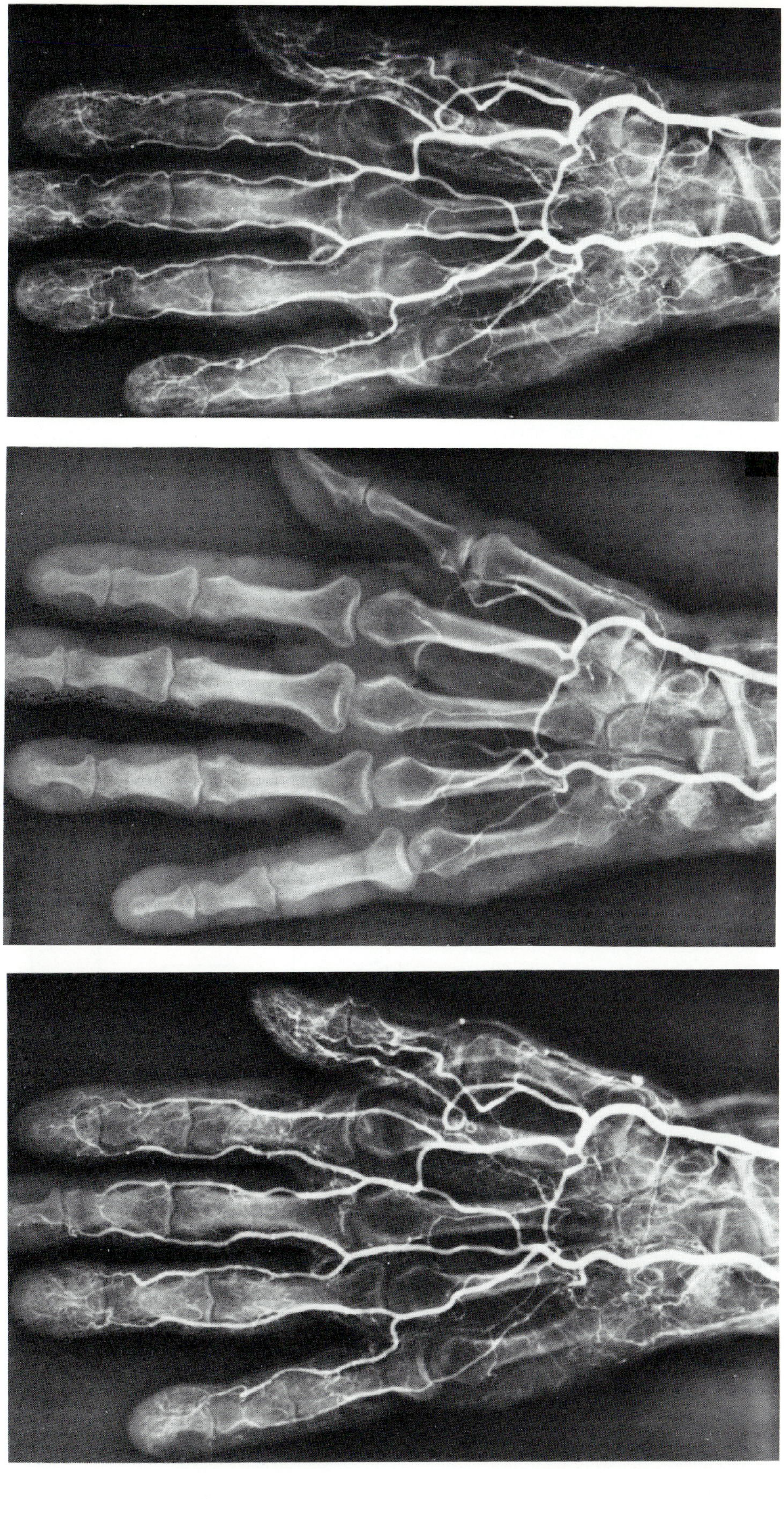

A B C

FIGURE 57-2. (*A*) Hand arteriogram at room temperature of patient with spastic Raynaud's syndrome. No arterial obstruction is present. (*B*) Same patient after hand cold exposure. Marked vasospasm is seen. (*C*) Same patient after hand cold exposure 48 hours after intraarterial reserpine showing complete prevention of cold-induced vasospasm by adrenoreceptor blockade.

end stage arteritis associated with collagen vascular disease. Obstruction of flow to both arteries of a digit is both necessary and sufficient to cause cold sensitivity (16). This explanation predicts that any person with significant palmar and digital arterial obstruction will experience Raynaud's attacks on pronounced cold stimulation. In our experience this is true.

In contrast to the relatively straightforward and quantitative relationship between arterial occlusive disease and Raynaud's syndrome, the pathophysiology of spastic Raynaud's syndrome remains incompletely understood. Plethysmographic and angiographic studies in affected patients clearly demonstrate complete digital artery closure after cold stimulation despite previously normal finger systolic pressures and the absence of arterial obstruction (17–19) (Figure 57-2). These patients clearly have a markedly increased force of cold-induced arterial constriction, a condition Sir Thomas Lewis termed ''local vascular fault'' over a half century ago. The pathophysiology of this increased constrictive force is not understood. Evidence for enhanced adrenergic neuroeffector activity has been suggested by the successful use of sympathetic blocking agents and experimentally by radioisotope clearance studies. Normal fingers subjected to hypothermia will show a decrease in arteriovenous shunt flow without disturbing the nutritional capillary flow. In patients with Raynaud's syndrome, however, both capillary and shunt flow is reduced at low temperatures, an effect which can be blocked by pretreatment with oral reserpine (20,21). These findings suggest that enhanced adrenergic neuroeffector activity is a major factor in the pathophysiology of Raynaud's syndrome. However, many of these findings may also be explained on the basis of a local fault which involves the neuromuscular junction.

The existence of a local fault resulting in intermittent vasospasm is suggested by several observations. The persistence or recurrence of vasospastic symptoms often seen following sympathectomy may be explained by an unaltered defect in the vessel wall, possibly responding to circulating catecholamines. Furthermore, vasospastic events typically occur in isolated and seemingly unrelated vessels, producing such disparate clinical events as variant angina, classic migraine, abdominal migraine, and Raynaud's syndrome. Indeed, in patients with variant angina, Raynaud's syndrome has been observed with five times the frequency seen in a control population (22). Plethysmographic studies have demonstrated an abnormal arterial waveform which appears between attacks in patients with Raynaud's syndrome (23), suggesting a fundamental abnormality of digital artery elasticity.

Alteration of the alpha-adrenergic receptors in vascular smooth muscle, possibly by repeated exposure to cold temperature, has also been implicated (24). Recent evidence in support of this theory has been the demonstration of significantly elevated levels of alpha-2 adrenergic receptors in circulating platelets of patients with vasospastic Raynaud's syndrome when compared to both patients with obstructive Raynaud's syndrome and normal controls as shown in Figure 57-3 (25). While the relationship between receptor levels in platelet membranes and vascular smooth muscle remains to be quantitated in humans, extrapolation from other experimental and clinical models suggests a direct correlation. The existence of an altered adrenergic receptor population may prove to be the fundamental lesion through which any one of a number of factors, such as neurogenic activity, immunologic mediators, or elevated serotonin levels, may result in vasospasm.

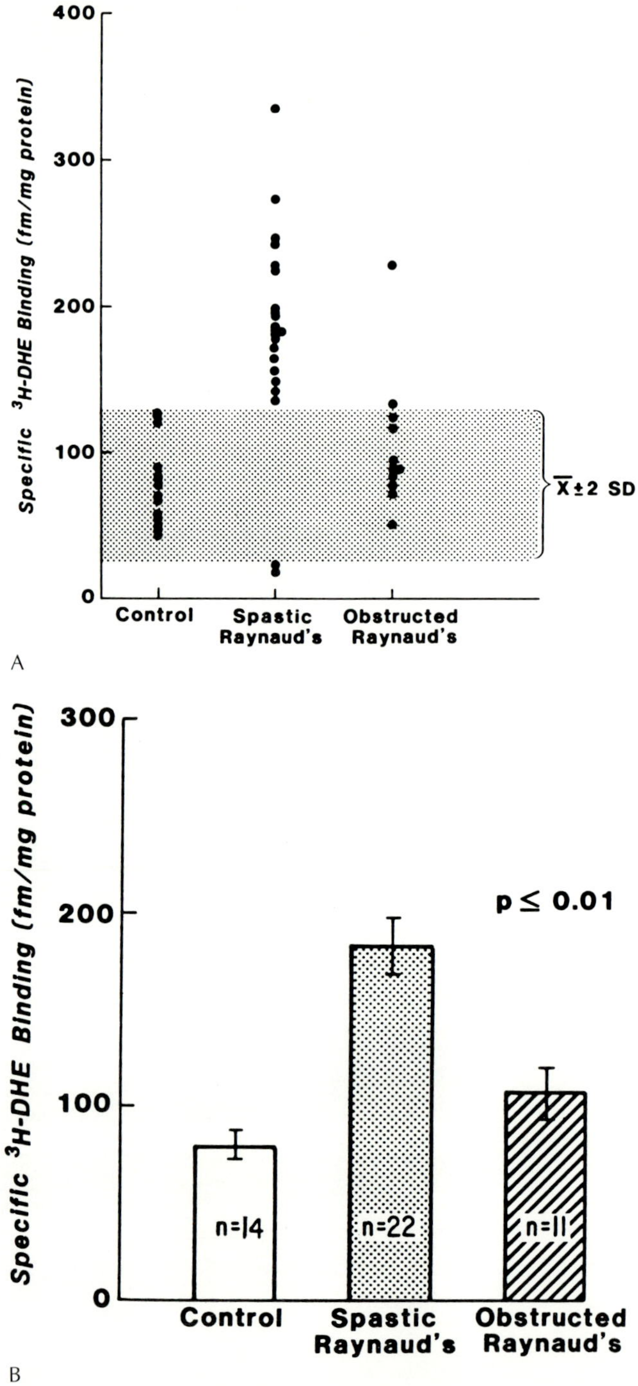

FIGURE 57-3. Range *(A)* and means *(B)* of alpha-2 adrenoreceptor concentration in platelets from normal controls and from patients with Raynaud's syndrome. Note that patients with spastic Raynaud's syndrome have a marked increase of the adrenoreceptor level. [Reprinted with permission of JM Porter, EJ Keenan: Alpha-2 adrenergic receptors in platelets from patients with Raynaud's syndrome (25).]

This may also explain the observation that sympathetic nerve transection is not as effective as adrenergic receptor blockade in relief of symptoms.

Many other factors have been considered in the pathophysiology of Raynaud's syndrome. Alterations in blood viscosity

(26,27), abnormal serum proteins (27–29), elevated serotonin levels (30), and altered arterial shear stress (31,32) have all been demonstrated on occasion in Raynaud's patients. While any of these factors may be significant in isolated cases, their presence is uncommon, inconsistent, and unlikely to be a major factor in the pathogenesis of Raynaud's syndrome in a large majority of patients (8,24,33).

Clinical Presentation

Raynaud's syndrome consists of episodic digital color changes brought on by cold or emotional stimulation. In a classic attack, the sudden cessation of arterial blood flow causes digital pallor (sometimes referred to as "white finger"). Cyanosis appears as a trickle of rapidly desaturated blood enters the subdermal veins. Last, the reactive hyperemia which follows brief periods of ischemia may cause the digits to turn red. Only a few patients experience triphasic digital color changes. Most note only transient digital pallor or cyanosis. Mild pain and paresthesias are frequent complaints, but severe pain is rare. In a typical attack the color change will persist as long as cold exposure continues. Upon rewarming, symptoms generally subside within 10 to 30 minutes. Raynaud's syndrome is generally limited to the upper extremities, although the feet are occasionally involved. Rarely, the toes are the exclusive site of episodic digital color changes.

Raynaud's syndrome may coexist with persistent or chronic forms of digital ischemia. Depending on the associated condition present, persistent digital cyanosis, or painful digital ischemic ulceration occasionally dominates the clinical picture and may be the presenting complaint in patients with long-standing Raynaud's syndrome. Conversely, previously asymptomatic patients presenting with the abrupt onset of hand ischemia, as seen in hypersensitivity angiitis, for example, frequently experience chronic Raynaud's syndrome following resolution of the initial ischemic symptoms (34). It is important to note that digital ulceration is never caused by vasospasm alone. Ulceration always implies widespread palmar and digital arterial obstruction.

Associated Diseases

While episodic digital ischemia defines Raynaud's syndrome, much of its significance relates to its frequent association with other disease processes. The thoroughness with which these associated conditions are sought affects one's perceptions of the clinical importance of Raynaud's syndrome. Episodic digital ischemia may be the first symptom of a systemic illness which may otherwise be silent in the early phase and which may be suggested initially only by subtle alterations in sensitive diagnostic tests. A list of the diseases which have been reported in association with Raynaud's syndrome is found in Table 57-1.

In some instances the relationship between the associated disease and Raynaud's syndrome is clearly causal, while in others they merely share some common pathophysiologic mechanism. In some circumstances the association may be coincidental. The immunologic and connective tissue diseases are by far the most frequent of associated diseases and are found in approximately 50 percent of referral populations (6,8,35). Approximately one-third of the patients in this group will have scleroderma, while mixed connective tissue disease, systemic lupus erythematosus (SLE), rheumatoid arthritis, Sjögren's syndrome, polyarteritis nodosa, polymyositis, and dermatomyositis are present in a smaller percentage of patients. A significant portion of this group, perhaps one-fourth of the total, presents with undifferentiated or overlap connective tissue disorders (i.e., evidence of target organ or tissue involvement without the pattern of a classically described syndrome) or with significant and persistent serologic abnormalities suggestive of immunologic disease but without initially identifiable end-organ involvement. Raynaud's syndrome is present in about 80 percent of patients with scleroderma or mixed connective tissue disease, 25 percent of rheumatoid arthritics, and 20 percent of patients with SLE (6,36,37). The associated diseases found in our most recently tabulated 307 patients with Raynaud's syndrome are shown in Table 57-2.

The pathophysiology of Raynaud's syndrome in patients with autoimmune diseases appears to vary among patients and even in the same individual at different points in the illness. Vasospasm is often seen early in the course of the disease. Patients with long-standing autoimmune disease frequently have a significant degree of palmar and digital arterial obstruction, presumably from associated vasculitis with direct destruction of the arterial wall. The role of circulating factors such as antigen-antibody complexes in producing cold sensitivity is entirely speculative at the present time but may eventually prove to be highly significant.

Large-vessel arterial obstructive disorders form another important category of associated diseases, seen in approximately 10 percent of referred patients with Raynaud's syndrome (38). Atherosclerosis is widespread in the general population and may

TABLE 57-2. Associated Disorders Found in 309 Patients with Raynaud's Syndrome, 1970–1981

Number of patients	307
Connective tissue disease:	
Scleroderma/CREST syndrome	57
Mixed connective tissue disease	12
Systemic lupus erythematosus	9
Rheumatoid arthritis	3
Sjögren's syndrome	6
Polyarteritis nodosa	2
Undifferentiated connective tissue disease/overlap syndrome	27
Suspected connective tissue disease	30
Total	146
Obstructive disease without immunologic disturbance	22
Trauma	23
Medication-induced	4
Miscellaneous causes	24
Idiopathic Raynaud's syndrome	88

cause episodic cold-induced digital ischemia if sufficiently severe to cause decreased resting digital pressure. Buerger's disease presents with upper extremity symptoms including Raynaud's syndrome in 20 percent of cases (39). Digital vasospasm is seen occasionally in thoracic outlet syndrome (9) and may be either spastic or obstructive. The spastic variety may result from irritation of sympathetic nerves. Obstructive Raynaud's syndrome in this setting may result from palmar or digital artery emboli from subclavian artery injury or aneurysm which occasionally accompanies thoracic outlet syndrome.

Vascular trauma from a variety of sources may result in symptoms of intermittent digital ischemia. The pathophysiology in such cases is usually poorly understood. While severe injury such as blunt trauma or frostbite generally causes arterial occlusions, both vasospastic and obstructive lesions likely have a role in more subtle trauma, such as that associated with vibration injury or chronic cold exposure (40–43).

Several pharmaceutical agents have been reported to cause or exacerbate Raynaud's syndrome. Both ergot preparations and beta-adrenergic blocking drugs may cause or exacerbate Raynaud's symptoms in certain patients. The pathophysiology of Raynaud's syndrome in patients taking cytotoxic drugs or birth control pills is not well established. In the case of birth control pills, the association may have been coincidental, devoid of any cause-and-effect relationship.

There are a variety of other conditions, as noted in Table 57-1, which have been found in smaller numbers of patients with Raynaud's syndrome. Most of these disorders are capable of producing certain alterations of coagulation, hemorrheology, or vessel reactivity which may occasionally induce Raynaud's syndrome. Therefore, while the pathogenetic relationships have not always been established with certainty, a causal association is still presumed to exist in the large majority of these conditions.

Finally, a significant minority of patients will still have an apparently idiopathic form of Raynaud's syndrome without any associated disease process. This group invariably has spastic Raynaud's syndrome. In our recent experience 30 percent of Raynaud's patients fall into this group. The overall prognosis for idiopathic Raynaud's syndrome appears quite good. However, this category of disease still requires longitudinal study, because occasional patients will prove to have significant systemic illness following a long period of supposedly uncomplicated episodic digital vasospasm.

Ischemic Digital Ulceration

Ischemic digital ulceration occurs infrequently. In the course of treating over 500 patients with Raynaud's syndrome in the past decade, we have encountered 48 patients with ischemic digital ulceration. The associated diseases seen in this patient group are listed in Table 57-3. It is clear that digital ulceration never results from vasospasm alone. The existence of ulceration always implies widespread palmar and digital arterial obstruction. In our experience, the three most common causes of such hand arterial obstruction are hypersensitivity angiitis, arteriosclerosis, and scleroderma including the CREST (Chondrocalcinosis, Raynaud's, Esophageal motility disturbance, Sclerodactyly, Telangiectasias) variant. Hypersensitivity angiitis, originally described from this institution as a cause of isolated hand ischemia, may constitute a variant of Buerger's disease (34).

TABLE 57-3. Associated Disorders Found in 48 Patients with Ischemic Digital Ulceration

Scleroderma	20
Hypersensitivity angiitis	18
Arteriosclerosis	8
Other	2

Occasional patients may develop digital ischemic ulcers as a result of emboli from proximal arterial lesions, including such sources as proximal subclavian arteriosclerosis, subclavian stenosis or aneurysm from thoracic outlet syndrome, or axillary or brachial atherosclerotic disease. Even in this setting, however, the digital ulceration results from occlusion of the palmar and digital arteries from embolic debris. Proximal arterial disease without distal embolization rarely, if ever, produces digital ulceration.

Diagnostic Studies

Since the only requirement for the diagnosis of Raynaud's syndrome is a history of cold or emotionally induced episodic digital color changes, diagnostic studies should be directed toward precise quantification of the degree of ischemia and the identification of associated disorders. The history is the most important aspect of the initial interview and will substantially direct the course and extent of additional investigations. A history of arthralgias, tight skin, rashes or telangiectasias, dysphagia, xerostomia, or xerophthalmia may suggest a connective tissue disorder. Symptoms of large-vessel peripheral vascular disease, exposure to trauma, or history of malignancy should be sought. A complete medication profile is essential. The physical examination is frequently normal, but attention should be directed to the quality of the pulses, the presence of digital ulcerations, joint changes, telangiectasias, or skin tightening.

The occlusive digital hypothermic challenge test (18) is useful in confirming the diagnosis of Raynaud's syndrome. This test measures digital blood pressure after local cooling. A decrease of digital blood pressure of 20 percent or greater is considered positive. The test is 90 percent sensitive and 90 percent specific for Raynaud's syndrome.

A minimal laboratory evaluation is important in the initial evaluation of patients with Raynaud's syndrome. A complete blood count and erythrocyte sedimentation rate should be obtained, as well as a urinalysis and chemistry profile. A serum rheumatoid factor and screening antinuclear antibody test are of sufficient value to be included in the baseline evaluation. The antinuclear antibody test is most sensitive when performed on two separate substrates (44). Roentgenograms of the hands are most helpful in detecting sclerodactyly, tuft resorption, arthritis, and calcinosis and should be included as part of the initial evaluation.

Additional laboratory studies should be performed selectively, based upon the results of the initial evaluation. These may include quantitative serum immunoglobulin or complement determination, cine-esophagography, or nerve conduction studies in selected patients. Arteriography of the upper extremity is commonly employed in patients undergoing evaluation in referral centers. The relative degrees of vasospasm and arterial obstruction and the response to various forms of treatment can easily be demonstrated by this procedure (19). However, because of the extremely good correlation between arteriography and noninvasive studies (45), the role of angiography is currently limited to the diagnosis of more proximal arterial disease for which surgical correction is contemplated.

Hand arteriography, while not mandatory in patients with Raynaud's syndrome, should be routinely obtained in the evaluation of patients with digital ischemic ulceration. Arteriography in this setting is not obtained to document the palmar and digital arterial occlusions known to be present, but to detect any proximal arterial lesions which may be a source for distal emboli and which may be amenable to arterial reconstruction.

Digital plethysmography with digital blood pressure determination is extremely useful in the evaluation and management of patients with Raynaud's syndrome. These tests are essential in differentiating spastic from obstructive Raynaud's syndrome. The noninvasive vascular studies provide valuable information on the mechanisms of disease and the effects of treatment in a cost-effective fashion (46).

Medical Therapy

Regardless of the presence of underlying disease which may also warrant treatment, most patients with Raynaud's syndrome will require some form of therapy directed specifically to their episodic digital ischemia. The majority of patients with mild to moderate symptoms will respond to cold and tobacco avoidance occasionally supplemented with pharmacologic support during the winter. While the role of cold exposure in the causation of episodic digital vasospasm is uncertain, the avoidance of low temperatures and the wearing of warm gloves during the winter months clearly constitute an important part of the treatment of Raynaud's syndrome. A permanent change of climate or occupation is seldom indicated; however, those persons with prominent occupational exposure to cold temperatures may not respond symptomatically until the exposure is reduced. The use of ergot preparations or beta-blocking drugs is relatively contraindicated in patients with Raynaud's syndrome, especially when an equally effective alternative medication is readily available (47–49).

Sympatholytic drugs have traditionally formed the mainstay of the pharmacologic treatment of Raynaud's syndrome. The effectiveness of these medications, as well as that of others used in the treatment of episodic digital ischemia, is limited by the presence of advanced arterial occlusive disease and by the appearance of side effects related to the nonselectivity of these agents with respect to their site of action. Spastic Raynaud's syndrome traditionally and predictably responds much better to medication than does the obstructive syndrome.

Oral reserpine, in daily doses of 0.25 to 0.5 mg, has had the widest clinical use, having been first used in the treatment of Raynaud's syndrome in 1960 (50). Oral doses up to 1.0 mg daily have been used successfully (51). Other sympatholytics, such as methyldopa, 1.5 to 2.0 mg/day, or tolazoline, 150 to 200 mg/day, have been relatively effective oral agents (52,53), but the large doses frequently required have often produced unpleasant side effects. Similarly, the potent drugs guanethidine, 30 to 50 mg/day, and phenoxybenzamine in variable dosages have been used successfully (54,55) but have frequently produced significant side effects at the doses required when used as a single agent. Prazosin is a new agent with alpha-1 adrenergic blocking activity and has been used effectively at the relatively low dose of 1.0 mg twice daily (56). In an effort to reduce the incidence and severity of side effects, investigators have used a combination of low doses of guanethidine (10 mg/day) and prazosin (1 to 2 mg/day) with satisfactory results for both episodic and persistent digital ischemia with ulcer formation (16,57). It is critical to note that the described drug benefits in Raynaud's syndrome rest almost exclusively on anecdotal data, usually the patient's subjective impression of benefit. Only a few double-blind trials have been reported, and these have generally shown disappointing results. Unfortunately there is currently no test allowing the objective assessment of drug benefit.

The use of the direct vasodilators in the treatent of Raynaud's syndrome has been generally unsuccessful. Evaluation of agents such as isoxsuprine and griseofulvin, an antifungal agent with direct vasodilating properties (58), has yielded inconsistent results (59,60). Other vasodilators such as papaverine and niacin have been studied in large-vessel peripheral vascular disease of the lower extremity but have not been used widely in the management of Raynaud's syndrome. Drugs with beta-adrenoreceptor stimulating properties have been tried, but without substantial benefit. The use of these drugs may actually result in a net reduction in cutaneous blood flow (61).

Nifedipine is a potent vasodilator belonging to the relatively recently introduced group of compounds described as calcium channel blocking agents. Subjective improvement has been noted in 50 to 60 percent of patients with doses between 30 and 60 mg/day in two reports (62,63), with confirmation by objective measurement of vasospastic response to cold reentry documented in a controlled double-blind study (64). Nifedipine is currently our single agent of choice in the treatment of spastic Raynaud's syndrome.

While the large majority of patients with mild to moderate digital vasospastic symptoms require no treatment beyond general supportive measures and the oral pharmacologic agents discussed above, the small group of patients with severe disease, including persistent digital ischemia, has prompted investigation of unconventional forms of therapy. One should note, however, that many patients with severe digital ischemia including finger

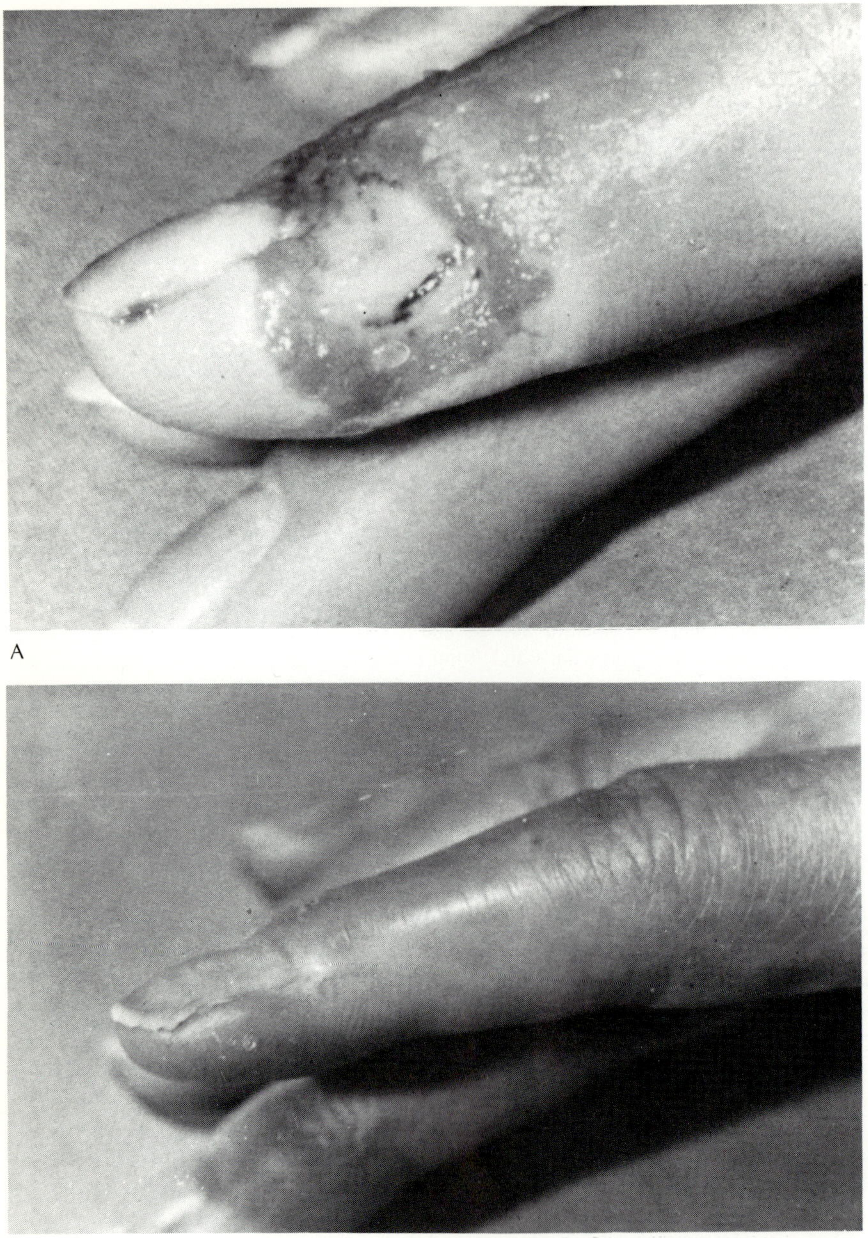

A

B

FIGURE 57-4. *(A)* Painful digital ulcer in patient with obstructive Raynaud's syndrome with widespread palmar and digital arterial obstruction. *(B)* Same patient 3 months later showing complete healing following conservative treatment with soap and water scrubs and antibiotics.

ulcerations still respond to traditional conservative management when this is applied with patience and careful attention to established surgical principles (Figure 57-4). For these patients, the most critical factor in their prognosis has unequivocally been their ability to refrain from further use of tobacco (57).

Historically, the intraarterial injection of reserpine, 0.5 mg, has had the longest clinical use of any of the more aggressive nonsurgical therapies, being first introduced in 1967 (65). Since then, several studies have confirmed the effectiveness of intraarterial reserpine in the treatment of Raynaud's syndrome, although claims for the duration of effect have ranged from a few days to several months (66–69). This procedure has been used both in patients with severe vasospasm as well as in those with persistent digital ischemia who have severe pain, cyanosis, or ulceration, conditions which always imply arterial obstruction. While the actual pharmacologic vasodilatory effect is probably limited to a few days, symptomatic improvement may persist once the spasm is relieved or the ulcer is healed.

To circumvent the problems associated with intraarterial injections, a technique for the regional administration of reserpine has been evaluated in which intravenous reserpine, 0.5 to 1.0 mg, is used (70). In a fashion analogous to the Bier block administration of regional anesthetics, the reserpine is injected into an exsanguinated, tourniquet-controlled extremity and allowed to diffuse into the local tissues before the tourniquet is released. Results achieved with this procedure have been equivalent to those with intraarterial reserpine. No one has ever convincingly demonstrated vasospasm in patients with ischemic digital ulcerations, which are always caused by arterial occlusive disease; therefore, the widespread use of vasodilator drugs in this setting does not rest on a solid pathophysiologic foundation.

The prostaglandins are a relatively new group of therapeutic agents which may have a limited role in the treatment of digital ischemia. Prostaglandin E_1 is a potent vasodilator and platelet antiaggregation agent which has been employed specifically for severe upper extremity vasospasm and arterial occlusive disease with anecdotal salutary effects in some patients so treated (71). Prostacyclin (prostaglandin I_2) is both a vasodilator and an inhibitor of platelet aggregation synthesized in the wall of normal blood vessels and has been shown to be of modest benefit in patients with ischemic lesions of the lower extremities (72). No trials have yet been reported, however, using prostacyclin for the treatment of upper extremity vasospastic disease. The utility of the prostaglandins is currently limited not only by lack of selectivity but also by lack of an oral preparation. Furthermore, intravenous infusion produces a severe local inflammatory response necessitating the use of a central venous catheter.

Anecdotal reports have indicated occasional benefit from the use of various agents which reduce blood viscosity, fibrinogen concentration, or platelet activity (73–77). Plasmapheresis has also been used in some patients with Raynaud's syndrome with satisfactory results, causing a reduction in whole blood viscosity and an improvement in erythrocyte deformability index (78). All of these modalities presume a significant pathogenetic role for hemorrheologic factors, a finding which has not been common in well-studied patients in large series. Reports of anecdotal improvement following treatment for a disease which is episodic in its natural history must be interpreted cautiously.

Ischemic digital ulcers are best managed with gentle soap and water scrubs, antibiotics as determined by culture reports, and conservative surgical debridement. The effect of vasodilator therapy has never been precisely determined, since the importance of any episodic arteriospasm in the setting of widespread small-artery occlusion is unknown. Vasodilators are frequently administered in the treatment of digital ischemic ulceration, but their use in such a setting remains anecdotal. We routinely prescribe nifedipine, 10 mg three times daily, for this condition. Intravenous Bier block reserpine frequently appears anecdotally beneficial.

Surgical Therapy

Sympathetic denervation of the upper extremity has been practiced for several decades as part of the treatment of Raynaud's syndrome. The second through fourth or fifth thoracic ganglia are usually removed, with care being taken to preserve the stellate ganglion and the cervical sympathetic chain. The fundamental drawback to this procedure has been the recurrence of symptoms following early improvement (79–81). Presumably, the well-known phenomenon of hypersensitivity to circulating catecholamines following denervation plays some role in the reappearance of vascular instability. Regeneration of sympathetic nerves has also been considered but never demonstrated. More likely, a complete sympathetic denervation of the upper extremity is rarely, if ever, actually accomplished. Residual autonomic fibers to the arm may be carried with the first thoracic nerve as well as the lower thoracic nerves and the presence of these fibers may preclude a thorough sympathectomy (82–84).

The reported rate of improvement following sympathectomy for Raynaud's syndrome has varied widely in different series. The surgical series have been quite variable depending upon the severity of symptoms, the duration of follow-up, the presence of associated disease, and the clinical criteria by which success is judged. Most observers have noted better results for idiopathic Raynaud's syndrome, while the presence of an associated connective tissue disorder greatly diminishes the prospect for long-term improvement (6,80,85). Curiously, the reported outcome does not appear to be influenced by the relative degrees of vasospasm and arterial obstruction (6,80). In general, patients with milder symptoms respond best to sympathectomy, while those patients with severe disease derive the least long-term benefit. The experience with surgery, as related to severity of disease, has generally paralleled the results of conservative medical management. When sympathectomy is applied to those patients with persistent digital ischemia and finger ulcers, the operation is generally deemed successful if the ulcer resolves. However, in our experience, a similar number of patients with digital ulcers respond to local debridement and pharmacologic therapy (57,70). Furthermore, the frequent recurrence of ulcers in patients with severe Raynaud's syndrome or persistent digital ischemia requires medical management anyway in the previously sympathectomized patient. These considerations have compelled us to abandon cervicothoracic sympathectomy as a rational or effective therapeutic option for upper extremity ischemia.

Microsurgical techniques have been used to achieve a localized sympathectomy in patients with Raynaud's syndrome. Digital artery sympathectomy, involving division of the terminal branches of the sympathetic nerves and adventitial stripping of the digital arteries, has been described (86,87). Since this procedure, like proximal sympathectomy, does not address the fundamental pathophysiology at the receptor level, the rationale is difficult to comprehend. Obstructive arterial lesions distal to the brachial artery have also been directly approached with microsurgical procedures (88). Vein interposition grafts to occluded portions of radial, ulnar, and palmar arteries have been associated with healing of ischemic lesions (87,89) However, the similar good results of medical therapy and the problems with long-term patency of microvascular bypass grafts will undoubtedly relegate this procedure to a very small role in the treatment of hand ischemia.

The only patients for whom gratifying surgical results may be expected constitute that small subgroup with digital ischemia on the basis of some proximal source of vascular insufficiency. Proximal obstruction from atherosclerosis, trauma, neoplasms, thoracic outlet syndrome, or other causes generally responds satisfactorily to appropriate revascularization techniques (88,90).

Overview

Raynaud's syndrome defines a clinical condition characterized by episodic digital vasospasm as manifested by digital color changes of pallor or cyanosis. The condition appears extraordinarily common in western civilization, affecting to some degree as much as 20 percent of the population in areas with cool, damp climates. Current evidence indicates two different pathophysiologic mechanisms in the production of Raynaud's attacks. In some patients an attack results from an increased force of cold-induced digital artery muscular contraction. New evidence suggests that the primary abnormality in such patients may reside in the neuromuscular end plate with an abnormal preponderance of alpha-2 adrenoreceptors. In other patients digital artery spasm appears to result from a normal constrictive response to cold occurring in an artery with diminished intraluminal pressure resulting from proximal arterial obstructive disease.

Associated disease accompanies Raynaud's syndrome in about 70 percent of affected patients who are sufficiently symptomatic to present for treatment, with the collagen vascular diseases being the most frequently associated conditions detected. Digital ischemic ulceration does not result from vasospasm. Such ulcerations always imply the coexistence of widespread palmar and digital artery obstructive disease.

Drug treatment of Raynaud's syndrome is infrequently required. The most effective agent in our experience is oral nifedipine, which produces subjective improvement in 50 to 60 percent of patients treated. Surgical sympathectomy appears of little benefit in these patients and is not currently recommended for either the treatment of Raynaud's syndrome or the digital ischemic ulceration.

References

1. Raynaud M: On local asphyxia and symmetrical gangrene of the extremities. In *Selected Monographs*. London, New Sydenham Society, 1888.
2. Hutchinson J: Raynaud's phenomena. Med Press Circular 1901, 123:402–405.
3. Allen EV, Brown GE: Raynaud's disease: A critical review of minimal requisites for diagnosis. Am J Med Sci 1932, 183:187–200.
4. Lewis T, Pickering GW: Observations upon maladies in which the blood supply to digits ceases intermittently, and upon bilateral gangrene of digits. Observations relevant to so-called "Raynaud's disease." Clin Sci 1933, 1:327–366.
5. Gifford RW Jr, Hines EA Jr: Raynauds disease among women and girls. Circulation 1957, 16:1012–1021.
6. deTakats G, Fowler EF: Raynaud's phenomenon. JAMA 1962, 179:99–106.
7. Olsen N, Nielsen SL: Prevalence of primary Raynaud phenomena in young females. Scand J Clin Lab Invest 1978; 37:761–764.
8. Porter JM, Rivers SP, Anderson CJ, Baur GM: Evaluation and management of patients with Raynaud's syndrome. Am J Surg 1981, 142:183–189.
9. Spittell JA Jr: Raynaud's phenomenon and allied vasospastic conditions. In Fairbairn JF, Juergens JL, Spittell JA Jr (eds): Allen-Barker-Hines *Peripheral Vascular Diseases*. Philadelphia, Saunders, 1972, pp 387–419.
10. Holling HE: Digital ischemia. In Holling HE (ed): *Peripheral Vascular Disease: Diagnoses and Management*. Philadelphia, Lippincott, 1972, pp 137–161.
11. Taylor W, Pelmear PL: Raynaud's phenomenon of occupational origin: An epidemiologic survey. Acta Chir Scand 1976, 465(Suppl):27–32.
12. Chatterjce DS, Petrie A, Taylor W: Prevalence of vibration-induced white finger in Hourspar miners in Weardale. Br J Ind Med 1978, 35:208–228.
13. Mackiewisz A, Piskorz A: Raynaud's phenomenon following long-term repeated action of great differences of temperature. J Cardiovasc Surg 1977, 18:151–154.
14. Hirai M: Cold sensitivity of the hand in arterial occlusive disease. Surgery 1979, 85:140–146.
15. Downs AR, Gaskell P, Morrow I, Munson CL: Assessment of arterial obstruction in vessels supplying the fingers by measurement of local blood pressures and the skin temperature response test—correlation with angiographic evidence. Surgery 1975, 77:530–539.
16. Rivers SP, Porter JM: Clinical approach to Raynaud's syndrome. Vasc Diag Ther 1983, 4:15–24.
17. Krahenbuhl B, Nielsen SL, Lassen NA: Closure of digital arteries in high vascular tone states as demonstrated by measurement of systolic blood pressure in the fingers. Scand J Clin Lab Invest 1977, 37:71–76.
18. Nielsen SL, Lassen NA: Measurement of digital blood pressure after local cooling. J Appl Physiol 1977, 43:907–910.
19. Rosch J, Porter JM, Gralino BJ: Cryodynamic hand angiography in the diagnosis and management of Raynaud's syndrome. Radiology 1977, 55:807–814.
20. Coffman JP, Cohen AS: Total and capillary fingertip blood flow in Raynaud's phenomenon. N Engl J Med, 1971, 285:259–263.
21. Coffman JD: Total and nutritional blood flow in the finger. Clin Sci 1972, 42:243–250.
22. Miller D, Waters DD, Warnica W, Szlachcic J, Kreeft J, Theroux P: Is variant angina the coronary manifestation of a generalized vasospastic disorder? N Engl J Med 1981, 304:763–766.
23. Sumner DS, Strandness DE Jr: An abnormal finger pulse associated with cold sensitivity. Am Surg 1972, 175:294–298.
24. Jamieson GG, Ludbrook J, Wilson A: Cold hypersensitivity in Raynaud's phenomenon. Circulation 1971, 44:254–264.
25. Keenan EJ, Porter JM: Alpha-2 adrenergic receptors in platelets from patients with Raynaud's syndrome. Surgery 1983, 94:204–209.
26. Goyle KG, Dormancy JA: Abnormal blood viscosity in Raynaud's phenomenon. Lancet 1976, 1:1317–1318.
27. Tietjen GW, Chien S, Leroy C, Gavras I, Gavras H, Crump FE: Blood viscosity, plasma proteins, and Raynaud's syndrome. Arch Surg 1975, 110:1343–1346.
28. O'Reilly MJG, Talpos G, Robert VC, White JM, Cotton LT: Controlled trial of plasma exchange in treatment of Raynaud's syndrome. Br Med J 1979, 1:1113–1115.
29. Okada A, Yamashita T, Nagano C, Ikeda T, Yachi A, Shibata S: Studies on the diagnosis and pathogenesis of Raynaud's phenomenon of occupational origin. Br J Ind Med 1971, 28:353–357.
30. Halpern A, Kuhn PH, Shaftel HE, Samuels SS, Shaftel N, Selman D, Birch HG: Raynaud's disease, Raynaud's phenomenon, and serotonin. Angiology 1960, 11:151–167.
31. Nerem RM: Vibration-induced arterial shear stress: The relationship to Raynaud's phenomenon of occupational origin. Arch Environ Health 1973, 26:105–110.
32. Schmid-Schonbein H: Critical closing pressure or yield shear stress as the cause of disturbed peripheral circulation? Acta Chir Scand 1976, 465(suppl):10–19.
33. Halperin JL, Coffman JD: Pathophysiology of Raynaud's disease. Arch Intern Med 1979, 139:89–92.
34. Baur GM, Porter JM, Bardana EJ, Wesche DH, Rosch J: Rapid

onset of hand ischemia of unknown etiology: Clinical evaluation and followup of ten patients. Ann Surg 1977, 186:184–189.
35. Velayos EE, Robinson H, Porciuncula FU, Masi AT: Clinical correlation analysis of 137 patients with Raynaud's phenomenon. Am J Med Sci 1971, 262:347–356.
36. Strandness DE Jr: Episodic digital ischemia. In Strandness DE Jr (ed): *Peripheral Arterial Disease: A Physiologic Approach*. Boston, Little, Brown, 1969, 265–278.
37. Porter JM, Bardana EJ Jr, Baur GM, Wesche DH, Andrasch RH, Rosch J: The clinical significance of Raynaud's syndrome. Surgery 1976, 80:756–764.
38. Rivers SP, Porter JM: Management of Raynaud's syndrome. In Bergan JJ (ed): *Clinical Surgery International*. New York: Churchill Livingstone, 1984, pp 185–200.
39. Hill GL, Moelino J, Tumewee F, Brataamadja D, Tohardi A: The Buerger syndrome in Java: A description of the clinical syndrome and some aspects of its aetiology. Br J Surg 1973, 60:606–613.
40. James PB, Galloway RW: Arteriography of the hand in men exposed to vibration. In Taylor W, Pelmear PL (eds): *Vibration White Finger in Industry*. London, Academic, 1975, pp 31–41.
41. Azuma T, Ohhashi T, Salsaguchi M: An approach to the pathogenesis of "white finger" induced by vibratory stimulation: Acute but sustained changes in vascular responsiveness of canine hindlimb to noradrenaline. Cardiovasc Res 1980, 14:725–730.
42. Adams T, Smith RE: Effect of chronic cold exposure on finger temperature responses. J Appl Physiol 1962, 17:317–322.
43. Buchanan JL, Cranley JJ Jr, Linton RR: Observations on the direct effect of cold on blood vessels in the human extremity and its relation to peripheral vascular disease. Surgery 1952, 31:62–73.
44. Anderson CJ, Bardana EJ, Porter JM, Bennett RM: Anticentromere and other antinuclear antibodies in Raynaud's syndrome. Clin Res 1980, 28:76A.
45. Yao JST, Gourmos C, Paypathanasiou K, Iruine WT: A method for assessing ischemia of the hand and fingers. Surg Gynecol Obstet 1972, 135:373–378.
46. Holmgren K, Baur GM, Porter JM: The role of digital plethysmography in the evaluation of Raynaud's syndrome. Bruit 1981, 5:19–24.
47. Henry LG, Blackwood JS, Couley JE, Bernhard VM: Ergotism. Arch Surg 1975, 110:929–932.
48. Muller-Schweinitzer E: Responsiveness of isolated canine cerebral and peripheral arteries to ergotamine. Arch Pharmacol 1976, 292:113–118.
49. Frolich ED, Tarayi RC, Duston HP: Peripheral arterial insufficiency a complication of beta-adrenergic blocking therapy. JAMA 1969, 208:2471–2472.
50. Peacock JH: The treatment of primary Raynaud's disease of the upper limb. Lancet 1960, 2:65.
51. Kontos HA, Wasserman AJ: Effect of reserpine in Raynaud's phenomenon. Circulation 1969, 39:259–266.
52. Coffman JD: Effect of vasodilator drugs in vasoconstricted normal subjects. J Clin Pharmacol 1968, 8:302–308.
53. Varadi DP, Lawrence AM: Suppression of Raynaud's phenomenon by methyldopa. Arch Intern Med 1969, 124:13–18.
54. Gifford RW Jr: Reserpine and Raynaud's phenomenon (editorial). N Engl J Med 1971, 285:290–291.
55. Leroy EC, Downey JA, Cannon PJ: Skin capillary blood flow in scleroderma. J Clin Invest 1971, 50:930–939.
56. Waldo R: Prazosin relieves Raynaud's vasospasm. JAMA 1979, 241–1037.
57. Taylor LM Jr, Baur GM, Porter J: Finger gangrene caused by small artery occlusive disease. Ann Surg 1981, 193:453–461.
58. Rubin A: Coronary vascular effects of griseofulvin. JAMA 1963, 185:971.
59. Wesseling H, denHeeten A, Wouda AA: Sublingual and oral isoxuprine in patients with Raynaud's phenomenon. Eur J Clin Pharmacol 1981, 20:329–333.
60. Charles CR, Cormick ES: Skin temperature changes in Raynaud's disease after griseofulvin. Arch Dermatol 1970, 101:331–336.
61. Coffman JD: Vasodilated drugs in peripheral vascular disease. N Engl J Med 1979, 300:713–718.
62. Kahan A, Weber S, Amor B, Saporta L, Hodara M, Degeorges M: Nifedipine and Raynaud's phenomenon (letter). Ann Intern Med 1981, 94:546.
63. Tyburczy J, Porter J: Nifedipine treatment of Raynaud's syndrome, unpublished data, 1983.
64. Rodeheffer RJ, Rommer JA, Wigley F, Smith CR: Controlled double-blind trial of nifedipine in the treatment of Raynaud's phenomenon. N Engl J Med 1983, 308:880–883.
65. Abboud FM, Eckstein JW, Lawrence MS, Hoak JC: Preliminary observations on the use of intra-arterial reserpine in Raynaud's phenomenon. Circulation 1967, 2:49.
66. Nobin BA, Nielsen SL, Eklov B, Lassen NA: Reserpine treatment of Raynaud's disease. Ann Surg 1978, 187:12–16.
67. Willerson JT, Thompson RH, Hookman P, Herdt J, Decker JL: Reserpine in Raynaud's disease and phenomenon: Short-term responses to intraarterial injection. Ann Intern Med 1970, 72:17–27.
68. Acevedo A, Reginato AJ, Schnell AM: Effect of intra-arterial reserpine in patients suffering from Raynaud's phenomenon. J Cardiovasc Surg 1978, 19:77–84.
69. Tindall JP, Whalen RE, Burton EE Jr: Medical uses of intra-arterial injections of reserpine: Treatment of Raynaud's syndrome and of some vascular insufficiencies of the lower extremities. Arch Dermatol 1974, 110:233–237.
70. Taylor LM Jr, Rivers SP, Keller FS, Baur GM, Porter JM: Treatment of finger ischemia with Bier block reserpine. Surg Gynecol Obstet 1982, 154:39–43.
71. Clifford PC, Martin MFR, Sheddon EJ, Kirby JD, Baird RN, Dieppe PA: Treatment of vasospastic disease with prostaglandin E_1. Br Med J 1980, 281:1031–1034.
72. Szczeklik A, Cryglewski RJ, Nizankowski R, Skawinski S, Ghiszki P, Korbut R: Prostacyclin therapy in peripheral arterial disease. Thromb Res 1980, 19:191–199.
73. Holti G: The effect of intermittent low molecular dextran infusions upon the digital circulation in systemic sclerosis. Br J Dermatol 1965, 77:560–568.
74. Jarrett PEM, Morland M, Browse NL: Treatment of Raynaud's phenomenon by fibrinolytic enhancement. Br Med J 1978, 2:523–525.
75. Ehrly AM: Treatment of patients with secondary Raynaud's syndrome. Acta Clin Scand 1976, 465(suppl):92–95.
76. Fitzgerald DE, Butterfield WJH: A case of increased platelet antiheparin factor in a patient with Raynaud's phenomenon and gangrene treated by aspirin. Angiology 1969, 20:317–324.
77. Perzanowski A, My'sliwiec M: Platelet adhesiveness fibrinolysis in Raynaud's disease. Wiad Lek 1972, 25:771–774.
78. Dodds AJ, O'Reilly MJG, Yates CJP, Cotton LT, Flute PT, Dormandy JA: Haemorrheological response to plasma exchange in Raynaud's syndrome. Br Med J 1979, 2:1186–1187.
79. Gifford RW Jr, Hines EA Jr, Craig WM: Sympathectomy for Raynaud's phenomenon: Follow-up study of 70 women with Raynaud's disease and 54 women with secondary Raynaud's phenomenon. Circulation 1958, 17:5–13.
80. Johnson ENM, Summerly R, Birnstingl M: Prognosis in Raynaud's phenomenon after sympathectomy. Br Med J 1965, 1:962–964.
81. Wellington JL, Lynn RB: Raynaud's syndrome. Angiology 1969, 20:129–135.
82. Telford ED: The technique of sympathectomy. Br J Surg 1935, 23:448–450.
83. Ray BS, Hinsey JC, Geohegan WA: Observations on the distribution of the sympathetic nerves to the pupil and upper extremity as determined by the stimulation of the anterior roots in man. Ann Surg 1943, 118:647–655.

84. Ellis H: Transaxillary sympathectomy in the treatment of hyperhidrosis of the upper limb. Am Surg 1979, 45:546–551.
85. Hall KV, Hillestad LK: Raynaud's phenomenon treated with sympathectomy: A follow-up study of 28 patients. Angiology 1960, 11:186–189.
86. Flatt AE: Digital artery sympathectomy. J Hand Surg 1980, 5:550–556.
87. Wilgis EFS: Evaluation and treatment of chronic digital ischemia. Ann Surg 1981, 193:693–698.
88. McNamara MF, Takaki HS, Yao JST, Bergan JJ: A systematic approach to severe hand ischemia. Surgery 1978, 83:1–11.
89. Silcott GR, Polich VL: Palmar arch arterial reconstriction for the salvage of ischemic fingers. Am J Surg 1981, 142:219–225.
90. Schmidt FE, Hewitt RL: Severe upper limb ischemia. Arch Surg 1980, 115:1188–1191.

PART EIGHT

Venous and Lymphatic Disease

Chapter 58

VARICOSE VEINS

AKSEL G. NORDESTGAARD and RUSSELL A. WILLIAMS

Varicose veins and their complications are common in western countries; up to 25 percent of the adult population may be affected. The prevalence of varicose veins increases with age; they are twice as common in women, and in the United States more than 20 million people are affected (1). Treatment imposes a major burden on health care resources, and disability from them results in much loss of labor-power. In contrast to the high prevalence in western countries is the relative rarity of varicose veins in the more traditional communities of the third world (2).

Varicose veins are normal veins that have become elongated, dilated, and tortuous. The term is generally applied to the superficial veins affected in the lower limb, but similar changes may occur in the lower esophageal area, the anorectal region (hemorrhoids), and the left spermatic cord veins (varicocele). The present chapter focuses on varicosities of the lower extremities, which are classified as primary varicose veins, that is, those of unclear etiology; secondary varicose veins, the aftermath of deep vein thrombosis; and those developing in pregnancy. Varicosities occurring with an arteriovenous fistula will be dealt with elsewhere (Chapter 69).

Pathophysiology

People have developed anatomic structures that functionally aid the return of blood from the extremities to the heart against gravity. The "muscle pump" compresses the veins and propels blood toward the heart, its efficiency enhanced by one-way valves placed at strategic points in the venous system. If competent, these valves also protect the venous system below from the wave of pressure generated by coughing, straining, lifting, standing, or other exertion. The venous valves become incompetent due to dilatation of the veins or destruction after deep venous thrombosis, altering venous hemodynamics with the resultant formation of varicose veins.

In the recumbent position, blood flows to the heart because of the negative pressure within the chest, the abdominal venous pump, and arterial pressure; the effect of gravity is almost the same throughout the vascular system. When upright, blood below the heart is returned against a hydrostatic pressure, decreased by the negative respiratory pressure and the abdominal venous pump which is enhanced by standing (3); but the main effector is the peripheral venous muscle pump of the legs.

The musculovenous pump in the lower extremities has been called the peripheral heart. The muscles, enveloped by a strong fascial sheath, generate high pressures during contraction, and the "chambers," especially the small venules or sinusoids in the soleus and gastrocnemius muscles, are tightly compressed. These venules contain no valves, but since there is less resistance in the proximal great veins than in the distal capillaries, blood is delivered into the proximal, valved veins.

During muscular systole the pressure can reach 250 mmHg in the leg and 115 mmHg in the thigh; in diastole the venous pressure in the deep system falls below that of the superficial veins, drawing blood in from them and from the capillaries of the surrounding muscles and the distal veins (4,5).

Normal and pathologic pressure patterns of the venous system are demonstrated using a small needle placed in a dorsal vein of the foot, taped in place, and attached to a transducer, amplifier, and strip recorder. When supine and resting this is between 5 and 10 mmHg in normal people and those with venous insufficiency but without significant obstruction (which may raise the ankle venous pressure slightly). Upon standing the pressure rises to a baseline level, between 100 and 110 mmHg at the ankle, equilibrating after about 20 s. For patients with venous insufficiency the rise of the pressure upon standing is rapid (less than 20 s), but the resting standing pressure is not different from the normal (Figure 58-1).

During walking or rhythmic standing on tiptoes the venous pressure is lowered to between 20 and 40 mmHg, because of the valves acting in concert with the musculovenous pump of the calf and thigh. However, when the valves are incompetent, the ambulatory venous pressure is considerably higher, and there are striking differences between patients with primary varicose veins with or without insufficiency of the perforating veins and patients with postthrombotic syndrome (6)(Figure 58-1). It has been said that regardless of the state of the perforator vein valves, venous hypertension during ambulation in patients having primary varicose veins is caused by retrograde flow through the saphenous main channel; at rest the flow in the main saphenous channel is zero (7,8).

An ambulatory venous pressure of 20 to 40 mmHg is essential for normal function of the microcirculation, but a continued high venous pressure, especially in the postthrombotic syndrome, disrupts the equilibrium in the microcirculation that normally redistributes tissue fluids.

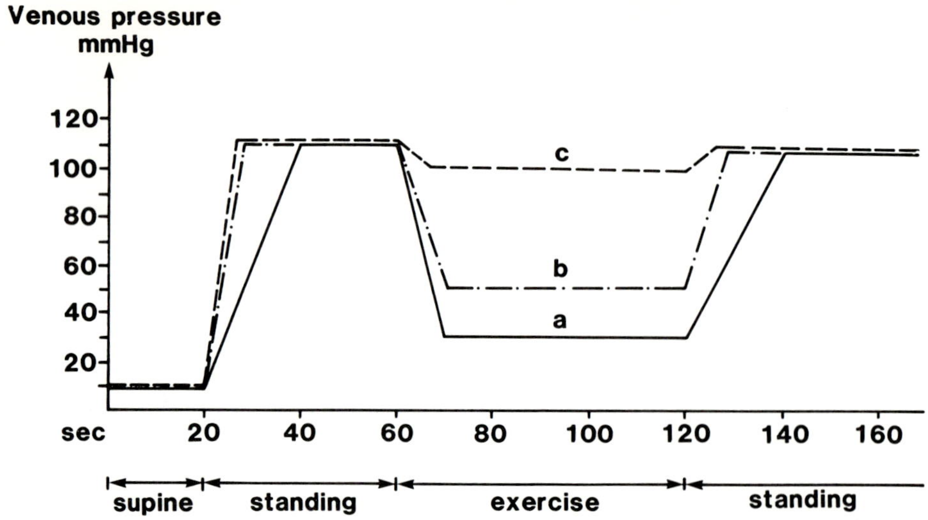

FIGURE 58-1. Venous pressure patterns, recorded on the dorsum of the foot, in normal persons (a), patients with primary varicose veins (b), and patients with postthrombotic syndrome (c).

Etiology and Pathogenesis

The precise cause of primary varicose veins is unknown; however, there is agreement that venous varicosities result from incompetence of the one-way valves that are indispensable for the efficient working of the musculovenous pump. An inherited weakness in the structure of the vein wall or valves is one theory, and a family history of varicose veins has been reported in more than 50 percent of patients (9). Other postulated etiological factors include the human's upright posture, coupled with occupations involving prolonged standing, pregnancy, obesity, age, and being of the female sex.

Newer epidemiological studies show that the difference in prevalence of varicose veins between western and third world countries is related to economic development (2,10,11). Several authors (2,12) consider raised intraabdominal pressure an important cause of varicose veins, and Burkitt (2) proposed that the low-residue western diet, depleted in fiber-rich plant foods as it is, underlies the difference.

No disease of the valves was found in a study of the proximal end of primary varicose saphenous veins (13). Rather, it was believed, separation of the valve commissures and incompetence result from dilatation of the vein. The varicose changes develop because intravenous pressures exceed the ability of the vein wall to withstand deformation. Transiently raised intraabdominal pressure, transmitted to the venous system, expands the saphenofemoral junction, producing incompetence of the femorosaphenous valve, a process that spreads successively downward, along the long saphenous veins, affecting its tributaries and the perforating veins, augmented by retrograde blood flow and increased venous pressure during exercise (7).

The short saphenous vein and its tributaries are similarly, but less often, affected; in some cases incompetent subcutaneous communications form between them and a varicose long saphenous vein, rendering the saphenopopliteal valve incompetent.

Valvular incompetence of the perforating veins is the underlying cause of secondary varicose veins. It is most often the result of earlier deep vein thrombosis, but very rarely a young patient may appear with typical findings of a single incompetent ankle perforator. Perforating vein incompetence leads to the secondary development of valvular incompetence of the long or short saphenous veins; however, in up to 5 percent, incompetence of the perforating veins with or without the postphlebitis syndrome is the only finding (14,15).

The effects of increased blood flow and venous hypertension build up over several years; the saphenous trunks dilate, and their walls become elongated and tortuous with loss of elasticity and of irregular thickness. These changes occur also, and to a greater degree, in the smaller, weaker walled superficial veins and venules.

Anatomy

The constancy of the arterial anatomy contrasts with the venous system, which varies greatly, an important consideration when operating on varicose veins. In the leg the three groups of veins are superficial, deep, and perforating; the superficial and deep veins, separated by the deep fascia, are linked by the perforating veins.

SUPERFICIAL (SUBCUTANEOUS) VEINS

The superficial veins have relatively thick, muscular walls and are grouped as small venules, veins of moderate size which form most of the prominent superficial varices, and the main venous trunks (long and short saphenous veins).

The long saphenous vein begins as an extension of the medial dorsal venous arch at the dorsomedial aspect of the foot and courses upward through the medial aspect of the leg and thigh to end in the common femoral vein by passing through the hiatus saphenous (foramen ovale). It is occasionally duplicated from the knee to the groin. The long saphenous vein has two important sets of tributaries, one pair joining at the knee and the other at the foramen ovale.

In the lower two-thirds of the leg above the ankle, the long saphenous vein is notably thick walled and closely accompanied by the saphenous nerve. In the thigh, twigs of the medial femoral cutaneous nerve run in the vicinity of the vein, and throughout its entire course it is accompanied by lymphatic trunks.

The short saphenous vein originates on the posterolateral aspect of the ankle, passing directly proximally to penetrate the deep fascia in the upper third of the leg. The point of entry into the popliteal vein is variable but is often near the superior aspect of the popliteal space.

In the distal third of the leg the short saphenous vein is in close relation to the sural nerve, in the proximal two-thirds with the medial sural cutaneous nerve, and throughout with lymphatic vessels. Throughout their courses, the long and short saphenous veins are connected particularly by the posteromedial vein of the thigh and unnamed tributaries.

DEEP VEINS

The main deep veins of the lower limb follow the arteries and are the paired posterior tibial, anterior tibial, and peroneal veins, which usually drain into the single popliteal and femoral veins of the thigh. These veins receive venous sinusoids from the calf muscles and communications from the superficial system.

PERFORATING VEINS

The perforating veins pierce the deep fascia and form a communication system between the superficial and deep system. They are most prevalent in the lower leg and may become incompetent, causing varicosities of the superficial veins. These are discussed in detail in Chapter 60.

Symptoms

Symptoms are not necessarily related to the size of the varicose veins or associated degree of incompetence. Severely involved legs may not produce symptoms, whereas numerous subjective complaints can arise from patients with minimal varicosities. Many, especially women, seek treatment for cosmetic reasons.

Initially the superficial veins with raised venous pressure are tense and may be palpated rather than seen, unless the legs have little subcutaneous tissue. Subsequently they are visibly dilated and then tortuous, often with progression of symptoms.

The most common symptom with any type of varicose veins is a dull, heavy, bursting ache that develops typically after prolonged standing (9). This aching sensation is relieved by elevation of the legs or using elastic support bandages or hose. Swelling and heaviness of the leg are common symptoms also relieved by elevation, and often occur with saphenofemoral, saphenopopliteal, or ankle perforator incompetence. A cyclic premenstrual exacerbation of complaints is not uncommon, and less frequent subjective symptoms are itching, burning, fatigue, cramps, and restless legs.

Gross varicose veins have a capacity of several hundred milliliters, the filling of which sometimes results in postural syncope.

Complications

Complications are not uncommon and in most cases progress while the venous disease remains untreated. Their basis is almost always venous hypertension, and the more severe complications are usually associated with secondary varicose veins where there is incompetence of one or more of the ankle perforators.

Venous stasis is most manifest in the skin and subcutaneous tissue of the lower third of the leg and the ankle. The postphlebitis syndrome of pigmentation, dermatitis (eczema), cellulitis, superficial phlebitis, ulceration, and hemorrhage is described in more detail in Chapter 60.

Pigmentation, often the earliest sign of chronic venous insufficiency, is caused by diapedesis of red blood cells or actual rupture of capillaries with deposition of hemosiderin in the dermis.

Dermatitis is uncommon early, when there is mild irritation or itch, but scratching aggravates the condition and may end with a chronic, scaly neurodermatitis or a weeping, raw dermatitis. With eczema or ulceration, natural protection against infection by the intact skin is lost, and the deeper tissues are liable to infection. An acute cellulitis caused by *Streptococcus pyogenes* or *Staphylococcus aureus* can develop, producing systemic symptoms, and antibiotic treatment may be necessary.

Superficial thrombophlebitis in a varicose vein presents with localized pain, cordlike induration, periphlebitis with reddish-brown skin discoloration and may originate from minimal trauma. Pulmonary embolism rarely supervenes but is made more likely by the spread of the thrombophlebitis to the deep veins.

Venous ulceration in a leg with varicose veins is the end stage of venous hypertension. Treatment of the veins and particularly the incompetent perforators, ideally before the skin ulcerates, will in all likelihood prevent skin breakdown. The ulcer is typically small, superficial, very painful because of exposure of nerve endings, and located above the medial malleolus (gaiter area).

Hemorrhage from varicose veins is not uncommon and has even been fatal (16). Spontaneous or traumatic bleeding is associated with either acute perforative or chronic ulceration. Spontaneous bleeding is more likely in elderly patients, almost half occurring from small, acute venous ulcers, not associated with chronic trophic changes (16). Subcutaneous bleeding is more common in young women.

Examination and Diagnosis

Lumbar nerve root irritation can cause an itching sensation of the calf which may mimic varicose disease. Osteoarthritis or internal derangements of the hip and knee, and arterial insufficiency, especially intermittent claudication or rest pain with trophic changes, may also be mistaken for varicose disease. Abnormalities of peripheral pulses raise the suspicion that arterial disease may be the basis of the symptoms. A burning sensation of the calf may also be due to peripheral neuritis from diabetic or alcoholic neuropathy.

Earlier deep vein thrombosis is important to discover, and its occurrence may be gleaned from a history of other illness, accidents, fractures, and operations, particularly if these were complicated. Previous treatment for varicose veins such as sclerotherapy, ligation, stripping, or elastic support is important to note.

The existence of cardiovascular, pulmonary, constitutional, infectious, or peripheral arterial disease may contraindicate or limit treatment for the varicose veins.

INSPECTION

A thorough physical examination is facilitated by good light and having the patient stand on a platform with his or her legs fully exposed. The examination should include the abdomen for abdominal tumors, pregnancy, or the scars of abdominal operations. Dilated suprapubic veins are evidence of previous iliofemoral or inferior vena cava thrombosis. In the legs, the location of varicosities suggests whether they are associated with the long or short saphenous vein. Sometimes an incompetent perforator is obvious from the subcutaneous bulging of its accompanying varicose vein. Other signs of chronic venous disease are noted.

PALPATION

Palpation with the pulp of the fingers is most helpful in detecting hidden varicosities, especially in fat legs where they can be difficult to see. The veins may be tender due to inflammation or thrombosis, or they may be fibrous. A defect in the deep fascia with or without an overlying prominent vein suggests in all likelihood that it is the site of a perforating, incompetent vein. This is best felt with the patient supine and the leg passively elevated to relax the muscles.

COUGH IMPULSE TEST

The cough impulse test is rapidly performed with the patient standing. The surgeon places the pulps of his or her fingers on the long saphenous vein 4 to 5 in below the saphenofemoral junction, and the patient coughs. An expansile impulse, usually with a thrill, indicates incompetence of the terminal saphenous valve at the junction with the femoral vein.

RETROGRADE-FILLING TEST (BRODIE-TRENDELENBURG TOURNIQUET TEST)

The retrograde-filling test demonstrates valvular incompetence in the saphenous veins, helping differentiate valvular from perforator incompetence. In the supine patient the veins are emptied by elevating the legs and stroking them firmly toward the groin. A rubber tourniquet is applied to occlude the superficial veins below the saphenofemoral junction; then the patient stands up quickly while the examiner notes the pattern of superficial venous refilling. If the superficial veins below the tourniquet fill quickly, perforators or the short saphenous vein is incompetent; if on the other hand the superficial veins remain empty, filling when the tourniquet is released, the saphenofemoral junction valve is incompetent. Remember, normal venous flow will fill the varicose veins within 30 to 60 s. Tourniquets simultaneously applied to the thigh and below the knee demonstrate short saphenous valvular incompetency.

PERTHE'S TEST

Perthe's test gives information about the perforating and deep venous systems. A tourniquet is applied to compress the superficial veins immediately below the knee, and the patient walks for 1 minute while the ankle veins are observed. If they become less prominent and less tense, the perforator and the deep vein valves are normal; should they remain the same size, the valves of the perforators are incompetent. Finally, if the veins become more prominent during the exercise and the patient complains of leg pain, deep venous insufficiency with incompetent perforating veins is suspected. Table 58-1 summarizes the usefulness of these three tests.

TABLE 58-1. Diagnostic Tests

Test	Information Given	Problems
Cough impulse	Positive result, expansive cough impulse usually with a thrill, indicates saphenofemoral incompetence	Less accurate than the retrograde filling test. False positive can be due to a strong cough impulse in the femoral vein, or a slight jerk of muscular contraction.
Retrograde filling test	Differentiates valvular incompetence of the saphenous veins from perforator incompetence	Incorrectly applied tourniquet, fat legs, and legs with multiple sites of incompetence may give unreliable and possible misleading results.
Perthes test	Gives information about the perforating and deep venous systems	Difficult test to perform and assess without practice

Patients with varicose veins limited to the long or short saphenous system, minimal swelling, no history of deep venous thrombosis, and no pigmentation or skin changes to suggest chronic venous insufficiency may be presumed to have primary varicose veins, and further diagnostic studies are not necessary. A history suggestive of deep venous thrombosis and extensive skin changes of chronic venous insufficiency requires evaluation to demonstrate whether or not there is deep venous insufficiency. This often includes noninvasive tests such as photoplethysmography, impedence plethysmography, phleborheography, and the use of a directional Doppler. Phlebography is invasive, but it is the most accurate method for anatomic identification of deep venous thrombosis and it gives information about the site of incompetent perforating veins. It is the "gold standard" against which other tests are compared.

Treatment

Primary varicose veins are not preventable; there are no certain etiological factors. However, prophylaxis and thrombolytic therapy for peripheral deep vein thrombosis will reduce the number of patients who develop secondary varicose veins.

Since varicose veins develop because of defective valves between the superficial and deep vein system, a rational basis for treatment is repair of these valves or interruption of incompetent pathways, by operation or in some cases sclerotherapy. Done well, this restores to normal the pressure fall recorded in the subcutaneous veins on exercise.

An extensive operation produces considerable discomfort, requires several days in hospital and an extended convalescence, and at times the incisions heal with a cosmetically unacceptable appearance. Sclerotherapy is more likely to be accepted by patients (17,18). Discomfort is less, and it is done on an ambulatory basis, interfering little with the patient's normal activities. Another point to bear in mind is that some patients may later need harvesting of the long saphenous vein trunk for arterial revascularization or coronary bypass.

Long-term results for treatment are improved with proper selection and treatment based on clinicopathological findings (19): group I patients (30 percent), those with dilated superficial veins only, are well treated by injection-compression therapy (sclerotherapy); group II patients (5 to 10 percent), those with incompetence of the lower leg perforating veins, are similarly treated with sclerotherapy; and group III patients (60 percent), those with involvement of either or both the long and short saphenous system require surgical treatment, and residual varicosities can be treated by sclerotherapy.

The severity of the venous problem, and the need for curative treatment is weighed against the patient's overall medical condition; varicose disease is very slowly progressive, not lethal, and rarely totally disabling.

Conservative Treatment

Minimal varicosities for which curative treatment is not indicated or desired can be made symptom-free by elastic support stockings. Conditions for which surgery or sclerotherapy is contraindicated, such as constitutional disease with a poor prognosis, advanced age with symptomatic varicosities, obesity, and pregnancy with abnormally distended veins, are all suitable for conservative treatment.

Elastic support relieves symptoms and may prevent the condition from worsening, but it does not cure the disease. External compression assists venous return by compressing dilated superficial veins, enhancing the efficiency of the calf-muscle pump. Compression increases the tissue pressure and promotes return of the extracellular fluid into the capillary venous system, decreasing edema and stasis complications. The support must be adequate with a proper pressure distribution profile that decreases from distally to proximally. In general, bigger and more distally located veins have a greater degree of venous insufficiency and need firmer support for control.

Elastic support of the leg is provided by elastic stockings or elastic bandages. The latter are generally the more versatile and effective and can be applied with varying degrees of compression as required. But with the different types of elastic stockings, some custom-made, now available, it is possible to properly fit the majority of patients. For men, elastic stockings should be knee length with an open toe and closed heel.

The support is put on in the morning before rising and removed on retiring at night. During daytime the patient is encouraged to walk or perform other activities such as swimming, bicycling, or dorsiflexion of the foot to activate the calf-muscle pump. It is recommended that he or she avoid long periods of standing, and even change occupation to accomplish this. Patients with complications from venous hypertension are advised to elevate their legs to reduce the hydrostatic pressure in the foot to zero. The leg is positioned approximately 20 in above the heart level several times daily. This is incorporated indefinitely in the daily routine, e.g., following each mealtime. Patients unable to do this can lie in bed with elevated legs to achieve the same effect.

Sclerotherapy

Sclerotherapy has been used in the treatment of varicose veins for over a century. Many of the earlier sclerosants produced undesirable side effects and results were variable, thus bringing the method into disfavor, particularly since they coincided with the evolution of improved surgical techniques.

With the introduction of sodium tetradecyl sulfate—a more active and less toxic agent—and refinement of techniques, sclerotherapy again attracted attention, and Fegan's modified continuous compression-sclerotherapy technique revived its popularity (20,21). Sodium tetradecyl sulfate (3% solution), a detergent, causes localized destruction of the venous intima, with less perivascular inflammatory response than previous agents. It also has a strong thrombogenic effect.

The best result is obtained if the veins are emptied, then compressed, so as not to refill with blood following injection of the sclerosant, ensuring close intimal contact and minimal luminal thrombus. If a thrombus forms, canalization eventually reopens the vein. For injection therapy to succeed, especially in large veins, several authors advise that the vein walls need to be compressed together for up to 6 weeks to prevent blood and thrombi collecting before permanent obliterative fibrosis has occurred (19,22). Newer studies question the need for this long bandaging time (23,24).

Sclerotherapy is not advised when there is either saphenofemoral or saphenopopliteal incompetence because these are treated by operation. Varicosities in the thigh are unsatisfactory for sclerotherapy because proper compression bandaging of the thigh is not possible and the thrombus may propagate into the femoral vein.

Contraindications to sclerotherapy are allergy to the sclerosing agent, pregnancy, severe postphlebitic conditions, excessive obesity, constitutional disease with poor prognosis, any condition where the patient is immobile and incapable of active movement immediately after injection, and extensive limb eczema or an infected ulcer. The latter is treated first by conservative means, and any varicose veins are managed by sclerotherapy after healing.

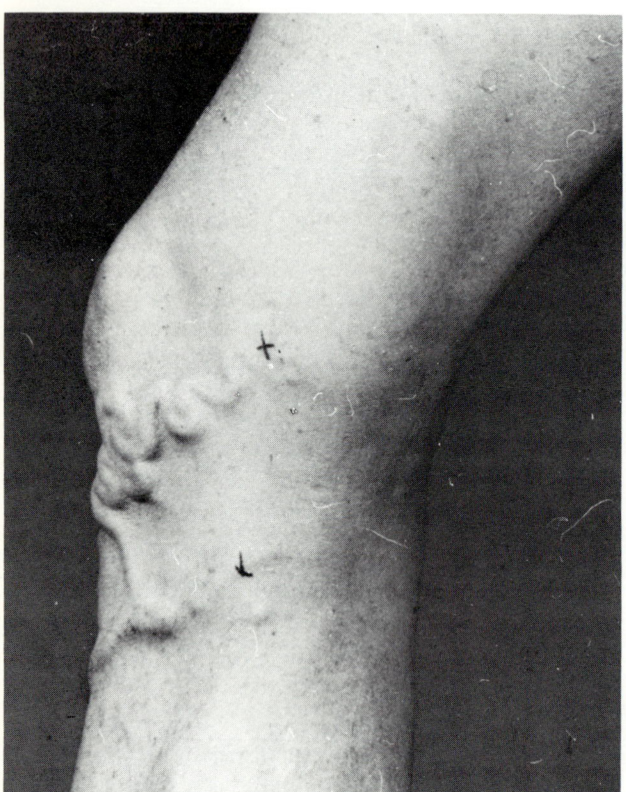

FIGURE 58-2. Large varicose tributaries, originating from the long saphenous vein, with the points of control marked.

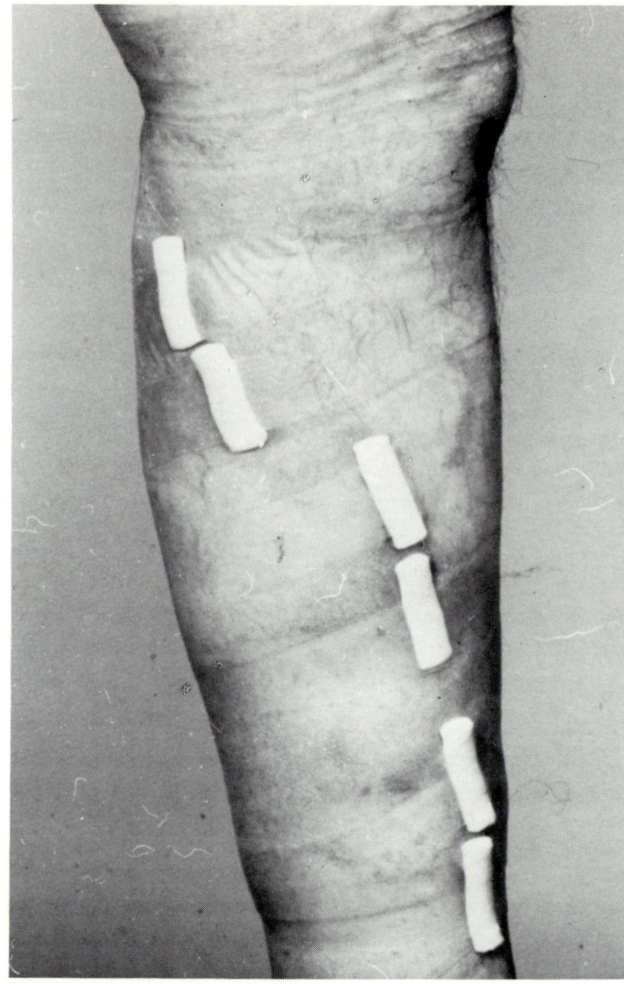

FIGURE 58-3. Cotton pads taped in place over the injection sites.

TECHNIQUES OF SCLEROTHERAPY

The extent of the varicosities is determined, and the "points of control," found by inspection and palpation, are marked precisely with a felt-tipped pen before injection (Figure 58-2). These should include all sites at which incompetent perforating veins join the superficial veins and selected points along the remaining varicose veins to ensure endosclerosis of that venous segment.

One technique to ensure that "empty" veins are injected is for the patient to lie down with the varicose vein–bearing limb hanging over the bedside so the veins are filled and distended and easier to puncture with the needle. Each injection (0.5 mL of 3% solution) is done with a disposable 2-mL syringe and 25-gauge 16-mm needle, which is inserted and taped at the premarked points of control while the leg is dependent; up to 15 injections may be given at any one treatment. The leg is then elevated above heart level to empty the vein, which is aspirated to confirm that the needle remains within its lumen; then the sclerosant is injected. Pulsation or bright red blood suggests that the needle is in an artery and should be removed at once. Starting with the most distal syringe, sclerosant is injected slowly and retained in a short segment of the adjacent 5 cm of vein by

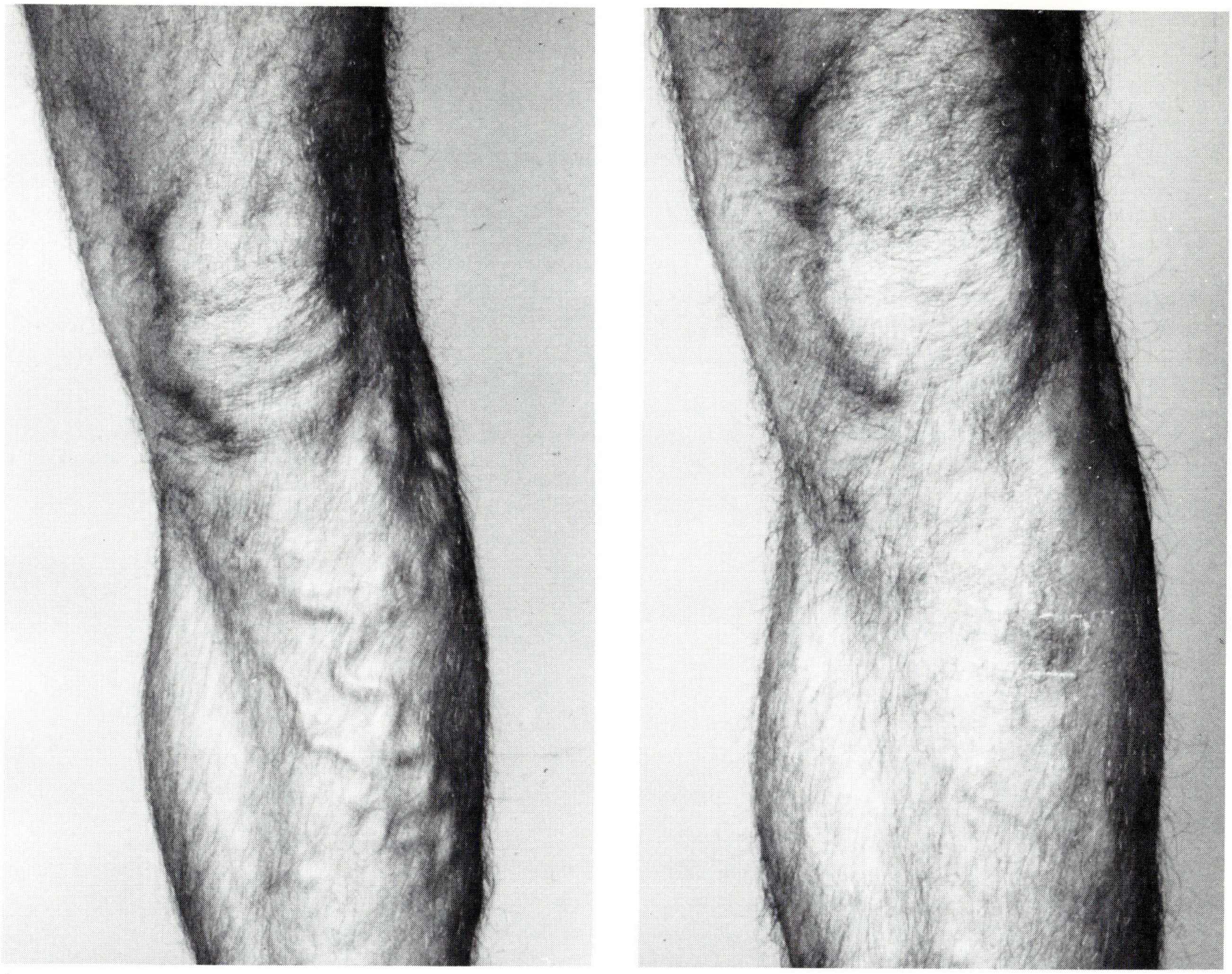

A B

FIGURE 58-4. Appearance before *(A)* and after sclerotherapy *(B)*.

compressing with the fingers above and below the injection site for 1 minute. Pain or moderate discomfort indicate an extravenous injection is being made, which is stopped at once.

After removing the needle, but before the compressing fingers are released, a small pressure dressing pad is placed over the injection site and adjacent vein and retained with a strip of tape (Figure 58-3). After completing all injections, and while the leg is still elevated, the leg is firmly bandaged with limited-stretch 7.5- and 10-cm cotton crepe bandages; first, the 7.5-cm bandage is applied from the metatarsal heads to the proximal injection site and then the 10-cm bandage over it. The correct application of the bandage is important and needs to be smooth with progressively reduced pressure up the leg. Finally, the bandages are covered by a lightweight elastic stocking or a length of flesh-colored elasticized stockinet. The bandages may need to be reapplied because they frequently become displaced and are the major source of complaints, especially in warm climates. The patient walks immediately and continues to do as much walking as possible during the succeeding weeks.

Hobbs (19) and Fegan (22) believe compression, maintained for 6 weeks after sclerotherapy, is important to ensure that permanent obliterating fibrosis develops, giving the best permanent result. However, it has been shown that the bandages need to be reapplied every 6 to 8 hours to maintain the correct pressure (25). Another study showed no difference in the results after 6 weeks between one group bandaged for only 8 hours and another for 6 weeks after sclerotherapy (23). Our practice is to bandage for 1 week, and then at a second visit to inject any residual veins, aspirate any "intravenous hematomas," and rebandage for a further 2 weeks (Figure 58-4).

COMPLICATIONS OF SCLEROTHERAPY

Complications of sclerotherapy are uncommon with the technique described. Rarely seen is a local allergic response with itching, swelling, and erythema, or a systemic allergy with swelling of the lips and tongue and mild bronchospasm. Anaphylactic reaction is extremely uncommon but has been reported, so facilities for treatment should be immediately available.

Excessive injections (more than 15) given at a single visit can result in an overdose, producing malaise with thirst, shivering, headaches, and sometimes chest pain or epigastric discomfort. A transient reddish-brown color of the urine has been thought to be a hemolytic reaction.

Intraarterial injection, mostly to the posterior tibial artery, causes immediate severe pain, and usually significant ischemic damage and gangrene of portions of the foot (26). Immediate treatment with heparin and low-molecular-weight dextran may be of value. A wise precaution is to not inject veins in the area below and behind the medial malleolus and avoid this serious complication.

Leakage from the injected vein or injection into the subcutaneous tissue may result in an ulcer from necrosis of fat or skin. This can leave yellowish-brown skin staining or permanent scars which are especially displeasing to a patient receiving cosmetic treatment, so it may be prudent not to use this technique for cosmetic therapy if such an outcome is unacceptable to the patient.

Injection into a peripheral nerve has been reported, particularly the sural, saphenous, or musculocutaneous nerves. The patient feels sudden severe pain; however the effects seldom last for more than a week.

Mild localized phlebitis is very common and is treated with analgesics or anti-inflammatory agents. Ascending thrombophlebitis can occur, especially when injections are made into the main tributaries or trunk of a large, long saphenous vein, particularly in the thigh. Deep venous thrombosis and pulmonary embolism have also been described, although there was no evidence that deep vein thrombosis occurred in a group of patients treated by the foregoing technique and studied with noninvasive venous studies (27). Injection into thigh veins is not recommended to avoid bandaging difficulties and to minimize the likelihood of the thrombus propagating into the femoral vein and embolizing.

An intravascular hematoma (clot) may cause persistent tenderness and may remain for many months as a palpable fibrotic cord. At the 1-week follow-up visit the hematoma is evacuated using a large-bore needle and syringe or via a small scapel point incision, with relief of symptoms. The small local pressure pad is reapplied.

A new growth of venules sometimes occurs over a recently treated site, possibly associated with a persistent incompetent perforating vein.

Surgery

Local excision or ligation treatment of varicose veins has been done for more than 2000 years, but general anesthesia and aseptic surgery make a more extensive, definitive operation possible, with a high likelihood of success.

In 1891 Trendelenburg introduced the technique of ligating the long saphenous vein above large varices in the thigh, and this was modified several years later by W. Thelwall Thomas who claimed a better result if the long saphenous vein was ligated at its termination. The prototype of intraluminal strippers that are now in wide use was introduced by Babcock in 1907 (4).

The modern operation of "flush ligation" and stripping treats the cause and removes the varicose veins themselves. Flush ligation disconnects the deep veins and more central veins of the abdomen from the superficial veins, eliminating the high-pressure backflow. The ligation is done at the saphenofemoral or saphenopopliteal junction, and in addition, any incompetent perforating veins in the thigh or leg are ligated. If the long or short saphenous vein is varicose, it is removed by stripping; additional varicosities can be avulsed through multiple, small incisions, or they may be treated by sclerotherapy later.

Surgical treatment is recommended for incompetence of either the long or short saphenous vein (19). Contraindications to surgery are almost the same as for sclerotherapy and include diseases with a poor prognosis, arterial occlusive disease of the lower extremities which would impede or even lead to failure of wound healing, a severe postphlebitic condition, immobility or likelihood of being incapable of active movement after the treatment, excessive obesity, and pregnancy. Infection or ulcer in the limb is healed before any operation on the veins.

If only flush ligation of either of the saphenous veins is the operation, it can be carried out under local anesthesia as an outpatient procedure. Stripping of varicose veins is done under general or spinal anesthesia, and an overnight hospital stay is usually necessary. Commonly, if both legs are affected, they are treated at the same operation, unless the veins are unusually large and widespread when one leg per session might be advisable.

Sclerotherapy should not be used on an unconscious patient to complement the vein surgery. Most surgeons remove as many varicosities as possible at the operation, ideally leaving no residual veins that would need to be managed by sclerotherapy at a follow-up outpatient visit.

Before vein surgery a complete physical examination and routine tests are carried out to evaluate the patient's fitness for anesthesia. With the patient standing on a platform, the operating surgeon marks all varicosities with a surgical indelible marking pen, including varicose tributaries to the saphenous veins and incompetent perforating veins. Even though injection therapy may be added later, the "points of control" are determined and marked because these can be stripped out or avulsed at operation.

During operation the table is tilted to elevate the patient's legs 10 to 15°, reducing the venous pressure and minimizing blood loss. The skin is prepared, avoiding excess rubbing so as not to remove the markings. To obtain a good cosmetic result, the incisions are small and placed in Langer's lines, which are parallel to the inguinal ligament in the groin, horizontal around the knee, and vertical on the anterior aspect of the legs.

THE LONG SAPHENOUS VEIN

The saphenofemoral junction is 2.5 to 3.5 cm below and lateral to the pubic tubercle. Using the saphenofemoral junction as its center, a 5- to 8-cm incision made parallel to the inguinal ligament exposes the long saphenous vein in the subcutaneous fat on the deep fascia as it joins with the femoral vein. The saphenofemoral junction and its usual five tributaries are exposed;

this final dissection is done very cautiously using a round-tipped scissor and vascular dissecting forceps to avoid damage to the delicate vein walls. It is advisable to securely ligate the venous tributaries rather than use vascular clips because these may dislodge and the venous bleeding can be massive and serious. To identify anatomic variations, good exposure of the saphenofemoral junction is required. Occasionally a superficial vein joins the femoral vein directly, within 1 cm of the saphenofemoral junction, instead of joining the long saphenous vein.

Recurrent varicosities may occur because tributaries are overlooked, hence the emphasis on identifying and dividing them. Of the two normal larger tributaries, the anterolateral vein of the thigh is easiest to locate and sometimes when large and straight, it can be mistaken for the long saphenous vein. The posteromedial vein of the thigh normally joins the long saphenous vein within 5 to 10 cm of its termination and is important because it connects with the short saphenous vein. Failure to ligate the posteromedial vein may cause recurrent varicosities of the short saphenous vein system.

The superficial external pubic artery runs beneath the termination of the long saphenous vein; however, it may pass superficially to it, in which case it needs to be excised because it conceals and hinders access to the superficial epigastric vein and the saphenofemoral junction.

When all tributaries are defined and divided, the saphenous vein is ligated flush with the femoral vein with simple and transfixion ligatures. If the only treatment is ligation, another simple ligature is placed distally and the vein divided. The wound is usually closed with subcutaneous and subcuticular sutures.

To minimize the risk of damage to the saphenous nerve, which is closely applied to the long saphenous vein at the ankle, and the lymphatic vessels, the long saphenous vein is stripped downward from the groin to a point 5 to 8 cm above the ankle (28–30). The distal portion of the vein is mobilized, and the smaller tip of the stripper is passed into the saphenous vein, gently directing it distally, its course noted by inspection and palpation. It should follow the previously marked saphenous vein. Negotiating its passage through the remains of the valves and the varices is occasionally difficult but can usually be done by gently withdrawing and advancing it several times. If the vein is very varicose, stretching the skin so the vein lies in the line of the stripper may help. Sometimes complete passage of the stripper is not possible, and a second stripper is passed downward from that part of the vein or even upward to that site from the ankle region. Once in the desired position, a small incision is made over the tip of the stripper to extract it after division and ligation of the distal long saphenous vein. The larger head of the stripper is then firmly tied in the divided distal vein in the groin and the incision closed. If the saphenous vein in the leg is not varicose, it may be sufficient to terminate stripping at a point below the knee.

Before the vein is stripped out, treatment of the remaining varicosities is completed. These include veins located away from the course of the stripper and which are unlikely to be avulsed by its passage. Some surgeons use the "worming" technique to remove these, which is done through very small incisions made by stabbing the skin over the vein with a number 11 scalpel blade. A fine mosquito artery forceps passed through the stab is used to find the varicose vein, opening the forceps jaws once or twice until the white vein wall is sighted, and grasped; with side-to-side movements, quite long lengths of the tortuous vein can be withdrawn through each site. Bleeding is controlled by pressure applied over the operation site for several minutes. No sutures are needed for these incisions, which are taped closed, ensuring a good postoperative appearance. Obvious or grossly incompetent perforating veins are exposed through small vertical incisions and ligated at the deep fascia.

Once treatment of the remaining varicosities and incompetent veins is completed, the stripper, previously secured in the vein, is gently and firmly drawn distally. To reduce bleeding, pressure is applied along the stripper's track by the assistant for some minutes, supplemented by firmly bandaging the leg, advancing with the bandages immediately behind the stripper head. Alternately all wounds are closed and dressed, the leg is bandaged, and the stripper is then extracted using the same technique.

THE SHORT SAPHENOUS VEIN

The short saphenous vein is dealt with similarly to the long saphenous vein. This may immediately follow ligating and stripping of the long saphenous vein. The patient needs to be repositioned in the prone position, with the knee slightly flexed to obtain good exposure. It can also be done with the patient remaining in the supine position while an assistant holds up the leg.

A 4- to 5-cm incision in one of the transverse lines of the popliteal fossa skin, about level with the knee joint, exposes the saphenopopliteal junction and its tributaries under the deep fascia. Care is taken to identify the adjacent nerves, retracting them out of the field. An important anatomical variation of the saphenopopliteal junction is the posteromedial branch of the long saphenous vein, which occasionally is large and almost replaces the normal saphenopopliteal junction. Another significant variation is the short saphenous vein ending in one of the gastrocnemial veins instead of the popliteal vein. With this anomaly the saphenous vein is ligated at its junction with the gastrocnemial vein.

The short saphenous vein is ligated flush with the popliteal vein, using the same technique as for the long saphenous vein; if only ligation is needed, it is divided between the ligatures, and the wound is closed by suturing the deep fascia together with subcutaneous and subcuticular skin stitches.

With the same technique as for the long saphenous vein, the stripper is gently passed distally, often to a point below the lateral malleolus where the vein originates. Its tip is secured through a small transverse incision. The vein and the closely related sural nerve are separated by blunt dissection to assure preservation of the nerve. Remaining varicosities or incompetent perforating veins are again treated by techniques described previously before the vein is stripped out.

Following surgery, the compression bandages are removed the next morning and replaced by small dressings on each incision. A strong elastic stocking is placed on the leg, and the patient is encouraged to walk hourly, sit with the leg elevated, and avoid standing and is discharged home that day to resume normal activities. At home the stockings are taken off at night. Any sutures are removed about 1 week later, and if there is no edema, the stocking is discarded. Not uncommonly bruising is seen along the course of the stripped vein; it resolves over several weeks.

Postoperative Complications

Complications after striping seldom occur and are usually relatively mild.

BLEEDING

Ecchymosis is the most common complication and usually appears 3 to 5 days after operation (30). Normally the discoloration is absorbed within 3 to 4 weeks. Postoperative bleeding rarely occurs and is easily controlled by adding a compression bandage and keeping the leg elevated for several hours. If they enlarge or become infected, hematomas in the femoral incision are evacuated. However, careful surgical technique, elevation of the leg during operation, and proper bandaging minimize the chance of these complications occurring.

EDEMA

Leg edema is common in the early postoperative period; in most cases the edema subsides spontaneously or with pressure bandaging, and usually lasts no more than a few weeks. Rarely it persists. Lymphatic disruption does occur with varicose vein surgery, but to what extent it is responsible for the postoperative leg edema is not known (29).

NERVE DAMAGE

About 50 percent of the patients after vein stripping have limited areas of hypoesthesia or total loss of skin sensation around and slightly proximal to the ankle incisions (30). Damage to the saphenous and sural nerves is less likely if they are dissected from the vein adventitia and if the smaller head on the stripper is used, stripping the long saphenous vein distally from the groin (28). Hypoesthesia caused by neuropraxia usually recovers within some months, but avulsion of branches of the nerves does not.

WOUND INFECTIONS

Wound infection occurs in less than 1 percent of patients. However, stripping the veins of a patient with an unhealed ulcer of the leg greatly increases the incidence of wound infection, so, if possible, stripping should not be done before the ulcer is healed.

THROMBOEMBOLIC DISEASE

Deep vein thrombosis and embolism are no more frequent after these operations than after other operations.

INDURATION OF THE STRIPPER TRACK

Fibrous tissue formation and induration along the stripper track may lead to complaints of a stiff feeling down the inside of the thigh. It disappears, usually after 1 or 2 months.

DEEP VEIN OR ARTERIAL STRIPPING

Extremely rarely, the stripper may enter the deep vein system, and failure to recognize this could cause irreparable damage to the deep vein system. Accidental stripping of the artery has also been described, with leg amputation the outcome.

Pregnancy

Varicose veins appearing or becoming worse during pregnancy are common, but most resolve within 3 to 4 months after delivery. Pregnancy is probably more an aggravating than a causative factor (2), and the explanation is the increasing blood flow through the pelvic veins and the increasing bulk of the pregnant uterus in the pelvis, which progressively obstructs the veins until it rises out of the pelvis after the third month. This may account for the observation that during the later months of pregnancy the veins regress along with the symptoms. Hormonal effects have also been proposed, and estrogens have a relaxant action on smooth-muscle cells in the vessel wall, which may be particularly related to the formation of spider hemangiomas or nevi.

Three distinct varieties of varicose veins are seen in pregnancy: (1) primary varicose veins, (2) vulval and pudendal varicose veins, and (3) multiple capillary nevi.

PRIMARY VARICOSE VEINS

Women who already have varicose veins usually find that they increase in size, with more symptoms, especially during the first part of the pregnancy. Mild primary long or short saphenous incompetence will often increase, returning to normal after delivery; but sometimes complete resolution does not occur after repeated pregnancies.

If treatment is necessary during pregnancy, it should be with elastic stockings and elevation. If the varicosities remain 3 to 4 months after delivery, surgery or sclerotherapy can then be considered.

VULVAL AND PUDENDAL VARICOSE VEINS

During pregnancy the increased blood flow and venous pressure in the internal iliac vein extends along its two tributaries, the internal pudendal and obturator veins, which dilate and may present as a "small bunch of black grapes" in the vulva. These usually never give rise to any serious complications during pregnancy and delivery, regressing to normal postpartum. During pregnancy no treatment is advisable, but if they still persist and give rise to symptoms after delivery, they can be removed by the surgical "worming" technique (4).

MULTIPLE CAPILLARY NEVI (SPIDER NEVI)

These small, dilated venules probably occur because of the estrogen influence on the smooth-muscle cells in the vein wall in certain susceptible individuals. They are seen in other conditions where the estrogen level is raised, such as cirrhosis of the liver and estrogen-producing tumors, and in women taking oral contraceptives. If possible the treatment is directed at the cause. If not too small, persistent spiders can be treated with sclerotherapy; diathermy laser and electrolysis are also used, but complications such as unsightly brown scars may give an even less acceptable appearance.

References

1. Coon WW, Willis PW III, Keller JB: Venous thromboembolism and other venous disease in the Tecumseh community health study. Circulation 1973, 48:839–846.
2. Burkitt DP: Varicose veins. Arch Surg 1976, 111:1327–1332.
3. Fegan WG, Milliken JC, Fitzgerald DE: Abdominal venous pump. Arch Surg 1966, 92:44–46.
4. Cockett FB, Dodd H (eds): *The Pathology and Surgery of Veins of the Lower Limb,* ed 2. New York, Churchill Livingstone, 1976.
5. Keane TFL, Fegan WG: Physiology of the calf veins. Angiology 1969, 20:489–495.
6. Johnson G Jr, Burnham SJ, Keagy BA: Varicose veins, postphlebitic syndrome, and chronic venous insufficiency. In Moore WS (ed): *Vascular Surgery*. New York, Grune & Stratton, 1983.
7. Bjordal R: Simultaneous pressure and flow recordings in varicose veins of the lower extremity. Acta Chir Scand 1970, 136:309–317.
8. Bjordal RI: Circulation patterns in incompetent perforating veins in the calf and in the saphenous sytem in primary varicose veins. Acta Chir Scand 1972, 138:251–261.
9. Lofgren EP: Present-day indications for surgical treatment of varicose veins. Mayo Clin Proc 1966, 41:515–523.
10. Burkitt, DP: Varicose veins, deep vein thrombosis, and haemorrhoids. Epidemiology and suggested aetiology. Br Med J 1972, 2:556–561.
11. Burkitt DP, Townsend AJ, Patel K, Skaug K: Varicose veins in developing countries. Lancet 1976, 2:202.
12. Adams JC: Etiological factors in varicose veins of the lower extremities. Surg Gynecol Obstet 1939, 69:7 17–725.
13. Edwards JE, Edwards EA: The saphenous valves in varicose veins. Am Heart J 1940, 19:338–351.
14. Doran FSA, White M: A clinical trial designed to discover if the primary treatment of varicose veins should be by Fegan's method or by an operation. Br J Surg 1975, 62:72–76.
15. Hobbs JT: Surgery and sclerotherapy in the treatment of varicose veins. Arch Surg 1974, 109:793–796.
16. Evans GA, Evans DMD, Seal RME, Craven JL: Spontaneous fatal haemorrhage caused by varicose veins. Lancet 1973, 2:1359–1362.
17. Jakobsen BH: The value of different forms of treatment for varicose veins. Br J Surg 1979, 66:182–184.
18. Hobbs JT: The treatment of varicose veins. Br J Surg 1968, 55:777–780.
19. Hobbs JT: The management of varicose veins. Surg Ann 1980, 12:169–186.
20. Reiner L: The activity of anionic surface active compounds in producing vascular obliteration. Proc Soc Exp Biol 1946, 62:49–54.
21. Cooper WM: Clinical evaluation of sotradecol, a sodium alkyl sulfate solution, in the injection therapy of varicose veins. Surg Gynecol Obstet 1946, 83:647–652.
22. Fegan WG: Continuous compression technique of injecting varicose veins. Lancet 1963, 2:109–112.
23. Raj TB, Makin GS: A random controlled trial of two forms of compression bandaging in outpatient sclerotherapy of varicose veins. J Surg Res 1981, 31:440–445.
24. Batch AJG, Wickremesinghe SS, Gannon ME, Dormandy JA: Randomised trial of bandaging after sclerotherapy for varicose veins. Br Med J 1980, 2:423.
25. Raj TB, Goddard M, Makin GS: How long do compression bandages maintain their pressure during ambulatory treatment of varicose veins? Br J Surg 1980, 67:122–124.
26. Fegan WG, Pegum JM: Accidental intra-arterial injection during sclerotherapy of varicose veins. Br J Surg 1974, 61:124–126.
27. William RA, Wilson SE: Sclerosant treatment of varicose veins and deep vein thrombosis. Arch Surg 1984, 119:1283–1285.
28. Cox SJ, Wellwood, JM, Martin A: Saphenous nerve injury caused by stripping of the long saphenous vein. Br Med J 1974, 1:415–417.
29. vanBellen B, Gross WS, Verta MJ Jr, Yao JST, Bergan JJ: Lymphatic disruption in varicose vein surgery. Surgery 1977, 82:257–259.
30. Keith LM Jr, Smead WL: Saphenous vein stripping and its complications. Surg Clin North Am 1983, 63:1303–1312.

Chapter 59

DEEP VEIN THROMBOSIS: PREVENTION AND MANAGEMENT

LAZAR J. GREENFIELD

Deep vein thrombosis is a serious and potentially life-threatening disorder. The magnitude of the problem is suggested by the fact that an estimated 180,000 to 250,000 patients per year are diagnosed clinically as having deep vein thrombosis, while twice this number may suffer from venous stasis ulcers and as many as 7 million may have lower extremity stasis changes and edema on a chronic basis. In addition to the disability associated with the postphlebitic syndrome, the mortality from the most serious complication of deep vein thrombosis, pulmonary thromboembolism, has been estimated to be in the range of 200,000 deaths per year in which it is either the sole cause or a major contributing factor (1,2).

The frequency of deep vein thrombosis itself is difficult to determine since it may remain clinically silent or may be misdiagnosed when nonspecific lower extremity signs and symptoms are present. Using the very sensitive ^{125}I-labeled fibrinogen scanning test in a series of unselected general surgical patients, Kakkar et al. found that 30 percent of them developed positive scans in the calf in the postoperative period (3). The diagnosis was confirmed by venography, and in 35 percent of them, the abnormality disappeared within 72 hours. In 23 percent, there was propagation of the thrombus into more proximal veins and in half of these patients, pulmonary thromboembolism occurred. The consequences of untreated deep vein thrombosis, then, are sufficiently serious to warrant aggressive diagnosis and management.

Historical Perspective

Our present knowledge of the causes of deep vein thrombosis and its relationship to pulmonary thromboembolism can be traced to the early work of Virchow who in 1856 introduced the term *thrombosis* and suggested three possible mechanisms which remain the foundation of our approach to the etiology of the disorder: stasis, hypercoagulability, and endothelial damage (4). Despite years of investigation, efforts to identify a common coagulation factor abnormality in patients with venous thrombosis have not been successful (5). However, in 1962, Seeger and Marciniak identified a naturally occurring inhibitor of activated factor X which was subsequently named antithrombin III (6). The subsequent finding of a congenital deficiency of this substance in a small group of patients was correlated with a strong predisposition to the development of venous thrombosis (7). Antithrombin deficiency has also been associated with arterial thrombosis in patients following vascular surgery (8). The classical association between venous thrombosis and malignancy as pointed out originally by Trousseau (9) has also been found to provide an early sign of an occult cancer, most commonly involving lung, gastrointestinal tract, breast, and uterus (10). Additional clinical correlations have demonstrated significantly increased risk of venous thrombosis in patients with hyperlipoproteinemia (11), oral contraceptive use, smoking history, and obesity (12). Less well-documented evidence exists for enhanced risk in the presence of advanced age, heart disease, trauma, sepsis, and non-O blood type (13).

Etiology and Pathophysiology

In surgical patients, stasis is probably the most important factor since there is a significant reduction in lower extremity venous flow following induction of general anesthesia which persists throughout the procedure. There is also a relationship between the duration of bed rest and the incidence of venous thrombosis which provides the stimulus for early ambulation. Vessel wall injury also can occur in collapsed vessels when the intimal walls are in contact, and some intimal injury can be demonstrated after hypoxemia. Although routine histological examination of veins containing thrombi fails to show an inflammatory response consistent with vessel wall injury, ultrastructural study shows leukocytic attachment between endothelial intercellular junctions in areas of venous stasis after trauma at a remote site. These changes can become the nidus for the formation of a propagating thrombus. Once a nidus of thrombus begins in the presence of stasis, the substances that promote platelet aggregation including acti-

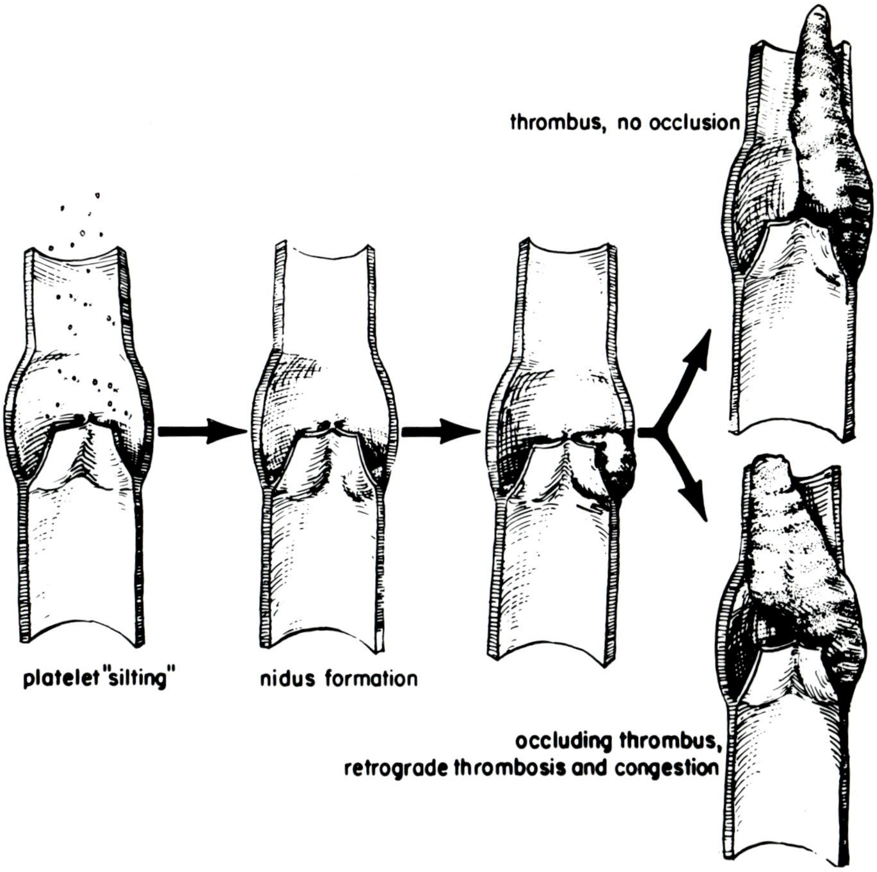

FIGURE 59-1. Venous thrombosis begins when stagnant flow permits platelets to set in a valvular sinus, forming a nidus of thrombus. The cycle of fibrin retraction and thrombin release aggregates more platelets as the thrombus either propagates upstream without occlusion or occludes the vein with retrograde thrombosis. [By permission of J Hardy (ed): *Hardy's Textbook of Surgery,* 1983, p 971.]

vated factor X, thrombin, fibrin, and catecholamines remain at high concentration in that area. Opposing this process is the fibrinolytic system of the blood and vein walls. The endothelium of the vein wall contains an activator that converts plasminogen into plasmin which lyses fibrin. As might be expected, however, the fibrinolytic system is inhibited after surgery and trauma, and there is also less activity in the veins of the lower extremity than in the upper extremity.

When contrast medium is injected in supine, immobilized patients, it may remain in venous valve sinuses for as long as 1 hour, confirming the stasis which exists in the soleal veins. This is the favored location for the formation of a nidus of thrombus as described. Successive layering of platelets, fibrin, red cells, and leukocytes produces an organized white thrombus which is more adherent to the vein wall than the propagating red thrombus which extends into the venous stream (Figure 59-1). The latter free-floating thrombus is much less likely to cause symptoms and more likely to result in embolism. If the original thrombus becomes attached to the opposite wall, it causes interruption of flow, retrograde thrombosis, and signs of venous stasis in the extremity. Subsequent edema formation within the confines of the deep fascia produces pain and a characteristic Homans' sign elicited by forcible dorsiflexion of the foot.

The site of venous obstruction determines the level at which swelling is observed clinically. Swelling at the thigh level always implies obstruction at the level of the iliofemoral system, while swelling of the calf or foot suggests obstruction at the femoropopliteal level. Autopsies suggest that it is more common for thrombi to originate in the soleus veins and then propagate proximally, but there is also evidence of primary thrombosis of femoral and iliac venous tributaries. Resolution of deep vein thrombosis with recanalization will affect the competence of the valves within the veins and can result in the postphlebitic syndrome as discussed in Chapter 60. Complete spontaneous lysis of large thrombi is relatively uncommon, and even when patients are treated adequately with heparin to prevent further thrombosis, complete lysis occurs in less than 20 percent of cases. It seems likely that complete dissolution of small asymptomatic calf-vein thrombi is a more common occurrence, but the actual frequency is unknown.

Diagnosis

Major venous thrombosis involving the deep venous system of the thigh and pelvis produces a characteristic clinical picture of pain, extensive pitting edema, and blanching that has been termed *phlegmasia alba dolens,* or "milk leg." Association with pregnancy may relate to hormonal effects on blood, relaxation of vessel walls, or mechanical compression of the left iliac vein at the pelvic brim, resulting in the term "milk leg of pregnancy." It was originally believed that the blanching was caused by spasm and compromise of arterial flow, but arteriograms fail to confirm this, and efforts to achieve sympatholysis to overcome "vasospasm" are ill-advised, since it is usually the subcutaneous edema that is responsible for the blanching. In addition to pregnancy, other mechanical factors that can affect the left iliac vein include compression from the right iliac artery or an overdistended bladder and congenital webs within the vein. These factors are responsible for the observed 4:1 preponderance of left versus right iliac vein involvement.

With further progression of venous thrombosis to impede most of the venous return from the extremity, there is a danger of limb loss from cessation of arterial flow. The clinical picture is characteristic, with sufficient congestion to produce phlegmasia cerulea dolens, or a blue leg. With the loss of sensory or motor function, the diagnosis can be made on clinical grounds and treatment started. Venous gangrene is likely unless an aggressive approach is utilized to remove the thrombus by open thrombectomy and to restore blood flow. A variant of this disorder associated with malignant disease occurs peripherally in the leg and has a high mortality rate.

As indicated earlier, these major complications represent less than 10 percent of the patients with venous thrombosis. In fact, only 40 percent of patients with venous thrombosis have any clinical signs of the disorder. In addition, false-positive clinical signs occur in up to 50 percent of patients studied (14). Because of this there has been a great deal of interest in the development of screening tests that could reveal thrombi before they became evident clinically. Of course, contrast venography provides direct evidence of both occlusive and nonocclusive thrombi, but it is invasive and requires the patient to move to a radiography suite. Ideally, the screening test would be accurate, noninvasive, and performed at the bedside. Although the ideal has not been achieved, there are a number of tests which have proved useful as documented more completely in Chapter 11.

ULTRASOUND

The Doppler probe can be used to advantage to detect major venous thrombi with a high degree of accuracy, but it is a subjective form of testing dependent on the examiner's experience. The principle is straightforward, based on the impairment of an accelerated flow signal produced by intraluminal thrombi (15). The examination begins at the ankle with identification of the posterior tibial vein signal adjacent to the artery. The flow signal should be altered by distal and proximal compression producing, respectively, augmentation and interruption of flow which also can be produced by the Valsalva maneuver. The same maneuvers are repeated over the superficial and deep femoral veins and can be done over the popliteal vein. Failure to augment flow on compression below or release of interruption of flow above the probe suggests venous thrombi. The sensitivity of the test exceeds 90 percent, but the specificity is 5 to 10 percent lower because of the possibility of other mechanical problems (Baker's cyst, hematoma, etc.) interfering with venous flow. A negative Doppler ultrasound examination is reassuring, but a positive or equivocal test should be confirmed by contrast venography. A negative test is *not* reassuring when major thromboembolism is suspected since the thrombus may have been evacuated from the extremity.

IMPEDANCE PLETHYSMOGRAPHY

The impedance plethysmography (IPG) method measures the volume response of the extremity to temporary occlusion of the venous system. The diagnosis of venous thrombosis depends on the changes in venous capacitance and rate of emptying after release of the occlusion. A proximal thigh cuff is inflated to 40 to 50 mmHg pressure for 50 to 120 s or until maximum filling has occurred by plateau of the electrical signal. The inflation cuff is then rapidly deflated, allowing rapid outflow and reduction of volume in a normal limb. Prolongation of the outflow wave suggests major venous thrombosis with 95 percent accuracy and is much more reliable than any voluntary technique of venous occlusion. The deficiency with this technique as with all of the noninvasive methods is in the detection of calf vein thrombosis or the definition of new pathology in patients with old thrombotic sequelae. The strain-gauge plethysmograph can be used in a similar fashion. A positive IPG test can be used to make therapeutic decisions in the absence of clinical conditions which can produce false-positive tests such as cardiac failure, constrictive pericarditis, hypotension, arterial insufficiency, or external compression of veins.

RADIOACTIVE-LABELED FIBRINOGEN

Clinical application of labeled fibrinogen has been facilitated by the development of portable scintillation counters for bedside use. After iodine blockage of the thyroid gland, the counts are obtained from marked locations on the lower extremities and expressed as a percentage of the radioactivity measured by counting over the heart. An increase of 20 percent or more in one area indicates the presence of an underlying thrombus. The test permits sequential scanning of the extremities over a period of days and is most sensitive to thrombi forming in the veins of the calves shortly after an operative procedure (16). It does not permit detection of thrombi in pelvic veins, and it cannot be used in an extremity in which there is a healing wound, fracture, cellulitis, arthritis, edema, ulceration, or superficial thrombophlebitis where false-positive results are likely. It is also contraindicated in patients under 30 years of age and in women of childbearing age. In the absence of these conditions it is quite accurate, however, showing a 90 percent correlation with contrast venograms. A negative correlation usually is explained by cessation of active thrombosis and failure to incorporate the tagged fibrinogen, making the test useful in discriminating between old and new venous thrombi.

VENOGRAPHY

The injection of contrast material for direct visualization of the venous system of the extremity is the most accurate method of confirming the diagnosis of venous thrombosis and the extent of the involvement. Injection is usually made into the foot while the superficial veins are occluded by tourniquet. A supplementary injection into the femoral veins may be required to visualize the iliofemoral system. Both filling defects and nonvisualization can be found and provide an assessment of the threat of a thrombus such as one seen to be floating free and extending into the iliofemoral system (Figure 59-2). Potential false-positive examinations may result from external compression of a vein or washout of the contrast material from collateral veins. The procedure can also be performed with isotope injection using a gamma scintillation counter to record flow of the isotope. Delayed imaging of persistent "hot spots" may also reflect isotope retention at the sites of thrombus formation. A perfusion lung scan can also be obtained for baseline comparison and to detect silent embolism. There is less definition of deep vein thrombi with this technique than with contrast venography, but it is a valuable technique for sequential study of patients and avoids the potential thrombogenesis of the injection of contrast medium.

ASSAY OF FIBRIN OR FIBRINOGEN PRODUCTS

The degradation of intravascular fibrin can be detected by measuring the plasma products of the lysis of fibrin or fibrinogen. Both fibrinopeptide A and fibrin fragment E can be detected by radioimmunoassay but are not specific for acute venous thrombosis. A negative test could conceivably have some value in excluding the diagnosis, but the tests are difficult and will require more investigation and simplification.

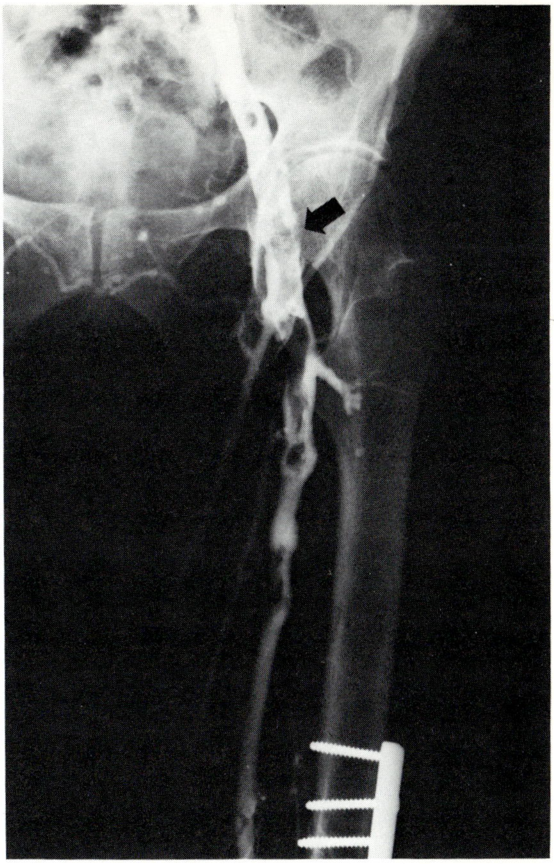

FIGURE 59-2. Contrast venogram shows a thrombus originating in a femoral vein tributary (*screws*) and extending to the level of the groin (*arrow*). Such a thrombus might well be asymptomatic. [By permission of J Hardy (ed): *Hardy's Textbook of Surgery*, 1983, p 972.]

Prophylaxis

Theoretically it should be possible to prevent formation of venous thrombi either by eliminating or reducing venous stasis or by altering blood coagulability. The belief that early ambulation prevents stasis and reduces the formation of thrombi has been controversial, and studies using tagged fibrinogen have not supported this assumption. One explanation for this is that early ambulation often consists of having the patient walk to a chair and sit, subjecting the legs to even more stasis. Other efforts, including electrical stimulation of calf muscles and passive motor-driven flexion of the foot, are under investigation, but discomfort, type of operative procedure, and cost remain obvious limitations.

There has been more interest in the prophylactic use of anticoagulant drugs and, more recently, drugs such as aspirin and dipyridamole which inhibit platelets. The latter drugs are under evaluation for this role, but preliminary reports have not shown adequate protection. However, there are good data to support the use of preoperative oral anticoagulant therapy with warfarin derivatives in high-risk patients. Unfortunately, this increases the risk of hemorrhage, and with the added difficulties of laboratory control of prothrombin time, there has not been widespread acceptance of this approach. The administration of dextran 40, which produces a variety of effects on platelets and clotting factors, has been demonstrated to reduce the incidence of detectable thrombi, but it too can produce hemorrhagic problems as well as allergic reaction and, in older patients, congestive failure.

In an effort to minimize the problems associated with anticoagulant prophylaxis, there has been renewed interest in administration of heparin, prior to and following surgery in low ("mini") doses that do not alter the laboratory clotting profile. Generally, a 5000-USP dose is given subcutaneously 2 hours preoperatively and then every 8 or 12 hours postoperatively for 6 days. This appears to provide protection for most high-risk groups with the exception of those undergoing orthopedic procedures. The beneficial effect may be from the enhancement of heparin cofactor (antithrombin III) as a natural inhibitor of activated factor X. Although some studies have failed to show protection, Kakkar et al. in a randomized series of 4121 patients showed protection against fatal pulmonary embolism as well as deep venous thrombosis (DVT) (17). There is a higher incidence of bleeding and wound complications associated with three times daily heparin prophylaxis, and since its major benefit appears to be in reducing the incidence of calf vein thrombosis, which is of questionable clinical significance, the question of optimal prophylaxis remains unresolved. For the general population of surgical patients under the age of 40 years, the risk of DVT is low and prophylaxis can be limited to early ambulation with or without graduated compression stockings. For patients over age 40 with major surgical procedures, the risk is moderate and prophylaxis should be considered, such as intermittent pneumatic compression or low-dose heparin administered subcutaneously twice daily. The patients at highest risk are those over age 40 who are obese and have or have had malignant disease, a history of DVT, or major trauma; these patients need more protection, which might include low-dose heparin, intermittent pneumatic compression, oral anticoagulants, or dextran (18). Low-dose heparin should not be used in neurosurgical patients because of the consequences of any intracranial bleeding. For these patients, external pneumatic compression is the prophylaxis of choice.

Treatment

The approach to management of the patient with DVT is based on minimizing the risk of pulmonary embolism, limiting further thrombosis, and facilitating resolution of existing thrombi to avoid the postphlebitic syndrome.

Initially, the patient is placed at bed rest with the foot of the bed elevated 8 to 10 inches. Generally, pain, swelling, and tenderness resolve over a 5- to 7-day period, at which time ambulation can be permitted with continued elastic stocking support. Standing still and sitting should be prohibited in order to avoid the increased venous pressure and stasis.

ANTICOAGULATION

The foundation of therapy for DVT is adequate anticoagulation, initially with heparin and then with warfarin derivatives for prolonged protection against recurrent thrombosis. Unless there are specific contraindications, heparin should be administered in an initial dose of 100 to 150 units per kilogram intravenously. Heparin is an acid mucopolysaccharide that neutralizes thrombin, inhibits thromboplastin, and reduces the platelet release reaction. It should be administered by continuous intravenous infusion regulated by whole blood or partial thromboplastin clotting time. Bleeding complications can be minimized by doses of heparin that prolong the laboratory clotting determinations in the range of twice normal with no loss of effectiveness. Continuous intravenous infusion regulated by an infusion pump seems to minimize the total dose required for control and is associated with a lower incidence of complications.

The side effects associated with heparin treatment include bleeding, thrombocytopenia, hypersensitivity, arterial thromboembolism, and osteoporosis. Bleeding is more likely to occur in elderly females, in patients treated with aspirin, or in patients who have had recent surgery or trauma. It has been well demonstrated that bleeding can occur when the results of laboratory monitoring tests are within the therapeutic range, which may be because of its effect on platelets.

Arterial thromboembolism can complicate heparin administration by any route and is more common in the elderly. It tends to occur after 7 to 10 days of therapy and is associated with thrombocytopenia. This complication carries a high morbidity and mortality rate and requires immediate cessation of heparin treatment. Thrombocytopenia as a complication may be caused by an immune reaction but is rapidly reversed when heparin is stopped, usually within 2 days. Hypersensitivity to heparin may take the form of a skin rash or rarely may produce anaphylaxis. Subcutaneous injections which show urticaria may become necrotic as an unusual form of sensitivity. Osteoporosis has been seen in patients on long-term heparin therapy in excess of 6 months. This is probably caused by a direct effect on bone resorption and can be avoided by shorter periods of treatment and dosage less than 15,000 units per day.

Oral administration of anticoagulants is begun shortly after initiation of heparin therapy, since several days usually are required to bring the prothrombin time within the therapeutic range of 2 to 2.5 times the control value and to provide the maximal antithrombotic effect. The warfarin derivatives block the synthesis of several clotting factors, and prolongation of the prothrombin time beyond the range suggested is associated with an increased incidence of bleeding complications. The nonhemorrhagic side effects are uncommon but include skin necrosis, dermatitis, and a syndrome of painful blue toes. Skin necrosis is heralded by painful erythema in areas of large amounts of subcutaneous fat and is reversible if the drug is stopped. Fortunately, the administration of vitamin K usually can restore the prothrombin time rapidly.

After an episode of acute DVT, anticoagulation should be maintained for a minimum of 3 months; some investigators favor 6 months for thrombi in the larger veins. There are many drugs, such as barbiturates, that interact with the warfarin derivatives, and therefore a routine for regular monitoring of prothrombin time is essential after the patient leaves the hospital. Oral anticoagulants are teratogenic and should not be used during established or planned pregnancy. In the pregnant patient, heparin is the drug of choice, and for long-term management, subcutaneous self-administration should be taught. This regimen allows a normal delivery and can be continued postpartum.

FIBRINOLYSIS

There has been great interest in the use of fibrinolytic agents to activate the intrinsic plasmin system. Both streptokinase and urokinase have been used and found to be effective, although they are associated with an incidence of 25 to 30 percent of hemorrhagic complications and fever (19). In 10 percent of patients, streptokinase is also associated with allergic reactions which vary from urticaria to anaphylaxis and can produce an adult respiratory distress syndrome (20). In addition, fibrinolytic agents have no advantage over heparin in the treatment of recurrent venous thrombosis or when thrombosis has existed for over 72 hours, and the lytic agents are contraindicated in the postoperative or posttraumatic patient.

SURGICAL APPROACHES

Operative Thrombectomy

A direct surgical approach to remove thrombi from the deep veins of the leg via the common femoral vein has been employed and facilitated by the use of Fogarty venous balloon catheters and an elastic wrap for milking the extremity. Although the operative results are impressive, venograms obtained prior to discharge from the hospital show rethrombosis in the majority of patients, and there does not seem to be any lesser incidence of the postphlebitic syndrome. Consequently, the procedure is now usually reserved for limb salvage in the presence of phlegmasia cerulea dolens and impending venous gangrene.

Vena Cava Interruption

Adequate anticoagulation usually is effective in managing DVT, but if recurrent pulmonary embolism occurs during anticoagulant therapy or if there is a contraindication to anticoagulation, then a surgical approach is necessary. Operation is also indicated as prophylaxis against recurrence of embolism for the patient who has required pulmonary embolectomy and in some high-risk patients who could not tolerate recurrence (Table 59-1).

Early surgical efforts to prevent recurrence of pulmonary embolism were directed to the common femoral vein, which was ligated bilaterally. This resulted in a high incidence of sequelae due to stasis in the lower extremity and an unacceptable rate of recurrent pulmonary embolism. The next approach was ligation of the inferior vena cava below the renal veins, which added the adverse effect of a sudden reduction in cardiac output. This effect, coupled with stasis sequelae and recurrent embolism through dilated collateral veins, led to efforts to compartmentalize the vena cava by means of sutures, staples, and external clips in order to provide filtration without occlusion.

Since these procedures required general anesthesia and laparotomy, the next logical step was to devise a transvenous approach that could be performed under local anesthesia. The Mobin-Uddin "umbrella" unit was the first to be inserted from the jugular vein and positioned under fluoroscopy below the renal veins, where it usually produced thrombosis of the vena cava [70 percent of cases (21)]. It also has been associated with complications of proximal thrombus formation and lethal migration into the pulmonary artery.

The Greenfield cone-shaped filter was developed to maintain patency after trapping emboli and to permit continued flow to avoid stasis and facilitate lysis of the embolus (Figure 59-3). It can be inserted from either the jugular vein or the femoral vein, the latter reserved for instances where there is an inadequate size of the jugular vein or an open wound of the neck (22). The recurrent embolism rate with this device has been 2 to 4 percent, and its long-term patency rate of 95 percent allows it to be placed above the renal veins when necessary for embolism control such as when there is thrombus within the renal veins or vena cava (23) (Figure 59-4). Another device, the Hunter balloon, occludes the vena cava after positioning it below the renal veins and contributes to stasis sequelae.

TABLE 59-1. Indications for Insertion of a Vena Caval Filter

1. Recurrent thromboembolism despite adequate anticoagulation
2. Thromboembolism in a patient who has a contraindication to anticoagulation
3. Complication of anticoagulation forcing therapy to be discontinued
4. Chronic pulmonary embolism with associated pulmonary hypertension and cor pulmonale (class V patient)
5. Immediately following pulmonary embolectomy
6. Relative indications: Patient with more than 50% of the pulmonary vascular bed occluded (class III) who would not tolerate additional embolism; patient with a large iliofemoral thrombus despite anticoagulation; septic embolism despite control of focus and antibiotics

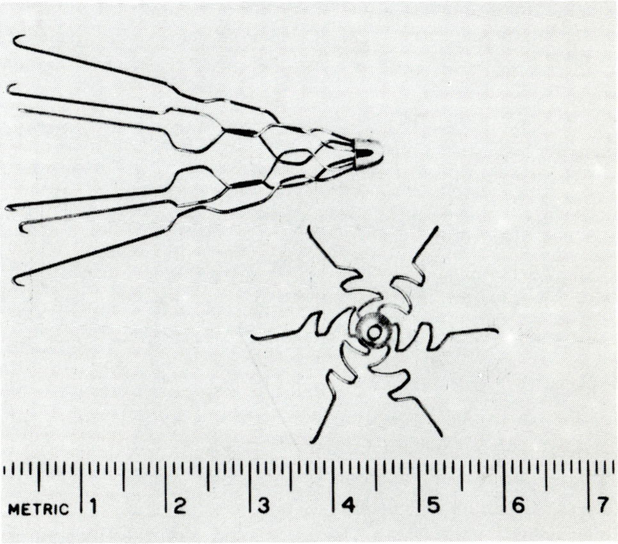

FIGURE 59-3. The Greenfield filter is made of stainless steel and is cone-shaped to preserve flow after an embolus is trapped. Flow preservation provides continued filtration, minimizes stasis sequelae, and facilitates lysis of the trapped thrombus.

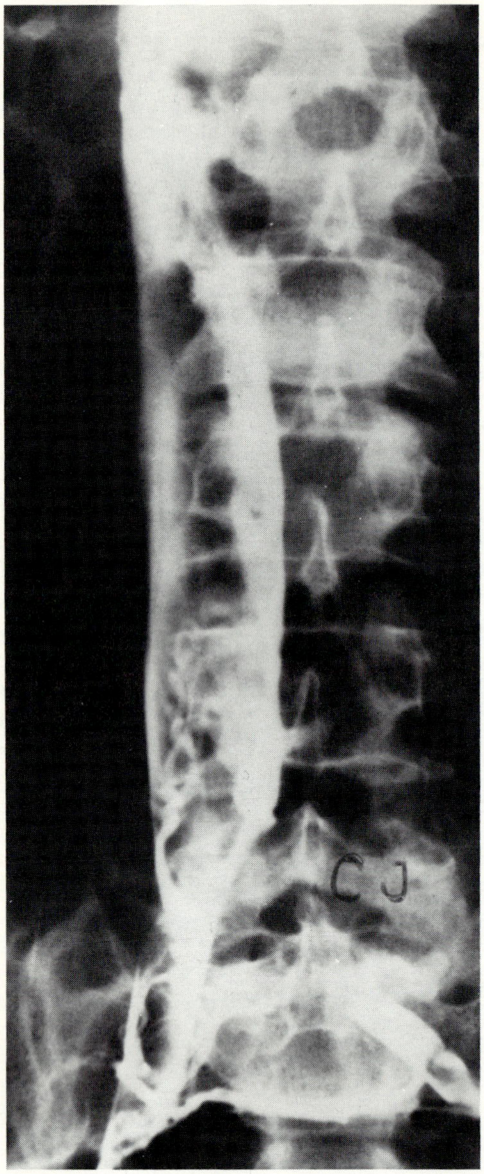

FIGURE 59-4. Contrast study of the vena cava showing a large thrombus in the inferior vena cava. Control of this "widow-maker" thrombus requires placement of the Greenfield filter above the level of the renal veins (L1).

The complications of filter insertion range in severity from minor wound hematomas caused by early resumption of anticoagulation to potentially lethal migration of the device into the pulmonary artery as documented with the Mobin-Uddin umbrella. The most common complication with the Greenfield filter has been misplacement in 7 percent of cases (23). When misplacement occurs below the diaphragm, the patient has inadequate protection, but the location in the renal or iliac vein poses no circulatory problem. A second filter can be placed in the appropriate location or the misplaced filter can be retrieved using a guide wire (24). This is always advocated for misplacement into the right heart. Air embolism can occur during jugular insertion, but the risk is minimized by having the patient hold his or her breath while the vein is open. In some patients the veins may be too small or fragile to permit insertion of the carrier catheter, and rarely the patient may be too obese to permit fluorocopy.

Recurrent embolism after filter placement has been seen in 2 to 4 percent of cases and may be caused by a source of thrombus outside the filtered flow region such as the upper extremities or the right atrium. Secondary infection of the Mobin-Uddin umbrella has been reported and required removal of the device. Secondary infection of captured thrombus within a Greenfield filter has been produced experimentally, but it was possible to sterilize the stainless steel filter and thrombus with antibiotic therapy (25). The capture of a very large embolus within a filter has the potential to suddenly occlude the vena cava with a precipitous fall in blood pressure. In a patient with known prior pulmonary embolism, this event can be mistaken for recurrent pulmonary embolism with disastrous results from vasopressor therapy. The basic distinction between functional hypovolemia and right ventricular overload can be made by the measurement of central venous pressure and Pa_{O_2}. The response to volume resuscitation for the patient with sudden vena caval occlusion should be dramatic.

There is one circumstance where migration of a Greenfield filter is possible after discharge. This occurs when there is failure to flush heparinized saline through the cylindrical carrier and a thrombus forms within it during the period of positioning under fluoroscopy. The thrombus can then tether the limbs of the filter, preventing their expansion and fixation to the wall of the vena cava. Only one such episode has been reported to the author, and it remains a totally preventable complication, much less likely to occur with the use of a guide wire to facilitate insertion and minimize the time that the carrier is used (22). For optimal protection a continuous drip of heparinized saline can be attached by intravenous tubing directly to the insertion catheter.

Other Thrombotic Disorders

The term *thrombophlebitis* should be restricted to the disorder of the superficial veins characterized by a local inflammatory process which is usually aseptic. The cause in the upper limb is usually acidic fluid infusion or prolonged cannulation. In the lower extremities it is usually associated with varicose veins and may coexist with DVT. The association with the injection of contrast material can be minimized by washout of the contrast material with heparinized saline.

THROMBOPHLEBITIS MIGRANS

This condition of recurrent episodes of superficial thrombophlebitis has been associated with visceral malignancy, systemic collagen vascular disease, and blood dyscrasias. Involvement of the deep veins and the visceral veins had also been described.

SUBCLAVIAN VEIN THROMBOSIS

This disorder is most likely to be secondary to an indwelling catheter and can occur in the pediatric age group. It may also occur as a primary event in a young, athletic person ("effort thrombosis"), presumably as a result of injury or congenital constriction at the thoracic inlet. When the diagnosis is made early, thrombolytic agents and a venogram should be obtained to determine whether operative decompression of the vein is indicated. First rib resection by anterior or axillary approach has been successful in preventing rethrombosis. When the diagnosis is made 3 or more days after the event, there is usually a good response to elevation and anticoagulation, although some venous insufficiency and discomfort with exercise may persist.

ABDOMINAL VEIN THROMBOSIS

Thrombosis of the inferior vena cava can result from tumor invasion or propagating thrombus from the iliac veins. Most commonly, however, it results from ligation, plication, or insertion of occluding caval devices. Thrombosis of the renal vein is most likely to occur in association with the nephrotic syndrome. It can be a source of thromboembolism and has been treated successfully by suprarenal placement of the Greenfield filter (26).

Portal vein thrombosis can occur in the neonate, usually secondary to propagating septic thrombophlebitis of the umbilical vein. Collateral development leads to the occurrence of esophageal varices. Thrombosis of the portal, hepatic, splenic, or superior mesenteric vein in the adult can occur spontaneously, but usually is associated with hepatic cirrhosis. Thrombosis of mesenteric or omental veins can stimulate an acute abdomen but usually results in prolonged ileus rather than intestinal infarction.

Hepatic vein thrombosis (Budd-Chiari syndrome) usually produces massive hepatomegaly, ascites, and liver failure. It can occur in association with a congenital web, endophlebitis, or polycythemia vera. Although some success has been reported using a direct approach to the congenital webs, the usual treatment is a side-to-side portacaval shunt to allow decompression of the liver. The development of pelvic sepsis after abortion, tubal infection, or puerperal sepsis can lead to septic thrombophlebitis of the pelvic veins and septic thromboembolism. Ovarian vein and caval ligation has been used traditionally, but the emphasis should be on drainage or excision of the abscesses and appropriate antibiotic therapy. We have also used the Greenfield filter in this situation, since it is inert stainless steel and avoids the development of an intraluminal abscess which can occur after the traditional approach of ligation of the vena cava (25).

Pulmonary Thromboembolism

OVERVIEW

The clinical significance of major pulmonary embolism can be appreciated by reference to the annual mortality attributed to it, which has been estimated to be 90,000 deaths in the United States alone. It is estimated that 5 of every 1000 adults undergoing major surgery will die from massive pulmonary embolism. Since it represents the most important complication of DVT, it is of particular concern to surgeons whose patients are prone to develop deep vein thrombosis in the immediate postoperative period. The full spectrum of the disorder ranges from asymptomatic minor embolism to sudden death from massive embolism.

DIAGNOSIS

The signs and symptoms of an embolic episode obviously depend primarily on the quantity of embolus involved and to a lesser extent on the cardiopulmonary status of the patient. In the classic presentation, the patient suddenly develops chest pain, cough, dyspnea, tachypnea, and marked anxiety. Although hemoptysis has traditionally been associated with pulmonary embolism, it is actually an uncommon sign; when present it usually occurs late in the course and probably represents pulmonary infarction. Objectively, the patient with major embolism usually shows tachycardia, an increased pulmonary second sound, cyanosis, prominent jugular veins, and varying degrees of hypotension. Less commonly, there may be wheezing, a pleural friction rub, splinting of the chest wall, rales, low-grade fever, ventricular gallop, and wide splitting of the pulmonic second sound. The incidence of these findings is shown in Table 59-2.

The differential diagnosis includes esophageal perforation, pneumonia, septic shock, and myocardial infarction. Since all of these entities are life-threatening, it is mandatory that an orderly approach be formulated to confirm or reject the working diagnosis. Laboratory studies in general are not very helpful in the differential diagnosis, although a white blood cell count of less than 15,000/mL may be suggestive when a pulmonary infiltrate is present to help rule out pneumonitis. The following determinations are particularly useful in the evaluation of suspected major embolism.

TABLE 59-2. Clinical Manifestations of Major Pulmonary Embolism

Symptoms	Incidence, %	Signs	Incidence, %
Dyspnea	80	Tachypnea	88
Apprehension	60	Tachycardia	63
Pleural pain	60	Accentuated P_2	60
Cough	50	Rales	51
Hemoptysis	27	S_3 or S_4	47
Syncope	22	Pleural rub	17

SOURCE: Adapted from the Urokinase Pulmonary Embolism Trial (30).

Electrocardiography

The most common electrocardiographic change associated with pulmonary embolism is nonspecific ST and T wave changes (66 percent of patients). More specific signs of right ventricular overload such as the often quoted S_1, Q_3, T_3 pattern are seldom seen. Consequently, the primary value of the electrocardiogram is to exlude the presence of a myocardial infarction. Unfortunately, the finding of a myocardial infarction does not exclude the diagnosis of pulmonary embolism, and in some cases a lung scan or pulmonary angiogram may be required to clarify the problem.

Chest Radiography

Although the chest radiograph may suggest the diagnosis of pulmonary embolism because of central vascular enlargement, asymmetry of the vascular markings with segmental or lobar ischemia (Westermark's sign), or pleural effusion, these signs are nonspecific. The chest radiograph then serves to exclude other diagnostic possibilities such as pneumonia, pneumothorax, esophageal perforation, or congestive heart failure. It also is essential in the interpretation of a lung scan, since any radiographic density or evidence of chronic lung disease makes a perfusion defect in that area less likely to represent pulmonary embolism. Chronic lung disease also reduces the applicability of lung scanning to the diagnosis.

Arterial Blood Gases

Blood gas and pH determinations can provide support for the diagnosis of pulmonary embolism. Hypoxemia with Pa_{O_2} less than 60 mmHg is found in the majority of patients and felt to be due to shunting by overperfusion of nonembolized lung and a widened alveolar-arterial oxygen gradient due to reduced cardiac output. The reduction in arterial P_{CO_2} that follows major embolism is the most discriminating finding since hypoxemia can be seen in several disorders likely to be misdiagnosed as massive embolism, e.g., septic shock (27). In the absence of hypoxemia and hypocarbia the diagnosis of major embolism in the severely ill patient can be excluded with moderate confidence, and an alternative diagnosis should be sought.

Central Venous Pressure

In the patient with systemic hypotension, the central venous pressure can provide valuable information as well as access for the administration of drugs and fluids. Low central venous pressure virtually excludes pulmonary embolism as the primary cause of the hypotension, since massive embolism almost always is accompanied by right ventricular overload and elevated right atrial pressures. Elevated right ventricular filling pressures may be transient, however, as hemodynamic accommodation occurs, and in subacute or chronic embolism, the central venous pressure may be normal.

Lung Scan

Availability and widespread usage of lung photoscanning has led to overemphasis of this test and a tendency to overdiagnosis pulmonary embolism. In the presence of a normal chest radiograph in a nonhypotensive patient, the lung scan is a valuable screening test that has increasing validity as the size of the perfusion defect approaches lobar distribution. Smaller peripheral perfusion defects are much more difficult to interpret, since pneumonitis, atelectasis, or other ventilation abnormalities alter pulmonary perfusion. A normal lung scan, on the other hand, essentially excludes the diagnosis of pulmonary embolism. Adding a ventilation scan for combined ventilation-perfusion imaging increases the accuracy of the diagnosis of thromboembolism, provided that there is a large area of ventilation-perfusion mismatch, but matched defects do not rule out embolism (28). The assumption that the underperfused regions of the lung after embolism will remain normally ventilated producing the mismatch in the scans is clouded by the known physiological effect of bronchoconstriction produced by embolism. Adding the additional variable of wide variance in scan interpretation among observers makes the diagnosis much more reliable when based on arteriography (Figure 59-5) (2). An alternative approach to the patient with suspected embolism and an abnormal perfusion scan is to perform venography and initiate anticoagulation if it is positive (28). If negative, pulmonary angiography would be required to exclude the diagnosis of embolism (Figure 59-6).

Pulmonary Arteriography

Selective pulmonary arteriography is the most accurate method of confirming the presence, size, and distribution of pulmonary emboli. The procedure is invasive, requiring passage of a cardiac

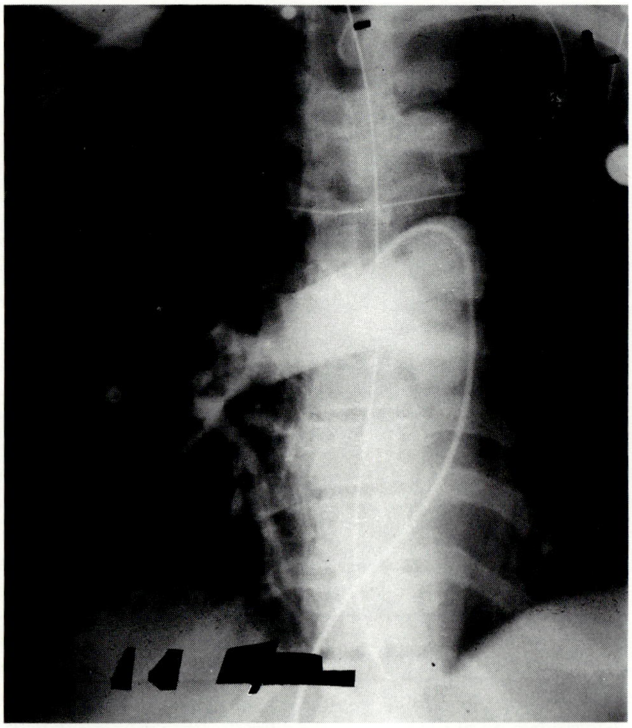

FIGURE 59-5. Selective pulmonary arteriogram with injection of contrast medium into the right main pulmonary artery. A coiled thrombus can be seen obstructing flow to the upper and lower lobes.

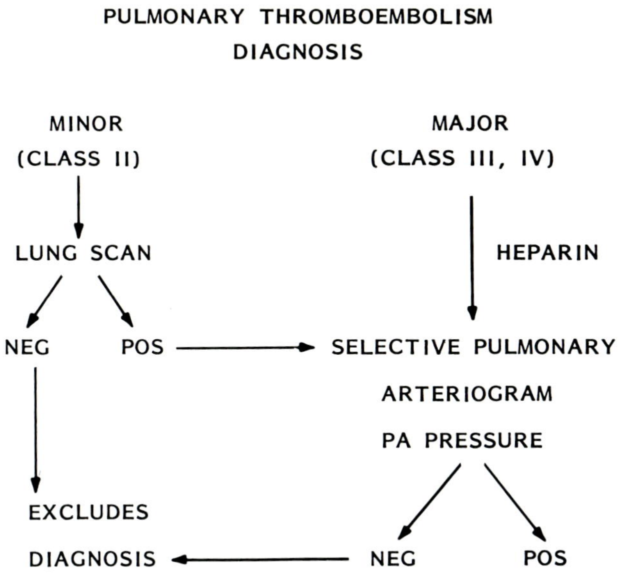

FIGURE 59-6. Schematic approach to the expeditious diagnosis of pulmonary thromboembolism based on clinical status. As an alternative to pulmonary arteriography in the patient with a positive lung scan, a venogram can be obtained to demonstrate DVT and justify anticoagulation.

catheter into the main pulmonary artery for injection of a bolus of contrast medium. A rapid film changer produces a series of radiographs that outline areas of decreased perfusion and usually show filling defects or the rounded trailing edge of impacted emboli (Figure 59-5). Straight cutoffs of the smaller pulmonary arteries are more difficult to interpret, particularly if there is associated chronic lung disease that tends to obliterate pulmonary vessels. The procedure can be performed at low risk, although this is the most hazardous group of patients for this type of study, which usually carries a 0.5 percent mortality rate (29). Avoidance of main pulmonary artery injection of contrast medium minimizes the complication rate. Additional useful information is obtained prior to contrast medium injection by measurement of pulmonary arterial (PA) pressures. A normal pulmonary angiogram excludes the diagnosis of pulmonary embolism in acutely ill patients. Although the resolution rate for pulmonary emboli is unpredictable, it is unrealistic to assume that a negative arteriogram within a week of the clinical event might miss the diagnosis because of rapid fibrinolysis. In the Urokinase Pulmonary Embolism Trial report, the earliest complete resolution was not seen before 14 days (30).

PATHOPHYSIOLOGY

Although DVT precedes pulmonary embolism, less than 33 percent of patients with documented pulmonary embolism show signs of venous thrombosis. Despite this, it is estimated that 85 to 90 percent of all pulmonary emboli originate from the veins of the lower extremity, while the remainder arise from the right side of the heart or other veins. In fact, the lower incidence of DVT after embolism may reflect the evacuation of the thrombus from the lower extremity. In addition, the emboli tend to be multiple, fragmenting either in the right side of the heart or during impaction into the pulmonary vascular bed. Older thrombi, however, contain laminated fibrin layers that make them more solid and more difficult to lyse.

Once the embolus has lodged and interrupted pulmonary blood flow, the ratio of regional ventilation to perfusion increases, and the lung responds by bronchoconstriction to reduce wasted ventilation. This response is mediated by local reduction in CO_2 output, since it can be prevented by ventilation with increased concentration of CO_2. Some experimental studies also suggest a generalized neural reflex vasoconstriction, but even if this occurs in humans, it is not likely to be as significant a factor in survival as the mechanical effect of major vascular occlusion. Similarly, the effects of vasoactive humoral agents can be demonstrated in animals, and there is good documentation that serotonin is elaborated from platelets adherent to the embolus, which also contributes to the bronchoconstriction observed. The ability of heparin to inhibit the release of serotonin adds further justification to the early use of this drug. Other vasoactive agents such as histamine and prostaglandins may play a role in humans, but the net effect is a reduction in size of peripheral airways, reduced lung volume, and reduced static pulmonary compliance.

The hypoxemia that characterizes major embolism is thought to be caused by a ventilation-perfusion imbalance secondary to the ventilation changes described above, although the findings in some patients resemble true arteriovenous shunting. The latter becomes anatomically possible if there is an unobliterated foramen ovale that opens in the presence of elevated right atrial pressures. Such an opening can also allow passage of a venous embolus into the systemic circulation, which then is termed *paradoxical embolism*. Although there may be some improvement in Pa_{O_2} after supplemental oxygen is administered, the effects usually are minimal. The return of pulmonary blood flow effected by embolectomy restores respiratory gas exchange, but the ischemia appears to result in some loss of capillary integrity, causing interstitial pulmonary edema or overt pulmonary hemorrhage.

Pulmonary infarction as a consequence of embolism is relatively rare and associated clinically with problems of poor systemic perfusion such as shock or congestive heart failure. In these patients the symptoms include pleuritic chest pain, dyspnea, cough, and hemoptysis. The signs include fever, tachycardia, splinting, and occasionally friction rub. There is usually prominent leukocytosis, an elevated lactic dehydrogenase level, and bilirubinemia. A wedge-shaped density usually is seen on the chest film.

The pulmonary vascular and cardiac effects of embolism are a direct consequence of the degree of obstruction of the pulmonary vascular bed. Occlusion of more than 30 percent of the vascular tree is required to begin to elevate mean PA pressure, and usually more than 50 percent occlusion is required to reduce systemic pressure. The degree of pulmonary hypertension produced is proportional to the extent of angiographic vascular occlusion, but in a previously normal patient, the limit of mean pressure generated by the right ventricle is approximately 40 torr. The fate of pulmonary emboli in human patients is not easy to predict, although a great deal of experimental work in animals has been reported. Injection of autologous thrombi into the pulmonary circulation of dogs is followed by relatively rapid recovery of pulmonary function and objective evidence of lysis over a period of weeks. Activation of plasminogen to plasmin,

TABLE 59-3. **Classification of Pulmonary Thromboembolism**

Class	Symptoms	Gases	PA Occlusion, %	Hemodynamics
I	None	Normal	<20	Normal
II	Anxiety, hyperventilation	Pa_{O_2} < 80 torr Pa_{CO_2} < 35 torr	20–30	Tachycardia
III	Dyspnea, collapse	Pa_{O_2} < 65 torr Pa_{CO_2} < 30 torr	30–50	CVP elevated, $\overline{PA}$ > 20 torr
IV	Shock, dyspnea	Pa_{O_2} < 50 torr Pa_{CO_2} < 30 torr	>50	CVP elevated, $\overline{PA}$ > 25 torr BP < 100 torr
V	Dyspnea, syncope	Pa_{O_2} < 50 torr Pa_{CO_2} < 30–40 torr	>50	CVP elevated, $\overline{PA}$ > 40 torr, low cardiac output

NOTE: CVP = central venous pressure; $\overline{PA}$ = mean pulmonary artery pressure; BP = blood pressure.

which is found in high concentration in the pulmonary circulation, promotes this fibrinolytic effect. Unfortunately, the resolution of aged thrombi proceeds more slowly and is hampered further by impaction of the embolus and isolation from pulmonary blood flow. Consequently, resolution after massive embolism in patients is unpredictable and often incomplete. It is not unusual to find residual fibrin strands or webs in the pulmonary arteries at autopsy as remnants of prior embolism.

CLASSIFICATION AND MANAGEMENT

The hemodynamic variables mentioned above provide a means of classification of patients that employs five grades of severity and is a useful guide to therapy and prognosis (Table 59-3). The minor degrees of embolism (classes I and II) usually can be managed by anticoagulants alone with a satisfactory outcome. Heparin is selected for initial treatment in a dose range designed to prolong the partial thromboplastin time to at least twice normal. At this dosage of approximately 150 units per kilogram there is adequate protection against further attachment of thrombi and platelets to the embolus. Many clinicians also begin oral anticoagulation therapy with warfarin derivatives shortly after starting heparin administration in order to allow several days' overlap of the drugs as prothrombin time is extended into the therapeutic range.

In some patients, however, anticoagulants cannot be used because of associated problems (e.g., peptic ulcer disease), and management must be directed to a mechanical means of protection against recurrent embolism as outlined previously. Other patients, in whom anticoagulation appears to be adequate, sustain recurrent embolism and become candidates for surgical intervention. The third indication for a surgical procedure is to protect against recurrent embolism in a patient who has sustained massive pulmonary embolism requiring open or catheter embolectomy. In these patients, even though a satisfactory embolectomy of the pulmonary circulation has been performed, the original focus of venous thrombosis remains untreated and is very likely to promote recurrent embolism, usually of major size.

There are additional relative indications for vena caval procedures to prevent embolism. One is in the high-risk patient over 40 years of age who is obese, has a serious associated medical illness (e.g., heart disease), or malignant disease, with a history of recent DVT and who is about to undergo a major surgical procedure or requires cessation of anticoagulation. Another relative indication exists in the patient with a long, free-floating thrombus at the groin level. The final relative indication is in the patient in whom 40 to 50 percent of the vascular bed has been occluded by embolism (class III) and who would most likely not be able to tolerate an additional embolus, particularly if there is associated cardiac or pulmonary disease.

Pulmonary emboli may accumulate gradually over a prolonged period if they are small enough to produce microembolism rather than macroembolism. The clinical picture in this case is then one of chronic cor pulmonale because significant pulmonary hypertension results from obliteration of the pulmonary vascular bed (class V). The presentation may be subtle with only dyspnea or syncope on exertion, but there is a loud P_2 and right ventricular strain on the ECG. The sequence may also not be accompanied by significant respiratory symptoms and may explain the etiology in some of the patients considered to have primary pulmonary hypertension. When the diagnosis is made, there is a very limited life expectancy, and the patient may benefit from a vena caval procedure to prevent further embolism even if the disorder is primary pulmonary hypertension (31). The rationale is that these patients develop right heart failure predisposing to DVT and pulmonary embolism which is lethal even if small. When acute cardiopulmonary decompensation occurs in these patients after embolism, they are not good candidates for embolectomy because of fixation of the older thrombi to the pulmonary arterial wall. They should be classified separately (class V) and managed by long-term anticoagulation and filter placement (Figure 59-7).

In cases in which the emboli originate from a septic focus, usually the pelvis in a female, the classic treatment has been vena caval ligation with ligation of the ovarian or spermatic veins. It must be recognized, however, that large collateral veins develop as a consequence of vena caval occlusion and may then become the avenues of recurrent embolism. For this reason, we have used the Greenfield filter at either suprarenal or infrarenal level in conjunction with antibiotic therapy.

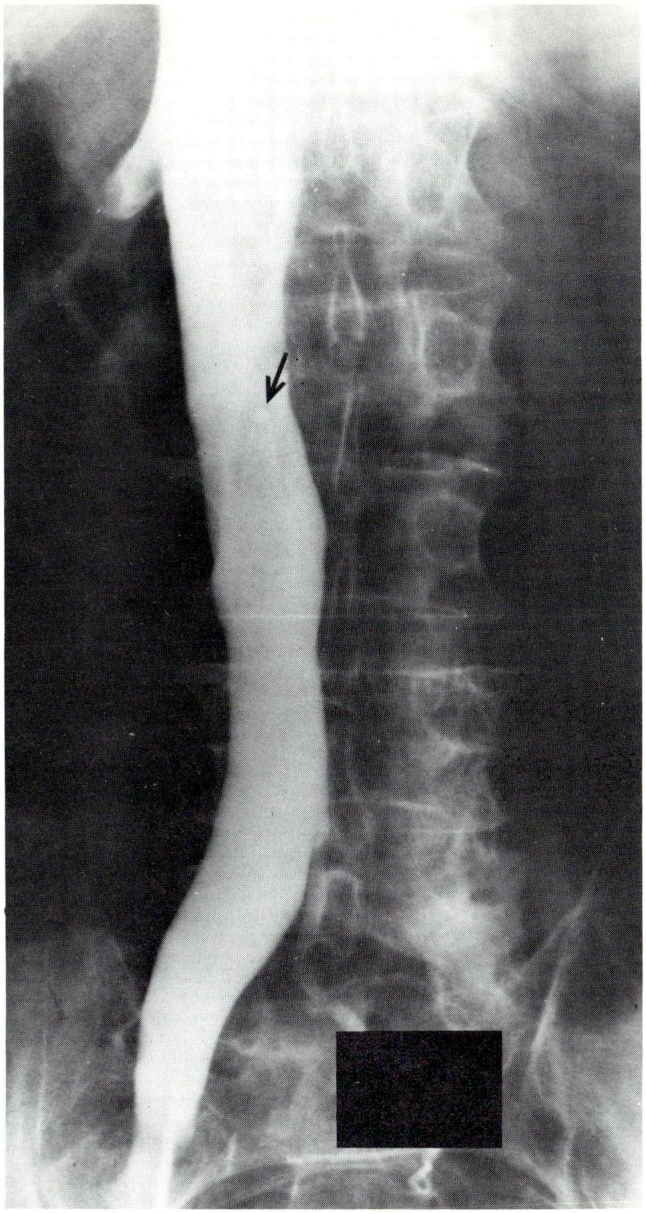

FIGURE 59-7. Vena cava study showing free flow of contrast medium through the Greenfield filter (*arrow*) placed in an infrarenal location at L3.

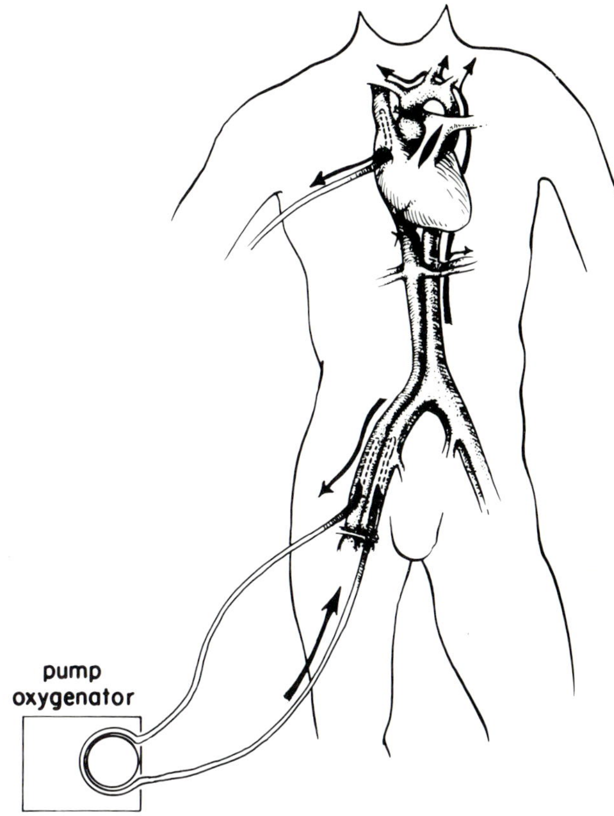

FIGURE 59-8. Following massive pulmonary embolism with shock (class IV), the patient who fails to respond to resuscitation must be supported by partial venoarterial bypass using the femoral vessels which can be cannulated under local anesthesia. Then, after general anesthesia and sternotomy, a second cannula in the superior vena cava allows total bypass for open embolectomy through the main pulmonary artery. [By permission of J Hardy (ed): *Hardy's Textbook of Surgery*, 1983, p 981.]

PULMONARY EMBOLECTOMY

For those patients who sustain massive embolism (classes III and IV), management must be a coordinated and rapidly responsive effort, since survival may be only a matter of minutes. As indicated earlier, it is critical to document the presence of massive pulmonary embolism by pulmonary arteriography since the clinical diagnosis, regardless of "classic" appearance, often is in error. The initial approach to patients who have either transient collapse (class III) or persistent systemic hypotension (class IV) should include full heparinization and administration of inotropic drugs if necessary to support the circulation while the diagnosis is confirmed. Isoproterenol (4 mg in 1000 mL 5% dextrose in water) is useful initially because of its bronchodilator and vasodilator effects as well as its positive inotropic cardiac effect. It may provoke arrhythmias, however, and necessitate the use of dopamine. For the class II patient who responds to heparin and does not require vasopressors for systemic pressure or urine output, careful monitoring is essential to determine whether anticoagulation alone will control the disorder.

The very high mortality rate associated with the Trendelenburg procedure (32) prompted the use of extracorporeal circulation to bypass the impacted pulmonary circulation. Embolectomy during cardiopulmonary bypass was reported first by Sharp in 1962 (33). Since then partial bypass support has also been utilized (Figure 59-8). Local anesthesia is used, and the femoral artery and vein are cannulated for venoarterial bypass. Once the sternotomy is performed, the partial bypass can be converted to total bypass by insertion of a superior vena caval catheter; the pulmonary emboli are then removed through a pulmonary arteriotomy.

Open pulmonary embolectomy still carries a high mortality rate, however, and the most serious complication is uncontrollable pulmonary hemorrhage which may follow restoration of pulmonary perfusion (34). Consequently, an alternative approach utilizing local anesthesia has been suggested by Greenfield et al. for transvenous removal of pulmonary emboli (35). A cup device attached to a steerable catheter* is inserted in the femoral or jugular vein, and the cup is positioned adjacent to the embolus seen on arteriography (Figure 59-9). The position is verified by injection of contrast medium through the catheter. Then syringe suction is applied to aspirate the embolus into the cup where it is held by suction as the catheter and captured embolus are withdrawn. Clinical experience with the technique reported in 1982 in 19 patients showed that emboli could be extracted in 16 of them (84 percent) with an overall survival of 73 percent (36). Emboli could not be removed when they had been impacted for more than 72 hours or if the patient arrested at the time of angiography, in which case open embolectomy was required. Placement of a Greenfield vena caval filter after removal of sufficient emboli to produce near normal hemodynamics protected the patients from recurrent embolism.

CHRONIC PULMONARY EMBOLISM AND PULMONARY HYPERTENSION

Recurrent thromboembolism may lead to progressive obliteration of the pulmonary vascular bed if the thrombi fail to undergo lysis. The resultant pulmonary hypertension produces exertional dyspnea and signs of right heart strain with cor pulmonale. With further progression of right heart overload tricuspid insufficiency may develop. This disorder may be difficult to distinguish from primary pulmonary hypertension, although the latter is more likely to be found in women under 20 years of age without a history of deep venous thrombosis.

Open thrombectomy for chronic occlusion was first performed by Allison et al. in 1958 and remains a possibility for improving pulmonary blood flow (37). Unfortunately, to be eligible for this procedure, the occlusion must involve the proximal portion of the pulmonary arterial tree and the distal bed must be patent. The physiological basis for continued distal patency after proximal occlusion is via bronchial arterial collateral flow. The procedure also has a significant mortality rate, reported at 38 percent by Cabrol et al. in a series of 16 patients (38). The complications of the procedure reported by these authors include hemorrhagic pneumonitis, cardiac failure, persistent pulmonary hypertension, pulmonary edema, hemothorax, empyema, and pulmonary infarction. The long-term results in surviving patients have been

*Medi Tech, Inc., Watertown, Massachusetts 02172.

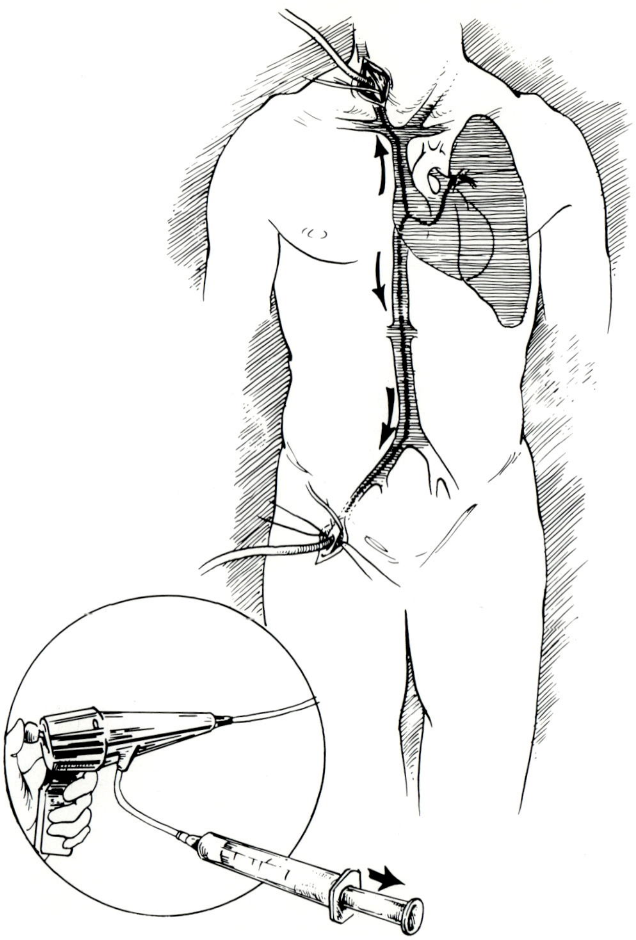

FIGURE 59-9. For the class IV patient who responds to resuscitation but remains hypotensive, catheter embolectomy can be performed under local anesthesia through the jugular or femoral vein. The steerable cup catheter is positioned under fluoroscopy adjacent to the embolus and syringe suction applied to capture the thrombus in the cup where it is held by sustained suction as the catheter is withdrawn. Repeat passage and control medium injection are used to clear all unattached emboli from branches of the pulmonary arteries.

favorable with improved respiratory function and relief of pulmonary hypertension. For the majority of patients with severe pulmonary hypertension, however, the outlook is poor unless they receive maximum protection from recurrent embolism, which in our experience has required both anticoagulation and vena caval filter placement (31).

References

1. Coon WW, Willis PW III, Keller JB: Venous thromboembolism and other venous disease in the Tecumseh Community Health Study. Circulation 1973, 48:839.
2. Davies GC, Salzman EW: The pathogenesis of deep vein thrombosis. In Joist JH, Sherman LA (eds): *Venous and Arterial Thrombosis*. New York, Grune and Stratton, 1978, pp 1–22.
3. Kakkar VV, Flanc C, Howe CT, Clarke MB: Natural history of postoperative deep vein thrombosis. Lancet 1969, 2:230.
4. Virchow R: *Gesammelte Abhandlungen zur Wissenschaftlichen Medizin*. Frankfurt, Meidinger Sohn, 1856, p 219.
5. Patterson JC, McLachlin JA: Precipitating factors in venous thrombosis. Surg Gynecol Obstet 1954, 98:96.
6. Seeger WH, Marciniak E: Inhibition of antiprothrombin C activity with plasma. Nature (London) 1962, 193:1188.
7. Ekberg O: Inherited antithrombin deficiency causing thrombophilia. Thromb Diath Haemorrh 1965, 13:576.

8. Towne JB, Bernhard VM, Hussey C, Garancis JC: Antithrombin deficiency—A cause of unexplained thrombosis in vascular surgery. Surgery 1981, 89:735.
9. Trousseau A: Phlegmatia alba dolens. In *Clinique Medicale de l'Hotel-Dieu de Paris,* ed 2, vol 3. Paris, JB Bailliere, 1865, pp 654–712.
10. Gore JM, Appelbaum JS, Greene HL, Dexter L, Dalen JE: Occult cancer in patients with acute pulmonary embolism. Ann Intern Med 1982, 96:556.
11. Hanson EC, Levine FH: Hyperlipoproteinemia as a significant risk factor for pulmonary embolism in patients undergoing coronary artery bypass grafting. Ann Thorac Surg 1982, 33:593.
12. Petitti DB, Wingerd J, Pellegrin F, Ramcharon S: Risk of vascular disease in women. JAMA 1979, 242:1150.
13. Jick H, Porter J: Thrombophlebitis of the lower extremities and ABO blood type. Arch Intern Med 1978, 138:1566.
14. Hirsh J, Hull R: Comparative value of tests for the diagnosis of venous thrombosis. World J Surg 1978, 2:27.
15. Strandness DE, Schultz RD, Sumner DA, Rushmer RF: Ultrasonic flow detection. A useful technique in the evaluation of peripheral vascular disease. Am J Surg 1967, 113:311.
16. Flanc C, Kakkar VV, Clarke MB: The detection of venous thrombosis of the legs using ^{125}I-labeled fibrinogen. Br J Surg 1968, 55:742.
17. Kakkar VV, Corrigan TP, Spindler JR, Fossard DP, Flute PT, Crellin RO: Efficacy of low doses of heparin in prevention of deep vein thrombosis after major surgery: A double-blind, randomized trial. Lancet 1972, 2:101.
18. Bonnar J, Walsh J: Prevention of thrombosis after pelvic surgery by British dextran 70. Lancet 1972, 1:614.
19. Bell WR, Meek AG: Guidelines for the use of thrombolytic agents. N Engl J Med 1979, 301:1266.
20. Martin TR, Sandblom RL, Johnson RJ: Adult respiratory distress syndrome following thrombolytic therapy for pulmonary embolism. Chest 1983, 83:151.
21. Cimochowski GE, Evans RH, Zarius CK, Lee CT, DeMeester TR: Greenfield filter versus Mobin-Uddin umbrella, the continuing quest for the ideal method of vena caval interruption. J Thorac Cardiovasc Surg 1980, 79:358.
22. Greenfield LJ, Stewart JR, Crute S: Improved technique for Greenfield vena caval filter insertion. Surg Gynecol Obstet 1983, 156(2):217–219.
23. Greenfield LJ, Peyton R, Crute S, Barnes R: Greenfield vena caval filter experience: Late results in 156 patients. Arch Surg 1981, 116:1451.
24. Greenfield LJ, Crute SL: Retrieval of the Kimray-Greenfield® vena caval filter. Surgery 1980, 88(5):719.
25. Peyton JWR, Hylemon MB, Greenfield LJ, Crute SL, Sugerman HJ, Quershi GD: Comparison of Greenfield filter and vena caval ligation for experimental septic thromboembolism. Surgery 1983, 93:533–537.
26. Stewart JR, Peyton JWR, Crute SL, Greenfield LJ: Clinical results of suprarenal placement of the Greenfield vena cava filter. Surgery 1982, 92:1–4.
27. Goodall RJR, Greenfield LJ: Clinical correlations in the diagnosis of pulmonary embolism. Ann Surg 1980, 191(2):219–223.
28. Hull RD, Hirsh J, Carter CJ, Jay RM, Dodd PE, Ockelford MB, Coates G, Gill GJ, Turpie AG, Doyle DJ, Buller HR, Raskob GE: Pulmonary angiography, ventilation lung scanning, and venography for clinically suspected pulmonary embolism with abnormal perfusion scan. Ann Intern Med 1983, 98:891.
29. Bell WR, Simon TL: A comparative analysis of pulmonary perfusion scans with pulmonary angiograms—From a national cooperative study. Am Heart J 1976, 92:700.
30. Urokinase Pulmonary Embolism Trial: A national cooperative study. Circulation 1973, 47(suppl II):47.
31. Greenfield LJ, Scher LA, Elkins RC: KMA-Greenfield® filter placement for chronic pulmonary hypertension. Ann Surg 1979, 189:560.
32. Trendelenburg F: Uber die operative behandlung der embolie der lumgenarterie. Arch Klin Chir 1908, 86:686.
33. Sharp EH: Pulmonary embolectomy: Successful removal of a massive pulmonary embolus with the support of cardiopulmonary bypass: A case report. Ann Surg 1962, 156:1.
34. Brown S, Muller D, Buckberg G: Massive pulmonary hemorrhagic infarction following revascularization of ischemic lungs. Arch Surg 1974, 108:795.
35. Greenfield LJ, Peyton MD, Brown PP, Elkins RC: Transvenous management of pulmonary embolic disease. Ann Surg 1974, 189:461.
36. Greenfield LJ, Stewart J, Crute S: Results of surgical management of pulmonary thromboembolism. J Clin Surg 1982, 1:194–199.
37. Allison PR, Dunhill MS, Marshall R: Pulmonary embolism. Thorax 1980, 15:273.
38. Cabrol C, Cabrol A, Acar J, Gandjbakhch I, Giraudon G, Laughlin L, Mattei MF, Godeau P: Surgical correction of chronic postembolic obstruction of the pulmonary arteries. J Thorac Cardiovasc Surg 1968, 76:742.

Chapter 60

CHRONIC VENOUS INSUFFICIENCY

GEOFFREY H. WHITE

The terms *chronic venous insufficiency* (CVI) and *venous insufficiency syndrome* describe a syndrome of limb symptoms including edema, pigmentation, pain, and disability which often progresses to chronic ulceration. Since there is a spectrum of severity ranging from asymptomatic to severe, and a variety of etiological processes, numerous terms may be encountered in the literature and in clinical practice. Thus the terms *postphlebitic syndrome* or *postthrombotic leg* are used because of the proven association with prior deep venous thrombosis (DVT), (1,2), whereas "deep venous insufficiency" differentiates these patients from those who have superficial varicose veins.

A classification of the various forms of chronic venous insufficiency is given in Table 60-1. From this table it can be seen that the two important mechanisms producing insufficiency are venous obstruction and valvular incompetence. However, this classification can be misleading since in most cases there are degrees of both of these processes. Assessment of the relative importance of these factors may not be possible with the standard ascending venogram which gives good anatomical detail, but little functional information. However, recent advances in noninvasive and invasive investigation techniques have made possible hemodynamic documentation of the pathophysiological processes and have led to a surge of renewed interest in the field of venous problems, which had previously been somewhat neglected in comparison to other aspects of vascular surgery.

Incidence and Significance

Venous ulcers were described by Hippocrates, who noted an association with varicose disease. Medical writings of the eighteenth and nineteenth centuries also emphasized the associated varicose veins and used the term varicose ulcer. However, Gay in 1867 noted that ulcers were associated with serious lesions of the deep veins and described abnormalities of the perforating veins and deep veins seen in patients with the postphlebitic syndrome (3). Homans in 1917 showed that recanalization of the vein with destruction of valves was probably very common after DVT and that ulcers of the leg followed (4). Proof of the relationship to previous DVT became possible after the introduction of venography by Dos Santos in 1938 (5). Bauer demonstrated that more than 50 percent of patients with DVT developed leg ulcer over a 10-year period (6), while Dodd and Cockett's analysis of various similar studies showed that between 30 and 87 percent of patients with venous ulcer had a history suggestive of DVT (1).

It has recently been estimated that 10 to 35 percent of the U.S. adult population has some form of venous disorder (7), and venous diseases are the seventh most common in incidence among 28 chronic diseases (8). Data from the Tecumseh Community Health Survey have been extrapolated to show that 5 percent of U.S. adults have stasis changes in the skin of the leg, and more than 500,000 suffer from venous ulcers (9). A Swedish study showed that 2.2 percent of the population aged over 18 had postphlebitic sequelae (10).

Approximately 90 percent of all leg ulcers are due to venous disease (11), and anyone associated with a vascular clinic is only too well aware of the immense demand placed upon facilities and staff if these patients are to be efficiently assessed and cared for. Conservative treatment is palliative but not curative; however, this has been the mainstay for centuries. Recent advances in surgical management are directed toward reversing hemodynamic deficits and may achieve better long-term results.

Anatomy

There are three principal systems of veins of the lower limb, named according to their anatomical relationship to the deep fascia: (1) *superficial veins*, which are external to the deep fascia; (2) *deep veins*, which are internal to the deep fascia; (3) *perforating veins*, which pierce the deep fascia as a communication between the superficial and deep systems.

SUPERFICIAL VEINS

These veins run in the subcutaneous plane as a freely communicating network.

Long Saphenous Vein

This is the important superficial vein of the anterior and medial aspects of the leg. The major trunk of the long saphenous vein receives four to five named tributaries in the upper thigh and terminates by penetrating the deep fascia at the fossa ovalis to enter the deep system. The course is discussed in more detail in Chapter 58.

Posterior Arch Vein

This vein or group of veins (Figure 60-1) runs on the posteromedial side of the calf, forming a posterior arch of tributaries

TABLE 60-1. Classification: Forms of Chronic Venous Insufficiency

Valvular Incompetence:
Primary:
Congenital valvular aplasia or incompetence
Hereditary varicose veins
Secondary:
Perforator vein incompetence
Deep vein incompetence
Superficial vein incompetence
Venous obstruction:
Chronic iliac vein occlusion
Femoropopliteal vein occlusion
Multisegment venous obstruction
Others:
Venous malformations
AV fistula

of the distal long saphenous vein. This vein has considerable importance with regard to the pathophysiology and surgery of the postphlebitic syndrome because of three reasonably constant perforating veins, which form a direct communication between the posterior arch veins and the posterior tibial veins of the deep system (12).

Short Saphenous Vein

This is the principal superficial network of the posterior and lateral aspects of the calf. After a course running up across the popliteal fossa, the short saphenous similarly drains into the deep system at the saphenopopliteal junction by penetrating the deep fascia.

DEEP VEINS

Venae Comitantes of the Named Arteries

These major veins run in the intermuscular planes deep to the deep fascia, in close association with the branches of the femoropopliteotibial arterial tree. Below the popliteal level, each artery is usually accompanied by two or three venous channels, interconnected by a plexus of smaller veins.

Intramuscular Venous Sinuses

These are large, thin-walled, valveless venous plexuses within the soleal and gastrocnemius muscles, which act as capacitance chambers and drain into the popliteal and tibial veins. Usually the site of entry of these sinuses into the deep veins is at a point where one of the perforating veins also joins the deep system (1).

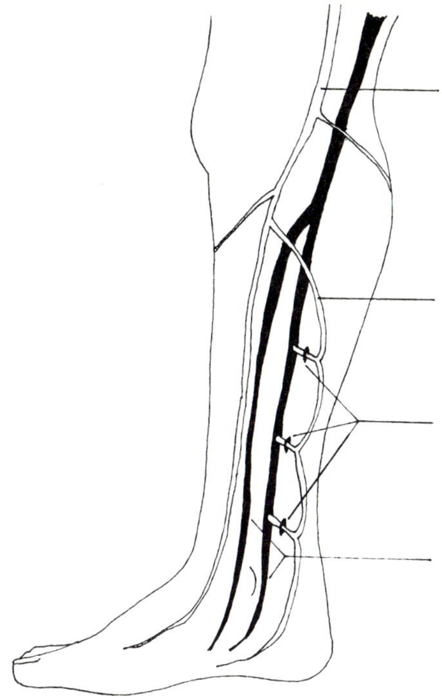

FIGURE 60-1. Relationship between the main superficial and deep veins of the leg, and the perforating veins that connect them.

PERFORATING VEINS

Although often referred to as "communicating veins" by anatomists, most of the surgical literature uses the term *perforating veins* to describe those veins which pierce the deep fascia, forming an anastomotic channel between the superficial and deep systems (13) (Figures 60-1 and 60-2). Anatomical studies reveal a great number of small veins which fulfill this function. However, only a relatively small number have surgical significance. These are often given eponyms, honoring the surgeons who first described their relevance to the postphlebitic syndrome.

The most important are on the medial side of the lower leg (Cockett's perforators) (14), joining the posterior arch vein to the posterior tibial plexus, and at the adductor level in the thigh (Dodd's perforator) (15), joining tributaries of the long saphenous vein and the femoral vein (Figure 60-3). Another surgically important vein is the lateral ankle perforator, found just above the external malleolus (16). Other sites of lesser significance are shown in Figure 60-2, including veins draining the gastrocnemius and soleus muscles (17).

Valves of the Leg Veins

All veins distal to the common iliac vein contain bicuspid valves, with the greatest frequency of valves in the more distal veins (18). In general the deep veins contain more valves than do the superficial veins (19). There is usually a valve in the principal vessel just distal to each entering branch and one near the mouth of the entering vein as well (19). The valves within the deep system of veins direct blood proximally toward the vena cava and heart, whereas blood within the superficial system is directed both proximally (up the vein itself) and internally, via the perforating veins, to the deep system. Exceptions to this are found within the foot, hand, and forearm, where blood is directed from the deep to superficial systems (17).

The perforating veins contain up to three valves, all found within their subfascial segment (20). The important roles of these valves are to prevent reflux of blood from the deep to superficial veins, thus preventing superficial venous hypertension, and to contribute to the venous "muscle pump" mechanism.

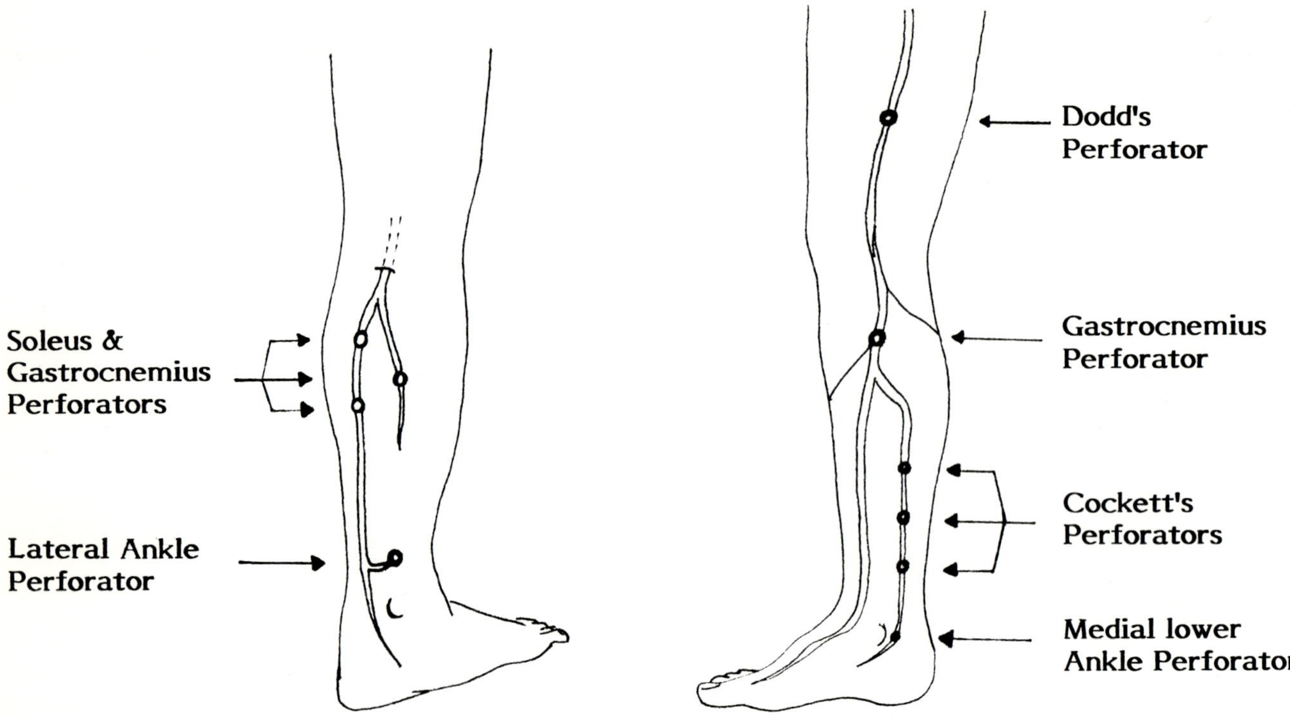

FIGURE 60-2. The important perforating veins of the medial and lateral sides of the leg.

Venous Hemodynamics: The Calf Muscle Venous Pump

NORMAL VENOUS HEMODYNAMICS

Venous pressure measurements taken from a vein in the foot demonstrate a static pressure of approximately 10 to 15 mmHg in the supine position at rest. This pressure is dependent primarily on the hydraulic pressure of blood. However, in the upright position, gravitational hydrostatic forces are added, increasing the measured pressure to that of a column of blood from the foot vein up to the level of the heart (i.e., approximately 90 to 100 mmHg) (17).

With exercise, the tight compartmental fascial linings allow the leg muscles to act as a ''pump,'' compressing the intramuscular venous sinuses and deep intermuscular veins. With competent valvular function, venous blood in these capacitance vessels is pumped progressively up the leg veins. The deep valves prevent retrograde flow down the leg, and perforator vein valves prevent outward flow into the superficial venous system. With sustained exercise, such as walking or foot dorsiflexion by repeatedly standing on tiptoes, there is a rapid fall in venous pressure to a level of approximately 30 mmHg (21,22). With cessation of exercise, there is a gradual rise of the venous pressure back up to the resting value over 20 to 30 s (23) (Figure 60-4). Thus during exercise, venous return is increased significantly, and since the capillary hydrostatic pressure is reduced along with venous pressure, there is less tendency for fluid flow out of the capillaries into the tissues.

The muscle pump has been demonstrated to have a period of ''diastole'' (i.e., phase of relaxation of the calf muscles during walking or cycling) which favors flow of venous blood in from the subcutaneous tissues around the ankle via the perforating veins (24).

ABNORMAL VENOUS HEMODYNAMICS DUE TO CHRONIC VENOUS INSUFFICIENCY

An intact valve mechanism is an integral requirement for efficient function of the venous muscle pump. In the postphlebitic leg, resolution of the thrombotic process not only renders incompetent many of the valves in the deep and perforating veins, but it also leaves a variable element of venous obstruction (2). Blood from the deep veins flows out through incompetent perforators into the superficial veins. Muscle contracture accentuates this outflow via the perforators and drives blood retrogradely in the incompetent deep system (25). As a result, there is only a minimal fall in peripheral venous pressure during leg exercise (26), resulting in a state of relative ''local ambulatory venous hypertension'' (1).

Venous pressure measurements in these patients with valvular incompetence demonstrate significantly less pressure fall during exercise compared to the normal leg and an abnormally rapid rise back up to resting pressure after cessation of exercise (22). The patient with perforator vein incompetence or deep vein incompetence will usually show a pressure drop of only 15 to 25 percent (the normal is approximately 70 percent)—the worst pressure profiles tend to be found in patients with evidence of both perforator and deep vein incompetence (see Figure 60-13). Pressures may be checked with the saphenous system occluded by a tourniquet cuff to judge whether saphenofemoral incompetence is worsening the situation. The milder exercise pressure changes seen in patients with primary varicose veins alone will be prevented by this maneuver (27), whereas failure of the cuff to restore the fall to normal proves some degree of calf-pump incompetence.

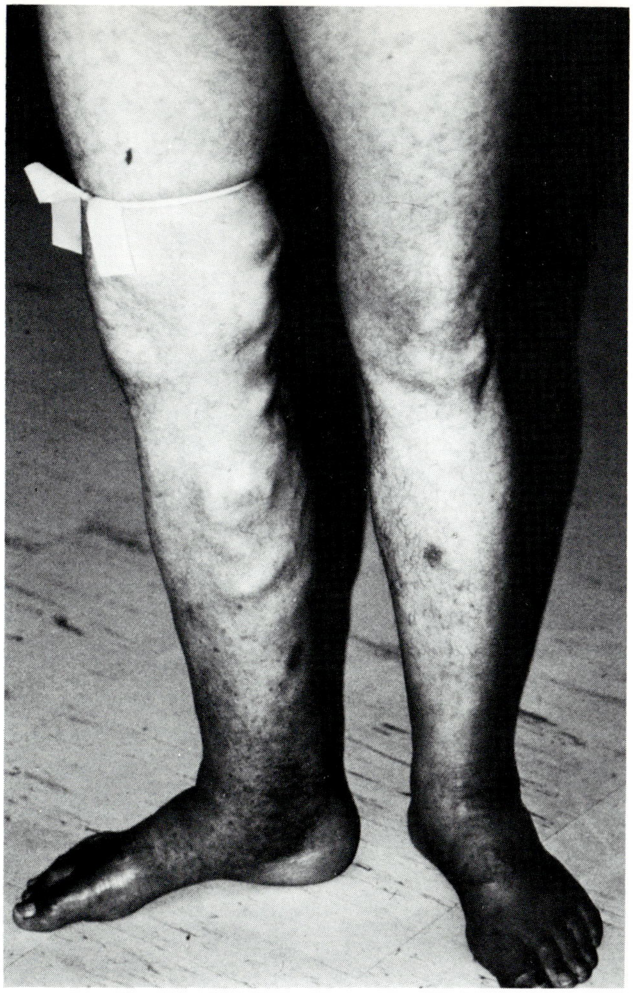

FIGURE 60-3. Thigh tourniquet occluding long saphenous vein (Trendelenburg test) does not prevent rapid refilling of an incompetent Dodd's perforator vein with leg dependent.

Clinical Features

The "typical" clinical picture of the patient with chronic venous insufficiency is that of an edematous leg with an area of skin thickening and dermatitis involving the medial side of the lower half of the leg, with associated pigmentation and inflammation. This progresses to a state of cellulitis, subcutaneous and dermal fibrosis, and ulceration (Figure 60-5).

There will often be a past history of documented DVT, or good presumptive evidence such as major trauma, operation, or previous episodes of leg swelling or pain consistent with DVT. Occasionally there will be a known history of causative conditions such as arteriovenous malformation. Frequently the leg is painful, although this is often little more than vague aches or night cramps, aggravated by dependency and relieved by elevation. If there is cellulitis or ulceration, the pain may be more severe and particularly localized to the affected area. Less commonly, a disabling throbbing or bursting pain may be experienced throughout the leg during walking, which has been referred to as venous claudication. This type of pain usually indicates major venous obstruction, with raised intracompartmental pressures (28). Obviously arterial insufficiency must be excluded in these rare cases.

The swelling is usually described as a brawny edema or induration and is caused by high venous pressure. Dilated vessels form an ankle flare (or "blowout") (12). This venous hypertension also results in increased hydrostatic pressure at the capillary level, causing diapedesis of erythrocytes via intercellular spaces in the capillary endothelial lining. Capillary rupture may also occur. Deposits of hemosiderin from these erythrocytes cause a brownish purple skin pigmentation. Histological study of the pigmented tissue has also implicated excessive melanocytic activity, secondary to inflammation (29). This feature is sometimes described as "senile purpura" (1). Combination of this pigmentation with the dermatitis caused by poor skin nutrition ("venous eczema") leads to severe itching, and patients often are first seen by a dermatologist (Figure 60-6). Venous spiders, stars, or telangiectasias may occur in association with CVI or with primary varicose veins (30). These are asymptomatic but may be treated by sclerotherapy (31) or laser (32) for cosmetic reasons.

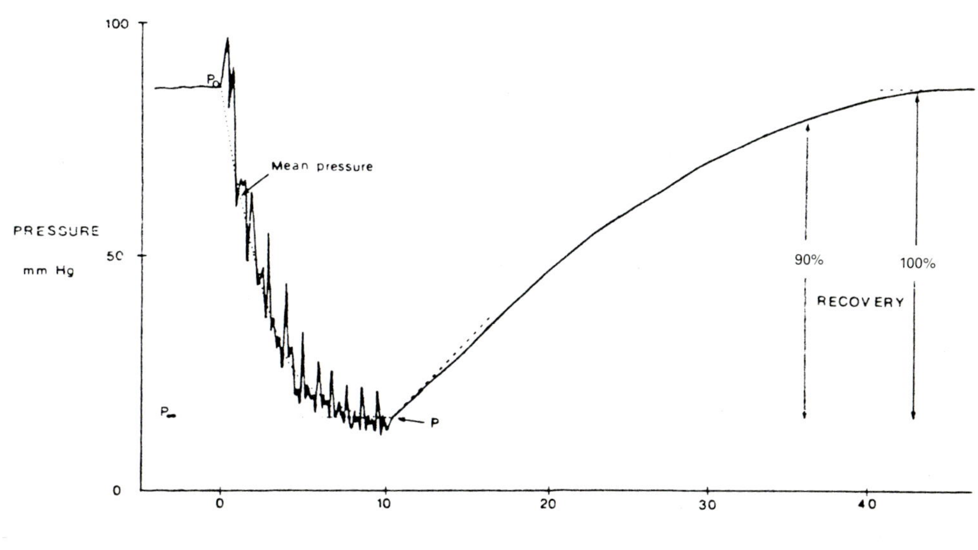

FIGURE 60-4. Recording of venous pressure of a normal limb during exercise (10 heel-raise movements) and during recovery phase. Note the rapid fall in pressure and the long recovery time (RT). P = initial resting pressure; P_∞ = mean exercise asymptotic value. [Reprinted with permission from Nicolaides AN et al (89).]

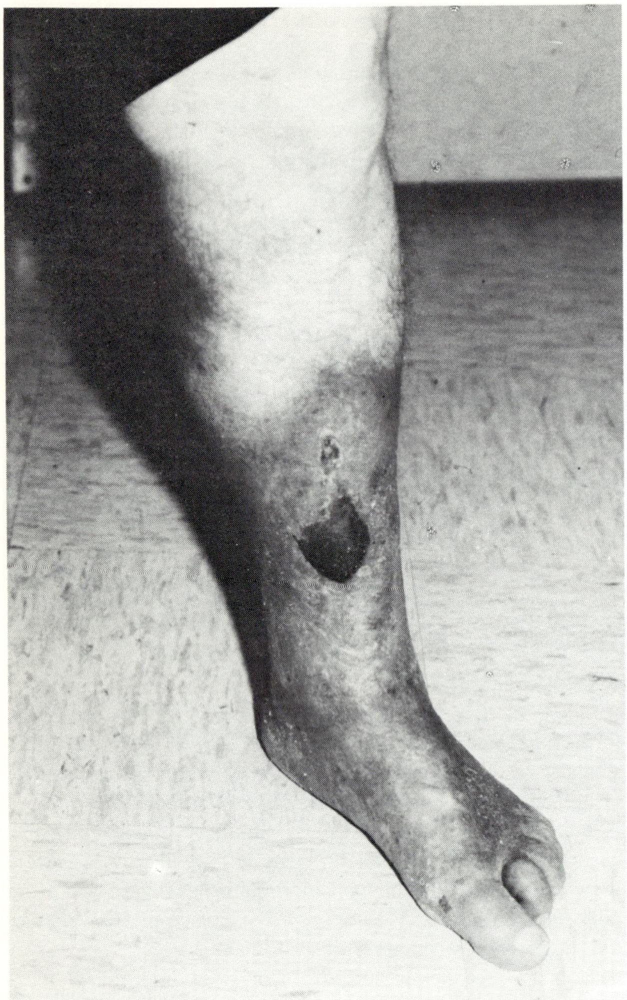

FIGURE 60-5. Typical distribution of pigmentation, trophic changes, eczema, and ulceration.

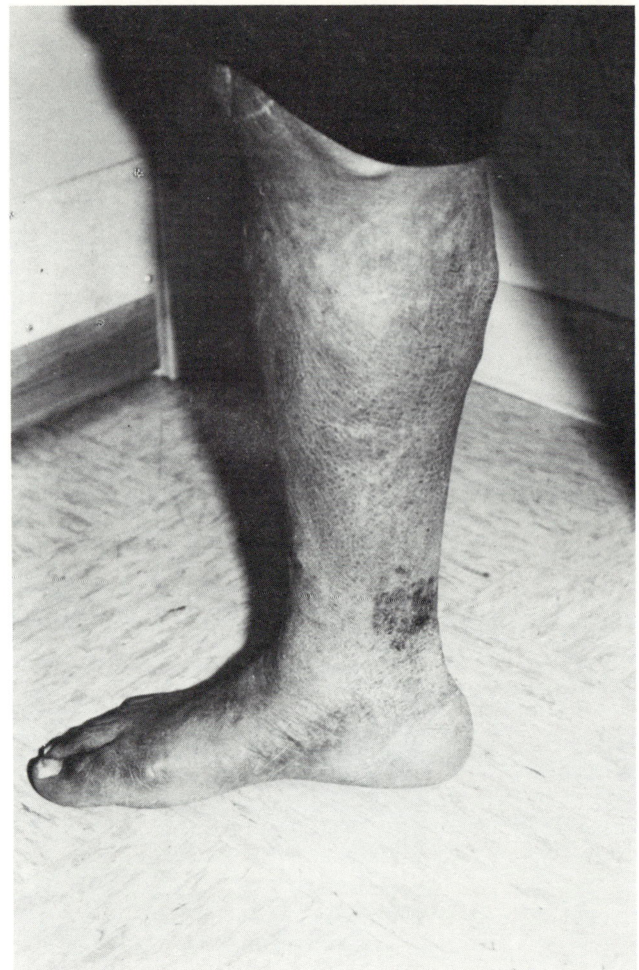

FIGURE 60-6. Prominent venous dermatitis, with dry, pruritic, scaly skin and old healed ulcer.

Hyperpigmentation and edema are usually the earliest signs of CVI, following DVT within 2 years. Other skin changes and ulceration more commonly take between 2 to 5 years to develop. An ulcer precursor state was described by Cockett (12). The skin initially becomes thin and atrophic due to hypoperfusion at the tissue level. Subsequent thickening occurs after the sustained high interstitial pressures have caused fat necrosis and fibrosis (1). However, since the histological appearance of this abnormal subcutaneous tissue is different from fat necrosis elsewhere in the body, the term *lipodermatosclerosis* has been proposed to describe the changes occurring in both skin and subcutaneous layers (33). Calcification may ultimately occur and can be detected radiologically (34), as shown in Figure 60-7.

In severe cases, muscle atrophy also occurs. The combination of this muscle atrophy with the presence of an overlying tight band of thickened, fibrosed tissue can give the leg an appearance described as the ''inverted champagne bottle.'' Neglected cases may progress to the stage of muscle contractures, with equinus deformity, pes cavus, and claw toes (1).

Varicose veins may be associated. If there is concurrent superficial vein incompetence, gross varicosities will be present. However, in most cases there are only mild secondary varicosities of the lower leg, or there are no varicose veins at all—this was noted by Gay as early in 1867 (3), and later reemphasis of this feature by Homans (4,19) stimulated investigation into the quite separate etiology of this syndrome, which had previously been considered a direct complication of varicose veins.

VENOUS ULCER

These so-called stasis ulcers or gravitational ulcers (Figure 60-8) occur in the gaiter distribution of the lower third of the leg and are almost always centered posterior and superior to the medial malleolus of the ankle. [This is the area where the subcutaneous and superficial venous pressure is highest due to the proximity of incompetent perforator veins (12) (Figure 60-9).] Typically these are oval or serpiginous in shape with sloping walls and are frequently multiple. The indurated skin surrounding the ulcer shows pigmentation and may have the scars of

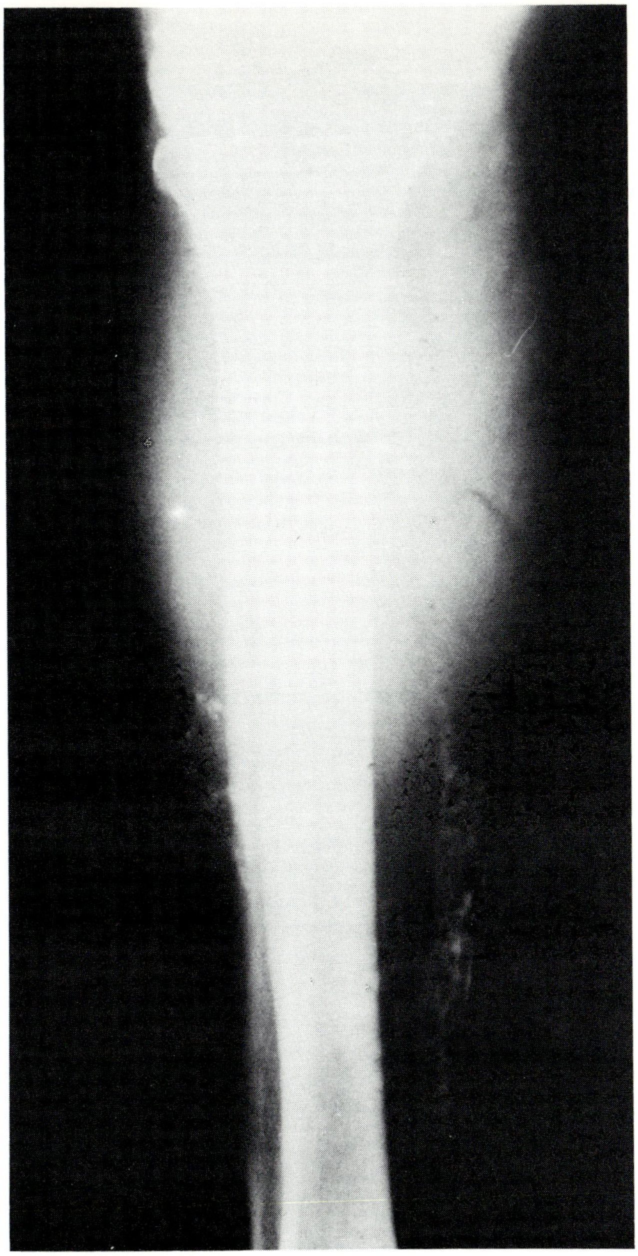

FIGURE 60-7. Subcutaneous calcification seen on x-ray of ''post-phlebitic'' leg.

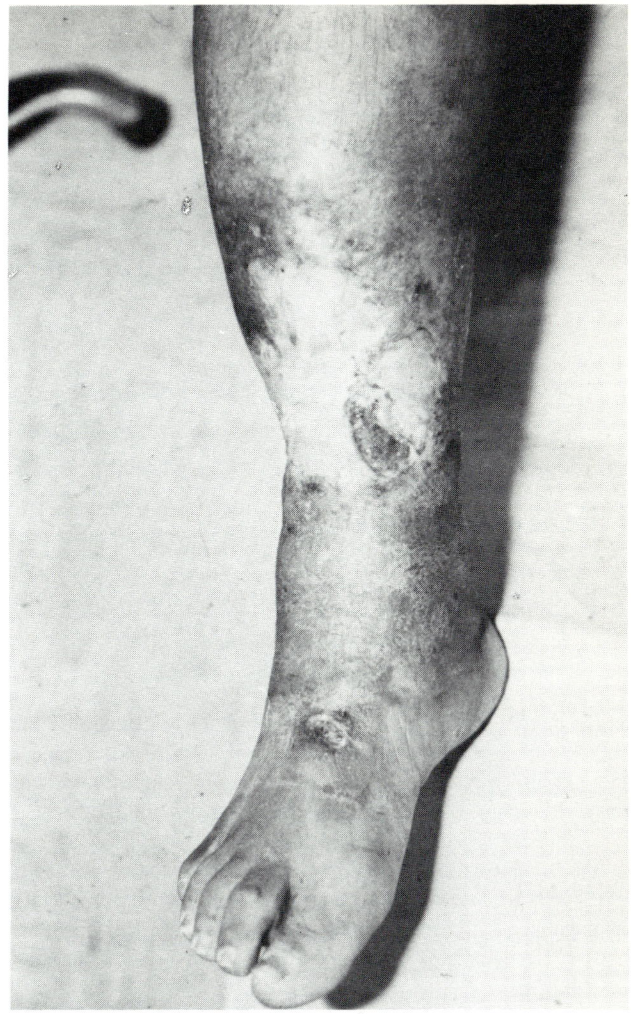

FIGURE 60-8. Venous ulcer which had healed and recurred many times with conservative treatment.

previous healed ulcers. The base is flat and covered with necrotic debris or infected slough. The tissue beneath the ulcer is also stiff and thickened. If infected, there is usually a surrounding area of cellulitis. Signs of healing are the presence of healthy vascular granulation tissue in the base, with a pink rim of new epithelium at the edges. Squamous-cell carcinoma may develop in a long-standing venous ulcer (Marjolin's ulcer) (35).

Venous ulcer may also occur in a corresponding area on the lateral side of the ankle and in the severe state may encricle the ankle (Figure 60-10). They are not found on the foot.

The ulcer is not usually intensely painful, unless infected. Pain is relieved by elevation.

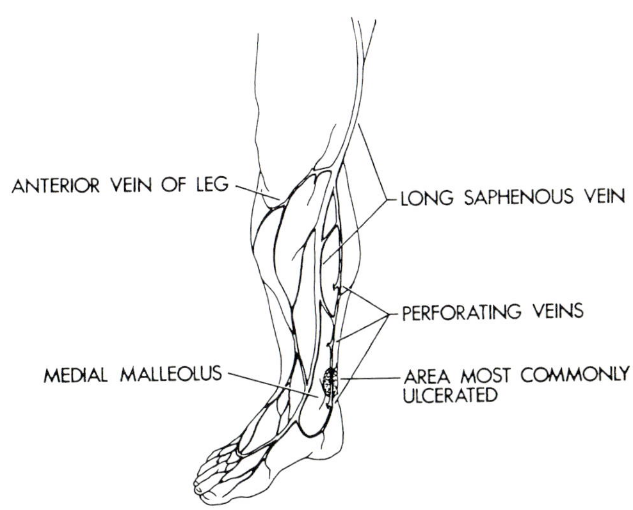

FIGURE 60-9. The area most commonly involved by venous ulcer is drained primarily by the perforating veins into the deep system. [From Hyde GL et al (109).]

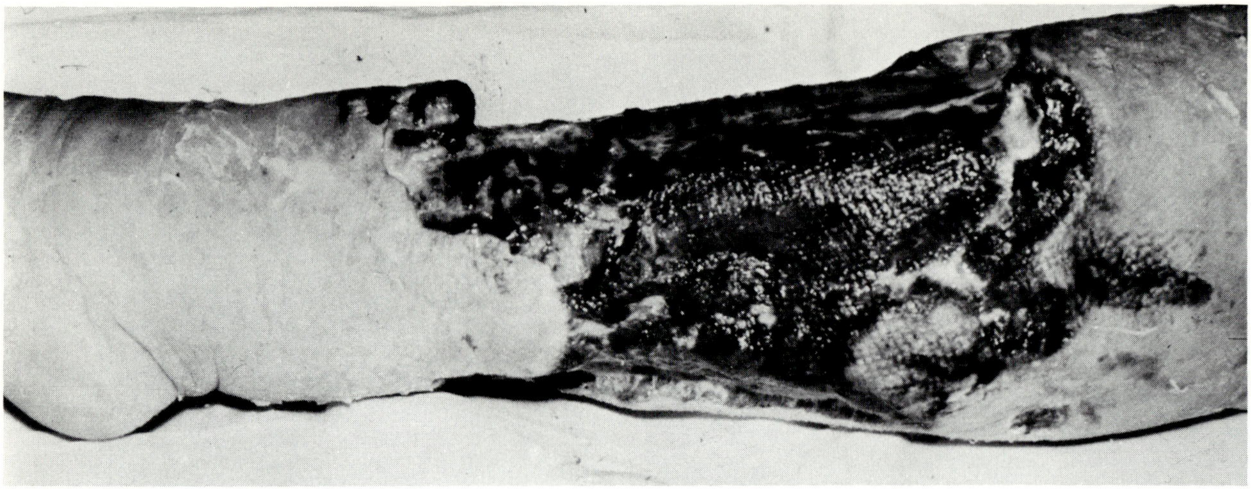

FIGURE 60-10. Severe venous ulcers, complicated by multiple episodes of infection and fibrosis, may encircle the ankle.

CLINICAL PICTURE OF CHRONIC VENOUS OBSTRUCTION

In the patient with chronic venous obstruction, especially in the iliofemoral position, ulceration does not usually occur unless there is also incompetence of the perforating veins. Many will have little more than intermittent leg edema and aching, relieved by elevation, since venous outflow may be quite adequate via collaterals or partial recanalization. However, there are a number of patients who never recanalize occluded segments, particularly in the iliac, common femoral, or superficial femoral position, and are frequently troubled by thigh and calf edema and by disabling pain (36). Case reports of venous claudication (37) theorize a mechanism of venous obstruction, with overdistention of the leg brought about by hyperemia during exercise (38). Elevated interstitial-fluid pressures in the muscle and fascial compartments have been documented (28). Extensive venous collaterals will usually be obvious over the thigh, genitalia (collaterals running from the groin of the affected limb across to the other groin), and lower abdominal wall. Most of the other features of CVI will be seen to a lesser or greater extent in the afflicted leg, depending on the length and position of the occluded segment and the degree of coexisting valvular incompetence of deep and superficial venous systems.

Venography is of great importance in these patients to accurately delineate the site of obstruction and for planning reconstructive surgery (36).

Patient Examination and Assessment

Patients are asked to stand for several minutes to allow for filling of the leg veins, and examination is performed initially in the erect position. The presence or absence of clinical features of CVI is noted, and sites of varicose veins are recorded. Saphenofemoral incompetence is judged by the presence of saphena varix or cough impulse, and confirmed by tourniquet (39) or Doppler probe testing (40). The short saphenous system is examined similarly for saphenopopliteal incompetence. Perforators may be identified by tourniquet testing and by palpating a localized fascia defect or tenderness at the relevant anatomical sites. Confirmation by Doppler probe may also be carried out (41,42). Clinical detection of incompetent perforators by palpation requires experience, since superficial varicose veins of the medial leg may feel like dilated perforators (43).

The examination includes an assessment of arterial adequacy, and if the patient has symptoms which may be due to neurological, muscular, or arthritic conditions, these must be excluded by further clinical testing or special investigations. The differential diagnosis for leg edema and leg ulcers is given in Tables 60-2 and 60-3.

Etiology of Chronic Venous Insufficiency: Classification of Causes

The causes of chronic venous insufficiency include

1. Perforator vein incompetence
2. Deep vein incompetence
3. Proximal venous obstruction
4. Superficial vein incompetence
5. Congenital venous malformations
6. Arteriovenous fistula
7. Calf muscle dysfunction

The most thoroughly documented factor in the etiology of chronic venous insufficiency is incompetence of the perforator

TABLE 60-2. Differential Diagnosis of Chronic Venous Insufficiency: Causes of Leg Edema

Unilateral:
Congenital:
AV malformation
Hereditary:
Milroy's disease
Traumatic:
Fracture, hematoma, burns, frostbite, chemical irritants, stings
Infective:
Cellulitis, abscess, osteomyelitis
Venous obstruction:
Acute deep venous thrombosis, chronic venous insufficiency
Tumors:
Soft tissue sarcomas, bone malignancies
Lymphatic obstruction:
Primary or secondary
Arthritis:
Acute gout, rheumatoid, osteoarthritis
Allergic:
Angioneurotic edema
Nutritional deficiency
Bilateral:
Congestive cardiac failure
Renal failure (nephrotic syndrome)
Lymphedema
Myxedema
Inferior vena cava obstruction
Hypoproteinemia (starvation, malabsorption, cirrhosis)
Toxemia of pregnancy

vein valves (1,44). In most cases this is secondary to destruction of these valves following deep venous thrombosis (45). Recently, increasing attention is being focused on abnormalities of the deep veins (46–48).

Any classification of the causes of venous insufficiency simplifies the often multifactorial etiology—for example, many patients with perforating vein incompetence will also have deep vein incompetence, because both are usually secondary to deep venous thrombosis (see Table 60-4).

TABLE 60-3. Differential Diagnosis of Chronic Venous Insufficiency: Causes of Leg Ulcer

Venous ulcer
Arterial insufficiency
Lymphatic obstruction
Neuropathic:
Diabetes, alcoholism, hemiplegia, polyneuritis, leprosy, tabes dorsalis
Traumatic:
Injury, burn, radiation, sclerotherapy
Vasculitic:
Systemic lupus erythematosus, polyarteritis nodosa, scleroderma, rheumatoid arthritis, allergic vasculitis
Infective:
Tropical ulcer (anaerobic infections, *Borrelia vincentii*, etc.)
Syphilitic (ulcerated gummas)
Tuberculous
Fungal (blastomycosis, sporotrichosis, actinomycosis)
Phagedemic ulcer (mixed infection due to neglect or starvation)
Others (amebiasis, chancroid, yaws, kalaazar, tularemia, granuloma inguinale, leishmaniasis)
Neoplastic:
Squamous-cell carcinoma (SCC) (Marjolin's ulcer = SCC in chronic venous ulcer)
Basal-cell carcinoma
Melanoma
Lymphoma (mycosis fungoides)
Pyoderma gangrenosum:
Associated with inflammatory bowel disease

TABLE 60-4. Patterns of CVI

1. Perforator vein incompetence (60%):
Alone
With superficial incompetence
With deep vein incompetence
2. Deep vein incompetence (32%):
With perforator vein incompetence
Alone
3. Deep vein obstruction (3%)
4. Incompetent saphenous system alone (5%)

This relationship is further complicated by the fact that dysfunction of perforator valves may be due either to local effects following destruction by thrombosis and subsequent recanalization in the veins of the lower part of the leg, or may be a remote secondary effect of pressure changes following destruction of the valves of deep veins higher in the leg (popliteal or femoral level). In the latter case the resultant raised pressure in the deep system is thought to cause dilatation of the perforator veins, rendering incompetent their stretched valves.

Varicose veins may accompany the other clinical features of CVI but are usually not involved in the causation (49). However, exceptions to this rule may occur in patients with large primary varicose veins of the long saphenous or short saphenous systems which have been left untreated for many years (49,50). However, the misconception that leg ulcer is a common sequel to varicose veins still prevails.

Reliable histological evidence for postphlebitic damage of the deep veins was provided by Edwards in 1937 (45) and confirmed by Bauer's phlebographic studies, published in 1940 (51). Bauer found that more than 50 percent of patients known to have DVT developed venous ulceration within 10 years, with less severe manifestations such as edema and pigmentation occurring in 72 percent at the same interval (52).

The venous drainage of the ankle "gaiter area" is via local superficial veins, many of which communicate either directly, or via the posterior arch veins, with the perforating veins on the medial side of the leg (12) (Figure 60-9). When there is valve destruction in the perforator veins, with or without associated deep vein incompetence, a state of "local ambulatory venous hypertension" is created and the usual beneficial effects of exercise in lowering venous pressure are considerably diminished.

There are probably also forms of intrinsic deficiency of the deep veins, similar to that of primary varicose superficial veins. Cases of congenital absence or malformation of the venous valves have been identified, and Kistner has described a condition of primary valve incompetence where valve elongation and prolapse have occurred, without evidence of phlebitis (53). This is of special significance when the femoral and popliteal valves are affected, since surgical repair or replacement may be beneficial (54).

Proximal venous obstruction may be due to extrinsic causes (compression by tumor, postirradiation fibrosis, or, on the left side, compression by the overriding right common iliac artery) or intrinsic causes (thrombosis or ligation). When DVT occurs, the usual course of events includes recanalization of the major channels, usually over several months. However, recanalization of the whole venous tree does not always occur, and the patient may be left with a chronic occlusion of the iliac or femoral vein, or both (55). Often collateral venous flow will be sufficient and symptoms may be absent or mild. Other patients have severe symptoms, usually including chronic edema and pain. This clinical picture cannot be accurately differentiated from the other forms of CVI since coexisting postphlebitic valve dysfunction often further complicates the picture. Noninvasive testing or venography is necessary for confirmation of the diagnosis when venous obstruction is suspected. Halliday has demonstrated that a significant percentage of patients who present with symptoms suggestive of venous claudication, even with minimal physical signs of chronic venous disease, can be shown to have iliac vein occusion after further investigation (36).

Congenital venous malformations such as the Klippel-Trènaunay syndrome (56,57) and arteriovenous fistulas are not common but may result in a similar syndrome of chronic venous problems. Occult arteriovenous fistula should be suspected in cases of venous ulcers which are resistant to conventional treatment.

One aspect which has not yet been resolved is the relative importance of impairment of the venous pump mechanism due to dysfunction of the calf muscles themselves. It seems likely that some neuromuscular disorders would cause this. Similarly, the muscle atrophy that occurs with severe CVI may become part of a vicious cycle preventing restoration of the venous pump (58) and thwarting attempts at healing.

Theories of Pathogenesis

A state of "ambulatory venous hypertension" exists, associated either with venous obstruction, perforator incompetence, or deep vein incompetence. There are several theories to explain how this condition results in venous ulceration.

VENOUS STASIS THEORY

This theory states that high pressure on the venous side of the capillary beds at the ankle level slows the functional blood flow through the cutaneous capillary network, causing deoxygenation of blood on a chronic basis. Edema also decreases arterial flow into this area of tissue. According to Homans (4), an area of local ischemia results with decreased supply of nutrients, such as oxygen, glucose, amino acids, and fats, and impaired cellular metabolism. The products of anaerobic metabolism further impair cell function, leading to eventual cell death and tissue breakdown, especially if minor trauma or infection occurs (19). Fibrosis of the subcutaneous tissues around the ulcer further compromises circulation, so that healing is unlikely without treatment.

The simplicity of this theory is appealing, and it has remained the stock explanation for many years (59,60). However, there has never been any evidence that a state of blood stasis truly occurs—to the contrary recent evidence suggests that local flow may in fact be increased.

ARTERIOVENOUS FISTULA THEORY

This theory states that there are multiple small arteriovenous (AV) fistulas in the subcutaneous layer and skin of the ulceration area, with shunting of blood away from the skin, reducing tissue oxygenation (61,62). This may explain why several early studies showed high oxygen concentration in blood draining an ulcerated area of skin (63). However, evidence of AV fistulas has not been shown anatomically.

OXYGEN DIFFUSION BLOCK THEORY

Following the identification of pericapillary fibrin cuffs in the affected tissues, careful experiments by Browse and Burnand (64,65) have led to the concept of fibrinogen escaping via venular and capillary pores (due to the high pressure), with accumulation of the fibrin being encouraged by an associated reduced fibrinolytic activity of the blood, tissues, and vein walls in patients with venous ulceration (66). This fibrin cuff acts as a diffusion block, preventing access of oxygen and other nutrients into the tissues, thus causing the condition of "lipodermatosclerosis" (previously termed fat necrosis or tissue fibrosis) and leading to cell death.

Evidence for this theory has been further supported by a double-blind trial which demonstrated the clinical effectiveness of stanozolol, an anabolic steroid drug which promotes natural fibrinolysis (67).

PHYSIOLOGICAL SHUNT THEORY

Recent studies using positron emission tomography have shown reduced oxygen utilization in the area of ulceration, despite increased blood flow and increased oxygen (68). This "physiological" shunt may be seen as evidence for the oxygen diffusion block theory or may be attributed to anatomical AV fistulas.

THEORY OF LYMPHATIC DEFICIENCY

Moyer (69) postulated a process of obliterative cutaneous lymphangitis, based on histological studies in which dermal lymphatics were found to be obliterated in the skin adjacent to "stasis" ulcers but were present and dilated following successful therapy by skin grafting. However, it seems likely that these changes were in fact secondary to the ulceration and infection, rather than causative. Kinmonth (70) has shown that the leg lymphatics are normal in most cases.

Noninvasive Investigations

Noninvasive vascular laboratory tests for venous diseases are discussed in detail in Chapter 11. This section will summarize the clinical applications of these techniques in the management of patients suspected of having chronic venous insufficiency. In many cases the diagnosis is made on history and examination alone, so that noninvasive tests are not necessary but may be employed to provide objective proof of the diagnosis, especially if surgery is contemplated. In other cases the diagnosis is not straightforward, and noninvasive testing may be invaluable as a screening procedure to prove or disprove underlying venous disease—examples of such cases include the patient with edematous leg but no other signs of CVI (71), leg pains which may be venous in origin, or the atypical leg ulcer (72). In these patients, noninvasive tests may demonstrate valvular insufficiency (by Doppler exam) or venous obstruction (by plethysmography). The severity of CVI may also be gauged by the use of photoplethysmography (72), which correlates closely with the results obtained from venous cannulation and direct measurement of ambulatory venous pressures (73).

DOPPLER ULTRASOUND

A 5- or 12-mHz Doppler probe may be used to detect venous flow and give an assessment of velocity. Patency of the leg veins is indicated by detection of spontaneous venous signals, modified by respiration and augmented by the Valsalva maneuver or squeezing the distal leg. Valvular incompetence is demonstrated by the presence of retrograde flow after compression of the abdomen or following release of calf compression. False results may be due to flow within major collateral vessels or to user inexperience. The Doppler probe is also an accurate aid for the localization of incompetent perforators (Figure 60-11) (74).

VOLUME-OUTFLOW PLETHYSMOGRAPHY

The various forms of plethysmography measure volume changes and may be used to demonstrate the normal changes in volume due to venous flow variations with respiration (see Figure 11-6), or following venous occlusion with a tourniquet. The most valuable application is the demonstration of venous outflow obstruction, as evidenced by delayed emptying. After placing a proximal venous tourniquet, a steady increase in leg volume is observed. When the tourniquet cuff is released, there is normally a rapid release to baseline with 50 percent of emptying occurring in the first 2 s (75). In the case of proximal vein obstruction there will be a decreased volume rise with inflation of the tourniquet cuff and greatly prolonged emptying time (see Figure 11-5).

Air plethysmography (phleborheography) measures these changes via air-inflated cuffs placed around the leg, whereas *strain-gauge plethysmography* measures changes in calf circumference.

Impedance plethysmography (IPG) is considered to be the most accurate method, with a sensitivity and specificity of approximately 95 percent (76). This technique depends on the fact that in the limbs electrical resistance is directly proportional to volume, so that small changes in electrical impedance represent corresponding changes in the leg volume. Electrodes applied to the skin are used to determine the venous outflow rate after the veins have been filled to capacitance. The advantages of IPG are that it is inexpensive and rapid and may be done at the bedside without the need for a highly experienced operator for interpretation. Disadvantages include the need for careful patient positioning and unreliable results below the level of the knee.

VENOUS REFLUX PLETHYSMOGRAPHY

Photoplethysmography (PPG) is a technique introduced by Barnes to record the blood content of the skin (77). The degree of venous reflux can be quantitated by measurement of the rate of venous capillary refill following emptying with exercise (78). Infrared light is emitted by a transducer into the underlying tissue, and the backscattered light is received by an adjacent photodetector, providing a strip-chart record of cutaneous blood content in the capillary network (72). Patients with CVI show a markedly shortened refilling time due to reflux (79), comparable to the results obtained via ambulatory venous pressure measure-

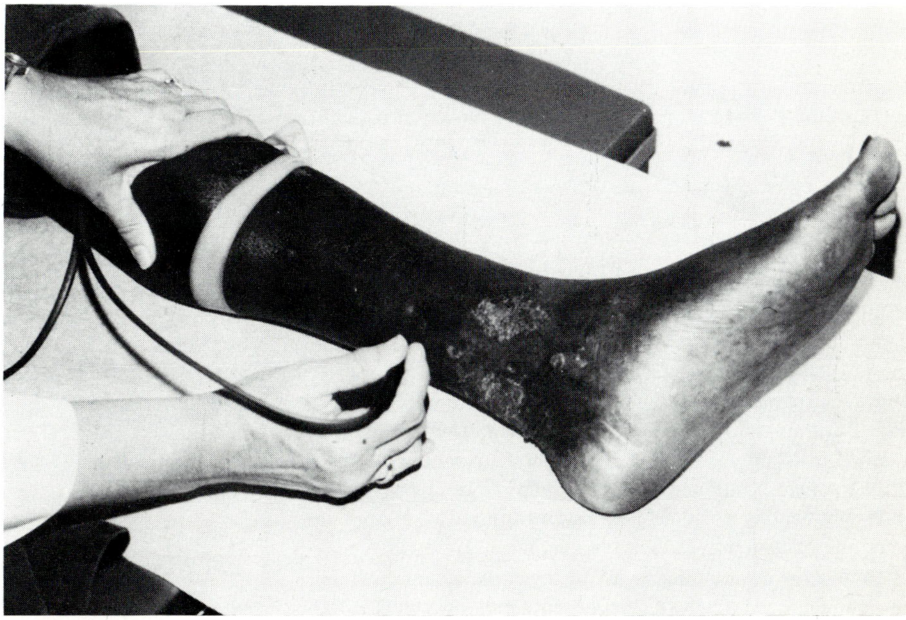

FIGURE 60-11. Reflux via incompetent deep veins or perforating veins may be detected with the Doppler probe when the upper calf is compressed.

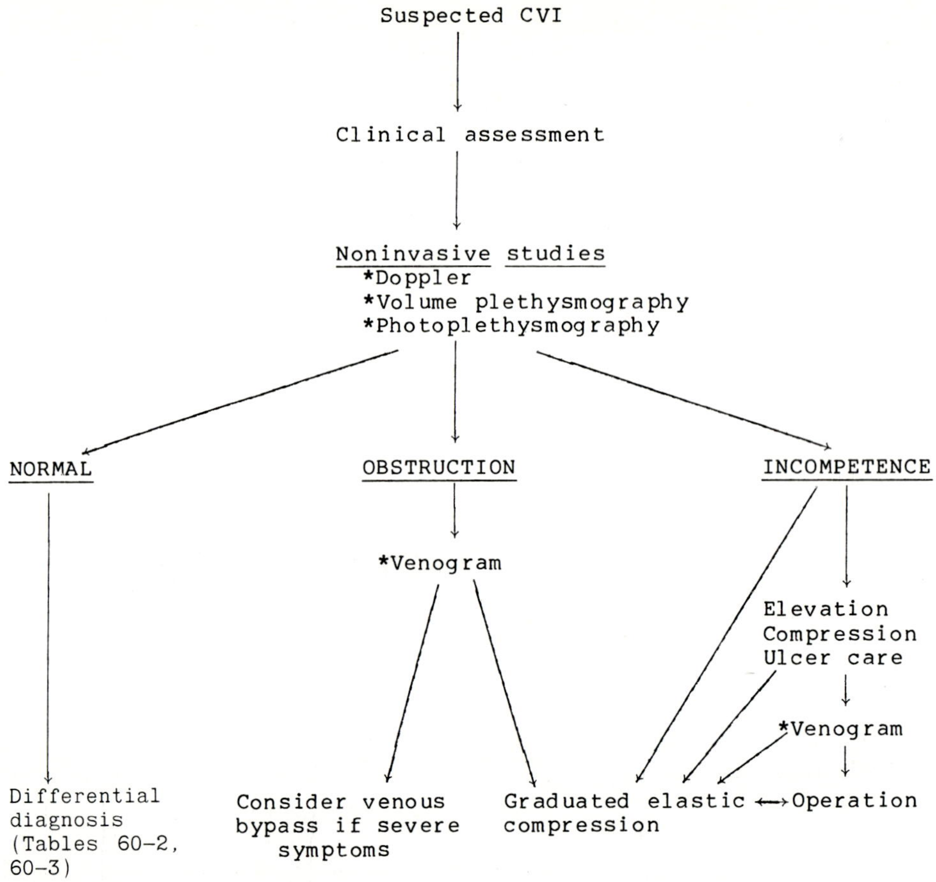

FIGURE 60-12. Algorithm for management of chronic venous insufficiency (CVI). [Adapted from Barnes RW (81).]

ment (73) (see Figure 11-9). Venous refilling is usually much quicker with deep insufficiency than with superficial (80), and this differentiation can be confirmed by using a tourniquet. However, the technique does not differentiate between incompetence in the proximal deep veins, calf deep veins, or perforator veins.

CLINICAL USES

Objective evaluation of the relative contribution of venous outflow obstruction and venous valvular incompetence in patients with CVI is provided via these noninvasive investigations (81), most of which will also readily differentiate normal from abnormal limbs. If the patient's noninvasive evaluation is normal, conditions other than venous disease should be considered as the cause of symptoms. Chronic venous outflow obstruction is uncommon, but its detection should lead to venography and consideration for surgery. Similarly, venous reflux can be confirmed by these techniques and appropriate therapy instituted. An algorithm for the management of CVI, including the role of noninvasive investigation, is shown in Figure 60-12.

Invasive Investigations

VENOGRAPHY

This is the method of investigation that has been used most extensively and is justifiably regarded as the conventional diagnostic standard for assessment of chronic venous insufficiency. Ascending phlebograms are obtained after injection of a contrast medium into a dorsal vein of the foot. The technique is described in detail elsewhere (82). The study may be performed with the patient positioned supine, upright, or semiupright in a non-weight-bearing position, and views are usually obtained in several planes (anterior, lateral, oblique, etc.). Tourniquets may be placed at the ankle or higher up the leg to prevent preferential flow into the superficial venous system, thus providing good visualization of the deep system and allowing identification of incompetent perforators carrying contrast medium from deep to superficial veins.

Although not indicated for investigation of uncomplicated varicose veins or CVI, venograms should be obtained in severe cases, especially if surgery is contemplated or if noninvasive studies have shown evidence of proximal obstruction which might be amenable to surgical treatment. Ascending venograms in those patients may demonstrate any of the following changes:

1. Structural changes in the deep or superficial systems, including varicosities
2. Presence of thrombus or other occlusion
3. Recanalized veins (83)
4. Presence of incompetent perforating veins

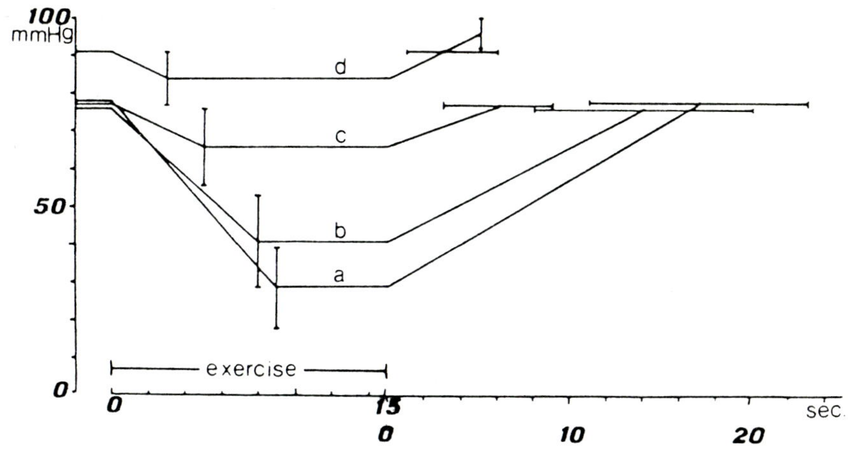

FIGURE 60-13. Ambulatory venous pressure measurements recorded in (a) normal volunteers; (b) patients with primary varicose veins; (c) patients with incompetent perforating veins; (d) combined deep and perforator incompetence, or venous obstruction. [Reprinted with permission from Kriessmann A: Ambulatory venous pressure measurements. In Nicolaides AN, Yao JST (eds): *Investigation of Vascular Disorders*. New York, Churchill Livingstone, 1981.]

5. Presence of proximal venous obstruction
6. Absence of valve cusps, or valvular deformity
7. Collateral vessels

These changes will allow confirmation of diagnosis and especially localize areas of possible surgical relevance such as the sites of perforators and areas of obstruction. However, competency of the deep vein valves cannot be accurately assessed without further studies.

Complications of venography include burning pains with infusion of the contrast medium, minor reactions such as urticaria and nausea (84), and in a small number of cases induction of thrombosis, due to hyperosmolar solutions. The incidence of CVT after these studies can be lowered by flushing out the contrast medium with a heparinized dextrose solution or by the use of newer nonionic, low osmolality contrast materials (85). More serious complications such as anaphylactic reaction or ulceration at the site of extravasation of contrast medium are uncommon.

DESCENDING VENOGRAPHY

Accurate determination of the function of deep vein valves requires study via a descending venogram or by dynamic ascending cinephlebography (86). Descending venography is performed in a semiupright position following placement of an angiogram catheter in the femoral vein. Contrast medium is injected slowly to allow observation for reflux of contrast medium down the femoral veins. A grading system has been devised to describe the severity of reflux (87). Interpretation requires experience, since in normal limbs there may be some degree of physiological reflux.

AMBULATORY VENOUS PRESSURE MEASUREMENTS

A needle placed in a vein on the dorsum of the foot gives accurate representations of deep venous pressures, since pressure changes occurring with positioning and exercise are almost identical in the superficial system and deep system (24). These pressure measurements can be recorded via a pressure transducer and amplifier connected to a potentiometric pen recorder (88). Measurements are taken first in a resting upright position, then during ankle dorsiflexion standing on tiptoes, and finally during recovery (89). Venous pressure in the leg falls during exercise and recovers gradually to the resting value when walking stops. After initiating exercise, with each successive calf muscle contraction the pressure normally becomes lower and lower until a steady state is reached. Nicolaides (89) termed this point the asymptotic value. A recording from a normal limb is shown in Figure 60-5, where the resting pressure of 90 mmHg in the upright position falls to the steady-state pressure of approximately 30 mmHg in less than 10 s, and then recovers slowly. Additional information is obtained by repeating these measurements with pneumatic cuff tourniquets applied at the ankle level alone or at several points on the leg to occlude the superficial veins and to demonstrate the contribution to altered physiological function due to superficial or perforator vein incompetence.

In pathological venous states, the pressure drop with exercise is markedly diminished, and the subsequent rate of refilling is rapid, producing a short recovery time. Nicolaides has demonstrated that those values can be correlated with the severity of incompetence symptoms, so that if the ambulatory venous pressure can be brought below 45 mmHg, the risk of ulceration is zero, whereas if the pressure stays above 60 mmHg, the risk is greater than 50 percent (89). The pressure drop with primary varicose veins is only mildly impaired, whereas the presence of incompetent perforators, deep valve incompetence, or outflow obstructions (due to proximal occlusion) causes relatively severe ambulant venous hypertension (Figure 60-13). In these studies the highest exercise pressures were seen in patients who have a combination of both deep valve incompetence and proximal occlusion. These techniques are used more for research than for clinical practice and are especially valuable for gauging the severity of physiological disturbance in various forms of CVI and for monitoring the effects of surgical procedures (90). A summary of the abnormal venous dynamics seen in CVI is given in Table 60-5.

TABLE 60-5. Venous Hemodynamics

	Normal	Abnormal
Static pressure (erect)	90–100 mmHg	90–100 mmHg
Ambulatory venous pressure (AVP), drop from static pressure	20–30 mmHg (80% drop)	45–90 mmHg (drop < 55%)
Venous refilling time (VRT)	> 20 s	< 18 s
Doppler testing of valves	Competent (no reflux)	Incompetent (reflux)

Nonoperative Treatment of Venous Ulcer

PROPHYLAXIS

Ideally the incidence of CVI would be reduced by measures which prevent DVT or by reduction of the valve damage caused by thrombotic processes. Currently accepted regimens such as the use of subcutaneous heparin, intermittent calf compression, compressive stockings, and Dextran-70 infusions have all been shown to be effective to a variable degree for prophylaxis of DVT, and by extension for CVI. Recently, attempts at early treatment of established DVT have been trialed, with the aim of lowering the incidence of sequelae such as embolism and CVI. Early venous thrombectomy (91) (with or without formation of an AV fistula to maintain flow) (92) and fibrinolytic therapy remain experimental (93,94). Unfortunately, in a recent trial by Kakkar (unpublished data; presented at National Symposium on Venous Disease in Phoenix, Oct. 1984), 100 patients whose DVT was treated with fibrinolytic therapy showed no beneficial late effects—the incidence of CVI was not significantly different from that in a group of conventionally treated DVT patients.

Patients presenting with early symptoms and signs of CVI Should be instructed in the use of measures to avoid deterioration—i.e., skin care, avoidance of prolonged standing without calf muscle exercise, leg elevation wherever possible, and use of compression stockings. Unfortunately, in many cases the patient's occupation makes it impossible to avoid prolonged standing, or an attitude of neglect allows progression of skin changes, leading to eventual ulceration. The long-term results depend heavily on continuity of care and follow-up, attempting to improve patient compliance by frequent reinforcement (95). There is a significant role for nurse practitioners, special ulcer dressing clinics, and home nursing care.

MEASURES TO REDUCE LIMB VENOUS HYPERTENSION

Posture

The pathophysiology of ambulatory venous hypertension should be explained to the patient in terms which she or he is likely to understand. It is important to avoid prolonged standing whenever possible, or to exercise the calf muscle whenever prolonged standing is unavoidable, to have the legs elevated on a chair or stool whenever sitting, and to have the legs elevated above the level of the heart when in bed. Elevation of the foot of the bed is preferable to placing a pillow under the legs. Specially designed tip-back chairs, which allow for efficient leg elevation (while working) have been recommended for those in a sedentary occupation.

Graded Compression Stockings

Custom-fitted, pressure-graduated compression stockings are required. These should ideally provide a compression pressure of 30 to 50 mmHg at the ankle and should be designed so as to allow a graduated pressure profile going up the leg, thus encouraging venous return (96). In most cases, it is sufficient that these stockings be of below-knee design, especially since these are more comfortable, encouraging patient compliance. Many poorly fitting, low compressive stockings are marketed, but these have inadequate elasticity and do not provide sufficient compression to be of benefit to this group of patients. Non-custom-made, graded elastic stockings with an average compression of 24 mmHg at the ankle have been shown to decrease leg volume, circumference, and pain in mildly symptomatic patients but are not adequate treatment for most cases of lymphedema, phlebitis, or CVI (97). Stockings usually require replacement every 6 months because of loss of elasticity.

CARE OF SKIN AND ULCER CARE

Venous eczema (venous dermatitis) is very common and presents as dry, flaky, fragile skin. Patients with this condition should be instructed in the use of skin emollients to prevent cracking that may progress to infection or ulcer. Troublesome itching will often respond to a short course of corticosteroid cream, especially when combined with elastic support. The avoidance of trauma to the imperiled area is also important. Episodes of cellulitis and edema should be treated early.

Ulcer Dressings

Cellulitis surrounding an ulcer should be treated with systemic antibiotics (as well as rest, elevation, and compression). Abscess may require incision and drainage, or wide debridement. Many preparations and materials have been recommended for dressing these ulcers. Preparations such as normal saline, sodium hypochlorite solutions, 3% peroxide, and povidone-iodine are all satisfactory. Topical antibiotic applications do little but change the skin flora and are generally not recommended because of possible local allergic reactions. A nonstick dressing material should be placed over the cleansed ulcer, and the leg wrapped from the metatarsal level up beyond the ulcer. A sponge-rubber pad may be applied over the area of the ulcer to aid compression. The whole dressing is then covered by elastic bandaging from toes to knee to provide compression and to reduce edema (Figure 60-14).

Occlusive dressings such as the Unna boot have been the mainstay for treatment of chronic leg ulcers for centuries. There are many proprietary forms of these gelatin and zinc paste-impregnated bandages, which allow for localized compression from forefoot to knee while the patient remains ambulant. Occlusive dressings of this form are of particular benefit for treatment of patients who are unable to perform their own dressings because of debilitating illness, infirmity, or neglect. Exudate is absorbed by the dressing, which is usually changed each week. Infected ulcers are not suitable for this technique because of the requirement for more frequent dressings. Refractory ulcers should be biopsied to exclude malignancy, and hospitalization of the patient might be required for adequate elevation and frequent dressing changes.

OTHER MEASURES

Local Fibrinolysis Enhancement

On the basis that fibrin deposition around small vessels of the area of venous ulcer causes an oxygen diffusion block, Browse

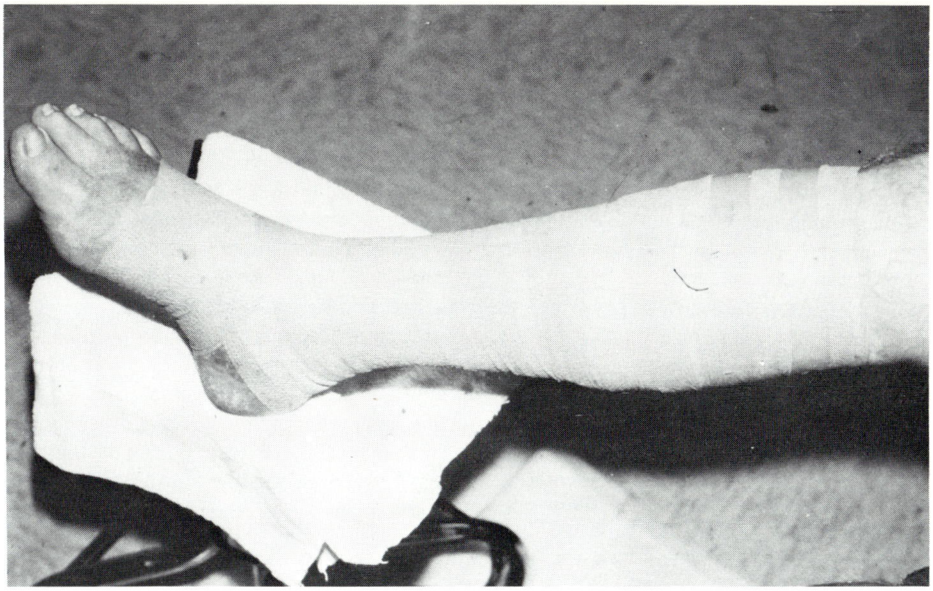

FIGURE 60-14. Recommended ulcer dressing technique, with the leg wrapped to the upper calf. Outer layer elastic bandage is applied next.

has recommended the use of a fibrinolytic enhancing medication (stanozolol) (98).

Treatment of Concurrent Medical Problems

Healing is aided by the management of medical conditions such as heart failure, diabetes mellitus, obesity, poor nutrition, and dermatitis.

INJECTION SCLEROTHERAPY

Details of the technique of injection sclerotherapy are discussed in detail in the previous chapter. The role of sclerotherapy in patients with CVI is somewhat controversial. Incompetent perforators can certainly be effectively treated, especially if they are dilated and visible at the skin surface (99) (Figure 60-15). The injection may be placed directly into the perforator itself or into an associated nearby superficial vein. However, in many instances the perforators are not easily located on the skin surface, so that accurate injection requires considerable experience. Injury to the posterior tibial artery has been reported in such cases, resulting in distal gangrene (100). Others feel that sclerotherapy in this group of patients results in an unacceptably high early recurrence rate (101).

Sclerotherapy of perforators may be combined with sclerotherapy of coexistent varicose superficial veins, although saphenofemoral or saphenopopliteal incompetence is more effectively treated by flush ligation (102). For example, good results have been achieved by employing surgical ligation of the long saphenous vein in conjunction with compression sclerotherapy of perforators and major superficial control points (103).

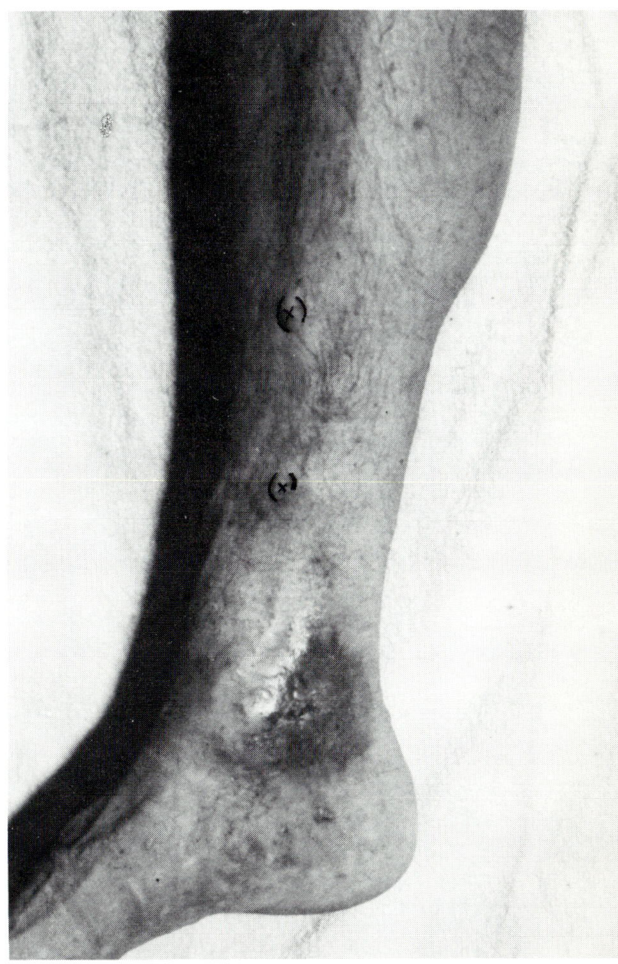

FIGURE 60-15. Leg of 30-year-old male with 10-year history of ulcer following DVT. Visible and easily palpable perforators. Ulcer healed 3 weeks following sclerotherapy and compression bandaging.

Surgical Treatment of Venous Ulcer

The surgical management of this problem will be considered under four groups. Following investigation, the cause of the ulcer may generally be classified into one of these groups, although in many cases the etiology will include aspects of several of the groups: (1) general principles for surgery of venous ulcer; (2) surgical treatment of incompetent perforators; (3) surgical treatment of proximal venous obstruction; and (4) surgical treatment of valve incompetence in the deep veins.

GENERAL PRINCIPLES FOR SURGERY OF VENOUS ULCER

If operation is contemplated, then the following general measures should be followed. Gross infection or cellulitis should first be controlled, and edema should be reduced by the measures outlined above. It is preferable to have the ulcer healed or as close to healed as possible at the time of operation to lower the chances of contamination of surgical incisions. On the occasions when there are significant associated varicose veins of the long saphenous or short saphenous systems, then those should be treated also, according to the principles outlined in the previous chapter. If there is combined venous and arterial insufficiency, arterial bypass should be performed initially (104), as skin grafting or other measures are likely to fail without adequate blood supply.

Excision and Grafting of Ulcer

If an ulcer is particularly chronic with very thick underlying tissue, then excision of the ulcer followed by skin grafting may be necessary. This may be done at the same time as division of the perforating veins or other surgical procedures or may follow as a secondary procedure. Wide excision of the ulcer base and surrounding abnormal tissue (including local dilated veins) has been advocated as a primary treatment, with acceptable results. In one series so treated, a 5-year recurrence-free rate of 77 percent was reported (105). Traditionally, grafting has been by the Thiersch "split-skin" grafting technique (Figure 60-16). However, in recent years the technique of mesh grafting has afforded considerable advantages for coverage of infected or contaminated area. "Postage-stamp" application of small areas of harvested skin may also be employed.

Occasionally when there has been exposure of bone or tendons, these methods of grafting will not be satisfactory, and a myocutaneous flap of tissue must be constructed. Following recent advances in microsurgery, it is now possible to use a vascularized free flap harvested from the inguinal area. Bone defects may be reconstructed by transfer of a portion of iliac crest, with attached muscle, based on the deep circumflex iliac vessels (106).

OPERATIONS FOR PERFORATOR VEIN INCOMPETENCE (Figure 60-17)

Individual Ligation of Perforators

In limbs with skin changes of minor degree or where a number of incompetent perforators can be readily identified by examination or investigation, ligation of the perforators may be performed through small separate incisions (107,108).

Extrafascial Ligation of Perforators (Cockett's Procedure)

This operation, not commonly employed today, aims to clear all the extrafascial enlarged veins and to divide perforating veins,

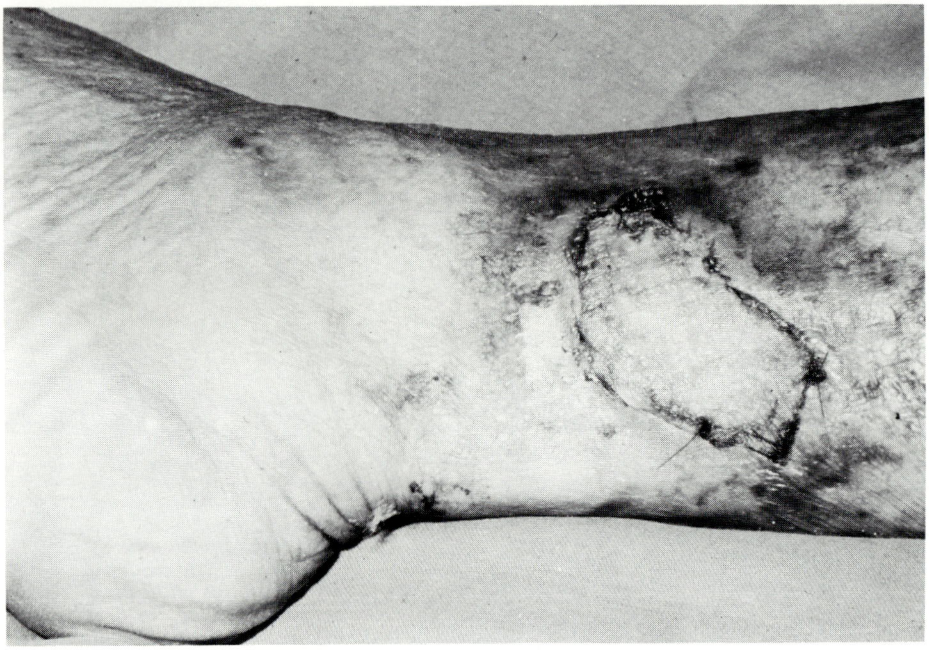

FIGURE 60-16. Successful skin graft on venous ulcer following sclerotherapy of incompetent perforators.

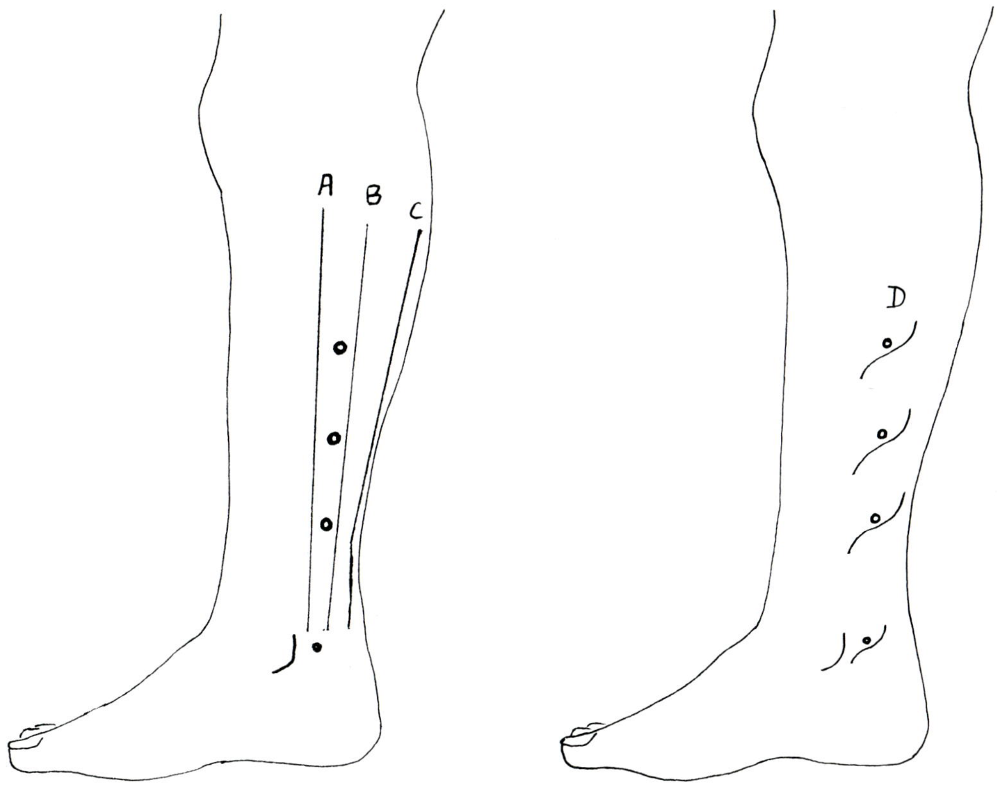

FIGURE 60-17. Incisions for ligation of perforators: A, medial approach; B, posteromedial approach; C, posterior approach; D, multiple incisions for individual ligations.

thus preventing transmission of the high venous pressure in the deep system out to the subcutaneous tissues and skin (12). The incision is usually made about 2 to 3 cm posterior to the medial border of the tibia, from about half-way down the calf to just above the medial malleolus. In some cases the incision will pass through ulcer, especially if simultaneous excision of the ulcer (and grafting) is planned (14). However, the perforating veins may be difficult to accurately locate in this plane (109), and dissection tends to be traumatic because of the adherence of subcutaneous fat and connective tissue to the fascia.

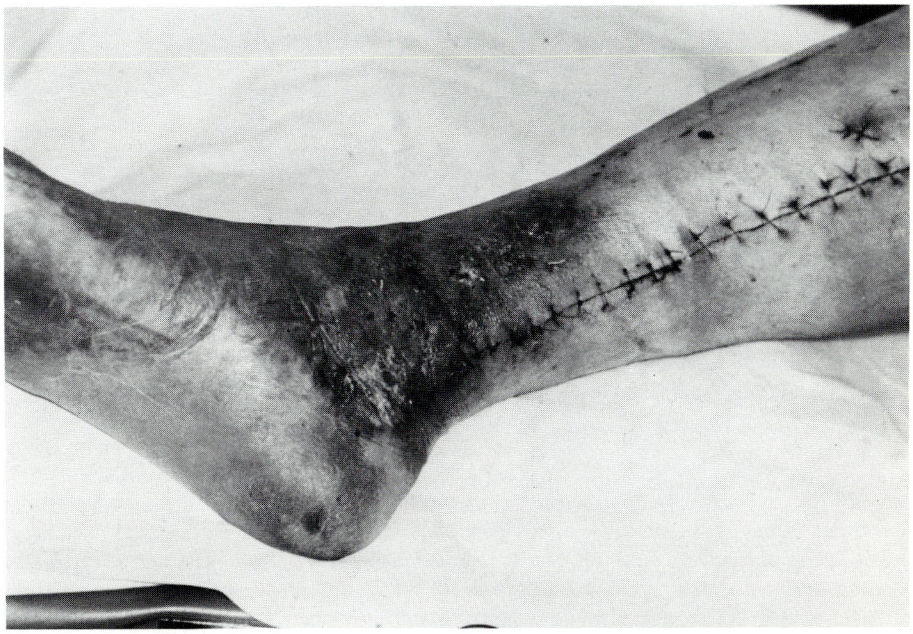

FIGURE 60-18. Early satisfactory result from Linton's procedure, with healing of chronic ulcer.

Subfascial Ligation of Perforators (Linton's Procedure)

A subfascial division technique was described by Homans in 1916 (19), and he then referred to the use of similar flap procedures by Madelung during the 1880s (110). However, it was Linton's classic publications in 1938 and 1953 that popularized subfascial ligation (44,111), although his recommended procedure also included flush ligation and stripping of the long saphenous vein, excision of the ulcer, and ligation of the femoral vein (44). Today "Linton's operation" has come to mean the modified method by which a subfascial incision is used to approach and divide the perforating veins (112,113) (Figure 60-18). The incision, made 1 in (3 cm) posterior to the medial border of the tibia, commences in the upper third of the calf, is continued down to a level several centimeters proximal to the medial malleolus, and is modified to avoid scarred or ulcerated areas (Figure 60-17). The incision is deepened through the subcutaneous fat and deep fascia without separating the layers (to avoid undermining), thus opening an accessible plane where the perforating vessels are readily identified and easily divided between ligatures. The subfascial approach minimizes traumatic handling of the skin and subcutaneous tissues (19). In closing, the deep fascia is reapproximated with absorbable interrupted or continuous sutures, and the skin is closed with great care using interrupted Prolene or nylon. Poor healing of this incision is a common complication but can be reduced by avoiding badly scarred tissue, by using meticulously atraumatic technique, and by resolving all infection before operation. Alternative incisions may be employed to avoid the ulcer area. A popular alternative is the posteromedial approach (114) (Figure 60-17).

Posterior Approach (Rob Procedure)

If perforators on the lateral side of the leg are also implicated, then a posterior "stocking-seam" incision allows access to both sides of the leg for subfascial ligation (115,116). This incision is carried longitudinally from below the popliteal fossa down to the Achilles tendon and is curved medially or laterally at the distal end (117) (Figures 60-17 and 60-19). The short saphenous vein may be ligated through the same incision, with care taken to avoid injury to the sural nerve. This procedure is most conveniently done with the patient in the prone position, which affords the advantage of an area of relatively good skin vitality away from areas of ulceration (118). For this reason the same approach may be preferred for ligation of medial perforators alone. The incompetent perforators are ligated and divided in the subfascial plane as in the modified Linton's procedure, with exploration in this plane being possible as far laterally as the fascial attachment to the fibula without excessive retraction (118). The incidence of wound infection and necrosis is lower with this incision (4 to 26 percent), and healing is usually prompt.

Results of Subfascial Ligation of Perforators

Whether a medial, posteromedial, or posterior incision is used, the incidence of recurrent ulcer is generally reported in the range of 4 to 20 percent after a period of 2 to 5 years (117–120). Field reported on 57 patients treated by this method, with only one recurrence (112), whereas Bowen reported 24 recurrences following surgery on 77 patients (113). Ligation of perforators gives excellent results if the perforators alone are incompetent (121); however, results are less favorable when this abnormality is combined with incompetence of the deep veins (122,123), which in fact seems to be the case in slightly less than half of all patients with perforator incompetence (114). Negus reported recurrence-free healing in 85 percent of 108 treated ulcers after 3 years and stressed that good postoperative results could also be achieved, even in this group with combined deep vein incompetence, by the use of permanent, knee-length, graduated,

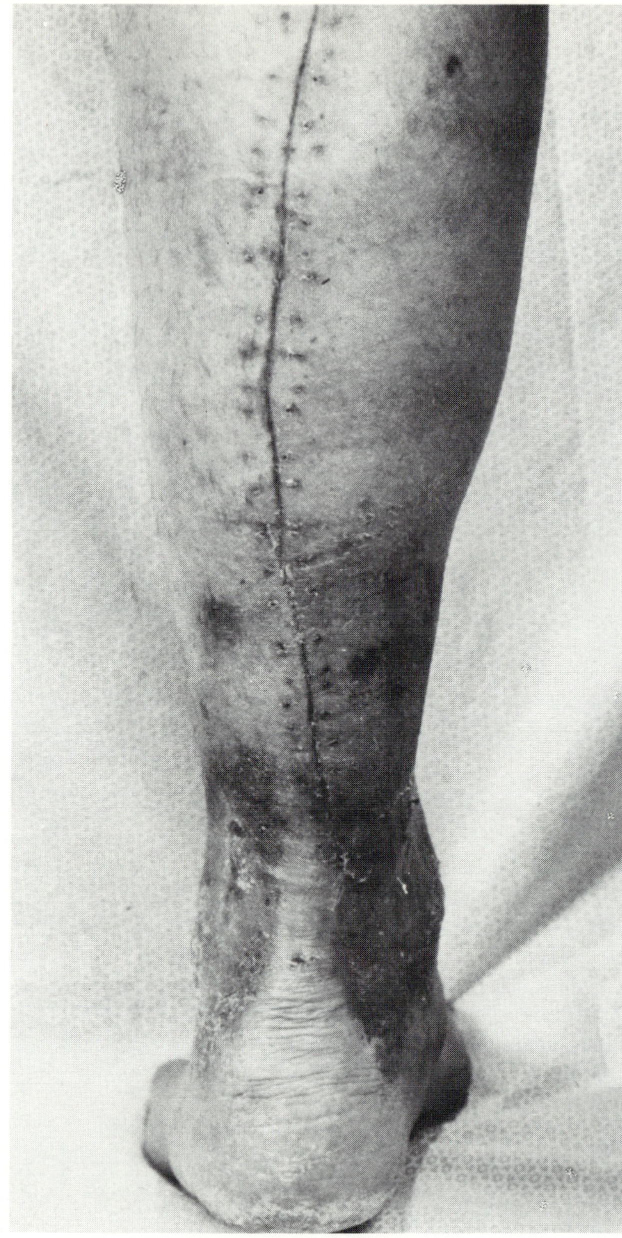

FIGURE 60-19. Medial and lateral ankle ulcers associated with multiple incompetent perforators have healed 1 month following bilateral subfascial ligation via posterior incision. Excellent result continues 1 year later with permanent compression stockings.

elastic compression stockings (119). DePalma also emphasized the need for continuous elastic support, especially if the leg remained edematous or symptomatic, and he reported that 46 of 50 operated cases were free of recurrent ulcer after follow-up for up to 12 years (120). Schanzer (114) also reported excellent results, with improvement in 22 of 25 cases after 3 years. In this group, ambulatory venous pressure measurements also improved in all cases postoperatively but were returned to the normal level in only five instances. It appears therefore that good results can be achieved, even though the total physiological defect is not corrected. Hull and Hyde (109,124) and Halliday (125) recommend subfascial ligation in all instances of severe stasis dermatitis with demonstrable perforator vein incompetence, even in the absence of ulceration, to prevent future ulceration.

Results are likely to be less satisfactory in several identified groups of patients. These are

1. Patients with rheumatoid arthritis or other forms of vasculitis, especially those taking steroid medications (126).
2. Patients with severe deep vein incompetence (123,127).
3. Patients with coexistent arterial insufficiency (120).
4. Patients with proximal venous obstruction (36,124).

OPERATIONS FOR VENOUS OBSTRUCTION

Femoral Vein Crossover Grafts (Palma Operation)

Surgical bypass of iliofemoral venous thrombosis utilizing the contralateral saphenous vein as a crossover graft was first described by Palma in 1960 (128). The diagnosis of iliac vein thrombosis may be obvious on clinical examination and is confirmed on ascending venography, which in most cases will also reveal recanalized postthrombotic damage in the femoropopliteal or calf veins (36). However, there are patients with strongly suggestive symptoms but only minimal signs of chronic venous disease in whom noninvasive studies or venogram will reveal this diagnosis (36).

Treatment is initially conservative, and bypass is reserved for a selected group of patients with disabling symptoms at least 6 months after the thrombotic episode. Exception may be made if the obstruction is due to external compression by tumor, etc., when earlier bypass is warranted. The saphenous vein is carefully mobilized from the contralateral leg, and the distal end is then divided and brought across via a subcutaneous tunnel to the femoral vein of the affected limb. An end-to-side anastomosis is performed after systemic heparinization, and postoperative anticoagulation is usually maintained orally with warfarin (Coumadin) for 3 to 6 months. An alternative technique is the use of a free vein graft (129).

Results. Cumulative patency of 75 percent at 5 years has been reported (36). A patent bypass relieves venous claudication but may not be sufficient to heal ulceration or relieve swelling if extensive postthrombotic change damage has occurred in the calf veins. However, ligation of the perforators may then further improve this situation. Some reports suggest that long-term patency is more likely if a distal arteriovenous fistula is constructed simultaneously and closed after several months (130).

Saphenopopliteal Vein Bypass (Husni Operation)

This procedure involves bypass of an occluded femoral vein segment by anastomosis of the saphenous vein into the distal popliteal vein. This operation was originally described by Warren in 1954 (131) and was later advocated and popularized by Husni (132), who described conditions required for successful outcome. Ideally, a venogram will demonstrate a patent saphenous vein with competent valves in a leg with venous disease limited to a segment extending from the common femoral to the popliteal vein. This situation is uncommon, and even then the procedure is considered only after failure of other measures such as anticoagulation, compression stockings, and ligation of incompetent perforators.

The surgical technique requires atraumatic handling of the vein and anticoagulation with heparin. A temporary peripheral AV anastomosis between the posterior tibial artery and distal saphenous vein may improve long-term patency (133).

Results. Patency rates of 66 to 75 percent have been reported, but significant symptomatic and functional improvement is achieved in less than 50 percent (134).

VENOUS VALVE SURGERY

Surgical correction of incompetent venous valves was first reported by Kistner in 1975 (87). Despite considerable enthusiasm for the concept of correcting deep vein incompetence, these procedures are still regarded as experimental. Direct repair of the incompetent valve may be possible (valvuloplasty) (87), or alternatively a segment of vein containing a competent valve may be transposed into the femoral or popliteal position (58,135).

The rationale for these procedures is supported by the finding that perforator vein division was less likely to be therapeutically beneficial in those patients who had serious abnormalities of the deep veins associated with incompetent perforators (122). The operation is applicable only to a small percentage of patients who have a severe degree of venous insufficiency with major deep vein reflux demonstrated on descending venography and in whom other methods of medical and surgical treatment have failed.

Venous Valvuloplasty

If the valves of the femoral vein are incompetent but not destroyed, a repair procedure may be possible. At operation, incompetence is first confirmed by a milking test, and the valve leaflets are then exposed through a venotomy placed either longitudinally through the commissure of the valve (87) or transversely immediately above the valve (136). The cusps are plicated and the vein is closed with fine Prolene sutures. Competency is then checked as before. Systemic heparinization is employed to prevent thrombosis, and spasm is treated with papaverine. If the valve is deemed unsuitable for repair, the surgeon may proceed to a vein segment transfer.

Vein Segment Transposition

This procedure has most often been used for treatment of incompetence of the superficial femoral vein and recently the popliteal (58). A portion of vein containing competent valve may be transposed from the saphenous or profunda position, or from the arm.

Results. There have been encouraging results in several series (58,114), with clinical improvement seen in up to 75 percent of patients. However, it may be difficult to differentiate the effects of the valve procedure from the effects of concurrent treatment such as compression stockings and bed rest while recovering from the operation. Johnson reported disappointing results and suggested that the transfer of a single valve was not sufficient to significantly alter long-term function (90). In this report, there was significant improvement in dynamic venous pressures and photoplethysmographic recovery time soon after vein segment transfer procedures, but this improvement was lost after 12 to 18 months and concomitant perforator vein ligation was considered a necessary adjunctive procedure. Ferris and Kistner reported on 46 patients, with good to excellent outcome in 80 percent (137), most of whom had also had perforator interruption in addition to the valve repair. Taheri (58) reported improvement in 75 percent of 43 cases of valve transposition performed for edema or pain. Despite symptomatic benefit, there was sometimes only slight improvement in ambulatory venous pressure. In the same series, 18 patients were treated for venous ulcer, and 17 healed following operation, whereas 5 valvuloplasty cases showed no improvement.

Procedures Which Are No Longer Recommended

Various techniques enjoyed a short vogue but have now been abandoned due to mediocre or detrimental results. These include popliteal vein ligation (138), ligation of the common femoral (139) or superficial femoral vein (140), and lumbar sympathectomy (139).

Patient Selection for Surgery

The traditional view has been that surgical intervention is indicated only when conservative measures are not successful and that nonoperative management should be pursued for at least 3 to 6 months before considering a surgical solution. Certainly the short-term results of conservative treatment for venous ulcer and symptoms are often good; on the other hand the long-term results are often dismal, with the mean duration of each episode of ulceration being 23 months in one large trial (141) and multiple recurrences occurring in at least 70 percent of patients. These results may be improved by the adjunctive use of a fibrinolysis-enhancing medication as advocated by Browse (64), but this treatment has not received wide acceptance.

In addition, the role of surgery is very dependent on the population being treated. Accurate compliance is vital for successful conservative management, but this compliance is dependent on many factors. For example, failure is more likely in the patient whose occupation denies the ability to avoid prolonged standing or precludes the wearing of compression stockings. In warm climates, stocking wearing is impractical, and the elderly or infirm patient may not be able to achieve adequate skin hygiene or put on compression stockings.

For these reasons, many practitioners are reconsidering the role of earlier surgery for these patients. With the excellent long-term results achieved after subfascial ligation of incompetent perforators (119), it seems that early surgery should be recommended in symptomatic patients who have been proved to have perforator incompetence (109)—in experienced hands injection compression sclerotherapy can be expected to offer similar success (102). These patients should continue wearing compression stockings, although the less comfortable high-pressure type may not be necessary if there is no deep vein reflux. This is certainly preferable to years of ulcer dressings or occusion bandages. The small group of patients in whom unsatisfactory results can be anticipated have already been discussed.

The guiding principles of surgical judgment can be summarized as follows:

1. Correction of the major arterial occlusion should be made before treatment of the venous ulcer in those patients in whom both are present (120).
2. In the small group of CVI patients who have no abnormality apart from severe saphenofemoral or saphenopopliteal incompetence, high ligation and stripping gives excellent results (114).
3. When there is perforator incompetence alone, perforator ligation (or sclerotherapy) can be expected to give good long-term results (119).
4. If perforator incompetence is combined with deep vein incompetence, achievement of good results depends on the treatment of the perforators followed by permanent use of knee-length, graduated elastic compression stockings (119).
5. Venous valve transposition and repair procedures may benefit patients with deep vein incompetence, although it remains to determine what is the ideal site and number of valves to be corrected (90).
6. Venous "claudication" suggests outflow obstruction, which may be relieved by venous bypass grafting (36).

References

1. Dodd H, Cockett FB: The post-thrombotic syndrome and venous ulceration. In Dodd H, Cockett FB (eds): *Pathology and Surgery of the Veins of the Lower Limb*, ed 2. Edinburgh, Churchill Livingstone, 1976.
2. Sumner DS: Applied physiology in venous problem. In Bergan JJ, Yao JST (eds): *Surgery of the Veins*. Orlando, Florida, Grune & Stratton, 1985.
3. Gay J: On varicose diseases of the lower extremities. Lettsomian lectures of 1867. London, Churchill, 1868.
4. Homans J: The etiology and treatment of varicose ulcer of the leg. Surg Gynecol Obstet 1917, 24:300–311.
5. Dos Santos JC: La phlebologie directe. Conception, technique, premiers resultats. J Int Chir 1938, 3:625.
6. Bauer G: Division of popliteal vein in the treatment of so-called varicose ulceration. Br Med J 1950, 2:318–321.
7. Widmar LK, Mall TH, Martin H: Epidemiology and sociomedical importance of peripheral venous disease. In Hobbs JT (ed): *The Treatment of Venous Disorders*. Philadelphia, Lippincott, 1977.

8. Borschberg E: *The Prevalence of Varicose Veins in the Lower Extremities*. Basel, Karger, 1967.
9. Coon WW, Willis PW, Keller JB: Venous thromboembolism and other venous diseases in the Tecumseh Community Health Survey. Circulation 1978, 48:839–846.
10. Gjores JE: The incidence of venous thrombosis and its sequelae in certain districts of Sweden. Acta Chir Scand 1956, 206 (suppl).
11. Boyd AM, Jepson RP, Ratcliff AH, Rose SS: The logical management of chronic ulcers of the leg. Angiology 1952, 3:207.
12. Cockett FB, Jones BE: The ankle blow-out syndrome: A new approach to the varicose ulcer problem. Lancet 1953, 1:17–23.
13. Straubesand J: Some problems presented by the anatomy of the perforating veins—introduction. In May R, Partsch H, Straubesand J (eds): *Perforating Veins*. Baltimore, Urban and Schwartzenberg, 1981.
14. Cockett FB: The pathology and treatment of venous ulcers of the leg. Br J Surg 1955, 43:260–278.
15. Dodd H: The varicose tributaries of the superficial vein passing into Hunter's canal. Post Med J 1959, 35:18–23.
16. Bassi G: Le varici arti inferiori. Minerva Med 1962.
17. Ludbrook J, Jamieson GG: Disorders of veins. In Sabiston DC (ed): *Davis-Christopher Textbook of Surgery*, ed 12. Philadelphia, Saunders, 1981.
18. May R: Nomenclature of the surgically most important connecting veins. In May R, Partsch H, Straubesand J (eds): *Perforating Veins*. Baltimore, Urban and Schwartzenberg, 1981.
19. Homans J: The operative treatment of varicose veins and ulcers based upon a classification of the lesions. Surg Gynecol Obstet 1916, 22:143–58.
20. Pimer F: On the valves of the perforating veins. In May R, Partsch H, Straubesand J (eds): *Perforating Veins*. Baltimore, Urban and Schwartzenberg, 1981.
21. Pollack AA, Wood EH: Venous pressure in the saphenous vein in the ankle in man during exercise and changes in posture. J Appl Physiol 1949, 1:649.
22. Nicolaides AN, Hoare M, Miles CR, et al: Value of ambulatory venous pressure in the assessment of venous insufficiency. Vasc Diag Ther 1982, 3:41–45.
23. Nicolaides AN, Zukowski A, Lewis R, Kyprianou P, Malouf GM: Venous pressure measurements in venous problems. In Bergan JJ, Yao JST (eds): *Surgery of the Veins*. Orlando, Florida, Grune & Stratton, 1985.
24. Hojensgard JC, Sturup H: Static and dynamic pressures in superficial and deep veins of the lower extremity in man. Acta Physiol Scand 1953, 27:49.
25. Arnoldi CC: Venous pressure measurements in patients with valvular incompetence of the veins of the lower limb. Acta Chir Scand 1966, 132:628.
26. Randhawa GK, Dhillon JS, Kistner RL, Ferris EB: Assessment of chronic venous insufficiency using dynamic venous pressure studies. Am J Surg 1984, 148:203–209.
27. Walker AJ, Longland C: Venous measurement of the foot in exercise as an aid to investigation of venous diseases in the leg. Clin Sci 1950, 9:101.
28. Taheri SA, Yacobucci GN, Williams J, Elias S: Deep posterior compartment pressure in the evaluation of venous insufficiency of the lower extremity: A preliminary report. Angiology 1984, 35:173–176.
29. Chatard H, Dufour H: A note on the mixed haematic and melanic nature of pigmentations in phlebology. Phlebologie 1983, 36:303.
30. Bean WB: *Vascular Spiders and Related Lesions of the Skin*. Springfield, Illinois, Charles C Thomas, 1958.
31. Ouvry PA, Davy A: The sclerotherapy of telangiectasia. Phlebologie 1982, 35:349.
32. Browse NL, Jarrett PEM, Morland M, Burnand K: Treatment of liposclerosis of the leg by fibrinolytic enhancement: A preliminary report. Br Med J 1977, 2:434–435.
33. Landthaler M, Haina D, Waidelich W, Braun-Faks O: Laser therapy of venous lakes and telangiectasias. Plast Reconstr Surg 1984, 73:78.
34. Lippmann HI, Goldin RR: Subcutaneous ossification of the legs in chronic venous insufficiency. Radiology 1960, 74:279.
35. Marjolin's Dictionnaire de Medecine (1852). Quoted by Aird I (ed): *A Companion in Surgical Studies*, ed 2. Edinburgh, Livingstone.
36. Halliday JP, Harris JP, May J: Femoro-femoral crossover grafts (Palma operation): A long-term follow-up study. In Bergan JJ, Yao JST (eds): *Surgery of the Veins*. Orlando, Florida, Grune & Stratton, 1985.
37. Bjordal RI: intermittent venous claudication: A report of two cases. Acta Chir Scand 1970, 136:641.
38. Tripolitis AJ, Milligan EB, Bodily KC, Strandness DE: The physiology of venous claudication. Am J Surg 1980, 139:447–448.
39. Trendelenburg F: Ueber die Unterbindung der Vena saphena magna bei Unterschenkelvaricen. Beitr Klin Chir 1890, 7:195.
40. Large J: Doppler testing as an important conservation measure in the treatment of varicose veins. Aust NZ J Surg 1984, 54:357–359.
41. Miller SS, Foote AV: The ultrasonic detection of incompetent perforating veins. Br J Surg 1974, 61:653.
42. O'Donnell TF, Burnand KG, Clemenson G, Lea Thomas M, Browse NL: Doppler examination vs. clinical and phlebographic detection of the localisation of incompetent perforating veins. Arch Surg 1977, 112:31–35.
43. Beasley WH, Fegan WG: An investigation into the localisation of incompetent perforating veins. Br J Surg 1970, 57:30–32.
44. Linton RR: The post-thrombotic ulceration of the lower extremity. Its etiology and surgical treatment. Ann Surg 1953, 138:415–432.
45. Edwards EA, Edwards JE: The effects of thrombophlebitis on the venous valve. Surg Gynecol Obstet 1937, 65:310–320.
46. Recek F: A critical appraisal of the role of ankle perforators for the genesis of venous ulcers in the lower leg. J Cardiovasc Surg 1971, 12:45.
47. Burnand KE, Lea Thomas M, O'Donnell E, Browse NL: Relation between postphlebitic changes in the deep veins and results of surgical treatment of venous ulcers. Lancet 1976, 1:936–938.
48. Shull KC, Nicolaides AN, Fernandes JF, Miles C, Horner J, Needham T, Cooke ED, Eastcott FHG: Significance of popliteal reflux in relation to ambulatory venous pressure and ulceration. Arch Surg 1979, 114:1304–1306.
49. Hoare MC, Nicolaides AN, Miles CR, Shull K, Jury RP, Needham T, Dudley HAF: The role of primary varicose veins in venous ulceration. Surgery 1982, 92:450–453.
50. Henry ME, Fegan WG, Pegum JM: Five year survey of the treatment of varicose ulcers. Br Med J 1971, 2:493.
51. Bauer G: A venographic study of thromboembolic events. Acta Chir Scand 1940, 84(suppl):61.
52. Bauer G: The etiology of leg ulcers and their treatment by resection of the popliteal vein. J Int Chir 1948, 8:937–960.
53. Kistner RL: Surgical repair of the incompetent femoral vein valve. Arch Surg 1975, 110:1336–1342.
54. Kistner RL: Venous valve surgery. In Bergan JJ, Yao JST (eds): *Surgery of the Veins*. Orlando, Florida, Grune & Stratton, 1985.
55. Cockett FB, Negus D: Iliac vein compression—Its relation to iliofemoral thrombosis and the post-thrombotic syndrome. Br Med J 1967, 2:14–19.
56. Servelle M: Klippel and Trenaunay's syndrome. 768 operated cases. Ann Surg 1985, 201:365–373.
57. Baskerville PA, Ackroyd JS, Thomas ML, Browse NL: The Klippel-Trenaunay syndrome: Clinical, radiological and haemodynamic features and management. Br J Surg 1985, 72:232–236.
58. Taheri SA, Lazar L, Elias S, Marchand P, Heffner R: Surgical treatment of postphlebitic syndrome with vein valve transplant. Am J Surg 1982, 144:221–224.

59. De Takats G, Quint H, Tillotson R: The impairment of the circulation in the varicose extremity. Arch Surg 1929, 18:671–676.
60. Cutler BS, et al (eds): *Manual of Clinical Problems in Surgery*. Boston, Little, Brown, 1984.
61. Pratt GH: Arterial varices: A syndrome. Am J Surg 1949, 77:456–460.
62. Brewer AC: Arteriovenous shunts. Br Med J 1950, 2:270.
63. Blalock A: Oxygen content of blood in patients with varicose veins. Arch Surg 1929, 19:895–905.
64. Browse NL, Burnand KG: The cause of venous ulceration. Lancet 1982, 2:243–245.
65. Burnand KG, Whimster I, Naidoo A, Browse NL: Pericapillary fibrin in the ulcer bearing skin of the lower leg: The cause of lipodermatosclerosis and venous ulceration. Br Med J 1982, 285:1071–1072.
66. Browse NL, Gray L, Jarrett PEM, Morland M: Blood and vein wall fibrinolytic activity in health and vascular disease. Br Med J 1977, 1:478–481.
67. Burnand KG, Clemenson G, Morland M, Jarrett PEM, Browse NL: Venous lipodermatosclerosis: Treatment by fibrinolytic enhancement and elastic companion. Br Med J 1980, 280:7–11.
68. Hopkins NFG, Spinks T, Rhodes CG, Ranicar ASO, Jamieson CW: Positron emission tomography in venous ulceration and liposclerosis: Study of regional tissue function. Br Med J 1983, 286:333–336.
69. Moyer CA, Butcher HR: Stasis ulcers: An evaluation of three methods of therapy and the implication of obliterative cutaneous lymphangitis as a credible etiologic factor. Ann Surg 1955, 141:577–588.
70. Kinmonth JB: Lymphangiology in clinical surgery. Ann R Coll Surg Engl 1954, 15:300.
71. Bergan JT, Flinn WR, Yao JST: Clinical application of noninvasive testing in venous disease. In Kempczinski RF, Yao JST (eds): *Practical Non-invasive Vascular Diagnosis*. Chicago, Year Book Medical Publishers, 1982.
72. Flinn WR, O'Mara CS, Peterson LK, Blackburn D, Yao JST: The use of photoplethysmography in the assessment of chronic venous insufficiency. In Kempczinski RF, Yao JST (eds): *Practical Non-invasive Vascular Diagnosis*. Chicago, Year Book Medical Publishers, 1982.
73. Abramowitz HB, Queral LA, Flinn WA, Nora PF, Peterson LK, Bergan JJ, Yao JST: The use of photoplethysmography in the assessment of venous insufficiency: A comparison to venous pressure measurement. Surgery 86:434, 1979.
74. O'Donnell TF, Burnand KG, Clemanson G, Lea Thomas M, Browse NL: Doppler examination vs clinical and phlebographic detection of the localisation of incompetent perforating veins. Arch Surg 1977, 112:31–35.
75. Nicolas GG, Miller FT Jr, Demuth WE Jr, Waldhansen JA: Clinical vascular laboratory diagnosis of deep venous thrombosis. Ann Surg 1977, 186:213–218.
76. Wheeler HB, Anderson FA: Impedance plethysmography. In Kempczinski RF, Yao JST (eds): *Practical Non-invasive Vascular Diagnosis*. Chicago, Year Book Medical Publishers, 1982.
77. Barnes RW, Garrett WV, Hummell BA, Hoak JC: Photoplethysmographic assessment of altered cutaneous circulation in the postphlebitic syndrome. Proc Assoc Adv Med Instrum (abstract) 1978, 13:25.
78. Norris CS, Beyrau A, Barnes RW: Quantitation plethysmography in the assessment of C.V.I.: A new method of noninvasive estimation of ambulatory venous pressure. Surgery 1983, 94:758–764.
79. Arnoldi CC, Linderholm H: Venous blood pressure in the lower limb at rest and during exercise in patients with idiopathic dysfunction of the venous pump of the calf. Acta Chir Scand 1969, 135:701.
80. Holm JSE: A simple plethysmographic model for differentiating primary from secondary varicose veins. Surg Gynecol Obstet 1976, 143:609.
81. Barnes RW: Noninvasive tests for chronic venous insufficiency. In Bergan JJ, Yao JST (eds): *Surgery of the Veins*. Orlando, Florida, Grune & Stratton, 1985.
82. Lea Thomas M: *Phlebography of the Lower Limb*. New York, Churchill Livingstone, 1982.
83. Linton RR: Modern concepts in the management of the postphlebitic syndrome with ulcerations of the lower extremity. Angiology 1952, 3:341.
84. Lea Thomas M, MacDonald LM: Complications of phlebography of the leg. Br Med J 1978, 2:307.
85. Widrich WC, Robbins AH, Rommel AJ, Andrews R: Iopamidol: A nonionic contrast agent for peripheral arteriography. Radiology 1982, 145:53–55.
86. Kakkar VV: Phlebology and cinephlebography. In Verstraete M (ed): *Methods in Angiology*. Boston, Martinus Nijhoff, 1980.
87. Kistner RL: Surgical repair of the incompetent femoral vein valve. Arch Surg 1975, 110:1336–1342.
88. Schull KC, Nicolaides AN, Fernandes e Fernandes J, Miles C, Horner J, Needham T, Cooke FD, Eastcott FHG: Significance of popliteal reflux in relation in ambulatory venous pressure and ulceration. Arch Surg 1979, 114:1304.
89. Nicolaides AN, Zukowski A, Lewis R, Kyprianou P, Malouf GM: Venous pressure measurements in venous problems. In Bergan JJ, Yao JST (eds): *Surgery of the Veins*. Orlando, Florida, Grune & Stratton, 1985.
90. Johnson ND, Querel LA, Flinn WR, Yao JST, Bergan JJ: Late objective assessment of venous valve surgery. Arch Surg 1981, 116:1461–1466.
91. Mahorner H: Thrombectomy for massive venous thrombosis. Mayo Clin Proc 1965, 40:809–814.
92. Eklof B, Einarsson E, Plate G: Role of thrombectomy and temporary arteriovenous fistula in acute iliofemmoral venous thrombosis. In Bergan JJ, Yao JST (eds): *Surgery of the Veins*. Orlando, Florida, Grune & Stratton, 1985.
93. Albrechtsson U, Anderson J, Einarsson E, Eklof B, Norgren L: Streptokinase treatment of deep venous thrombosis and the postthrombotic syndrome. Follow-up evaluation of venous function. Arch Surg 1981, 116:33–37.
94. Persson AV, Robichaux WT, Jaxheimar EC, DiPronio EM: Burst therapy: A method of administering fibrinolytic agents. Am J Surg 1984, 147:531–536.
95. Ruckley CV, Dale JJ, Callam MJ, Harper DR: Causes of chronic leg ulcer. Lancet 1982, 2:615–616.
96. Horner J, Fernandes e Fernandes J, Nicolaides AN: Value of graduated compression stockings in deep vein insufficiency. Br Med J 1980, 280:820–821.
97. Pierson S, Pierson D, Swallow R, Johnson G: Efficacy of graded elastic compression in the lower leg. JAMA 1983, 249:242–243.
98. Browse NL, Jarrett PEM, Morland M, Burnand K: Treatment of liposclerosis of the leg by fibrinolytic enhancement: A preliminary report. Br Med J 1977, 2:434–435.
99. Hobbs JT: Surgery and sclerotherapy in the treatment of varicose veins. Arch Surg 1974, 109:793–796.
100. Fegan WG: Treatment of varicose veins by injection compression. In Hobbs JT (ed): *The Treatment of Venous Disorders*. Philadelphia, Lippincott, 1977.
101. Lofgren EP: Treatment of long saphenous varicosities and their recurrence: A long-term follow-up. In Bergan JJ, Yao JST (eds): *Surgery of the Veins*. Orlando, Florida, Grune & Stratton, 1985.
102. Hobbs JT: A random trial of the treatment of varicose veins by surgery and sclerotherapy. In Hobbs JT (ed): *The Treatment of Venous Disorders*. Philadelphia, Lippincott, 1977.
103. Sladen JG: Compression sclerotherapy: Preparation, technique, complications and results. Am J Surg 1983, 146:228–232.

104. De Palma RE: Surgical therapy for venous stasis: Results of a modified Linton operation. Am J Surg 1979, 117:810–813.
105. Ackermann LV: *Surgical Pathology*, chap 26, ed 6. St Louis, CV Mosby, 1981, p 1545.
106. Davies DM: Microvascular surgery. Br Med J 1985, 290:910–912.
107. De Palma RE: Surgical therapy for venous stasis. Surgery 1974, 76:410.
108. Haeger K: The problem of radicality in surgery for venous incompetence of the leg. Vasa 1972, 1:127.
109. Hyde GL, Litton TC, Hull DA: Long-term results of subfascial vein ligation for venous stasis disease. Surg Gynecol Obstet 1981, 153:683–686.
110. Madelung: Ueber die Auschaelung cirsoider varicen an den unteren Extremilaeten. Verhanndel deutsch Gesellsch Chir, 1884, xiii, 114.
111. Schanzer H, Pierce EC II: A rational approach to surgery of the chronic venous stasis syndrome. Ann Surg 1982, 195:25–29.
112. Field P, Boxel PV: The role of the Linton flap procedure in the management of stasis dermatitis and ulceration in the lower limbs. Surgery 1971, 70:920.
113. Bowen FH: Subfascial ligation (Linton operation) of the perforating leg veins to treat post-thrombophlebitic syndrome. Am Surg 1975, 41:148.
114. Schanzer H, Peirce EC II: A rational approach to surgery of the chronic venous stasis syndrome. Ann Surg 1982, 195:25–29.
115. Felder DA, Hardy TO: A posterior subfascial approach to the communicating veins of the leg. Surg Gynecol Obstet 1955, 100:730.
116. Blumenberg RM, Gelfland ML: The posterior stocking seam approach to radical subfascial clipping of perforating veins. Am J Surg 1978, 136:202.
117. Healey PJM, Healey EH, Wong R, Schaberg FJ: Surgical management of the chronic venous ulcer: The Rob procedure. Am J Surg 1979, 137:556.
118. Almgren B, Bowald S, Eriksson I, Forsberg O: The posterior approach for subfascial ligation of perforating veins. Acta Chir Scand 1982, 148:243–245.
119. Negus D, Friedgood A: The effective management of venous ulcerations. Br J Surg 1982, 70:623–627.
120. DePalma R: Surgical therapy for venous stasis: Results of a modified Linton operation. Am J Surg 1979, 137:810–813.
121. Felder DA, Bernstein EF: A re-evaluation of the posterior subfascial approach for the ligation of the communicating veins in the leg. Surgery 1960, 47:349–352.
122. Burnand KG, O'Donnell TF, Lea Thomas M, Browse NL: The relative importance of incompetent communicating veins in the production of varicose veins and venous ulcers. Surgery 1977, 82:9–14.
123. Burnaud KG, Lea Thomas M, O'Donnell TF, Browse NL: Relationship between postphlebitic changes in the deep veins and results of surgical treatment of venous ulcers. Lancet 1976, 1:936–938.
124. Hull DA, Hyde GL: Early subfascial ligation of perforating veins in prevention of venous ulceration. Am Surg 1965, 31:313–317.
125. Halliday P: The place of subfascial ligation of perforating veins in the treatment of the post-phlebitic syndrome. Br J Surg 1971, 58:104–111.
126. Negus D: Perforating vein interruption in the postphlebitic syndrome. In Bergan JJ, Yao JST (eds): *Surgery of the Veins*. Orlando, Florida, Grune & Stratton, 1985.
127. Browse NL, Burnand KG: The causes of venous ulcerations. Lancet 1982, 2:243–245.
128. Palma ER, Esperon R: Vein transplants and grafts in the surgical treatment of the postphlebitic syndrome. J Cardiovasc Surg 1960, 1:94–107.
129. Hardin CA: Bypass saphenous grafts for the relief of venous obstruction of the extremity. Surg Gynecol Obstet 1962, 115:709–712.
130. Johnson V, Eiseman B: Evaluation of arteriovenous shunt to maintain patency of venous autograft. Am J Surg 1969, 118:915–920.
131. Warren R, Thayer T: Transplantation of the saphenous vein for postphlebitic stasis. Surgery 1954, 35:867–876.
132. Husni EA: In situ saphenopopliteal bypass graft for incompetence of the femoral and popliteal veins. Surg Gynecol Obstet 1970, 130:279–284.
133. Gruss JD, Bartels D, Tsafardakis F, Kawai S: The AV fistula operation technique. In May R, Weber J (eds): *Pelvic and Abdominal Veins*. Amsterdam, Excerpta Medica, 1981, p 215.
134. Gruss JD: The saphenopopliteal bypass for chronic venous insufficiency (May-Husni operation). In Bergan JJ, Yao JST (eds): *Surgery of the Veins*. Orlando, Florida, Grune & Stratton, 1985.
135. Kistner RL, Sparkuhl MD: Surgery in acute and chronic venous disease. Surgery 1979, 85:31–43.
136. Raju S: Venous insufficiency of the lower limb and stasis ulceration. Changing concepts and management. Ann Surg 1983, 197:688–697.
137. Ferris EB, Kistner RL: Femoral vein reconstruction in the management of chronic venous insufficiency. Arch Surg 1982, 117:1571–1579.
138. Bauer G: Division of the popliteal vein in the treatment of so-called varicose ulceration. Br Med J 1950, 2:318–321.
139. Robinson JR, Moyer CA: Comparison of late sequelae of common and superficial femoral vein ligations. Surgery 1954, 35:690–697.
140. Buxton RW, Ferris JM, Moyer CA, Coller FA: Surgical treatment of long-standing deep phlebitis of the leg. Surgery 1944, 15:749–756.
141. Callan MJ, Ruckley CV, Dale JJ, Harper DR: The natural history of chronic leg ulceration (abstract). Br J Surg 1984, 71:990.

Chapter 61

VENOUS RECONSTRUCTIVE SURGERY

LUIS A. QUERAL

Venous disease of the lower extremities is a clinical entity that is commonly encountered in the practice of medicine. Diagnosing the condition is easy, but effectively treating it is both vexing and challenging. Venous insufficiency is vexing because a cure is rarely achieved, and it is challenging because only through proper therapeutic maneuvers can it be ameliorated. From the physician's perspective, success in the management of patients with venous disease depends largely on two factors: (1) identification of the pathophysiology involved, and (2) institution of therapy that will normalize the aberrant physiology. Therefore, the thrust of this chapter is to emphasize a thorough physiological investigation of the patient and then to present alternative modes of treatment with particular emphasis on venous reconstructive surgery.

Historical Perspective

Venous disease of the lower extremities has probably afflicted human beings from the time the erect stance was first developed. It is therefore not surprising that the history of treatment of venous stasis begins in antiquity. Hippocrates noted that venous varicosities were a postpubertal phenomenon and were more likely to afflict those who spent much time with their feet dangling down from horse mounts (1). His therapeutic advice was to elevate the leg and to use compressive bandages: "In the case of an ulcer, it is not expedient to stand; more specially if the ulcer is situated in the leg" (Hippocrates, 460–377 B.C.).

Much was written about venous disease of the lower extremities during Roman times. Aurelius Cornelius Alsus (25 B.C. to A.D. 50) advised that plaster, linen roll, and bandages be used to treat leg ulcers. Varicose veins were to be treated by exposure, followed by avulsion with a blunt hook with a touch of the cautery. Claudius Galen (AD 130 to 200) treated varicose veins in a similar fashion and liked to apply wine to venous ulcers (2).

The generally salubrious methods of the Greco-Roman period were forgotten during the Middle Ages. Instead, Galen's theory that varicose veins were filled with deleterious "humors" was applied to venous disease of the lower extremities for nearly 15 centuries with disastrous results. Attempts at compression were thought to lead to madness or death since the humors were squeezed back into the body. Furthermore, ulcerations were believed to be natural "drains" for otherwise toxic humors.

The humoral theory became obsolete after William Harvey wrote of his discovery of the circulation of the blood in 1628. Harvey understood the effect of muscular contractions in assisting the flow of venous blood, and, therefore, he studied the valves and the veins (2). As a result, by the eighteenth century, external compression was reinstituted as an effective mode of therapy for venous ulceration. It is remarkable that, in modern times, the only important addition to compression therapy has been the introduction of elastic adhesive bandages.

The surgical treatment of varicose veins was originally described by Alsus and Galen (2). They bluntly tore out varicosities. A refinement of technique, ligation, was instituted by Aetuys of Amida, a Byzantine physician (A.D. 502 to 575) (2). Ligation was later practiced by Ambroise Paré in the sixteenth century (3). Today greater saphenous ligation is usually associated with Frederick Trendelenburg (1844 to 1924) (3). The extirpation of the vein with the stripper was suggested by Mayo in 1904 and, in association with ligation, is today a standard of therapy (4).

In the nineteenth century a more aggressive approach of ulcer debridement and split-thickness skin grafting was described by Homans (5). Soon it was recognized that this achieved temporary relief for the patient but no permanent cure. Linton and Hardy sought to modify the underlying pathophysiology of the venous ulcer by ligation of the superficial femoral vein with concomitant saphenous vein stripping (6). This was only moderately successful, and, 6 years later, Linton and Cockett both suggested ligation of calf perforating veins (7,8). Unfortunately, this approach has not been permanently successful in all patients. In 1963 a novel attempt at recreating a competent valve in the deep venous system was first suggested by Psathakis (9). He approached the problem of venous insufficiency by drawing the gracilis tendon surgically between the popliteal vein and artery and suturing to the biceps tendon. In doing so, the tendon was to act as a pinch valve to prevent venous reflux. This attempt to correct venous pathophysiology by direct venous reconstruction was ingenious; however, Psathakis's work has not been confirmed in other clinics.

Recently, Kistner has attempted to treat venous insufficiency by directly repairing a previously incompetent femoral valve (10). He theorized that the establishment of one competent valve in the deep venous system of the lower extremity is all that is needed to reverse abnormal venous hemodynamics. This concept stimulated us to treat patients with chronic venous insufficiency by valvular transposition (11). The solution was only partially successful, with a majority of patients reverting to their preoperative status (12). Nevertheless, those patients successfully treated here have led us to believe that this modality of treatment may offer relief in selected cases.

A modification of valvular transposition has been proposed by Taheri and termed "valve transplantation" (13). This technique consists of harvesting a brachial vein segment harboring a competent valve and transplanting it to the proximal popliteal vein. Taheri reports that 78 percent of patients improved after surgery. However, his results have not been reproduced elsewhere.

The above described operations for venous insufficiency were developed to recreate lost valvular competency. However, venous postthrombotic disease can also be caused by obstruction to the venous outflow of the lower extremities. In 1960 E. C. Palma originated a techique for relieving unilateral iliac vein obstruction (14). He described mobilizing the greater saphenous vein from the normal limb and tunneling it suprapubically to the affected limb where it was anastomosed to the femoral vein. This femorofemoral crossover graft has been reported by Halliday to have a 75 percent 5-year patency (15) and is clearly effective in appropriately selected patients. Superficial femoral vein obstruction can also be treated by anastomosing the ipsilateral greater saphenous vein to the popliteal vein just distal to the obstruction. This procedure was described by Husni (16) in 1970, but its long-term effectiveness is still not clearly established.

The variety of surgical approaches described to treat the patient with venous disease of the lower extremities is quite bewildering. In order to choose the appropriate one, the surgeon must have a clear understanding of the pathophysiology to be corrected.

Anatomy and Pathophysiology

A range of indiviudal variation exists in the anatomy of the veins of the lower extremities. Nevertheless, an overall pattern of venous drainage can be described to emphasize salient tenets.

The walls of veins are composed of three layers: intima, media, and adventitia. Special characteristics of the media make veins liable to dilate and become tortuous and varicosed in response to sustained elevated intravascular pressures. The intima has endothelial folds that create valves which direct blood flow proximally toward the heart. These valves are quite delicate and subject to injury.

The veins of the lower extremity can be grouped into three systems: superficial, deep, and perforating. The superficial veins lie in the subcutaneous fat shallow to the muscular fascia. These veins can empty into the popliteal vein through the lesser saphenous system or into the femoral vein through the greater saphenous system. Deep veins travel in proximity to the major arteries and are therefore deep to the fascia. Perforating veins carry blood directly from the superficial to the deep veins and are usually located along the medial aspect of the distal thigh and calf.

Unidirectional venous valves are profuse in the lower extremities and are of great importance in permitting the muscle-powered antigravitational return of blood to the heart. Destruction of the valves leads to ineffiency in venous return and, eventually, to edema, hyperpigmentation, and ulceration. The key to treating such venous incompetence is to establish the anatomical location of the valvular malfunction and/or obstruction. Only then can rational therapeutic maneuvers be instituted to correct or ameliorate the venous abnormality.

The importance of competent valves in the major veins of the lower extremity must be understood physiologically to fully appreciate the results to their malfunction. Venous return from the leg upon the assumption of the upright position is dependent on what has been termed the "musculovenous pump" (17). Muscular calf contraction compresses the deep veins and, therefore, squeezes blood toward the heart. This contraction can only happen when valvular integrity exists. The emptying of the deep veins decreases their intraluminal pressure, and blood from the relatively hypertensive superficial system is "sucked" along a pressure gradient through perforating veins into the deep veins. Such centripetal flow of blood is a particularly important means for decreasing superficial venous pressure in the ankle region. Failure of the musculovenous pump will result in ankle skin changes that range from eczema to frank ulcerations. It appears, therefore, that the skin of the lower limbs does not withstand persistent venous engorgement well and that it is normally protected from this engorgement by competent valves and active calf muscular activity.

The etiology of venous valvular malfunction is either congenital or secondary to deep venous thrombosis. The former accounts for primary varicose veins, and the latter is the cause of the widespread valvular destruction often seen in patients with chronic venous disease of the lower extremities. It appears that the delicate unidirectional valves are destroyed during the process of recanalization that follows deep venous thrombosis. However, this process is sometimes incomplete, and then chronic venous obstruction results. Patients with venous occlusions are dependent on collaterals to provide drainage or "outflow" of blood from their lower extremities. When collaterals are inadequate, edema and discomfort result. Sometimes, the venous engorgement responsible for the edema occurs acutely as a direct consequence of exercise. Such patients have enough venous outflow at rest but cannot handle the increase in arterial inflow that is a normal response to exercise. The resultant sudden pooling of blood in the lower extremity (or extremities) is subjectively described as either an "aching" or a "heaviness." This phenomenon has been called venous claudication and is important because its treatment is a surgical venous bypass of the obstruction.

Patient Evaluation

Patients burdened with venous disease of the lower extremities have a variety of complaints. Those afflicted with primary varicose veins most often find fault with the cosmetic appearance of their lower extremities. On the other hand, patients with deep venous insufficiency and/or incompetent perforators complain of ankle edema, hyperpigmentation, and sometimes ulcerations.

Logically the greater the valvular destruction of the veins, the more severe the presenting symptoms. Whatever the clinical presentation, the diagnosis of venous disease can readily be established, even by a novice. The challenge lies in the treatment, and the key to therapeutic success is a thorough evaluation of the patient.

The physical findings of patients with venous disease confirm the historically obtained diagnosis and often delineate the severity of the problem. However, the simple examination of patients does not reliably establish the site(s) of valvular malfunction and/or obstruction. Instead, the noninvasive laboratory has been found to best establish what valves are incompetent and what veins are thrombosed. Patients can initially be screened with a continuous-wave Doppler and impedance plethysmography (IPG). The Doppler can reliably establish the site of abnormal bidirectional flow and also can detect deep venous thrombosis when the normal respiratory variation of venous flow is absent (18). IPG is very helpful in establishing the presence of deep venous thrombosis and the lack of collateral flow around the site of occlusion (19). However, as helpful as these two testing modalities are, neither establishes in a quantitative fashion the degree of valvular malfunction present. This can be done by directly measuring venous pressure or by other noninvasive techniques.

Normally, the venous pressure in the subcutaneous veins of the foot and ankle falls rapidly during exercise and then rises slowly to its previous resting level. The time required for the pressure to return to baseline is called recovery time. Patients with varicose veins (superficial venous insufficiency) inhibit a shallow drop in pressure and a rapid return to the baseline volume. Patients with severe deep venous insufficiency display a minimal drop in pressure during exercise and a very short recovery time (20).

The measurement of venous pressure accurately quantitates venous dynamics but is clinically cumbersome. Patients object to needle cannulation of their foot veins, and doctors find the process lengthy and the instrumentation unwieldy. Fortunately, there are two relatively simple noninvasive techniques that record accurately lower extremity venous dynamics: strain-gauge plethysmography (SGP) and photoplethysmography (PPG).

SGP allows precise monitoring of the calf volume. Exercise is an activation of the musculovenous pump and causes blood to leave the leg and thus a decrease in calf volume. Cessation of exercise results in the return to a volumetric baseline. The latter can be measured in minutes and is termed the recovery time. A 15-s recovery time denotes valvular malfunction, and a prolonged recovery time denotes valvular integrity.

PPG is a technique that utilizes infrared light to monitor capillary volume directly. Changes in capillary filling parallel changes in venous pressure, and recovery times have been shown to be identical for both techniques (21). This method requires minimal effort and is very reliable.

Although both of the above described techniques can effectively quantitate abnormal venous dynamics, PPG is less cumbersome and allows for easier differentiation of patients. It appears that after using both, PPG is the technique of choice for the noninvasive laboratory quantification of venous insufficiency (22). PPG can help in patient selection and can be used to better assess the hemodynamic success of any venous reparative procedure (Figure 61-1).

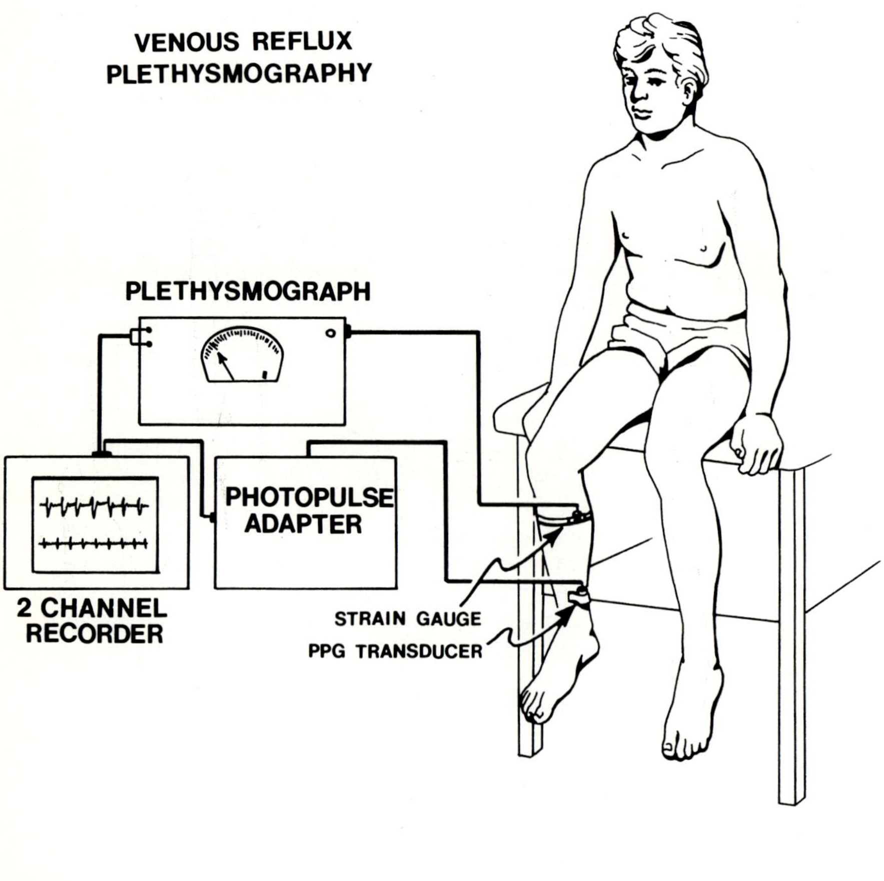

FIGURE 61-1. A patient is seen with a strain gauge applied around the calf and a PPG transducer near the medial malleolus. Calf muscular contractions are then carried out by the patient and changes recorded. Each of these techniques quantitates the degree of valvular competency.

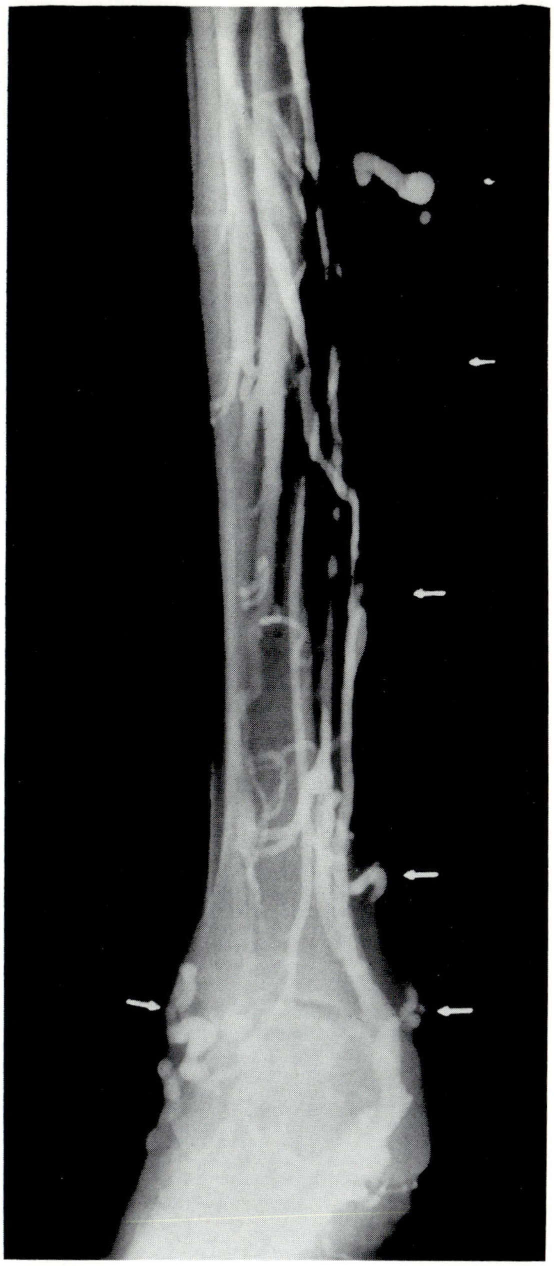

FIGURE 61-2. This ascending venogram clearly illustrates incompetent perforating veins (highlighted by arrows) mostly along the medial aspect of the calf. No evidence of acute deep venous thrombosis is noted.

Both noninvasive techniques quantitate the severity of valvular malfunction and enhance the management of patients significantly. However, the precise anatomical locaton of the incompetent valves can best be identified by venography. Contrast material injected into a subcutaneous foot vein is driven into the deep system by an ankle tourniquet. The contrast material then quickly fills the veins of the leg and, later, those in the thigh and pelvis. Loss of valves in the deep veins and in the incompetent perforators can be identified readily (Figure 61-2). Venography can also be performed in a descending fashion by injecting contrast material into the external iliac vein with the patient standing semierect. Patients with malfunctioning femoral valves have retrograde filling of the more distal veins. The incompetence of these valves can be seen clearly on the study (Figure 61-3).

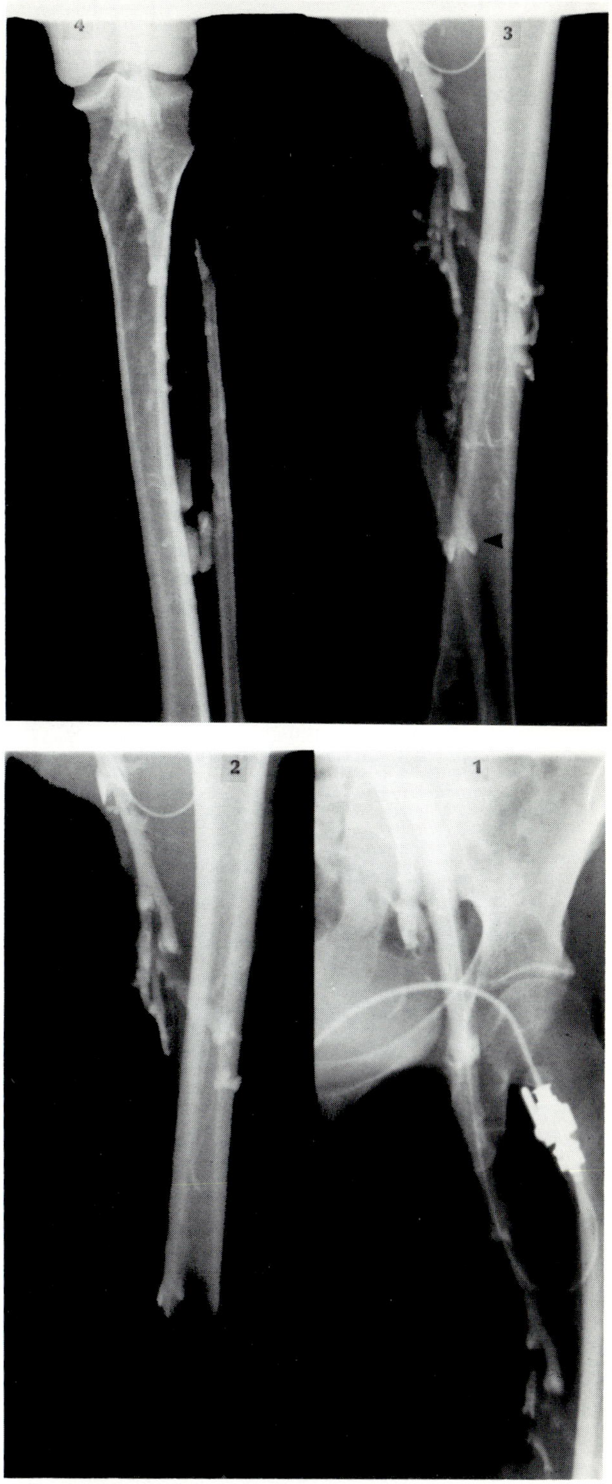

FIGURE 61-3. In these sequential descending venogram films a number of incompetent valves can be seen. The arrowhead on the portion marked 3 clearly illustrates abnormal retrograde reflux.

Therapeutic Maneuvers

Severe venous insufficiency is uniformly curable by bed rest and lower extremity elevation. So long as the patient's ankles are positioned higher than the heart, the normally deleterious effect of gravity is reversed and intraluminal venous pressure is lowered. As a direct consequence, edema is reduced and tissue healing ensues shortly thereafter. The disadvantage of this treatment modality is obvious: a normal lifestyle is hardly possible from a supine position. Nevertheless, patients can be effectively temporarily treated by a regimen of bed rest and leg elevation.

External compression therapy has been utilized effectively since the time of the Roman Empire (2) and, to this day, remains as the bulwark of all methods of nonoperative management. External compression reduces edema, thereby maintaining venous channels empty. Furthermore, the bandages used can protect an ulcerated area from external contamination and repeated trauma. We have successfully employed two types of bandages:

1. A nonmedicated and nonadhesive elastic bandage which provides high pressure (40 mmHg) at the ankle level and lower pressure at the calf level. This bandage is available commercially as a stocking (e.g., Ace bandage).

2. A medicated bandage containing zinc oxide, gelatin, and glycerin (e.g., the Unna paste boot) with an additional compression elastic bandage applied around it.

External compression has the advantage of allowing treatment of the patient without hospitalization. Therefore, strict bed rest and elevation are recommended only if the less expensive and less burdensome external compression applicances fail to significantly improve the venous condition of the patient.

Although leg elevation and compression therapy are effective, they only provide symptomatic relief and recurrence follows shortly after cessation of their application. A variety of procedures have been proposed in an attempt to correct the underlying abnormal hemodynamics (Table 61-1). All of these methods can provide significant relief to a given patient. Yet choosing a particular procedure for a given patient requires knowledge of the underlying pathophysiology and how the procedure will affect it. The indications for and effectiveness of each of the procedures will be discussed.

TABLE 61-1. Various Surgical Reconstructive Techinques

Sclerotherapy
Superficial venous ligation and stripping
Perforating vein interruption
Valvular transposition or transplantation
Venous bypasses

Sclerotherapy

Sclerotherapy is practiced commonly in Europe and has been reported to be quite effective. The principle of injection therapy is to place a sclerosant agent in a superficial vein and obliterate the lumen without a thrombus occurring. The latter is prevented by the application of compression bandages immediately after the injection. A variety of sclerosant agents can be used, but the most popular are 5% sodium morrhuate and 3% sodium tetradecyl sulfate, with the latter being most effective. Fegan (23) has reported that 91 percent of a series of 340 patients were cured or improved with this method. However, varices caused by saphenofemoral or saphenopopliteal incompetences should not be treated by injection-compression therapy. Such varices are very difficult to maintain compressed, and intraluminal thrombi almost invariably result from the sclerosant agent injection. Hobbs (24) has estimated that incompetence of the saphenofemoral junction is present in about 60 percent of patients with varicose veins, and the saphenopopliteal junction is involved in at least 20 percent. Thus, it appears as if a large number of patients with superficial varices cannot be effectively treated with sclerotherapy.

Those patients who are not excluded by the above listed criteria can be effectively treated by adherance to several basic principles. (1) The sclerosant should be injected into an empty vein, which is then compressed by an elastic bandage to avoid thrombus formation. (2) Great care should be taken to avoid the extravasation of the sclerosant into the extravascular tissues. (3) Compression bandages should not be removed for at least 48 hours.

The main complications from this technique appear to be allergic reaction to the sclerosant and tissue necrosis from infiltration of the same. Hobbs (24) claims that these complications are rare and more likely to occur when the technique is being perfected. Sclerotherapy appears to be most effective when done for cosmetic reasons, and perhaps it is because of this that it has not achieved much popularity in the United States. Nevertheless, we have found in our clinic that sclerosing large ''feeding'' veins near an ulcer crater allows for rapid healing of the area.

Ligation and Stripping

Superficial varicosities are a very common clinical entity. Coon et al. (25) have estimated that approximately 12 percent of the adult population (24 million persons) of the United States has significant varicosities. Patients so afflicted can be quite asymptomatic, or more commonly they complain of aching, heaviness, swelling, and cramping. Varicosities are believed to develop from the sequential retrograde breakdown of the venous valve which begins at the saphenofemoral juncture (26), or less often from incompetent perforating veins.

The diagnosis of varicose veins is readily made by physical examination. Their etiology can often be established by obtaining a good history from the patient. When the patient has suffered from deep venous thrombosis in the past, the cause of the varicosities is frequently either an insufficient deep venous system and/or incompetent perforating veins (secondary varicosities). Other patients have a positive family history and an insidious onset without any other pathology affecting the deep veins of the lower extremities (primary varicosities). The latter group are particularly well suited to surgical ligation and stripping.

The treatment of primary varicose veins by ligation of the saphenofemoral junction and stripping of the greater saphenous vein was popularized by Dr. Charles H. Mayo in 1904 (4). This surgical procedure continues to be widely practiced today and is a very effective way of treating superficial varicosities. The surgical techique is well described in nearly every surgical atlas and therefore will not be repeated in this chapter. The long-term results (10 years after surgery) have been reported to be good to excellent in 86 percent of patients (27).

From a hemodynamic perspective the surgical extirpation of the greater saphenous system can be quite effective in reducing ambulatory venous hypertension. Patients whose varcosities contribute adversely to the venous dynamics of the lower extremity can be noninvasively identified. These individuals, who have abnormally short PPG recovery times corrected (lengthened) by a superficial tourniquet, are ideal candidates for ligation and stripping. In a series of 22 patients studied at the University of Maryland the use of a tourniquet normalized the recovery time in 30 limbs. All of these patients underwent ligation and stripping. After surgery, the PPG recovery time reverted to normal in 28 limbs with only 2 limbs remaining abnormal.

When the PPG recovery time is normalized, the relief of symptoms is dramatic and patient contentment is nearly always achieved. Furthermore, the noninvasive selection of surgical candidates helps to decrease the number of greater saphenous veins needlessly removed. This point is quite important since this vein is the best arterial substitute for myocardial or lower extremity arterial revascularization.

Subfascial Ligation of Perforating Veins

Perforating veins in the lower extremity normally carry blood from the superficial to the deep system and are also called communicating veins. Such centripetal flow can be disrupted should the valves in the perforating veins become incompetent. Then blood flow is reversed, and the result is superficial ambulatory venous hypertension, which leads to edema, stasis, hyperpigmentation, and eventually ulceration. The surgical interruption of these communicating veins has been popular ever since originally proposed by Linton (8) and by Cockett (7) in the mid-1950s. A number of investigators were quite enthusiastic and reported a success rate of around 90 percent (28). However, more recently others have reported rather disappointing results (29). The question that has yet to be answered is: Who should have interruption of perforating veins?

Our own experience with subfascial ligation of perforators has been good because of a high degree of patient selectivity. Patients with superficial venous insufficiency have a ligation and stripping prior to an interruption of the perforating veins. Furthermore, patients with deep venous insufficiency are not subjected to a Linton procedure. This approach has also been successfully employed and reported by Negus (28).

The techique for interrupting incompetent communicating veins is straightforward. A long vertical incision is made in the leg, usually along its medial aspect with the inferior portion of the wound going posterior to the medial malleolus. Dissection is sharply carried directly down to the deep fascia, which is then incised and widely undermined. It is important to avoid dissection in the subcutaneous areas since tissue necrosis can then occur. All communicating veins are identified, ligated, and divided. The fascia is then closed with a running absorbable suture and the skin stapled shut. No sutures are placed in the subcutaneous area. Finally, an Unna paste boot and elastic bandage are applied in the operating room. This last part is important in preventing edema in the postoperative period. Edema is the chief culprit in causing tissue breakdown and wound disruption. This complication should be feared and avoided.

Unfortunately, the above described operation is very likely to fail if the deep venous system is incompetent. It can be logically theorized that new perforating veins eventually reappear in the postoperative period as a result of persistent deep venous hypertension. Clearly, patients who have the misfortune of harboring deep valvular incompetence have the best chance of improvement if the causative venous insufficiency is somehow corrected.

Valvular Transposition

The key element in venus disease of the lower extremity is valvular incompetence. Stripping venous insufficiency can be treated with ligation and stripping. Perforating veins that are incompetent can be interrupted by subfascial ligation. However, the question that remains unanswered is how to treat deep venous insufficiency.

Surgical correction of an incompetent femoral venous valve was initially performed in 1968 by Kistner (30), and the first series of repairs was reported in 1975 (10). These patients were treated by the direct surgical repair of an incompetent or leaking femoral venous valve—valvuloplasty. This work was pioneering in its concept but not widely applicable since very few patients can be found to need a valvuloplasty. However, the concept of a competent femoral valve markedly improving patients stimulated our approach to the problems of venous disease and our interest in the effect of a competent valve at the femoral level. To test this concept a number of valvular transpositions have been performed (11). This procedure is performed by transsecting the superficial femoral vein and anastomosing the distal end to a competent saphenous or profunda vein (Figure 61-4). Such transposition places a competent valve in the deep venous system of the lower extremity. Results were very encouraging initially, but several years later a number of patients regressed to their previous condition (20). Patients who benefit from the transposition without regressing were noted to be relatively young and, for the most part, free from distal venous disease (Figures 61-5

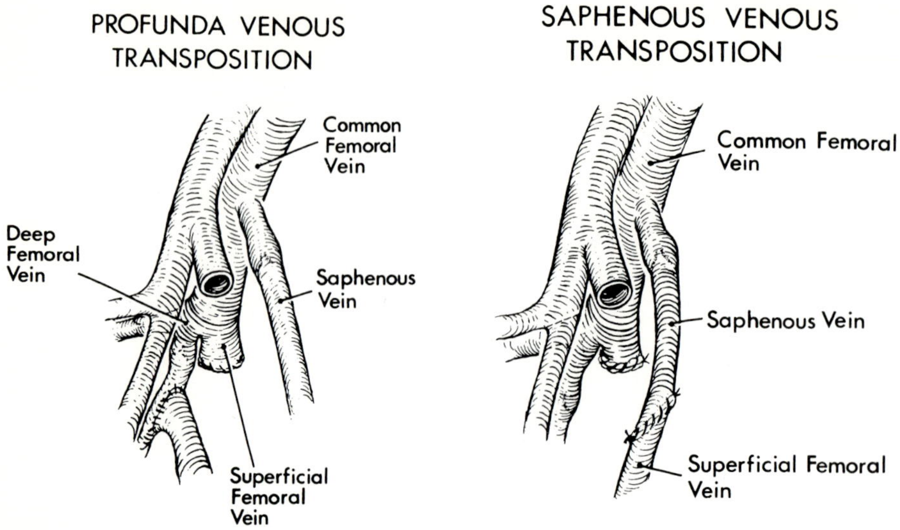

FIGURE 61-4. Femoral valve transposition can be achieved by anastomosing the transected and incompetent superficial femoral vein to either the saphenous or deep femoral veins—both of which are competent.

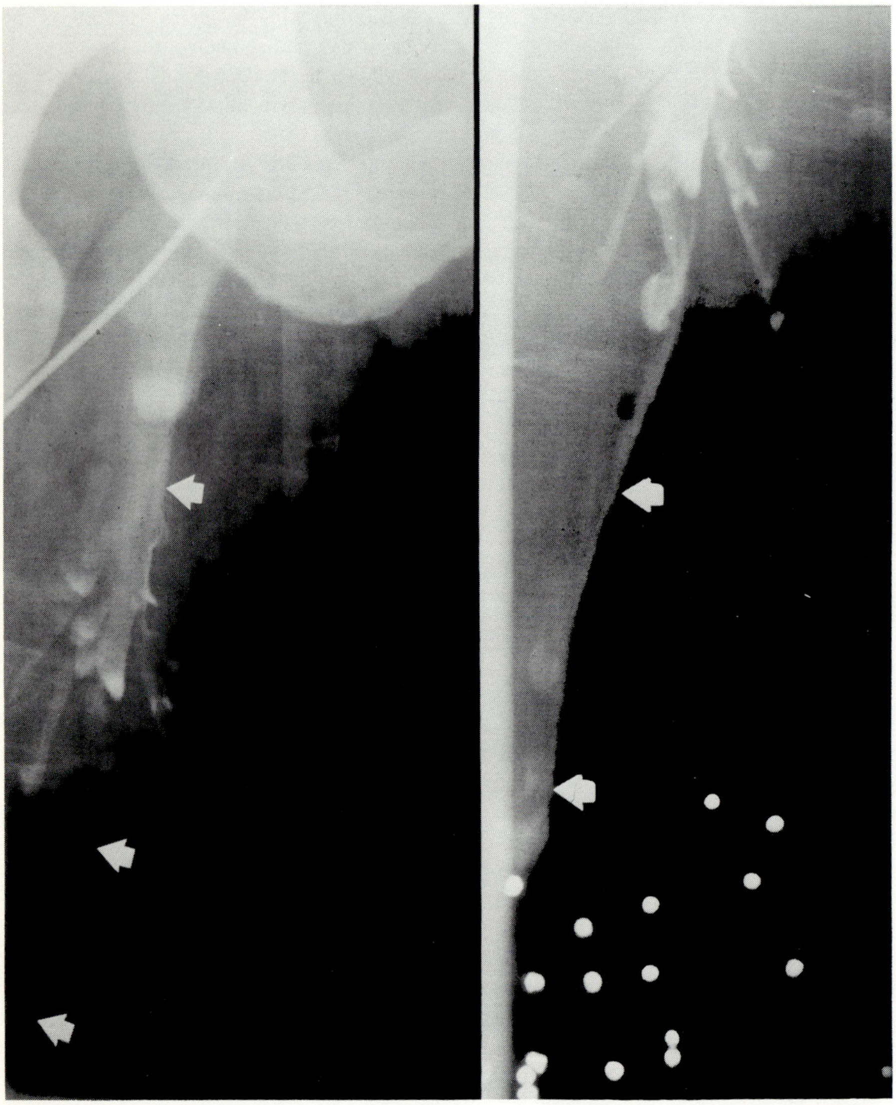

FIGURE 61-5. This descending venogram was performed on a patient with superficial femoral venous incompetence (*arrows*) caused by a gunshot wound.

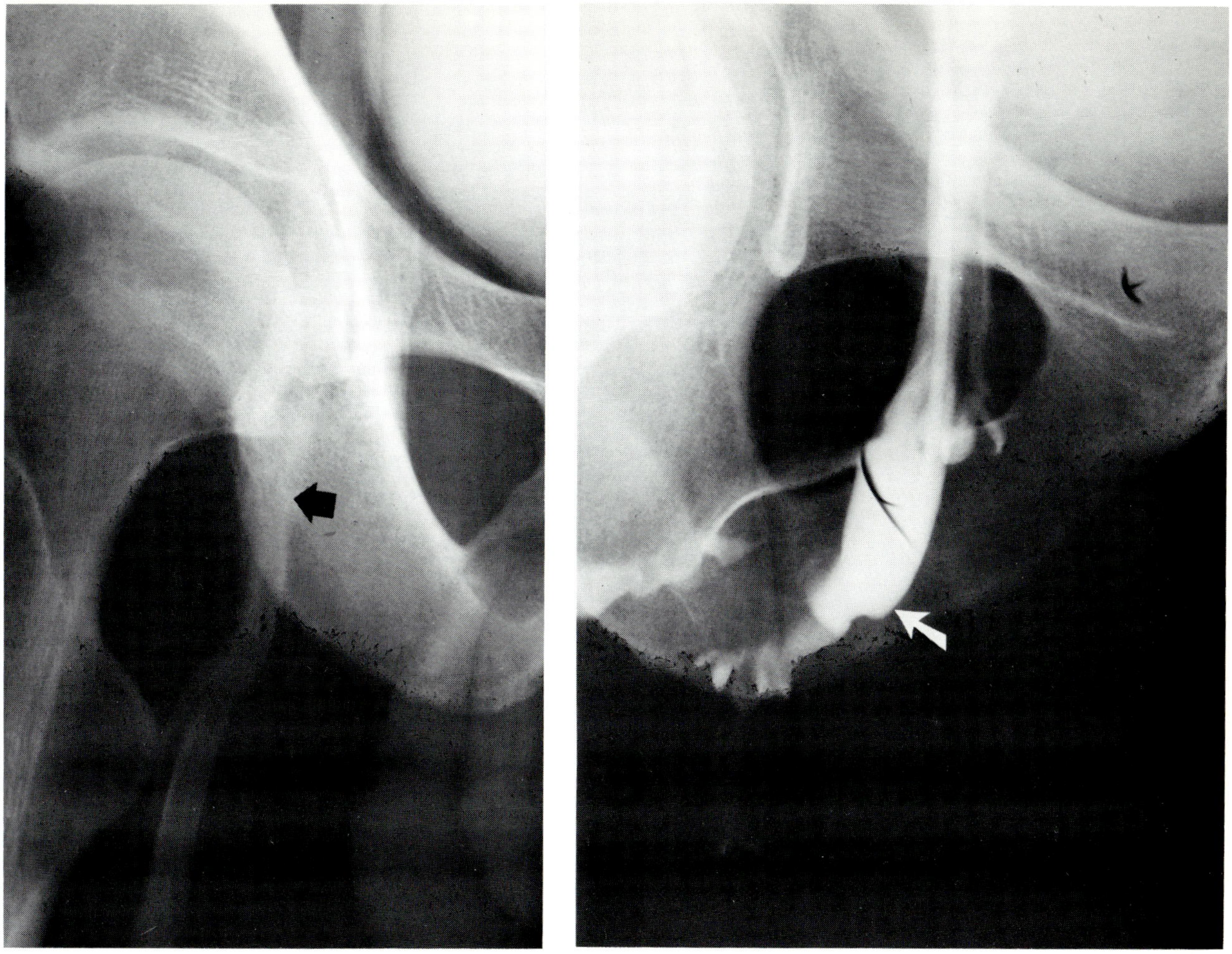

FIGURE 61-6. The patient described in Figure 61-5 had a saphenous vein transposition, and the post-operative ascending venogram illustrates (*dark arrow*) patency of the transposition. A descending venogram illustrates competency (*light arrow*).

and 61-6). It appears, therefore, that a competent valve at the femoral level can improve patients who do not have extensive distal destruction of valvular integrity in the lower extremity.

More recently, Taheri (13) has suggested that a competent valve transplanted from the arm into the proximal popliteal vein markedly improves patients with deep venous insufficiency. His results are preliminary and lack long-term follow-up. Nevertheless, the concept of a competent valve inserted more distally in the venous system is appealing. It is hoped that other medical centers will attempt to reproduce Taheri's optimistic results.

Venous Bypasses

Venous disease of the lower extremities is usually due to loss of valvular integrity. However, a minority of patients with the postthrombotic syndrome suffer from venous occlusion. In a recent report of 147 patients with clinically suspected venous insufficiency, Raj (31) found only 13 percent with predominantly obstructive disease. The site(s) of obstruction varies, and surgical procedures have been described for correction of iliac vein and superficial femoral vein thromboses.

Chronic obstruction of the iliac vein may cause edema and pain. The degree of presenting symptoms is dependent on the abundance of bridging collaterals. The fewer the collaterals the more pronounced the symptoms. Such patients are candidates for surgically bypassing the thrombosed large venous channel. An occluded iliac vein can be bypassed by utilizing the contralateral saphenous vein as a crossover graft. This procedure was originally described by Palma (14) and was popularized in the United States by Dale (32). The long-term patency of this bypass has been reported by Halliday et al. (15) to be 75 percent. Perhaps this patency can be improved by the addition of a temporary arteriovenous fistula as depicted in Figure 61-7.

A bypass of an obstructed superficial femoral vein was described by Husni (16) in 1970 and coined "sapheno popliteal bypass." This procedure is done by dissecting the greater saphenous vein in the distal thigh and terminally anastomosing it to the side of the popliteal vein just beyond the site of superficial femoral obstruction. The results of this operation have not been

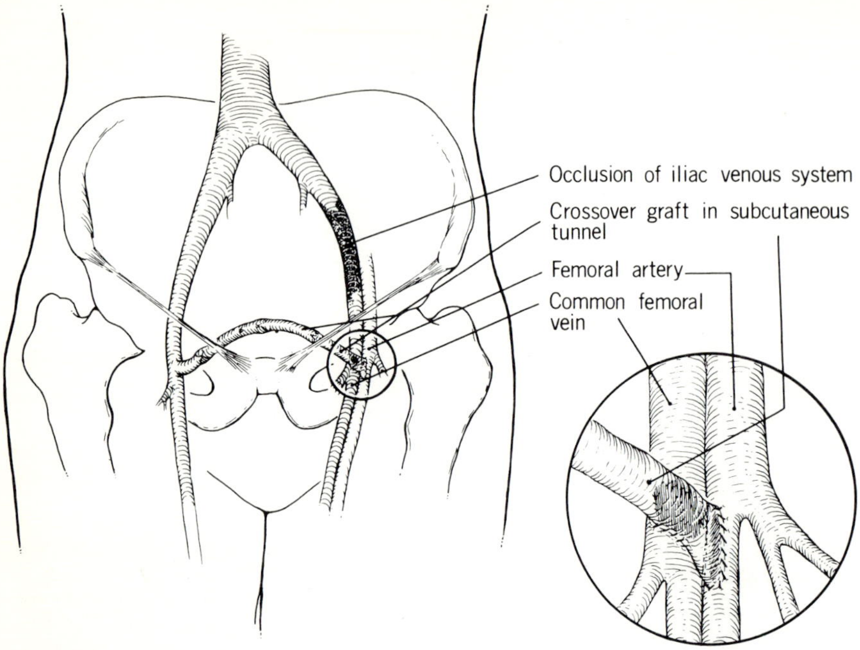

FIGURE 61-7. This is an illustration of a femorofemoral venous bypass performed for an occluded *left* iliac vein. An optional arteriovenous fistula has been depicted in the circular inset. A nonabsorbable suture is usually left around the fistula to facilitate better interruption of the fistula.

as favorable as those obtained from a crossover femorofemoral graft. Gruss (33) has reported that out of 12 patients only 5 have obtained significant symptomatic relief.

The selection of patients for bypass surgery merits careful attention. Most patients with venous stasis disease suffer from valvular incompetence. A minority are burdened with a high resistance to venous return because of a paucity of collateral pathways. Differentiating incompetence from obstruction is difficult. A history of venous claudication coupled with an abnormal IPG exam strongly suggests an obstructive etiology. This select group contains ideal candidates for the above described venous bypasses.

Key Points in Surgical Judgment

1. Establish underlying pathophysiology by the following mechanisms: (a) Doppler, (b) IPG, (c) PPG, (d) venography.

2. Establish nonsurgical treatment of leg elevation and elastic compression.

3. Should conservative measures fail, choose a surgical procedure seeking to improve aberrant venous dynamics (insufficiency or obstruction).

4. Monitor patients hemodynamically postoperatively so as to correctly gauge success.

References

1. Major RH: *A History of Medicine*, vol 1. Oxford, Blackwell, 1954.
2. Anning ST: The historical aspects. In Dodd H, Cockett FB (eds): *Surgery of the Veins of the Lower Limb*. New York, Churchill Livingstone, 1976.
3. Foote RR: *Varicose Veins*, ed 2. St. Louis, Butterworth, 1954.
4. Mayo CH: The surgical treatment of varicose veins. St Paul Med J 1904, 6:695.
5. Homans J: The etiology and treatment of varicose ulcers of the leg. Surg Gynecol Obstet 1917, 24:300.
6. Linton RR, Hardy FB: Post-thrombotic syndrome of the lower extremity—treatment by interruption of the superficial femoral veins and ligation and stripping of the long and short saphenous veins. Surgery 1948, 24:452.
7. Cockett FB: The pathology and treatment of venous ulcers of the leg. Br J Plast Surg 1955, 43:260.
8. Linton RR: The post-thrombotic ulceration of the lower extremity: Its etiology and surgical treatment. Ann Surg 1953, 138:415.
9. Psathakis N: Has the ''substitute valve'' at the popliteal vein solved the problem of venous insufficiency of the lower extremity? J Cardiovasc Surg 1968, 9:64.
10. Kistner RL: Surgical repair of the incompetent femoral vein valve. Arch Surg 1975, 110:1336–1342.
11. Queral LA, Whitehouse WM, Flinn WR, Nieman HL, Yao JST, Bergan JJ: Surgical correction of chronic deep venous insufficiency by valvular transposition. Surgery 1980, 87:688–695.
12. Johnson JD, Queral LA, Flinn WR, Yao JST, Bergan JJ: Late objective assessment of venous valve surgery. Arch Surg 1981, 116:1461–1466.
13. Taheri SA, Heffner R, Meenaghan MA, Budd T, Albian B, Elias SM, Pollack LH, Pendergast DR, Shores RM: Technique and results of venous valve transplantation. In Bergan JJ, Yao JST (eds): *Surgery of the Veins*, New York, Grune & Stratton, 1985.
14. Palma EC, Esperon R: Vein transplants and grafts in the surgical treatment of the post-phlebitic syndrome. J Cardiovasc Surg 1960, 1:94–107.
15. Halliday P, Harris J, May J: Femoro-femoral crossover grafts (Palma

operation): A long term follow-up study. In Bergan JJ, Yao JST (eds): *Surgery of the Veins*. New York, Grune & Stratton, 1985.

16. Husni EA: In situ saphenopopliteal bypass graft for incompetence of the femoral and popliteal veins. Surg Gynecol Obstet 1970, 130:279.
17. Strandness DE: Applied venous physiology in normal subjects and venous insufficiency. In Bergan JJ, Yao JST (eds): *Venous Problems*. Chicago, Yearbook Medical Publishers, 1978.
18. Barnes RW, Russell HE, Wilson MR: *Doppler Ultrasonic Evaluation of Venous Disease, A Programmed Audiovisual Instruction*, ed 2. Iowa City, University of Iowa, 1975.
19. Wheeler HB, Patwardham NA: Evaluation of venous thrombosis by impedance plethysmography. In Madden J, Hume M (eds): *Venous Thromboembolism: Prevention and Treatment*. New York, Appleton-Century-Crofts, 1976.
20. Pearce WH, Ricco JB, Queral LA, Flinn WR, Yao JST: Hemodynamic Assessment of Venous Problems. Surgery 1983, 93:715–721.
21. Abramowitz HB, Queral LA, Flinn WR, Nova PF, Peterson LK, Bergan JJ, Yao JST: The use of photoplethysmography in the assessment of venous insufficiency: A comparison to venous pressure measurements. Surgery 1979, 86:434–441.
22. Linhardt GE, Queral LA, Dagher FJ: Noninvasive evaluation of venous insufficiency: Photoplethysmography vs. strain gauge plethysmography. Curr Surg 1982, 39:319–322.
23. Fegan WG: Treatment of varicose veins by injection as practiced in Dublin. In Hobbs JT (ed): *Treatment of Venous Disorders of the Lower Limb*. Lancaster, MTP Press, 1978.
24. Hobbs JT: The treatment of varicose veins by sclerotherapy. In Rutherford RB (ed): *Vascular Surgery*, ed 2. Philadelphia, Saunders, 1984.
25. Coon WW, Willis PW III, Keller JB: Venous thromboembolism and other venous disease in the Tecumseh Community Health Study. Circulation 1973, 48:839.
26. Ludbrook J: Aspects of Venous Function in the Lower Limbs. Springfield, Illinois, Charles C Thomas, 1966.
27. Larson RH, Lofgren EP, Meyers TT, Lofgren KA: Long-term results after vein surgery: Study of 1,000 cases after 10 years. Mayo Clin Proc 1974, 49:114.
28. Negus D: Perforating vein interruption in the post-phlebitic syndrome. In Bergan JJ, Yao JST (eds): *Surgery of the Veins*. New York, Grune & Stratton, 1985.
29. Browse NL, Burnard KG: The causes of venous ulceration. Lancet 1982, 2:243–245.
30. Kistner RL: Surgical repair of the incompetent femoral vein valve. Arch Surgery 1975, 110:1336–1342.
31. Raju S: Venous insufficiency of the lower limb and stasis ulceration: Changing concepts and management. Ann Surg 1983, 197:688–697.
32. Dale WA: Crossover vein grafts for relief of iliofemoral venous block. Surgery 1965, 57:608–612.
33. Gruss JD: Der Hentige Stand der rekonstructiven. Venenchirurgie Schwerpunktmed 1983, 6:31.

Chapter 62

PORTAL VENOUS HYPERTENSION

MARSHALL J. ORLOFF

Portal hypertension is the complication of liver disease that most frequently requires surgical treatment. In normal subjects at rest, portal pressures range from 60 to 140 mm saline (4 to 10 mmHg), while inferior vena caval pressures range from 7 to 55 mm saline (0.5 to 4 mmHg). Clinically meaningful portal hypertension may be defined as a pressure in the portal vein that is 200 mm saline or greater, when the pressure in the inferior vena cava is normal. Stated in other terms, clinically meaningful portal hypertension exists when the difference between portal and inferior vena caval pressure (called the *corrected* portal pressure) exceeds 150 mm saline (11 mmHg) (1). More important, portal hypertension may be defined in terms of the pathologic disturbances it produces that compromise health and threaten life. Some of these disorders, such as bleeding esophageal varices and hypersplenism, are a direct reflection of the high pressure in the portal circulation and its collateral communications. Others, such as ascites, hepatic coma, peptic ulcers, and renal failure, are complicated manifestations of a number of factors including the portal hypertension, the underlying liver disease, and the required treatment.

Etiology of Portal Hypertension

The causes of portal hypertension are shown in Table 62-1. Except for the rare splanchnic arteriovenous fistulas, obstruction to portal blood flow is the mechanism by which all of the conditions produce portal hypertension. The various diseases may be divided into two categories: those that originate in the blood vessels outside the liver and those within the liver.

TABLE 62-1. Causes of Portal Hypertension

Extrahepatic Disease
Portal Vein Obstruction
1. Thrombosis due to infection or trauma
2. Cavernomatous transformation
3. Congenital atresia or stenosis
4. Extrinsic compression
Hepatic Vein (Outflow) Obstruction
1. Budd-Chiari syndrome
2. Constrictive pericarditis
Excessive Portal Blood Flow
1. Arteriovenous fistula between hepatic artery and portal vein
2. Arteriovenous fistula between splenic artery and vein
Intrahepatic Obstructive Disease
1. Alcoholic cirrhosis
2. Posthepatic cirrhosis
3. Biliary cirrhosis (primary and secondary)
4. Toxic (chemical or drug) cirrhosis
5. Metabolic (genetic) cirrhosis (hemochromatosis)
6. Nutritional cirrhosis (after intestinal bypass)
7. Other forms of cirrhosis (cryptogenic, congestive, etc.)
8. Alcoholic hepatitis
9. Neoplasms and granulomas
10. Schistosomiasis
11. Venoocclusive disease
12. Congenital hepatic fibrosis
13. Hepatoportal sclerosis

Extrahepatic obstruction of the portal vein is responsible for less than 5 percent of cases of portal hypertension. It is most often caused by thromobsis. Neonatal omphalitis is a relatively frequent cause of portal vein thrombosis, but often the event responsible for thrombosis cannot be determined. Cavernomatous transformation is the end result of thrombosis, and recanalization of the portal vein. Congenital atresia of the portal vein and extrinsic compression are rare causes of portal hypertension. Extrahepatic portal hypertension usually develops in childhood or early adult life. Furthermore, the patients usually do not have liver damage, are otherwise in good health, and usually tolerate both the complications of their circulatory disorder and the required surgical therapy quite well.

Extrahepatic obstruction of the hepatic venous outflow system occurs in a group of uncommon conditions called the Budd-Chiari syndrome. The obstruction is usually due to inflammatory or neoplastic thrombosis or fibrosis of the hepatic veins and, sometimes, of the adjacent inferior vena cava. The etiology of the process is often obscure, although some cases are associated with the use of oral contraceptives, polycythemia vera, and neoplasms. Marked hepatomegaly and massive ascites are the most striking clinical findings. When the occlusion is confined to the hepatic veins, the condition has been relieved consistently by construction of a side-to-side portacaval shunt.

Intrahepatic obstructive diseases account for more than 95 percent of cases of portal hypertension. Of these, cirrhosis associated with chronic alcoholism is by far the most common cause in the United States. Cirrhosis due to viral hepatitis is a fairly common cause of portal hypertension, whereas the incidence of biliary cirrhosis due to extrahepatic bile duct obstruction or primary intrahepatic disease is low. The other forms of intrahepatic obstruction are uncommon in the United States. Because cirrhosis is largely a disease of adulthood and, particularly with alcoholic cirrhosis, because it develops slowly over many

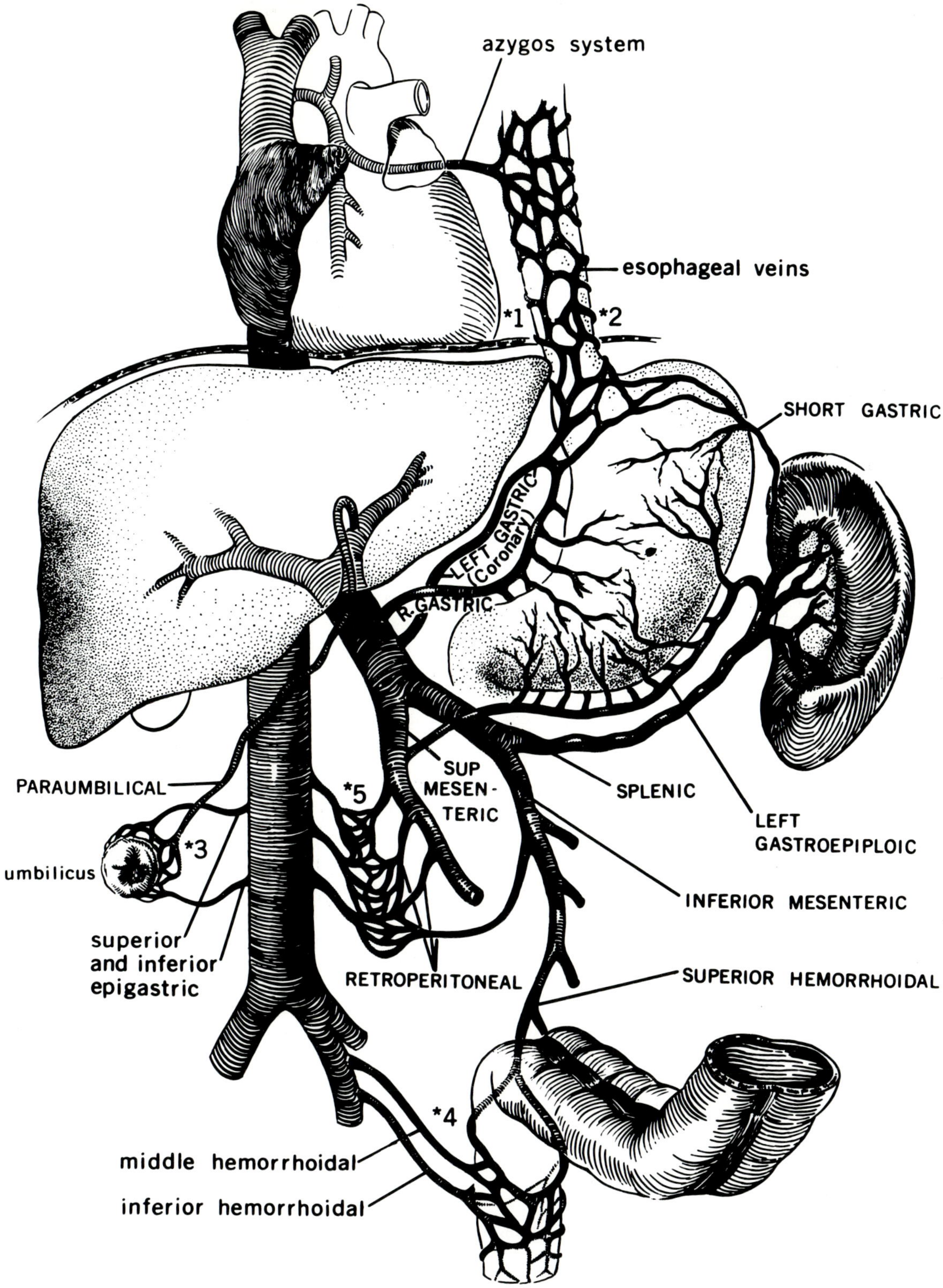

FIGURE 62-1. Sites of portal-systemic anastomoses, labeled *1 to *5 [From Orloff MJ: The liver. In Sabiston DC (ed): *Davis-Christopher Textbook of Surgery*, ed. 12. Philadelphia, Saunders, 1981.]

years, patients with portal hypertension of the intrahepatic type are most often in the fifth or sixth decade of life. Moreover, they are usually in poor health because of the underlying liver disease, and the risk of operative treatment is significant.

The etiologic agents that cause cirrhosis of the liver produce widespread destruction of the hepatic parenchyma, which leads to an overgrowth of fibrous tissue and the formation of regenerative nodules in a pathologic rearrangement of liver architec-

TABLE 62-2. Results of Two Studies of the Survival Rates of Patients Admitted to General Hospitals because of Cirrhosis

Authors (Ref.)	Sources of Cases and Years	No. of Cases	Manifestations of Cirrhosis	Survival, %		
				1 Year	2 Years	5 Years
Ratnoff, Patek (5)	Five New York hospitals (1916–1938)	296	Ascites	32	17	7
		245	Jaundice	26	23	5
		106	Hematemesis	28	25	20
Boston Interhospital Liver Group (6)	Seven Boston hospitals (1959–1961)	467	Varices	34	21	5.5
		288	Varices without bleeding	43	25	8
		179	Varices with bleeding	21	14	1.5

ture (2). As a result, the hepatic blood vessels are compressed and distorted. Because of their low pressure and thin protective coat of connective tissue, the branches of the hepatic vein are affected more than the other components of the vasculature, and hepatic venous outflow obstruction develops. Our studies have shown that this postsinusoidal obstruction is the fundamental hemodynamic lesion in the common forms of cirrhosis (3). Outflow obstruction leads to an increase in sinusoidal pressure, which, in turn, is reflected in an elevation of portal pressure and a decrease in portal blood flow to the liver. In extreme stages of postsinusoidal obstruction, the valveless portal vein may become an outflow tract and conduct blood in a retrograde manner away from the liver, leaving the heptic artery alone to nourish the parenchyma. An additional consequence of the disruption of hepatic integrity is the development of communications between the intrahepatic branches of the hepatic artery and portal vein, and between the tributaries of the portal vein and hepatic vein. The arteriovenous shunts contribute to the portal hypertension. Moreover, both types of shunts divert blood away from the hepatic parenchyma and compromise the nutrition of the liver cells. In an unsuccessful attempt to compensate for the reduction in portal flow to the liver, hepatic artery flow increases and the liver becomes dependent upon the hepatic artery for a major portion of its blood supply.

The elevated pressure in the portal vein leads to an enlargement of all the collateral venous connections between the portal and systemic circulations, and to the development of varicosities (Figure 62-1). In addition, splenomegaly develops. Blood flow through the collaterals is away from the liver, which further impairs hepatic nutrition. Despite their large size, the portal-systemic anastomoses are insufficient to accommodate the volume flow of portal blood and to overcome portal hypertension. Most prominent among the collaterals are those in the submucosa of the lower esophagus and upper stomach, and those around the umbilicus and anterior abdominal wall. Rupture of the esophageal varices often causes massive hemorrhage and is associated with a high mortality rate.

Currently in the United States cirrhosis of the liver is the sixth leading cause of death and ranks eighth in economic cost among the major illnesses (4). In subjects older than 40 years it is the fourth ranking cause of death. Furthermore, during the past three decades the mortality rate from cirrhosis increased more than that of any of the other common causes of death. Chronic alcoholism, the most frequent cause of cirrhosis, has been estimated to involve 10 million people in the United States. During the past decade there has been an increase of 3 million chronic alcoholics, so that alcoholism is now one of the largest social, economic, and public health problems in our country. The social cost of alcoholism was estimated to amount to 43 billion dollars in the year 1975.

Table 62-2 shows the results of two studies of the survival rates of patients admitted to general hospitals because of cirrhosis. In the classic study of Ratnoff and Patek (5), who examined in retrospect the histories of 386 patients admitted to five New York hospitals between 1916 and 1938, only a third of the patients with ascites were alive after 1 year and only a few survived for 5 years. Survival rates for patients with jaundice and hematemesis were similar. In the more recent prospective study of the Boston Interhospital Liver Group (6), 79 percent of the patients who bled from esophageal varices were dead within 1 year of bleeding, and in the entire group of 467 patients, with and without bleeding, only 26 lived for 5 years. The exact mortality rate from alcoholic cirrhosis in the United States today is difficult to determine because studies of this matter have involved different populations of patients, but there is no question that it is a highly lethal disease. The results of the two studies shown in Table 62-2 indicate that once a patient entered the hospital for treatment of cirrhosis, the chances of living for 1 year were similar to those of a patient with acute lymphocytic leukemia, and the chances of surviving 5 years were about the same as those observed in most untreated cancers.

The causes of death in patients with cirrhosis and varices were tabulated by the Boston Group. Hemorrhage from esophageal varices was responsible for a third of the deaths, hepatic failure accounted for a third, renal shutdown for 11 percent, infection for 9 percent and miscellaneous causes for the remainder. These figures, which are similar to those obtained in other studies, clearly show that varix bleeding is a major cause of death in cirrhosis. This complication in particular has occupied the attention of surgeons and is the major indication for surgical therapy.

Emergency Treatment of Bleeding Esophageal Varices Due to Cirrhosis

The most frequent cause of death from upper gastrointestinal bleeding is rupture of an esophageal varix with hemorrhage. Until recently, approximately three out of four cirrhotic patients who entered the hospital with their first episode of bleeding varices failed to leave the hospital alive. Table 62-3, which shows the results of a number of studies conducted during the past 40 years, indicates that as of 1962 the immediate mortality rate of the first variceal hemorrhage averaged 73 percent (7–13).

TABLE 62-3. Mortality Rate of First Episode of Bleeding from Esophageal Varices in Patients with Cirrhosis

Authors (Ref.)	Year Reported	Type of Hospital	No. of Patients	Mortality Rate, %
Ratnoff, Patek (5)	1942	Five private-teaching	106	40
Higgins (9)	1947	City indigent	45	76
Atik, Simeone (7)	1954	City indigent	59	83
Nachlas, O'Neal, Campbell (11)	1955	City indigent	102	59
Cohn, Blaisdell (8)	1958	City indigent	456	74
Taylor, Jontz (12)	1959	Veterans	102	45
Merigan, Hollister, Gryska, Starkey, Davidson (10)	1960	City indigent	74	76
Orloff (13)	1962	City indigent	87	84
		Total	1031	Mean 73

From these statistics, it is apparent that the emergency treatment of bleeding esophageal varices is the single most important aspect of the therapy of portal hypertension.

The precipitating cause of rupture of esophageal varices is uncertain. It has been proposed that erosion of the mucosa by reflux acid–peptic esophagitis is involved. However, in a gross and microscopic study of the distal esophagus in 20 patients at the time of bleeding, we found esophagitis in only one patient (14). Moreover, bleeding from esophageal varices has been reported in patients with proven gastric achlorhydria. The evidence strongly suggests that increased hydrostatic pressure is responsible for "blowout" rupture of esophageal varices (14,15). It is important to point out that finding esophageal varices in a patient with cirrhosis does not mean that the patient will develop bleeding. In fact, only 25 to 35 percent of patients with proven varices ultimately bleed from the varices (6). However, once bleeding has occurred, the patient is almost certain to bleed again, usually within a year of the first bleeding episode. The prognosis and therapeutic implications of esophageal varices depend on whether or not bleeding has occurred.

EMERGENCY DIAGNOSIS

In most patients who enter the hospital with upper gastrointestinal hemorrhage, the diagnosis of bleeding esophageal varices depends on affirmative answers to three questions. Does the patient have cirrhosis? Does the patient have portal hypertension and esophageal varices? Are the varices the site of the bleeding, rather than some other lesions such as a duodenal or gastric ulcer, gastritis, or hiatus hernia? Information sufficient to answer these questions usually can be obtained within a few hours of the patient's admission to the hospital by means of an organized diagnostic plan that includes some or all of the following steps:

1. *History and Physical Examination.* A history of chronic alcoholism, hepatitis, jaundice, previous bleeding episodes, melena, abdominal swelling, edema, and mental abnormalities, and the absence of symptoms of peptic ulcer suggests the diagnosis of cirrhosis. The most important physical findings are hepatosplenomegaly, spider angiomas, palmar erythema, collateral abdominal veins, muscle wasting, jaundice, ascites, edema, and neurologic signs such as tremor and asterixis. In many patients, not all of these classic signs are present. Confirmation of gastrointestinal bleeding by aspiration of the stomach through a nasogastric tube and by gross and chemical examination of the stool is an essential early measure and should really be considered part of the physical examination. A nasogastric tube should be inserted in all patients.

2. *Blood Studies.* Blood samples for typing and cross matching and for studies are drawn immediately on hospital admission. Initial studies include a complete blood count; liver function tests [sodium sulfobromophthalin (Bromsulphalein) (BSP) or indocyanine green excretion (ICG), prothrombin, bilirubin, alkaline phosphatase, albumin, globulin, glutamic-oxaloacetic transaminase, glutamic-pyruvic transaminase]; and determinations of urea nitrogen, electrolytes, pH, arterial blood gases, and blood alcohol. The liver tests that are most consistently abnormal and of greatest value are the BSP or ICG excretion, if performed in the absence of marked jaundice and after hypovolemic shock has been corrected. The prothrombin and serum bilirubin measurements also are often abnormal. It is not unusual for the other liver function tests to be normal in the presence of advanced cirrhosis.

3. *Esophagogastroduodenoscopy.* With the development of the flexible fiberoptic esophagogastroscope, endoscopy has become a well-tolerated, relatively simple procedure that can be performed rapidly at the bedside in the emergency room. It is the best diagnostic measure for demonstrating varices in the esophagus or stomach and for determining with certainty the presence or absence of gastritis and of the uncommon Mallory-Weiss syndrome. In combination with confirmatory roentgenographic studies, it makes possible the diagnosis of esophageal varices with a high degree of confidence (16).

4. *Upper Gastrointestinal X-Rays.* As soon as shock is corrected and the patient's condition stabilized, it is our practice to perform a barium contrast upper gastrointestinal series. Roentgenographic studies are directed at determining the presence or absence not only of esophageal varices, but also of other lesions such as a duodenal ulcer, gastric ulcer, or hiatus hernia. The literature contains many statements which suggest that esophageal varices are demonstrated in only 50 to 60 percent of patients who have them. Our experience indicates that a skillful and interested radiologist can accurately demonstrate varices at the time of bleeding in more than 90 percent of cirrhotic patients (Figure 62-2).

5. *Hepatic Vein Catheterization.* This simple procedure, which has become a routine diagnostic measure in our institution, is used to determine wedged hepatic venous pressure, free hepatic venous pressure, and inferior vena caval pressure. He-

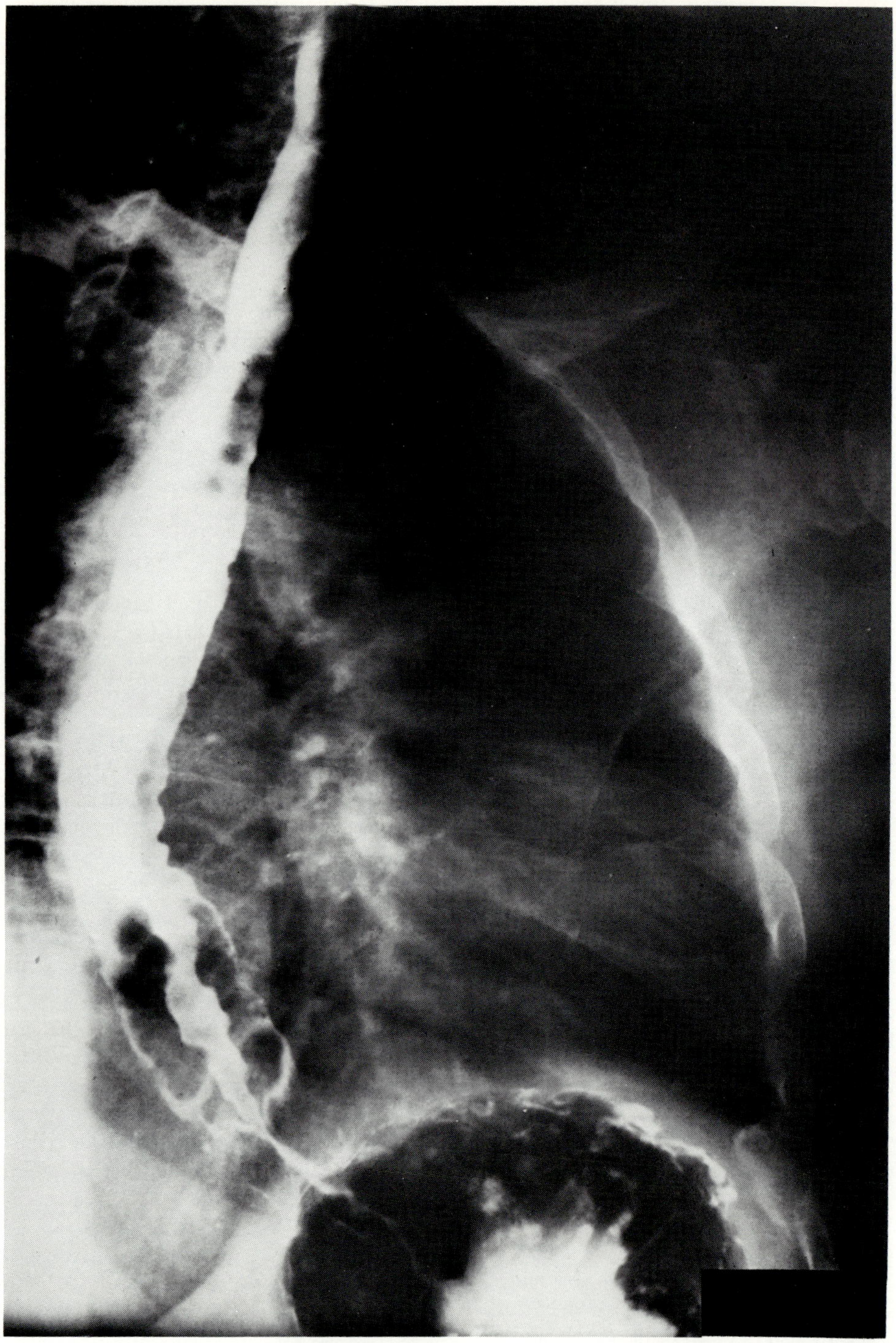

FIGURE 62-2. Barium contrast upper gastrointestinal reoentgenogram showing large esophageal varices. [From Orloff MJ: The liver. In Sabiston DC (ed): *Davis-Christopher Textbook of Surgery,* ed. 12. Philadelphia, Saunders, 1981.]

patic venography is usually added to the studies, although it is not essential and does not yield information that is as important as that obtained from the pressure measurements. The main purpose of venography is to determine the direction of flow in the portal vein. Wedged hepatic venous pressure (WHVP) accurately reflects portal pressure in the common forms of cirrhosis and establishes the diagnosis of portal hypertension with certainty.

The emergency diagnosis of bleeding esophageal varices has been made accurately from information obtained in these first five steps in more than 99 percent of our patients (13,17). It has been regularly possible to complete these diagnostic measures within 5 hours of the patient's admission to the emergency room.

6. *Splenoportography and Splenic Manometry.* Visualization of the portal venous system is not usually required for emergency diagnosis of varix hemorrhage in patients with cir-

rhosis. In the few patients with normal liver function in whom extrahepatic portal obstruction is suspected, splenoportography provides crucial information about the site of obstruction and patency of the portal venous system. Some years ago we regularly performed splenoportography as part of the emergency diagnostic workup in all patients. However, we discontinued use of the procedure in most patients with cirrhosis because it failed to yield information not provided by other, less invasive diagnostic tests. Splenic manometry is usually combined with splenoportography and offers an alternative to hepatic vein catheterization. If desired, the splenic pulp pressure can be determined readily at the bedside by percutaneous puncture of the spleen under local anesthesia. Although this procedure does not determine the site of bleeding, it indicates the presence or absence of portal hypertension. Bleeding from esophageal varices infrequently occurs with a splenic pulp pressure below 250 mm saline and rarely occurs with a pressure below 200 mm saline.

7. *Splenic, Hepatic, Celiac, Left Gastric, and Superior Mesenteric Arteriography.* Percutaneous selective catheterization and visualization of the splanchnic arteries provide interesting hemodynamic information about the status of the circulation in cirrhosis (18). With proper timing, injection of contrast media into the splenic artery or superior mesenteric artery provides delayed visualization of the portal vein and its collateral connections, a technique known as indirect portography. Arteriography and indirect portography have largely replaced splenoportography as the initial approach to visualization of the portal system because the risk and incidence of complications are somewhat lower. It is particularly useful in patients whose spleen has been removed previously. We have found that selective injection of the left gastric artery frequently produces excellent delayed visualization of esophageal varices. Selective arteriography is not an essential or routine emergency diagnostic procedure in cirrhotic patients with varix hemorrhage. After performing the procedure as a regular part of the emergency diagnostic workup in all patients over a period of 7 years, we discontinued its routine use because it did not provide essential information.

The differential diagnosis of upper gastrointestinal bleeding in 99 percent of cirrhotic patients is confirmed to a consideration of six lesions in addition to ruptured varices. Three of these lesions—hemorrhagic gastritis, duodenal ulcer, and gastric ulcer—are common. The other three lesions—gastric cancer, hiatus hernia, and the Mallory-Weiss syndrome—are infrequent causes of bleeding. Each of these conditions produces characteristic symptoms, and each can be ruled in or out by the combination of esophagogastroduodenoscopy and barium contrast upper gastrointestinal x-rays. Bleeding in cirrhotic patients originates from lesions other than esophageal varices in 20 to 25 percent of cases. While this statistic should serve to alert the clinician to a spectrum of etiologic considerations, it should not be interpreted as an indication that the diagnosis of varix hemorrhage is particularly complicated or cannot be made with accuracy. In point of fact, once esophageal varices are demonstrated, the chance that another lesion is responsible for the bleeding is not more than 10 percent. Furthermore, if instances of mild bleeding in cirrhotic patients with proven varices are eliminated, gastrointestinal hemorrhage will be found to arise from rupture of the varices in over 95 percent of patients. Thus, demonstration of esophageal varices in a cirrhotic patient with significant upper gastrointestinal bleeding provides overwhelming odds that the varices are the source of the hemorrhage.

GENERAL MEASURES OF EMERGENCY TREATMENT

Cirrhosis of the liver is a severe, debilitating disease with remote manifestations, only one of which is bleeding from esophageal varices. Death after varix rupture is frequently due to hepatic decompensation, renal failure, or infection, rather than to exsanguination. Although control of bleeding is of primary importance, the effectiveness of therapy of the underlying liver disease often determines the outcome. Therefore, there are certain general measures of treatment that apply to all patients, regardless of the specific forms of therapy used to stop the hemorrhage.

1. *Prompt Restoration of Blood Volume.* Vigorous replacement of blood loss with whole blood transfusion is essential. Large-bore intravenous catheters should be inserted in each arm at the start of therapy. Every effort is made to obtain fresh blood less than 12 hours old for administration because of the serious defects in coagulation associated with liver disease as well as those superimposed by multiple transfusions. Bleeding cirrhotic patients usually have thrombocytopenia in addition to abnormalities of the protein blood clotting factors. In addition, recent evidence indicates that the red blood cells of cirrhotic patients are deficient in 2,3-diphosphoglyceric acid, a substance that mediates the dissociation of oxygen from hemoglobin. The use of fresh blood has been recommended to correct the abnormality in oxygen transport. When fresh blood cannot be obtained, an acceptable alternative is the use of a combination of packed red blood cells, fresh-frozen plasma, and platelet transfusions.

2. *Prevention of Hepatic Coma.* Although the nervous disorders associated with liver disease are diverse and poorly understood, the encephalopathy observed in patients with bleeding esophageal varices sometimes appears to be due to the absorption of large quantities of ammonia directly into the systemic circulation through portal-systemic collateral veins. For this reason, measures directed at destroying ammonia-forming bacteria and eliminating all nitrogen from the gastrointestinal tract are initiated promptly. These include removal of blood from the stomach by lavage with iced saline through a nasogastric tube, instillation of cathartics (60 mL magnesium sulfate) and neomycin (4 g) into the stomach, and thorough and repeated cleansing of the colon with enemas containing neomycin (4 g per liter of water). The fear that insertion of a nasogastric tube will perforate the varices is unfounded, and such a tube should be placed at the start of the diagnostic workup. Although ammonia-binding agents, such as sodium glutamate and arginine, and ion exchange resins have been used, we have obtained no evidence that agents of this sort are of value.

3. *Support of the Failing Liver.* Parenterally administered hypertonic glucose solutions containing therapeutic doses of vitamins K, B, and C are included in the initial treatment regimen. Appropriate amounts of electrolytes are added to the parenteral fluids. In general, administration of sodium is avoided because patients with advanced cirrhosis usually have an increase in total body sodium and a tendency to retain salt and water.

4. *Frequent Monitoring of Vital Functions.* The usual techniques are used to determine the magnitude of bleeding and adequacy of blood volume replacement. These include measurements of vital signs; of urine output by way of an indwelling

catheter; of central venous pressure by a polyethylene catheter threaded through an arm cutdown into the superior vena cava; of hematocrit; and of rate of blood loss by continuous suction through a nasogastric tube. Serial measurements of arterial blood pH and blood gases are facilitated by insertion of an indwelling catheter into the radial artery, which also makes possible continuous recordings of blood pressure. Because of the systemic circulatory abnormalities and hyperdynamic state that frequently exist in bleeding cirrhotic patients, we have added serial determinations of cardiac output by the dye dilution technique using indocyanine green to our monitoring regimen, and occasionally we measure the pulmonary artery wedge pressure by percutaneous insertion of a Swan-Ganz pulmonary artery catheter.

5. *Correction of Hypokalemia and Metabolic Alkalosis.* Most of the more than 1000 bleeding cirrhotic patients that we have studied have had significant hypokalemia and metabolic alkalosis preoperatively (19). The deleterious effects of hypokalemia are well known. In addition, alkalosis has a number of harmful consequences that include (a) interference with the release of oxygen to the tissues by shifting the oxyhemoglobin dissociation curve to the left; (b) in combination with hypokalemia, precipitation of cardiac arrhythmias, particularly in patients taking digitalis; (c) potentiation of ammonia toxicity by elevating the tissue concentration of ammonia, and increasing the passage of ammonia across the blood-brain barrier; and (d) production of tetany by lowering the level of ionized calcium in extracellular fluid. Correction of hypokalemia and metabolic alkalosis is undertaken soon after admission to the hospital and consists of parenteral administration of large quantities of potassium chloride, supplemented, occasionally, by infusion of an acidifying agent such as arginine hydrochloride or hydrochloric acid. Administration of potassium is usually required for several days in amounts occasionally as high as 500 meq/day.

6. *Treatment of Hyperdynamic Cardiovascular State.* Many studies have shown that patients with cirrhosis and portal hypertension frequently have a hyperdynamic state that consists of a decrease in vascular tone and peripheral resistance, an increase in cardiac output, and an increase in venous oxygen saturation with widespread peripheral arteriovenous shunting and marked pulmonary arteriovenous admixture (20–22). These abnormalities are sometimes intensified by bleeding from esophageal varices or performance of a portacaval shunt, and high-output cardiac failure may develop, particularly in older patients and those with far-advanced liver disease. For this reason we perform serial measurements of cardiac output in all patients both preoperatively and postoperatively. Patients with a hyperdynamic state and a cardiac output of 6 L/min or higher are digitalized over a 48-hour period, beginning preoperatively, before any signs of cardiac failure develop. Vigorous correction of hypovolemia is undertaken simultaneously. Once blood volume is restored, fluids are restricted to avoid circulatory overload, and diuretics are used if there are any signs of overhydration. Positive inotropic drugs are used when appropriate.

SPECIFIC EMERGENCY MEDICAL THERAPY

Emergency medical treatment used specifically to stop varix bleeding includes esophageal balloon tamponade, systemic intravenous administration of vasopressin (posterior pituitary extract), selective mesenteric intraarterial administration of vasopressin, endoscopic sclerotherapy, and percutaneous transhepatic obliteration of varices. Although each of these measures is capable of temporarily controlling bleeding varices, there is no solid evidence that they have significantly influenced the mortality rate of varix hemorrhage in cirrhotic patients.

Esophageal Balloon Tamponade

The most widely used nonoperative measure of therapy has been esophageal balloon tamponade. As shown in Table 62-4, balloon

TABLE 62-4. Results of Esophageal Balloon Tamponade in Cirrhotic Patients with Bleeding Varices

Authors (Ref.)	Year Reported	Type of Study	No. of Patients	Initial Control, %	Ultimate Control, %	Mortality Rate, %
Ludington (23)	1958	Retrospective selective	58	75	43	—
Conn (24)	1958	Retrospective selective	50	70	—	82
Read et al. (25)	1960	Retrospective selective	38	84	24	74
Orloff et al. (26)	1962	Prospective unselective	45	56	20	82
Villanueva, Magnenat (27)	1964	Retrospective selective	64	64	—	69
Hermann, Traul (28)	1970	Retrospective selective	75	87	60	64
Pitcher (29)	1971	Prospective selective	50	92	82	36
Johansen, Baden (30)	1973	Retrospective selective	91	88	45	—
Novis et al. (31)	1976	Retrospective selective	42	85	46	60
Teres et al. (32)	1978	Prospective selective	79	86	38	26
			Total 592	Mean 76	Mean 46	Mean 59

TABLE 62-5. **Results of Systemic Intravenous Vasopressin Therapy in Cirrhotic Patients with Bleeding Varices**

Authors (Ref.)	Mode of Administration	No. of Patients	No. of Trials	Initial Control, %	Ultimate Control, %	Mortality Rate, %
Schwartz et al. (34)	Bolus	11	27	89	Infrequent	—
Merigan et al. (35)	Bolus	15	22	73	Infrequent	93
Shaldon, Sherlock (36)	Bolus	8	25	100	37	75
Johnson et al. (37)	Continuous infusion	11	11	64	64	45
Chojkier et al. (38)	Continuous infusion	10	10	50	30	70
Orloff (39)	Bolus	180	180	95	Immediate operation	42
		84	84	95	Immediate operation	17
		38	38	87	18	—

tamponade undoubtedly stops varix bleeding initially in a large percentage of the patients in whom it is used (23–32). However, the results have been discouraging because many of the patients have resumed bleeding when the balloons were deflated. Moreover, we and others have observed frequent and sometimes lethal complications of balloon tamponade, which include perforation of the esophagus, asphyxiation from regurgitation of the balloon into the pharynx, and aspiration pneumonia (24,26,33). The ultimate mortality rate of cirrhotic patients treated by balloon tamponade is difficult to determine because most reports have failed to include such information; moreover, almost all reports have been based on retrospective reviews of the medical records of highly selected patients. Nevertheless, no data indicate that balloon tamponade has measurably influenced the mortality rate of bleeding esophageal varices during a trial of 35 years. For these reasons, we have abandoned the use of balloon tamponade as a definitive form of treatment and use it only on infrequent occasions as a temporary measure to prepare patients for operation when massive bleeding cannot initially be controlled by other means.

Systemic Intravenous Vasopressin

In both experimental animals and humans, vasopressin (posterior pituitary extract) reduces portal pressure and blood flow by constricting the splanchnic arterioles. The response is directly related to the dose and rapidity of injection, and in the usual clinical dosage range has a duration of 1 hour or less. However, as shown in Table 62-5, the transient reduction of portal pressure is sufficient to stop varix hemorrhage temporarily in a large percentage of patients (34–39). Unfortunately, most of the patients bleed again unless operation is performed within 8 hours of treatment, and subsequent administration of the drug is much less effective in stopping bleeding. Recently, continuous rather than bolus intravenous infusion of vasopressin in low doses has been tried in an attempt to lengthen the period of hemostasis. It is apparent, however, that vasopressin alone is not a definitive form of treatment but may be of considerable immediate value while other measures are being readied or the patient is being prepared for operation. Every patient with bleeding esophageal varices is given vasopressin soon after admission to our institution. The agent is administered intravenously over a 15- to 20-minute period in a dose of 20 units of posterior pituitary extract (Pituitrin) diluted in 200 mL of solution. We have not observed any cardiac abnormalities from a single-dose bolus infusion of posterior pituitary extract, but prolonged infusion may be hazardous in patients with coronary artery disease. Recent studies have shown that adding nitroprusside (40) or nitroglycerin (41) to the administration of vasopressin reduces the deleterious cardiac effects of vasopressin while maintaining the beneficial reduction of portal pressure. Posterior pituitary extract is as effective in controlling bleeding as pure vasopressin. This measure of therapy has largely replaced esophageal balloon tamponade as our means of obtaining immediate control of hemorrhage.

Selective Mesenteric Intraarterial Vasopressin

Continuous infusion of vasopressin into an indwelling catheter inserted in the superior mesenteric artery was introduced by Nusbaum et al. (42) in 1967 to control bleeding esophageal varices. Since that time, the technique has been widely used and rather uncritically accepted. The objective of the method is to obtain prolonged effects of vasopressin on the splanchnic circulation without systemic hemodynamic effects. However, a number of recent studies have shown that continuous selective mesenteric intraarterial infusion of vasopressin often is accompanied by a decrease in cardiac output, a fall in femoral arterial P_{O_2}, and a rise in arterial blood pressure, so that the systemic effects of the drug clearly are not avoided (43,44). Moreover, portal venous P_{O_2} regularly falls during infusion, an undesirable side effect. Table 62-6 shows results of this form of therapy (38,45–51). Initial control of varix bleeding has been good, but it has not been superior to that obtained with much simpler and less invasive systemic intravenous administration of vasopressin. Most important, in the several prospective controlled clinical trials that have been performed recently, infusion of vasopressin into the superior mesenteric artery has been no more effective than systemic intravenous administration and has been associated with a higher incidence of complications (40,48). Moreover, it was found that mesenteric intraarterial infusion of vasopressin failed to influence the mortality rate from varix hemorrhage when compared with conventional therapy. When the potential and actual complications of indwelling catheterization of the superior mesenteric artery are added to these recent findings, there is little to indicate that the selective intraarterial technique is worthwhile.

TABLE 62-6. Results of Selective Mesenteric Intraarterial Vasopressin Therapy in Cirrhotic Patients with Bleeding Varices

Authors (Ref.)	Year Reported	No. of Patients	Initial Control, $	Ultimate Control, %	Mortality Rate, %
Murray-Lyon et al. (45)	1973	17	65	24	65
Nusbaum et al. (46)	1974	41	98	—	61
Conn et al. (47)	1975	17	71	41	53
Johnson, Widrich (48)	1976	49	69	53	71
Kaufman et al (49)	1977	39	79	59	49
Getzen et al. (50)	1978	23	52	—	74
Chojkier et al. (38)	1979	12	50	33	75
Sherman et al. (51)	1979	28	71	43	48
		Total 226	Mean 73	Mean 47	Mean 61

Endoscopic Sclerotherapy

Injection of sclerosing solutions into or around bleeding esophageal varices through an esophagoscope was first reported in 1939, but the technique was discarded in the 1950s in favor of portal-systemic shunting. In the early 1970s, however, there was a revival of endoscopic sclerotherapy, and, currently, there is widespread interest in this mode of treatment (52–65). Sclerotherapy has been used most often as emergency treatment for bleeding varices, but recently there has been an increasing use of serial sclerotherapy as the sole form of long-term treatment (54,55,58,60–65). Some results of emergency endoscopic sclerotherapy, often followed by long-term serial injection treatment, in patients with liver diseases of various types are presented in Table 62-7.

Uncontrolled, predominantly retrospective evaluations of heterogeneous groups of selected patients indicate that emergency endoscopic sclerotherapy has controlled acute variceal hemorrhage in 71 to 96 percent of patients. Recurrent bleeding has been frequent, however, and the hospital mortality rate has been substantial in patients with the types of liver disease common in the United States. Two randomized controlled trials in selected patients of long-term sclerotherapy aimed at obliterating all esophageal varices have shown a reduction in the frequency of subsequent bleeding episodes, but no improvement in survival compared to conventional medical treatment (54,58,62). To date both the early and long-term results of endoscopic sclerotherapy are significantly inferior to our results of emergency portacaval shunt in patients with cirrhosis (see later, Table 62-11).

Sclerotherapy has been associated with a substantial number of complications, including necrosis and perforation of the esophagus and esophageal stricture. The safety of the procedure is difficult to assess because reported complication rates have varied widely. Complication rates have been higher in prospective studies (e.g., 30, 51, and 63 percent) than in retrospective reviews (10 to 46 percent) At least 10 to 15 percent of patients have had a serious complication of the procedure. Questions about the safety of endoscopic sclerotherapy remain unanswered.

Obviously, randomized clinical trials are needed to determine the efficacy and safety of endoscopic sclerotherapy. The role of this procedure, if any, in the treatment of bleeding varices in patients with cirrhosis remains to be established.

Percutaneous Transhepatic Obliteration of Varices

Recently, some radiologists have attempted to obliterate esophageal varices by percutaneous transhepatic catheterization of the

TABLE 62-7. Emergency Endoscopic Sclerotherapy for Bleeding Varices in Patients with Liver Disease

Authors (Country, Year, Ref.)	Type of Series	No. of Patients (Follow-up)	Rebleeding, %	Early Deaths, %	Total Deaths, %	Complications, %
Johnston, Rodgers (Ireland, 1973; 52)	Retrospective selective	87 (3 mo–15 yr)	Many	40	58	7
Paquet et al (Germany, 1978; 53)	Retrospective selective	200 (6 mo–8 yr)	?	21	41	10
Kjaergaard et al. (Denmark, 1982; 56)	Retrospective selective	61 (1–48 mo)	55	31	65	46
Alwmark et al. (Sweden, 1982; 57)	Prospective unselective	50 (1–36 mo)	?	14	51	?
MacDougall et al. (England, 1982; 58)	Prospective selective	51 (1–44 mo)	43	2	22	51
Goodale et al. (United States, 1982; 59)	Retrospective selective	42 (4–33 mo)	48	19	60 (6 mo)	33
Barsoum et al. (Egypt, 1982; 60)	Prospective selective	50 (1–4 yr)	32	26	30	30
Soehendra et al. (Germany, 1983; 61)	Retrospective selective	120 (6–48 mo)	15	37	58	?
Terblanche et al. (South Africa; 1983, 62)	Prospective selective	38 (1–6 yr)	58	33	62 (5 yr)	63

portal vein and its branches and injection of blood clots, hemostatic polymers, or sclerosing solutions into the coronary vein and the varices (66–73). This method has been used in actively bleeding patients as emergency treatment, and as elective therapy in patients who have recovered from a bleeding episode. Substantial experience with the percutaneous transhepatic technique has accumulated, although many of the results reported in the literature are anecdotal. The incidence of rebleeding has been high, and there has been a substantial number of complications directly related to the procedure. Moreover, the procedure has failed to improve the survival rate of patients with varix hemorrhage. There is little question that the varices, if obliterated, will invariably recur; hence, the potential of this approach lies in the temporary control of active hemorrhage in the expectation of preparing the patient for definitive treatment. While opinion may differ on the likelihood that this techique will succeed, it is important to emphasize that it is an invasive and potentially dangerous measure that should not be widely attempted unless careful trials demonstrate its efficacy. The ultimate and essential test of any new therapeutic modality is its influence on the high mortality rate of the disease.

Oral Propranolol Therapy

Propranolol has not been used in the emergency treatment of bleeding varices. However, chronic oral administration of propranolol to patients with cirrhosis produces a sustained reduction in portal venous pressure, mainly, but perhaps not entirely, by decreasing cardiac output. This observation led Lebrec and his colleagues to conduct a 4-year, randomized clinical trial in which they compared chronic propranolol treatment (38 patients) with placebo (36 patients) in good-risk, ambulatory cirrhotic patients who had recovered from an episode of bleeding from esophageal varices or acute gastric erosions (74,75). The patients were largely in Child's risk class A and did not have jaundice or ascites. In their final report in 1984, Lebrec et al. concluded that propranolol therapy produced a highly significant reduction in the incidence of recurrent bleeding and a significant decrease in mortality rate (75). However, Conn has challenged these conclusions by pointing out that the use of different, and what he considers more appropriate, statistical methods to analyze the data of Lebrec et al. results in no difference in mortality rate between the control and treatment groups (76). Furthermore, in another randomized clinical trial involving 48 cirrhotic patients, Burroughs et al. found no differences in the incidence of rebleeding or the mortality rate between patients treated with propranolol and those given placebo (77).

A number of questions about the efficacy and safety of propranolol therapy of bleeding varices in cirrhotic patients remain to be answered. Will it be effective in patients with advanced and decompensated cirrhosis who make up the bulk of those who bleed from esophageal varices? Will it have an adverse effect on ascites and increase the incidence of encephalopathy? Will the reduction in cardiac output adversely affect hepatic function? What are the side effects of propranolol in patients with liver disease of various types and degrees of severity, and is it a safe drug for lifelong use in such patients? More information must be obtained before conclusions can be drawn about the efficacy of this form of drug therapy.

SPECIFIC NONSHUNTING EMERGENCY SURGICAL THERAPY

During the past 35 years, the widely accepted approach to the treatment of bleeding varices in patients with cirrhosis has involved the use of temporary nonsurgical emergency measures directed at stopping the hemorrhage so as to permit the deliberate and methodical preparation of the patients for an elective portal systemic shunt. This approach has been based on the belief that, on the one hand, it is often possible to stabilize and improve the underlying liver disease and, on the other hand, cirrhotic patients will not tolerate major operations performed under emergency circumstances in the face of hemorrhage. Considerable evidence indicates that this approach has not substantially influenced survival of the bleeding cirrhotic population, since two-thirds to three-fourths of the patients have died during the initial bleeding episode and only 10 to 20 percent have become eligible for elective therapy. Because of the failure of the "conventional" approach, there has been considerable recent interest in emergency surgical management. Experience is insufficient as yet to establish definite criteria for selection of patients for operation. Although it is clear that the risk of operation is great in patients with decompensated cirrhosis, it is also certain that such patients have little chance of surviving with nonoperative therapy. Currently, emergency operative treatment is largely confined to the use of three types of operations: (1) direct suture ligation of the bleeding varices, (2) esophagogastric devascularization procedures, and (3) emergency portal-systemic shunt. All three operations control varix bleeding initially in most patients. However, a major potential problem associated with all emergency operations is hepatic decompensation, which may result when a critically ill patient with a severely damaged liver is subjected to anesthesia and major trauma, in addition to hemorrhage.

Transesophageal Varix Ligation

Although transesophageal ligation (Figure 62-3) of esophageal varices was first described 36 years ago, the reported experience with this procedure has not been large (78–81). The mortality rate has ranged from 15 to 86 percent. The largest reported series has involved 72 selected patients with an operative mortality rate of 50 percent. Because the value of this procedure was not clearly established, some years ago we undertook a prospective comparison of emergency transesophageal varix ligation and medical therapy (82). Every cirrhotic patient admitted to the hospital with varix bleeding was included in the study with no attempt at selection. The diagnostic workup was completed within 6 hours and, in the surgical group, the operation was performed within 8 hours of admission to the hospital. The study was conducted in comparable groups of chronic alcoholics with advanced cirrhosis and massive varix hemorrhage. Approximately one-half the patients in each group had jaundice and ascites, and one-fourth had hepatic encephalopathy. When feasible, the patients who survived emergency surgical or medical therapy were prepared for and underwent an elective portacaval shunt at a later date.

The results of this study are included in the summary presented in Table 62-13. Emergency transesophageal varix ligation consistently controlled bleeding. The early survival rate was 54

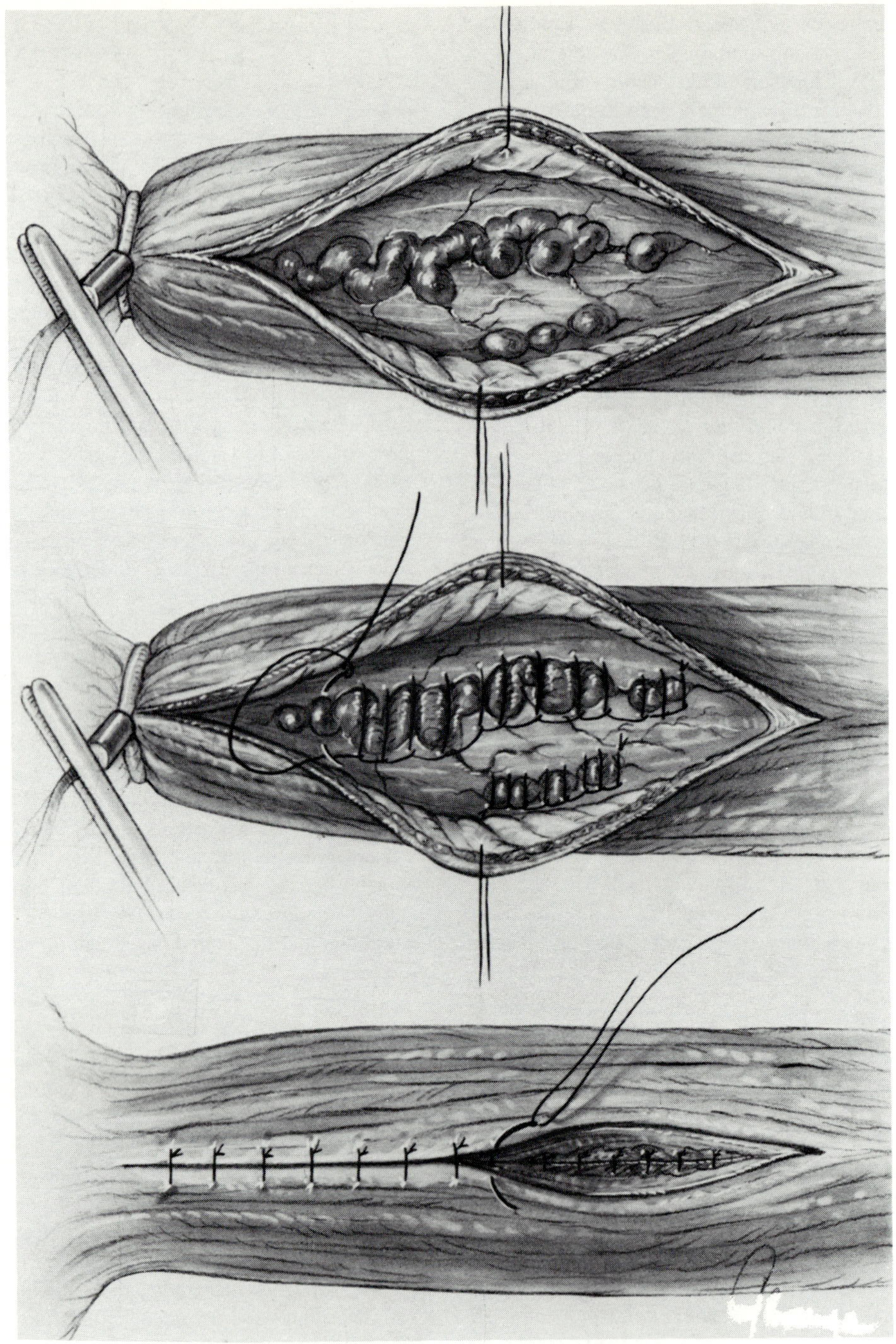

FIGURE 62-3. Technique of transesophageal varix ligation. (Orloff, 82.)

percent following operative ligation compared with 14 percent in the medically treated patients. The 5-year survival rate was 21 percent in the surgical group and 3 percent in the medical group, and the 10-year survival rates were 11 percent and 0, respectively. Our experience showed that varix ligation is not a definitive procedure but rather must be considered the first of two stages in treatment, the second stage of which is an elective portacaval shunt. The refusal of some patients to undergo an elective shunt was invariably associated with rebleeding and played a major role in the declining survival rate. Moreover, in evaluating the long-term results of both varix ligation and medical therapy, the mortality rate from the subsequent elective portacaval shunt must be included.

A major reason for considering transesophageal varix ligation as emergency treatment for bleeding varices is the belief that it is an effective procedure of lesser magnitude than other emergency operations. Our experience has shown that such is not the case. The time required to perform the operation, the magnitude of the trauma, the metabolic response, and the effects on liver function are similar to those associated with emergency porta-

TABLE 62-8. **Results of Esophageal Transection for Bleeding Varices in Patients with Liver Diseases of Various Types**

Authors (Country, Year, Ref.)	No. of Patients (Follow-up)	Timing of Operation	Operative Mortality Rate, %	Total Mortality Rate, %	Rebleeding Rate, %
Johnston (Ireland, 1982; 88)	70 (1–6 yr)	Elective, 51 Emergency, 19	16	36	20
Osborne, Hobbs (England, 1981; 89)	20 (6–20 mo)	Emergency	25	35	33
Kirby et al. (England, 1975; 90)	45 (3–13 yr)	Emergency	27	1 yr, 58 2 yr, 68	33
Pugh et al. (England, 1973; 85)	37 (1–6 yr)	Emergency	57	1 yr, 76 2 yr, 84	57
George et al. (England, 1973; 91)	30 (1 mo–7 yr)	Emergency	53	73	64
Wanamaker et al. (United States, 1983; 92)	20 (10–60 mo)	Elective, 5 Emergency, 15	60	75	40

caval shunt. While varix ligation appears to have distinct advantages over medical therapy, it does not appear to be the best emergency surgical procedure available.

Esophagogastric Devascularization Procedures

Various esophagogastric devascularization procedures have been used as both emergency and elective treatment of bleeding esophageal varices (83–97). Included among these are (1) gastric or esophageal transection and reanastomosis, most recently done with the aid of a stapling gun, which is sometimes combined with splenectomy and extensive ligation of the veins around the distal esophagus and upper stomach; (2) esophagogastrectomy and pyloroplasty with or without interposition of a segment of colon or jejunum, and with or without ligation of collateral veins and splenectomy; (3) splenectomy alone or with coronary vein ligation; and (4) ligation of the hepatic, left gastric, and splenic arteries. By and large, these operations involve transection of the esophagus and/or resection of parts of the lower esophagus and upper stomach and/or extensive ligation of collateral veins that connect with the esophageal varices. The results of the various esophagogastric devascularization procedures are difficult to evaluate because most of the series are small, involve highly selected patients with many types of portal hypertension, and are retrospective in nature. By far the greatest experience with these operations has been in Japan, where surgeons have largely abandoned portal-systemic shunting in favor of esophagogastric devascularization, which they have performed prophylactically, electively, and emergently (83,86,87,95). The Japanese have reported favorable results, but their reports do not lend themselves readily to analysis, and the results have not been verified in other countries. Moreover, in several reports the long-term survival rate of cirrhotic patients has been low. In the United States, esophagogastric devascularization procedures in cirrhotic patients have been associated with substantial mortality rates and a high incidence of recurrent varix bleeding. Table 62-8 shows the results of esophageal transection in patients with various types of liver disease. Table 62-9 shows the results of esophagogastric devascularization used under a variety of circumstances in patients with a wide range of hepatic diseases. The results are

TABLE 62-9. **Retrospective Studies of Esophagogastric Devascularization for Bleeding Varices in Patients with Cirrhosis of Various Types**

Authors (Country, Year, Ref.)	Type of Series	No. of Patients (Follow-up)	Operative Mortality Rate, %	Overall Mortality Rate, %	Rebleeding Rate, %
Koyama et al. (Japan, 1980; 93)	Selective Elective or emergency or prophylactic	68 (1 mo–7 yr)	13	Total, 35 1 yr, 35 5 yr, 62	20
Sugiura et al. (Japan, 1979; 83)	Selective Elective or emergency or prophylactic	196 (1 mo–10 yr)	6	Total, 21	5
Yamamoto et al. (Japan, 1976; 87)	Selective Elective or emergency	64 (2–12 yr)	11	Total, 38 1 yr, 19 5 yr, 35	16
Johnson et al. (United States, 1969; 94)	Selective Elective or emergency	55 (1–17 yr)	45	Total, 71 1 yr, 50 5 yr, 60	50
Umeyama et al. (Japan, 1983; 95)	Selective Elective or emergency	60 (1–13 yrs)	16	5 yr, 57	24
Mir et al. (Spain, 1982; 96)	Selective Elective or emergency	30 (1–6 yr)	57	Total, 63	23
Van Beek et al. (United States, 1984; 97)	Selective Elective or emergency	34 (21–61 mos)	56	Total, 65	27

difficult to analyze because the data have not been adequately categorized.

EMERGENCY PORTACAVAL SHUNT

Author's Prospective Study

Portal-systemic shunt is the only available definitive treatment for portal hypertension and esophageal varices. Numerous studies have shown that a technically satisfactory portacaval shunt will permanently solve the problem of bleeding varices in the vast majority of patients. The obvious potential advantage of performing this procedure under emergency circumstances is that, unlike other forms of treatment, it can be expected to provide both immediate and prolonged control of varix hemorrhage. The question is, can cirrhotic patients tolerate an operation of this magnitude when it is performed as an emergency in the face of bleeding? To answer this question, we have been conducting a prospective study of emergency portacaval shunt, similar to our comparative evaluation of varix ligation and medical therapy (98–105). The study is distinguished from all other reported studies of emergency treatment in that it has involved *every* cirrhotic patient admitted with varix bleeding, regardless of his or her condition on admission. Between 1963 and 1983, 264 consecutive unselected patients underwent emergency portacaval shunt within 8 hours of admission to the emergency room. Follow-up study has been conducted in a special clinic, and the current status of 97 percent of the patients is known.

TABLE 62-10. Emergency Portacaval Shunt in Unselected Patients with Cirrhosis: Characteristics of Early Group (n = 180) and Recent Group (n = 84)

	Early Group, %	Recent Group, %
Pathologic Manifestations		
Hematemesis	98	94
Jaundice on admission	49	48
Ascites on admission	53	42
Encephalopathy on admission	19	18
Severe muscle wasting	30	42
Hyperdynamic cardiovascular state	82	90
Liver dye retention ≥21%	95	92
Varices on endoscopy	98	100
Varices on x-ray	95	97
Cirrhosis on liver biopsy	100	100
Portal hypertension by direct measurement	100	100
Treatment		
Temporary control by IV vasopressin	95	95
Permanent control by portacaval shunt	98	100
Blood transfusions:		
<5000 mL	61	69
5000–7000 mL	16	21
>7000 mL	23	10
Type of shunt:		
Side-to-side	83	74
End-to-side	15	26
Other	2	0
Skin-to-skin operating time:		
<4 hours	45	57
4–5 hours	42	31
>5 hours	13	12
Gradient across shunt <50 mm	86	98

We have divided our 264 unselected patients into two groups: an early group of 180 patients operated upon from 1963 up to 1978, and a recent group of 84 patients operated upon from 1978 through 1983. The characteristics of the two groups were similar and are shown in Table 62-10. Almost all of the patients were chronic alcholics, and all had cirrhosis on liver biopsy. On admission, about half of the patients in each group had jaundice and ascites; 19 percent had frank encephalopathy or coma; 30 and 42 percent, respectively, had severe muscle wasting; and 82 and 90 percent, respectively, had a hyperdynamic state. Systemic intravenous posterior pituitary extract temporarily controlled the varix bleeding in 95 percent of the patients and allowed sufficient time to complete the diagnostic workup. Emergency portacaval shunt promptly and permanently stopped the varix hemorrhage in 98 and 100 percent of the patients, respectively. The requirement for blood transfusion before and during operation for the two groups averaged 5.1 and 3.7 L, respectively. Side-to-side portacaval shunt was performed in 83 and 74 percent of the patients, respectively; end-to-side shunt in 15 and 26 percent; and another type of shunt in three patients in the early group. There was no difference in survival rate between patients with side-to-side anastomosis and those with end-to-side anastomosis. The "skin-to-skin" operating time, which included various measurements of splanchnic pressures and blood flows, averaged 4.1 hours and was less than 5 hours in 87 and 88 percent of each group. All patients had portal hypertension with corrected free portal pressures, obtained by subtracting the inferior vena caval pressure, which averaged 267 mm saline. The portacaval anastomosis reduced the portal pressure to normal in all patients.

Table 62-11 summarizes the long-term results of emergency portacaval shunt. In the early group, 58 percent of the 180 patients survived the operation, and the 5- and 12-year survival rates were 38 and 30 percent, respectively. In contrast, 83 percent of the recent group of 84 patients survived the shunt, and the 5-year survival rate is 72 percent. One-third of the patients in each group had a documented history of encephalopathy before the shunt (105). After the shunt, 31 percent of the early group and 16 percent of the recent group have had encephalopathy at one time or another. The lower incidence in the recent group may be due to the fact that they have not been followed up for as many years as the early group. Severe encephalopathy requiring chronic dietary protein restriction occurred in only 7 percent of the patients. At the time of discharge, 95 percent of patients in the early group and 99 percent of patients in the recent group could tolerate a diet containing 80 g of protein per day.

TABLE 62-11. Emergency Portacaval Shunt in Unselected Patients with Cirrhosis: Results of Long-Term Follow-up of Early Group ($n = 180$) and Recent Group ($n = 84$)

Results	Early Group, %	Recent Group, %
Operative survival (30 days or longer)	58	83
5-year survival	38	72
Actuarial 12-year survival	30	—
Encephalopathy:		
Before shunt	33	36
After shunt	31	16
Patency of shunt by yearly catheterization	99	100
Abstinence from alcohol	48	70
General status after 5 years:		
Excellent or good	62	69
Fair	29	24
Poor	9	7
Liver function after 5 years:		
Improved	44	52
Unchanged	33	35
Worse	22	13

Long-term shunt patency has been demonstrated by yearly angiography in 99 percent of the early patients and 100 percent of the recent patients. The two thrombosed shunts in the early group were of the end-to-side type. Forty-eight percent of the survivors in the early group and 70 percent of the recent group have not consumed alcohol at any time during the follow-up period. Again, the recent group has not been followed up for as long as the early group. After 5 years, the general status of the survivors in the early group and recent group, respectively, is excellent or good in 62 and 69 percent, fair in 29 and 24 percent, and poor in 9 and 7 percent; all but one patient in the poor category have resumed heavy alcohol consumption. Sixty percent of the survivors have been gainfully employed or doing full-time housework during part or all of the follow-up period. Five years after the shunt operation, results of liver function tests showed an improvement over preoperative results in 44 percent of the early group and 52 percent of the recent group; no change in 33 and 35 percent, respectively; and worsening in 22 and 13 percent, respectively.

Beginning with the moment of admission and continuing through the lifelong follow-up visits, detailed data on every patient were recorded on standard forms and entered continuously into a computer analysis program. Since our study involved unselected patients, we carefully analyzed all factors present on admission that might have influenced survival, in the hope of identifying criteria for future selection of patients for operation. Table 62-12 summarizes the preoperative findings obtained from the history, physical examination, and diagnostic workup that were associated with a statistically significant decrease in survival rate in the early group and, therefore, can be considered to be risk factors. Six such risk factors were identified: (1) presence of ascites on admission; (2) serum glutamic oxaloacetic transaminase (SGOT) level of 100 units per deciliter or higher; (3) sodium sulfobromophthalein (BSP) retention greater than 50 percent in 45 minutes; (4) hypokalemic alkalosis with an arterial blood pH of 7.50 or greater and a serum potassium level below 3.5 meq/L; (5) requirement of 5 L or more of blood transfusion before and during operation; and (6) consumption of alcohol within 7 days prior to admission. Because the presence of these risk factors was associated with survival rates of from 36 to 53 percent, they cannot be considered contraindications to emergency shunt. Age; sex; jaundice; encephalopathy; severe muscle wasting; a small liver; a large spleen; a history of delirium tremens; and the blood levels of bilirubin, albumin, and prothrombin did not have a statistically significant influence on survival.

In 17 patients (9 percent of our series), jaundice, ascites, encephalopathy, and severe muscle wasting were present concurrently on admission. All these patients had markedly disturbed liver function, and 9 had an SGOT level above 100 units per deciliter. The operative survival rate of these patients with the most advanced stage of alcoholic cirrhosis was 47 percent, a rate similar to that of patients with ascites alone. However, 1

TABLE 62-12. Preoperative Risk Factors That Significantly Decreased Survival of the Early Group of 180 Unselected Cirrhotic Patients Treated by Emergency Portacaval Shunt

Risk Factors	Percent of Group	Survival, %	Significance, p
Ascites:			
Present	53	46	<0.01
Absent	47	72	
SGOT:			
$\geq$100 units/dL	34	43	<0.01
$<$100 units/dL	66	70	
BSP retention:			
$>$50%	21	36	<0.01
$\leq$50%	79	66	
Hypokalemic alkalosis:			
pH >7.5; K^+ <3.5	29	42	<0.05
pH ≤7.5; K^+ ≥3.5	71	67	
Blood transfusion:			
$\geq$5 L before and during operation	39	41	<0.001
$<$5 L before and during operation	61	70	
Last drank alcohol:			
$\leq$7 days before admission	71	53	<0.05
$>$7 days before admission	29	71	

TABLE 62-13. Comparison of Results of Emergency Portacaval Shunt, Transesophageal Varix Ligation, and Medical Treatment in Unselected Patients with Cirrhosis and Bleeding Varices

			Emergency Shunt	
Clinical Factors and Survival Rates	Medical Treatment*	Varix Ligation*	Early Group	Recent Group
Number of patients	59	28	180	84
Jaundice on admission, %	42	57	49	48
Ascites on admission, %	41	50	53	42
Encephalopathy on admission, %	25	25	19	18
Mean liver index on admission	2.8	2.8	2.4	2.6
Admission hemoglobin 11 g/dL or less, %	70	71	71	74
Varices demonstrated, %	95	100	100	100
Mean volume of blood transfused, L	7.2	4.2	5.0	3.7
Early survival (30 days), %	17	54	58	83
5-year survival, %	3	21	38	72
12-year survival, %	0	11	30	—

*Followed by elective portacaval shunt when possible.

year after operation only 18 percent were still alive, and 5 years postoperatively the survival rate was only 12 percent, so the outlook for these patients is grim under any circumstances. Nevertheless, without portacaval shunt, these preterminal cirrhotics rarely survive beyond 2 years.

Table 62-13 compares the results of the three forms of emergency treatment of bleeding varices that we evaluated prospectively in unselected patients during the past 22 years, and Figure 62-4 compares the cumulative survival curve of the early group of shunted patients with the survival curves resulting from the other two types of emergency therapy. Although these three groups of patients were not studied concurrently, they are similar from every standpoint. Early survival rates produced by the two forms of surgical therapy were substantially greater than that resulting from emergency medical treatment. Five- and twelve-year survival rates, both actual and actuarial, were significantly greater following emergency shunt than after either of the other two types of emergency therapy.

Figure 62-5 compares the cumulative survival curve of the 84 patients in the recent group with that of the 180 patients in the early group. As our experience with emergency portacaval shunt has increased, there has been a striking improvement in results. In unselected patients, all comers included, the operative survival rate has increased from 58 to 83 percent, and the 5-year survival rate has almost doubled from 38 to 72 percent. It should be emphasized that *no* patient who came to us with bleeding varices was excluded from the emergency shunt program. Nonetheless, the 5-year survival rate of emergency shunt in *unselected* patients is now the same as or better than the 5-year survival rate of elective shunt in *highly selected* patients reported by others.

The results of our studies indicate that emergency portacaval

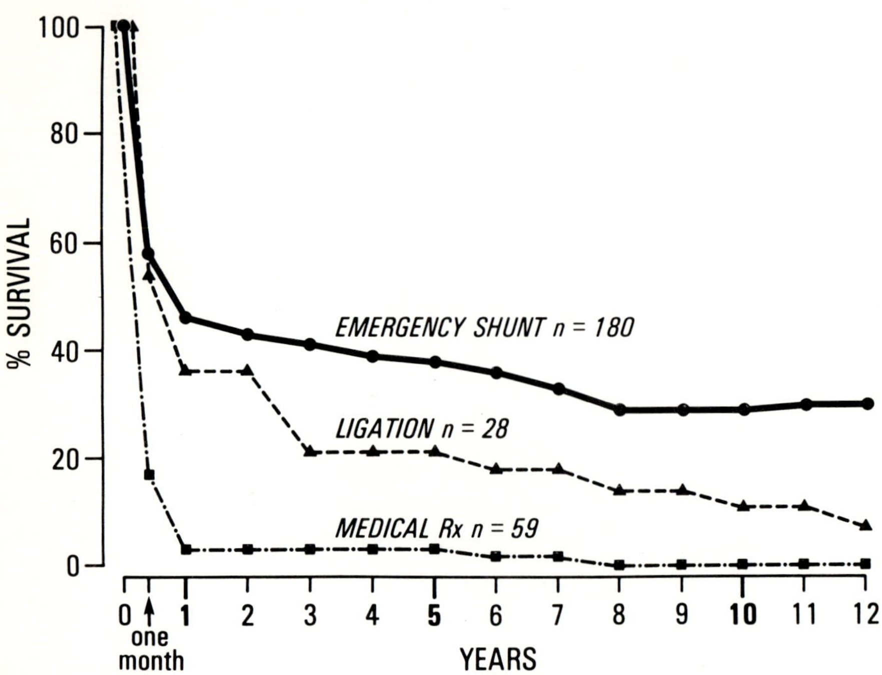

FIGURE 62-4. Cumulative 5-year survival rates of patients with cirrhosis and varix hemorrhage following emergency portacaval shunt (early group), transesophageal varix ligation, and medical treatment.

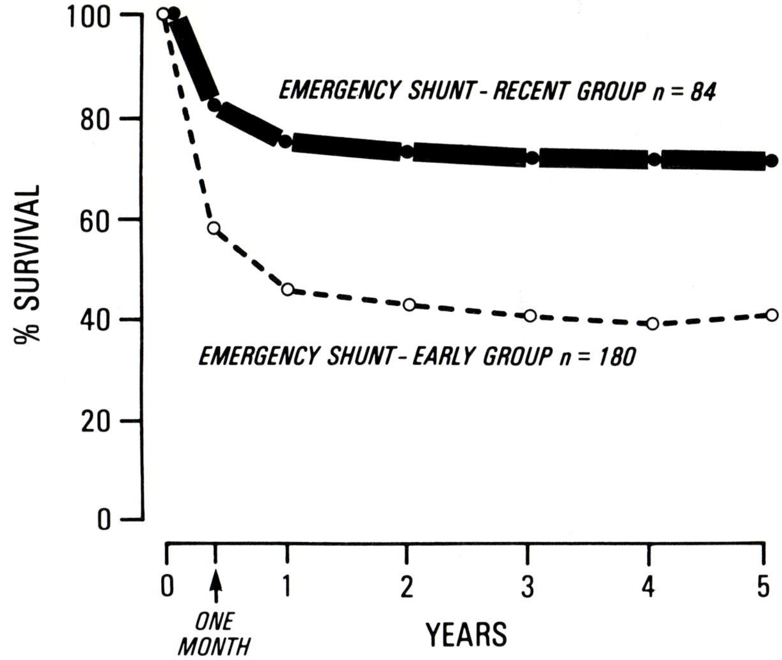

FIGURE 62-5. Cumulative survival rate of 84 unselected patients with cirrhosis who underwent emergency portacaval shunt in the recent group, as compared with the cumulative survival rate of 180 patients in the early group.

shunt has improved both the immediate and long-term survival rates of cirrhotic patients with bleeding esophageal varices. As is true of survival statistics for cancer and other lethal disorders, the absolute survival rate is of limited meaning unless it is viewed in the context of the natural history of the disease. The 5- and 12-year survival rate in our experience to date are many times greater than those associated with emergency medical therapy followed by elective portacaval shunt in the relatively small number of patients who survive. Undoubtedly, some patients with advanced cirrhosis will not survive with any form of therapy currently available. The problem is that criteria for identifying such patients are not yet known. The development of sound criteria for selecting patients for various forms of treatment unquestionably will improve the results of operative management. Until such guidelines are developed by well-controlled, prospective studies, or until alternative effective therapy is devised, emergency portacaval shunt appears to be the therapy of choice for most cirrhotic patients who bleed from esophageal varices.

Postoperative Care following Emergency Portacaval Shunt

Patients with liver disease who bleed from esophageal varices are among the most seriously ill patients in any hospital, regardless of the specific therapy used to control the bleeding. In those who undergo emergency portacaval shunt, the expertness of the postoperative care is a major factor in determining survival. All such patients should be admitted to an intensive care unit with equipment and personnel geared to managing the complicated problems associated with hepatic disease. A description of specific prophylactic and therapeutic aspects of postoperative care follows.

MONITORING. Careful monitoring of vital signs, central venous pressure, urine output, arterial pH, arterial and alveolar gases, fluid balance, body weight, and abdominal girth are essential. Serial electrocardiograms and determinations of cardiac output and peripheral resistance often are very helpful. Measurement of the pulmonary artery wedge pressure with a Swan-Ganz catheter is indicated occasionally but not routinely. Serial measurements of liver function; of the formed elements in the blood, including platelets; of blood coagulation; of serum electrolytes; and of renal function must be done.

PARENTERAL FLUID THERAPY. Patients with cirrhosis are often water-logged even before the onset of bleeding from varices, and they have a markedly impaired capacity to excrete water loads. The bleeding episode and the operation intensify renal sodium and water retention and exaggerate the already existing fluid intolerance. Parenteral fluid therapy should be calculated to maintain such patients on the dry side. Fluid losses are replaced by a solution of 10% dextrose in water containing vitamins B, C, and K. The total volume usually amounts to 1500 to 2000 mL/day, based on daily losses of 500 mL nasogastric aspirate, 500 to 1000 mL urine, 800 to 1000 mL insensible water, and a gain of 250 to 400 mL from endogenous water formation. Sodium is given only to replace nasogastric losses, which rarely exceed 30 to 40 meq/day. Parenteral potassium therapy is started as soon as urine output is adequate and is given in whatever amounts are necessary to maintain the serum potassium concentration between 4 and 5 meq/L. Usually the requirement is 150 to 200 meq/day, but doses as high as 500 meq/day may be necessary. If metabolic alkalosis develops, as is often the case, it usually responds to repletion of potassium with large quantities of parenteral potassium chloride. In addition to crystalloid fluid therapy, it is often necessary to add colloid to replace continuing losses of blood and plasma. Transfusions of fresh blood are given for blood loss or a hematocrit below 30 percent. Type-specific, single-donor plasma, fresh-frozen plasma, or salt-poor concentrated albumin is given for losses of fluid into the operation site and peritoneal cavity (acute ascites), as determined by the combined measurements of abdominal girth, central venous pressure, urine output, body weight, and hematocrit showing hemoconcentration.

Pulmonary Therapy. Pulmonary complications, particularly infection and wet lung, are a major cause of morbidity and mortality in patients with cirrhosis and bleeding varices. In about 2 percent of our cases it has been necessary to maintain the patient on a respirator for several days postoperatively. In such cases, mechanical ventilatory support usually can be provided through an endotracheal tube that may be left indwelling for 48 to 72 hours. Occasionally, it is necessary to perform a tracheostomy for ventilation and tracheobronchial toilet, but it should be recognized that complications of tracheostomy, particularly bleeding, are more frequent in cirrhotic patients than in others. Portable chest x-rays are obtained daily in patients on respirators or those having pulmonary problems. The decision to taper off and then discontinue mechanical ventilatory support is based on measurements of arterial blood and alveolar gases, ventilatory volumes, chest x-rays, and physical findings.

All patients not on a respirator are given continuous oxygen therapy by nasal catheter, nasal prongs, or mask for 5 to 7 days postoperatively because of the frequent cardiovascular abnormalities and arteriovenous shunting that exist in cirrhosis. From the start, all patients receive intensive respiratory therapy that consists of intermittent tracheobronchial aspiration, postural drainage, chest physiotherapy, intermittent positive-pressure respiration, frequent turning, encouragement to cough and breathe deeply, and the use of blow bottles and a humidifier. Diuretics may be of value in the treatment of pulmonary edema due to left heart failure or infection.

Hyperdynamic Cardiovascular State. As mentioned previously, cirrhotic patients regularly have a hyperdynamic cardiovascular state and sometimes develop high output cardiac failure. In fact, 82 percent of our early group of patients who underwent emergency portacaval shunt, and 90 percent of our recent group had a cardiac output of 6 L/min or higher before and/or after operation. All such patients are digitalized over a period of 48 hours, parenteral fluid therapy is restricted to avoid circulatory overload, and inotropic drugs are given if myocardial performance is not satisfactory.

Delirium Tremens. Alcoholic cirrhotic patients frequently have delirium tremens following hemorrhage alone or in combination with a portacaval shunt or other operation. In the absence of bleeding or an operation, delirium tremens by itself is associated with a substantial mortality rate (106,107). When added to the stress of hemorrhage or a major operation, the mortality rate is even higher. Initial treatment consists of administration of a central nervous system depressant. We prefer intramuscular magnesium sulfate in doses of 2 g every 2 to 4 hours. If magnesium sulfate therapy is not rapidly effective, chlordiazepoxide hydrochloride (Librium) is added in a dose of 25 to 50 mg intramuscularly every 4 hours. Supportive treatment in the form of adequate parenteral fluids containing concentrated glucose and vitamins, antipyretic agents, and pulmonary therapy is important. This hyperactive, hypermetabolic disorder must not be confused with hepatic encephalopathy, because a central nervous system depressant may be lethal in patients with hepatic encephalopathy. Intravenous alcohol is a severe hepatotoxin, and no basis exists for its use in cirrhotic patients with postoperative delirium tremens. Parenteral paraldehyde has no advantages over other hypnotic drugs and, in the author's opinion, should not be used because of the frequent soft tissue abscesses and noxious odor it produces.

Hepatic Failure. The majority of patients appear to be in surprisingly good condition immediately following an emergency portacaval shunt. However, by the second or third postoperative day some deterioration of liver function is noted in almost all patients. In many patients, the liver dysfunction stabilizes and then improves, but in some it progresses to hepatic coma and the full syndrome of hepatic failure, with jaundice, severe abnormalities of blood coagulation, ascites, and renal insufficiency. Liver failure is the most frequent cause of death in cirrhotic patients who bleed from esophageal varices, whether or not they have had a portacaval shunt. The hepatic coma that occurs during the immediate postoperative period is due to liver cell failure and is not related to ammonia intoxication or systemic shunting of nitrogenous substances absorbed from the intestines (108–110). Unfortunately, there is no specific therapy for hepatic failure, and all that can be done is to provide parenteral nutritional support and symptomatic therapy of the individual abnormalities that arise. There is no evidence that exchange transfusion, hemodialysis, or extracorporeal perfusion of the blood through a pig, baboon, or human liver are of value in this situation. Spontaneous recovery sometimes occurs.

Because it is rarely possible to remove all of the blood from the gastrointestinal tract preoperatively, neomycin therapy (1 g every 6 hours by nasogastric tube), cathartics (60 mL magnesium sulfate per day by nasogastric tube), and a daily neomycin enema (4 g in 1 quart of water) are continued for 3 days postoperatively. If continued beyond 3 days, troublesome diarrhea usually follows. With this regimen, significantly elevated blood ammonia levels or signs of nitrogen-related encephalopathy rarely occur within the first postoperative week.

Gastric Acid Hypersecretion. Inconclusive evidence suggests that, following portacaval shunt, gastric acid hypersecretion develops and is associated with an increased incidence of peptic ulcer disease (111,112). To protect against this potential complication, nasogastric suction is continued for 3 or 4 days postoperatively and cimetidine is given throughout the stay. As soon as the nasogastric tube is removed, the patient is given hourly antacid therapy until the oral dietary intake is satisfactory, and then the antacid schedule is changed to between meals and at bedtime. An antacid that does not contain sodium is used. Antacid and cimetidine therapy are discontinued 3 months postoperatively.

Renal Failure. Two common forms of renal dysfunction follow varix hemorrhage and portacaval shunt. The first is acute tubular necrosis, which results from a period of hypotension and consequent renal ischemia. It is manifested by oliguria, azotemia, hyperkalemia, a low fixed urine specific gravity and osmolality, substantial quantities of sodium in the urine, and a urine sediment containing casts and red blood cells. Treatment consists of stringent fluid restriction, measures to reduce serum potassium, and, if necessary, hemodialysis. The second renal disorder is spontaneous renal failure associated with hepatic decompensation, the so-called hepatorenal syndrome (111–115). It is more insidious in onset than acute tubular necrosis and is manifested initially by progressive azotemia without striking oliguria. In contrast to acute tubular necrosis, the urine specific gravity in the hepatorenal syndrome is variable and ranges up to 1.020, there is almost no sodium in the urine, the osmolality of the urine is high, and the urine sediment is normal. There is no specific treatment for spontaneous renal failure, and therapy is directed at reversing the hepatic decompensation, minimizing dilutional hyponatremia, and correcting problems as they appear. There is no indication for the use of diuretics, and, in fact, they may intensify the renal abnormality. Numerous vasoactive agents have been used for the purpose of improving renal blood flow, but none has influenced the outcome. Hemodialysis has created more problems than it has solved. The mortality rate of the combined syndrome of hepatic and renal decompensation is very high.

INFECTION. Substantial evidence indicates that patients with cirrhosis have a high incidence of infection, perhaps because of their debilitated general condition. Surprisingly, wound and intraperitoneal infections following emergency portacaval shunt have been uncommon in our experience, occurring in only 3 percent of our patients. However, pulmonary infections have been common and urinary tract infections not infrequent. The value of prophylactic antibiotic therapy in this condition is uncertain. Appropriate antibiotics are given for proven infections, always on the basis of bacterial cultures and antibiotic sensitivity tests. We routinely obtain cultures of tracheal aspirates and urine during the early postoperative period to avoid delays in therapy should infection develop.

NUTRITION. Nutritional therapy is very important in liver disease (116). Oral diet is started as soon as the patient tolerates removal of the nasogastric tube for 24 hours, usually on the fifth or sixth postoperative day. Initially, a 200-mg-sodium, 4000-calorie, high-carbohydrate, regular fat, 20-g-protein, bland diet is introduced. There is no basis for restricting fat, and doing so only makes the diet unpalatable. The protein content of the diet is increased in 20-g increments every 3 days up to 80 g, and the patient is carefully observed and tested each day for signs of encephalopathy. If the patient tolerates 80 g of protein per day, she or he is discharged on a 60-g-protein diet after having received a diet list and specific instructions from a dietician. Rigorous sodium restriction is continued for several months, and, even after a year has elapsed, sodium intake is not allowed to advance above 2.5 g/day. Daily therapeutic doses of vitamins B and C are added to the diet.

ALCOHOLISM. A factor that influences long-term survival following portacaval shunt is success or failure in abstaining from alcohol. It is vitally important that a frank discussion be held with the patient regarding the serious dangers of further ingestion of alcohol. The help of psychiatrists and social workers should be obtained while the patient is in the hospital and continued after discharge. It is incumbent upon the surgeon to exploit the special relationship with the patient in a long-term effort to cure the underlying cause of the patient's liver disease.

FOLLOW-UP. A lifelong program of follow-up evaluation and treatment is a crucial part of the care of cirrhotic patients who have undergone portacaval shunt. The liver disease cannot be cured, but it can be stabilized to the point of permitting a long and productive life in reasonable comfort. After discharge from the hospital, outpatient visits are scheduled weekly for the first 8 weeks, monthly for the remainder of the first postoperative year, and every 3 months thereafter for the remainder of the patient's life.

Elective Portal-Systemic Shunt for Bleeding Esophageal Varices Due to Cirrhosis

INDICATIONS AND SELECTION CRITERIA

Elective surgical treatment directed at overcoming portal hypertension is indicated in patients who have not undergone an emergency portacaval shunt and have recovered from an episode of bleeding esophageal varices, provided there is a reasonable likelihood that the patient will survive the elective operation. Table 62-14 shows the results of two prospective studies of the fate of cirrhotic patients who recovered from a bleeding episode and qualified for surgical therapy but were deliberately not subjected to operation (117,118). Over 90 percent of the patients bled again from esophageal varices and died. In our study, all of the patients were dead within 2 years of their first bleeding episode. The only consistently effective treatment for portal hypertension is the portal-systemic shunt, which, when performed properly, will protect more than 90 percent of patients against subsequent varix hemorrhage. Therefore, a single episode of varix bleeding is an indication for elective shunt therapy in all cirrhotic patients, unless they have hepatic decompensation. Unfortunately, only 10 to 20 percent of bleeding cirrhotic patients survive nonsurgical emergency therapy and recover sufficient hepatic function to become eligible for elective shunt.

TABLE 62-14. Prospective Studies of the Fate of Cirrhotic Patients Who Survived an Episode of Bleeding Esophageal Varices and Did Not Undergo Portacaval Shunt

Author (Ref.)	No. of Patients	Criteria for Inclusion in Prospective Study	Rebleeding from Varices, %	Mortality Rate, %	
				2-year	5-year
Mikkelson (117)	35	Child's risk class A; recovered from one or more bleeding episodes, qualified for shunt	95	50	100
Orloff (118)	27	Unselected, all Child's risk classes; recovered from one (first) bleeding episode; qualified for shunt	93	100	—

What criteria can be used to predict the likelihood of a patient surviving an elective shunt procedure without serious sequelae? The answer is not known with any degree of certainty and is particularly difficult because the decision not to operate is tantamount to accepting a lethal outcome. Extensive efforts have been directed toward identifying biochemical, hemodynamic, morphologic, and clinical criteria for selecting patients for elective portal-systemic shunt (103,119–133). The results of liver function tests, such as the level of serum albumin or bilirubin, the amount of BSP or indocyanine green retention, or the magnitude of prothrombin deficiency, do not correlate with the response to shunt except at the extremes. Hemodynamic studies involving angiography and pressure measurements have been of little predictive value, mainly because of the lack of a practical technique for measuring the capacity of hepatic arterial blood flow to compensate for the diversion of portal venous flow. It has been proposed that the presence of acute alcoholic hepatitis, acute hyaline necrosis, or many Mallory bodies on liver biopsy is a contraindication to operation (117,124,127). However, in our recent study of liver biopsies from 164 patients with alcoholic cirrhosis who underwent emergency portacaval shunt, there was no correlation between survival and the finding of any or all of these features of acute alcoholic hepatitis (134).

In the final analysis, the decision whether to operate is based on a composite of many clinical features of a patient's disease, determined during a period of intensive medical treatment in the hospital. Certain features are ominous; thus, the presence of persistent jaundice, of ascites that cannot be stabilized, of repeated bouts of encephalopathy, of advanced muscle wasting, and of a poor appetite indicate that operation should not be undertaken. If these general critieria have been followed, the operative mortality rate has been in the acceptable range of 10 percent. Whenever possible, patients are prepared for an elective operation during a 3- to 6-week period in the hospital with a regimen directed at improving nutrition, slowly restoring blood volume and red cell mass, correcting electrolyte and acid-base abnormalities, and unloading excess fluid.

RESULTS OF OPERATION

Table 62-15 shows some results of elective portal-systemic shunt performed for varix bleeding in patients with cirrhosis (133,135–143). Beyond any doubt, the portal-systemic shunt prevents subsequent varix bleeding in the vast majority of patients. Moreover, 39 to 70 percent of highly selected patients subjected to elective treatment have survived 5 years.

The crucial question regarding the value of elective, therapeutic portal-systemic shunt concerns whether a comparable, selected group of patients who are treated medically rather than surgically will survive as long or as well. Unfortunately, despite use of the shunt operation for 40 years, this question has not yet been answered. Four prospective clinical trials have been reported, three of them suggesting an advantage of shunt operations and one of them indicating no advantage (Table 62-16) (117,139–149). However, all four trials involved small numbers of highly selected patients and had a number of serious shortcomings in design and conduct, so that the results do not warrant a conclusive answer. On the basis of our current knowledge, and until conclusive information to the contrary is available, the elective portacaval shunt is indicated in patients who have bled one or more times from esophageal varices.

There are several untoward sequelae of the portal-systemic anastomosis. The most important of these is postshunt encephalopathy, which presumably is due to shunting of ammonia, or some nitrogenous substance absorbed from the intestine, directly into the systemic circulation. The reported incidence of this disturbing complication has varied considerably but has been in the range of 15 to 30 percent of patients. Because ammonia is formed by the action of bacteria on nitrogenous substances in the terminal ileum and colon, encephalopathy usually can be controlled by limiting the protein content of the diet and by the use of intestinal antibiotics such as neomycin or agents such as lactulose. If these measures fail, operative exclusion of the colon by ileostomy or ileosigmoidostomy may be effective. It is important to recognize that a substantial number of patients who have not

TABLE 62-15. Results of Elective Portal-Systemic Shunt in Highly Selected Patients with Cirrhosis

Authors (Ref.)	No. of Patients	Type of Shunt	Operative Mortality Rate, %	Varix Rebleeding, %	5-Year Survival, %
Voorhees et al. (141)	404	324 portacaval, 80 splenorenal, & other	12	7	51
McDermott et al. (138)	237	166 splenorenal, 71 portacaval	23	15	54
Barnes et al. (135)	173	103 portacaval, 70 splenorenal	13	14	39
Mikkelson et al. (139)	173	All portacaval	12	7	44
Linton et al. (137)	169	129 splenorenal, 47 portacaval	12	19	50
Turcotte, Lambert (133)	147	All portacaval	21	—	35
Ottinger (143)	140	All splenorenal	12	10	41
Bismuth et al. (136)	120	72 central splenorenal, 48 portacaval	2	3	66
Wantz, Payne (144)	97	All portacaval	11	5	68 (4-year)
Walker et al. (142)	50	All portacaval	6	12	70
Orloff (140)	612	All portacaval	2	0.5	60

TABLE 62-16. Prospective Controlled Clinical Trials of Elective Therapeutic Portacaval Shunt in Highly Selected Patients with Cirrhosis

Authors (Ref.)	Year Reported	No. of Patients Randomized	Operative Mortality Rate, %	Actuarial Survival, %		Encephalopathy, %
				3 years	5 years	
Jackson et al. (145)	1971	Surgical, 67	8	61	52	34
		Medical, 77 (26)*	—	42	31	44
Resnick et al. (146)	1974	Surgical, 46	13	—	57	20
		Medical, 25 (7)*	—	—	48	35
Mikkelson et al. (139)	1974	Surgical, 37	5	70	60	—
		Medical, 38 (3)*	—	37	10	—
Rueff et al. (147)	1976	Surgical, 31	19	47	—	32
		Medical, 49 (18)*	—	56	—	44

*Figures in parentheses represent the number of patients in the medical group who subsequently underwent portacaval shunt for rebleeding, often as an emergency procedure.

had a surgical shunt have portal-systemic encephalopathy, as shown so clearly in the medical groups of the controlled clinical trials reported in Table 62-16. Therefore, studies of portal-systemic shunt that report a low or no incidence of encephalopathy are of doubtful validity.

The development of peptic ulcer is another potential complication of portal-systemic shunt. Hepatic bypass of a potent intestinal hormone that stimulates gastric acid hypersecretion is a regular consequence of a portacaval anastomosis. It would seem prudent to institute antacid therapy, cimetidine, and a dietary ulcer regimen following shunt operations.

Venous shunt therapy, of course, represents treatment of the complications of cirrhosis and has no direct beneficial effect on the liver disease itself. In contast to the effects of portacaval shunt in experimental animals with normal livers, the influence of the operation on liver function in humans with cirrhosis and portal hypertension is variable. In our studies comparing hepatic function 5 years after shunt with preoperative function, there was either moderate improvement or no change in 85 percent of patients. Deterioration of hepatic function has been related more closely to whether or not the patient resumed the ingestion of alcohol than to any other factor.

CHOICE OF PORTAL-SYSTEMIC SHUNT

Because the portal venous system contains no valves, it is possible to decompress it at various points, provided the anastomosis with the low pressure systemic venous system is of sufficient size to accommodate a large flow of blood. Several types of portal-systemic shunts are available for relief of portal hypertension (Figure 62-6). Descriptions of these shunts follow.

Direct Portacaval Shunt

The most commonly used shunt procedures are the direct end-to-side and side-to-side anastomoses between the portal vein and inferior vena cava. The *end-to-side portacaval* shunt accomplishes splanchnic decompression by shunting all splanchnic venous blood into the inferior vena cava, and, at the same time, it decompresses the liver sinusoid by eliminating the contribution of portal venous blood to hepatic inflow and pressure. However, it rarely lowers hepatic sinusoidal pressure to normal, and sinusoidal hypertension often persists because hepatic arterial blood continues to encounter difficulty in leaving the liver through the obstructed hepatic venous outflow system. The *side-to-side portacaval* shunt produces splanchnic decompression equivalent to the end-to-side anastomosis, but it accomplishes significantly greater hepatic decompression by allowing egress of liver blood in a retrograde direction through the portal vein into the low-pressure vena cava. The side-to-side shunt converts the portal vein into an outflow tract, and portal blood does not continue to perfuse the liver. An important question about the side-to-side anastomosis concerns the theoretical possibility that it creates an intrahepatic arteriovenous fistula in which hepatic arterial blood leaves the liver via the portal vein without having made contact with the hepatic cells and having contributed to hepatic nutrition and metabolism. Studies in experimental animals suggest that arteriovenous shunting occurs to some degree but is compensated for by an increase in afferent hepatic arterial blood flow so that hepatic nutrition is not compromised (150).

Although the two types of direct portacaval shunt produce similar splanchnic decompression and are equally effective in relieving and preventing varix hemorrhage, the overall hemodynamic effects of the two procedures are distinctly different. Hence, there has been a continuing controversy regarding the comparative advantages and disadvantages of the end-to-side and side-to-side anastomoses (151–154). In a series of studies, we have compared the effects of the two types of shunt on hepatic blood flow, liver function, liver morphology, and ammonia tolerance in dogs with experimental cirrhosis, and on hepatic function, ammonia tolerance, the 5-year incidence of encephalopathy, and the 5-year survival rate in cirrhotic humans who were operated on for bleeding esophageal varices (155,156). There were no significant differences between end-to-side and side-to-side portacaval shunt in any of the parameters evaluated. We have concluded that there is no demonstrable advantage of one

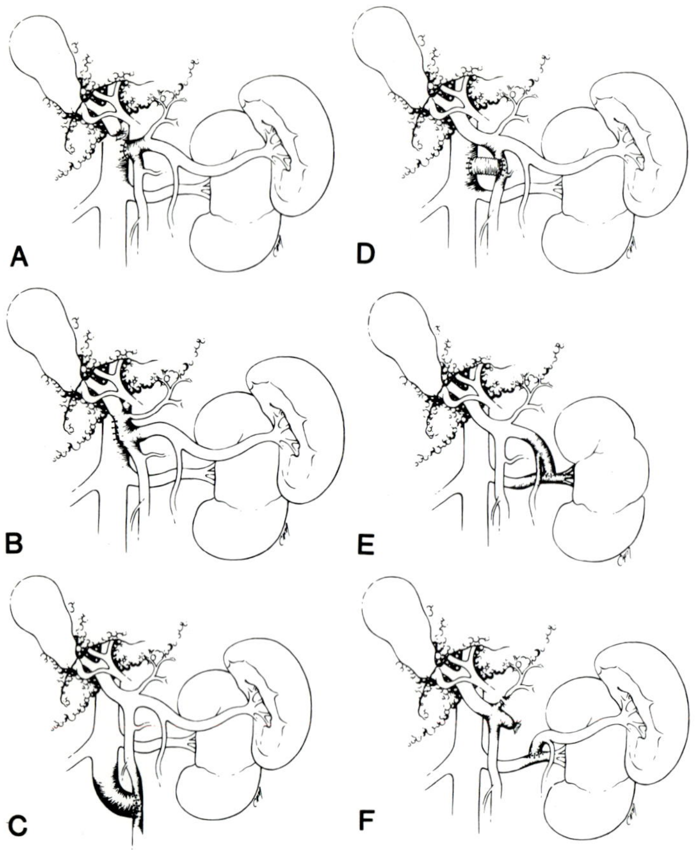

FIGURE 62-6. Common types of portal-systemic venous shunts used to relieve portal hypertension. *(A)* End-to-side portacaval; *(B)* side-to-side portacaval; *(C)* mesocaval; *(D)* interposition mesocaval H-graft; *(E)* conventional splenorenal; *(F)* selective distal splenorenal. [From Orloff MJ: Portal hypertension: Portacaval anastomosis. In Dudley H, Pories WJ, Carter DC (eds): *Smith's Operative Surgery. 2. Alimentary Tract and Abdominal Wall,* ed 4. London, Butterworths, 1983.]

type of direct portacaval shunt over the other under most circumstances. The one exception may be the unusual patient with severe hepatic outflow obstruction manifested by a pressure on the hepatic side of a clamp occluding the portal vein (hepatic occluded portal pressure, or HOPP) that is higher than the free portal pressure (FPP). Such patients may have reversal of portal flow, and they have been known to develop intractable ascites following an end-to-side portacaval shunt, which eliminates the portal vein as an outflow tract and thereby may increase sinusoidal hypertension (157). Although clear documentation of this phenomenon does not exist, a side-to-side portacaval shunt would seem to be the procedure of choice in such cases.

Conventional Splenorenal Shunt

The *splenorenal anastomosis* is a variant of the side-to-side, in-continuity shunt. It utilzies tributaries of the portal vein and vena cava that, obviously, are of smaller size than the parent vessels. It is followed by a lower incidence of protein-related portal-systemic encephalopathy than the direct portacaval anastomosis because it shunts a small volume of nitrogen-containing portal blood into the systemic circulation. At the same time, it does not decompress the portal bed as effectively as the direct portacaval shunt, is associated with a significant incidence of varix rebleeding, and has a high incidence of thrombosis. In the author's opinion it is the procedure of choice only in infrequent instances when severe and intractable hypersplenism complicates portal hypertension and requires splenectomy, or when previous operations in the right upper quadrant of the abdomen make it technically difficult to perform a direct portacaval shunt. Also, splenorenal shunt is indicated when it is desirable to avoid dissection of the portal vein and inferior vena cava because orthotopic liver transplantation at some time in the future is being contemplated. The most commonly used type of splenorenal shunt involves removal of the spleen and anastomosis of the end of the splenic vein to the side of the left renal vein. However, a central side-to-side splenorenal shunt can be done in continuity without splenectomy and is our choice of operation whenever a splenorenal shunt must be done. This variant has been said to permit continued portal venous perfusion of the liver, but it is doubtful that such is the case since the principles that govern the hemodynamics of a valveless system dictate that flow is in the direction of the area of lowest pressure, i.e., the splenorenal anastomosis.

Mesocaval Shunt and Mesocaval H-Graft

The *mesocaval shunt* is an anastomosis between the superior end of the divided inferior vena cava and the side of the superior mesenteric vein. In principle, it is hemodynamically similar to the side-to-side portacaval shunt. In patients with extrahepatic portal hypertension due to occlusion of the portal vein, this type of shunt is very effective. However, in adult cirrhotic patients it is doubtful that this procedure represents a first choice. Cirrhotic patients retain salt and water, and division of the inferior vena cava may lead to intractable edema of the lower extremities.

The use of H-grafts between the intact portal or superior mesenteric vein and inferior vena cava, introduced 35 years ago, recently has attracted renewed interest (158–165). Synthetic prostheses of Dacron and Teflon, autogenous jugular vein, and homologous vena cava have been used for this purpose. The *interposition mesocaval or portacaval H-graft* is a relatively minor technical variation of the direct side-to-side portacaval shunt and, despite claims to the contrary, the two procedures are hemodynamically identical. The major advantage claimed for the H-graft procedure is that it is technically less difficult to perform than conventional shunts. The major potential disadvantage is the possibility of thrombosis, particularly of the synthetic prostheses. In general, the use of grafts in the venous system has a long history of failure, so there is justifiable skepticism about the possibility of consistent long-term patency of the H-graft. Short-term results of interposition shunts involving a collective total of some 400 patients have been reported from 15 centers. The operative mortality rate in this heterogeneous collection of patients has been about 15 percent, which is not lower than that associated with conventional portacaval shunts. The short-term incidence of thrombosis has ranged from 5 to 20 percent, which is unacceptable when compared with the less than 2 percent long-term occlusion rate of direct portacaval anastomoses in experienced hands. The incidence of postshunt encephalopathy has been similar to that following direct portacaval shunt, as expected.

Selective Distal Splenorenal Shunt

An unsettled issue of great importance regarding the use of portacaval shunt concerns its effect both on liver cell function, presumably related to liver blood flow, and on portal-systemic encephalopathy, presumably related to hepatic bypass of nitrogenous substances absorbed from the intestines. When portal blood is completely shunted away from the liver, further liver damage might be anticipated unless there is a compensatory increase in hepatic arterial blood flow. It is not possible by any currently available, practical method to predict the adequacy of hepatic arterial compensation prior to performance of a portacaval shunt. It has been proposed that a worsening of liver function or outright hepatic failure following portacaval shunt is due to a sudden diversion of needed blood away from the liver. The familiar hepatic dysfunction that follows creation of a portacaval shunt (Eck fistula) in the dog with a normal liver is cited as evidence for this proposal. The absence of significant hepatic dysfunciton in patients with extrahepatic occlusion of the portal vein, either before or after portal-systemic anastomosis, is thought to result from the combination of a long period of adaptation to diminished portal flow and an initially normal hepatic parenchyma.

On the basis of preoperative and intraoperative measurements made in a small group of subjects, it has been proposed that cirrhotic patients with normal or near-normal portal blood flow, who often appear to be the best-risk patients with the least severe liver disease, are intolerant of sudden shunting of portal blood, and often die of progressive hepatic failure. On the other hand, it has been proposed that patients with substantially reduced portal blood flow tolerate a portacaval shunt well because the bypass produces little further reduction in the blood supply to the liver. Finally, it has been suggested that calculations of maximal portal perfusion pressure from intraoperative pressure measurements reflect portal blood flow and permit a prediction of the response to portacaval shunt. The logic of this simple hypothesis is attractive, even though it ignores the vital role of the hepatic arterial blood supply in compensating for portal diversion and the complex nature of the hepatic circulation. However, substantial recent data obtained by five separate groups from preoperative and intraoperative measurements of both pressure and blood flow in the portal vein in large numbers of patients failed to show a correlation between any hemodynamic measurements performed prior to portacaval shunt and survival, hepatic function, or development of encephalopathy after shunt (119,120,122,129,130). The results of our study of this matter are shown in Table 62-17. There was no statistically significant correlation between preshunt maximum perfusion pressure and postshunt survival, liver function, hepatic failure, or development of encephalopathy. Contrary to the hypothesis, patients with the lowest preshunt maximum perfusion pressure had the lowest survival rate, whereas patients with the highest preshunt maximum perfusion pressure had the highest survival rate and the lowest incidence of encephalopathy following portacaval shunt. The only hemodynamic parameter that has been shown to correlate with the response to portacaval shunt is the magnitude of compensatory increase in hepatic artery flow, determined in retrospect after performance of the shunt. In a significant study, Burchell et al. (120) demonstrated, by direct intraoperative blood flow measurements immediately after portacaval shunt, that survival and incidence of encephalopathy were directly related to the amount of increase in hepatic artery flow. Unfortunately, there is no currently available practical method of predicting this increase preoperatively.

On the presumption that portacaval shunt injures the liver and increases portal-systemic encephalopathy in patients with a large hepatorenal portal flow, Warren and his associates (166) proposed in 1967 a modified shunting procedure that they believed would selectively decompress esophageal varices while, at the same time, preserving blood flow to the liver and avoiding systemic shunting of intestinal blood. The operation consists of a *distal splenorenal shunt,* in which the splenic side of the divided splenic vein is anastomosed to the intact left renal vein, and *gastrosplenic isolation* aimed at diverting the gastroesophageal venous flow through the shunt. Gastrosplenic isolation is accomplished by ligating the coronary, right gastric, and right gastroepiploic veins and by dividing the gastrohepatic, gastrocolic, and splenocolic ligaments. The objectives of the selective shunt were to produce better results than those achieved with direct portacaval shunt by (1) preventing recurrent bleeding (and death from such bleeding) as effectively as direct portacaval shunt; (2) improving the immediate and long-term survival rate by decreasing the number of deaths from liver failure; and (3) improving the quality of life by reducing the incidence of encephalopathy. Interest in distal splenorenal shunt has been widespread since its introduction 18 years ago. Table 62-18 shows some current results of the operation (167–181).

TABLE 62-17. Relationship of Maximum Portal Perfusion Pressure before Portacaval Shunt to Survival and Encephalopathy after Shunt

Maximum Portal Perfusion Pressure, (mm saline)	No. of Patients	Survival, %	Encephalopathy at Any Time in Survivors, %
≤100	83	53	32
101–200	42	64	44
201–300	29	62	28
>300	20	70	28

TABLE 62-18. Results of Elective Therapeutic Distal Splenorenal Shunt in Highly Selected Patients with Liver Diseases

Authors (Ref.)	Year of Report	Type of Series	No. of Patients	Underlying Disease	Child's Risk Class	Operative Mortality Rate, %	Years of Follow-up	Total Mortality Rate, %	Encephal-opathy, %	Rebleeding, %	Known Shunt Occlusion, %
Vang et al. (175)	1976	Retrospective, selected patients	25	Cirrhosis of various types	A-13 B-9 C-2	16	2.4–5.5	58	56	29	8
Martin et al. (170)	1978	Retrospective, selected patients	50	Cirrhosis of various types	A-12 B-32 C-6	10	Variable	24 (3-yr)	18	26	2
Zeppa et al. (177)	1978	Retrospective, selected patients	91	Cirrhosis (52 alcoholic, 39 nonalcoholic)	Mostly A	1	0.5–6	43 (5-yr actuarial)	?	?	?
Rikkers et al. (171)	1978	Prospective, randomized, selected patients	26	Cirrhosis of various types	A	12	2–6	38 (3-yr)	13	13	10
Bhalerao et al. (167)	1978	Retrospective, selected patients	52	Liver disease of various types	?	40	0.5–4	52	0	11	16
Langer et al. (168)	1980	Prospective, randomized, selected patients	27	Cirrhosis of various types	A-6 B-16 C-5	19	1–7	33	14	9	10
Turcotte, Eckhauser (174)	1980	Retrospective, selected patients	55	Cirrhosis of various types	?	16	1–7	31	?	?	?
Fischer et al. (178)	1981	Prospective, randomized, selected patients	23	Cirrhosis (22 alcoholic, 1 nonalcoholic)	A-13 B-8 C-2	4	1–5	22	9	14	27
Warren et al. (179)	1982	Retrospective, selected patients	348	Cirrhosis (198 alcoholic, 150 nonalcoholic)	86% A & B	4	1–10	41 (5-yr actuarial)	4	?	7

Distal splenoral shunt has been used almost exclusively as an elective procedure in patients who have survived one or more episodes of varix hemorrhage. By and large the operation has been reserved for good-risk subjects with various forms of mild-to-moderate liver disease, good hepatic function, and excellent liver blood flow. Ascites has been considered a contraindication to the operation by most surgeons, although ascites that promptly responds to diuretic therapy has recently been removed by some workers from the list of contraindications. It is important to recognize that the highly selected patients who have undergone distal splenorenal shunt are not representative of the spectrum of bleeding cirrhotics admitted to a general hospital.

Has the distal splenorenal shunt accomplished the objectives that Warren and his colleagues (166) believed it would accomplish? Although it is still too early to draw firm conclusions, available data provide the following impressions: (1) The operation effectively prevents bleeding from varices in most patients. However, compared with direct end-to-side or side-to-side portacaval shunts performed electively in similar patients, it appears to be associated with higher incidences of recurrent varix hemorrhage, persistence of varices, and occlusion of the shunt. In two series, rebleeding occurred in 29 and 26 percent of the patients, respectively (170,175). (2) Although the operative mortality rate in almost every institution has been high during the initial phase when the procedure was being learned, it has declined progressively as experience with the operation has increased. Nevertheless, the operative mortality rate appears to be somewhat higher than that of direct end-to-side or side-to-side portacaval anastomoses performed electively in comparable good-risk patients. It is generally agreed that distal splenorenal shunt is technically the most difficult of all the commonly used shunt procedures. (3) The 5-year survival rate does not appear to be different from that associated with direct portacaval shunt in similar patients; if anything, the long-term survival rate is somewhat lower following distal splenorenal shunt, but available data are inconclusive. (4) The incidence of encephalopathy during the first few years after distal splenorenal shunt is lower than the incidence following direct portacaval shunt, and encephalopathy tends to be milder. Thus, the advantage or disadvantage of distal splenorenal shunt compared with direct portacaval shunt during the first 5 years postoperatively depends on the relative importance given to a lower incidence and severity of encephalopathy on the one hand, and to apparently higher rates of recurrent varix hemorrhage, shunt occlusion, operative mortality, and, perhaps, long-term mortality on the other hand.

There is reason to raise the possibility that, with the passage of time following distal splenorenal shunt, the incidence of encephalopathy will increase and the survival rate will decrease compared with statistics for direct portacaval shunt. Accumulating evidence from detailed studies during prolonged follow-up shows that liver function deteriorates, the incidence of death from liver failure increases, hepatic blood flow decreases, collateral vessels connecting the portomesenteric and gastrosplenic sides of the portal circulation develop, and portal perfusion of the liver is lost with diversion of portomesenteric blood through the splenorenal shunt (180,181). Furthermore, recent reports of studies in patients with distal splenorenal shunt have identified a substantial incidence of thrombosis of the portal vein which, of course, eliminates the main objective of the operation, namely, continued perfusion of the liver (180). The theoretical attractiveness of the distal splenorenal shunt for a selected segment of the bleeding cirrhotic population is undeniable, but its value remains to be established by long-term studies from several centers of survival rates, incidence of shunt thrombosis, frequency of rebleeding, and incidence of liver failure and encephalopathy.

Portacaval Shunt with Arterialization

In the hope of improving liver blood flow after end-to-side portacaval shunt, in 1968 Maillard et al. (182,183) proposed a procedure that *combined portacaval shunt with arterialization of the hepatic stump of the portal vein.* In 1974, Maillard et al. (183) summarized the experience of others using this approach in 46 patients, and described in detail their own experience with 36 patients. Maillard et al. used the splenic artery to arterialize the hepatic stump of the portal vein, and performed the procedure electively in good-risk patients (Child's groups A and B). The operative mortality rate was 17 percent, and 1 month postoperatively 30 percent of the arteriovenous anastomoses had thrombosed. After 1 year, the majority of the patients studied had developed thromboses of either the anastomosis or the intrahepatic branches of the portal vein. The incidence of encephalopathy in the patients with patent anastomoses was 17 percent. On the basis of these results, there is little to recommend serious consideration of this operation.

Other (Uncommon) Shunts

None of the several other techniques for creating connections between the portal and systemic venous systems are used widely or are established therapy for portal hypertension. The left gastric vena caval shunt, developed by Inokuchi and his colleagues (184) in Japan, is based on the concept of selectively decompressing esophageal varices through the left gastric (coronary) vein while maintaining portal perfusion of the liver similar to the distal splenorenal shunt. The small left gastric vein is connected to the inferior vena cava by an interposed graft of autogenous saphenous vein or superficial femoral vein. Splenectomy, ligation of the tributaries of the splenic vein, and ligation of the connections between the right and left gastric veins are added to the shunt procedure. By 1978, Inokuchi et al. had performed the operation electively in 103 patients with postnecrotic or posthepatitic cirrhosis, 32 patients with idiopathic portal hypertension, and 5 patients with extrahepatic portal hypertension. The shunt was done as a therapeutic procedure for bleeding varices in 97 patients and as a prophylactic operation in 43 patients. In the therapeutic shunt group, the operative mortality rate was 5 percent, the cumulative mortality rate during 3 months to 5 years of follow-up was 29 percent, the incidence of shunt occlusion 1 month postoperatively was 11 percent, and the frequency of rebleeding was 10 percent. That none of the patients was observed to have encephalopathy after operation is remarkable in light of the consistent observation that many unoperated upon cirrhotic patients have encephalopathy. The results of left gastric vena caval shunt have not been confirmed by other workers.

The portarenal shunt is a form of in-continuity shunt similar to the side-to-side portacaval shunt (185). The left renal vein is transected, and the vena caval end is anastomosed to the side of the portal vein, superior mesenteric vein, or splenic vein. Alternatively, the portal vein may be divided and its splanchnic end anastomosed to the end of the transected renal vein, which is hemodynamically similar to an end-to-side portacaval shunt. Under most circumstances the portarenal shunt has no advantages over conventional portacaval shunts.

Shunts have been devised that utilize the reopened umbilical vein which connects with the portal vein, but they are not promising because of the small size of the vessel. Included in this category are the omphalocaval shunt and the saphenoumbilical shunt (186).

PROPHYLACTIC PORTAL-SYSTEMIC SHUNT

Because of the very high mortality rate associated with varix bleeding, some workers have advocated prophylactic portacaval shunt in patients with demonstrable varices who have never bled. Although a patient who has bled from esophageal varices is almost certain to bleed again, nothing suggests that the mere demonstration of varices in a patient with no history of bleeding permits one to predict the likelihood of varix rupture. In fact, recent statistics indicate that only one-fourth to one-third of patients with esophageal varices who have no history of bleeding will subsequently have varix hemorrhage. Thus, two-thirds to three-fourths of the patients subjected to prophylactic portacaval shunt would undergo an operation to prevent a complication that would not have developed had they not received surgical therapy. Herein lies the fallacy of prophylactic shunt.

Prophylactic portacaval shunt has been compared with medical therapy in three prospective studies conducted in selected cirrhotic patients with esophageal varices that had not bled (187–190). All three studies showed that while protecting the patients against bleeding, prophylactic shunt had no influence on survival of selected patients. These results are not surprising. When a major operation is performed in seriously ill patients to prevent a complication that might develop in only one-fourth of these patients if they did not have the operation, the results can hardly be expected to be good. Therefore, there is no indication for the prophylactic operation. However, it is important to emphasize that the results of prophylactic portacaval shunt are in no way applicable to the treatment of bleeding esophageal varices by therapeutic portacaval shunt because these patients have already developed the complication of bleeding, which is almost certain to recur unless the portal hypertension is relieved.

Treatment of Bleeding Esophageal Varices Due to Extrahepatic Portal Obstruction

Portal hypertension due to extrahepatic portal obstruction is a strikingly different condition from intrahepatic portal hypertension (191–201). The patients are usually much younger and most often are children. They do not have liver disease, and, consequently, they have a much greater tolerance for bleeding and for operations. Except in infancy, they rarely have ascites, and hepatic coma due to liver cell failure does not develop. Because the portal vein is usually obliterated, a direct portal vein to vena cava anastomosis cannot be performed for portal decompression. Finally, age and the related technical matter of adequate vessel size influence treatment.

Patients with extrahepatic portal obstruction come to the attention of the surgeon usually because of bleeding from esophageal varices or splenomegaly. Although hematemesis is the most common symptom, the bleeding sometimes presents as melena. Exsanguinating hemorrhage does not occur nearly as often as in cirrhosis. On physical examination, splenomegaly is almost always found, but the liver is not palpable. Dilated collateral veins in the abdominal wall may be striking. Liver function tests usually are normal, but hematologic studies often reveal peripheral cytopenia that reflects hypersplenism. The hypersplenism is infrequently severe. Upper gastrointestinal x-rays and esophagogastroscopy demonstrate varices. Because the obstruction is presinusoidal, hepatic vein catheterization shows a normal wedged hepatic vein pressure. Ultrasonography of the abdomen regularly shows occlusion of the portal vein. Splenic or superior mesenteric arteriography, with indirect portography, provides crucial information about the site of the portal obstruction and the size of the vessels available for portal decompression. Splenoportography with manometry is equally, and sometimes more, effective in demonstrating the obstruction, but it is a diganostic procedure of second choice because of the small risk of bleeding from the spleen that might require a precipitant and premature operation.

The definitive treatment of extraheptic portal obstruction is the portal-systemic venous shunt. However, for technical reasons related to the size of the vessels required for the shunt, temporizing hemostatic measures may have to be used in infants and young children until they have grown to the point at which an adequate anastomosis is feasible. A mesocaval shunt usually should not be performed before the age of 4, and a splenorenal shunt is often not feasible before the age of 7 or 8. We have preferred to delay operation until the age of 10 if at all possible. Consequently, the emergency treatment of varix bleeding in infants and young children consists of blood transfusions and, when necessary, medical measures such as esophageal balloon tamponade and intravenous vasopressin. Failure to control bleeding is an indication for endoscopic sclerotherapy or transesophageal varix ligation. Rebleeding following these temporizing measures is the rule, but it is usually well tolerated and controllable until the child reaches a suitable age.

The types of portal-systemic anastomosis used in patients with an obliterated portal vein are the superior mesenteric vein–inferior vena cava shunt and the splenorenal shunt. When the splenorenal shunt is used, we prefer the central side-to-side splenorenal anastomosis with preservation of the spleen. The mesocaval shunt has been followed by a lower incidence of rebleeding and is the procedure of choice. Both operations have been associated with operative mortality rates below 5 percent. Other operative procedures, such as esophagogastrectomy with intestinal interposition, are associated with a substantial mortality rate and incidence of failure, and are indicated only when a portal-systemic shunt is impossible and the patient has severe and recurrent bleeding. In our experience and that of most other workers, hepatic encephalopathy rarely occurs following shunt operations for extrahepatic portal hypertension.

Other Uses of Portal-Systemic Shunt in Patients with Portal Hypertension

INTRACTABLE ASCITES

Ascites is a frequent and serious complication of cirrhosis. Although several factors are involved in the pathogenesis of ascites, substantial evidence indicates that increased pressure within the liver plays a major role in ascites formation and is the primary mechanism responsible for transudation of ascitic fluid (202–205). Moreover, evidence suggests that the intrahepatic hypertension in cirrhosis is a result of hepatic venous outflow obstruction.

In most cirrhotic patients, ascites disappears in response to a regimen consisting of abstinence from alcohol, a nourishing diet, salt restriction, and one or more of a variety of diuretic and antialdosterone drugs. Nevertheless, in a small but disturbing group of patients, ascites is refractory to these measures. It is for this group that the surgeon has attempted to devise operative measures of relief. If it is assumed, on the basis of substantial evidence, that increased hydrostatic pressure within the liver is important in the pathogenesis of ascites, it should be possible to relieve ascites by reducing intrahepatic pressure. Theoretically, decompression of the obstructed hepatic vascular bed may be accomplished, to a greater or lesser degree, by reducing the inflow of blood to the liver or by improving the outflow of blood from the liver. Inflow-reducing procedures include ligation of the hepatic artery and end-to-side portacaval shunt, both of which have been used in the treatment of cirrhotic ascites. Hepatic artery ligation no longer merits serious consideration, because it is an unpredictable operation that is associated with a high mortality rate. Improving the outflow of blood from the liver by a direct attack on the hepatic veins is not possible. However, numerous studies have demonstrated that the valveless portal vein is capable of serving as an outflow tract and that the objective of hepatic decompression is realized by a side-to-side portacaval shunt.

In a series of experiments, we evaluated the effects of portacaval shunts on ascites (206–211). These studies showed that side-to-side portacaval shunt relieved ascites, overcame intrahepatic hypertension, eliminated the hypersecretion of aldosterone that follows hepatic outflow occlusion, and reduced the markedly augmented thoracic duct lymph flow to normal. End-to-side portacaval anastomosis was much less effective than the lateral anastomosis in relieving the sequelae of increased pressure in the liver.

On the basis of these experimental observations, we have performed a side-to-side portacaval shunt in 18 selected patients with alcoholic cirrhosis and truly intractable ascites. All our patients failed to respond to prolonged and intensive medical treatment for ascites before operation was considered. Sixteen of the eighteen patients (89 percent) survived the operation, and all the survivors have been relieved of ascites, salt retention, and hyperaldosteronism for periods ranging from 3 to 13 years. The most notable feature of the response to operation, other than relief of ascites, has been a striking improvement in nutrition and vigor accompanied by substantial gains in lean tissue mass and body fat. Our small but consistent experience has led to the conclusion that side-to-side portacaval shunt is of lasting benefit when used in carefully selected cirrhotic patients with truly intractable ascites who have failed to respond to vigorous and expert medical management. It must be emphasized that the number of such patients is small.

BUDD-CHIARI SYNDROME

The Budd-Chiari syndrome (BCS) is a group of disorders in which obstruction to hepatic venous outflow results from occlusion of the hepatic veins and/or the adjacent inferior vena cava (IVC) (212–215). Over 700 cases of BCS have been reported, and the condition is being recognized with increasing frequency. Although in many cases of BCS no etiologic or predisposing condition can be identified, in recent years an underlying disorder has been found in more than half of the cases. The most common conditions that predispose to BCS are hematologic disorders with thrombotic tendencies such as polycythemia rubra vera and paroxysmal nocturnal hemoglobinuria (approximately 18 percent of cases); use of oral contraceptives (approximately 10 percent of cases); pregnancy and the postpartum period (approximately 10 percent of cases); malignant neoplasms that invade the IVC and hepatic veins from adjacent organs (approximately 10 percent of cases); and infections of the liver such as amebic abscess, hydatid cyst, and schistosomiasis (approximately 10 percent of cases). In Japan, India, and South Africa a common chronic form of BCS is membranous obstruction of the vena cava (MOVC), an idiopathic condition that probably results from acquired thrombosis and recanalization of the IVC (216–220). The "membrane" has been found to vary from very thin to several centimeters thick, and sometimes has occluded a long segment of retrohepatic IVC.

The pathologic lesion of BCS is thrombosis of the major hepatic veins and/or the IVC, which results in hepatic venous outflow obstruction, intrahepatic and portal hypertension, dilatation of the liver sinusoids, intense centrilobular congestion of the hepatic parenchyma, and ischemia, pressure necrosis, and atrophy of the parenchymal cells in the center of the liver lobule. Early in the course of BCS, these lesions are reversible if the obstruction is relieved. However, persistence of the high pressure and congestion within the liver results in irreversible damage, hepatic fibrosis, and progression to cirrhosis, often within a matter of months. The two paramount dangers in BCS are development of irreversible liver damage and extension of thrombosis from the hepatic veins into the IVC.

The clinical course of BCS is most commonly acute, with rapid progression of liver disease and its consequences over periods ranging from a few weeks to a few months. In some patients, however, BCS develops insidiously and progresses over months or years. The usual clinical manifestations are abdominal distension due to ascites, hepatomegaly, abdominal pain, weakness, wasting, and anorexia. Some patients additionally have splenomegaly, mild jaundice, and distension of the superficial veins of the anterior abdominal wall. When the IVC is obstructed, an important additional sign is edema of the lower extremities and lower trunk. In the chronic forms of BCS, all of the manifestations of cirrhosis of the liver are found.

The diagnosis of BCS in the initial weeks and months is based on finding the typical symptoms and signs combined with abnormal results of several diagnostic studies, the most important of which are angiographic examination of the IVC and hepatic veins with pressure measurements, and percutaneous needle liver biopsy. In BCS confined to the hepatic veins, IVC studies show a patent IVC and normal pressure for patients with ascites, whereas in BCS involving the IVC, cavography demonstrates an area of IVC obstruction and IVC pressure is elevated. Hepatic venography shows occlusion of the major hepatic veins and wedge injection demonstrates a distinctive "spider web pattern" of venous collaterals. Wedged hepatic vein pressure is markedly elevated. Liver biopsy reveals the typical lesion of obstruction to hepatic venous outflow, namely, intense centrilobular congestion and centrilobular loss of parenchyma and necrosis. Other diagnostic studies that may be helpful are (1) hepatic scintiscanning, which demonstrates decreased and nonhomogeneous hepatic uptake of radiocolloid and sometimes shows central localization of radiocolloid, the so-called central hot spot; (2) computed tomography, which shows absence of opacification of the major hepatic veins; (3) ultrasonography, which shows absence of normal hepatic veins; and (4) liver function tests such as BSP and indocyanine green dye clearance, serum alkaline phosphatase, and serum albumin, which invariably show significant hepatic dysfunction.

In patients who are operated upon, the clinical manifestations and results of diagnostic studies are confirmed at operation by the findings of massive ascites; an enlarged, congested liver; splenomegaly; extensive portal-systemic collateral veins; normal IVC pressure; portal hypertension; and a markedly elevated hepatic occluded portal pressure, which sometimes is higher than the free portal pressure.

Nonoperative therapy of BCS includes infusion of thrombolytic agents such as streptokinase and urokinase in the hope of dissolving the thrombi in the hepatic veins and/or IVC; anticoagulant therapy to prevent propagation of the thrombi; and control of ascites by the usual diuretic regimen. None of these measures has been effective, and nonoperative therapy has been associated with an almost uniformly poor prognosis. Most patients have died within a few months of onset of symptoms, and the small number who have survived the acute phase have almost all died from the complications of cirrhosis within a few years.

Side-to-side portacaval shunt has proven to be the most effective therapy of BCS caused by thrombosis of the hepatic veins. Its use is based on substantial evidence demonstrating that it converts the valveless portal vein into an outflow tract, thereby decompressing the obstructed hepatic vascular bed. In an experimental evaluation of portacaval shunt in dogs with BCS, we found that the side-to-side anastomosis decompressed the liver and cured ascites in 96 percent of the dogs, reduced liver size to normal, reversed the pathologic lesions in the liver often to normal, and resulted in long-term survival of many of the dogs (221). On the basis of these experimental findings, we have performed a side-to-side portacaval shunt early in the course of 12 patients with BCS with one operative death and one long-term death. The 11 survivors of the operation have lived free of ascites without diuretic therapy for from 1 to 13 years (Table 62-19). The shunt has remained patent in all patients. Liver function has returned to normal, hepatosplenomegaly has disappeared, and there has been no encephalopathy. Serial liver biopsies performed 2 to 10 years postoperatively showed substantial reversal of the pathologic lesions of BCS. Our experience demonstrates the importance of performing a side-to-side portacaval shunt early in the course of BCS in order to reverse the liver damage and prevent extension of thrombosis from the hepatic veins into the IVC.

A side-to-side portacaval shunt is contraindicated when BCS is caused by thromobosis or occlusion of the IVC. Under such circumstances a mesoatrial shunt has been used with some short-term success, although there has been a high incidence of thrombosis of the bypass graft (222). It is possible that the results of therapy can be improved by substituting for mesoatrial shunt the combined procedure of side-to-side portacaval shunt and caval-atrial bypass.

Orthotopic liver transplantation is indicated in patients with chronic BCS who have progressive hepatic failure, and in patients who have had an unsuccessful portal-systemic shunt unless the underlying cause of BCS is uncontrollable (223,224). In 14 patients with advanced and decompensated liver disease due to BCS, liver transplantation has resulted in a 71 percent 1-year survival rate and a 54 percent actuarial 3-year survival rate.

Other surgical procedures of uncertain value in BCS are thoracic transposition of the spleen, peritoneovenous shunt, and percutaneous transluminal angioplasty. Peritoneovenous shunt is a palliative procedure that should not be used as primary treatment of BCS because it does not decompress the liver or influence the ongoing hepatic damage. Percutaneous transluminal

TABLE 62-19. Long-Term Results of Side-to-Side Portacaval Shunt in 12 Patients with Budd-Chiari Syndrome Treated by the Author

			Follow-up					
Case	Predisposing Condition	Duration Onset to Operation, weeks	Years	Ascites	Need for Diuretics	Liver Function Tests	Encephalopathy	Current Status
1	Unknown	6	13	0	0	Normal	0	Alive
2	Unknown	14	12	0	0	Normal	0	Alive
3	Oral contraceptives	7	10	0	0	Normal	0	Alive
4	Unknown	9	9	0	0	Normal	0	Alive
5	Unknown	4	7	0	0	Normal	0	Alive
6	Polycythemia vera	14	Died, 6 days	—	—	—	—	Died, 6 days
7	Behçet's disease	25	2	0	0	Abnormal	0	Died, 2 years
8	Oral contraceptives	15	5	0	0	Normal	0	Alive
9	Unknown	17	4	0	0	Normal	0	Alive
10	Polycythemia vera	8	3	0	0	Normal	0	Alive
11	Oral contraceptives	9	2	0	0	Normal	0	Alive
12	Unknown	78	1	0	0	Abnormal	0	Alive

angioplasty has had some short-term success in five patients with chronic BCS due to stenosis of the IVC.

Several surgical procedures have been used by Japanese surgeons to treat the chronic form of BCS caused by membranous obstruction of the vena cava (MOVC) (216–218). When the area of IVC obstruction has been short, fracture of the "membrane" by transcardiac membranotomy has been the principal treatment and has had a short-term success rate of greater than 70 percent. Percutaneous transluminal angioplasty also has been successful in a few patients observed for short periods of follow-up. When the area of IVC obstruction has been long, treatment has consisted of direct excision and repair of the involved area of IVC, or cavoatrial bypass graft. Both of these procedures have had some success but have been associated with a substantial incidence of failure and a high mortality rate. Finally, patients with MOVC have undergone a variety of operations of uncertain value that are designed to create portosystemic or portopulmonary collateral venous connections.

VENOOCCLUSIVE DISEASE

Venoocclusive disease (VOD) is a group of disorders in which hepatic venous outflow obstruction is due to subendothelial sclerosis of the sublobular hepatic veins and terminal hepatic venules within the liver (225–227). VOD is caused by ingestion of plants containing pyrrolizidine alkaloids, antineoplastic drugs, irradiation of the liver, and bone marrow transplantation. Extensive occlusion of the small hepatic veins results in centrilobular hemorrhagic necrosis of the liver parenchyma which progresses to diffuse fibrosis and then cirrhosis. Although VOD can occur at any age, it has been observed most often in children in whom, after a prodromal febrile illness, there is an acute onset of abdominal distension due to ascites, abdominal pain, hepatosplenomegaly, weakness, and sometimes mild jaundice and peripheral edema. Some patients recover from the acute stage of VOD, but approximately one-fifth die and the remainder go on to rapidly develop cirrhosis with all of its clinical manifestations. The most important diagnostic study in VOD is percutaneous needle liver biopsy, which demonstrates the specific abnormality of extensive occlusion of the small hepatic veins within the liver as well as centrilobular hemorrhagic necrosis. The results of hepatic scintiscanning, liver function tests, and wedged hepatic vein pressure (WHVP) measurements are similar to those found in BCS, but angiographic studies are not very helpful because the major hepatic veins and IVC are normal in VOD. Experience with treatment of VOD has been reported only in patients who have the disorder as a result of ingestion of pyrrolizidine alkaloids (228). When such patients are seen in the acute stage, supportive medical therapy is used. Side-to-side portacaval shunt is indicated during the acute stage if bleeding esophageal varices develop or if the clinical and liver biopsy signs of hepatic venous outflow obstruction do not subside after 4 to 8 weeks. In the chronic phase of VOD, when the usual manifestations of cirrhosis have developed, side-to-side portacaval shunt is recommended even before varix hemorrhage has occurred. The mortality rate from chronic VOD is high, and the major cause of death is bleeding esophageal varices.

References

1. Reynolds TB, Ito S, Iwatsuki S: Measurement of portal pressure and its clinical application. Am J Med 1970, 49:649.
2. Popper H: Pathologic aspects of cirrhosis, a review. Am J Pathol 1977, 897:228.
3. Bell RH Jr, Miyai K, Orloff MJ: Response of cirrhotic patients with acute alcoholic hepatitis to emergency portacaval shunt for bleeding varices. Gastroenterology (abstract) 1982, 82:1015.
4. Noble EP (ed): Third Special Report to the U.S. Congress on Alcohol and Health. Rockville, Maryland, US Department of Health, Education, and Welfare, 1978.
5. Ratnoff OD, Patek AJ Jr: Natural history of Laennec's cirrhosis of the liver. Analysis of 386 cases. Medicine 1942, 21:207.
6. Garceau AJ and the Boston Inter-Hospital Liver Group: The natural history of cirrhosis. I. Survival with esophageal varices. N Engl J Med 1963, 268:469.
7. Atik M, Simeone F: Massive gastrointestinal bleeding: A study of 296 patients at City Hospital of Cleveland. Arch Surg 1954, 69:355.
8. Cohn R, Blaisdell FW: The natural history of the patient with cirrhosis of the liver with esophageal varices following the first massive hemorrhage. Surg Gynecol Obstet 1958, 106:699.
9. Higgins WH Jr: The esophageal varix: A report of one hundred and fifteen cases. Am J Med Sci 1947, 214:436.
10. Merigan TC Jr, Hollister RM, Gryska PF, Starkey GWG, Davidson CS: Gastrointestinal bleeding with cirrhosis: Study of 172 episodes in 158 patients. N Engl J Med 1960, 263:579.
11. Nachlas MM, O'Neil JE, Campbell AJA: The life history of patients with cirrhosis of the liver and bleeding esophageal varices. Ann Surg 1955, 141:10.
12. Taylor FW, Jontz JG: Cirrhosis with hemorrhage. Arch Surg 1959, 78:786.
13. Orloff MJ: Emergency treatment of bleeding esophageal varices in cirrhosis. Curr Probl Surg, July 1966, pp. 13–28.
14. Orloff MJ, Thomas HS: Pathogenesis of esophageal varix rupture: A study based on gross and microscopic examination of the esophagus at the time of bleeding. Arch Surg 1963, 87:301.
15. Liebowitz HR: Pathogenesis of esophageal varix rupture. JAMA 1961, 175:874.
16. Hoare AM: Comparative study between endoscopy and radiology in acute upper gastrointestinal hemorrhage. Br Med J 1975, 1:27.
17. Orloff MJ: Emergency portacaval shunt for bleeding esophageal varices. In Fiddian-Green RG, Turcotte JG (eds): *Gastrointestinal Hemorrhage*. New York, Grune & Stratton, 1980, pp 295–310.
18. Viamonte M Jr, Warren WD, Fomon JJ, Martinez LO: Angiographic investigations in portal hypertension. Surg Gynecol Obstet 1970, 130:37.
19. Sloop RD, Orloff MJ: An important syndrome of metabolic alkalosis in patients with cirrhosis, bleeding varices, and portacaval shunt. Surg Forum 1966, 17:37.
20. Del Guercio LRM, Coommaraswamy RP, Feins NR, Woolman SB, State D: Pulmonary arteriovenous admixture and the hyperdynamic cardiovascular state in surgery for portal hypertension. Surgery 1964, 56:74.
21. Siegel JH, Greenspan M, Cohn JD, Del Guercio LRM: The prognostic implications of altered physiology in operations for portal hypertension. Surg Gynecol Obstet 1968, 126:249.
22. Siegel JH, Williams JB: A computer based index for the prediction of operative survival in patients with cirrhosis and portal hypertension. Ann Surg 1969, 169:191.
23. Ludington AG: A study of 158 cases of esophageal varices. Surg Gynecol Obstet 1958, 106:519.

24. Conn HO: Hazards attending the use of esophageal tamponade. N Engl J Med 1958, 259:701.
25. Read AE, Dawson AM, Kerr DNS, Turner MD, Sherlock S: Bleeding oesophageal varices treated by oesophageal compression tube. Br Med J 1960, 1:227.
26. Orloff MJ, Halasz NA, Lipman CA, Schwabe AD, Thompson JC, Weidner WA: The complications of cirrhosis of the liver. Ann Intern Med 1967, 66:165.
27. Villanueva A, Magnenat P: Resultats du traitement des hemorrhagies oesophagogastriques sur varices par la sonde de Sengstaken-Blakemore. Gastroenterologia 1964, 102:242.
28. Hermann RE, Traul D: Experience with the Sengstaken-Blakemore tube for bleeding esophageal varices. Surg Gynecol Obstet 1970, 130:879.
29. Pitcher JL: Safety and effectiveness of the modified Sengstaken-Blakemore tube: A prospective study. Gastroenterology 1971, 61:291.
30. Johansen TS, Baden H: Re-appraisal of the Sengstaken-Blakemore balloon tamponade for bleeding esophageal varices, results in 91 patients. Scand J Gastroenterol 1973, 18:181.
31. Novis BH, Duys P, Barbezat GO, Clain J, Bank S, Terblanche J: Fiberoptic endoscopy and the use of the Sengstaken tube in actue gastrointestinal hemorrhage in patients with portal hypertension and varices. Gut 1976,17:258.
32. Teres J, Anastasio C, Bordas JM, Rimola A, Bru C, Rodes J: Esophageal tamponade for bleeding varices. Controlled trial between the Sengstaken-Blakemore tube and the Linton-Nachlas tube. Gastroenterology 1978, 75:566.
33. Conn HO, Simpson JA: Excessive mortality associated with balloon tamponade of bleeding varices. JAMA 1967, 202:587.
34. Schwartz SI, Bales HW, Emerson GL, Mahoney EB: Use of intravenous Pituitrin in treatment of bleeding esophageal varices. Surgery 1959, 45:72.
35. Merigan TC, Plotkin GR, Davidson CS: Effect of intravenously administered posterior pituitary extract on hemorrhage from bleeding varices. N Engl J Med 1962, 266:134.
36. Shaldon S, Sherlock S: The use of vasopressin (Pitressin) in the control of bleeding from oesophageal varices. Lancet 1960, 2:222.
37. Johnson WC, Widrich WC, Ansell JE, Robbins AH, Nasbeth DC: Control of bleeding varices by vasopressin: A prospective randomized study. Ann Surg 1977, 186:369.
38. Chojkier M, Groszmann RJ, Atterbury CE, Bar-Meir S, Blei AT, Frankel J, Glickman MG, Kniaz JL, Schade R, Taggart GJ, Conn HO. A controlled comparison of continuous intraarterial and intravenous infusions of vasopressin in hemorrhage from esophageal varices. Gastroenterology 1979, 77:540.
39. Orloff MJ: Emergency treatment of variceal haemorrhage. Can J Surg 1979, 22:550.
40. Mols P, Hallemans R, Van Kuyk M, Melot C, Lejeune P, Ham H, Vertongen F, Naeje R: Hemodynamic effects of vasopressin, alone and in combination with nitroprusside, in patients with liver cirrhosis and portal hypertension. Ann Surg 1984, 199:176.
41. Groszmann RJ, Kravetz D, Bosch J, Glickman M, Bruix J, Bredfeldt J, Conn HO, Rodes J, Storer EH: Nitroglycerin improves the hemodynamic response to vasopressin in portal hypertension. Hepatology 1982, 2:757.
42. Nusbaum M, Baum S, Sakiyalak P, Blakemore WS: Pharmacologic control of portal hypertension. Surgery 1967, 62:299.
43. Barr JW, Lakin RC, Rösch J: Similarity of arterial and intravenous vasopressin in portal and systemic hemodynamics. Gastroenterology 1975, 69:13.
44. Millette B, Huet PM, Lavoie P, Viallet A: Portal and systemic effects of selective infusion of vasopressin into the superior mesenteric artery in cirrhotic patients. Gastroenterology 1975, 69:6.
45. Murray-Lyon I, Pugh RNH, Nunnerley HB, Laws JW, Dawson JL, Williams R: Treatment of bleeding oesophageal varices by infusion of vasopressin into the superior mesenteric artery. Gut 1973, 14:59.
46. Nusbaum M, Younis MT, Baum S, Blakemore WS: Control of portal hypertension. Selective mesenteric arterial infusion of vasopressin. Arch Surg 1974, 108:342.
47. Conn HO, Ramsey GR, Storer EH, Mutchnick MG, Joshi PH, Phillips MM, Cohen GD, Fields GN, Petroski D: Intra-arterial vasopressin in the treatment of upper gastrointestinal hemorrhage: A prospective, controlled clinical trial. Gastroenterology 1975, 68:211.
48. Johnson WC, Widrich WC: Efficacy of selective splanchnic arteriography and vasopressin perfusion in diagnosis and treatment of gastrointestinal hemorrhage. Am J Surg 1976, 131:481.
49. Kaufman SL, Harrington DP, Barth KH, Maddrey WC, White RI Jr: Control of variceal bleeding by superior mesenteric artery vasopressin infusion. Am J Roentgenol 1977, 126:567.
50. Getzen LC, Brink RR, Wolfman EF Jr: Survival following infusion of Pitressin into the superior mesenteric artery to control bleeding esophageal varices in cirrhotic patients. Ann Surg 1978, 187:337.
51. Sherman LM, Shenoy SS, Cerra FB: Selective intraarterial vasopressin: Clinical efficacy and complications. Ann Surg 1979, 189:298.
52. Johnston GW, Rodgers HW: A review of 15 years experience in the use of sclerotherapy in the control of acute haemorrhage from oesophageal varices. Br J Surg 1973, 60:797.
53. Paquet KJ, Oberhammer E: Sclerotherapy of bleeding oesophageal varices by means of endoscopy. Endoscopy 1978, 10:7.
54. Terblanche J, Northover JMA, Bornman P, Kahn D, Barbezat GO, Sellars SL, Saunders SJ: A prospective evaluation of injection sclerotherapy in the treatment of acute bleeding from esophageal varices. Surgery 1979, 85:239.
55. Di Magno EP, George L, Gores A, Carlson GL: Does sclerotherapy alter the natural history of bleeding esophageal varices? (abstract) Gastroenterology 1983, 84:1137.
56. Kjaergaard J, Fischer A, Miskowiask J, Lindahl F, Baden H: Sclerotherapy of bleeding esophageal varices. Long-term results. Scand J Gastroenterol 1982, 17:363.
57. Alwmark A, Bengmark S, Borjesson B, Gullstrand P, Joelsson B: Emergency and long-term transesophageal sclerotherapy of bleeding esophageal varices. A prospective study of 50 consecutive cases. Scand J Gastroenterol 1982, 17:409.
58. MacDougall BRD, Theodossi A, Westaby D, Dawson JL, Williams R: Increased long-term survival in variceal haemorrhage using injection sclerotherapy. Results of a controlled trial. Lancet 1982, 1:124.
59. Goodale RL, Silvis SE, O'Leary JF, Gebhard R, Mjollnes L, Johnson M, Fryd D: Early survival after sclerotherapy for bleeding esophageal varices. Surg Gynecol Obstet 1982, 155:523.
60. Barsoum MS, Bolous FI, El-Rooby AA, Rizk-Allah MA, Ibrahim AS: Tamponade and injection sclerotherapy in the management of bleeding oesophageal varices. Br J Surg 1982, 69:76.
61. Soehendra N, deHeer K, Kempeneers I, Runge M: Sclerotherapy of esophageal varices: Acute arrest of gastrointestinal hemorrhage or long-term therapy? Endoscopy 1983, 15:136.
62. Terblanche J, Kahn D, Campbell JAH, Bornman PC, Jonker MAT, Wright J, Kirsch R: Failure of repeated injection sclerotherapy to improve long-term survival after oesophageal variceal bleeding. Lancet 1983, 1:1328.
63. Westaby D, Williams R: The history of injection sclerotherapy for esophageal varices. Gastrointest Endosc 1983, 29:303.
64. Conn HO: Endoscopic sclerotherapy: An analysis of variants. Hepatology 1983, 3:769.
65. Health and Public Policy Committee, American College of Physicians: Position paper. Endoscopic sclerotherapy for esophageal varices. Ann Intern Med 1984, 100:608.

66. Lunderquist A, Vang J: Transhepatic catheterization and obliteration of the coronary vein in patients with portal hypertension and esophageal varices. N Engl J Med 1974, 291:646.
67. Passariello R, Rossi P, Simonetti G, Ciolina A, Rovighi L: Emergency transhepatic obliteration of bleeding varices. Cardiovasc Radiol 1979, 2:97.
68. Lunderquist A, Borjesson B, Owman T, Bengmark S: Isobutzl-2-cyanoacrylate (Bucrylate) in obliteration of gastric coronary vein and esophageal varices. Am J Roentgenol 1978, 130:1.
69. Turner WW Jr, Ellman BA: Transhepatic embolization in patients with acute variceal hemorrhage. Am J Surg 1981, 142:731.
70. Bengmark S, Borjesson B, Hoevels J, Joelsson B, Lunderquist, A, Owman T: Obliteration of esophageal varices by PTP. A follow-up of 43 patients. Ann Surg 1979, 190–549.
71. Smith-Laing G, Scott J, Long RG, Dick R, Sherlock S: Role of percutaneous transhepatic obliteration of varices in the management of hemorrhage from gastroesophageal varices. Gastroenterology 1981, 80:1031.
72. Sos TA: Transhepatic portal venous embolization of varices; Pros and cons. Radiology 1983, 148:569.
73. Benner KG, Keefe EB, Keller FS, Rösch J: Clinical outcome after percutaneous transhepatic obliteration of esophageal varices. Gastroenterology 1983, 85:146.
74. Lebrec D, Poynard T, Hillon P, Benham JP: Propranolol for prevention of recurrent gastrointestinal bleeding in patients with cirrhosis. A controlled study. N Engl J Med 1981, 305:1371.
75. Lebrec D. Poynard T, Bernuau J, Bercoff E, Nouel O, Capron J-P, Poupon R, Bouvry M, Rueff B, Benhamou J-P: A randomized controlled study of propranolol for prevention of recurrent gastrointestinal bleeding in patients with cirrhosis: A final report. Hepatology 1984, 4:355.
76. Conn HO: Propranolol in portal hypertension: Problems in paradise? Hepatology 1984, 4:560.
77. Burroughs AK, Jenkins WJ, Sherlock S, Dunk A, Walt RP, Osvafor TOK, Mackie S, Dick R: Controlled trial of propranolol for the prevention of recurrent variceal hemorrhage in patients with cirrhosis. N Engl J Med 1983, 309:1539.
78. Boerema I: Bleeding varices of oesophagus in cirrhosis of the liver and Banti's syndrome. Arch Chir Neeri 1949, 1:253.
79. Ottinger LW, Moncure AC: Transthoracic ligation of bleeding esophageal varices in patients with intrahepatic portal obstruction. Ann Surg 1974, 179:35.
80. Rothwell-Jackson RL, Hunt AG: The results obtained with emergency surgery in the treatment of persistent haemorrhage from gastrooesophageal varices in the cirrhotic patient. Br J Surg 1971, 58:205.
81. Wirthlin LS, Linton RR, Ellis DS: Transthoracoesophageal ligation of bleeding esophageal varices. A reappraisal. Arch Surg 1974, 109:688.
82. Orloff MJ: A comparative study of emergency transesophageal ligation and nonsurgical treatment of bleeding esophageal varices in unselected patients with cirrhosis. Surgery 1962, 52:103.
83. Futagawa S, Sugiura M, Hidai J, Shima F: Emergency esophageal transection with paraesophagogastric devascularization for variceal bleeding. World J Surg 1979, 3:229.
84. Johnston GW: Treatment of bleeding varices by oesophageal transection with the SPTU gun. Ann R Coll Surg Engl 1977, 59:404.
85. Pugh RNH, Murray-Lyon PM, Dawson JL, Pietroni MC, Williams R: Transection of the oesophagus for bleeding oesophageal varices. Br J Surg 1973, 60:646.
86. Sugiura M, Futagawa S: Further evaluation of the Sugiura procedure in the treatment of esophageal varices. Arch Surg 1977, 112:1317.
87. Yamamoto S, Hidemura R, Sawada M, Takeshige K, Iwatsuki S: The late results of terminal esophagoproximal gastrectomy (TEPG) with extensive devascularization and splenectomy for bleeding esophageal varices in cirrhosis. Surgery 1976, 80:106.
88. Johnston GW: Six years' experience of oesophageal transection for oesophageal varices using a circular stapling gun. Gut 1982, 23:770.
89. Osborne DR, Hobbs KEF: The acute treatment of haemorrhage from oesophageal varices: A comparison of oesophageal transection and staple gun anastomosis with mesocaval shunt. Br J Surg 1981, 68:734.
90. Kirby R, Burke FD, Jones JDT: Emergency and elective surgical treatment of portal hypertension. Ann Roy Coll Surg Engl 1975, 57:148.
91. George P, Brown G, Ridgway G, Crofts B, Sherlock S: Emergency oesophageal transection in uncontrolled variceal haemorrhage. Brit J Surg 1973, 60:635.
92. Wanamaker SR, Cooperman M, Carey LC: Use of the EEA stapling instrument for control of bleeding esophageal varices. Surgery 1983, 94:620.
93. Koyama K, Takagi Y, Ouchi K, Sato T: Results of esophageal transection for esophageal varices. Am J Surg 1980, 139:204.
94. Johnson G Jr, Womack NA, Gabriele OF, Peters RM: Control of the hyperdynamic circulation in patients with bleeding esophageal varices. Ann Surg 1969, 169:661.
95. Umeyama K, Yoshikawa K, Yamoshita T, Todo T, Satake K: Transabdominal oesophageal transection for oesophageal varices: Experience in 101 patients. Br J Surg 1983, 70:419.
96. Mir J, Ponce J, Juan M, Garrigues V, Pina R, Berenguer J: Esophageal transection and paraesophagogastric devascularization performed as an emergency measure for uncontrolled variceal bleeding. Surg Gynecol Obstet 1982, 155:868.
97. Van Beek DF, Gleysteen JJ, Malangoni MA, Klamer TW, Lewis JD: Mortality and rebleeding after hypertensive variceal disconnections. Arch Surg 1984, 119:446.
98. Orloff MJ: Emergency portacaval shunt: A comparative study of shunt, varix ligation and nonsurgical treatment of bleeding esophageal varices in unselected patients with cirrhosis. Ann Surg 1967, 166:456.
99. Orloff, MJ: Emergency treatment of bleeding esophageal varices. In Markoff NG (ed): *The Therapy of Portal Hypertension*. Stuttgart, Georg Thieme Verlag, 1968, p 211.
100. Orloff MJ: Emergency treatment of bleeding esophageal varices in alcoholic cirrhosis. In Sardesai VM (ed): *Biochemical and Clinical Aspects of Alcohol Metabolism*. Springfield, Illinois, Charles C Thomas, 1969, p 288.
101. Orloff MJ, Chandler JG, Charters AC, Condon JK, Grambort DE, Modafferi TR, Levin SE: Emergency portacaval shunt for bleeding esophageal varices. Prospective study in unselected patients with alcoholic cirrhosis. Arch Surg 1974, 108:298.
102. Orloff MJ, Chandler JG, Charters AC, Condon JK, Grambort DE, Modafferi TR, Levin SE: Portacaval shunt as emergency procedure in unselected patients with alcoholic cirrhosis. Surg Gynecol Obstet 1975, 141:59.
103. Orloff MJ, Bell RH Jr, Hyde PV, Skivolocki WP: Long-term results of emergency portacaval shunt for bleeding esophageal varices in unselected patients with alcoholic cirrhosis. Ann Surg 1980, 192:325.
104. Orloff MJ, Bell RH Jr: Improved survival of unselected cirrhotic patients with bleeding esophageal varices treated by emergency portacaval shunt. Gastroenterology 1983, 84:1389 (abstract).
105. Bell RH Jr, Hyde PVB, Skivolocki WP, Brimm JE, Orloff MJ: Prospective study of portasystemic encephalopathy after emergency portacaval shunt for bleeding varices. Am J Surg 1981, 142:144.
106. Isbell H, Fraser HF, Wikler A, Belleville RE, Eisenman AJ: An experimental study of the etiology of ''rum fits'' and delirium tremens. Q J Stud Alcohol 1955, 16:1.

107. Nielson, J: An intensive one year study of delirium tremens in Copenhagen. Acta Psychiatr Scand [Suppl 187] 1965, 41:32.
108. Fischer JE: Heaptic coma in cirrhosis, portal hypertension, and following portacaval shunt. Its etiologies and the current status of its treatment. Arch Surg 1974, 108:325.
109. Schenker S, Breen KJ, Hoyumpa AM Jr: Hepatic encephalopathy. Current status. Gastroenterology 1974, 66:121.
110. Zieve L, Nicoloff DM: Pathogenesis of hepatic coma. Ann Rev Med 1975, 26:143.
111. Clark JS, Ozeran RS, Hart JC, Cruze K: Peptic ulcer following portacaval shunt. Ann Surg 1958, 148:551.
112. Phillips MM, Ramsby GA, Conn HO: Portacaval anastomosis and peptic ulcer: A nonassociation. Gastroenterology 1975, 68:121.
113. Papper S: Renal failure in cirrhosis (the hepatorenal syndrome). In Epstein M (ed): *The Kidney in Liver Disease*. New York, Elsevier, 1976, pp 91–112.
114. Wilkinson SP, Williams R: Renal failure in cirrhosis: Current views and speculations. Adv Nephrol 1977, 7:15.
115. Wong PY, McCoy GC, Spielberg A, Milara RV, Balint JA: The hepatorenal syndrome. Gastroenterology 1979, 77:1326.
116. Gabuzda GJ: Nutrition and liver disease. Practical considerations. Med Clin North Am 1970, 54:1455.
117. Mikkelson WP: Therapeutic portacaval shunt. Preliminary data on controlled trial and morbid effects of acute hyaline necrosis. Arch Surg 1974, 108:301.
118. Orloff MJ: Elective therapeutic porta-caval shunt. In Orloff MJ, Stipa S, Ziparo V (eds): *Medical and Surgical Problems of Portal Hypertension*. London, New York, Academic Press, 1980, p 127.
119. Burchell AR, Moreno AH, Panke WF, Nealon TF: Hemodynamic variables and prognosis following portacaval shunt. Surg Gynecol Obstet 1974, 138:359.
120. Burchell AR, Moreno AH, Panke WF, Nealon TF Jr: Hepatic artery flow improvement after portacaval shunt: A single hemodynamic clinical correlate. Ann Surg 1976, 184:289.
121. Campbell DS, Parker DE, Anagnostopoulos CE: Survival prediction in portacaval shunts: A computerized statistical analysis. Am J Surg 1973, 126:748.
122. Charters AC, Brown BN, Sviokla S, Knox D, Orloff MJ: The influence of portal perfusion on the response to portacaval shunt. Am J Surg 1975, 130:226.
123. Child CG III, Turcotte JG: Surgery and portal hypertension. In Child CG III (ed): *The Liver and Portal Hypertension*. Philadelphia, Saunders, 1964, p 1.
124. Eckhauser FE, Appelman HD, O'Leary TJ, Palley TZ, Block DM, Turcotte JG: Hepatic pathology as a determinant of prognosis after portal decompression. Am J Surg 1980, 139:105.
125. Kanel CC, Kaplan MM, Zawacki JK, Callow AD: Survival in patients with postnecrotic cirrhosis and Laennec's cirrhosis undergoing therapeutic portacaval shunt. Gastroenterology 1977, 73:679.
126. Kessler RE, Tice DA, Soloway AC, Zimmon DS: Clinical vs hemodynamic classification of cirrhosis. Surg Forum 1975, 26:417.
127. Mikkelson WP, Kern WH: The influence of acute hyaline necrosis on survival after emergency and elective portacaval shunt. Major Probl Clin Surg 1974, 14:233.
128. Orloff MJ, Duguay LR, Kosta LD: Criteria for selection of patients for emergency portacaval shunt. Am J Surg 1977, 134:146.
129. Price JB Jr, Britton RC, Voorhees AB Jr: The significance and limitations of operative hemodynamics in portal hypertension. Arch Surg 1967, 95:843.
130. Steegmuller KW, Marklin H-M, Hollis HW Jr: Intraoperative hemodynamic investigations during portacaval shunt. Arch Surg 1984, 119:269.
131. Siegel JH, Goldwyn RM, Farrell EJ, Gallin P, Friedman HP: Hyperdynamic states and the physiologic determinants of survival in patients with cirrhosis and portal hypertension. Arch Surg 1974, 108:282.
132. Smith GW: Use of hemodynamic selection criteria in the management of cirrhotic patients with portal hypertension. Ann Surg 1974, 179:182.
133. Turcotte JG, Lambert MJ III: Variceal hemorrhage, hepatic cirrhosis, and portacaval shunts. Surgery 1973, 73:810.
134. Bell RH Jr, Miyai K, Orloff MJ: Outcome in cirrhotic patients with acute alcoholic hepatitis after emergency portacaval shunt for bleeding esophageal varices. Am J Surg 1984, 147:78.
135. Barnes BA, Ackroyd FW, Battit GE, Kantrowitz PA, Schapiro EH, Strole WE, Todd DP, McDermott WV Jr: Elective portosystemic shunts: Morbidity and survival data. Ann Surg 174:76, 1971.
136. Bismuth H, Franco D, Hepp J: Portal-systemic shunt in hepatic cirrhosis. Does the type of shunt decisively influence the clinical result? Ann Surg 1974, 179:209.
137. Linton RR, Ellis DS, Geary JE: Critical comparative analysis of early and late results of splenorenal and direct portacaval shunts performed in 169 patients with portal cirrhosis. Ann Surg 1961, 154:446.
138. McDermott WV, Pallazzi H, Nardi GL, Mondet A: Elective portal systemic shunt. N Engl J Med 1961, 264:419.
139. Mikkelson WP, Turrill FR, Pattison AC: Portacaval shunt in cirrhosis of the liver. Clinical and hemodynamic aspects. Am J Surg 1962, 104:204.
140. Orloff MJ: Portal hypertension: Portacaval anastomosis. In Dudley H, Pories WJ, Carter DC (eds): *Rob and Smith's Operative Surgery*, ed 4. London, Butterworths, 1983, pp 546–569.
141. Voorhees AB Jr, Price JB Jr, Britton RC: Porta-systemic shunting procedures for portal hypertension. Twenty-six year experience in adults with cirrhosis of the liver. Ann Surg 1970, 119:501.
142. Walker RM, Shaldon C, Vowles KD: Late results of portacaval anastomosis. Lancet 1961, 2:727.
143. Ottinger LW: The Linton splenorenal shunt in the management of the bleeding complications of portal hypertension. Ann Surg 1982, 196:664.
144. Wantz GE, Payne MA: Experience with portacaval shunt for portal hypertension. N Engl J Med 1961, 265:721.
145. Jackson FC, Perrin ED, Felix WR, Smith AG: A clinical investigation of the portacaval shunt. V. Survival analyses of the therapeutic operation. Ann Surg 1971, 174:672.
146. Resnick RH, Sher FL, Ishihara AM, Chalmers TC, Zimmerman H, The Boston Inter-Hospital Liver Group: A controlled study of the therapeutic portacaval shunt. Gastroenterology 1974, 67:843.
147. Rueff B, Degos F, Degos JD, Maillard JN, Prandi D, Sicot C, Fauvert R, Benhamou JP: A controlled study of therapeutic portacaval shunt in cirrhosis. Lancet 1976, 1:655.
148. Conn HO: Therapeutic portacaval anasotmosis: To shunt or not to shunt. Gastroenterology 1974, 67:1065.
149. Grace ND, Muench H, Chalmers TC: The present status of shunts for portal hypertension in cirrhosis. Gastroenterology 1966, 50:684.
150. Tamaki A, Golby M, Orloff MJ: Effects of side-to-side portacaval shunt on hepatic hemodynamics and metabolism. Surg Forum 1968, 19:324.
151. Reynolds TB, Hudson NM, Mikkelson WP, Turrill FL, Redeker AG: Clinical comparison of end-to-side and side-to-side portacaval shunt. N Engl J Med 1966, 274:706.
152. Iwatsuki S, Mikkelson WP, Redeker AG, Reynolds TB, Turrill FL: Clinical comparison of the end-to-side and side-to-side portacaval shunt: Ten year follow-up. Ann Surg 1973, 178:65.
153. Panke WF, Rousselot LM, Burchell AR: A sixteen-year experience with end-to-side portacaval shunt for variceal hemorrhage: Analysis of data and comparison with other types of portasystemic anastomoses. Ann Surg 1968, 168:956.

154. Turcotte JG, Wallin VW Jr, Child CG II: End-to-side versus side-to-side portacaval shunts in patients with hepatic cirrhosis. Am J Surg 1969, 117:108.
155. Bernstein JE, Nutting RO, Orloff MJ: Comparison of the effects of end-to-side and side-to-side portacaval shunts on liver function, liver blood flow, and ammonia metabolism in dogs and man. Surg Forum 1968, 19:328.
156. Orloff MJ, Chandler JG, Charters AC, Condon JK, Grambort DE, Modafferi TR, Levin SE: Comparison of end-to-side and side-to-side portacaval shunt in dogs and human subjects with cirrhosis and portal hypertension. Am J Surg 1974, 128:195.
157. Charters AC, Chandler JG, Condon JK, Grambort DE, Levin SE, Modafferi TR, Orloff MJ: Spontaneous reversal of portal flow in patients with bleeding varices treated by emergency portacaval shunt. Am J Surg 1974, 127:25.
158. Cameron JL, Zuidema GD, Smith GW, Harrington DP, Maddrey WC: Mesocaval shunts for the control of bleeding esophageal varices. Surgery 1979, 85:257.
159. Dowling JB: Ten years' experience with mesocaval grafts. Surg Gynecol Obstet 1979, 149:518.
160. Drapanas T: Interposition mesocaval shunt for treatment of portal hypertension. Ann Surg 1972, 176:435.
161. Drapanas T, LoCicero J III, Dowling JB: Hemodynamics of the interposition mesocaval shunt. Ann Surg 1975, 181–523.
162. Graziano JL, Sullivan HJ: Portal decompression: Clinical experience with the "H" graft. Ann Surg 1973, 178:109.
163. Thompson BW, Read RC: Interposition "H" grafting for portal hypertension. Arch Surg 1974, 108:502.
164. Mulcare RJ, Halleran D, Gardine R: Experience with 49 consecutive Dacron interposition mesocaval shunts. Am J Surg 1984, 147:393.
165. Reznick RK, Langer B, Taylor BR, Lossing A, Blendes LM, Colapinto RF: Results and hemodynamics changes after interposition mesocaval shunt. Surgery 1984, 95:275.
166. Warren WD, Salam AA: Surgery for the portal hypertension of cirrhosis; The need for change. Major Prob Clin Surg 1974, 14:127.
167. Bhalerao RA, Pinto AC, Bapat RD, Shetty SV, Bhide PD, Wainganker VS, Kirtane JM, Mehendale VG, Shetty SD: Selective transplenic decompression of oesophageal varices by distal splenorenal and splenocaval shunt. Gut 1978, 19:831.
168. Langer B, Rotstein LE, Stone RM, Taylor BR, Patel SC, Blendis LM, Colapinto RF: A prospective randomized trial of the selective distal splenorenal shunt. Surg Gynecol Obstet 1980, 150:45.
169. Maillard J, Flamant YM, Hay JM, Chandler JG: Selectivity of the distal splenorenal shunt. Surgery 1979, 86:663.
170. Martin EW Jr, Molnar J, Cooperman M, Pace WG, Thomford NR, Casey LC: Observations on fifty distal splenorenal shunts. Surgery 1978, 84:379.
171. Rikkers LF, Rudman D, Galambos JT, Fulenwider JT, Millikan WJ, Kutner M, Smith RB, Salam AA, Jones PJ Jr, Warren WD: Randomized controlled trial of the distal splenorenal shunt. Ann Surg 1978, 187:271.
172. Rotstein LE, Mahowka L, Langer B, Blendis LM, Stone RM, Colapinto RF: Thrombosis of the portal vein following distal splenorenal shunt. Surg Gynecol Obstet 1979, 149:847.
173. Salam AA, Warren WD, Le Page Jr, Viamonte MR, Hutson D, Zeppa R: Hemodynamic contrasts between selective and total portal-systemic decompression. Ann Surg 1971, 173:827.
174. Turcotte JG, Eckhauser FE: Elective portosystemic shunts. In Fiddian-Green RG, Turcotte JG (eds): *Gastrointestinal Hemorrhage*. New York, Grune & Stratton, 1980, p 311.
175. Vang J, Simert G, Hansson JA, Thylen V, Bengmark S: Results of a modified distal spleno-renal shunt for portal hypertension. Ann Surg 1976, 184:224.
176. Warren WD, Salam AA, Hutson D, Zeppa R: Selective distal splenorenal shunt. Technique and results of operation. Arch Surg 1974, 108:306.
177. Zeppa R, Hensley GT, Levi JU, Bergstresser PR, Hutson DG Sr, Livingstone AS, Schiffer, Fink P: The comparative survival of alcoholics versus nonalcoholics after distal splenorenal shunt. Ann Surg 1978, 187:510.
178. Fischer JE, Bower RH, Atamian S, Welling R: Comparison of distal and proximal splenorenal shunts. A randomized prospective trial. Ann Surg 1981, 194:531.
179. Warren WD, Millikan WJ Jr, Henderson JM, Wright L, Kutner M, Smith RB III, Fulenwider JT, Salam AA, Galambos JT: Ten years portal hypertensive surgery at Emory. Ann Surg 1982, 195:530.
180. Henderson M, Millikan WJ Jr, Chipponi J, Wright L, Jones PJ, Meier L, Warren WD: The incidence and natural history of thrombus in the portal vein following distal splenorenal shunt. Ann Surg 1982, 196:1.
181. Belghiti J, Grenier P, Nouel O, Nahum H, Fekete F: Long-term loss of Warren's shunt selectivity. Angiographic demonstration. Arch Surg 1981, 166:1121.
182. Maillard JN, Benhamou JP, Rueff B: Arterialization of the liver with portacaval shunt in the treatment of portal hypertension due to intrahepatic block. Surgery 1970, 67:883.
183. Maillard JN, Rueff B, Prandi D, Sicot C: Hepatic arterialization and portacaval shunt in hepatic cirrhosis. An assessment. Arch Surg 1974, 108:315.
184. Inokuchi K: Selective decompression of esophageal varices by a left gastric venacaval shunt. Surg Ann 1978, 10:215.
185. Baird RJ, Tutassaura H, Miyagishma RT: Use of the left renal vein for portal decompression. Ann Surg 1971, 173:551.
186. Sobel S, Kaplitt MJ, Popowitz L, Girardet RE, Adamsons RD: Omphalocaval shunt: A new procedure for portal decompression. Surgery 1970, 68:456.
187. Conn PO: Prophylactic portacaval shunts. Ann Intern Med 1969, 70:859.
188. Conn PO, Lindenmuth WW: Prophylactic portacaval anastomosis in cirrhosis patients with esophageal varices. Interim results with suggestions for subsequent investigations. N Engl J Med 1968, 279:725.
189. Jackson FC, Perrin, EB, Smith AG, Dagradi AE, Nadal HM: A clinical investigation of the portacaval shunt. II. Survival analysis of the prophylactic operation. Am J Surg 1967, 115:22.
190. Resnick RH, Chalmers TC, Ishihara AM, Garceau AJ, Callow AD, Schimmel EM, O'Hara ET, Boston Inter-Hospital Liver Group: A controlled study of the prophylactic portacaval shunt. A final report. Ann Intern Med 1969, 70:675.
191. Clatworthy HW Jr, Boles ET Jr: Extrahepatic portal bed block in children: Pathogenesis and treatment. Ann Surg 1959, 150:371.
192. Clatworthy HW Jr, DeLorimer AA: Portal decompression procedures in children. Am J Surg 1964, 107:447.
193. Fonkalsrud EW, Myers NA, Robinson MJ: Management of extrahepatic portal hypertension in children. Ann Surg 1974, 180:487.
194. Grauer SE, Schwartz SI: Extrahepatic portal hypertension. A retrospective analysis. Ann Surg 1979, 189:566.
195. Mikkelsen WP: Extrahepatic portal hypertension in children. Am J Surg 1966, 111:333.
196. Voorhees AB Jr, Price JB Jr: Extrahepatic portal hypertension. A retrospective analysis of 127 cases and associated clinical implications. Arch Surg 1974, 108:338.
197. Walker RM: Treatment of portal hypertension in children. Proc R Soc Med 1962, 55:770.
198. Bismuth H, Franco S: Portal diversion for portal hypertension in children. The first ninety patients. Ann Surg 1980, 192:18.
199. Belli L, Puttini M, Marni A: Extrahepatic portal obstruction.

Clinical experience and surgical treatment in 105 patients. J Cardiovasc Surg 1980, 21:439.

200. Webb, LJ, Sherlock S: The aetiology, presentation and natural history of extra-hepatic portal venous obstruction. J Med 1979, 58:627.

201. Alvarez F, Bernard O, Brunelle F, Hadchouel P, Odievre M, Alagille D: Portal obstruction in children. II. Results of surgical porto-systemic shunts. J Pediatr 1983, 103:703.

202. Hyatt RE, Smith JR: The mechanism of ascites. Am J Med 1954, 16:434.

203. Lieberman FL, Denison EK, Reynolds TB: The relationship of plasma volume, portal hypertension, ascites, and renal sodium retention in cirrhosis. The overflow theory of ascites formation. Ann NY Acad Sci 1970, 170:202.

204. Madden JL, Lore JM Jr, Gerold FP, Ravid JM: The pathogenesis of ascites and a consideration of its treatment. Surg Gynecol Obstet 1954, 99:385.

205. Sherlock S, Shaldon S: The aetiology and management of ascites in patients with hepatic cirrhosis. A review. Gut 1963, 4:95.

206. Orloff MJ, Ross TH, Baddeley RM, Nutting RO, Spitz BR, Sloop RD, Neesby TM, Halasz NA: Experimental ascites. VI. The effects of hepatic venous outflow obstruction and ascites on aldosterone secretion. Surgery 1964, 56:83.

207. Orloff MJ, Spitz BR, Wall MH, Thomas HS, Halasz NA: Experimental ascites. IV. A comparison of the effects of end-to-side and side-to-side portacaval shunts on intractable ascites. Surgery 1964, 56:784.

208. Orloff MJ, Wright PM, DeBendetti MJ, Halasz NA, Annetts DL, Musicant ME: Experimental ascites. VII. The effects of external drainage of the thoracic duct on ascites and hepatic hemodynamics. Arch Surg 1966, 93:119.

209. Orloff MJ: Surgical treatment of intractable cirrhotic ascites. In Longmire WP Jr (ed): *Portal Hypertension*. Curr Probl Surg, July 1966, p 28.

210. Orloff MJ: Effect of side-to-side portacaval shunt on intractable ascites, sodium excretion, and aldosterone metabolism in man. Am J Surg 1966, 112:297.

211. Orloff MJ: Pathogenesis and surgical treatment of intractable ascites associated with alcoholic cirrhosis. Ann NY Acad Sci 1970, 170:273.

212. Parker RGF: Occlusion of the hepatic veins in man. Medicine (Baltimore) 1959, 38:369.

213. Powell-Jackson PR, Melia W, Canalese J, Pickford RB, Portmann B, Williams R: Budd-Chiari syndrome: Clinical patterns and therapy. Q J Med 1982, 201:79.

214. Mitchell MC, Boitnott JK, Kaufman S, Cameron JR, Maddrey WC: Budd-Chiari syndrome: Etiology, diagnosis and management. Medicine (Baltimore) 1982, 61:199.

215. Orloff MJ: Budd-Chiari syndrome and veno-occlusive disease. In Blumgart LH (ed): *Surgery of the Liver and Biliary Tract*. Edinburgh, Churchill Livingstone, In press.

216. Yamamoto S, Yokoyama Y, Takeshige K, Iwatsuki S: Budd-Chiari syndrome with obstruction of the inferior vena cava. Gastroenterology 1968, 54:1070.

217. Hirooka M, Kimura C: Membranous obstruction of the hepatic portion of the inferior vena cava. Arch Surg 1970, 100:656.

218. Khuroo MS, Datta DV: Budd-Chiari syndrome following pregnancy. Report of 16 cases with roentgenologic, hemodynamic and histologic studies of the hepatic outflow tract. Am J Med 1980, 68:113.

219. Semson IW: Membranous obstruction of the inferior vena cava and hepatocellular carcinoma in South Africa. Gastroenterology 1982, 82:171.

220. Okuda K: Membranous obstruction of the inferior vena cava: Etiology and relation to hepatocellular carcinoma. Gastroenterology 1982, 82:376.

221. Orloff MJ, Johansen KH: Treatment of Budd-Chiari syndrome by side-to-side portacaval shunt: Experimental and clinical results. Ann Surg 1978, 188:494.

222. Cameron JL, Herlong HF, Sanfey H, Boitnott J, Kaufman SL, Gott VL, Maddrey WC: The Budd-Chiari syndrome. Treatment by mesenteric-systemic venous shunts. Ann Surg 1983, 198:335.

223. Starzl TE, Iwatsuki S, Shaw BW Jr, Van Thiel DH, Gartner JC, Zitelli BJ, Malatack JJ, Schade RR: Analysis of liver transplantation. Hepatology 1984, 4:47s.

224. Schenker S: Medical treatment vs transplantation in liver disorders. Hepatology 1984, 4:102s.

225. Bras G, Jelliffe DB, Stuart KL: Veno-occlusive disease of the liver with non-portal type of cirrhosis occurring in Jamaica. Arch Pathol 1954, 57:285.

226. Bras G, McLean E: Toxic factors in veno-occlusive disease. Ann NY Acad Sci 1963, 111:392.

227. Stuart KL, Bras G: Veno-occlusive disease of the liver. Q J Med 1957, 26:291.

228. Gore DO, Stuart KL, Bras G: Veno-occlusive disease of the liver: Surgical aspects. Surgery 1961, 49:334.

Chapter 63

THE LYMPHATIC SYSTEM

TIMOTHY A. MILLER and LYGIA STEWART

Lymphedema: Significance of the Problem

Lymphedema, or the presence of an abnormally large amount of fluid in the intercellular spaces of the body occurring because of lymphatic dysfunction, is as yet a very poorly understood entity in medicine. Its causes can be congenital or acquired. Chronic lymphedema has no real medical or surgical cure, although various means are available to control the extent of the swelling. It can have serious complications such as recurrent celluitus and, in rare instances, lymphangiosarcoma. A thorough understanding of the normal anatomy, physiology, pathophysiology, and current treatment options along with their complications is essential to finding a solution to this problem.

Historical Aspects

Lymphedema was probably encountered clinically from the earliest beginnings of medical history. Hippocrates wrote of edema of the skin (1); Paul of Aegina and Aretaeus of Cappodocia described "dropsy," elephantiasis, and chronic pedal edema (2,3).

But while causes of edema secondary to infections and renal and vascular etiologies were identified as separate entities (4), lymphedema, as such, was not recognized until much later (5). Perhaps one reason for this is the largely microscopic nature of lymphatics, making them difficult to study or even recognize. And it was not until after the lymphatic system was described that the concept of lymphedema became known. There is evidence that the ancients saw lymph, but they did not correlate it with edema. Hippocrates and Aristotle spoke and wrote of "white blood" and "colorless fluid," but they knew nothing of a lymphatic system which was first described in 1627 by Gaspare Aselli. More than a century later Mascagni published the first systemic description of the lymphatic system in 1787. Hewson in 1774 and Cruikshank in 1789 were the first to postulate the involvement of this newfound lymphatic system in various pathological conditions and to suggest that its obstruction could lead to lymphedema. Sterling in 1894 put forth his theories on filtration and absorption which explained the pathophysiological process of lymphedema (5). The first mention of congenital lymphedema was in 1892 when Milroy described Milroy's disease (6), and surgical causes of lymphedema were first noted by Halstead in 1921 (7).

It is difficult to date the various medical approaches to the problem, but surgical approaches can be more easily documented. Lymphangioplasty, the first surgical procedure described in modern literature, appeared in 1908 by Handley (8). Kondoleon suggested excision of muscle fascia, and in 1912 Charles described excision of skin and subcutaneous tissue with grafting (9). In 1917, Sistrunck (10) described a successful approach of subcutaneous and skin excision beneath flaps, and this was reintroduced in 1936 by Homans (11). Thompson (12) suggested the de-epithelialized dermal flap in 1962, Goldsmith (13) the omental flap in 1967, and Rivero (14) the lymphatic-venous anastomosis technique in the 1960s. Finally O'Brien proposed microsurgical reanastomosis in 1976 (15).

Pathophysiology

To have a complete understanding of lymphedema pathophysiology an understanding of the anatomy and normal physiology of the lymphatic system is essential.

ANATOMY OF THE LYMPHATIC SYSTEM

It is generally agreed that lymphatics and lymph nodes arise from endothelial sprouting of the primordial venous system (16,17). This development begins in four areas: the paired jugular and iliac sacs, the cisterna chyli, and the retroperitoneal system. These sacs develop peripherally between the third and eighth week of embryonic life and invade almost all tissues of the body with the major exceptions of the central nervous system, bone marrow, coating of the eye, internal ear, and intralobar portions of the liver. The thoracic duct results from the fusion of the cisterna chyli and the left jugular buds. The lymphatic channels and regional nodes of each extremity are eventually formed by this peripheral growth and drained either into the cisterna chyli (lower extremities) or directly into the thoracic ducts (upper extremities), which return lymph to the venous system.

The lymphatics are similar to capillaries; however, the basement membrane which is present in capillaries is absent in lymphatics. The lymphatic capillaries progress in size into collecting lymphatics. These form a valved system which connects to the original lymph nodes. The collecting lymphatics have intimal, medial, and adventitial layers with elastic fibers and smooth muscle in the media in direct proportion to lymphatic size.

Leg Lymphatics

The subcutaneous compartment (in which lymphedema occurs) is drained by three groups of lymphatics: a dermal plexus, collecting channels, and superficial lymphatic trunks. The intradermal lymphatics do not have valves and drain into the valved system lying in the deepest dermal level at the subcutaneous junction (16). By means of collecting channels the dermal plexus drains into main lymphatic trunks located on the surface of the muscle fascia. These lymphatics then drain proximally into the lymph node system. It is these lymphatics that are seen in lymphangiograms.

There is a separate deep lymphatic system which drains the compartments and several channels located near bone. There is general agreement that the superficial and deep lymphatic systems are separate and communicate only under abnormal conditions, such as proximal obstruction (18,19).

As the deep vessels ascend, they maintain a constant diameter and valves can be seen at regular intervals. About four vessels normally drain into the popliteal lymph nodes in the posterior knee, and four to six vessels ascend the thigh medially in the deep subcutaneous system to drain into the deep inguinal nodes.

The superficial lymphatic system, which can more easily be studied by lymphangiography, drains into two pathways closely corresponding to the venous drainage of the leg. One system courses parallel to the saphenous vein and a second along the lesser saphenous system. These trunks are also valved. They bifurcate, rejoin, and maintain the same diameter as they ascend the extremity. Some evidence exists that lymphatic channels draining the lower leg do not receive tributaries from the thigh. Lymphangiographic studies have shown that the skin and subcutaneous tissue of the thigh drains into the superior inguinal lymph nodes, while the lower leg drains into the more inferior inguinal nodes (20). Because of this, in some patients with acquired lymphedema, the swelling may be limited to the lower leg.

The inguinal nodes are divided into two groups: superficial (around the fossa ovalis) and deep (around the fatty tissue of the femoral sheath). These nodes drain proximally into the nodes around the iliac vessels. Although virtually all lymphatic flow passes through the inguinal nodes, it has been shown that lymph drainage can bypass these nodes and drain directly into the iliac area (21).

Arm Lymphatics

The superficial lymphatic channels appear anatomically similar to those in the leg, coursing along the general pattern of the basilic (medial aspect) and cephalic (lateral aspect) veins. At times they may join each other, but normally they course separately until they drain into axillary nodes.

PHYSIOLOGY OF THE LYMPHATIC SYSTEM

The lymphatic system serves a number of functions: drainage of a fraction of the macromolecular protein loss from the capillary circulation; removal of bacteria and foreign material; and transport of specific substances, such as vitamin K, from the gastrointestinal tract. Lymphatics at the capillary level are extremely permeable and have a low hydrostatic pressure compared to interstitial fluid (21–24). Because of the marked permeability and hydrostatic differences as well as the valved nature of the system, lymph normally passes proximally and does not usually accumulate within the interstitium. Lymph is essentially an ultrafiltrate somewhat similar to plasma; it forms as a transudate resulting from the relatively high hydrostatic pressure of the arterial system. Over a 24-hour period approximately 50 percent of the circulating albumin can be lost from the arterial-capillary system (24). Although the vast majority of that protein loss is resorbed into the venules by a combination of osmotic and hydrostatic forces, a minimal amount (approximately 0.1 percent) is not resorbed (20). The lymphatic system is responsible for the return of this fraction of the macromolecular capillary loss. In the normal extremity, lymph contains 0.1 to 0.5 g of total protein per 100 mL as compared to 6 g of protein per 100 mL in blood. Interestingly, in this dilute protein concentration there is a disproportionately high ratio of albumin to globulin because of the higher molecular weight of globulin. This emphasizes the fact that lymph results from an ultrafiltration process across a semipermeable membrane. Once lymph enters a lymphatic from the extracellular spaces, it is not appreciably altered or concentrated (25).

Lymph flow proximally results from a combination of factors: interstitial pressure; the negative and positive fluctuation in the intraabdominal and intrathoracic cavities; and the adjacent compression of the arterial pulsations in muscular activity. The valves promote proximally directed flow. It is likely that compression of arterial pulsations and muscular contractions are particularly influential on the flow within the deep lymphatic system.

There is some question as to whether lymphatic flow is assisted by an intrinsic contracture mechanism within the vessels themselves. The lymphatic vessels are known to contain muscle fibers as well as nerve endings. Several investigators have shown that the lymphatics of various laboratory animals respond to a variety of a hormonal and chemical influences, and it seems likely that some function similar to peristalsis does exist (26–30).

LYMPHEDEMA

Lymphedema has several causes, but in all types there is impaired transcapillary fluid exchange and impaired transport of lymph. This ultimately results in an edematous, and, later, fibrotic, indurated extremity. Different factors characterize the acquired and primary (congenital) types of this condition, but in both, lymph drainage fails to keep up with production, resulting in accumulation of a relatively protein rich interstitial fluid. In chronic lymphedema, total protein may be as high as 5 g per 100 mL, compared to the normal value of 0.1 to 0.5 g per 100 mL and the value of 0.9 g per 100 mL in cardiac failure (25). The high osmotic pressure secondary to the high protein concentration will further attract even greater amounts of fluid. A new balance of pressures is established at a higher level, and the increase in interstitial pressure in surrounding tissue compliance tends to increase lymph flow.

Fibrosis of the extremity is caused by two factors: (1) that resulting from the protein-rich edema fluid, and (2) that due to depression of macrophage activity. The protein-rich environment results in the formation of edema by two mechanisms. First, edema occurs in areas of poorly oxygenated, stagnated fluid with accumulation of metabolic products. These metabolic disturbances induce the formation of fibrin and fibrous tissue. Second, the protein-rich environment favors the deposition of collagen, thus shifting the usual balance between collagen lysis and deposition toward deposition (31). As mentioned, depression of macrophage activity is the second factor causing tissue fibrosis. In normal tissue macrophages play a role in inducing collagen lysis. Studies show that macrophages in lymphedematous tissue are in a depressed state, and thus collagen lysis is also decreased. All these factors combine to cause tissue fibrosis, which in itself further inhibits the ability of the lymphatic vessels to clear the excess fluid, and a cycle of further lymphedema and tissue fibrosis is perpetuated (31).

Clinical Presentation

Lymphedema can be caused by several factors which can generally be categorized under acquired or primary (congenital) etiologies. Lymphedema is most commonly acquired from infections or parasitic etiologies; from trauma to lymphatic channels secondary to burns, radiation, surgery, or direct injury; from allergic reactions resulting in lymphedema; after a trauma; and from malignant etiologies. Patients designated as having primary lymphedema are born with a reduced number of lymphatics or lymphatics which are structurally abnormal.

Though the etiologies vary, the clinical picture is similar but can vary from mild extremity swelling to seriously disabling or life-threatening complications such as recurrent cellulitis and lymphangiosarcoma.

Early edema fluid accumulation results in a soft pitting type of edema, usually beginning in the ankle and gradually ascending. Modest increases in extremity diameter can be associated with substantial weight increases. Such patients typically complain of fatigue in the involved extremity. Corresponding with the duration of the lymphedema, the protein concentration of the edema fluid gradually increases. The combined lymphatic stasis and accumulation of interstitial fluid provide an ideal culture medium for bacteria. As many as 25 percent of patients have recurrent episodes of lymphangitis (28). Attacks of lymphangitis account for a significant morbidity in some patients and can occur several times a year, often without preceding trauma. With progressive edema there is increased fibrosis of the connective tissue elements within the subcutaneous tissue in skin. The lymphangitis accelerates the process of fibrosis. In chronic lymphedema (elephantasis, for example) the skin is thick and hyperkeratotic and the entire extremity is indurated with nonpitting edema.

PRIMARY LYMPHEDEMA

As mentioned, primary lymphedema results from lymphatic abnormalities present at birth. This group of edemas can be categorized in several ways. Two methods of classification are (1) by age of onset, and (2) by lymphangiographic findings. These will be discussed below. A third category comprising benign tumors of lymphatics will be dealt with separately.

Classification by Age of Onset

This is a purely arbitrary distinction first employed by Kinmonth (32) in which primary lymphedema is categorized into congenital lymphedema, lymphedema praecox, and lymphedema tarda based on the age of onset. While it is a useful classification, it may not be a true distinction pathophysiologically.

Congenital lymphedema includes all forms of lymphedema present at birth. Presumably this would also include benign lymphatic tumors which are usually present at birth. These are considered separately below. Milroy's disease is a specific subset of this category with the following characteristics: (1) it represents about 2 percent of the primary lymphedemas; (2) it has a familial pattern with an autosomal dominant inheritance pattern, thus affecting males and females almost equally; (3) its lymphangiographic pattern is usually one of hypoplasia; and (4) it usually affects the lower extremities (32).

Lymphedema praecox is generally manifest during adolescence, and it accounts for approximately 80 percent of patients with primary lymphedema. This may represent another form of congenital lymphatic system disease but with a later onset of symptoms (32).

Lymphedema tarda presents in middle age or after age 35. It is quite likely that the general category designated as "primary lymphedema" probably encompasses several conditions with varying and incompletely understood etiologies.

Classification by Lymphangiographic Findings

Three general anatomic patterns of the lymphatic system have been described in patients with primary lymphedema: aplasia, hypoplasia, and hyperplasia (varicose) (33). The most common lymphangiographic finding is hypoplasia, seen in 70 percent of cases with primary lymphedema. In this form of lymphedema, when blue dye is injected, it spreads slowly into the web space. Occasionally a single superficial lymphatic channel can be seen. On radiographic examination after injection of contrast medium there is typically one or two slightly enlarged lymphatic vessels.

In the aplastic form (approximately 15 percent) the blue dye diffuses readily through the dermal plexus but remains confined to the dorsum of the foot and rarely extends above the ankle. Numerous dilated, tortuous channels that easily fill with contrast medium can be seen radiologically. Dermal backflow is almost always evident. The varicose type is thought to be the consequence of incompetent lymphatic valves.

Lymphangiographic findings generally correlate with the age of onset (30). In those individuals who have the congenital form or an early onset of edema the aplastic lymphangiographic form is usually found. The hypoplastic form predominates in patients with a lymphedema praecox. Although most evidence seems to indicate that some anatomical abnormality is likely to be present in patients who have lymphedema, it is becoming apparent that this correlation is not absolute. In a lymphangiographic study of 200 patients it was impossible to correlate the pathological lymphatic patterns and the clinical severity of the condition (34). In patients who have unilateral lymphedema, abnormal lymphangiographic findings on the clinically normal side are characteristic (35), and although a substantial number of patients eventually develop bilateral swelling, others do not. It is therefore possible that in addition to an anatomical abnormality some functional derangement within the lymphatics must exist.

BENIGN TUMORS OF LYMPHATICS

Lymphangiomas are generally divided into three types: (1) lymphangioma simplex, composed of small capillary-sized lymphatic channels; (2) cavernous lymphangioma, comprising dilated lymphatic channels often with fibrous adventitial covering; and (3) cystic lymphangioma, or cystic hygroma. All three are felt to have their origin in the embryologic development of the lymphatic system. Sabin (36) and later Goetsch (37) postulated that during the development of the lymphatic system, cell buds of lymphatic primordium occasionally fail to establish communication with veins, therefore resulting in isolated lymphatic spaces. Portions of the lymphatic system can become sequestered and retain the ability to produce lymph and form endothelial cysts. These lymphatic cysts slowly enlarge and infiltrate the surrounding tissues by pushing other structures aside.

The tumors are all benign. The majority are present at birth, and 90 percent can be identified by the end of the first year of life (38,39). They tend to grow in proportion to the growth of the child. They can greatly enlarge at times of infection.

The most common of the three types of lymphangioma is the cystic hygroma. Hygromas appear as soft, cystic, discrete nontender masses that transilluminate. They vary in size from a few millimeters to several centimeters. They can be located on any portion of the body; however, the majority are found in the head and neck region. Hygromas of the neck, tongue, and intraoral regions can present significant problems with respiration in the newborn and on occasion require emergent excision.

These lesions must be distinguished from hemangiomas, branchial cleft cysts, lipomas, and occasionally neoplasms such as rhabdomyosarcoma (40).

ACQUIRED LYMPHEDEMA

The removal or destruction of the axillary or inguinal nodes by surgery, radiation, infection, tumor invasion, or other inflammation can produce lymphedema. The most common worldwide cause is direct infestation of the lymph nodes by the filarial parasite *Wuchereria bancrofti* (30,32,41); however, the occurrence of permanent lymphedema complicating other infectious or inflammatory processes is unusual. Approximately 10 to 15 percent of the patients undergoing radical mastectomy develop significant postoperative arm swelling (39,42,43). There is a higher incidence in those patients undergoing radiation therapy, in obese patients and in patients who have postoperative problems with wound healing. The swelling may not become clinically evident for as long as 1 year. This delay is the result of the ongoing fibrotic process which further constricts and obstructs lymphatic drainage. The swelling generally begins in the upper arm and eventually may become massive.

Lymphangiographic studies in acquired lymphedema demonstrate a varicose-type pattern with dilation of the lymphatic vessels and blockage at the area of the involved nodes.

Lymphedema caused by malignant disease generally occurs late in the disease process after there is extensive spread of tumor.

Differential Diagnosis

In the vast majority of patients the diagnosis of lymphedema can and should be made by history and physical examination. The gradual onset of edema beginning at the ankle and proceeding proximally over a period of several months unassociated with other symptoms is characteristic. In females, swelling classically occurs at a time of menarche or pregnancy.

A major diagnostic problem is determining whether leg swelling is due to lymphatic or venous causes. The distinction can usually be made on clinical evidence. Edema secondary to venous disease demonstrates decreased capillary perfusion, characteristic dark brawny edema, and ulceration of the skin secondary to impaired perfusion and tissue anoxia. In lymphedema, capillary perfusion is unimpaired, ulceration is extremely rare; and the deep brown discoloration of venous problems is extremely unusual.

Following a period of bed rest, lymphedema typically resolves in several days, whereas venous edema tends to improve within hours.

In very difficult diagnostic situations venography is generally more informative than lymphangiography and considerably easier and safer to perform. Lymphangiography is tedious, difficult, and hazardous. In general, lymphangiographic findings will not influence the eventual medical or surgical management.

Noninvasive Studies

Several approaches are available for evaluation of the edematous extremity. The size can be evaluated by circumferential measurements and water volume displacement. Circumferential measurements, to be meaningful, should be standardized. Ideally, this involves taking the measurement after a full day's activities from a bony reference point on the extremity. It should be emphasized that small variations in the circumference of the extremity represent substantial changes in fluid accumulation and weight. Water volume measurements are more accurate, although also more cumbersome (26).

Lymphatic function has been evaluated by the clearance of various radioisotopes including gold (^{198}Au), technetium-labeled dextran, and radioiodinated serum albumin (^{131}I), (RIHSA). In normal individuals approximately 80 percent of RIHSA injected into the web space will be cleared in 24 hours (44). In those with lymphedema the percentage is approximately half (24,45,46). RIHSA clearance has also been used to document postoperative improvement in lymphatic function (10,45–47). The contralateral extremity should not be used as a control in primary lymphedema because of the high incidence of bilateral lymphatic abnormalities. Variables such as volume of isotope injected, patient activity during the test, extremity position, and monitoring techniques (size of counter, time) must also be rigidly controlled and standardized.

These studies should be carried out preoperatively and postoperatively (as treatment) with standard techniques to best evaluate the effect of any therapeutic modality.

Lymphangiography

What is known of the gross anatomy of the peripheral lymphatics, in both normal and disease states, is defined through direct cannulation of the lymphatics (48). The technique involves injecting 5 mL of an equal mixture of methylene blue and 1% lidocaine into the web spaces of the extremity. In the normal individual the dermal lymphatics are outlined by this concentration of the dye. Once the superficial lymphatics are outlined by the blue dye, a transverse incision is made 2 to 3 inches proximal to the site of injection and the lymphatic channels are cannulated with a 27- to 30-gauge needle. Contrast material [such as ethiodized oil (Ethiodol)] is then injected slowly into the lymphatic system. No more than 10 mL per leg or 5 mL per arm is given. Multiple x-rays are then obtained over the next 24 hours to visualize the lymphatics.

Since the superficial and deep lymphatics do not normally communicate, the deep lymphatics must be visualized separately. This is done in a similar fashion, except that the approach to the deep lymphatic chain is slightly posterior to the medial malleolus near the area of the posterior tibial vessels (32).

While lymphangiograms are helpful, an experienced observer can gain considerable information simply from the rate of diffusion and the pattern of the methylene blue distribution.

Potential complications of a lymphangiograph are many and include lymphangitis, wound infection, cellulitis, allergic reaction to the injected contrast material, pulmonary embolism of contrast material, and long-term straining of the extremity. Fever, chills, headache, nausea, vomiting, and arthralgia are common after this test. While a lymphangiograph can provide helpful information, it should not be considered a routine diagnostic procedure in evaluating lymphedematous patients and should be performed only with a specific goal in mind. At this time a lymphangiogram has no possible therapeutic use.

Medical Treatment

Most patients with lymphedema are adequately managed without surgical intervention. The medical treatment is oriented toward the inciting event. Infectious causes, in the acute phase, are often managed with the appropriate antibiotic regime combined with the principles of limb elevation and compression. Parasitic causes such as *Wuchereria bancrofti* and *Brugia malayi* are first treated with diethylcarbamazine, which eliminates the organisms from the blood. An anti-inflammatory and/or antihistamine is usually administered concurrently to control the allergic reactions to the dying parasite (49). Also, as with all forms of lymphedema, limb elevation and compression should be used. Allergic causes are managed by withdrawal of the inciting agent and with antihistamines and anti-inflammatory agents. In cases of chronic lymphedema, however, neither the medical nor the surgical approach can provide a cure for the process. It is, therefore, imperative that the patient understand the chronicity of the condition as well as the importance of controlling the edema and preventing infection. Medical management can only attempt to improve lymphatic drainage by combining limb elevation, external compression, and the judicious use of diuretics and other selected medications such as steroids and benzopyrones (31,50,51).

Certain measures can be taken by the patient. The patient should be instructed to avoid any unnecessary standing for long periods of time, to elevate the foot of the bed with 15-cm wood blocks, and to wear elastic stockings conscientiously. The stocking should fit tightly, and the measurements of the individual patient should be taken after a period of bed rest when the extremity is smallest in diameter. A full-length stocking or leotard is often discarded by the patient because of inconvenience and discomfort. For most patients a knee-length stocking is an excellent compromise. Intermittent compression machines of various types have been successful when used conscientiously, but they require a great deal of time and dedication (52). They are no substitute for continuous compression stockings.

Diuretics are occasionally effective in reducing the interstitial water load associated with lymphedema. To be most beneficial, diuretics should be taken intermittently, particularly in the premenstrual period. It is recommended that longer acting thiazides be used combined with a potassium-sparing diuretic over a 4-day period.

Other medications such as steroids injected into lymphatics and benzopyrones have been reported to be useful in lymphedema (31,50). Benzopyrones are known to stimulate macrophages (31) and thus, theoretically, they could act to increase lysis of collagen through this mechanism. Clinical trials of benzopyrones show softening of lymphedematous tissue as well as modest decreases (0.5 cm over a 10-month average) in the size of extremities with long-term use. In all trials patients report subjective improvement in symptoms (31,51,53,54). This approach certainly deserves further examination.

Generally infection cannot be avoided. The patient should be instructed in meticulous foot care to avoid fungal infections. In patients with recurrent infectious episodes of unknown origin, prophylactic penicillin is the drug of choice; *Streptococcus* is the most common etiological agent.

When infection occurs, it must be treated early and aggressively. The patient should be restricted to bed rest, the extremity elevated, and antibiotics administered. Each inflammatory process exacerbates the fibrosis.

Operations

The operative approach to lymphedema must be considered in two categories: (1) operations to control chronic lymphedema, and (2) the surgical approach to tumors of the lymphatic system.

Surgical intervention should be considered only after medical management has been attempted and has failed. Indications for surgery include functional impairment, cosmetic reasons, and recurrent lymphangitis. Patients frequently complain of fatigue related to the weight of the swollen extremity and an inability to control the size of the extremity. Cosmetic indications are strongest in adolescent females where severe psychological problems can be present.

The frustration encountered in the surgical management of lymphedema is reflected in the numerous procedures described over the last 70 years.

There are two main categories of procedures: physiologic and excisional (see Table 63-1). The physiologic operations attempt to reconstruct lymphatic drainage either by introducing distant or local pedicle tissue or by microvascular techniques. The excisional operations remove varying amounts of subcutaneous tissue and skin. It should be emphasized that most pedicle flap procedures include a significant amount of excision.

PHYSIOLOGIC OPERATIONS

Direct Lymphatic Reconstruction

Lymphangioplasty was first proposed by Handley in 1908 (8). He implanted silk threads in the subcutaneous tissues in hopes of creating new lymphatic channels. In successive years various other synthetic materials have been used without success (19,30,36,55,56). Their failure was largely related to the high incidence of infection and extrusion. It is difficult to conceive how valveless channels formed around a foreign body could ever drain lymph against gravity.

Lymphaticovenous shunts were first proposed by Rivero in 1967 (14) when he surgically approximated a hemisectioned lymph node to the side of a vein. Early results were encouraging; however, fibrous ingrowth has consistently been noted within the first postoperative year (57,58). Currently work is still being done on lymphaticovenous anastomoses with clinical trials to evaluate the long-term patency (59–66). Direct microvascular repair of lymphatics was proposed by O'Brien (15). This approach is obviously the most direct method of lymphatic reconstruction in patients with obstructive or secondary lymphedema. Early results are promising (67–70), but some feel this approach may not attack all the problems of chronic lymphedema (71). This method certainly deserves further investigation.

TABLE 63-1. Procedures for the Surgical Management of Lymphedema Described during the Last 70 Years

I. Physiological Operations
   A. Direct lymphatic reconstruction
      1. Alloplastic implants
      2. Microlymphatic repair
      3. Lymph node–venous anastomosis
   B. Pedicle flaps
      1. Local skin flap
      2. Buried dermal flaps
      3. Omental flap
II. Excisional Operations
   A. Total subcutaneous excision and skin grafting (the Charles procedure)
   B. Subcutaneous excision beneath flaps

Pedicle Flap Reconstruction

Local skin flaps have been used, but they have not been successful, probably because only the dermal lymphatic plexus is transferred (72,73).

The simple excision of deep muscle fascia was one of the first operations attempted by Kondoleon in the hope that the involved subcutaneous tissue would drain into the normal muscle and deep lymphatics (9). This was unsuccessful because of rapid fascia regrowth (74). Thompson, however, introduced a procedure in which a de-epithelialized dermal flap was buried into the muscle with the expectation of achieving a permanent lymphatic communication between the subcutaneous tissue and uninvolved muscle compartment (12). Favorable results have been reported (75,76). In fact, RIHSA clearance studies have documented improvement postoperatively (19). However, it is important to note that a substantial amount of skin and subcutaneous tissue is excised in this procedure (19,30,77). It is therefore difficult to know how much of the postoperative improvement is due to the dermal flap versus the simple excision.

A pedicle of omentum has been employed to serve as a new conduit for lymphatic flow (13,34,48). Initial reports were encouraging; however, laboratory experiments have shown that no communication between the omentum and extremity develops (78,79). The omentum appears to be surrounded by a smooth bursalike sac at reoperation (46). The lack of valves in the omental lymphatic system makes this an unlikely candidate for successful reconstruction. Moreover, the incidence of postoperative complications is significant.

EXCISIONAL OPERATIONS

Total Subcutaneous Excision

Originally described by Charles in 1912 (80) and commonly used since then (81), the Charles operation is an extensive procedure that removes all skin subcutaneous tissue and deep fascia in the leg except in the foot. The bared muscle is covered by a split-

or full-thickness graft. Split-thickness grafts initially appear satisfactory, but late scarring is extreme and the grafts are likely to be injured easily. They ulcerate frequently and develop a severe, hyperkeratotic, weeping, chronically infected dermatitis. The end result is almost always far worse than the original problem of lymphedema, and therefore we strongly oppose the use of split-thickness graft resurfacing after subcutaneous excision (82). The full-thickness grafts taken from the excised tissue are considerably more durable (10), although it is a formidable challenge to achieve a complete take of full-thickness skin grafts over such a large area. Even when the grafts are successful, substantial scarring and chronic breakdown of these areas are not uncommon. In chronic long-standing lymphedema where there is a substantial element of fibrosis, this may, however, be the only technically feasible procedure available.

Staged Subcutaneous Excision Beneath Flaps

Staged subcutaneous excision beneath flaps was originally described by Sistrunk in 1917 (10) and later popularized by Homans (11). Improvement is directly related to the amount of skin and subcutaneous tissue removed and the postoperative care given by each patient. The procedure is described to patients as a means of facilitating management of lymphedema and not as a cure, but results have been favorable. During the operation as much subcutaneous tissue and skin are removed as possible while attempting to maintain a viable skin flap and achieve primary wound healing (83–86).

Operative Technique

Preoperative Care. Patients are placed at bed rest with extremity elevation until edema has largely resolved. This is usually begun at home, but the patient is admitted at least 4 days preoperatively. It generally takes 5 to 14 days for edema resolution, and this rate is dependent on the chronicity of the condition and amount of fibrosis present.

Procedure in the Leg. All procedures utilize a pneumatic tourniquet placed as proximally as possible. Subcutaneous excision of the leg is done in two stages. The medial side is usually done first and involves the largest amount of resection. Anteriorly and posteriorly based skin flaps approximately 1.5 to 2 cm in thickness are elevated from the medial side of the extremity. The subcutaneous tissue is completely resected down to and including the muscle fascia. After excising the subcutaneous fat from the periosteum of the tibia, the deep fascial compartment of the calf is entered, affording a relatively avascular plane of dissection above the gastrocnemius muscle. Posteriorly the sural nerve is identified and preserved. Dissection then proceeds superiorly over the knee and inferiorly to the ankle region above the fascia. The flap should not be developed beyond the anterior border of the medial malleolus. Because of the potential for avascular necrosis, ankle flaps are rarely longer than 6 cm. Substantial amounts of redundant skin (6 to 10 cm) and subcutaneous fat (400 to 900 g) can be removed. The wound is then closed over a rubber suction drain which is left in place a minimum of 5 days. Interrupted and continuous 4-0 nylon is used for closure without placement of any subcutaneous or dermal sutures.

The second stage is done 2 to 3 months later on the lateral aspect of the leg in similar fashion, taking care to preserve muscle fascia and the perineal nerve or the sensory branches (superficial peritoneal nerve) leading to the dorsum of the foot. These pierce the deep fascia about 4 to 6 cm above the extensor retinaculum of the ankle. Specific areas of ankle swelling can be excised several months later through a separate incision.

Procedures in the Arm. These are most commonly performed on postmastectomy patients. A medial excision is carried out from an incision extending from the distal ulna across the medial epicondyle through the posteromedial upper arm. Flaps about 1 cm thick are elevated to the midsagittal aspect of the forearm and tapered distally and proximally. The deep fascia is undisturbed. During the lateral dissection, which is usually done as a second stage, the dorsal sensory branches of the ulnar and radial nerves are identified and preserved. Considerable amounts of fat can be excised from the upper arm, and flaps can be thicker (1.5 to 2 cm) in this area. Wide bands of redundant skin can be excised, and this can be carried up into the axilla with removal of the tourniquet. Suction catheters are placed as in the leg, and skin closure performed as previously described.

Postoperative Care. With both the procedure in the leg and the arm, the extremity is immobilized in a gauze dressing reinforced with a posterior splint and is kept elevated, 5 days for the arm and 8 days for the leg. The patient is measured for a form-fitting elastic stocking, and Ace wraps are used prior to this. After elevation the arm can be placed in a sling, and dependency of the leg is begun on the ninth day and ambulation by the eleventh day, but only with either a firm leg wrapping or elastic stockings in place (87).

SURGICAL TREATMENT OF BENIGN LYMPHATIC TUMORS

These tumors have already been described under "Clinical Presentation." Here, we will deal with the treatment of these lesions.

Spontaneous remission of cystic hygroma, the most common form of lymphatic tumor, is extremely rare. Percutaneous aspiration of hygromas is usually followed by prompt recurrence and occasionally hemorrhage or development of infection. Introduction of sclerosing agents has been proposed, but the multiloculated nature of most hygromas makes this therapy unfeasible. Excision subsequent to sclerosis is technically difficult (43). Radiation therapy has no place in the treatment of cystic hygroma.

Treatment of cystic hygromas should be surgical excision, taking care to preserve all normal structures in the area. At times a staged excision is appropriate. These lesions are nonmalignant, and care should be taken to preserve all normal anatomy. Excision is usually deferred until the age of 6 months if there is no compression of the trachea or respiratory difficulty (38,39).

Lymphangioma simplex is similar in behavior to the cystic hygroma; however, it is more evenly distributed throughout the body, occurring more frequently in the extremities and trunk. Treatment is the same as for the cystic hygroma. Cavernous lymphangiomas likewise are amenable to surgical resection, usually when the child is a few years old. Often, they must be excised in stages. Lymphangiomas have also been reported in the small bowel, lungs, and solid viscera of the abdomen. Resection is necessary only if the lesions produce symptoms.

Outcome

Eighty-five percent of patients treated by staged skin and subcutaneous excision have at least a 50 percent reduction in extremity size (87). In addition, there is a decreased incidence of postoperative cellulitis (18 percent) and infection (4 percent). All patients have some recurrence of swelling after a full day's work, with progressive swelling in 6 percent (87).

One year after surgery a twofold increase in the clearance of RIHSA has been documented, suggesting that the excision of substantial amounts of subcutaneous tissue somehow improves lymphatic function (46,47,87). The mechanism and explanation of this improvement, however, is unclear at this time. Extensive surgical dissection may establish lymphatic venous anastomoses during the process of healing; the procedure may favorably alter the balance of lymph flow by effectively reducing the amount of lymph-forming tissue; the excision of substantial tissue and skin may result in external compression, effecting an increase in interstitial pressure much like elastic stockings, thus improving lymph flow.

The discouraging fact remains that no procedure cures lymphedema. A degree of edema inevitably follows any operative procedure. In our opinion compared to all available methods of surgical management, skin and subcutaneous excision is the most reliable, consistently beneficial, and uncomplicated means of surgically managing the symptoms of lymphedema.

Complications

Complications of lymphedema can be categorized under those relating to the disease and those relating to the treatment of the disease (i.e., surgical complications).

COMPLICATIONS OF LYMPHEDEMA

These complications have already largely been described under "Clinical Presentation" and include such entities as recurrent cellulitis, lymphangitis, and fibrosis of the subcutaneous tissue. Lymphangiosarcoma can also be a complication of lymphedema.

Lymphangiosarcoma

Stewart and Treves described the association between postmastectomy lymphedema and lymphangiosarcoma in 1948 (88). The malignant lesion of the lymphatics is nearly always associated with lymphedema, most commonly with postmastectomy lymphedema, but also with filariasis (24,35,67,80,89–91). The lesion generally appears approximately 10 years after the onset of lymphedema and pursues an aggressive malignant course. Average survival is 19 months following initiation of treatment. The lesion is described as a reddish purple discoloration or nodule and has been confused with Kaposi's sarcoma. Satellite lesions are occasionally found, but the tumor spreads primarily by a hematogenous route.

The mainstay of therapy has traditionally been radical amputation (90). Because of the very small number of these tumors, it is impossible to study the effects of various forms of therapy in randomized fashion.

Successful treatment of other soft tissue sarcomas with preoperative radiation therapy and chemotherapy, with surgical excision, and with postoperative adjunct chemotherapy (91) makes a similar approach in lympangiosarcoma justified. There is, however, insufficient evidence to strongly recommend any one form of therapy for this highly malignant tumor, and prognosis remains poor.

COMPLICATIONS OF SURGICAL TREATMENT

Each surgical approach carries with it its own unique set of complications. Lymphangioplasty has the usual complications of infection and extrusion; lymphatic-venous anastomosis has the complications of fibrous ingrowth which ultimately results in failure, and omental flaps have been found to develop a bursa about the omentum. All of these complications result in failure of the approach. Approaches shown to be successful also have associated complications. The Charles technique of complete skin and subcutaneous tissue removal followed by grafting can have the serious complications of late scarring, ulceration, and development of a hyperkeratotic, weeping, chronically infected dermatitis in the split-thickness grafted extremities. This can progress to the serious complication of amputation if not handled adequately (82). Full-thickness skin-grafted extremities can have failure of total graft vascularization, which depending on severity can have significant morbidity.

Complications associated with staged subcutaneous excision beneath flaps are not as serious as those associated with the Charles procedure. These include ischemic necrosis of areas of the flap (6 percent in our series) and varying degrees of decreased sensitivity about 3 cm on either side of the incision. No alteration in hand or foot sensation or motor function has been noted in our series, although this is a possible complication (87).

Recurrence of edema to some extent is a complication of all lymphedema operations. This incidence and relative occurrence in all approaches has been previously described.

References

1. Adams F: *The Genuine Works of Hippocrates*, vol 196. London, The Sydenham Society, 1849.
2. Adams F: *The Seven Books of Paulus Degineta*, 3 vols, 1:188, 3:504, 529 London, 1844–47.
3. Adams F: *The Extant Works of Aretaeus the Cappadocion*. London, 1856, p 344.
4. Mettler A: *History of Medicine*. Philadelphia, Blakiston, 1947, pp 344, 493, 529, 662, 717, 743.

5. Battezzafi M, Donini I: History of the lymphatic system and of clinical investigation of lymph circulation. In *The lymphatic system*. New York and Toronto, John Wiley and Sons, 1972.
6. Milroy WF: An undescribed variety of hereditary oedema. NY Med J 1892, 56:505.
7. Halstead WS: The swelling of the arm after operations for cancer of the breast. Elephantiasis chirurgica: Its cause and prevention. Bull Johns Hopkins Hospital 1921, 32:309.
8. Handley WS: Lymphangioplasty: A new method for the relief of the brawn arm breast cancer and for similar conditions of lymphatic oedema: Preliminary note. Lancet 1908, 1:783.
9. Kondoleon E: Die operative behandlung der elephantiastischen Oedeme. Zentralbl Chir 1912, 39:1022.
10. Sistrunck WE: Further experiences with the Kondoleon operation for elephantiasis. JAMA 1918, 71:800.
11. Homans J: The treatment of elephantiasis of the legs: A preliminary report. N Engl J Med 1036, 215:1099.
12. Thompson N: Surgical treatment of chronic lymphedema of the lower limb. Br Med J 1962, 5519:1567.
13. Goldsmith HS, de los Santos R: Omental transposition in primary lymphedema. Surg Gynecol Obstet 1967, 125:607.
14. Rivero OR, Calnan JS, Reis ND, Taylor LM: Experimental peripheral lymphovenous communication. Br J Plast Surg 1967, 20:124.
15. O'Brien B: Replantation and reconstructive microvascular surgery. Ann R Coll Surg Engl 1976, 58:87, 171.
16. Crockett DJ: Lymphatic anatomy and lympho-edema. Br J Plast Surg 1965, 18:12.
17. Sabin FR: The development of the lymphatic system. In Keibel F, Mall FP (eds): *Manual of Human Embryology*, vol 2. Philadelphia, Lippincott, 1912.
18. Malek P, Belan A, Kocandrle VL: The superficial and deep lymphatic system of the lower extremities and their mutual relationship under physiological and pathological conditions. J Cardiovasc Surg 1964, 5:686.
19. Thompson N: The surgical treatment of chronic lymphoedema of the extremities. Surg Clin North Am 1967, 47:445.
20. Rodbard S, Feldman P: Functional anatomy of the lymphatic fluids and pathways. Lymphology 1975, 8:49.
21. Selkurt E (ed): *Physiology*. Boston, Little, Brown, 1966.
22. Casley-Smith JR: The fine structure and functioning of tissue channels and lymphatics. Lymphology 1980, 13:177.
23. Guyton AC, Barber BJ: The energetics of lymph formation. Lymphology 1980, 13:173.
24. Yoffey JM. Courtice FC: *Lymphatics, Lymph and Lymphoid Tissue*. Cambridge, Massachusetts, Harvard University Press, 1956.
25. Taylor GW, Kinmonth JB, Rollinson E, Rotblat J, Frances GS: Lymphatic circulation studies with radioactive plasma protein. Br Med J 1957, 1:133.
26. Acevedo D: Motor control of the thoracic duct. Am J Physiol 1943, 139:600.
27. Olszewski WL, Engaset A: Intrinsic contractility of prenodal lymphatic vessels and lymph flow in human leg. Am J Physiol 1980, 239:775.
28. Roddie IC, Mawhinney HJD, McHale NG, Kirkpatrick CF, Thornburg K: Lymphatic motility. Lymphology 1980, 13:173.
29. Rusznyak I: Recent experiments on the physiology and pathology of the lymphatic circulation. Minerva Med 1954, 43:1468.
30. Stone EJ, Hugo NE: Lymphedema. Surg Gynecol Obstet 1972, 135:625.
31. Pillar NB: Lymphedema, macrophages and benzopyrones. Lymphology 1980, 13:109.
32. Kinmonth JB: *The Lymphatics*. London, Edward Arnold Publishers, 1982, pp 105–144.
33. Kinmonth JB, Taylor GW, Tracey GD, Marsh JD: Primary lymphedema: Clinical and lymphangiographic studies of a series of 107 patients in which the lower limbs were affected. Br J Surg 1957, 45:1.
34. Pflug JJ, Calnan JS: The normal anatomy of the lymphatic system in the human leg. Br J Surg 1971, 58:925.
35. Buonocore, Young JR: Lymphangiographic evaluation of lymphedema and lymphatic flow. Am J Roentgenol Radium Ther Nucl 1965, 95:751–765.
36. Sabin FR: Direct growth of veins by sprouting. In *Contributions to Embryology*, vol 14. Washington, DC, Carnegie Institute of Washington, 1922, p 1.
37. Goetsch E: Hygroma colli cysticum and hygroma axillere: Pathologic and clinical study and report of twelve cases. Arch Surg 1938, 36:394.
38. Bill AH Jr, Sumner DS: A unified concept of lymphangioma and cystic hygroma. Surg Gynecol Obstet 1965, 120:79.
39. Fonkalsrud EW: Surgical management of congenital malformation of the lymphatic system. Am J Surg 1974, 128:152.
40. Fonkalsrud EW: Malformation of the lymphatic system and hemangiomas In Holder TH, Ashcraft KW (eds): *Pediatric Surgery*. Philadelphia, WB Saunders, 1980.
41. Dale A: The swollen leg. Curr Probl Surg, September 1973.
42. Fitts WT, Keuhnelian JG, Ravdin IS, Schor S: Swelling of the arm after radical mastectomy. Surgery 1954, 35:460.
43. Treves N: An evaluation of the etiological factors of lymphedema following radical mastectomy. Cancer 1957, 10:444.
44. Schirger A, Harrison EG, Janes JM: Idiopathic lymphedema. Review of 131 cases. JAMA 1962, 182:14.
45. Emmett AJ, Barron JN, Veall N: The use of I^{131} albumin tissue clearance measurements and other physiological tests for the clinical assessment of patients with lymphoedema. Br J Plast Surg 1967, 20:1.
46. Miller TA, Harper JD, Longmire WP Jr: The management of lymphedema by staged subcutaneous excision. Surg Gynecol Obstet 1973, 136:1.
47. Miller TA: Surgical management of lymphedema of the extremity. Plast Reconstr Surg 1975, 56:633.
48. Goldsmith HS, de los Santos R, Beattie EJ: Relief of chronic lymphedema by omental transposition. Ann Surg 1967, 166:572.
49. *Harrison's Principles of Internal Medicine*. New York, McGraw-Hill Book Company, 1980, p 895.
50. Fyfe NCM, Ruth DL, Edwards JM, Kinmonth JB: Intralymphatic steroid therapy for lymphedema. Preliminary studies. Lymphology 1982, 15:23.
51. Clodius L, Deak L, Piller NB: A new instrument for the evaluation of tissue tonicity in lymphedema. Lymphology 1976, 9:1.
52. Zeliolrouski A: Lympha-press. A new pneumatic device for treatment of lymphedema of the limbs. Lymphology 1980, 13:68.
53. Piller NB, Clodius L: The use of a tissue tonometer as a diagnostic aid in extremity lymphedema: A determination of its conservative treatment with benzopyrones. Lymphology 1976, 9:127.
54. Piller NB: Conservative treatment of acute and chronic lymphedema with benzopyrones. Lymphology 1976, 9:132.
55. Handley WS: Hunterian lectures on the surgery of the lymphatic system. Br Med J 1910, 1:922.
56. Silver D, Puckett C: Lymphangioplasty: A ten year evaluation. Surgery 1976, 80:748.
57. Calnan JS, Reis ND, Rivero OR, Copenhagen HF, Taylor LM: The natural history of lymph node-to-vein anastomosis. Br J Plast Surg 1967, 20:134.
58. Puckett C: Evaluation of lymphovenous anastomosis in obstructive lymphedema. Plast Reconstr Surg 1980, 66:116.
59. Baxter TJ, Gilbert A, O'Brien B McC, Sykes PJ, Vorrath JW, Bennett RC: The histopathology of microlymphatic venous anatomosis. Aust NZ J Surg 1980, 50:320.
60. Fox U, Montersi M, Romagnoli G: Microsurgical treatment of lymphedema of the limbs. Int Surg 1981, 66:53.

61. O'Brien B, Shafiroff BB: Microlymphaticovenous and resectional surgery in obstructive lymphedema. World J Surg 1979, 3:3.
62. Puckett CL, Jacobs ER, Hurritz JS: Evaluation of lymphovenous anastomosis in obstructive lymphedema. Plast Reconstr Surg 1980, 66:116.
63. Degni M: New technique of lymphaticovenous anastomosis for the treatment of lymphedema. J Cardiovasc Surg 1978, 19:577.
64. Degni M: New microsurgical technique of lymphatico-venous anastomosis for the treatment of lymphedema. Lymphology 1981, 14:61.
65. Jamal S: Lymphovenous anastomosis in filarial lymphedema. Lymphology 1981, 14:64.
66. Huang G: Microlymphaticovenous anastomosis for treating lymphedema of the extremities and external genitalis. J Microvasc Surg 1981, 3:32.
67. Shafiroff BB, Nightingale G, Baster JJ, O'Brien B: Lymphatico lymphatic anastomosis. Ann Plast Surg 1979, 3:199.
68. O'Brien B. Mc Black MJ, Pagdestram I: Role of microlymphaticovenous surgery in obstrectro lymphedema. Clin Plast Surg 1978, 5(2):293.
69. Krylov V: Microlymphatic surgery of secondary lymphedema of the upper limb. Ann Chir Gynecol 1982, 71:77.
70. Daniller A: *Microlymphatic Surgery*. In Serafin D, Buncke HJ (eds): Microsurgical composite tissue transplantation. St. Louis, Mosby, 1979.
71. Clodius L, Piller NB, Casley-Smith JR: The problems of lymphatic microsurgery for lymphedema. Lymphology 14:69, 1981.
72. Gillies H, Fraser FR: The treatment of lymphoedema by plastic operation: A preliminary report. Br Med J 1935, 1:96.
73. Smith JW, Conway H: Selection of appropriate surgical procedures in lymphedema: Introduction of hinged pedicle. Plast Reconstr Surg 1954, 14:347.
74. Peer LA, Shahgholi M, Walker JD Jr, Mancusi-Ungaro A: Modified operation for lymphedema of leg and arm. Plast Reconstr Surg 1954, 14:347.
75. Sataguchi S: Surgical treatment of chronic lymphedema of the extremities. Lymphology 1979, 12:45.
76. Tanape T: The surgical treatment of chronic lymphedema of the extremity. Lymphology 1979, 12:47.
77. Larson DL, Coers CR, Doyle JE, Rappaport AS, Kloehn R, Lewis SR: Lymphedema of the lower extremity. Plast Reconstr Surg 1966, 38:293.
78. Danese CA, Papaioannou AN, Morales LE, Mitsuda S: Surgical approaches to lymphatic blocks. Surgery 1968, 56:821.
79. Goldsmith HS: Long-term evaluation of omental transporation for chronic lymphedema. Ann Surg 1974, 180:847.
80. Charles RH: *A System of Treatment*, vol 3. London, Churchill, 1912.
81. Dellon AL: The Charles procedure for primary lymphedema. Plast Reconstr Surg 1977, 60:589.
82. Miller TA: Charles procedure for lymphedema: A warning. Am J Surg 1980, 139:290.
83. Gilbson T, Tough JS: A simplified one-stage operation for the correction of lymphedema of the leg. Arch Surg 1955, 71:809.
84. Fonkalsrud EW, Coulson WF: Management of congenital lymphedema in infants and children. Ann Surg 1973, 177:280.
85. Fonkalsrud EW: Surgical management of congenital lymphedema in infants and children. Arch Surg 1979, 114:1133.
86. Song R: Surgical treatment of lymphedema of the lower extremity. Clin Plast Surg 1982, 9(1):113.
87. Miller TA: Lymphedema. In Grabb WC, Smith JW (eds): *Plastic Surgery*. Boston, Little, Brown, 1979.
88. Stewart FW, Treves N: Lymphangiosarcoma in postmastectomy lymphedema: A report of six cases in elephantiasis. Chirurgia. Cancer 1948, 1:64.
89. Unruh H, Robertson DI, Karasewich E: Postmastectomy lymphangiosarcoma. Can J Surg 1979, 22:586.
90. Woodward AH, Ivins JC, Soule EH: Lymphangiosarcoma arising in chronic lymphedematous extremities. Cancer 1972, 30:562.
91. Rosenberg SA, Suit HD, Baker LH, Rosen E: Sarcomas of the soft tissues and bone. In Devita VT Jr, Hellman S, Rosenberg SA (eds): *Cancer: Principles and Practice of Oncology*. Philadelphia, JB Lippincott, 1982.

PART NINE

Vascular Trauma

Chapter 64

TRUNCAL VASCULAR TRAUMA: AORTA, INNOMINATE VESSELS, VENA CAVA, PORTAL VEIN, AND VISCERAL ARTERIES

KENNETH L. MATTOX and DAVID V. FELICIANO

In the chest, the major challenges in truncal vascular injury relate to the innominate artery and descending thoracic aorta. Three vascular systems within the abdomen present challenges to the trauma surgeon: (1) the aorta and its branches, (2) the vena cava and its tributaries, and (3) the portal venous system. Abdominal aortic injuries are subdivided into injuries to the suprarenal aorta, infrarenal abdominal aorta, visceral arteries, renal arteries, and iliac arteries. Trauma to the vena cava is subdivided into injuries to the iliac vein, infrarenal vena cava, suprarenal vena cava, and the hepatic veins. Portal venous injury encompasses trauma to the inferior mesenteric vein, superior mesenteric vein, splenic vein, and portal vein.

Abdominal vascular injury rarely occurs alone. In more than one-third of all abdominal vascular injuries multiple associated vascular injuries occur. Furthermore, there is a high incidence of associated injury to the liver, spleen, pancreas, stomach, duodenum, small bowel, and colon. The surgeon, therefore, must develop treatment priorities for both associated vascular injuries and the constellation of solid organ and enteric trauma often encountered.

Historic Considerations

Historic contributions to the development of vascular surgery technique are covered in other chapters of this book. Although isolated case reports of truncal cardiovascular trauma sprinkle the literature prior to 1960, only during the last 20 years have significant series of such injuries emerged from civilian trauma centers in Houston, San Francisco, Dallas, New York, New Orleans, and other cities (1–8). The reports of vascular injuries in World War I, World War II, the Korean War, and the Vietnamese Vascular Trauma Registry contain too few cases of truncal vascular injury to provide statements involving new modes of therapy (9–12).

Since 1960, blunt injury to the innominate and subclavian arteries and the thoracic aorta has been seen with increasing frequency (13–16). Major evolutionary steps in the treatment of such injuries involve (1) cardiopulmonary bypass; (2) considerations for heparinless shunts; and (3) finally, direct repair following clamping proximal and distal to the affected injury with subsequent revascularization (15–18). These contributions parallel pioneering work in the field of elective vascular repair of these major arteries (19–22). The recent increased incidence in truncal vascular injury parallels the increased incidence of drunk driving, narcotic trafficking, availability of handguns, and violent crimes (23–26).

Pathophysiology

The etiology of truncal vascular injuries is most often penetrating trauma except for blunt injury to the hepatic veins, thoracic outlet, and descending thoracic aorta. A few isolated cases of blunt injury to the abdominal aorta have been reported. Injuries to the main or peripheral branches of the iliac arteries and veins may occur secondary to pelvic fracture. Iatrogenic injuries to the iliac arteries and veins, the subclavian artery and veins, and, at times, visceral arteries are a subset of penetrating injury. Since truncal vessels carry large volumes of blood, injury to any large truncal vessel produces early exsanguinating hemorrhage, hypovolemia, and all the clinical symptoms associated with shock. In rare instances, an untreated injury may result in a traumatic arterial aneurysm or an arteriovenous fistula.

Clinical Presentation

Patients with penetrating truncal vascular injury usually present with multisystem organ trauma. The history of the penetrating wound usually is known, with the entrance and/or exit sites readily identifiable. In the chest, symptoms of thoracic outlet obstruction with hematoma formation may be present, and respiratory embarrassment is common when hemothorax is present. With concomitant cardiac or pericardial injury, the classic symptoms of pericardial tamponade may be present. With penetrating abdominal wounds, vascular injury may occur at locations quite distant from the wound entrance site. Such patients usually are hypovolemic with clear signs indicating the need for laparotomy. Victims of stab wounds may require peritoneal lavage to confirm the presence of a hemoperitoneum.

Fifty percent of patients with blunt injury to the trunk who are subsequently determined to have thoracic vascular injury have no signs of external vascular trauma (19). Physical findings strongly suggestive of injury to the innominate artery and/or descending thoracic aorta include (1) alterations in upper extremity pulse or blood pressure, (2) loss of pulses in the lower extremity (pseudocoarctation syndrome), (3) paraplegia at the T3 to T6 level, (4) intrascapular murmur, (5) hematoma at the thoracic outlet, and (6) large bruises on the chest wall indicative of marked deceleration (see Table 64-3).

Symptoms on presentation may be *time-related*. A patient with a major truncal vascular injury who is not seen in the emergency room until 1 or more hours after injury will have a greater constriction in blood volume than the patient who arrives in the emergency center within 10 to 20 minutes of injury. When transportation is delayed or transport between two to three hospitals occurs, the patient is pale, apprehensive, hypoxemic, and hypovolemic. Hypotension and hypothermia may be noted, and the patient may complain of abdominal and/or chest pain and is frequently asking for pain medication. The apprehension may be a manifestation of hypoxemia and shock, and opiates should not be administered prior to stabilization, resuscitation, and full evaluation. The clinical symptoms, likewise, can change unfavorably unless expeditious emergency center workup followed by rapid transport to the operating room is accomplished.

The natural history of major truncal vascular injury is well established. Blunt injury to the aortic arch or innominate artery rarely results in rupture into the pericardial or pleural spaces, and exsanguinating hemorrhage is very uncommon. Instead, hematoma occurs at the thoracic outlet and may produce airway and superior caval obstruction. On x-ray, the hematoma is seen at the thoracic outlet rather than at the isthmus (Figure 64-1). Injuries in this location may result in early death from airway obstruction or hypovolemia. Untreated innominate artery injury victims surviving the immediate insult subsequently develop chronic traumatic aneurysms which continue to enlarge, producing pressure symptoms on adjacent organs such as the trachea, esophagus, vena cava, and nerve structures. On rare occasions, such traumatic aneurysms may "necessitate" producing external exsanguinating hemorrhage.

In both Parmley's 1958 classic series of autopsied cases and a recent 2-year review in Houston of blunt injuries to the descending thoracic aorta, only 15 percent of patients who sustained such deceleration injuries reached a medical treatment facility alive (26,27). Seat belts, passive restraints, Emergency Medical Services (EMS) systems, air ambulance transportation, and even trauma centers have been ineffectual in preventing and/or reducing the prehospital mortality from this injury. The increasing reported incidence of this injury has paralleled the development of lighter weight vehicles and continued high incidence of drunk driving accidents. Of the 15 percent of patients with blunt injury to the descending thoracic aorta reaching a hospital alive, the untreated 48-hour in-hospital mortality is 50 percent. Five percent of untreated patients will develop chronic traumatic aneurysms of the descending thoracic aorta. Three to ten percent of patients with this injury will have multiple injuries to the descending thoracic aorta (28). Blunt injuries to the descending thoracic aorta may cause partial intimal tears or complete transections. The expanding hematoma is held by a very thin layer of parietal pleura which may lose its containment at any time during transport, in the emergency department, during arteriography, at the time of the skin incision, during insertion of the chest retractor, or even just prior to the application of proximal and distal controlling vascular clamps. A few patients may even develop medial dissection and delayed onset of paraplegia. With a pseudocoarctation syndrome, renal failure and mesenteric ischemia may ensue.

The natural history of penetrating wounds to the abdominal major vessels is dependent upon the vessel injured. Within 4 hours of injury, the manifestations consist of exsanguinating hemorrhage, hypovolemia, profound shock, and death. Patients who survive this initial period have a contained or partially contained hematoma. A contained hematoma of the vena cava (a rare phenomenon) may be self-limited, since late-appearing venous aneurysms or thrombosis of the vena cava have not been

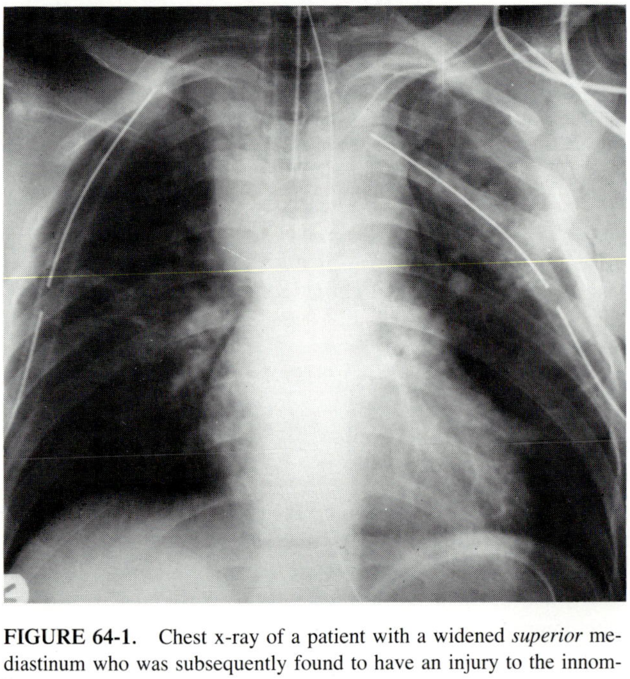

FIGURE 64-1. Chest x-ray of a patient with a widened *superior* mediastinum who was subsequently found to have an injury to the innominate artery.

described. Chronic traumatic aneurysms of the aorta and its major branches have been described. Less than 5 percent of patients with untreated penetrating truncal vascular injury will develop arteriovenous fistula and late-appearing traumatic aneurysms (29).

Noninvasive Studies

The noninvasive studies available to the surgeon evaluating a patient with potential penetrating or blunt truncal injury include chest x-ray, intravenous pyelogram, digital subtraction angiography, and computerized axial tomography. The latter two studies have not been extensively evaluated for vascular trauma and will not be elaborated upon other than to comment that such advanced radiographic techniques may hold great promise in the future, especially if incorporated into the resuscitation rooms and operative suites of trauma centers. Ultrasonography, liver and spleen scans, and other such noninvasive studies have no place in evaluating potential truncal vascular injury.

With blunt thoracic injury as well as penetrating truncal wounds, the chest x-ray is the single most important evaluation performed in the emergency center. Ideally, it should be accomplished in the shock room and not in a radiographic suite some distance from the resuscitation area. Entrance sites for penetrating wounds should be marked with radiographic clips. One initially looks for signs of hemopneumothorax and the presence of foreign bodies (bullets). The possibility of a bullet embolus to the heart, pulmonary artery, or even distally in the arterial tree must be considered. With blunt injury to the innominate artery, hematoma at the thoracic outlet occurs and may extend to both pleural caps (Figure 64-1). With potential injury to the descending thoracic aorta, a large number of radiographic suggestive signs have been described (Table 64-1). These signs do not suggest only great vessel injury but should also elicit suspicion of an injury to the descending thoracic aorta and strong consideration for either immediate operation or arteriography. Arteriography is preferred unless the hematoma is extremely large and in imminent risk for rupture (Figure 64-2). Clues suggesting an intravascular migratory missile have also been described (Table 64-2). Routine chest x-ray is performed to determine the presence of a pneumothorax, hemothorax, or hemopneumothorax. In the stable patient with an initially appearing normal x-ray it is important to obtain a second x-ray after 4 hours and again after 12

TABLE 64-1. Radiographic Signs Suggestive of Injury to the Descending Thoracic Aorta

Widening superior mediastinum >8 cm
Depression of left main stem bronchus >140°
Obliteration of aortic knob
Deviation of trachea to right
Deviation of nasogastric tube in esophagus to right
Fracture of first and/or second ribs
Fracture of scapula and/or sternum
Fracture/dislocation of thoracic spine
Loss of aortopulmonary "window" on lateral chest x-ray
Anterior displacement of trachea on lateral chest x-ray
"Calcium layering" in aortic arch or knob
Left pleural "cap hematoma"
Multiple fracture of left ribs
Massive left hemothorax

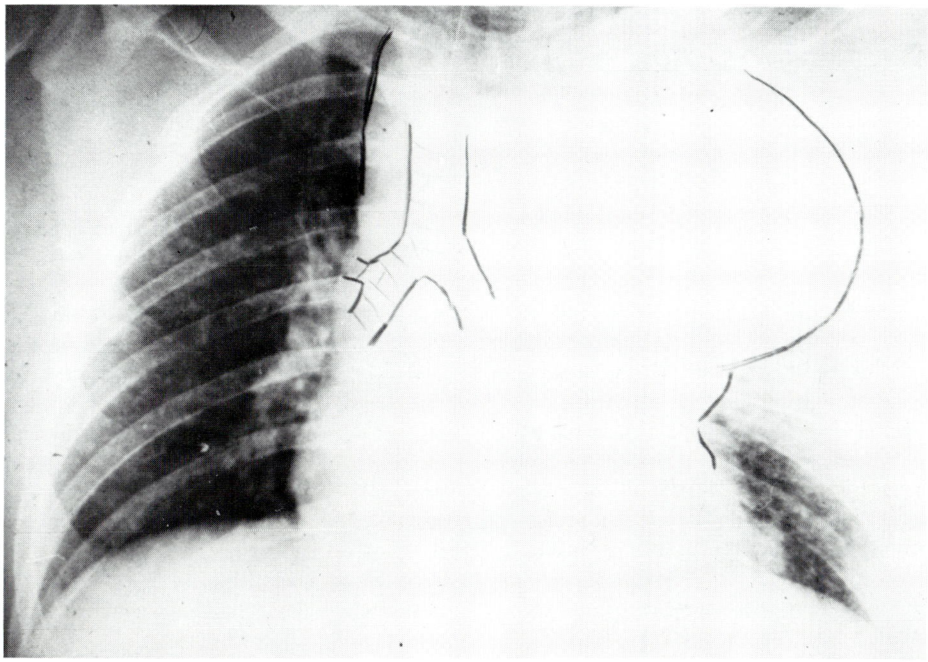

FIGURE 64-2. Chest x-ray of a patient with a massive traumatic aneurysm of the descending thoracic aorta and high risk of immediate rupture.

TABLE 64-2. Clues Suggestive of Intravascular Migrating Missile

Confusing "course" of bullet
Single entrance site or bullet not seen on initial x-ray
Missile out of "focus" over cardiac silhouette
Clinical symptoms less than expected from predicted course of bullet
Bullet changing locations on serial x-rays

TABLE 64-3. Clinical Signs and Symptoms Suggestive of Great Vessel Injury

Upper extremity hypertension
"Steering wheel" mark on anterior chest
Intrascapular murmur
Intermittent or permanent paralysis in legs
History of lower body sensory loss
Absent or decreased femoral pulses
Back pain (thoracic)
Hematoma palpable at thoracic outlet
History suggestive of massive energy transfer

to 18 hours. If the patient is hypovolemic and the chest x-ray is normal (and no major extremity injury is present), major abdominal injury must be presumed.

In the shock room at the time of insertion of a large-bore intravenous needle, blood is drawn for type and cross match and a double-dose bolus of intravenous pyelogram dye is injected. With radiopaque marking clips at the site of penetrating wounds, a flat plate of the abdomen is obtained 3 to 5 minutes later. This single-shot intravenous pyelogram study demonstrates a potential course of bullet traverse, the presence or absence of free air in the abdomen, and a nephrogram. With penetrating wounds, the objective is to look for a functioning contralateral kidney in case a nephrectomy is required. With blunt injury, if renal artery trauma is suspected, arteriography is preferable to an intravenous pyelogram. Drip nephrotomograms and multiple views on the intravenous pyelogram do not adequately evaluate vascular injury. The kidneys and ureters may be deviated laterally and anteriorly when retroperitoneal hematoma is present. With pelvic hematoma from iliac and/or hypogastric artery injury, the bladder may be deviated and/or abnormally positioned.

Arteriography is mandatory in stable patients with suspected vascular injuries of the thoracic outlet, the great vessels of the chest, and the descending thoracic aorta. A long list of clinical symptoms and radiographic clues may prompt the initial evaluating physician and subsequent surgeons to consider diagnostic angiography (Table 64-3). In patients with rapidly expanding hematomas or exsanguinating hemorrhage but with potential for salvage, immediate thoracotomy in the operating room should be performed without angiography. In stable patients, angiography may be safely performed through a retrograde femoral approach as long as the catheter and guide wire are not advanced with force. Once the catheter is in the aorta, other angiographic abdominal studies in the multisystem injured patient may be obtained. Abdominal angiography for suspected abdominal arterial injury, especially to the renal artery, might be considered if facilities are immediately available and delay of definitive treatment does not result. In instances of blunt injury to the pelvic vasculature, angiography is therapeutic. Injection of thrombosing coils or clot serves as an adjunct to the operative management of pelvic vascular injuries. In the hypovolemic, hypotensive patient, the routine nonselective use of angiography is contraindicated. Angiography is mandatory when late complications of vascular trauma such as arteriovenous fistulas and traumatic aneurysms occur. Patients with such diagnoses are not hypovolemic and are not in danger of exsanguinating hemorrhage during angiography.

Medical Treatment

The nonoperative treatment of patients with suspected truncal vascular injuries is merely preparatory to operation and involves treatment of shock. If time is a critical issue, type-specific, uncross-matched blood may be given with a significant degree of safety (30). In the patient with a suspected abdominal or thoracic aortic injury and nonexpanding hematoma with a blood pressure in the range of 80 to 100 mmHg systolic, the administration of blood and large volumes of crystalloids should be reserved until just before the skin incision is made. Elevation of the blood pressure to normotensive and/or hypertensive levels may cause further bleeding into the hematoma and release the tamponading effect. Although experimentally induced aortic injuries have been treated with g suits and antishock garments, the effectiveness of increasing cardiac afterload using such garments has not been demonstrated clinically in human beings in any prospective randomized trials. Increasing the afterload below an area of aortic injury may actually perpetuate bleeding rather than impede it. The use of such medical antishock garments for pelvic hematoma from blunt injury and possibly iliac artery and vein injuries may have some physiologic basis. In patients with blunt injury to the descending thoracic aorta and in whom operation on the thoracic aorta is deemed impossible, the use of antihypertensive agents and afterload reduction agents has been proposed (31,32), but this form of therapy has not received wide acceptance.

Recycling of scavenged shed blood is ideally applicable to victims of vascular trauma. Autotransfusion may be accomplished using a variety of commercially available devices, for example, the Haemonetics Cell Saver.* Autotransfusion complements, but does not replace, the use of homologous banked blood. Autologous blood contaminated with enteric contents (even if extensively washed) should not be used if compatible homologous blood is available. With suspected vascular trauma, prophylactic antibiotics should be administered prior to surgery and continued for 36 to 48 hours.

*Haemonetics Corporation, 17 Erie Drive, Natick, Massachusetts 01770.

Operative Therapy

Operative therapy for patients with vascular trauma is part of a continuum requiring surgical decision making and surgical skill from the initial phases in the emergency center as well as in the arteriogram suite, the operating room, the intensive care unit, and rehabilitation. The surgeon should not abdicate the role as primary decision maker at any level to an emergency room or critical care consulting physician. Especially in areas of truncal vascular trauma, *one* physician orchestrates *all* suggested consultant interventions.

Operative therapy begins with a rapid but complete assessment in the emergency department and insertion of adequate large-bore central venous lines. Should innominate artery injury with concomitant innominate venous or superior vena caval injury be suspected, at least one large venous line is placed in the lower extremity. Should potential for hepatic vein or inferior vena cava injury be present, at least one large-bore intravenous line is inserted in the upper extremity.

With exsanguinating hemorrhage and penetrating thoracic trauma, urgent thoracotomy, in either the emergency center or the operating room, may be life-saving in a patient with hypovolemic cardiac arrest (33,34). Since the survival rate following emergency center thoracotomy for blunt injury to the thoracic great vessels is less than 5 percent, its use is discouraged (35). Emergency center thoracotomy for intraabdominal bleeding from major vascular injury (such as the abdominal aorta) has been recommended by some trauma centers. It is, however, effective in less than 5 percent of all cases, even when applied in the more aggressive trauma centers to injuries limited to the aorta or iliac arteries (35). Emergency center thoracotomy for intraabdominal vascular injury, even coupled with emergency center laparotomy, has an extremely low success yield (36).

Transfemoral insertion of occluding balloon catheters into the inferior vena cava, descending thoracic aorta, or abdominal aorta seems an attractive alternative but is time-consuming, may cause injury to the femoral artery or vein, and may be unnecessary if a suspected injury to the aorta, vena cava, or mesenteric vasculature is not present. Furthermore, the blind insertion of such catheters may result in protrusion of balloon-tipped catheters through the injury into the hematoma, thereby making the hemorrhage worse.

Proper choice of *incision* is mandatory for achieving proximal and distal control and expeditiously repairing the vascular injury. Innominate artery injuries are best approached through a median sternotomy with a right cervical extension. Injuries to the descending thoracic aorta are best approached through a posterolateral fourth interspace incision. All major abdominal vascular injuries are best approached through a liberal, long, midline abdominal incision.

Injuries to the innominate artery are repaired via bypass grafting from the ascending aorta to the distal innominate artery utilizing Dacron tube graft. Using a partially occluding clamp, a graft is fashioned to the ascending aorta and flushed with blood to allow clotting in the interstices of the graft. The area of injury is not entered, and the distal innominate artery is isolated just prior to its bifurcation to the subclavian and the right carotid. A vascular clamp is placed just proximal to the bifurcation to allow collateral flow from the subclavian to the brain by way of the right common carotid. When end-to-end anastomosis is accomplished between the graft and the distal innominate artery, neither hypothermia, shunt, nor heparin is required. Adequate flushing is accomplished to prevent fibrin clot or air embolism at the time the clamps are released. The area of injury and hematoma is now entered and the rent, usually just at the aortic arch, is oversewn, sometimes with the use of pledgets (Figure 64-3) (14).

Blunt injury to the descending thoracic aorta is approached through a fourth or fifth intercostal space, posterolateral incision. The surgeon must consider the circulation distal to the occluding clamps to areas of the spinal cord, kidneys, liver, abdominal viscera, and lower extremities. Beginning in the late 1950s and continuing through early 1970, the use of pump bypass and total-body heparinization with a left atrial or left ventricular to descending thoracic aorta or left femoral artery bypass was considered the best method for protecting these organs. During the early 1970s temporary nonclotting shunts received popularity. In the late 1970s and building upon experience developed for elective aneurysms of the descending thoracic aorta, simple clamp/repair procedures began to be the procedure of choice. With close communication between the anesthesiologist and surgeon and with the use of vasodilators, cardiac strain can be prevented. The simple clamp and repair technique seems to afford the best results with respect to mortality rates and incidence of paraplegia (Table 64-4) (37–44). The chronic cases include some patients with nontraumatic aneurysms; however, the principles of therapy should be identical for both traumatic and degenerative chronic aneurysms.

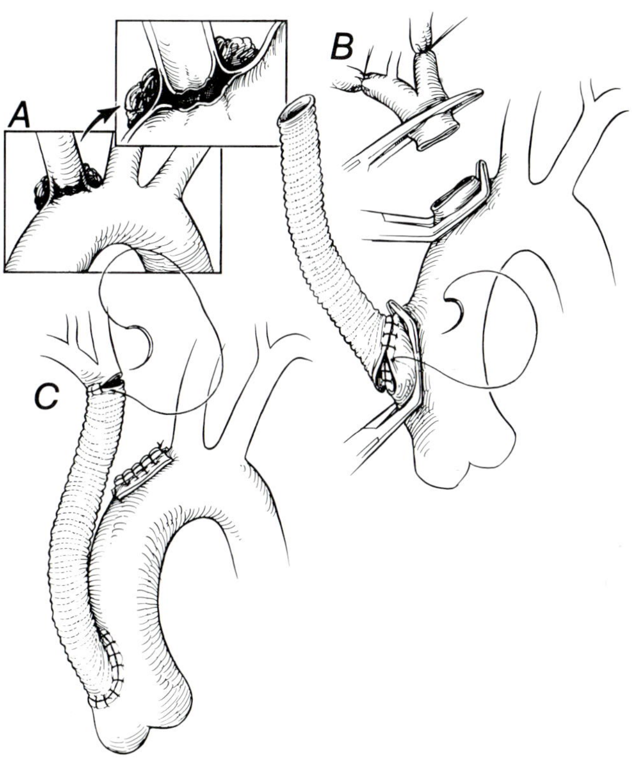

FIGURE 64-3. Drawing demonstrating technique of bypass grafting for innominate artery injury. [Copyright © Baylor College of Medicine 1981. Used with permission.]

TABLE 64-4. Survival and Paraplegia as a Function of Repair Techniques during Surgery for Blunt Injury to the Descending Thoracic Aorta

	Pump			Clamp			Shunt			Total		
Author (Ref.)	No.	Para.*	Died	No.	Para.	Died	No.	Para.	Died	No.	Para.	Died
Acute Repair												
Applebaum (37)	9	1	1	7	0	0	2	0	1	18	1	2
Turney (38)	2	0	1	6	0	0	23	1	5	31	1	2
Ketonen (39)	8	0	1	1	0	1	—	—	—	9	0	2
Vasco (40)	12	0	7	5	0	0	2	0	0	19	0	7
Kirsh (19)	10	0	5	0	0	0	27	1	2	37	1	7
Wilson (41)	4	0	1	3	0	1	0	0	0	7	0	2
Akins (42)	24	0	9	1	0	0	12	1	0	37	1	9
Pickard (15)	8	1	4	8	1	2	1	0	0	17	2	6
Subtotal	77	2	29	31	1	4	67	3	8	175	6	41
% of total		2.6	37.7		3.2	12.9		4.5	11.9		3.4	23.4
Chronic Repair												
Applebaum (37)	2	0	0	0	0	0	5	1	0	17	1	0
Finkelmeier (43)	2	0	0	1	0	0	7	2	0	10	2	0
Crawford (16)	0	0	0	86	2	10	37	2	8	123	4	18
Vasco (40)	5	0	1	1	0	0	2	0	0	7	0	1
Wilson (41)	3	0	0	0	0	0	0	0	0	3	0	0
McCollum (44)	38	0	2	9	0	0	2	0	0	49	0	2
Subtotal	50	0	3	97	2	10	53	5	8	200	7	21
% of total		0	6		2.1	10.3		9.4	15.1		3.5	10.5
Grand Total	127	2	32	128	3	14	120	8	16	375	13	62
% of Total		1.6	25.2		2.3	10.9		6.7	13.3		3.5	16.5

*Para. = paraplegia.

After entering the pleural cavity, the parietal pleura over the descending aorta distal to the injury is encircled with an umbilical tape. Using blunt dissection and taking care not to injure the phrenic, vagus, or recurrent laryngeal nerves, the transverse aortic arch between the left carotid and the subclavian artery is encircled with umbilical tape. The left subclavian artery is encircled in the same manner. On rare occasions it may be necessary to place the encircling tape between the innominate and left carotid arteries. Close cooperation between the surgeon and anesthesiologist assures control of pharmacologic agents. Vascular clamps are applied proximal and distal to the injury and on the left subclavian artery. The hematoma is entered and any backbleeding from intercostal vessels may be controlled with either partially occluding clamps, occluding balloon catheters, or ligation. Any torn intercostal vessels involved in the transection must be sacrificed. One may accomplish the repair either by an end-to-end anastomosis using a polypropylene monofilament 3-0 or 4-0 suture or using a short segment of appropriately sized Dacron graft. The safe operative time for performing this anastomosis is thought to be 30 to 45 minutes (37,45,46).

Exposure, proximal and distal control, and repair are complex when injuries involve the aorta, vena cava, iliac arteries and veins, mesenteric arteries, and portal venous system; and each of these injured areas must be approached separately. Injuries to the aorta are further subdivided between suprarenal and infrarenal locations, with the approach and management being entirely different, depending on location.

Although abdominal vascular injuries rarely occur alone, definitive therapy of nonvascular system injuries usually is delayed until after the vascular repair. Temporary closure of enteric contamination from the stomach, small bowel, and colon is indicated prior to entering the hematoma associated with a vascular injury. Placing laparotomy packs around hepatic injuries controls hemorrhage from the liver while the more life-threatening vascular injury is controlled.

Rarely is a fountain of blood encountered in the abdomen of a patient with an intraabdominal vascular injury. Hypotension, however, will occur as the abdomen is entered and clotted and unclotted blood in the peritoneal cavity is encountered, as well as a hematoma in the region of the vascular injury. The surgeon or assistant should occlude the aorta at the esophageal hiatus by manually compressing the aorta against the spine. At this point, the surgeon pauses to determine a procedural plan before plunging into the retroperitoneal or mesenteric hematoma. Consideration is given to extending the incision, preparing for autotransfusion, requesting additional assistance, and planning the proper exposure technique. Type and cross matching for extra blood may be deemed necessary, as well as application of gentle pressure over the hematoma to impede continued hemorrhage. Baseline blood gases are determined, and temporary closure or isolation of colon injuries is indicated.

The suprarenal aorta is best approached laterally through a generous midline abdominal incision, by rotating the abdominal viscera, including the left colon, spleen, kidney, and stomach to the right. This maneuver is accomplished by sharply incising the lateral peritoneal reflection and using blunt dissection to re-

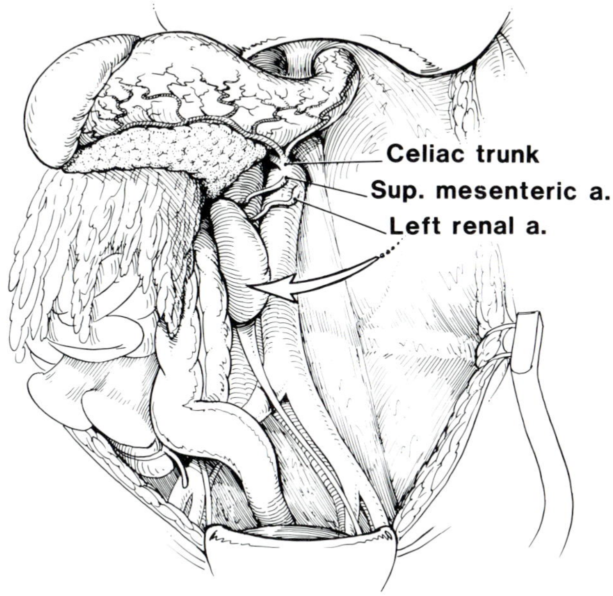

FIGURE 64-4. Maneuver to expose abdominal aorta in plane behind kidney with medial rotation of viscera. [Copyright © Baylor College of Medicine 1981. Used with permission.)

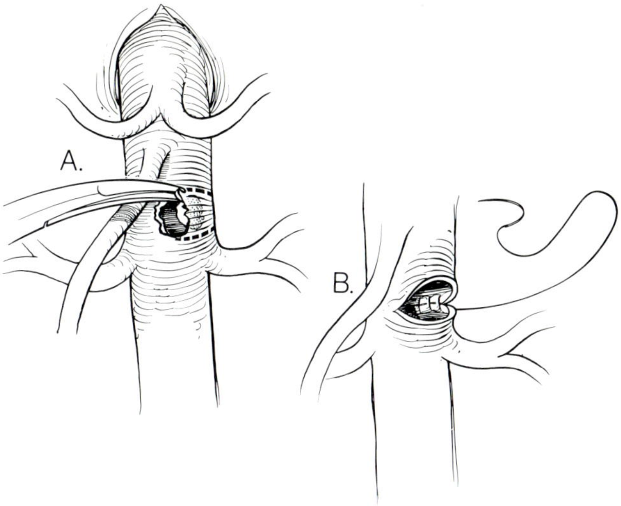

FIGURE 64-5. Drawing depicting two holes in abdominal aorta. The holes have been joined to facilitate aortorrhaphy. [Copyright © Baylor College of Medicine 1984. Used with permission.]

flect the colon, spleen, pancreas, and kidney to the midline by developing a plane along transversus abdominis fascia just anterior to the psoas muscle (Figure 64-4). Sharp division of the ligaments between the diaphragm and spleen hilum may be necessary. The left renal artery is reflected anteriorly with the left kidney. With the dissecting finger placed on top of the aorta and using blunt dissection, the aorta may be exposed from the crura of the diaphragm to the iliac arteries. The left crus may be incised if necessary, exposing the aorta from as high as T6. Precise control with vascular clamps placed immediately adjacent to the injury is then possible. Care is taken to minimize injury to lumbar arteries. If iatrogenically injured, these segmental arteries are suture-ligated following repair of the major injury. If anterior and posterior holes are present in the aorta, they are joined (Figure 64-5). Then lateral repair through a running suture line of 4-0 polypropylene is accomplished if possible. Often mobilization is difficult; therefore, an interposition graft of knitted Dacron or polytetrafluoroethylene (PTFE) is chosen to prevent marked narrowing of an anastomosis (Figure 64-6). When this repair technique for injuries of the suprarenal aorta is used, entering the chest to cross clamp the descending thoracic aorta can be avoided.

Injuries to the infrarenal abdominal aorta may be approached through the root of the transverse mesocolon just as an infrarenal abdominal aneurysm is electively approached. A ''super'' Kocher maneuver, swinging the cecum and entire right colon to the left (Figure 64-7) is another exposure technique which may be used. The iliac veins, right iliac vessels, vena cava, and abdominal aorta are then exposed down to the location of the renal arteries. With most penetrating wounds of the infrarenal abdominal aorta, an end-to-end anastomosis or lateral repair is possible, although the surgeon should not hesitate to use an appropriately sized Dacron or PTFE interposition graft.

Injuries to iliac arteries and veins produce significant exsanguinating hemorrhage because the surrounding peritoneum may

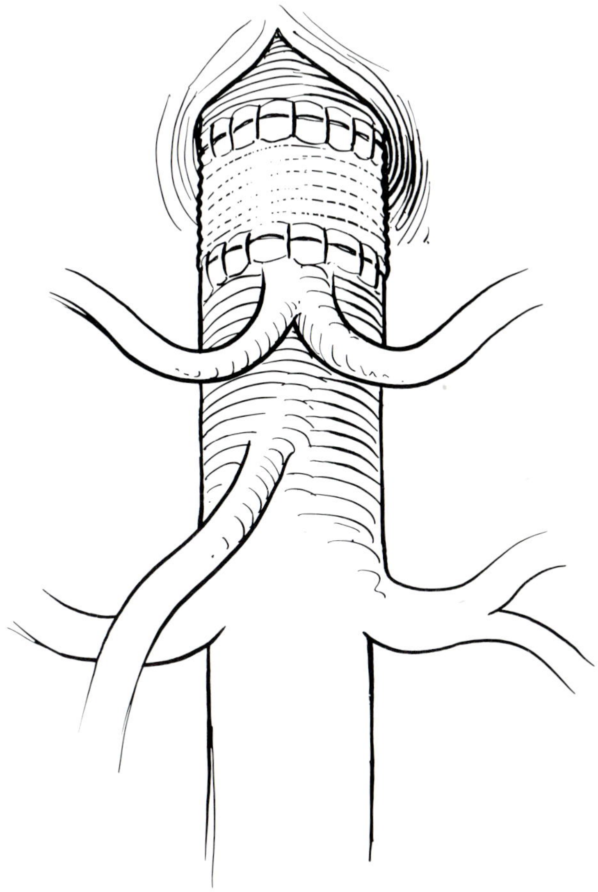

FIGURE 64-6. Drawing depicting Dacron tube graft interposition for abdominal aortic injury. [Copyright © Baylor College of Medicine 1984. Used with permission.]

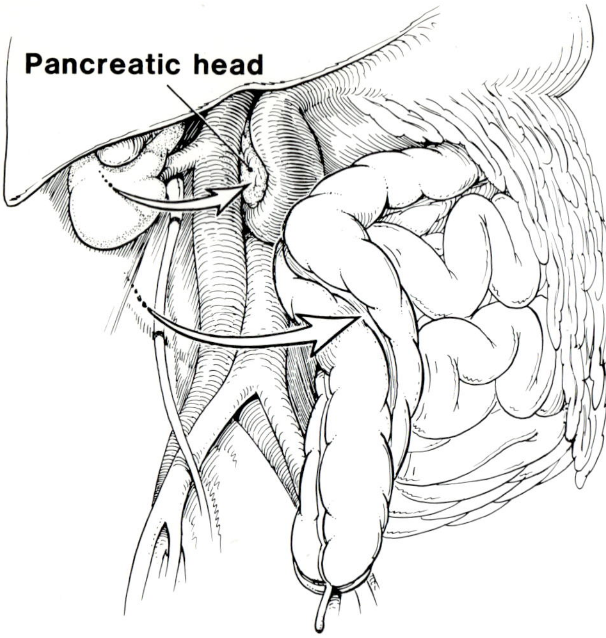

FIGURE 64-7. Drawing depicting exposure of the inferior vena cava and infrarenal abdominal aorta by use of an extended liberal Kocher maneuver. [Copyright © Baylor College of Medicine 1981. Used with permission.]

easily distend, allowing large volumes of blood to collect in the retroperitoneal space without creating a tamponading effect. Exposure is achieved by reflecting the right or left colon and entering the hematoma directly. Care is taken not to injure the ureter which crosses the iliac artery at the bifurcation of the common into the internal and external iliac arteries. Ideally, a large, partially occluding vascular clamp is placed deep in the wound in the area of rapid exsanguination, simultaneously clamping the artery, vein, and even ureter until control can be achieved. As the area of injury is isolated, additional clamps can be placed above and below the partially occluding clamp. Injuries to the bifurcation of the iliac artery and/or vein can be difficult to expose, and the assisting surgeon must use occluding sponge sticks to press firmly against the pelvis (see Figure 64-10). Blindly plunging into the hematoma and placing alligator clamps on the vessels may produce additional and irreparable injury to the adjacent iliac veins. Approximately 60 percent of all iliac injuries may be repaired primarily by lateral arteriorrhaphy or end-to-end anastomosis, and an interposition substitute conduit will be required in approximately 10 percent. On rare occasions, ligation of the common or external iliac artery may be life-saving. The internal iliac artery may be ligated with impunity. With extensive contamination from concomitant injuries to the colon, ligation of the iliac artery at the aorta and distal to the injury may be the treatment of choice. Following closure of the abdomen, a femoral-femoral crossover graft away from the area of contamination provides extraanatomic routing, eliminating the possibility of a contaminated graft and ensuing complications of thrombosis, pseudoaneurysm, and substitute conduit blowout with exsanguinating hemorrhage.

Renal artery injuries resulting from blunt trauma may be revascularized by using the splenic artery, saphenous vein, or synthetic prostheses. The chance of salvage following an intimal tear to the renal artery is remote when treatment is delayed for several hours. Diagnosis is made by intravenous pyelography followed by arteriography (47).

Injuries occurring at the origin of the celiac axis may be controlled by the maneuver described for repairing suprarenal aortic injuries. Following exposure and digital control, temporary control of celiac axis injuries may be accomplished by placing a 3-0 polypropylene suture in the area of brisk arterial bleeding. A decision can then be made to bypass or primarily repair this injury. Frequently, following ligation, pulsations from the superior mesenteric and hepatic artery collaterals are present, and no further therapy is necessary (48). Ligation of the splenic artery near its origin may result in splenic infarction and might necessitate a splenectomy. However, with good collaterals and a rich vasabrevia blood supply to the spleen, splenic infarction may not occur. Injuries to the common hepatic artery should be repaired by end-to-end anastomosis or interposition of a 5- or 6-mm PTFE graft. If the common hepatic artery is ligated, significant hepatic dysfunction results. The right or left hepatic artery may be directly ligated when the injury is restricted only to these vessels. When the right hepatic artery is ligated, cholecystectomy is performed because the cystic artery most often arises from this branch. Injuries to the distal branches of the superior mesenteric artery may be ligated. Injuries to the proximal superior mesenteric artery should be repaired if at all possible. Control may be achieved through the medial rotation of the viscera previously described for repair of injury to the suprarenal aorta. One may then cross clamp the superior mesenteric artery at its origin from the aorta. This artery is approached through the root of the mesentery by following the middle colic artery down to the superior mesenteric artery, with the colon reflected up toward the xyphoid. Thus, the superior mesenteric artery is approached from just above the duodenum and over the spine. The superior mesenteric artery emerges from behind the pancreas. If the injury is in the intrapancreatic portion, it is best ligated, and a bypass graft, preferably a 5- or 6-mm PTFE, is accomplished by swinging the graft from the infrarenal abdominal aorta away from the area of concomitant pancreatic injury. This vessel should then be covered with peritoneum and isolated from enteric structures by placing omentum between the prosthetic graft, duodenum, and small bowel to prevent the development of a graft to enteric fistula. An interposition graft should not be placed in the area of a pancreatic injury, because breakdown of the anastomosis may result. If possible, at least two of the three visceral arteries should be patent following treatment for abdominal vascular trauma. Mesenteric ischemia is common if only one of the three vessels remains patent. Injuries to the inferior mesenteric artery may be repaired if repair can be easily accomplished, but ligation (especially near the origin of the inferior mesenteric artery) may be performed.

Penetrating wounds to the iliac veins result in marked exsanguinating hemorrhage. The flow and volume of blood through the iliac veins equal that of the iliac arteries. Control is sometimes very difficult, requiring maximum exposure and innovative control techniques, including partially occluding clamps, compression with sponge forceps containing folded sponges, and at times digital compression (Figure 64-8). Although lateral repair and end-to-end anastomosis are desirable, ligation of the iliac veins including the common and external iliac vein is some-

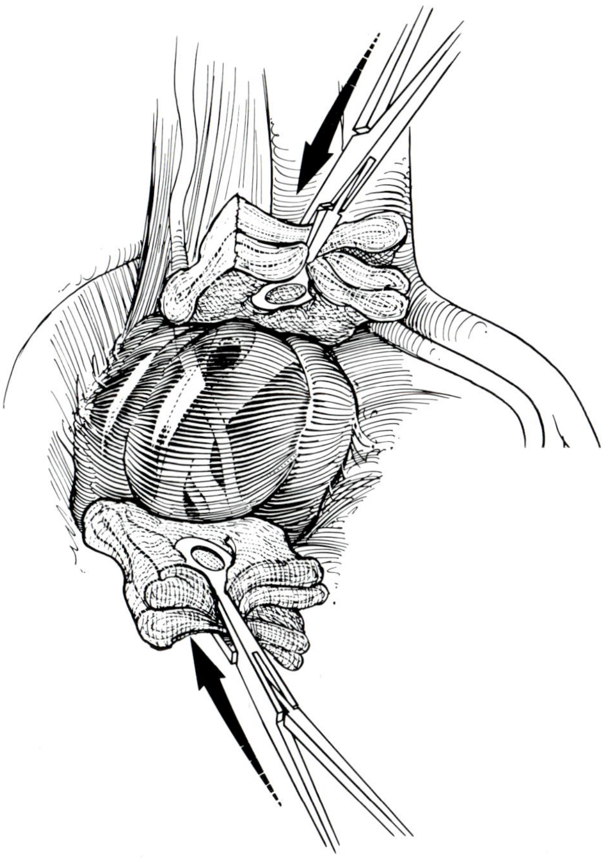

FIGURE 64-8. Drawing depicting temporary control of iliac venous injury using folded sponges above and below the injury and compressed against the posterior pelvis by the surgical assistant. [Copyright © Baylor College of Medicine 1984. Used with permission.]

times necessary to achieve control of exsanguinating hemorrhage. Injuries at the bifurcation of the iliac veins or where the iliac veins join the inferior vena cava are especially difficult to control. As with iliac artery injuries, repair should be accomplished with a 4-0 polypropylene suture. The large needle used with larger suture material produces additional holes in the vessel.

Injuries to the infrarenal inferior vena cava are approached through a liberal Kocher maneuver, rotating the appendix, cecum, right colon, and duodenum to the midline, and exposing the iliac vessels and vena cava to above the kidneys (see Figure 64-7). In most instances, direct lateral venorrhaphy may be accomplished with a running 4-0 polypropylene suture. If there is both an anterior and a posterior hole in the vena cava, occluding clamps can be placed in the area of the injury, the anterior hole lengthened, and the posterior hole sutured through the anterior hole. Subsequent closure of the anterior hole is then accomplished in a similar running fashion (Figure 64-9). The vena cava should not be rotated to expose the posterior hole. Such a maneuver would tear fragile lumbar veins which will retract into the paravertebral tissue and make control of hemorrhage very difficult. Contained, nonpulsatile retrohepatic vena caval injuries should not be explored. However, if not contained, the injuries are exposed by taking down the triangular ligaments of the liver, rotating the right lobe of the liver up and out of the abdomen to

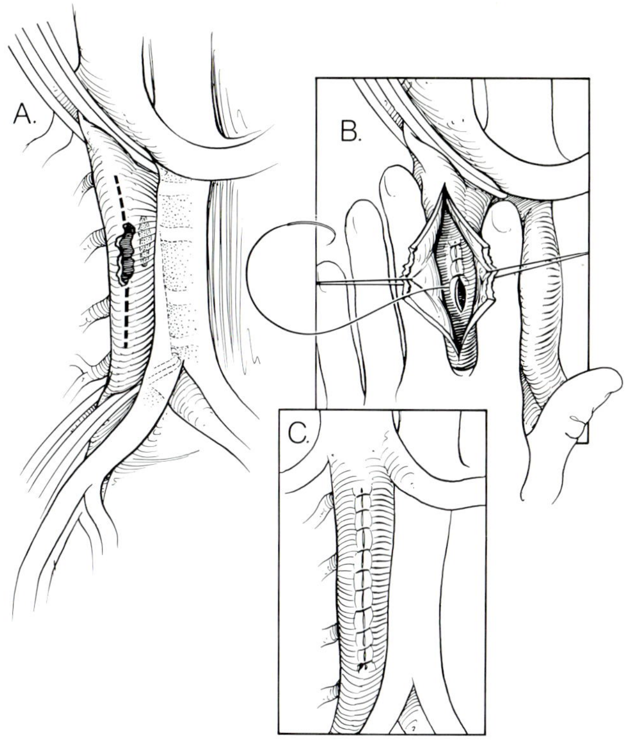

FIGURE 64-9. Drawing depicting method of exposure and closure of a posterior inferior vena cava injury by deliberate enlargement of the anterior injury. [Copyright © Baylor College of Medicine 1984. Used with permission.]

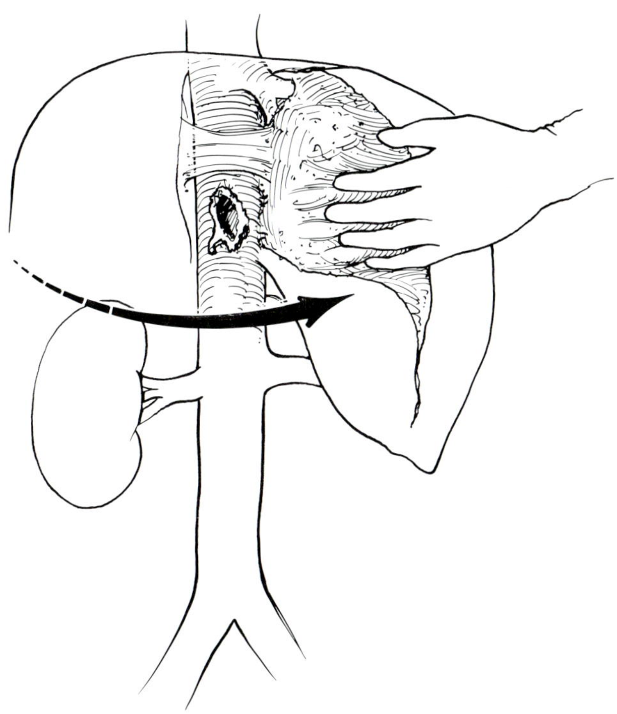

FIGURE 64-10. Drawing depicting a liver which has been rotated up and out of the abdomen (after lysing the coronary ligaments) to facilitate exposure of the retrohepatic inferior vena cava. [Copyright © Baylor College of Medicine 1984. Used with permission.]

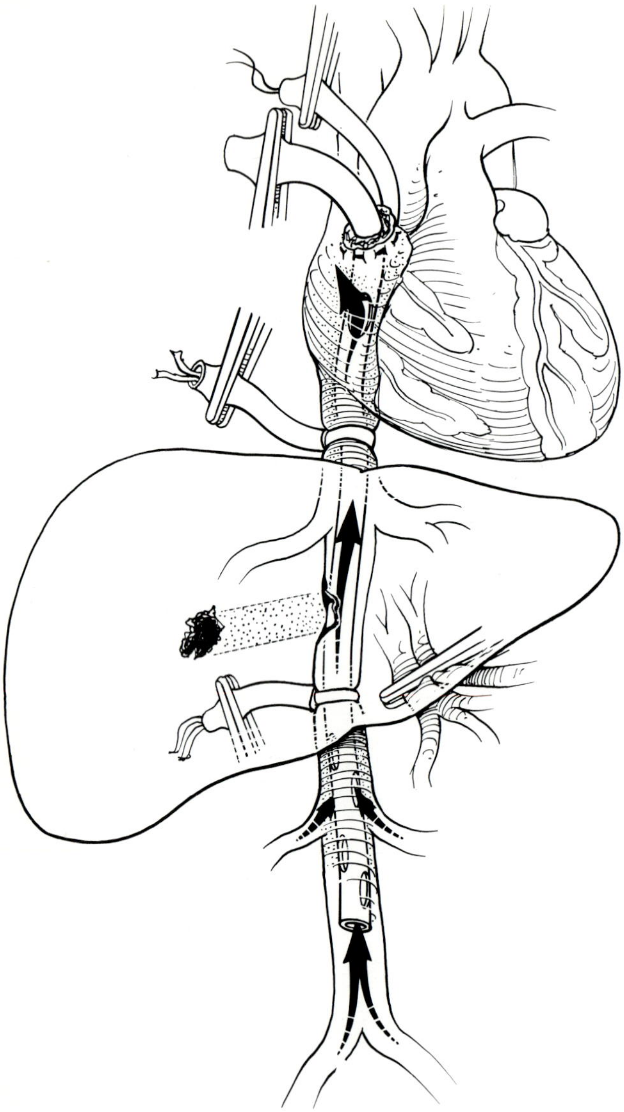

the left, and exposing direct venous drainage from the liver into the vena cava as well as the intrahepatic portion of the vena cava (Figure 64-10). Frequently, lateral repair may be easily achieved if the injury is not in the intrahepatic portion of the vena cava. When this maneuver does not achieve exposure, hemorrhage from the liver and vena cava is controlled by tamponading laparotomy packs, and a median sternotomy is performed. The diaphragm is divided laterally to the right atrium and ventricle, carrying the incision down to the area of the vena cava. With both an abdominal and a thoracic retractor in place, a purse-string suture is placed in the right atrial appendage, a chest tube is inserted through this purse string into the inferior vena cava, and an extra hole is cut in the chest tube upon its entrance into the right atrium (Figure 64-11). A clamp is placed across the open end of the chest tube near its entrance into the right atrial appendage (49). Occluding ligatures are placed around the intrapericardial portion of the inferior vena cava and around the inferior vena cava just above the renal veins. A vascular clamp is placed across the porta hepatis, thereby creating a vascular isolation to the liver (Figure 64-12). Injuries to the hepatic veins and the intrahepatic and retrohepatic portion of the inferior vena cava may thus be repaired precisely. Pilcher (50) has described a technique of inserting a bypass tube (via the groin) with a circumferential occluding balloon. Although a 30-mL Foley balloon may be inserted from the infrarenal inferior vena cava to occlude a hole in the suprarenal inferior vena cava, such total interruption of blood flow to the right heart often results in hypovolemia and hypotension (Figure 64-13).

An alternative technique of approaching a contained right lateral retrohepatic venous injury is merely to pack the abdomen

FIGURE 64-11. Drawing depicting an intracaval shunt inserted via a purse string in the right atrial appendage. Note an extra hole has been placed in the intraatrial portion of the shunt. Also note the location of occluding ligatures. [Copyright © Baylor College of Medicine 1984. Used with permission.]

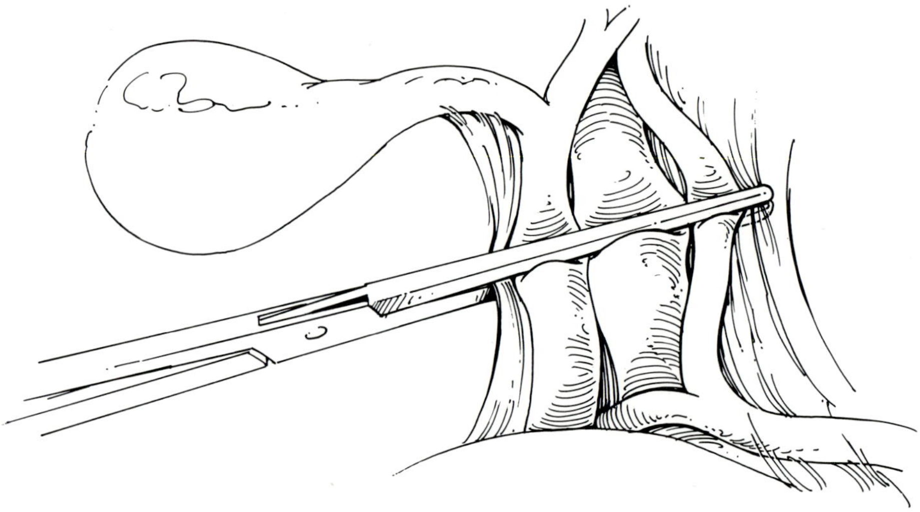

FIGURE 64-12. Drawing depicting the use of a noncrushing vascular clamp to accomplish complete, total occlusion of the hepatic artery and portal vein (Pringle maneuver.) [Copyright © Baylor College of Medicine 1984. Used with permission.]

and liver with laparotomy packs. If hemorrhage control is achieved, the abdomen should be closed, and the patient made normovolemic and normothermic in the intensive care unit. The patient is then either sent to a level one trauma center or operated upon 3 to 5 days later in a semielective mode with a plan of how the area of injury should be approached if rebleeding occurs (51).

Portal venous injuries are difficult to recognize, expose, and repair (52). Injuries to the inferior mesenteric vein and the splenic vein may be treated by simple ligation using a large suture such as 3-0 or 4-0 polypropylene. Distal injuries of the superior mesenteric vein, likewise, are best treated by ligation. However, injuries of the proximal superior mesenteric vein, the splenic vein between the inferior mesenteric vein and the portal vein, and the portal vein proper are especially difficult to manage. There is a high association of concomitant associated vascular injury, which is usually of a higher priority than the portal venous injury (52). Digital pressure will usually control bleeding from the portal vein until exposure is complete. Injuries to the portal vein or the confluence of the splenic vein and superior mesenteric vein area should not be mass-ligated but should be exposed precisely. With the transverse mesocolon retracted superiorly and the fourth portion of the duodenum and small bowel retracted inferiorly, the middle colic vein may be traced down to the root of the mesentery. The superior mesenteric vein can be exposed while digital compression is achieved to prevent exsanguinating hemorrhage. In approximately 50 percent of the

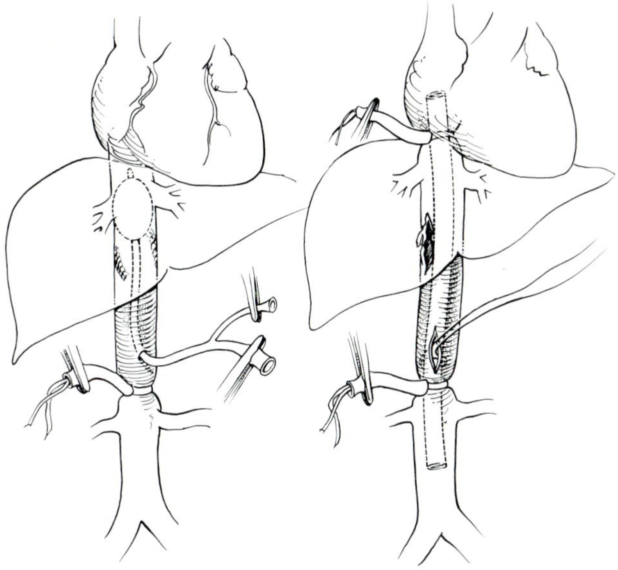

FIGURE 64-13. Drawing depicting balloon tamponade of a retrohepatic inferior vena cava injury by using a 30-mL Foley balloon inserted via a purse string in the infrarenal inferior vena cava. [Copyright © Baylor College of Medicine 1984. Used with permission.]

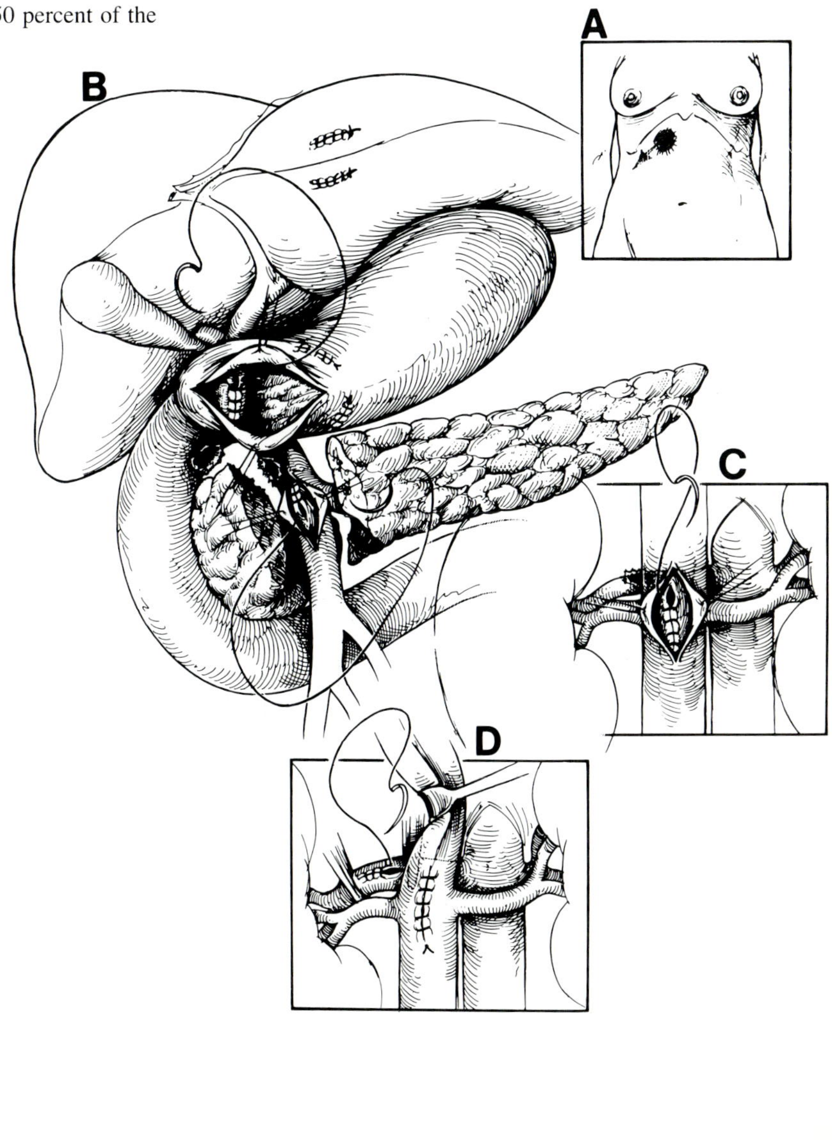

FIGURE 64-14. Drawing depicting deliberate division of the neck of the pancreas to facilitate exposure of an injury at the confluence of the splenic and superior mesenteric veins to form the portal veins. [Copyright © Baylor College of Medicine 1980. Used with permission.]

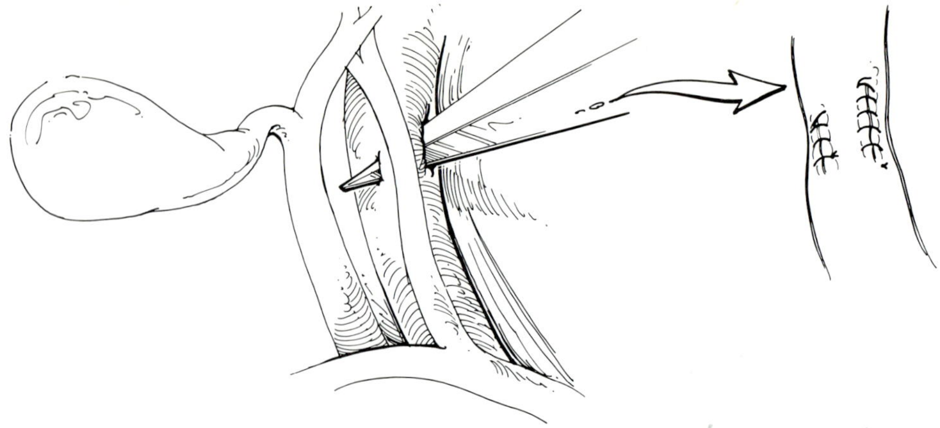

FIGURE 64-15. Drawing depicting lateral portal venorrhaphy using 4-0 or 5-0 polypropylene. [Copyright © Baylor College of Medicine 1984. Used with permission.]

cases, the superior mesenteric vein can be exposed all the way to its junction with the splenic vein underneath the inferior edge of the pancreas. Should the injury be higher, exposure is best achieved by entering the lesser sac through the gastric colic omentum. A concomitant injury in the neck of the pancreas overlying the portal vein is frequently seen. In such instances exposure is very difficult but may be enhanced considerably with deliberate division of the pancreas (Figure 64-14). At times the posterior hole can be sutured by enlarging the anterior hole after precise vascular control has been achieved with vascular clamps. Injuries to the portal vein in the porta hepatis are best approached through a Kocher maneuver, rotating the duodenum and pancreas to the left. Care is taken not to injure the hepatic artery and the common bile duct. A Pringle maneuver or a double Pringle maneuver may be necessary to prevent hemorrhage while the dissection proceeds. The preferred method of repair is lateral portal venorrhaphy (Figure 64-15). Portal venous injuries have also been reconstructed with prosthetic material of PTFE and Dacron. Stone has suggested that ligation of the portal vein can be tolerated, although others have had a high mortality rate when using this form of therapy (52,53). Should ligation be used to control hemorrhage in the portal vein, a portal decompressive procedure might be considered, i.e., a mesocaval shunt, at the time of the original operation or subsequently if portal hypertension develops.

Results

MORTALITY RATES

The 5 percent mortality rates associated with operative repair of innominate artery injuries is related to multisystem trauma, not to the innominate injury itself. In a large series of innominate artery injuries, Graham et al. (14) reported only a 13 percent operative mortality rate and no neurologic sequelae in patients where simple bypass techniques without shunts, pumps, or heparinization were utilized for innominate artery injuries or who underwent ligation of the innominate vein. Five patients in this group had chronic innominate artery conditions such as arteriovenous fistula and false aneurysms which were likewise managed by the bypass exclusion technique without hypothermia pumps or shunts. Isolated single case reports of innominate artery repair using deep hypothermia and shunting procedures have likewise had acceptable results with a low mortality rate (54–56).

Among patients undergoing surgery for blunt injury to the descending thoracic aorta, the reported mortality rates range from 5 to 25 percent in those series large enough for analysis and which include all patients presenting to a major trauma center (15–22). In referral hospitals where the patients with significant head injuries are excluded, the mortality rate among patients with a contained hematoma is 0 to 5 percent. The operative mortality rate also varies with the technique of management (see Table 64-4). The mortality rate, likewise, is associated with multisystem trauma, with death occurring secondary to head injury, infection, respiratory insufficiency, and renal insufficiency.

The most dreaded complication following operation for transection of the descending thoracic aorta is paraplegia. Paraplegia has been reported to be associated with hypotension, radiographic dye injection to the aorta, embolization of autologous clot into the intercostal or bronchial arteries for hemoptysis, injury or ligation of single or multiple intercostal arteries, and direct trauma to intercostal arteries (57,58). Contrarily, patients have had extremely long segments of the thoracic and abdominal aorta replaced as well as numerous intercostal arteries ligated without the development of paraplegia (22). The blood supply to the anterior spinal artery is multiple and segmental. This variable anatomy dictates that the occurrence of paraplegia is random and unpredictable. Although patients with thoracoabdominal injury have tolerated aortic cross clamping in excess of 75 minutes without hepatic, renal, or neurologic impairment, a 30- to 45-minute cross-clamp time to accomplish the vascular reconstruction has been recommended by numerous authors (45,46,59). Techniques to allegedly protect the spinal cord have been discussed previously under pathophysiology. In all cases, the cord supplied by intercostal arteries between the cross clamps

TABLE 64-5. Mortality Rate from Suprarenal Abdominal Aortic Injury

Author (Ref.)	Year	No. of Cases	Mortality Rate, %
Brinton (65)	1982	3	0
Kashuk (64)	1982	9	44
Allen (66)	1972	16	75
Lim (63)	1974	17	71
Mattox (61)	1975	28	64

TABLE 64-6. Mortality Rate from Infrarenal Abdominal Aortic Injury

Author (Ref.)	Year	No. of Cases	Mortality Rate, %
Brinton (65)	1982	12	50
Kashuk (64)	1982	9	53
Lim (63)	1974	15	53
Allen (66)	1972	21	62

remains at risk. Reports containing enough data for analysis using the three techniques of repair reveal that the incidence of paraplegia is lowest when cardiopulmonary bypass or simple cross-clamp repair is utilized (see Table 64-4). Techniques of measuring evoked nerve potentials during surgery reveal that alterations are measurable during times of aortic cross clamping and hypothermia. Following release of the cross clamp, however, these potentials return with variable results, including no neurologic deficit whatsoever (60). Therefore. the interpretation of the meaning of the neurologic evoked potentials has yet to be clarified.

The mortality rate for patients with suprarenal abdominal aortic injuries exceeds 50 percent, with the majority of deaths being from exsanguinating hemorrhage or multisystem trauma (Table 64-5) (61–65). The mortality rate for patients undergoing surgical repair of infrarenal abdominal aortic injuries also exceeds 50 percent (Table 64-6) (66,67).

The mortality rate for patients undergoing operation for iliac artery injury ranges from 38 to 60 percent (Table 64-7) (68–70). Complications of infection are common due to the high associated rate of injury to the ureters and sigmoid colon. Thrombosis of repaired iliac arteries and the abdominal aorta is rare. However, if thrombosis of the iliac artery does occur, claudication is extremely uncommon. The mortality rate for isolated injuries to the iliac veins is 6 percent (71). Following ligation for iliac vein injury, venous insufficiency may produce incapacitating chronic venous hypertension (72,73).

The operative mortality rate for injuries to the inferior vena cava depends on location (Figure 64-16), and causes of death include hemorrhagic shock, multisystem injury, and respiratory insufficiency (74). Of special consideration are patients with combined injuries to the aorta and inferior vena cava. When both injuries occur at once, the operative mortality rate is 60 to 75 percent (75). The operative mortality rate among patients with injuries to the portal venous system is dependent upon the location and the mechanism of injury (Table 64-8).

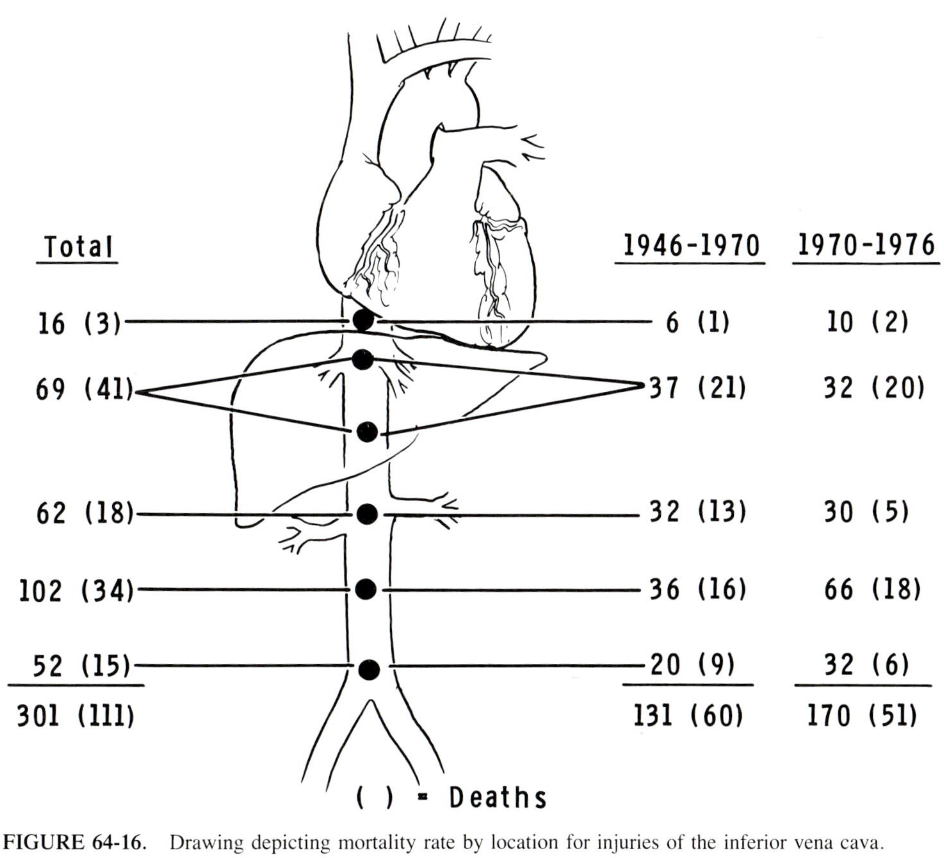

FIGURE 64-16. Drawing depicting mortality rate by location for injuries of the inferior vena cava.

TABLE 64-7. **Mortality Rate from Iliac Artery Injury**

	Common		Internal		External		Total	
Author (Ref.)	No.	Mortality, %	No.	Mortality, %	No.	Mortality, %	No.	Mortality, %
Buscaglia (11)*							9	11
Morris (70)*							17	29
Kashuk (64)*							19	53
Sirinek (69)	13	46	—	—	7	0	20	30
Mattox (68)	33	52	22	36	28	25	83	39

*No breakdown as to specific iliac artery site.

TABLE 64-8. **Mortality Rate from Portal Venous Injury**

	Portal Vein		SMV*		SV†		IMV‡		Total	
Author (Ref.)	No.	Percent	No.	Percent	No.	Percent	No.	Percent	No.	Percent
Graham (74)	37	52	45	32	7	0	9	0	98	33
Kashuk (64)	9	67	10	20	1	0	3	33	23	39
Sirinek (69)	5	100	12	25	—		—		17	47
Stone (52)	41	46	37	27	—		—		78	37

*Superior mesenteric vein.
†Splenic vein.
‡Inferior mesenteric vein.

COMPLICATIONS

Operative and early complications have been presented earlier in this chapter. Delayed in-hospital complications, in general, are those relating to infection from associated injuries. With multisystem injury, especially to the colon, spleen, kidney, liver, stomach, and major vascular structures, subphrenic abscess is extremely common. With uncontrolled infection, late-appearing respiratory insufficiency or stress bleeding is common.

Delayed complications relating to the vascular repair include false aneurysm, arteriovenous fistula, thrombosis, and vascular infection (29,76). Though rarely occurring with truncal vascular trauma, false aneurysm has been reported, especially in descending thoracic aorta and iliac artery repairs. Arteriovenous fistula most often occurs because of an originally missed injury rather than a breakdown of repair. Thrombosis of a major repair is most common in the iliac vein and inferior vena cava. Although thrombosis of the inferior vena cava has been seen following many primary repairs of the inferior vena cava where venography was performed, lower extremity venous hypertension is not as common as in patients with thrombosis of the iliac veins (Figure 64-17). Delayed thrombosis of external iliac arteries has been reported, although claudication does not occur if collaterals have developed.

Following vascular reconstructive procedures of the superior

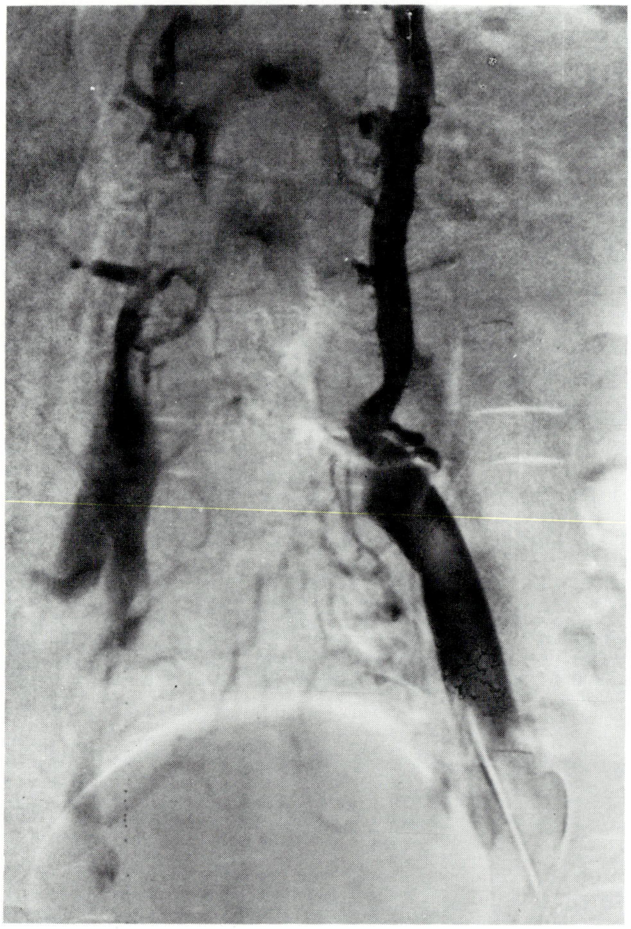

FIGURE 64-17. Venogram illustrating total occlusion of the inferior vena cava following a simple venacavorrhaphy for a single stab wound. Note collateral venous return via ascending lumbar veins toward the azygous system.

mesenteric artery, breakdown of the repair may occur if it is in close proximity to the pancreatic fistula or drainage. Erosion from intraabdominal arterial grafts may produce a late-appearing graft to enteric fistula. In such instances, a sentinel bleeding episode usually occurs, and endoscopy fails to reveal a bleeding point in the stomach or proximal duodenum. In this event, the surgeon exposes the area of prosthesis for control and repair.

It has been the experience at Baylor College of Medicine and Ben Taub General Hospital that perivascular infections following trauma occur mainly in the iliac and extremity locations. An infected vascular repair occurred twice in patients with a primary end-to-end anastomosis and once in a patient in whom Dacron was inserted in the external iliac position. Both cases were successfully managed by removal of the area of infection, ligation of the iliac artery, and reconstruction by femoral-femoral crossover bypass.

Key Points to Surgical Judgment

1. The surgeon caring for the patient with potential truncal vascular injury must become involved early in the evaluation, stabilization, control, and treatment of such injuries. This involvement includes care in the prehospital phase, emergency department, operating room, and intensive care unit.

2. The chest x-ray is the single most significant diagnostic test in the emergency center to determine major intrathoracic truncal vascular injury or confirm a normal chest x-ray in a patient who is markedly hypovolemic, thereby indicating major intraabdominal pathology.

3. A hematoma at the thoracic outlet is indicative of injury to the innominate artery, whereas a hematoma at the thoracic aortic isthmus is more indicative of injury to the descending thoracic aorta just distal to the subclavian artery.

4. The proper choice of incision is mandatory for adequate exposure and control of truncal vascular injuries.

5. Innovative exposure techniques through rotation of the viscera to the right or left and exposing the aorta or vena cava from the lateral approach reduce the need for banked blood, decrease the time required for exposure and control, and allow for orderly reconstructive procedures. Autotransfusion in the emergency center and intraoperatively has great utility in the patient with truncal vascular injury and should be considered in all such cases.

6. The use of synthetic substitute vascular conduits for reconstructive vascular procedures speeds up the operation and has been shown to be effective in all areas of truncal vascular injury.

References

1. Dillard BM, Nelson DL, Norman HG Jr: Review of 85 major traumatic arterial injuries. Surgery 1968, 63:391–395.
2. Drapanas T, Hewitt RL, Weichert RF, et al: Civilian vascular injuries: A critical appraisal of three decades of management. Ann Surg 1970, 172:351–360.
3. Patman RD, Poulos E, Shires GT: The management of civilian arterial injuries. Surg Gynecol Obstet 1964, 118:725–738.
4. Rapaport A, Feliciano DV, Mattox KL: An epidemiologic profile of urban trauma in America—Houston style. Tex Med 1982, 78:44–50.
5. Cheek, RC, Pope JC, Smith HF, et al: Diagnosis and management of major vascular injuries: A review of 200 operative cases. Am Surg 1975, 41:755–760.
6. Perry MO, Thal ER, Shires GT: Management of arterial injuries. Ann Surg 1971, 173:403–408.
7. Buscaglia LC, Blaisdell FW, Lim RC: Penetrating abdominal vascular injuries. Arch Surg 1969, 99:764–769.
8. Treiman RL, Doty D, Gaspar MR: Acute vascular trauma. A fifteen year study. J Surg 1966, 111:469–473.
9. Makins GH: *Gunshot Injuries to the Blood Vessels*. Bristol, England, John Wright & Sons, 1919.
10. DeBakey ME, Simeone FA: Battle injuries of the arteries in World War II: An analysis of 2,471 cases. Ann Surg 1946, 123:534–579.
11. Hughes CW: Arterial repair during the Korean War. Ann Surg 1958, 147:555–561.
12. Rich NM, Baugh JH, Hughes CW: Acute arterial injuries in Vietnam: 1000 cases. J Trauma 1970, 10:359–369.
13. Graham JM, Feliciano DV, Mattox KL, et al: Management of Subclavian Vascular Injuries. J Trauma 1980, 20:537–544.
14. Graham JM, Feliciano DV, Mattox KL: Innominate vascular injury. J Trauma 1982, 22:647–655.
15. Pickard LR, Mattox KL, Espada R: Transection of the descending thoracic aorta secondary to blunt trauma. J Trauma 1977, 17:749–754.
16. Crawford ES, Palamara AE, Salem SA, et al: Aortic aneurysms: Current status of surgical treatment. Surg Clin North Am 1979, 59(4):597–636.
17. Wolfe WG, Kleinman LH, Sabiston DC Jr: Heparin coated shunts for lesions of the descending thoracic aorta. Arch Surg 1977, 112:1481–1486.
18. Beall AC Jr, Arbegast NR, Ripepi AC: Aortic laceration due to rapid deceleration. Arch Surg 1969, 98:595–601.
19. Kirsh MM, Behrendt DM, Orringer MB: The treatment of acute traumatic rupture of the aorta. Ann Surg 1976, 184:308–316.
20. Gott VL: Heparinized shunts for thoracic vascular operations. Ann Thorac Surg 1972, 14:219–220.
21. Wakabayashi A, Connolly JE: Prevention of Paraplegia Associated with Resection of Extensive Thoracic Aneurysms. Arch Surg 1976, 111:1186–1189.
22. Crawford ES, Rubio PA: Reappraisal of adjuncts to avoid ischemia in the treatment of aneurysm of descending thoracic aorta. J Thorac Cardiovasc Surg 1973, 66:693–704.
23. Trunkey DD: Trauma. Sci Am 1983, 249:28–33.
24. Robertson LS: Highway injury. Tex Med 1983, 79:48–50.
25. Baker SP, Spitz WU: Age effects and autopsy evidence of disease in fatally injured drivers. JAMA 1970, 213:1079–1083.
26. Parmley LF, Mattingly TW, Manion WC, et al: Non-penetrating traumatic injury of the aorta. Circulation 1958, 17:1086–1101.
27. Mattox KL: Invited commentary, blunt thoracic aortic injury. World J Surg 1980, 4:551–552.
28. Fisher RG, Hadlock F, Ben-Manachem Y: Laceration of the thoracic aorta and brachiocephalic arteries by blunt trauma. Radiol Clin North Am 1981, 19:91–110.
29. Rich NM, Hobson RW II, Collins CJ Jr: Traumatic arteriovenous

fistulas and false aneurysms: A review of 558 lesions. Surgery 1975, 78:817–828.

30. Blood and fluid replacement in shock. In Walt AJ (ed): Philadelphia, *Early Care of the Injured Patient*. WB Saunders, 1982, pp 9–27.
31. Akins CW, Buckly MJ, Dagett W: Acute traumatic disruption of the thoracic aorta: A ten year experience. Ann Thorac Surg 1981, 31:305–309.
32. Pezzella AT, Effler DB, Levy I: Non-operative management of unusual blunt traumatic rupture of the thoracic aorta. Tex Heart Inst J 1982, 9:359–362.
33. Mattox KL, Beall AC Jr, Jordan GL Jr, et al: Cardiorrhaphy in the emergency center. J Thorac Cardiovasc Surg 1974, 68:886–895.
34. Moore EE, Moore JB, Galloway AC, et al: Post-injury thoracotomy in the emergency department: A critical evaluation. Surgery 1979, 86:590–598.
35. Bodai BI, Smith JR, Ward RE, et al: Emergency thoracotomy in the management of trauma. JAMA 1983, 249:1891–1896.
36. Mattox KL, Allen MK, Feliciano DV: Laparotomy in the emergency department. J Am Coll Emer Phys 1979, 8:180–183.
37. Appelbaum A, Karp RB, Kirkland JW: Surgical treatment for closed thoracic aorta injuries. Surg Clin North Am 1979, 59:597–636.
38. Turney SZ, Attar A, Cowley RA, et al: Traumatic rupture of the aorta: A five year experience. J Thorac Cardiovasc Surg 1976, 71:458–460.
39. Ketonen P, Jarvinen A, Luosto R, et al: Traumatic rupture of the thoracic aorta. J Thorac Cardiovasc Surg 1977, 72:727–734.
40. Vasco JS, Raess DH, William TE Jr, et al: Nonpenetrating trauma of the thoracic aorta. Scand J Thorac Cardiovasc Surg 1977, 72:727–734.
41. Wilson RF, Arbulu A, Bassett JS, et al: Acute mediastinal widening following blunt chest trauma. Surgery 1977, 82:400–406.
42. Akins CW, Buckley MJ, Dagett W: Acute traumatic disruption of the thoracic aorta: A ten year experience. Ann Thorac Surg 1980, 31:305–309.
43. Finkelmeier BA, Mentzer RM Jr, Kaiser DL, et al: Chronic traumatic thoracic aneurysm. J Thorac Cardiovasc Surg 1982, 84:257–266.
44. McCollum CH, Graham JM, Noon GP, et al: Chronic traumatic aneurysms of the thoracic aorta: An analysis of 50 patients. J Trauma 1979, 19:248–252.
45. Najafi H, Javio H, Hunter J, et al: Descending aortic aneurysmectomy without adjuncts to avoid ischemia. Ann Thorac Surg 1980, 30:326–335.
46. Lerberg DB, Bahnson HT: Surgical treatment of thoracic aortic aneurysms. Bergan JJ, Yao JST (eds): *Aneurysms Diagnosis and Treatment*. New York, Grune & Stratton, 1982, pp 119–129.
47. Brown MF, Graham JM, Mattox KL, et al: Renovascular Trauma. Am J Surg 1980, 140:802–806.
48. Graham JM, Mattox KL, Beall AC Jr, et al: Injuries to the visceral arteries. Surgery 1978, 84:835–839.
49. Schrock T, Blaisdell W, Mathewson C: Management of blunt trauma to the liver and hepatic veins. Arch Surg 1968, 96:698–704.
50. Pilcher DB, Harman PD, Moore EE: Retrohepatic vena cava balloon shunt introduced via the sapheno-femoral junction. J Trauma 1977, 17:837–841.
51. Feliciano DV, Mattox KL, Jordan GL Jr: Intra-abdominal packing for control of hepatic hemorrhage: A reappraisal. J Trauma 1981, 21:258–290.
52. Graham JM, Mattox KL, Beall AC Jr: Portal venous system injuries. J Trauma 1978, 18:422–429.
53. Stone HH, Fabian TC, Turkleson ML: Wounds of the portal venous system. World J Surg 1982, 6:335–340.
54. Lim LT, Saletto JD, Flanigan DP: Subclavian and innominate artery trauma. Surgery 1979, 86:890–897.
55. Magilligan DJH, Davila JC: Innominate artery disruption due to blunt trauma. Arch Surg 1979, 114:307–309.
56. Murray GF, Brawley RK, Gott VL: Reconstruction of the innominate artery by means of a temporary heparin-coated shunt bypass. J Thorac Cardiovasc Surg 1971, 62:34–42.
57. Crawford ES, Beall AC Jr, Moyer JH: Complications of aortography. Surg Gynecol Obstet 1957, 104:129–141.
58. Kardjiev V, Simeonov A, Chankov I: Etiology, pathogenesis and prevention of spinal cord lesions in selective angiography of the bronchial and intercostal arteries. Radiology 1974, 112:81–83.
59. Garcia-Rinaldi R, Defore WW, Mattox KL, et al: Unimpaired renal, myocardial, and neurologic function after cross-clamping of the thoracic aorta. Surg Gynecol Obstet 1976, 143:249–252.
60. Coles JG, Wilson GJ, Sima AF, et al: Intraoperative detection of spinal cord ischemia using somatosensory cortical evoked potentials during thoracic aortic occlusion. Ann Thorac Surg 1982, 34:299–306.
61. Mattox KL, McCollum WB, Beall AC Jr, et al: Management of penetrating injuries of the suprarenal aorta. J Trauma 1975, 15:808–815.
62. Yeo MT, Domanskies EJ, Bartlett, RH, et al: Penetrating injuries of the abdominal aorta. Arch Surg 1974, 108:838–842.
63. Lim RC, Trunkey DD, Blaisdell FW: Acute abdominal aortic injury. Arch Surg 1974, 109:706–711.
64. Kashuk JL, Moore EE, Millikan JS, et al: Major abdominal vascular trauma—A unified approach. J Trauma 1982, 22:672–679.
65. Brinton M, Miller SE, Lim RC Jr, et al: Acute abdominal aortic injuries. J Trauma 1982, 22:481–486.
66. Allen TW, Reul GJ, Morton JR, et al: Surgical management of aortic trauma. J Trauma 1972, 12:862–868.
67. Fromm SH, Carrasquilla C, Lucas C: The Management of gunshot wounds of the aorta. Arch Surg 1970, 101:388–390.
68. Mattox KL, Rea J, Ennix CL, et al: Penetrating injuries to the iliac arteries. Am J Surg 1978, 136:663–667.
69. Sirinek KR, Gaskill HB, Root HD, et al: Truncal vascular injury—Factors influencing survival. J Trauma 1983, 23:372–377.
70. Morris GC, Beall AC Jr, Roof WR, et al: Surgical experience with 220 acute arterial injuries in civilian practice. Am J Surg 1960, 99:775–781.
71. Ryan W, Snyder W, Bell T, et al: Penetrating injuries of the iliac vessels. Am J Surg 1982, 144:642–645.
72. Rich NM, Collins GJ Jr, Andersen CA, et al: Venous trauma: Successful venous reconstruction remains an interesting challenge. Am J Surg 1977, 134:226–230.
73. Rich NM, Collins GJ, Andersen CA, et al: Autogenous venous interposition grafts in repair of major injuries. J Trauma 1977, 17:513–520.
74. Graham JM, Mattox KL, Beall AC Jr, et al: Traumatic injuries of the inferior vena cava. Arch Surg 1978, 113:413–418.
75. Mattox KL, Whisennand HH, Espada R, et al: Management of acute combined injuries to the aorta and inferior vena cava. Am J Surg 1975, 130:720–724.
76. Feliciano DV, Mattox KL: Traumatic aneurysms, in *Vascular Surgery*, Rutherford RB (ed). Philadelphia, Saunders, 1984, pp 848–855.

Chapter 65

POSTTRAUMATIC PAIN SYNDROMES: CAUSALGIA AND MIMOCAUSALGIA

WILSON V. GARRETT, JESSE E. THOMPSON, C. M. TALKINGTON, and BERTRAM L. SMITH

The orderly and predictable healing of wounds following injury can be anticipated in almost all instances. The return of function, normalization of vasomotor tone, and relief of pain normally accompany the healing process. Occasionally, however, despite uncomplicated treatment of the wound and in the absence of any obvious precipitating factors, a posttraumatic pain syndrome may develop. The pain may be severe and unrelenting even after minor injury. Accompanying the pain will be varying degrees of vasomotor and sudomotor dysfunction. Disuse leads to trophic changes which may ultimately become irreversible.

In 1864, Mitchell, Morehouse, and Keen (1) described a syndrome subsequently referred to as *causalgia* (*kausos,* heat; *algos,* pain). Their observations were made in the course of treating soldiers suffering gunshot wounds of extremity nerves. The description remains a classic:

> The great mass of sufferers described this pain as superficial, but others said it was also in the joints, and deep in the palms. If it lasted long, it was referred finally to the skin alone.
>
> Its intensity varies from the most trivial burning to a state of torture, which can hardly be credited, but which reacts on the whole economy, until the general health is seriously affected.
>
> The part itself is not subject to an intense burning sensation but becomes exquisitely hyperesthetic so that a touch or a tap of the finger increases the pain. Exposure to the air is avoided by the patient with a care which seems absurd, and most of the bad cases keep the hands constantly wet, finding relief in moisture rather than in the coolness of the application. . . .
>
> As the pain increases, the general sympathy becomes more marked. The temper changes and grows irritable, the face becomes anxious and has a look of weariness and suffering. The sleep is restless, and the constitutional condition reacting on the wounded limb exasperates the hyperesthetic state, so that rattling of a newspaper, a breath of air, another's step across the ward, the vibration caused by military band, or the shock of the feet in walking, gives rise to increase of pain. At last the patient grows hysterical if we may use the only term which covers the fact. He walks carefully, carries the limb tenderly with a sound hand, he is tremulous, nervous and has all kinds of expedients for lessening the pain.

The proportion of causalgia cases to the total number of nerve injuries varies but ranges from 1.8 to 12 percent (2). The injuries are usually partial to major mixed nerves, particularly the sciatic, tibial, and median. The pain syndrome produced is characteristically severe and debilitating.

Following the report of Homans (3), who coined the term "minor causalgia," clinicians were made aware of this milder but similar syndrome in which no obvious or demonstrable nerve injury had occurred. Many other terms have been used to describe this entity, including posttraumatic sympathetic dystrophy, reflex dystrophy, Sudeck's atrophy, and others (4). These descriptive terms were usually based upon the trophic changes observed. In the interest of simplicity, these terms can be discarded in favor of *mimocausalgia* since the symptoms mimic causalgia (5).

Clinical Manifestations

In most cases of causalgia, pain begins early, within hours following injury. Many patients describe a burning pain, although in some a superficial tingling or stinging is more prominent. Other deeper components produce a tearing, crushing, stabbing, or aching sensation. The pain is felt into the hand or foot in the distribution of the involved nerve. Hyperalgesia is severe, and patients go to great lengths to prevent even minimal contact with the affected area. Any form of stimulus to the limb, such as movement, contact, heat, or cold, can precipitate agonizing pain. The arm is diligently protected, often covered, and postured to prevent even venous congestion which can increase the pain. Auditory, visual, or emotional stimuli can also lead to sudden, intense discomfort. The immobilization of the part leads to the characteristic trophic changes of edema, osteoporosis, and stiffness. The skin of the palms or soles is glossy and shiny, and the terminal pads of the fingers atrophy, producing a tapering appearance. Vasomotor and sudomotor changes are seen as well, and the skin becomes cold, cyanotic, and moist. The application of warmth may provide relief. Less commonly, vasodilation is seen with erythematous mottling and scaling of the skin. Relief in these cases may be obtained by cooling the extremity.

Unless successful therapy intervenes, progressive atrophic changes with fibrosis, contractures, arthritic changes, or stiffening of the joints will lead to irreversible and crippling deformities. Mitchell (1) emphasized the psychiatric sequelae:

> Perhaps few persons who are not physicians can realize the influence which long-continued and unendurable pain may have upon both body and mind . . . under such torments the temper changes, the most amiable grow irritable, the soldier becomes a coward, and the strongest man is scarcely less nervous than the most hysterical girl.

In mimocausalgia, a similar syndrome develops, although in most cases the symptoms are less severe and more responsive to conservative treatment. Pain, sympathetic overactivity with vasoconstriction and hyperhidrosis, delayed functional recovery, and trophic changes are characteristic. The symptoms are disproportionately severe when compared to the initial injury which may have been seemingly innocuous.

For the syndrome to develop, three factors must be present: a painful injury or operation, a "susceptible" individual, and an abnormal autonomic nervous system response to the injury. The immobilization following injury appears to play a great role in initiating a vicious cycle leading eventually to functional impairment (6) (Figure 65-1). Such immobility may often be purposeful with secondary gain considerations. The malingerer cannot be successfully treated until compensation litigation has been resolved (2). It has been suggested that a certain dependent, emotionally labile personality predisposes to the development of the syndrome, although psychological testing has not proved this susceptibility to be the case (7). Owens (8) has demonstrated that almost 70 percent of causalgia patients give a history of sympathetic overreactivity. Evans (9) also suggests that vasomotor instability is a common predisposing factor.

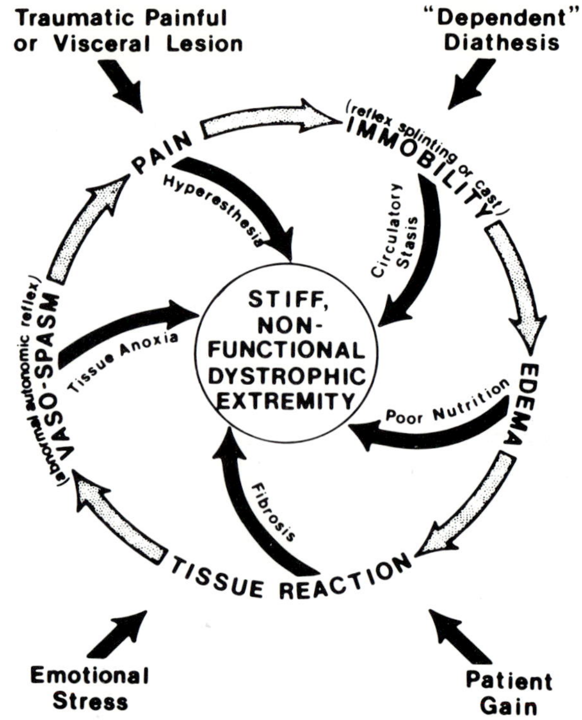

FIGURE 65-1. Vicious cycle: Graphic representation of various factors contributing to pathogenesis of stiff, swollen, painful, dystrophic extremity. (Lankford and Thompson, Ref. 6.)

Etiology

Three possible sites have been suggested for the origin of the pain impulses in causalgia: (1) the peripheral tissues where the pain is felt, (2) the damaged segment of the nerve, and (3) the central nervous system.

Lewis (10) theorized that pain-producing vasodilator substances were released at the site of injury, leading to a stimulation of sensory afferents as well as a lowering of their threshhold. He felt, as did DeTakats (11), that a "washing away" of these substances occurred after sympathectomy. Doupe (12) proposed that a cross-linkage occurred between sympathetic efferents and sensory afferents at both the site of injury and distally in the skin subjected to nutritional changes. Leriche (13) felt that the pain was secondary to vasospasm.

Pain impulses can originate at the site of nerve damage in several ways. Structural changes in nerves may distort conduction; scarring and neuroma formation could produce a trigger point stimulating sensory afferents; a failure of insulating properties of injured nerve fibers might allow the spread of sensory afferent stimuli; and artificial synapses between sympathetic efferents and sensory afferents and between motor and sensory nerves might occur at the site of injury (14). Pain fibers of the C group have a lower threshhold to such cross-stimulation. Melzack and Wall (15), in a refinement of the earlier fiber dissociation concept of Noordenbos (16), suggested a theory in which certain cells (T cells) in the substantia gelatinosa of the dorsal horn of the spinal cord function as a gate for incoming sensory impulses. Impulses traveling along myelinated nerve fibers (A delta fibers) tend to close the gate for incoming C fiber impulses. If myelinated fibers were damaged selectively at the site of injury, C fiber impulses would predominate, opening the gate for central transmission of nervous stimuli interpreted as burning pain.

Livingston (17) suggested an important role of the central nervous system, proposing the presence of an abnormal level of activity or increased stimulation of the internuncial neuronal pool located in the posterior horn of the spinal cord. These central effects produce peripheral changes such as spasms and vasomotor disturbances. These then stimulate once again the sensory afferents, setting up a perpetual cycle. Sunderland (18) extended this thesis and proposed that the abnormal foci of the dorsal horn not only have a localized segmental effect but affect transmission all the way to the cerebral cortex, causalgia being the terminal event of this disorderly activity on the sensorium. This is the basis of his so-called turbulence hypothesis.

All of these different mechanisms may be operative in producing the symptoms of causalgia. The sympathetic nervous system certainly plays a key role in the process since interruption of sympathetic innervation to the involved part characteristically provides relief.

Treatment

Drucker (19) divided the progress of causalgia and mimocausalgia into three stages:

I. Acute: Constant, immediate, aching, burning, disproportionate pain; edema; increased hair and nail growth, hyperalgesia; hyperhidrosis; patchy osteoporosis after 1 to 2 months.

II. Dystrophic: By 3 months, edema becomes indurated; cool, pale, cyanotic skin; cracked, brittle nails; continuous pain; x-ray: diffuse osteoporosis.

III. Atrophic: Pain spreads beyond the area of injury; skin and fingertips wasted; joint contractures; x-ray: marked demineralization and ankylosis.

When the findings have progressed to stage III, irreversible changes are likely, and treatment will fail. Therefore, the first order of treatment is preventive, early intervention. To prevent the syndrome following hand surgery, a common precipitating event, Urbaniek and Roth (20) recommended that the tourniquet should be released before wound closure. Tight dressings should be avoided in favor of a thick, bulky hand dressing. Postoperative elevation to minimize edema is crucial. If undue pain occurs after casting, the cast must be split to the skin.

When early sympathetic dystrophic changes appear, pain relief and active use of the hand, arm, or leg are instituted. Passive motion by the therapist should be avoided as it may increase pain and edema. Narcotics should be avoided. Splinting the hand in a functional position may be helpful, and dynamic splinting may be added as improvement occurs. Desensitization of the hyperalgesic area should be begun, first stroking the area with wisps of cotton and slowly progressing to coarser objects. Trigger points should be injected with local anesthetic or steroid mixtures. A nonsteroidal anti-inflammatory agent is begun and continued long-term. A short course of high-dose steroids may be helpful as well (21). Amitriptyline hydrochloride (Elavil) is recommended by Benson (22) in a dose of 50 to 75 mg nightly or up to 150 mg divided during the day. He also advises a phenothiazine such as fluphenazine hydrochloride (Prolixin) which potentiates narcotics, possesses an analgesic property of its own, and depresses the response to peripheral stimuli. The recommended dosage is 1 mg three times daily, but doses up to 10 mg daily can be administered. A sympatholytic drug such as phenoxybenzamine (Dibenzyline) should be begun at 10 mg daily and increased to 40 mg daily as tolerated.

A transcutaneous electrical nerve stimulation (TENS) unit may be applied. This device was invented to predict the response to dorsal column stimulation. Its application of more proximal nerve stimulation has met with varied and short-lived success (18). Success or failure of this device in the hands of an experienced examiner will be apparent by the third to fifth treatment (9).

Regional medical sympathectomy can be attempted. Chuinard (23) reported relief of symptoms in 21 of 25 patients treated by injecting a solution of reserpine in a modification of the Bier regional intravenous anesthetic block. Reserpine is a catecholamine depletor and inhibits adrenergic nerve endings. One milligram is diluted in 50 mL of normal saline for the upper extremity; 2 mg is diluted in 100 mL normal saline for the lower. An intravenous catheter is inserted into a vein of the forearm, hand, or foot. The extremity is exsanguinated with an Esmarch's rubber bandage, and an above-elbow or above-knee tourniquet is inflated to 300 mmHg for 15 minutes to allow tissue fixation. Placing the reserpine in 0.25% bupivacaine (Marcaine) or 0.1% lidocaine (Xylocaine) will decrease the discomfort accompanying injection of the solution. A warm and painless extremity may result for several days, allowing intensification of physical therapy. Hannington-Kiff (24) and others (25) have made similar observations using a solution of guanethidine, an agent unavailable in this country in a parenteral form.

In 1930, Spurling (26) reported relief of a case of causalgia treated by cervicothoracic sympathectomy. Experiences during

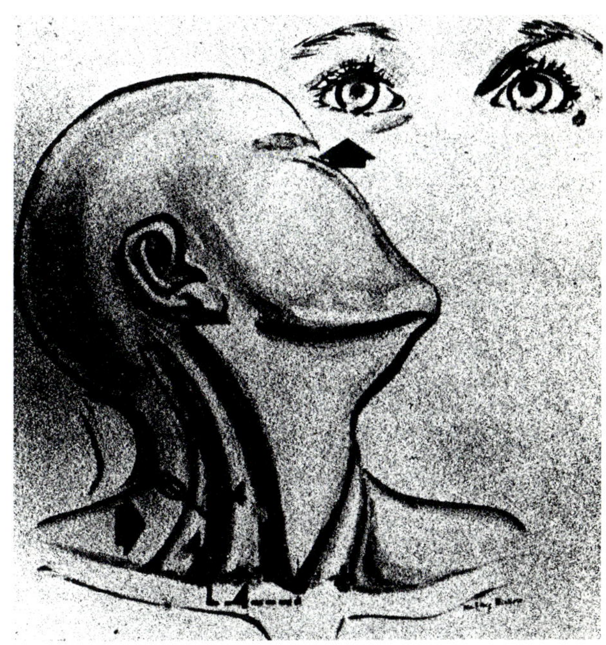

FIGURE 65-2. Technique of stellate ganglion block. A 23-gauge needle is directed medially and slightly inferiorly at a point 4 cm lateral and 4 cm superior to the sternal notch, to a depth of 4 cm, with the patient's head extended and rotated to the opposite side. (Lankford and Thompson, Ref. 6.)

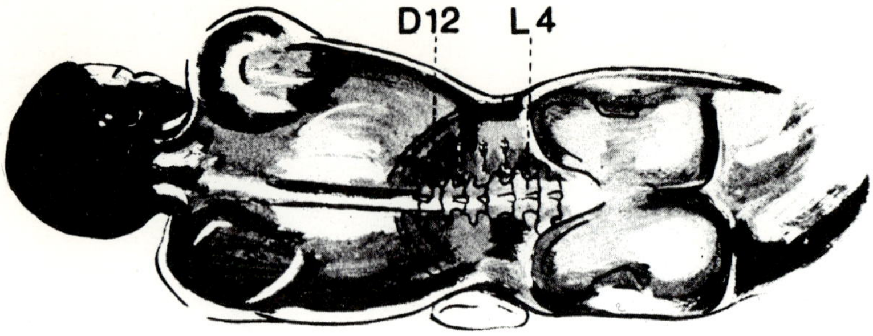

FIGURE 65-3. Lumbar sympathetic block with three-needle technique. The patient is lying on his side with the involved side uppermost. See text for details. (Lankford and Thompson, Ref. 6.)

World War II demonstrated clearly the place of sympathetic block and sympathectomy as definitive therapy for patients with causalgia (27,28). If the patient has true causalgia or if symptoms are not relieved promptly by the measures just listed, one should proceed directly to sympathetic blocks, which are both diagnostic and therapeutic. In early cases, relief of pain may well last beyond the duration of the block and even be curative. Repeated blocks should be performed until pain is controlled. If the results of sympathetic block are equivocal, a control block with normal saline may be performed. If relief from repeated sympathetic blocks becomes less effective or static, and the initial response is dramatic but of short duration, surgical sympathectomy should be considered. Early sympathectomy will prevent the occurrence of irreversible trophic changes, as well as obviate the establishment of fixed pain patterns which may become refractory even to sympathectomy if the syndrome is allowed to be prolonged without definitive therapy.

Stellate ganglion blocks, using 1% lidocaine or 0.25% bupivacaine, bathe the stellate ganglion, which lies at the level of C7–D1. A satisfactory technique for stellate ganglion block of the upper extremity is as follows (Figure 65-2). With the patient's head extended and turned away from the operator, the needle is inserted at a point 4 cm lateral to the midline and 4 cm cephalad from the clavicle to a depth of 4 cm in the neck. The needle is directed medially and inferiorly toward the lateral bony mass of C7–D1. Ten milliliters of local anesthetic solution is injected. Prompt development of Horner's syndrome with warming and drying of the hand and relief of pain indicates a successful block.

Lumbar block is more difficult. Three needles are placed 5 cm lateral to the midline opposite the transverse processes of L1, L2, and L3, or L2, L3, and L4 (Figure 65-3). When the transverse processes are encountered, the needles are redirected above or below and inserted to a depth of 3.5 to 4 cm so that their tips encounter the sympathetic trunk, lying along the anterolateral border of the lumbar vertebrae. Ten milliliters of 1% lidocaine is injected through each needle. Within a few moments a sympathetic effect should appear, with warming and drying of the foot and relief of pain.

When surgical sympathectomy is found to be necessary for the upper extremity, the D2 and D3 ganglia are removed. Several approaches may be employed. The classic posterior approach of Smithwick through the bed of the third rib in the extrapleural plane may be used. With this operation, Horner's syndrome should be easily avoided, and this degree of sympathectomy is adequate. Cervicothoracic sympathectomy can be performed by a transaxillary approach, either through a third interspace thoracotomy or via the bed of the excised first rib. A supraclavicular approach may be utilized as well, although at least a temporary Horner's syndrome may be more likely to occur. Lumbar sympathectomy is performed by a standard lumbar approach, and the L2 and L3 ganglia are removed. Following sympathectomy, physical therapy and all other ancillary measures should be diligently continued to ensure optimal results.

Results of Treatment

A series of 236 patients treated by the authors has been reviewed. Thirty-eight had causalgia, whereas 198 demonstrated changes consistent with mimocausalgia. Among patients with causalgia, definitive therapy in all instances was surgical sympathectomy. Among patients with mimocausalgia, 99 were managed by sympathetic blocks alone. Between one and five blocks were performed on consecutive or alternating days. Eighty-seven patients with mimocausalgia underwent sympathectomy. Twelve patients required only intensification of medical management, principally physical therapy, to obtain relief.

The results of treatment are shown in Table 65-1. In the causalgia group, 89.5 percent had excellent results, 2.6 percent had good results, and 7.9 percent had poor results. Residual symptoms remained with 36.8 percent; most of these patients had experienced satisfactory relief of pain but continued to have residual disability.

Among 198 patients with mimocausalgia, 78.8 percent had excellent relief of pain and edema, 15.6 percent had good results, and 5.6 percent had poor results. Significant residual symptoms remained with 28.2 percent; these symptoms were usually secondary irreversible contractures and stiffness. The most common cause of failure of sympathectomy or blocks was delay between the onset of symptoms and institution of appropriate therapy.

TABLE 65-1. Results of Treatment

Classification	No. of Cases	Excellent	Good	Poor	Residual Symptoms
Causalgia	38	34 89.5%	1 2.6%	3 7.9%	14 36.8%
Mimocausalgia	198	156 78.8%	31 15.6%	11 5.6%	56 28.2%
Totals	236	190 80.5%	32 13.5%	14 6.0%	70 29.6%

Summary

The history, clinical manifestations, etiology, and treatment of causalgia and mimocausalgia have been reviewed. Newer concepts of etiology and therapy are evolving, but sympathetic ablation, either medically or surgically, still remains the most important therapeutic modality. Delayed therapy caused by misdiagnosis accounts for most of the treatment failures.

References

1. Mitchell SW, Morehouse GR, Keen WW: *Gunshot Wounds and Other Injuries of Nerves*. Philadelphia, Lippincott, 1964.
2. Bergan JJ, Conn J: Sympathectomy for pain relief. Med Clin North Am 1968, 52:147–159.
3. Homans J: Minor causalgia: A hyperesthetic neurovascular syndrome. N Engl J Med 1940, 222:870–874.
4. Garrett WV, Thompson JE, Talkington CM, et al: Causalgia and its allied problems. In Bergan JJ, Yao JST (eds): *Evaluation and Treatment of Upper and Lower Extremity Circulatory Disorders*. Orlando, Florida, Grune & Stratton, 1984, pp 499–508.
5. Thompson JE: The diagnosis and management of post-traumatic pain syndromes (causalgia). Aust NZ J Surg 1979, 3:299–304.
6. Lankford LL, Thompson JE: Reflex sympathetic dystrophy, upper and lower extremity: diagnosis and management, AAOS Instructional Course Lectures 1977, 26:163–178.
7. Wilson RL: Management of pain following peripheral nerve injuries. Orthop Clin North Am 1981, 12:343–359.
8. Owens JC: Causalgia. Am Surg 1957, 26:417–426.
9. Evans WA: Reflex sympathetic dystrophy: Report on 57 cases. Ann Intern Med 1947, 26:417–426.
10. Lewis T: *Pain*. New York, Macmillan, 1942.
11. DeTakats G: Causalgic states in peace and war. JAMA 1945, 128:699.
12. Doupe, J, Cullen CH, Chance GQ: Post-traumatic pain and causalgic syndrome. J Neurol Neurosurg Psychiatry 1944, 7:33–48.
13. Leriche R: *The Surgery of Pain*, Young A (trans and ed): London, Baillere, Tindall, and Cox, 1939.
14. Barnes R: The role of sympathectomy in the treatment of causalgia. J Bone Joint Surg 1953, 35B:172–180.
15. Melzack R, Wall PD: Pain mechanisms: A new theory. Science 1965, 150:971–979.
16. Noordenbos W: *Pain*. Amsterdam, Elsevier, 1959.
17. Livingston WK: *Pain Mechanisms: A Physiological Interpretation of Causalgia and Its Related States*. New York, Macmillan, 1943.
18. Sunderland S: *Nerves and Nerve Injuries*, ed 2. Edinburgh, Churchill Livingstone, 1978, pp 381–420.
19. Drucker, WR, Hubay CA, Holden WD, et al: Pathogenesis of post-traumatic sympathetic dystrophy. Am J Surg 1959, 97:454–465.
20. Urbaniek JR, Roth JH: Office diagnosis and treatment of hand pain. Orthop Clin North Am 1982, 13:477–495.
21. Kozin F, Ryan LM, Carerra GF, et al: The reflex sympathetic dystrophy syndrome (RSDS). III. Scintigraphic studies, further evidence for the efficacy of systemic corticosteroids and proposed diagnostic criteria. Am J Med 1981, 70:23–30.
22. Benson WF: Discussion of presentation by RG Chuinard at annual meeting. American Society for Surgery of the Hand. Atlanta, Georgia, 1980.
23. Chuinard RG, Dabezies EJ, Gould JS, et al: Intravenous reserpine for treatment of reflex sympathetic dystrophy. South Med J 1981, 74:1481–1484.
24. Hannington-Kiff JG: Relief of causalgia in limbs by regional intravenous guanethidine. Br Med J 1979, 2(6186):367–368.
25. Glynn CJ, Basedow RW, Walsh JA: Pain relief following postganglionic sympathetic blockage with i.v. guanethidine. Br J Anaesth 1981, 53:1297–1302.
26. Spurling RG: Causalgia of the upper extremity: Treatment by dorsal sympathetic ganglionectomy. Arch Neurol Psych 1930, 23:784.
27. Kirklin JW, Chenoweth AE, Murphey F: Causalgia: A review of its characteristics, diagnosis, and treatment. Surgery 1947, 21:321.
28. Shumacker HB, Abramson DI: Post-traumatic vasomotor disorders. Surg Gynecol Obstet 1949, 88:417.

Chapter 66

VASCULAR INJURIES IN THE NECK AND THORACIC OUTLET

MALCOLM O. PERRY

Trauma is the fourth leading cause of death in the United States; over 50 million injuries occur each year, and more than 100,000 people die as a result of these injuries. Although these patients frequently have multiple injuries, wounds of major vessels are the sole cause, or a major contributing cause, in many of the deaths (1).

In most situations there is little difficulty in ascertaining that the patient has a serious injury. Many of these people have multiple wounds, and a careful assessment of all injuries is required in order to establish priorities of care. This is particularly true in penetrating wounds of the brachiocephalic vessels since not only is hemorrhage a threat, but also interruption of blood flow to the brain may produce serious neurological problems as well.

Etiology

Major vascular wounds can occur in any environment, but the greatest incidence is seen in urban areas where violence is endemic. Penetrating trauma caused by knives and bullet wounds is more common than blunt trauma, although in some cases vascular wounds as a result of blunt trauma can be more difficult to diagnose and to treat. Certain varieties of blunt trauma are particularly likely to result in vascular injury: steering wheel injuries, deceleration forces, falls, and crushing blows to the chest and root of the neck can be followed by serious vascular wounds.

Mechanisms of Injury

Most penetrating injuries are caused by stabbing or bullets traveling at a low velocity, and the damage is mainly confined to the wound tract. Knife wounds usually cause punctures, lacerations, and occasionally transections, while bullets are more likely to sever the artery. The blast effect caused by high-velocity missiles may cause widespread damage since the cavitation produced by a missile traveling at 1500 to 3000 ft/s is capable of damaging vessels remote from the wound tract. When such a blast cavity collapses, a suction effect is generated which can draw surface structures such as bits of skin, clothing, or dirt along the wound tract.

A high-velocity bullet or metal fragment can produce a great deal of tissue damage, especially if it strikes bone and all of the bullet's energy is dissipated in the target. Moreover, splinters of bone may become secondary missiles and injure other structures. Such widespread damage may not be suspected on initial inspection since there may be only a small entrance and exit wound.

Brachiocephalic Arterial Injuries

Most wounds of the cervical vessels and the thoracic outlet are caused by penetrating trauma (2–5), and the common carotid artery is usually involved, the left more than the right (Table 66-1). There are special problems encountered in these patients when there is a vascular injury and a neurological deficit; there also may be wounds of the pharynx, esophagus, trachea, and major nerves. The neurological deficit associated with some of these injuries presents a unique and often perplexing problem. It appears that the outcome in most patients depends on the extent of the initial preoperative neurological deficit unless some technical problems occur during resuscitation and repair.

TABLE 66-1. Brachiocephalic Arterial Injuries

Innominate	8
Subclavian	38
Axillary	43
Aorta	11
Common carotid	53
Internal carotid	17
External carotid	19
Vertebral	7
Total	196

Injuries of vessels in the thoracic outlet, at the base of the neck, present major problems regarding the surgical exposure since it may be necessary to open the chest in order to obtain proximal control of the great vessels arising from the arch of the aorta. The decision to open the chest early can be an important part of the management. There are a number of vital structures in this area, and the danger of combined injuries of large arteries and veins is apparent. Wounds to vessels in these two areas will be considered separately because of the technical requirements.

Carotid Injuries

It is helpful to divide carotid arteries into three groups for evaluation: Group I—the first and largest group contains those patients who have injuries of the common and internal carotid artery (ICA), but who have no neurological deficit (6). Group II patients have a mild neurological deficit, and group III patients have a severe neurological deficit which includes coma and hemiplegia.

A significant number of these patients have other injuries such as closed head trauma which especially can distort the diagnostic picture. Such combined problems are particularly confusing when the indications for surgery are being considered—a precise neurological evaluation is mandatory before an operation is begun. The results of most studies strongly support surgical repair of all penetrating carotid artery injuries in patients who have either no neurological deficit or only a mild neurological deficit; thus, all of the patients in groups I and II would undergo repair of isolated carotid artery wounds (6–8). This decision is easy to reach when the artery is bleeding briskly, but it may be more difficult to decide what to do when there is complete carotid artery occlusion and no neurological symptoms, or occlusion plus a profound stroke. In such a situation technical problems encountered during surgery could conceivably produce additional brain damage, although in the reported experience this has been rare (9–11).

Failure to visualize an artery with arteriograms does not always mean that the vessel is occluded. A very slow flow of blood through a small channel may not be visualized even with good arteriographic techniques, but rapid sequence computerized tomographic scanning or nuclear magnetic resonance studies should clarify such situations. These studies will be especially important in patients who have sustained blunt trauma and in whom there may be hyperextension injuries of the distal internal carotid artery. In this situation the ICA is forcibly stretched over the transverse process of C3 and the body of C2, a mechanism of injury which causes multiple transmural tears that predispose to thromboembolic events (Figure 66-1). Until a neurological problem appears in these patients, there may be little evidence of carotid artery injury. If such a lesion is untreated, it is likely to progress to complete occlusion, sometimes with extension of the clot into the cerebral arteries, producing a massive stroke. Thromboembolism may supervene; middle cerebral artery emboli have been observed in such patients.

EVALUATION AND PREOPERATIVE PREPARATION

The basic management of penetrating trauma to the neck is straightforward: wounds which pierce the platysma muscle require surgical exploration (12). It may be useful to divide penetrating wounds of the neck into three zones as suggested by Monson, Saletta, and Freeark (13). Although the exact levels vary according to the authorities who have suggested them, the modification proposed by Snyder is simple (14). Zone III extends from the base of the skull to the angle of the mandible, zone II from the angle of the mandible to 1 cm above the head of the clavicle, and zone I from 1 cm above the head of the clavicle inferiorly to include the thoracic outlet. By clinical examination it may be difficult to determine if injuries in zones I and III have damaged major vascular structures such as the carotid artery. In these situations, if the patients are hemodynamically stable, preoperative biplane arteriography is extremely useful. In selected patients with penetrating injuries in zone II who have no neurological deficit, operation may be performed without arteriography, although preoperative arteriography is helpful in the management of these patients as well. If there is a neurological deficit, a careful arteriographic study which includes biplane intracranial films is required.

DIAGNOSIS

Those signs and symptoms which suggest arterial injury of vessels in the extremities apply equally to the neck, but unfortunately the cervical arteries are not directly accessible for examination of pulses, especially in patients with blunt trauma. Jernigan and Gardner (15) have described features suggesting that the patient has sustained blunt trauma to the carotid artery (Table 66-2). There may be very few signs of injury in these people, since less than half of the patients will have superficial evidence of blunt trauma (Figure 66-2). Unless these patients present with neurological symptoms, blunt trauma to the carotid artery may not be apparent for several hours, or even much longer in some cases. Preoperative arteriograms are needed in these situations to expose such injuries, and arteriography should be used liberally in patients who have blunt or penetrating trauma to the neck and thoracic outlet.

OPERATIVE MANAGEMENT

Patients who have carotid artery injuries and continued prograde blood flow are candidates for surgical repair (6). A patient who has complete occlusion of the ICA as a result of blunt trauma, who is not bleeding, and who has a severe neurological deficit accompanied by coma and hemiplegia may be best treated by nonoperative techniques or by ligation of the ICA if operation is required for other reasons. The complete removal of thrombus in these situations is often difficult, and leaving behind residual clots may predispose to embolization which extends the neurological damage.

With isolated carotid wounds extensive monitoring is not required usually, but a radial arterial line is helpful for measure-

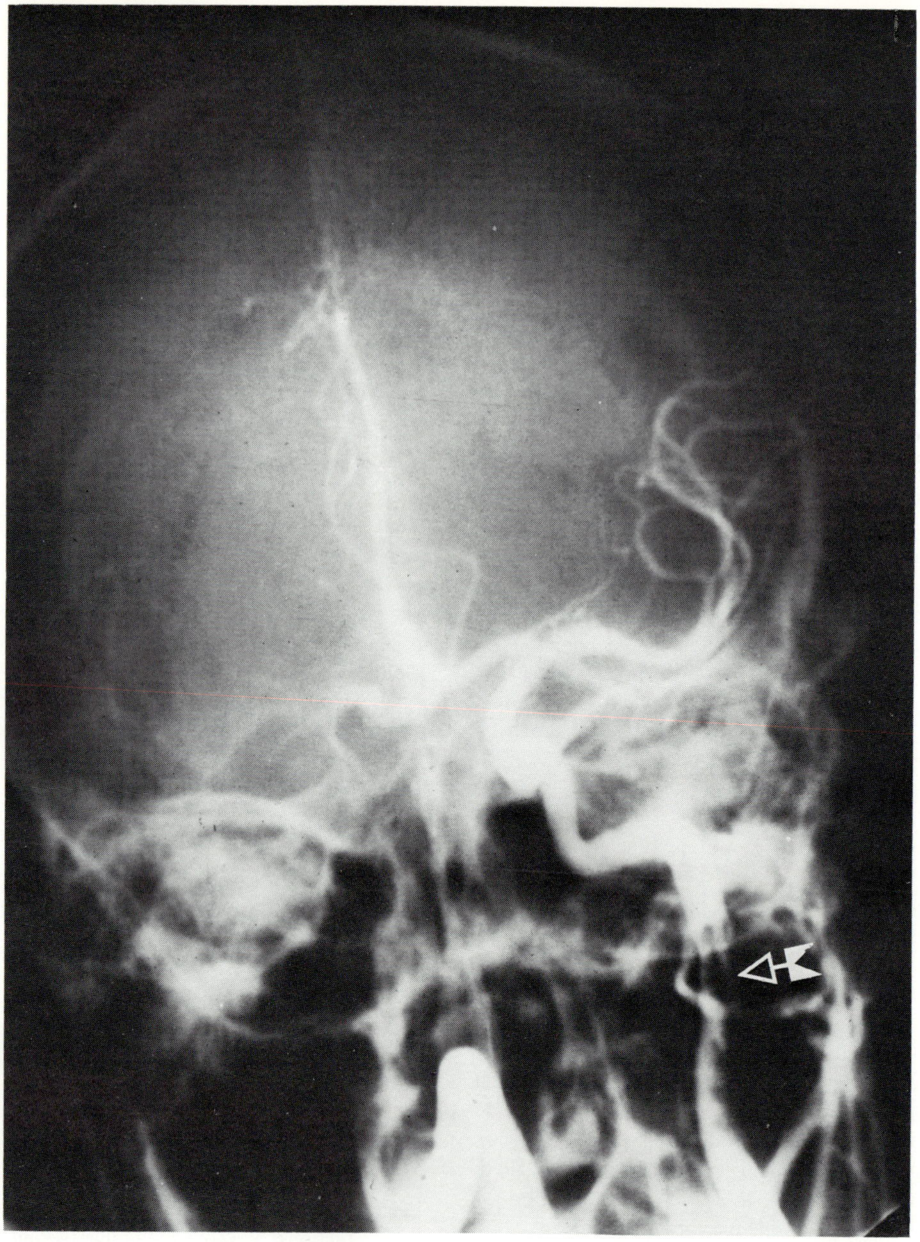

FIGURE 66-1. The hyperextension injury of the internal carotid artery predisposes to thrombosis. The arrow marks the presence of a large mural clot in the distal ICA in a patient who had sustained blunt trauma. Resection and vein graft replacement were required.

TABLE 66-2. **Blunt Trauma—Carotid Artery Injuries**

Clinical Features
Hematoma of neck
Horner's syndrome
Transient attack of ischemia
Lucid interval
Limb paresis in an alert patient

SOURCE: Modified from Jernigan and Gardner (15).

ments for arterial blood pressure and blood-gas tensions. General anesthesia, hypercapnea, and some neurological wounds interfere with cerebral autoregulation, and cerebral blood flow then will respond directly to changes in systemic arterial pressure. The maintenance of normal blood pressure is an important concept in the correct management of these situations.

As in almost all cases of cervical trauma the induction of anesthesia must be accomplished gently to prevent the dislodgment of tamponading clots which might cause recurrence of bleeding or embolize into the intracranial circulation (14). A variety of anesthetic agents are effective and safe, and the final

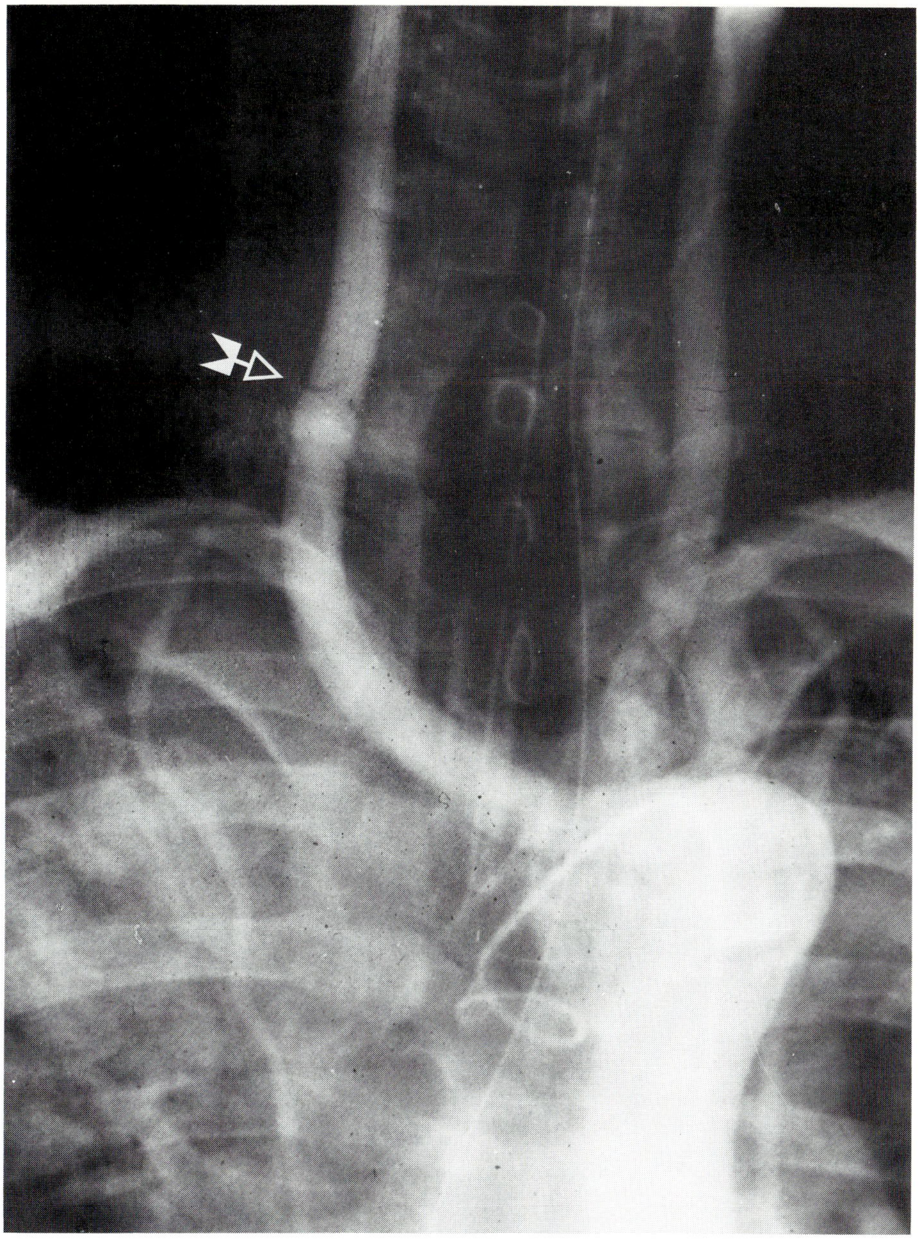

FIGURE 66-2. A blow to the neck caused the intimal fracture and transmural damage which produced a small fusiform aneurysm (*arrow*). Graft replacement of this section of the artery was necessary.

choice rests with the anesthesiologist, but drugs which are likely to cause hypotension are not desirable and should be avoided. Endotracheal intubation is required in these patients, and preoperative knowledge of laryngeal nerve function is essential; if this information is not known before the patient reaches the operating room, the vocal chords can be directly inspected during tracheal intubation.

If the wound has not been accurately identified by preoperative arteriography, wide surgical exposure will be needed for exploration. The neurovascular structures are reached through the customary carotid incision made along the anterior border of the sternomastoid muscle, approaching the artery slightly from the anterolateral aspect to initially obtain control of the common carotid artery proximal to the area of suspected injury. Once the arterial wound is exposed, gentle digital pressure will usually control bleeding without clamping the vessel, thus minimizing the time of carotid artery occlusion. Injuries of the external carotid artery are usually clamped, and repaired or ligated as indicated, and unless there is evidence that the external carotid artery is functioning as a major cerebral collateral, it often is sacrificed. It is usually neither grafted nor shunted during repair.

Once the bleeding is controlled, the internal carotid artery backflow is assessed. Brisk, pulsatile backflow is usually evidence of adequate cerebral perfusion, but measurements of ca-

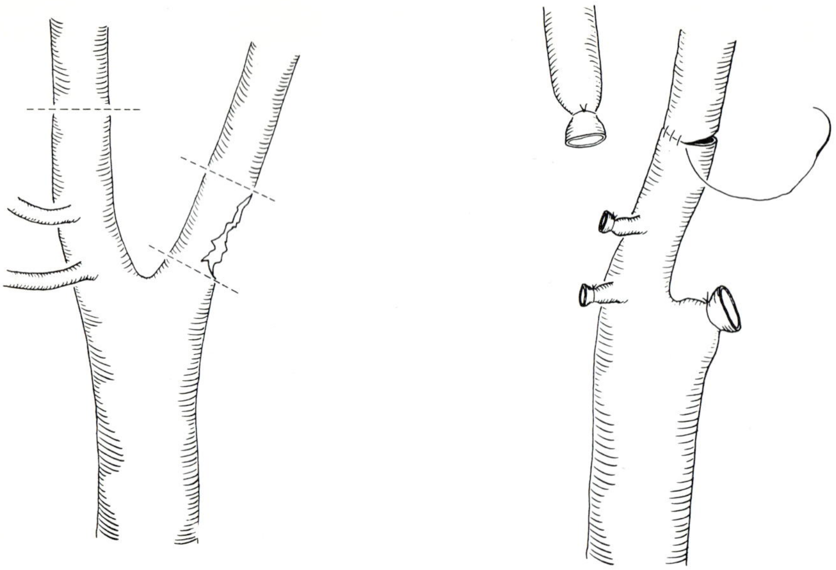

FIGURE 66-3. It may be possible to substitute the external carotid artery for the ICA in some situations. [From Perry (1).]

rotid artery stump pressures may be helpful. It has been suggested that back pressures greater than 70 mmHg indicate adequate cerebral perfusion, and thus such patients do not require additional support of cerebral circulation during the period of carotid artery occlusion necessary for repair (1,11,14). Moreover, if the pressures are above 70 mmHg and the distal carotid cannot be cleared of clots, and ligation is necessary, this pressure should be adequate to prevent major stroke unless thromboembolism supervenes.

If the pressures are low or the backflow from the ICA is scanty and shunts are selected, a variety of techniques may be used, but the simple inlying straight tube shunt is readily available. Unless the patient has multiple injuries, or has injuries of the eye, central nervous system, or multiple fractures, most surgeons use systemic heparin when shunts are in place, although it would seem more important to heparinize the patients if the distal carotid artery is filled with a stagnant pool of blood. Most studies of shunting and intraoperative heparinization during the repair of carotid artery injuries have failed to delineate clearly the need for and results of these maneuvers (6–8).

In repair of arterial injuries, standard vascular techniques are used, but because of the importance of securing a smooth intimal surface in the carotid artery, resection and anastomosis are favored. This is especially important with blunt trauma because the mural damage is likely to be extensive. After resection, a repair without tension is required or an interposition graft is needed. Customarily the saphenous vein from the ankle is chosen to restore continuity in the carotid artery. If the defect in the proximal ICA is small, the distal external carotid can be ligated and this vessel substituted for the origin of the ICA as illustrated in Figure 66-3. If, because of low pressures or scanty backflow, a shunt is selected and a graft is also needed, the graft can be placed over the shunt prior to insertion; the shunt is then removed just before the anastomosis is completed, as shown in Figure 66-4.

Penetrating injuries of the ICA at the base of the skull are very difficult to expose, but division of the digastric muscle, resection of the styloid process, and, on occasion, temporary anterior dislocation of the mandible usually will permit visual-

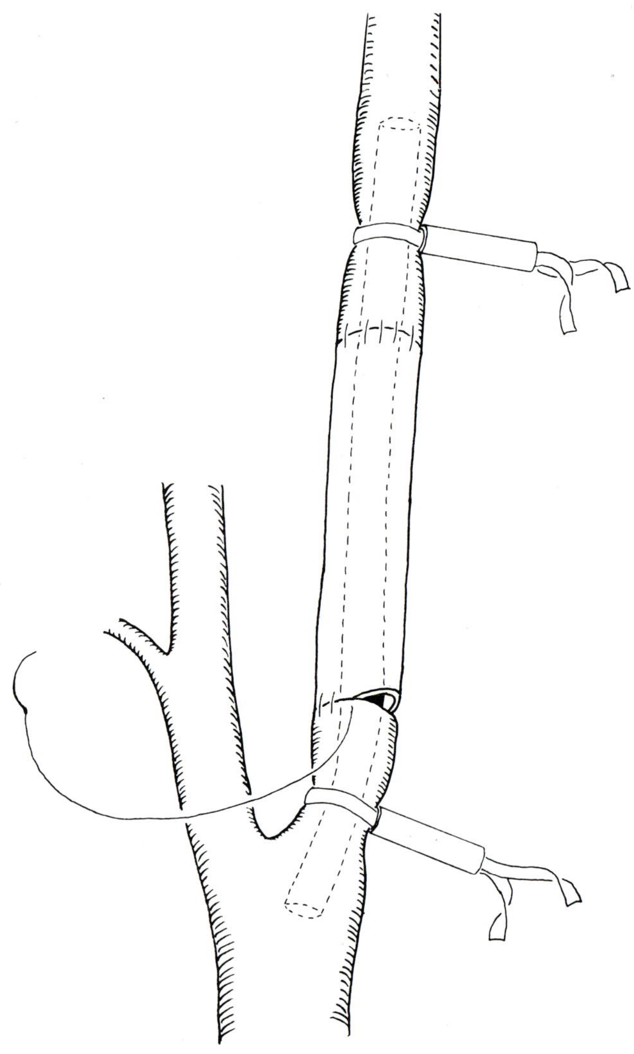

FIGURE 66-4. When temporary inlying carotid shunts are needed in conjunction with vein grafting, this method is useful. The shunt also acts as a stent during the repair. [From Perry (1).]

ization of the carotid as it enters the skull. Lacerations at the carotid foramen which are too high to allow placing a vascular clamp distally can be controlled by inserting a balloon-tipped catheter through a separate incision in the artery, then advancing the catheter beyond the laceration and gently inflating the balloon to control backbleeding (1). Soft Fogarty catheters with an attached three-way stopcock can be used, or special balloon occlusion catheters designed for the carotid artery are available.

Vertebral Artery Injuries

Wounds of the vertebral arteries are rare—the vessels enter the bony canal at the C6 level and exit at C2—and apparently are protected from many injuries. In the past, without preoperative arteriograms, vertebral artery damage was probably undetected unless discovered because of bleeding during exploration. Treatment consisted of proximal ligation, packing, and, on rare occasions, direct exposure and suture ligation (10,11,13).

Since preoperative arteriography is employed more frequently to assess the damage accurately and to evaluate the collateral circulation, more vertebral artery wounds will probably be discovered (11). Direct repair, even in the bony canal, is possible with modern vascular techniques. A penetrating injury to a dominant or single vertebral artery should be considered for repair. Continued bleeding or the late development of a false aneurysm or arteriovenous fistula are serious complications of such wounds.

Traumatic occlusion of a small vertebral artery in a patient with normal connections into the circle of Willis is not likely to cause serious problems and usually can be left alone. In such circumstances treatment at operation customarily would be ligation only; therefore, the patient can be spared a rather difficult surgical exposure. With multiple injuries (carotid and vertebral) carotid repair is more important, and if the patient has the more common cerebral vascular architecture, this should suffice (1,14). In some patients the vertebral artery may be occluded by a percutaneously placed balloon.

POSTOPERATIVE CARE

Although any vascular repair is susceptible to bleeding, it is unusual in patients with vertebral artery injuries unless there are multiple injuries or coagulation defects. Drains are not commonly employed in treating isolated wounds of the carotid arteries, but in selected patients with multiple cervical injuries, drains may be used for 12 hours or so to prevent an accumulation of blood which, if under tension, might cause compression of the artery. Postoperatively the patients must be carefully monitored for the appearance of neurological symptoms, since any change is an indication for repeat arteriography to evaluate the status of repair and to assess the possibility of cerebral thromboembolism. Although postoperative carotid artery occlusion rarely occurs, if it does the patient should be returned immediately to the operating room for thrombectomy, correction of any technical errors, and immediate reestablishment of cerebral blood flow. In such situations it is best not to delay for arteriography since thrombosis and the possibility of stroke require immediate surgery. An expeditious restoration of flow is usually successful in preventing permanent neurological problems (1).

It now appears that carotid ligation will be needed in only a small group: patients with complete ICA occlusion and severe neurological deficits including coma and hemiplegia (6,7,10). Revascularization, with repair of all the damaged artery and complete removal of all clots, is seldom possible in patients who have total ICA occlusion as a result of blunt trauma (9). If repair is attempted, but incomplete, progressive neurological deterioration and death may occur. Restoration of flow to the carotid without clearing the distal artery is dangerous. In these patients carotid ligation is probably best, perhaps complemented by constructing an extracranial-to-intracranial bypass to maintain distal cerebral perfusion (11).

Venous Injuries in the Neck

Wounds of major veins frequently cause more troublesome bleeding than some arterial injuries (2). The thin walls, numerous fragile tributaries, and susceptibility to operative damage continue to present technical problems in isolation and control. Direct finger pressure, suction, and packing are usually effective methods to reduce the bleeding, while more precise control is obtained with vascular clamps. Since there are few guidelines to assist in preoperative diagnosis, the extent of injury is known only at surgery (12).

Ligation is almost always the treatment of these wounds. In a few situations (bilateral internal jugular, innominate and proximal subclavian vein injuries) suture repair may be chosen. Lateral or tangential sutures are effective in controlling the low-pressure bleeding and, if placed with care, will not seriously narrow the large vein if only a clean puncture or laceration is present. More extensive damage usually requires suture ligation since there are often associated injuries which take priority, and delays for complicated vein repairs are contraindicated.

Injuries of Vessels of Root of the Neck

The diagnosis of vascular injuries is obvious in the presence of specific findings such as profuse bleeding, large hematomas, weak or absent distal pulses, and continued intrathoracic hemorrhage, but up to one-third of these patients have no specific diagnostic signs (Figure 66-5). Those findings which suggest injuries to the great vessels as listed in Table 66-3 may be of help in establishing the diagnosis. Most of the patients with penetrating wounds at the base of the neck and concomitant

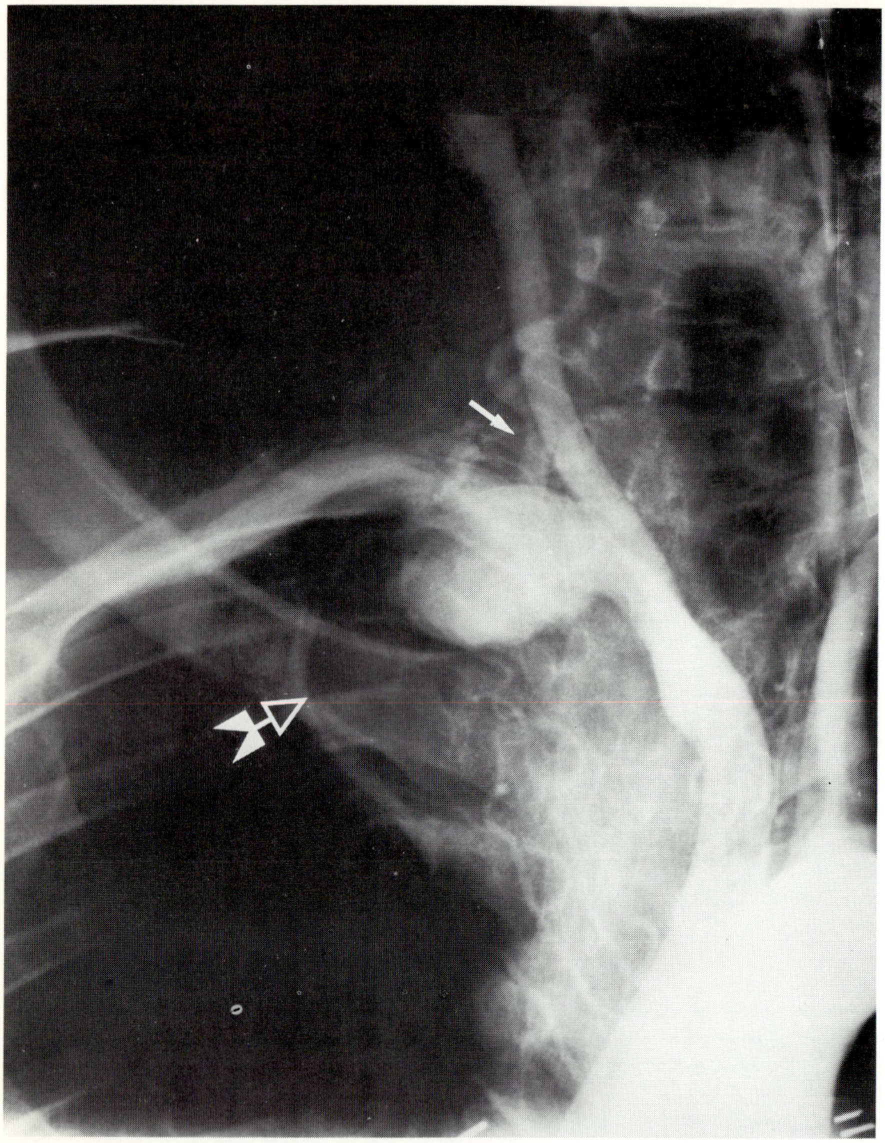

FIGURE 66-5. The large arrow points to the false aneurysm of the right subclavian artery. The aneurysm is partially filled with laminated clot. The vertebral artery (*small arrow*) arises from the posterior wall of the artery. Vein graft repair of the subclavian artery was performed.

major arterial injuries have large hematomas, or a wide mediastinum, but in some cases the signs may be more subtle. Persistent bleeding in the chest may be the only sign of injury to one of the great vessels. If the injured patient is stable, arteriography is helpful in precisely defining the extent and location of the wounds, but obtaining good biplane pictures of the arch and the great vessels is difficult because of overlapping images. Arteriography is not as reliable in these patients in excluding arterial penetration as it is in the extremities. Nevertheless, arteriograms are strongly recommended in patients who have injuries in zones I and III, not only to aid in diagnosis, but also to plan the operation.

TABLE 66-3. Injuries of Great Vessels in the Chest

Clinical Features
Cardiac arrest
Persistent or recurring hypotension
Cardiac tamponade
Wide mediastinum
Recurrent hemothorax
Posterior fracture—dislocation of first rib

OPERATIVE MANAGEMENT

Injuries to major vessels in zone III may be particularly difficult to evaluate since the wound is not readily accessible for examination, and yet direct exposure of a major vascular injury without obtaining proximal control can lead to fatal hemorrhage (2,3,5). If the penetrating wound in zone III is thought to have injured the great vessels, proximal control via a middle sternal splitting incision is recommended before mobilizing a vascular wound. Some authorities even suggest making a sternal splitting incision for all penetrating wounds at the base of the neck which enter below the cricoid cartilage or below C6; others suggest a more moderate approach. Most surgeons support the view that if a major vascular wound of the great vessels is strongly suspected,

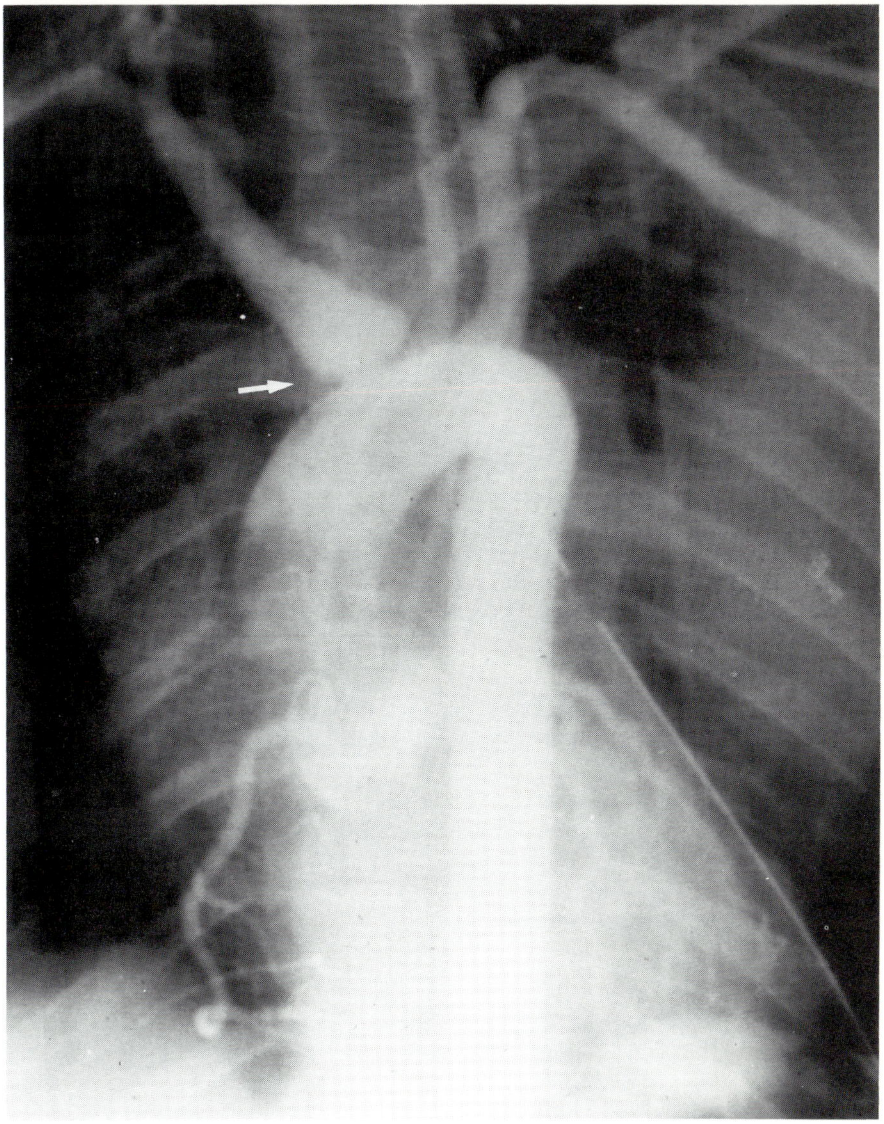

FIGURE 66-6. Blunt chest trauma–caused lung contusion and near-avulsion of the innominate artery (*arrow*). Through a middle sternal splitting incision, a 10-mm knitted Dacron graft was sewed end-to-side to the ascending aorta, and end-to-end to the undamaged distal innominate artery. The innominate origin was oversewn.

early thoracotomy is needed (5). Similarly, if during the course of cervical exploration of the carotid vessels, bleeding, hematoma, or blood staining of the carotid sheath at the root of the neck are encountered, an immediate sternal splitting incision should be made to obtain control since this may be the only sign of a proximal common carotid artery injury. With the exception of the left subclavian artery all of the vessels from the aortic arch can be reached easily through this middle sternal incision, but if necessary the sternal splitting incision can be extended into the second or third interspace, or a separate left thoracotomy incision may be opened to control the left subclavian artery at its origin.

Direct control of bleeding usually can be accomplished by the common techniques of digital pressure until a vascular clamp can be put in place proximal to the injury. In some cases, in fact, small lacerations of large vessels can be controlled with direct finger pressure and then repaired by simply passing the vascular sutures beneath the occluding finger. In other situations where the wounds are not easily controlled, a balloon-tipped catheter may be inserted directly through the wound, inflated, and gently retracted to temporarily control bleeding while proximal vascular clamps are put in place.

Once control is obtained, standard vascular techniques of repair are used. Lateral repair occasionally can be successful in large vessels, but if the wound cannot be closed without narrowing the artery, patch-graft angioplasty with autogenous tissue is indicated. More extensive wounds of the great vessels require resection and anastomosis, and in many instances an interposition plastic graft will be needed since suitably sized autografts are rarely available (Figure 66-6). Unless there is heavy direct bacterial contamination, such plastic grafts are satisfactory substitutes; but if there is heavy contamination and direct repair is deemed risky, a temporary remote bypass (axillary-axillary, subclavian-carotid, carotid-carotid) can be constructed to restore blood flow.

Temporary shunt procedures to maintain cerebral perfusion while innominate and common carotid arteries are being repaired have been used infrequently, and although several reports allude

TABLE 66-4. Mortality Rate for Penetrating Injuries of the Carotid Artery

	Neurological Status on Admission	Number	Died
Group I	No deficit	49	0
Group II	Mild deficit	8	1
Group III	Severe deficit	15	5

TABLE 66-5. Carotid Artery Injuries—Blunt Trauma Mortality Rate

	Number	Died	Percent
All cases	17	4	23
All carotid operations	14	2	14
Immediate successful operation	7	0	0

to these maneuvers, none describe the indications or document the basis for their use (2–5). As with the carotid artery, it appears that if there is a back pressure of 70 mmHg or greater in the common carotid or the innominate artery, temporary shunting procedures will not be required during the short time necessary to perform a direct repair. Similarly, heparinization has not been used with great frequency in these situations because of the presence of multiple wounds in many patients. The local installation of heparin solutions (100 U.S.P. units of heparin per 10 mL of saline) has been found to be satisfactory in retarding local thrombosis during temporary occlusion while repairs are completed. Postoperatively few surgeons use systemic anticoagulation in these patients.

RESULTS

Accurate diagnosis obtained with arteriography and computerized tomographic scanning, combined with an aggressive surgical approach to these patients, has produced quite satisfactory results. As shown in Table 66-4 penetrating carotid artery injuries often can be successfully managed if they are identified and repaired prior to the appearance of a neurological deficit. Blunt trauma to the cervical carotid vessels continues to present more difficult problems, but Table 66-5 lists the results obtained in the author's series. In this small group of patients early surgical repair appears effective and relatively safe. Although some of the patients die as a result of hemorrhage, the majority of the problems which occur in these patients who have been successfully resuscitated are caused by neurological damage which occurred prior to treatment.

Injuries of major vessels at the root of the neck continue to be formidable problems; the major threat remains exsanguination either before or during operation. In stable patients preoperative arteriography should reduce these risks, and perhaps innovative techniques such as nuclear magnetic resonance imaging will further improve diagnostic accuracy. Such methods, followed by an aggressive surgical approach with wide exposure to ensure control of hemorrhage, should result in continued improvement in care.

References

1. Perry MO: *The Management of Acute Vascular Injuries.* Baltimore, Williams and Wilkins, 1981.
2. Flint LM, Snyder WH, Perry MO, Shires T: Management of major vascular injuries in the base of the neck. Arch Surg 1973, 106:407.
3. Hewitt RL, Smith AD, Becker ML, Lindsey ES, Dowling JB, Drapanas T: Penetrating vascular injuries of the thoracic outlet. Surgery 1974, 76:715.
4. Lim LT, Saletta JD, Flanigan DP: Subclavian and innominate artery trauma. Surgery 1979, 86:890.
5. Reul GJ, Beall AC, Jordan GL, Mattox KL: The early operative management of injuries to the great vessels. Surgery 1973, 74:862.
6. Thal ER, Snyder WH, Hays RJ, Perry MO: Management of carotid artery injuries. Surgery 1974, 76:955.
7. Liekweg WG, Greenfield LJ: Management of penetrating carotid arterial injury. Ann Surg 1978, 188:587.
8. Bradley EL: Management of penetrating carotid injuries: An alternative approach. J Trauma 1973, 13:248.
9. Yamada S, Kindt GW, Youmans JR: Carotid artery occlusion due to nonpenetrating injury. J Trauma 1967, 7:333.
10. Perry MO, Snyder WH, Thal EW: Carotid artery injuries caused by blunt trauma. Ann Surg 1980, 1:74.
11. Fry RE, Fry WJ: Extracranial carotid artery injuries. Surgery 1980, 88:581.
12. Roon AJ, Christensen N: Evaluation and treatment of penetrating carotid injuries. J Trauma 1979, 19:391.
13. Monson DO, Saletta JD, Freeark RJ: Carotid vertebral trauma. J Trauma 1969, 9:987.
14. Snyder WH, Thal ER, Perry MO: Peripheral vascular injuries, in Rutherford RR (ed): *Vascular Surgery.* Philadelphia, Saunders, 1983.
15. Jernigan WR, Gardner WC: Carotid artery injuries due to closed cervical trauma. J Trauma 1971, 11:429.

Chapter 67

VASCULAR COMPLICATIONS RELATED TO DRUG ABUSE

RICHARD A. YEAGER, ROBERT W. HOBSON II, and CREIGHTON B. WRIGHT

Drug abuse in the United States is endemic to all areas of society. The expansion of parenteral drug abuse provides surgeons with a challenging array of pulmonary, cardiac, and vascular complications, either directly or indirectly related to the drug injections (1). The compulsion and ingenuity of drug abusers allows any part of the body to be a potential injury site (1–4). Even the repeated intracardiac injection of illicit drugs has been reported (5).

Heroin is the most commonly abused intravenous drug, but the list includes cocaine, other narcotics, barbiturates, nonnarcotic analgesics, and amphetamines (1,6). In addition to the systemic effects of these drugs, direct injections can cause vascular injury and limb ischemia by a variety of mechanisms, including local vascular trauma and infection, distal emboli, as well as chemical injury. Often the excipients (talc, cornstarch, or fillers) of oral preparations, or the agent used to "cut" the heroin (quinine, barbiturates, or lactose) do as much or more vascular damage than the drug itself (6,7). Surgeons should be aware of the myriad of vascular problems associated with drug abuse and be prepared to manage them. This chapter will review the spectrum of vascular injuries related to parenteral drug abuse including pathophysiology, clinical presentation, and management.

Overview of the Clinical Problem

The drug abuse population presents several difficult management problems. History concerning time factors, type of drug, method of preparation, and mode of injection may be lacking or inaccurate. This often is due to either the patient's deceptive behavior or the clouded sensorium related to chronic drug usage. Outpatient therapy and follow-up is inconsistent due to poor patient compliance, which may compromise treatment protocols. For instance, deep venous thrombosis due to drug injection is best treated by hospitalization and heparinization for 2 weeks (8), since shorter courses of heparin followed by outpatient warfarin therapy are not feasible in this noncompliant patient population.

Peripheral venous access for phlebotomy or drug therapy is usually not available due to dermal scars and peripheral venous sclerosis secondary to repeated injections. Often the patient is knowledgeable about his or her own best available venous access, and this information should be solicited. Furthermore, when surgical repair of drug-related vascular injuries is required, autogenous veins are often not available for interposition grafting and patch angioplasty (9). Consideration should be given for the use of autogenous arterial grafts (10,11) in this situation, although common synthetic prostheses such as polytetrafluoroethylene (PTFE) or Dacron are also utilized. However, the use of synthetic materials may be associated with attendant problems of infection in an already immunologically compromised host (12) (Figure 67-1).

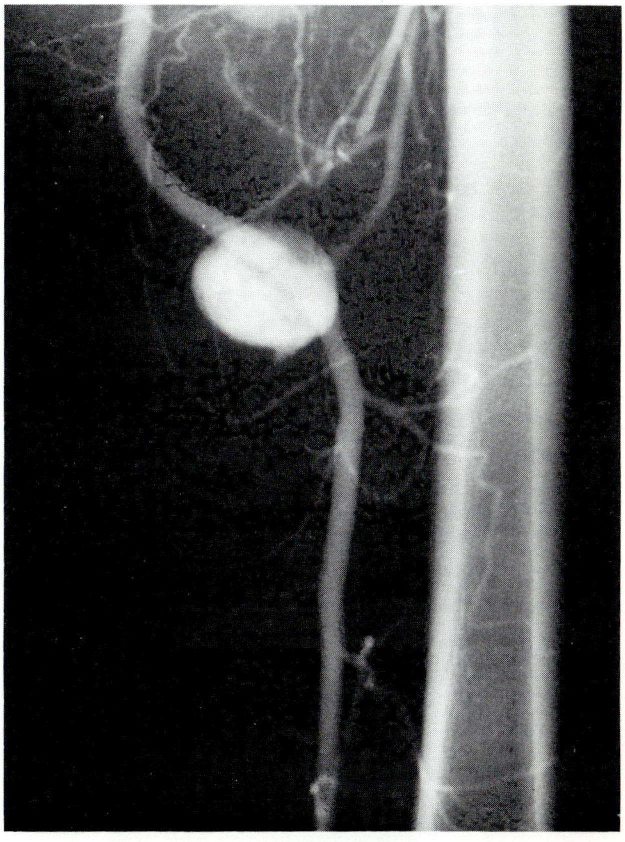

FIGURE 67-1. Infected pseudoaneurysm at PTFE-superficial femoral arterial anastomosis in drug abuser with obturator foramen bypass.

The drug abuser may present as a diagnostic problem with vague complaints of abdominal distress, low-grade fever, as well as evidence of systemic organ (hepatic, renal, pulmonary) impairment. When this is the case, endocarditis should be considered in the differential diagnosis. Bacterial and fungal endocarditis has a significant incidence in the drug abuse population

(3,13,14). Furthermore, the liberal use of arteriography as a diagnostic tool in difficult cases is suggested, since occult vascular lesions such as arteritis, arteriovenous fistula, or mesenteric mycotic aneurysm have been identified angiographically in this group (15–17).

Heroin nephropathy with renal failure is often encountered in the drug addict (18). Vascular shunts created for hemodialysis access, as well as other subcutaneous vascular grafts, are frequently adapted for drug abuse injections by this population. Eventual graft infections commonly occur, necessitating removal of the prosthesis. For this reason, peritoneal dialysis is considered an alternative to hemodialysis in any renal-failure patient with a history of drug abuse. Consequently, the drug-abuse patient presents many unique and challenging management problems that demand innovative diagnostic and therapeutic approaches. It is hoped that a better understanding of the potential clinical problems and management alternatives will improve medical and surgical care for this group.

Vascular Complications Related to Intravenous Drug Injection

The intravenous abuse of drugs can lead to several local venous complications including superficial vein thrombosis, deep vein thrombosis, septic thrombophlebitis, and infected venous pseudoaneurysms. Furthermore, pulmonary vascular complications can occur as a direct result of venous injections.

SUPERFICIAL VENOUS THROMBOSIS AND ASSOCIATED "PUFFY HAND"

Repeated injections into the superficial veins causes sclerosis and thrombosis of the veins due to chronic mechanical and chemical trauma. Although lymphatic obstruction due to injected particulate debris is of primary importance (19), the eventual obliteration of the entire superficial venous drainage is a contributing factor in causing the "puffy hand" syndrome described in drug addicts (2). Other causes for acute hand swelling in the drug addict include infection, lesions related to "skin popping" (20), compartment syndrome (21), bullous skin lesions related to barbiturate overdose (22), and acute arterial injection (23). After ruling out other causes, treatment for acute puffy hand should include elevation, antibiotics, and anticoagulation. A number of these patients will develop intractable hand and arm swelling for which compression support sleeves are useful.

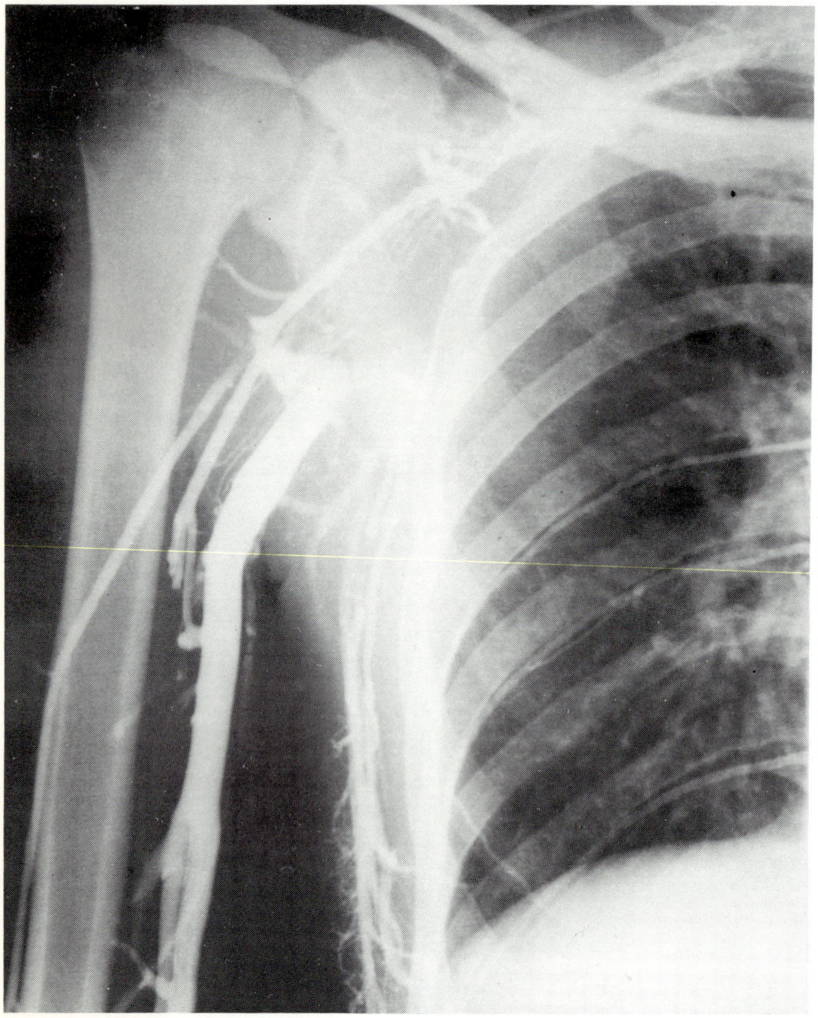

FIGURE 67-2. Axillary venous thrombosis related to illicit drug injection.

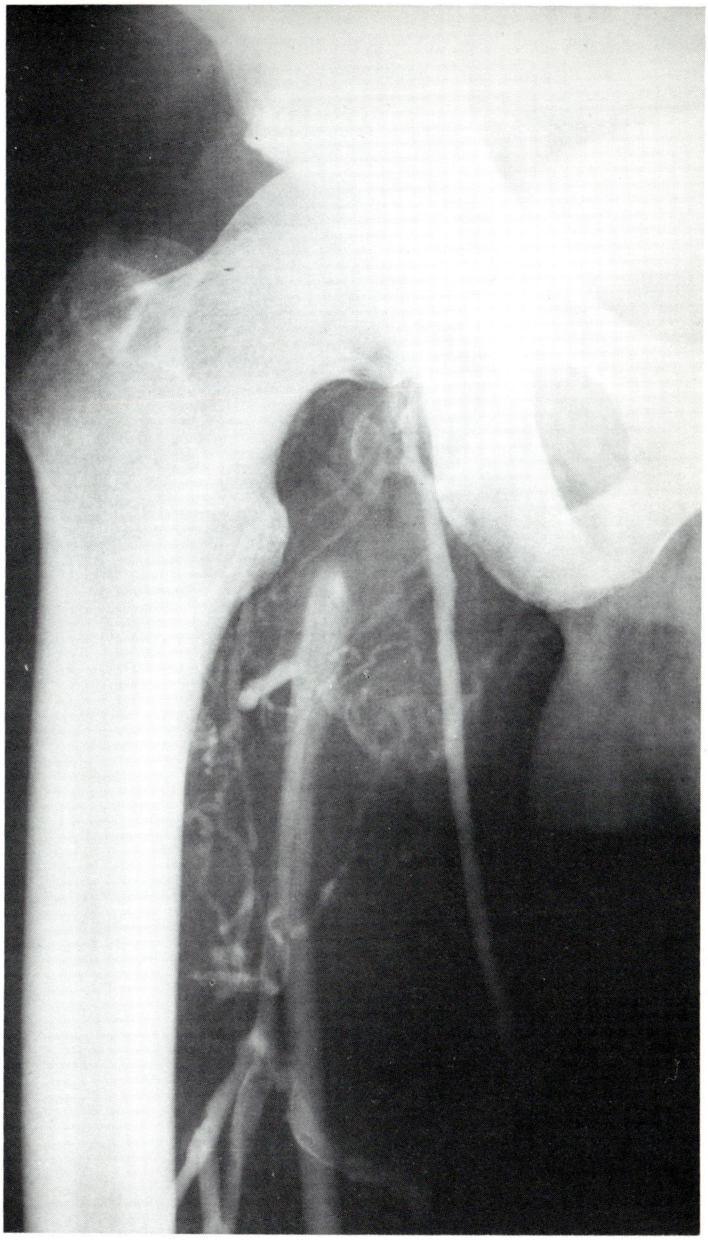

FIGURE 67-3. Femoral venous thrombosis related to illicit drug injection.

DEEP VEIN THROMBOSIS

Once the drug abuser has sclerosed all superficial veins, she or he resorts to injecting the deep veins. The most popular sites are the femoral, axillosubclavian, and jugular veins. The repeated mechanical and chemical trauma to the venous wall ultimately leads to thrombus formation (Figures 67-2 and 67-3). Treatment includes elevation and heparin anticoagulation for 2 weeks. Long-term outpatient warfarin therapy is not a practical alternative in this population.

SEPTIC THROMBOPHLEBITIS

Venous thrombosis with a superimposed infection is a more complex problem. Septic thrombophlebitis results when local venous injury occurs with either thrombosis or hemorrhage associated with hematoma formation. Organisms are then introduced into or around the thrombus, usually at the time of drug injection. In general most infections seen in addicts appear to be related to their injection habits and not due to the contamination of heroin or drug paraphernalia (24–26). *Staphylococcus aureus* is the most common causative organism for septicemia in these cases. Skin contamination is a likely source for the sepsis. The incidence of staphylococcal carriers among people who undergo chronic drug injections is reported to be high (26). Sterile preparation of the skin prior to drug injection is seldom practiced. Furthermore, addicts often use saliva or unsterile water as a mixing medium for their drugs. The addict is prone to develop infections since chronic narcotism can inhibit phagocytosis and lymphocyte-mediated immunity (1,2,27).

The natural history of untreated septic thrombophlebitis includes persistent bacteremia as well as septic pulmonary emboli resulting in lung abscesses. The incidence of infected pulmonary emboli associated with septic thrombophlebitis has been reported to be 7 to 30 percent (28,29). Persistent bacteremia can also lead to endocarditis with its attendant complications. One series of 100 patients with septic thrombophlebitis was characterized as being 46 percent drug abusers. Local pain was the most common (83 percent) complaint, while erythema or edema constituted the most common physical signs (63 percent) (28). Experience from burn centers (30) confirms that septic thrombophlebitis can be difficult to detect, often presenting as occult septicemia. Blood cultures are often positive, while the diagnosis of venous thrombosis generally requires contrast venography. A high index of suspicion for septic thrombophlebitis should be maintained when managing a drug abuser.

The treatment of septic thrombophlebitis depends on whether the infection involves the superficial or deep venous system. A superficial suppurative phlebitis is managed with excision of the vein, systemic antibiotics, and open wound drainage. Delayed primary wound closure is recommended. Initial management of deep venous septic thrombophlebitis includes heparin anticoagulation and antibiotics. If clinical improvement is observed in 24 hours, therapy is continued. If clinical response is lacking, the involved vein is explored and either excised or ligated (31,32). Weinberg and Pasternak (32) recommended ligation of the subclavian vein at the junction with the internal jugular vein for septic thrombophlebitis involving the subclavian vein. Extraction of infected thrombus by balloon thrombectomy has also proved beneficial in clearing the sepsis. Gram's stain and culture of the thrombus assists with diagnosis. In cases involving intrathoracic veins, positive diagnosis based on thrombectomy may indicate thoracotomy or sternotomy for venous exploration, drainage, or venous ligation (31). The use of transvenous infrarenal vena caval filters may be considered in cases of septic thrombophlebitis (33,34); however, it should be employed probably only if venous ligation is not feasible.

INFECTED VENOUS PSEUDOANEURYSMS

The combination of local infection and repeated needle trauma can destroy the venous wall with eventual pseudoaneurysm formation. Venous pseudoaneurysms are occasionally utilized as preferred sites for repeated drug injections. Two patients in our practice presented with expanding purulent groin masses, associated with surrounding cellulitis and induration. Aspiration of the mass demonstrated sanguinopurulent content. Arteriography failed to confirm an arterial false aneurysm. Both patients were explored and found to have infected femoral venous pseudoaneurysms (35). Venography prior to exploration may have demonstrated the extent of pathology as well as the venous anatomy. Surgical treatment consists of drainage of associated abscess, proximal and distal venous ligation, with excision of involved vein, and extraction of septic thrombi (36).

ANGIOTHROMBOTIC PULMONARY HYPERTENSION

Pulmonary hypertension and cor pulmonale reportedly occur with intravenous drug abuse. Chronic pulmonary arterial embolization of particulate debris is the pathogenesis. The classic "blue velvet syndrome," as documented by Wendt and coauthors (37), involves the intravenous injection of paregoric and talc containing tripelennamine (Pyribenzamine) hydrochloride. Pathologic study of the lungs confirmed angioocclusive lesions associated with a diffuse pulmonary vascular sclerosis as well as intravascular talc crystals. Other reports have documented pulmonary granulomatosis resulting from intravenous injection of talc-containing drugs intended for oral use (38,39). The tablets most commonly used for intravenous injection after crushing and dissolving are methylphenidate (Ritalin), methadone, tripelennamine (Pyribenzamine), propoxyphene hydrochloride (Darvon), phenmetrazine (Preludin), and amphetamines (38). Pathophysiologically, these conditions are comparable to the injection of excipients into the extremity arterial circulation.

Dyspnea is the usual symptom resulting from the pulmonary talc granulomatosis (38). A normal chest roentgenogram does not rule out the presence of extensive pulmonary talc granulomatosis. Even with total obliteration of the lumina of many smaller pulmonary arteries, pulmonary infarcts are infrequent (38). The diagnosis should be considered in any drug addict with cardiopulmonary distress. Lung biopsy will often confirm the diagnosis.

Arterial Injury and Extremity Gangrene Related to Drug Abuse

Repeated attempts at deep venous injection will result commonly in inadvertent arterial puncture. Brachial or femoral arterial injections are most frequent. Upper extremity arterial injections result in the syndrome referred to as a "hand trip." Maxwell and coauthors (3) accurately describe this as a burning pain in the region supplied by the injected artery. A hyperemic flush is noted in the same region. Signs and symptoms of ischemia predominate with pain, edema, cyanosis, and gangrene. The etiology of the ischemia and gangrene has been the focus of much interest and some controversy.

Ischemia can be related to direct mechanical arterial wall injury resulting in intimal flap, arteriovenous fistula, or pseudoaneurysm. Other pathophysiologic mechanisms for ischemia related to the drugs or excipients include chemical endarteritis, vasospasm, and particulate embolization. The end result is distal arterial thrombosis and ischemic necrosis. The degree of tissue loss is often dependent on the type of drug injected, the concentration, and the time delay before treatment.

PATHOPHYSIOLOGY

Vasoconstriction

VanderPost (40) is credited with first reporting the damaging effects due to intraarterial drug injection. He reported digital gangrene related to an inadvertent ulnar artery injection of 10%

thiopental sodium during anesthesia. Others have reported various extremity complications related to intraarterial barbiturate injections (41,42). The early clinical reports stimulated experimental work on the pathophysiology of arterial drug injections. An early hypothesis proposed vasoconstriction as a primary factor resulting in gangrene. However, studies done by Kinmonth and Shepherd (43) demonstrated that the vasoconstriction seen with injections of 5% thiopental lasted only about 30 s. Using a rabbit-ear model, the investigators found that sympathectomy and heparin were of benefit in decreasing the area of tissue necrosis, while vasodilators were of no benefit. Tissue necrosis was related to thiopental concentration.

A contrasting report by Burn (44) suggested that thiopental provoked a release of norepinephrine from the arterial wall causing vasoconstriction. In a model measuring gangrene in the mouse tail, pretreatment with reserpine resulted in a decrease in the observed amount of tissue necrosis. However, Ellertson and coworkers (45) studied a rabbit-ear model with angiography and could identify no spasm of the central artery of the ear with proximal ligation and injection of 10% thiopental. They did notice venospasm and venous thrombosis which they felt could play a role in the development of gangrene. Alix and coworkers (46) and then Wright and colleagues (6) studied flow alterations after various drug injections in the hind limb of a canine model as well as the lower extremity of a subhuman primate. Barbiturates, amphetamines, narcotics, and narcotic analgesics were studied. Most drugs caused an increase in femoral arterial blood flow unaccompanied by any evidence of vasoconstriction. Some species variation was noted in that amphetamine caused vasoconstriction in the dog but had no effect on limb blood flow in the subhuman primate.

Chemical Endarteritis

Some drugs have a direct toxic effect on the artery, resulting in endothelial destruction and interstitial edema (47,48). Engler (49) observed early arterial wall inflammation associated with canine femoral arterial drug injections. These findings have led to work investigating the effect of steroids on arterial drug injection. Enloe and coworkers (50) used a rabbit-ear model as described by Kinmonth and measured the effect of intraarterial hydroxyzine to produce gangrene. They found the immediate injection of lidocaine or papavarine was of some benefit, but intraarterial dexamethasone prevented gangrene. In addition, Buckspan and coinvestigators (47) found pharmacologic doses of dexamethasone (Decadron) significantly reduced gangrenous changes due to intraarterial thiopental sodium (sodium Pentothal) in a rabbit-ear model. The reported clinical experience of Maxwell and coauthors (3) invoked a chemical endarteritis with barbiturate injections causing endothelial damage of capillaries, arterioles, and arteries. They did not use steroids in their treatment regimen; however, Gaspar and Hare (48) utilized dexamethasone in their series of patients with gangrene due to drug injection.

Particulate Embolization

Particulate embolization is an important factor concerning the degree of tissue loss secondary to an intraarterial drug injection (6,7). When oral preparations are mixed with water and injected, the excipients (talc, cornstarch, fillers, emulsives) are often more injurious than the drug itself. Wright and coinvestigators (6) found that intraarterial injections of suspensions of cornstarch and talc produced reductions of femoral arterial flow in the subhuman primate. Sequential femoral arteriograms demonstrated microvascular obstruction in digital arteries with proximal propagation of thrombus. Polarizing microscopy of gangrenous tissues from drug addicts has documented numerous refractile bodies in the small arteries (7). Additionally, retinal circulation emboli have been reported in drug addicts (51).

Barbiturate Crystallization

Certain classes of drugs may have unique biochemical features which augment the pathophysiology. For instance, barbiturates in aqueous solution are alkaline (pH 10.6 to 11.4). However, with a decrease of the pH into the physiologic range, crystallization occurs. Brown and coinvestigators (52) studied various in vitro preparations and concluded that, following barbiturate injection into blood, acid crystals form which cause intimal damage and initiate red cell hemolysis and platelet aggregation. The higher the concentration of the barbiturate, the more likely was crystal formation. It has been suggested that these crystals cause a mechanical block of small arterioles (52,53). The frequency of vascular complications related to barbiturates may be underestimated, since barbiturate is often used to "cut" heroin (3). Maxwell and coauthors (3) proposed a schematic representation for the pathophysiology of intraarterial barbiturate injection (Figure 67-4).

Summary of Pathophysiology

Ischemia and gangrene related to intraarterial drug injection involve several mechanisms simultaneously. Unfortunately, critical factors affecting the degree of tissue loss cannot be controlled by the surgeon, namely, the type of drug injected, the concentration, and the time delay before treatment. Nevertheless, an understanding of the pathophysiology will help the surgeon design a proper management protocol. An arterial injection may be followed by a transient period of arterial or venous spasm associated with microembolization of particulate matter and secondary distal thrombosis. Most reported data do not support arterial spasm as a significant factor in the pathophysiology of untoward effects caused by intraarterial drugs of abuse (6,43), although Ryan and coauthors (5) emphasize that by prolonging endothelial drug exposure even transient vasospasm may be of importance. A chemical arteritis often occurs, resulting in endothelial cell injury and subsequent vascular thrombosis (3,49,50). Other factors which may relate to the degree of tissue loss include prolonged tourniquet time or extremity arterial compression due to abnormal posturing during an obtunded state. Also, systemic drugs may cause hypotension which will further reduce extremity blood flow and possibly contribute to local drug exposure.

MANAGEMENT

Management of an acute intraarterial drug injection includes initial resuscitation with normalization of cardiac output and peripheral perfusion, tetanus prophylaxis, and elevation for edema, as well as extremity immobilization. The early evaluation should

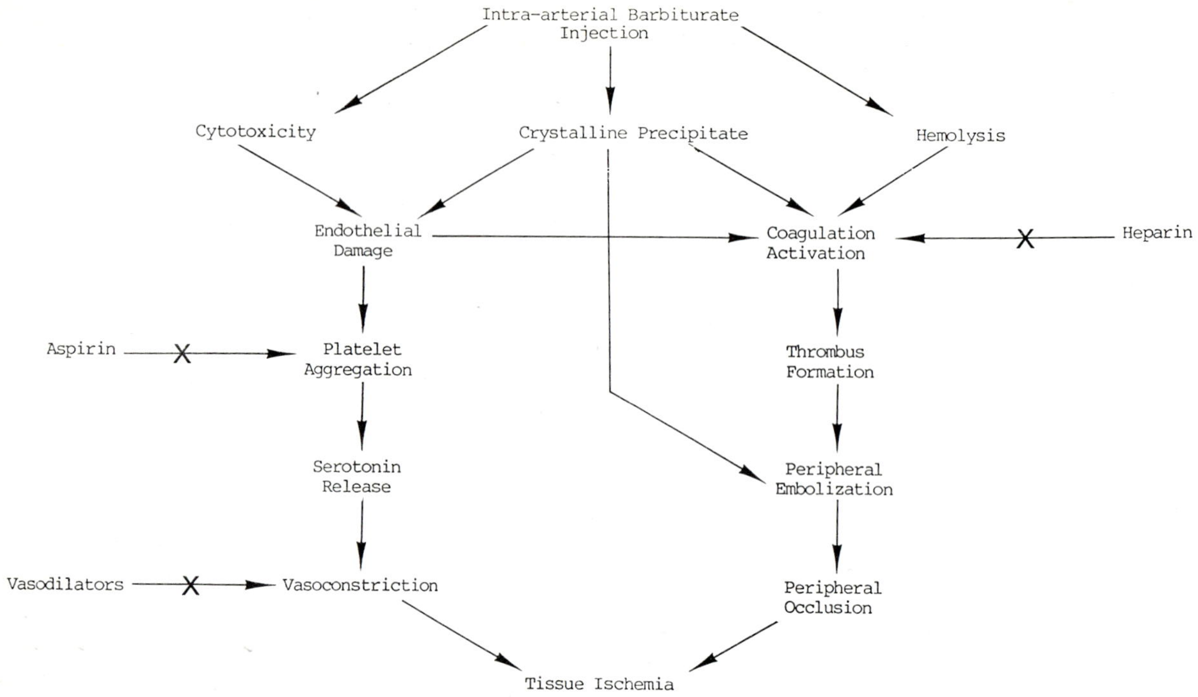

FIGURE 67-4. Schematic representation of pathophysiology of intraarterial barbiturate injection. (From Maxwell TM, Olcott C, Blaisdell FW: Vascular complications of drug abuse. Arch Surg 105:875–882, 1972. Reprinted by permission. Copyright 1972, American Medical Association.)

include segmental ultrasonic Doppler pressures of the extremities as well as Doppler evaluation of the palmar or pedal arches and digits. Compartment pressures should be measured as clinically appropriate (21), and if elevated, fasciotomy performed. Early arteriography is indicated to rule out arterial injury or thrombosis at the injection site and to evaluate distal arterial spasm or occlusion. If an arterial injury is identified at the site of injection (thrombosis, intimal flap, pseudoaneurysm, arteriovenous fistula), either early or delayed surgical repair is planned, depending on the type of injury, the degree and etiology of the distal ischemia, and the extent of local sepsis. For instance, a major arterial thrombosis accompanied by severe distal ischemia obviously requires prompt surgical intervention; however, management of a small arteriovenous fistula may be delayed until resolution of infection and local edema has occurred.

Generally most arterial drug injections with accompanying distal ischemia should be acutely managed with intravenous heparin anticoagulation which will maintain patent collaterals and inhibit further propagation of thrombus. Albo and coworkers (54) have recommended intraarterial heparin for digital and small arterial thromboses; however, the efficacy of this mode of treatment has not been proved. Najjar and colleagues (55) did treat one patient with digital arterial microemboli, combining vasodilators with open arteriotomy and heparinized saline irrigations. The patient improved, although no follow-up was obtained. Additionally, individual cases treated with low-molecular-weight Dextran have been reported with mixed results (7,48,56). The clinical use of vasodilators has had variable results as well (3,7). If the patient is seen within a few hours of injection and spasm is noted angiographically, vasodilators would seem indicated.

Stellate ganglion and brachial plexus blocks have been recommended by some authors (43,56,57). Brachial plexus block provides analgesia as well as sympathetic blockade. Regional block can result in local hematomas when the patient is anticoagulated (54). Ryan and coauthors (57) recommend a continuous brachial plexus block with an indwelling catheter in a heparinized patient. Another therapeutic modality to consider in the treatment of drug-related vascular injury includes a thrombolytic agent such as streptokinase (58), which was used successfully in one of our patients to lyse distal thrombi following radial arterial drug injection (35). Furthermore, there is some experimental evidence that intraarterial steroids may be of benefit (47,50), and additional clinical trials seem indicated.

Often a drug addict will present late following intraarterial drug injection with demarcating tissue necrosis. Treatment at this time involves antibiotics, tetanus prophylaxis, local debridement, and even amputation designed to preserve maximal tissue function.

Arterial Infections Related to Drug Abuse

Koch (59) in 1851 described a patient with an infected aneurysm involving the superior mesenteric artery, but it was Osler (60) who introduced the term *mycotic aneurysm* in 1885 to describe peripheral aneurysms resulting from embolization due to endocarditis. Although the term mycotic aneurysm is still used to describe arterial infections of all types, the recommended classification of Wilson and coauthors (61) retains Osler's original term only for those arterial infections resulting from emboli of endocardial origin. Most extremity arterial infections encountered in drug addicts are accurately classified as traumatic infected pseudoaneurysms (61).

CLINICAL PROBLEM

Infectious complications are the major cause for hospitalization of drug addicts and account for 15 percent of their deaths (62). The infected pseudoaneurysm is a serious vascular complication that most commonly involves the femoral or brachial artery. These are sites of repeated needle injections. The process usually involves direct mechanical arterial injury either by simple needle puncture, arterial wall laceration, or arterial wall injection with transmural necrosis. Secondary infection then occurs from the initial or subsequent contaminated needle injection. The association of chronic needle use and a heightened incidence of chronic staphylococcal carrier states has been previously discussed (26). Less commonly, direct extension of a groin abscess can occur, resulting in arterial wall destruction and development of an infected false aneurysm. Furthermore, septicemia may result in arterial wall seeding either through the vasa vasorum or into injured endothelium. As a result, mesenteric and other visceral mycotic aneurysms occur in the drug addict after repeated episodes of sepsis or endocarditis.

Huebl and Read (63) reported on three heroin addicts with infected pseudoaneurysms (two femoral, one iliac). All three were successfully managed with arterial ligation and drainage. Several reports have followed (1,3,13,64–70) documenting numerous anatomical sites of involvement. Besides femoral and brachial infected pseudoaneurysms, other arterial infection sites reported in drug addicts include superior mesenteric (68), carotid (66), subclavian (69), radial (70), pulmonary (1), external iliac (70), inferior mesenteric (17), and abdominal aorta (71).

Clinical presentation of an extremity arterial infection usually includes local pain and swelling at the site (70). Infected femoral pseudoaneurysms are usually larger than simple groin abscesses (64), and they exhibit expansile pulsation laterally (64,67). An obvious danger with infected pseudoaneurysms, particularly in the groin, is that the diagnosis will not be considered and the surgeon will proceed with incision and drainage, followed by profuse hemorrhage which may be very difficult to control. A high index of suspicion is urged. Preoperative arteriography can be very useful in confirming the diagnosis. For instance, in one series of mycotic aneurysms (70), abnormalities were noted in 29 of 30 arteriograms performed.

According to our experience and others (70) *Staphylococcus aureus* continues to be the most common causative organism cultured in these patients. In one series (70), infection was caused by this organism in more than 70 percent of the cases. Initial aspiration and Gram's stain will help in antibiotic selection prior to the culture report. The emergence of methicillin-resistant *Staphylococcus* makes the use of antibiotic sensitivities mandatory.

Mesenteric and other visceral mycotic aneurysms that occur in the drug addict are generally related to endocarditis. Clinical suspicion for bacterial or fungal endocarditis should be high in any drug abuser (3,72–76). Cardinal clinical findings with endocarditis include positive blood cultures and a changing heart murmur. However, with right-sided endocarditis, septic pulmonary emboli commonly can occur in the absence of cardiac murmurs. Left-sided endocarditis often presents with peripheral emboli resulting in peripheral arterial seeding. This can result in mycotic aneurysms at sites throughout the circulation, including visceral arteries such as the superior (68) and inferior (17) mesenteric arteries. One of our patients, with an unsuspected mycotic aneurysm of the superior mesenteric artery, died as a result of acute mesenteric arterial thrombosis and a small bowel infarction (35). This patient initially presented as a diagnostic problem with vague abdominal complaints. Arteriography should be used liberally as a diagnostic tool in such drug abuse patients, since prompt diagnosis of mesenteric and other visceral mycotic aneurysms may result in earlier surgical intervention.

MANAGEMENT

Arteriography should be utilized liberally when a patient presents with an inflamed mass located near a major artery. In addition, needle aspiration of fluctuant groin masses prior to incision and drainage is recommended. Blood-tinged aspirate or clinical presentation of a pulsatile mass are definite indications for preoperative arteriography. Infected venous pseudoaneurysms should be suspected in the presence of similar physical findings and a normal arteriogram. Venography may be helpful in establishing this diagnosis.

Surgical management of infected pseudoaneurysms of the brachial or femoral artery should include proximal and distal arterial ligation with drainage or excision of the involved artery. In the case of infected femoral pseudoaneurysm, proximal control can often be obtained at the level of the inguinal ligament. However, if the inflamed mass extends above the inguinal ligament, proximal control of the external iliac artery through a right lower quadrant extraperitoneal incision is recommended. The artery is divided and ligated at this level. If feasible, distal control of the superficial femoral artery is obtained before entering the infected aneurysm and controlling the profunda femoris artery from within (9). Ligation of normal uninvolved arterial segments is recommended. In the experience of Johnson and coauthors (70), rebleeding following excision in five of six patients was due to failure of a ligature placed on infected arterial segments. Attempts at vascular reconstruction should be made only after simple excision of the aneurysm has resulted in signs of limb-threatening ischemia. Johnson (70) reported severe ischemia in 9 of 28 (32 percent) patients who underwent excision of the common femoral artery alone or with its bifurcation. Subsequent management of these cases would include either obturator foramen bypass (64) or other extraanatomical bypass (77), usually with a synthetic prosthesis through clean tissue planes. Limb-threatening ischemia of the upper extremity is not as likely since involvement usually is distal to the profunda brachii artery (71). If use of autogenous tissue grafts is possible, this can be accomplished by placing the autograft through the area of infection (67).

Ledgerwood and Lucas (66) reported on the management of three patients (two drug addicts) with aneurysmal abscess involving the carotid artery. Patients were treated with antibiotics and proximal carotid arterial ligation followed by delayed distal ligation and drainage. No patient experienced a neurological deficit. Measurement of carotid stump pressure is useful in determining the safety of carotid arterial ligation. A systolic stump pressure in excess of 70 mmHg indicates adequate collateral hemispheric blood flow, and carotid arterial ligation under these circumstances is acceptable (78). In cases of lower stump pressures, autogenous reconstruction is recommended if feasible (11).

Vasculitis Related to Drug Abuse

Drug abuse has recently been reported to cause several forms of arteritis. Citron (15) reported a series of drug abusers who developed a necrotizing angiitis indistinguishable from periarteritis nodosa. Most of these patients abused methamphetamine alone or in combination with heroin or *d*-lysergic acid diethylamide. These patients developed pancreatitis, renal failure, hypertension, pulmonary edema, and/or neuropathy. Arteriography demonstrated arterial aneurysms and sacculations in various organ systems including kidney, liver, pancreas, and small bowel. Biopsy demonstrated a panarteritis of small- and medium-sized arteries with fibrinoid necrosis and luminal thrombosis (15). Other links between drug abuse and arteritis include a cerebral arteritis reportably attributed to the abuse of amphetamines (79–81), as well as heroin alone (82) or in combination with D-lysergic acid diethylamide (83).

The pathogenesis of drug abuse vasculitis may relate to the presence of circulating immune complexes and their deposition on blood vessel walls (84–87). This leads to complement activation, migration of polymorphonuclear leukocytes, and release of lysosomal enzymes which results in arterial wall damage (86). The diagnosis should be suspected in any patient with a drug history presenting with signs and symptoms suggesting involvement of the renal, hepatobiliary, gastrointestinal, or central nervous systems. Treatment obviously includes cessation of the drugs. A resolution of drug-related renal arteritis with prednisone therapy has been reported (84).

Ergotism

During the Middle Ages, ergotism occurred in epidemics across central and eastern Europe (88). Its etiology was later found related to the ingestion of rye bread contaminated by the fungus *Claviceps purpurea,* an ergot-producing mold. Symptoms included diarrhea, abdominal cramps, vomiting, headache, convulsion, coma, and peripheral ischemia (89). The characteristic burning sensation in the feet and hands associated with ergotism came to be known as "St. Anthony's Fire" (90). Present-day ergot poisoning is an iatrogenic disease related to an overuse of medications containing ergot alkaloids prescribed for migraine headaches or postpartum hemorrhage. The pathophysiology of ergotism is related to vasoconstriction. The classification of the ergot derivatives and their pharmacologic properties have been tabulated by Merhoff and Porter (88) (Table 67-1). Common among these is ergotamine tartrate (Cafergot), a migraine headache medication. Additionally, methysergide maleat (Sansert) is a semisynthetic ergot alkaloid which is prescribed for migraine headaches and can cause severe vasoconstriction. Bagby (91) has described three clinical settings in which ergot intoxication may occur. They include the chronic ingestion of therapeutic doses, the acute ingestion of excessive amounts, and the acute ingestion of small amounts by individuals with hypersensitivity to the drug.

Symptomatic vasospasm is most common in the extremities, although it may involve any organ system (88). Ergot-induced vasospasm involving the renal (92), carotid (93), mesenteric (94), and coronary (95) arteries has been reported. A high index of suspicion is necessary to make the diagnosis of ergot-induced vasospasm since many patients will not volunteer a history that headache medication was taken. Arteriography usually demonstrates involvement of large- and medium-sized arteries with abruptly tapered smooth stenosis (89) associated with significant

TABLE 67-1. Pharmacologic Properties of Ergot Derivatives

Class	Action			
	Vasoconstriction	Oxytocic	α-Blocker	Sympatholytic
Amino acid alkaloids (ergotamine tartrate)	Most active	Highly active but of delayed onset, not active orally	Active	Active
Dihydrogenated amino acid alkaloids				
(Dihydroergotamine)	Active but less than above	Active on pregnant human uterus	Most active	Most active
(Dihydroergotoxine)	None			
Amino alkaloids				
(ergonovine & methylergonovine)	Slight	Most active	None	?

SOURCE: From Merhoff GC, Porter JM: Ergot Intoxication: Historical review and description of unusual clinical manifestations. Ann Surg 180:733–779, 1974. Reprinted by permission.

collaterals (96). Arterial thrombosis is uncommon, while extremity arterial spasm is usually bilateral and symmetrical (97). In the lower extremities, spasm may begin at the level of the common iliac arteries, although the femoral and popliteal arteries are more commonly involved (97).

Central to the treatment of ergotism is discontinuance of the drug. Improvement can be expected in a matter of days once metabolism of the drug is complete (88). In the presence of severe ischemia and impending tissue loss, heparinization is recommended to assist in the maintenance of patent collaterals, thereby preventing propagation of thrombus (88). Parenteral use of vasodilators is controversial since ergotamine is bound to the alpha receptors, and attempts to experimentally displace it with phenoxybenzamine have been unsuccessful (88,98). Nevertheless, there have been successful clinical reports utilizing intravenous niacin sodium (99), intravenous alcohol (100), papaverine (101), intravenous sodium nitroprusside (102), and intraarterial tolazoline (89,103). Recently a successful clinical experience utilizing a calcium channel blocker was reported (104). Ergotamine has been shown to be a vasoconstrictor even in the sympathectomized limb (105), although direct sympathetic blockade using conduction anesthetic techniques as well as regional sympathectomy have both been reported to be of clinical benefit (101,106,107).

References

1. Jaffe RB, Koschmann EB: Intravenous drug abuse pulmonary, cardiac and vascular complications. Am J Roentgenol Radium Ther Nucl Med 1970, 109:107–120.
2. Geelhoed GW, Joseph WL: Surgical sequelae of drug abuse. Surg Gynecol Obstet 1975, 139:749–755.
3. Maxwell TM, Olcott C, Blaisdell FW: Vascular complications of drug abuse. Arch Surg 1972, 105:875–881.
4. Ritland D, Butterfield W: Extremity complications of drug abuse. Am J Surg 1973, 126:639–648.
5. Ryan JJ, Hoopes JE, Jabaley ME: Drug injection injuries of the hands and forearms in addicts. Plast Reconstr Surg 1974, 53:445–451.
6. Wright CB, Lamoy RE, Hobson RW II: Hemodynamic effects of intra-arterial injection of drugs of abuse. Surgery 1976, 79:425–431.
7. Lindell TD, Porter JM, Langston C: Intra-arterial injections of oral medications. A complication of drug addiction. N Engl J Med 1972, 287:1132–1133.
8. Dale WA, Lewis MR: Heparin control of venous thromboembolism. Arch Surg 1970, 101:744–755.
9. Feldman AJ, Berguer R: Management of an infected aneurysm of the groin secondary to drug abuse. Surg Gynecol Obstet 1983, 157:519–522.
10. Wiley EJ: Vascular replacement with arterial autografts. Surgery 1965, 57:14–21.
11. Ehrenfeld WK, Wilbur BG, Olcott CNIV, Stoney RJ: Autogenous graft replacement of infected prosthetic grafts in the femoral position. Surgery 1983, 93:39–45.
12. Orangio GR, Pitlick SD, Latta PD, Mandel LJ, Marino C, Guarneri JJ, Giron JA, Margolis IB: Soft tissue infections in parenteral drug abusers. Ann Surg 1984, 199:97–100.
13. Joseph WL, Fletcher HS, Giordano JM, Adkins PC: Pulmonary and cardiovascular implications of drug addiction. Ann Thorac Surg 1973, 15:263–274.
14. Halpern M, Rho Y: Death from narcotics in New York City. Incidence, circumstances and post mortem findings. NY State J Med 1966, 66:2391–2408.
15. Citron BP, Halpern M, McCarron M, Lundberg GD, McCormick R, Pincus IJ, Tatter D, Haverback BJ: Necrotizing angiitis associated with drug abuse. N Engl J Med 1970, 283:1003–1011.
16. Gabow P, deTorrente A, Holt S, Kelly GL: Arteriovenous fistula from drug abuse. Implications for hemodialysis. JAMA 1976, 235:2220–2221.
17. Lau J, Mattox KL, DeBakey ME: Mycotic aneurysm of the inferior mesenteric artery. Am J Surg 1979, 138:443–445.
18. Sreepada Rao TK, Nicastri AD, Friedman EA: Natural history of heroin-associated nephropathy. N Engl J Med 1974, 290:19–23.
19. Neviaser RJ, Butterfield WC, Wieche DR: The puffy hand of drug addiction. A study of pathogenesis. J Bone Joint Surg 1972, 54-A:629–633.
20. Dunne JH, Johnson WC: Necrotizing skin lesions in heroin addicts. Arch Dermatol 1972, 105:544–547.
21. Owen CA, Mubarak SJ, Hargens AR, Rutherford L, Garetto LP, Akeson WH: Intramuscular pressures with limb compression. Clarification of the pathogenesis of the drug-induced muscle-compartment syndrome. N Engl J Med 1979, 300:1169–1172.
22. Beveridge GW, Lawson AAH: Occurrence of bullous lesions in acute barbiturate intoxication. Br Med J 1965, 1:835–837.
23. Daniel DM: The acutely swollen hand in the drug user. Arch Surg 1973, 107:548–551.
24. Moustoukas NM, Nichols RL, Smith JW, Garey RE, Egan RR: Contaminated street heroin. Relationship to clinical infections. Arch Surg 1983, 118:746–749.
25. Tuazon CU, Hill R, Sheagren JN: Microbiologic study of street heroin and injection paraphernalia. J Infect Dis 1974, 129:327–329.
26. Tuazon CU, Sheagren JN: Staphylococcal endocarditis in parenteral drug abusers: Source of the organism. Ann Intern Med 1975, 82:778–780.
27. Reynolds AK, Randall LO: *Morphine and Allied Drugs*. University of Toronto Press, Toronto, 1957, p 65.
28. Baker CC, Petersen SR, Sheldon GF: Septic phlebitis: A neglected disease. Am J Surg 1979, 1381:97–103.
29. Warden GD, Wilmore DW, Pruitt BA: Central venous thrombosis: A hazard of medical progress. J Trauma 1973, 13:620–626.
30. Stein JM, Pruitt BA: Suppurative thrombophlebitis. A lethal iatrogenic disease. N Engl J Med 1970, 282:1452–1455.
31. Winn RE, Tuttle KL, Gilbert DN: Surgical approach to extensive suppurative thrombophlebitis of the central veins of the chest. J Thorac Cardiovasc Surg 1981, 81:564–568.
32. Weinberg G, Pasternak BM: Upper-extremity suppurative thrombophlebitis and septic pulmonary emboli. JAMA 1978, 240:1519.
33. Greenfield LJ, Peyton R, Crute SL, Barnes R: Greenfield vena caval filter experience. Late results in 156 patients. Arch Surg 1981, 116:1451–1456.
34. Peyton JWR, Hylemon MB, Greenfield LJ, Crute SL, Sugerman HJ, Quershi GD: Comprison of Greenfield filter and vena caval ligation for experimental septic thromboembolism. Surgery 1983, 93:533–537.
35. Yeager RA, Hobson RW II, Padberg FT, Lynch TG, Chakravarty M: Vascular complications related to drug abuse. J Trauma (submitted).
36. Johnson JJ, Lucas CE, Ledgerwood AM, Jacobs LA: Infected venous pseudoaneurysm. A complication of drug addiction. Arch Surg 1984, 119:1097–1098.

37. Wendt VE, Puro HE, Shapiro J, Mathews W, Wolf PL: Angiothrombotic pulmonary hypertension in addicts. "Blue velvet" addiction. JAMA 1964, 188:137–139.
38. Waller BF, Brownlee WJ, Roberts WC: Structure-function correlations in cardiovascular and pulmonary diseases (CPC) self-induced pulmonary granulomatosis. A consequence of intravenous injection of drugs intended for oral use. Chest 1980, 78:90–94.
39. Robertson CH, Reynolds J, Wilson JE III: Pulmonary hypertension and foreign body granulomatosis, in intravenous drug abusers: Documentation by cardiac catheterization and lung biopsy. Am J Med 1976, 61:657–663.
40. VanderPost CWH: Report of case of mistaken injection of Pentothal sodium into an aberrant ulnar artery. S Afr Med J 1942, 16:182.
41. Cohen SM: Accidental intra-arterial injection of drugs. Lancet 1948, 2:311–371.
42. Stone HH, Donnelly CC: The accidental intra-arterial injection of thiopental. Anesthesiology 1961, 22:995–1005.
43. Kinmonth JB, Shepherd RC: Accidental injection of thiopentone into arteries. Studies of pathology and treatment. Br Med J 1959, 2:914–918.
44. Burn JH: Why thiopentone injected into an artery may cause gangrene. Br Med J 1960, 2:414–416.
45. Ellertson DG, Lazarus HM, Auerbach R: Patterns of acute vascular injury after intra-arterial barbiturate injection. Am J Surg 1973, 126:813–817.
46. Alix EC, Bogumill GP, Wright CB: Intra-arterial injection of abused drugs. Cardiovasc Res 1975, 9:266–271.
47. Buckspan GS, Franklin JD, Novak GR, Bennett BD, Lynch JB, Dean RH: Intra-arterial drug injury: Studies of etiology and potential treatment. J Surg Research 1978, 24:294–301.
48. Gaspar MR, Hare RR: Gangrene due to intra-arterial injection of drugs by drug addicts. Surgery 1972, 72:573–577.
49. Engler HS, Freeman RA, Kanavage CB, Ogden LL, Moretz WH: Production of gangrenous extremities by intra-arterial injections. Am Surg 1964, 30:602–607.
50. Enloe G, Sylvester M, Morris LE: Hazards of intra-arterial injections of hydroxyzine. Can Anaesth Soc J 1969, 16:425–428.
51. Atlee WE Jr: Talc and cornstarch emboli in eyes of drug abusers. JAMA 1972, 219:9–51.
52. Brown SS, Lyons SM, Dundee JW: Intra-arterial barbiturates. A study of some factors leading to intravascular thrombosis. Br J Anaesth 1968, 40:13–19.
53. Waters DJ: Intra-arterial thiopentone: A physico-chemical phenomenon. Anaesthesiology 1966, 21:346–356.
54. Albo D Jr, Cheung L, Ruth L, Snyder C, Reemtsma K: Effect of intra-arterial injections of barbiturates. Am J Surg 1970, 120:676–678.
55. Najjar FB, Bridi G, Rizk G: Management of micro-emboli of the digital arteries. Leb Med J 1974, 27(4):467–471.
56. Hamer R, Phelps D: Inadvertent intra-arterial injection of phentaramine: A complication of drug abuse. Ann Emerg Med 1981, 10(3):148–150.
57. Ryan JJ, Hoopes JE, Jabaley ME: Drug injection injuries of the hands and forearms in addicts. Plast Reconstruct Surg 1974, 53:445–451.
58. Lloyd WK, Porter JM, Lindell TD, Rosch J, Dotter CT: Accidental intra-arterial injection in drug abuse. Am J Roentgenol Radium Ther Nucl Med 1973, 117:892–895.
59. Koch L: Ueber aneurysma der arteriae mesenterichae superioris, in inaug dural-abhandlung. Erlangen, J.J. Barfus' Schen Universitats, Buchdruckerei, 1851, pp 5–23.
60. Osler W: The Gulstonian lectures on malignant endocarditis. Br Med J 1855, 1:467.
61. Wilson SE, VanWagenen P, Passaro E Jr: Arterial infection. Curr Probl Surg 1978, 15:6–89.
62. Hau T, Kallick CA: Surgical infections in drug addicts. World J Surg 1980, 4:403–413.
63. Huebl HC, Read RC: Aneurysmal abscess. Minn Med 1966, 49:11–16.
64. Fromm SH, Lucas CE: Obturator bypass for mycotic aneurysm in the drug addict. Arch Surg 1970, 100:82–83.
65. Willoughby CP, Evans E, Stoker TAM, Gabriel R: Arterial hemorrhage in a drug addict. Br Med J 1973, 2:307–308.
66. Ledgerwood AM, Lucas CE: Mycotic aneurysm of the carotid artery. Arch Surg 1974, 109:496–498.
67. Anderson CB, Butcher HR Jr, Ballenger WF: Mycotic aneurysms. Arch Surg 1974, 109:712–717.
68. Yellin AE: Ruptured mycotic aneurysm. A complication of parenteral drug abuse. Arch Surg 1977, 112:981–986.
69. Ho KL, Rasseich ZS: Mycotic aneurysm of the right subclavian artery. Complication of heroin addiction. Chest 1978, 74:116–117.
70. Johnson JR, Ledgerwood AM, Lucas CE: Mycotic aneurysm: New concepts in therapy. Arch Surg 1983, 118:577–582.
71. Collins GJ Jr, Rich NM, Hobson RW II, Andersen CA, Green D: Multiple mycotic aneurysms due to *Candida* endocarditis. Ann Surg 1977, 186:136–139.
72. Louria DB, Hensle T, Rose J: The major medical complications of heroin addiction. Ann Intern Med 1967, 67:1–22.
73. Cherubin CE, Baden M, Kavaler F, Lerner S, Cline W: Infective endocarditis in narcotic addicts. Ann Intern Med 1968, 69:1091–1098.
74. Ramsey RG, Gunnar RM, Tobin JR Jr: Endocarditis in the drug addict. Am J Cardiol 1970, 25:608–618.
75. Stimmel B, Donoso E, Dack S: Comparison of infective endocarditis in drug addicts and non drug users. Am J Cardiol 1973, 32:924–929.
76. Scalcini MC, Sanders CV: Endocarditis from human-to-human transmission of *staphylococcus aureus*. Arch Intern Med 1980, 140:111–112.
77. Leather RP, Karmody AM: A lateral route for extra-anatomical bypass of the femoral artery. Surgery 1977, 81:307–309.
78. Ehrenfeld WK, Stoney RJ, Wylie EJ: Relation of carotid stump pressure to safety of carotid artery ligation. Surgery 1983, 93:299–305.
79. Halpern M, Citron BP: Necrotizing angiitis associated with drug abuse. Am J Roentgenol Radium Ther Nucl Med 1971, 111:663–671.
80. Margolis MT, Newton TH: Methamphetamine ("speed") arteritis. Neuroradiology 1971, 2:179–182.
81. Rumbaugh CL, Bergeron RT, Fang HCH, McCormick R: Cerebral angiographic changes in the drug abuse patient. Radiology 1971, 101:335–344.
82. King J, Richards M, Tress B: Cerebral arteritis associated with heroin abuse. Med J Aust 1978, 2:444–445.
83. Lignelli GJ, Buchheit WA: Angiitis in drug abusers. N Engl Med 1971, 284:111.
84. Heazlewood JJ, Bochner F, Craswell PW: Hallucinogenic drug induced vasculitis. Med J Aust 1981, 1:359–360.
85. McAllister HA Jr, Mullick FG: The cardiovascular system. In Riddel RH (ed): *Pathology of Drug-Induced and Toxic Disease*, New York, Churchill Livingstone, 1982, pp 201–228.
86. Fauci AS, Haynes BF, Katz P: The spectrum of vasculitis: Clinical, pathologic, immunologic, and therapeutic considerations. Ann Intern Med 1978, 89:660–676.
87. Alarcon-Segovia D: The necrotizing vasculitides: A new pathogenetic classification. Med Clin North Am 1977, 61(2):241–260.
88. Merhoff GC, Porter JM: Ergot intoxication: Historical review and description of unusual clinical manifestations. Ann Surg 1974, 180:773–779.
89. Henry LG, Blackwood JS, Conley JE, Bernhard VM: Ergotism. Arch Surg 1975, 110:929–932.

90. Fitzgerald B: Saint Anthony's fire or carpal tunnel syndrome? (A case of iatrogenic ergotism). Hand 1978, 20:82–86.
91. Bagby RJ, Cooper RD: Angiography in ergotism: Report of two cases and review of the literature. Am J Roentgenol Radium Ther Nucl Med 1972, 116:179–186.
92. Fedotin MS, Hartman C: Ergotamine poisoning producing renal artery spasm. N Engl J Med 1970, 283:518–520.
93. Richter AM, Banker VP: Carotid ergotism, a complication of migraine therapy. Radiology 1973, 106:339–340.
94. Berman JK, Brown HM, Foster RI, Grisell TL: Massive resection of the intestine. JAMA 1947, 135:918–919.
95. Goldfischer JD: Acute myocardial infarction secondary to ergot therapy. N Engl J Med 1960, 262:860–863.
96. Yater WM, Cahill JA: Bilateral gangrene of feet due to ergotamine tartrate used for pruritis or jaundice. JAMA 1936, 106:1625–1631.
97. Ancalmo N, Ochsner JL: Peripheral ischemia secondary to ergotamine intoxication. Arch Surg 1974, 109:832–834.
98. Innes IR: Identification of the smooth muscle excitatory receptors for ergot alkaloids. Br J Pharmacol 1962, 19:120–128.
99. Thompson WS, McLure WW, Landowne M: Prolonged vasoconstriction due to ergotamine tartrate. Arch Intern Med 1950, 85:691–698.
100. Ahlgren I, Haeger K, Nylander G: Imminent gangrene of the leg after ergot poisoning. Angiology 1968, 19:354–361.
101. London M, Magora F, Rogel S: Acute ergot poisoning. Angiology 1970, 21:515–567.
102. Carliner NH, Denune DP, Finch CS, Soldberg LI: Sodium nitroprusside treatment of ergotamine-induced peripheral ischemia. JAMA 1974, 227:308–309.
103. Cranley J, Kause R, Strasser E: Impending gangrene of all four extremities secondary to ergotism. N Engl J Med 1963, 269:727–729.
104. Dagher FJ, Pais SO, Richards W, Queral LA: Severe unilateral ischemia of the lower extremity caused by ergotamine: Treatment with nifedipine. Surgery 1985, 97:369–375.
105. Bluntschli HJ, Goetz RH: The effect of ergot derivatives on the circulation in man with special reference to two new hydrogenated compounds (dihydroergotamine and dihydroergocornine). Am Heart J 1948, 35:873–894.
106. Hudgson P, Hart JAL: Acute ergotism: Report of a case and review of the literature. Med J Aust 1964, 2:589–591.
107. McLoughlin MG, Sanders RJ: Ergotism causing peripheral vascular ischemia. Rocky Mt Med J 1972, 69:45–49.

PART TEN

Arteriovenous Fistula

Chapter 68

PRINCIPLES OF VASCULAR ACCESS SURGERY

RUSSELL A. WILLIAMS, LAWRENCE HOLLANDER, ROBERT S. BENNION, and SAMUEL E. WILSON

From the beginning, the full potential of hemodialysis for the long-term treatment of patients with chronic renal failure was limited by the lack of a means for repeated access to the vascular system. At the outset, it was necessary for repeated cutdowns to be made on an artery and vein for each dialysis, following which, the vessels were ligated. The duration of a course of dialysis was, therefore, limited to the treatment of acute renal failure. W. J. Kolff, the designer of the first practical dialysis machine, observed, in 1944, "When a preparation of the arteries was necessary (all veins being ruined) very persistent hemorrhages arose from the subcutaneous tissue owing to the heparine. . . . After the 12th dialysis became a failure, the artery being damaged, the urea percentage of the blood rapidly rose to 640 mg percent whereupon death followed" (1).

Scribner, Dillard, and Quinton (an internist, a surgeon, and an engineer) in 1960 introduced the first successful apparatus for provision of reasonably long term cannulation of an artery and vein using an external Silastic shunt (2) (Figure 68-1). This was widely adopted over the succeeding 6 years, up to the time Cimino and coworkers reported their success in 1966, with the autologous, subcutaneous arteriovenous fistula (3). This "arterialized" superficial arm vein could be repeatedly cannulated, and it has stood the test of time, remaining today still the best method for provision of long-term vascular access.

The availability of vascular access is now also an important consideration in the treatment of patients needing long-term administration of anticancer medication and other drugs, for total parenteral nutrition, and for the treatment of patients by means of plasmapheresis.

Physiology of Arteriovenous Fistulas

An arteriovenous (AV) fistula has local and systemic, hemodynamic and nonhemodynamic effects. These vary, depending on whether the fistula is acute or chronic, and are modified by the anatomical configuration of the fistula and by how far proximally or distally it is sited on the vascular tree.

A fistula may be formed directly between an adjacent artery and vein or, if these vessels are separated, by connecting them with conduit limb of variable diameter or length. When the connecting limb is very short, such as in a Cimino fistula, the flow through the fistula, when plotted in relation to the fistula di-

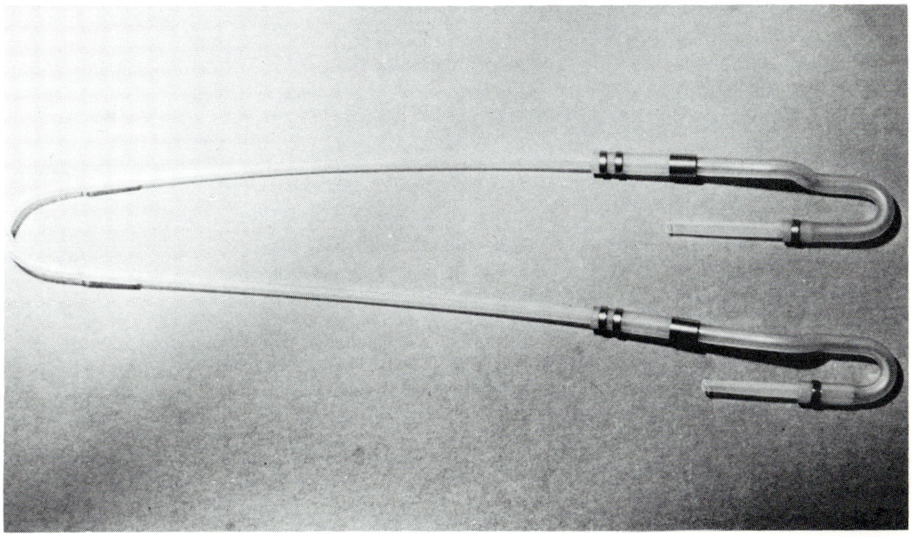

FIGURE 68-1. Early form of Quinton-Dillard-Scribner shunt in which metal bands were used to hold components together. [From Wilson and Owens (4).]

ameter, increases following a sigmoid curve with increasing diameter of the fistula (4). There is little flow through the fistula until its diameter exceeds 20 percent of that of the proximal artery. From then onward, flow increases rapidly with small changes in fistula diameter, until the diameter reaches 75 percent of the proximal arterial diameter. Following that, there are only small increases in flow with increasing fistula diameter.

In all fistulas, the direction of blood flow in both the proximal artery and vein is normal. With small fistulas (by definition, these have a diameter less than 75 percent of the proximal arterial lumen) the blood flow in the distal vein and artery is in the normal direction. However, this is usually reversed in large fistulas (diameter greater than 75 percent of the arterial lumen).

Fistulas that are to be utilized for therapeutic purposes are constructed so that they are of the large variety. This ensures the greatest blood flow and decreases the likelihood of fistula clotting. Fistulas formed between the radial or posterior tibial artery and a vein have blood flow rates of 150 up to 500 mL/min. Grafts attached to larger arteries such as the femoral or axillary have flow rates of 500 to 1500 mL/min through them.

When a fistula is opened, there is a fall in peripheral resistance which leads to a decrease in the proximal fistula artery pressure and which is compensated for by an increase in cardiac output. Proximal arterial flow then increases, and, accompanying this, there is an increase in proximal venous outflow that is not accompanied by a significant rise in central venous pressure because of the large capacity of the venous system.

The highest blood pressure in the distal artery is usually only about two-thirds of systemic pressure, which is nevertheless higher than that at the fistula opening. Therefore, flow is often retrograde in the distal artery. Valves in the veins direct blood flow cardiad and result in an initially high peripheral venous pressure. "Arterialization" of the veins leads to dilation and valvular incompetence, which may cause distal venous hypertension.

Blood in the distal fistula vein flows retrograde until at some point the valves are able to withstand the pressure. The blood in the distal vein is carried cardiad by venous collaterals which open off the vein. With time, there is significant increase in the number of collateral vessels formed between the proximal and distal arteries and the proximal and distal veins. In the arterial system, these are stimulated by the pressure differences across the bed, and in the venous system, they hypertrophy to accommodate the large retrograde flow. Ligation of the distal fistula artery reduces the degree of development of collateral arterial vessels.

Venous collaterals develop more extensively than do arterial ones, and they accommodate the considerable retrograde venous flow that follows as incompetence of the valves occurs.

Ligation of the proximal fistula artery decreases flow through the fistula and peripheral vascular bed, an effect that is much less pronounced with a chronic fistula in which large collaterals have been stimulated to develop. These maintain blood flow through the distal vascular bed and the fistula to a much greater extent than does flow through the proximal fistula artery.

In small fistulas, there is a gradual buildup of platelets and fibrin along the fistula tract; these are replaced by smooth muscle and fibrous tissue and eventually result in fistula closure. With time, in larger fistulas, there is lengthening and dilation of the proximal and distal veins and the proximal artery in addition to the vascular collaterals. The proximal artery develops smooth-muscle hypertrophy in addition to dilation, and then it elongates. Later the muscle atrophies, and the vessel becomes tortuous and aneurysmal. In the vein, there is an increase in smooth-muscle and fibrous tissue of the subintimal layer. Eventually it may develop atherosclerosis. The vein dilates for up to 8 months following construction of an AV fistula.

In addition to the foregoing changes, there is an increase in the temperature of the tissues surrounding an AV fistula because of increased flow in the adjacent collaterals. AV fistulas have been used to treat discrepancies in limb lengths in children. The increased collateral flow stimulates bone growth.

A large AV fistula may produce congestive cardiac failure. To compensate for the increased fistula flow, the pulse, stroke volume, and cardiac output increase, and there is increased vasoconstriction of other parts of the vascular bed.

Blood may be "stolen" from the vascular bed peripheral to the fistula, producing symptoms of ischemia. This happens when fistula blood flow equals about one-third of the prefistula cardiac output. Heart failure occurs when the fistula flow is 20 to 50 percent of the cardiac output.

Short-Term Vascular Access

EXTERNAL AV SHUNT

The external AV shunt is commonly referred to as the Scribner shunt and was initially the only means for facilitating long-term vascular access in patients with chronic renal failure (2). It has been reported to have an average patency rate ranging from 2 up to 15.6 months.

The Scribner shunt is occasionally useful because it can be used immediately and may still be utilized for patients with acute renal failure or for those with chronic renal failure requiring immediate dialysis. It can also be used to treat patients with acute poisoning, and rarely in an individual who cannot tolerate frequent needle puncture.

The shunt is composed of an arterial and a venous cannula tip and Silastic tubing that connects these cannulas. The cannula tips are chosen to be as large as possible so as to provide good flow through the shunt, yet if too large, they may crimp the intima of the fistula artery, hindering flow (Figure 68-2). This shunt is most commonly placed between the radial artery and adjacent cephalic vein at the wrist or in the ankle region between the posterior tibial artery and saphenous vein.

Atherosclerotic arteries are avoided, as these limit inflow to the shunt, increasing the likelihood of it clotting. Venous outflow must be unimpeded, making a leg with chronic venous stasis or a limb with acute phlebitis, unsuitable for insertion of the Scribner shunt. Under optimal conditions, the shunt is constructed in the operating room, although at times, in very ill patients, it may be necessary to construct it at the bedside of an intensive care unit.

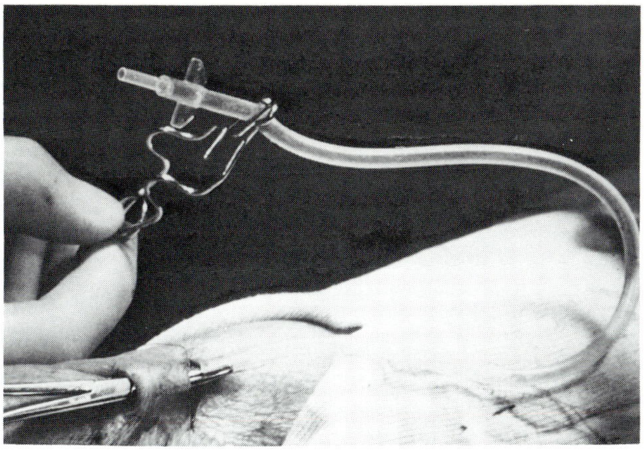

FIGURE 68-2. A modification of the Scribner shunt with Silastic wings attached to prevent rotation of the cannula tip within the vessels. [From Wilson and Owens (4).]

This shunt is usually placed in the nondominant arm. However, if the plan is for the patient to also have a more permanent subcutaneous fistula, then the subcutaneous fistula is placed in the nondominant arm and the external shunt in the dominant arm.

Before utilizing the radial artery for a Scribner shunt, a determination is made that the ulnar artery will maintain the hand circulation. This is done by compressing both the radial and ulnar arteries at the wrist and elevating the hand, which becomes pale. Release of pressure over the ulnar artery normally reestablishes the hand perfusion.

The radial artery must be of an adequate size to deliver blood at a sufficient rate to prevent clotting and maintain patency of the shunt. In patients with advanced atherosclerosis—particularly diabetic patients—the radial artery may be too diseased for use.

A suitably sized vein adjacent to the radial artery is selected to accommodate the venous cannula. A tourniquet is used to demonstrate the vein, which is then marked with an indelible skin pen, for subsequent location during the operation.

Under local infiltration anesthesia or a brachial plexus block, a longitudinal skin incision is made adjacent to the radial artery, 3 to 4 cm proximal to the skin creases at the wrist. This sites the shunt to avoid kinking and displacement of the cannula and tubing with flexion of the wrist. If the radial artery is found to be atherosclerotic at the wrist, the longitudinal skin incision can be extended cephalad and the larger, more proximal radial artery utilized for construction of the shunt. Once the shunt is inserted in the artery, flow through it is tested by releasing the clamp. The shunt is filled with heparinized saline and reclamped to prevent clotting of any blood within its lumen. The vein is cannulated in a fashion similar to the artery.

After completion of vessel cannulation, redundant Silastic tubing is cut off and the two cannulas are connected with a Teflon connector. This connector is placed on the straight part of the tube rather than at the apex of the loop, avoiding kinking of the shunt tubing. The tubing is left long enough to allow easy connection to the artificial kidney (Figure 68-3). Blood flow rate through the fistula is roughly judged as adequate if the bubble that remains in the connecting tube washes around the loop in 2 to 3 s.

The arm is loosely dressed to avoid kinking of the shunt, and a segment of the loop is left visible to detect any clotting. Particular attention is paid to dressing the shunt loosely so no pressure is applied to the arm that would produce venous outflow obstruction and lead to shunt clotting. Application of a tourniquet or pneumatic cuff for venisection or blood pressure measurements is forbidden on the operated arm. Ideally, the shunt is left for up to 48 hours to allow some healing to occur. If it must be used immediately for dialysis, an attempt is made to avoid excess heparinization and so reduce the risk of hematoma formation. It is unwise to use the shunt for the administration of medications, because these may produce phlebitis and venous occlusion, followed by clotting of the shunt.

The ulnar or brachial arteries are alternative vessels on which to base the shunt if the radial artery is unsuitable. A suitable adjacent vein is selected similarly. The shunt usually fails from clotting on the venous side of the circuit, and it may be salvaged by relocating the venous cannula.

Should the patient require long-term dialysis, a subcutaneous Cimino fistula can be constructed at the same operation, or a short time later in the opposite arm. If the Scribner shunt remains patent, there are techniques for converting the cannulated artery and vein to a more proximal Cimino fistula.

In the leg, a similar method is used for making a Scribner shunt between the posterior tibial artery and the saphenous vein. The posterior tibial artery is, however, likely to be unsuitable in older patients with atherosclerosis. Because of the location of the posterior tibial artery, it is more convenient to use a curved Silastic rather than a straight connector, which directs the shunt tubing proximally so it lies on the leg, avoiding the foot. This curved Silastic tubing is more difficult to declot than the straight tubing.

The most common complication arising with the Scribner shunt is thrombosis. It may be recognized when clot and serum are seen separated in the tubing. At times, the patient notices the disappearance of the pulsation within the shunt. The shunt is declotted by disconnecting the two limbs. Arterial pressure may extrude the thrombus from the arterial side, or it may be aspi-

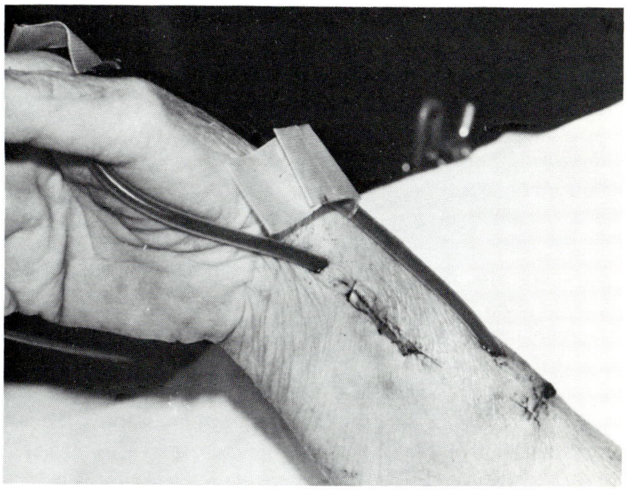

FIGURE 68-3. Scribner external shunt. The tubing is left sufficiently long for easy connection to hemodialysis and exits from the skin after a short course through the subcutaneous tissues. [From Wilson and Owens (4).]

rated out using a syringe and heparinized saline. Failing this, a small (size number 3) Fogarty catheter is inserted into the arterial cannula, taking particular care to not distract and dislodge the cannula through overinflation of the balloon.

On the venous side, a Fogarty catheter is more likely to successfully remove the clot than is simple aspiration. At times, the venous clot may be pushed into the venous circulation. If, after reconnecting the tubing, flow through the declotted shunt appears inadequate, a ''shuntogram'' is obtained by injecting contrast material to determine if the venous outflow is restricted or if an intimal flap has been raised in the artery.

The other major problem that occurs with a Scribner shunt is infection of the subcutaneous tract. This may be managed by systemic antibiotics and seems to be tolerated fairly well, because the shunt acts like a surgical drain through the limb tissues.

Bleeding can occur if the cannula tip extrudes from the artery because it is inadequately secured by ligatures or if the shunt tubing becomes disconnected. At times, there is bleeding if the cannula tip erodes through the vessel in which it is placed. This is more likely when infection is present.

If the tissues overlying the cannula are stretched and taut, there is a risk of skin erosion by the cannula. This is avoided by ensuring that there is an adequate loose coverage of the cannula by subcutaneous tissue at the time of construction. In addition, placing the skin incision directly over the intended line of the cannula is avoided.

The shunt tubing lies on the forearm and needs to be carefully guarded by the patient to prevent dislodgement. A Scribner shunt can severely restrict a patient's activities.

PERCUTANEOUS CENTRAL VENOUS CANNULATION TECHNIQUES

One drawback to the construction of a Scribner shunt is it utilizes vessels which are potentially available for more permanent vascular access sites. Catheters, which provide suitable blood flow for hemodialysis, are now available for percutaneous cannulation of the femoral or subclavian veins. These are used commonly, where a Scribner shunt would have been used in the past, preserving vessels for permanent vascular access. Blood is withdrawn from the cannulated vein, passed through the dialyzer, and returned to the patient by a peripheral vein or via the second lumen of a double-lumen catheter.

The indications for the use of percutaneous venous cannulation are, again, for acute renal failure, for exogenous poisoning, and, in addition, for patients with chronic renal failure who require emergency dialysis as their initial treatment because of advanced uremia. This technique is also available for patients who have a permanent vascular access site which has developed a complication such as thrombosis or infection. These patients are thus maintained while a further permanent site is constructed or the failed site is salvaged.

Percutaneous subclavian vein catheterization was first reported by Aubaniac, a French military surgeon, in 1952 (5). Since *Vascular Access Surgery* was published in 1980 (6), many changes in technique and armamentarium have evolved in the field of central venous access. Initially, central venous lines were used for intravenous (IV) access, central venous pressure monitoring (7), and total parenteral nutrition (8). In addition to these three functions, this list has been expanded to include venous access for chemotherapy infusion, left heart and pulmonary artery pressure monitoring, temporary dialysis, and multiple lumen vascular access channel catheters for complicated medical and surgical critical care patients.

Anatomy

A thorough knowledge of the structures of the thoracic inlet is necessary to proceed with percutaneous central venous catheterization. The subclavian vein meets the internal jugular vein behind the sternoclavicular joint bilaterally. On the right side this confluence forms the superior vena cava. On the left side it forms the innominate vein, which carries the left-sided venous blood, entering the superior vena cava just cephalad to the right atrium. The cephalic vein lies uniformly in the deltopectoral groove and joins the subclavian vein in such a way that it is difficult to direct a guide wire or catheter into the proximal subclavian vein. Generally, the cephalic vein or external jugular vein is used for access by cutdown approach (Figure 68-4).

The anterior scalene muscle separates the subclavian artery and brachial plexus, which are posterior to this muscle, from the subclavian vein which lies anterior to the muscle (Figure 68-5). The scalene muscle helps protect the subclavian artery and brachial plexus from injury during needle insertion. The thoracic duct enters the left subclavian vein near its confluence with the left internal jugular vein. The lymphatic vessel on the right enters in the same position but is much smaller.

Topographically, the subclavian vein lies on a straight line between the sternal notch and the junction of the medial and middle third of the ipsilateral clavicle immediately dorsal (posterior) to the clavicle. The vein enters the thorax between the clavicle and first rib. The internal jugular vein may be found lateral to the carotid pulse and enters the thorax between the sternal and clavicular heads of the sternocleidomastoid muscle bilaterally. These surface landmarks are essential to know for safe percutaneous central venous catheter placement.

Approaches

There are two approaches to percutaneous central venous access. In the direct approach the catheter enters the subclavian vein through a direct percutaneous puncture site. In the indirect ap-

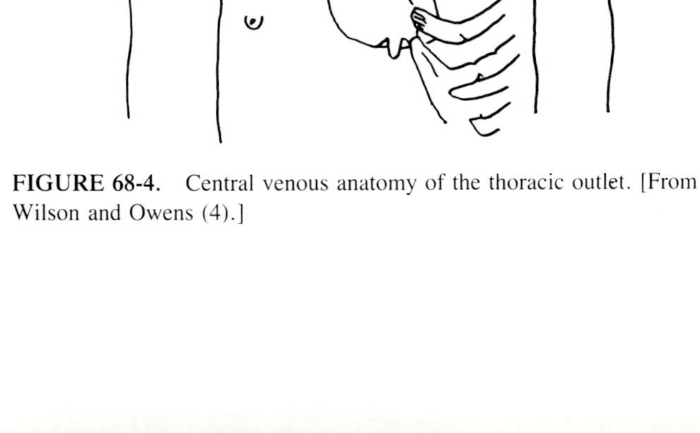

FIGURE 68-4. Central venous anatomy of the thoracic outlet. [From Wilson and Owens (4).]

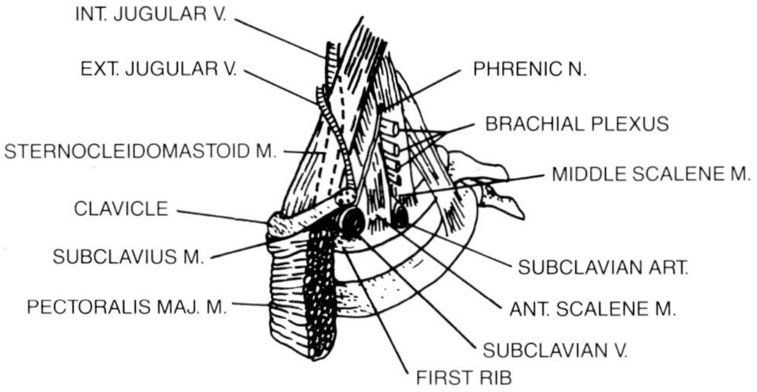

FIGURE 68-5. Costoclavicular scalene triangle demonstrating position of subclavian vein between clavicle and first rib.

proach the catheter enters the subclavian vein from a subcutaneous tunnel.

Direct Approach. Direct central venous access is obtained by cannulating the subclavian or internal jugular vein percutaneously with a polyethylene, polyurethane, or Teflon catheter and advancing the catheter into the superior vena cava. A Seldinger guide wire may or may not be used, depending on the equipment being utilized. The Seldinger technique involves percutaneous vascular access by threading a catheter over a previously placed thin guide wire. The wire is advanced through a small needle that has been inserted through the skin into a vessel (artery or vein). The indication for direct vascular approach includes the following: monitoring of central venous pressure; pulmonary artery pressure; hyperalimentation; temporary dialysis; and intravenous access in patients with poor peripheral veins or critical care patients in need of multiple intravenous portals. The available armamentarium includes single-, double-, or triple-lumen catheters, each with its appropriate indication and insertion technique.

The 16-gauge catheter was the first one commonly used for direct percutaneous central venous access. This polyethylene cateter was inserted through a 14-gauge needle into the subclavian or internal jugular vein and advanced into the superior vena cava. Recently, this catheter has been used less frequently for several reasons. The insertion needle is 14-gauge and is potentially dangerous because of its large size. The catheter which is inserted through the needle may be accidentally sheared off by the sharp edges of the needle. The catheter is quite brittle and less flexible, creating a situation that predisposes to the formation of a fibrin sheath around the catheter (9). These catheters are considered to increase the risk of thromboembolic phenomena.

Direct subclavian vein venipuncture is usually performed in a minor-surgery room under local anesthesia with the patient sedated and the operative site prepared and draped to maintain sterile conditions. An operating room table is useful to maintain the patient in the Trendelenburg position so as to distend the subclavian vein or internal jugular vein. If possible, IV fluid is administered to expand the venous compartment to ensure that the patient is normovolemic. A useful sign in the head-down position is that the intravascular volume is adequate if the operator can see the external jugular vein dilated with blood. A pillow may be placed in the midline of the patient's back to drop the shoulders posteriorly and to position the central veins anteriorly.

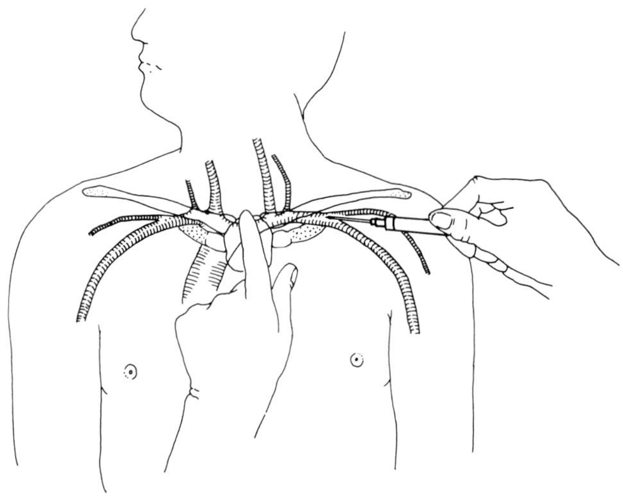

FIGURE 68-6. Technique for percutaneous puncture of subclavian vein. [From Wilson and Owens (4).]

The patient's head is turned to the opposite side. The operator's index finger is placed in the sternal notch, and the thumb is placed under the clavicle at a point between the medial and middle third of the clavicle (Figure 68-6). A cutaneous wheal of local anesthetic is made at this area. The distance between the index finger and the thumb represents the proximal subclavian vein and its union with the internal jugular vein to form the superior vena cava behind the sternoclavicular joint.

The 14-gauge needle is connected to a 10-mL syringe without a Luer lock. The needle is inserted into the skin at the wheal, directed medially toward the sternal notch, while posteriorly sliding the needle under the clavicle and aspirating on the syringe as the needle is advancing. When the subclavian vein is entered, a ''flashback'' of venous blood fills the syringe. One stops for a second to be quite sure the blood is dark red and the piston of the syringe is not rising as it would if the subclavian artery were entered. The bevel of the needle is turned down, and the patient performs a Valsalva maneuver. This increases the central venous pressure and prevents air from entering the needle when the syringe is disconnected. The syringe is removed, and the intracatheter is inserted into the needle and advanced, gently rotating the catheter as it progresses into the subclavian vein. When the catheter is in place, the 14-gauge needle is withdrawn from the skin and the plastic needle guard is immediately snapped on to protect the needle from lacerating the catheter. Now the metal stylet is removed from inside the catheter, and the catheter is connected to IV fluids. When the IV bag is lowered beneath the level of the operating room table, blood will be seen in the IV tubing if the catheter is properly placed. In addition, flow rates of the IV will tell the operator if the catheter is properly positioned. The plastic needle guard is sutured to the skin with 3-0 monofilament suture, and the insertion site is dressed. A postinsertion x-ray is always taken to be sure the catheter is in the superior vena cava and not turned upward into the jugular vein. In addition, one must be sure that a pneumothorax has not been created with the needle insertion.

The technique for placing the catheter in the superior vena cava from the internal jugular vein is similar. The index finger is placed in the space between the sternal and clavicular heads of the sternocleidomastoid muscle just cephalad to the clavicle. A wheal of local anesthetic is made approximately a third of the way up into the neck at the lateral border of the sternocleidomastoid muscle. The needle is inserted in the wheal at the lateral border of the muscle aimed at the index finger just deep to the clavicle. All other aspects of internal jugular cannulation are identical to the infraclavicular subclavian approach. The internal jugular approach is easier and safer because the risk of pneumothorax is less. The patients, however, find it very uncomfortable because there is catheter motion with head movement. To prevent the catheter motion, the patient's neck must be splinted, which becomes quite uncomfortable after a short period of time.

The direct subclavian vein catheterization may be accomplished utilizing the Seldinger technique. Some of the newer percutaneous central venous catheters are made from soft, pliable, nonthrombogenic Silastic or Teflon which is so supple that it must be inserted into position over a thin guide wire (Figure 68-7). Either the subclavian vein or internal jugular vein may be used, but because these catheters are tolerated for long periods of time, the subclavian approach is favored. There are many kits available that contain all the required equipment. These catheters may contain single, double, or triple lumens for dialysis or critical care patients in need of IV access. These catheters are placed, using x-ray or preferably C arm control. The patient is prepared and draped as noted above, including Trendelenburg position, running IV, pillow in the back midline, head turned away from operative side, and having the patient perform a Valsalva maneuver when the needle hub is exposed to room air. The external jugular vein is used as a measurement of intravascular volume.

A wheal of local anesthetic is made in the dermis, sited just caudal to the junction of the middle and medial third of the clavicle, and an 18-gauge needle on a syringe is inserted into the skin through this wheal, aimed medially toward the sternal notch and angled posteriorly, deep to the clavicle. As the needle is advanced, bevel downward, negative pressure is placed on the syringe until there is a "flashback" of dark venous blood in the syringe. The piston of the syringe will not self-rise if the needle is in the vein.

The patient is now asked to perform a Valsalva maneuver, and the syringe is removed from the needle. The J-shaped soft end of the guide wire, which is Teflon-coated, is straightened by a plastic tip deflector and is inserted into the 18-gauge needle and advanced into the subclavian vein, rotating the wire as it is advanced. At this point, an x-ray or C arm is used to assure the correct position of the guide wire in the superior vena cava. After appropriate maneuvering of the wire into proper position, both the tip deflector and the insertion needle are removed. Using a venotomy dilator inserted over the guide wire, or a number 11 blade, the skin opening is enlarged to permit the catheter to enter the skin. The venotomy dilator is then removed, and the Silastic or Teflon catheter is inserted over the guide wire. If a multiple-lumen catheter is used, it is important to have either heparinized saline, 100 units per milliliter, or IV fluids prepared for all the IV portals. The catheter is also advanced using a rotational motion. Before attempting to advance the catheter over the guide wire, care must be taken to see that the guide wire reaches the IV connector side of the catheter for both traction and protection from pushing the wire into the venous system, while the catheter is being advanced over it. When the catheter is in appropriate position, the guide wire is then removed and the catheter is secured with a monofilament suture and connected to the appropriate IV tubing.

Recently a breakaway or peel-away Teflon sheath has been made available to introduce over the guide wire, allowing a catheter to be inserted into the sheath after the guide wire is removed. This sheath is then pulled apart and removed. Although there is little advantage to this technique, where direct percutaneous access is performed, the breakaway or peel-away sheath is indispensable when inserting buried reservoirs, infusion pumps, Hickman catheters, or pacemakers by the percutaneous central venous method (Figure 68-8).

Indirect Approach. The indirect percutaneous catheter insertion technique to catheterize the central venous system evolved through pacemaker technology. When pacemakers were placed in subcutaneous pouches, the pacemaker lead had to be inserted under direct vision into the peripheral vein, such as the cephalic vein in the deltopectoral groove, the external jugular vein, or the internal jugular vein. Occasionally, the cephalic vein was too small to accept the lead wire, or the lead wire could not be placed and advanced from the external jugular vein into the superior vena cava. At this point, a cutdown to reach the subclavian or internal jugular veins was necessary. The problem was solved with the development of the breakaway–peel-away sheath, which permitted percutaneous insertion of the pacemaker lead into the superior vena cava from the subclavian vein entry point and then allowed complete coverage of the lead in the subcutaneous pocket.

The percutaneous technique has become so popular that the cutdown technique for placing a pacemaker lead in the cephalic vein under direct vision is losing its appeal as surgeons become more comfortable with the percutaneous subclavian vein catherterization technique. The technique is now used for routine insertion of Hickman catheters through a subcutaneous tunnel for chemotherapy, hyperalimentation, or vascular access, and in the near future will be used for self-contained infusion pumps for systemic constant infusion of heparin, insulin, morphine, or chemotherapy.

The initial procedure is similar, no matter which device is being inserted. A permanent pacemaker lead introducer set with breakaway or peel-away sheath is necessary. The patient is prepared and draped as noted previously. The head of the bed is lowered until the vein can be seen to fill. A wheal of local anesthetic is placed in the dermis caudal to the juntion of the middle and medial third of the clavicle, and an 18-gauge needle is inserted into the skin and aimed medially toward the sternal notch and posteriorly deep to the clavicle.

The J-shaped soft end of the Teflon-coated guide wire is straightened by a plastic tip deflector and inserted into the 18-gauge needle and advanced into the subclavian vein, rotating the wire as it is advanced. At this point an x-ray or C arm is used to assure the correct position of the guide wire in the superior vena cava. The patient should have electrocardiogram monitoring, for the guide wire may cause ventricular arrhythmias if it is advanced into the right ventricle. At this point, the insertion needle and the guide wire tip straightener are removed and the wire is left alone, care being taken not to pull it out.

A pocket or tunnel must be made for the specific device that is being inserted. For the pacemaker, self-contained reservoir,

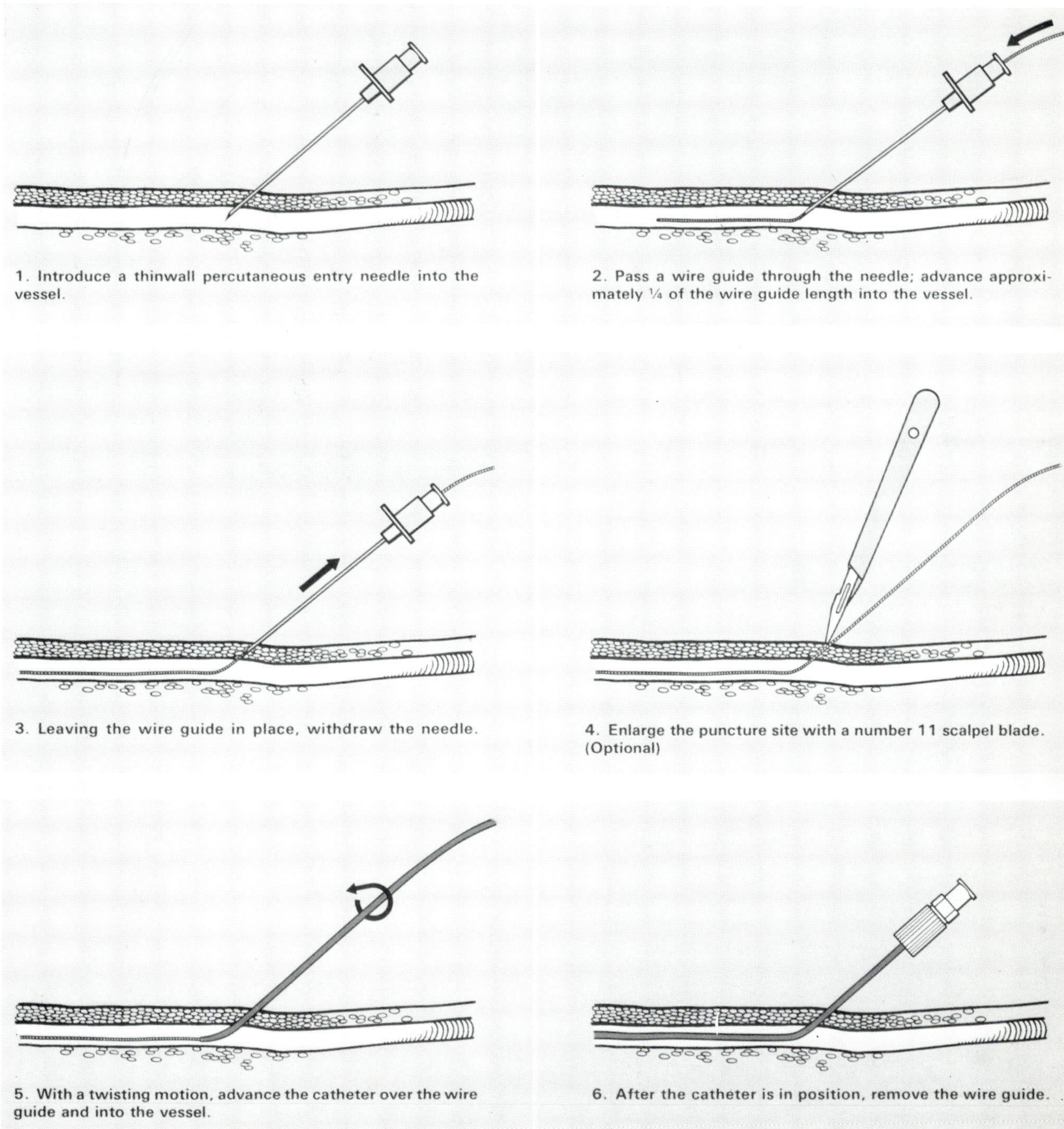

FIGURE 68-7. Seldinger technique for introducing catheters. [From Wilson and Owens (4).]

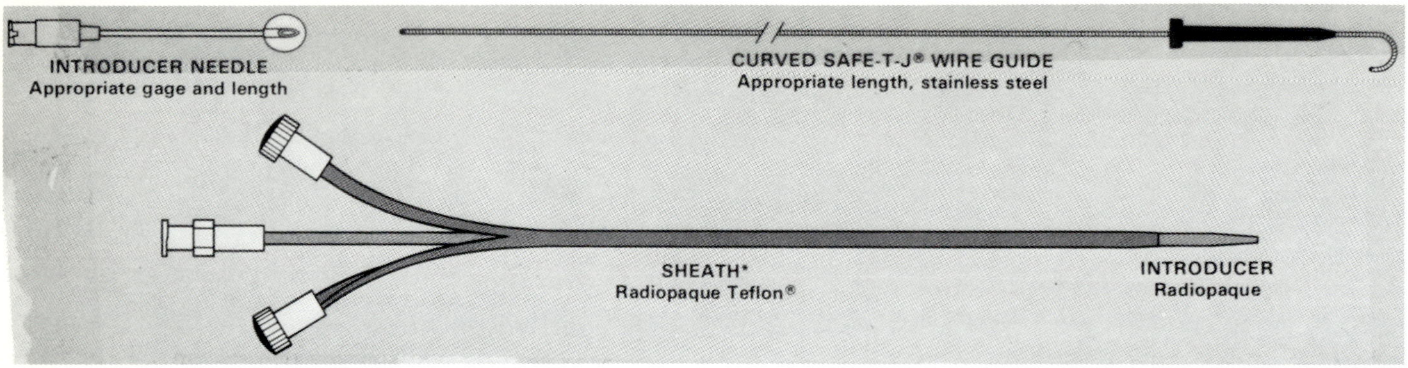

FIGURE 68-8. Needle, guide wire, and catheter introduced. The sheath is peeled off the catheter after introduction.

or self-contained infusion pump, a subcutaneous pocket is created on the ipsilateral pectoral region. The pocket should be caudad to the incision so that the device will lie below the incision when the wound is closed and the patient is upright.

The Hickman catheter is a 90-cm, silicone rubber catheter with a Dacron cuff 30 cm from the Luer lock end. The Dacron cuff is buried in a subcutaneous tunnel so that fibrous tissue will grow into the cuff for stabilization and to retard septic complications.

Two stab wounds are required to create a subcutaneous tunnel for the Hickman catheter. A stab wound is made on the precordium and at the exit site near the guide wire. Using local anesthesia, a tunnel is created between the two stab wounds. The Hickman catheter, which has been irrigated with heparinized saline, 100 U.S.P. per milliliter, is inserted into the precordial stab wound and brought out of the stab wound near the guide wire. The catheter is advanced so that the Dacron cuff is in the subcutaneous tunnel. The Hickman catheter is now measured and cut so that the tip of the catheter following the course of the subclavian vein (plus innominate vein on the patient's left side) and superior vena cava will lie at the level of the right third rib.

With the apparatus in position (pacemaker, reservoir, pump, or Hickman catheter) attention is again turned to the guide wire. Over the guide wire, insert the sheath introducer assembly. Using a twisting motion, advance the sheath introducer assembly over the guide wire. Leaving the sheath in place, remove the guide wire and the introducer. Venous blood will come out from inside the sheath.

From the pocket or tunnel develop a subcutaneous path for the lead or catheter to enter the breakaway sheath. This may require a small incision where the sheath enters the skin. Introduce the lead or catheter into the sheath and advance into position (Figure 68-9). Break the sheath by pulling it apart. Withdraw the sheath as the peeling continues. If the lead or catheter withdraws from the sheath as the sheath is being peeled and withdrawn, reinsert the catheter gently and continue peeling. The wounds are now closed with interrupted subcuticular absorbable sutures (Figure 68-10). Patients are placed on prophylactic antibiotics immediately prior to and 24 hours postoperatively. The Hickman catheter, reservoir, or pump is aspirated and irrigated with heparinized saline to ensure proper function.

When using the percutaneous subclavian approach for central venous access, care must be taken when patients are obese, emphysematous, or hypovolemic. The side of a patient with a healed clavicular fracture or mastectomy should be avoided for attempts at percutaneous subclavian vein access. Occasionally, a patient will be seen with occlusion of the superior vena cava. These patients are obviously poor candidates. A preoperative venogram should be performed if the surgeon feels there is a risk of superior vena cava occlusion. It is probably best to avoid a side of the chest that has previously undergone radiation therapy.

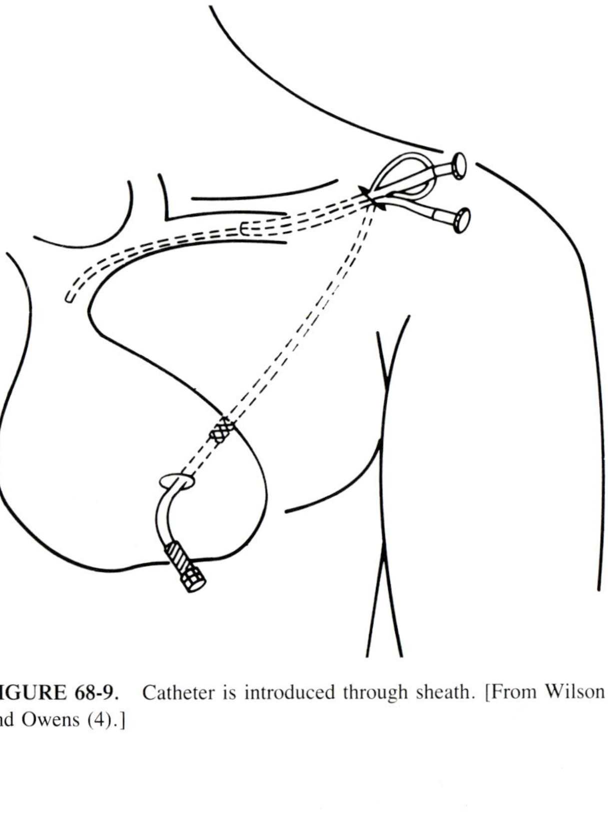

FIGURE 68-9. Catheter is introduced through sheath. [From Wilson and Owens (4).]

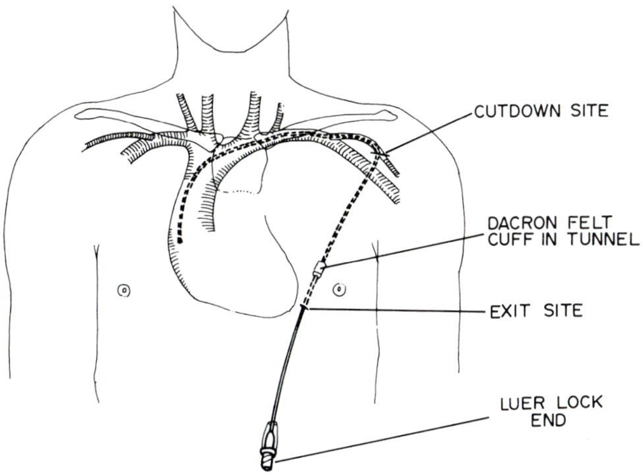

FIGURE 68-10. Position of central venous catheter suitable for hyperalimentation placed via cephalic vein for long-term access. [From Wilson and Owens (4).]

TABLE 68-1. Complications of Percutaneous Vascular Access

Early	Late
Thoracic:	Catheter obstruction
Pneumothorax	Thoracic:
Tension pneumothorax	Hydrothorax
Subcutaneous emphysema	Hydromediastinum
Hemothorax	Venous:
Hydrothorax	Air embolism
Hemomediastinum	Central vein thrombosis
Hydromediastinum	Superior vena cava syndrome
Arterial:	Hepatic vein thrombosis
Subcutaneous hematoma	Cardiac:
Arterial laceration	Arrhythmia
Pseudoaneurysm	Coronary sinus thrombosis
Venous:	Lymphatic:
Venous laceration	Lymphatic fistula
Air embolism	Chylothorax
Catheter embolism	Septic:
Lymphatic:	Catheter sepsis
Thoracic duct laceration	Septic thrombosis
Cardiac:	Suppurative thrombophlebitis
Arrythmia	
Perforation and tamponade	
Neurologic injury:	
Brachial plexus	
Phrenic nerve	
Vagus nerve	
Recurrent laryngeal nerve	
Catheter misplacement	

Complications

Early complications of percutaneous central venous catheterization are due to technique. Pneumothorax is the most often seen. Later complications are usually related to sepsis or central venous thrombosis. Septic complications are more common in multiple lumen catheters and less frequent in vascular access devices that are completely buried, as compared to the Hickman catheter which exits from the patient. Catheter sepsis may be heralded only by fever, tachycardia, or glucose intolerance. Treatment of catheter-related bacterial infection usually requires removal of the foreign body. Subclavian vein thrombosis is generally not symptomatic.

Other complications are listed in Table 68-1.

Other Sites

The percutaneous access sites used for emergency hemodialysis or other procedures may include the femoral vessels. The femoral vein is cannulated in the groin using local infiltration anesthesia. Following insertion of a 16-gauge cannula into the vein, a guide wire is threaded through the cannula into the common iliac vein or the inferior vena cava. The guide wire should not be forced. If resistance is met, it is withdrawn a little and a further attempt at free passage made. The catheter is then passed over the free end of the guide wire into the iliac vein or inferior vena cava.

Percutaneous venous cannulation provides a means for the immediate dialysis of a patient. The external catheter may be removed following the course of dialysis, reducing the chance of infection. Catheter thrombosis between dialyses is prevented by infusion of low-dose heparin for the duration of the catheter's use.

Blood flows of up to 200 mL/min can be achieved via these catheters, making this method of dialysis as efficient as others. The technique does not increase cardiac workload, unlike external AV shunts or internal AV fistulas.

These catheters may be changed after a period of days by reinsertion of the guide wire along the existing catheter, withdrawal of the older catheter, and its replacement with a clean catheter by the Seldinger technique. With the development of Silastic catheters, which reduce the likelihood of catheter thrombosis and because of the lower risk of infection of a catheter placed in the subclavian vein rather than in the groin, subclavian catheters can be left in situ or replaced and provide dialysis access over an interval of several weeks. This obviates the need for repeated needle punctures.

Long-Term Vascular Access

The best long-term access is made by utilization of the patient's own vessels to construct an autogenous subcutaneous AV fistula. Failing this, biological conduits such as bovine carotid artery heterograft or human umbilical vein or synthetic materials such as PTFE (polytetrafluorethylene) are used to bridge the distance between suitable arteries and veins.

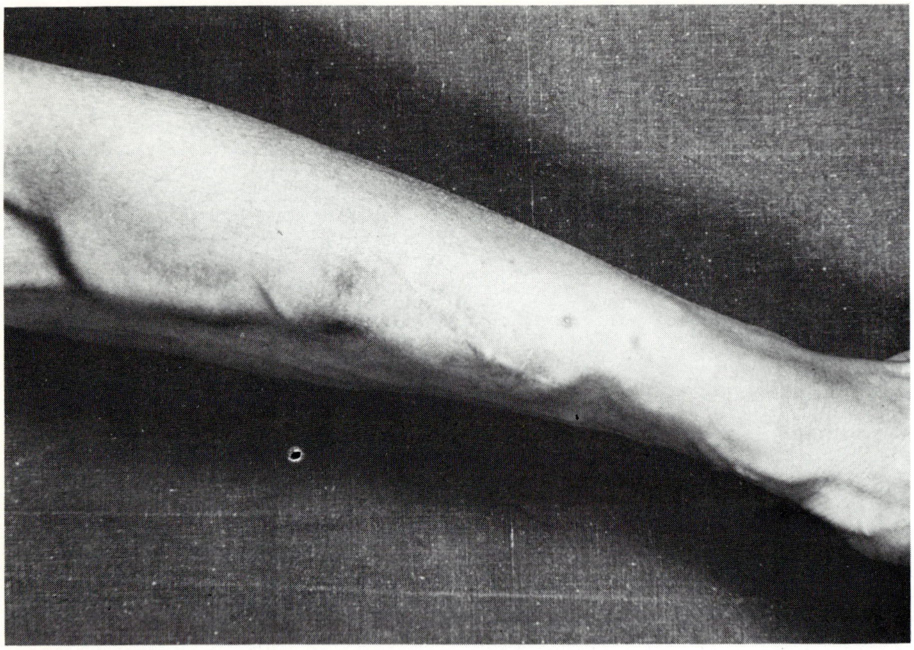

FIGURE 68-11. Well-developed (''arterialized'') Cimino fistula. [From Wilson and Owens (4).]

SUBCUTANEOUS AV FISTULA

The autogenous AV fistula of the Cimino type is associated with the longest useful patency and lowest rate of infection, and is least likely to thrombose. For construction, it requires an artery large enough to support a high rate of blood flow and veins that will ''arterialize'' and thus dilate. The fistula is unobtrusive and does not interfere significantly with patient activities, unlike the Scribner shunt. It does, however, require 3 to 5 weeks following its construction for maturation of the veins into large, thick-walled vessels that can be repeatedly and reliably punctured (Figure 68-11).

It may not be feasible to construct a Cimino fistula in a patient who has small fragile veins or a paucity of veins, possibly as the result of previous episodes of thrombophlebitis or sclerosis following intravenous injections. It is also difficult to construct in patients who have an obese arm. The fistula is easier to construct and more likely to remain patent in a patient who has prominent veins, such as a manual worker. The radial artery may not be large enough to maintain flow through the fistula in patients with advanced atherosclerosis. This is a pertinent consideration in the diabetic patient with renal failure. Again, as with the Scribner shunt, it should be determined before construction that the hand circulation can be maintained by the ulnar artery alone, using the maneuver described previously.

Cimino fistulas have up to a 90 percent useful patency rate at 12 months, which falls to about 75 percent at 4 years. Once failure occurs, they can, uncommonly, be surgically revised for extended longevity. Fistulas may clot during an episode of hypotension or because of restriction of the venous outflow of the arm by clothing, a sphygmomanometer cuff, or a tourniquet. In addition, flow through the fistula is reduced by advancing atherosclerosis in the feeding artery and can ultimately fall to a critically low level at which the fistula thromboses.

Following construction of an AV fistula in the arm, swelling may be seen in the hand. This is usually easily managed by elevating the hand on a pillow for a time. Rarely, severe venous hypertension follows the development of valvular incompetence in the distal fistula venous bed. Very uncommonly a forearm fistula ''steals'' blood from the distal arterial circulation, leading to hand ischemia.

The fistula is constructed using local infiltration anesthesia or alternatively a brachial plexus nerve block. Patients with progressive renal failure may have their fistula formed and matured beforehand, in anticipation of the need for maintenance hemodialysis. This is done when their creatinine clearance falls to 10 mL/min.

Before constructing a Cimino fistula, the arm pulses are carefully palpated, and a sphygmomanometer cuff is applied around the upper arm to restrict venous outflow and aid visualization of the venous anatomy. The veins are marked out using an indelible pen. It is preferable to construct the Cimino fistula in the nondominant arm. This aids training the patient for regular home dialysis, should this eventuate.

At operation, a longitudinal incision is made in the skin overlying the radial artery. The cephalic vein is dissected out from the subcutaneous fat, ligating any tributaries as necessary so that it lies alongside the radial artery without kinking or producing any stenosis. Following this, the radial artery is dissected and mobilized, taking care not to avulse any of its smaller branches since this produces a periarterial hematoma, which can interfere with the construction of an adequate fistula.

The artery and vein are anastomosed together in one of four configurations (Figure 68-12). (1) The side-to-side anastomosis is the easiest to do well and is associated with the highest fistula flow rate. (2) The arterial end to vein side reduces turbulence and the likelihood of distal arterial steal but is associated with a lower flow rate. (3) The vein end to arterial side results in the highest proximal venous flow and minimal distal venous hypertension but is technically more difficult to construct. (4) The

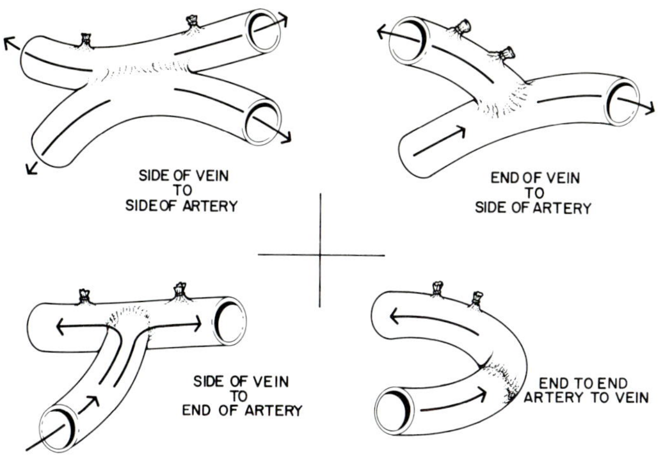

FIGURE 68-12. Configurations of artery and vein in Cimino fistula. [From Wilson and Owens (4).]

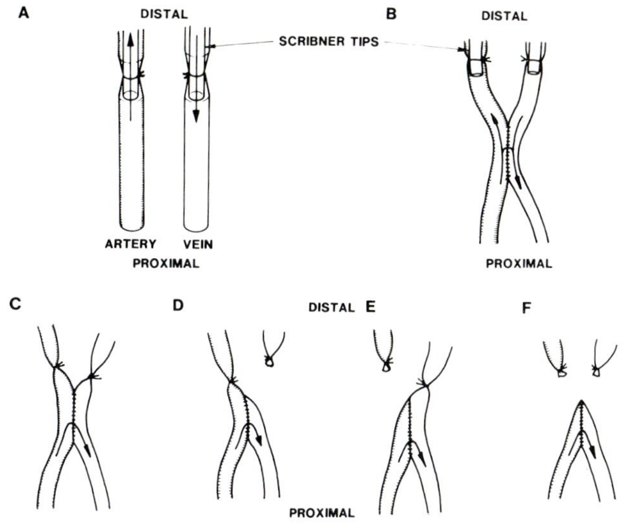

FIGURE 68-13. *(A–F)* Methods for conversion of functioning Scribner shunt to AV fistula. [From Wilson and Owens (4).]

end-to-end anastomosis combines the least likelihood of development of distal arterial steal and venous hypertension with the lowest fistula flow rate of the four configurations.

The fistula is made utilizing about a 1-cm-long venotomy and arteriotomy. If valves are present in the vein at the site of the venotomy, they are resected with small scissors. Fine suture material such as 7.0 prolene is used for the anastomosis, taking care to tie the knots on the outside of the vessels. A continuous suturing technique is employed, starting at the midpoint of the posterior wall, with the side-to-side anastomosis.

Before completing the anastomosis, a coronary artery dilator is passed proximally in the artery and vein to ascertain no stenosis has been produced by suturing at the vessel junctions. Any bleeding occurring after the vascular clamps have been released is usually controlled by the application of firm pressure with a swab for several minutes. Only if this fails is the bleeding site controlled by insertion of additional fine sutures. These can lead to further bleeding from the needle tracks and increase the likelihood of inadvertently narrowing the anastomosis.

After the operation is successfully completed, a strong thrill should be palpable. If there is vigorous arterial pulsation but no thrill, outflow obstruction is suspected and one should confirm that there is no stenosis in the vein. Part of the anastomosis is dismantled and a small, simple rubber or Fogarty catheter is passed into the vein. If a stricture is felt, it may be dilated by bougies or by blowing up the balloon on the Fogarty catheter.

In some patients, it is not possible to construct the standard Cimino fistula at the wrist. If the patient is thin, the proximal cephalic vein is easily seen at the elbow and may be used for anastomosis to the brachial artery in the cubital fossa. A transverse incision is made a little proximal to the cubital fossa, and the brachial artery is mobilized distally to the level of the bicipital tendon. The median nerve lies medial and posterior to the artery and should be protected. The anastomosis between the artery and vein is limited to about a length of 5 to 7 mm to reduce the chances of developing a steal syndrome, which is more likely here.

At times, the basilic vein can be mobilized from the level of the wrist to the middle of the forearm and then tunneled subcutaneously for anastomosis to the radial artery. It is also possible to anastomose the basilic vein to the ulnar artery, but this should not be done if there has been a previous radiocephalic fistula in that arm because of the high chance of compromising the circulation to the hand, since the radial artery is usually occluded.

In patients who have a functioning Scribner shunt, the shunt can be converted to a more permanent subcutaneous arteriovenous fistula. This is done by locating the cephalic vein about 5 cm above the Scribner shunt incision (Figure 68-13). The operation is done in a site free from any residual operative tissue induration. The arterialized cephalic vein and the artery are mobilized and anastomosed side-to-side. Following this, the distal artery and vein leading to the cannula tips are ligated and the Silastic tubing and cannulas are removed. In patients who had a functioning Scribner shunt, the arterialized veins, converted to a Cimino fistula, can often be used for dialysis earlier than in a newly formed subcutaneous fistula.

The Cimino fistula may function for many years. Eventually it may fail due to sclerosis of the veins as a result of repeated venipuncture or following renal transplant, when changes occur in the blood that restore coagulation to normal. It is not wise to discard an AV fistula following renal transplant because dialysis may be necessary during episodes of acute rejection or if there is failure of the kidney. Reoperation to salvage a failed Cimino fistula is commonly unsuccessful. Failure is usually most expeditiously managed by construction of a further access site. If another Cimino fistula cannot be constructed or the old site revised, then a prosthetic bridge fistula is made.

BRIDGE FISTULAS

Bridge fistulas constructed from graft materials are a good alternative to the radiocephalic fistula. They can be formed between almost any artery and vein, are easily accessible under the skin for reliable needle puncture, and can be used for dialysis earlier than the AV autogenous fistula.

These fistulas take on various configurations. If the vein and artery are close to each other, the bridge material may run in a loop or lie in a U configuration. If the artery and vein are some distance apart, the bridge graft lies in a straight or curved line. Care should be taken to avoid kinking of the fistula material, and in particular, it should not pass over joints where flexion will restrict flow and lead to graft clotting. One-year patency rates of 75 to 80 percent, comparable to those of the Cimino fistula, have been reported with polytetrafluoroethylene (PTFE) grafts.

The larger the artery used to provide flow through the fistula, the lower the rate of fistula thrombosis. For this reason, thigh fistulas, using the common or superficial femoral artery, are less likely to clot. In addition, they can be easily utilized by the patient, who has both hands free, for home dialysis, but they have the major disadvantage of a higher postoperative infection rate. *Location of the fistula in the arm is almost always the first-choice site* and is the mandatory position in the older patient with significant leg vessel artherosclerosis or the obese patient who has dermatitis in the groin.

A variety of biological and prosthetic materials have been used for bridge fistula construction. These include bovine carotid artery, human umbilical vein, homologous saphenous vein (10), and synthetic materials. In the latter group, the PTFE graft has proved particularly successful and is currently the most commonly used material for bridge fistulas.

The bovine heterograft was developed over a decade ago, by enzyme debridement of fresh bovine carotid arteries, followed by tanning with dialdehyde (11). A 6- to 10-mL internal diameter graft about 40 to 50 cm long results. The material is pliable and easily sutured. At one time, it was thought bovine heterografts should be utilized primarily rather than a Cimino fistula. However, some 5 years after introduction of bovine grafts, it was evident that they were prone to infection and aneurysm formation. Progressive degeneration of the graft material occurs so that the whole graft tends to undergo aneurysmal dilation or forms nonanastomotic aneurysms. This was seen more often in grafts anastomosed between proximal larger vessels, probably due to the increased material damage associated with higher blood flow rates. These grafts also develop stenosis at the venous anastomosis in company with other prosthetic materials, which leads to graft blood flow restriction and then clotting. The early enthusiasm for bovine heterografts has now waned.

The human umbilical vein graft was prepared in the hope that it would overcome the deficiencies of bovine carotid grafts (12). It was believed it would be nonimmunogenic. The graft is prepared by tanning the human umbilical vein, collected atraumatically at the time of infant delivery, with either dialdehyde starch or glutaraldehyde, which converts it into a more rigid collagen tube. The material retains a critical surface tension level similar to that of autogenous saphenous vein. Thus, it was thought that it would also be more resistant to thrombus formation than synthetic grafts or modified bovine grafts. Electron microscopy has indeed demonstrated very few defects in the subintimal lining or internal elastic lamina that would expose the potentially thrombogenic materials of the media.

Results of long-term patency are not available. A reported high rate of thrombosis was blamed on excessive pressure application over the graft following needle withdrawal. This graft has been found to develop inflow and outflow stenosis with resultant thrombosis and has also undergone aneurysmal dilation.

Dacron velour, employed in vascular surgery for many years, has also been used for constructing bridge fistulas. This material has relatively large pores, which permit good ingrowth of tissue with formation of a firmly adherent inner lining. This may explain the relatively lower infection and thrombosis rate that has been found with Dacron velour bridge fistulas. Cumulative patency rates of about 80 percent have been found at 24 months (13).

In a laboratory study in which Dacron velour fistulas were punctured three times weekly for sham dialysis, there was no evidence of anastomotic intimal hyperplasia, pseudoaneurysm formation, or thrombosis. These results were also found in one clinical study, while another reported a 19 percent incidence of thrombosis and 5 percent incidence each of pseudoaneurysm formation and graft infection. Despite these encouraging reports, Dacron has not gained widespread favor for use as a fistula material, probably because it is somewhat resistant to easy needle penetration.

Expanded PTFE is now the most commonly used material for construction of bridge fistulas. PTFE handles well, does not require preclotting, is widely available, and has a long shelf life and high patency rate. PTFE bridge fistulas are consistently found to have a 24-month percentage cumulative patency rate of slightly less than 70 percent, compared with slightly more than 70 percent for a Cimino autogenous fistula. The figure for bovine heterografts, at the same time, is about 35 percent (14).

The average incidence of complications per 100 graft months of follow-up, excluding death or occlusion, is 0.69 for autogenous Cimino-Brescia fistulas. For PTFE grafts, it is approximately double that for Cimino fistulas (1.5), and for bovine heterografts it is slightly more than three times the Cimino figure (2.4). Twenty to thirty percent of patients cannot have an autogenous fistula constructed, and at present, in the majority, this is resolved by using PTFE for construction of a bridge fistula.

Should thrombosis develop in a PTFE graft, it can be relatively easily treated by thrombectomy (see "Complications"). Infection of PTFE grafts occurs in up to 10 percent. Over two-thirds of these infections are found within the first 4 months of use, and the majority require removal of the graft for resolution. To minimize chances of bacterial seeding and infecting the replacement fistula, the infected graft is removed some days before establishing another bridge fistula elsewhere. If the infection involves the anastomosis, it is not uncommon that the artery will need to be ligated, and if this is the common femoral or brachial artery with the anastomosis immediately proximal to the bifurcation, multiple vessels may need to be tied off, exposing the patient to the risk of limb ischemia.

The diameter of the bridge graft is selected to be larger than that of the supply artery to ensure maximum fistula flow. The size, if too large, also increases the likelihood of developing high-output cardiac failure and distal limb ischemia. Experience has shown that grafts of 6 mm in diameter provide good flow and retain their patency while being uncommonly associated with the foregoing complications. In the arm, a 6-mm graft is usually selected, so that the large graft to artery ratio provides maximal flow.

Distal limb tissue perfusion is also affected by the degree of atherosclerosis that has developed in the distal arterial tree, and this is a significant consideration in the older patient who is being prepared for a thigh bridge fistula. If this is a concern, then a preoperative angiogram may be helpful in planning further patient management. However, if the patient's ankle blood pressure is 80 percent or more of his or her brachial blood pressure and he or she has no history of claudication, then distal ischemia is unlikely to follow if a bridge fistula is constructed.

Bridge fistulas have been formed between most of the suitably sized superficial arteries and veins. After subcutaneous implantation, the prosthesis can be readily palpated and punctured. Puncture should, if possible, be delayed until the prosthesis has been incorporated in the surrounding tissue. The puncture sites then tend to "heal," making extravasation and perigraft hematoma formation less likely than in the unincorporated prosthesis (Figure 68-14). Puncture of a graft in the first 24 h after implantation is not only possible but often necessary. For patient comfort, ease of handling by the patient or nurse, and safety, bridge fistulas are best placed in the arm.

In the arm, a bridge fistula can be constructed between the radial artery and cephalic or basilic vein in the cubital fossa (straight) (Figure 68-15), the cephalic or basilic veins and the brachial artery (loop) (Figure 68-16), and the axillary vein and brachial artery (straight) (Figure 68-17). The conduit is tunneled through the subcutaneous tissue on the radial side of the forearm to allow the arm to lie comfortably during dialysis.

Bridge fistulas in the arm have a shorter useful patency than those in the thigh, since clotting is more likely because of the lower fistula flow rates. On the other hand, bridge fistulas in the arm are less likely to become infected than thigh fistulas, which

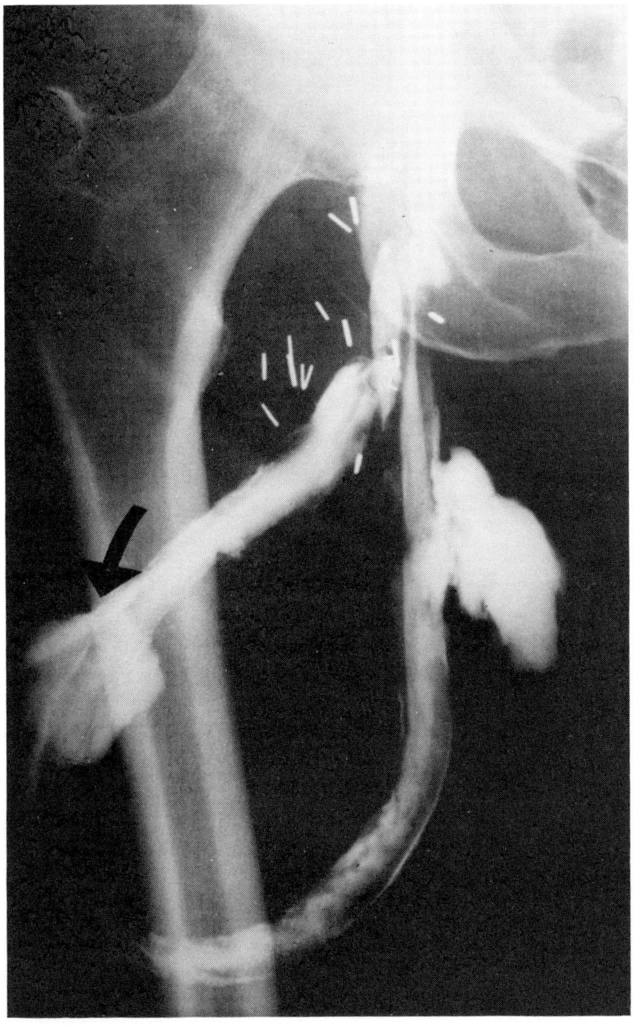

FIGURE 68-14. Perigraft hematoma—the result of early puncture (*arrow*) before the graft was tissue-incorporated.

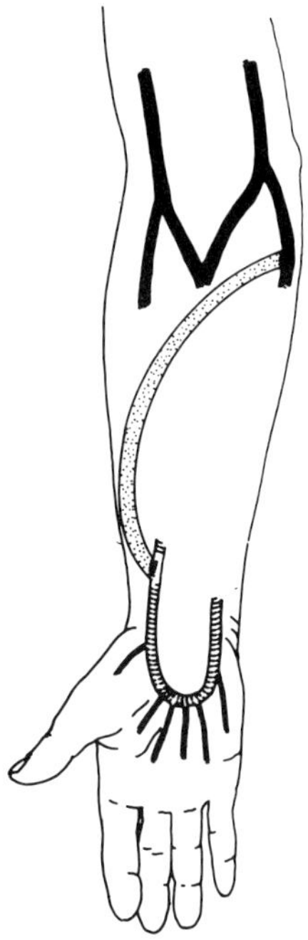

FIGURE 68-15. PTFE bridge fistula between radial artery and cephalic or basilic vein in cubital fossa. [From Wilson and Owens (4).]

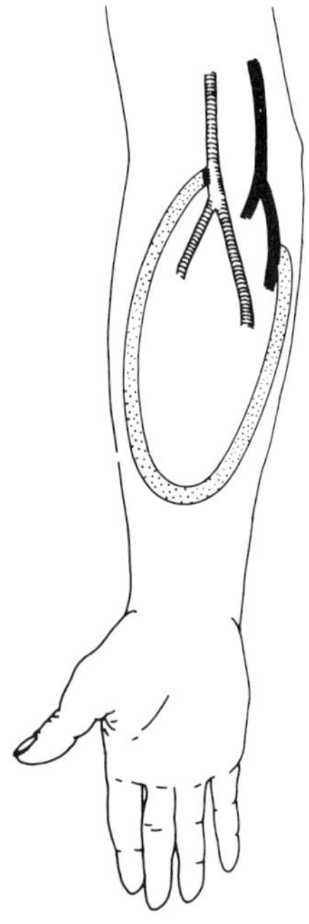

FIGURE 68-16. PTFE bridge fistula between brachial artery and cephalic or basilic veins. [From Wilson and Owens (4).]

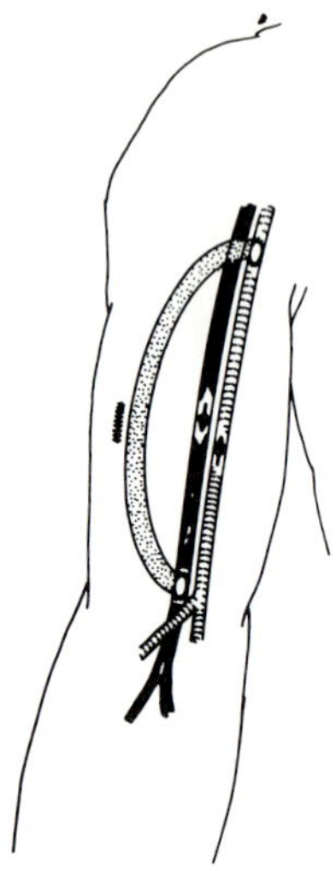

FIGURE 68-17. PTFE bridge fistula between brachial artery and axillary vein. [From Wilson and Owens (4).]

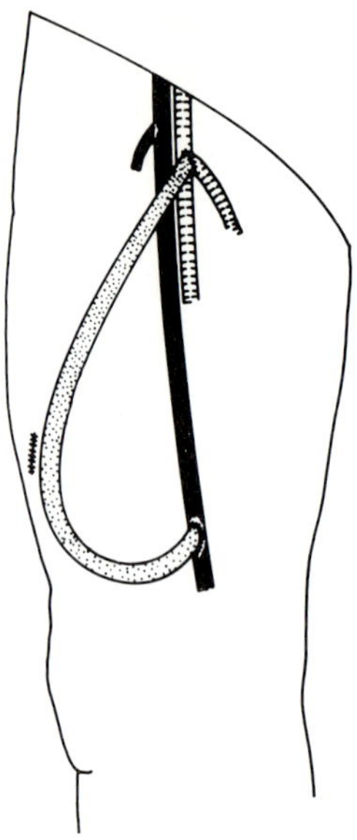

FIGURE 68-18. Position of femorosaphenous bridge fistula. [From Wilson and Owens (4).]

are in proximity to the bacteria of the heavily colonized groin skin.

In the thigh, the initial bridge fistula is constructed between the femoral artery proximal to its exit from the adductor canal and the proximal saphenous or femoral vein (Figure 68-18). Upon failure, the arterial end of the fistula can be moved to the more proximal femoral artery.

With long-term hemodialysis, the surgeon can be called on to create multiple vascular access sites, because each will eventually fail. It is conceivable that some patients could potentially outlive their available limb access sites. Then, an AV fistula between the axillary vein and artery has been employed. Complications in this central site are serious and difficult to manage.

Complications of AV Fistulas

THROMBOSIS

The most common complication is fistula or graft thrombosis. The likelihood of this occurring depends on the type of shunt, the site of the AV anastomosis, the prosthetic material used, and the diameter of patient's veins and arteries.

The autogenous Cimino fistula thromboses early following construction in about 10 to 15 percent of patients. This may be due to poor vessels (an atherosclerotic radial artery or small veins) or technical factors such as obstruction at the venous anastomosis. With time, the Cimino fistula is more likely to remain patent than a bridge fistula. However, in the initial period, the bridge fistula has a higher patency rate. Thrombosis occurring 3 months or later following construction of a Cimino fistula is commonly due to fibrosis of the veins, following the repeated trauma of needle punctures. Late thrombosis of a prosthetic graft, however, is usually due to "intimal hyperplasia" producing stenosis of the venous outflow.

When late clotting of a Cimino fistula occurs, it may be most expedient to convert it to a bridge prosthetic fistula. Late thrombosis of a graft due to intimal hyperplasia in the vein adjacent to the prosthetic venous anastomosis occurs with PTFE and other prosthetic materials. Differences in compliance between the vein and the prosthetic material result in turbulence and hydraulic trauma to the vein.

At times, outflow obstruction is appreciated early before the graft thomboses by the dialysis nurse who observes a rise in pressure at the venous end of the conduit or notes that the blood in the venous chamber is becoming dark during dialysis. Following this observation, a "shuntogram" is obtained. This is a radiography in which contrast material is injected into the conduit.

Thrombosis of a bridge fistula after a satisfactorily long period of use is managed with a thrombectomy, which salvages about 40 percent of grafts. Thrombectomy is done through an incision sited at the venous end of the graft. A graft which has been in situ for a long time often has a well-formed, fibrous capsule, and dissection of this can lead to tearing of the PTFE material. A 2-cm-long incision is made in the graft just proximal to the venous anastomosis. The patient is heparinized, and a small Fogarty embolectomy catheter is passed into the vein to remove any thrombus. This maneuver has dislodged clot into the venous and pulmonary circulation.

If this fails to restore good flow in the graft, it is then necessary to explore the arterial end to remove clots. If these maneuvers result in good flow and good pulsation with a strong thrill, then the operation may be terminated. However, if this does not occur, then an angiogram should be obtained to determine if there is any correctable stenosis at the arterial or venous ends of the fistula. Such a lesion at the venous anastomosis is managed by a patch angioplasty or constructing a more proximal venous anastomosis or grafting from the fistula to a more proximal vein. Percutaneous transluminal angioplasty in selected cases has not been successful in management of venous runoff stenosis in our experience.

INFECTION

Infection is second to cardiovascular disease as a cause of mortality and morbidity in patients on chronic dialysis. The highest rate of infection is found with Scribner external shunts, while the lowest is with the Cimino fistula. Needling of fistulas can produce a hematoma which then becomes infected with skin organisms. Involvement of the anastomatic site with infection may lead to endovasculitis, septicemia, and metastatic abscess formation.

Grafts may become infected at the time of implantation from skin organisms and poor aseptic technique. To lower the likelihood of this, perioperative antibiotics effective against skin organisms, particularly *Staphylococcus epidermidis* and *S. aureus*, are routinely used. On occasion, a superficial soft tissue infection overlying a graft will resolve; however, graft infections usually require removal of the prosthetic material for complete resolution. Grafts are thought to be more resistant to infection once they have become incorporated and a pseudointimal lining has formed.

When a graft is infected and is to be removed for control of the infection, plans are made for implantation of a new graft at a different site. An interval of a few days should be allowed between removal and implantation of the new graft for resolution of the associated bacteremia and cellulitis, thus reducing the chances of "seeding" and infecting the new graft.

In some cases of graft infection limited to a needle puncture site, a length of the graft may be excised and a replacement segment tunneled through uninfected tissues to join the remaining proximal and distal ends.

CONGESTIVE HEART FAILURE

With a large AV communication fed by a moderately large artery, there is a considerable increase in venous return to the heart, which maintains the increased cardiac output necessary to sustain fistula flow. This can eventually lead to heart failure. When cardiac failure develops, it may be treated quite simply by "banding" of the fistula. This is done by encircling the prosthetic graft with a 1-cm cuff of Teflon. The arterial end of the prosthesis may be narrowed by placing several interrupted sutures to achieve the same effect. The flow through the graft is reduced to a level of 300 to 400 mL/min. Reduction of the blood flow to lower levels is likely to lead to graft thrombosis.

VASCULAR INSUFFICIENCY

A vascular steal syndrome occurs uncommonly. It is seen with side-to-side fistulas constructed at the wrist. Reversed flow in the distal radial artery increases as the fistula ages, and the collaterals hypertrophy between the proximal and distal arteries, elevating the blood pressure in the distal artery. Thus, a significant pressure gradient develops between the distal artery and fistula itself, stealing blood from the more peripheral muscle beds.

The patient experiences ischemic pain in the hand, which is often more severe during hemodialysis. Vascular steal has also been observed in patients with fistulas formed between the femoral artery and saphenous vein in the leg. The steal may be corrected in the hand by ligation of the radial artery immediately distal to the fistula, converting it from a side-to-side to an end-to-side anastomosis.

VENOUS HYPERTENSION

An AV fistula is a planned means for raising pressure locally in the venous system. However, venous hypertension may occur in the tissues distal to the fistula. In the time immediately following construction of the fistula, occurrence of a significant elevation of pressure in the distal venous channels is prevented by competent venous valves. With the valvular incompetence that eventually develops, there is retrograde distal venous flow, and the higher pressure is transmitted distally up to a null point where there is no venous flow and the valves are competent. The pressure is dissipated by the opening of a large venous collateral bed. In some patients, there is marked swelling of the hand, discoloration, and pigmentation of the skin comparable to that seen in venous stasis disease in the leg. In long-standing cases, venous stasis ulceration may be seen. The treatment is ligation of the vein immediately distal to the fistula.

An end-vein-to-side-artery fistula, which is slightly more difficult to construct, would obviate development of this problem. However, many surgeons prefer initially to make a side venous anastomosis, reasoning that should the extremely rare problem of venous hypertension develop, the distal vein can then be easily ligated. Massive edema of the entire extremity after construction of an AV fistula signifies proximal major venous obstruction.

VASCULAR ACCESS NEUROPATHY

A small number of patients with a Cimino fistula report symptoms of the carpal tunnel syndrome. These symptoms are especially noticeable during the night. If this syndrome is suspected, its existence may be proved by nerve conduction velocity studies. There will be a reduction in median nerve conduction time across the carpal ligament.

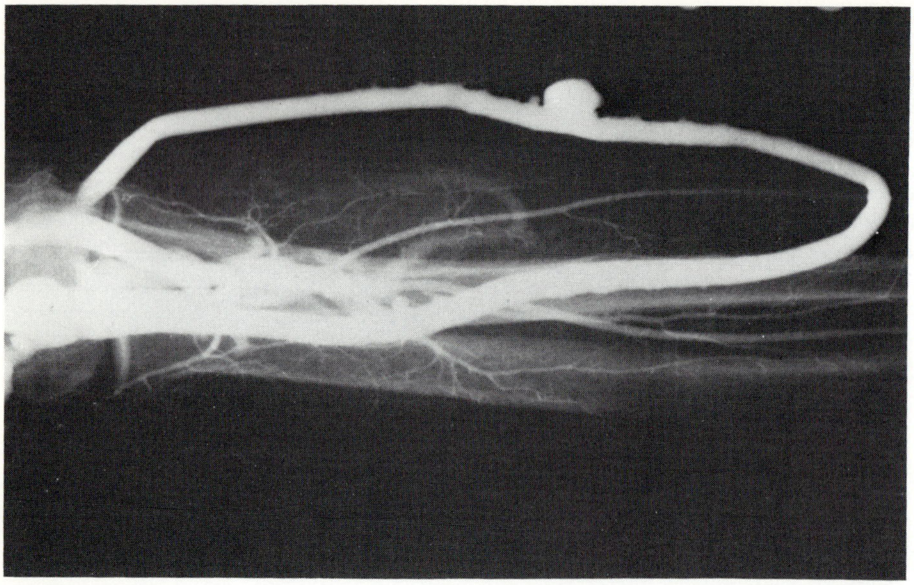

FIGURE 68-19. Pseudoaneurysms may develop at needle puncture sites as shown in this 2-year-old PTFE graft.

The carpal tunnel syndrome possibly arises because of increased venous pressure in the hand, leading to tissue edema and compression of the median nerve. Another theory is that it is due to a vascular steal, producing ischemia of the nerve. Some evidence for this etiology comes from the observation that ligation of the radial artery distal to the AV fistula has improved the symptoms. This syndrome has been managed in a few patients by division of the carpal ligament similar to the proven treatment for the median nerve compression occurring in patients not on dialysis.

ANEURYSMS

Vascular prostheses may develop pseudoaneurysms secondary to needle puncture and perigraft hematoma (Figure 68-19) formation or true aneurysmal dilation of the whole graft. The latter is thought to be the result of degeneration and "fatigue" of the graft material itself.

If the pseudoaneurysm is not infected, it can be managed by local excision and repair of the graft or excision of the graft segment with interportion position of a new length of material.

References

1. Graham·WB: Historical aspects of hemodialysis. Transplant Proc 1977, 9:1.
2. Quinton WE, Dillard D, Scribner BH: Cannulation of blood vessels for prolonged hemodialysis. Trans Am Soc Artif Intern Organs 1960, 6:104.
3. Brescia MJ, Cimino JE, Appel K, Hurwich BJ: Chronic hemodialysis using venipuncture and surgically created arteriovenous fistula. N Engl J Med 1966, 275:1089.
4. Owens ML, Bower RW: Physiology of arteriovenous fistulas. In Wilson SE, Owens ML (eds): *Vascular Access Surgery*. Chicago, Year Book Medical Publishers, 1980.
5. Aubaniac R: L'injection intraveineuse sousclaviculaire: Advantages et technique. Presse Med 1952, 60:1456.
6. Wilson SE, Owens ML: *Vascular Access Surgery*. Chicago, Year Book Medical Publishers, 1980.
7. Wilson JN, Grow JB, Demong CV, Prevedel AE, Owens JC: Central venous pressure in optimal blood volume maintenance. Arch Surg 1962, 85:563.
8. Dudrick SJ, Ruberg RL: Principles and practice of parenteral nutrition. Gastroenterology 1971, 61:901.
9. Peters WR, Bush WH Jr, McIntyre RD, Hill LD: The development of fibrin sheath on indwelling venous catheters. Surg Gynecol Obstet 1973, 137:43.
10. May J, Tiller D, Johnson J, Ross Sheil AG: Saphenous vein arteriovenous fistula in regular dialysis treatment. N Engl J Med 1969, 280:770.
11. Sterling WA, Hazel LT, Diethelm AG: Vascular access for hemodialysis by bovine graft arteriovenous fistulas. Surg Gynecol Obstet 1975, 141:69.
12. Dardik H, Ibrahim IM, Dardik I: Arteriovenous fistulas constructed with modified human umbilical cord vein graft. Arch Surg 1976, 111:60.
13. Jamil Z, O'Donnell JA, Merk EA, Hobson RW: A comparison of knitted Dacron velour and bovine heterografts for hemodialysis access. J Surg Res 1979, 26:423.
14. Haimov M, Burrows L, Shanzer H, Neff M, Baez A, Kwun K, Slifkin R: Experience with arterial substitutes in the construction of vascular access for hemodialysis. J Cardiovasc Surg 1980, 21:149.

Chapter 69

CONGENITAL ARTERIOVENOUS FISTULA

MARCELLO A. BORZATTA and STANLEY R. KLEIN

An arteriovenous fistula is an abnormal communication between an arterial and a venous channel, short-circuiting the intervening capillary bed. Arteriovenous fistulas are usually characterized as acquired or congenital. Acquired arteriovenous fistulas may be the result of trauma, usually penetrating, causing injury to a juxtaposed artery and a vein; spontaneous rupture of an arterial aneurysm into a neighboring vein; or transmural erosion of the involved vessels caused by an infection or a neoplastic process (1,2). In contrast, abnormalities of the embryology of the circulatory system represent the single etiology of congenital arteriovenous fistulas. It is essential to delineate congenital from acquired arteriovenous fistulas because the clinical manifestations, therapeutic implications, and prognosis differ considerably.

Congenital arteriovenous fistulas encompass a broad spectrum of clinical manifestations including small cutaneous lesions which are barely perceptible; large conglomerates of engorged, tortuous arteries and veins yielding disfiguring skin lesions or even grossly deforming an extremity; and visceral lesions which can affect multiple organs. In the past a variety of classifications have been used to describe and catalog the multiple clinical sigmata of congenital arteriovenous fistulas including angioma arteriale racemosum, cirsoid aneurysm, serpentine aneurysm, hemangioma cavernosum, and angioma telangectaticum. Because of the myriad of clinical presentations and frequent complexity of these lesions, congenital arteriovenous fistulas continue to represent a challenge to the most experienced clinician despite the relative rarity of spectacular systemic manifestations observed with the acquired arteriovenous lesion.

Historical Aspects

The Florentine Guido Guidi (1500–1559) was the first to describe the appearance of a congenital arteriovenous fistula, followed by Lealis Lealis in 1707 who reported on a single fistula between spermatic artery and vein (3,4). Most subsequent case reports, series, and investigations addressed the acquired arteriovenous fistula. In 1757, William Hunter wrote of a traumatic arteriovenous fistula secondary to phlebotomy, noting the accompanying thrill, bruit, and engorged tortuosity of the proximal artery (5). In 1833 Breschet treated two patients with traumatic arteriovenous fistula by ligating the artery proximal to the fistulous communication, but in both cases such treatment resulted in gangrene (6). Reports concerning the presentation and management of arteriovenous fistulas became more numerous in the latter part of the nineteenth century. In 1843 Norris successfully performed a double artery ligation. Nicoladoni in 1875 and Branham in 1890 described the deceleration of the pulse rate which followed compression of the proximal artery, a phenomenon which bears their names as an eponym (7–9). In 1920 Collander was responsible for the first complete and critical review of the literature, reporting on a total of 447 cases of arteriovenous fistulas of which only 3 were definitely of congenital origin (10). Beginning in 1920, Holman conducted extensive investigative studies which ultimately clarified the local and systemic physiologic sequelae of an acquired arteriovenous fistula (11).

The extensive clinical experience developed as a consequence of the large military conflicts of the twentieth century, combined with the laboratory investigations of Holman and others who constructed fistulas in renal failure patients, has greatly expanded our knowledge of the hemodynamic effects of acquired arteriovenous fistulas (12–16).

Malan and Puglionise (17,18) and Szilagyi et al. (19) have collected a large series of congenital arteriovenous fistulas, stressing the differences between congenital and acquired lesions. By identifying unique management problems and formulating the first comprehensive classifications regarding congenital arteriovenous fistulas, a foundation for future investigation has been firmly established.

Classification

The diverse variety of manifestations of congenital arteriovenous fistulas has led to much confusion regarding the nature of the lesion and an organization of a logical classification. Many nomenclatures have been suggested in an attempt to provide a framework inclusive of the numerous clinical variants. Two of these proposals provide a relatively simple, yet complete, catalog encompassing the myriad of clinical manifestations of congenital arteriovenous fistulas.

In 1961, Malan and Puglionisi divided congenital vascular malformations with an abnormal arteriovenous communication into truncular arteriovenous fistulas (local or diffuse, more or less active) and arteriovenous angiomas (single or diffuse, more or less active) (17,18). The truncular arteriovenous fistula consists of a communication, either single or multiple, between an arterial trunk and one or more venous channels. Szilagyi et al. devised another simple classification of congenital arteriovenous fistulas based on the embryology of the peripheral circulatory system (19,20). The developmental sequence of the extremity vasculature was well described by Woollard, who identified three stages: (1) stage of undifferentiated capillary network (2) retiform stage, and (3) vascular maturation stage (21) (Figure 69-1). The arrest or misdirection of development at any or all of the three stages is responsible for the varied clinical manifestations. Hemangiomas result from the arrest of development during the stage of undifferentiated capillary network, while arteriovenous aneurysms are a consequence of misdirection of development during the retiform stage. An arteriovenous aneurysm may consist of "macrofistulous communications," demonstrable by angiography, or of "microfistulous anastomoses" that are typically absent in angiographic studies. If vascular maturation (stage 3) remains incomplete, anomalous mature vascular channels are the result. Port-wine stains represent an example of an aberration occurring during stage 3 (22–24).

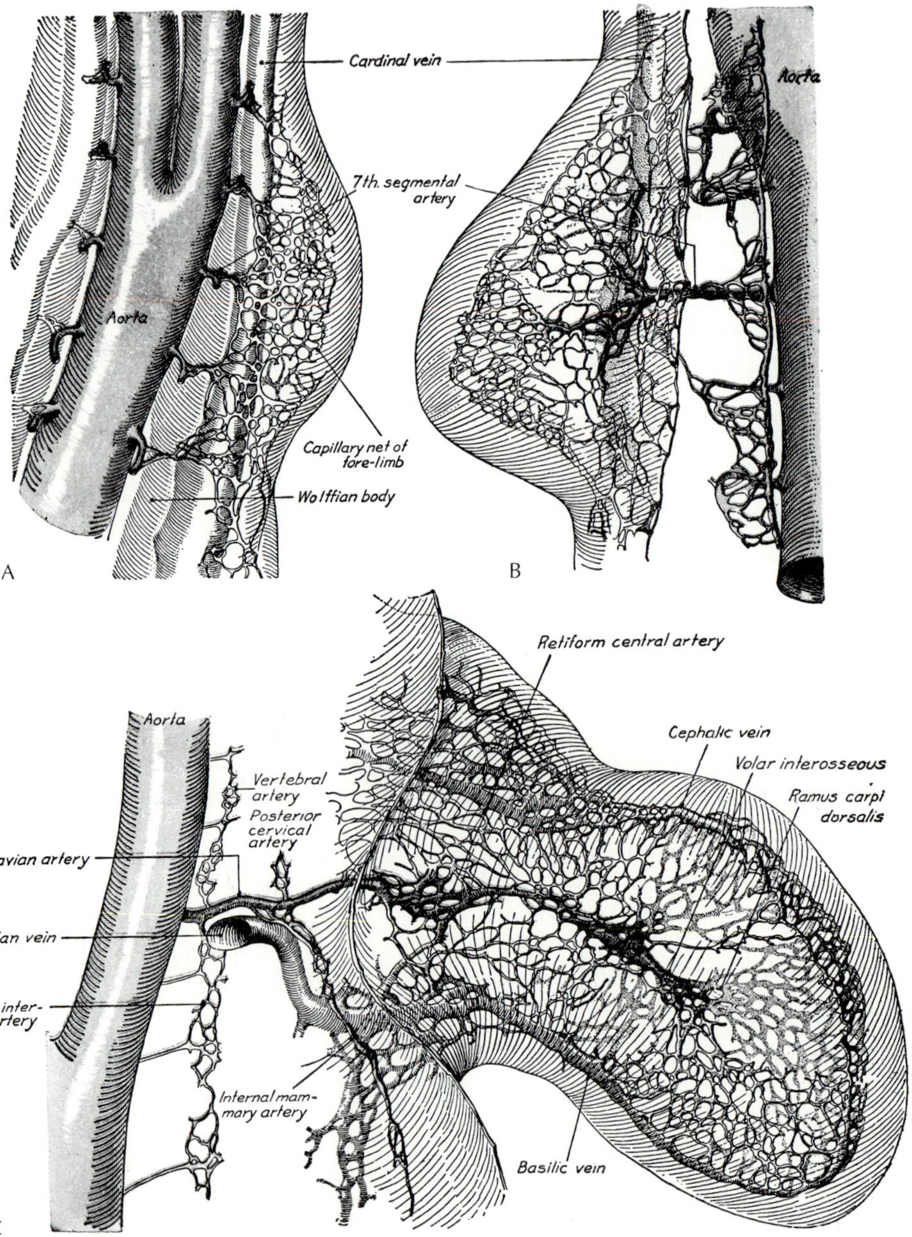

FIGURE 69-1. Drawings from injected pig embryos showing three stages in early development of blood vessels of the anterior appendage bud. [After Woollard (21).] (*A*) Embryo of 4.5 mm (equivalent to 4-week-old human embryo). (*B*) Embryo of 7.5 mm (equivalent to 5-week-old human embryo). (*C*) Embryo of 12 mm (equivalent to 6-week-old human embryo). (Reprinted with permission from Patten BM: *Human Embryology*, ed 2. New York, McGraw-Hill, 1953.)

Pathophysiology

The hemodynamic consequences associated with an arteriovenous fistula are the result of the shunting of arterial blood into the low-resistence, high-capacitance venous channel(s), thus bypassing an intervening capillary bed. The magnitude of the local peripheral and systemic effects is dependent upon the location, diameter, and number of vascular communication(s).

Locally there is increased flow in the proximal (afferent) artery(ies), which becomes markedly enlarged and tortuous. The distal arterial circulation is deprived of a substantial proportion of blood volume and, depending on the size of the fistulous communication and relative resistances, may act as an afferent artery for the fistula. The venous circulation is subjected to substantial hypertension resulting in gross elongation and tortuosity of the entire surrounding bed.

Each vein is "arterialized," a process in which the smooth muscle in the vessel wall hypertrophies but no elastic laminas appear. Several local sequelae of venous hypertension include distal venous stasis, loss of valvular competence, and occasional reversal of direction of flow (25–28).

The peripheral effects of an arteriovenous fistula are again directly related to the magnitude of the shunt. The "steal" of arterial blood flow through the fistula results in decreased perfusion of the peripheral tissues with potential ischemic problems, while increased venous pressure at the site of the shunt produces the previously enumerated manifestations (29,30). The systemic effects of arteriovenous connections include increased cardiac output, increased heart rate, dilatation, and, to a lesser degree, hypertrophy of the heart, a decrease in diastolic blood pressure with an increase in the pulse pressure, and an increase in the blood volume. If the flow through the fistula is large, the increase in cardiac output resulting from an increase in the heart rate and myocardial contractility might not meet the demand and high-output cardiac failure follows (31).

Peripheral and central effects are usually more marked with acquired than congenital arteriovenous fistulas. Although the total cross-sectional area of the congenital communication is large, it is a sum of multiple small connections, each at a relatively high resistance (19,32,33). Consequently, the overall volume of shunted arterial blood is less than that measured in an acquired arteriovenous fistula of the same cross-sectional area with a single communication between an artery and a vein.

Therefore, congenital arteriovenous fistulas very seldom are the cause of significant systemic hemodynamic perturbation. One exception is the large congenital arteriovenous fistula which affects the central nervous system or liver of an infant and may well produce fulminant cardiac failure (34,35).

Location

Congenital arteriovenous fistulas may occur almost anywhere in the body, usually involving all tissues in a given anatomic region (36). Most commonly they involve the extremities, lower more frequently than upper. Among the fistulas of the extremities, those involving the femoral vessels are the most common (19) (Figure 69-2). Congenital arteriovenous fistulas have also been described in the head and neck, where they consist of multiple vascular channels and often result in significant craniofacial deformity (37) (Figure 69-3). The central nervous system is also affected by arteriovenous malformation in both the cerebral and spinal locations, often with dramatic manifestations, which are extensively described in the neurosurgical literature. Although rare, pelvic arteriovenous fistulas represent challenging therapeutic problems for they are usually quite extensive and present with either symptoms of compression of viscera or vaginal bleeding (38). Among the visceral congenital arteriovenous fistulas, lesions in the lungs, kidneys, and alimentary tract have been described (39,40). The arteriovenous fistulas of the lungs derive their blood supply either from pulmonary or systemic arterial sources but almost always empty into the pulmonary veins. Fistulas of the celiac and mesenteric circulation have also been described and represent an uncommon, but treatable, cause of portal hypertension (41).

Clinical Presentation

SUBJECTIVE SYMPTOMS

Almost two-thirds of the congenital arteriovenous fistulas are complex lesions originating from errors in any of the three developmental stages of the extremity circulatory system (20). Although the vast majority of these fistulas are present at birth, they frequently become clinically evident during the second or third decade of life, following puberty, pregnancy, or trauma (42). The subjective manifestations differ with the location of the fistula. Cutaneous arteriovenous malformations or lesions affecting the head and neck may be disfiguring, and the patient's primary concern is usually of a cosmetic nature (Figure 69-4). Patients with arteriovenous fistulas of the limbs often describe pain, swelling, deformity, or abnormal growth of the involved extremity (Figure 69-5). The presence of prominent superficial unilateral varicosities or their location in an unusual site should alert the physician to the possibility of an underlying arteriovenous fistula. If the fistula is hemodynamically significant, the patient might describe systemic manifestations including dyspnea on exertion or easy fatigability.

Visceral arteriovenous fistulas, when symptomatic, may present with local or systemic consequences. For example, arteriovenous fistulas of the gastrointestinal tract often present with hemorrhage (Figure 69-6), and renal lesions may give rise to hematuria or hypertension.

OBJECTIVE FINDINGS

The large variety of objective clinical findings reflects the diverse extent and loci of these lesions. Below, important features are grouped by fistula location.

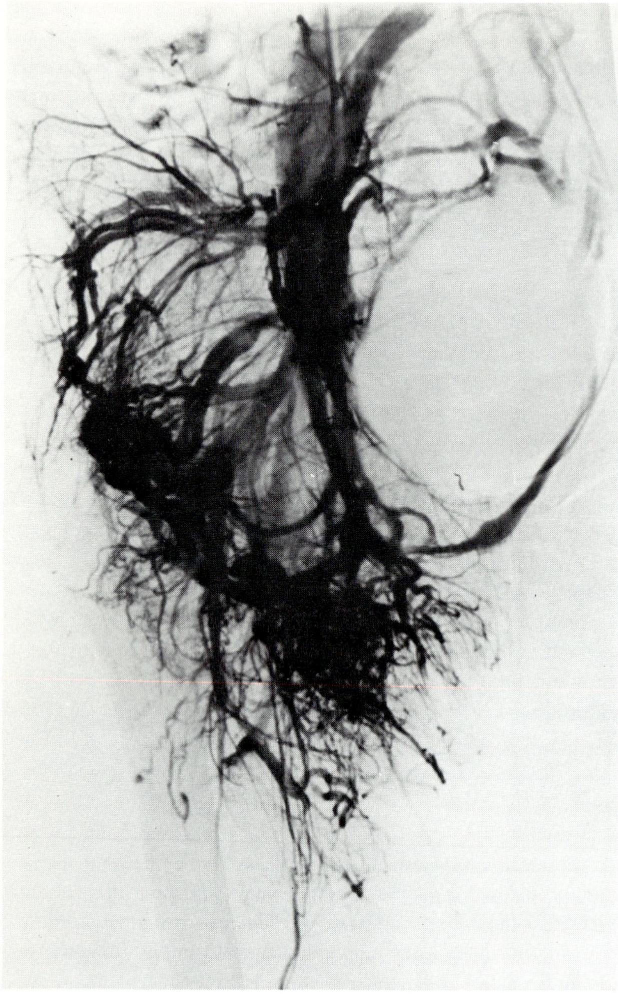

FIGURE 69-2. Congenital arteriovenous fistula originating from the right iliofemoral vessels: angiographic appearance.

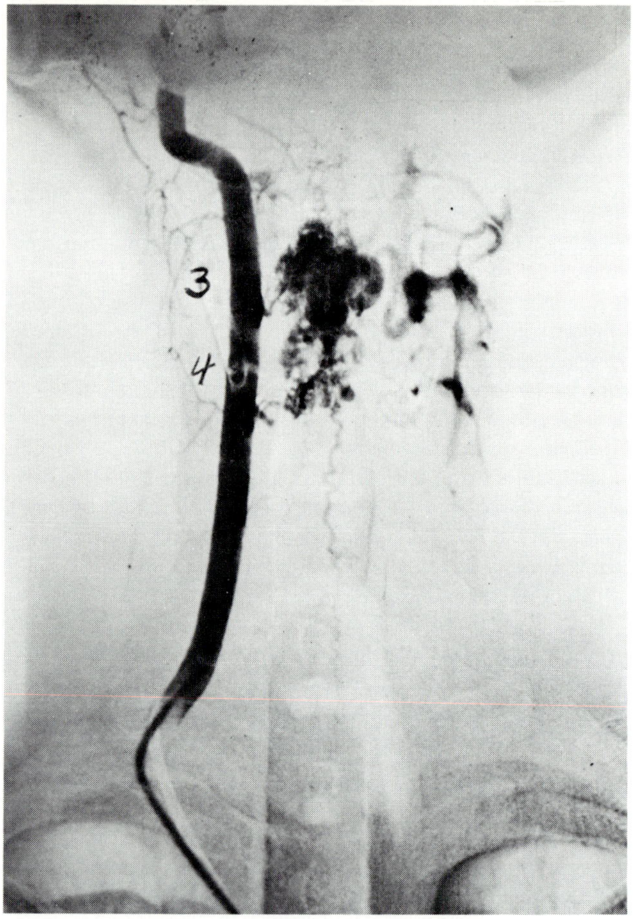

FIGURE 69-3. Arteriographic demonstration of cervical spinal arteriovenous malformation. The patient, a 30-year-old Hispanic female, presented with recurrent subarachnoid hemorrhage. The arteriovenous malformation originates from the right vertebral artery; two major feeding branches are identified at cervical level 3 and 4.

Superficial Arteriovenous Fistulas

CUTANEOUS APPEARANCE. Arteriovenous fistulas are frequently associated with cutaneous manifestations. Fifty percent of the lesions confined to the extremities are associated with "birthmarks." The Parkes Weber and Klippel-Trenaunay syndromes both describe a clinical complex of arteriovenous fistulas of the limb and port-wine stains (22) (Figure 69-7).

SKIN TEMPERATURE. Temperature is usually increased in the affected limb, although if the peripheral perfusion is compromised by the shunt, the temperature in distal areas might be lower than other tissues.

DERMAL APPENDAGES. Increased sweating and hair growth often both occur.

VENOUS HYPERTENSION. Signs of chronic venous insufficiency such as edema, thickening of the skin, ulceration, and gangrene may occur. The ulcerations usually affect the distal extremity and are not located in the perimalleolar area as expected of isolated venous insufficiency. Evidence of dilated, serpiginous veins is almost invariably present in conjunction with congenital arteriovenous fistulas.

TURBULENT CIRCULATION. A palpable thrill and auscultative bruit (which is usually continuous, "machinery-like," with systolic augmentation) are frequently, but not always, associated with a congenital arteriovenous fistula.

BRANHAM-NICOLADONI SIGN. Pulse deceleration with compression of the fistula can be present but is frequently absent given the limited systemic effects of congenital fistulas.

DISPARATE LIMB DEVELOPMENT. An increase in length and/or girth of the affected limb may be present. The hypertrophy usually involves both soft tissue and osseous structures. The lengthening is seldom marked (2 to 5 cm), although sufficient to produce pelvic asymmetry and low back pain.

Visceral Arteriovenous Fistulas

Pulmonary arteriovenous fistulas may receive their blood supply from the pulmonary or systemic arterial circulation (39). Of the fistulas originating from the pulmonary system, only 10 percent are symptomatic (Figure 69-8). They are usually diagnosed in the third or fourth decade of life and occur twice as frequently in females as in males. Approximately 60 percent are associated with Osler-Rendu-Weber syndrome (Figure 69-9). Approximately 60 percent of the lesions are located in the lower lobe

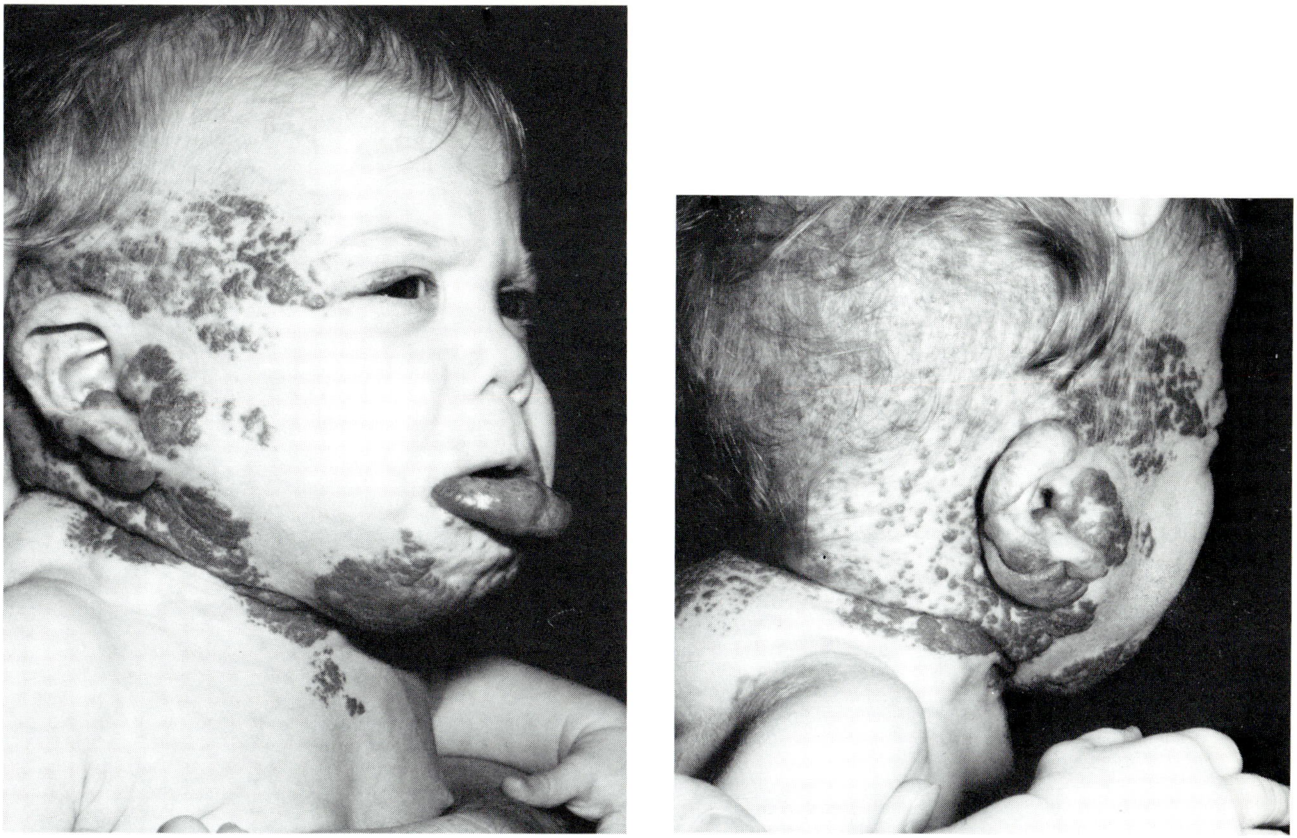

A B

FIGURE 69-4. Female caucasian infant with disfiguring hemangiomas of the face: (*A*) involvement of the right side of the face and tongue; (*B*) extension to the scalp and deformity of the lobe of the right ear.

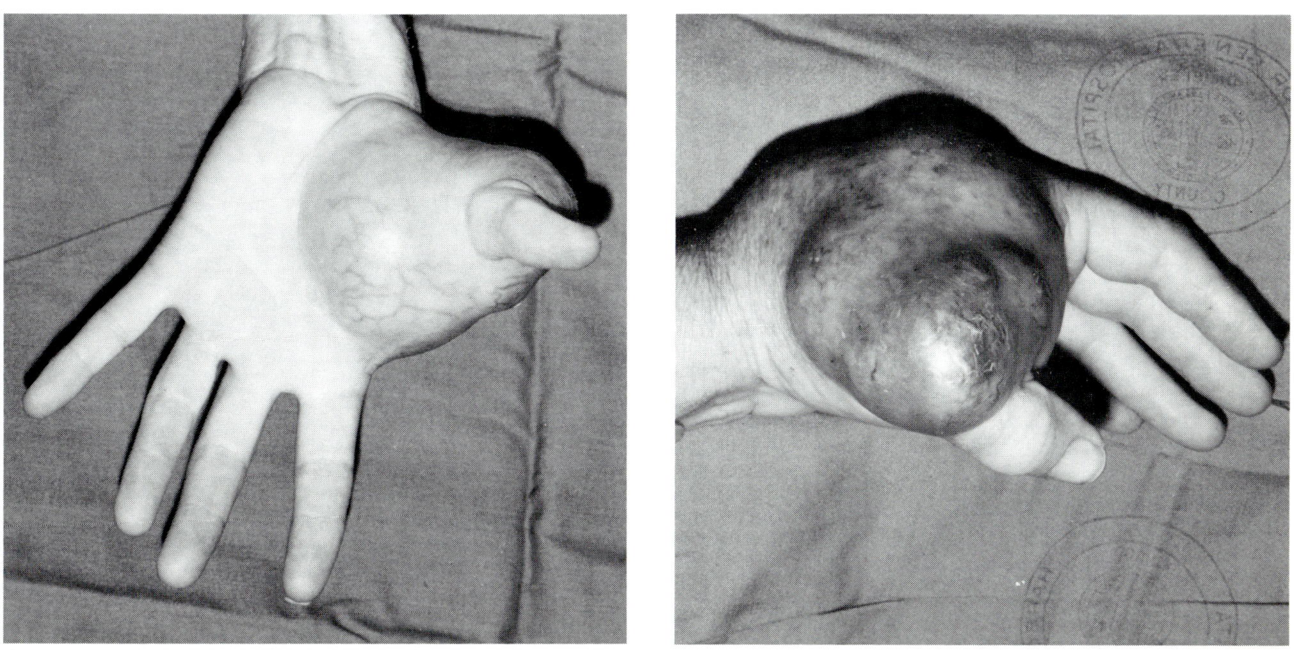

A B

FIGURE 69-5. Twenty-six-year-old Hispanic female affected by congenital arteriovenous malformation of the left thenar eminence: (*A*) volar aspect; (*B*) some ischemic complications on the dorsal aspect.

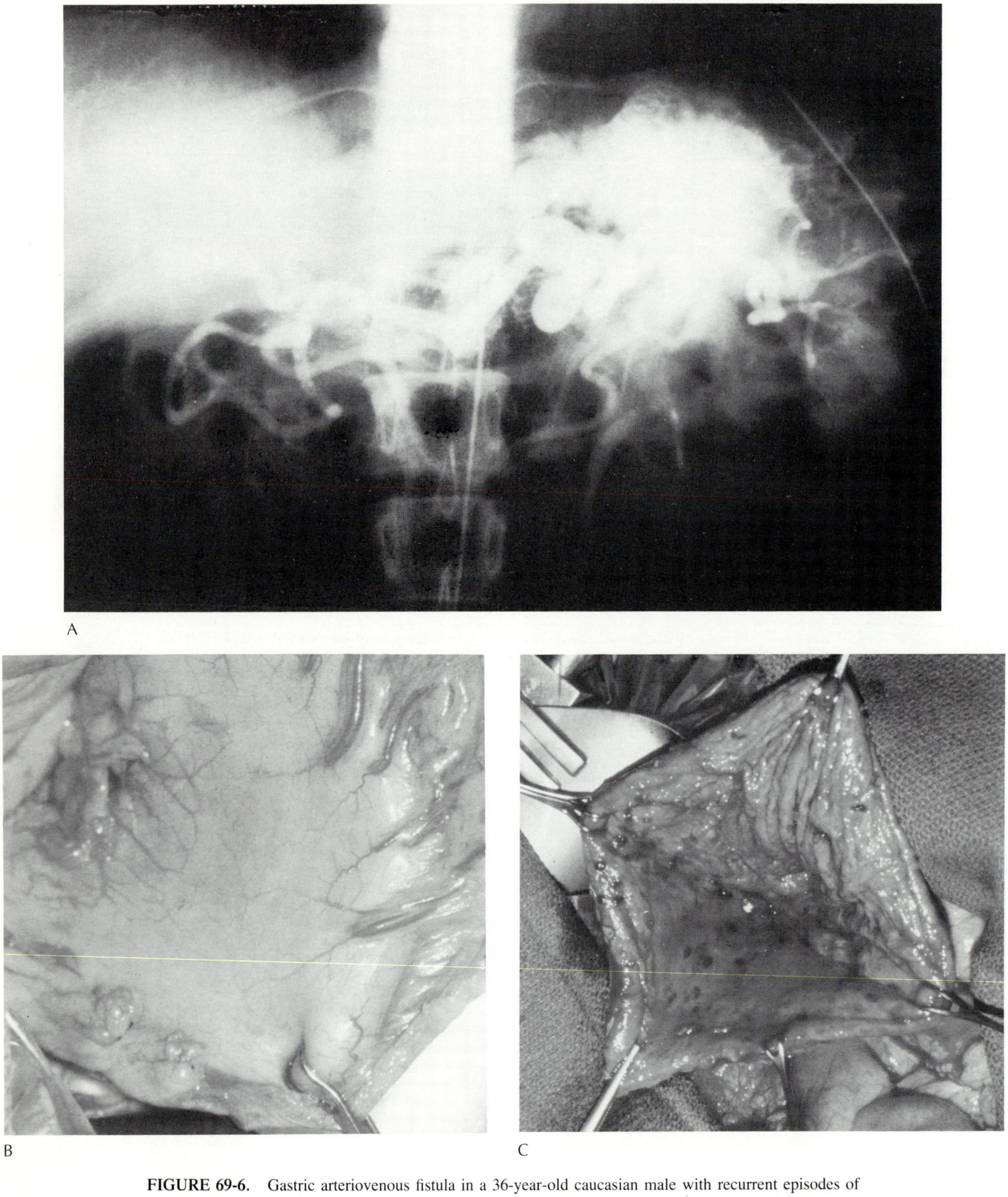

A

B

C

FIGURE 69-6. Gastric arteriovenous fistula in a 36-year-old caucasian male with recurrent episodes of hematemesis: (*A*) arteriographic appearance; (*B*) intraoperative evidence of tortuous, engorged venous and arterial channels along both the lesser and greater curvature of the stomach; (*C*) mucosal aspect with evidence of superficial ulcerations.

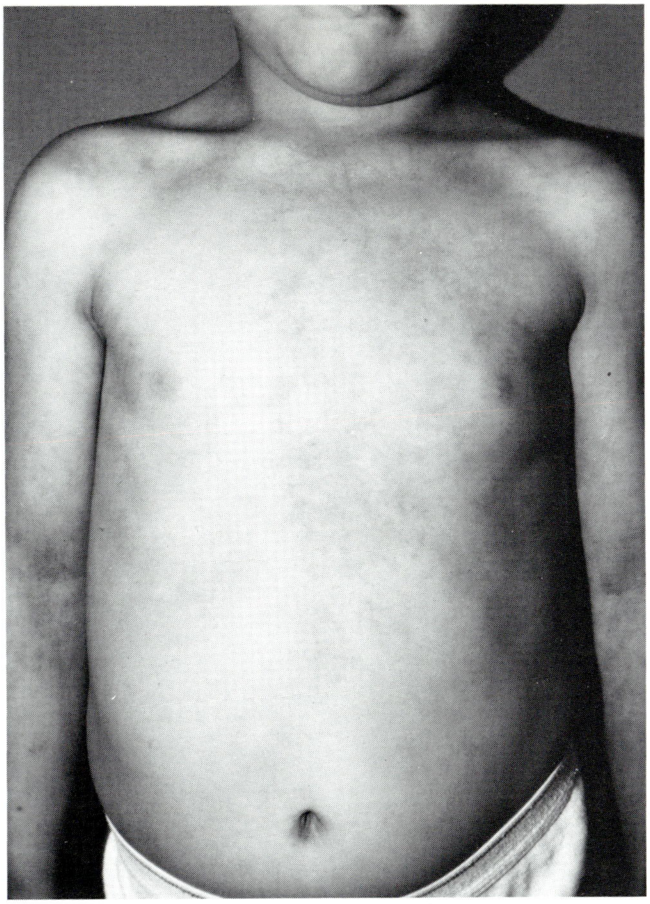

A

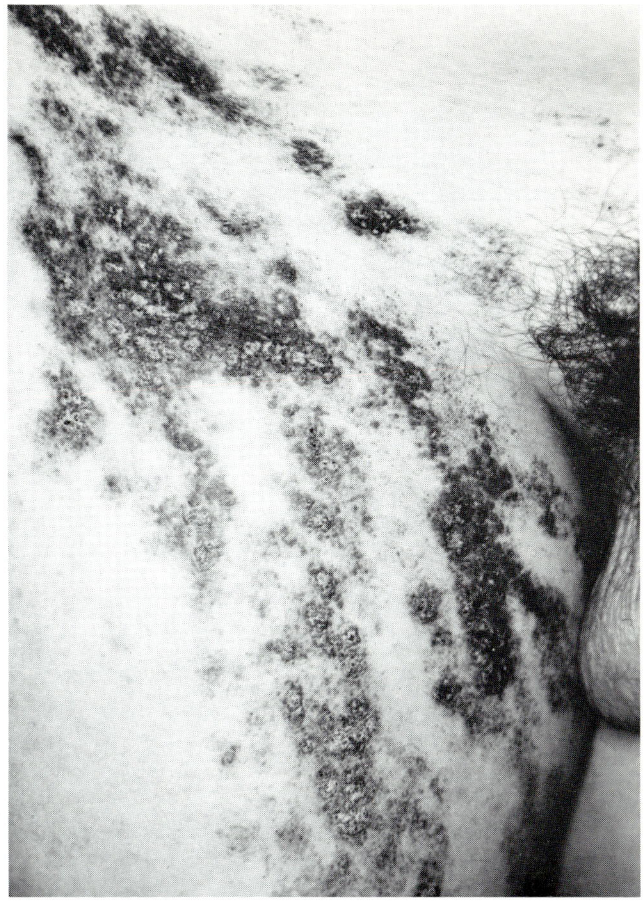

B

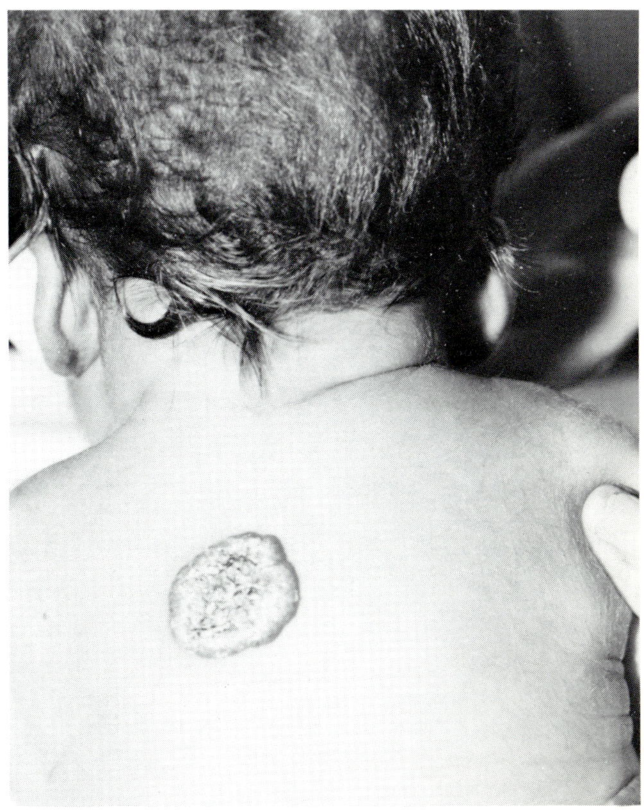

C

FIGURE 69-7. Cutaneous appearance of vascular malformation: (*A*) 7-year-old male with cutaneous hemangiomas of chest and upper extremities; (*B*) congenital hemangiomatosis of the lower extremity; (*C*) 1-month-old male with capillary hemangioma of the back.

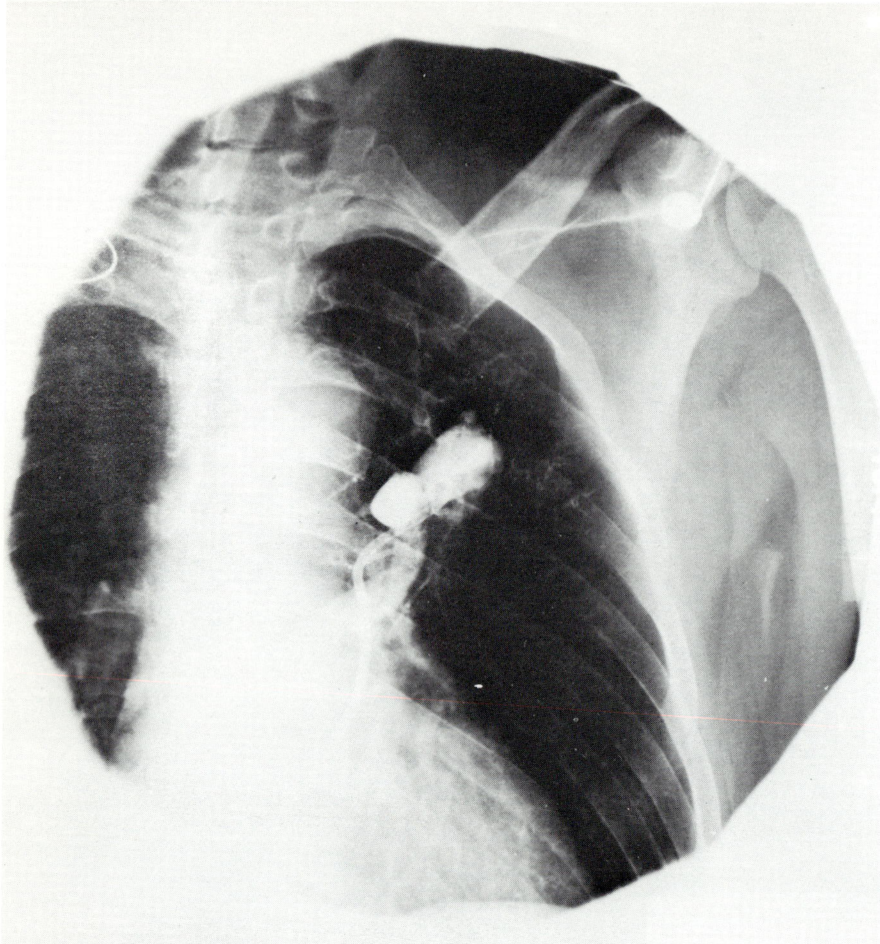

FIGURE 69-8. Thirty-three-year-old caucasian male with recurrent hemoptysis. Arteriographic demonstration of congenital arteriovenous fistula of the left lung originating from the pulmonary arterial circulation.

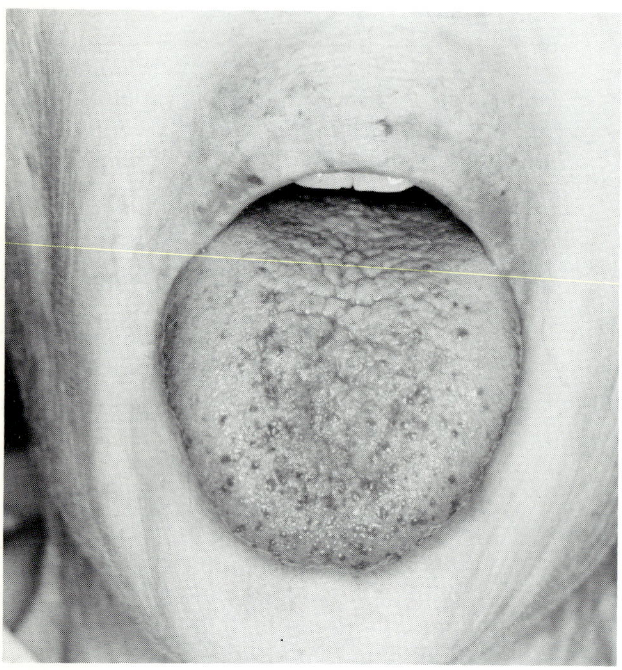

FIGURE 69-9. Osler-Rendu-Weber disease: mucosal telangiectasia.

just beneath the visceral pleura. Their presence produces a right-to-left cardiac shunt but characteristically does not result in a readily documented effect on systemic hemodynamics. Presenting symptoms are usually exertional dyspnea and easy fatigability. In 20 percent of the cases they can result in complications which include brain abscess, cerebral vascular accident, hemoptysis, and hemothorax. On physical examination evidence of cyanosis and clubbing is often found along with an extracardiac murmur increasing during inspiration. The chest x-ray usually discloses a single circumscribed, noncalcified lesion (75 percent), located in the medial third of the lower lobe, without associated cardiomegaly. The pulmonary fistulas with systemic blood supply are very rare. They derive their arterial flow from the bronchial arteries, the internal mammary artery, the intercostals, or directly from the aorta. In contrast to fistulas with pulmonary arterial supply, these cause a left-to-right shunt and are often hemodynamically significant, leading to cardiomegaly and left ventricular hypertrophy. A chest x-ray may show rib notching due to the extensive collateral circulation.

Among the other visceral arteriovenous fistulas, those in the kidney present with hematuria and hypertension in 50 percent of patients. An intraabdominal bruit is usually found on physical examination. Arteriovenous fistulas in the mesenteric or celiac circulations may present with portal hypertension, ascites, or gastrointestinal bleeding. Arteriovenous fistulas between the hepatic artery and vein are extremely rare. Reported cases included findings of hepatomegaly, jaundice, and fulminant cardiac failure (43).

Diagnosis

The diagnosis of arteriovenous fistulas, especially of the extremities, is usually conclusively made on clinical grounds alone. At times, diagnostic procedures may help in a complex situation but are always important in delineating the nature and extent of the lesion prior to initiation of treatment. Among the noninvasive procedures, oscillometry, a segmental measure of the volume of the arterial pulsation, demonstrates an increased amplitude in the proximity of the fistulous communication with decreased oscillometric values distally (44,45). Digital plethysmography (pulse-volume recording) also provides useful information. Determinations at the site of a congenital arteriovenous fistula will show an increase in the pulse-volume and digital volume, directly proportional to the size of the shunt (44). Directional Doppler scanning has been useful especially in identifying microfistulous anastomoses not visualized by an angiogram (46).

Additional invasive diagnostic modalities include determination of the venous P_{O_2} in the efferent venous drainage. Contrast echocardiography has also been employed for the detection of echoes in the systemic venous system following arterial injection of indocyanine green, which indicates an arteriovenous communication. This modality is particularly useful in confirming the suspected diagnosis of a visceral arteriovenous fistula or in assessing the residual arteriovenous shunt following an attempted surgical excision (47). Nuclear isotope studies have been employed in the past but are essentially obsolete at present (48). Contrast and subtraction techniques of angiography, often using highly selective catheterization procedures, are unequivocal proof of the lesion and frequently provide a "road map" during the course of treatment. Enhanced computerized axial tomography and digital subtraction angiography are being utilized more frequently. The presence and extent of a congenital arteriovenous fistula are often easily demonstrated with digital subtraction angiography (49,50). However, this technique has the shortcomings of not depicting necessary anatomic detail and failing to permit application of interventional therapeutic radiographic methods. The enhanced computerized axial tomogram accurately reveals the three-dimensional anatomy encompassed by an arteriovenous fistula (51–54). It has an application for head and neck, truncal, and extremity lesions.

The classic finding on the standard arteriogram is the presence of a cluster of anomalous arterial trunks with numerous, rapidly filling communications with the venous system (Figure 69-10). In congenital arteriovenous fistulas, it is not always possible to demonstrate the arteriovenous communications radiographically. In many patients (approximately 40 percent), despite the clinical evidence of a congenital arteriovenous fistula, the arteriogram fails to demonstrate any gross arteriovenous connection. In these cases the indirect angiographic evidence of the existence of arteriovenous fistulas becomes of diagnostic significance. Suggestive findings include increased flow in the afferent artery or arteries, tortuosity and hypertrophy of the proximal artery or arteries, premature filling of the venous trunks, accumulation of the contrast medium at the area of the fistula, and depletion of contrast medium in the distal arterial tree (20).

Treatment

While standard methods of vascular reconstruction for the involved structures are the accepted therapy for acquired arteriovenous fistulas, the treatment of congenital arteriovenous fistulas, in contrast, continues to represent a difficult problem for even the experienced clinician (28,31,44). The nature of congenital arteriovenous fistulas, where a single arteriovenous com-

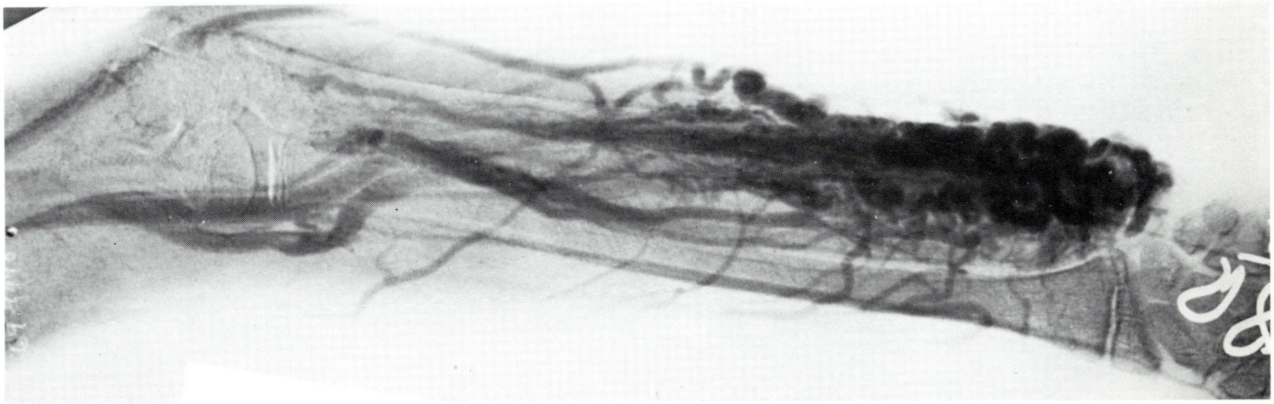

FIGURE 69-10. Twenty-five-year-old male with congenital arteriovenous fistula of the upper extremity demonstrating the classic arteriographic findings: cluster of tortuous, engorged vessels with rapid venous filling.

munication is rare and extensive lesions with numerous macro- and microfistulous connections are instead the rule, forms the basis for this therapeutic challenge (Figure 69-11). At the outset it is important to point out that not all congenital arteriovenous fistulas require treatment. For example, cutaneous lesions such as capillary or cavernous hemangiomas will often undergo spontaneous involution. This is a gradual process usually occurring during the first 3 years with complete or near complete regression achieved by the seventh year of life (22,55). Camouflage of cutaneous lesions with cosmetics may provide significant improvement, but applicability is limited and often represents an unacceptable burden for the patient (22). Supportive measures such as protective and compressive garments are often successful in controlling lesions affecting the extremities (20).

Several definite indications for specific treatment of superficial arteriovenous fistulas can be identified: (1) superficial lesions causing significant cosmetic disability; (2) lesions involving an extremity and causing disfigurement or impaired function; (3) hemorrhage; (4) ulceration or infection; (5) the rare case of a fistula producing systemic hemodynamic embarrassment. When formulating a plan for the treatment of a congenital arteriovenous fistula, accurate delineation of the location and extent of the lesion in conjunction with the demonstration of the arteriovenous connections and of the feeding vessels is of paramount importance. The extent of the collateral circulation should necessarily also be assessed. Arteriography and directional Doppler studies, if microfistulous connections are suspected, usually provide the necessary information. Unfortunately, even though the arteriogram reveals a well-localized lesion, these are often found to be much more extensive at the time of surgery. If a localized congenital arteriovenous fistula is depicted, radical excision, with or without preoperative intraarterial embolization to reduce intraoperative bleeding, is the treatment of choice (19,20,44). Complete excision of an extensive congenital arteriovenous fistula is seldom possible. Partial excision, proximal artery ligation, or dissection and interruption of multiple arterial branches supplying the fistula have been attempted with discouraging results because the lesion usually rapidly recurs and complications such as distal ischemia and gangrene are frequent (19,20,42,44). Fry et al. have performed with some success, in selected patients, total or near-total excision of congenital arteriovenous fistulas of the extremities in staged operations, often employing reconstructive procedures to obliterate large defects (56). Given the poor results achieved with isolated surgical management, other treatment modalities have been applied, including radiotherapy, sclerosing agents, thrombosing agents, electrocoagulation, and cryotherapy, with limited success (57–59). Dermabrasion and surgical tattooing of cutaneous lesions have also been employed with variable results (60,61). The destruction of the ectatic vessels with a laser beam is a recently introduced, but an extremely promising, therapeutic modality especially applicable to skin lesions (62–64).

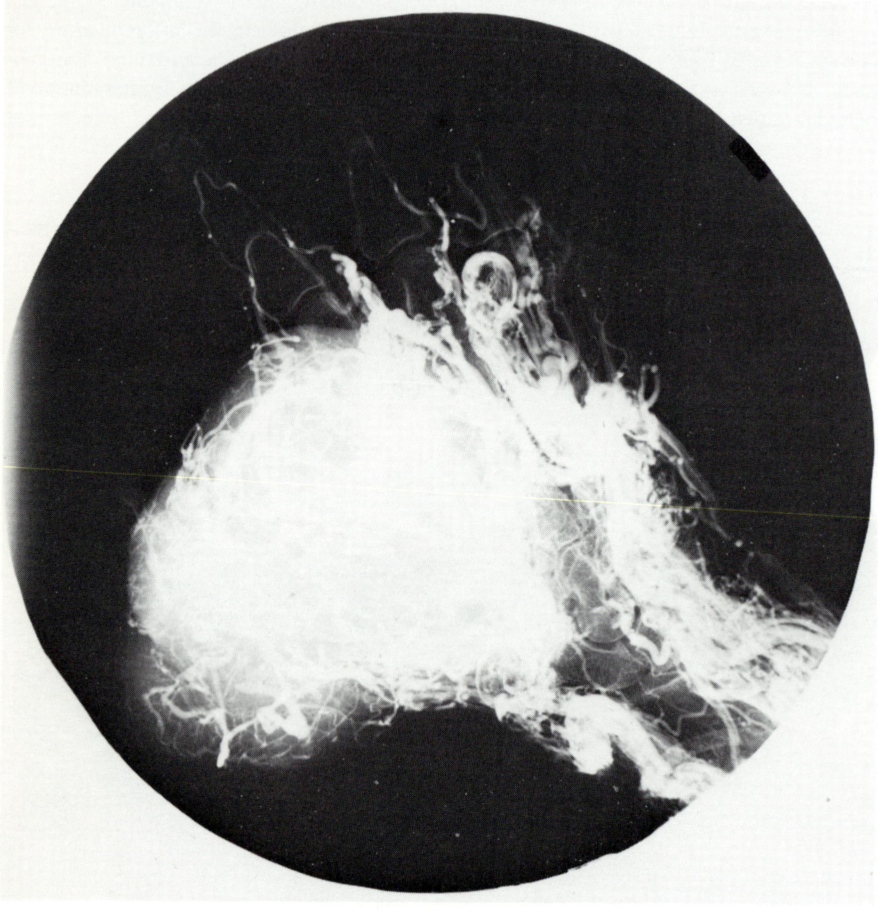

FIGURE 69-11. Numerous macrofistulous communications in an extensive congenital arteriovenous fistula of the right hand of a 23-year-old female complaining of disfigurement and impaired function.

Interventional radiologic techniques of embolization have offered a relatively safe modality which can accomplish complete obliteration of the fistulas in few cases and at least control of the symptoms and complications in many other instances (65,66). This technique has the objective of minimizing the remaining shunt while preserving the named axial arteries and major collateral circulation responsible for peripheral perfusion. Serial embolizations are usually required, and the major, although rare, complications include distal ischemia and systemic and pulmonary embolization (67,68). When intraarterial embolization is ineffective alone, a subsequent limited surgical resection, employing one of the above-mentioned precedures, may provide temporary palliation. Finally, amputation at times is required to control either local or systemic effects secondary to an extensive congenital arteriovenous fistula of the extremities (44).

The management of visceral arteriovenous fistulas is generally more aggressive, especially since the manifestations of these lesions are always dramatic and often life-threatening. Radical excision is again the treatment of choice and at times will require partial or total resection of the affected organ. Pulmonary, renal, or gastrointestinal lesions can often be treated in this manner following accurate preoperative localization. In the case of extensive visceral involvement which precludes simple extirpation, the combination of intraarterial embolization with or without surgery represents an effective and relatively safe modality (69–71). Arteriovenous malformations of the central nervous system, in both the intracranial and spinal locations, are approached with similar objectives in that when in an accessible location and of limited extension, they should be completely excised (72,73) (Figure 69-12). If they are not amenable to isolated surgical treatment because of extensive size or deep location, embolization via percutaneous arteriography or stereotactic radiotherapy has been successfully employed (74–77).

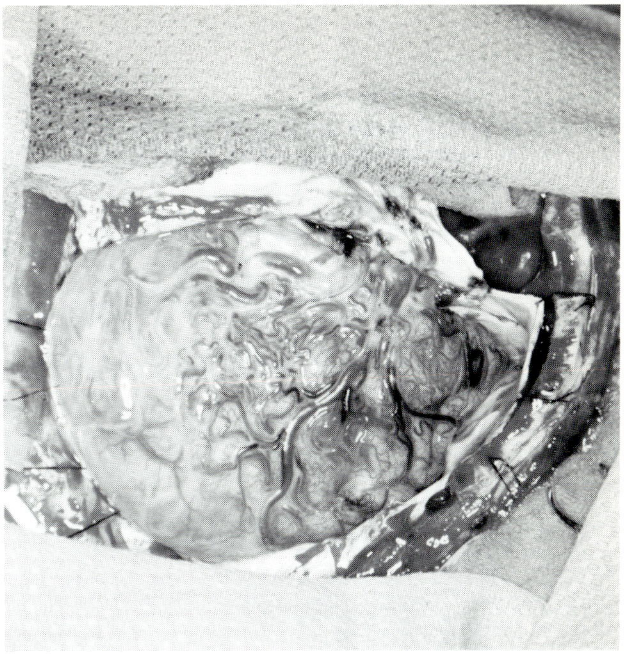

FIGURE 69-12. Intraoperative appearance of a frontoparietal arteriovenous malformation. Note the large tortuous, feeding, angular arterial branches.

Summary

Congenital arteriovenous fistulas can be located anywhere in the body, but more frequently affect the extremities. They are often extensive lesions with multiple macro- and microfistulous arteriovenous connections. Systemic effects are distinctly rare with congenital arteriovenous fistulas. When the lesion is well localized, radical excision is the treatment of choice; when the lesion is extensive, early conservative management is recommended. If supportive measures such as protective and compressive garments are ineffective in controlling the lesion or if complications such as bleeding or cardiac failure occur, selective intraarterial embolization might be employed. Many newer therapeutic modalities have been recently introduced, but experience is too limited to accurately portray their indication. When intraarterial embolization fails to provide control of the lesion or its complications, only then should palliative surgical procedures such as limited excision or ligation of feeding vessels be considered, keeping in mind the limited efficacy and potential severe complications. Amputation should be limited to extensive arteriovenous fistulas producing life-threatening conditions or severe compromise of the quality of life when all of the above measures have failed.

References

1. Dardik H, Dardik I, Strom MG, et al: Intravenous rupture of arteriosclerotic aneurysms of the abdominal aorta. Surgery 1976, 80:647–651.
2. Yater WM, Luckett WF, Leonard BW: Mycotic arteriovenous fistula: Report of a case. Med Ann DC 1940, 9:439–441:454.
3. Vidius Vidus. In Virchow R: *Pathologie des tumeurs*. Germer-Balliere, Paris, 1876.
4. Lealis Lealis quoted in Malan E et al: J Cardiovasc Surg 1965, 6:4, note 2.
5. Hunter W: The history of an aneurysm of the aorta with some remarks on aneurysms in general. Trans Med Obstet Soc Phys London 1757, 1:323.
6. Breschet G: Memoire sur les anevrysmes, Mem Acad Med (Paris) 1833, 3:101.
7. Norris GW: Varicose aneurysm at the bend of the arm; Ligature of the artery above and below the sac; Secondary hemorrhages with a return of the aneurysmal thrill at the tenth day; Cure. Am J Med Sci 1833, 5:27.
8. Nicoladoni C: Phlebarteriectasie der rechten obern extremitat. Arch Klin Chir 1875, 18:252.

9. Branham HH: Aneurysmal varix of the femoral artery and vein following a gunshot wound. J Surg 1890, 3:250.
10. Collander CL: Study of arteriovenous fistula with an analysis of 449 cases. Johns Hopkins Hosp Rep 1920, 19:259.
11. Holman E: *Abnormal Arteriovenous Communications: Peripheral and Intracardiac, Acquired and Congenital*, ed 2. Springfield, Illinois, Charles C Thomas, 1968.
12. Reid MR: The effect of arteriovenous fistula upon the heart and blood-vessels: An experimental and clinical study. Bull Johns Hopkins Hosp 1920, 31:43–50.
13. Reid MR: Studies on abnormal arteriovenous communications, acquired and congenital. I. Report of a series of cases. Arch Surg 1925, 10:601–638.
14. Gundermann W: Kriegschirurgischer Bericht aus der Giessener Klinik: uber die ersten 5 Monate des Krieges. Beitr Klin Chir 1915, 97:479–537.
15. Nanu I, Alexandrescu-Dersca C, Lazeanu E: Les troubles cardiaques consecutifs aux anevrismes arterio-veineux. Arch Mal Coer 1922, 15:829–840.
16. Kennedy JA, Burwell CS: Measurements of the circulation in a patient with multiple arteriovenous connections. Am Heart J 1944, 28:133–148.
17. Malan E, Puglionisi A: Congenital angiodysplasias of the extremities. (Note I: Generalities and classification; venous dysplasia.) J Cardiovasc Surg 1964, 5:87.
18. Malan E, Puglionisi A: Congenital angiodysplasias of the extremities. (Note II: Arterial, arterial and venous, and hemolymphatic dysplasias.) J Cardiovasc Surg 1965, 6:255.
19. Szilagyi DE, Elliot JP, DeRusso FJ, et al: Peripheral congenital arteriovenous fistulas. Surgery 1965, 57:61–80.
20. Szilagyi DE, Smith RF, Eliott JP, et al: Congenital arteriovenous anomalies of the limbs. Arch Surg 1976, 111:423–429.
21. Woollard, HH: The development of the principal arterial stems in the forelimb of the pig. Contr Embryol 1922, 14:141–154.
22. Wisnicki JL: Hemangiomas and vascular malformations. Ann Plast Surg 1984, 12(1):41–59.
23. Mulliken JB, Glowacki J: Hemangiomas and vascular malformations in infants, children: A classification based on endothelial characteristics. Plast Reconstr Surg 1982, 69:912.
24. Mulliken JB, Murray JE: Natural history of vascular birthmarks. In William HB (ed): *Symposium on Vascular Malformations and Melanotic Lesions*. St Louis, CV Mosby, 1983, pp 58–73.
25. Ingebrigtsen R, Krog J, Leraand S: Velocity and flow of blood in the femoral artery proximal to an experimental arteriovenous fistula. Acta Chir Scand 1962, 124:45.
26. Schenk WG Jr, Bahn RA, Cordell AR, Stephens JG: The regional hemodynamics of experimental acute arteriovenous fistulas. Surg Gynecol Obstet 1957, 105:733.
27. Ingebrigtsen R, Wehn PS: Local blood pressure and direction of flow in experimental arterio-venous fistula. Acta Chir Scand 1960, 120:142.
28. Strandness DE Jr, Sumner DS: Arteriovenous fistulas. In *Hemodynamics for Surgeons*. New York, Grune & Stratton, 1975, pp 621–663.
29. Elkin DC, Warren JV: Arteriovenous fistulas: Their effect on the circulation. JAMA 1947, 134:1524.
30. Reid MR: Abnormal arteriovenous communications, acquired and congenital. III. The effects of abnormal arteriovenous communications on the heart, blood vessels, and other structures. Arch Surg 1925, 11:25–42.
31. Sumner DS: Hemodynamics and pathophysioloy of arteriovenous fistulas. In Rutherford RB (ed): *Vascular Surgery*. Philadelphia, Saunders, 1977, pp 733–765.
32. Cross FS, Glover DM, Simeone FA, Oldenburg FA: Congenital arteriovenous aneurysms. Ann Surg 1958, 148:649.
33. Pemberton J, Saint JH: Congenital arteriovenous communications. Surg Gynecol Obstet 1928, 46:470.
34. Crocker DW, Cleland RS: Infantile hemangioendothelioma of the liver: Report of three cases. Pediatrics 1957, 19:596.
35. Levine OR, Jameson AG, Nellkaus G, Gold AP: Cardiac complications of cerebral arteriovenous fistula in infancy. Pediatrics 1962, 30:563.
36. Horton BT, Chormley RK: Congenital arteriovenous fistula. Proc Staff Meet Mayo Clin 1933, 8:773–776.
37. Devine KD, Beahrs OH, Lovestedt SA, et al: Congenital arteriovenous fistulas of the face and neck. Plast Reconstr Surg 1959, 23:273–282.
38. Pritchard DA, Maloney JD, Bernatz PE, et al: Surgical treatment of congenital pelvic arteriovenous malformation. Mayo Clin Proc 1978, 53:607–611.
39. Prager RL, Laws KH, Bender HW: Arteriovenous fistula of the lung. Ann Thorac Surg 1983, 36(2):231–239.
40. Maldonado JE, Sheps SG, Bernatz PE, et al: Renal arteriovenous fistula: A reversible cause of hypertension and heart failure. Am J Med 1964, 37:499–513.
41. Linder F, Vollmar J, Krumhaar D: Die arteriovenosen Fisteln des Pfortadergebietes. Langenbecks Arch Klin Chir 1968, 320:50–63.
42. Lindehauer MS: Congenital arteriovenous fistula. In Rutheford RB (ed): *Vascular Surgery*. Philadelphia, Saunders, 1977, pp 793–800.
43. Graham WP III, Eiseman B, Pryor R: Hepatic artery aneurysm with portal vein fistula in a patient with familial hereditary telangiectasia. Ann Surg 1964, 159:362–367.
44. Malan E, Tardito E, Sala A: Arteriovenous fistulas. In Haimovici H (ed): *Vascular Surgery: Principles and Techniques*. New York, McGraw-Hill, 1976, pp 533–550.
45. Zetterquist S, Bergvall U, Linde B, et al: The validity of some conventional methods for the diagnosis of obliterative arterial disease in the lower limb as evaluated by arteriography. Scand J Clin Lab Invest 1971, 28:409–421.
46. Pisko-Dubienski ZA, Baird RJ, Bayliss CED, et al: Identification and successful treatment of congenital microfistulas with the aid of directional Doppler. Surgery 1975, 78:564–572.
47. Pritchard DA, Maloney JD, Sekard CB, et al: Peripheral arteriovenous fistula. Detection by contrast echocardiography. Mayo Clin Proc March 1977, 52:186–190.
48. Handa J, Handa H, et al: Radioisotopic study of arteriovenous anomalies. AJR 1972, 115:751.
49. Seeger JF, Commody RF: Digital subtraction angiography of the arteries of the head and neck. Radiol Clin North Am 1985, 23:(2)193–210.
50. Picus D, Totty WG: Iatrogenic femoral arteriovenous fistulae evaluation by digital vascular imaging. AJR 1984, 142:567.
51. Webb RW: CT of solitary pulmonary vascular lesions. Semin Roentgenol 1984, 19:189.
52. Hayward RD: Intracranial arteriovenous malformations. Observations after experience with computed tomography. J Neurol Neurosurg Psychiatry 1976, 39:1027.
53. Leblanc R, Ethier R, Little JR: Computerized tomography findings in arteriovenous malformations of the brain. J Neurosurg 1979, 51:765.
54. Terbrugge K, Scotti G, Eithier R, et al: Computed tomography in intracranial arteriovenous malformations. Radiology 1977, 122:703.
55. Wallace HJ: The conservative treatment of hemangiomatous nevi. Br J Plast Surg 1953, 6:78.
56. Fry WJ: Surgical considerations in congenital arteriovenous fistulas. Surg Clin North Am February 1974, 54(1):165–174.
57. Riche MC, Hadjean E, Tran-Ba Huy P et al: The treatment of capillary-venous malformations using a new fibrosing agent. Plast Reconstr Surg 1983, 71:607.
58. Ogawa Y, Inoue K: Electrothrombosis as a treatment of cirsoid

angioma in the face and scalp and varicosities of the leg. Plast Reconstr Surg 1982, 70:310.

59. Hidano A, Ogihara Y: Cryotherapy with solid carbon dioxide in the treatment of nevus flammeus. J Dermatol Surg Oncol 1977, 3:213.
60. Conway H, McKinney P, Climo M: Permanent camouflage of vascular nevi of the face by intradermal injection of insoluble pigments (tattooing): Experience through twenty years with 1022 cases. Plast Reconstr Surg 1967, 40P:457.
61. Brown JB, Cannon B, McDowell A: Permanent pigment injection of capillary hemangiomata. Plast Reconstr Surg 1946, 1:106.
62. Apfelberg DB, Maser MR, Lash H: The argon laser for cutaneous lesions. JAMA 1981, 245:2073.
63. Cosman B: Clinical experience in the laser therapy of port-wine stains. Lasers Surg Med 1980, 1:133.
64. Noe JM, Barsky SH, Geer DE, et al: Port-wine stains and the response to argon laser therapy: Successful treatment and the predictive role of color, age and biopsy. Plast Reconstr Surg 1980, 65:130.
65. Phillips JF, Yao JST: Congenital vascular malformations. In Neiman HL, Yao JST (eds): *Angiography of Vascular Disease.* New York, Churchill Livingstone, 1985, pp 393–419.
66. Pevsner PH: Micro balloon catheter for superselective angiography and therapeutic occlusion. AJR 1977, 128:225.
67. Olcott C, Newton TH, Stoney RJ: Intra-arterial embolization in the management of arteriovenous malformations. Surgery January 1976, 79(1)3–12.
68. Demuth RJ, Miller SK, Keller F: Complications of embolization treatment for problem cavernous hemangioma. Ann Plast Surg August 1984, 13(20):135–144.
69. Rosch J, Dotter CT, Brown MJ: Selective arterial embolization: A new method for control of acute gastrointestinal bleeding. Radiology 1972, 102:303.
70. Kerber CW, Freeny PC, Cromwell L, et al: Cyanoacrylate occlusion of renal arteriovenous fistula. AJR 1977, 128:663.
71. Bookstein JJ, Chlosta RM, Foley D, et al: Transcatheter hemostasis of gastrointestinal bleeding using modified autogenous clot. Radiology 1974, 113:277.
72. Stein BM: General techniques for the surgical removal of arteriovenous malformations. In Wilson CB, Stein BM (eds): *Intracranial Arteriovenous Malformations.* Current Neurosurgical Practice. Baltimore, Williams and Wilkins, 1984.
73. Wolpert SM, Stein BM: Catheter embolization of intracranial arteriovenous malformations as an aid to surgical excision. Neuroradiology 1975, 10:13.
74. Stein BM, Wolpert SM: Surgical and embolic treatment of cerebral arteriovenous malformations. Surg Neurol 1977, 7:359.
75. Hilal SK, Sane P, Maward ME, et al: Therapeutic interventional radiologic procedures in neuroradiology. In Abrams H (ed): *Abrams Angiography,* ed 3. Boston, Little, Brown, 1983.
76. Backlund EO, Arnt J, Dahlin H, et al: Radiosurgery in intracranial arteriovenous malformations. Int Congr Neurol Surg 1978, 433:162.
77. Steiner L, Backlund EO, Greitz T, et al: Radiosurgery in intracranial arteriovenous malformations. Int Congr Neurol Surg 1978, 433:168.

PART ELEVEN

Infection, Amputation, Transplantation, and Sexual Function

Chapter 70

THE PREVENTION AND MANAGEMENT OF PROSTHETIC GRAFT INFECTION

JOHN A. C. BUCKELS and SAMUEL E. WILSON

Infection of a prosthetic graft is the most serious complication of vascular reconstructive surgery. Even though graft sepsis is uncommon, it carries grave consequences with significant risk of loss of life or limb. The prevention and treatment of prosthetic graft infection has therefore become a major topic of concern for vascular surgeons.

Significance

The incidence of graft infection reported in the literature varies between 1.5 and 6 percent (1–5). The highest incidences were seen in some of the earliest reports, and several authors have noted that with experience there is a reduction in the incidence. (1,2). Nonetheless the majority of reports indicate a continuing incidence of 2 to 3 percent over the last two decades (Table 70-1). The reported mortality rate of graft sepsis varies between 20 and 75 percent (1–5). The mortality rate is highest if the aortic anastomosis is involved and lowest for distal infections. Conversely the amputation rate is highest for cases with distal sepsis.

TABLE 70-1. Incidence of Prosthetic Graft Infections

Author (Ref.)	Study Period	Number of Grafts	Number of Infections
Hoffert et al. (4)	1955–1962	201	12 (6%)
Conn et al. (3)	1959–1969	435	22 (5%)
Szilagyi et al. (2)	1952–1971	2145	33 (1.5%)
Bouhoutsos et al. (12)	1957–1972	532	14 (2.6%)
Goldstone et al. (1)	1959–1973	566	14 (2.5%)
Jamieson et al. (11)	1955–1973	664	15 (2.3%)
Liekweg et al. (5)	1965–1974	859	22 (2.6%)

One difficulty in reviewing earlier results is the lack of definition in reporting, with some authors not differentiating between graft and wound infections. Szilagyi and colleagues (2) divided incisional infections into three grades according to depth of involvement. Grades I and II involved skin and subcutaneous tissue, and grade III was reserved for infections involving the arterial prosthesis itself. However, in order to accurately classify graft infections it is important to further specify type of graft material, graft site, and whether the graft alone or anatomoses (proximal or distal) are involved, as well as the time of presentation (early or late). Recently Bunt (6) has proposed a classification of graft infection (GIF), graft enteric erosion (GEE), graft enteric fistula (GEF), and aortic stump sepsis (ASS), and these terms will be used in this text.

Historical Note

In 1912 Alexis Carrel demonstrated that blood flow through a prosthetic tube was possible on a long-term basis and so laid one of the foundations of vascular surgery. Nevertheless it was many years before clinical arterial bypass was undertaken, and initially arterial homografts were used. It was not until 1951 that a synthetic prosthesis (Vinyon N) was inserted (7). Shortly afterward the first secondary aortoenteric fistula originating from an aortic bifurcation homograft was reported (8), and in 1956 came the first account of a secondary aortoenteric fistula occurring after aortic aneurysm replacement with a nylon graft (9). Since then over 500 cases of graft infection have been recorded. These recommendations are based on the principles of surgical management which have been evolved by earlier workers together with recommendations from our own experiences.

Pathophysiology

The three main postulated mechanisms of infection of prosthetic grafts are operative contamination, mechanical erosion, and bacteremia, and these will be considered in turn.

OPERATIVE CONTAMINATION

Potential sources of contamination at the time of graft insertion include natural skin flora, divided lymphatics and lymph nodes in the presence of distal sepsis, intestinal bag contents, aneurysm contents, lack of aseptic technique during emergency procedures, and concurrent nonvascular surgery.

Operative contamination from skin flora is most likely during groin procedures due to the proximity of the prosthesis to the skin and the high bacterial counts in the inguinal region (10). Several authors (2,11,12) have noted a significant reduction in graft sepsis if the distal anastomosis is above rather than below the inguinal ligament, though factors other than skin bacterial count can be implicated. Vertical groin incisions tend to gape when the hip is flexed, and in obese patients the wound lies buried between two moist skin surfaces. Hence wound breakdown and hematoma formation are not uncommon, and both predispose to secondary infection of the prosthetic graft.

Divided lymphatics and lymph nodes in the presence of distal sepsis have often been quoted as sources of graft contamination (1,13), though there is little experimental data to support this view. Bouhoutsos et al. (12) were unable to culture bacteria from groin lymph nodes in patients with culture-positive distal sepsis, and in a similar unpublished study (Buckels) we have had the same findings.

Cultures from Lahey bag effluents during aortic surgery have yielded positive growth in 2.5 to 14 percent of cases (14–16), though no related episodes of graft sepsis were recorded. Positive cultures from aneurysm contents may be of greater significance. Several reports have documented a 10 to 23 percentage of positive cultures from the aneurysm wall or contents (15,16); one report showed that the incidence was greater in symptomatic and ruptured aneurysms, though only one related graft infection occurred. Recently Buckels et al. (17) reported a significantly higher incidence of graft infections if the aneurysm contents culture was positive than if it was negative, and they recommend routine cultures with prolonged antibiotic therapy if positive cultures are obtained.

Emergency procedures, particularly repair of ruptured aortic aneurysms, have been accompanied by higher graft infection rates (11,13). This may in part be due to failure to adhere strictly to aseptic techniques, though other factors such as fitness of the patient and the high incidence of positive bacterial cultures from ruptured aneurysms can also be implicated.

The practice of concurrent nonvascular procedures during vascular reconstruction cannot be commended. Some authors have reported patients undergoing additional procedures such as cholecystectomy, appendectomy, gastrectomy, and even colonic resection without incident (18,19). However Goldstone and Moore (1) noted a predisposing factor in 7 of their 14 cases of graft sepsis of which 2 had undergone incidental appendectomy, and Becker and Blundell (13) noted 3 of their 14 patients with graft infection had undergone concomitant surgery, one gastrectomy and two cholecystectomies. A recent review of aneurysm patients undergoing a second surgical procedure found a higher complication rate among patients who had an additional cholecystectomy, though the overall mortality rate was unchanged (20).

MECHANICAL EROSION

The pathogenesis of graft enteric erosion (GEE) is generally accepted to be caused by mechanical erosion by a pulsatile graft into locally adherent bowel. However opinion is divided as to the etiology of graft enteric fistula (GEF). GEF also was initially considered to be caused by simple mechanical factors, though two recent reports have produced clinical and experimental evidence supporting a primary infectious etiology of at least some fistulas (21,22). Moreover Busuttil et al. (22) found that 5 of 11 GEFs communicated via a pseudoaneurysm, Buchbinder et al. (23) noted that 7 of 16 GEFs did so; and the former proposed that graft infection at the aortic suture line led to pseudoaneurysm formation which subsequently eroded into the bowel. Further, though indirect, support for a primary infectious etiology comes from Wilson et al. (24) who noted a high incidence of gram-positive aerobic cocci (not normal duodenal or small-bowel flora) in GEFs presenting within the first postoperative year.

BACTEREMIA

Bacteremia as a source of clinical graft infection has been reported infrequently, though the true incidence of this mechanism is difficult to assess. Goldstone and Moore (1) documented a single instance in 14 patients with graft sepsis, and Szilagyi et al. (2) reported an incidence of 1 in 40. More recently Cormier et al. (25) postulated a bacteremic origin for 4 of their unit's 8 cases of graft infection. It is likely that this route of graft infection has been underdiagnosed because the bacteremic seeding occurs some time before clinical recognition of graft sepsis and therefore the initial bacteremic episode is not identified.

Most of the evidence for bacteremic infection comes from animal studies. Malone et al. (26) placed Dacron aortic grafts in dogs given intravenous infusions of 1×10^7 *Staphylococcus aureus* at successive time intervals. They found graft infection rates of 100 percent during the first 2 weeks, but this was reduced to 57 percent at 3 months and to 30 percent at 1 year. Histological studies showed that infection occurred at areas of absent or incomplete pseudointima, with an infection rate of 95 percent for those with an incomplete lining compared to 0 percent for those fully lined. Other studies have shown that percutaneous infection of grafts in dogs could spread to the proximal or distal anastomoses if the graft was not well incorporated into the surrounding tissues (27).

Clinical Presentation

ONSET

The majority of vascular graft infections occur early in the postoperative period with up to half being evident in the first month and three-quarters in the first 3 months (1,2,12). It is of interest that reports of graft sepsis with a high incidence in the first 3 postoperative months contain a high proportion of distal bypass infections (2,12), compared to reports of predominantly proximal bypass infections which occurred much later at mean times of 8 to 15 months (1,28). The presentation of GEFs is even later, with a mean postoperative interval of 32 months (24).

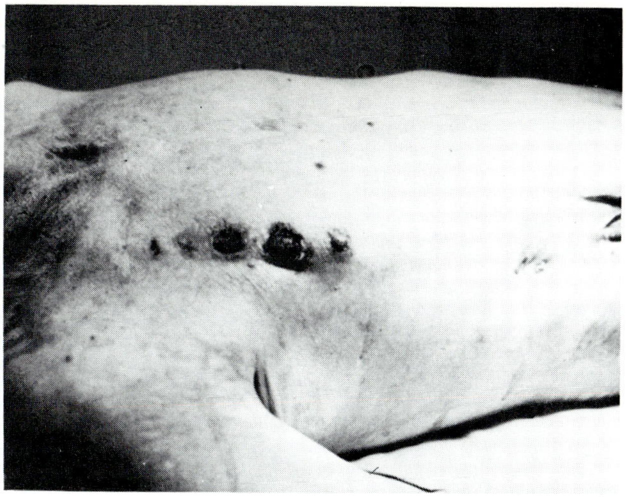

FIGURE 70-1. Skin necrosis overlying infected axillofemoral prosthesis.

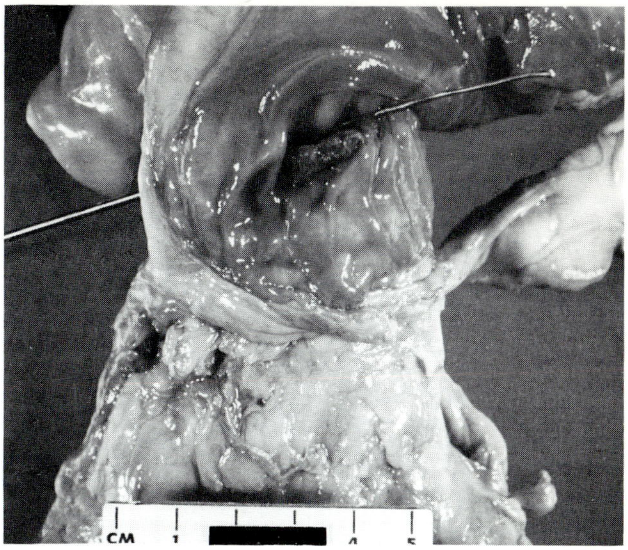

FIGURE 70-2. Postmortem specimen of aortoduodenal fistula. Prosthesis is lying behind duodenum with probe passed through fistulous opening. Note adherent clot in duodenal lumen.

SYMPTOMS AND SIGNS

Early infections usually present around the superficial portions of the graft with wound erythema leading to wound breakdown and discharge of pus. The inguinal incision is the site of graft infection in 57 to 77 percent of cases (1,2). Moreover, procedures which necessitate an inguinal incision have a two to three times greater likelihood of graft sepsis than those which do not. Szilagyi et al. (2) found that aortobifemoral graft procedures had an incidence of graft sepsis of 1.6 percent compared to 0.7 percent for aortoiliac bypass, and Jamieson et al. (11) noted a graft infection rate of 3.2 percent for operations with an inguinal incision compared to 0.9 percent for operations without an inguinal wound.

Drainage of a wound abscess over a superficial portion of an infected graft usually leads to either a persistent sinus or wound breakdown with exposure of the prosthesis (Figure 70-1). Presentation can occur at any time up to 6 months with the prosthetic infection manifesting as a small sinus tract in the inguinal incision, occasionally mistaken for a stitch abscess. Other associated events can include thrombosis and septic embolization. If the anastomosis is involved, false aneurysm formation and major hemorrhage are likely.

Intraabdominal graft infections tend to be more occult in the early stages. Fever, rigors, raised leukocyte count, or unusual symptoms may be early clues to graft infection. Later developments include abdominal pain with or without false aneurysm formation and eventually hemorrhage. This may be intraperitoneal, or if a GEE or GEF is present, major gastrointestinal bleeding (Figure 70-2). This is not usually immediately fatal, and many patients have an initial small "herald bleed" allowing planned treatment.

Diagnosis

A high index of suspicion is the key to the early diagnosis of graft infection. Any patient with a vascular prosthesis who develops signs of sepsis should be considered to have a graft infection until proved otherwise. Furthermore any patient with a prosthetic intraabdominal or retroperitoneal graft who develops gastrointestinal bleeding should be managed as a case of GEE or GEF until proved otherwise.

Grafts in the femoropopliteal or axillofemoral areas can be monitored for local signs of infection such as wound erythema, discharge, or hematoma formation. If there is a possibility of deep wound infection or graft involvement, exploration and drainage or removal should be undertaken as a diagnostic procedure and appropriate cultures can be taken for bacteriological identification. One difficulty that can arise is hemorrhage in the early postoperative period which may be due to infection or to technical problems such as graft or suture failure or poor host tissues. This can only be delineated by subsequent bacteriological identification from deep wound cultures, and the advisability of vascular defect repair usually has to be judged by local factors. Venous and "downstream" arterial blood cultures are unlikely to be helpful unless a GEE or GEF is present.

Specific diagnostic techniques that have been used include sinography, ultrasound, needle aspiration, intravenous urography, arteriography, isotope and computerized tomography (CT) scanning, and in cases of suspected GEE and GEF, barium contrast studies and endoscopy.

If a sinus exists, sinography can demonstrate involvement of the graft (Figure 70-3) and also the extent of graft infection (Figure 70-4). Ultrasonography can demonstrate cystic areas around a graft and even pseudoaneurysm formation, though neither is specific for graft infection. Ultrasonography is more useful in the femoral region or where a graft lies superficially since minor collections around the aorta or its branches can be difficult to detect because of overlying intestinal gas. Ultrasonography is

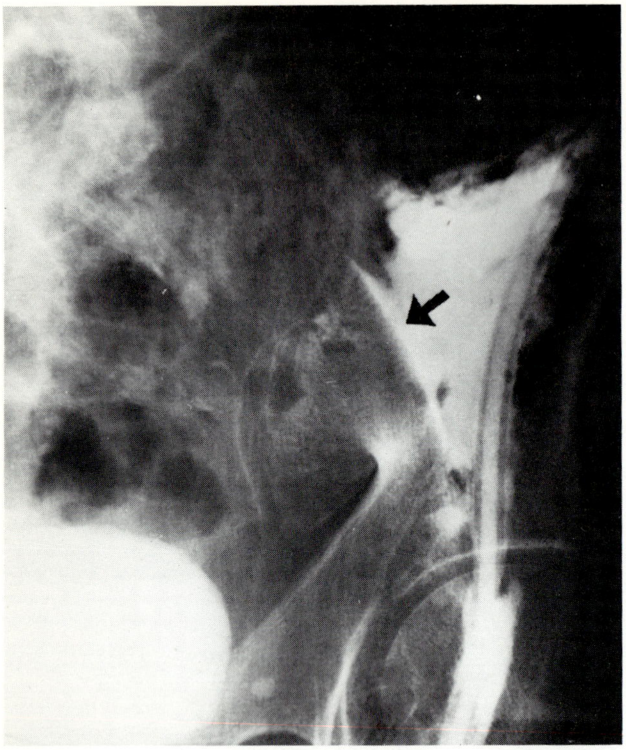

FIGURE 70-3. Contrast injected through groin sinus overlying femoral limb of a bifurcation graft showing typical coiled-spring appearance of the crimped prosthesis (*arrow*).

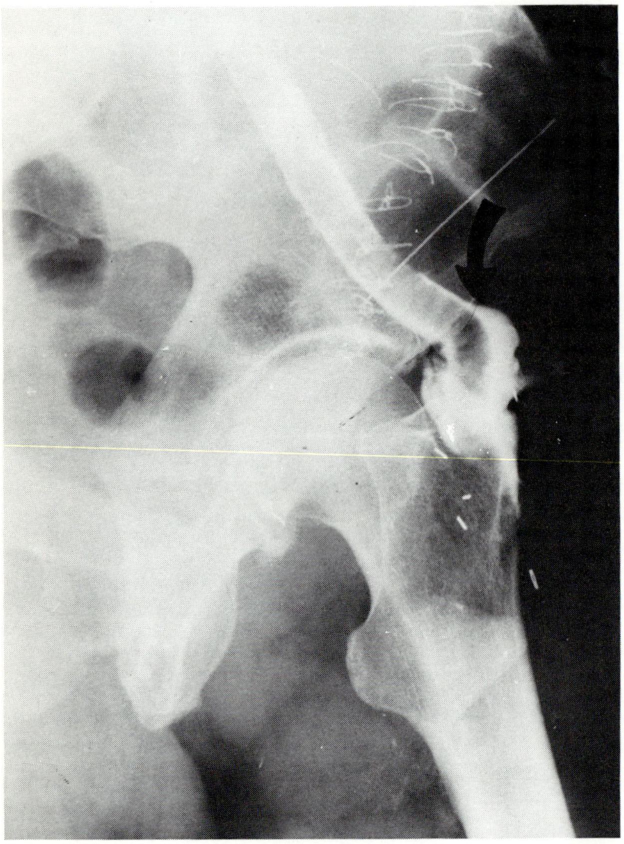

FIGURE 70-4. Sinogram showing involvement of retroperitoneal portion of left limb of bifurcation graft.

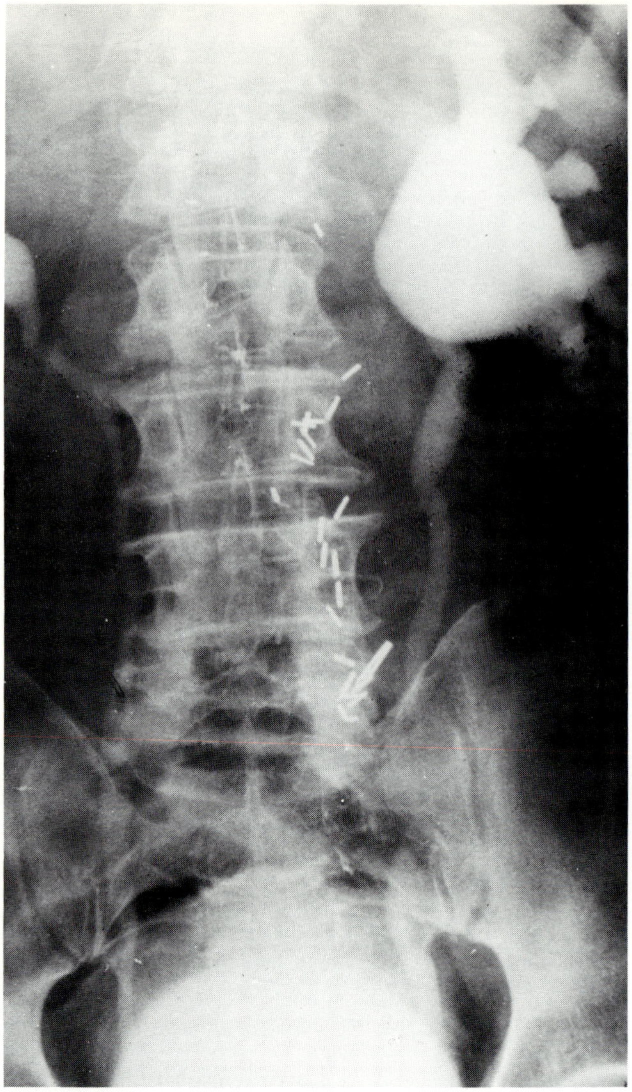

FIGURE 70-5. Intravenous urogram showing left hydronephrosis in a patient with an infected aortic graft.

particularly useful in aiding needle aspiration of any collection around a graft, which is then cultured and if positive enables precise antibiotic therapy.

With suspected infection of a retroperitoneal graft, an excretory urogram may show ureteral obstruction on the side of the infected limb (Figure 70-5). Arteriography has been advocated but is only useful in detecting thrombus or pseudoaneurysm formation. This is clinically useful but not diagnostic of infection. However if performed during active bleeding caused by a GEF, confirmation of a communication between the bloodstream and the intestine can be made (Figure 70-6). Isotope scanning using gallium-67, technetium-99m, and indium-111 has been used. Indium-111–labeled leukocytes seem to be the most specific, though false-positive scans do occur (29). A major limitation with isotopes is that a false-positive scan is more likely if the test is performed within the first postoperative month. Contamination of the white blood cells with platelets may lead to focal isotope uptake in the graft due to platelet deposition in the pseudointima, yielding a falsely positive study. CT scanning can delineate periaortic abnormalities, and the finding of "gas pock-

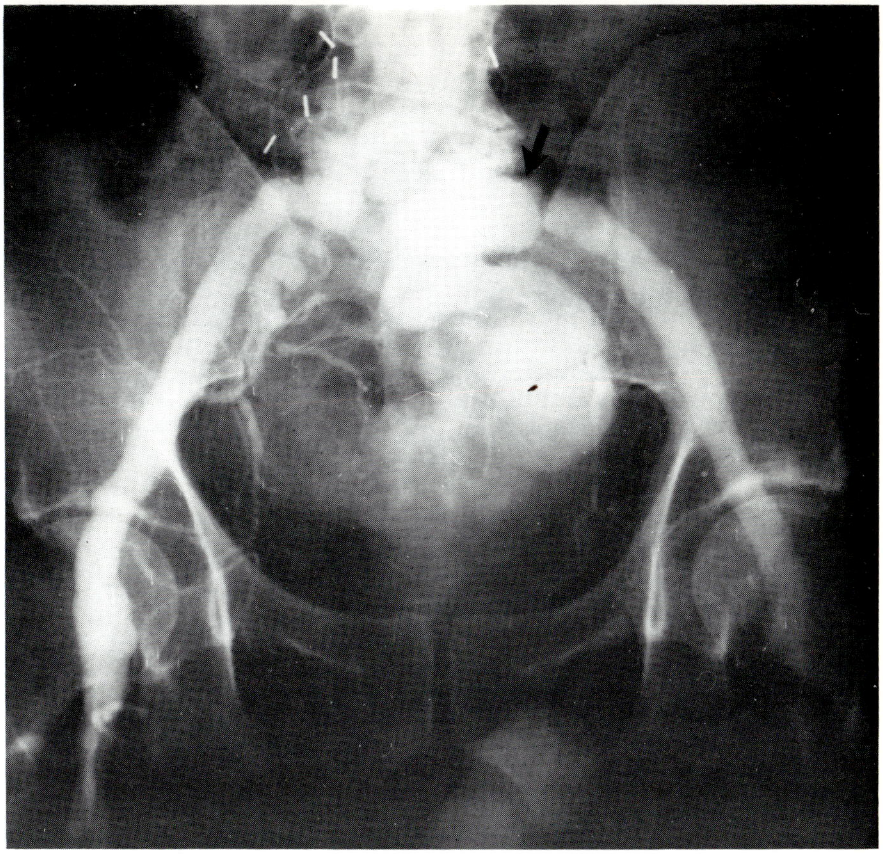

FIGURE 70-6. Arteriogram demonstrating graft enteric fistula. Contrast is seen in the rectum coming from the proximal anastomosis of a left iliofemoral bypass graft.

ets'' in the location of the graft is diagnostic of infection. Because the majority of infecting organisms are nonenteric, this sign is likely to be helpful in only a minority of cases. CT scanning can detect small periaortic fluid collections and false aneurysms, and this approach should prove to be increasingly useful in the earlier diagnosis of aortic graft infections.

Barium studies can be helpful in patients with a GEE or GEF who do not require emergency surgery. Though a negative result does not exclude graft involvement, barium outlining the crimped pattern of the graft producing a ''coiled-spring'' appearance is diagnostic of GEE or GEF. Other findings include duodenal obstruction, suggesting compression from a false aneurysm. Patients who present with massive gastrointestinal bleeding require immediate laparotomy and aortic control.

Upper gastrointestinal endoscopy is useful in patients who present with an initial ''herald'' bleed which stops or who have a slow rate of bleeding. This should be carried out in the operating room with the patient and surgeon prepared for immediate laparotomy. Cases have been recorded of graft visualization or bleeding from the third or fourth part of the duodenum which is diagnostic of a GEE or GEF. Other proximal lesions may be seen even in the presence of a GEE or GEF, and only if these are actively bleeding is the diagnosis of GEE or GEF unlikely.

Prevention

PERIOPERATIVE PREVENTION TECHNIQUES

An obsessional adherence to strict aseptic techniques at all times is good surgical practice but is mandatory for vascular prosthetic operations. The preparation of a wide expanse of skin is frequently necessary in complex reconstructions, and in these cases a plastic adhesive drape impregnated with povidone-iodine is a useful adjunct. Other aspects of perioperative management are important in the prevention of graft infections. In an extensive review of surgical wounds, Cruse and Foord (30) found an overall infection rate for ''clean'' wounds of 1.8 percent, though the rate for ''clean'' vascular wounds was 3.7 percent. Delaying skin shaving from the night before an operation to immediately before surgery reduced the wound infection rate from 2.3 to 0.9 percent. Skin preparation with soap and alcohol carried a wound infection rate of 2.0 percent versus 1.2 percent with povidone-iodine and chlorhexidine. The same authors also found that increasing the length of preoperative hospitalization increased the risk of wound sepsis from 1.1 percent for less than 24 hours, to 2 percent for more than 1 week, and to 4.3 percent for more than 2 weeks. The duration of surgery increased the rate from 1.4 percent for less than 1 hour, to 2.8 percent for 1 to 2 hours, and to 4.4 percent for 2 to 3 hours.

Preoperative angiography has been implicated as another risk factor. Landreneau and Raju (31) found that transfemoral angiography during the week prior to surgery was associated with an increase in groin wound infections of which 81 percent occurred on the side of arterial puncture.

OPERATIVE PREVENTION TECHNIQUES

A number of operative techniques have been advocated to reduce the risk of graft infection. Most are recommended, even though unproved, because they are based on sound theory and their success can be judged by the low incidence of graft sepsis reported by many of their proponents.

The higher incidence of wound infections if inguinal anastomoses are employed supports the view that suprainguinal anastomoses should be constructed if anatomically sound. If an inguinal anastomosis is required, an oblique rather than a vertical incision is recommended in order to reduce the likelihood of superficial wound disruption.

Several techniques have been proposed to isolate the aortic anastomosis from the intestine in addition to reconstituting the peritoneum over the grafts, or in patients with an aneurysm, closure of the sac. These include covering the aortic anastomosis with a cuff of graft (32), mobilizing the duodenum to the right and not replacing it over the graft (33), and covering the graft with omentum (34). Avoidance of any bowing of the graft has led some surgeons to routinely use an end-to-end aortic anastomosis, and Sauvage (35) recommends a common tailored low-profile anastomosis made from the two limbs to reduce the bulky common lumen of the prosthesis.

Prophylaxis

Though there are sound theoretical grounds for using prophylactic systemic antibiotics (implant of foreign body and serious consequences if graft infection ensues), there are minimal controlled data to support their administration. Given the low incidence of graft sepsis, very large numbers of patients would be required to reach any statistically valid conclusion, and such a study has yet to be reported. Several authors have recorded admirably low graft sepsis rates without the routine use of antibiotics. However, several prospective well-controlled large studies show reduced wound infection rates with antibiotic prophylaxis (36,37), though the small numbers of infections precluded a statistically significant effect on graft infection rates. Because the incidence of wound infection overall is approximately 5 percent and is likely to lead to graft infection in some cases, prophylaxis against the common pathogens is recommended and it is our practice to use antibiotics (e.g., a cephalosporin) active against *S. aureus* and the common gram-negative organisms during the perioperative period. Moreover if positive cultures are obtained from distal septic lesions or aneurysm contents, organism-specific antibiotics should be given on a therapeutic basis. Details of the pathogens most commonly isolated from infected grafts are given in Table 70-2.

TABLE 70-2. Bacteria Isolated from Infected Grafts

	Graft Infection	Graft Enteric Erosion	Graft Enteric Fistula
Patients studied	205	32	85
Organisms:			
S. aureus	43%	10%	13%
S albus	14%	—	4%
Escherichia coli	17%	27%	23%
Proteus	8%	3%	6%
Klebsiella	4%	10%	7%
Pseudomonas	10%	17%	3%
Streptococci	—	23%	20%
Anaerobes	—	3%	13%
Other	4%	7%	11%

SOURCE: Data compiled from Bunt (6) and Wilson et al. (24).

Antibiotic impregnation or bonding of the prosthetic graft, akin to the aminoglycoside-containing cement used in arthroplasty, is an attractive concept which may have future applications in the prevention and management of graft infection. This has been effective in animal models, providing protection from both topical contamination (38) and bacteremic challenge (39), and clinical results are awaited.

Treatment and Outcome

A review of the literature reveals that the greatest likelihood of a successful outcome requires graft excision with extraanatomic revascularization if distal ischemia is present, together with antibiotic therapy (Table 70-3). The techniques of graft excision and revascularization depend on the site of graft infection, extent of graft involvement, and type of graft infection, i.e., GIF, GEE, or GEF.

Local care has been advocated by Kwaan and Connolly (40), who reported that 9 of 10 cases with femoral graft infection treated by wound debridement and povidone-iodine irrigation functioned for 1 to 4 years. These were a selected group, and though wound cultures were positive, it is difficult to know if the graft matrix itself was infected. This form of therapy might be considered for high-risk patients if there is no evidence of proximal infection, blood cultures are negative, and there is no history of bleeding and no anastomotic involvement; otherwise conventional methods of graft excision and revascularization should be used.

FEMOROPOPLITEAL GRAFTS

These carry lower mortality rates though higher amputation rates than most other graft infections. Infected prosthetic femoropopliteal grafts should be excised. Revascularization, if required, should be performed either in situ using autogenous ma-

TABLE 70-3. **Treatment and Outcome of Prosthetic Graft Infection**

	Local Treatment		Graft Excision		Graft Excision Plus Bypass	
Site	A, %	M, %	A, %	M, %	A, %	M, %
Femoropopliteal	16	16	48	4	33	16
Aortoiliac	—	50	23	45	8	33
Aortofemoral	6	29	27	35	11	20
GEE	—	73	—	70	—	18
GEF	—	94	—	74	—	46

KEY: A = amputation, M = mortality.
SOURCE: Data compiled from Bunt (6).

terial (41) or using a polytetrafluoroethylene (PTFE) graft inserted as an extended extraanatomical bypass, avoiding the infected field such as a femorotibial or crossover femoropopliteal-femorotibial graft as appropriate. The mortality rate for this mode of treatment is around 10 to 15 percent, but the amputation rate can be zero in such cases (42). Patients treated by graft excision alone have a low mortality but higher amputation rate. Local care has been advocated (40), but as discussed earlier, it is unlikely that many of the cases were true grade III graft infections.

AORTOILIAC GRAFTS

Patients with infection of aortoiliac grafts not associated with intraabdominal or gastrointestinal hemorrhage (i.e., not anastomotic and not GEE or GEF) should be started on broad-spectrum or organism-specific antibiotics prior to surgery. Because the body of the graft is usually involved, total graft removal is required. If the original anastomoses were end-to-side, the vessel defects can be closed by simple approximation or with autogenous vein patches. If the original aortic anastomosis was end-to-end, the aortic stump should be closed in two layers with monofilament sutures and then buttressed with prevertebral fascia. Debridement of the infected tissues around the graft site is then performed and the retroperitoneum drained with catheters which can be used for local antibiotic irrigation. The aortic stump should finally be covered with omentum which will not prevent aortic blowout but can prevent subsequent aortoduodenal fistulization.

In patients in whom graft thrombosis has occurred, or those in which the original grafting was for occlusive disease, immediate reconstruction is not usually required. If the graft is patent or the original pathology was aneurysmal disease, a decision about immediate revascularization should be made on clinical grounds aided by Doppler and pulse-volume recordings (43). The most satisfactory reconstructive procedure is axillofemoral or bifemoral bypass (44). Recurrent graft infection can occur, and revascularization should be delayed if possible. We see no advantage in routinely employing extraanatomic bypass procedures prior to removal of infected aortic grafts since bacteremic infection or operative contamination of the new graft is possible. In some patients revascularization before excision of the infected prosthesis may be necessary.

When aortoiliac infection is associated with hemorrhage, the first priority is to obtain proximal aortic control operatively. At laparotomy infrarenal aortic clamping is often difficult due to periaortic adhesions, and more proximal control by clamping the aorta at the diaphragmatic hiatus should be used. In patients with a large pseudoaneurysm, intraaortic tamponade using a Foley catheter or Fogarty venous thrombectomy catheter can be effective. The principles of management as outlined above are then followed with additional closure or excision of any involved viscus in cases of GEE or GEF.

Untreated aortoiliac graft infections are uniformly fatal. Graft excision without revascularization carries a 50 to 75 percent mortality rate, and the greatest likelihood of survival has been with graft excision and revascularization. Though the overall mortality rate in reported cases has been around 40 percent, recent series have shown survival rates up to 84 percent (21). Early diagnosis has a major bearing on outcome, and in a recent report of GEFs there was a significant difference in timing of operative therapy between survivors (2.2 days) and nonsurvivors (12.4 days) (45).

AORTOFEMORAL GRAFTS

The main differences between aortofemoral infections and aortoiliac infections (as outlined above) are the occurrence of sepsis involving only one limb of a graft and the means of providing reconstruction through a noninfected field. For unilateral groin infection we recommend retroperitoneal detachment of the affected limb with inguinal excision (46). If the leg remains viable, delayed reconstruction is performed as a crossover femorofemoral or femoropopliteal graft. Should immediate revascularization be required, we recommend either an obturator bypass or a crossover graft brought through a clean operative field and anastomosed at a point distal to the original graft insertion.

AXILLOFEMORAL GRAFTS

Infection of an axillofemoral graft is a particularly grave complication because the original indication was likely to have been either vascular bypass for limb salvage in a high-risk patient or following excision of an infected intraabdominal graft. Patient survival requires removal of the infected graft, and in some cases an intraabdominal graft can be inserted, though the amputation and mortality rates for these patients are high. Such cases emphasize the need for a prosthesis which is truly infection-resistant.

Summary

1. Prosthetic graft infection is uncommon (less than 3 percent) but carries unacceptably high morbidity and mortality rates.

2. Treatment is graft excision, and revascularization, when required, should be delayed if possible and performed through an extraanatomic route.

3. Earlier diagnosis improves outcome, and a high index of suspicion should be maintained at all times. Late infections may present with unusual symptoms.

4. Prevention is better than cure. In addition to a strict aseptic technique, we recommend prophylactic antibiotics for all patients receiving prosthetic grafts.

5. Future developments such as antibiotic graft impregnation may be useful in high-risk patients and may help in the management of patients with established graft sepsis.

References

1. Goldstone J, Moore WS: Infection in vascular prostheses. Am J Surg 1974, 118:225–233.
2. Szilagyi DE, Smith RF, Elliott JP, Vrandecic MP: Infection in arterial reconstruction with synthetic grafts. Ann Surg 1972, 176:321–333.
3. Conn JH, Hardy JD, Chavez CM, Fain WR: Infected arterial grafts. Ann Surg 1970, 171:704–712.
4. Hoffert PW, Gensler S, Haimovici H: Infection complicating arterial grafts. Arch Surg 1965, 90:427–435.
5. Liekweg WG, Greenfield LJ: Vascular prosthetic infections: Collected experience and results of treatment. Surgery 1977, 81:335–342.
6. Bunt TJ: Synthetic vascular graft infections. Surgery 1983, 93:733–746.
7. Voorhees AB, Jaretzki A, Blakemore AH: The use of tubes constructed from Vinyon "N" cloth in bridging arterial defects. Ann Surg 1952, 135:332–336.
8. Brock RC: Aortic homografting—A report of six successful cases. Guys Hosp Rep 1953, 102:204–228.
9. Claytor H, Birch L, Cardwell ES, Zimmerman SL: Suture line rupture of a nylon aortic bifurcation graft into the small bowel. Arch Surg 1956, 73:947–950.
10. Ulrich JA: Dynamics of bacterial skin populations. In Maibach HI, Hildick-Smith G (eds): *Skin Bacteria and Their Role in Infection*. New York, McGraw-Hill, 1965.
11. Jamieson GG, DeWeese JA, Rob CG: Infected arterial grafts. Ann Surg 1975, 181:850–852.
12. Bouhoutsos J, Chavatzas D, Martin P, Morris T: Infected synthetic arterial grafts. Br J Surg 1974, 61:108–111.
13. Becker RM, Blundell PE: Infected aortic bifurcation grafts: Experience with fourteen patients. Surgery 1976, 80:544–549.
14. Russell HE, Barnes RW, Baker WA: Sterility of intestinal transudate during aortic reconstructive procedures. Arch Surg 1975, 110:402–404.
15. Ernst CB, Campbell HC, Daugherty ME, Sachatello CR, Griffen WO: Incidence and significance of intra-operative bacterial cultures during abdominal aortic aneurysmectomy. Ann Surg 1977, 185:626–633.
16. Scobie K, McPhail N, Barber G, Elder R: Bacteriologic monitoring in abdominal aortic surgery. Can J Surg 1979, 22:368–371.
17. Buckels JAC, Black J, Fielding JWL, Ashton F, Slaney G: The significance of positive bacterial cultures from aortic aneurysm contents. Br J Surg 1985, 72:440–442.
18. DeBakey ME, Ochsner J, Cooley DA: Associated intraabdominal lesions encountered during resection of aortic aneurysms. Dis Colon Rectum 1960, 3:485.
19. Hardy JD, Tomkins WC, Chavez CM, Conn JH: Combining intraabdominal arterial grafting with gastrointestinal or biliary tract procedure. Am J Surg 1973, 126:598–600.
20. Bickerstaff LK, Hollier LH, VanPeenen HJ, Melton LJ, Pairolero PC, Cherry KJ: Abdominal aortic aneurysm repair combined with a second surgical procedure—Morbidity and mortality. Surgery 1984, 95:487–491.
21. Perdue GD, Smith RB, Ansley JD, Constantino MJ: Impending aortoenteric hemorrhage: The effect of early recognition on improved outcome. Ann Surg 1980, 192:237–243.
22. Busuttil RW, Rees WR, Baker JD, Wilson SE: Pathogenesis of aortoduodenal fistula: Experimental and clinical correlates. Surgery 1979, 85:1–13.
23. Buchbinder D, Leather R, Shah D, Karmody A: Pathologic interactions between prosthetic aortic grafts and the gastrointestinal tract. Am J Surg 1980, 140:192–198.
24. Wilson SE, Bennion RS, Serota AI, Williams RA: Bacteriological implications in the pathogenesis of secondary aortoenteric fistulas. Br J Surg 1982, 69:545–548.
25. Cormier JM, Ward AS, Lagneau P, Janneau D: Infection complicating aortoiliac surgery. J Cardiovasc Surg 1980, 21:303–314.
26. Malone JM, Moore WS, Campagne J, Bean B: Bacteremic infectability of vascular grafts: The influence of pseudointimal integrity and duration of graft function. Surgery 1975, 78:211–216.
27. Weber TR, Lindenauer SM, Miller TA, Salles CA, Ramsburgh S, Gleich P: Focal infection of aortofemoral prostheses. Surgery 1976, 79:310–312.
28. Fry WJ, Lindenauer SM: Infection complicating the use of plastic arterial implants. Arch Surg 1967, 94:600–609.
29. Serota AI, Williams RA, Rose JG, Wilson SE: Uptake of radiolabelled leukocytes in prosthetic graft infection. Surgery 1981, 90:35–40.
30. Cruse PJE, Foord R: A five-year prospective study of 23,649 surgical wounds. Arch Surg 1973, 107:206–210.
31. Landreneau MD, Raju S: Infections after elective bypass surgery for lower limb ischemia: The influence of preoperative transcutaneous arteriography. Surgery 1981, 90:956–961.
32. Sapirstein W: A method of reinforcing vascular prosthetic anastomosis. Surgery 1971, 70:744–745.
33. Miller DR: Prevention of aortoduodenal fistula by duodenal reflection. Am J Surg 1979, 138:332–333.
34. Javid H, Julian OC, Dye WS, Hunter JA: Complications of abdominal aortic grafts. Arch Surg 1962, 85:650–662.
35. Sauvage LR: A crimped external velour knitted Dacron prosthesis for aortoiliac replacement or bypass. In Wright CB, Hobson RW, Hiratzka LR, Lynch TG (eds): *Vascular Grafting*. Boston, John Wright PSG, 1983.
36. Kaiser AB, Clayson KR, Mulherin JL, Roach AC, Allen TR, Edwards WH, Dale WA: Antibiotic prophylaxis in vascular surgery. Ann Surg 1978, 188:283–289.
37. Chester JF, Fergusson CM, Chant AD: The effect of cephadrine prophylaxis on wound infection after arterial surgery through a groin incision. Ann R Coll Surg Engl 1983, 65:389–390.
38. Greco RS, Harvey RA, Henry R, Prahlad A: Prevention of graft infection by antibiotic bonding. Surg Forum 1980, 31:29–30.

39. Moore WS, Chvapil M, Seiffert G, Keown K: Development of an infection resistant vascular prosthesis. Arch Surg 1981, 116:1403–1407.

40. Kwaan JH, Connolly JE: Successful management of prosthetic graft infection with continuous povidone-iodine irrigation. Arch Surg 1981, 116:716–720.

41. Ehrenfeld WK, Wilbur BC, Olcott CN, Stoney RJ: Autogenous tissue reconstruction in the management of infected prosthetic grafts. Surgery 1979, 85:82–92.

42. Greenfield LJ, Liekweg WG: Management of vascular prosthetic infections. In *Graft Materials in Vascular Surgery*. Miami, Florida, Symposium Specialists, Inc., 1978.

43. O'Donnell TF, Crossman D, Callow AD: Noninvasive intraoperative monitoring: A prospective study comparing Doppler systolic occlusion pressure and segmental plethysmography. Am J Surg 1978, 135:539–546.

44. Blaisdell FW, Hall AD: Axillary-femoral artery bypass for lower extremity ischemia. Surgery 1963, 54:563–568.

45. Kleinman LH, Towne JB, Bernhard VM: A diagnostic and therapeutic approach to aortoenteric fistulas: Clinical experience with twenty patients. Surgery 1979, 86:868–880.

46. Bennion RS, Hiatt JR, Williams RA, Wilson SE: Surgical management of unilateral groin infection after aortofemoral bypass. Surg Gynecol Obstet 1983, 156:724–728.

Chapter 71

AMPUTATIONS IN THE DYSVASCULAR PATIENT

GEOFFREY H. WHITE

Indications for Amputation

Vascular disease is the primary indication for amputation in more than 80 percent of cases (1,2). Most of these patients are more than 60 years of age, and the ratio of males to females is 9:1 (3). However, the concept of limb salvage by vascular bypass surgery has received considerable attention during recent years, and with advances in surgical techniques, prosthetic bypass materials, and patient selection criteria, the severely ischemic limb can often be saved (4–7). In other instances the amputation level can be improved by lower extremity revascularization (8). For example, prior or simultaneous arterial reconstruction may allow for local amputation of a toe or forefoot in the patient who might otherwise have required major amputation at the below-knee or above-knee level. If vascular reconstruction is not possible, then a local resection of the toe or forefoot will usually be successful only if there is localized small-vessel disese such as that due to diabetic arterial disease, microemboli from proximal vessel atherosclerotic plaques, vasospastic disorders (9), vasculitis (10), or blood hyperviscosity (11). In these conditions there may be clear-cut demarcation of necrotic tissue, with the rest of the foot being unaffected. This is the ideal indication for local resection. The presence of severe ischemia of the foot, marked dependency rubor, or widespread infection contraindicates local amputation (12).

In general terms the indications for amputation in the dysvascular patient are (1) incapacitating pain at rest, (2) ulceration, (3) gangrene, (4) uncontrolled sepsis, and (5) failed minor amputation. In some cases it is difficult to decide whether a complicated bypass graft, as opposed to a primary amputation, should be attempted in a limb with poor distal runoff (13,14). Previously, primary amputation was favored in many of these patients because it was felt that the mortality and morbidity of complicated bypass procedures was prohibitive, especially if several bypass operations may have become necessary due to early failure. In some of these patients, sympathectomy is an acceptable alternative, either by surgical lumbar sympathetic chain division (15) or by phenol injection block (12).

Recent studies indicate that in the high-risk patient, the risks of a peripheral bypass and of a major amputation are about equal (12). In other words the same high-risk patients tend to do poorly following either bypass grafting or amputation. If arteriograms do not demonstrate distal vessels suitable for bypass, or if for other reasons it is not anticipated that a bypass graft would remain patent for at least 6 months to 1 year, then early amputation may be preferred (16). However, with the recent tendency toward attempts at limb salvage, other options include exploration of the popliteal artery for on-table arteriography to define previously undetected distal vessels (14,17) or exploration of the tibial vessels themselves as a prelude to distal bypass. Sometimes even the vessels of the foot may be revascularized. Such heroic attempts are pointless if the patient does not have the ability to ambulate on the extremity once healing is achieved or if the anticipated required level of amputation will not be significantly improved.

A further factor is the available bypass material. If the patient has a good saphenous vein, then attempts at revascularization of vessels distal to the popliteal are more likely to meet with long-term success than if a prosthetic material will be required (18,19). However, if the indication for bypass is a nonhealing ulceration rather than rest pain, then healing may occur before the graft occludes and amputation is avoided in a significant number of these patients (16).

In general the mortality of the various procedures depends not so much on the procedure itself but on the presence or absence of severe risk factors, although above-knee amputation does carry a higher operative mortality risk than below-knee amputation (20,21). The most important risk factors are ischemic heart disease, previous myocardial infarction, cardiac arrhythmia, congestive cardiac failure, severe pulmonary disease, and uncontrolled hypertension (13).

AMPUTATION FOR ACUTE ISCHEMIA

Acute ischemia causing tissue necrosis presents a special management problem. If the patient has presented late, with irreversible tissue loss accompanied by systematic intoxication or myoglobinuria (due to myonecrosis), then arterial reconstruction is not warranted and urgent amputation is indicated. This also applies if there is extensive or invasive infection.

Limbs with lesser degrees of acute tissue ischemia may often be salvageable by arterial bypass or embolectomy, usually combined with compartment fasciotomy. Therefore if the signs of ischemia are not irreversible, then the patient should be studied by preoperative or operative angiography with a view to proceeding to thromboembolectomy or bypass if possible. In some of these cases limb salvage is not totally achieved, but the patient may at least become suitable for amputation at a more favorable level.

Determination of the preferred level of amputation is difficult in the presence of acute ischemia. If there are no indications for urgent operation, then the ischemic areas may be observed for signs of improvement due to developing collateral blood flow. Heparin anticoagulation or thrombolytic therapy are employed in selected patients with evidence of acute thrombosis (22).

AMPUTATION IN THE DIABETIC PATIENT

Diabetics are at special risk of developing leg ischemia and gangrene. In fact, gangrene is more than 50 times as frequent in diabetic patients over 40 years of age than in nondiabetic patients of the same age (23). The combination of large-vessel atherosclerosis, small-vessel angiopathy, and neuropathy causes a high incidence of lower extremity ischemia, often with infection. Gibbons reported that more than 80 percent of diabetic patients who had presented to the hospital with foot sepsis had limb-threatening infections (24). Fearon et al. studied 100 diabetics who required a below-knee amputation and found that 93 percent had severe ischemia and 79 percent had significant infection (25). Twenty percent of these patients had previously undergone arterial reconstructive procedures.

Bacterial cultures of infected lesions in diabetic patients usually yield multiple organisms, with a mixture of anaerobes and aerobes. The principle pathogens are usually *Staphylococcus*, *Enterococcus*, other streptococcal organisms, *Pseudomonas*, *Proteus*, and *Escherichia coli*. Underlying osteomyelitis is frequently present at the time of presentation (26). Because of the virulence and invasiveness of foot infections in the diabetic, delay in surgical control can lead to loss of the foot or fatal sepsis (25). The foot should be carefully examined for deep infection. Areas with abscess, suppuration, or invasion of tendon sheaths and plantar fascia should be treated urgently by incision and drainage, wide debridement, or local amputation. If the vascularity of the foot is good, then usually no further procedure will be necessary (Figure 71-1). However, with irretrievable, poor vascularity, definitive amputation may then be carried out after the septic condition has been controlled. In some cases when the heel or the proximal tissues are already involved, primary below-knee amputation is indicated, rather than local procedure (Figure 71-2).

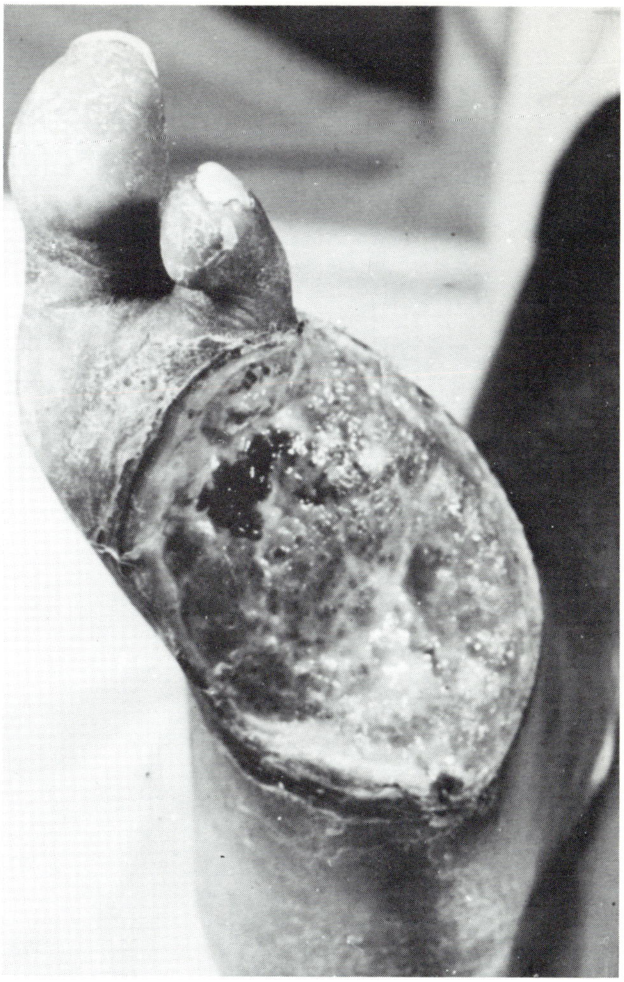

FIGURE 71-1. Local amputation of infected, gangrenous toes in a foot with otherwise good vascular supply resulted in successful salvage of the foot.

In general, surgical wounds in diabetics tend to have a higher incidence of infection (27) and delayed healing (26,28) than in nondiabetic patients. However, the presence of diabetes does not seem to significantly affect the rate of amputation stump healing or infection (29). In fact, diabetics without concomitant large-vessel atherosclerosis are more successful in achieving primary stump healing than nondiabetic atherosclerotic patients (30,31).

Preoperative Management

Preoperative care involves treatment of the affected limb, stabilization of the patient's general medical condition, and preparation for a prosthesis, including exercises if practical.

The patient should be restricted to bed rest, and the foot should be protected from trauma and pressure ulceration by the use of a bed cradle and sheepskin or foam rubber heel protectors. The foot is washed with soap and water at least twice daily and carefully dried. Povidone-iodine (Betadine) is applied to necrotic or ulcerated areas, and weeping toes are separated with gauze swabs or cotton wool. Cellulitis and lymphangitis are treated with intravenous antibiotics, while abscesses or closed-space infections require early drainage and debridement. Pain should be treated adequately with narcotic analgesics.

A thorough assessment is made of the patient's cardiac, res-

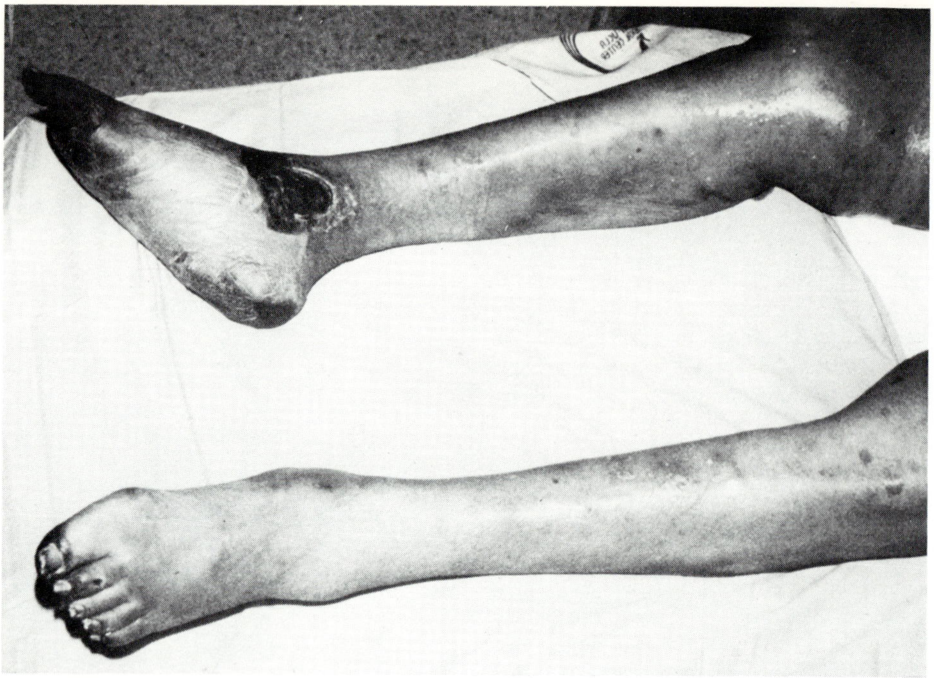

FIGURE 71-2. Ulceration or necrosis of the heel or ankle are contraindications to local amputation. Below-knee amputation was necessary.

piratory, and renal systems. Even if urgent amputation is required, a period of 4 to 8 hours for the stabilization of diabetes, cardiac failure, and fluid and electrolyte imbalance can be invaluable. Diabetes is frequently out of control and may be best managed by a sliding-scale insulin regime or insulin infusion together with intravenous fluid replacement. If longer preoperative time is available, this process of stabilization of the patient's general medical condition is a priority. A full assessment is made of the risk factors for surgery, and in selected cases where limb salvage or an improved level of amputation may be possible with revascularization, angiography is performed complemented by noninvsive vascular investigation. These investigations may also give valuable information concerning the likelihood of primary wound healing at a selected level of amputation. However, the angiogram findings do not contribute to the determination of amputation level.

The patient is informed of the plans for prosthesis and, if practical, should be seen by the prosthetist and physical therapist before surgery. Limb and joint mobilization exercises and strengthening procedures are commenced at this stage. A team approach to rehabilitation introduced at this stage fosters a positive attitude between staff and patient, stressing the expectations for restoration of ambulation.

Principles of Amputation Surgery

The commonly used major lower-limb amputations are shown in Figure 71-3. The main guiding philosophy is that amputation, when necessary, should be performed at the most distal possible site where healing is likely to occur and that the knee joint should be preserved in as many cases as possible. In comparison to amputations below the level of the knee joint, above-knee amputation has a higher operative mortality rate (21), with a far lower rate of patient independence and return to ambulation (with a prosthesis). The loss of mobility caused by absence of the flexible knee joint and the loss of proprioceptive sense from the joint lining renders the use of a prosthesis far more difficult and doubles the amount of energy that needs to be used for mobilization (32). Even when lying in bed, the above-knee amputee is at a disadvantage because the added length of the below-knee procedure enables greater leverage for movement and rolling. A list of the principal amputations used in dysvascular patients is given in Table 71-1.

A tourniquet should never be used during amputation in the dysvascular patient because of the risk of further compromising the arterial supply to the area of the amputation stump. Intraoperative hemorrhage is usually not troublesome because of the nature of the patient's vascular disease. Antibiotic prophylaxis is always employed because of the risk of anaerobic infection in the severely ischemic limb, including gas gangrene. If a patient has gross infection of the limb at the time of surgery, then intense therapeutic antibiotic regimes should be followed. Infected areas and necrotic tissue should be well wrapped and protected at the time of operation to prevent direct contamination of the amputation wound. Perioperative antibiotics also decrease preoperative bacteremia and infection dissemination during operative transection of contaminated lymphatics (33).

In making the skin incision the surgeon must take care to avoid undermining and hence devascularizing the skin, especially if a flap technique is being followed. The tissues should

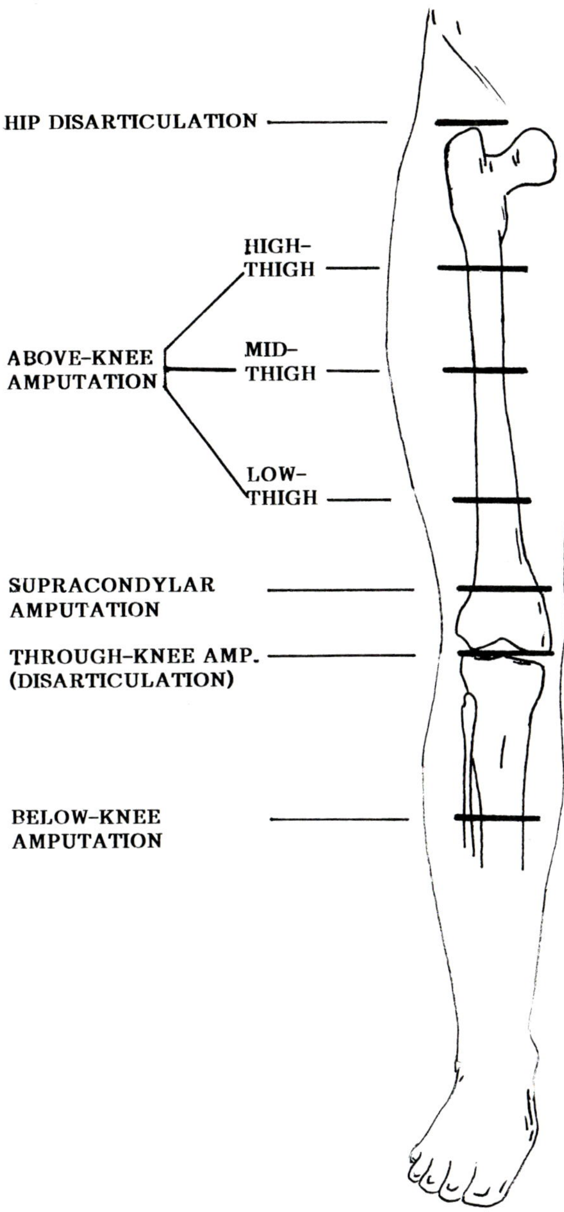

FIGURE 71-3. Common levels for major amputations of the lower limb.

TABLE 71-1. Principal Amputations Used in the Dysvascular Patient

Toe amputation:
  Transphalangeal
  Transmetatarsal

Forefoot amputation—transmetatarsal
Amputation at the ankle—Syme amputation
Below-knee amputation
Through-knee amputation

Above-knee amputation:
  Supracondylar
  Midthigh
  High-thigh

be handled gently at all times, avoiding the use of traumatic instruments such as firm clamps, retractors, or sharp forceps on the skin and muscle areas. Long plantar flaps are used in the calf, foot, and toes because of the superior blood supply to the plantar aspect of the lower leg. Bone is always transected several centimeters proximal to the other structures, at a level high enough to permit the soft tissue to approximate, producing a good covering. Sharp, bony spicules are smoothed from the edge with a file or rasp. Surrounding muscle bulk is used to cover and protect the bone end, especially for weight-bearing stumps. The muscle bulk is transected slightly proximal to the fascial and skin layers to allow for wound closure without bulging or tension. Nerves are ligated and divided as high as possible to help prevent formation of amputation neuroma.

Hemostasis should be meticulous so that wound drains will not be necessary, as these probably increase the incidence of wound infection and wound breakdown (21,29,34). The skin must never be sutured under tension and may be left open if there is local infection.

Intensive efforts are made toward early limb and joint mobilization postoperatively, and rehabilitation should commence as soon as the patient has recovered from the operation, aided by preoperative instruction, preparation, and exercises.

Surgical Techniques of Amputation

AMPUTATION OF THE TOE (TRANSPHALANGEAL LEVEL)

Well-demarcated gangrene of the tip of a single toe or of several toes may be allowed to proceed naturally to autoamputation in many cases. However, localized amputation is preferable if the involved toe is painful or if there is infection in the form of cellulitis, discharging ulceration, or osteomyelitis. This may be done at the transphalangeal level when there is no spread of infection or necrosis into the forefoot and when the arterial supply to the rest of the foot is adequate for wound healing. Often arterial bypass will be necessary prior to amputation.

The skin incision may be circular or may incorporate anterior and posterior or lateral flaps (see Figure 71-4*A*). Access to the line of incision is provided by retracting adjacent toes with a rolled gauze (rather than traumatizing the tissue with metal retractors) and gripping the toe with a towel forceps. The initial incision is made to the depth of the bone, avoiding undermining the skin. The bone is then cleared of attached tendons and is usually divided midway through the proximal phalanx using bone cutters or bone rongeurs. The bone may require further shortening to allow closure of the skin without tension.

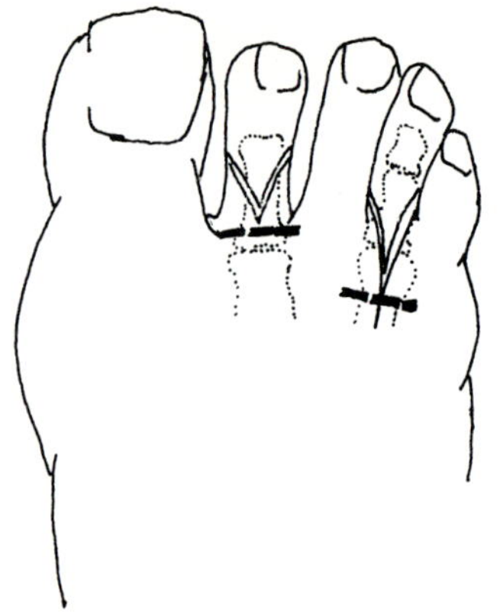

A

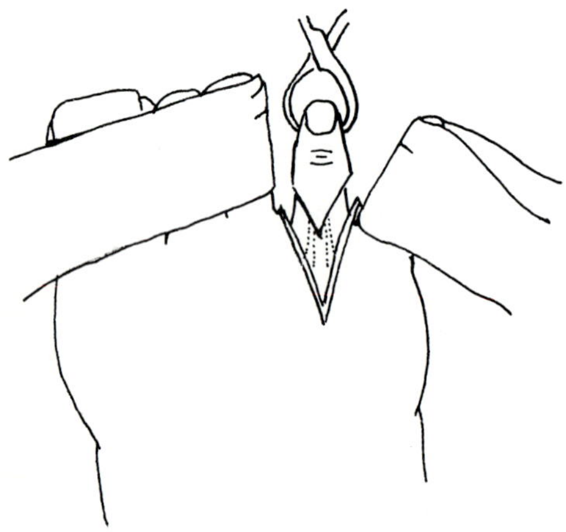

B

FIGURE 71-4. (*A*) Incisions for transphalangeal and transmetatarsal amputation of the toe (levels of bone division indicated). (***B***) Ray amputation incision onto the dorsum of the foot to expose head of metatarsal.

If infection is present, it is preferable not to close the wound; otherwise the skin may be loosely approximated with interrupted sutures, usually nylon or polypropylene.

In most cases the patient may commence ambulation on the day following surgery.

RAY AMPUTATION OF THE TOE (TRANSMETATARSAL LEVEL)

When infection or necrosis of a single toe involves the whole of the skin of the toe or a small part of the adjacent forefoot, then a ray (or wedge) amputation is indicated. Usually this applies to a single toe alone; however, occasionally two adjacent toes may be amputated using this method. The initial incision should be planned so as to conserve all viable skin, to allow for closure of the wound without tension. In the usual case the plantar skin tends to be spared because of its more adequate blood supply. The incision, often referred to as a racquet incision, skirts the necrotic skin of the toe and is then continued a short distance on the dorsum of the foot to allow exposure of the metatarsal head (see Figure 71-4*B*). This incision is similarly taken directly down to the bone, dividing tendons and ligaments without undermining the skin. The metatarsal is cleared of tendons using a periosteal elevator, taking great care to avoid injury to adjacent digital arteries. The bone is then divided through the distal part of the metatarsal, and the affected bone and soft tissues are excised free by a combination of sharp dissection with a scalpel and cutting with heavy scissors. Occasionally, unsuspected infection of the tendon sheaths or fascial planes may be detected extending into the foot at the time of operation; this usually necessitates more proximal amputation. At the conclusion of the procedure, the wound is loosely approximated with interrupted sutures, but it may be best left open if there has been infection.

During both of these techniques of toe amputation, hemostasis should be achieved mainly by gentle pressure, since excessive use of the cautery will encourage further necrosis.

TRANSMETATARSAL AMPUTATION OF THE FOREFOOT

Transmetatarsal amputation is usually employed if there is gangrene involving several toes, especially if one of these is the great toe or if the ischemic or infective process extends too far proximally up the foot to allow for healing of a ray amputation. Once again the ischemic process is usually more severe on the dorsal surface, so the skin incision is designed to allow for a longer plantar flap (Figure 71-5). The line of the dorsal aspect of the skin incision is positioned slightly distal to the line of metatarsal division. The incision is continued down to the metatarsals, and when these are cleared of tendon and ligament, the bones are divided with bone shears or an electric saw. A thick pad of subcutaneous tissue is preserved on the plantar aspect, and the other tissues are dissected away using a scalpel. Further trimming of bone and exposed tendon is performed as necessary to allow for closure of the wound by the plantar flap without tension.

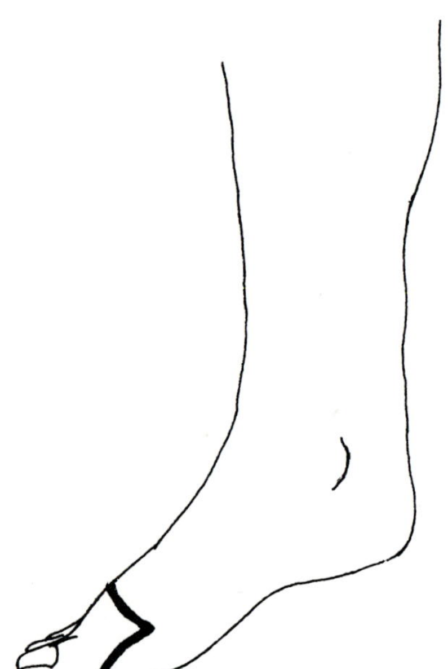

FIGURE 71-5. Incision for transmetatarsal amputation of the forefoot, incorporating plantar flap.

As with all amputations for vascular disease, the skin should always be handled gently, avoiding the use of forceps wherever possible. Interrupted sutures are placed loosely, and the wound may be drained using soft Penrose tubing. A stump dressing is fashioned using gauze pads and elasticized bandage, or a plaster of paris backslab may be applied with the aim of later converting this to a short leg cast to allow early ambulation. Following healing of the transmetatarsal amputation, the patient is usually able to walk satisfactorily without significant disability.

Following recovery the patient's shoe can be modified by padding and arch support.

AMPUTATION AT THE ANKLE (SYME AMPUTATION)

This technique, which is a modification of disarticulation through the ankle joint, was originally described by Syme in 1862 (35). The operation involves excision of the distal joint surface of the tibia and fibula, with a flap of skin from the heel being used to cover the transected bone. This provides a weight-bearing end to the stump and leaves a leg which is only several inches shorter than normal, thus allowing the patient to walk for short distances without a prosthesis. Because of the high potential for ischemic complications, patients should be carefully selected for this procedure. Contraindications include ischemia, ulceration, or infection of the heel. The main indication for this procedure is the presence of well-demarcated gangrene of the forefoot which extends too far up the foot to allow for a successful transmetatarsal procedure but in which there is a well-preserved vascularity of the ankle region and the heel pad. Presence of the popliteal or posterior tibial pulse is very favorable for healing (36,37).

Little (20) advocates this procedure for treatment of the diabetic who has severe infection of the forefoot associated with small-vessel disease but in whom the ankle pulses are often preserved. In these cases the Syme procedure may be best performed as a secondary amputation following earlier local resection of all infected or ischemic tissue. The incision is shown in Figure 71-6*A*. The upper, horizontal line begins on the lateral side of the ankle just below the lateral malleolus and is brought across the front of the ankle joint in a straight line to a point just below the medial malleolus. The lower, vertical part of the incision is carried down across the sole of the foot in front of the heel in a straight line to join the posterior aspects of the ends of the upper incision. The whole of this incision is carried down to bone, carefully avoiding skin undermining and preserving a maximum length of posterior tibial artery. The ankle joint is entered through its anterior aspect, and division of the tendons and ligaments across the front of the ankle allows disarticulation of the talus. The next part of the procedure involves dissecting out the calcaneus with great care to avoid damage to the soft tissue and skin of the heel pad. This is performed using sharp dissection with a scalpel around the calcaneus, staying close to the bone, and dissecting off surrounding fibrous tissue, ligament, and fat. This is usually described as a subperiosteal removal of the calcaneus; however, because of the absence of easily identifiable planes, it is very difficult to stay within a true subperiosteal plane. Completion of excision of the calcaneus is best achieved with the partially disarticulated foot reflected down to allow better exposure. When the calcaneus has been excised, the anterior flap is gently retracted, allowing access to the distal end of the tibia and fibula (Figure 71-6*B*). The articular cartilage is removed with a saw, dividing directly across the lower end of both bones at a level just above the joint. Hemostasis is achieved, and the heel pad is angled up and secured across the cut end of the bones and held in place by closure of the skin, using interrupted sutures of nylon or Prolene which can be left in place for several weeks. The wound may be dressed with layers of gauze held in place by elasticized bandaging, applied with gentle compression so as to minimize edema. Alternatively the stump may be placed within a well-padded plaster of paris cast, which can later be fitted with a rubber stop to allow partial weight bearing.

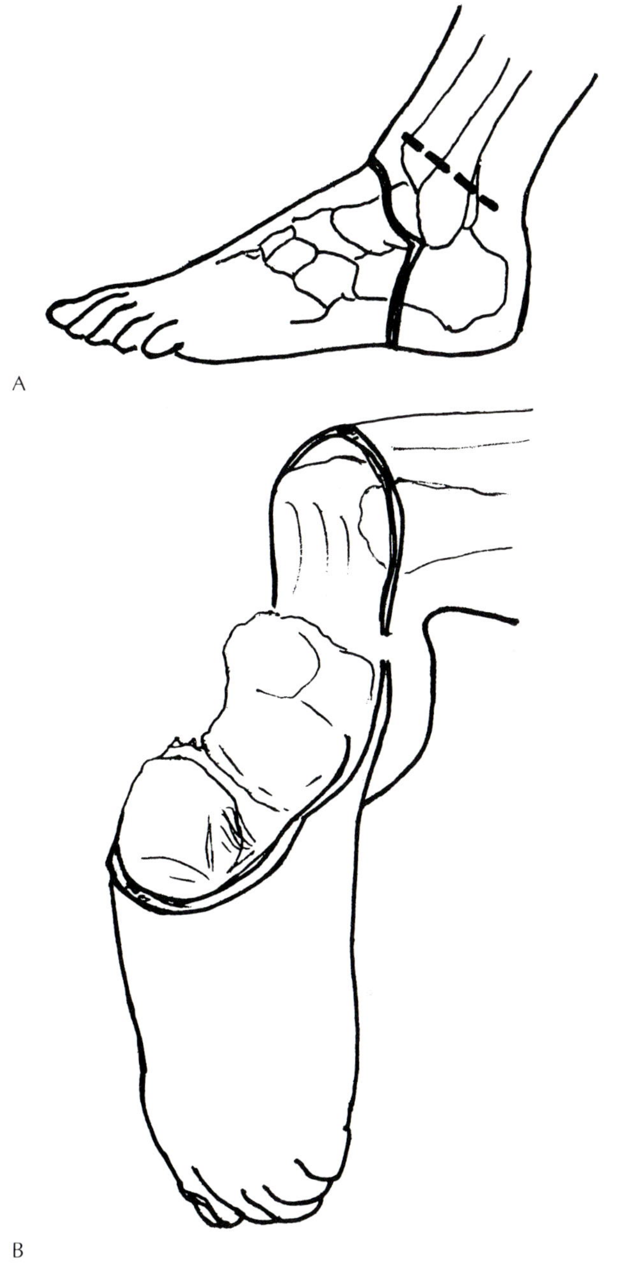

FIGURE 71-6. Syme's amputation. (*A*) Skin incision. (*B*) The disarticulated foot is retracted downward after the joint has been entered and the calcaneus dissected.

BELOW-KNEE AMPUTATION

The general rule that amputation stumps should be as long as possible does not apply for the below-knee amputation, since fitting a prosthesis is more difficult and stump complications are increased if the below-knee stump is too long. The problems of weight bearing and retaining adequate soft tissue to cover the stump are increased with a longer tibia, and since the more distal tissues will tend to have a less adequate blood supply, stump ulceration and pain will be more common. The anterior margin of the tibia is usually beveled (Figure 71-7), and there must be enough solid tissue with good blood supply to cover it, as provided by a long posterior flap. The optimum length of stump is between 5 and 7 in (12 to 18 cm) as measured from the tibial tubercle. However, as little as 2 to 3 in is sufficient for prosthesis fitting, so shorter available length does not dictate above-knee level. As the fibula does not bear the pressure of a prosthesis well, it should be amputated several centimeters higher than the tibia.

Prior to 15 years ago, most amputations for vascular disease were performed at the above-knee level. However, since that time it has been shown that between 70 and 85 percent of all vascular amputations may be performed below the knee with satisfactory healing rates (38,39). Clinical judgment concerning the state of the circulation and nutrition of the skin both preoperatively and intraoperatively has been shown to be an important factor in predicting healing of a below-knee stump (40). If there is good bleeding noted at the time of operation, then the chance of wound healing has been shown to be greater than 90 percent (41) and even in the case where there is little or no bleeding, eventual healing still occurred in 69 percent of cases. It is therefore preferable to decide on the level of amputation, both by clinical judgment and perhaps by special investigations, before the time of surgery, rather than to commence with a below-knee incision with the idea of immediately moving to the above-knee level if necessary.

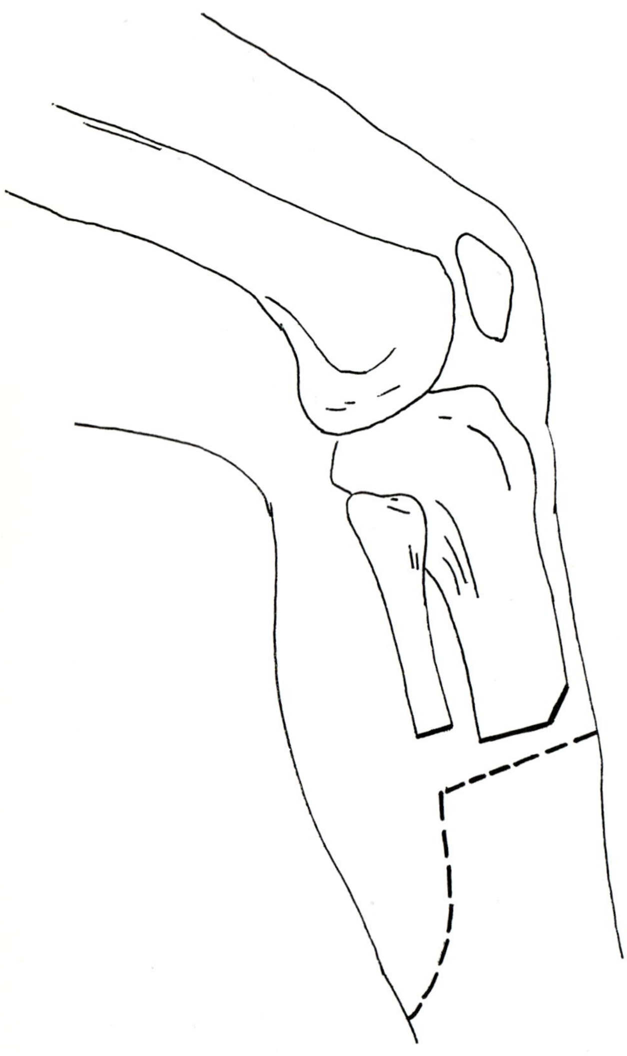

FIGURE 71-7. Posterior myocutaneous flap incision and level of bone section for below-knee amputation.

There are several conditions which dictate that a below-knee amputation should not be performed (Table 71-2). These are

1. Severe joint contractures of the knee or hip. These make prosthesis fitting virtually impossible, and even if this is possible, the functional result will not be satisfactory.
2. Leg spasticity or rigidity due to previous stroke.
3. Severe arthritic changes of the knee. Painful arthritic knee joints will usually not be worth saving because of poor functional result.
4. Skin ulceration or infection extending above the below-knee amputation level. Similarly, questionable or borderline skin viability in the patient confined to bed should prompt selection of a higher level.
5. Deep infection or necrosis of the muscle compartments extending above the midcalf level.
6. Peripheral neuropathy with sensory loss at the amputation level. This will make ulceration of weight-bearing areas of the stump very likely.

In these cases, through-knee amputation is often an acceptable alternative to the above-knee procedure.

There are several incisions described for the below-knee amputation. These include (1) the circumferential, no-flap incision; (2) short, equal anterior and posterior flaps; and (3) long posterior flap (Figure 71-7). As we have used the long posterior flap technique in most cases, the following description will be of this method. The scar for end-bearing stumps should preferably be anterior or posterior to the end of the stump; however, this is not usually applicable to the below-knee amputation where most prostheses are not of the end-bearing type. We have preferred the long posterior myoplastic flap or myocutaneous flap because the superior blood supply of the posterior compartment leads to a higher rate of primary healing and because the muscle bulk of the gastrocnemius gives a good cover for the end of the tibia.

TABLE 71-2. Contraindications to Below-Knee Amputation

Joint contracture of knee or hip
Leg spasticity or rigidity
Severe knee arthritis
Skin ulceration or infection at BKA incision level
Infection or necrosis of leg muscle compartment
Sensory nerve loss at BKA incision level

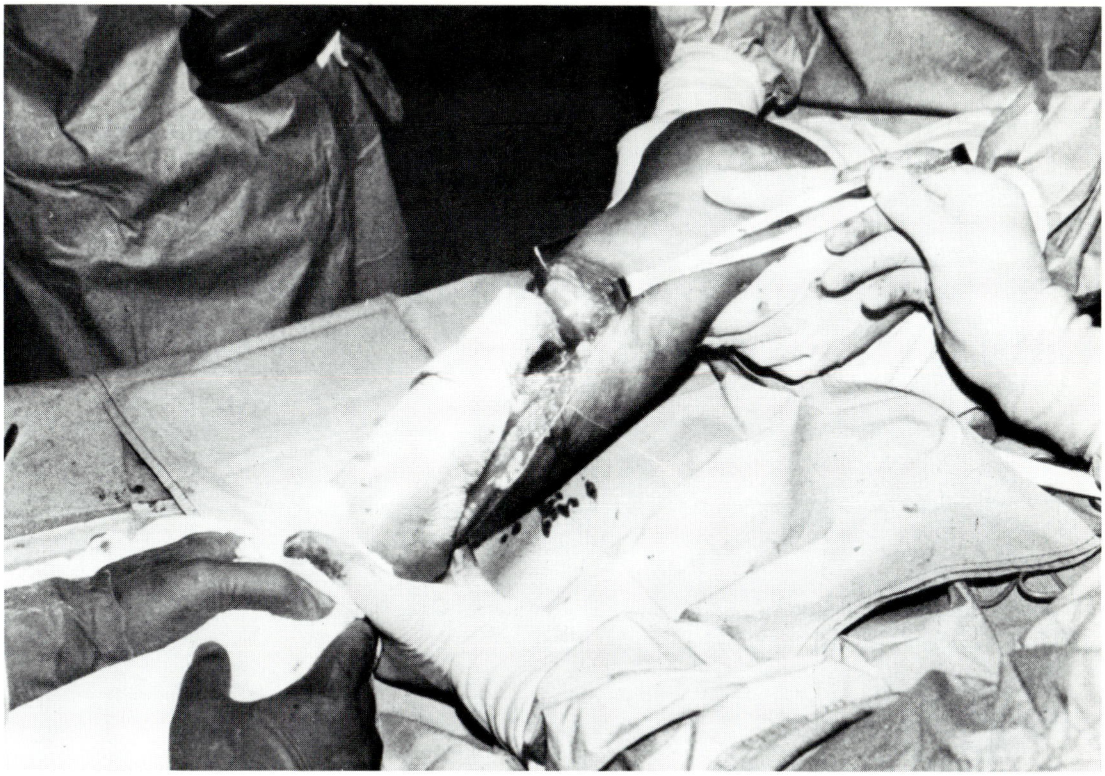

FIGURE 71-8. The bone is sectioned with a saw while the skin is gently retracted.

The incision for this procedure is demonstrated in Figure 71-8. The operation may be performed with general anesthetic, spinal anesthesia, or an epidural. Following skin preparation and draping, the incision is marked on the skin with a marking pen. The anterior or horizontal aspect of the incision continues back to a point just behind the fibula laterally and to the corresponding point on the medial side of the leg, and from these points the posterior or vertical line of the incision is taken down to form a long, curved, posterior flap of a length sufficient to cover the stump. The skin incision is deepened through the deep fascia in a single cut perpendicular to the skin so as to avoid undermining. The two saphenous veins and several tributaries are ligated. The incision is then deepened through the muscle of the anterior compartment at a level several centimeters distal to the proposed line of division of the tibia.

Either the tibia or the fibula may be divided first, depending on the surgeon's preference. If the tibia is to be divided first, then the surrounding muscles are divided in the same line as the skin incision back to the level of the posterior border of the tibia. The anterior tibial neurovascular bundle is identified and the vessels ligated prior to section. The bone is cleared of muscle on all sides using a scalpel and a periosteal elevator. The tibia may then be divided using a hand saw, Gigli saw, or electric saw. The anterior surface is usually beveled prior to sectioning the main part of the bone. The fibula is similarly cleared of muscle, and the posterior tibial neuromuscular bundle and peroneal vessels are ligated when exposed (Figure 71-9). At this stage the main muscle bulk of the leg will have been divided in a line perpendicular to the skin (Figure 71-8), and the posterior myocutaneous flap may now be completed using a long amputation knife to divide obliquely the soleus and gastrocnemius muscles. Bleeding vessels and venous sinuses are ligated; it is important to achieve good hemostasis to avoid the formation of postoperative hematomas. Nerves are stretched down, ligated and divided, and allowed to retract.

The bone ends are smoothed with a file, then the wound is irrigated and closed in two layers, approximating first the layers of the deep fascia by bringing the posterior flap forward over

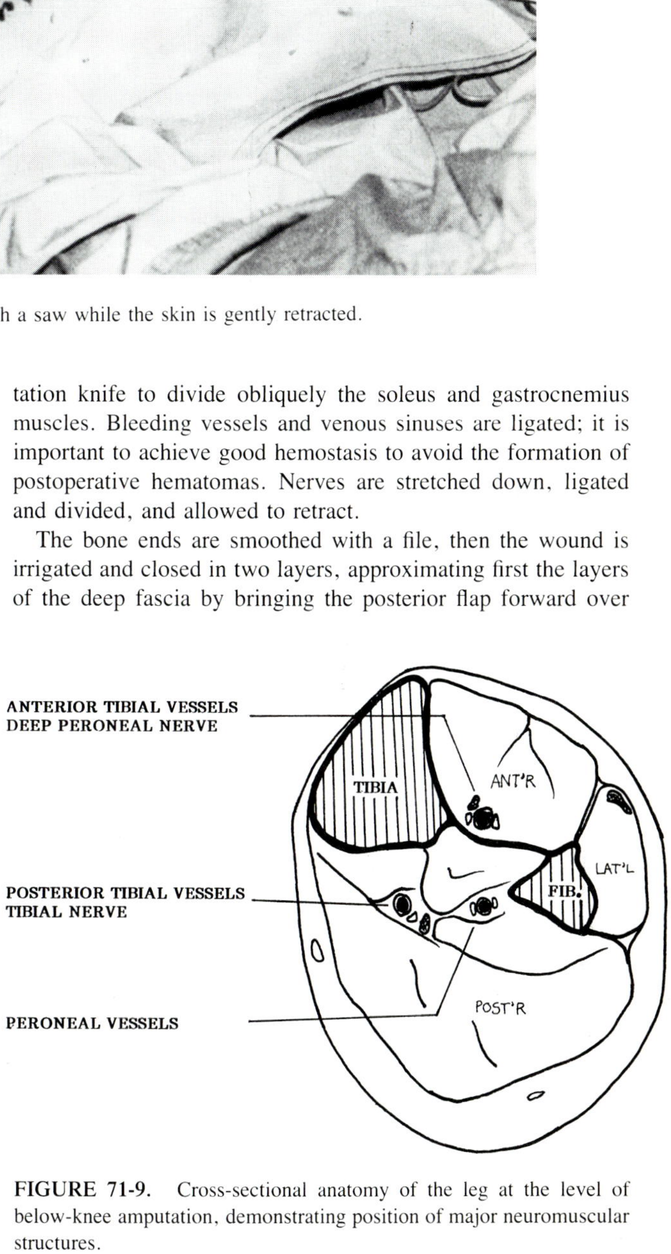

FIGURE 71-9. Cross-sectional anatomy of the leg at the level of below-knee amputation, demonstrating position of major neuromuscular structures.

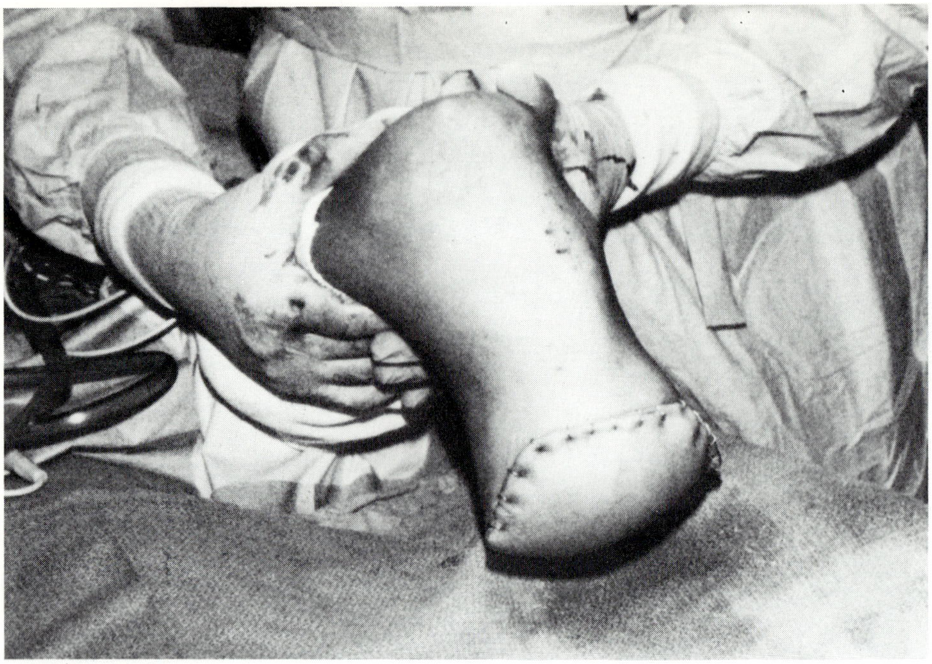

FIGURE 71-10. The stump is closed without tension, allowing dog ears to mold into the shape of the stump over several weeks.

the ends of the bone to be sutured to the thin anterior fascia and to the periosteum and finally closing the skin with interrupted sutures, avoiding tension (Figure 71-10). Skin apposition must be precise, since delay of epitheliazation is likely if there are any gaps between the skin edges because of the reduced vascularity. No attempt is made to trim dog ears as these will mold into the general shape of the stump after several weeks. Closed suction drains may be used but are generally not necessary. A thick dressing of gauze pads and cotton wool bandaging is then applied, and the final layer may be elastic Ace bandages or a plaster of paris cast.

ABOVE-KNEE AND THROUGH-KNEE AMPUTATION

Many techniques of the above-knee amputation have been reported—in general these are all variations of a similar operative procedure. The distal supracondylar amputation and Gritti-Stokes techniques have lost popularity because of the realization that the through-knee amputation has the advantage of preserving proprioceptive areas of the joint and affords greater bone length which makes manipulation of prosthesis simpler. Otherwise the general rule for above-knee amputation is that the maximum bone length should be conserved within the bounds of the patient's vascular problem.

Myodesis procedures, where the muscles are sutured or otherwise fixed to holes drilled in the bone, are generally not encouraged in the dysvascular patient because these are longer, more complicated procedures which are probably no more effective in the long term in these patients. It is far simpler to divide the muscles distal to the site of bone division and then to suture antagonistic groups over the end of the bone stump, anchoring them to each other and to periosteum. This allows for preservation of muscle activity and gives a good covering for the bone.

The skin incision usually employs equal anterior and posterior flaps (fish-mouth incision) as shown in Figure 71-11; however, a circumferential skin incision is just as effective.

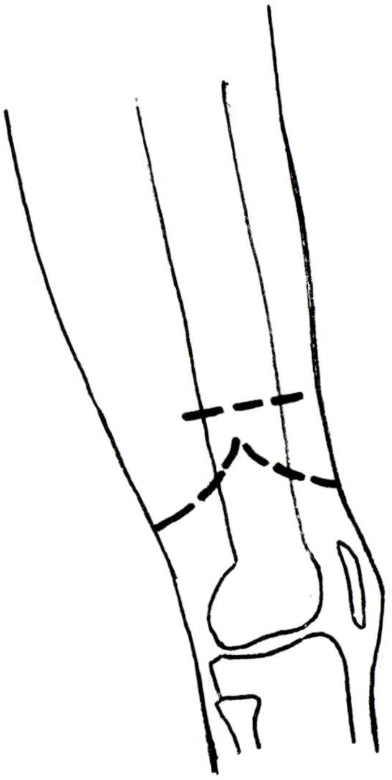

FIGURE 71-11. Anterior-posterior "fish-mouth" incision for above-knee amputation.

Through-Knee Amputation

If a through-knee amputation is to be performed, the skin incision must be distal to the knee joint by 4 to 5 cm and the patella and patellar tendon are usually preserved and sutured over the exposed femoral condyles. The incision is deepened straight through to the depth of bone, perpendicular to the skin, and divides the muscles and tendons attached to the upper part of the tibia (sartorius, gracilis, semitendinosus, quadriceps expansion, and gastrocnemius). The patellar tendon is separated from the tibial tubercle, and the knee joint is entered anteriorly, dividing the collateral ligaments, cruciate ligaments, and menisci. With the knee bent and the tibia brought forward, the posterior capsule of the joint may be divided, giving access to the popliteal neurovascular structures. The artery and vein are suture-ligated, and the nerves are brought down, ligated, and then allowed to retract up into the muscle bulk to avoid later pressure. The patella is reflected back over the femoral condyles and may be held in place by suturing the infrapatellar tendon to the posterior capsule; however, if there is insufficient length, then the suturing may be to the stumps of the cruciate ligaments. The divided tendons are also sutured to the knee capsule.

The wound is closed in two layers; if the circumferential skin incision was used, then usually the skin closure will be transverse across the end of the stump. Amputation dressing is then applied, with or without a plaster cast.

Above-Knee Amputation

This procedure is done with the aim of always preserving the maximum possible bone length. We have usually used anterior and posterior flaps, but a circumferential incision is also suitable. Short flaps are preferred because of the possibility of jeopardizing blood supply in long flaps. The incision passes through skin, subcutaneous tissue, and deep fascia without undermining, and then is continued obliquely through the muscle layers, in toward the anticipated line of bone section. As the major vessels are almost certainly occluded, hemorrhage is rarely a problem. The main dissection usually commences on the medial aspect of the leg to expose the femoral vessels which are clamped and ligated as they are encountered (Figure 71-12). The sciatic nerve is exposed more posteriorly and ligated after being pulled down, so that it will then retract up into the muscle bulk and be protected from direct pressure. Ligation of this nerve is important because of the artery which accompanies it. The bone is sectioned using a hand or electric saw, and the ends are smoothed with a file. Opposing muscle groups are then sutured over the end of the bone, with special attention being given to fixation of the rectus femoris and hamstrings to each other and to the periosteum, to preserve balance of contractile function. The adductor magnus and fascia lata are sutured to each other transversely over the bone. Careful approximation of muscle layers also obliterates dead space within the wound. The fasciae of the anterior and posterior flap are then approximated with interrupted, absorbable sutures. If necessary, wound drainage may be instituted with a closed suction drain or a Penrose tissue drain placed at the base of the flaps. The skin is carefully approximated without tension. The amputation dressing is then applied, and a plaster of paris cast may be applied, especially if an immediate prosthesis is to be used.

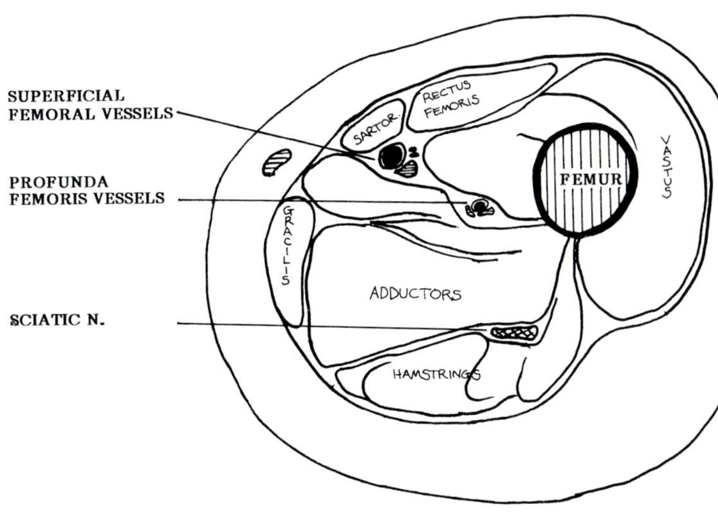

FIGURE 71-12. Cross-sectional anatomy of the thigh at the level of above-knee amputation.

Determination of Amputation Level

In the ideal situation, it would be possible to determine preoperatively whether or not an amputation would heal at a chosen level, so that an inappropriately high level of amputation could be avoided, and revision of an amputation to a higher level would never be necessary. Many special investigative techniques have been advocated for this purpose (Table 71-3). Of these the most reliable are transcutaneous P_{O_2} determination and measurement of skin clearance of ^{133}Xe, with helpful but less dependable information derived from segmental Doppler blood pressures and skin perfusion pressures. Factors which have been shown to have little predictive value include angiographic appearance and level of the most distal pulse (42).

Skin circulation is the single most important factor in determining amputation healing (43). In experienced hands, clinical

TABLE 71-3. **Preoperative Determination of Amputation Level**

Clinical judgment of skin viability and nutrition
Transcutaneous P_{O2} measurement
Skin clearance of ^{133}Xe
Segmental Doppler blood pressures
Segmental skin perfusion pressures
Skin temperature measurement (thermography)
Photoplethysmography

judgment (based on factors such as skin viability, nutritional changes, and physical signs of ischemia) has been shown to be accurate, so that in many cases the noninvasive investigations may merely serve to reinforce this judgment. In any case most series now record a healing rate of up to 85 percent for below-knee amputation, so it is not unreasonable to attempt salvage of the knee in almost all cases that do not have specific contraindications such as ulceration or infection extending above this level or contracture of the knee joint. Prediction of healing potential of forefoot amputations may be particularly difficult on clinical grounds, whereas these noninvasive techniques may provide more exact information and allow for accurate selection of patients who will require a revascularization procedure to achieve primary healing at the lower amputation level.

Burgess (44) has pointed out that no single technique can be expected to unfailingly predict the outcome of an amputation because of the effects of variables such as surgical technique (tissue handling, flap length, wound tension); alterations in blood flow caused by the procedure itself; and postoperative problems such as pressure from dressings, intercurrent diseases, wound infection, and malnutrition which may compromise eventual healing. For these reasons, it is easier to predict failure due to circulatory deficiency than it is to predict success.

TRANSCUTANEOUS P_{O_2} MEASUREMENT

It has been demonstrated than transcutaneous oxygen tension (Ptc_{O_2}) measurements, taken with a skin sensor electrode at a temperature of 45°C, are an accurate indication of the severity of vascular disease, depending on blood oxygen content and local blood flow (45,46). Recent studies have shown that the transcutaneous P_{O_2} of the anterior and posterior skin at the level of amputation correlates well with eventual success or failure. Katsamouris et al. found that healing was very likely if local Ptc_{O_2} exceeded 40 mmHg and that failure always occurred for Ptc_{O_2} less than 20 mmHg (47). Burgess (48) also found that transcutaneous oxygen tension levels correlated well with healing outcome for below-knee amputation but did not identify a definite threshold value. However, all patients with Ptc_{O_2} less than 26 mmHg failed to heal.

^{133}Xe CLEARANCE

The rate of clearance of an injected dose of ^{133}Xe at the proposed site of amputation may be calculated as a measure of local skin blood flow. Moore and Malone (49–51) have reported that when skin blood flow was found to be greater than 2.6 mL per 100 g per minute by this technique, successful primary wound healing occurred in all cases, whereas only 50 percent of cases healed when the skin blood flow was between 2.0 and 2.6 mL per 100 g per minute. Other studies of this technique have shown less correlation with healing rates, with some failures being seen in the presence of blood flow measured up to 7.5 mL per 100 g per minute (52).

SEGMENTAL BLOOD PRESSURE

Segmental blood pressure and flow waveforms as measured by Doppler ultrasound have not in general shown good correlation with healing (25), probably because of the high proportion of diabetics who tend to have incompressible, calcified arteries which give false pressure measurements (53). There is little agreement as to what pressure is necessary for primary healing; Verta reported failure of transmetatarsal amputation with ankle pressures less than 35 mmHg (54), whereas Barnes and Baker reported that 60 mmHg was the minimal ankle pressure associated with successful healing (55,56).

When the ankle-to-brachial systolic index is considered, it seems likely that healing will occur with values greater than 0.35 to 0.45 (54,57). This technique does not give a good indication of the status of circulation in collateral vessels, and there is a significant incidence of successful healing in the presence of extremely low or undetectable segmental pressures (44).

Other techniques which have been reported include skin temperature measurement (58,59), photoplethysmography (60), digital plethysmography (61,62), and skin perfusion pressures (63,64). Most of these techniques suffer from lack of widespread availability or excessive variability in results, such as those obtained in skin temperature measurements by thermography which have been found to be dependent on variants other than blood flow, including ambient temperature, patient exercise, and presence or absence of infection.

Postoperative Care

Following any of these amputation procedures, the leg is initially elevated on several pillows to help prevent swelling. The dressing is usually not disturbed for 3 or 4 days, unless there is significant pain or fever suggestive of complications. In the cases where drainage tubes are necessary, they are removed as soon as possible, preferably within 24 hours. We prefer not to suture the drains in place, so that they may be gently removed without disturbing the dressing. The elastic stump bandage helps prevent swelling, while allowing for passive and active exercise in order to avoid contractures. If a plaster cast has been applied, flexion contractures will not occur, but there may be some loss of joint mobility.

Conditions such as diabetes, hypertension, heart disese, and chronic respiratory disorders require close monitoring and control during the postoperative period. Systemic antibiotics should be continued for several days if there was infection; in the absence of infection several prophylactic doses of antibiotic are sufficient. Early mobilization of the patient is encouraged, either

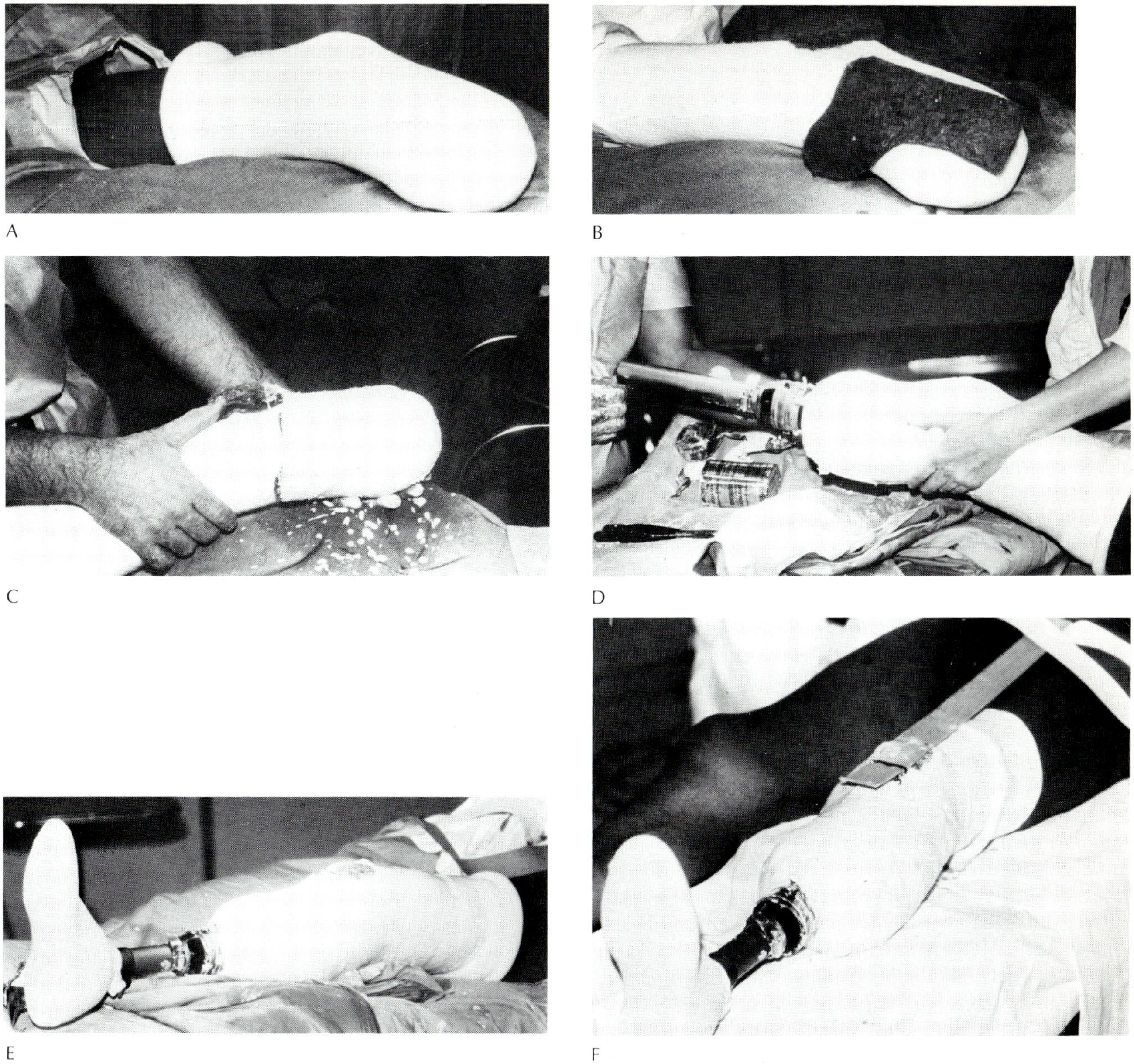

FIGURE 71-13. Techniques of immediate postoperative prosthesis fitting. (*A*) Stump sock. (*B*) Relief pads to protect bony prominences. (*C*) Application of plaster cast. (*D*) Attachment plate incorporated into the plaster, with adjustable-length pylon tube. (*E*) Completed prosthesis with foot attached. (*F*) Suspension strap and waist belt attached to prosthesis.

by the use of a temporary pneumatic air-splint (65,66) with crutches or a walking frame, or by the technique of immediate postoperative prosthesis application, as outlined below. The rehabilitation of the patient commences as soon as possible and is best achieved using a multidisciplinary approach involving regular instructions and supervision by a physiotherapist, occupational therapist, prosthetist, and surgeon.

Once the wound is healing satisfactorily, a stump dressing consisting solely of an elastic Ace bandage can be employed to prevent stump edema and to aid in molding the shape. The patient is instructed in the proper technique of bandage application and should reapply the bandage several times per day. After the first few days, the patient should not be allowed to lie in bed with the stump propped up on pillows, since this tends to allow the development of contractures. Sutures should usually be left in place for at least 2 weeks and sometimes for longer. Narcotic analgesia will usually be required for several days, however, complaints of severe pain are suggestive of a major complication and should precipitate removal of the dressing and inspection of the wound. The possible occurrence of phantom limb pain should be explained to the patient. Postoperative confusion is common because of the generally elderly population that one is dealing with and because of factors such as infection, analgesia, and multiorgan disease. If the patient is confused, then steps must be taken to prevent him or her from trying to get out of bed, which often precipitates injury to the amputation stump.

Immediate Postoperative Prosthesis Fitting

The concept of improved amputation stump healing and accelerated rehabilitation brought about by immediate postoperative prosthesis fitting dates back to the 1960s (67). The main benefits claimed for this technique are a faster rehabilitation of the patient with improved patient morale and motivation, coupled with early acceptance of the procedure and conditioning to accept and use the prosthesis. Other advantages have been noted with early prosthesis fitting, including better control of edema of the stump, less pain, perhaps earlier healing, protection of the wound from trauma, and prevention of contractions. The earlier mobilization is thought to be associated with a lower incidence of venous thromboembolic episodes and respiratory complications such as atelectasis and pneumonia. Patients have been noted to regain strength and to show earlier learning of balance control due to the increased proprioceptive input from muscles and joints of the involved limb which occur with early mobilization, exercise, and partial weight bearing.

Obviously, all patients will not be suitable for this technique, especially those who had been severely debilitated by sepsis or long-term illness. There is also the potential for compromising wound healing in the patient with severe vascular disease. However, with correct selection of amputation level, by avoiding weight bearing, and by transferring weight onto the proximal parts of the limb rather than the amputation stump, wound-healing problems can be avoided. As this technique involves the patient wearing a plaster cast over the amputation stump for 2 to 3 weeks, it should not be used for patients in whom ischemic wound breakdown or possible infection are anticipated, since the stump will not be accessible for inspection. Early involvement of the prosthetist is essential. Preferably she or he will see the patient before the operation and will assist at the time of surgery in the application of the cast. The surgical technique of amputation does not differ from that described above, except that after the initial wound dressing is applied, the immediate fitting technique (Figure 71-13) involves application of a rigid cast socket made up of an inner layer (the stump sock), appropriate protection of bony prominences by padding (the relief pads), a polyurethane cap or pad applied over the end of the stump, followed by application of the plaster cast (68). A suspension strap with belt is incorporated in the plaster cast and placed around the patient's waist. Finally, an attachment plate is incorporated into the distal end of the plaster; the pylon tube and prosthetic foot will later be fitted into this attachment plate. Often a window is made in the cast over the patella to protect this area from pressure sores. If the patient is well enough, mobilization may commence on the first postoperative day, initially allowing the patient to sit and to exercise the limb and then progressing to standing while supported by a walking frame or crutches, without placing weight on the prosthesis. The team of prosthetist, physical therapist, and surgeon supervises and encourages the patient with most of the early exercises and use of the prosthesis. This is best supervised in the physical therapy department where special equipment for ambulation such as parallel bars is available. The patient progresses from standing and balancing with limited ambulation through progressive weight bearing over several weeks. During this time the patient should never put full weight on the prosthesis because of the risk of wound problems. The plaster cast is usually changed after 14 or 21 days, at which time the sutures are removed. After this time the patient may be discharged and have further rehabilitation as an outpatient. The patient makes use of this temporary prosthesis until full wound healing and molding of the stump have occurred, at which time the permanent prosthesis may be measured and manufactured.

Complications of Amputation

The complications of these procedures may be divided into those which are specific for the operation and those which are due to the high incidence of severe cardiopulmonary diseases and diabetes seen in this patient population. Several follow-up studies have shown that approximately 50 percent of amputee patients die within 2 to 3 years of the operation, usually because of cardiac or cerebrovascular problems, and that, of the survivors, a further 30 to 50 percent eventually require amputation of the contralateral leg within the same time span (69–71). Until recent years the operative mortality rate among those with amputations below the knee was approximately 10 percent, and among those with through-knee or above-knee amputation, the usual rates were 20 to 30 percent (21). With recent improvements in patient preparation for surgery, anesthetic techniques, and intensive care capabilities, there should now be a mortality rate of 5 percent or less for below-knee and perhaps 10 percent for above-knee operations. Bodily and Burgess (71) recently reported a series of 55 patients who had major amputations, with an operative mortality rate of only 1.5 percent, and Fearon and Wheelock reported a 3 percent mortality rate for below-knee amputation in 100 diabetics (25). There is also a relatively high incidence of postoperative cardiovascular and cerebrovascular complications such as myocardial infarction, stroke, or respiratory failure (72). The long-term survival prospects for diabetics is significantly worse than for nondiabetics (73).

If the amputation was performed for the treatment of sepsis, then infective complications including septicemia and multiorgan failure are also common. A high incidence of postoperative venous thrombosis has been reported, particularly for amputation above the knee (20). This is most likely related to the prolonged hospitalization of the patient both before and after operation and to the generally poor medical condition of these patients. Neurological changes such as confusion, disorientation, and reactive depression frequently occur and may be difficult to manage as well as rendering rehabilitation difficult. Care of the skin wound is compromised in these patients, and they may require special observation to prevent accidents such as falling out of bed, which often leads to breakdown of the stump. Other common general complications include urinary tract infection and urinary retention, gastrointestinal bleeding, and renal failure.

The main complications of the procedure itself are infections and nonhealing of the wound due to ischemia. These problems can be avoided with good selection of amputation level, with preoperative treatment for infected ischemic limbs, and with the use of antibiotic prophylaxis. However, even with ideal management, episodes of skin-flap ischemia and suture-line infections cannot always be avoided. Wound breakdown may be a primary problem due to ischemia or may occur secondary to excessive pressure applied from the dressing, plaster cast, or poorly fitting prosthesis or from excessively early weight bearing on a prosthesis. Small areas of wound breakdown will often heal with conservative management. However, ischemic failure with or without infection usually requires revision. A failed below-knee amputation may often be revised to a higher level while still retaining the knee joint or may necessitate above-knee amputation.

Phantom pain occurs frequently, and the patient should be warned of this possibility before surgery. Usually the symptoms are not severe and no specific treatment is necessary, but occasionally narcotic or antidepressant medication may be required. Any severe pain occurring in the region of the stump should be investigated by careful inspection of the wound for complications such as ischemia, infection, or hematoma. Occasionally neuroma formation occurs at the divided nerve endings. Other important local complications include joint contractures. The main way to avoid this complication is to ensure that joint and leg exercises are commenced early in the postoperative period and that rehabilitation begins immediately with the patient being ambulated in a non-weight-bearing fashion with crutches or a walking frame. Adequate treatment of wound and stump pain in the early postoperative period aids early mobility.

Failure to rehabilitate should also be regarded as a complication since a major aim of good amputation care is to achieve eventual ambulation and independent mobility. Recent experience suggests that at least 75 percent of amputees who have been fitted with a prosthesis will make daily use of it, although a significant proportion of these do not use the prosthesis outside of their home (74).

Conclusions

The guiding principle in amputation surgery is to obtain maximal restoration of function. This requires preservation of joints wherever this is compatible with healing. Early ambulation is optimal and may best be achieved by the use of immediate prosthesis techniques in suitable patients. Amputation should thus be regarded from the rehabilitation perspective as a reconstructive procedure designed to restore function and allow the patient to return to an independent lifestyle. With the combination of low-

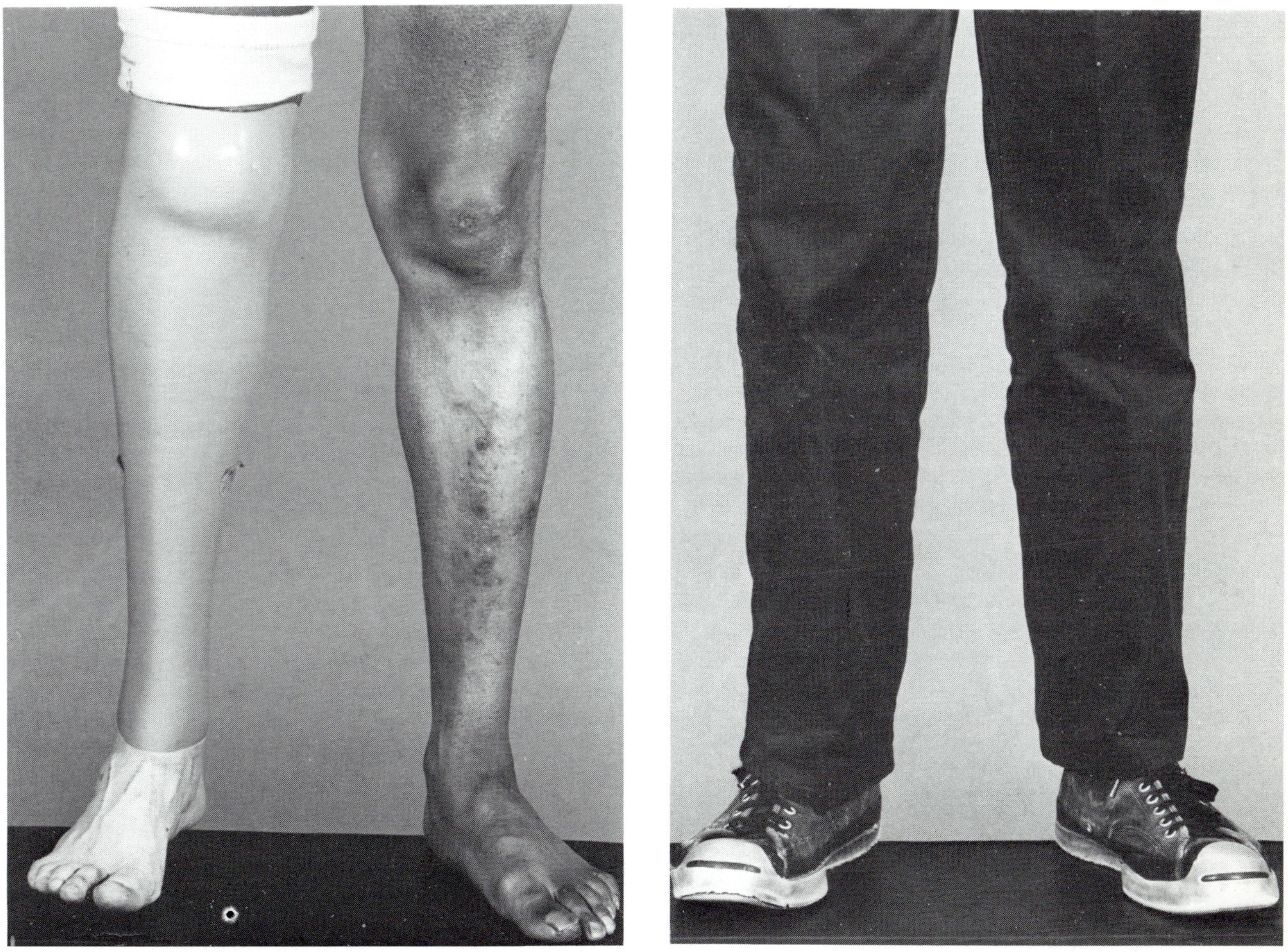

FIGURE 71-14. Modern lightweight, functional below-knee prosthetic limb (*A*) may be very difficult to differentiate from normal limb (*B*).

level, joint-preserving amputations and efficient, light, functional prostheses (Figure 71-14), amputation is no longer regarded simply as removal of dead tissue but as a true reconstructive procedure which is one alternative among many in the treatment of severe limb ischemia. Attitudes toward amputation and subsequent rehabilitation should emphasize that return to ambulation is the expected outcome.

References

1. Glattly HW: Aging and amputations. Artif Limbs 1966, 10:1.
2. Stoney RJ: Ultimate salvage for the patient with limb-threatening ischemia: Realistic goals and surgical considerations. Am J Surg 1978, 136:228–232.
3. Kay HW, Newman JD: Relative incidence of new amputations. Statistical comparisons of 6000 new amputations. Orthot Prosthet 1975, 29:3–9.
4. Perdue GD, Smith RB, Veazey CR, Ansley JD: Revascularization for severe limb ischemia. Arch Surg 1980, 115:168–171.
5. Auer AI, Hurley JJ, Binnington HB, Nunnelee JD, Hershey FB: Distal tibial vein grafts for limb salvage. Arch Surg 1983, 118:597–602.
6. Dardik H, Ibrahim IM, Dardik JJ: The role of the peroneal artery for limb salvage. Ann Surg 1979, 189:184–198.
7. O'Mara HO, Flinn WR, Neiman HL, Bergan JJ, Yao JST: Correlation of foot arterial anatomy with early tibial bypass patency. Surgery 1981, 89:743–752.
8. Johansen K, Burgess EM, Zorn R, Holloway GA, Malchow D, Bach A: Improvement of amputation level by lower extremity revascularisation. Surg Gynecol Obstet 1981, 153:707–709.
9. Hoyle SJ, Teitlembaum S, Gore I, Warren R: Atheromatous embolisation: A factor in peripheral gangrene. N Engl J Med 1959, 261:128–131.
10. Peng TF, Davis JA, Somer T, Kaplan L, Bluestone R: A clinical approach to systemic vasculitis. Semin Arthritis Rheum 1980, 9:248–304.
11. McGrath MA, Tracy GD, Lord RSA, Penny R: Peripheral ischemia caused by blood hyperviscosity. Aust NZ J Surg 1973, 43:109–113.
12. Tracy GD, Lord RSA, Hill DA, Graham AR, McGrath MA: Management of ischemia of the foot beyond arterial reconstruction. Surg Gynecol Obstet 1982, 155:377–379.
13. Gregg RO: Bypass or amputation? Concomitant review of bypass arterial grafting and major amputations. Am J Surg 1985, 149:397–402.
14. McAnena OJ, Kiely FA, O'Donnell JA: Evaluation of the benefits of intraoperative prereconstructive angiography. Vasc Surg 1984, 18:211–216.
15. Szilagyi DE, Smith RF, Scarpella JR, Hoffman K: Lumbar sympathectomy: Current role in the treatment of atherosclerotic occlusive disease. Arch Surg 1967, 95:753–757.
16. Yeagher RA, Hobson RW, Janil Z, Lynch TE, Lee BC, Jain K: Differential patency and limb salvage for polytetrafluoroethylene and autogenous saphenous vein in severe lower extremity ischemia. Surgery 1982, 91:99–103.
17. Flanigan DP, Williams, LF, Keifer T, Schuler JJ, Behrend AJ: Prebypass operative arteriography. Surgery 1982, 92:627–633.
18. Bergan JJ, Veith FJ, Bernhard VM, Yao JST, Flinn WR, Gupta SK, Scher LA, Samson RH, Towne JB: Randomisation of autogenous vein and polytetrafluoroethylene grafts in femoral-distal reconstruction. Surgery 1982, 92:921–930.
19. Edwards WH, Mulherin JL: The role of graft material in femorotibial bypass grafts. Am Surg 1980, 191:721–726.
20. Little JM: *Major Amputations for Vascular Disease*. Edinburgh, Churchill Livingstone, 1975.
21. Otteman MG, Stahlgren LH: Evaluation of factors which influence mortality and morbidity following major lower extremity amputation for atherosclerosis. Surg Gynecol Obstet 1965, 120:1217–1220.
22. Hargrove WC, Barker CF, Berkowitz HD, Perloff LJ, McLean G, Freiman D, Ring EJ, Roberts B: Treatment of acute peripheral arterial and graft thromboses with low-dose streptokinase. Surgery 1982, 92:981–993.
23. Bell ET: Atherosclerotic gangrene of the lower extremities in diabetic and non-diabetic persons. Am J Clin Pathol 1957, 28:27–35.
24. Gibbons GW: Management of pre- and postoperative infection in the diabetic patient. Host Pathogen News 1983, 1:1–5.
25. Fearon J, Campbell DR, Hoar CS, Gibbons GW, Rowbotham JL, Wheelock FC: Improved results with diabetic below-knee amputations. Arch Surg 1975, 120:777–780.
26. Sizer JS, Wheelock FC: Digital amputations in diabetic patients. Surgery 1972, 72:980–989.
27. Cruse J, Foord RA: A five year prospective study of 23,649 surgical wounds. Arch Surg 1973, 107:206–210.
28. Kitter A: A technique for salvage of the diabetic gangrenous foot. Orthop Clin North Am 1973, 1:21–30.
29. Tripses D, Pollak FW: Risk factors in healing of below-knee amputation. Am J Surg 1981, 141:718–720.
30. Moore WS, Hall AD, Lim RC: Below the knee amputation for ischemic gangrene. Am J Surg 1972, 124:127–134.
31. Cranley JJ, Krause RJ, Strasser ES, Hafner CD: Below the knee amputation for arteriosclerosis obliterans. Arch Surg 1969, 98:77–80.
32. Wu Y, Flanigan DP: Rehabilitation of the lower extremity amputee. In Bergan JJ, Yao JST (eds): *Gangrene and Severe Ischemia of the Lower Extremities*. New York, Grune & Stratton, 1978.
33. Jamieson CW, Hill D: Amputation for vascular disease. Br J Surg 1976, 63:683–690.
34. Beraldi RS, Keonin Y: Amputations in peripheral vascular occlusive disease. Am J Surg 1978, 135:231–234.
35. Syme J: *Observations in Clinical Surgery*. Edinburgh, Edmondson and Douglas, 1982.
36. Rosenman CD: Syme amputation for ischemic disease in the foot. Am J Surg 1969, 118:194–199.
37. McCollough NC, Shea JD, Warren WD, Sarmiento A: The dysvascular amputee: Surgery and rehabilitation. In *Current Problems in Surgery*. Year Book Medical Publishers, Chicago, 1971.
38. Wray CH, Still JM, Moretz WH: Present management of amputations for peripheral vascular disease. Am Surg 1972, 38:87–92.
39. Sarmiento A, Warren WD: A re-evaluation of lower extremity amputations. Surg Gynecol Obstet 1969, 129:799–802.
40. Little JM, Stewart GR, Niesche FW, Williams C: A trial of flapless below-knee amputation for arterial insufficiency. Med J Aust 1970, 1:883–886.
41. Kiln RB, Warren R, Baske GW: The geriatric amputee. Ann Surg 1972, 176:305–314.
42. Silbert S, Haimovici H: Results of midleg amputations for gangrene in diabetics. JAMA 1950, 144:454–458.
43. Burgess EM: Major lower extremity amputations following arterial reconstruction. Arch Surg 1974, 108:655–660.
44. Burgess EM, Matsen FA: Determining amputation levels in peripheral vascular disease. J Bone Joint Surg 1981, 63A:1493–1497.
45. White RA, Nolan L, Harley D, Long J, Klein S, Tremper K,

Nelson R, Tabrisky J, Shoemaker W: Noninvasive evaluation of peripheral vascular disease using transcutaneous oxygen tension. Am J Surg 1982, 144:68–75.
46. Eickhoff JH, Jacobsen F: Correlation of transcutaneous oxygen tension to blood flow in heated skin. Scand J Clin Lab Invest 1980, 40:761–765.
47. Katsamouris A, Brewster DC, Megerman J, Cina C, Darling RC, Abbott WM: Transcutaneous oxygen tension in selection of amputation level. Am J Surg 1984, 147:510–515.
48. Burgess EM, Matsen FA, Wyss CR, Simmons CW: Segmental transcutaneous measurement of pO_2 in patients requiring below-the-knee amputation for peripheral vascular insufficiency. J Bone Joint Surg 1982, 64:378–382.
49. Moore WS: Determination of amputation level. Measurement of skin blood flow with ^{133}xenon. Arch Surg 1973, 107:798–802.
50. Malone JML, Moore WS, Goldstone J, Malone SJ: Therapeutic and economic impact of a modern amputation program. Ann Surg 1979, 189:798–802.
51. Moore WS, Henry RE, Malone JM, Daly MJ, Patton D, Childers SJ: Prospective use of ^{133}xenon clearance for amputation level selection. Arch Surg 1981, 116:86–88.
52. Holloway GA, Burgess EM: Cutaneous blood flow and its relation to healing of below-knee amputation. Surg Gynecol Obstet 1978, 146:750–756.
53. Gibbons GW, Wheelock FC, Siembieda C, Hoar CS, Rowbotham JL, Persson AB: Non-invasive prediction of amputation level in diabetic patients. Arch Surg 1979, 114:1253–1257.
54. Verta MJ, Gross WS, van Bellen B, Yao JST, Bergan JJ: Forefoot perfusion pressure and minor amputation for gangrene. Surgery 1976, 80:729–734.
55. Barnes RW, Shanik GD, Slaymaker EE: An index of healing in below-knee amputation: Leg blood pressure by Doppler ultrasound. Surgery 1976, 79:13–20.
56. Baker WH, Barnes RW: Minor forefoot amputation in patients with low ankle pressure. Am J Surg 1977, 133:331–332.
57. Wagner FW: Amputation of the foot and ankle. Current status. Clin Orthop 1977, 122:62–69.
58. Lee RY, Trainor FS, Karner D, McCann WJ, Madden JL: Noninvasive hemodynamic evaluation in selection of amputation level. Surg Gynecol Obstet 1979, 149:241–244.
59. Henderson HP, Chir B, Hackett MEJ: The value of thermography in peripheral vascular disease. Angiology 1978, 29:65–67.
60. Abramowitz HB, Queral LA, Flinn WR, Nora PF, Peterson LK, Bergan JJ, Yao JST: The use of photoplethysmography in the assessment of chronic venous insufficiency: A comparison to venous pressure measurement. Surgery 1979, 86:434–439.
61. Strandress DE, Sumner DS: Current research review. Noninvasive methods of studying peripheral arterial function. J Surg Res 1972, 12:419–430.
62. Barnes RW, Thornhill B, Nix L, Rittgers SE, Turley G: Prediction of amputation wound healing: Roles of Doppler ultrasound and digit plethysmography. Arch Surg 1981, 116:80–83.
63. Holstein P, Sager P, Lassen NA: Wound healing in below knee amputations in relation to skin perfusion pressure. Acta Orthop Scand 1979, 50:49–58.
64. Faris I, Duncan H: Skin perfusion pressure in the prediction of healing in diabetic patients with ulcers or gangrene of the foot. J Vasc Surg 1985, 2:536–540.
65. Little JM: A pneumatic weight-bearing temporary prosthesis for below-knee amputees. Lancet 1971, 1:271–273.
66. Kerstein MD: Utilisation of an air-splint after below-knee amputation. Am J Phys Med 1974, 53:119–126.
67. Burgess EM, Romano RL: The management of lower extremity amputees using immediate postsurgical prosthesis. Clin Orthop 1968, 57:137–146.
68. Russek AS: Amputation, immediate postoperative fitting, and early ambulation. In Haimovici H (ed): *Vascular Surgery: Principles and Techniques,* ed 2. Norwalk, Connecticut, Appleton-Century-Crofts, 1984.
69. Couch NP, David JK, Tilney NL, Crane C: Natural history of the leg amputee. Am J Surg 1977, 133:469–473.
70. Mazet R: The geriatric amputee. Artif Limbs 1967, 11:35–41.
71. Bodily KC, Burgess EM: Contralateral limb and patient survival after leg amputation. Am J Surg 1983, 148:280–282.
72. Castronuovo JJ, Deane LM, Deterling RA, O'Donnell TF, O'Toole DM, Callow AD: Below-knee amputation. Is the effort to preserve the knee joint justified? Arch Surg 1980, 115:1184–1187.
73. Burgess EM: Amputations for ischemia. In Kempczinski RF (ed): *The Ischemic Leg*. Chicago, Year Book Medical Publishers, 1985.
74. Finch DR, MacDougal M, Tibbs DJ, Morris PJ: Amputations for vascular disease. The experience of a peripheral vascular unit. Br J Surg 1980, 67:233–237.

Chapter 72

REHABILITATION OF THE AMPUTEE

RICHARD A. SULLIVAN

Rehabilitation medicine provides a comprehensive team approach to the problems of disability, whatever the etiological cause. The need for such an approach should be obvious to the physician when facing the number of potential underlying medical, social, and psychological problems associated with the diagnosis of peripheral vascular disease. The term *dysvascular amputee* connotes a basic underlying group of medical diseases with the secondary symptom being that of vascular insufficiency endangering the viability of the leg. The problems are further compounded by the advanced age of the average patient population and their susceptibility to fear and depression because of the threat of amputation to their lifestyle and independence.

It is imperative, therefore, that a comprehensive, multidisciplinary analysis of the patient's needs precede the actual amputation itself if such a time frame is medically feasible. The modern-day approach with the surgical attempts for limb salvage often allows the time for the total evaluation. The need for and the positive results of such preplanning cannot be overstressed. The end result affects more than merely the site of the amputation. It also affects the end result of the rehabilitation process, which is the attainment of a patient population, well-adjusted and well-trained, and better able to cope with their disability in a social environment most in line with their former lifestyle.

The program of rehabilitation should, therefore, begin in the preoperative stage and proceed from there to achieve the goals of physical health, independence of function, and a satisfying lifestyle commensurate with the patient's potential.

The Rehabilitation Team

The problems inherent in the diagnosis of dysvascular disease with the necessity to proceed to amputation strongly suggest the need for a holistic approach to achieve the best possible end result for the patient. The total rehabilitation team concept is best capable of handling these problems. The spectrum of problems is too broad for single physician management.

The rehabilitation team consists of the following members.

THE PHYSICIANS

The Surgeon

It is the responsibility of the surgeon to evaluate and treat the problem of vascular insufficiency vigorously in the hope that amputation can be avoided. This can be accomplished by conservative means in some cases or by surgical bypass procedures resulting in limb salvage. When such intervention is not feasible or fails to correct the problem, a proper level of amputation must be determined and carried out.

The Physiatrist

The physiatrist is a specialist in rehabilitation medicine who can supply the surgeon not only with medical expertise but also with a complete team of rehabilitation specialists to better evaluate the complexity of problems. In the uncomplicated case requiring amputation, the physiatrist can proceed promptly with the program of physical restoration, prosthetic fitting, and training. The physiatrist is specially trained in the prescription of exercise routines taking into consideration the tolerance of the patient, the use of modalities to reduce or abolish pain, programs of training to improve functional capacity and independence in daily living activities, and the prescription of and training in the use of prosthetic devices and ambulation aids. The therapeutic team working together under the direction and prescription of the physiatrist provides a comprehensive approach to the patient's physical, prosthetic, psychological, and social needs. The decisions in each case are specific to the individual needs and problems. Decisions as to programs and prostheses are the responsibility of the team physician.

THE NURSE

The nurse provides care, both preoperatively and postoperatively with a total understanding of the problems with which the patient presents. The nursing staff must be fully aware of the need for personal warmth and emotional support and understanding at this most difficult time in the patient's life. They must be aware of all the problems inherent in the diagnosis of dysvascular disease and amputation, affecting as it does not only the involved extremity but also the other limb and the entire cardiovascular system.

THE PHYSICAL THERAPIST

The physical therapist is a well-trained professional knowledgeable in the techniques and considerations of exercise physiology and tolerance, energy conservation, the use of modalities to relieve pain, gait training, and prosthetic care and management. They are directed in their treatment by the prescription of the team physician. They treat the patient as well as observe the patient's reaction to the program, keeping the physician and other team members abreast of any developments which could affect the general health of the patient. Their observations and recommendations can alter the therapeutic program, ultimately reducing the chances of complications.

THE OCCUPATIONAL THERAPIST OR ACTIVITIES OF DAILY LIVING THERAPIST

These are professionally trained team members involved in preparing the patient for a return to independent living. Either one of these professionals is available as part of the team, depending upon the staffing pattern of the facility. They are responsible for retraining the patient in the activities of daily living. This includes dressing, bed activities, toileting, bathing, transfer safety with or without a prosthesis, as well as prosthetic management. They recommend the devices and equipment needed to achieve the highest level of independence at home, and a prescription for the devices is then provided by the physician after consultation. Both the family and the patient are trained in device and equipment use. Visits to the patient's home are provided, if necessary, to assess architectural barriers and provide solutions for such barriers.

THE PROSTHETIST

The trained technician assists the team in making the final judgmental considerations regarding the prosthetic components to be used in the permanent prosthesis to provide the patient with the greatest function and safety. It is the prosthetist's responsibility to fabricate the prosthesis once it is prescribed by the physician. Any further adjustments are carried out after fabrication, as needed. The inclusion of the prosthetist as a primary team member allows prompt attention to problems of fit, suspension, and safety during the initial period of training as well as keeping the prosthetist aware of the need for additional considerations in view of the patient's general physical or cardiac status.

THE PSYCHOLOGIST

The expertise of the psychologist may or may not be necessary in each case but should be available to the team on a consultative basis to aid in the interpretation and handling of serious emotional problems and depressions. The care and treatment of any preamputation or postamputation mental disorders that could adversely affect the achievement of a rehabilitation goal of self-care and independence are essential. The psychologist, through the process of testing and interview, can follow with counseling sessions that can improve the functional result in some cases.

THE SOCIAL WORKER

The social worker should be available as a consultant to evaluate the social milieu of the patient and help the team determine if a return to the former lifestyle and home environment is feasible in view of the complication of amputation and diminished personal independence. The patient and the family's strengths and weaknesses must be assessed by the worker through interview. The social community agencies available to the patient must be considered and offered to provide solutions to problems relating to care and assistance needs to allow the patient to return home. Aid in institutional placement is also provided, if necessary.

THE VOCATIONAL COUNSELOR

Many dysvascular patients are still of an employable age. They can often require an evaluation of their previous work experiences to determine if a return to their former employment is indicated or feasible in the face of the amputation. There is a need for counseling as well as for a review of the former job specifications. The employer often must be contacted and encouraged to reemploy the patient. If a return to the former job is not possible, assistance in seeking a new position or evaluation for and retraining in a new type of work may be needed. All of these services are available through the rehabilitation center's vocational services section.

The Evaluation Process

Each of the team members should be available to the patient and the team in order to fully provide the amputee with the services needed to achieve the most optimal rehabilitation result.

In the preoperative period, when it becomes obvious that the limb must be ablated, the vascular surgeon and the physiatrist, each representing his or her individual area of expertise, should work together and plan the site of the amputation. Many factors should be considered at this time. The present concept of saving the knee at all costs must be weighed against the danger of potential failure of the below-knee amputation, especially in the elderly and the diabetic, and the effect of failure on the patient physically and psychologically.

It is at this point that a comprehensive evaluation of the case should be made by the physiatrist and pertinent members of the rehabilitation team to assess the total needs of the patient. The entire spectrum of physical, social, psychological, and economic problems has to be evaluated. The team must determine whether the potential danger to the health and longevity of the patient justifies subjecting the patient to the below-knee level of amputation with its inherent dangers of nonhealing, infection, pain, and debility, which can lead to prolonged hospitalization and possible further amputation surgery. The dangers of these complications can further shorten the already compromised life expectancy of the patient in addition to negatively affecting the quality of life in these terminal years.

A thorough evaluation could result in a decision to proceed with an immediate above-the-knee amputation, resulting in a speedier recovery without the danger of excessive morbidity. The limited potential of the patient as assessed preoperatively can often justify such a conclusion and treatment plan even in this day of advanced surgical techniques. The limited use of the above-the-knee prosthesis with the prerequisite safety components is often preferable from the functional and social point of view. Limited household ambulation either at home or in an institution for toileting and other basic needs can be achieved for the above-the-knee amputee with the proper prosthesis assisted by a walker or cane. Some limited ambulation is also possible with a walker even without a prosthesis when the functional goals are limited. The final decision entails assessment of the cardiovascular status of the patient prior to the present complication, as well as the presence of other secondary medical diseases adversely affecting the patient's potential.

There are many acceptable systems of evaluation which can help the team assess the patient. Several weighted-scale systems have been developed to formalize the results of the total assessment. One such method is called PULSES (1). The letters stand for

P: Physical condition—the presence of coexisting disease

U: Upper limb function

L: Lower limb function

S: Sensory condition—sensation, communication, speech, hearing, vision

E: Excretory function

S: Social history—intellectual and emotional adaptability, housing, family support, finances

Scoring for each component ranges from 1 for intact and independent, to 4 for fully dependent. The subscores are then tallied to give an overall measure of functional independence. Scores can range from a low of 6 to a high of 24. The higher the score, the greater the dependence of the patient. A score of 12 suggests a severe limitation in at least two functional areas. The final figure resulting from such a comprehensive analysis can assist in developing achievable goals.

The Site of the Amputation

ABOVE-THE-KNEE AMPUTATION

The preferred site in the above-knee amputation is approximately 4 in above the knee joint. This allows space for the mechanism of the prosthetic knee joint to be attached without resulting in knee length differentials when the patient is seated. Longer lengths are possible if the polycentric knee joint is used, but this is seldom the mechanical joint of choice in this age group.

Any further shortening of the residual limb above the 4-in level can readily be prosthetically accommodated but can increase the workload of the patient by shortening the lever arm and reducing the muscle bulk available to the patient to operate the prosthesis.

Knee disarticulation amputations and the Gritti-Stokes type of amputation, which involves the fusion of the patella to the shortened femur, have little advantage for the patient except for the easier surgery in the case of the knee disarticulation since no bone cutting is involved. The end result can be prosthetically handled and fitted but is poorer both cosmetically and functionally. In addition, failures of the Gritti-Stokes fusions are not infrequent with time and often require the patient to undergo further surgery for revision.

BELOW-THE-KNEE AMPUTATION

The preferable site for the below-knee amputation is at the juncture of the upper and middle third of the tibia. The fibula should be shortened and beveled to better accommodate the prosthetic socket shape. A long posterior skin flap is preferred with the suture line anterior to the tibia and superior to the end of the tibia. Any further sparing of the length of the tibia is of no functional value and causes problems of prosthetic fit. Nonhealing of the stump can also result secondarily to the poor vascularity at lower levels.

The Syme's amputation at the foot with the removal of the malleoli and the preservation of the heel pad has a place in isolated cases of the dysvascular patient but is certainly not a common site. The classic Chopart and Pirogoff amputation sites, amputation of the foot with tarsal sparing in the former and sparing of the calcaneus in the latter, are no longer recommended because of their tendency to develop fixed ankle and forefoot flexion-inversion deformities and painful callouses.

Transmetatarsal and digital amputations remain acceptable and are manageable with minimal prosthetic intervention in most cases.

At the time of surgery it is imperative for the surgeon to remove all the ischemic and necrotic tissue if healing is to be achieved promptly. The need for a good blood supply to obtain healing must be considered since a greater supply of blood is required to achieve healing than for tissue viability. The rewarding end result of attending to these tenets is the development of a well-healed, painless stump which can be quickly fitted with an adequate prosthesis following a short stay of hospitalization (2,3).

BILATERAL AMPUTATIONS

The best result is obtained for the below-knee amputee if equal lengths are developed. Obviously this is not done if the initial amputation site was excessively high. The combined above-knee on one side and below-knee on the other side is advantageous to the patient functionally if surgically feasible.

The bilateral above-the-knee amputation favors long stumps of almost equal lengths if possible. The potential for limited prosthetic ambulation must not be ruled out. Even if ambulation is not a consideration, the leg lengths provide improved sitting stability for the patient.

The Immediate Postoperative Period

This period is vital to the development of a healthy functional residual limb or stump. It is essential that the patient maintain a healthy psychological outlook as well as good physiological health through the administration of an adequate diet and the control of diabetic or cardiac status with good medical and nursing management (4). Wound and other secondary infections must be avoided. Dressing needs must be attended to, depending on the surgeon's use of a rigid or nonrigid dressing at the conclusion of the surgery. Both are acceptable means of maintaining controlled stump pressure, avoiding swelling of the stump, and maintaining a hematoma-free state. Dressing changes and pressure bandaging rewrapping of the stump require great care. In the case of the rigid dressing, the cast must be evaluated daily for signs of odor or drainage that can suggest underlying problems. The condition of the other limb must also be carefully monitored since the problem of vascular insufficiency is seldom unilateral. The opposite limb can be fragile and in danger of ulcer development due to mismanagement during periods of bed rest and position changes. Edema of the stump should be avoided at all costs.

In the below-knee amputation, the knee should be kept extended at the outset, with or without the use of a splint, depending upon the patient's ability to cooperate. Upon removal of the dressing several days postoperatively, gentle range of motion exercises should be instituted. The patient should be encouraged to move about the bed more freely, including standing at the side of the bed or transferring to a chair. Dressings must be applied uniformly and without undue pressure on the healing suture line.

There is a need for immediate postoperative limb immobilization to avoid trauma to the operative site and pressure. There must be an appreciation of the fact that though more comfortable for the patient at the time, repositioning of a stump with a pillow beneath the hip or knee can result in a much more serious long-term functional outcome to a much greater degree than the temporary pain of the moment (i.e., flexion contractures).

The team nurse must be expert in stump wrapping techniques with the ability to quickly recognize the symptoms of limb strangulation and swelling secondary to improper wrapping procedures. The nurse must also be aware of the effects of abnormal pressure on the operated limb at the incision, especially if the added problems of sensory loss and mental confusion intervene to alter the patient's ability to cooperate in positioning and exercise. The nurse must alert the team when there is evidence of a developing problem that further team cooperative effort can avoid or substantially minimize.

Proper observation, positioning, and skin and nail care for the opposite limb are also nursing responsibilities.

PREPROSTHETIC TRAINING (5)

Positioning

To avoid contractures, do not

1. Put a pillow under the hip or knee
2. Put pillows between the thighs
3. Sit in the wheelchair with knee bent
4. Rest amputated leg on crutch handle or arm of wheelchair
5. Hang amputated limb, flexed, over the side of the bed
6. Lie with knee bent
7. Ambulate with the hip of the amputated side flexed forward or the the knee flexed

Bandaging

Elastic (Ace) bandages are used to prevent or reduce swelling and assist in uniform shrinkage and shaping of the stump.

1. The bandage should be applied with moderate tension.
2. Only figure 8 wraps should be used: avoid circular turns which could strangle the stump.
3. The stump should be wrapped day and night.
4. In order to achieve the most shrinkage at the stump end, apply most pressure at the bottom in an upward and outward direction and reduce pressure as you go up the stump.
5. Rewrap at least two times daily or if bandage loosens or becomes uncomfortable.

The stump shrinker is an elastic shaped covering. It is of lesser value since the tension cannot be altered or directed to a certain area such as the base of the stump. It can be used, however, if the patient is incapable of managing the bandage, endangering the stump. This may be especially true in the elderly diabetic with reduced vision and sensation.

Bandaging should be continued during the period of temporary prosthesis use to achieve as much shrinkage and shaping as possible. Its continued use at night is recommended once a permanent prosthesis is received until one is assured of stabilization of the stump.

Care of the Residual Limb

1. Wash daily with soap and rinse well. Wash with moderate vigor to remove dry skin. Avoid excessive rubbing over bony prominences. Pat dry and lightly powder the stump.
2. Do not soak the stump unnecessarily.
3. Examine the stump daily for evidence of rash or skin irritation.

Physical Therapy

When the patient is medically stable, ambulation under the guidance of the physical therapist should be started either in the parallel bars or with a walker. General conditioning exercises and positional exercises on the exercise mats can be started to improve overall strength and endurance to offset the physical deterioration which may have occurred during the preoperative period or during the postoperative bed confinement. The patient is mobilized and prepared to receive the temporary prosthesis.

EXERCISES

1. Range of motion to hips and knees.
2. General conditioning and resistive exercises on the mats. These positional exercises redevelop the strength and coordination needed to move about in bed, achieve and maintain a static and dynamic sitting balance, and standing and transfer skills with and without the prosthesis.
3. Resistive exercises to all four extremities and trunk can require the use of weighted dumbbells, wall pulleys, and more modern resistive exercise machines such as the Cybex and Kinetron.
4. Ambulation training with and without the prosthesis starting in the parallel bars and proceeding to walkers and canes. All the exercises are gradually increased to attain overall strength improvement and functional endurance for the patient.
5. Training in self-care activities—dressing, bathing, grooming, safely donning and removing the prosthesis, and transfer skills—wheelchair propulsion and management may also be necessary.

This process should proceed smoothly and quickly unless there are physical or stump complications. The individual patient's condition best determines when exercises can be increased in intensity and gait training started.

Wheelchair ambulation should be encouraged early to maintain strength and avoid prolonged bed confinement between periods of treatment. The patient should be encouraged to maintain ranges of motion and to avoid flexed postures. Muscle setting exercises are introduced before wound healing.

There are special seat boards available for wheelchairs which have projection on the amputated side to maintain the amputated knee in extension during periods of wheelchair use. The special boards have hinges which allow the projection to be bent when the patient wants to transfer out of the chair (Figure 72-1*A* and 1*B*).

There are special rear-weighted wheelchairs available for the double amputee to avoid tipping of the chair due to weight imbalances secondary to the amputations. If a wheelchair is needed, it is a prescription item which should be individually chosen for the patient to allow the maximum of independence.

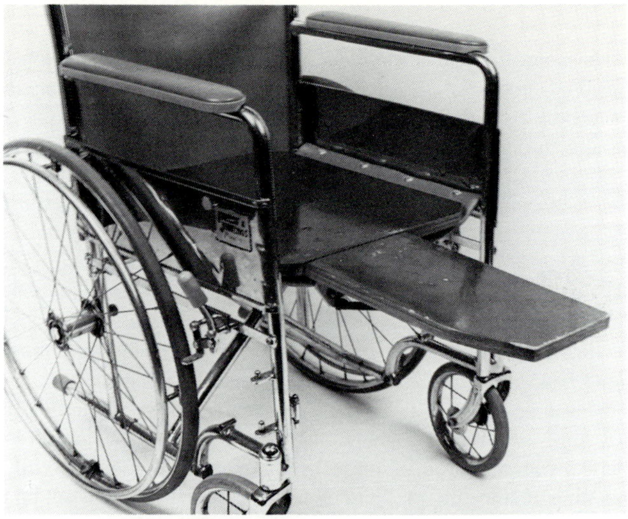

A

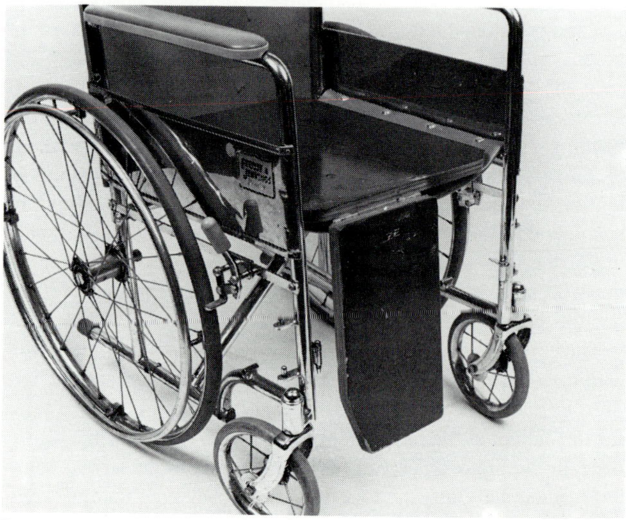

B

FIGURE 72-1. *(A)* Wheelchair board in extension to maintain knee extension. *(B)* Wheelchair board in flexion to allow knee flexion and transfers.

The Painful Stump

The problem of the painful stump when present can be a difficult and frustrating experience both for the patient and for the treatment team. A painful scar or suture line, neuroma, ill-fitting prosthesis, prosthetic malalignment, too little flexion built into the socket, and neuropathy are many of the causes. In addition, the psychological affect of nonacceptance of the amputation and depression can compound the problem.

In all cases of painful stumps, pressure areas in the socket should be sought and relieved promptly, and suspension should be reevaluated and adjusted if necessary. Prolongation of such problems can lead to painful stumps. The patient should be encouraged to continue the program. The psychologist can assist in problem cases. Psychosocial causes and reactive depression can exaggerate and prolong the problem. Pain can be an attention-getting mechanism or a tool to manipulate the family or the team. A thorough evaluation of all possible causes is mandatory before finalizing one of neuroma.

PHANTOM LIMB

Very few amputees fail to note the phantom limb sensation (6,7,8). It can vary greatly in intensity. In traumatic and crush injuries the patient usually has the sense of the extremity in its deformed and mangled state. The dysvascular amputee phantom will often mimic the prior painful state. Phantom limb sensation (7) is the conscious feeling that a limb is still present after amputation. Phantom limb pain (7) is the conscious feeling that a very painful limb is still present even after amputation.

There are three main theories attempting to describe the mechanism of the phantom limb pain.

1. *Gate Theory*. Following the theories of Melzack and Wall (9), Melzack suggests that the loss of sensory input after amputation decreases the self-sustaining neural activity of the gate, thereby causing pain. This theory supports the use of electrical stimulation and the transcutaneous electrical nerve stimulation (TENS) units as a method of treatment.

2. *The Peripheral Theory*. This theory proposes that persistent sensations from nerve endings in the stump continue to represent the parts originally innervated by the severed nerve. However, complete analgesia of the peripheral nerve or even rhizotomies have failed to relieve the pain, thus weakening this concept's plausibility.

3. *Psychological Theory*. This theory holds that there is a "wish fulfillment" resulting from the denial of the loss of a part, and the pain results from the denial of affect associated with the loss, as well as hostility and guilt—emotional responses to the loss of an important body part that is significant to the patient's relationship with others. Pain may result from self-punishment for such hostile and guilty emotions.

The patient should be encouraged to think of the condition as a normal one and a temporary one. If the complaint is severe and disabling, application of a TENS apparatus often provides temporary relief as well as a gradual reduction in the overall discomfort. In most cases the patient tolerates the sensation well. A prosthetic fitting, which "fills the gap," and ambulation with the prosthesis almost always eliminate or significantly reduce the problem. Constant positive reinforcement as to the problem being only temporary and readily controlled is essential.

Neurosurgery, dorsal column stimulation, and biofeedback techniques are other treatment modalities that have gained and lost favor over the years. The combination of electrical stimulation, prompt fitting, and ambulation with psychological support continues to provide the best results.

NEUROMA

A neuroma is a tumor or new growth largely made up of nerve fibers. It is thought to be secondary to the trauma of amputation surgery with continued regeneration of the nerve fibers resulting in a mass of nerve tissue. This is often painful and suggested as the cause of a painful stump.

The diagnosis of neuroma as the cause is overused and results in frequent unnecessary surgical interventions. Neuromas are rare.

The use of the TENS apparatus, ultrasound, and whirlpool baths to ease the discomfort plus positive emotional support by the treating team can often solve the problem and avoid unnecessary surgery.

The Rehabilitation Period

THE CLINIC

Once the acute postoperative period is passed, the patient proceeds to the next level of care, which is usually provided at the rehabilitation center. Here the patient can be treated either on an inpatient or on an outpatient basis, depending on the patient's physical capacity at the time of discharge from the acute hospital.

The clinic team is composed of the physician, the physical therapist, the prosthetist, and, of course, the patient. The clinic should also have available to it consultative services in occupational therapy, psychology, social services, and vocational services. These services are available on a case by case basis as the need presents itself. Driver education with the ability to provide the substitute devices necessary to compensate for the amputation should also be available.

The team members should meet on a weekly scheduled basis to assess patient progress in the therapeutic program as well as to assess the prosthetic and treatment needs of new admissions. Joint discussions between the team members resolve the problems that develop in the process of retraining, taking advantage of the expertise of the individual members of the team.

The clinic setting should provide privacy and an atmosphere of concern and dedication to the needs of the patient. It is here that the prescriptions of both the temporary and the permanent prostheses are made to meet the specific needs of the patient. Stump problems are assessed and treated as are problems of pain. Assistive devices such as crutches, canes, and walkers are provided (Figure 72-2) as the experience of the treating therapists indicates their need. The time of discharge from the clinic is determined by the team when the patient has achieved the goals set at the outset or lesser results because of intervening problems suggesting maximal improvement. Follow-up recommendations and appointments are provided, assuring the patient that the clinic remains there to serve him or her at any time in the future should the need arise.

THE TREATMENT PROGRAM

This phase actually began during the immediate postoperative period. It is continued at the rehabilitation facility or in the therapy department of the hospital. There is a gradual increase in the intensity of the program of physical restoration to achieve reconditioning and improve mobility to prepare the patient for prosthetic fitting and ambulation training. Usually within 2 weeks the patient is seen in the amputee clinic and the temporary prosthesis is prescribed (10).

In the case of the below-knee amputee, the socket is fabricated in the method similar to that of the permanent prosthesis. It is individually prepared. There is an initial casting of the stump followed by the preparation of the socket using molded plastics such as Polysar. It is then fitted to a pylon, a solid ankle cushion heel (SACH) foot and supracondylar cuff are attached, and the prosthesis is aligned. A cosmetic cover is then applied. The patient can be ambulated with either the hard socket or a soft insert.

The prosthesis is suspended by a leather supracondylar cuff secured by a buckle. A fork strap and waist belt may be added to assist suspension. Occasionally, if needed for knee stabilization or because of proprioceptive deficits, a thigh corset is applied. Attention should be given to any associated problems

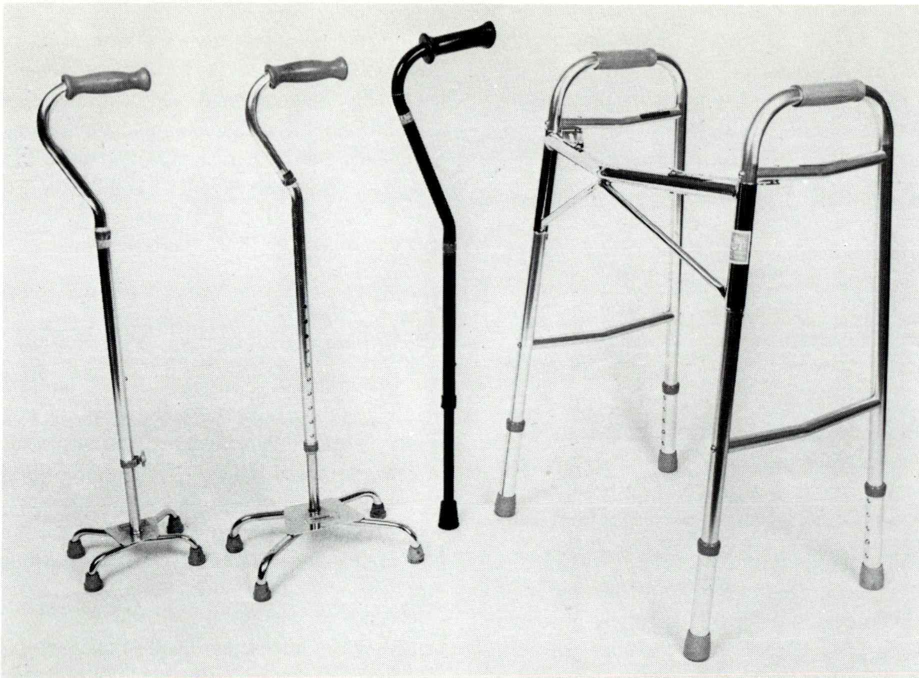

A B C D

FIGURE 72-2. Assistive ambulation devices. *(A)* Small-based quad cane. *(B)* Wide-based quad cane. *(C)* Straight cane. *(D)* Walker.

with the contralateral leg and foot. Special shoes should be supplied if needed (Figure 72-3).

In the above-knee amputee, a similar socket is fabricated following casting of the thigh. A single-axis knee joint with a manual knee locking merchanism is then applied. For reasons of safety and stability many patients need to begin ambulation training with the prosthetic knee locked. A SACH foot is also provided and the prosthesis aligned. The usual suspension mechanism for the temporary above-knee prosthesis is a hip joint and pelvic belt (Figure 72-4*A* and 4*B*).

The advantages of prescribing temporary prosthetic fitting are as follows:

Shrinkage and shaping of the stump can be achieved through the addition of stump socks to compensate for the shrinkage as it occurs.

Early ambulation results in greater safety for the patient and the amputated limb since the prosthesis is individually prepared and fitted.

Should excessive shrinkage be required, it is simple and inexpensive to replace the socket to achieve full results.

Adjustments in alignment are easily carried out as needed.

A more definitive decision can be made as to the knee and ankle-foot mechanism best suited for the patient in the permanent prosthesis.

The patient, once trained, can be discharged and returned to home and even to employment using the temporary prosthesis while still progressing toward complete shrinkage and shaping.

The permanent prosthesis can be prescribed and fabricated while the patient is fully functional and active at home or work.

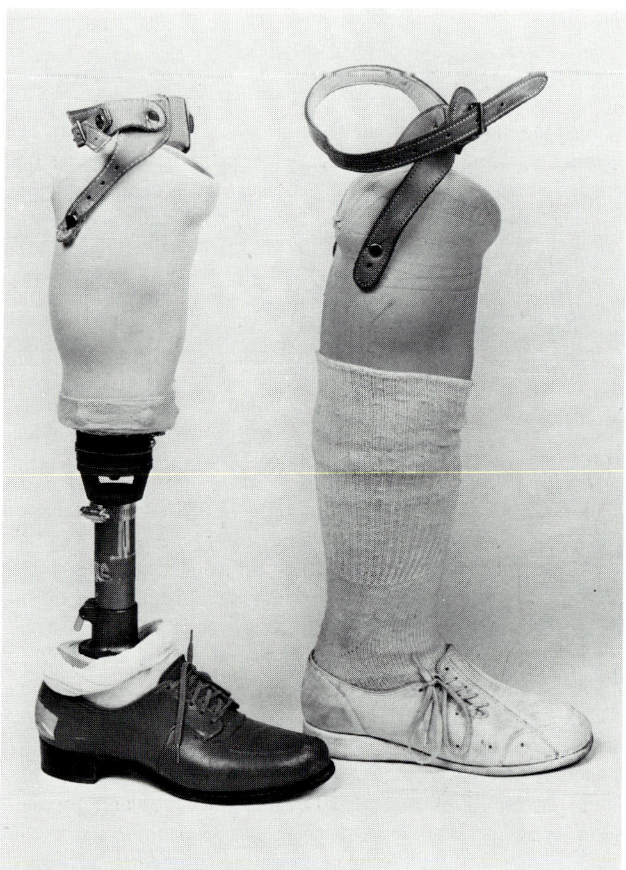

FIGURE 72-3. The temporary below-knee prosthesis with and without cosmetic cover.

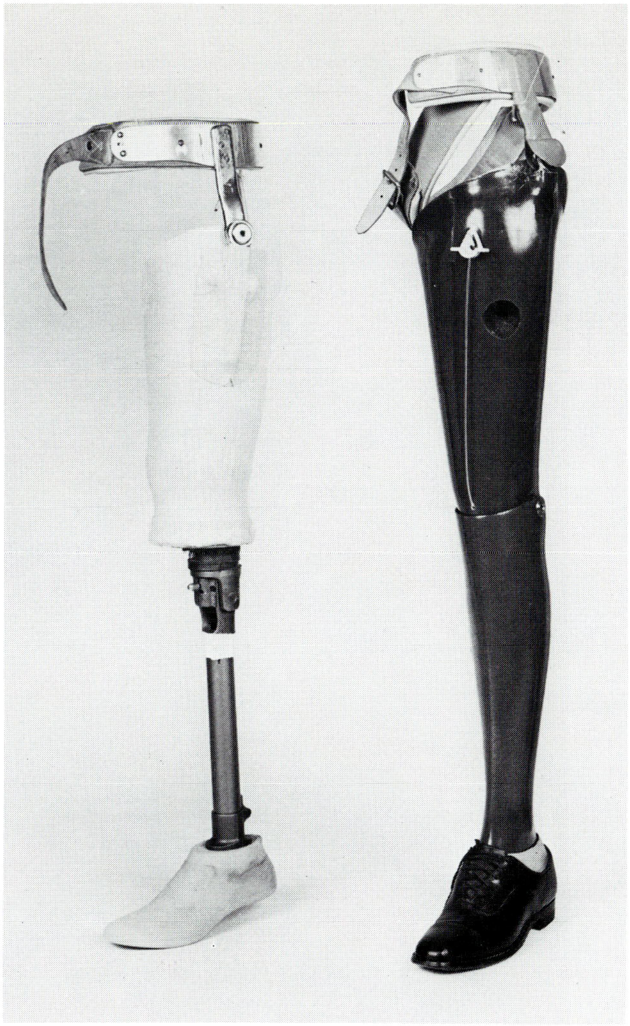

FIGURE 72-4. *(A)* The temporary above-knee prosthesis. *(B)* The permanent above-knee prosthesis with manual knee lock.

Upon receiving the permanent prosthesis, the patient is fully trained and confident.

The permanent prosthesis has a much longer life expectancy since only minimal further shrinkage is seen, assuring longer socket fit.

The temporary is less costly to fabricate, cosmetically acceptable, and fully functional.

The training period with the temporary prosthesis can determine the feasibility of permanent prosthetic fitting by establishing whether the patient has the physical and mental capacity to handle a prosthesis with safety.

COMPLICATIONS THAT CAN AFFECT THE PROCESS OF PROSTHETIC FITTING AND TRAINING

1. There can be significant weight loss during the preamputation period, and as this weight is regained, fitting problems can develop. The normal weight of the patient minus the amputated leg should be assessed, and, since this weight is usually regained, the prescription and fitting of the permanent prosthesis should be delayed for a reasonable time to note the pattern of weight regaining.

2. Interval problems of stump swelling should be attended to with a discontinuation of prosthetic use to avoid stump irritations, ulcers, and pain. Stump wrapping should be reinstituted and continued throughout the day and night until the stump can be once again safely inserted into the socket. The techniques of stump wrapping and care of the stump should be well taught. This includes the donning and management of stump socks.

3. Pressure areas should be promptly observed and socket modifications carried out or any other cause attended to to avoid ulcerations.

4. Flexion contractures of the hips or knees should be compensated for in the prosthetic alignment or by building greater amounts of flexion in the socket at the time of fabrication.

5. The skin of the stump should be observed daily for any sign of skin rash and immediate corrective measures taken to correct the problem.

6. A painful stump should be evaluated as to cause and corrected. A neuroma is a rare problem and often overdiagnosed as the cause of pain in the stump. Other, simpler causes should be ruled out first.

7. The problem of phantom limb can be cared for best by prompt fitting of the limb with a prosthesis and the start of gait training. The patient should be counseled and reassured that the problem is usually temporary. Prompt psychological counseling should be started if the problem remains or worsens.

8. A painful stump after total evaluation can be treated using the modalities available to the therapist. Ultrasound to achieve deep heating, whirlpool bath for superficial heating and massage, as well as the TENS apparatus should be tried. Each has been successful in easing as well as eradicating pain.

9. An unhealed suture line or ulcerated area of the stump requires immediate and aggressive management. Meticulous cleanliness must be observed. Debridement should be complete to remove infected and necrotic tissue, allowing a clean surface for healing. Cultures can provide an insight into the infective agent and precise antibiotics given. Sterile dressings are used, and the continued use of the elastic bandages is necessary to avoid edema which impedes healing. Whirlpool baths with Betadine or pHisoHex added can be used to debride and cleanse. Prosthetic use is usually contraindicated during the healing period (11).

The Permanent Prosthesis

THE PROSTHETIC PRESCRIPTION

Below-Knee Prescriptions

The usual prescription for the standard below-knee amputee is a patellar tendon-bearing prosthesis with supracondylar medial wedge suspension in the soft insert, and SACH foot.

Variations include

Suprapatellar strap and cuff suspension

Thigh corset with knee joint and waist belt and fork strap

Single-axis foot

Multiaxis foot

In most cases the standard prescription provides the optimal result. The multiaxis foot-ankle mechanism is gaining in popularity now that many of its mechanical defects have been corrected. It provides the patient with a more normal gait pattern since it allows a greater amount of plantar flexion and dorsiflexion as well as some medial and lateral mobility of the ankle and foot. The SACH foot provides a less mobile action in dorsiflexion and plantar flexion and some limited medial-lateral motion. Its motion is a result of layers of cushioned rubber and a toe break in the forefoot.

The use of the thigh corset and waist belt is seen less and less frequently in amputee clinics. There is some use in the case of the elderly and/or sensory-deficient patient to provide a feedback as to position to improve security and ambulation safety. When a thigh corset is used, the waist belt and fork strap are necessary for suspension to avoid stump pistoning.

Another use of the corset and knee joint is to provide a greater control of the unstable knee joint. This can also be provided by the supracondylar fit with a high anterior wall (suprapatellar), however. Genu recurvatum can also be controlled.

The soft insert which is placed in the socket is again almost always provided. Some physicians still feel, however, that in the dysvascular, sensory-deficient stump the use of the hard socket is preferred. A five-ply stump sock is then used. This technique is also sometimes used to offset the problem of weight gain or swelling of the stump which does not allow penetration of the stump into the prosthesis with the insert in place. It is usually a temporary device to allow continued ambulation while the problem is being rectified. If the condition is permanent, a new socket would be provided.

Above-Knee Prescriptions

The usual prescription for the standard above-knee amputee is a pelvic band suspension with hip joint, semisuction quadrilateral socket, safety knee, and single-axis foot-ankle mechanism.

Variations include

Suction socket with silesian belt suspension

Hydraulic knee

Single-axis knee with manual knee lock (see Figure 72-4*B*).

SACH foot

The suction socket with silesian belt suspension is usually prescribed for the younger patient because of the difficulty in donning and removing the prosthesis. The semisuction socket is a reasonable substitute since it is easily donned and provides the feeling of lightness which is secondary to the suction received. This feeling of increased lightness has proved to be of great value to the elderly patient.

The hydraulic knee is often used in conjunction with the suction socket suspension and provides an excellent, more normal knee motion during gait. Many different types of hydraulic knees are available, each with differing characteristics.

The single-axis knee with the manual knee lock allows the patient to ambulate with the knee locked in extension. This increases safety and stability. For sitting the knee is easily unlocked with a pull strap.

The polycentric knee joint can be used and is more stable but less cosmetically acceptable. It is of value for the knee disarticulation level of amputation since its space requirements are minimal.

Numerous safety knees are also available. These knee mechanisms allow the patient to increase or decrease the friction at the knee, allowing more or less freedom of swing as well as stability at the joint during the stance phase of ambulation by locking the knee in position at heel strike, avoiding knee buckling.

The SACH foot is still prescribed in some clinics, but there is no question that the single-axis foot-ankle mechanism provides a better and safer gait for the above-knee amputee.

PROSTHETIC REPLACEMENT

It is unwise to change the prosthetic components when future limbs are fabricated. When the patient has successfully adjusted to a particular suspension, socket, knee mechanism, or ankle-foot, she or he usually finds any change in the prescribed part extremely difficult to adjust to. Changes in the components should be done only if there is a real need, not merely to modernize the prosthesis. Prosthetic rejection is high when such substitutions are attempted.

AMBULATION AIDS

The usual program of rehabilitation begins with the patient ambulating in the parallel bars as the patient progresses to full weight bearing on the limb and adjusts to the prosthesis. The patient can then proceed to ambulation with a walker, two canes, one cane, and eventually no assistive aids. It is usually recommended, however, that a cane of some type be used for outside ambulation for safety. The final aid required for an individual patient depends upon many variables and must be an individual decision.

In the retraining of gait for the more advanced patient, a treadmill is often used to improve the smoothness and cadence of gait.

There are many varieties of walkers and canes available to the patient, providing variable levels of safety and support. Again, the patient's individual needs must be assessed and the proper device then prescribed.

DRIVER TRAINING

In the case of the right-leg amputee, minor adjustments are required to the automobile to allow the patient to accelerate with the left leg. An accelerator extension is available and easily placed in the vehicle and retraining is minimal. The double amputee requires training in the use of hand controls, but again, retraining and driving are still reasonable goals.

THE DOUBLE AMPUTEE

The double below-knee amputee usually can be successfully ambulated for household activities and some limited functions outside the home. Once again, the amount of activity is limited by the patient's medical status, age, and level of amputation. Double amputations should not suggest nonambulation. Often, limited prosthetic use which allows the patient to perform a standing pivot transfer to bed, wheelchair, or commode can be of great help to the patient, allowing independence which might not be feasible if the prostheses were denied. The psychological effect of even such limited success cannot be ignored. In addition, the presence of the prosthetic legs even as a cosmetic effect while in the wheelchair can be of significant value to the patient and justify fitting.

Training in the activities of daily living from the wheelchair can be achieved and still allow complete independence. Transfers can be safely performed using a sliding board to move from bed, car, tub, or commode. In the bath, special benches and portable shower heads allow the patient to bathe independently.

When the double above-knee amputee is fitted prosthetically, function is limited. The psychological effect of the presence of the legs while in the wheelchair may be of value. Such prostheses may, however, limit the independence of the patient for wheelchair living because of their weight and bulk.

METABOLIC REQUIREMENTS OF AMBULATION

It is obvious that energy requirements increase as the level of amputation increases and if both extremities are involved. During normal walking speeds, energy consumption increases can vary from about 20 percent greater in the standard below-knee amputee to 65 percent greater in the middle-aged above-knee amputee (12). Retaining the knee joint greatly reduces the energy expenditure, and for this reason there continues to be a great effort made to save the knee at the time of surgery. Evaluations suggest that a bilateral below-knee amputee, who requires 40 percent more energy than a nonamputee, still requires about 25 percent less energy to function than a unilateral above-knee patient, who requires 65 percent more energy than a nonamputee.

Bilateral above-knee amputees use more than double the energy to ambulate. Tests suggest a 110 percent rise in energy requirements during ambulation (13).

Evaluations have shown that ambulation with one above-knee amputation and axillary crutches increases energy consumption up to 60 percent above normal at normal gait speeds. This can, therefore, be a good test of the patient's ability to successfully ambulate with a prosthesis since if the patient expending this energy without the added weight of the prosthesis has difficulty ambulating, then a prosthetic fitting which requires a greater energy expenditure is contraindicated.

One obvious way to reduce energy costs is to reduce the cadence. The average speed of ambulation with an above-knee prosthesis is 2.4 km/h; a below-knee amputee, 3.2 to 4 km/h; a normal adult ambulates at a speed of 4.8 km/h. Such reductions in cadence can equalize energy expenditures (14,15). Wheelchair ambulation requires an energy consumption average only 9 percent above that of normal walking and is therefore, from the energy standpoint, a better substitute for the elderly or the patient with advanced cardiopulmonary disease.

The life expectancy of the elderly or diabetic dysvascular amputee is usually limited because advanced disease in the extremity usually suggests a generalized problem. Studies suggest the average life expectancy to be about 1.5 years in dysvascular patients (16). In addition, progression to loss of the other limb is common and is seen in about 25 percent of cases (17).

In spite of these negative statistics, the improved quality of life provided for the medically stable patient justifies prosthetic fitting and training. It stresses the need for prompt training and fitting. Cases should be judged individually, giving weight to the psychological needs of the patient as well. When there is doubt as to success or failure, a trial with a temporary prosthesis will quickly provide the answer satisfying both the doctor and the patient more readily than a denial based on judgment alone.

References

1. Moskowitz E, McCann C: Classificaton of disability in the chronically ill and aging. J Chronic Dis 1957, 5:342.
2. Robinson K: Amputation in vascular disese. Ann R Coll Surg Engl 1980, 62:88.
3. Castronuovo JJ Jr., Deane LM, Deterling RA Jr., O'Donnell TF Jr., O'Toole DM, Callow AD: Below knee amputation: Is the effort to preserve the knee joint justified? Arch Surg 1980, 115:1184.
4. Rizzo N: Physical therapy management of diabetics undergoing lower extremity amputation. Diabetes Educ 1983, 8:24.
5. Sullivan RA, Tucker J, Taliaferro F: Manual for lower extremity amputees. Patient education publication. Kessler Institute, 1975.
6. Riding J: Phantom limb—Some theories. Anesthesia 1976, 31:102.
7. Feldman RC: Current theories and treatments related to phantom limb pain. Br J Med 1978, 9:26.
8. Sherman R, Teppons J: Suggested guidelines for treatment of phantom limb pain. Orthopedics 1982, 5:1595.
9. Melzack R, Wall PD: Pain mechanisms—a new theory. Science 1965, 150:971.
10. Sullivan RA, Tucker J: Amputee management using fitted temporary prosthesis: Preliminary report. Arch Phys Med Rehabil 1974, 55:409.
11. Horne G, Abramowicz J: The management of healing problems in the dysvascular amputee. Prosthet Orthot Int 1982, 6:38.
12. Traugh GH, Corcoran PJ, Royes RL: Energy expenditures of am-

bulation in patients with above-knee amputations. Arch Phys Med Rehabil 1975, 56:67.
13. Corcoran PJ: Energy cost of ambulation in bilateral lower extremity amputees in preparation. Arch Phys Med Rehabil 1974, 55:111.
14. Gonzalez EG, Corcoran PJ, Reyes RL: Energy expenditures in below-knee amputees: Correlation with stump length. Arch Phys Med Rehabil 1974, 55:111.
15. Waters RL, Perry J, Antonelli D, Hislop H: Energy cost of walking of amputees; influence of level of amputation. J Bone Joint Surg [Am] 1978, 58:42.
16. Hansson J: Leg amputee: Clinical follow-up study, Acta Orthop Scand [Suppl] 1964, 69:1.
17. Warren R, Kihn RB: Survey of lower extremity amputations for ischemia. Surgery 1968, 63:107.

Chapter 73

VASCULAR ASPECTS OF ORGAN TRANSPLANTATION

V. K. MITTAL and L. H. TOLEDO-PEREYRA

Vascular Aspects during Harvesting

Vascular factors of importance during organ harvesting relate to harvesting the organs from live or cadaveric donors, harvesting of multiple or single organs, and arterial anomalies.

KIDNEY HARVESTING

Kidneys can be procured for transplantation from cadaveric or live, related donors. In the case of cadaveric donors, both kidneys are procured en bloc or singly and may be a part of multiple organ harvesting (1–7). Once the decision is made to harvest the kidneys, a major concern is to prevent ischemic damage. If the donor's cardiovascular status and urine output cannot be maintained with intravenous fluids alone, dopamine, 5 to 10 μg/mL, should be given intravenously, titrated to increase renal blood flow and cardiac output (8,9).

Other agents have been used to stabilize the lysosomal membrane, including chlorpromazine and prednisolone, though their use is unproven. Chlorpromazine (50 mg) is administered intravenously about half an hour before the onset of warm ischemia, and methylprednisolone (1 g) is given intravenously at the same time (10–12). It is common practice to induce "full heparinization" about 10 minutes before clamping the aorta in order to minimize the risk of small-vessel thrombosis in the kidneys (1–3).

During the harvesting from a cadaveric donor, the surgeon makes every effort to identify and preserve multiple vessels arising from the aorta and occasionally from the iliac arteries. Damage to multiple vessels is less likely if the en bloc procedure is used. When the kidneys are to be removed singly, as is often done in multiple organ donors (2,4), the vessels are removed with a Carrell patch of either the aorta or the iliac vessels. Double renal veins are also not unusual.

In the case of a living donor, a preoperative arteriogram is mandatory (13,14). This demonstrates the vascular supply of the kidney and aids in determining which kidney is to be removed. It is preferable to remove a kidney with a single artery as it is imprudent to take a patch from the aorta in a living donor. A kidney with multiple arteries is only rarely considered for removal from a living donor.

After arteriography a reduction in the renal plasma flow and renal function has been noted in some patients; hence nephrectomy is usually deferred for a week or more. Preoperatively, the donor is well hydrated to ensure maintenance of a high renal blood flow during nephrectomy as this decreases the chance of postoperative acute tubular necrosis developing in both donor and recipient (15). Full heparinization is recommended by a few authors, but it creates unnecessary risks for the donor with little evidence of positive benefit to the recipient.

Technical considerations during harvesting include isolation of the gonadal vein on the left side, ligating it as it enters the left renal vein. On the right side, it usually enters the vena cava. Similarly the adrenal vein is identified, ligated, and divided on the left. The left renal vein is cleaned and traced up to the point it crosses the aorta, and lymphatics from the kidney are divided between sutures to prevent lymphocele formation in a live donor or the recipient. Renal arteries are identified as they enter the aorta and dissected free of adventitial tissue. A lumbar vein is often found joining the renal vein, especially on the left side, and is divided and ligated (Figure 73-1).

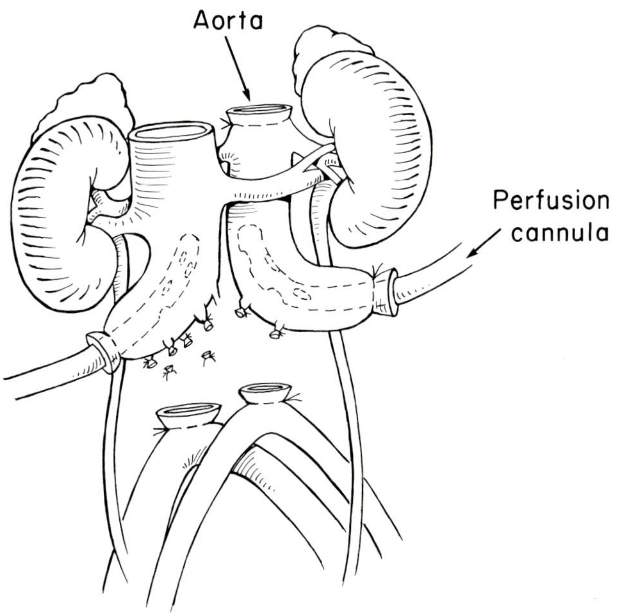

FIGURE 73-1. In situ perfusion of dissected kidneys.

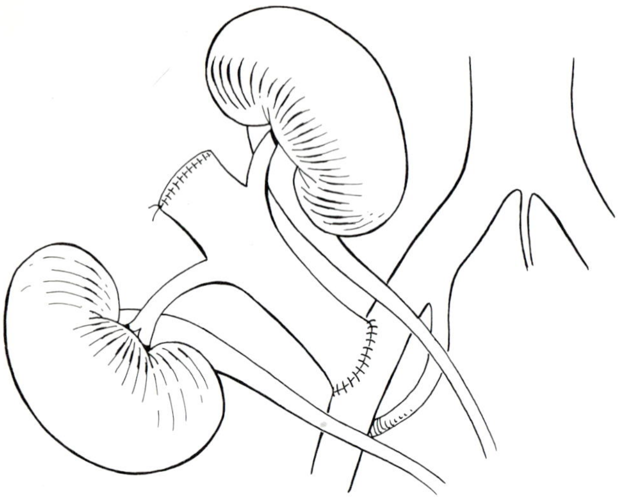

FIGURE 73-2. En bloc transplantation of pediatric kidneys to adult recipient.

Care is taken to minimize trauma to the renal artery. Injection of periadventitial lidocaine or 4% procaine (Novocain) may be helpful in preventing spasm. Excessive traction can lead to intimal damage, recognized by palpation of a weakness in the wall of the artery with associated periadventitial tissue hematoma. Rarely a vessel between the kidney itself and the adrenal gland may be encountered. The donor's renal artery and the renal vein stumps are oversewn with 3-0 or 4-0 vascular sutures to ensure hemostasis.

In pediatric cadaveric donors, both of the kidneys can be harvested en bloc and transplanted en bloc in an adult patient (Figure 73-2).

When the kidneys are harvested as a part of multiple organ harvesting, they are removed last, as they withstand a longer warm ischemia period than other organs and usually are perfused in situ with cold crystalloid solution (1,2,4).

PANCREAS HARVESTING

The entire pancreas can be harvested as a pancreaticoduodenal graft, or a portion of the organ as a segmental pancreatic graft. Only a segmental pancreas graft is harvested from a live donor (16,17). The main theoretical advantage of an entire pancreas graft is the larger mass of tissue taken, enhancing blood flow to the graft and possibly diminishing the incidence of thrombosis.

Whole pancreas donation may be combined with heart and kidney donation in the same donor, but when the liver is also harvested, only a segmental pancreatic graft is removed (1,2). When the liver is not used, the entire pancreas can be removed on a patch of aorta containing the celiac axis and superior mesenteric artery.

In harvesting the whole pancreas, the lesser sac is entered by dividing the branches of the gastroepiploic vessels. The spleen is then mobilized and the short gastric vessels divided as they enter the spleen. Small vessels from the gland to the mesocolon and the retroperitoneal tissues are secured. The inferior mesenteric vein is divided at its junction with the splenic vein. The splenic artery is dissected to its origin with the celiac axis. The left gastric artery is ligated and divided. Following this, the splenic vein is traced to its junction with the superior mesenteric vein and the origin of the portal vein.

If a segmental pancreatic graft is to be removed, then its vascular supply is dependent on the splenic vein and artery and the line of transection is at the level of superior mesenteric vessels. For a total pancreas graft the dissection is continued, and

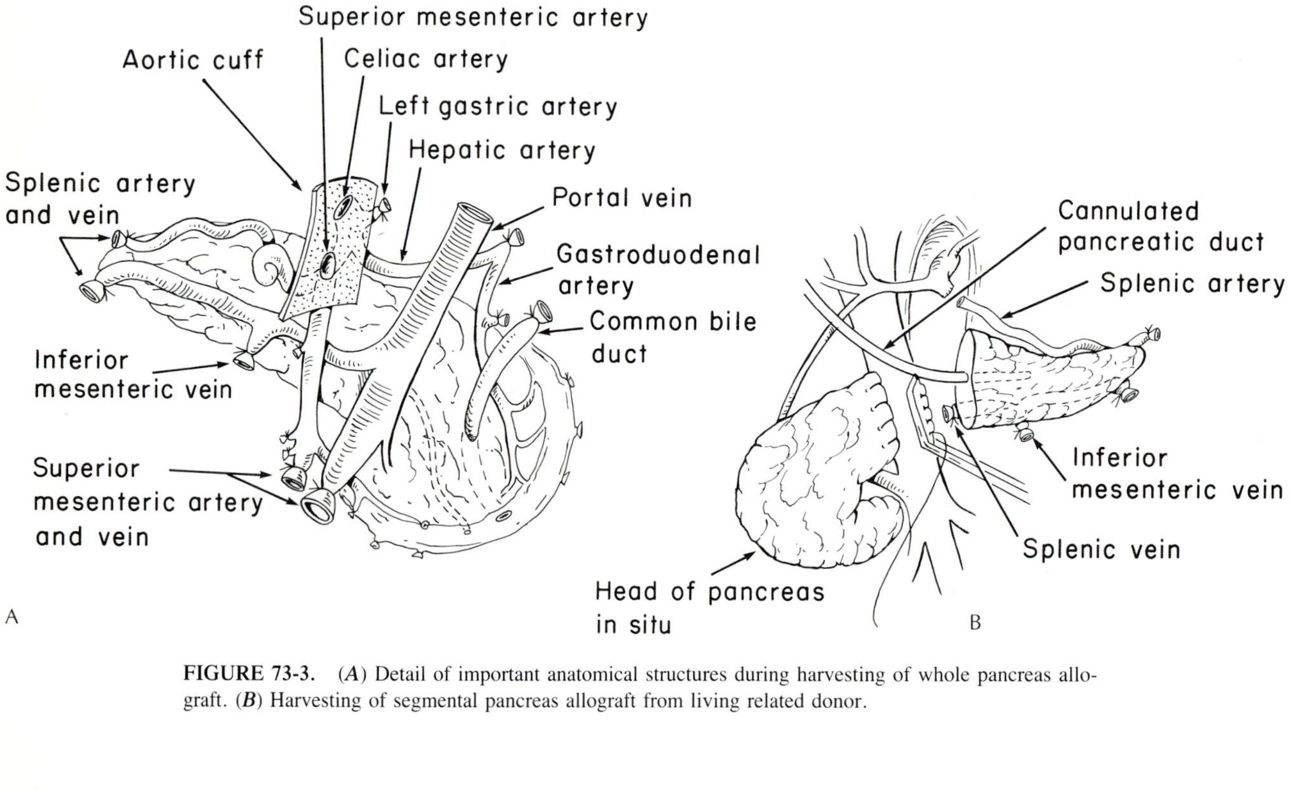

FIGURE 73-3. (*A*) Detail of important anatomical structures during harvesting of whole pancreas allograft. (*B*) Harvesting of segmental pancreas allograft from living related donor.

the duodenum is mobilized by the Kocher maneuver and the common bile duct ligated proximal to its entry into the pancreatic tissue. The hepatic artery is divided distal to the origin of the inferior pancreaticoduodenal artery; in this way, the arterial arcade is maintained for the head of the pancreas.

After full heparinization, the aorta is cross-clamped proximal to the celiac axis and distal to the superior mesenteric artery. The portal vein is cross-clamped away from the pancreas at its bifurcation, and the superior mesenteric vein is ligated below the inferior border of the pancreas. The blood flow of a total pancreas graft is dependent on a patch from the aorta including the origin of celiac axis and the superior mesenteric artery, and the portal vein (Figure 73-3*A*).

In the case of a segmental pancreatic graft harvested from a live, related donor (16,17), the splenic artery and vein are first ligated near the hilum of the spleen and the spleen is left in situ, supplied by the short gastric vessels. The inferior mesenteric vein is ligated and divided, as it joins the splenic vein. The vascular supply of the graft is then dependent on the splenic artery and the splenic vein, and these are divided along with the organ at its neck (Figure 73-3*B*).

Complications encountered in the living, related pancreas donor include (1) intraoperative bleeding, particularly during the dissection of the tail of the pancreas from the hilum of the spleen (this can be avoided by careful dissection, ligating the artery before the vein), and postoperative bleeding from the divided pancreas; (2) operative trauma to the spleen or short gastric vessels necessitating splenectomy; (3) pancreatitis of the residual head and body of the gland; (4) diabetes mellitus in the donor, which is the most serious complication; and (5) small bowel adhesions or obstruction.

LIVER HARVESTING

The liver is harvested as a part of multiple organ harvesting or as a single organ (17–19). As previously stated, the liver and a whole pancreatic graft cannot be harvested simultaneously from the same donor due to the common vascular supply, though a segmental pancreatic graft can be procured along with a liver (20).

A preoperative angiogram of the donor is helpful to determine the vascular supply of the liver and to identify accessory vessels, such as those arising from the superior mesenteric artery and left gastric artery (21). At a few centers a preoperative angiogram is done in the donor; otherwise anomalies are carefully sought at the time of harvesting. The left hepatic artery may arise from the left gastric artery or a right hepatic artery may arise from the superior mesenteric artery (Figure 73-4). The blood flow of the liver graft is dependent on the portal vein, the vena cava, and the celiac axis. After donor exploration, the hepatic artery is traced to the origin of the celiac axis. The gastroduodenal artery and the right gastric branch of the hepatic artery are both ligated and divided. The left gastric artery is divided along the lesser curvature of the stomach, leaving the main trunk behind protecting any branch to the liver from the left gastric artery. The celiac artery is followed to its origin, and the aorta at this site is dissected out for 2 to 3 cm above and below the celiac axis. The splenic artery is identified and divided.

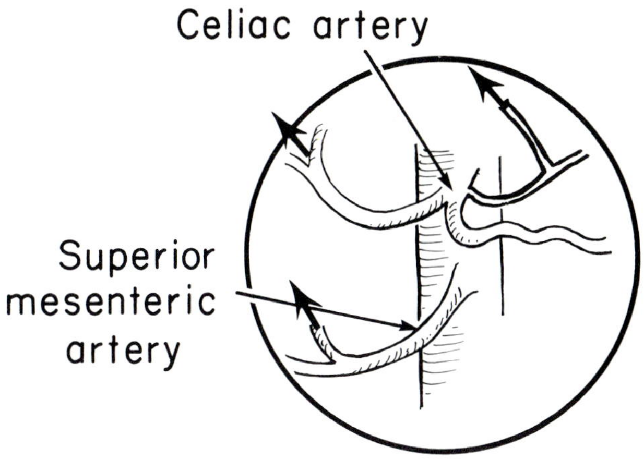

FIGURE 73-4. Common variations in hepatic arterial supply. In some donors (approximately 17 percent) an aberrant branch from the left gastric artery may supply the left lobe of the liver. Branches to the right lobe may arise from the superior mesenteric artery.

The inferior vena cava above and below the liver is mobilized, and the three phrenic veins that enter the suprahepatic vena cava are ligated and divided. Failure to do so will result in severe hemorrhage after reimplantation of the liver. During dissection of the liver, care is taken to preserve the blood supply to the gallbladder and the common bile duct, as in any surgical operation on the biliary tree. The neck of the pancreas provides easy access to the portal vein (Figure 73-5), and once the portal vein is exposed, the coronary vein can be identified, suture ligated, and divided. During the isolation of the infrahepatic vena cava the right adrenal vein is identified and ligated, as are the lumbar veins as they are encountered. During the mobilization of the suprahepatic vena cava, a rim of the diaphragm is left attached to the suprahepatic vena cava.

If in situ perfusion is to be carried out, then this can be done by a cannula inserted into the portal vein via the splenic or the superior mesenteric vein. Another cannula is inserted into the

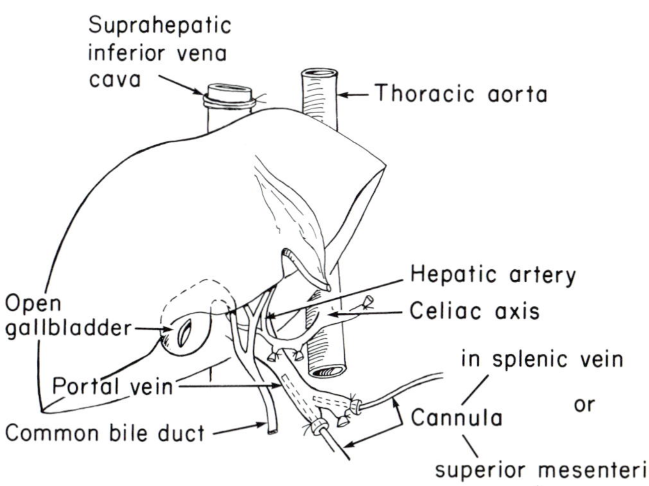

FIGURE 73-5. After dissection of the liver, it is cooled in situ by cannulation of the portal vein via the splenic or superior mesenteric vein.

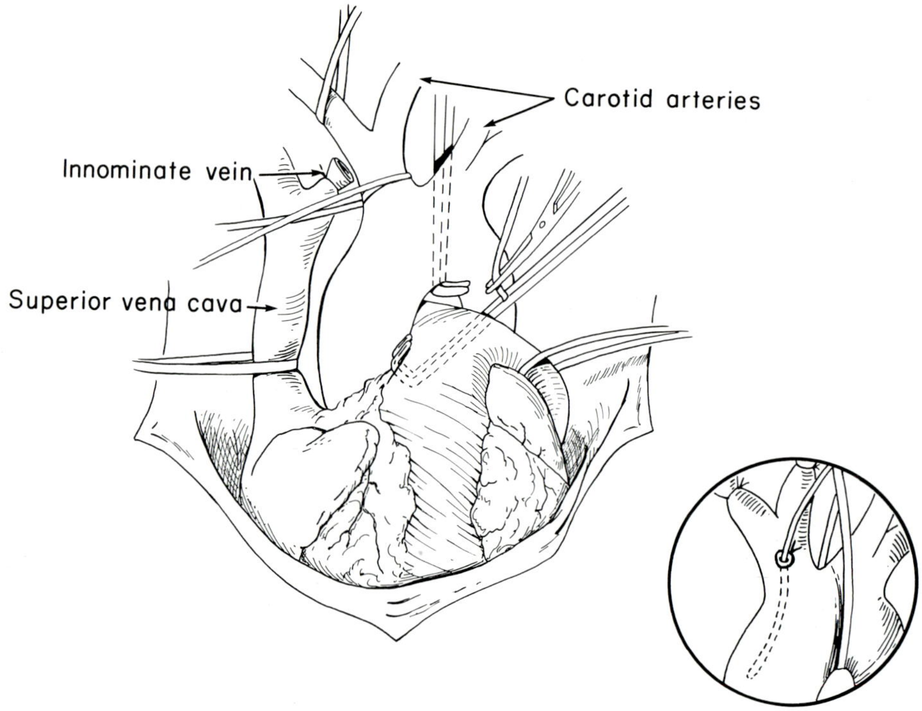

FIGURE 73-6. Detail of important structures during heart allograft dissection. Inset shows placement of catheter for cardioplegia through a purse-string suture in the innominate arterial trunk.

infrarenal aorta to perfuse the liver via the celiac axis and the kidneys via the renal arteries. The abdominal aorta at the level of the diaphragm is cross-clamped to commence the in situ perfusion.

The suprahepatic vena cava is divided at the right atrium and the aorta at the arch. The inferior vena cava is divided proximal to the entrance of the renal vein. The ligamentous attachments of the vena cava can be divided as the liver is removed.

CARDIAC HARVESTING

The heart can be harvested alone or as a part of multiple organ harvesting (1). A composite heart and lung graft has recently been introduced successfully. When the isolated heart is harvested, the organ is mobilized and the superior vena cava and the inferior vena cava are dissected free from the diaphragm to the right atrium. The left subclavian vein is divided, and the innominate artery is exposed. Following this, the innominate artery is completely mobilized to the region of the right carotid, and its branches are individually identified. The innominate artery is encircled between loops, and the dissection is carried along the aorta to its root. Finally the pulmonary artery is mobilized to its right and left main branches. The cardioplegic solution is placed through the innominate artery into the aorta.

Excision of the donor heart is started by dividing the venous inflow, the superior vena cava, cephalad to the junction of the right atrium and the inferior vena cava at the junction with the atrium. Following this, the aorta is divided immediately distal to the innominate artery with a TA50 stapling device (Figure 73-6). The pulmonary artery main branches are then divided, leaving the heart attached only by the pulmonary veins. As a last step in the harvesting of the heart, the pulmonary veins are divided at the level of their respective pericardial reflections (Figure 73-7).

LUNG HARVESTING

Lung transplantation is in its infancy. Initially, the lungs were isolated as a single organ and transplanted; however, there has not been long-term survival. The vascular supply of the lungs is

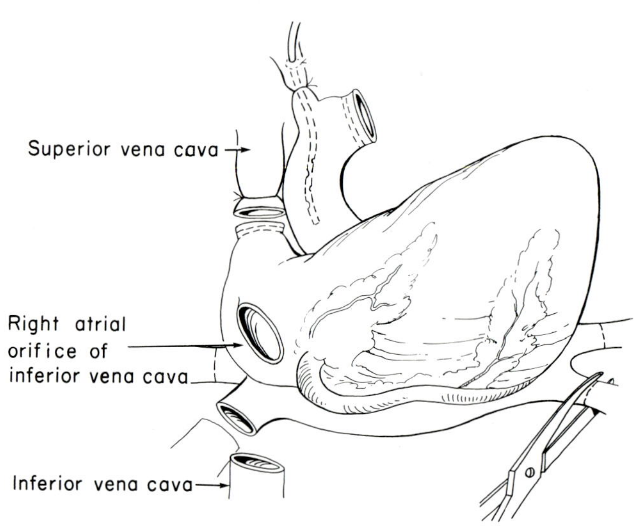

FIGURE 73-7. In the final steps of heart excision, the heart is lifted from the pericardial sac and the individual pulmonary veins are divided at the level of their respective pericardial reflections.

based on the pulmonary artery and left atrium immediately after the entrance of the pulmonary veins. Recently, combined heart and lungs harvesting has been carried out with improved results (1). In order to avoid malfunction of the donor lung prior to transplantation, it is important that periods of warm ischemia be avoided, and to achieve this, good cardiovascular function should be established, with fluid replacement.

Combined heart and lungs harvesting is being done more frequently with the vascular supply dependent on the aorta and the superior and inferior vena cavas.

Vascular Aspects during Transplantation

KIDNEY TRANSPLANTATION

All prospective recipients are carefully evaluated prior to kidney transplantation. This assessment includes seeking a history of cardiovascular disease, hypertension, congestive heart failure, cardiac arrythmia, uremic pericarditis, and valvular heart disease.

If the patient has severe coronary artery disease, a pretransplant coronary artery bypass may be considered and hypertension is controlled prior to transplantation. Unexplained episodes of hypotension during dialysis may be the first clue to the existence of ischemic heart disease or a silent myocardial infarction.

Extensive peripheral vascular occlusive disease may cause problems in performing acceptable graft vascular anastomoses. If there is occlusion of iliac vessels, this may necessitate use of other vessels for a renal transplant anastomosis. A correctable iliac vessel occlusion or aneurysm is treated before the transplantation procedure (Figure 73-8). Vascular occlusive disease or a previous reconstruction of the aortoiliac area may preclude renal transplantation. Any clinical suggestion of peripheral vascular occlusive disease is investigated by noninvasive vascular tests and, if indicated, by angiogram.

A prior history of venous disease may be associated with an increased incidence of postoperative venous thrombosis or renal vein thrombosis. The likelihood of this may be increased if the patient was taking estrogen or progesterone therapy before the transplant, especially in the female. If an iliac vein thrombosis is suspected, a preliminary venogram is done, as this might compromise the iliac vein anastomosis. When a history of thrombophlebitis is present or a deep vein thrombosis is found, patients are heparinized and treated before proceeding to their transplantation (22). Deep vein thrombosis, when documented, may be treated by placement of a preoperative inferior vena caval clip or filter.

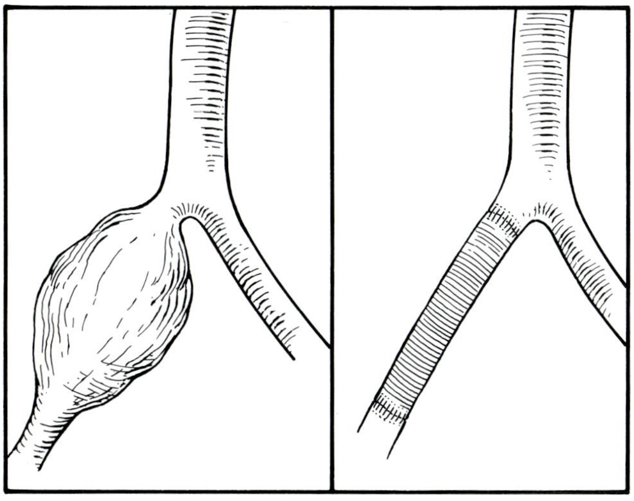

FIGURE 73-8. Correction of large arteriosclerotic aneurysm of common iliac artery prior to transplantation using Dacron graft.

Surgical Technique of Kidney Transplantation

The kidney is usually transplanted extraperitoneally into one of the iliac fossae. However, in juvenile diabetics, kidney tranplantation may be combined with pancreatic transplantation in the other iliac fossa (Figure 73-9). The surgical procedure after initial evaluation of the kidney consists of exposure and preparation of the iliac vessels and the construction of the anastomoses.

Preoperatively, a central venous pressure line is placed, particularly in patients who have a history of cardiovascular disease. Spinal anesthesia may be used. The iliac vessels are exposed retroperitoneally by making an oblique incision in the lower quadrant.

Extraperitoneal dissection should be minimal, and the perivascular lymphatics are carefully ligated to avoid forming a lymphocele. The inferior epigastric vessels are ligated and divided. The dissection of the iliac vessels is kept medial to the lymph nodes that underlie the inguinal ligament because most lymphoceles start here. For the vascular anastomoses the renal vein of the donor kidney is anastomosed to the external iliac vein in an end-to-side fashion with a 5-0 Prolene continuous suture. The renal vein is not unclamped until the arterial anastomosis is complete.

A short renal vein can be accommodated by ligation of the recipient hypogastric vein, thus freeing the common and external iliac vein which can then be mobilized for anastomosis to the renal vein of the donor kidney. In the case of the cadaver kidney with two renal veins, these may be anastomosed using a patch from the donor's inferior vena cava sutured to the external iliac vein in a side-to-side fashion. Small renal vein branches of the donor kidney can be ligated safely.

The arterial anastomosis may be done by either of two methods. An end-to-side technique, anastomosing the donor renal artery to the side of the external iliac artery of the recipient (Figure 73-10*A*) (23), minimizes the dissection of the lymphatic vessels and spares the hypogastric collateral blood supply to the genitalia. The other technique is end-to-end arterial anastomosis. The donor's renal artery is anastomosed end-to-end to the mobilized and divided hypogastric artery of the recipient (Figure 73-10*B*). This is particularly done when the donor renal artery has no patch as in the case of a living donor. Where there are extensive arteriosclerotic plaques, with severe stenosis of the common and internal iliac arteries, a localized endarterectomy can be performed and an end-to-side anastomosis done (24).

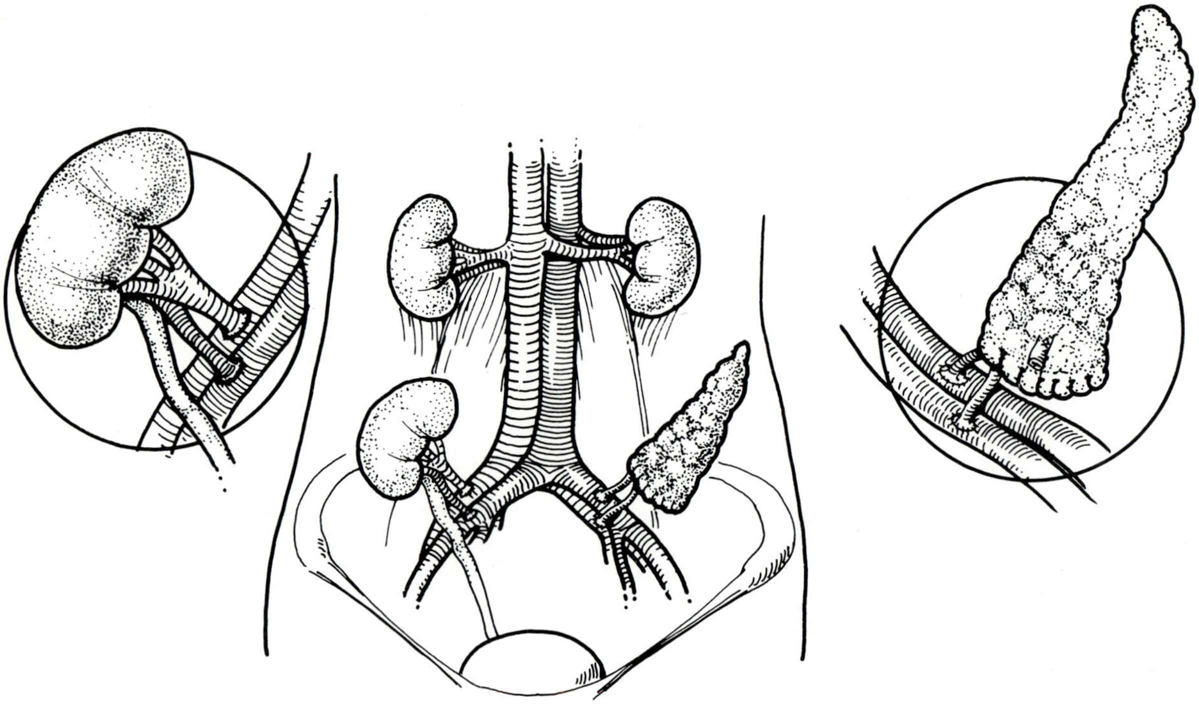

FIGURE 73-9. Simultaneous transplantation of kidney and pancreas allografts from same donor into iliac fossae of diabetic recipient. (Used with permission of the American College of Surgeons.)

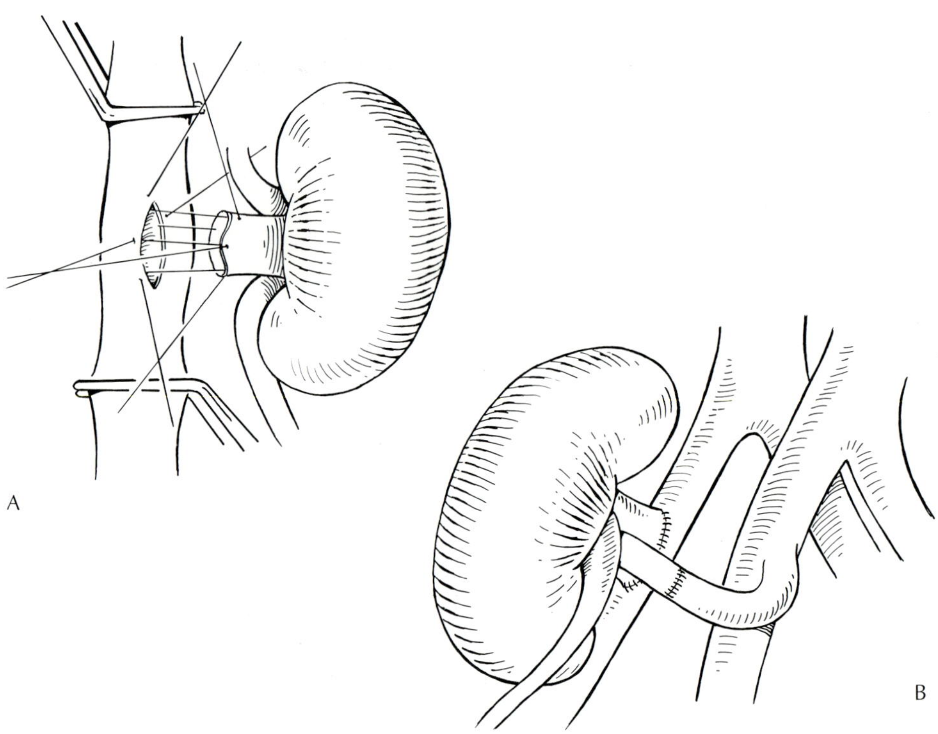

A

B

FIGURE 73-10. (*A*) Detail of end-to-side anastomosis of donor renal artery to external iliac artery of recipient. (*B*) End-to-end anastomosis of donor renal artery with hypogastric artery of recipient.

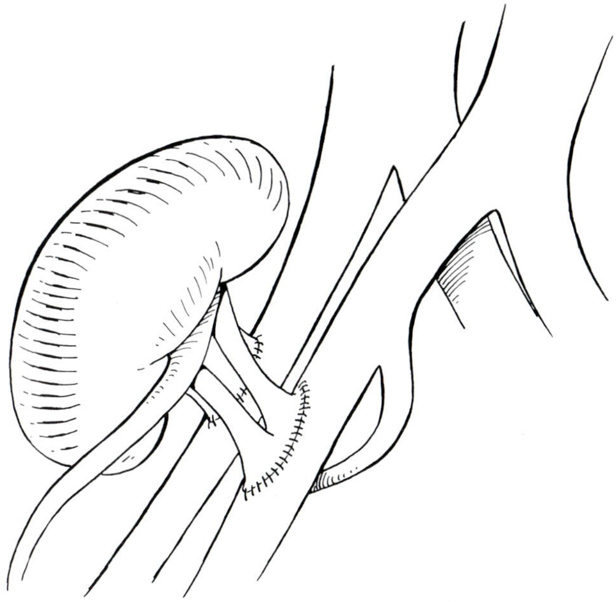

FIGURE 73-11. Handling of multiple renal arteries by end-to-side anastomosis of donor renal arteries with aortic patch with external iliac of recipient.

Multiple renal arteries are present in approximately 20 percent of all the kidneys. Inadvertent ligation can result in infarction and later in a caliceal-cutaneous fistula. Kidneys with multiple arteries from cadaver donors are harvested with an aortic patch and anastomosed in an end-to-side fashion with the external iliac artery (Figure 73-11).

In case of a pediatric donor, both the kidneys can be anastomosed en bloc using the aorta. With a living donor, where there are two renal arteries, both renal arteries may be anastomosed to each other, forming a single opening which is anastomosed in an end-to-end fashion to the hypogastric artery of the recipient (Figure 73-12*A* through *D*). A polar artery to the donor kidney may be anastomosed to the main artery of the kidney with interrupted sutures (Figure 73-12*E*). Rarely, the renal artery is very short and may be extended by either a donor arterial graft or prosthetic graft (Figure 73-12*F*). When both anastomoses are completed, renal perfusion is restored by taking the clamps off of the renal vein first and then the artery. The kidney should become pink within a few minutes.

Vascular Complications of Renal Transplantation

Postoperative Hemorrhage. This may occur from the wound, the transplanted kidney, or the vascular anatomosis (25). Local technical factors resulting in hemorrhage include unidentified and untied renal vessels, particularly with cadaveric donors. Common changes in clotting factors in renal failure patients include prolonged bleeding time, abnormal platelet count, and abnormal protein consumption. Thus meticulous hemostasis is required. The use of regional heparinization during hemodialysis should decrease this risk. Thrombosis of the renal artery or vein may also be responsible for infarction resulting in hemorrhage (26).

Spontaneous Rupture of the Renal Graft. This has been reported in 0.8 to 9.6 percent of the recipients, with a mean of 3.6 percent (27,28). One reason for graft rupture is uncontrolled acute rejection, though the cause is uncertain in most cases (29). When it occurs, rupture is usually in the first 3 weeks after transplantation. The kidney splits in a longitudinal direction along its convex border (30). A mass is palpable along with the signs of acute blood loss. Usually the diagnosis is made at exploration (28).

Although some groups have advocated transplant nephrectomy, an attempt to control the bleeding is made. However, uncontrolled bleeding necessitates immediate transplant nephrectomy (31).

Infection leading to secondary hemorrhage from the vascular anastomosis have been reported in 1.0 to 3.9 percent of patients with a mean of 1.9 percent (32,33). In most instances the infection arises from the transplanted kidney itself, and anastomotic breakdown usually occurs within 4 months after transplantation. The signs of infection are masked by immunosuppression (34). Secondary hemorrhage appears to be more common after end-to-side anastomosis compared to end-to-end anastomosis. Secondary hemorrhage is treated with arterial ligation and transplant nephrectomy. If required, the external or common iliac artery can usually be ligated without producing leg ischemia (35). If ischemia appears, then a bypass is performed (22). There have been isolated case reports of bleeding from mycotic aneurysms controlled by proximal ligation with retention of kidney, but this is not usually recommended.

Renal Artery Thrombosis. This is diagnosed by an arteriogram, or at the time of surgery, aided by the Doppler. Goldman and his colleagues reported only 6 cases in 525 transplants (36). Thrombosis was largely due to technical factors or multiple small-vessel anastomoses (37,38). The thrombosis may be due to an intimal flap or intimal damage produced during donor nephrectomy or at the time of vascular anastomosis.

A sudden slowing of the urinary output may indicate renal artery thrombosis. A decision to reexplore the patient is made on clinical grounds, as early exploration may avert the need for nephrectomy if a technical problem can be corrected. Delayed arterial thrombosis, however, is largely due to rejection, with low flow in the renal arteries.

Later arterial thrombosis may also be due to renal artery stenosis and surgery can be performed, excising the stenotic segments (Figure 73-13).

Renal Vein Thrombosis. This has been reported in 1 to 4 percent of clinical series and often occurs as a result of trauma sustained during nephrectomy, transplantation, or secondary to iliofemoral vein thrombosis, particularly on the left side (39). Symptoms suggesting renal vein thrombosis include swelling of the graft and heavy excretion of urinary proteins. In such cases, a venogram is performed to confirm the diagnosis (40).

Renal vein thrombosis may be partial, and conservative therapy may be advisable in these cases (41). With complete renal vein thrombosis it is more reasonable to carry out nephrectomy. The incidence of pulmonary embolism is high in these cases, and heparin should be used along with surgical therapy, if planned (42).

Arterial Stenosis. This has been reported in 0.6 to 13.5 percent of the recipients, but this may not reflect the real inci-

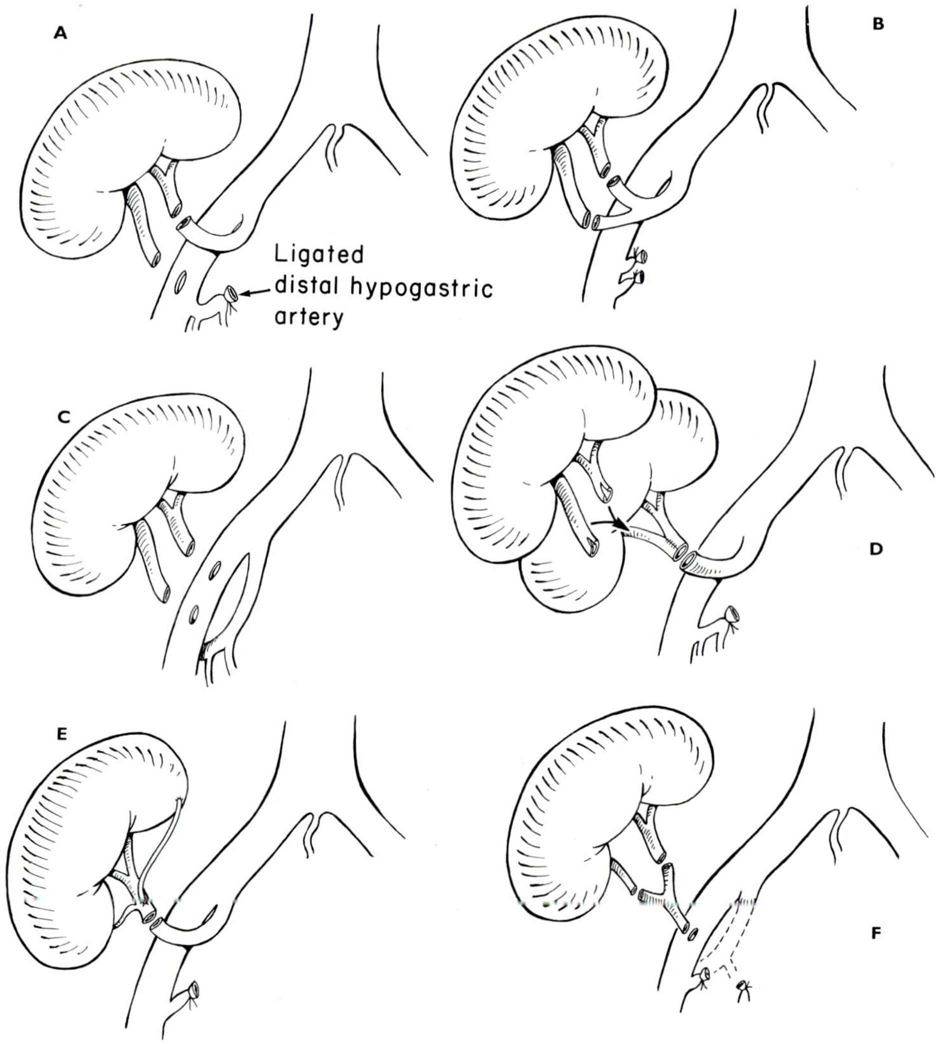

FIGURE 73-12. (*A–D*) In living, related donors, when two renal arteries are present, a variety of techniques may be used for anastomosis, using a combination of end-to-side external iliac and end-to-end hypogastric. The two renal arteries may also be sutured together. (*E*) In addition, the end of the smaller branch can be anastomosed to the side of the larger renal artery. (*F*) Rarely, extensive reconstruction is performed to accommodate unique anatomic variation.

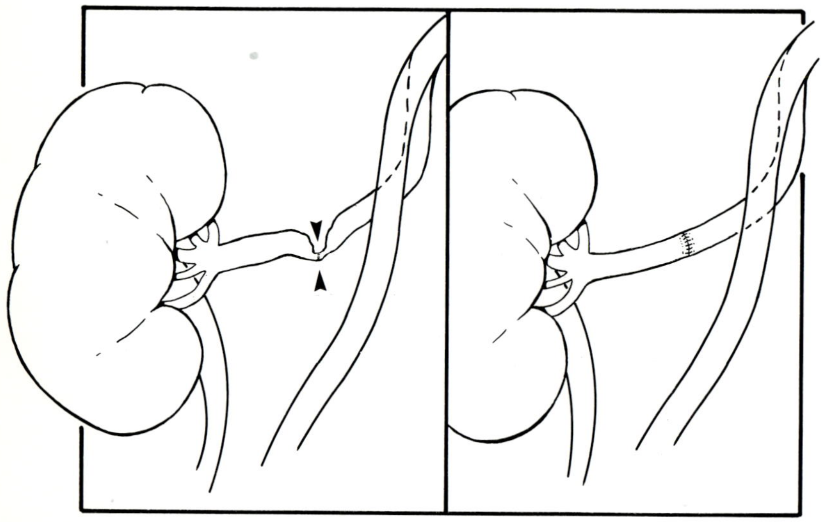

FIGURE 73-13. Correction of renal artery stenosis by excision of stenotic segment.

dence of arterial stenosis, as only the cases that develop hypertension after renal transplantation are investigated (43–49). Renal artery stenosis seems to be more frequent with an end-to-end anastomosis than with end-to-side (50).

Arterial stenosis is associated with hypertension (51,52) or a bruit over the grafted kidney and diminished renal function. Since hypertension can be controlled medically, only those cases not readily controlled by drugs or in whom the renal function deteriorates rapidly are investigated further (53). Renal biopsy excludes rejection or recurrent renal disease, though it may show features of chronic rejection with or without subintimal fibrosis, which may be the cause of the renal artery stenosis. Selective renal vein renin levels have been used to aid the diagnosis of a functional stenosis. An arteriogram of the graft displays the anatomy and sometimes the cause (54).

A critical stenosis reduces the vessel diameter by greater than 50 percent. The following types of renal artery stenosis have been described by Lacombe: (I) stenosis of the recipient iliac artery due to arteriosclerosis; (II) a localized stenosis of the suture line between the recipient and donor vessel or angulation caused by poor positioning of the kidney or vessels during transplantation; (III) more diffuse stenosis of the donor renal artery or its branches which may be due to immunological damage and is frequently associated with severe rejection in the kidney itself. Other causes of this stenosis where there is no evidence of kidney rejection may be related to damage during harvesting by the perfusion cannule or the snares used for perfusion.

Surgical correction is usually done using a transperitoneal approach as the vessels can be exposed more satisfactorily. Type I lesions are dealt with by endarterectomy with a vein patch or by vein bypass. Type II lesions are amenable to resection and direct reanastomosis, although transposition of the iliac artery as advocated by Lacombe may be of value in this complex situation. In a few cases an autogenous vein or Dacron graft may need to be used for a bypass procedure. Type III lesions are best treated by a vein patch or by a vein bypass. In complicated cases removal of the kidney with extracorporeal vascular repair and reimplantation can be utilized (55).

Another technique that has been used in renal artery stenosis is percutaneous transluminal dilatation, and good results have been reported in cases of native renal artery stenosis (56,57). Sneiderman and his colleagues (58) reported technically successful results in 11 of 14 attempts in 12 patients, with control of blood pressure for up to 13 months. These findings suggest percutaneous transluminal dilatation could precede consideration of surgery as a therapeutic procedure, although its role remains to be defined in transplanted kidneys.

Aneurysm. Aneurysms may be encountered during evaluation of a recipient, or they can be found in the prospective donor (59). In the donor, aneurysm of the aorta may involve the renal artery, or the renal artery itself may have an isolated aneurysm. An aortic aneurysm, per se, does not cause any problems in harvesting the kidneys. If a renal artery aneurysm is encountered during the evaluation in a living donor, the kidney should not be harvested (60). However, in the case of a cadaveric donor, if an incidental renal artery aneurysm is found, the kidney can be harvested and transplanted after excising the aneurysm (61).

In the recipient, if aneurysmal disease is found during evaluation, this aneurysm should be repaired prior to renal transplantation. The aneurysmal disease may involve the aorta, the iliac vessels, or an isolated iliac artery. Renal artery aneurysms encountered include saccular, fusiform, dissecting aneurysms as part of an aortic dissection, and a false aneurysm as a result of rupture of a diseased artery or from trauma (62).

After transplantation, an aneurysm of the renal artery itself or an aneurysm involving the anastomotic site can occur. These can be (1) an anastomotic aneurysm, (2) poststenotic aneurysm of the renal artery, and (3) a mycotic aneurysm. These can rupture, thrombose with distal embolization, or cause distal limb ischemia due to thrombosis and embolism of iliac vessels. The incidence of renal artery aneurysm is very low (63). In 965 autopsies, Erdsman found that it was 0.73 percent (64). The incidence of renal artery aneurysms or iliac artery aneurysms after renal transplantation is not documented (65).

Anastomotic aneurysms are false aneurysms that result from partial or total separation of the anastomosis and are located at the junction of the renal artery and the hypogastric or external iliac artery of the recipient (66,67). These can result because of suture failure, because the integrity of the anastomotic line may have been in question at implantation, or because of damage to the suture material from careless handling. In addition, a hematoma surrounding the anastomosis may later become infected, leading to a communication with the arterial lumen (68).

Clinically, these aneurysms present as a palpable, pulsatile mass or with a complication such as rupture, distal embolization, or thrombosis. When the iliac artery is involved, pressure symptoms may be present related to compression on surrounding organs, particularly the ureter.

Definitive diagnosis is made by an angiogram, and surgical repair is required, provided there is no infection at the anastomotic site. Management includes the control of the vessel proximally and distally, followed by excision of the whole area with reconstruction of the anastomosis. In a few cases, where the aneurysm is small, it can be excised with margins of the renal artery on each side and an end-to-end anastomosis performed.

A true postoperative aneurysm of the renal artery is the result of poststenotic dilation and differs from an anastomotic aneurysm as all the layers of the blood vessel are involved. The incidence of postoperative aneurysms is not known. They can present with postoperative hypertension (69), as a palpable pulsatile mass, or as one of the complications such as rupture, thrombosis, or embolism and should usually be investigated with an arteriogram.

The treatment is surgical excision and primary repair if there is no infection in that area. If the distance between the donor and recipient artery is too great, it can be reconstituted with a synthetic graft or autogenous saphenous vein.

Mycotic aneurysms develop as the result of septic embolization either to the bifurcation of an artery or its vasa vasorum or to an atheromatous plaque (70). Other causes include secondary infection of an atherosclerotic aneurysm, local direct infection of the artery, and infected pseudoaneurysm. A fungal aneurysm may be found both in long-term hemodialysis patients and in immunosuppressed patients after transplantation (71).

Mycotic aneurysms have been reported in the literature following the removal of an infected renal graft involving any blood vessel, but in renal transplant patients, usually involving the renal artery or the iliac vessels (72–74).

Usually the mycotic aneurysm presents as a rapidly enlarging, tender, warm, pulsatile mass, and the patients have a fever and leukocytosis. A systolic bruit may be heard over the mass. The diagnosis is made on a computerized tomography (CT) scan of the area, which shows gas bubbles and can be confirmed on arteriogram.

Principles of treatment include transplant nephrectomy and debridement of all infected tissue, aerobic and anaerobic cultures including culture for fungi, and the proper chemotherapy. Proximal and distal control of the vessels to be ligated is obtained, and the aneurysm is excised without reconstruction. An open drainage of the wound is preferred. Antibiotics are continued for 6 weeks.

The external iliac vessels may be ligated without need for revascularization, provided the collaterals are developed and not disturbed (i.e., the internal iliac artery, the circumflex artery, and the inferior epigastric artery). If limb ischemia appears at a later date, a femoral-femoral crossover bypass or an obturator bypass can be performed (75).

Any attempt to reestablish vascular flow because of limb ischemia, even though gross infection is not present, is often associated with persistent infection and a high incidence of rebleeding. An extraanatomic bypass procedure through a clean area is required in this situation (76).

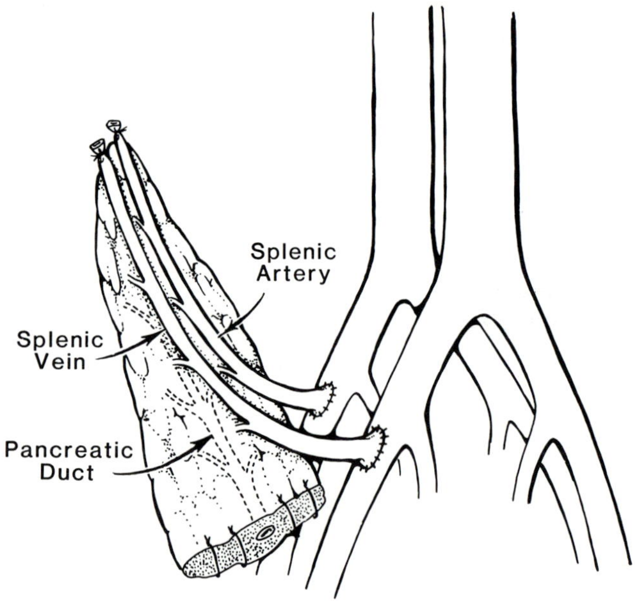

FIGURE 73-14. Segmental pancreas transplant to iliac fossa of recipient, with end-to-side anastomosis of splenic artery and vein to external iliac vessels. (Used with permission of John Wiley and Sons.)

PANCREAS TRANSPLANTATION—TECHNIQUES AND COMPLICATIONS

Pancreas transplantation is mainly offered to juvenile diabetics who have secondary complications of diabetes mellitus involving kidneys, eyes, and nerves (77). It is preferred, at the present time, that recipients with severe renal function impairment be considered for simultaneous pancreatic and kidney transplantation, or the pancreas transplantation can be done months after the kidney transplant (78–86).

Pancreatic transplantation is done as a segment or as a whole pancreas transplant (87). It has recently been recommended that a large mass of pancreas should be used to provide as much functional islet tissue and as large a vascular bed as possible. Smaller segmental pancreatic transplants may be more susceptible to vascular thrombosis than total pancreatic grafts. The segmental graft is done using half of the gland body and tail, with vascular anastomosis between the donor's splenic artery or celiac axis and the splenic or portal vein with the recipient's external iliac artery and vein, respectively (Figure 73-14) (88). The whole-organ pancreatic transplantation is done using the entire gland, with a patch of aorta containing the celiac and superior mesenteric artery and the portal vein, which are then anastomosed in an end-to-side fashion with the recipient's external iliac artery and vein, respectively (Figure 73-15) (89).

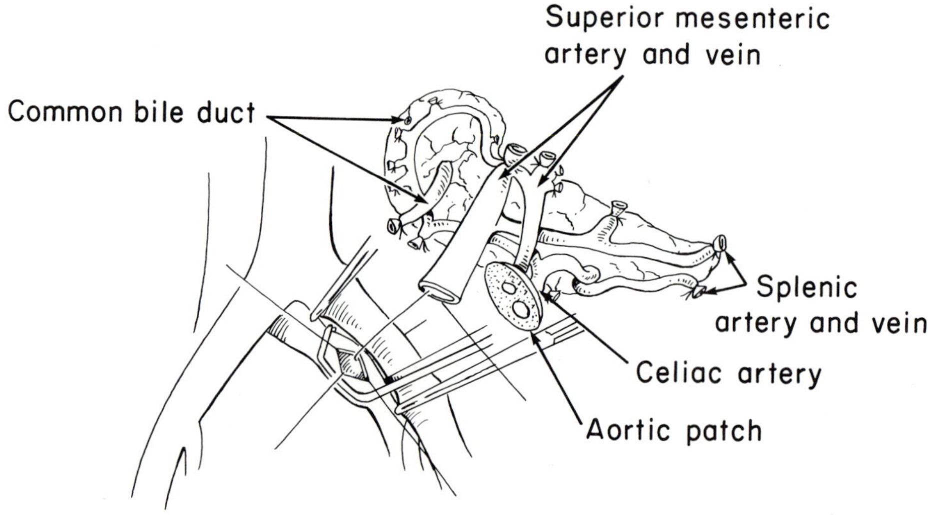

FIGURE 73-15. In whole organ pancreas transplantation an aortic patch is anastomosed end-to-side with the external iliac artery, and the portal vein is anastomosed to the external iliac vein.

Segmental pancreatic transplantation is performed either extra- or intraperitoneally, depending upon the preference of the team (90). At our center, segmental pancreatic transplantation is done similarly to kidney transplantation, by an extraperitoneal approach. The iliac vessels are identified and isolated, and then the splenic artery and the vein are anastomosed in an end-to-side fashion with 5-0 Prolene to the external iliac artery and vein of the recipient. After the anastomosis is complete, the clamps are removed and the organ becomes vascularized. These pancreatic grafts have been drained with a closed drain system. In several cases we have made a distal fistula between the splenic artery and the splenic vein to improve the vascular flow (91–93).

In the case of the whole pancreatic graft, the end of the donor portal vein is anastomosed to the side of the recipient common iliac vein using 5-0 Prolene suture, and an aortic patch containing the origins of the celiac and superior mesenteric artery is anastomosed to the common iliac arteries in an end-to-side fashion using 5-0 Prolene. The site of the venous anastomosis is kept slightly higher than the arterial anastomosis to prevent any kinking (94).

Vascular complications following pancreatic transplantation include bleeding, which may be from small vessels that have not been identified and left untied, or from coagulation defects secondary to the renal failure. Vascular thrombosis, more often seen in segmental pancreatic transplantation as the pancreas has a low blood flow, is less likely to occur in whole-organ transplantation, as the blood flow is greater. It may be suspected on a ^{99m}Tc pertechnatate scan and confirmed by arteriogram. The changes that follow pancreatic ischemia are irreversible and usually result in graft destruction.

These patients are also maintained on low-molecular-weight dextran intravenously in the early postoperative period to prevent platelet aggregation. The use of heparin and/or warfarin (Coumadin) is not advocated in general; however, a few centers have tried them with satisfactory results.

LIVER TRANSPLANTATION—TECHNIQUES AND COMPLICATIONS

The first successful liver transplantation was performed by Starzl in 1967 (95). Since then, more than 500 of these have been performed throughout the world (96,97). The indications for liver transplantation have been liberalized (98–107). A thorough preoperative evaluation of the recipient is performed, and from the point of view of the vascular system, it is important to ascertain the patency of the portal vein as occlusion contraindicates liver transplantation. For that, a CT scan or ultrasonography can be performed (108,109). Celiac angiography with a delayed phase will also demonstrate the portal vein, and very rarely, direct portal venography is performed. Preoperatively, central venous and arterial lines are placed to monitor the hemodynamic parameters and deficient coagulation factors are replaced (105,110).

The first part of the procedure for any liver transplantation is native hepatectomy, and in cases with portal hypertension bleeding is excessive from the retroperitoneal collaterals during the dissection. The spleen is not removed as liver blood flow would be reduced. As much suprahepatic vena cava, portal vein, hepatic artery, and intrahepatic vena cava as possible should be preserved. The vascular pedicle of the liver is dissected first to identify the hepatic artery, the common bile duct, and the portal vein. The falciform and triangular ligaments are divided. Following this, the phrenic veins entering the suprahepatic vena cava are identified, suture-ligated, and divided.

The infrahepatic inferior vena cava is now identified and mobilized, and the distal hepatic artery is divided to obtain the maximum length possible distal to the right gastric and the gastroduodenal branches. The portal vein and the infrahepatic vena cava are similarly divided close to the liver. The common bile duct is divided just distal to the cystic duct level, taking precautions not to injure its vascular supply.

The liver is lifted cephalad, and the right adrenal vein which enters the inferior vena cava is identified, ligated, and divided. Several lumbar veins may be encountered in the retrohepatic area; these are ligated and divided. The suprahepatic vena cava is dissected as close to the liver as possible to provide the maximum length of the suprahepatic vena cava cuff for subsequent anastomosis. At this point the vena cava is clamped along with the cuff of the diaphragm and divided, completing the native hepatectomy (Figure 73-16) (95).

During revascularization of the donor liver, the first anastomosis performed is that to the suprahepatic vena cava, starting with the posterior wall, which is closed with a running stitch from inside, retracting the anterior wall with stay sutures, and the anterior wall is then closed. The next anastomosis is that to the portal vein and is carried out by rotating the vascular clamp on the recipient portal vein to the left or to the right so that both sides of the portal vein can be reached. This anastomosis is done using Prolene 5-0 or 6-0 (Figure 73-17*A*). It is important to ensure that there is no redundancy of the portal vein which can cause kinking of the anastomosis. Before completion of the portal vein anastomosis, a small intravenous cannula is inserted to flush the liver with 400 to 500 mL of a warm Ringer's lactate solution, the fluid escaping into the inferior vena cava. When the portal vein anastomosis is completed, it is unclamped and blood is allowed to perfuse the liver, though the suprahepatic clamp is left in place until about 100 mL of blood has escaped from the infrahepatic vena cava of the donor. The infrahepatic clamp is reapplied and the suprahepatic clamp removed. In this way the metabolic products are flushed out of the liver (111).

Following this, the hepatic artery is anastomosed end-to-end using 6-0 Prolene suture. When multiple donor hepatic arteries are present, the largest is anastomosed end-to-end with the recipient hepatic artery, and the smaller can be anastomosed to the side of the recipient's hepatic artery (Figure 73-17*B*). When the right hepatic artery arises from the superior mesenteric artery, a segment of this is taken from the donor, the left hepatic artery is anastomosed to one branch of the superior mesenteric artery, and the main trunk is anastomosed to the recipient's hepatic artery (Figure 73-17*C*). In children, the donor's aorta is anastomosed in and end-to-side fashion to the host's aorta. The infrahepatic vena cava anastomosis is then performed with a running 4-0 Prolene suture. After the vascular anastomoses are completed, the biliary construction is done.

Intraoperative bleeding is often severe as most patients have portal hypertension and extensive portal systemic shunts are present with coagulation defects. Coagulation parameters including platelets, PT, PTT, and serum calcium must be maintained at normal levels. Vascular thrombosis either of the hepatic artery or portal vein can occur and is manifested postoperatively by

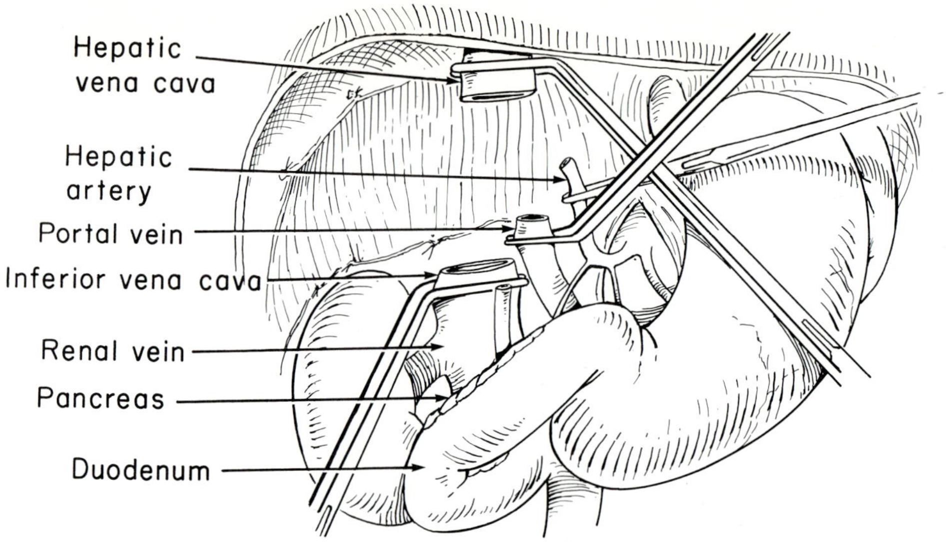

FIGURE 73-16. Completion of native hepatectomy on the recipient.

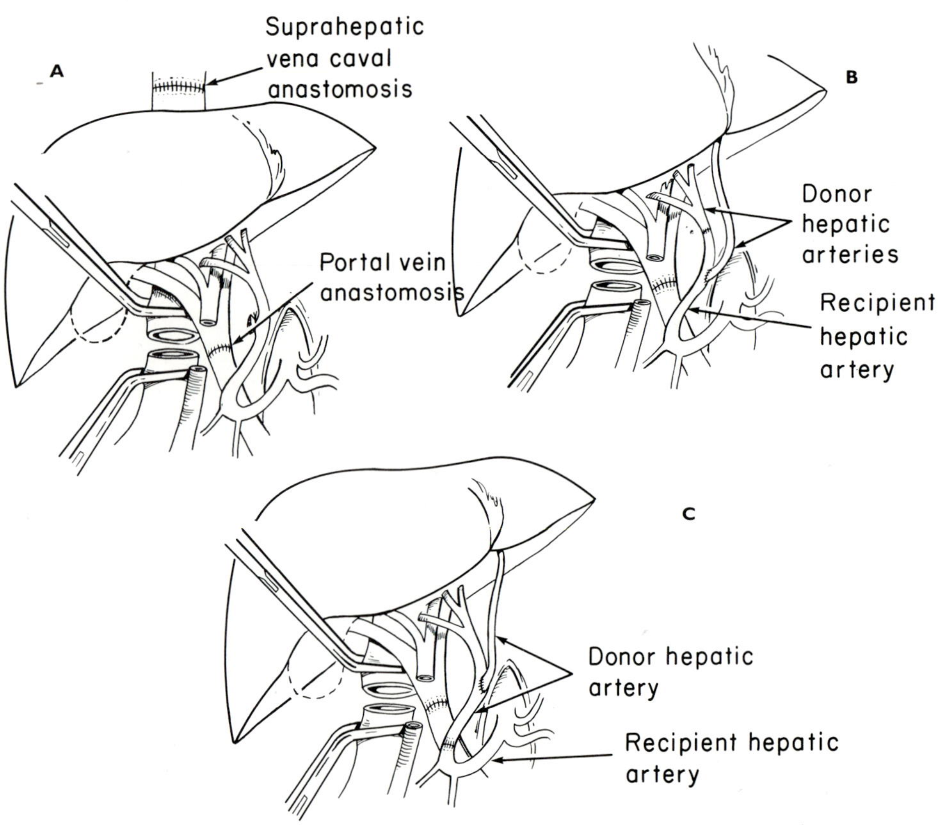

FIGURE 73-17. (*A*) Completed end-to-end anastomoses of suprahepatic vena cava and protal vein. (*B*) When double donor hepatic arteries are present, the end of the smaller artery may be anastomosed to the side of the recipient's hepatic artery, then the larger vessel is anastomosed to the end of the recipient's hepatic artery. (*C*) Alternatively, the smaller hepatic artery may be anastomosed to the larger donor hepatic artery with subsequent anastomosis of the larger vessel end-to-end with the recipient's hepatic artery.

increasing serum bilirubin and transaminase levels. This is more likely in pediatric patients with small vessels (112) and also in cases with multiple, anomalous vascular vessels to the donor liver. Starzl has reported patients who had delayed thrombosis of the portal vein or hepatic artery. When vascular thrombosis is diagnosed, urgent surgery is required to excise the necrotic liver tissue or possibly reconstruct the vessels (113,114).

Other complications may be vena cava occlusion, or thrombosis of the suprahepatic anastomosis, which may lead to lower trunk edema and renal insufficiency. A vena cavogram makes the diagnosis, and operative repair is undertaken. In delayed cases of stenosis a balloon angioplasty may be possible (115).

CARDIAC TRANSPLANTATION—TECHNIQUES AND COMPLICATIONS

During the evaluation, the recipients have a thorough physical examination of the extracardiac systems, especially for peripheral or cerebral vascular disease (116).

The first part of the operation is excision of the diseased heart, which is performed through a midline sternotomy. The patient is prepared for cardiopulmonary bypass by cannulating the aorta and the superior and inferior vena cava. The positions of the caval cannulas are particularly important since the distal ends must be left in the recipient during anastomosis to the donor's right atrium.

The ascending aorta is mobilized by dissection and a plane between it, and the pulmonary artery is made in preparation for application of the aortic cross clamp prior to removal of the recipient organ. After the patient is on cardiopulmonary bypass, the recipient's heart is excised, leaving the aortic cannula in place, along with the aortic cross clamp. The superior and inferior vena cava cannula and then the right atrial cuff and left atrial cuff are tailored for reimplantation of the donor heart at the interatrial septum.

During the implantation of the donor's heart, the left atrial anastomosis is done first. It begins at the point midway between the superior and inferior pulmonary veins on the left and is done with a Prolene suture superiorly and inferiorly to the level of the interatrial septum. The left atrial anastomosis is completed by finishing the anastomosis of the interatrial septum.

Following this the right atrium of the donor's heart is prepared for anastomosis to the recipient's cuff of the right atrium which is done with a continuous suture. The donor and the recipient aorta are tailored to an appropriate size to avoid tension or stenosis and are anastomosed in a single layer. Once the aortic anastomosis is near completion, warming is initiated (117).

Upon completion of the aortic anastomosis a stab wound is created in the ascending aorta, following placement of a button suture with a Teflon buttress which is left untied. This allows for air to be vented from the aortic root upon removal of the aortic cross clamp. The pulmonary artery is then anastomosed end-to-end. The completion of the implant is carried out by closing the atrial suture line, and then the aortic vent is closed by tying the buttress mattress suture. Following this, the superior vena cava and ascending aortic cannulas are removed, and a permanent atrial pacemaker is placed on the right atrial appendage (Figure 73-18).

One of the major complications of the cardiac transplant is rejection, be it acute or chronic. The other is arteriosclerosis of the graft coronary arteries, which is attributed to immune injury of the endothelial surface of the coronary vessels. This loss of integrity of the endothelial surface increases the likelihood of coronary vessel thrombosis. Microthrombi deposits in these sites and subsequent proliferation of intimal cells leads to a thickened

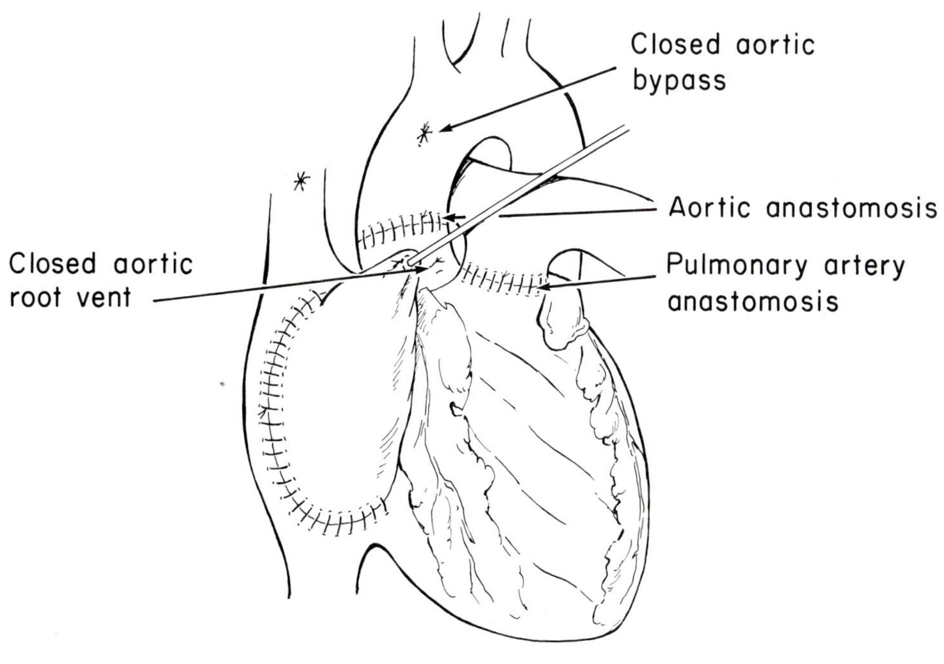

FIGURE 73-18. Completed cardiac transplant showing aortic, pulmonary arterial, and right atrial anastomoses. Cannulas have been removed from the ascending aorta and superior vena cava. A right atrial pressure monitoring line is placed through the right atrial appendage.

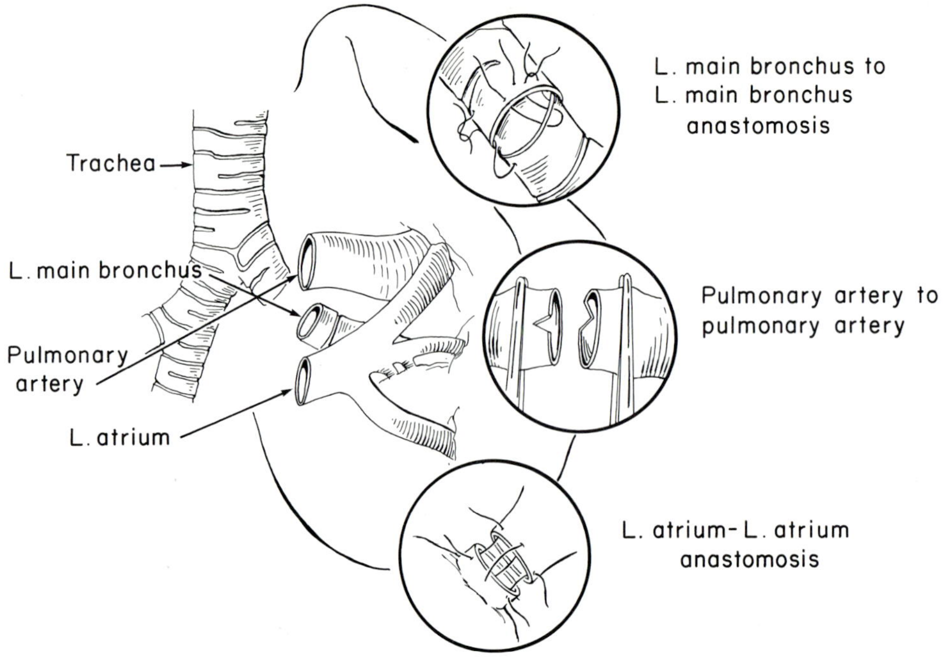

FIGURE 73-19. Detail of anastomoses in lung transplantation.

hyperplastic intima and formation of an atheromatous plaque (118). These changes are a manifestation of chronic vascular rejection in the coronary artery of the graft and may result in a silent and potentially fatal myocardial infarction (119).

Griepp and his associates (120) demonstrated a reduction in this complication after the introduction of a regimen consisting of dipyridamole, warfarin, and diet control of lipid levels. Warfarin has now been dropped from the regimen because of bleeding complications, and current prophylaxis consists of dipyridamole in combination with dietary lipid restriction (121,122).

LUNG TRANSPLANTATION—TECHNIQUE AND COMPLICATIONS

For lung transplantation, a posterolateral thoracotomy is performed on the recipient, the chest is entered through the fifth space, and the lung is carefully dissected similar to that undertaken for a pneumonectomy. The artery and the veins at the entrance of the left atrium and the main bronchus are also carefully dissected out. Special care should be taken not to destroy the lymphatic chains and peribronchial connective tissue. The lymphatics are tied off and divided if necessary. Heparin (2000 units) is given intravenously prior to cross clamping the vascular structures (123).

After the pulmonary vessels and the bronchus are dissected out, the left atrium is clamped with an avascular clamp to gain a sufficient length without obstructing the atrial flow at the same time. The venous anatomosis is done using a 5-0 Prolene suture. Following this, the pulmonary artery anastomosis is performed in an end-to-end fashion with a single layer of Prolene. Finally, the main bronchus anastomosis is carried out and reinforced with peribronchial and connective tissue (Figure 73-19) (124–130).

Once the anastomosis is completed, the tracheal clamps are opened, followed by the vascular clamps. Special attention is paid to the vascular flow to the transplanted lung, avoiding overload. Therefore, the vascular clamps are opened very slowly. The chest is closed in the usual fashion, and two chest tubes are left for drainage. Vascular problems in the postoperative period are similar to those of any other transplant and include postoperative hemorrhage and vascular thrombosis, which may be on the arterial or the venous side (131,132).

References

1. Toledo-Pereyra LH: Organ harvesting. In Toledo-Pereyra LH (ed): *Basic Concepts of Organ Procurement, Perfusion and Preservation for Transplantation*. New York, Academic, New York, 1982, pp 57–72.
2. Toledo-Pereyra LH: Multiple organ harvesting for transplantation. Surg Gynecol Obstet 1984, 158:572–576.
3. Zeichner WD, Toledo-Pereyra LH, MacKenzie GH, Wohlman MH: Cadaveric nephrectomy: Procurement, harvesting, preservation. *Contemp Surg* 1983, 22:53–62.
4. Starzl TE, Hakala TR, Shaw BW, Hardesty RL, Rosenthal TJ, Griffith BP, Iwatsuki S, Bahnson HT: A flexible procedure for multiple cadaveric organ procurement. Surg Gynecol Obstet 1984, 159:223.
5. Bjorken C, Lundgren G, Ringden O, Groth CG: A technique for

rapid harvesting of cadaveric renal and pancreatic grafts after circulating arrest. Br J Surg 1976, 63:517–519.
6. Report of the Ad Hoc Committee of the Harvard Medical School, 1968.
7. Conference of the Medical Royal Colleges and their Faculties in the United Kingdom. Diagnosis of brain death. Br Med J 1976, 2:1187–1188.
8. Green R, Boyer D, Halasz N, Collins GM: Pharmacological protection of rabbit kidneys from normothermic ischemia. Transplantation 1979, 28:131–134.
9. Luksza A: Brain dead kidney donors: Selection, care and administration. Br Med J 1979, 1:1316–1319.
10. Zincke H, Woods J: Donor pretreatment in cadaver renal transplantation. Surg Gynecol Obstet 1977, 145:183–188.
11. Chatterjee S, Berne T: The effect of furosemide on 24-hour hypothermic renal preservation. J Surg Res 1975, 19:357–361.
12. Chatterjee S, Berne T: Use of cellular membrane stabilizers to prevent ischemic damage to the kidneys. Surg Forum 1975, 25:335–336.
13. Jacobs S, McLoughlin A, HJalasz N: Living donor nephrectomy. Urology 1975, 5:175–177.
14. Weiland D, Sutherland DER, Chavers B, Simmons RL, Ascher NL, Najarian JS: Information on 628 living related kidney donors at a single institution with long-term followup in 472 cases. Transplant Proc 1984, 16:5.
15. Collins G, Green R, Boyer D, Halasz NA: Protection of kidneys from ischemic injury: Dosage and timing of mannitol administration. Transplantation 1980, 29:83–84.
16. Chinn PL, Sutherland DER, Goetz FC, Oliphant UJ, Elick BA, Najarian JS: Metabolic effect of hemipancreatectomy in living-related graft donors. Transplant Proc 1984, 16:11–17.
17. Sutherland DER, Goetz FC, Najarian JS: Living related donor segmental pancreatectomy for transplantation. Transplant Proc 1980, 12(suppl 2):19.
18. Starzl TE, Koep L, Schroter G, Halgrimson CG, Porter KA, Weil R̀: Liver replacement for pediatric patients. Pediatrics 1979, 63:825.
19. Starzl TE, Marchioro T, Von Kaulla K, Hermann G, Brittain RS, Waddell WR: Homotransplantation of the liver in humans. Surg Gynecol Obstet 1963, 117:659.
20. Calne RY, Williams R: Liver transplantation in man—Observation on technique and organization in five cases. Br Med J 1968, 2:535.
21. Calne RY, Williams R: Liver transplantation. In Ravilch M (ed): *Current Problems in Surgery*. Chicago, Year Book Medical Publishers 1979, p. 16.
22. Goldman M, Leapman S: Renal allograft rupture with ileofemoral thrombophlebitis. Arch Surg 1978, 113:304–305.
23. Bore P, Basu P, Rudge C, Sells RA: Contaminated renal allografts. Arch Surg 1980, 115:755–756.
24. Mosley J, Castro J: Arterial anastomoses in renal transplantation. Br J Surg 1978, 65:60–63.
25. Schweizer R, Lountz S, Belzer FO: Wound complications in recipients of renal transplants. Ann Surg 1973, 177:58–62.
26. Fernando O, Higgins A, Moorehead J: Secondary hemorrhage after renal transplantation. Lancet 1976, 2:368.
27. Lord R, Effeney D, Hayes J, Tracy GD: Renal allograft rupture. Ann Surg 1973, 177:268–273.
28. Susan L, Braun W, Banowsky L, et al: Ruptured human renal allograft. Urology 1978, 9:53–57.
29. Luna I, Leadbetter R, Gilbert D: Spontaneous rupture of the kidney: A complication of anticoagulation—Report of two cases. J Urol 1973, 109:788–789.
30. Homan W, Cheigh J, Kim S, Mouradian J, Tapia L, Riggio RR, Stenzel KH, Rubin AL, Stubenbord WT: Renal allograft fracture: Clinicopathological study of 21 cases. Ann Surg 1977, 186:700–703.
31. Dryburgh P, Porter K, Krom A, Uchida K, West JC, Weil R, Starzl TE: Should the ruptured renal allograft be removed? Arch Surg 1979, 114:850–852.
32. Kyriakides G, Simmons R, Najarian J: Wound infection in renal transplant wounds. Ann Surg 1975, 182:770–775.
33. Rubin RH: Infection in the renal transplant patient. In Rubin RH (ed): *Infection in the Compromised Host*. New York, Plenum (in press).
34. Matas A, Scheinman J, Patazzi L: Immunopathological studies of the ruptured human renal allograft. Transplantation 1976, 22:420–426.
35. Gorey T, Bulkley G, Spees E, Sterioff S: Iliac artery ligation: The relative paucity of ischemic sequelae in renal transplant patients. Ann Surg 1979, 190:753–757.
36. Goldman M, Vineyard G, Laks H, Kahan MG, Wilson RE: A twenty-year survey of arterial complications of renal transplantation. Surg Gynecol Obstet 1975, 141:758–760.
37. Venkateswara Rao, Smith E, Alexander J, Fidler JP, Pemmarāju SR, Pollack VE: Thrombo-embolic disease in renal allografts. Arch Surg 1976, 111:1086–1092.
38. Vidne B, Leapman S, Butt K, Kountz SL: Vascular complications in human renal transplantation. Surgery 1976, 79:77–81.
39. Doyle T. McGregor W, Fox P, Maddison FE, Rodgers RE, Kauffman HM: Homotransplant renal artery stenosis. Surgery 1975, 77:53–60.
40. Arruda J, Jonasson O, Gutierrez L, Pillay VKG, Kurtzman NA: Renal vein thrombosis in kidney allografts. Lancet 1973, 2:585–586.
41. Golden J, Stone R, Goldenberger L: Immune-related vein thrombosis in a renal allograft. Ann Intern Med 1976, 85:612–613.
42. D'Appuzo V, Bretscher D, Oetliker O, Nachbur B: Renal vein thrombosis after transplantation. Lancet 1973, 2:975–976.
43. Mendez-Picon G, Nghiem D, Lilly L, et al: Renal artery stenosis in transplant recipients. Proc Am Soc Transplant Surg (in press).
44. Woo K, Yeung C, D'Apice A, et al: Transplant renal artery stenosis. Aust NZ J Surg 1979, 49:613–616.
45. Zawada E, Maxwell M, Marks L, Lee DB, Kaufman JJ: The diagnostic and therapeutic uses of saralasin in renal transplant hypertension. J Urol 1980, 123:148–152.
46. Dautrebande J, Pirson Y, et al: Reversible renal artery stenosis in renal transplantation. Urology 1979, 13:529–531.
47. Jacquot C, Idatte J, Bedrossian J, Weiss Y, Safar M, Bariety J: Long-term blood pressure changes in renal homotransplantation. Arch Intern Med 1978, 138:233–236.
48. Lacombe M: Arterial stenosis complicating renal allotransplantation in man: A study of 38 cases. Ann Surg 1975, 181:283–288.
49. Lacombe J: Correction of renal transplant artery stenosis by transposing iliac arteries. Urology 1979, 13:21–23.
50. Henriksson C, Aurell M, Claes G, et al: Surgical correction of renal artery stenosis in renal transplantation. Scand J Urol Nephrol 1976, 38(suppl):139–144.
51. Bachy C, Alexandre G, van Yperselle de Strihou C: Hypertension after renal transplantation. Br Med J 1976, 2:1287–1289.
52. Tarazi R: Hypertension following renal transplantation. Arch Intern Med 1978, 138:906–907.
53. Jachuck S, Wilkinson R, Uldall P, Elliott RW, Taylor RMR, Hacking PM: Medical management of renal artery stenosis in transplant recipients. Br J Surg 1979, 66:19–22.
54. Nilson A, Henriksson C, Thoren O: Angiographic diagnosis and follow up of artery stenosis in renal transplantation. Scand J Urol Nephrol 1976, 38(suppl):131–138.
55. Eastcott HHG: *Arterial Surgery*, ed 2. Philadelphia, Lippincott, 1973.
56. Carr D, Quinn R, Hamilton D, Briggs JD, Junor BJR, Semple PF: Transluminal dilatation of transplant renal artery stenosis. Br Med J 1980, 2:196–197.

57. Gruntzig A, Vetter W, Meier B, Kuhlmann U, Lütolf U, Siegenthaler W: Treatment of renovascular hypertension with percutaneous transluminal dilatation of a renal artery stenosis. Lancet 1978, 1:801–802.
58. Sneiderman K, Sprayegen S, Sos T, et al: Percutaneous transluminal dilatation in renal transplant arterial stenosis for relief of hypertension. Proc Am Soc Transplant Surg (in press).
59. Barry WF, Kim SK: Renal artery aneurysms. Am J Roentgenol 1966, 98:132.
60. Hageman JH, Smith RF, Szilagyi DD, Elliott JP: Aneurysms of the renal artery. Problems of prognosis and surgical management. Surgery 1978, 84:563.
61. Szilagyi DE, Smith RF, Elliott JP, Hageman JH, Dall'Olmo CA: Anastomotic aneurysms after vascular reconstruction: problems of incidence, etiology and treatment. Surgery 1975, 78:800.
62. Citarelli F, Shin CS, Ippolito JJ, Das SP, Rubin B: Aneurysm of a polar renal artery. Surgery 1975, 78:660.
63. Hubert JP Jr, Pairolero PC, Kazmier FJ: Solitary renal artery aneurysm. Surgery 1980, 88:557.
64. Erdsman G: Angionephrography and suprarenal angiography. Acta Radiol (Stockholm) 1957, 155(suppl):104.
65. Farooki MA: Aneurysms in the United States and the United Kingdom. Int Surg 1973, 58:475.
66. Moore WS, Hall AD: Late suture failure in the pathogenesis of anastomotic false aneurysms. Ann Surg 1970, 172:1064.
67. Smith RF, Szilagyi DE, Colville JM: Surgical treatment of mycotic aneurysms. Arch Surg 1962, 85–663.
68. Knox GW: Peripheral vascular anastomotic aneurysms. Ann Surg 1976, 183:120.
69. Cummings KB, Lecky JW, Kaufman JJ: Renal artery aneurysms and hypertension. J Urol 1973, 109:144.
70. Kyriakides GK, Simmons RL, Najarian JS: Mycotic aneurysms in transplant patients. Arch Surg 1976, 111:472.
71. Blum L, Keefer EBC: Clinical entity of cryptogenic mycotic aneurysm. JAMA 1964, 188:505.
72. Anderson CB, Butcher HR, Ballinger WF: Mycotic aneurysms. Arch Surg 1974, 109:712.
73. Barker WF: Mycotic aneurysms. Ann Surg 1954, 139:84.
74. Cliff MM, Soulen RL, Finestone AJ: Mycotic aneurysms—A challenge and a clue. Review of ten-year experience. Arch Intern Med 1970, 126:977.
75. Fromm SH, Lucas CE: Obturator bypass for mycotic aneurysm in the drug addict. Arch Surg 1970, 100:82.
76. Nabseth DC, Deterling RA: Surgical management of mycotic aneurysm. Surgery 1961, 50:347.
77. Tchobroutsky G: Relation of diabetic control to development of microvascular complications. Diabetologia 1978, 15:143–152.
78. Gerrish EW: Final Newsletter, American College of Surgeons/National Institute of Health Organ Transplant Registry, June 30, 1977.
79. Gliedman ML, Tellis VA, Soberman R, Rifkin H, Veith FJ: Long-term effects of pancreatic transplantation in patients with advanced juvenile onset diabetes mellitus. Diabetes Care 1978, 1:1–9.
80. Kelly WD, Lillehei RC, Merkel FK, Idezuki Y, Goetz FC: Allotransplantation of the pancreas and duodenum along with the kidney in diabetic nephropathy. Surgery 1967, 61:827–837.
81. Lillehei RC, Ruiz JO: Pancreas. In Najarian JS, Simmons RL (eds): *Transplantation*. Philadelphia, Lea & Febiger, 1972.
82. Lillehei RC, Ruiz JO, Acquino C, Goetz FC: Transplantation of the pancreas. *Acta Endocrinol (Copenh)* 1976, 83(suppl 205):303–320.
83. Sutherland DER: Human Pancreas and Islet Transplant Registry Tabulation Newsletter, March 1981.
84. Sutherland DER, Goetz FC, Ramsay RC, Fryd DS, Najarian JS: Clinical and experimental kidney and pancreas transplantation for diabetics. In Little HL, Jack RL, Patz A, Rorsham PH (eds): *Diabetic Retinopathy*. New York, Thieme Stratton, 1983, pp 199–221.
85. Sutherland DER, Chinn PL, Goetz FC, Elick BA, Najarian JS: Minnesota experience with 85 pancreas transplants between 1978 and 1983. World J Surg 1984, 8:244–252.
86. Toledo-Pereyra LH: Pancreatic transplantation. Surg Gynecol Obstet 1983, 157:49–56.
87. Lillehei RC, Simmons RL, Najarian JS, Weil R, Uchida H, Ruiz JO, Kjellstrand CM, Goetz FC: Pancreaticoduodenal allotransplantation: Experimental and clinical experience. Ann Surg 1970, 172:405–436.
88. Sutherland DER, Goetz FC, Rynasiewicz JJ, Baumgartner D, White DC, Elick BA, Najarian JS: Segmental pancreas transplantation from living related and cadaver donors: A clinical experience. Surgery 1981, 90:159–164.
89. Connolly JE: Pancreatic whole organ transplantation. Surg Clin North Am 1978, 58:383–390.
90. Calne RY, McMaster P, Rolles K, Duffy TJ: Technical observations in segmental pancreas allografting: Observations on pancreatic blood flow. Transplant Proc 1980, 12(suppl 2):51–57.
91. Sutherland DER, Goetz FC, Elick BA, Najarian JS: Experience with 49 segmental pancreas transplants in 45 diabetic patients. *Transplantation* 1982, 34:330.
92. Gliedman ML, Gold M, Whittaker J, Rifkin H, Soberman R, Freed S, Tellis V, Veith FJ: Clinical segmental pancreatic transplantation with ureter-pancreatic duct anastomosis for exocrine drainage. Surgery 1973, 74:171–180.
93. Sutherland DER, Goetz FC, Najarian JS: Intraperitoneal transplantation of immediately vascularized segmental grafts without duct ligation: A clinical trial. Transplantation 1979, 28:485–491.
94. Merkel FK, Poticha SM, Nudelman EJ, Colwell JA, Bergan JJ: Pancreas transplantation in man: I. The donor and recipient operation. Arch Surg 1971, 103:205–210.
95. Starzl TE: Experience in Hepatic Transplantation. Philadelphia, Saunders, 1969.
96. Couch NP: Supply and demand on kidney and liver transplantation: A statistical survey. Transplantation 1966, 4:587.
97. Starzl TE, Koep LJ, Porter K, Schroter GPJ, Weil R, Hartley RB, Halgrimson CG: Decline in survival after liver transplantation. Arch Surg 1980, 115:815.
98. Abouna GM, Preshaw R, Silva J, et al: Liver transplantation in a patient with cholangiocarcinoma and ulcerative colitis.
99. Barnes BA, et al: Final Report of the Task Force on Liver Transplantation. Boston, Massachusetts, Department of Public Health, 1983.
100. Calne RY: Transplantation of the liver. Ann Surg 1978, 188:129.
101. Corman JL, Putnam CW, Iwatsuki S, et al: Liver allograft. Its use in chronic active hepatitis with macronodular cirrhosis, hepatitis B surface antigen. Arch Surg 1979, 114:75.
102. Daloze P, Corman J, Block P, et al: Enzyme replacement in Niemann-Pick's disease by liver homotransplantation. Transplant Proc 1975, 7:607.
103. MacDougall BRC, McMaster P, Calne RY, Williams R: Survival and rehabilitation after orthotopic liver transplantation. Lancet 1980, 1:1326.
104. Pichlmyer R, Braelich E, Neuhaus P, et al: Liver transplantation and impending hepatic failure. International Symposium on Liver Support, Hanover, Germany, June 1980 (abstract).
105. Putnam CW, Starzl TE: Transplantation of the liver. Surg Clin North Am 1977, 57:361.
106. Starzl TE, Koep LJ, Halgrimson CG, Hood J, Schroter GPJ, Porter KA, Weill R III: Liver transplantation—1978. Transplant Proc 1979, 11:240.

107. Van Wyk J, Halgrimson CG, Giles G, Lilly L, Martineau G, Starzl TE: Liver transplantation in biliary atresia with concomitant hepatoma. South Afr Med J 1972, 46:885.
108. Calne RY, Williams R, Lindop M, Farman JV, Tolley ME, Rolles K, MacDougall B, Neuberger J, Wyke RJ, Raftery AT, Duffy TJ, Wight DGD, White DJG: Improved survival after orthotopic liver grafting. Br Med J 1981, 283:115.
109. Calne RY, Williams R: Liver transplantation. In Ravilch M (ed): *Current Problems in Surgery*. Chicago, Year Book Medical Publishers 1979, p 16.
110. Jacoby I, Roth HP (eds): NIH Concensus Development Conference: Liver Transplantation, Bethesda, National Institute of Arthritis, Diabetes, and Digestive and Kidney Diseases, and the NIH Office of Medical Applications of Research, 1983.
111. Starzl TE, Marchioro TL, von Kaulla KN: Homotransplantation of the liver in humans. Surg Gynecol Obstet 1963, 117:659.
112. Starzl TE, Koep L, Schroter G, Halgrimson CG, Porter KA, Weil R: Liver replacement for pediatric patients. Pediatrics 1979, 63:825.
113. Starzl TE: Personal reflections in transplantation. Surg Clin North Am 1978, 58:879.
114. Starzl TE, Koep L, Halgrimson C, Hood J, Schroter PJ, Porter KA, Weil R: Fifteen years of clinical liver transplantation. Gastroenterology 1979, 77:375.
115. Starzl TE, Iwatsuki S, Van Thiel DH, Gartner JC, Zitelli BJ, Malatack JJ, Schade RR, Shaw BW, Hakala TR, Rosenthal JT, Porter KA: Evolution of liver transplantation. Hepatology 1982, 2:614.
116. Baumgartner WA, Reitz BA, Oyer PE, Stinson EB, Shumway NE: Cardiac homotransplantation. Curr Prob Surg 1979, 16:3.
117. Copeland JG, Salomon NW, Mammana RB, et al: Cardiac transplantation: A two year experience. Heart Transplant 1981, 1:67.
118. Diacoff CG, Allen PD, Streck CJ: Pulmonary vascular resistance following reimplantation and transplantation. Ann Thorac Surg 1970, 9:569.
119. Caves PK, Stinson EB, Billingham ME, Rider AK, Shumway NE: Diagnosis of human cardiac allograft rejection by serial cardiac biopsy. J Thorac Cardiovasc Surg 1973, 66:461.
120. Griepp RB, Stinson EB, Bieber CP, Reitz BA, Copeland JG, Oyer PE, Shumway NE: Control of graft arteriosclerosis in human heart transplant recipients. Surgery 1977, 81:262.
121. Oyer PE, Stinson EB, Jamieson SW, et al: One year experience with cyclosporine A in clinical heart transplantation. Heart Transplant 1982, 1:285–290.
122. Pennock JL, Oyer PE, Reitz BA, Jamieson SW, Bieber CP, Wallwork J, Stinson EB, Shumway NE: Cardiac transplantation in perspective for the future: Survival complications, rehabilitation, and cost. J Thorac Cardiovasc Surg 1982, 83:168.
123. Hardy JD, Webb WR, Dalton ML Jr, Walker GR: Lung homotransplantation in man. JAMA 1963, 186:1065.
124. Huggins CE: Reimplantation of lobes of the lung: An experimental technique. Lancet 1959, 2:1059.
125. Veith FJ, Richards K: Improved technique for canine lung transplantation. Ann Surg 1970, 171:553.
126. Benfield JR, Coon BS: The role of the left atrial anastomosis in pulmonary reimplantation. J Thorac Cardiovasc Surg 1976, 53:676.
127. Wildevuur, Heemstra H, Tammeling GJ, et al: Long-term observations of the changes in pulmonary arterial pressure after reimplantation of the canine lung. J Thorac Cardiovasc Surg 1968, 56:799.
128. Donnarel G, Lebreuil G, Sommer A, et al: Factors in the origin of pulmonary hypertension observed after lung transplantation. Lyon Mediterranee Med 1969, 5:51.
129. Veith FJ, Richards K: Mechanism and prevention of fixed high vascular resistance in autografted and allografted lungs. Science 1969, 163:699.
130. Veith FJ, Richards K: Lung transplantation with simultaneous contralateral pulmonary artery ligation. Surg Gynecol Obstet 1969, 129:768.
131. Stevens GH, Rangel DM, Yakeishi Y, Fonkalsrud EW: Technical problems in lung allotransplantation. Arch Surg 1969, 99:506.
132. Trummer MJ, Berg P: *Lung Transplantation*. Springfield, Illinois, Charles C Thomas, 1968, pp 6–10.

Chapter 74

SEXUAL FUNCTION AND VASCULAR SURGERY

RALPH G. DePALMA

Since arterial blood flow into the corpora cavernosa initiates and maintains penile erection, important relationships exist between sexual function and vascular surgery. Leriche's 1923 paper (1) listed impotence as the first symptom in men with the syndrome that has been named after him. In the last three decades highly successful operations were developed to correct aortoiliac occlusive and aneurysmal disease; however, these procedures themselves often provoked postoperative impotence and other sexual disabilities (2,3). Sexual dysfunction after these operations was caused by the failure to perfuse the internal iliac arteries or by destruction of genital autonomic nerves. Therefore, techniques of aortic reconstruction evolved which now minimize these complications (4–7). It is encouraging that these reconstructive methods also offer the prospect of restored sexual function in some men. The importance of intact internal iliac circulation was underscored with the recognition that a second renal transplant usually causes impotence when both of these arteries are divided for end-to-end anastomoses in kidney transplants (8). Recently methods to correct this complication have been described (9).

Along with methods to prevent or treat impotence due to aortoiliac occlusion, it was learned that small-vessel occlusion also causes vasculogenic impotence (10). Since 1980 (11) there has been increasing interest in the entity of vasculogenic impotence. Rapid progress in understanding this problem has occurred in the last 5 years, and recent data suggest an important relationship between arteriosclerotic risk factors and impotence due to vascular disease (12,13). Isolated arteriopathies of the pudendal arteries as well as pudendal disruptions caused by embolism or trauma can now be documented by selective internal iliac angiography. The detection of such lesions has stimulated interest in microvascular operations on the penile and pudendal arteries.

Physiology of Erection

The last several years witnessed increased understanding of the relationship between the nervous system and penile erection and its vascular physiology. Work by Michal (14), Virag (15), and Lue and associates (16,17) provided new information about the remarkable physiology of arterial blood flow increase during penile erection. Normal penile erection involves a neurally regulated increase in the arterial flow to the corpus cavernosum and the corpus spongiosum with obstruction of venous outflow from the corpus cavernosum. This process depends upon the *relaxation* of smooth muscle within the erectile tissue. This relaxation involves the trabeculae of the corpora cavernosa, the intracavernosal arteries, and arterioles. Venous outflow may be controlled by secondary venous compression or extravascular smooth muscle. The exact mechanism of venous occlusion during erection is not completely understood.

Both sympathetic and parasympathetic peripheral efferent pathways participate in stimulating erection. Investigations by Ottesen and associates (18) and Goldstein and colleagues (19) show that peripheral transmission is probably mediated by a vasoactive intestinal polypeptide (VIP) neurotransmittor. VIP causes relaxation of the vascular tissues of the penis, permitting a spectacular increase in blood flow through the pudendal arteries. In the process of erection, penile blood flow increases from a resting level of 10 mL/min to approximately 120 mL/min or more to initiate erection. A blood flow of 30 to 40 mL/min maintains erection. Contraction of the muscles of the pelvic floor also causes suprasystolic blood pressure in the corpora cavernosa, enhancing shaft rigidity (20). The magnitude of these flow and pressure changes shows that penile erection is a unique process within the circulatory system. In summary, normal penile erection depends upon adequate delivery of arterial blood to the corpora cavernosa; intact neural mechanisms ultimately mediating penile vascular relaxation; and a degree of venous outflow occlusion. Complete or partial dysfunction in one or more of these mechanisms results in erectile failure.

The recent discovery that an intracavernosal injection of papaverine, a smooth-muscle relaxant (21), or an alpha blocker such as phenoxybenzamine (22) produces an artificial erection provides important insights into the physiology of penile erection. Intracavernosal injection of pharmacologic agents is useful as a diagnostic and possibly therapeutic tool. With adequate arterial inflow, intracavernosal injections of these agents regularly produce erections in pure neurogenic impotence. Combined with a noninvasive evaluation of penile flow, intracorporal injection to produce artificial erection has been used in our vascular laboratory to select patients for highly selective internal iliac angiography which requires epidural anesthesia. Failure to erect suggests proximal arterial flow restriction. The advantages and precautions to be observed with this type of testing will be discussed.

Types of Impotence and Their Diagnosis

Middle-aged men can develop erectile dysfunctions which might result from complex interactions between vascular, neural, and psychogenic factors. The estimation of each component can be a complex clinical problem. In the interest of clarity the evaluation of each component will be considered separately.

VASCULOGENIC IMPOTENCE

The approach to the patient with vasculogenic impotence depends upon a careful history, physical examination, and noninvasive vascular laboratory testing. In considering a practical approach to patients with impotence from the standpoint of a vascular surgeon, the history is paramount. First the surgeon should estimate the importance of sexual function for each particular patient. Some older people are not concerned or do not desire return of sexual function. This should be recorded and also discussed with the patient's partner.

If sexual function is a concern, the four basic questions devised by Levine (23) should be answered. These are

1. What is the physiologic impairment? Is it the inability to obtain an erection, the inability to maintain an erection during intercourse, or some combination?
2. How firm does the penis become? Not firm at all, slightly firm but erection not self-supporting, decreased firmness with coitus still possible, or fully turgid?
3. Is the impairment constant or episodic? Under what circumstances is the pattern not present: with other partners, with masturbation, with sleep, upon awakening, during the day, when engaging in erotic activity?
4. What life events were occurring when the dysfunction appeared?

It is possible to gain an impression about the etiology of erectile dysfunction from the answers to these questions. For example, gradual loss of erectile ability under all circumstances in the absence of traumatic life events (such as a recent divorce) and associated with ischemic lower extremity symptoms or cardiac disease would suggest vasculogenic impotence.

The history must delineate risk factors which promote vascular disease including cigarette smoking, hyperlipidemia, glucose intolerance, and hypertension. Virtually every drug used to treat hypertension can cause impotence. In addition, tranquilizers, excess use of nasal inhalers, and alcohol and drug abuse can cause impotence. Patients with aortoiliac occlusive or aneurysmal disease do not usually present to the vascular surgeon with the complaint of impotence. They usually are referred for claudication or aneurysm repair. In our vascular laboratory only 3 of 128 cases screened for the chief complaint of impotence alone were found to have previously undiagnosed aortoiliac disease (13), but two of these men were found to have abdominal aortic aneurysms.

Selective arteriography is required to define lesions of the internal iliac or distal pudendal artery. In patients with symptomatic aortoiliac disease, conventional angiography is usually used; in these patients it is also possible to study the internal iliac circulation if the radiologist is alerted prior to the procedure. The diagnostic approach to impotent men depends upon a reasonable definition of the etiology of impotence, in particular dividing patients into subsets. Most vascular surgeons see patients with penile arterial insufficiency due to aortoiliac occlusive disease. Claudication, not impotence, is the chief complaint. However, the surgeon must be alert to detect those men with occlusions of the pudendal arteries alone. In patients with aneurysms there may have been embolization to the pudendal arteries, mechanical obstruction of internal iliac flow, or stretching of the periaortic and pelvic neural plexi. In these cases a discussion of sexual function is important preoperatively as are preoperative and postoperative vascular laboratory studies.

A group of men exist in whom erectile dysfunction is the sole presenting symptom of arterial disease. These cases are complex and require specialized investigations to differentiate organic from psychogenic causes. A history of trauma with associated pelvic fractures or disruption of the pudendal arteries in the perineum due to direct injuries is highly significant in a young man. Isolated arteriopathy occurs in the pudendal arteries of middle-aged men with risk factors for atherosclerosis. A syndrome of corpus cavernosum venous leakage (24) characterized by failure to maintain an erection in the presence of a high corpus cavernosal inflow has also been defined. The incidence of this disorder in middle-aged men is not known. Cavernosal leaks can cause primary impotence in young men (25). This diagnosis is confirmed by cavernosography using dilute contrast media. Diabetes is a common cause of impotence in middle-aged men. While diabetes is associated with vascular lesions, some diabetic patients respond with normal erections on intracavernosal injection of papaverine. This suggests a neurogenic dysfunction and has important therapeutic implications.

Vascular Laboratory Testing for Impotence

The vascular laboratory is useful in supporting the diagnosis of vasculogenic impotence. Many middle-aged men with an otherwise normal examination of the large peripheral vessels exhibit penile vascular abnormalities. Our laboratory uses both measurement of the penile-brachial index (PBI) from Doppler signals detected in the cavernosal arteries and penile pulse-volume recordings (26). Controversy exists regarding the ability of noninvasive testing to define vasculogenic impotence. A PBI of less than 0.6 is unequivocally associated with the complaint of failure of erectile function; a PBI in the range of 0.6 to 0.7 erectile function may or may not be satisfactory. Plethysmographic recording of the penile pulse volume (PVR) has been used by us to define these borderline cases. In examining individual characteristics of penile PVR, the duration of the rate of upstroke appears to be the most reliable measure correlating with the presence or absence of erectile function. Data showing a comparison of PBI and penile PVR and characteristic waveforms are shown in Figure 74-1. To further refine detection of a pelvic steal syndrome these tests can also be performed after exercise.

When an abnormal PBI or penile pulse-volume recording suggests possible small-vessel disease, the author now uses a carefully monitored intracorporal injection of 40 mg of papaverine and 2 mg of phentolamine. If this injection fails to elicit a normal erection, a diagnosis of proximal vascular occlusion is supported. One risk of this test is priapism with doses of the phar-

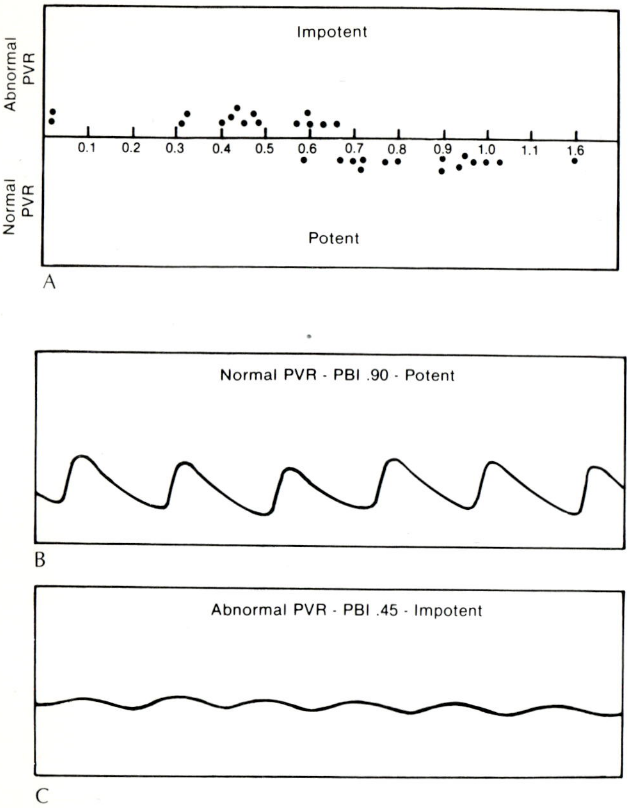

FIGURE 74-1. (*A*) Correlation of pulse-volume recordings with penile brachial indices. (***B,C***) Characteristic pulse-volume recordings and penile brachial indices in potent and impotent men. [From DePalma R: Prevention of sexual dysfunction in aorto-iliac surgery. In Jamieson C (ed): *Current Operative Surgery*. London, Bailliere Tindall, 1985. Reprinted with permission.]

macologic agents initially suggested (13,21,22). It is important that these patients be monitored carefully and that the pharmacologically induced erection subsides normally after 2 to 3 hours.

NEUROGENIC IMPOTENCE

The diagnosis of neurogenic impotence is usually made indirectly, although it is difficult to separate neural from vascular factors in some patients. Lumbosacral injuries and paraplegia are associated with overt neural injury. When diabetic neuropathy is the culprit, most diabetics exhibit peripheral neuropathy usually detected by clinical examination (27). The bulbocavernosus reflex latency time can be quantified by electrical stimulation with an electromyography (EMG) recording by an electrode inserted in the bulbocavernosus muscle (28). The more recently developed surface perineal electrode recording makes this test more widely applicable (29). In normal potent men the mean reflex latency time of this reflex is 35 + 1.2 ms. A time of over 40 ms is considered abnormal; however, the prolongation of the latency period does not necessarily indicate a direct cause and effect relationship to erectile failure according to Blaivas et al. (28). Cystometry has also been used to study diabetics since the detrusor muscle and the smooth muscles involved in erection are enervated from the same sacral nerve roots. Since these are closely interconnected, neurogenic bladder dysfunction indicates an abnormality of the nervous control of erection. Ellenberg has stressed this relationship in the examination of diabetic men (27). In men with neural disorders it is important to explain at the outset the need to accept a penile prosthesis if sexual function is an important consideration.

ENDOCRINE SCREENING

Other causes of impotence include endocrine abnormalities. Slag et al. (30) consider screening to include values of luteinizing hormone, follicle stimulating hormone, testosterone, thyroxine, triiodothyronine (T_3), T_3 resin uptake, and prolactin. Diabetes is the endocrine abnormality most often overlooked. This diagnosis must sometimes be clarified by a glucose tolerance test. In some diabetics calcification of the seminal vesicles appears on plain abdominal films. In general, with most patients presenting to our vascular clinic, we have yet to define endocrine abnormalities other than diabetes as dominant causes of impotence in middle-aged men.

PSYCHOGENIC IMPOTENCE

Normal erection is clearly a complex process with important psychic components. Wagner (31) has used visual erotic stimulation with measurement of curves obtained from circumferential strain gauges applied to the penis to detect diameter and pressure change. This test is logical in that the ability to erect in connection with sexual arousal is the problem requiring clarification. Wagner (31) also tests vibratory penile stimulation. These tests are best conducted in a multidisciplinary setting by trained psychiatrists and sexologists once the more obvious organic causes are excluded.

Nocturnal penile tumescence (NPT) is used to differentiate psychogenic impotence from organic impotence. This test adds considerably to the diagnosis of psychogenic erectile dysfunction when a completely normal erection occurs during sleep. To observe a normal erection, noctural monitoring should be conducted over two or three nights. When changes in tumescence are recorded, the patient is checked visually for erection and tested for penile shaft rigidity. This subject is well reviewed by Wagner (31). The "postage stamp test" in which the patient awakes to find broken postage stamps in the morning, presumably indicating a nocturnal erection, is crude. Portable NPT systems used at home, and which do not involve direct observation of erection, cannot differentiate changes in penile diameter or minimal tumescence from penile rigidity sufficient for vaginal penetration.

Prevention of Sexual Disturbances in Vascular Operations

The operative principles that can prevent sexual disabilities use dissections which preserve both vascular and neural elements of the erectile process. Vascular operations must then restore or maintain internal iliac flow, avoid atheroembolism, and minimize nerve injuries caused by extensive dissection. In young patients endarterectomy is favored when the disease is limited and lesions are soft atheromas with minimal calcification. A successful proximal endarterectomy maintains direct axial flow to the internal iliacs (Figure 74-2). In men with such limited early disease, the anatomy favors continued sexual function, probably because the disease is less advanced. Cases suitable for endarterectomy are said to be more frequent in a European experience (20).

While *erectile failure* is the most common postoperative sexual disability related to aortoiliac surgery, aortic dissection with interruption of the autonomic nervous fibers in the periaortic area also causes *ejaculatory dysfunction*. This phenomenon can be distressing for many men and their partners. In couples desiring pregnancy, anejaculation is a serious complication. *Anorgasmia* in the presence of normal penile erection is also a rare and distressing neural complication of aortoiliac dissection. For these reasons alone the use of nerve-sparing dissection techniques is clearly worthwhile.

Aortofemoral bypass can cause vasculogenic impotence when the external iliac arteries are occluded or severely stenotic and retrograde pelvic perfusion is prevented (32). Patients with hemodynamically significant external iliac disease are more likely rendered impotent when end-to-end proximal anastomoses are employed, since prograde flow into the internal iliac arteries may be decreased by division of the aorta. End-to-side aortofemoral bypass preserves distal flow through the native aorta but also may create a cul-de-sac of low flow in an area of severe distal atherosclerosis. The author prefers end-to-end aortic graft anastomoses with provisions to perfuse the internal iliacs (Figure 74-3). Femorofemoral bypass is an excellent option in properly selected cases. It avoids completely the need for aortic dissection. If a subcritical lesion exists in the donor iliac vessel, transluminal angioplasty can be chosen to render this vessel fit for a femorofermoral bypass (33) (Figure 74-4). Femorofemoral bypass provides long-term patency similar to that of aortoiliac reconstruction and can lead to satisfactory return of sexual function as documented historically and by vascular laboratory criteria.

In the author's experience, internal iliac artery patency on at least one side is needed for satisfactory erectile function. However, Flannigan et al. (34) described restoration of erection using extraanatomic bypasses with angiographic evidence of bilateral internal iliac artery occlusion. Important collaterals to the pudendal vessels arise from the medial circumflex femoral arteries which are often perfused via the deep femoral artery. It is therefore important to provide free flow into the deep femoral artery to perfuse these collaterals. Figure 74-5 shows how this may be accomplished in an axillobifemoral graft.

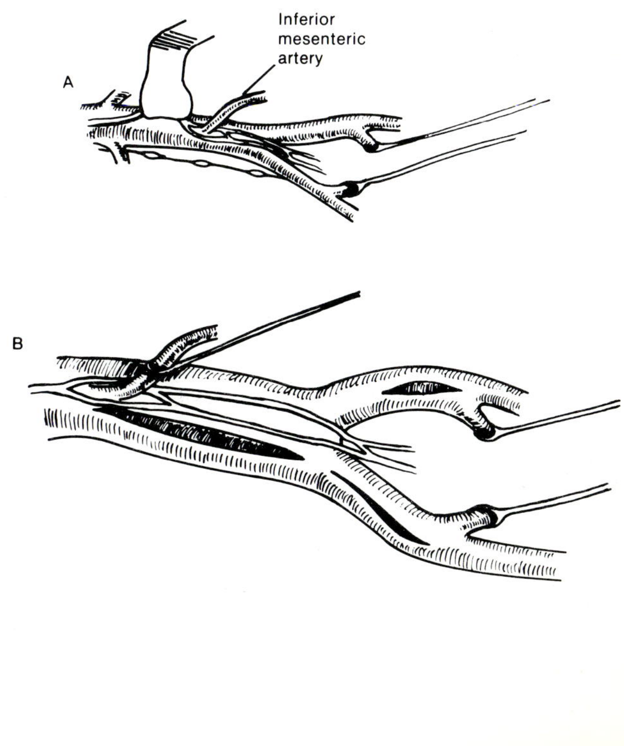

FIGURE 74-2. Technique of aortoiliac endarterectomy. (*A*) Exposure and (*B*) arteriotomy preserve inferior mesenteric artery and sympathetic nerves. [From DePalma R: Prevention of sexual dysfunction in aortoiliac surgery. In Jamieson C (ed): *Current Operative Surgery*. London, Bailliere Tindall, 1985. Reprinted with permission.]

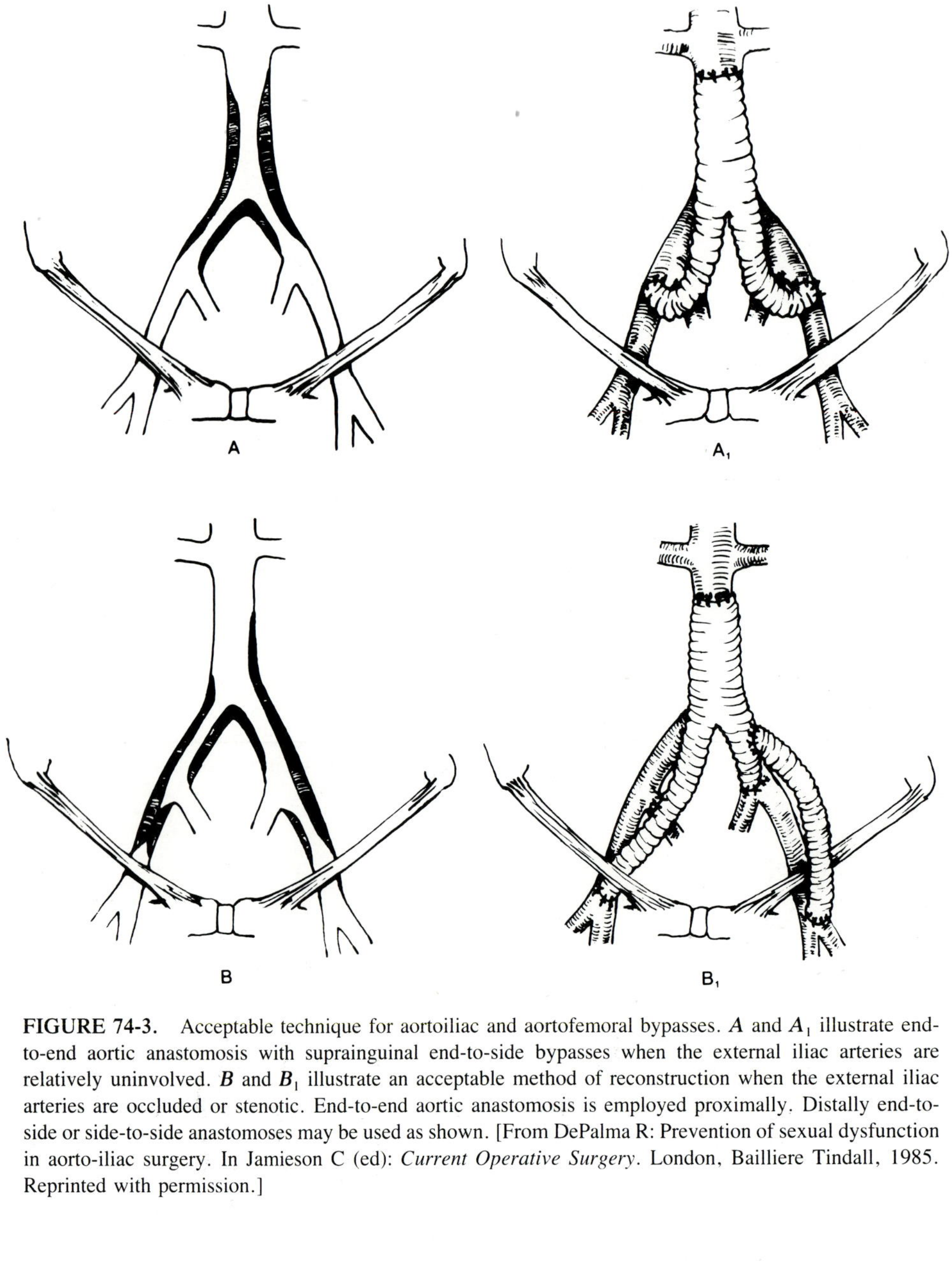

FIGURE 74-3. Acceptable technique for aortoiliac and aortofemoral bypasses. *A* and A_1 illustrate end-to-end aortic anastomosis with suprainguinal end-to-side bypasses when the external iliac arteries are relatively uninvolved. *B* and B_1 illustrate an acceptable method of reconstruction when the external iliac arteries are occluded or stenotic. End-to-end aortic anastomosis is employed proximally. Distally end-to-side or side-to-side anastomoses may be used as shown. [From DePalma R: Prevention of sexual dysfunction in aorto-iliac surgery. In Jamieson C (ed): *Current Operative Surgery*. London, Bailliere Tindall, 1985. Reprinted with permission.]

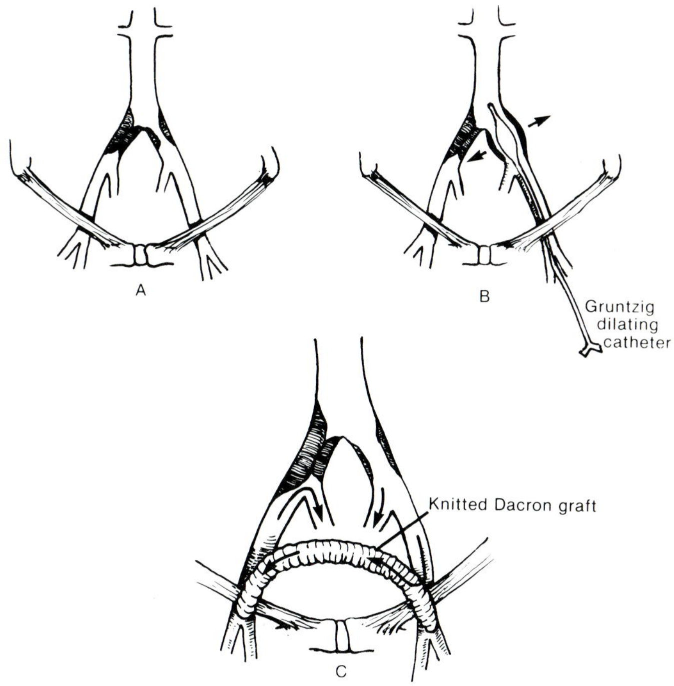

FIGURE 74-4. (*A,B*) Transluminal angioplasty combined with femorofemoral bypass for totally occluded right common iliac artery and stenotic left common iliac artery. (*C*) Bilateral internal iliac artery flow is improved. [From DePalma R: Prevention of sexual dysfunction in aorto-iliac surgery. In Jamieson C (ed): *Current Operative Surgery*. London, Bailliere Tindall, 1985. Reprinted with permission.]

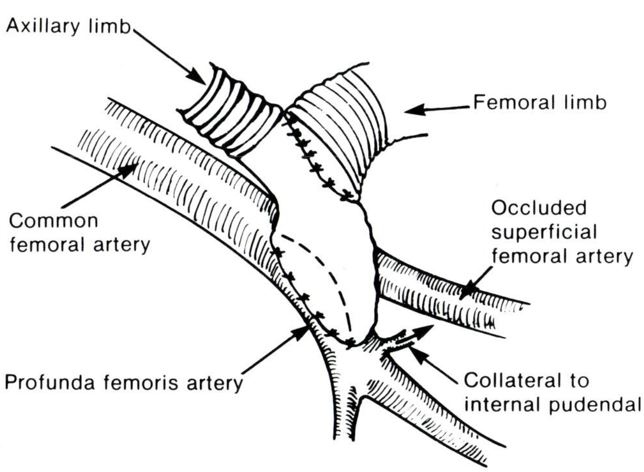

FIGURE 74-5. Technique of axillobifemoral graft with hood of the graft being extended over the stenotic origin of the deep femoral artery. [From DePalma R: Prevention of sexual dysfunction in aorto-iliac surgery. In Jamieson C (ed): *Current Operative Surgery*. London, Bailliere Tindall, 1985. Reprinted with permission.]

ABDOMINAL AORTIC REPAIR

An inlay technique for an abdominal aortic aneurysmectomy is preferred. This minimizes interference with neural fibers and preserves the collaterals of the inferior mesenteric artery. The application of atraumatic clamps to the iliac arteries with minimal dissection also simplifies these operations and minimizes neural disruption. In cases where the common iliac artery is aneurysmal, a pantaloon type of reconstruction can be used (Figure 74-6). Resection of the aneurysmal sac is not recommended. The incision in the aorta is made well to the right to avoid the pleural plexuses on the left side. The orifice of the inferior mesenteric artery is sutured from within.

In planning aortic aneurysm repair it is important to have information about the anatomy of the internal iliac arteries prior to operation. Thus, the author recommends aortography prior to aneurysm repair. This is also useful in detecting other abnormalities, e.g., accessory renal arteries or suprarenal aneurysmal involvement. Oblique views ensure adequate visualization of the internal iliac artery and its branches.

The minimal dissection required with the inlay type of aneurysm reconstruction expedites surgery. When the common iliacs are aneurysmal, it is usually possible to tailor the distal reconstruction so that blood flow perfuses the internal iliacs in some fashion. This can sometimes be done by incising the common iliac artery aneurysm to obtain a rim of normal arterial tissue proximal to the common iliac bifurcation. This stump can be sutured in a manner to preserve the internal iliac orifice and an anastomosis made to a normal external iliac artery. When both internal and external iliac arteries are aneurysmal, the anastomoses must be made in normal arterial tissue. Occasionally both internal iliac arteries must be sacrificed; this can lead to impotence. The surgeon can never guarantee normal postoperative sexual function because the main aim of these operations is to preserve life and limb.

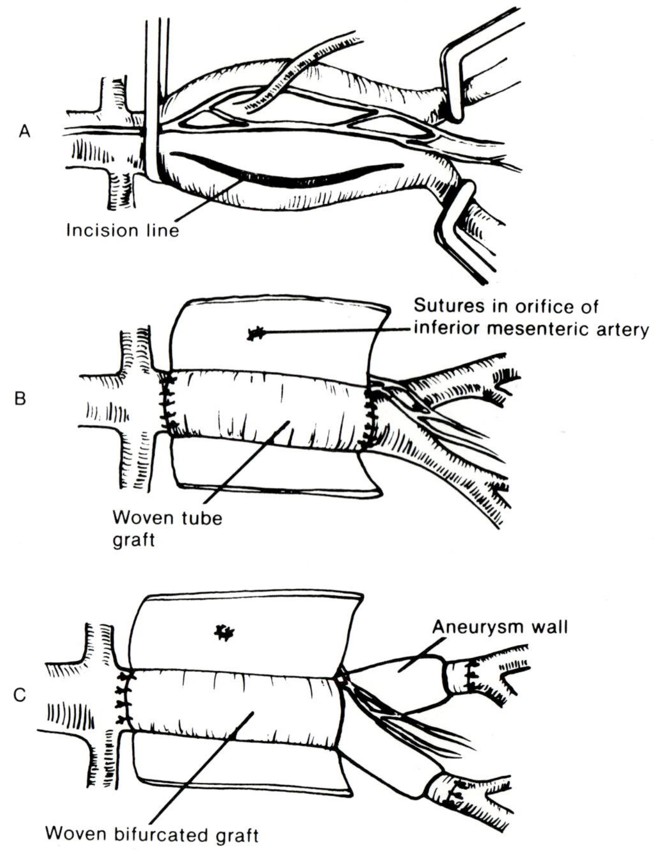

FIGURE 74-6. (*A*) Technique of aortic and aortoiliac aneurysm repair by the inlay method. Note incision in the right side of the aneurysm. The iliac arteries are clamped after minimal mobilization. (*B*) Straight graft sutured in place with minimal dissection of aneurysm wall. (*C*) Bifurcation graft placed to preserve nerves crossing left iliac artery. [From DePalma R: Prevention of sexual dysfunction in aorto-iliac surgery. In Jamieson C (ed): *Current Operative Surgery*. London, Bailliere Tindall, 1985. Reprinted with permission.]

Operations Specifically for Impotence

INTERNAL ILIAC ARTERY ENDARTERECTOMY

The segmental distribution of atherosclerosis rarely involves the internal iliac arteries. However, with selective angiography, isolated lesions of the main iliac internal artery or its divisions including the pudendal artery supplying the penis are being detected more frequently. Plaques in the main internal iliac artery lend themselves to endarterectomy. An extraperitoneal approach (Figure 74-7) provides excellent exposure of the internal iliac artery including its anterior and posterior divisions. The internal pudendal artery is not easily accessible as it courses in the buttock. It usually arises from the anterior division of the internal iliac artery and exits the pelvis at the lower border of the greater sciatic foramen. It crosses the ischial spine, then reenters the pelvis through the lesser sciatic notch, proceeds along the wall of the ischiorectal fossa, and emerges in the perineum about 4 cm anterior to the ischial tuberosity (Figure 74-8).

SMALL-VESSEL RECONSTRUCTIONS

Rarely an endarterectomy of the distal reaches of the internal iliac artery can be performed to include the origin of the pudendal artery at the greater sciatic notch. Bypasses have also been performed after renal transplantation to restore flow to a patent pudendal outflow tract (9). Since exposure of the course of the main internal pudendal artery is difficult in the pelvis or buttock, a variety of indirect approaches have been devised.

There is now considerable interest in operations for patients with isolated pudendal artery lesions. In their early evolutions, these procedures included vein grafts from the femoral artery or the use of the inferior epigastric artery to revascularize directly the corpus cavernosa. These efforts resulted in failure due to closure of the bypasses. The author has also used anastomoses of the inferior epigastric artery to a vein patch on the corpus cavernosum with apparent success in two patients. However,

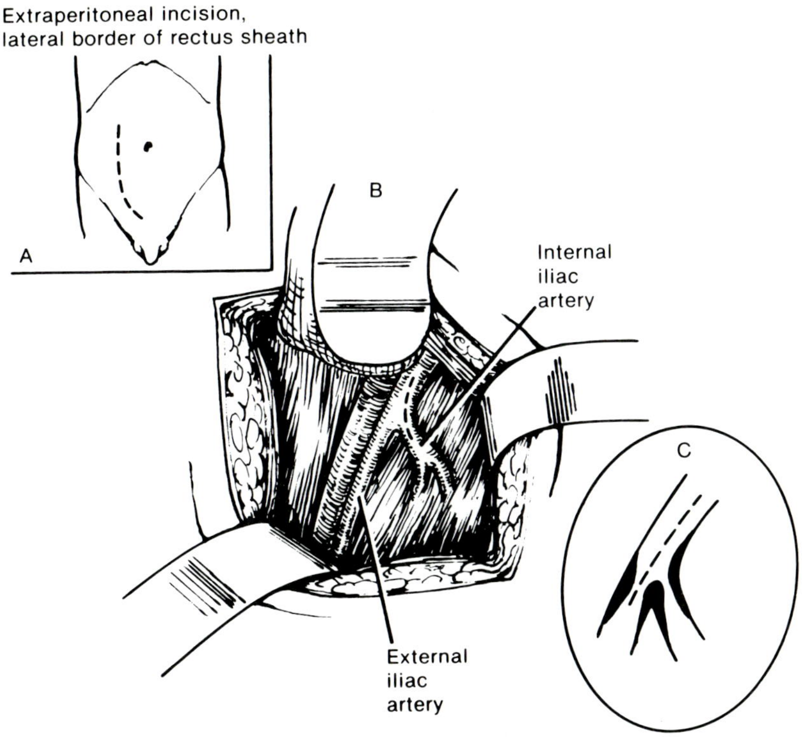

FIGURE 74-7. Technique of isolated internal iliac endarterectomy. (*A*) Incision. (*B*) Curved incision in internal iliac artery extending into common iliac. (*C*) Linear incision when external iliac artery is also involved. [From DePalma R: Prevention of sexual dysfunction in aorto-iliac surgery. In Jamieson C (ed): *Current Operative Surgery*. London, Bailliere Tindall, 1985. Reprinted with permission.]

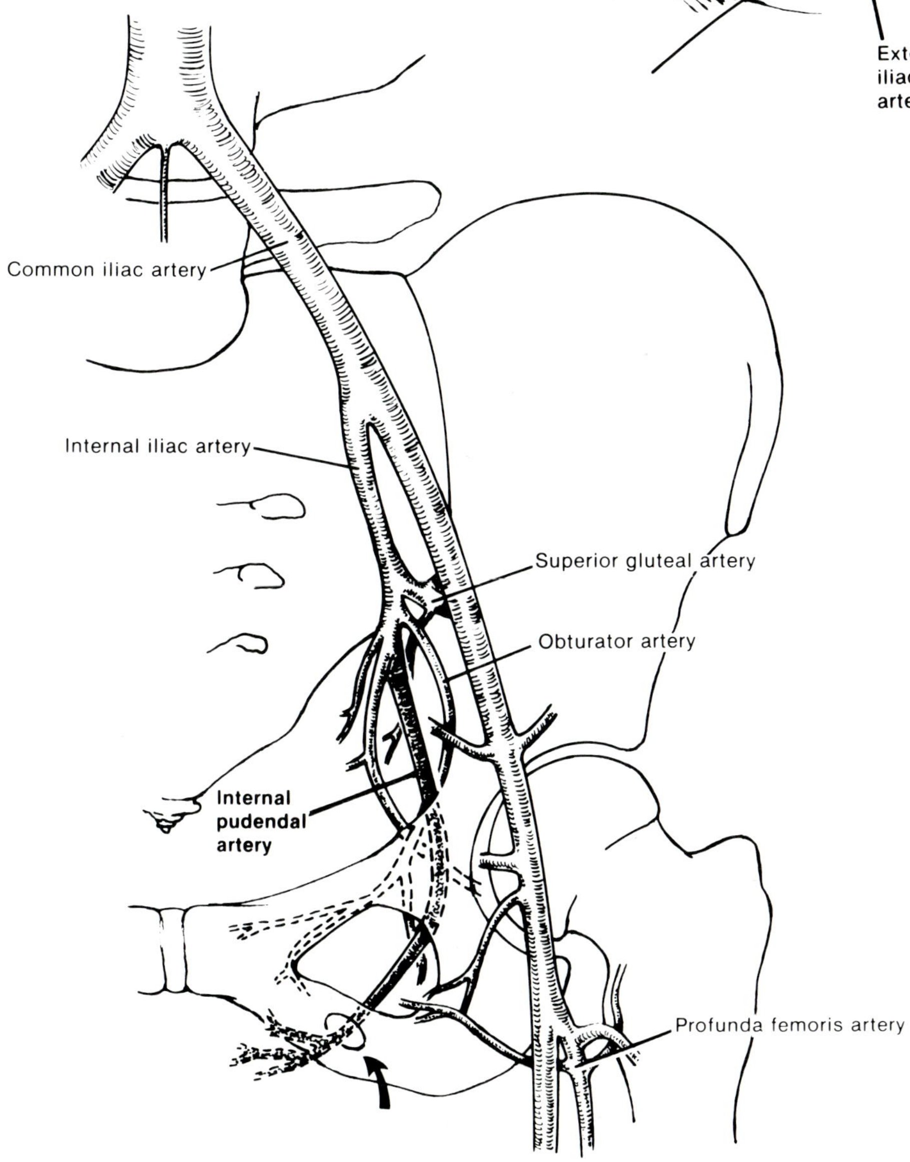

FIGURE 74-8. Diagram of internal iliac artery and internal pudendal artery.

serious priapism also occurred in two other cases and required ligation of the arterial graft. Priapism probably occurs because blood is delivered directly to the cavernous spaces without mediating neural conrol.

Artery bypass to the dorsal vein of the penis has also been described by Virag (35). End-to-end or end-to-side anastomoses of one inferior epigastric artery to one dorsal artery to provide retrograde perfusion of the deep cavernosal artery appear rational. These operations are done under magnification. Long-term follow-up is not available, but early results appear promising in young patients with traumatic lesions. Direct anastomoses to the deep cavernosal artery have also been described: the size of this vessel may in some cases preclude successful microvascular anastomosis.

Results of epigastric artery to dorsal penile artery anastomoses have been reported recently at meetings. No follow-up longer than $2\frac{1}{2}$ years is available. Goldstein and colleagues (36) described improved erectile function in 11 of 14 patients with traumatic occlusive disease. Puech-Leao and associates (37) record the early results of these procedures as well. Crespo and associates (38) have described multiple microvascular anastomoses to penile arteries using vein grafts. No long-term data exist on the patency of these bypasses, nor is long-term patency yet related to potency.

PROSTHESES

Inflatable or semirigid prostheses are important alternatives to direct microvascular reconstructions. These currently offer, in the author's opinion, a most reliable means of restoring erectile function. Patients with normal function several years following aortoiliac reconstruction may later develop loss of erectile function. Presumably this occurs due to progression of distal disease. In these cases inflatable prostheses yielded satisfactory results (39). It is important to recognize that some patients will not accept the prosthetic alternative. Once a prosthesis has been inserted, whatever normal tumesecence existed preoperatively is lost. There is also the prospect of infection or later mechanical failure. In spite of this, modern prostheses offer a most secure surgical alternative for men with impaired penile erection. The type of prosthesis should be determined by the preferences of both the urologic surgeon and the patient. From the standpoint of the postoperatively impotent patient, normal neural function is important for sensation, orgasm, and ejaculation. These functions will partly determine patient satisfaction after the insertion of a penile prosthesis.

General Medical Treatment

In screening over 200 patients at the George Washington University Clinic, our laboratory has detected men in whom impotence is the first signal of vascular disease involving coronary or other arteries. The proportion of such patients reporting to any clinic is determined by local referral patterns and biases introduced by clinical interests in this problem. Fully one-third of patients presenting to our vascular laboratory exhibit abnormal pulse-volume recordings. Some of these men respond to medical therapy. Most importantly, this includes complete cessation of smoking and the use of isoxuprine 10 mg four times daily. When improvement is reported clinically, pulse-volume recording often returns to a normal pattern. The significance and durability of such changes require further study. In occasional patients with renal hypertension, renal artery endarterectomy, bypass, or angioplasty can obviate the need for continued antihypertensive therapy. Patients suitable for this type of treatment are usually young and should have had renal hypertension for less than 3 years.

Conclusion

The diagnosis and treatment of impotence has become an important area of medicine which requires further study. Better methods to quantify erectile function will make this study more objective. The application of noninvasive vascular laboratory measurements and selective arteriography are important tools for vascular surgeons and urologists. Multidisciplinary interactions between neurophysiologists, urologists, and psychiatrists have added much new information about the normal physiology of erection. For the vascular surgeon, advances in the techniques of aortoiliac surgery minimize or prevent postoperative sexual dysfunction in most patients and restore function in others. The diagnosis and treatment of isolated pudendal artery occlusions are particular challenges, as is the elucidation of the etiology of these lesions and their relevance to arterial disease in other critical vessels such as the coronary arteries.

References

1. Leriche R: Des Obliterations Arterielle Hautes (Obliteration De LaTerminasion De L'aorte) Comme Causes Des Insuffisances Circulatoires Des Membres Inferieurs. Bull Mem Soc Chir 1923, 49:1404.
2. May AG, DeWeese JA, Rolo CG: Changes in sexual function following operation on the abdominal aorta. Surgery 1969, 65:41.
3. Sabri S, Cotton LT: Sexual function following aorto-iliac reconstruction. Lancet 1971, 2:121.
4. DePalma RG: Aorto-iliac dissection principles. In Zorgniotti A, Rossi G (eds): *Vasculogenic Impotence*. Springfield, Illinois, Charles C Thomas, 1980, pp 299–308.
5. DePalma RG, Kedia K, Persky L: Vascular operations for pres-

ervation of sexual function. In Bergan JJ, Yao JST (eds): *Surgery of the Aorta and Its Body Branches*. New York, Grune & Stratton, 1979, pp 277–296.
6. Weinstein MH, Machleder HI: Sexual function after aorto-iliac surgery. Ann Surg 1974, 181:787.
7. DePalma RG: Etiology and management of sexual problems related to aorto-iliac disease and surgery. In Veith FJ (ed): *Current Critical Problems in Vascular Surgery*. New York, Appleton-Century-Crofts, 1982, pp 429–443.
8. Gittes RF, Waters WB: Sexual impotence: The overlooked complication of a second renal transplant. J Urol 1979, 121:719.
9. Billet A, Dagher FJ, Queral LA: Surgical correction of vasculogenic impotence in a patient after bilateral renal transplantation. Surgery 1982, 91:108.
10. Ginestie JF, Romieu A: *Radiologic Exploration of Impotence*. The Hague, Martinus Nijihoff, 1978.
11. Zorgniotti AW, Rossi G (eds): *Vasculogenic Impotence*. Springfield, Illinois, Charles C Thomas, 1980.
12. Virag R, Bouilly D, Fryman D: Is impotence an arterial disorder: A study of arterial risk factors in 440 impotent men. Lancet 1985, 1:181.
13. DePalma RG, Edwards C: Non invasive evaluation of erectile dysfunction and intracorporal papaverine injections. In Virag R (ed): *Proceedings of First World Conference on Impotence*, 1985, in press.
14. Michal V, Simana J, Rehak J, Masin J: Haemodynamics of erection in man. Physiol Bohemoslov 1983, 32:497.
15. Virag R, Spencer PP, Frydman D: Artificial erection in diagnosis and treatment of impotence. Urology 1984, 24:157.
16. Lue TF, Takamura T, Schmidt RA, Palubinskas AJ, Tanagho EA: Hemodynamics of erection in the monkey. J Urol 1983, 130:1237.
17. Lue TF, Salim JZ, Schmidt RA, Tanagho EA: Neuroanatomy of penile erection: Its relevance to iatrogenic impotence. J Urol 1984, 131:273.
18. Ottesen B, Wagner G, Virag R, Fahrenkrug J: Penile erection: Possible role for vasoactive intestinal polypeptide as a neurotransmitter. Br Med J 1984, 288:9.
19. Goldstein I, Krane RJ, Ottesen B, Fahrenkrug J, Wagner G: Vasoactive polypeptide (VIP) release during pelvic nerve stimulated penile erections. Invest Urol, in press.
20. Michal V: Arterial disease as a cause of impotence. In *Clinics in Endocrinology and Metabolism*. Philadelphia, Saunders, 1982, pp 725–748.
21. Virag R, Virag H: L'Epreuve A La Papaverine Intracaverneuse Dans L'Etude de L'Impuissance: Perespectives therapeutiques. J Mal Vasc 1983, 8:293.
22. Brindley GS: Cavernosal alpha-blockade: A new technique for investigating and treating erectile impotence. Br J Psychiatry 1983, 143:332.
23. Levine SB: Marital sexual dysfunction: Erectile dysfunction. Ann Intern Med 1976, 85:342.
24. Virag R: Unstable erection due to venous insufficiency: Diagnosis and surgical correction: Ten cases with a mean follow-up of 12 months. *J Mal Vasc 1981*, 6(2):121.
25. Ebbehøj J, Wagner G: Insufficient penile erection due to abnormal drainage of cavernous bodies. Urology 1979, 13:507.
26. Stauffer D, DePalma RG: A comparison of penile-brachial index (PBI) and penile pulse volume recordings (PVR). Bruit 1983, 17:29.
27. Ellenberg M: Impotence in diabetes: The neurologic factor. Ann Intern Med 1971, 75:213.
28. Blaivas JG, O'Donnell TF Jr, Gottlieb P, Labib KB: Measurement of bulbocavernousus reflex latency time as part of a comprehensive evaluation of impotence. In Zorgniotti AW, Rossi G (eds): *Vasculogenic Impotence*. Springfield, Illinois, Charles C Thomas, 1980, pp 49–66.
29. Haldeman S, Bradley WE, Bhati NN, Johnson BK: Pudendal evoked responses. Arch Neurol 1982, 39:280.
30. Slag MF, Morley JE, Elson MK, Trence DL, Nelson CJ, Nelson AE, Kinlaw WB, Beyer HS, Nuttall FQ, Shafer RB: Impotence in medical clinic outpatients. JAMA 1983, 249:1736.
31. Wagner G: Methods for differential diagnosis of psychogenic and erectile failure. In Wagner G, Green R (eds): *Impotence: Physiological, Psychological, Surgical Diagnosis and Treatment*. New York, Plenum, 1981, pp 89–129.
32. Queral LA, Whitehouse WM, Flinn WR: Pelvic hemodynamics after aorto-iliac reconstruction. Surgery 1979, 26:799.
33. Merchant RF Jr, DePalma RG: The effects of femoro-femoral grafts on postoperative sexual function: Correlation with penile pulse volume recordings. Surgery: 90:962, 1981.
34. Flannigan DP, Schuler JJ, Kiefer T: Elimination of iatrogenic impotence and improvement of sexual function following aorto-iliac revascularization. Arch Surg 1982, 117:544.
35. Virag R, Frydmann D, Legman H, Bouily P: Possibilities chirurgicales dans l'impuissance vasculaire. Gaz Med France 1983, 90:2031.
36. Goldstein I, Mortara R, Krane RJ: Microsurgery for atherosclerotic and non-atherosclerotic occlusive disease. In Virag R (ed): *Proceedings of First World Conference on Impotence*, 1985, in press.
37. Puech-Leao LE, Puech-Leao P, Albers MTV: *Impotencia Sexual Vasculogenico*. Sao Paulo, Brazil, Sarvier, 1981.
38. Crespo E, Soltanik E, Bove D, Farrell G: Treatment of vasculogenic sexual impotence by revascularizing cavernous and/or dorsal arteries using microvascular techniques. Urology 1982, 20:271.
39. DePalma RG, Kedia K, Persky L: Surgical options in the correction of vasuclogenic impotence. Vasc Surg 1980, 14:92.

INDEX

Note: Page numbers in *italic* indicate illustrations or tables.